S0-AAZ-258

DIAGNOSIS OF BONE AND JOINT DISORDERS

VOLUME 3

Donald Resnick, M.D.

Chief,
Department of Radiology
Veterans Administration Medical Center
San Diego, California
and
Professor of Radiology
Department of Radiology
University of California, San Diego
San Diego, California

Gen Niwayama, M.D., D.Med.Sc.

Director, Autopsy Division
Department of Pathology
Brotman Medical Center
Culver City, California
and
Associate Clinical Professor
Department of Pathology
School of Medicine
University of California, Los Angeles

With Emphasis on Articular Abnormalities

W. B. SAUNDERS COMPANY
Philadelphia • London • Toronto • Mexico City • Rio de Janeiro • Sydney • Tokyo

W. B. Saunders Company: West Washington Square
Philadelphia, PA 19105

1 St. Anne's Road
Eastbourne, East Sussex BN21 3UN, England

1 Goldthorne Avenue
Toronto, Ontario M8Z 5T9, Canada

Apartado 26370 – Cedro 512
Mexico 4, D.F., Mexico

Rua Coronel Cabrita, 8
Sao Cristovao Caixa Postal 21176
Rio de Janeiro, Brazil

9 Waltham Street
Artarmon, N.S.W. 2064, Australia

Ichibancho, Central Bldg., 22-1 Ichibancho
Chiyoda-Ku, Tokyo 102, Japan

Library of Congress Cataloging in Publication Data

Resnick, Donald.

Diagnosis of bone and joint disorders.

1. Joints — Diseases — Diagnosis. 2. Joints — Radiography. 3. Bones — Radiography. 4. Bones — Diseases — Diagnosis. I. Niwayama, Gen, joint author. II. Title. [DNLM: 1. Bone diseases — Diagnosis. 2. Joint diseases — Diagnosis. 3. Joints — Abnormalities. R43d] RC932.R46 616.7′1′075 79-3791 ISBN 0-7216-7561-1

Diagnosis of Bone and Joint Disorders

ISBN 0-7216-7561-1 Volume 1
ISBN 0-7216-7562-X Volume 2
ISBN 0-7216-7563-8 Volume 3
ISBN 0-7216-7564-6 Set

Last digit is the print number: 9 8 7 6 5 4 3

CONTENTS

Section VIII DEGENERATIVE DISEASE

Section IX CRYSTAL-INDUCED AND RELATED DISEASES

Section X METABOLIC DISEASES

Section XI ENDOCRINE DISEASES

SECTION XIII

INFECTIOUS DISEASES

OSTEOMYELITIS, SEPTIC ARTHRITIS, AND SOFT TISSUE INFECTION: THE MECHANISMS AND SITUATIONS

by Donald Resnick, M.D., and Gen Niwayama, M.D.

60

Infection of bone and joint is a common and disturbing problem for children and adults alike, and it represents a diagnostic or therapeutic challenge to the pediatrician, internist, orthopedic surgeon, radiologist, and pathologist. Its manifestations are varied and are dependent upon the site of involvement, the initiating event, the infecting organism, and the acute or chronic nature of the illness. Early diagnosis is imperative, as it allows prompt treatment which can prevent many of the dreaded complications of the disease.

An adequate description of the radiographic and pathologic features of bone and joint infection must address the problem from several aspects. Fundamental to this description is an analysis of the mechanisms by which the organisms reach the osseous and articular structures, the pathogenesis of the infective process itself, and any specific situations or circumstances that can influence the incidence and pattern of such contamination; this analysis is accomplished in the present chapter. Equally germane to the description of radiographic and pathologic abnormalities of skeletal infection is a discussion of the specific agents that are capable of infecting bones and joints and of the specific osseous and articular sites that can become contaminated. These latter topics are addressed in Chapters 61 and 62.

TERMINOLOGY

Any discussion of bone and joint infection must utilize certain terms to describe the disease process. It is important that definitions of these terms be presented at the outset of the discussion so that the reader, in forging through the intricacies and complexities of the problem, does not become lost.

The term *osteomyelitis*, which was introduced by Nelaton[1] in 1844, implies an infection of bone and marrow. Osteomyelitis most commonly refers to bacterial infections, although fungi, parasites, and viruses can infect the bone and the marrow. As used in this chapter, *infective (suppurative) osteitis* indicates contamination of the bone cortex. Infective osteitis can occur as an isolated phenomenon or, more frequently, as a concomitant to osteomyelitis. Radiographic and pathologic differentiation of osteitis and osteomyelitis can be extremely difficult; however, such differentiation is possible on many occasions and can influence considerably the choice of an appropriate therapeutic regimen. Osteitis is not confined to infectious processes; inflammation of the cortex can be observed in numerous conditions, such as ankylosing spondylitis, psoriasis, and Reiter's syndrome, in which an infective etiology has not been firmly established. *Infective (suppurative) periostitis* implies contamination of the periosteal cloak that surrounds the bone. In this situation, a subperiosteal accumulation of organisms frequently leads to infective osteitis and osteomyelitis, to interruption of periosteal blood supply to the cortex, producing necrosis, or to disruption of the periosteum and the accumulation of pus in the soft tissues. Radiography is commonly unable to delineate the precise extent of the infection (suppurative periostitis, osteitis, or osteomyelitis). Furthermore, periostitis can be noted in the absence of infection, being evident in neoplastic, metabolic, inflammatory, and traumatic disorders. *Soft tissue infection* indicates contamination of cutaneous, subcutaneous, muscular, fascial, tendinous, ligamentous, and bursal structures. This may be seen as an isolated condition, as a forerunner to infective periostitis, osteitis, and osteomyelitis, or as a complication of periosteal, osseous, marrow, and articular infection. Soft tissue infection can lead to inflammation of adjacent periosteal tissue (periostitis) without necessarily implying that the periosteum is contaminated. *Articular infection* implies a septic process of the joint itself. Septic arthritis can occur as an isolated condition that may soon spread to the neighboring bone or as a complication of adjacent osteomyelitis.

The clinical stages of osteomyelitis are frequently designated as *acute*, *subacute*, and *chronic*. This does not imply that definitive divisions exist between one stage and another, nor does it signify that all cases of osteomyelitis progress through each of these phases. The rather abrupt onset of clinical symptoms and signs during the initial stage of infection clearly indicates the acute osteomyelitic phase; if this acute phase passes without complete elimination of infection, subacute or chronic osteomyelitis can become apparent. The transition from acute to subacute and chronic osteomyelitis can indicate that inadequate or inappropriate therapeutic measures have been employed or that the organisms are especially resistant to accepted modes of therapy. Viable organisms can persist in small abscesses or fragments of necrotic bone, resisting all attempts at eradication of the septic process. At intervals of months or even years, the residual organisms can produce flare-ups of osteomyelitis. In contrast to those patients who can be traced through each of the three clinical stages of osteomyelitis, other individuals reveal chronic osteomyelitis at the initial time of evaluation,[2] presenting with vague symptoms and signs on clinical examination and evidence of a long-standing process on radiographic evaluation.

Observations on large numbers of patients with infection underscore the difficulty in accurately differentiating among acute, subacute, and chronic osteomyelitis on the basis of clinical manifestations.[3] Some individuals with apparently acute disease reveal historical evidence suggesting indolent infections; alternatively, patients with documented osteomyelitis for many years can appear with acute exacerbations characterized by fever, pain, tenderness, and warmth. This difficulty is compounded by histological and radiologic examinations that demonstrate the simultaneous occurrence of changes compatible with both acute and chronic disease. This evidence indicates that the physician should beware of too rigorously applying the terms acute, subacute, and chronic osteomyelitis.

Descriptive terms have been applied to certain radiographic and pathologic characteristics that are encountered during the course of osteomyelitis. A *sequestrum* represents a segment of necrotic bone that is separated from living bone by granulation tissue. Sequestra may reside in the marrow for protracted periods of time, harboring living organisms that have the capability of evoking an acute flare-up of the infection. An *involucrum* denotes a layer of living bone that has formed about the dead bone. It can surround and eventually merge with the parent bone, or it can become perforated by *tracts or sinuses* through which the pus may escape. Sinuses leading to the skin surface are termed *fistulae.* Granulation tissue and sequestra can be discharged from the body spontaneously through the fistulous channels. A *bone abscess* (Brodie's abscess) is a sharply delineated focus of infection. It is of variable size, can occur at single or multiple locations, and represents a site of active infection. It is lined by granulation tissue and is frequently surrounded by eburnated bone. Occasionally, a sclerotic nonpurulent form of osteomyelitis exists, which is termed *Garré's sclerosing osteomyelitis.*[4] Although this term is carelessly applied to any form of osteomyelitis with severe osseous eburnation, it should be reserved for those cases in which intense proliferation of the periosteum leads to bony deposition and in which there is no necrosis or purulent exudate and little granulation tissue.[3] Sclerosing osteomyelitis of Garré is rare, is typically due to *Staphylococcus aureus*, and is most commonly seen in the mandible.[5, 287]

OSTEOMYELITIS

Routes of Contamination

It is convenient to consider the four principal routes by which osseous (and articular) structures can be contaminated.

1. Hematogenous spread of infection. Infection can reach the bone (or the joint) via the bloodstream. The vulnerability of any specific bone (or site within that bone) to infection is influenced by and dependent upon the anatomy of the adjacent vascular tree.

2. Spread from a contiguous source of infection. Infection can extend into the bone (or the joint) from an adjacent contaminated site. Cutaneous, sinus, and dental infections are three important examples in which a primary extraskeletal infective focus can subsequently involve neighboring osseous and articular structures.

3. Direct implantation of infection. In certain situations, infection is directly implanted into the bone (or the joint). Puncture and penetrating injuries represent important vehicles for this route of contamination.

4. Postoperative infection. In this age of aggressive orthopedic surgery, postoperative infection is becoming increasingly important. Although many examples of this type of infection relate to direct implantation, spread from a contiguous septic focus, or hematogenous contamination of the bone (or the joint), infection following surgery is so important that it deserves special emphasis.

In any particular individual, the exact mechanism of the infection may not be clear. Furthermore, in some individuals, more than one potential mechanism may be operational. Nonetheless, accurate interpretation of the radiographic and pathologic characteristics of osteomyelitis (and septic arthritis) requires an awareness of the potential pathways by which organisms may reach the osseous and the articular structures.

Hematogenous Spread of Infection

General Clinical Features. The general features of hematogenous osteomyelitis have been well outlined.[2, 3, 6-17] Traditionally, such osteomyelitis has been regarded as a disease of childhood (3 to 15 years of age),[18-20] although a rise in the incidence of hematogenous osteomyelitis in older patients has recently been noted.[3] Neonatal osteomyelitis is also well known.[13, 16, 21-25] There are major clinical (and radiologic) differences in the presentation and course of hematogenous osteomyelitis in the child, the infant, and the adult. Childhood osteomyelitis can be associated with a sudden onset of high fever, a toxic state, and local signs of inflammation, although this presentation is certainly not uniform.[3] In the infant, hematogenous osteomyelitis can lead to pain, swelling, and an unwillingness to move the affected bones; in this age group, infected indwelling umbilical venous and arterial catheters can become the source of septicemia, resulting in osteomyelitis at multiple sites.[26-29] The adult form of hematogenous osteomyelitis may have a more insidious onset with a relatively longer period between the appearance of symptoms and signs and accurate diagnosis. In all age groups, the prior administration of antibiotics for treatment of the febrile state can attenuate or alter the clinical (and radiologic) manifestations of the bone infection.[30] Most series indicate that in children, boys are affected more frequently than girls. A similar male dominance is observed in adults. In infancy, boys and girls are affected with approximately equal frequency.

Single or multiple bones can be infected; involvement of multiple osseous sites appears to be particularly common in infants.[31] In the younger age group, the long tubular bones of the extremities (femur, humerus, tibia) are especially vulnerable; in adults, osteomyelitis of the vertebral column is not infrequent.

Although the list of potential organisms that can cause hematogenous osteomyelitis is indeed long, certain species are frequently implicated. *Staphylococcus aureus* is responsible for the vast majority of cases, although its prevalence appears to be diminishing.[3] Gram-negative, mycobacterial, and fungal organisms, and, less commonly, *Hemophilus influenzae* and *Diplococcus pneumoniae* may be the responsible agents. In infants, group B Streptococcus has reemerged as a causative agent of osteomyelitis; typically, this organism involves a single bone, particularly the humerus.[15, 288, 289] A recent surgical procedure or concurrent soft tissue infection frequently is associated with staphylococcal septicemia and osteomyelitis[29]; disorders of the gastrointestinal and genitourinary tracts may initiate a gram-negative septicemia; and an acute or chronic respiratory infection is important in the pathogenesis of tuberculous, fungal, and pneumococcal osteomyelitis.[3]

VASCULAR ANATOMY

Overview. A distinct osseous circulation supplies the bone tissue and cells, the marrow, the perichondrium, the epiphyseal cartilage in the immature skeleton, and, in part, the articular cartilage.[32] The vascular supply of a tubular bone is derived from several points of arterial inflow, which become complicated sinusoidal networks within the bone (Fig. 60–1). Drainage is accomplished via venous channels that exit from multiple locations.

In tubular bones, one or two diaphyseal nutrient arteries pierce the cortex and divide into ascending and descending branches. As they extend to the ends of the bones, they repeatedly branch, becoming finer channels, and are joined by the terminals of metaphyseal and epiphyseal arteries. The metaphyseal arteries originate from neighboring systemic vessels, whereas the epiphyseal arteries arise from periarticular vascular arcades.

The arteries within the bone marrow form a series of cortical branches that connect with the fenestrated capillaries of the haversian systems. At the bony surface, the cortical capillaries form connections with overlying periosteal plexuses, which themselves are derived from the arteries of the neighboring muscles and soft tissues. The cortices of the tubular bones derive nutrition from both the periosteal and the medullary circulatory systems; the direction of blood flow in each of these systems and the specific contribution each makes in nourishing the cortex are controversial. Although it is frequently maintained that the periosteal vessels supply the outer one third of the cortex and that the medullary vessels supply the inner two thirds, the contribution of each may be age-dependent. Based upon animal studies, the direction of arterial blood flow in the mature skeleton is predominantly centrifugal and that of the venous drainage is centripetal; in the immature animal, the contribution of the periosteal network is greater.[290] The exuberant anastomoses between the two systems allow blood to flow in either direction according to physiologic conditions.

The central arterioles drain into a thin-walled venous sinus, which subsequently unites with veins that retrace the course of the nutrient arteries, piercing the cortex at various points and joining larger and larger venous channels.

At the ends of the tubular bones, the nutrient arteries of the epiphysis form a series of intraosseous anastomoses with branches that pass into the subchondral regions. A series of end-arterial loops pierces the subchondral bone plate and, occasionally, the calcified zone of articular cartilage before turning to enter the venous sinusoid of the epiphysis.

This blood supply to the diaphysis, metaphysis, and epiphysis of tubular bones is very much dependent upon the age of the patient (see discussion later in this chapter).[6, 32, 33] In the child, distinct epiphyseal and metaphyseal arteries can be distinguished on either side of the cartilaginous growth plate, and anastomoses between these vessels are either infrequent or absent. Furthermore, the periosteum of the bones of young patients is more vascular than that of adults; its vessels communicate more freely with those of the shaft, and also give rise to many metaphyseal vessels.[32]

The blood supply also varies from one bone to another. Although the vascular anatomy of the tubular bones of the extremities has been emphasized in the preceding discussion, anastomosing periosteal and nutrient vessels are also fundamental to the blood supply of large, irregular bones such as those of the pelvis and scapula, whereas periosteal vessels supply compact and cancellous bone as well as marrow in the carpal and tarsal areas.

Articulations receive blood vessels from periarterial plexuses that pierce the capsule to form a vascular plexus in the deeper part of the synovial membrane.[32] The blood vessels of the synovial membrane terminate at the articular margins as looped anastomoses (circulus articularis vasculosus). The epiphysis and the adjacent synovium share a common blood supply.[8, 34]

The Three Vascular Patterns of the Tubular Bones. The radiologic and pathologic features of osteomyelitis differ in the child, the infant, and the adult, a fact that is related in large part to peculiarities of the vascular anatomy of the tubular bones in each of these three age groups (Table 60–1). Al-

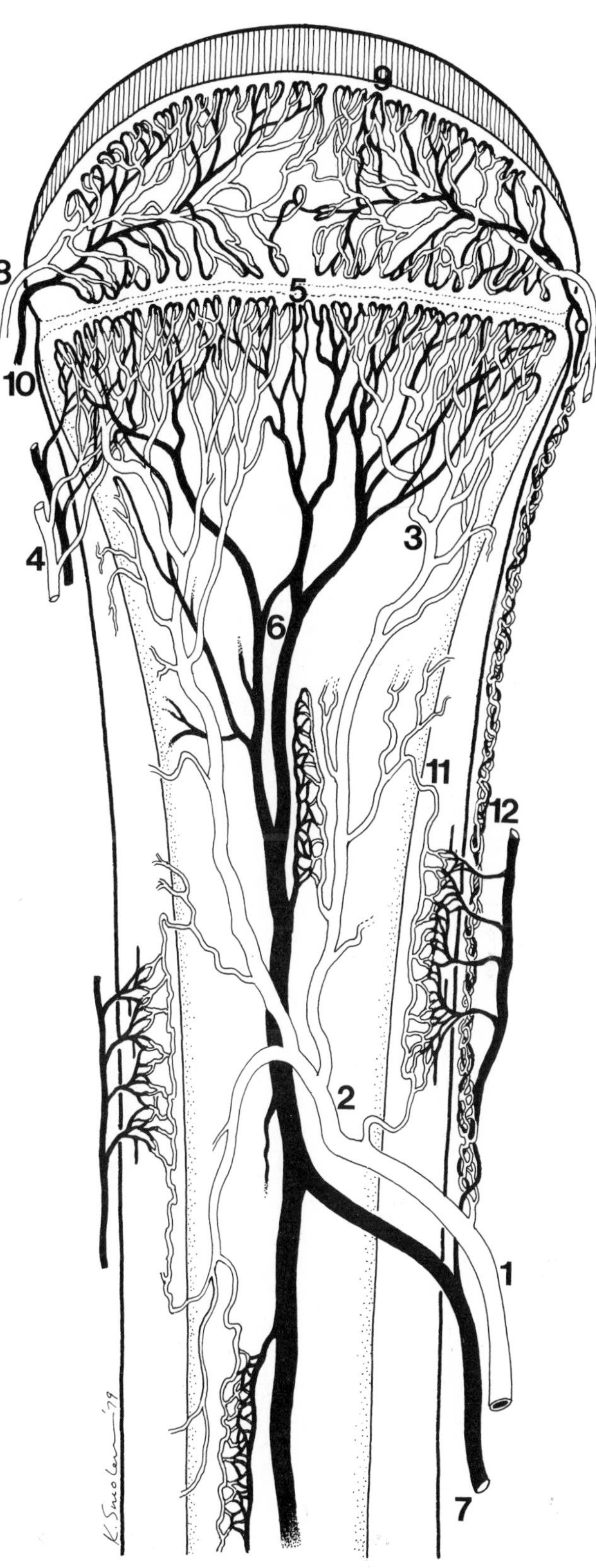

Figure 60–1. *Normal osseous circulation to a growing tubular bone. Nutrient arteries (1) pierce the diaphyseal cortex and divide into descending and ascending (2) branches. These latter vessels continue to divide, becoming fine channels (3) as they approach the end of the bone. They are joined by metaphyseal vessels (4) and, in the subepiphyseal (growth) plate region, they form a series of end-arterial loops (5). The venous sinuses extend from the metaphyseal region toward the diaphysis, uniting with other venous structures (6) and eventually piercing the cortex as a large venous channel (7). At the ends of the bone, nutrient arteries of the epiphysis (8) branch into finer structures, passing into the subchondral region. At this site, arterial loops (9) are again evident, some of which pierce the subchondral bone plate before turning to enter the venous sinusoid and venous channels of the epiphysis (10). At the bony surface, cortical capillaries (11) form connections with overlying periosteal plexuses (12). Note that in the growing child, distinct epiphyseal and metaphyseal arteries can be distinguished on either side of the cartilaginous growth plate. Anastomoses between these vessels either do not occur or are infrequent.*

Table 60–1
VASCULAR PATTERNS OF TUBULAR BONES

Pattern	Age	Characteristics
Infantile pattern	0–1 year*	Diaphyseal and metaphyseal vessels may perforate open growth plate
Childhood pattern	1–16 years†	Diaphyseal and metaphyseal vessels do not penetrate open growth plate
Adult pattern	>16 years	Diaphyseal and metaphyseal vessels penetrate closed growth plate

*Upper age limit is dependent upon specific local anatomic variations in the appearance and growth of the ossification center.
†Upper age limit is related to the time at which the open growth plate closes.

though the anatomic features outlined below are not without exception, it is extremely instructive to consider each of the three vascular patterns separately, for these anatomic principles govern the radiographic and pathologic characteristics of the disease process.[6, 18]

Childhood Pattern. Between the ages of approximately 1 year and the time when the open cartilaginous growth plates fuse, a childhood vascular pattern can be recognized in the ends of the tubular bones (Fig. 60–2*A*). Apart from those vessels in a narrow fringe at the periphery of the cartilage, the capillaries on the metaphyseal side of the growth plate are the terminal ramifications of a nutrient artery. It is here in the metaphysis that the vessels turn in acute loops to join large sinusoidal veins, which occupy the intramedullary portion of the metaphysis; and it is here that blood flow is slow and turbulent. The epiphyseal blood supply is distinct from that on the metaphyseal aspect of the plate, as the latter structure represents a barrier through which vessels do not pass. This anatomic characteristic combined with additional features to be discussed below, explains the peculiar predilection of hematogenous osteomyelitis to affect metaphyses and equivalent locations in the child.[10]

Infantile Pattern. A fetal vascular arrangement may persist in some tubular bones up to the age of 1 year with local variations corresponding to the time of full development of the epiphyseal bone nucleus (Fig. 60–2*B*). During fetal life, perichondral vessels progress toward the ends of the cartilaginous anlage, turning back when they reach the as yet unossified cartilaginous ends of the bone. In the terminal stages of intrauterine life and in the first 6 to 12 months following birth, when the growth cartilage is established but not yet limited by bone on its epiphyseal side, some vessels at the surface of the metaphysis penetrate the preexisting growth plate, ramifying in the epiphysis. After termination, they form large

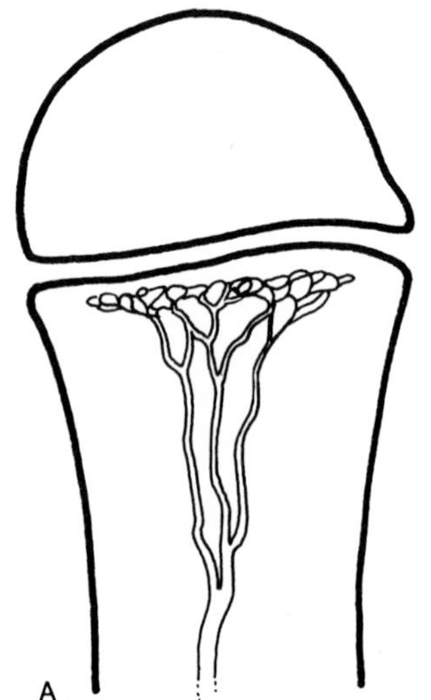

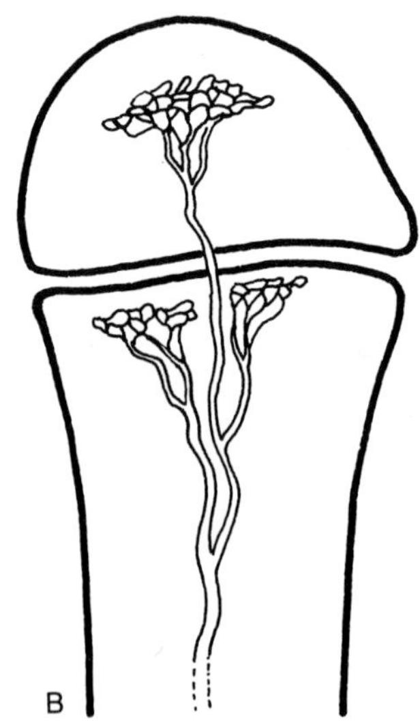

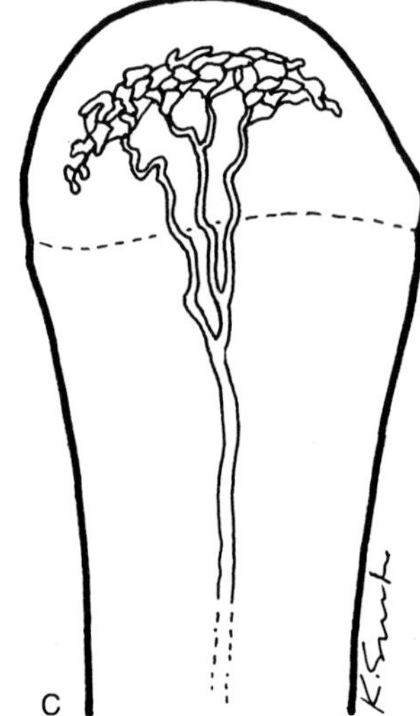

Figure 60–2. *Normal vascular patterns of a tubular bone in the child, the infant, and the adult.* **A,** *In the child, the capillaries of the metaphysis turn sharply, without violating the open growth plate.* **B,** *In the infant, some metaphyseal vessels may penetrate the open growth plate, ramifying in the epiphysis.* **C,** *In the adult, with closure of the growth plate, a vascular connection between metaphysis and epiphysis can be recognized.*

venous lakes not dissimilar to metaphyseal sinusoids. This arrangement affords a vascular connection between the metaphysis and epiphysis and explains the frequency of epiphyseal and articular infection in the infant.

Adult Pattern. With narrowing and closing of the epiphyseal growth plate, metaphyseal vessels progressively penetrate the diminishing cartilaginous structure, reestablishing a vascular connection between the metaphysis and the epiphysis (Fig. 60–2C). Blood within the nutrient vessels can then reach the surface of the epiphysis through large anastomosing channels, and organisms within these vessels can gain quick access to the ends of bones and the adjacent articulations.

HEMATOGENOUS OSTEOMYELITIS IN THE CHILD[2, 6, 18, 19, 35-49, 291] **(Table 60–2).** Hematogenous osteomyelitis reaches the metaphysis by way of the nutrient vessels; with intravenous injection of bacteria, organisms localize in the vascular spaces in the metaphysis as early as 2 hours following inoculation.[40] Metaphyseal location is related to (1) the peculiar anatomy of the vascular tree (Fig. 60–3*A*) in which the last ramifications of the nutrient artery negotiate sharp turns just short of the growth plate, emptying into a system of large sinusoidal veins; (2) the inability of vessels to penetrate the open epiphyseal plate; (3) the slow rate of blood flow in this region; (4) a decrease in phagocytic ability of neighboring macrophages; or (5) secondary thrombosis of the nutrient artery. These factors serve to create an ideal medium for the growth and multiplication of organisms (Fig. 60–4). The infection does not commonly localize in the metaphyseal or periosteal vessels, as these vessels do not possess a similar system of vascular loops proximal to the venous sinusoids.[6]

Inflammation in the adjacent bone is characterized by vascular engorgement, edema, cellular response, and abscess formation.[35] The peripheral portion of one or more abscesses may be heavily infiltrated with viable polymorphonuclear leukocytes, but in the more central portion of the abscess cavity, necrotic leukocytes can be detected.[2] Extensive involvement of the metaphyseal veins leads to early edema. Transudates extend from the marrow to the adjacent cortex. The inflammatory process enters the cortical bone and extends across it by way of its haversian and Volkmann's canals, especially in that area of the distal metaphysis in which the cortex is extremely thin.

Cortical porosity is produced, at least in part, by osteoclastosis, leading to enlargement of haversian canals, facilitating cortical penetration by the accumulating organisms. The inflammatory process soon reaches the outer surface of the cortex and abscesses develop, lifting the periosteum and disrupting the periosteal blood supply to the external cortical surface. Elevation of the periosteum is prominent in the immature skeleton because of its relatively loose attachment to the subjacent bone. The elevated periosteum lays down bone in the form of an involucrum that partially or completely surrounds the infected bone. Infection may penetrate the periosteal membrane, extending into the adjacent soft tissues and leading to single or multiple abscesses.

Cortical necrosis and sequestration can subsequently appear. Necrosis is facilitated by deprivation of blood supply to the inner portion of the cortex owing to thrombosis of the metaphyseal vessels and by interruption of periosteal blood supply to the outer portion of the cortex as a result of lifting of the periosteum.

With treatment of the infection, with spontaneous escape of pus into the soft tissues, or with surgical decompression, a reparative response may supersede. Apposition of new bone on the walls of the widened haversian canals and cortical thickening can be seen. Osteoclastic activity at the junction of living and dead bone can produce resorption or fragmentation of the necrotic tissue. The marrow cavity becomes filled with granulation tissue, which is later replaced by fibrous elements. Further healing is characterized by transformation of abscesses into cystic cavities and replacement of scar tissue either by cellular or fatty marrow.[2]

Hematogenous osteomyelitis of the child is not confined to tubular bones.[10, 13, 41] In flat or irregular bones, such as the calcaneus, the clavicle, and the

Table 60–2

HEMATOGENOUS OSTEOMYELITIS OF TUBULAR BONES

	Infant	Child	Adult
Localization	Metaphyseal with epiphyseal extension	Metaphyseal	Epiphyseal
Involucrum	Common	Common	Not common
Sequestration	Common	Common	Not common
Joint involvement	Common	Not common	Common
Soft tissue abscess	Common	Common	Not common
Pathologic fracture	Not common	Not common	Common*
Fistulae	Not common	Variable	Common

*In neglected cases.

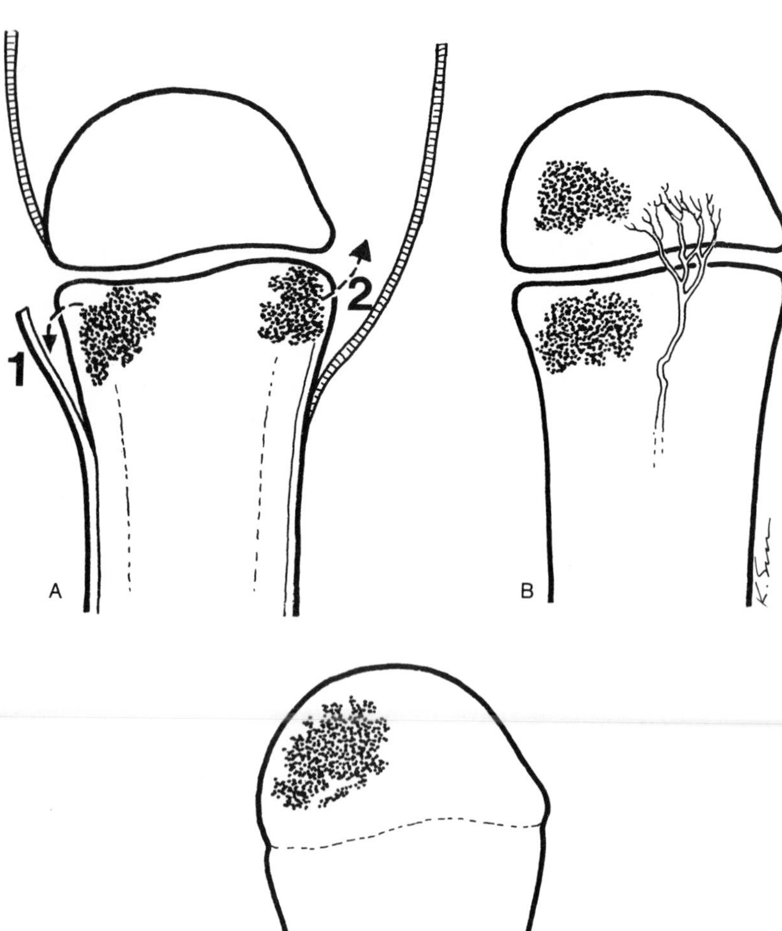

Figure 60–3. Sites of hematogenous osteomyelitis of a tubular bone in the child, the infant, and the adult. **A,** In the child, a metaphyseal focus is frequent. From this site, cortical penetration can result in a subperiosteal abscess in those locations in which the growth plate is extra-articular (1) or in a septic joint in those locations in which the growth plate is intra-articular (2). **B,** In the infant, a metaphyseal focus may be complicated by epiphyseal extension owing to the vascular anatomy in this age group. **C,** In the adult, a subchondral focus in an epiphysis is not unusual, owing to the vascular anatomy in this age group.

bones of the pelvis, childhood osteomyelitis may show predilection for metaphyseal-equivalent osseous locations adjacent to an apophyseal cartilaginous plate and epiphyseal-equivalent locations adjacent to articular cartilage.[10] Preferential involvement of these sites as well as of metaphyseal-equivalent locations of long bones (e.g., adjacent to the apophyses of the tibial tuberosity and femoral trochanters) is again related to regional vascular anatomy, which, in these areas, is similar to that of the metaphyses of the tubular bones.[42] Infection in these "unusual" sites (short or flat bones) may occur in 18 to 25 per cent of all cases of osteomyelitis.[43-45] The radiographic and pathologic characteristics of osteomyelitis in metaphyseal- and epiphyseal-equivalent areas are similar to those in the long bones.[43, 44]

Hematogenous Osteomyelitis in the Infant[6, 7, 14-16, 46, 47] **(Table 60–2).** Although there are fundamental similarities between the manifestations of hematogenous osteomyelitis in the infant and those in the child, certain differences are also apparent. As some of the vessels in the metaphysis penetrate the growth plate, a suppurative process of the metaphysis may extend into the epiphysis (Figs. 60–3*B* and 60–5). Epiphyseal infection can then result in articular contamination and damage the cells on the epiphyseal side of the growth cartilage, leading to arrest or disorganization of growth and maturation. Articular involvement is also facilitated by the frequent localization of infantile osteomyelitis to ends of the bone in which the growth plate is intra-articular (e.g., hip), allowing direct contamination of the joint space from a metaphyseal septic focus[7] (see discussion later in this chapter).

Profuse involucrum formation is also characteristic of osteomyelitis in the infant; exuberant cloaks of bone may extend around the metaphysis and diaphysis of a tubular bone, reflecting the ease with which the immature periosteum is lifted from the subjacent bone and the extreme richness of the periosteal vessels in infancy. The remarkable healing properties of osseous tissue in the first years of

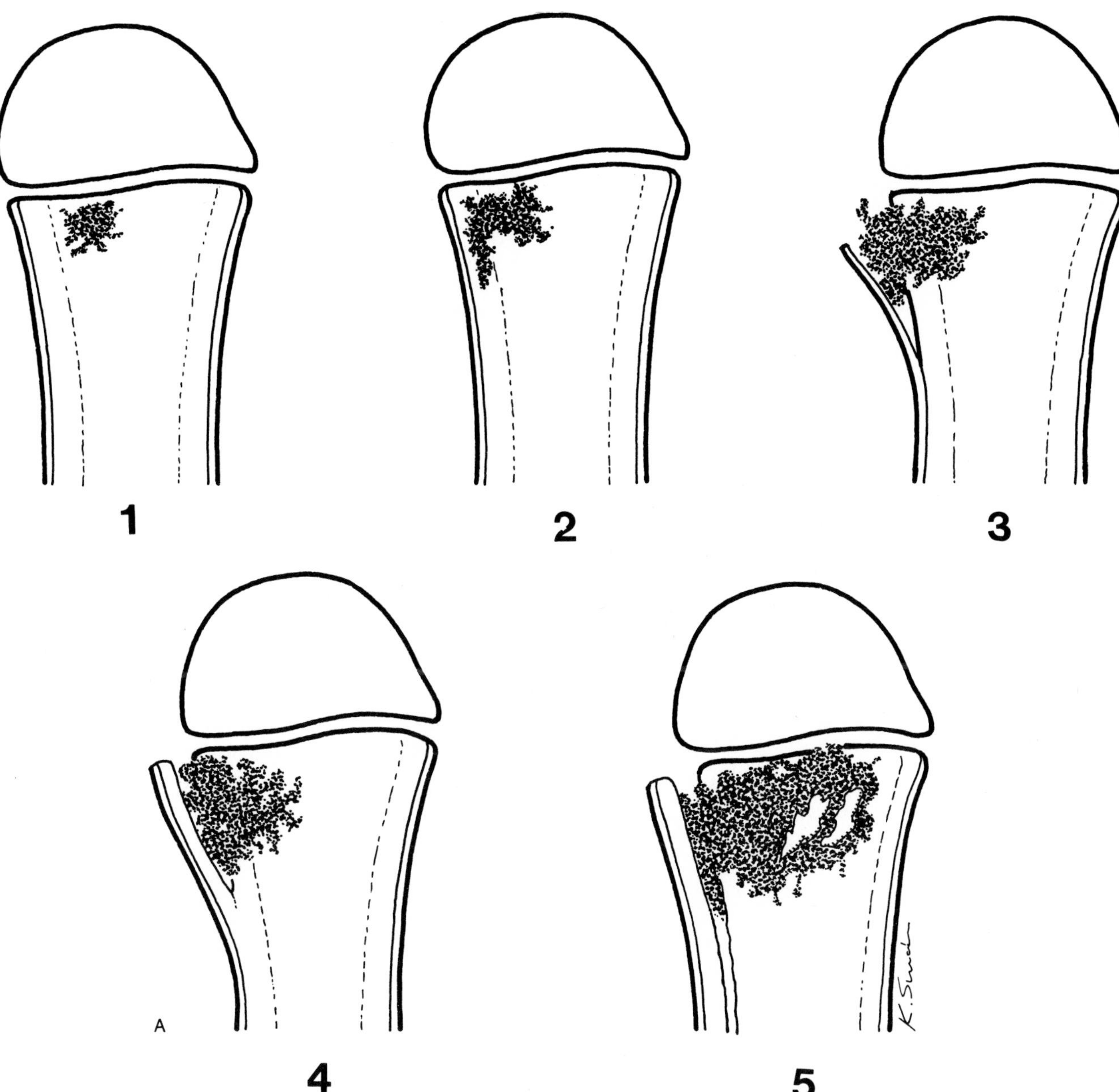

Figure 60–4. *Hematogenous osteomyelitis of a tubular bone in the child.*

A *Sequential steps in the initiation and progression of infection. 1, A metaphyseal focus is common; 2, the infection spreads laterally, reaching and invading the cortical bone; 3, cortical penetration is associated with subperiosteal extension and elevation of the periosteal membrane; 4, subperiosteal bone formation leads to an involucrum or shell of new bone; 5, the involucrum may become massive with continued infection.*

Illustration continued on the following page

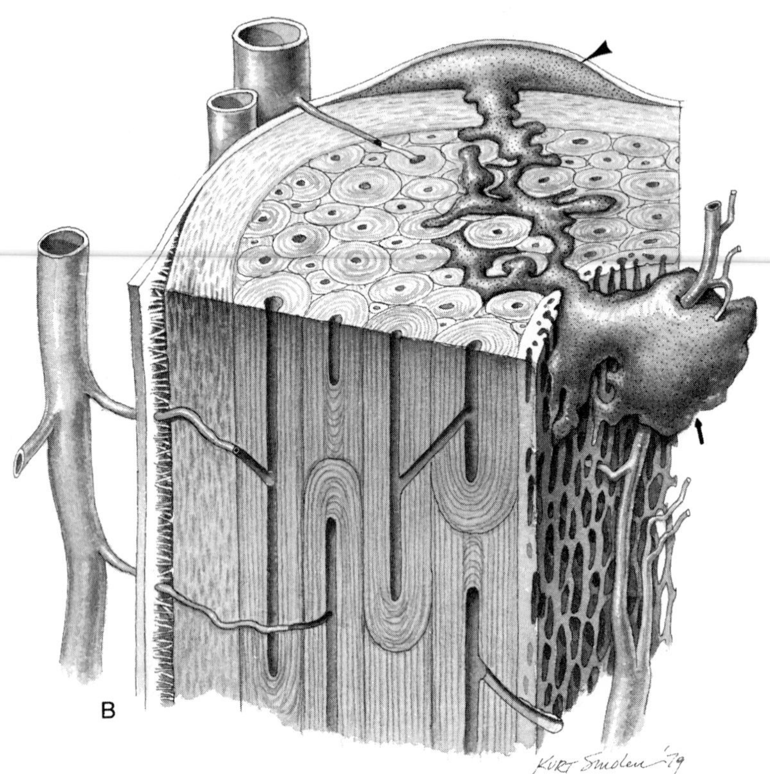

Figure 60–4. Continued

B *A diagram of the manner in which infection in the medullary canal (arrow) permeates the cortex and collects beneath the periosteal membrane (arrowhead).*

Illustration continued on the opposite page

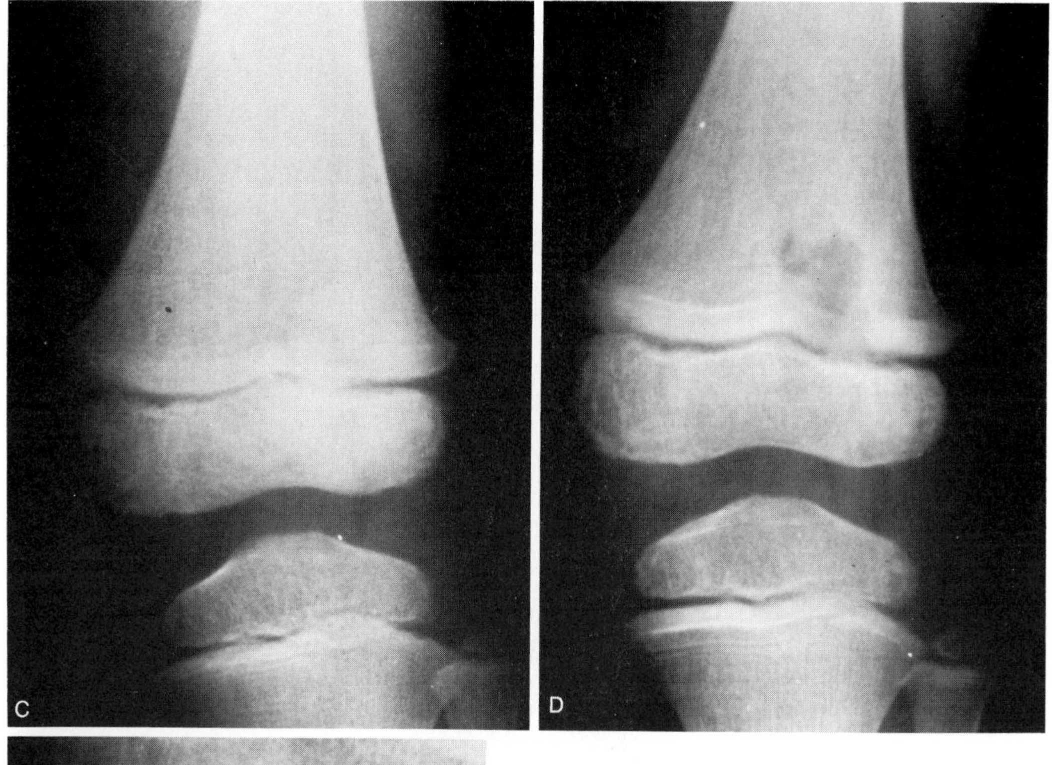

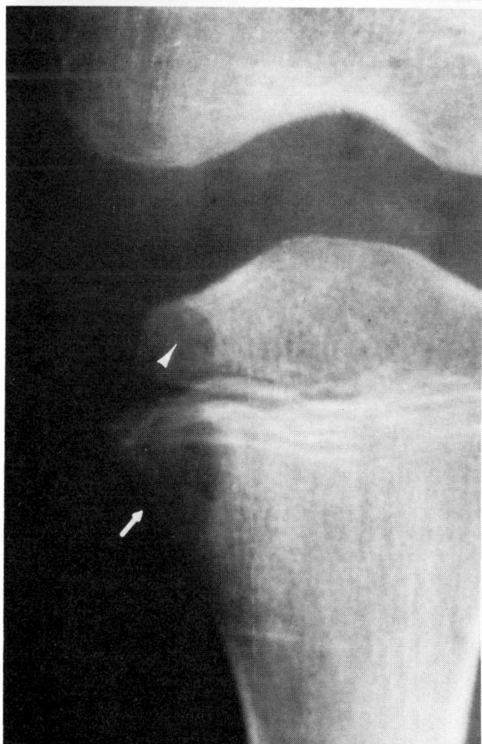

Figure 60–4. Continued

C, D *In this child with pain and swelling of the knee, initial radiographs at the time of clinical presentation do not reveal osseous destruction. Two weeks later, a lytic metaphyseal focus in the femur is readily apparent. It extends to the growth cartilage (causative organism is staphylococcus).*

E *Rarely, in the child, a metaphyseal infection (arrow) can violate the growth cartilage with epiphyseal involvement (arrowhead) (causative organism is staphylococcus).*

Illustration continued on the following page

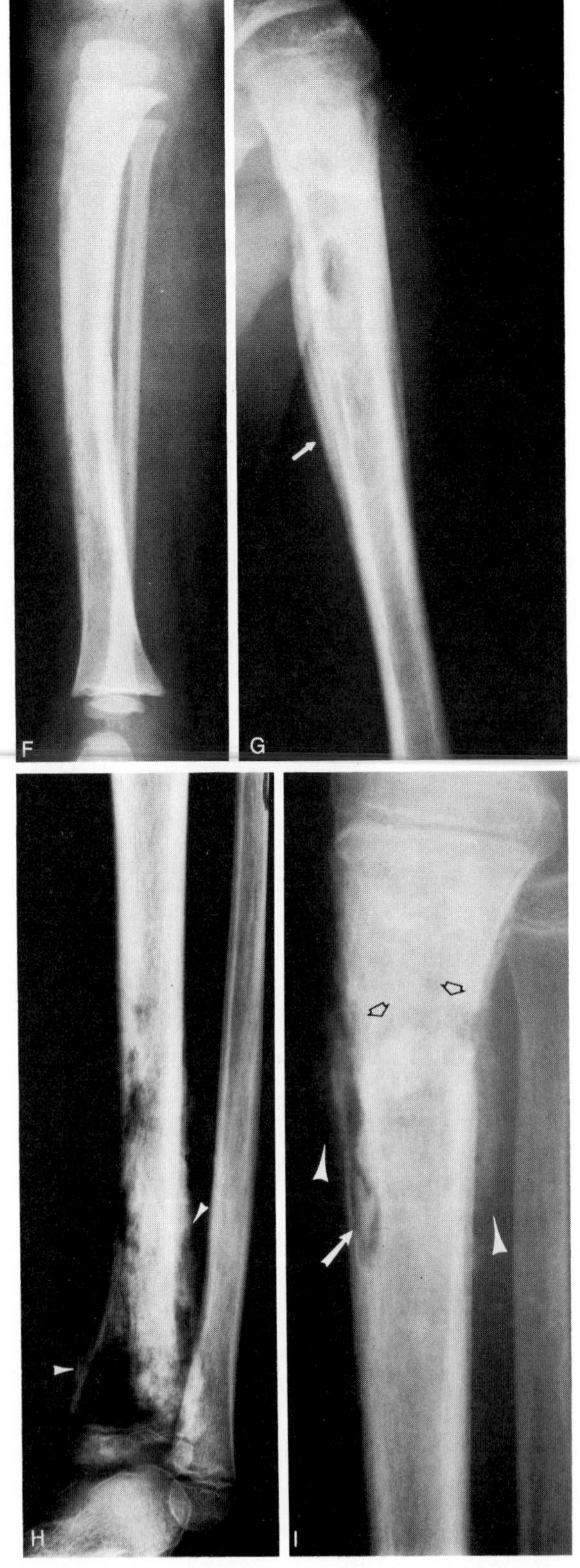

Figure 60–4. Continued

F *In this child with acute hematogenous osteomyelitis, widespread involvement of the metaphysis and diaphysis of the tibia, cortical penetration, and soft tissue swelling are evident.*

G *Note metaphyseal and diaphyseal medullary destruction as well as involucrum formation (arrow).*

H *Observe permeative bone destruction of the distal tibial metaphysis and diaphysis with periosteal bone formation (arrowheads).*

I *In this patient, the roentgenographic findings include medullary bone destruction of the metaphysis and diaphysis of the proximal tibia, cortical penetration with periostitis (arrowheads), a sequestrum (solid arrow), and a pathologic fracture (open arrows).*

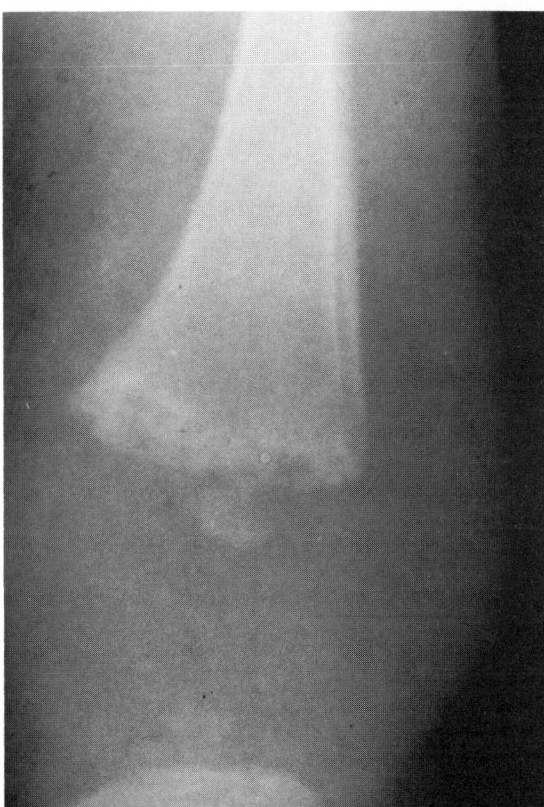

Figure 60–5. *Hematogenous osteomyelitis of a tubular bone in the infant. In this infant with acute staphylococcal osteomyelitis, metaphyseal and epiphyseal involvement of the distal femur is associated with periostitis and articular involvement.*

life are evidenced by the fact that the prominent involucrum commonly merges with cortex of the subjacent bone, eventually leaving little or no trace of previous osteomyelitis.

In addition to epiphyseal and joint involvement and massive involucrum formation, infantile osteomyelitis is associated with cortical sequestration and soft tissue alterations such as edema or abscess formation, which can lead to significant changes in the first days of the infection, prior to the appearance of osseous abnormalities.[9, 46] Apparently, in the younger age groups, infection more easily violates the adjacent periosteum, facilitating soft tissue contamination. Fistulae are relatively rare in infantile osteomyelitis.

HEMATOGENOUS OSTEOMYELITIS IN THE ADULT[6, 7, 18] **(Table 60–2).** Hematogenous osteomyelitis in the mature skeleton does not commonly localize in the tubular bones; hematogenous osteomyelitis of the spine, pelvis, and small bones is more common in the adult patient. In cases in which such localization is evident, the free communication of the metaphyseal and epiphyseal vessels through the closed growth plate allows infection to localize in the subchondral (beneath the articular cartilage) regions of the bone (Figs. 60–3C and 60–6). Joint contamination can complicate this epiphyseal location.

The fibrous and firm attachment of the periosteum to the cortex in the adult resists displacement and, therefore, subperiosteal abscess formation, extensive periostitis, and involucrum formation are relatively unusual in this age group. Furthermore, the intimacy of the periosteum and cortex in the adult assures adequate cortical blood supply in most individuals; extensive sequestration is not a common feature of adult-onset osteomyelitis. Rather, infection violates and disrupts the cortex itself, producing atrophy and osseous weakening, and predisposes the bone to pathologic fracture. Infection may also spread along the entire length of the tubular bone with involvement of large segments of the diaphysis; chronic osteomyelitis with fistulae is common.

ACUTE HEMATOGENOUS OSTEOMYELITIS — RADIOLOGIC AND PATHOLOGIC ABNORMALITIES (Table 60–3) (Fig. 60–7). Radiographic evidence of significant osseous destruction in hematogenous pyogenic osteomyelitis is delayed for a period of days to weeks. It is the insensitivity of this modality in the early diagnosis of bone infection that has prompted the utilization of other modalities such as scintigraphy for the prompt recognition of osteomyelitis (see discussion later in this chapter). However, initial and subtle roentgenographic changes in the soft tissues may appear within 3 days of bacterial contamination of bone.[9] Focal deep soft tissue swelling in the metaphyseal region of infants and children may be the first important roentgenographic sign. Such swelling, which is temporally related to the vascular changes and edema of the early osteomyelitic process, results in displacement of the lucent tissue planes from the underlying bone. A few days later, muscle swelling and obliteration of the soft tissue planes can be observed.[46, 48, 49] The deep muscles and soft tissues are affected first, followed later by involvement of the more superficial muscles and subcutaneous tissue.[9]

In pyogenic infection, radiographically evident bone destruction and periostitis can be delayed for 1 to 2 weeks following intraosseous lodgment of the organisms (Fig. 60–4C, D). At all early stages, the degree of bony involvement that is visible on the roentgenogram is considerably less than that which is evident on pathologic examination.[9] Eventually, large destructive lesions become evident on the radiograph. In the child, these lesions appear as enlarging, ill-defined lucent shadows of the metaphysis surrounded by varying amounts of eburnation; the lucent lesions extend to the growth plate and, on rare occasions, may violate it (Fig. 60–4E). In addition, destruction progresses horizontally, reaching the cortex, and periostitis follows (Fig. 60–4F,G).

In the infant, the epiphyses are unossified or only partially ossified so that radiographic recognition of epiphyseal destruction can be extremely

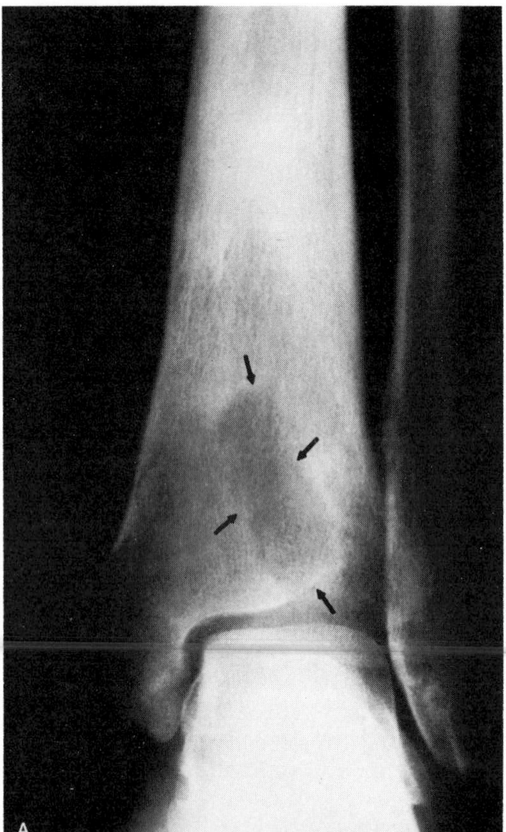

Figure 60–6. *Hematogenous osteomyelitis of a tubular bone in the adult.*

A *An epiphyseal localization is not infrequent in this age group. Observe the lytic lesion (abscess) with surrounding sclerosis extending to the subchondral bone plate (arrows). Metaphyseal and diaphyseal sclerosis is evident. The elongated shape of the lesion is typical of infection (causative organism is staphylococcus).*

B, C *On a radiograph and photograph of a coronal section of a humerus in an adult patient with osteomyelitis, note the metaphyseal and epiphyseal destruction with extension into the subchondral bone (arrows). Such destruction is frequent in this age group.*

Illustration continued on the opposite page

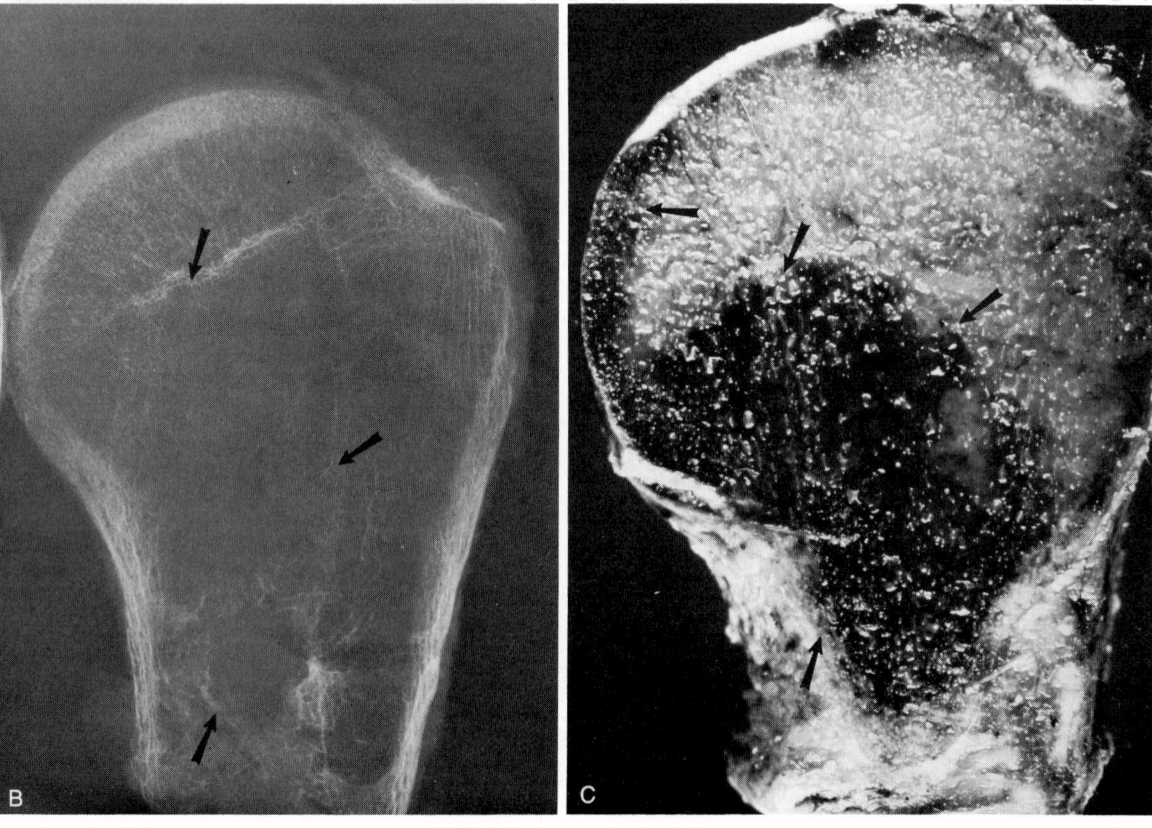

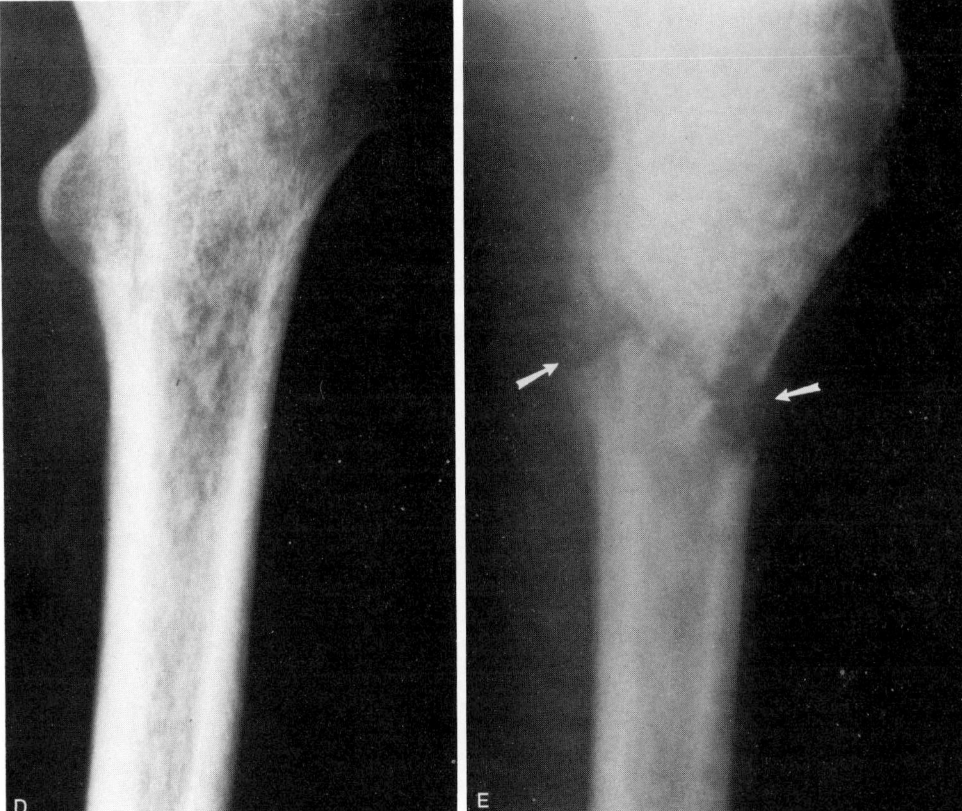

Figure 60–6. Continued
D, E *This 20 year old man developed acute osteomyelitis following an aortic valve replacement. The initial film* **(D)** *reveals mottled, ill-defined destruction of the metaphysis and diaphysis of the proximal femur with endosteal erosion. Four weeks later* **(E)**, *progressive lysis and sclerosis with a pathologic fracture (arrows) and soft tissue swelling are evident (causative organism is staphylococcus).*

Table 60–3

HEMATOGENOUS OSTEOMYELITIS: RADIOGRAPHIC–PATHOLOGIC CORRELATION

Pathologic Abnormality	Radiographic Abnormality
Vascular changes and edema of soft tissues	Soft tissue swelling with obliteration of tissue planes
Infection in medullary space with hyperemia, edema, abscess formation, and trabecular destruction	Osteoporosis, bone lysis
Infection in haversian and Volkmann's canals of cortex	Increasing lysis, cortical lucency
Subperiosteal abscess formation with lifting of the periosteum and bone formation	Periostitis, involucrum formation
Infectious penetration of periosteum with soft tissue abscess formation	Soft tissue swelling, mass formation, obliteration of tissue planes
Localized cortical and medullary abscesses	Single or multiple radiolucent cortical or medullary lesions with surrounding sclerosis
Deprivation of blood supply to cortex due to thrombosis of metaphyseal vessels and interruption of periosteal vessels, cortical necrosis	Sequestration
External migration of dead pieces of cortex with breakdown of skin and subcutaneous tissue	Fistulae

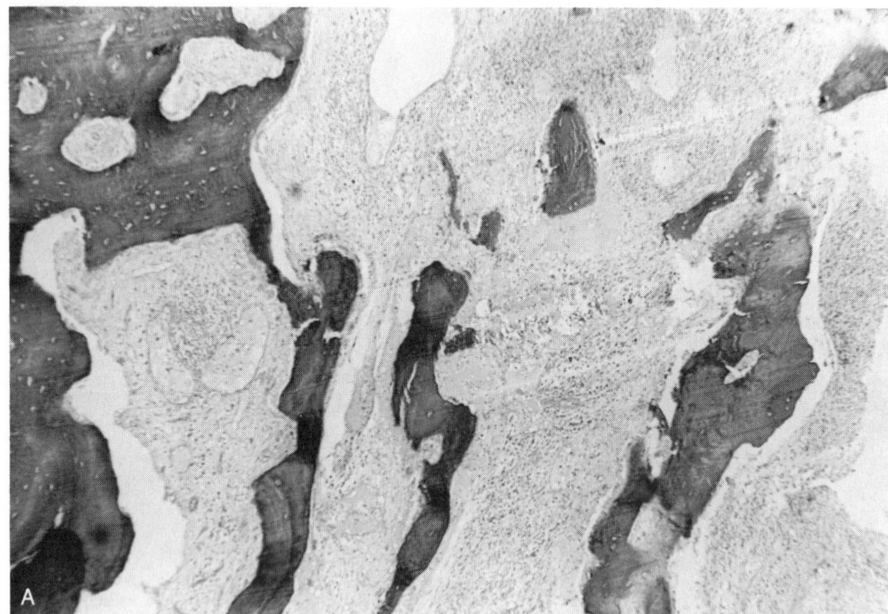

Figure 60–7. Hematogenous osteomyelitis: Pathologic abnormalities.

A Acute osteomyelitis. Note necrosis of multiple bony trabeculae and an acute inflammatory cellular infiltration in the marrow spaces (100×).

Illustration continued on the opposite page

difficult. Metaphyseal lucent lesions, periostitis, and a joint effusion are helpful radiographic clues (Fig. 60–5). Arthrography is frequently of additional aid; joint aspiration allows documentation of the infection, and opacification of the articulation can provide information regarding the integrity of the cartilaginous surface of the epiphysis.

In the adult, soft tissue alterations are more difficult to detect on roentgenographic examination. Epiphyseal, metaphyseal, and diaphyseal osseous destruction creates radiolucent areas of varying size, which are associated with mild periostitis (Fig. 60–6). Cortical resorption can be identified as endosteal scalloping, intracortical lucent regions or tunneling, and poorly defined subperiosteal bony defects or gaps.

Subacute and Chronic Hematogenous Osteomyelitis — Radiographic and Pathologic Abnormalities (Fig. 60–7)

Brodie's Abscess. Single or multiple radiolucent abscesses can be evident during subacute or chronic stages of osteomyelitis. These abscesses were initially described in the tibial metaphyses by Brodie in 1832[50, 51] in a study of eight male patients between the ages of 13 and 34 years. Although this investigator did not have the advantages of radiographic and bacteriologic techniques, his detailed descriptive analysis has been honored by the eponym "Brodie's abscess," which is still applied to the pyogenic lesions. Further descriptions of Brodie's abscesses belong to Brickner,[52] Henderson and Simon,[53] Brailsford,[54] and, more recently, Harris and Kirkaldy-Willis.[55] These abscesses are now defined as circumscribed lesions showing predilection for (but not confined to) the ends of tubular bones, characterizing subacute pyogenic osteomyelitis, usually of staphylococcal origin.

It has been suggested that bone abscesses develop when an infective organism has a reduced virulence or when the host demonstrates increased resistance to infection.[55] Brodie's abscesses are especially common in children, more typically boys. In this age group, they appear in the metaphysis, particularly that of the distal or proximal tibia. Less frequently, they occur in other tubular, flat, or irregular bones, including the vertebral bodies, and are diaphyseal in location.[2] Rarely, they traverse the open growth plate, affecting the epiphysis, although such extension does not commonly result in growth disturbance.[56] Abscesses vary from less than 1 cm to over 4 cm in diameter. The wall of the abscess is lined by inflammatory granulation tissue which is surrounded by spongy bone eburnation (Fig. 60–7*D,E*). The fluid in the abscess may be purulent or mucoid[2]; bacteriologic examination of the fluid may or may not reveal the infecting organisms.

Radiographs outline radiolucency with adjacent sclerosis (Fig. 60–8). This lucency is commonly located in the metaphysis, where it may connect with the growth plate by a tortuous channel. Radiographic detection of this channel is important; identification of a metaphyseal defect connected to the growth plate by such a tract assures the diagnosis of osteomyelitis. Furthermore, such channels usually indicate a pyogenic process and are uncommon in tuberculosis. In the diaphysis, the radiolucent abscess cavity can be located in central or subcortical areas of the spongiosa or in the cortex itself and may contain a central sequestrum.[57, 58, 281] When in the cortex, its radiographic appearance, consisting of a lucent lesion with surrounding sclerosis and perios-

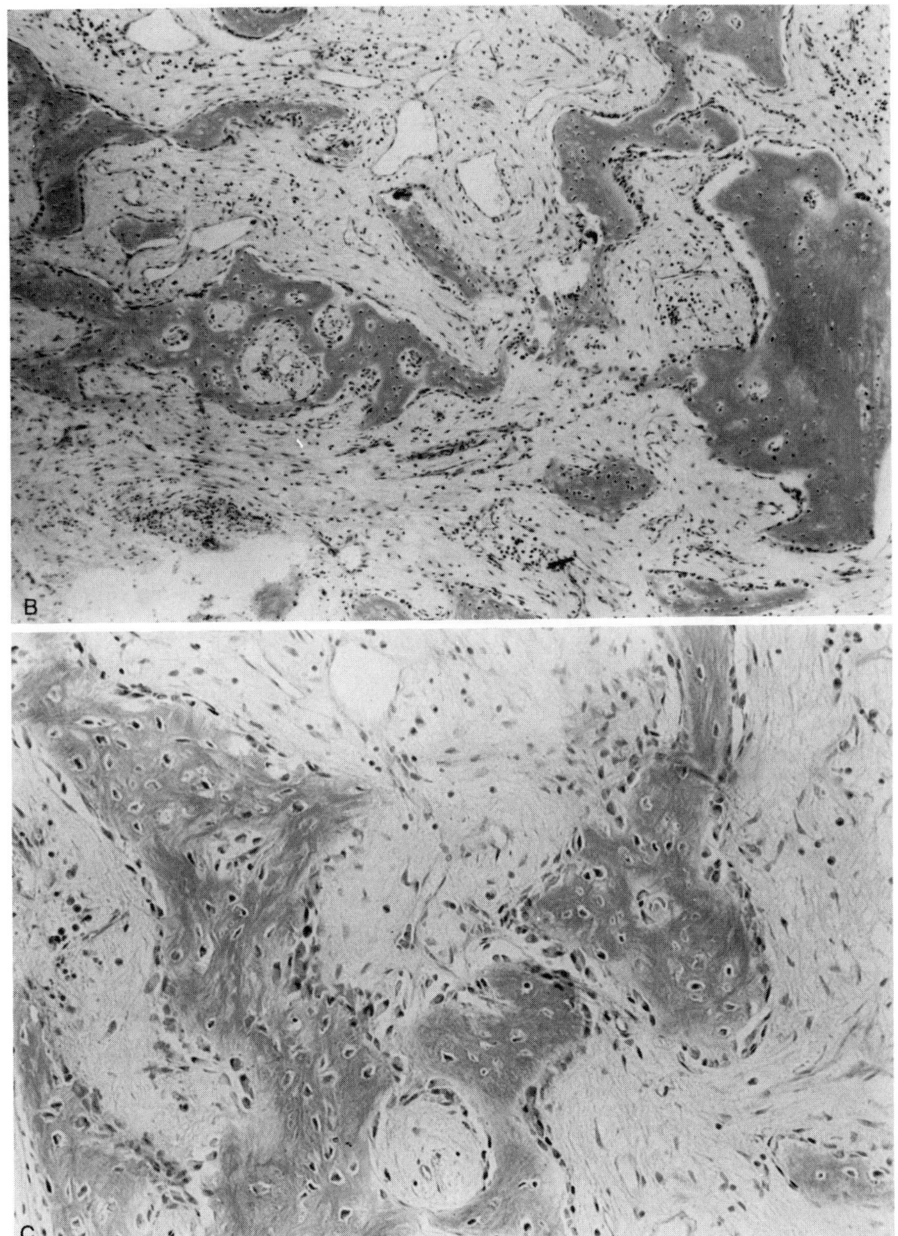

Figure 60–7. Continued
B, C *Chronic osteomyelitis. Low (100×) and high (250×) power photomicrographs reveal reactive bone formation in the vicinity of a chronic pyogenic inflammatory lesion. The normal hematopoietic marrow has been replaced by vascular connective tissue that contains lymphocytes and plasma cells. The newly formed woven bone is covered by large active osteoblasts.*

Illustration continued on the following page

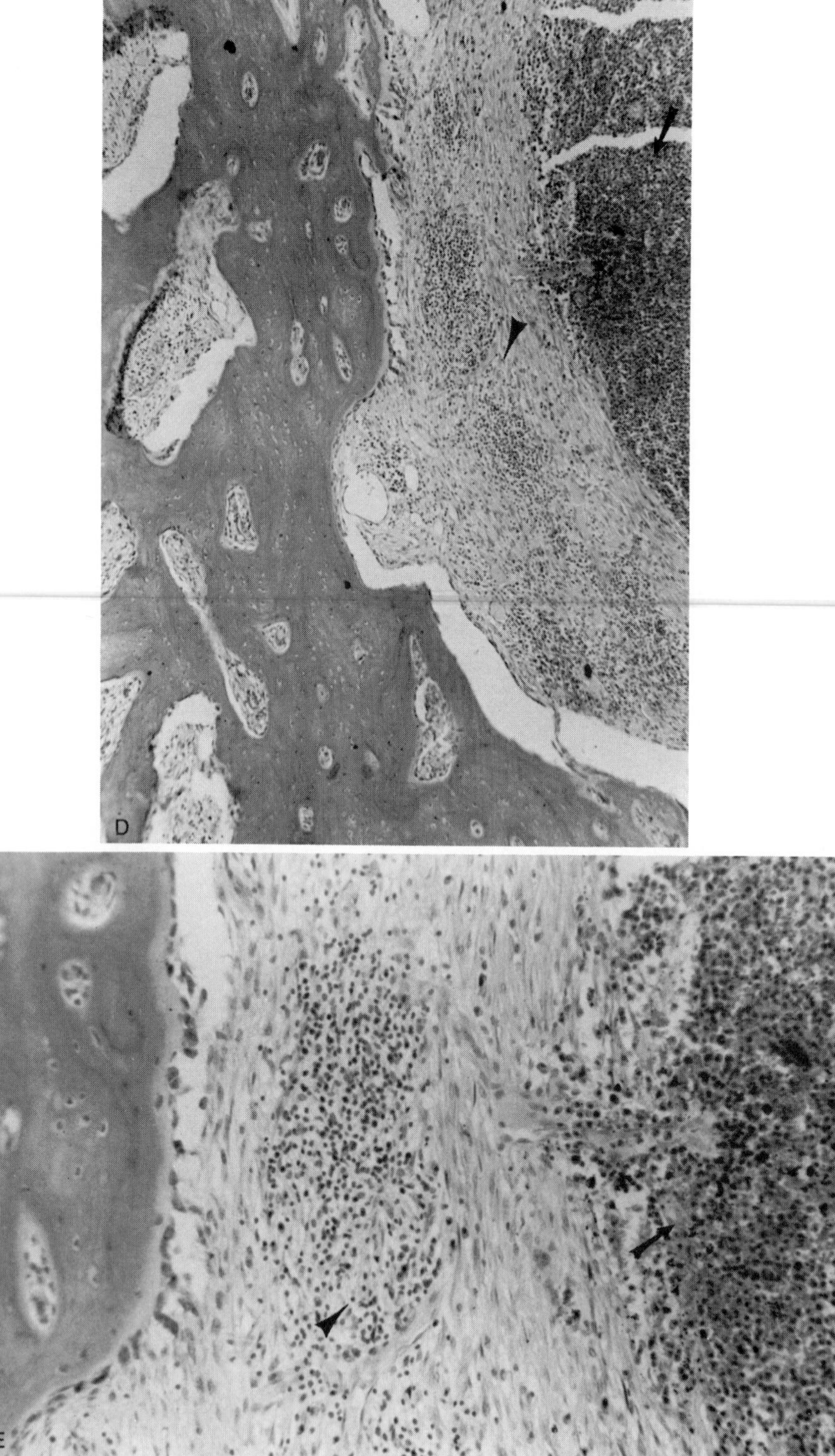

Figure 60–7. Continued

D, E *Brodie's abscess. On low power (100×) and high power (250×) photomicrographs, note the abscess mass consisting of cellular debris and neutrophils (arrow), a surrounding fibrotic reaction (arrowhead), and peripheral eburnated bone.*

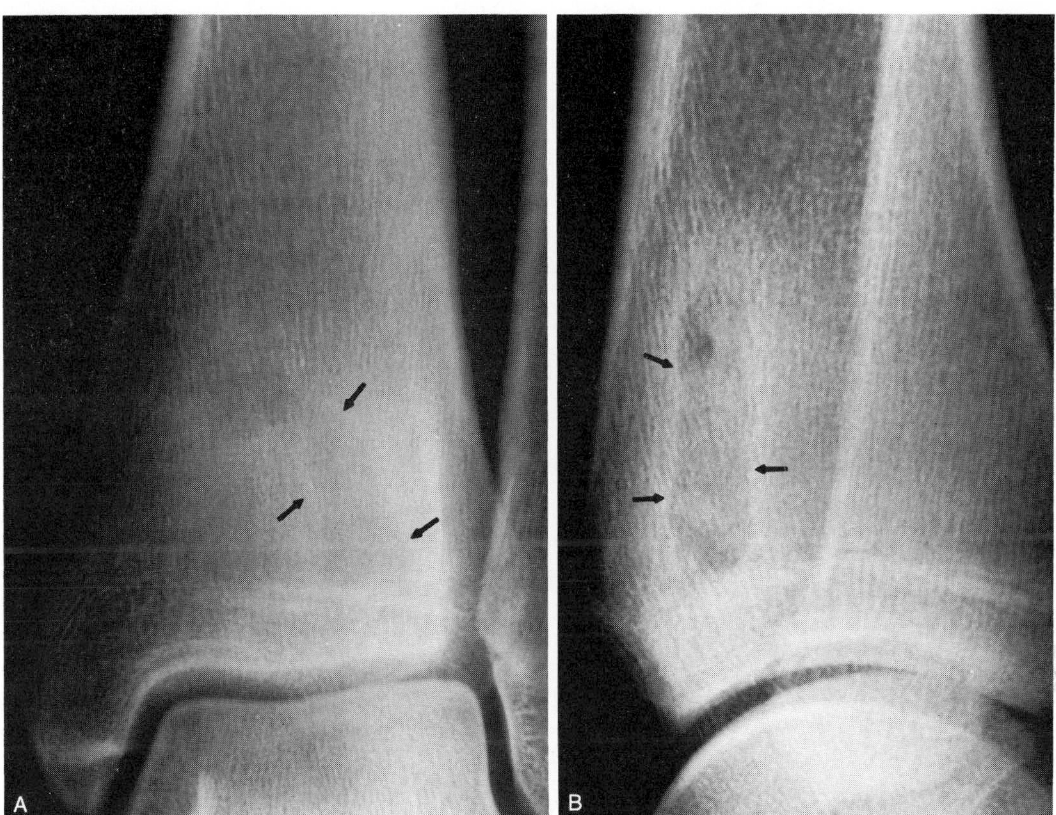

Figure 60–8. *Hematogenous osteomyelitis: Brodie's abscess.*

A, B *Anteroposterior and lateral radiographs outline a typical appearance of an abscess of the distal tibia due to staphylococci. Observe the elongated radiolucent lesion with surrounding sclerosis extending to the closing growth plate (arrows). The channel-like shape of the lesion is important in the accurate diagnosis of this condition.*

Illustration continued on the following page

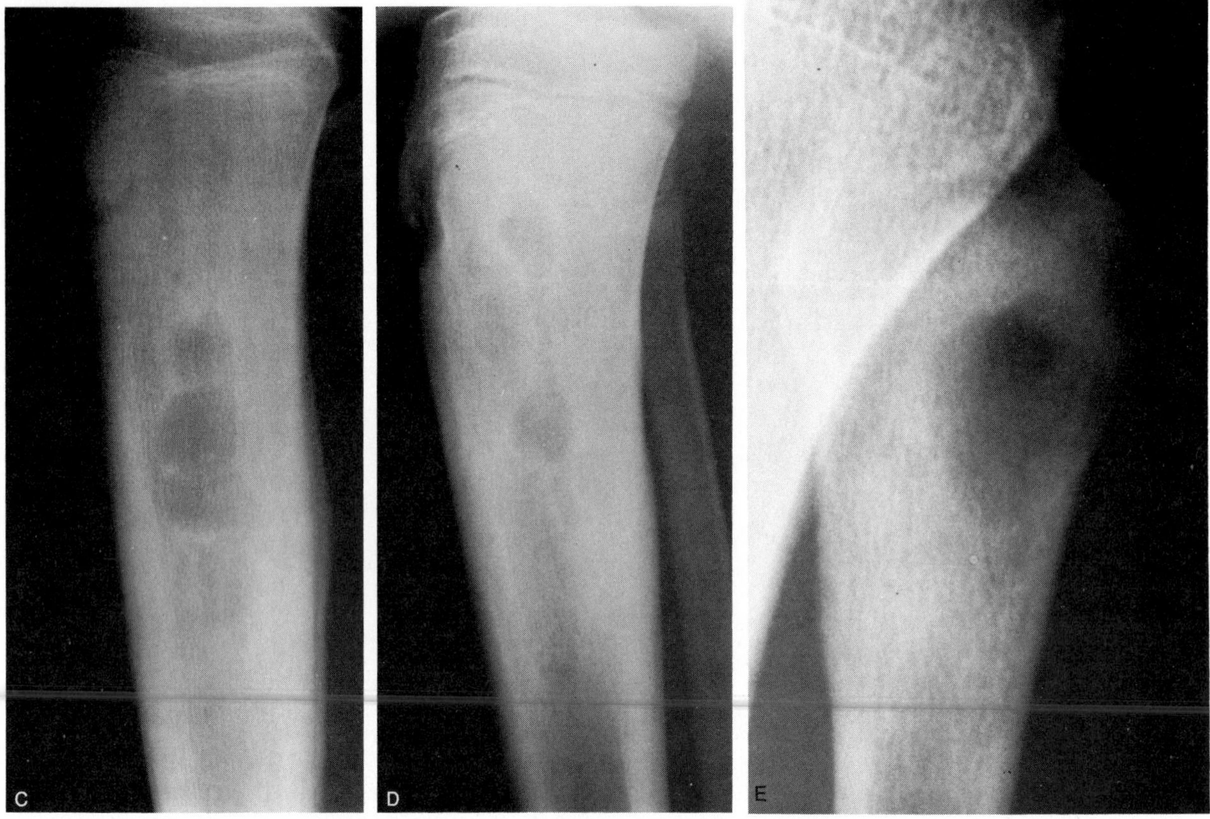

Figure 60–8. Continued

C *An example of an abscess of the proximal diaphysis of the tibia. Note its multiloculated appearance, surrounding sclerosis, and periosteal bone formation.*

D *In a different patient, a dumbbell-shaped lesion is evident. Note the channel-like characteristics of this abscess and surrounding bone eburnation of the tibia.*

E *This well-circumscribed abscess is located in the proximal fibula. It too is contained within sclerotic bone.*

titis, simulates that of an osteoid osteoma or a stress fracture. A circular or elliptical radiolucent lesion without calcification that is smaller or larger than 2 cm is characteristic of a cortical abscess; a circular lucent area with or without calcification smaller than 2 cm is typical of an osteoid osteoma; and a linear lucent shadow without calcification is characteristic of a stress fracture.

Sequestration. During the course of hematogenous osteomyelitis, cortical sequestration can become evident. One or more areas of osseous necrosis are commonly situated in the medullary aspect of a tubular bone (sequestration is less prominent in flat bones), where they create radiodense bony spicules (Fig. 60–9). The increased density is primarily related to the fact that a sequestrum does not possess a blood supply and does not participate in the hyperemia and resulting osteoporosis of the adjacent living bone. The sequestrum is frequently sharply marginated as it rests in a space surrounded by granulation tissue, and it varies in size from minute fragments to long necrotic segments. Sequestra may extrude through cortical breaks, extending into the adjacent soft tissues, where they may eventually be discharged through draining fistulae.[59] Tomography and fistulography are helpful procedures in documenting the presence and position of retained sequestra.

Sclerosing Osteomyelitis. In the subacute and chronic stages of osteomyelitis, considerable periosteal bone formation can surround the altered cortex, and an increased number and size of spongy trabeculae can reappear in the affected marrow,[2] indicating a healing response and leading to considerable radiodensity and contour irregularity of the affected bone (Fig. 60–10). It is not entirely accurate to designate these changes sclerosing osteomyelitis of Garré (see earlier discussion).

Spread from a Contiguous Source of Infection

General Clinical Features. Bone (and joint) contamination can result from spread of a contiguous source of infection. In most of the cases of osteomyelitis (and septic arthritis) arising from such a contiguous source, soft tissue infections are implicated (postoperative infection is discussed sep-

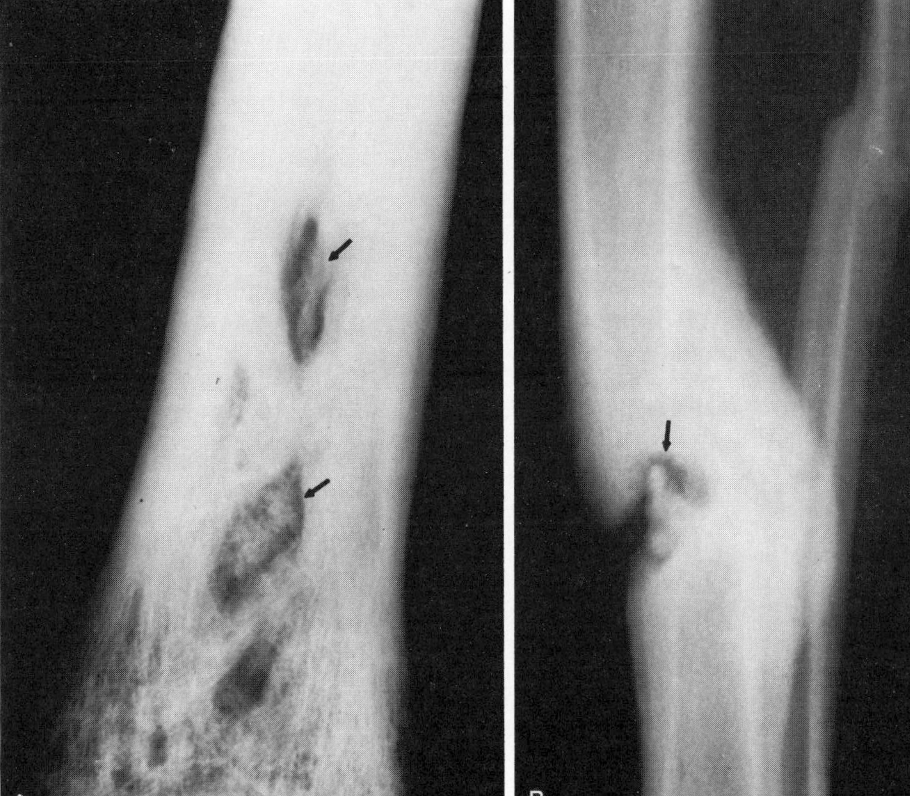

Figure 60–9. Chronic osteomyelitis: Sequestration.

A *In this femur, chronic osteomyelitis is associated with several radiodense, sharply marginated foci (arrows) within lucent cavities that contain granulation tissue.*

B *In a different patient, chronic osteomyelitis of a tibia followed a fracture. Note the well-defined sequestrum (arrow).*

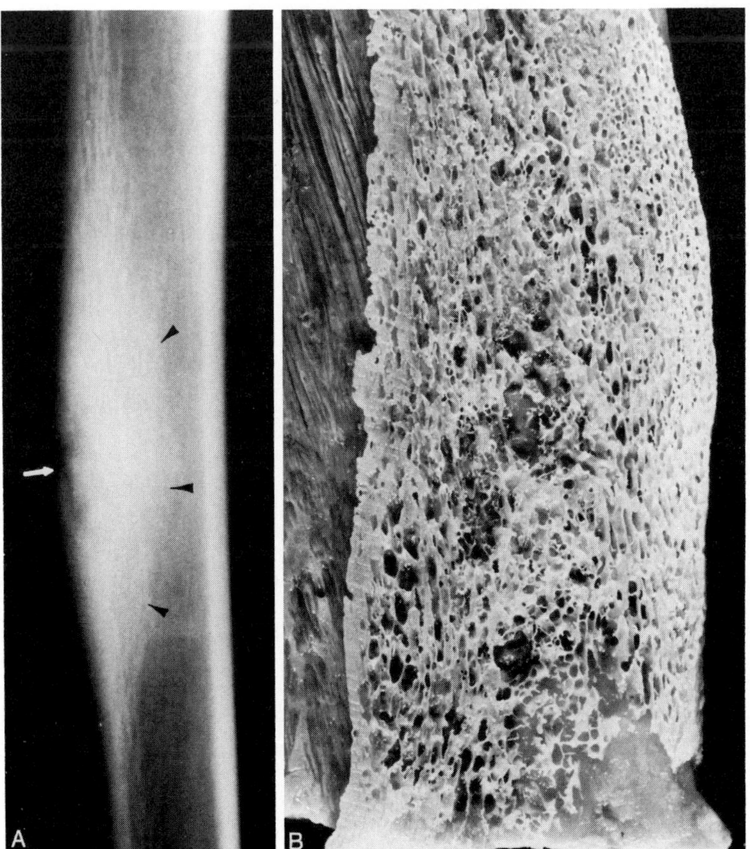

Figure 60–10. Chronic sclerosing osteomyelitis.

A *Chronic osteomyelitis can be associated with considerable new bone formation. In this patient, a cortical abscess contains a sequestrum (arrow) and is surrounded by sclerosis (arrowheads). The appearance is reminiscent of that of an osteoid osteoma.*

B *A macerated coronal section of a femur in a patient with chronic osteomyelitis indicates the considerable osseous expansion and trabecular thickening that can accompany infection.*

arately).[60] The contamination of bone from an adjacent soft tissue infection is particularly important in the hands, the feet, the mandible, and the skull.[61-63] The following discussion emphasizes the findings in the hands and the feet, although the importance of osteomyelitis of the mandible and maxilla in individuals with poor dental hygiene and of the frontal portion of the skull and face in individuals with chronic sinusitis is undeniable. The occasional occurrence of osteomyelitis of the cervical spine following dental extraction is reported,[295] although it is not certain if the infection reaches the bone via tissue planes, lymphatics, or bloodstream.

Soft tissue infections that lead to bone and joint contamination are frequent following trauma; animal and human bites[64-66] and puncture wounds[67-71] are especially troublesome in this regard. Diagnostic and therapeutic procedures such as venous puncture and catheterization can lead to secondary infection of soft tissue and bone.[72, 73] Irradiation and burns are other important sources of soft tissue and osseous contamination. Although the specific clinical manifestations vary with the site of soft tissue infection, local inflammatory symptoms and signs predominate and gram-positive or gram-negative bacterial organisms are usually evident. Human and animal bites are frequently deep and extensive, allowing direct inoculation of osseous and articular structures, and they are discussed later in the chapter.

General Radiographic and Pathologic Features (Table 60–4). Neglected soft tissue infections have a detrimental effect on neighboring osseous and articular structures. "The destruction of bone that takes place might be compared with the erosive action of a turbulent stream of water upon a wall of rock"[74]; whereas the direction of contamination in hematogenous osteomyelitis is from the bone outward into the soft tissue, the direction of contamination in osteomyelitis resulting from adjacent sepsis is from the soft tissues inward into the bone (or joint) (Fig. 60–11). Thus, early evidence of soft tissue suppuration is the rule. Organisms within soft tissues disrupt fascial planes and form abscesses. They extend into the periosteum by initially invading its outer and more fibrous portion. Displacement of the periosteum is more frequent and marked in children because of its looser attachment. Resulting periosteal bone formation is commonly the initial radiographic manifestation of osteomyelitis. However, it must be noted that following traumatic initiation of soft tissue infection, periostitis may appear early in response to injury and not reflect actual bone infection.[75] In addition, posttraumatic limitation of motion may produce osteoporosis with medullary radiolucent areas and intracortical tunneling ("pseudoperiostitis"), further simulating infection. New bone deposition can result also from stimulation of the periosteal membrane by adjacent infection.[76] Obviously, periostitis beneath suppurative soft tissues may not always indicate infective osteitis or osteomyelitis.

With further accumulation of pus, subperiosteal resorption of bone and cortical disruption ensue. The osseous response may be identical to that associated with soft tissue tumors.[77] As infection gains access to the spongiosa, it may spread in the marrow, producing lytic osseous defects on the radiograph.

Specific Locations

Hand

Pathways of Spread of Infection. There are three distinct routes available to organisms that become lodged in the soft tissues of the hand; infection may disseminate via tendon sheaths, fascial planes, or lymphatics[78] (Fig. 60–12).

Tendon Sheaths. As previously noted (see Chapter 15), synovial sheaths surround the flexor tendons of each digit of the hand; they extend from the terminal phalanges in a proximal direction to the palm.[79] In the first and fifth digits, connection with

Table 60–4

OSTEOMYELITIS DUE TO SPREAD FROM A CONTIGUOUS SOURCE OF INFECTION: RADIOGRAPHIC-PATHOLOGIC CORRELATION

Pathologic Abnormality	Radiographic Abnormality
Soft tissue contamination and abscess formation	Soft tissue swelling, mass formation, obliteration of tissue planes
Infectious invasion of the periosteum with lifting of the membrane and bone formation	Periostitis
Subperiosteal abscess formation and cortical invasion	Cortical erosion
Infection in haversian and Volkmann's canals of cortex	Cortical lucency and destruction
Contamination and spread in marrow	Bone lysis

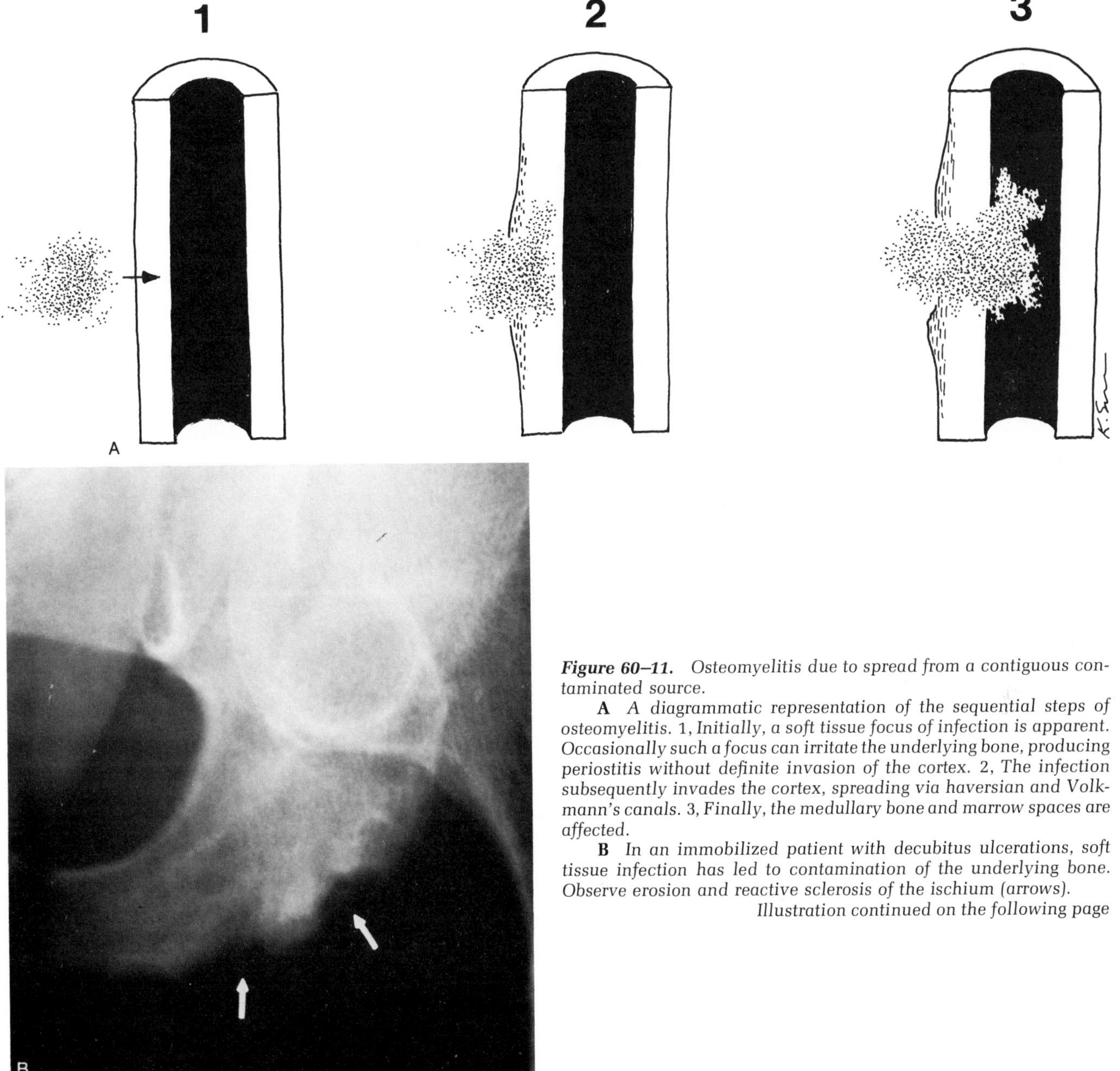

Figure 60–11. Osteomyelitis due to spread from a contiguous contaminated source.

A *A diagrammatic representation of the sequential steps of osteomyelitis. 1, Initially, a soft tissue focus of infection is apparent. Occasionally such a focus can irritate the underlying bone, producing periostitis without definite invasion of the cortex. 2, The infection subsequently invades the cortex, spreading via haversian and Volkmann's canals. 3, Finally, the medullary bone and marrow spaces are affected.*

B *In an immobilized patient with decubitus ulcerations, soft tissue infection has led to contamination of the underlying bone. Observe erosion and reactive sclerosis of the ischium (arrows).*

Illustration continued on the following page

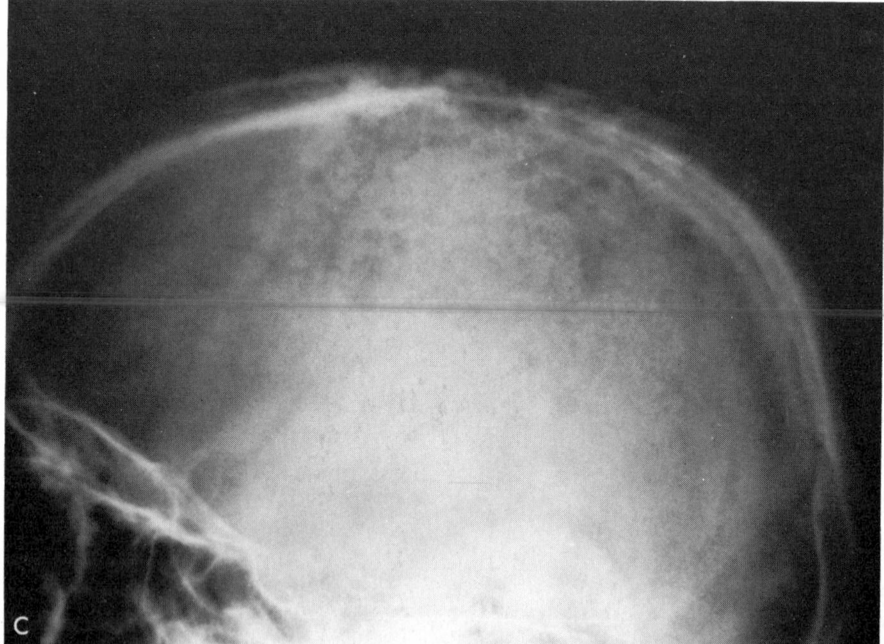
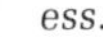

Figure 60–11. Continued

C–E *Following a hair transplantation, this patient developed swelling of the scalp, local tenderness, and fever. The radiograph of the skull* **(C)** *demonstrates multiple osteolytic foci involving predominantly the outer table and diploic space. A photograph* **(D)** *and radiograph* **(E)** *of the resected cranial vault indicate the extent of the infectious process.*

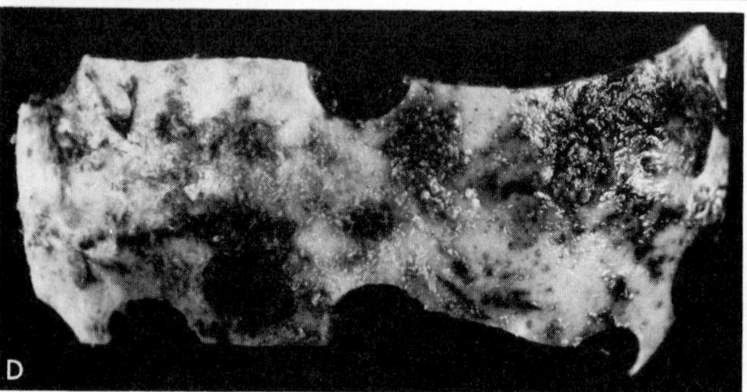

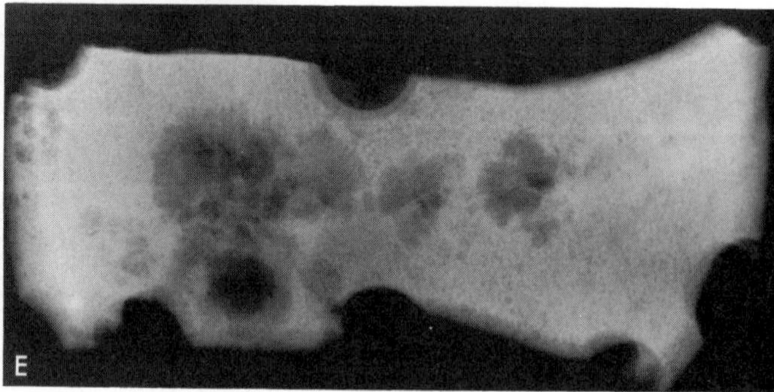

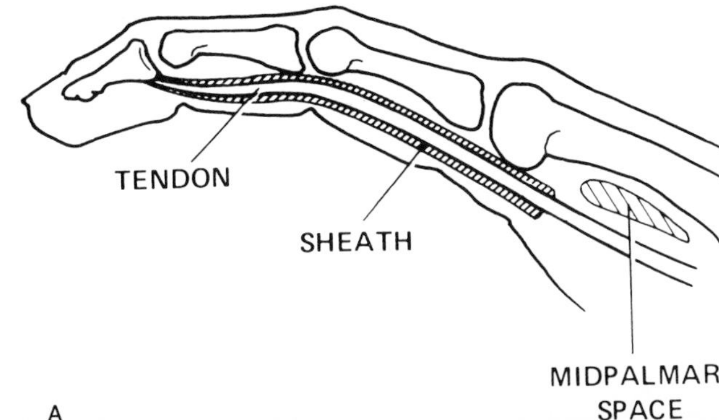

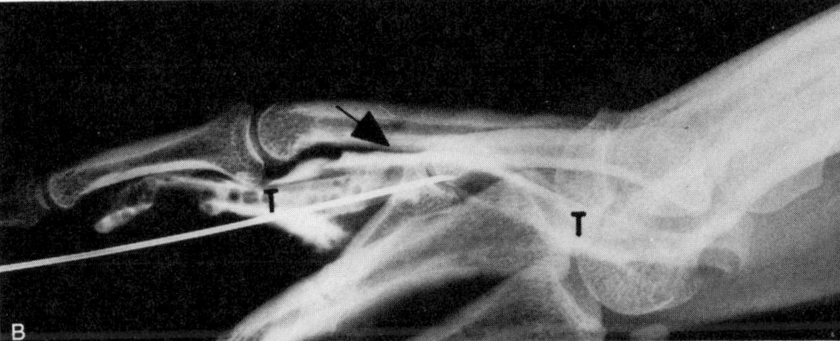

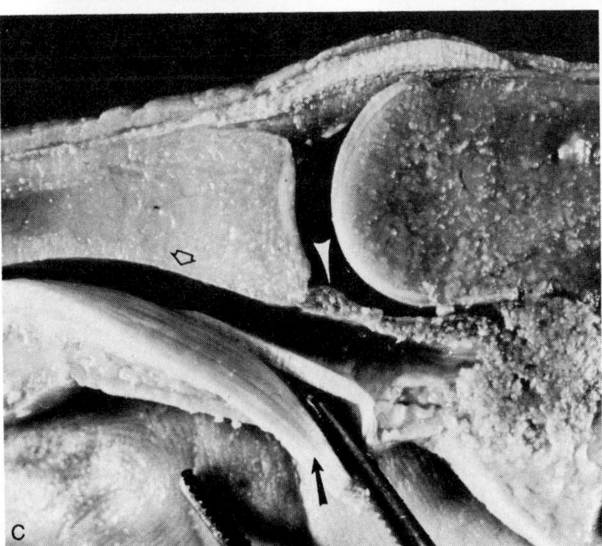

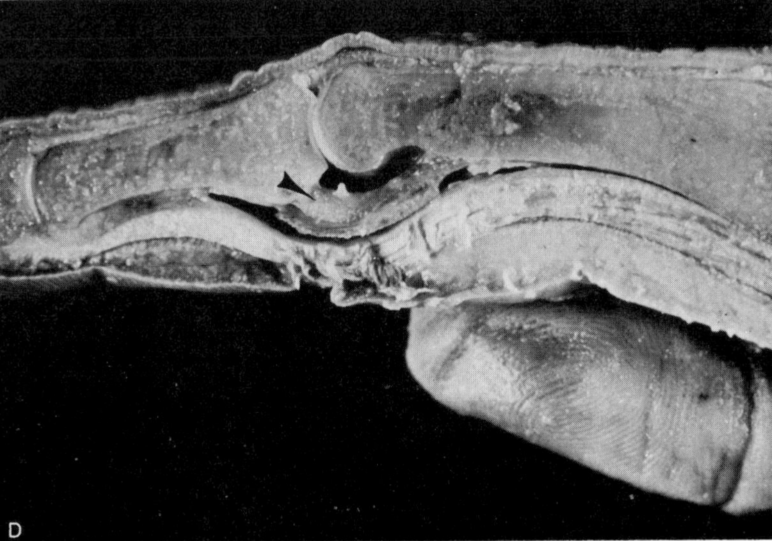

Figure 60–12. *Spread of infection in the hand: Available anatomic pathways.*

A *Digital tendon sheaths: The digital flexor tendon sheaths surround the tendon at its point of attachment to the terminal phalanx and extend proximally for a variable distance. In the second, third, and fourth fingers, they usually terminate just proximal to the metacarpophalangeal articulation in close proximity to the midpalmar space.*

B *Digital tendon sheaths: A digital tenogram outlines the tendon (T) within its sheath. Note the intimacy of the sheath to the proximal (arrow) and middle phalanges.*

C *Digital tendon sheaths: At the metacarpophalangeal joint, a sagittal section outlines the intimate relationship between the articulation and bones and the sheath. The tendon has been retracted (arrow) and is separated from the joint by a volar capsule (arrowhead). More distally, the sheath is adjacent to the proximal phalanx (open arrow).*

D *Digital tendon sheaths: A sagittal section through the proximal interphalangeal joint delineates the capsular tissue (arrowhead) that separates the articular cavity from the sheath and tendon.*

Illustration continued on the following page

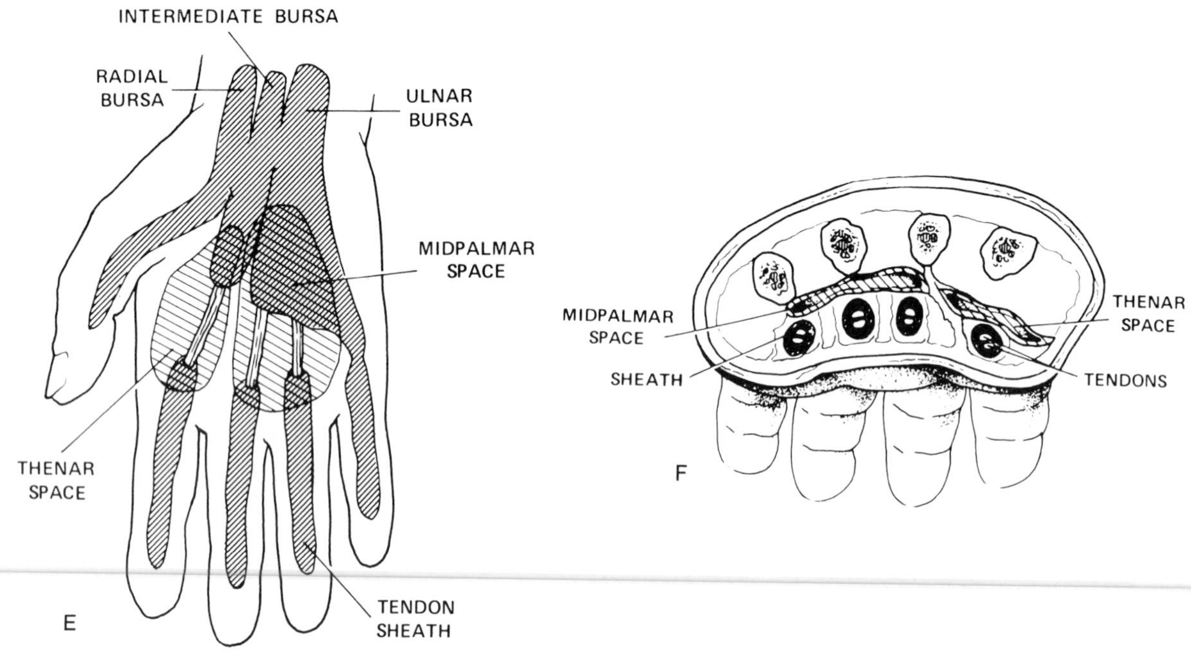

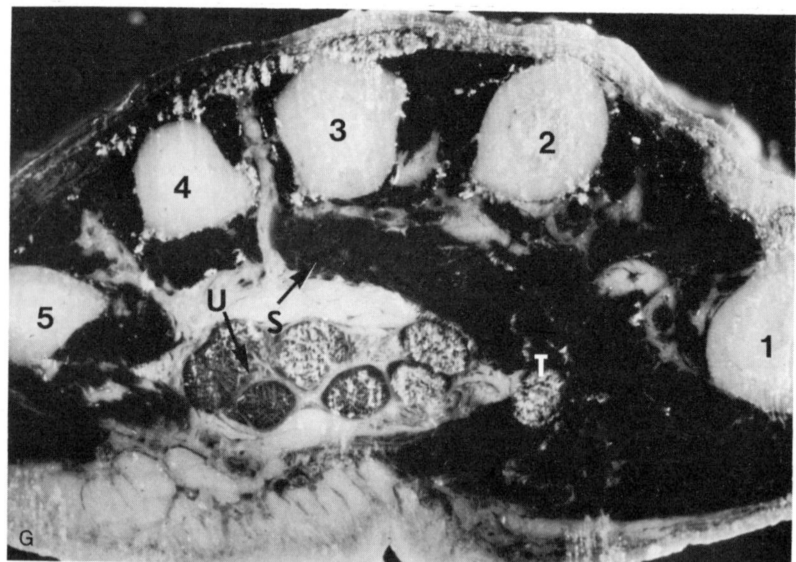

Figure 60–12. Continued

E *Fascial planes: A drawing demonstrates the relationships of the tendon sheaths, bursae, and fascial planes (thenar space, midpalmar space).*

F *Fascial planes: A drawing of a section through the metacarpals outlines two spaces, the midpalmar and thenar spaces, separated by a septum and located above the digital flexor tendon sheaths. Note the close relationship between the sheath of the index finger and thenar space and between the sheaths of the third, fourth, and fifth fingers and midpalmar space.*

G *Fascial planes: A cross section through the metacarpals demonstrates the ulnar bursa (U). The approximate position of the potential midpalmar space (S) is indicated. The flexor pollicis longus tendon (T) and sheath that continues proximally as the radial bursa are noted. (From Resnick D: J Can Assoc Radiol 27:21, 1976.)*

the radial and ulnar bursae, two synovial sacs on the volar aspect of the wrist, is frequently apparent. It is this communication that allows spread of infection from the first and fifth digits to the palm; such extension from the other digits is less constant. Sequential contamination of the fifth finger, ulnar bursa, radial bursa, and first finger produces a typical horseshoe abscess.[80] The initimate relationship of the tendon sheaths to the volar aspect of the phalanges and proximal interphalangeal and metacarpophalangeal articulations explains the occurrence of osteomyelitis and septic arthritis in cases of neglected tendon sheath infection.[81]

The extensor tendon sheaths extend in six compartments beneath the dorsal carpal ligament on the dorsum of the wrist (see Chapter 15). In this location, infection usually occurs in the subcutaneous or subaponeurotic space, whereas infective extensor tenosynovitis is less frequent. When present, such infection can contaminate the wrist[78] (Fig. 60–13).

Infective digital tenosynovitis can result from a puncture wound, particularly in a flexor crease of the finger, at which site skin and sheath are intimately related. Additional sources of infection are spread from the pulp space or dorsum of the hand or fingers.[82] The sheath infection may perforate into an adjacent bone or joint in the finger; the most characteristic site of such extension includes the proximal interphalangeal articulations and adjacent middle phalanx (Figs. 60–14 to 60–16). The metacarpophalangeal articulations are less commonly altered. Infection within the volar sheaths of the first and fifth digits may quickly spread to the ulnar and radial bursae, and from these latter areas into the wrist.[82] Such extensions more frequently involve the radial bursa. In the second, third, and fourth digits, the infective process can spill from the open proximal end of the sheath. Further extension along the lumbrical muscles would allow widespread contamination.

The diagnosis of tenosynovitis is accomplished from the four cardinal signs of Kanavel[81]: exquisite tenderness over the course of the sheath, semiflexed position of the finger, severe pain on extension, and symmetric swelling of the digit. On radiographs, diffuse soft tissue swelling is apparent. Osteoporosis and articular and osseous destruction, the latter commencing along the volar aspect of the bone, are evident.

Fascial Planes. Infections in the fascial planes of the hand are numerous but result in joint or bone alterations less frequently than those in the synovial sheaths. Although several fascial planes exist, two potential spaces dorsal to the volar sheaths and bursae are of particular importance.[81, 83] The midpalmar space extends in a triangular fashion along the ulnar aspect of the hand from the third metacarpal to the hypothenar eminence; the thenar space extends along the radial aspect of the hand from the third metacarpal to the thenar eminence (Fig. 60–12). The two are separated from each other by a firm septum. Utilizing injection studies, Kanavel[81] demonstrated the frequent spread of fluid from the flexor tendon sheath of the index finger into the thenar space. Less frequently, communication between this space and the flexor tendon sheaths of the first and third digits was noted. Common communications between the flexor tendon sheaths of the third, fourth, and fifth digits and the midpalmar space were seen.

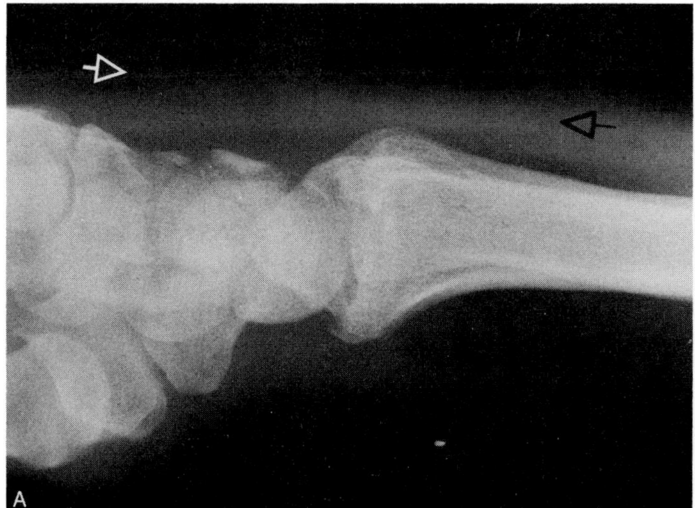

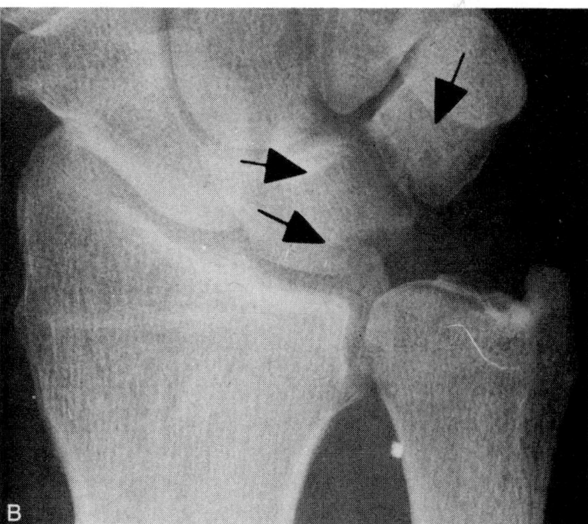

Figure 60–13. *Spread of infection in the hand: Extensor tenosynovitis and osteomyelitis. A 50 year old man noted pain and swelling on the dorsum of the wrist for 3 weeks following trauma. At surgery, a staphylococcal tenosynovitis and osteomyelitis were confirmed.*

A *Note the localized soft tissue swelling (arrows) on the dorsum of the wrist.*

B *Lytic lesions and apposing cortical irregularities of the lunate and triquetrum (arrows) are apparent. Shrapnel from a previous injury is seen.*

(From Resnick D: J Can Assoc Radiol 27:21, 1976.)

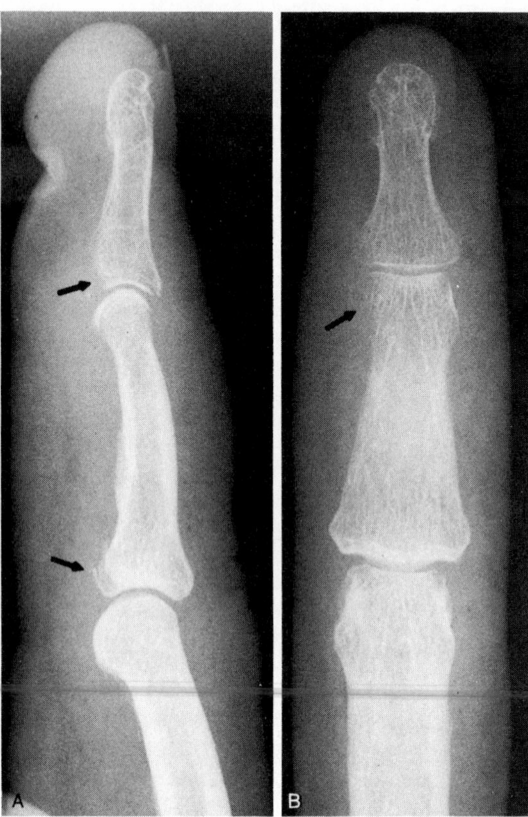

Figure 60–14. *Spread of infection in the hand: Digital flexor tenosynovitis. This man had a chronic infection on the flexor surface of the finger. Observe the characteristic soft tissue swelling, especially on the volar aspect of the digit, and the resulting osteomyelitis of the phalanges (arrows). The distal interphalangeal articulation became involved.*

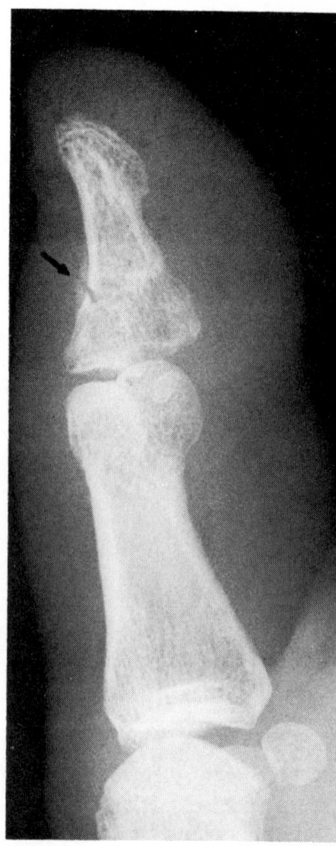

Figure 60–15. *Spread of infection in the hand: Digital flexor tenosynovitis. A neglected infected flexor tenosynovitis of the thumb has led to osteomyelitis and a pathologic fracture (arrow) of the terminal phalanx in addition to soft tissue swelling.*

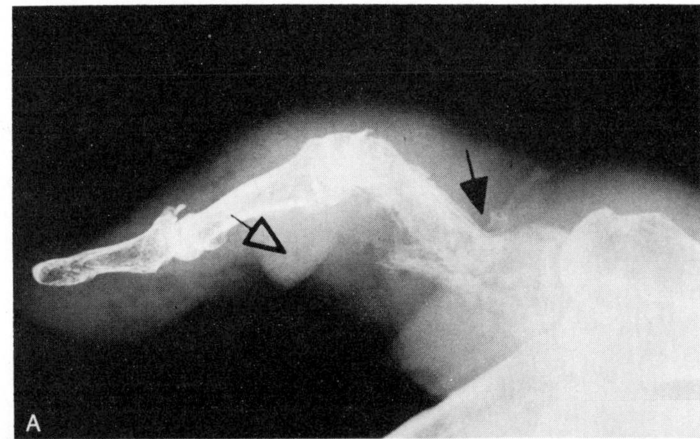

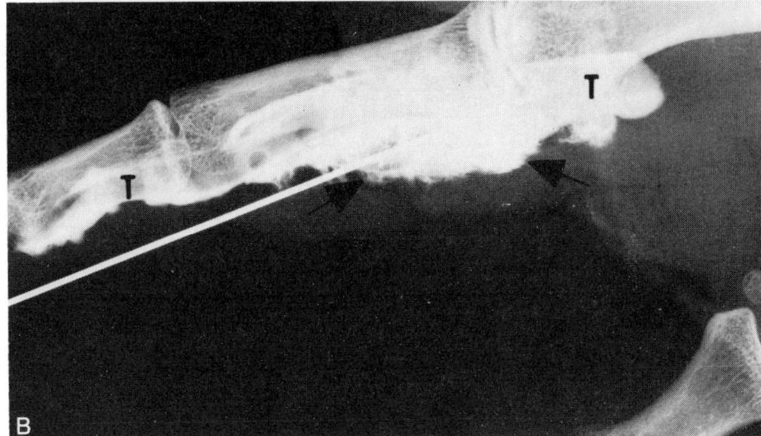

Figure 60–16. *Spread of infection in the hand: Digital flexor tenosynovitis.*

A *Following a neglected puncture wound, a 45 year old woman developed tenosynovitis and osteomyelitis. Note the soft tissue swelling, particularly along the volar surface of the proximal phalanx (open arrow), semiflexed position of the finger, and extensive permeative osseous destruction, with pathologic fracture (solid arrow) of the proximal phalanx.*

B *An experimental excessive pressure injection into the digital tendon sheath has resulted in extravasation of contrast material beneath the proximal phalanx (arrows). The tendon (T) within the sheath is apparent. Infection could disseminate in a similar fashion.*

(From Resnick D: J Can Assoc Radiol 27:21, 1976.)

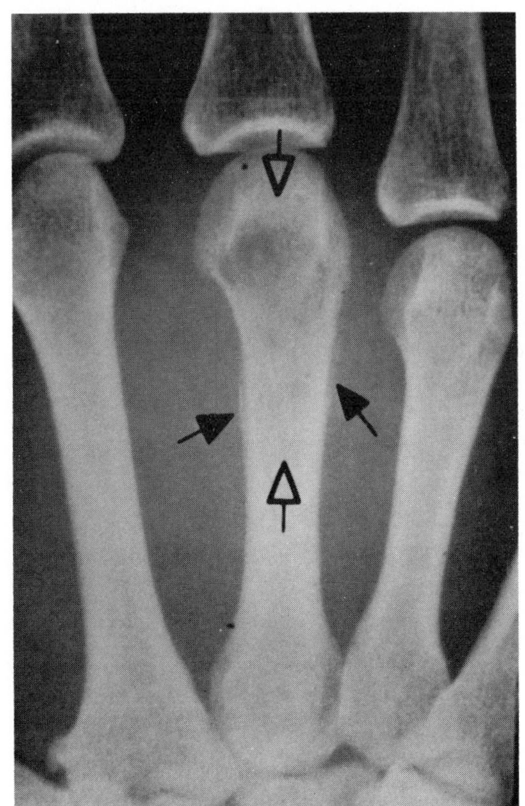

Figure 60–17. *Spread of infection in the hand: Midpalmar space infection. Osteomyelitis of the third metacarpal has resulted from spread of infection from the midpalmar space. A large lytic lesion (open arrows) may be noted and periostitis is seen (solid arrows). (From Resnick D: J Can Assoc Radiol 27:21, 1976.)*

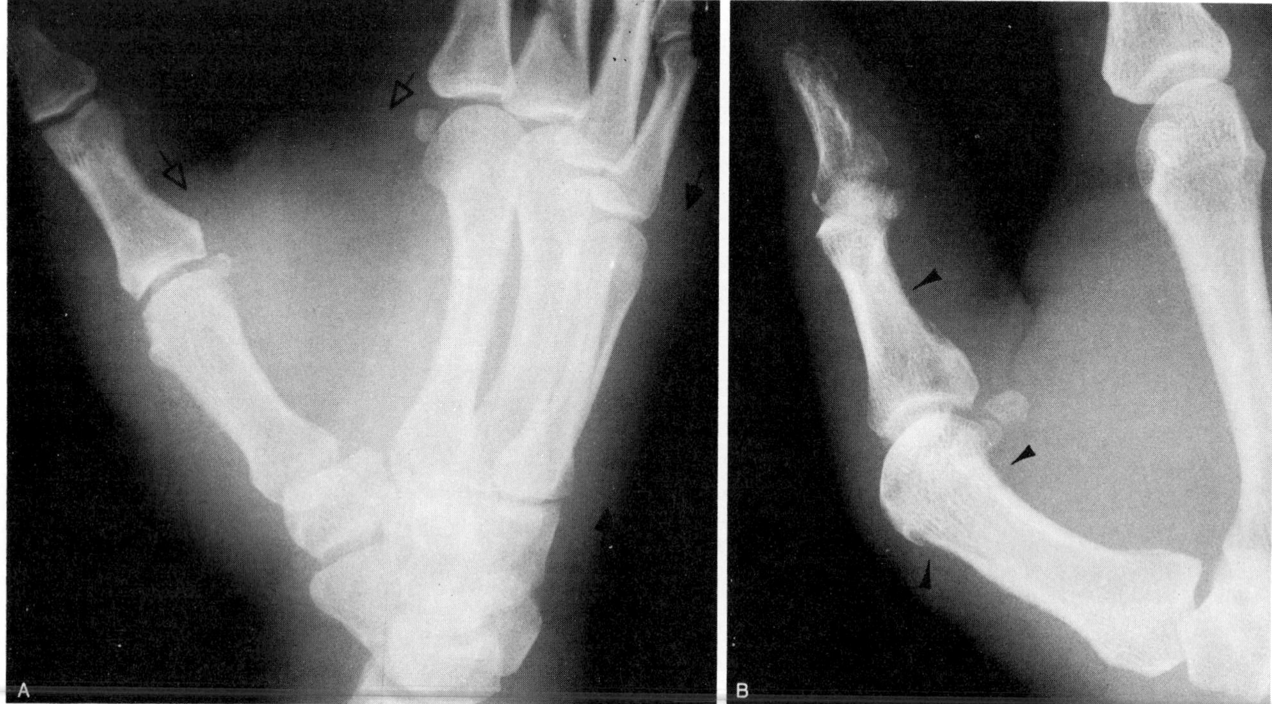

Figure 60–18. *Spread of infection in the hand. Thenar space infection.*

A *A thenar space infection has produced extensive soft tissue swelling (open arrows), forcing the thumb into abduction. Dorsal swelling (solid arrows) in these instances results from lymphedema.*

B *Two weeks later, osseous resorption and contamination of the metacarpal and proximal phalanx can be seen (arrowheads). The source of the infection, the soft tissues of the tip of the thumb, is evident on the film.*

(From Resnick D: J Can Assoc Radiol 27:21, 1976.)

Infection in the midpalmar space may result from direct implantation during injury or by extension from suppurative sheaths. The proximity of the midpalmar space to the third, fourth, and fifth metacarpals may promote osteomyelitis in neglected infections[78, 81] (Fig. 60–17). Palmar swelling, semiflexion of the fingers, and bony destruction are the accompanying clinical and radiologic manifestations. Neglected infection of the thenar space, resulting from direct implantation or extension from adjacent flexor tendon sheaths (usually the second) or from the midpalmar space, can also lead to osteomyelitis of the metacarpals (Fig. 60–18). Extensive swelling along the radial aspect of the hand forces the thumb into abduction.[82] Web-space infections between the volar and dorsal skin may ascend through lumbrical muscle sheaths into the thenar and the palmar spaces.[80] The dorsal subaponeurotic and dorsal subcutaneous spaces are less frequently involved in hand infections, although lymphatic vessels at the latter site may produce marked swelling and lymphedema in cases of palmar infections.[80]

LYMPHATICS. Lymphangitis may result from superficial injuries. Rapid extension can produce widespread swelling without clinical evidence of synovial sheath infection. In intense cases, complications, including tenosynovitis, septicemia, osteomyelitis, and septic arthritis, may be noted.[82]

Specific Entities

FELON. A felon results from infection in the terminal pulp space.[82-84] Bone involvement is not infrequent in neglected cases[85] because of the close proximity of the terminal phalanx (Fig. 60–19). In

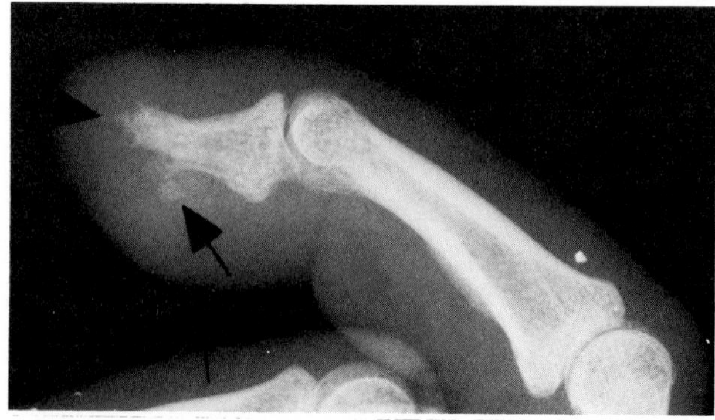

Figure 60–19. *Spread of infection in the hand: Felon. An infection in the pulp space has produced considerable soft tissue swelling (open arrows). Extension into the tuft and diaphysis of the terminal phalanx is apparent (solid arrows). Shrapnel from a previous injury can be seen. (From Resnick D: J Can Assoc Radiol 27:21, 1976.)*

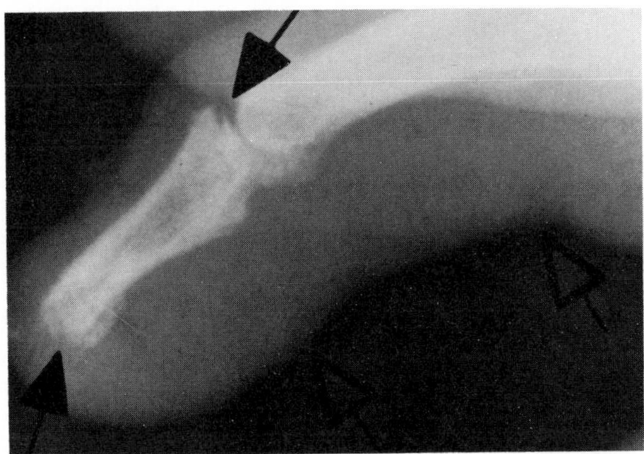

Figure 60–20. Spread of infection in the hand: Paronychia. Widespread infection of the pulp space, digital flexor tendon sheath, terminal tuft, and distal interphalangeal joint (solid arrows) resulted from an initial subcuticular abscess. Soft tissue swelling along the tendon sheath may be noted (open arrows). (From Resnick D: J Can Assoc Radiol 27:21, 1976.)

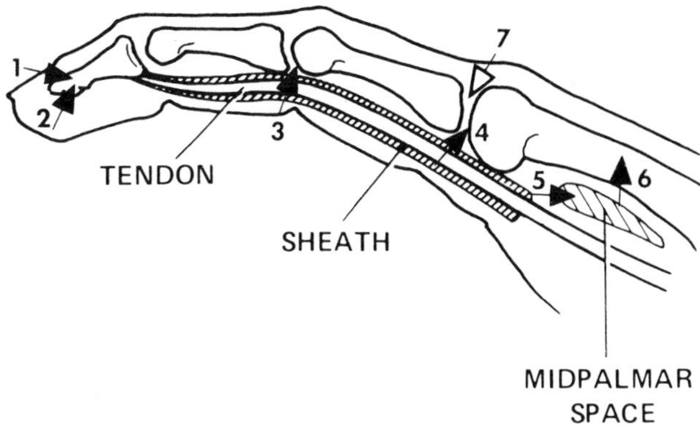

Figure 60–21. Spread of infection in the hand: Summary of pathways. A paronychia (1), may rarely invade the distal terminal phalanx. A felon (2) may produce destruction of the tuft and diaphysis of a distal phalanx. Suppurative tenosynovitis may spread to the proximal interphalangeal joint (3) and less frequently to the metacarpophalangeal joints (4). From the proximal end of the sheath of the third, fourth, and fifth digits, pus may reach the midpalmar space (5). Direct metacarpal invasion (6) is then possible. Puncture wounds of the metacarpophalangeal joint (7) are frequent during fist-fights (see text). (After Resnick D: J Can Assoc Radiol 27:21, 1976.)

addition to osteomyelitis, soft tissue edema adjacent to the bone can produce relative ischemia and bone necrosis.[86] The tuft and diaphysis of the terminal phalanx are characteristically destroyed, with relative sparing of the phalangeal base.[85, 86] Sequestra may be evident. Furthermore, pyarthrosis of the distal interphalangeal joints and involvement of the flexor tendon sheaths are occasionally noted.[82]

Paronychia. Subcuticular abscesses of the nail fold are termed paronychia.[82, 84] On rare occasions, osseous destruction of a terminal phalanx may be evident[85] (Fig. 60–20).

Incidence of Osteomyelitis and Septic Arthritis Following Hand Infections. The reported incidence of bone and joint involvement during the course of hand infection has varied. Resnick[78] noted such involvement in 10 per cent of 78 patients, although in one third of the infected individuals, the diagnosis of osteomyelitis and septic arthritis was not evident on radiographs and could be established only during surgery (Fig. 60–21). Previous reports have indicated a much higher incidence of bone and joint involvement,[85] but with earlier diagnosis and current antibiotic and surgical therapy, obvious reduction of this dreaded complication has occurred. A recent study has indicated a 17 per cent incidence of infective osteitis, tenosynovitis, or septic arthritis in an evaluation of 1400 cases of hand infection.[61]

The frequency of hand infections in drug addicts is noteworthy[78, 87]; infections commonly follow local injections with contaminated needles. However, bilateral swelling of the dorsum of the hand in addicts, the "puffy hand" syndrome, can relate not to infection but to lymphedema resulting from lymphatic destruction and fibrosis of the subcutaneous tissues.[88, 89]

Foot

Pathways of Spread of Infection. The plantar aspect of the foot is especially vulnerable to soft tissue infection. Foreign bodies, puncture wounds, or skin ulceration from weight-bearing can represent the portal of entry for various organisms. In a diabetic patient, soft tissue breakdown over certain pressure points (such as the metatarsal heads and calcaneus) leads to infection that is combined with vascular and neurologic abnormalities.[90-92]

There are three plantar muscle compartments — medial, intermediate, and lateral[93-96] (Fig. 60–22). These compartments are separated from each other by two intermuscular septa extending from the plantar fascia to the overlying osseous structures. The medial compartment contains the muscles to the great toe and the lateral compartment contains those to the fifth toe, with the intermediate compartment containing the remainder.

Cadaveric injection studies[97] have emphasized (1) that the intermediate compartment contains the greatest amount of potential space; when this compartment becomes filled, continued infusion of fluid will produce extravasation either into the medial compartment or more importantly along the flexor hallucis longus tendon into the lower leg (Fig. 60–22*D*, *E*); (2) that the lateral compartment has the least amount of potential space; extravasation from this area occurs into the dorsal compartment or plantar fat of the foot; and (3) that the medial compartment has a potential space somewhat greater than that of the lateral compartment and less than that of the intermediate compartment; extravasation from this area commonly occurs into the intermediate compartment.

These experimental observations can be applied to the evaluation of soft tissue infections on the plantar aspect of the foot. Initial contamination of skin and subcutaneous tissue at pressure points can soon lead to infective osteitis, osteomyelitis, and septic arthritis of adjacent bones and joints; this is especially frequent about the metatarsophalangeal articulations, calcaneus, and terminal phalanges. Soft tissue dissemination of infection can also occur via the medial, lateral, or intermediate compartment; in these instances, osteomyelitis and septic arthritis can be seen to be remote from the initial site of soft tissue contamination. Furthermore, the intermediate compartment provides a pathway by which the infection can spread from the plantar aspect of the foot into the lower leg; neglected foot infections may eventually require amputations at levels above or below the knee.

Specific Entities

PUNCTURE WOUNDS. Puncture wounds of the plantar aspect of the foot can lead to osteomyelitis and septic arthritis[67, 68, 70, 71, 292] (Fig. 60–23). These injuries are especially prominent in children who walk barefoot, exposing the unprotected foot to nails, glass, splinters and other sharp objects. The infective organisms can vary, but gram-negative agents such as *Pseudomonas aeruginosa* are frequently implicated[67, 68, 70, 98-100]; this is not surprising, as these organisms are usually found in the soil and may be normal inhabitants of skin.[70] Typically, local pain and swelling appear within days following a punc-

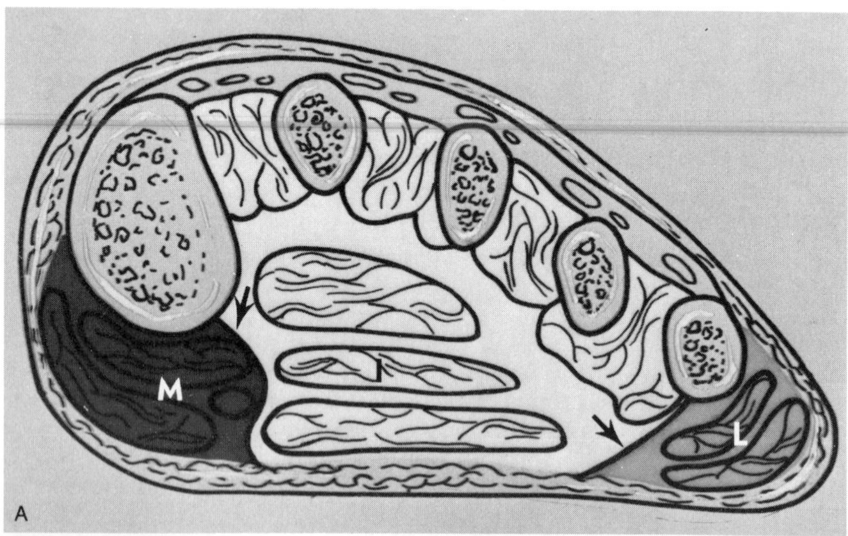

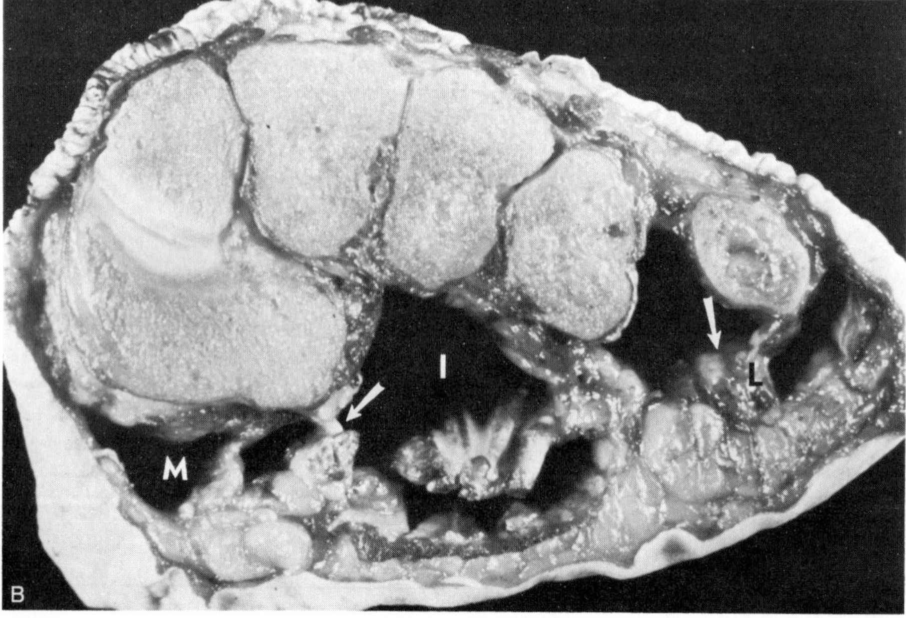

Figure 60–22. *Spread of infection in the foot. Available anatomic pathways.*

A, B *Plantar compartmental anatomy on cross sections of the foot. Note the medial (M), intermediate (I), and lateral (L) compartments separated by two intermuscular septae (arrows).*

Illustration continued on the opposite page

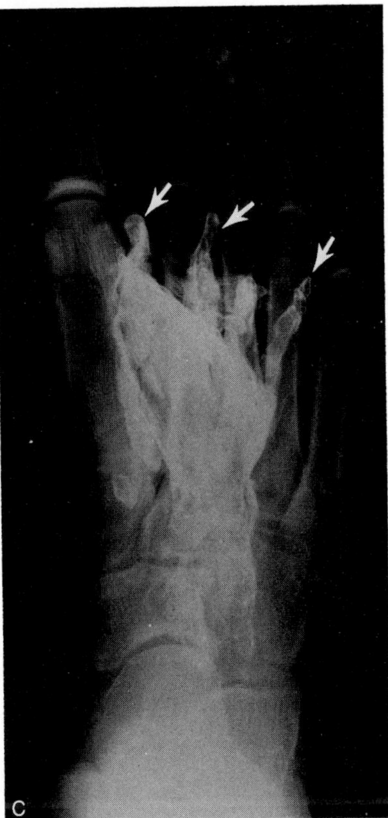

Figure 60–22. Continued

C *An injection into the intermediate plantar compartment reveals the extent of this space. Note the filling of the sheaths about the lumbrical muscles (arrows).*

D, E *A photograph and radiograph of a cross section of the leg 5 cm above the malleoli following overdistention of the intermediate plantar compartment with methylmethacrylate indicate that some of the material has reached the posterior muscles of the leg (arrows). This pathway is important in the dissemination of infection in the foot.*

*(***A, C–E,*** From Feingold M, et al: Invest Radiol 12:281, 1977.)*

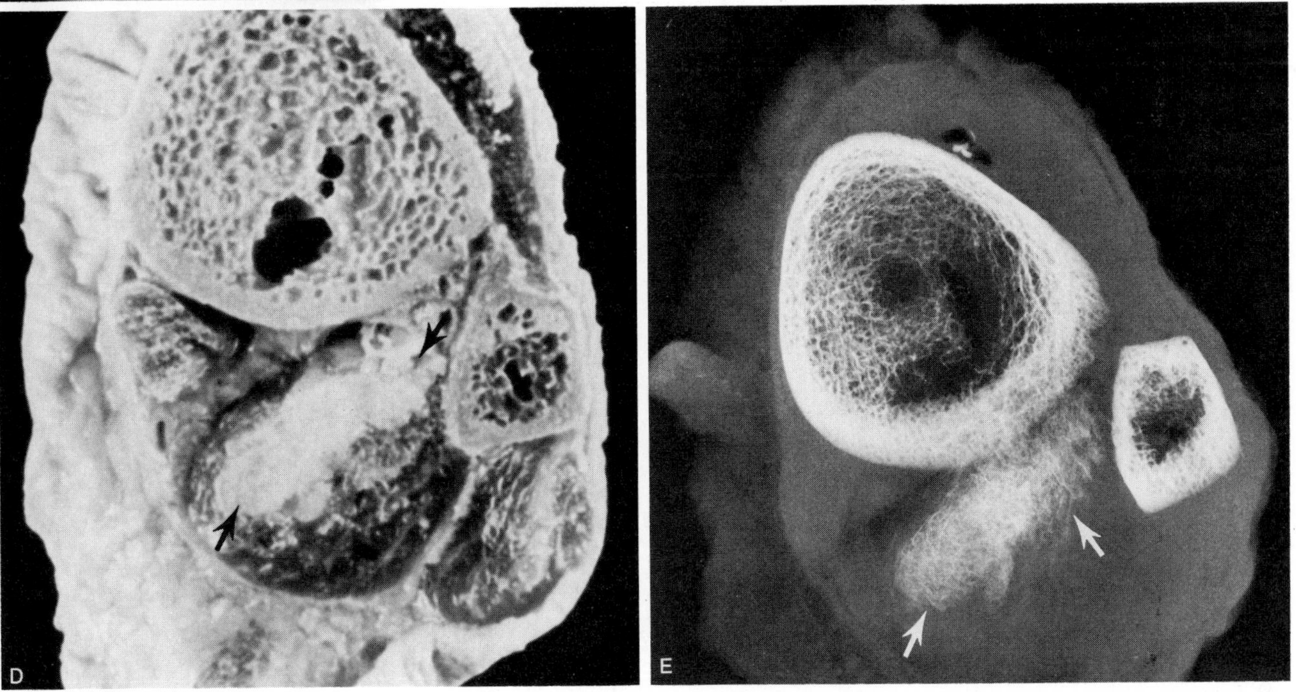

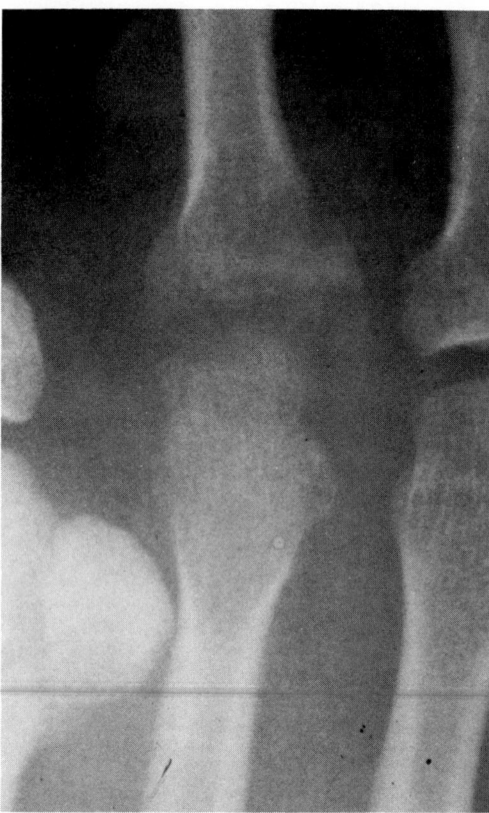

Figure 60–23. *Spread of infection in the foot: Puncture wounds. Following a puncture wound from a nail, this patient developed a plantar soft tissue infection which later led to osteomyelitis and septic arthritis. Observe osseous destruction of the metatarsal head and proximal phalanx, joint space narrowing, and soft tissue swelling.*

ture wound, although radiographs are usually normal at this time. Following a delay of 1 to 3 weeks, the roentgenograms reveal typical abnormalities of osteomyelitis or septic arthritis. It has been suggested that *Pseudomonas aeruginosa* has a propensity for infecting cartilage[67] with early evidence of cartilaginous destruction (articular or epiphyseal growth cartilage) following intra-articular or metaphyseal introduction of organisms; infective chondritis due to Pseudomonas can also be noted in the sternoclavicular joints, intervertebral discs, and ear. Johanson[98] contended that Pseudomonas infections do not develop in puncture wounds in noncartilaginous areas of the foot.

Wooden splinters and thorns can induce osseous and articular changes in the foot.[71] Areas of osteolysis, osteosclerosis, and periostitis may relate to secondary infection, simple irritation from the foreign body, or, perhaps, toxins within the thorns themselves.[325] The clinical course is characteristically protracted, and the accurate diagnosis of the clinical and radiologic manifestations may be difficult, as the remote history of a puncture wound may seem insignificant to the patient and not be reported to the physician.

Foot Infections in Diabetes Mellitus. Complete discussion of this common and complicated problem is beyond the scope of this book, and the interested reader should consult with other sources.[91] Instead, an overview is presented.

Clinical, radiologic, and pathologic characteristics of osteomyelitis (and septic arthritis) complicating foot infections in diabetic patients are modified by the associated problems of these individuals, including vascular insufficiency and neurologic deficit.[101] Clinical differentiation between infection and gangrene can be difficult, although both processes may coexist in the same individual. Systemic manifestations of sepsis are uncommon; local symptoms and signs dominate, including pain, swelling, erythema, and diminished peripheral pulses. Cellulitis and skin ulcerations are readily apparent.

The roentgenographic picture usually reveals significant soft tissue swelling and mottled osteolysis (Fig. 60–24). Osteosclerosis, fragmentation, and periostitis may be seen. Radiolucent areas within the soft tissues are commonly identified.[102] This finding can relate to the presence of air due to dissection around open wounds or following local debridement or to the presence of gas due to clostridial or nonclostridial infections. Although nonclostridial gas-producing infections can occur in nondiabetic as well as diabetic patients, there is a significantly higher incidence in the latter individuals. The responsible organisms may be either aerobic, such as *Escherichia coli, Aerobacter aerogenes, Klebsiella pneumoniae,* and non-hemolytic streptococci, or anaerobic, such as Bacteroides and anaerobic streptococci.[103-106] Cultures containing more than one organism, some of which are present in normal skin, are typical.[101]

In some diabetic patients with foot infections that are complicated by osteomyelitis and septic arthritis, pathologic fractures and subluxations are prominent. These findings can simulate those accompanying diabetic neuroarthropathy, and differentiation of neurologic and infectious processes can be very difficult. In fact, both infection and neuroarthropathy of the midfoot and forefoot frequently coexist in diabetic patients. The presence of ill-defined osseous contours is the most helpful radiologic clue to osteomyelitis.

Direct Implantation of Infection

General Clinical Features. This route of contamination is commonly combined with spread from a contiguous source of infection. Thus, puncture wounds of the hand and the foot can lead to osteomyelitis (and septic arthritis) by contaminating adjacent soft tissues or directly inoculating the bone or joint (Fig. 60–25). This latter complication is especially prevalent in the foot, at

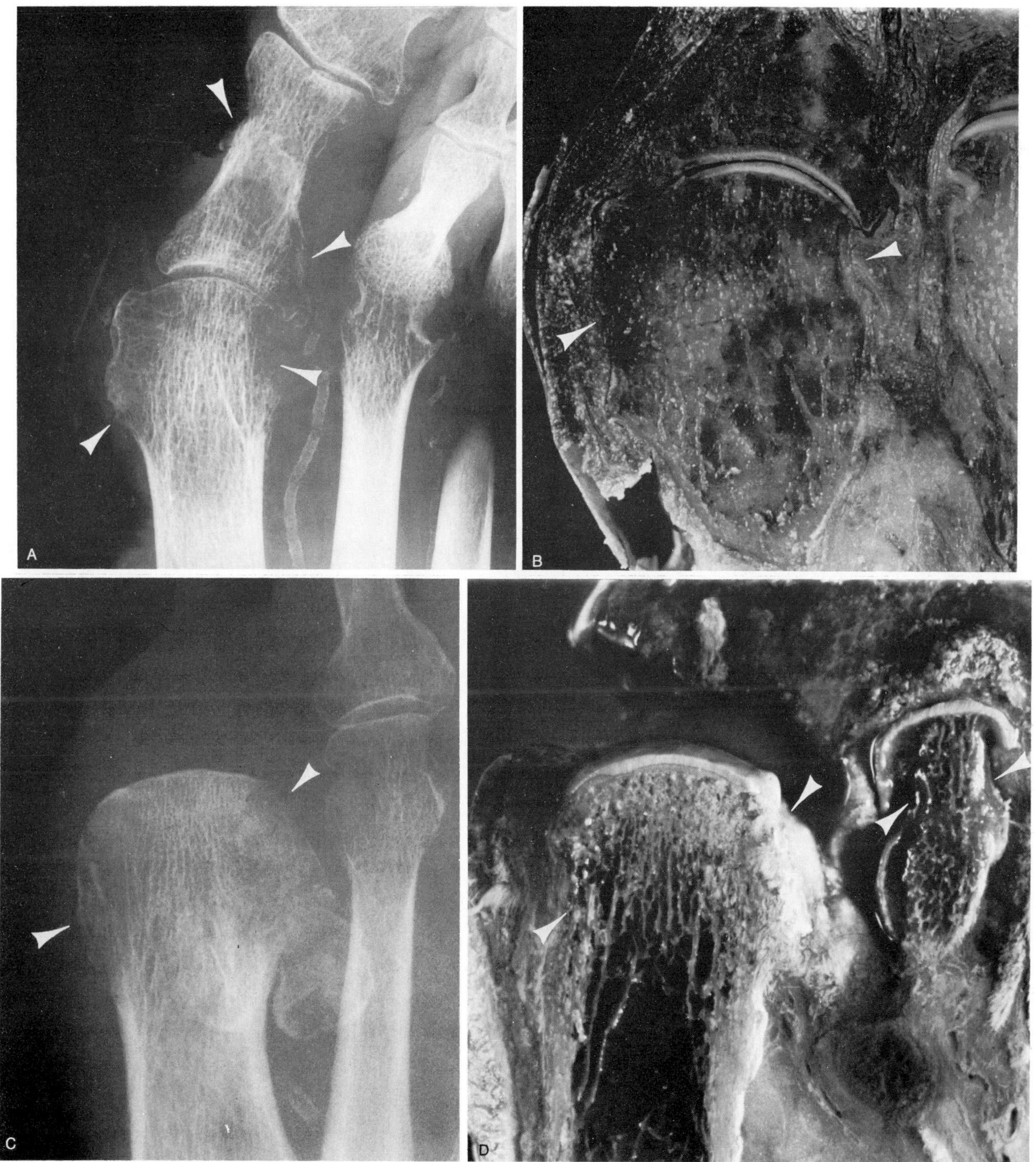

Figure 60–24. *Spread of infection in the foot: Diabetes mellitus.*

A, B *A radiograph and transverse sectional photograph reveal a soft tissue infection about the first metatarsophalangeal joint with ulcerations and with erosion of bone (arrowheads). Observe vascular calcification and alterations at the second metatarsophalangeal articulation.*

C, D *In a different diabetic patient who had had the first toe amputated for infection, a radiograph and transverse sectional photograph illustrate contamination of the first and second metatarsal heads with osseous erosion (arrowheads).*

Illustration continued on the following page

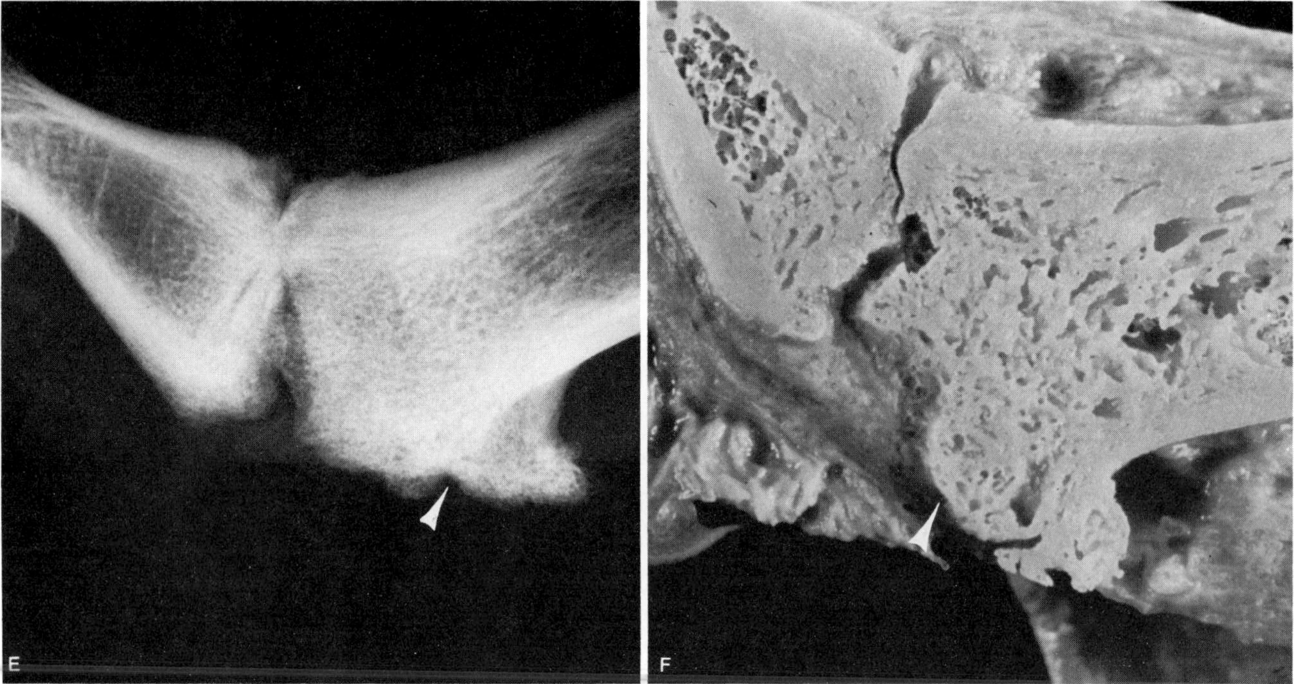

Figure 60–24. Continued

E, F *In this diabetic individual, a sagittal sectional radiograph and photograph illustrate a plantar soft tissue erosion with osteomyelitis and septic arthritis of the first metatarsophalangeal joint. Note the bone fusion between the sesamoid and the base of the metatarsal (arrowhead).*

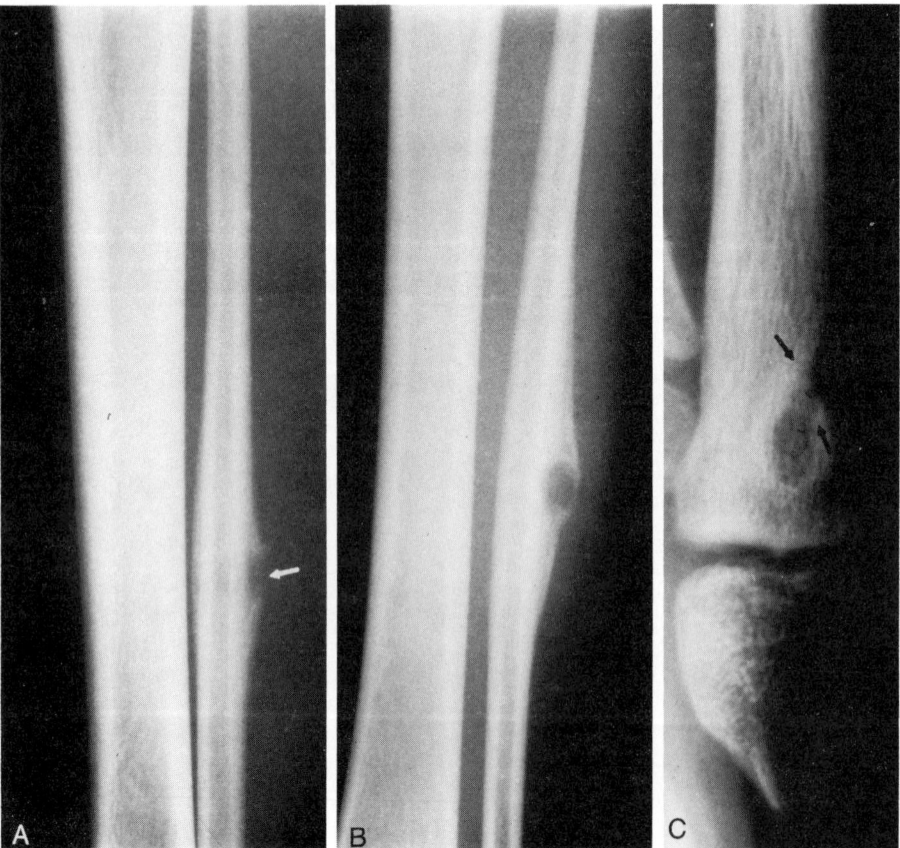

Figure 60–25. *Direct implantation of infection: Puncture wounds.*

A, B *Thorn granuloma. Following a puncture wound with a thorn, a lytic lesion of the fibula became evident. Cultures were repeatedly negative. Note the considerable periostitis and the eccentric location with violation of the cortex (arrow), indicating an external source. (**A, B,** Courtesy of Dr. W. Pogue, Grossmont Hospital, San Diego, California.)*

C *Following a puncture wound, an abscess of the distal fibula due to staphylococci developed. Note the tract running from the cortex to the lesion (arrows), indicating the nature of the original injury.*

which site nails, splinters, or glass can lead to deep puncture wounds, producing immediate bone (and joint) contamination; in the hand, at which site a human bite received during a fist fight can directly injure osseous and articular structures; and in any site following animal bites.

General Radiographic Features. The features of bone (and joint) involvement following direct implantation of infection are virtually identical to those following spread of infection from a contiguous contaminated source. Commonly, osseous destruction and proliferation lead to focal areas of lysis, sclerosis, and periostitis. Soft tissue swelling is common, related not to infection but to edema resulting from the injury itself.

Specific Entities

Human Bites. The significance of this injury is often overlooked, and the delay that frequently occurs in the patient's seeking a physician's aid can result in serious sequelae.[107-111, 293] The most common cause of injury is a fist-blow to the mouth resulting in laceration of the dorsum of the metacarpophalangeal articulation, although human bites are also frequent on the volar or dorsal aspect of the fingers. Joint infection is more common than bone infection in these cases. *Staphylococcus aureus* is the usual implicated organism. During a fist fight, the flexed metacarpophalangeal joint striking the opponent's teeth has little protective superficial tissue. As the hand is unclenched, the overlying tissue shifts and the organisms within the joint have no route of egress. The combination of *Bacillus fusiformis* and spirochetes does particularly well in this anaerobic setting; septic arthritis and osteomyelitis may be noted after a delay of days to weeks.[112] The radiographic findings include peculiar bony defects and fractures,[78] tooth fragments,[65] and osseous and articular destruction[78] (Fig. 60–26).

Animal Bites. Superficial animal bites or scratches can inoculate local soft tissues, later leading to infection of underlying bones and joints; and deep animal bites can introduce organisms directly into both osseous and articular structures.[64, 66, 113-116, 293, 294] The infecting organisms vary, but *Pasteurella multocida* is commonly implicated; this latter organism is a normal isolate in the oral

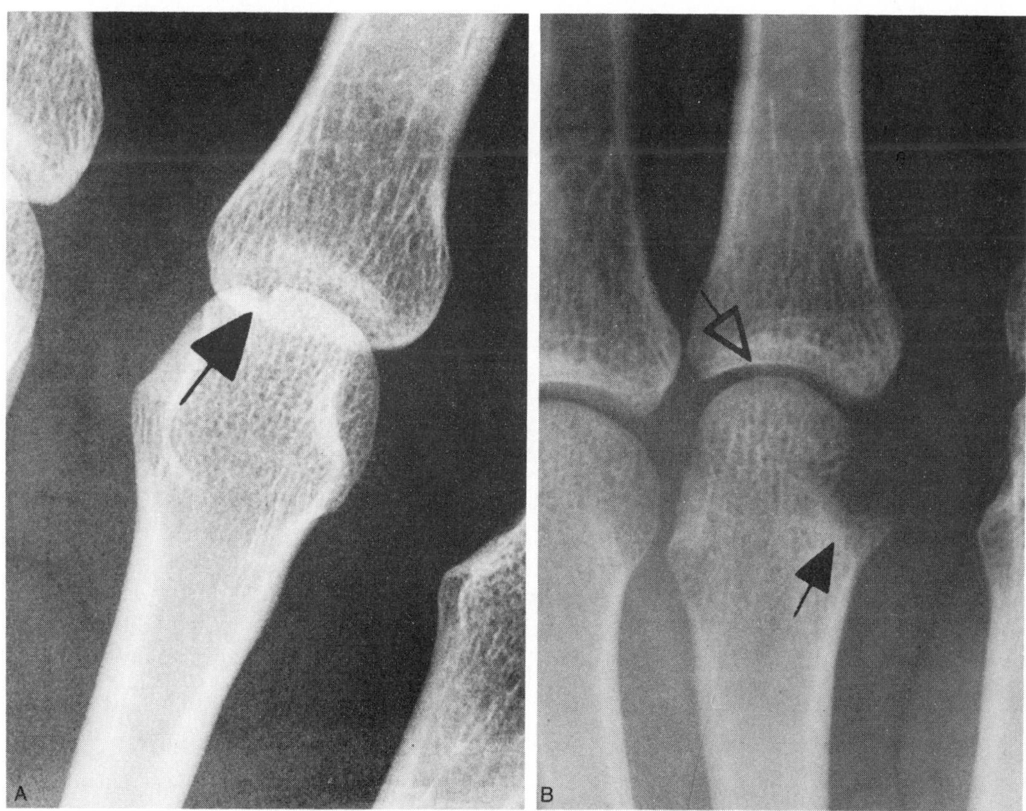

Figure 60–26. *Direct implantation of infection: Human bites.*

A *A small subchondral fracture of the metacarpal head (arrow) in this patient was produced by a fist-fight.*

B *Progressive destruction of the third metacarpal head (solid arrow) and narrowed metacarpophalangeal joint (open arrow) resulted from infection following a fist-fight in which the fist struck the opponent's teeth. (From Resnick D: J Can Assoc Radiol 27:21, 1976.)*

cavities of 12 to 54 per cent of dogs and 52 to 70 per cent of cats.[64, 117, 118] Other organisms include *Staphylococcus aureus* and *S. epidermidis* and Bacteroides species.[293]

Any anatomic site can be affected, although animal bites predominate in the hand, the arm, and the leg (Fig. 60–27). Inflammation with pain and swelling develops at the wound site in 1 to 3 days. Low-grade fever and lymphadenopathy can also be evident. In neglected cases, septicemia, infective synovitis, osteitis, osteomyelitis, and arthritis can develop.[66] Fractures may also be observed.[294]

Open Fractures and Dislocations. Whenever a fracture or dislocation is complicated by disruption of the overlying skin, direct inoculation of bones and joints can occur. This problem is especially relevant to injuries of the tibia; this is a superficially located bone, and extensive trauma at this site is frequently complicated by violation of the overlying soft tissues and skin. Despite the early administration of antibiotics, chronic osteomyelitis is frequent in this setting. Radiographic documentation of infection is not difficult; the ill-defined and irregular osseous destruction accompanying osteomyelitis is rarely confused with the manifestations of a nonsuppurative healing fracture (Fig. 60–28).

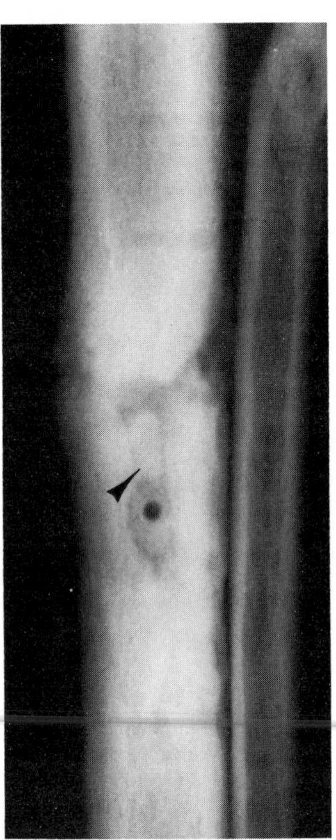

Figure 60–28. *Direct implantation of infection: Open fractures. This patient had a comminuted fracture of the tibia complicated by osteomyelitis. Operative intervention with application of a plate was also attempted, although the plate was removed because of continued drainage. Note a sequestrum in the tibia (arrowhead), fibrous union of the fracture, and the multiple osseous defects due to the removed screws.*

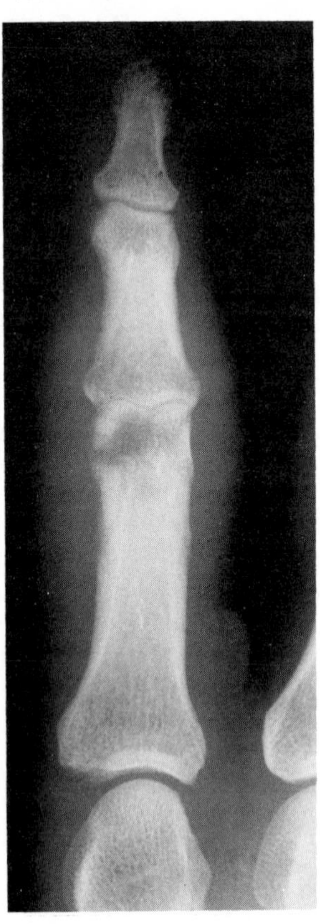

Figure 60–27. *Direct implantation of infection: Animal bites. Following a cat bite, this patient developed Pasteurella osteomyelitis and septic arthritis. Observe soft tissue swelling, osseous destruction of the proximal and middle phalanges, and joint space narrowing and flexion at the proximal interphalangeal joint.*

Postoperative Infection

Postoperative osteoarticular infections represent a problem of major concern, especially to the orthopedic surgeon. They may occur as a result of contamination of bones and joints from adjacent infected soft tissues, direct inoculation of osseous and articular tissue at the time of surgery, or, less frequently, hematogenous spread to an operative site from a distant location.[119, 120] Any surgical procedure can be complicated by osteomyelitis (and septic arthritis) (Fig. 60–29). Particularly troublesome are instances of infection following internal fixation of fractures, intervertebral disc surgery, and various types of arthroplasty.[60, 121-123] Clinically, considerable delay in diagnosis is not infrequent, as the signs of the infection are masked by the concomitant tissue injury or the suppressive effect of prophylactic agents,

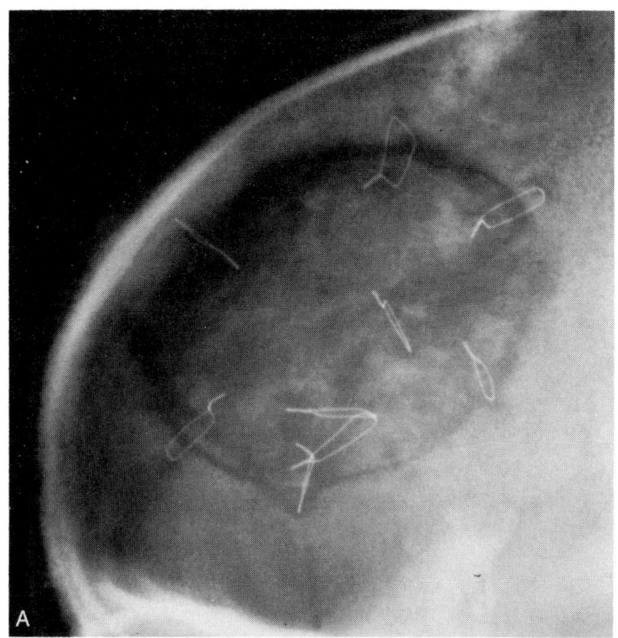

Figure 60–29. Postoperative infection.

A *An infection at a craniotomy site has resulted in considerable resorption of much of the osseous flap.*

B–D *Following an infection, the greater trochanter was removed. Subsequently, this patient developed aggressive osteomyelitis and septic arthritis of the hip, which eventually required amputation. A photograph of the removed bone* **(B)** *illustrates the destruction about the osteotomy site (arrow). A photograph of a macerated coronal section* **(C)** *illustrates some destruction of the outer aspect of the bone (arrows). This is also documented on the radiograph of the section (arrows)* **(D)**.

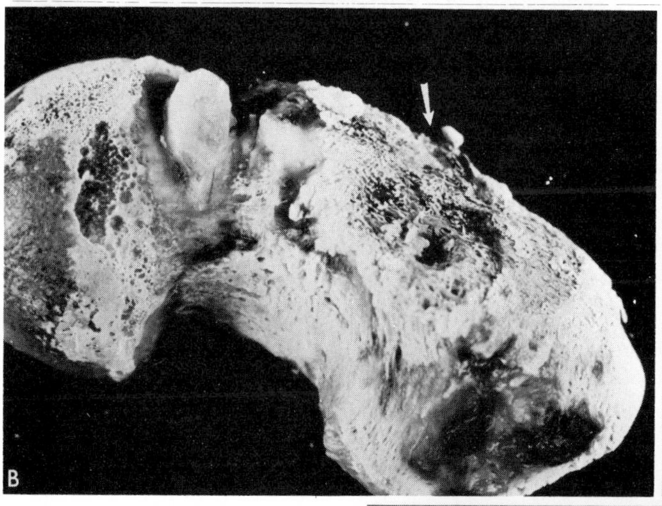

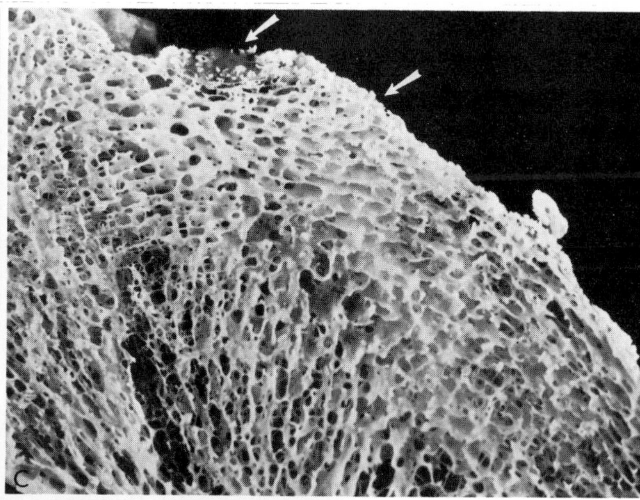

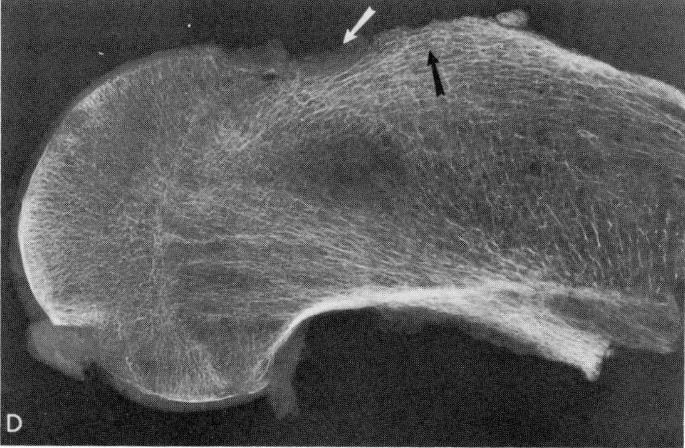

or the infecting organisms may be of limited pathogenicity. Any site can be affected, although the tibia and the femur are the most typical locations of infection following internal fixation of fractures; and the hip and the knee are the most typically infected sites following arthroplasty. One or more organisms may be implicated; *Staphylococcus aureus* is the most common pathogen.

Numerous radiographic techniques can be employed to evaluate postoperative infection. Routine radiography, tomography, fistulography, and arthrography can all be helpful; increasing osseous and cartilaginous destruction, periostitis, soft tissue swelling, and exaggerated "lucency" about cemented metallic prostheses can be recognized (see Chapter 25).

Complications

Severe Osteolysis. Although modern methods of diagnosis and treatment of infection usually assure proper therapy before too long a delay, this is not uniformly the case. Some individuals with osteomyelitis do not receive early or adequate treatment, and in these patients, severe osteolysis may ensue.[124, 125] Large foci of destruction can eventually lead to disappearance of long segments of tubular or flat bones (Fig. 60–30). Although institution of proper chemotherapeutic agents may reverse some of the deleterious effects of the infection, bizarre deformity consisting of osteosclerosis and osteolysis may require courageous reconstructive procedures.[282]

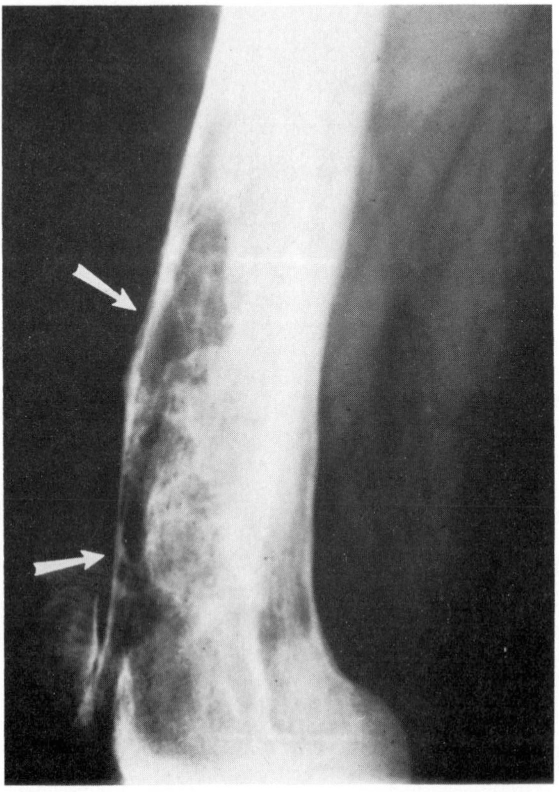

Figure 60–30. *Complications of osteomyelitis: Severe osteolysis. In this patient with chronic osteomyelitis, osteolysis of a large segment of the distal femur is evident (arrows).*

Epiphyseal Growth Disturbance. In the infant, infection that has spread to the epiphysis of a tubular bone can produce significant damage.[126-128] Injury to the cartilage cells on the epiphyseal side of the growth plate is irreparable,[129] and subsequent growth disturbances are to be expected. However, even with severe epiphyseal disintegration, some regeneration of the epiphysis can occur following eradication of the infection (Fig. 60–31).[130, 131, 299] Unfortunately, it is difficult to accurately predict the occurrence and extent of epiphyseal recovery following injury.[128] Thus, in all infants, the documentation of osteomyelitis with epiphyseal involvement must be accomplished at an early stage so that prompt therapy is instituted, and later complications, such as shortening of the limb and secondary degenerative arthritis, are avoided.

Neoplasm. Epidermoid carcinoma arising in a focus of chronic osteomyelitis is not uncommon[101] and may be evident in at least 0.5 per cent of patients with long-term draining infections of bone.[132] The latent period between the onset of osteomyelitis and the appearance of neoplasm is variable, although a time span of 20 to 30 years is typical. Neoplasm most frequently arises adjacent to the femur and the tibia, being evident clinically as pain, increasing drainage, onset of a foul odor from the fistula, a mass, and lymphadenopathy; and radiographically as progressive destruction of bone (Fig. 60–32).

An epidermoid carcinoma can develop at any site along the fistulous tract, although it is commonly quite deep; the epithelial lining of the tract undergoes repeated degeneration because of the presence of pus within the fistula.[2] It is in this setting that malignant degeneration occurs. The prognosis is guarded, as distant metastasis is not infrequent.

Although epithelial carcinoma is the most common neoplasm that is encountered in osteomyelitis,[132-138] fibrosarcoma,[133, 139, 140] angiosarcoma,[133] rhabdomyosarcoma,[133] reticulum cell sarcoma, adenocarcinoma,[141] basal cell carcinoma,[142] and plasmacytoma[143] have also been noted.[101] At times, the tissue consists of proliferative fibrous or granulation tissue and has been termed granulation tissue sarcoma.[144]

Amyloidosis. Secondary amyloidosis can complicate chronic osteomyelitis.[101] This complication has become less frequent, a fact that is attributable to improvement in the chemotherapy of infection. In studies of 105 cases of secondary amyloidosis, only five were associated with chronic osteomyelitis.[145-147]

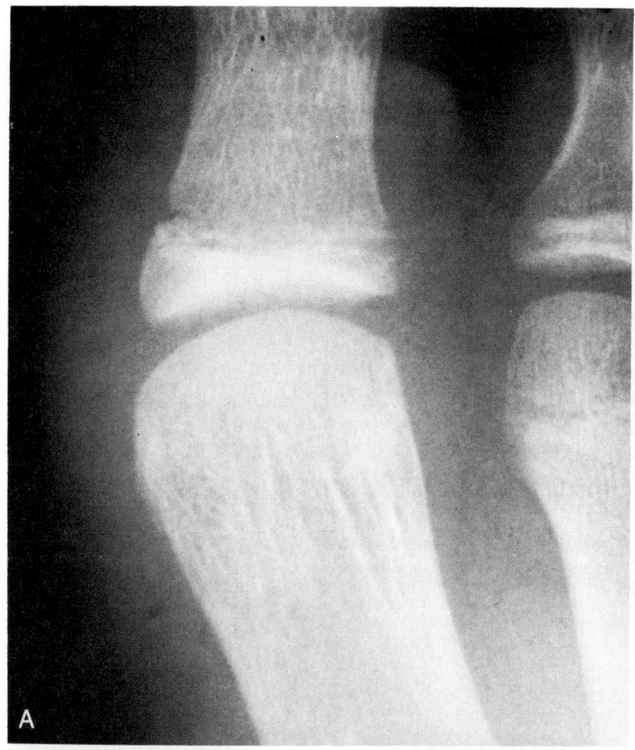

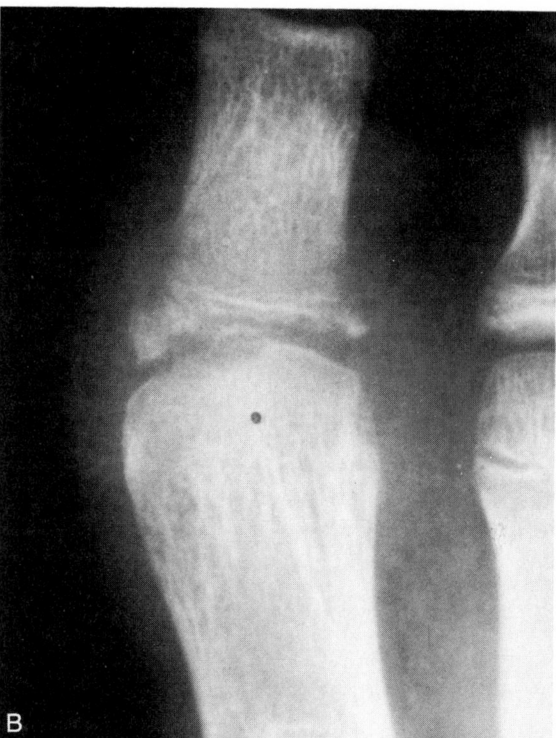

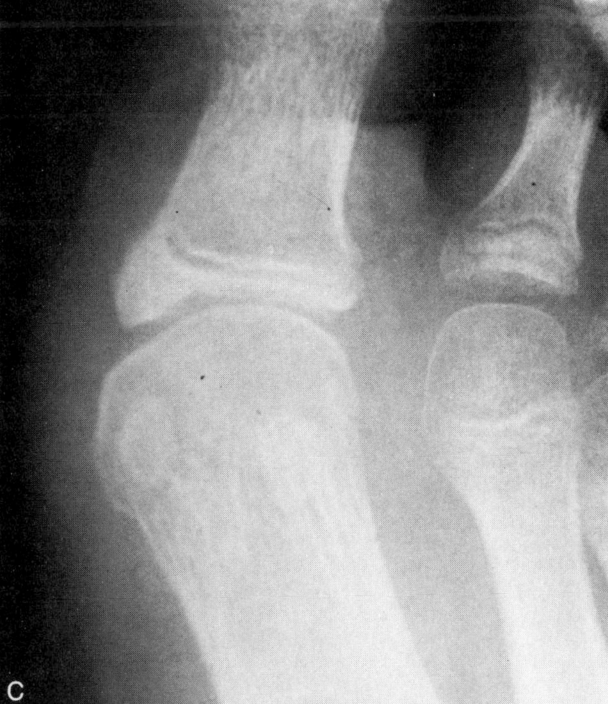

Figure 60–31. *Complications of osteomyelitis: Epiphyseal destruction. This 11 year old boy developed osteomyelitis and septic arthritis of the first metatarsophalangeal joint.*

A *An initial film reveals metaphyseal irregularity, soft tissue swelling, and a radiodense epiphysis of the proximal phalanx.*

B *One week later, the epiphysis has fragmented and largely disappeared, and osteolysis of both the metatarsal and the phalanx can be noted. Joint space narrowing is seen.*

C *Four weeks later, reconstitution of the epiphysis is seen.*

(Courtesy of Dr. T. Goergen, Palomar Memorial Hospital, Escondido, California.)

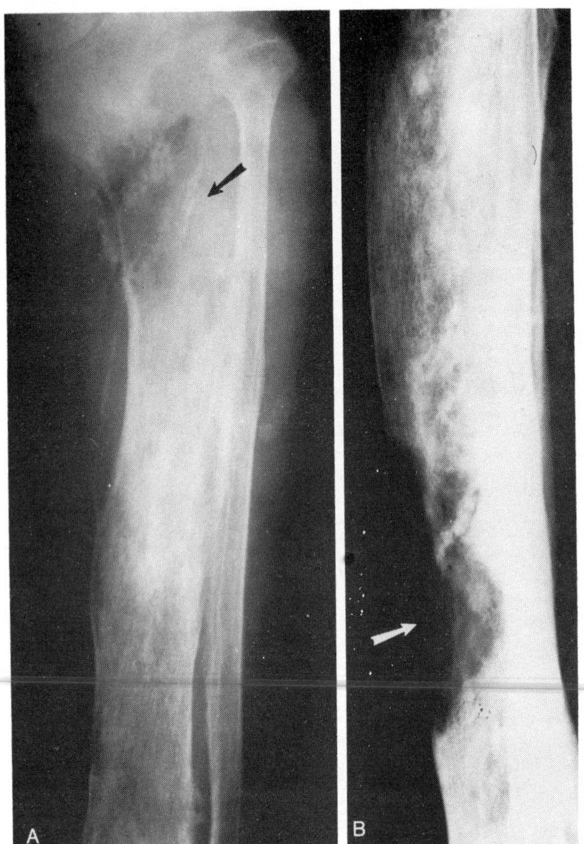

Figure 60–32. Complications of osteomyelitis: Neoplasm.

A Epidermoid carcinoma. This 63 year old man with chronic draining osteomyelitis developed a mass in the proximal tibia about a fistula. Superimposed on the radiographic changes of chronic infection of the tibia is a lytic lesion of the proximal aspect of the bone (arrow), which represented an epidermoid carcinoma invading the osseous tissue.

B Reticulum cell sarcoma. In this patient with chronic osteomyelitis of the tibia, the area of osseous destruction (arrow) was related to a reticulum cell sarcoma.

Modifications and Difficulties in Diagnosis

ANTIBIOTIC MODIFIED OSTEOMYELITIS. The previous discussion has concerned itself with the radiologic and pathologic findings of untreated osteomyelitis. In the modern era of sophisticated chemotherapeutic techniques, the infective process is often interrupted at a relatively early stage. If therapy is adequate, complete healing of the osseous abnormalities can occur, although clinical improvement is not initially paralleled by radiographic improvement. During the early healing phase of osteomyelitis, bone resorption continues as damaged osseous tissue is removed. Thus, radiographically evident increased destruction can occur at a time when the clinical picture is improving. Knowledge of this phenomenon assures that the clinician, alarmed at worsening roentgenograms, does not modify beneficial therapeutic regimens. Obviously, the patient, not the radiograph, must be treated. Soon the roentgenogram, too, will reveal evidence of osseous reconstitution, and the benefits of therapy become equally obvious to both the clinician and the radiologist.

Table 60–5

RADIOGRAPHIC SIGNS OF ACTIVITY IN CHRONIC OSTEOMYELITIS

Change from previous film
Ill-defined areas of osteolysis
Thin, linear periostitis
Sequestration

Inappropriate or inadequate chemotherapy can mask the clinical and roentgenographic manifestations of osteomyelitis for a period of time.[30] Most typically, acute lesions are obscured and the osteomyelitic process presents in a subacute or chronic form.

"ACTIVE" AND "INACTIVE" CHRONIC OSTEOMYELITIS. Although the radiographic features of chronic osteomyelitis are well established, differen-

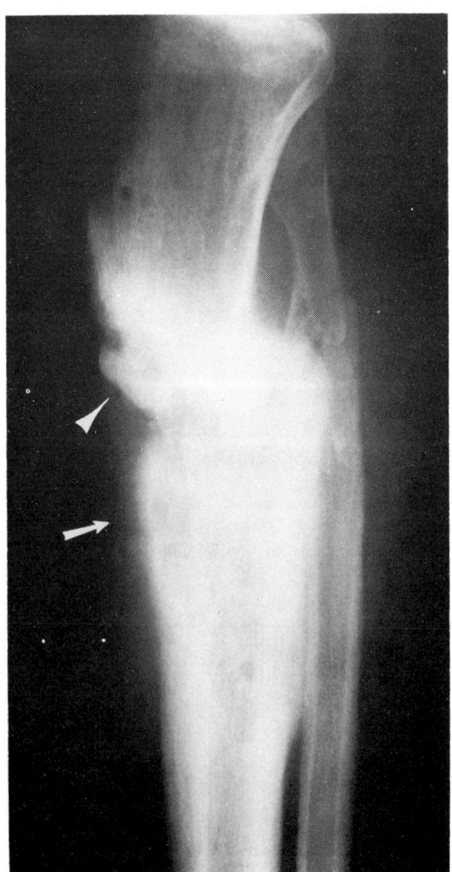

Figure 60–33. Activity in chronic osteomyelitis. In this patient with chronic osteomyelitis, the presence of ill-defined destruction, fluffy periostitis (arrow), and a sequestrum (arrowhead) indicates activity.

tiation of active and inactive chronic osteomyelitis by roentgenographic techniques can be extremely difficult (Table 60–5). The extensive osteolytic and osteosclerotic changes of a chronic osteomyelitic process that is dormant can obscure the changes of reactivation for a period of time. Other diagnostic modalities, such as magnification radiography or radionuclide examination utilizing technetium and gallium pharmaceuticals, can be helpful in this setting (see discussion later in this chapter). There are, however, certain indications on the radiograph that do allow differentiation of active and inactive chronic osteomyelitis. In cases of active infection, comparison with earlier available roentgenograms can detect a changing pattern or image that is characterized by new areas of destruction. Periostitis that is thin and linear in quality and separated from the subjacent bone suggests activity. Furthermore, ill-defined or fluffy periosteal excrescences extending into the adjacent soft tissues also indicate active infection (Fig. 60–33). Finally, the documentation of sequestration on routine radiography or tomography implies activity, as necrotic osseous fragments commonly harbor viable organisms.

Differential Diagnosis

General Features. The combination of clinical and radiologic characteristics in osteomyelitis usually assures correct diagnosis. Occasionally, aggressive bone destruction combined with periostitis and soft tissue swelling simulates the changes in malignant neoplasms, especially Ewing's or osteogenic sarcoma in the child, reticulum cell sarcoma in the young adult, and skeletal metastasis in the older individual. In neoplastic disorders and in infection, the pattern of osseous destruction is of "moth-eaten" appearance or permeative nature: The area of abnormality is not clearly separated or marginated from the adjacent normal bone; rather, the marginal characteristics of the lesion(s) are ill defined and the zone of transition from normal to abnormal bone extends over a relatively long distance. With very aggressive behavior, the lesion(s) may merge imperceptibly with the surrounding bony tissue.

Periostitis. The nature of the periosteal proliferation accompanying osteomyelitis is varied. In some patients, single or multiple osseous shells appear about the parent bone and later merge with it. This "onionskinning" is not specific for osteomyelitis as it may also be evident in malignant neoplasm such as Ewing's sarcoma. In cases of osteomyelitis in which a single thick layer of periosteal bone is seen, the changes are reminiscent of eosinophilic granuloma or traumatic periostitis.

Osteolytic Foci. The identification in a child of a metaphyseal radiolucent lesion abutting the growth plate or connecting with it by a channel certainly suggests the presence of an abscess. In these instances, the lucent focus is surrounded by sclerotic bone and may be accompanied by periostitis. Although osteogenic sarcoma is typically metaphyseal in location and Ewing's sarcoma may be metaphyseal, the osteolytic foci in these tumors are more poorly marginated, and with osteogenic sarcoma considerable neoplastic bone production may be evident. In an adult, osteolytic foci within an infected epiphysis can simulate the appearance of a giant cell tumor, intraosseous ganglion, or subchondral cyst.

Cortical lucent lesions can indicate an abscess, osteoid osteoma, or stress fracture. The nature of the lesion and the surrounding bony eburnation generally allows differentiation among these conditions (see earlier discussion).

Osteosclerosis. In some cases of osteomyelitis, exuberant bone formation produces widespread sclerosis. This may be of uniform quality or combined with mottled radiolucent shadows. The resulting radiographic picture can simulate malignant bone tumors (such as osteogenic sarcoma, Ewing's sarcoma, reticulum cell sarcoma, and chondrosarcoma), osteonecrosis, fibrous dysplasia, or Paget's disease. If the abnormal area does not extend down to the subchondral bone of an epiphysis in a tubular bone, the diagnosis of Paget's disease can be eliminated. The absence of large lytic areas, cortical disruption, soft tissue masses, and visible tumor matrix militates against the diagnosis of sarcomas.

Sequestration. Radiodense foci representing sequestra are reliable indicators of infection. Their occasional appearance in tumors (e.g., fibrosarcoma) does not significantly diminish the diagnostic nature of the finding.

Soft Tissue Masses and Swelling. Soft tissue prominence is a common finding in infectious and neoplastic conditions. In general, tumors are associated with circumscribed soft tissue masses that displace surrounding soft tissue planes and frequently contain visible tumor matrix. Infections lead to infiltration and obscuration of soft tissue planes. This differentiation is not uniformly reliable.

Soft tissue infections or neoplasms can infiltrate subjacent osseous tissue. The pattern of cortical and medullary destruction and associated periostitis accompanying the process is not usually specific enough to allow a single diagnosis.

SEPTIC ARTHRITIS

Routes of Contamination

The potential routes of contamination of articulations can be divided into the same categories as

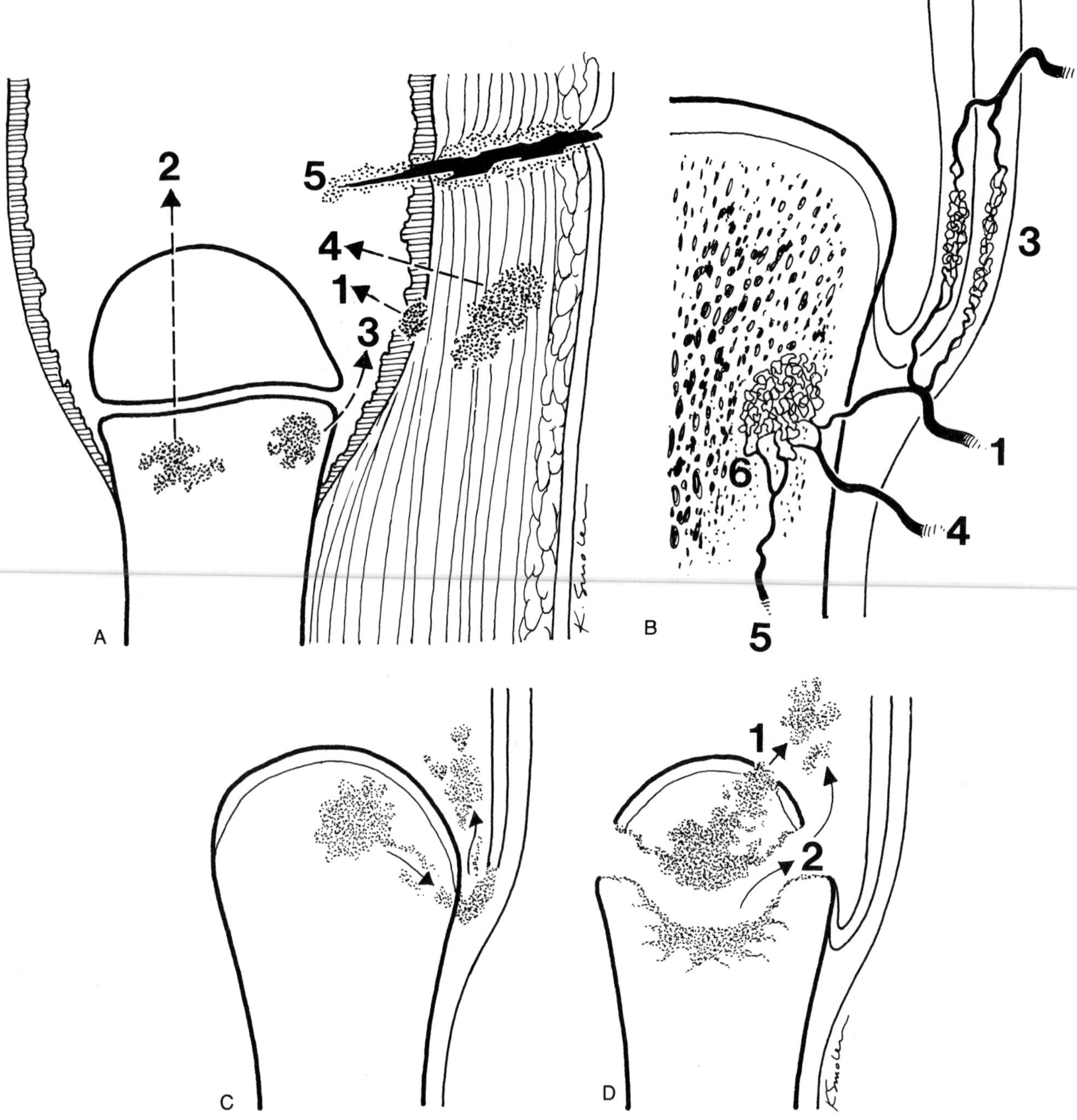

Figure 60–34. Septic arthritis: Potential routes of contamination.

A Hematogenous spread of infection to a joint can result from direct lodgment of organisms in the synovial membrane (1) or, as illustrated in **B**, direct vascular continuity between an infected epiphysis and the synovial membrane. Spread into the joint from a contiguous source can occur from a metaphyseal focus that extends into the epiphysis and from there into the joint (2); from a metaphyseal focus with extension into the joint when the growth plate is intra-articular (3); or from a contiguous soft tissue infection (4). Direct implantation following a penetrating wound (5) can also lead to septic arthritis.

B, C Hematogenous spread of infection to a joint can occur due to vascular continuity between the epiphysis and synovial membrane. In **B** the vessels shown include arterioles (1), venules (2), and capillaries (3) of the capsule, periosteal vessels (4), the nutrient artery (5), and metaphyseal-epiphyseal anastomoses (6). In this fashion, the synovial membrane may become infected from an osseous focus before the joint fluid is contaminated. In **C**, this sequence of events is diagrammed.

D Spread from a contiguous osseous surface can result from penetration of the cartilage (1) or pathologic fracture with articular contamination (2). In this situation, synovial fluid may become infected before the synovial membrane.

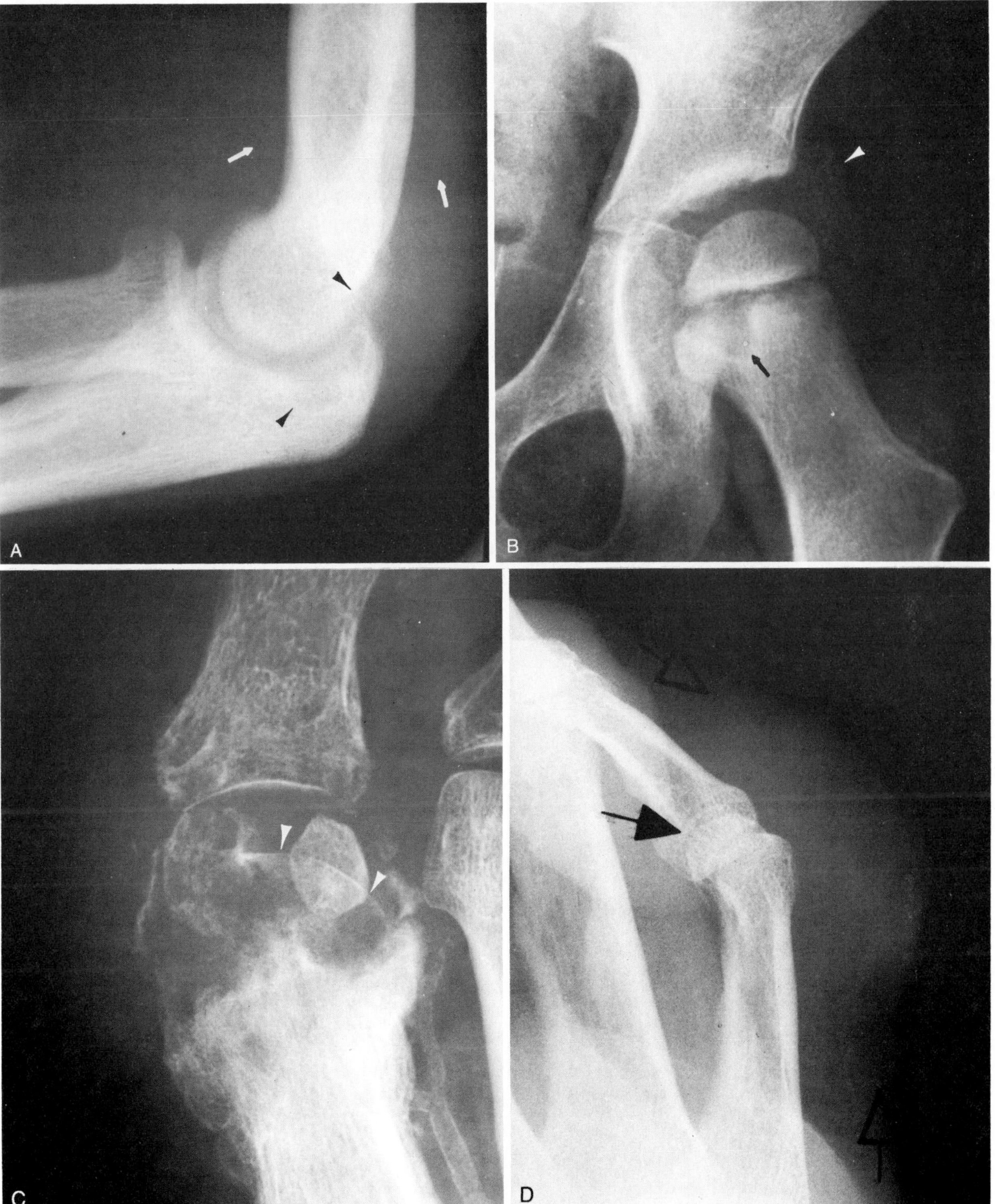

Figure 60–35. *Septic arthritis: Potential routes of contamination.*

A *Hematogenous spread of infection. Septic arthritis in this patient was related to implantation of organisms into the synovial membrane. An effusion with elevation of the fat pads (arrows) was evident long before osseous involvement occurred (arrowheads).*

B *Spread from a contiguous metaphyseal focus in a child. In the hip, the growth plate is an intra-articular structure. Thus, an osteomyelitic focus in the metaphysis (arrow) can lead to joint contamination, with widening of the articular space and soft tissue swelling (arrowhead).*

C *Spread from a contiguous epiphyseal focus in an adult. Osteomyelitis of the first metatarsal in this diabetic patient preceded the occurrence of joint infection. Note the collapse of the articular surface with depression of the subchondral bone (arrowheads) allowing contamination of the joint contents.*

D *Spread from a contiguous soft tissue infection. An infection in soft tissue (open arrows) following an injury led to contamination of the proximal interphalangeal joint of the fifth finger with bony erosion and joint space narrowing (solid arrow).*

Illustration continued on the following page

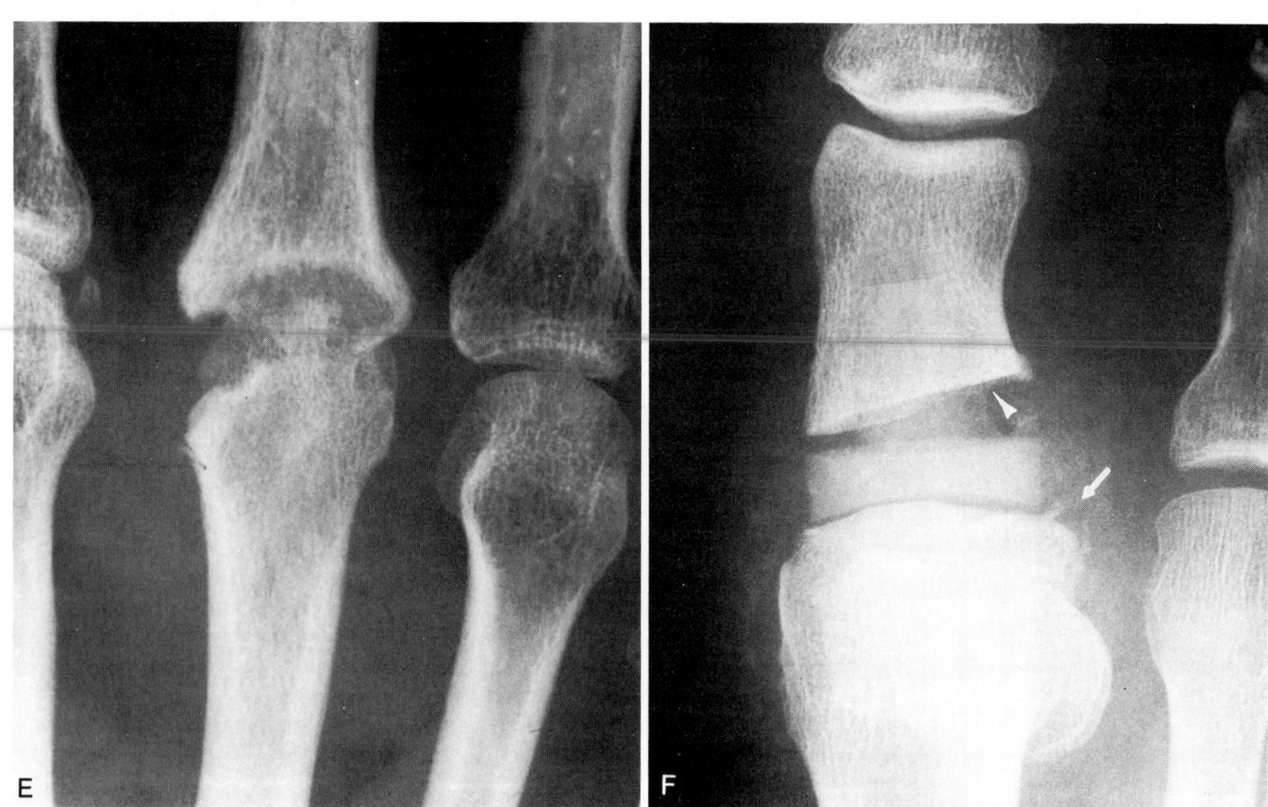

Figure 60–35. Continued

E *Direct implantation of infection of a metacarpophalangeal joint following a fist-fight in which the opponent's tooth penetrated the articulation. Observe soft tissue swelling, joint space narrowing, and ill-defined destruction of bone.*

F *Postoperative infection. Following the placement of a phalangeal prosthesis for degenerative joint disease, infection developed that required the removal of the prosthesis. Note soft tissue swelling and mild osseous erosion and fragmentation (arrow). Resorption of a small part of the phalangeal surface is also evident (arrowhead).*

were utilized in the previous discussion of osteomyelitis (Figs. 60–34 and 60–35).

Hematogenous Spread of Infection. Hematogenous seeding of the synovial membrane is due to either direct lodgment of organisms within the synovial vessels or spread from an adjacent epiphyseal focus of osteomyelitis by means of vascular continuity between the epiphysis and the synovial membrane.[8]

Spread from a Contiguous Source of Infection. A joint may become contaminated by intra-articular extension of osteomyelitis from an epiphyseal or metaphyseal focus, or of neighboring suppurative soft tissue processes.

Direct Implantation of Infection. Inoculation of a joint can occur during aspiration or following a penetrating wound.

Postoperative Infection. An intra-articular suppurative process can occur following any type of joint surgery.

Hematogenous Spread of Infection

Pathogenesis. Hematogenous spread of infection to a joint indicates that organisms lodge within the vasculature of the synovial membrane directly from a distant infected source or indirectly from an adjacent bone infection. In either case, infection of the synovial membrane precedes contamination of the synovial fluid.[8, 300] Thus, initial arthrocentesis may suggest bland inflammation of the articulation. Lodgment of organisms (bacteria) in the synovial membrane has been documented experimentally following their intravenous injection; similar studies have indicated that living bacteria obtain access to synovial fluid more readily than to spinal fluid, aqueous humor, or urine.[148]

The reaction of the synovial tissue to the contained organisms varies according to the local and general resistance of the patient, and the number, type, and virulence of the infecting agents. Thus, in some cases of infective arthritis, a limited and locally confined reaction of the synovial membrane is encountered; in other cases, severe tissue inflammation is seen. Although the precise pathogenesis of subsequent injury to intra-articular structures is not known, the appearance of fibrin deposition in septic arthritis may be important in this regard.[149] Fibrin deposits adherent to articular cartilage could interfere with proper cartilaginous nutrition from the adjacent synovial fluid and could also impede the release of metabolic products from the cartilage.[148] Fibrin could possibly attract leukocytes chemotactically; these cells phagocytize fibrin, and degranulation of the leukocytes and release of enzymes into the synovial fluid may accentuate the intra-articular inflammatory process.[148] If this mechanism is indeed operational, the elimination of fibrin clots through surgical drainage may afford some control over the extent of joint destruction.

As collagenase appears to be important in the pathogenesis of cartilage destruction in rheumatoid arthritis, this substance may also be important in the chondrolysis of infective arthritis.[150] Enzymatic release by the lysosomes in the leukocytes is probably important in cartilaginous injury in septic arthritis.[148] The possibility that further abnormalities in this process also result from an autoimmune response to damaged cartilage has been suggested.[151] The extent of articular destruction accompanying infective arthritis, whatever its pathogenesis, is influenced by the defense mechanisms of the host. Elderly patients, patients with serious chronic illnesses, patients who are receiving immunosuppressive therapy, and those with preexisting joint diseases have an increased incidence of articular infection.[152, 153]

General Clinical Features. Septic arthritis affects men and women of all ages, although it predominates in the young.[154-156, 296] Monoarticular involvement is the major pattern of presentation, especially in the younger age groups, although polyarticular localization is occasionally noted. The specific site(s) of infection are dependent upon the age of the patient, the organism, and the existence of an underlying disease or problem, although the knee, particularly in children, infants, and adults,[152,153] and the hip, especially in children and infants,[157-160] are frequently affected. With pyogenic infection, an acute onset with fever and chills is typical, although a prodromal phase of several days' duration with malaise, arthralgia, and low-grade fever can be encountered.[161] Pain, tenderness, redness, heat, and soft tissue swelling of the involved articulation are common. Leukocytosis and positive blood and joint cultures are important laboratory parameters of pyogenic arthritis. The most commonly implicated bacteria are *Staphylococcus aureus;* others include alpha- and beta-hemolytic streptococci, pneumococci, Hemophilus, Pseudomonas, gonococcus, *Escherichia coli,* and Serratia. Mycobacterial and fungal agents may also be implicated.

Radiographic-Pathologic Correlation (Table 60–6). In response to bacterial infection, the synovial membrane becomes edematous, swollen, and hypertrophied.[2, 162, 163] Increased amounts of synovial fluid are produced; the fluid may be thin and cloudy, contain large numbers of leukocytes, and reveal a lowered sugar level and elevated protein count. After a few days, frank pus accumulates in the articular cavity and destruction of cartilage begins[35] (Fig. 60–36). The early site of cartilaginous change is variable. Prominent abnormality may appear at the margins or central portions of articulations, accompanied by growth of the inflamed synovium across the surface of the cartilage or between cartilage and bone. Even or uneven cartilaginous erosion (from superficially located pannus) and disruption or sepa-

Table 60–6

SEPTIC ARTHRITIS: RADIOGRAPHIC-PATHOLOGIC CORRELATION

Pathologic Abnormality	Radiographic Abnormality
Edema and hypertrophy of synovial membrane with fluid production	Joint effusion, soft tissue swelling
Hyperemia	Osteoporosis
Inflammatory pannus with chondral destruction	Joint space loss
Pannus destruction of bone	Marginal and central osseous erosion
Fibrous or bony ankylosis	Bony ankylosis

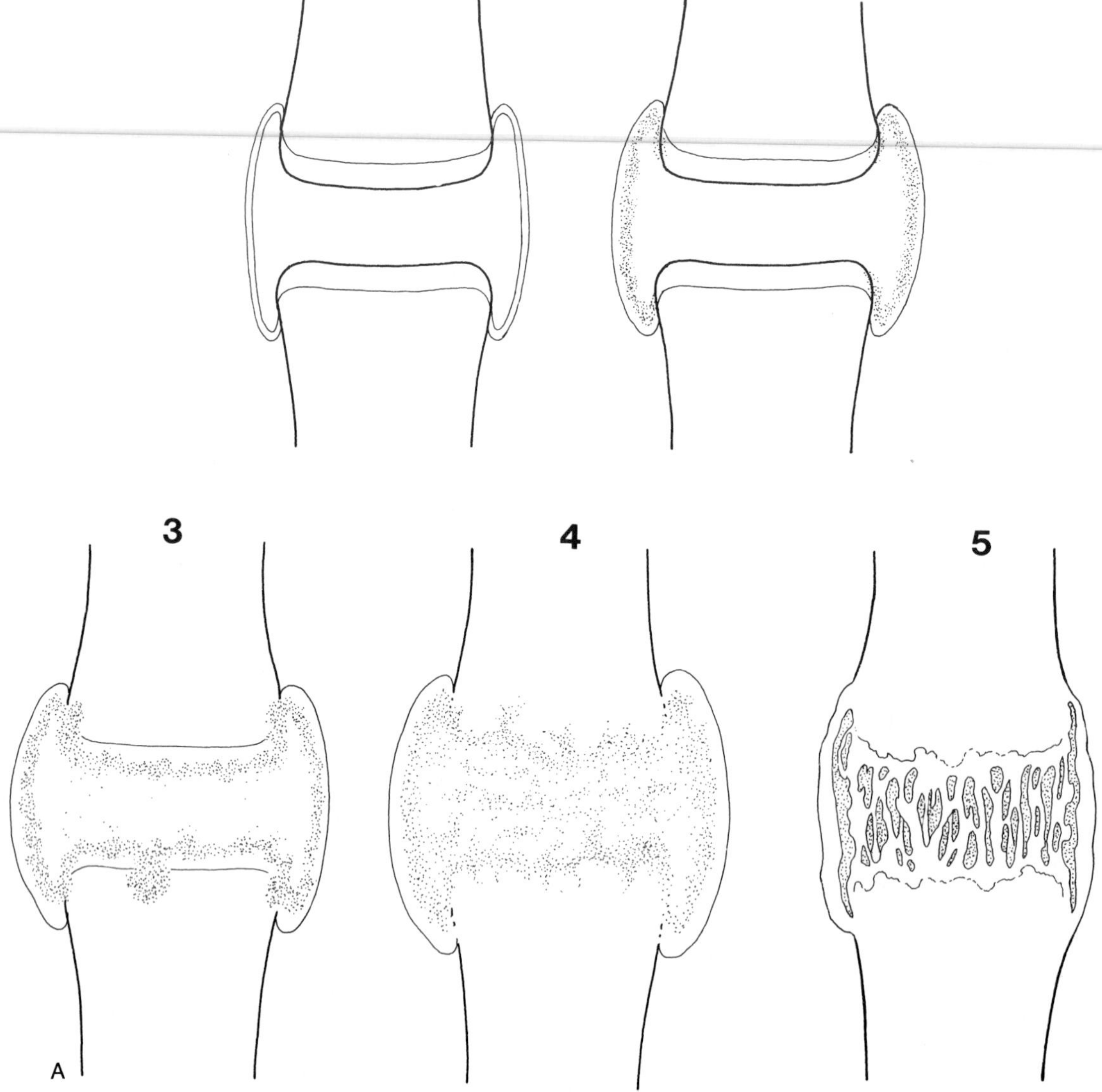

Figure 60–36. *Septic arthritis: Pathologic abnormalities.*

A *1, Normal synovial joint; 2, an edematous swollen and hypertrophic synovial membrane becomes evident; 3,4, accumulating inflammatory pannus leads to chondral destruction and to marginal and central osseous erosions; 5, bony ankylosis can eventually result.*

Illustration continued on the opposite page

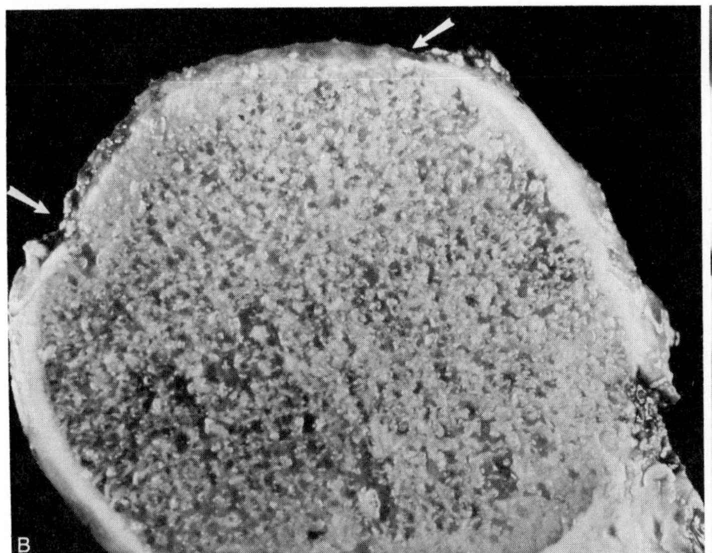

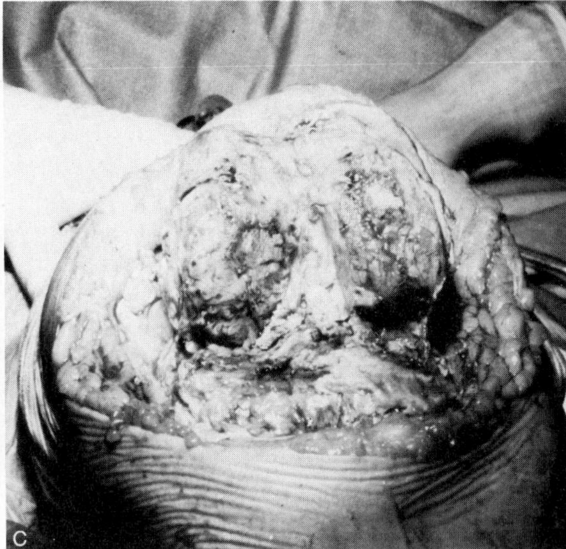

Figure 60–36. Continued

B *A photograph of a coronal section of a femoral head in a patient with a bacterial septic arthritis reveals erosion of cartilage and bone over the central portion of the head (between arrows).*

C *An operative photograph of the knee in a patient with a bacterial septic arthritis reveals extensive erosion and destruction of cartilaginous and osseous tissue of the femur with synovial proliferation. (***C,** *Courtesy of Dr. F. Richard Convery, University of California, San Diego, California.)*

ration (from subchondral pannus) can develop. With further accumulation of hypertrophied synovium and fluid, the capsule becomes distended, surrounding soft tissue edema is evident, and osseous abnormalities ensue. Superficial marginal and central bony erosions may progress to extensive destruction of large segments of the articular surface. Fibrous or bony ankylosis can eventually occur.

Radiographic abnormalities parallel the pathologic changes in pyogenic arthritis[164] (Fig. 60–37). Radiographically evident soft tissue swelling accompanies synovial hypertrophy. Interosseous space narrowing, which is frequently diffuse, reflects damage and disruption of the chondral surface. Osseous erosions at the edges of the articulation, related to the effects of diseased synovium on bone, lead to marginal defects that are similar in appearance and location to those of rheumatoid arthritis. They predominate at the unprotected osseous surfaces that do not possess cartilaginous coats at the periphery of the joint. Subchondral extension of pannus destroys the bone plate and adjacent trabeculae, leading to poorly defined gaps in the subchondral "white" line on the roentgenogram. Further destruction of bone becomes evident and, in late stages, bony ankylosis of the articulation may be seen.

These pathologic and radiographic abnormalities are modified in accordance with the infecting organism. Rapid destruction of bone and cartilage is characteristic of bacterial arthritis, whereas in tuberculosis and fungal diseases, articular changes occur more slowly. In tuberculosis, marginal osseous erosions with preservation of joint space and periarticular osteoporosis can be prominent. Pathologically, in this disease, subchondral extension of pannus, mass-like intra-articular protrusion of granulation tissue, and fibrous ankylosis, rather than bony ankylosis, can be evident.[2]

In all varieties of septic arthritis, involvement of adjacent osseous structures produces typical features of osteomyelitis. Poorly defined "moth-eaten" bony destruction and periostitis are seen. In some instances of pyogenic arthritis, calcification in and around the joint is observed.[165, 166] These deposits are more common in those patients with severe and lengthy illness, occur after a period of 4 to 12 weeks, and are probably related to dystrophic calcification in association with rupture of the joint capsule and extension of the infection into the adjacent soft tissue. They have been produced in experimental joint infections.[167, 168] In humans, soft tissue calcification may be responsible for residual pain owing to local mechanical factors.

Rarely, gas formation within a joint can complicate septic arthritis due to *Escherichia coli* and *Clostridium perfringens*[169-174] (Fig. 60–38). Much more frequently, the appearance of radiolucent collections in an infected articulation indicates that a prior arthrocentesis has been performed or that an open wound exists with communication between the joint and the skin surface.

Spread from a Contiguous Source of Infection

Pathogenesis. In certain age groups, osteomyelitis can be complicated by contamination of the

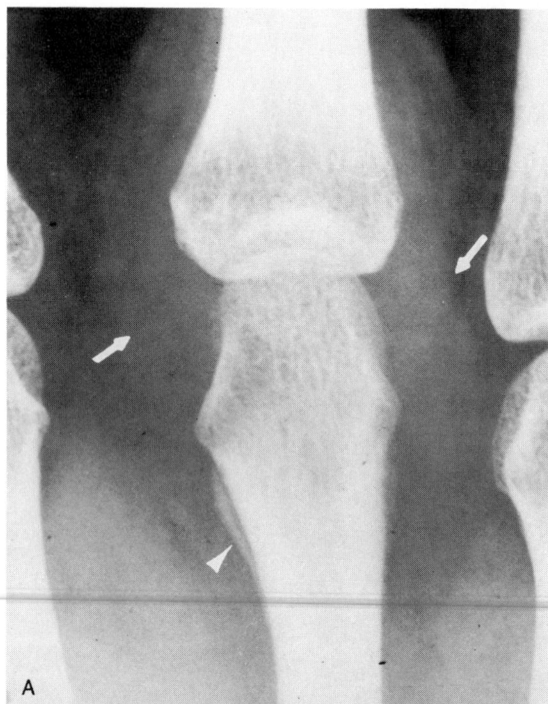

Figure 60–37. *Septic arthritis: Radiographic abnormalities.*

A *Soft tissue swelling. A low KV radiograph of an infected metacarpophalangeal articulation demonstrates soft tissue edema (arrows), osteoporosis, and periostitis (arrowhead). (***A,** *Courtesy of Dr. J. Weston, Lower Hutt, New Zealand.)*

B, C *Radiographs obtained 6 months apart in a neglected infection reveal the classic radiographic features of pyogenic septic arthritis. The initial film* **(B)** *demonstrates joint space narrowing and osseous erosions, which predominate at the margins of the talus (arrows). The latter film* **(C)** *shows spectacular destruction, with collapse of osseous surface. Note the absence of significant osteoporosis.*

Illustration continued on the opposite page

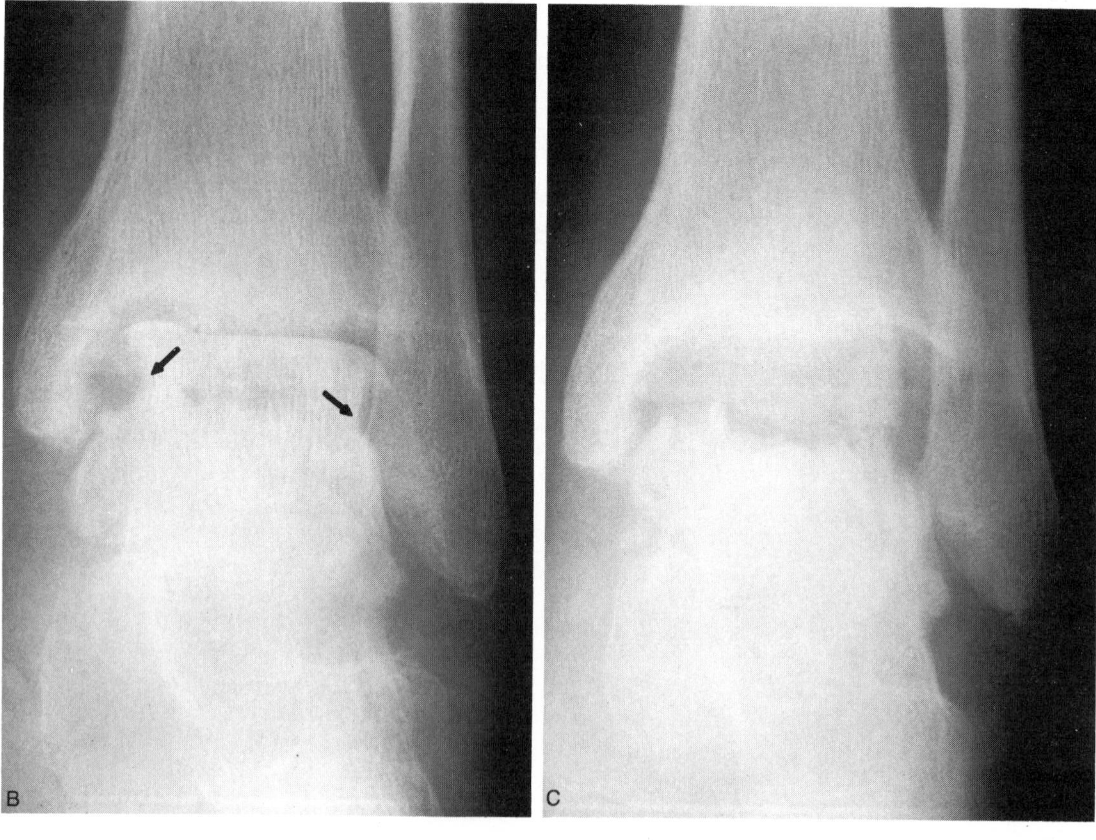

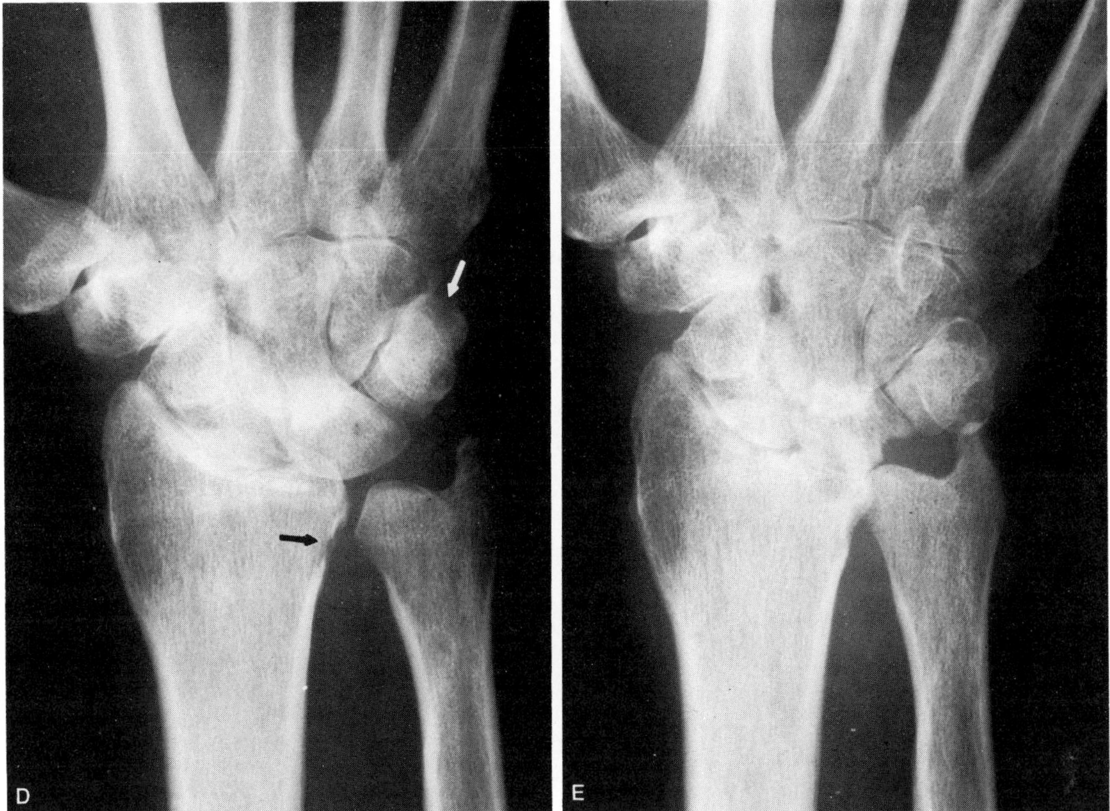

Figure 60–37. Continued

D, E *In this wrist, pyogenic arthritis has produced diffuse compartmental abnormalities. In the earlier film* **(D)**, *note joint space loss at the radiocarpal, midcarpal, and common carpometacarpal articulations, subtle osseous erosions (arrows), periarticular osteoporosis, and soft tissue swelling. In the later film* **(E)**, *progressive destruction is evident. The appearance is not unlike that in rheumatoid arthritis.*

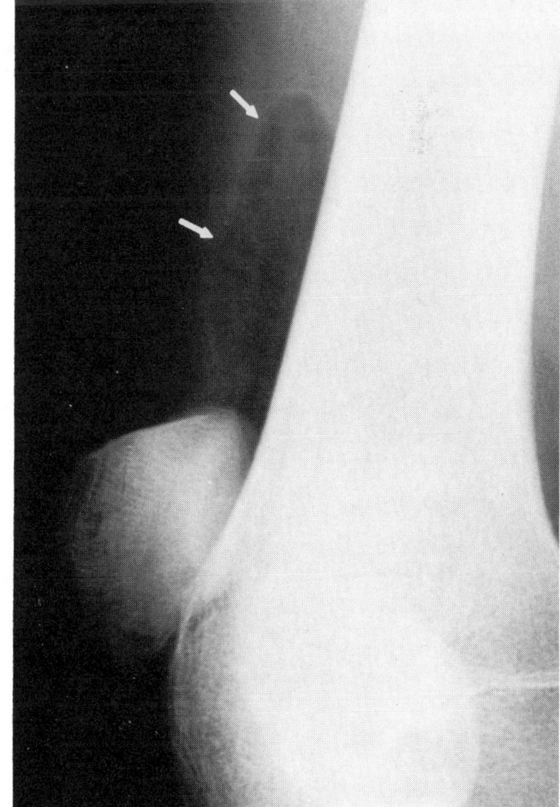

Figure 60–38. Septic arthritis: Intra-articular gas formation. Escherichia coli pyogenic arthritis can rarely lead to intra-articular "bubbly" collections of gas (arrows). Much more frequently, radiolucent collections within the joint relate to air introduced during arthrocentesis or via a tract that communicates with the skin.

adjacent articulation. In the infant the presence of vascular communication between metaphyseal and epiphyseal segments of tubular bones allows organisms within nutrient vessels to localize in the epiphysis and subsequently extend into the joint. This may occur via the common vascular pathways of the epiphysis and synovial membrane (hematogenous spread of infection) or as a result of transchondral extension directly into the articular cavity (spread from a contiguous source). In the latter situation, radiographic evidence of osteomyelitis generally precedes that of articular infection. In the adult, vascular connections between the epiphysis and metaphysis are reestablished as the growth plate closes. Hematogenous osteomyelitis can thus affect the epiphysis in this age group. Once again, subsequent joint contamination can occur via hematogenous pathways or through disruption of the chondral surface.

A second situation in which septic arthritis can occur as a result of contamination from a contiguous source is related to adjacent soft tissue infection or, more rarely, nearby visceral infection (e.g., vesicoacetabular or enteroacetabular fistulae)[175, 297] (Figs. 60–39 to 60–41). In these instances, the organisms are first evident in periarticular locations and only later penetrate the capsule to enter the synovial membrane and articular cavity.

A third situation in which joint infection develops due to extension from a surrounding suppurative process occurs in those locations in which the growth plate has an intra-articular location; the most important such site is the hip. Because of this anatomic arrangement, osteomyelitis localized to the metaphysis can enter the articulation by extending laterally without violating the growth plate. With penetration of the thin metaphyseal cortex, organisms can directly extend into the synovium or the articular cavity.

Radiographic-Pathologic Correlation. Generally, there is radiographic evidence that the infective process originates outside the articulation. This evidence may include soft tissue deficit, swelling, or gas formation; osteomyelitis with typical epiphyseal or metaphyseal destruction; and diverticulitis or cystitis with fistulization, detected on appropriate contrast examination. In certain situations, however, joint effusion and cartilaginous and subchondral osseous destruction are the first radiographic clues to infection; radiographic abnormalities in the adjacent structures may be subtle or entirely absent. In the infant in whom the epiphysis is unossified or only partially ossified, detection of primary osteomyelitis can be extremely difficult, and an enlarging effusion, displacement or subluxation of the ossified epiphyseal nucleus, or blurring of the subchondral white line on the opposite bone (e.g., acetabulum) may be the first evidence of sepsis. In the

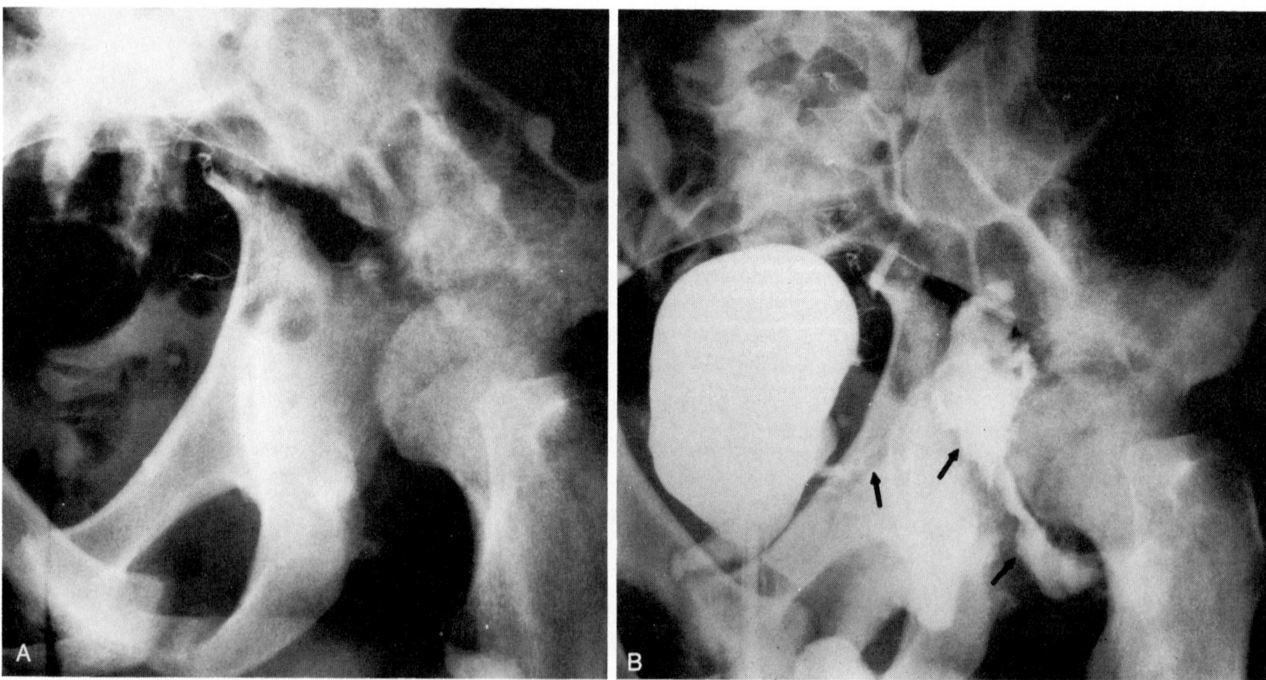

Figure 60–39. *Septic arthritis: Contamination from a contiguous source of infection. During an automobile accident, this patient sustained severe pelvic trauma resulting in fractures and injury to the bladder.*

A *A radiograph reveals, in addition to the obvious comminuted fractures of the pelvis, an ill-defined osteoporotic femoral head.*

B *A cystogram following an intravenous pyelogram demonstrates communication between the bladder and the hip, with contrast accumulation in the joint (arrows).*

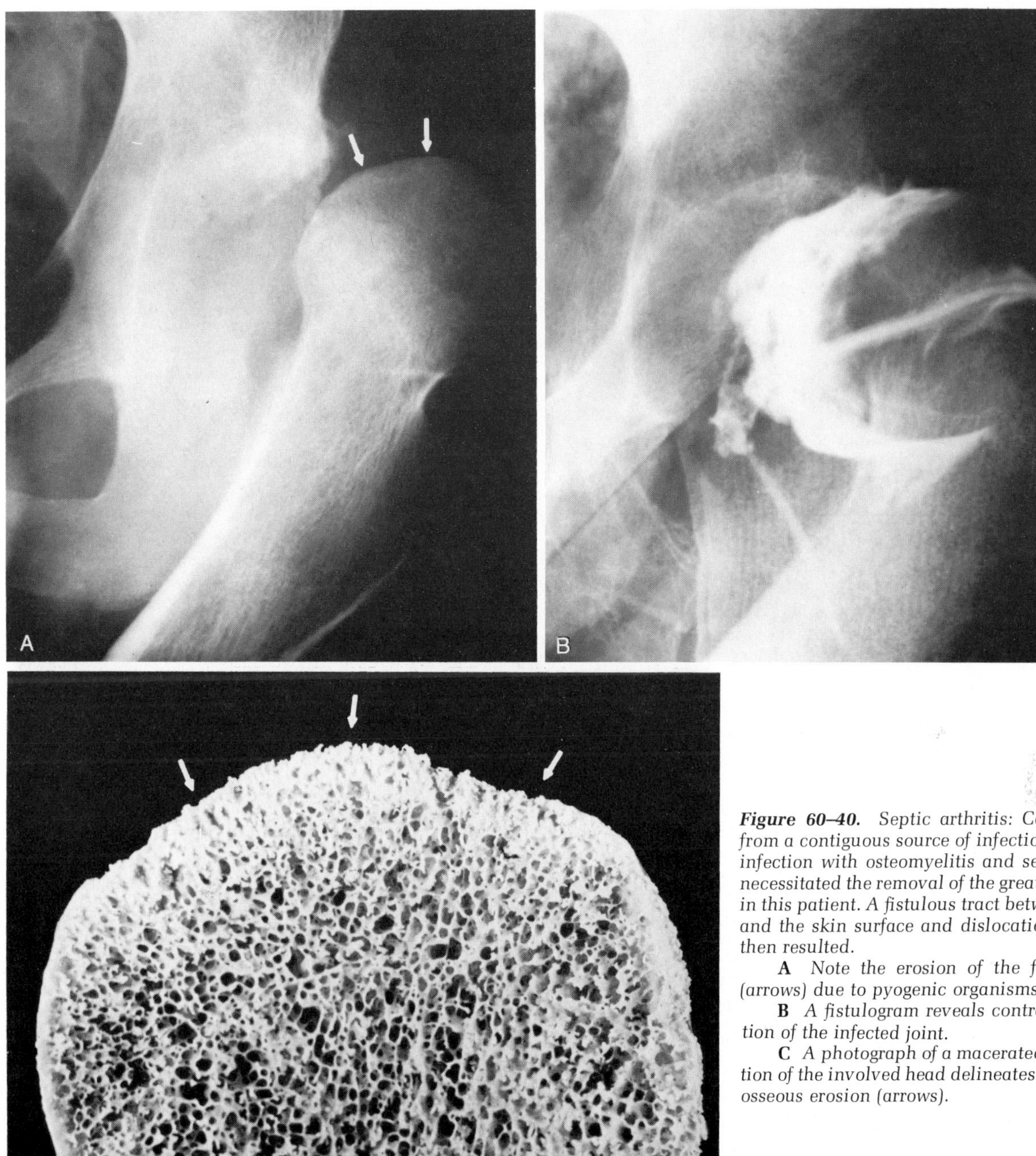

Figure 60–40. *Septic arthritis: Contamination from a contiguous source of infection. Soft tissue infection with osteomyelitis and septic arthritis necessitated the removal of the greater trochanter in this patient. A fistulous tract between the joint and the skin surface and dislocation of the hip then resulted.*

A *Note the erosion of the femoral head (arrows) due to pyogenic organisms.*

B *A fistulogram reveals contrast opacification of the infected joint.*

C *A photograph of a macerated coronal section of the involved head delineates the degree of osseous erosion (arrows).*

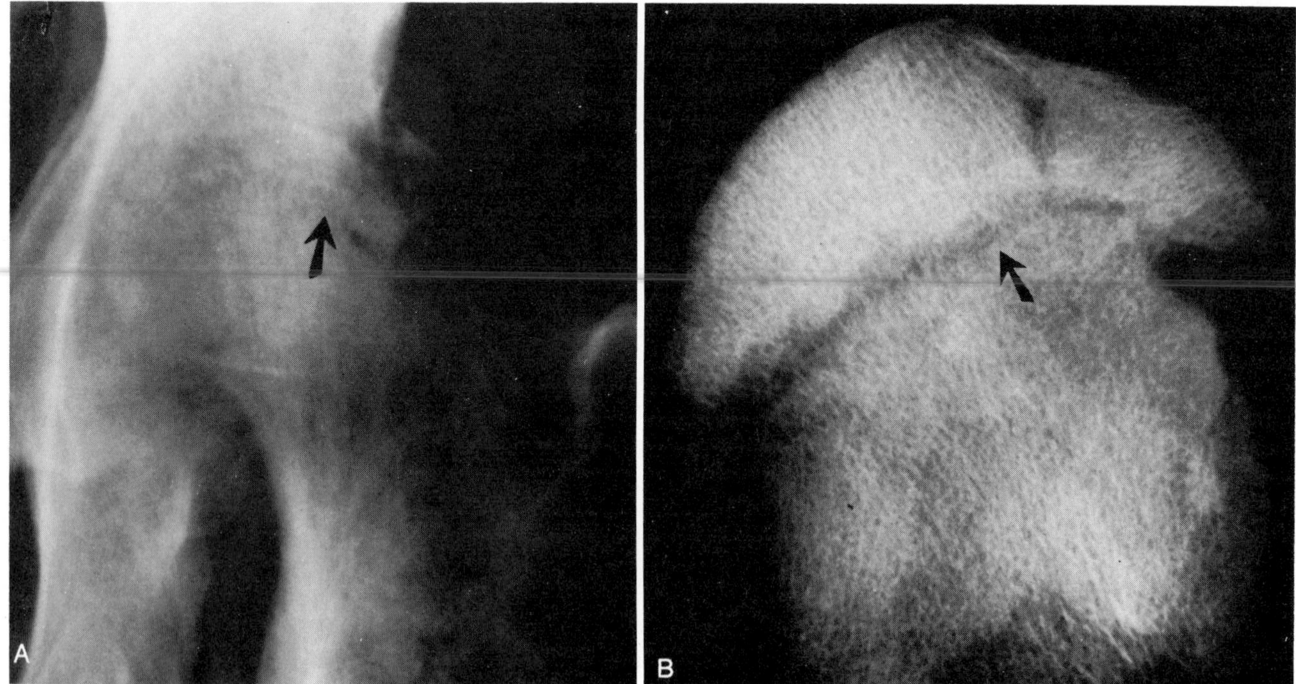

Figure 60–41. *Septic arthritis: Contamination from a contiguous source of infection. This 43 year old man with rheumatoid arthritis had undergone a laparotomy and bowel resection with a colostomy for sigmoid diverticulitis. A fistula developed between the bowel, left hip, and skin, which was related to* Escherichia coli *infection.*

A *A radiograph of the hip outlines the narrowed joint space and bony destruction. A radiolucent line can be seen in the femoral head (arrow).*

B *Following a modified Girdlestone procedure, a radiograph of the removed femoral head identifies the osseous destruction and fracture line (arrow).*

(From Resnick D: Radiology 114:581, 1975.)

adult with diabetes mellitus, joint space narrowing or marginal and central osseous erosion of the metatarsophalangeal or interphalangeal articulation may alert the physician to a clinically unsuspected septic arthritis.

Once the articulation has been violated, the radiographic and pathologic abnormalities of the infection are virtually identical to those associated with hematogenously derived suppurative joint disease. Soft tissue swelling, diffuse loss of joint space, poorly defined marginal and central osseous defects, periostitis, fragmentation, and calcification can be observed. In some cases, fistulography with retrograde injection of contrast material will opacify the articulation, providing definite evidence of communication of the joint and overlying skin surfaces.

SPECIFIC ENTITIES

Septic Arthritis of the Hip in Infancy and Childhood. Although additional mechanisms of hip infection in infants and children can include hematogenous seeding of the synovium and direct implantation following needle puncture when drawing blood from the femoral vessels,[176-178] the spread of infection into the hip from a metaphyseal (or epiphyseal) focus is well known, common, and of such importance that it deserves special emphasis.[159, 179-185]

Neonatal septic arthritis was first documented by Thomas Smith in 1874.[186] The hip is the most frequently affected joint, and *Staphylococcus aureus* is the most commonly implicated organism. In this age group, infection can reach this articulation by spreading from a metaphyseal focus of osteomyelitis either directly into the joint (the growth plate is intra-articular) or to the epiphysis by way of vascular channels that cross the growth plate and, from there, into the articulation. Clinically, infants with septic arthritis of the hip may reveal irritability, loss of appetite, and fever. Local symptoms and signs may be absent or minimal, complicating accurate diagnosis, although swelling in the thigh and a hip held in flexion, abduction, and external rotation are helpful clues.[187] Initial roentgenograms of the hip are frequently unremarkable. Soft tissue or capsular swelling[188] and a positive obturator sign[189] are not readily apparent on neonatal roentgenograms, although the findings, when present, may be more reliable in this age group than in adults[190, 298] (Fig. 60–42). With accumulation of intra-articular fluid, pathologic subluxation or dislocation of the femoral head can occur,[191] although the lack of ossification in most of the proximal capital femoral epiphysis makes this sign difficult to apply (Fig. 60–43). Helpful, however, is radiographically detectable osteomyelitis of the femoral metaphysis manifested as osteolysis, osteosclerosis, and periostitis.

The radiographic findings of hip infection in infants can simulate those accompanying other conditions. Displacement of the femoral head or metaphysis occurs in infants with congenital dislocation of the hip, neurologic deficits, and traumatic epiphyseal separations. Thus, aspiration of the joint is mandatory in firmly establishing the diagnosis of septic arthritis as well as in providing guidelines for adequate therapy. Appropriate antibiotic adminis-

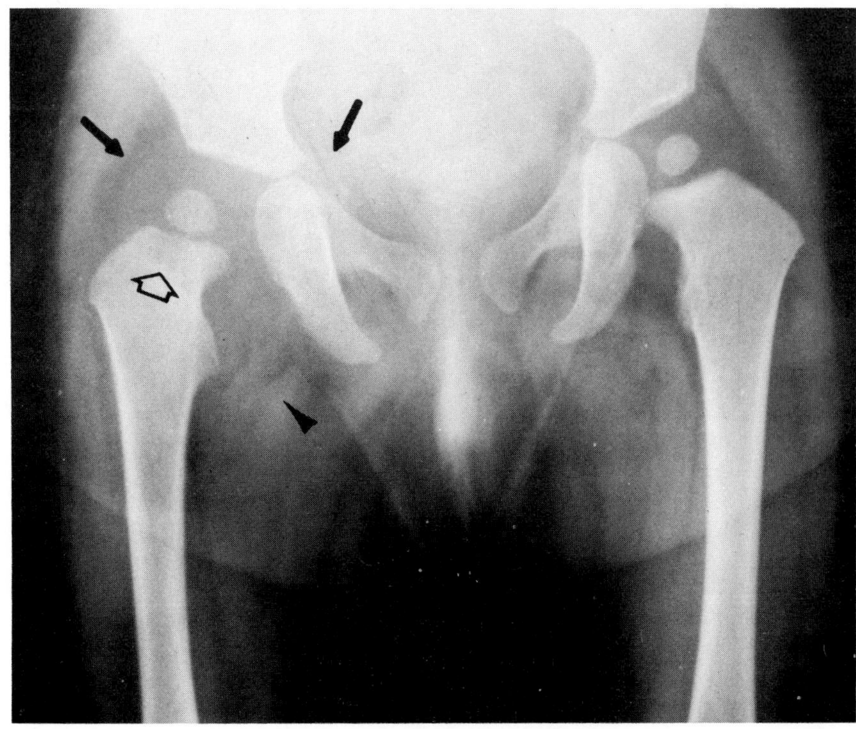

Figure 60–42. *Septic arthritis of the hip: Infancy. This infant developed septic arthritis of the right hip and osteomyelitis. Note displacement of the "capsular" and obturator fat planes (solid arrows), obliteration of the iliopsoas fat plane (arrowhead), and a metaphyseal focus of infection (open arrow). The femoral head is displaced laterally and is slightly enlarged. The soft tissue findings indicative of intra-articular fluid may be more helpful in diagnosis in this age group than in adults. (Courtesy of Dr. J. Weston, Lower Hutt, New Zealand.)*

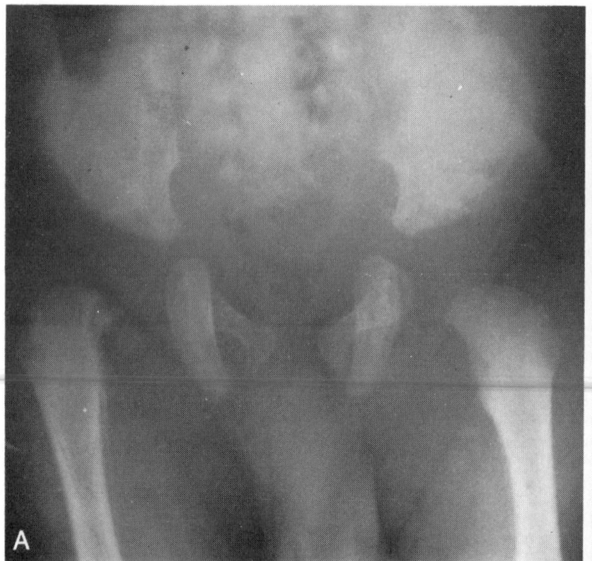

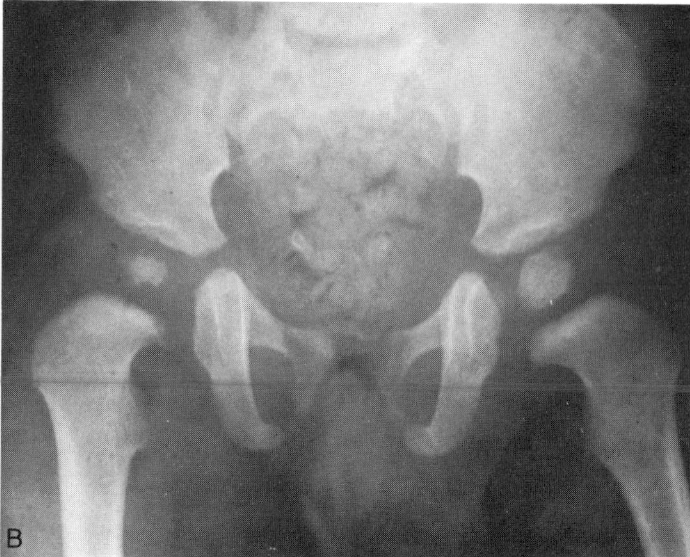

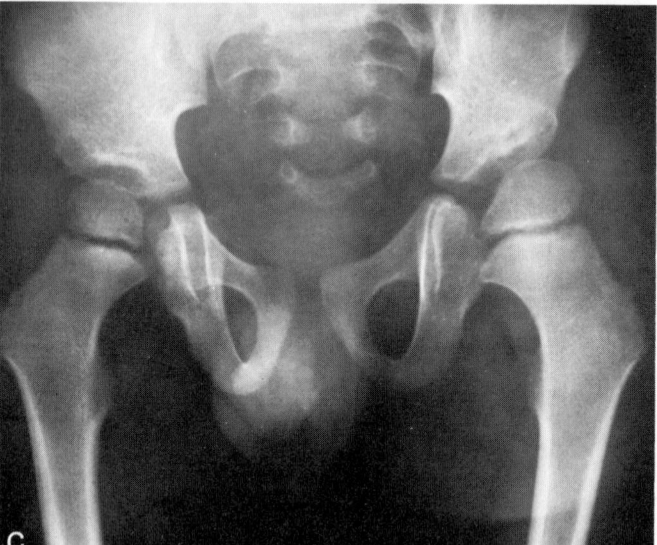

Figure 60–43. *Septic arthritis of the hip: Infancy. This 21 day old infant developed bilateral septic arthritis of the hips.*

A *The right hip is subluxed laterally and periosteal reaction is evident along the proximal femur. The left hip shows minimal lateral displacement.*

B *At 13 months of age, both hips are well located in the acetabulum. The left acetabulum is shallow, and the left epiphyseal ossification center is larger.*

C *At 3½ years of age, the right femoral head is small, and there is coxa magna on the left side. The shallow left acetabulum is again seen.*

Reproduced with permission from Freiberger RH, et al: Hip Disease of Infancy and Childhood. In RD Moseley Jr, et al: Current Problems in Radiology. Copyright 1973 by Year Book Medical Publishers, Inc, Chicago.)

tration combined with repeated aspiration or surgical drainage, or both, applied at an early stage of the septic process will diminish the likelihood of subsequent destruction of the cartilaginous femoral head and acetabulum. Only as the child develops and ossification of the immature skeleton proceeds will the degree of residual deformity become apparent (Fig. 60–44). Such deformities may include coxa magna, complete dissolution of the femoral head and neck with the lesser trochanter articulating with the acetabulum, or persistent dislocation of the femoral head or femoral shaft.[185, 324]

Septic arthritis of the hip is also frequent in the child, although the overall incidence of this problem and its devastating effects on local cartilage and bone are less prominent in children than in neonates. Furthermore, in the child, septic arthritis of the hip resulting from contamination by an adjacent focus of osteomyelitis is not so common as in the infant; the vascular channels that extend across the growth plate from metaphysis to epiphysis in the infant have become largely obliterated, and the increased cortical thickness of the child's metaphysis over that in the neonate may provide increased resistance to intra-articular spread from a metaphyseal infection.[22] A childhood hip infection may be associated with the acute onset of fever, pain, swelling, and limping, as well as with dramatic leukocy-

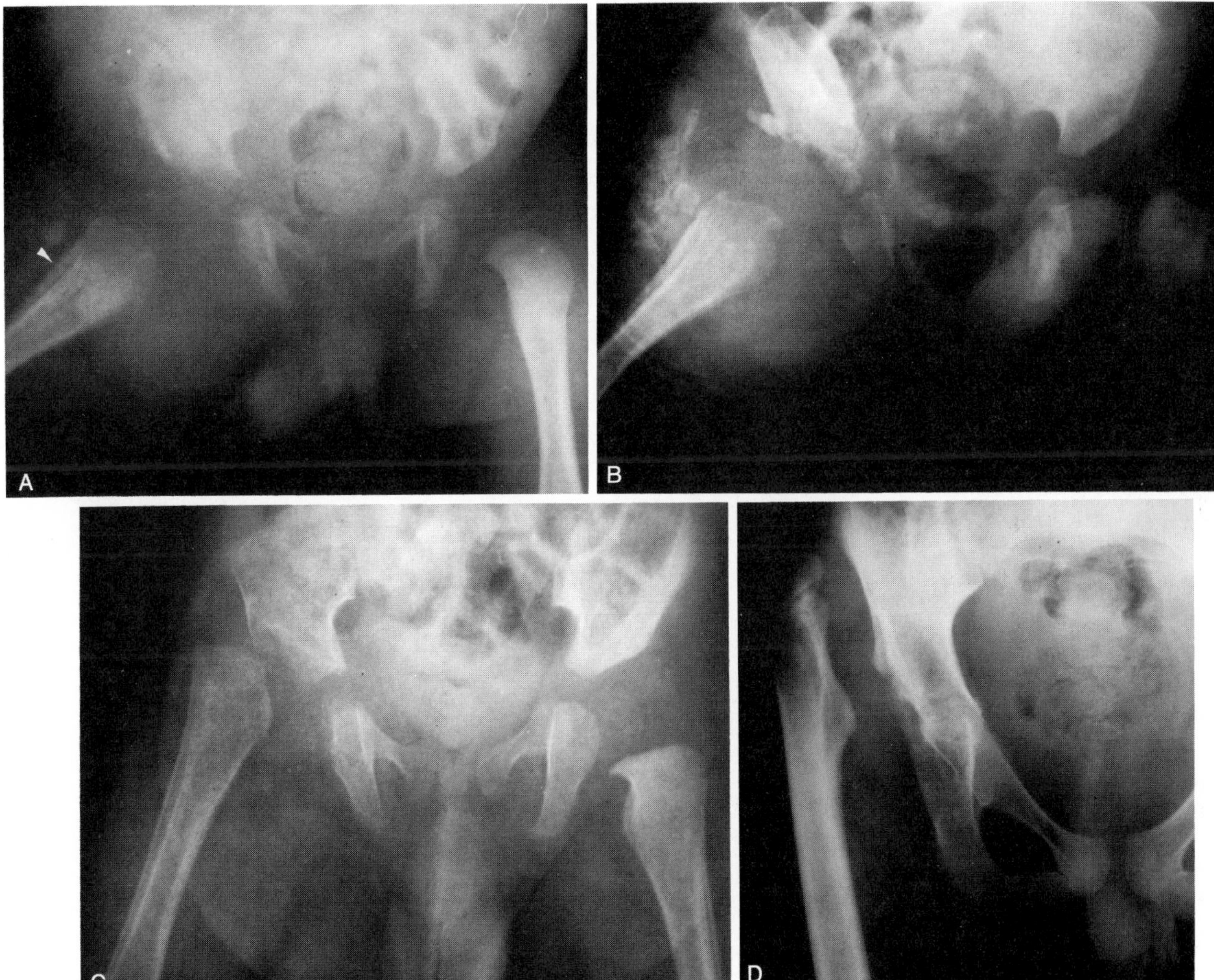

Figure 60–44. *Septic arthritis of the hip: Infancy. This neonate developed septic arthritis of the right hip.*

A *An initial radiograph reveals soft tissue swelling and periosteal reaction along the femur (arrowhead).*

B *Two weeks later, extensive periosteal reaction and soft tissue ossification are evident.*

C *At 2 months of age, superior subluxation of the femur is seen.*

D *At age 13 years, the ossification centers of the greater and lesser trochanter are apparent. Femoral dislocation, acetabular shallowness, and absence of epiphyseal ossification are evident.*

(Reproduced with permission from Freiberger RH, et al: Hip Disease of Infancy and Childhood. In RD Moseley Jr, et al: Current Problems in Radiology. Copyright 1973 by Year Book Medical Publishers, Inc, Chicago.)

tosis. On radiographs, accumulation of intra-articular fluid may produce soft tissue swelling, capsular distention and subtle lateral displacement of the ossified epiphysis (Fig. 60–45). Recognition of this latter finding is facilitated by comparison roentgenograms of the opposite hip. Concentric loss of joint space, subchondral osseous defects, and lytic foci of the femoral metaphysis can be evident.[192] Although the radiographs are eventually quite diagnostic of infection, initial abnormalities may be mistaken for those associated with juvenile chronic arthritis or Legg-Calvé-Perthes disease.[185] Joint aspiration is mandatory for definite diagnosis and appropriate treatment. The prognosis of septic arthritis of the hip for a child is far better than that for an infant, although growth disturbances (coxa vara or coxa valga, leg shortening or overgrowth),[193] fibrous or bony intra-articular ankylosis, and osteonecrosis of the femoral head[194, 195] can be observed.

Osteonecrosis of the femoral head following metaphyseal or epiphyseal infection in the child (or infant) is a very important complication of the disease (Figs. 60–46 and 60–47). In the hip, the vascular circle formed by the ascending branches of the circumflex femoral vessels is intimate with the capsular attachment. In the setting of proximal femoral osteomyelitis, these branches can become obliterated primarily by two mechanisms: septic thrombosis and compression by a sterile sympathetic effusion with a rise in intra-articular pressure.[195-197] In either case, aseptic ischemic necrosis may accompany the septic process of the neighboring bone, although the osteonecrotic epiphysis may subsequently become contaminated by the adjacent suppurative focus. Osteonecrosis of the epiphysis is usually not recognized until 6 to 8 weeks after the onset of infection. The epiphysis can reveal a generalized increase in radiodensity, followed by fragmentation and, less commonly, collapse. Persistent clinical and radiologic deformity can occur following healing of the osteomyelitis and septic arthritis.

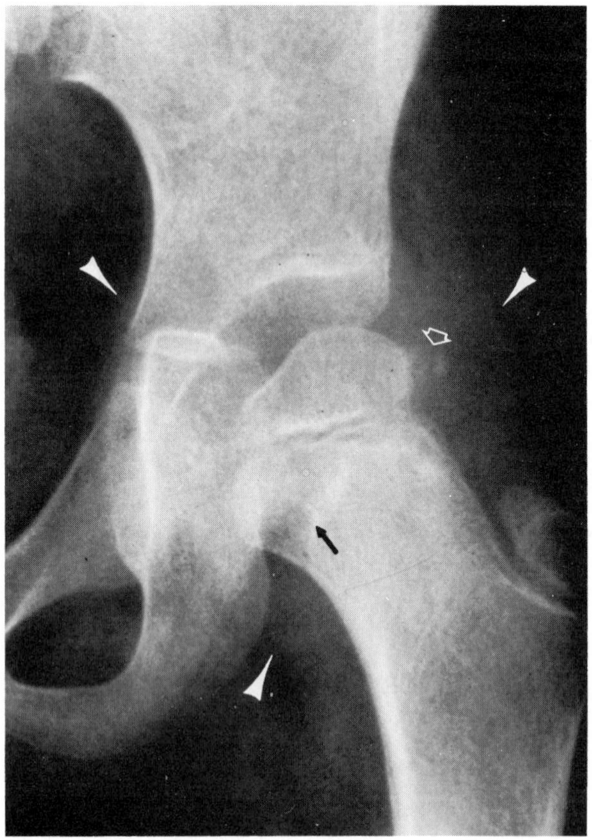

Figure 60–45. Septic arthritis of the hip: Childhood. Septic arthritis complicated metaphyseal osteomyelitis in this child. Observe osseous destruction (solid arrow), soft tissue swelling with displacement of fat planes (arrowheads), widening of the joint space due to lateral subluxation of the femoral head, and periarticular calcification or ossification (open arrow).

Direct Implantation of Infection

Direct inoculation of organisms into a joint can occur in many different clinical situations. Arthrocentesis accomplished for evaluation of synovial contents or utilized for arthrography can introduce gram-positive or gram-negative bacteria.[198] Similarly, penetrating injury, such as occurs in a fist-fight (see earlier discussion) or from a bullet, knife, nail, or other sharp object, can lead to septic arthritis. In these instances, articular abnormalities become evident in a variable period of time (which is determined by the type and virulence of the infective organism), with soft tissue swelling, joint space widening or narrowing, and osseous erosion.

Postoperative Infection

As previously outlined, articular surgery in the form of an arthrotomy, arthrodesis, arthroplasty, or other procedure can be complicated by joint infection in the postoperative period. This complication may occur in 1 to 10 per cent of patients, the incidence being related to many factors, including the type and length of surgery and the presence of an underlying disorder, such as rheumatoid arthritis, osteoarthritis, ankylosing spondylitis, and systemic lupus erythematosus. Infections occurring soon after the procedure are usually related to direct inoculation of the joint during the operation or to intra-articular spread from an adjacent contaminated focus (e.g., soft tissue abscess). Joint infection occurring long after surgery is frequently associated with obvious preceding sepsis elsewhere in the body and may relate to hematogenous spread to the articulation from this distant process.[199-202] The reported incidence of this latter phenomenon following total

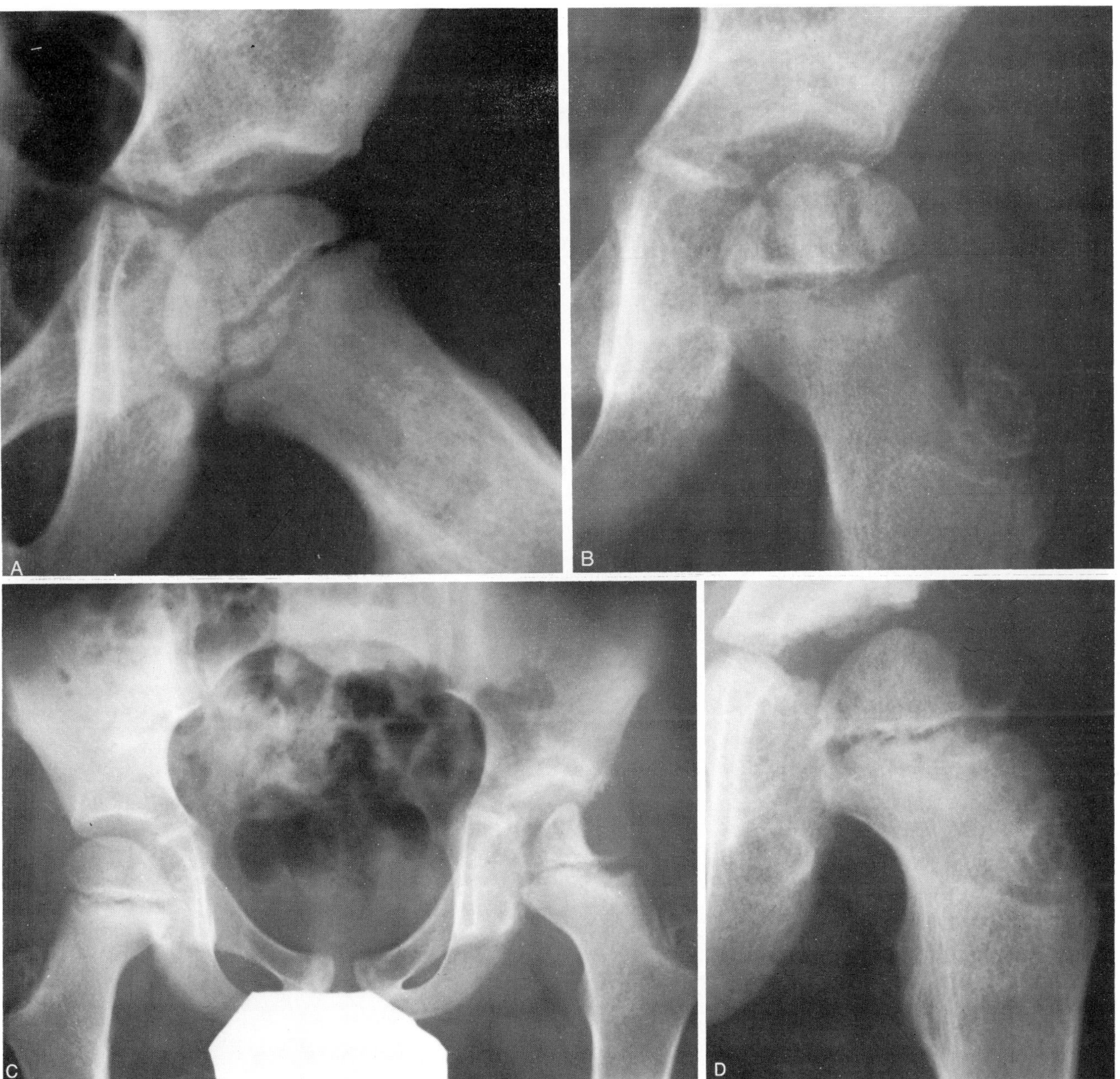

Figure 60–46. *Septic arthritis of the hip: Childhood. This 4½ year old boy developed suppurative arthritis of the left hip.*

A *An initial radiograph was normal except for soft tissue swelling.*

B *One month later, following incision and drainage as well as antibiotic therapy, lateral subluxation of the femoral head indicates reaccumulation of fluid. The fissuring and increased density of the head reflect osteonecrosis.*

C *Ten months later, lateral subluxation persists, and the lateral half of the epiphyseal ossification center has been resorbed.*

D *Three months later, some reconstitution of the femoral head has taken place.*

(Reproduced with permission from Freiberger RH, et al: Hip Disease in Infancy and Childhood. In RD Moseley Jr, et al: Current Problems in Radiology, Copyright 1973 by Year Book Medical Publishers, Inc, Chicago.)

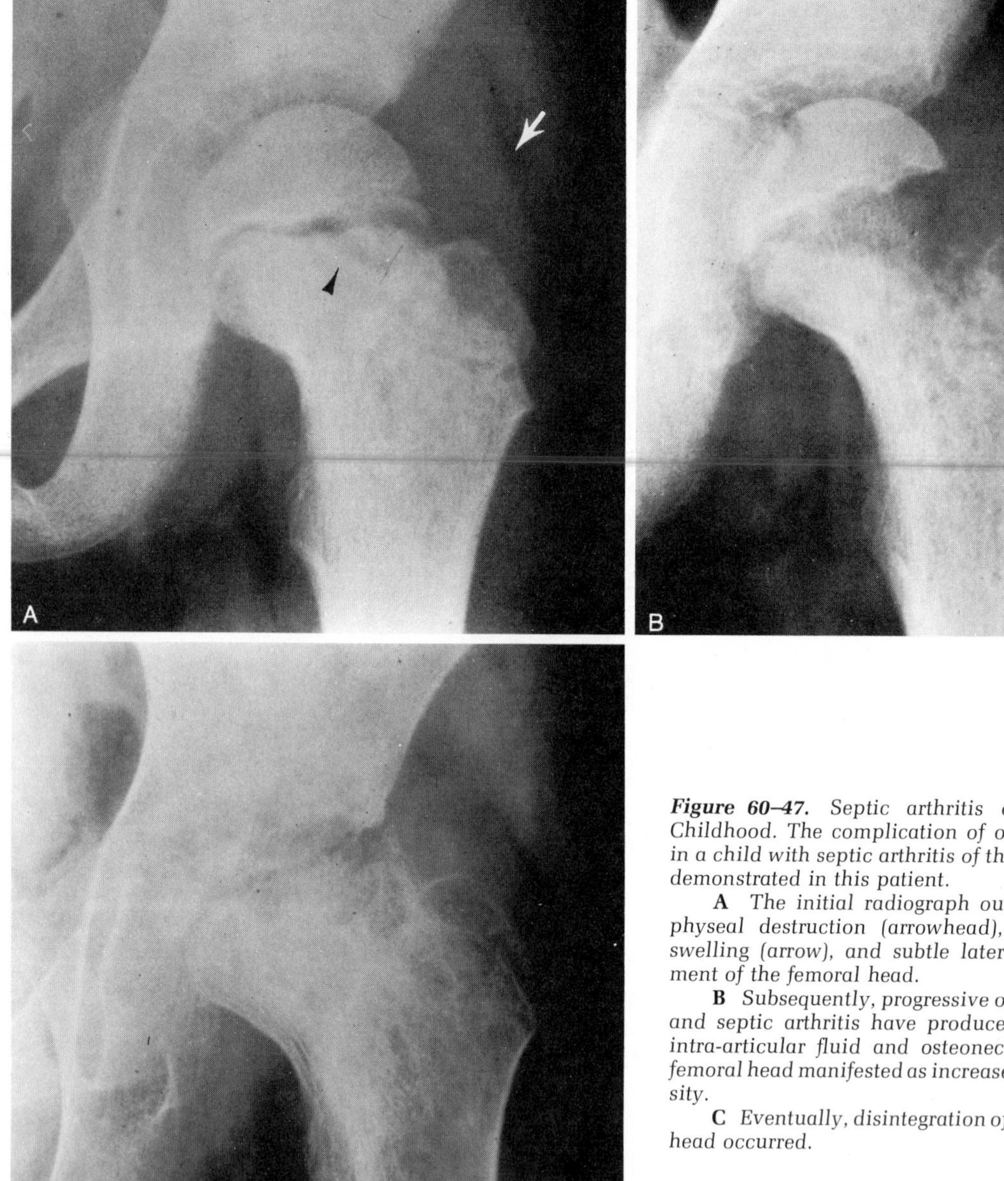

Figure 60–47. *Septic arthritis of the hip: Childhood. The complication of osteonecrosis in a child with septic arthritis of the hip is well demonstrated in this patient.*

A *The initial radiograph outlines metaphyseal destruction (arrowhead), soft tissue swelling (arrow), and subtle lateral displacement of the femoral head.*

B *Subsequently, progressive osteomyelitis and septic arthritis have produced increased intra-articular fluid and osteonecrosis of the femoral head manifested as increased radiodensity.*

C *Eventually, disintegration of the femoral head occurred.*

hip arthroplasty is approximately 0.3 per cent.[202, 203]

Radiographic evaluation of postoperative joint infection may be complicated by the presence of metallic implants and radiopaque or radiolucent cement. Increased radiolucency at the interfaces between metal and cement and between cement and bone can indicate a suppurative process, although similar abnormalities are encountered in asymptomatic patients, and in those with loose, noninfected prostheses. Additional evidence of endosteal erosion and of lysis and sclerosis of the medullary bone is strongly indicative of infection. Arthrography can be especially helpful in this situation; the puncture allows aspiration of intra-articular contents for laboratory evaluation, and the injected contrast material may dissect between the cement and osseous surface, fill abscess cavities, or reveal synovial irregularity and lymphatic vessels (see Chapter 25).

Complications

Several potential complications of septic arthritis, such as epiphyseal destruction and osteonecrosis, have already been discussed. Several others deserve emphasis.

Synovial Cysts. The incidence of synovial cyst formation in septic arthritis appears to be low, based upon the paucity of available literature on the subject. Occasionally, sepsis in a joint may become evident as distention and contamination of a communicating cyst. Rarely, synovial rupture of the cyst with or without fistula formation can be observed.[204, 205, 283] In patients with rheumatoid arthritis, fistulae about superficial articulations can result from superimposed articular infection[206] (see Chapter 26).

Soft Tissue and Tendon Injury. Septic arthritis can result in disruption of adjacent capsular, tendinous, and soft tissue structures. This complication has been well documented in the glenohumeral joint, at which site arthrography may indicate intra-articular synovial inflammation, tears of the rotator cuff, and soft tissue abscess formation[207, 208] (see Chapter 15). Similar phenomena are to be expected at other locations.

Osteomyelitis. Radiographic and pathologic evidence of osteomyelitis is commonly associated with septic arthritis. Bony abnormalities can antedate and be the source of the suppurative joint process or can indicate the contamination of adjacent bony surfaces from a primary joint infection.

Intra-articular Bony Ankylosis. Partial or complete osseous fusion may represent the residual findings of septic arthritis. This complication

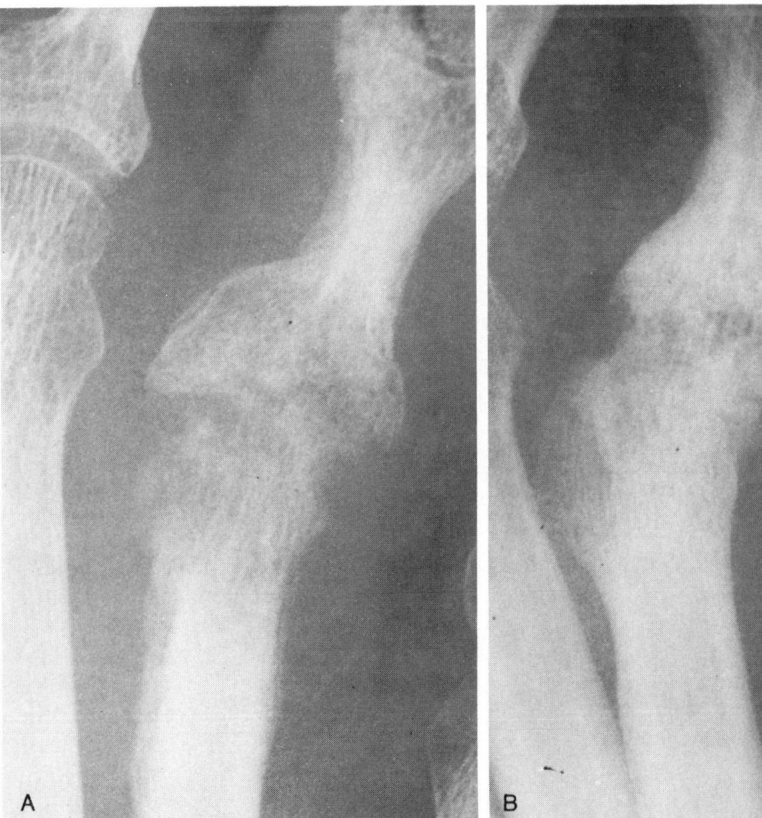

Figure 60–48. *Septic arthritis: Intra-articular bony ankylosis. Following pyogenic arthritis, partial or complete bony ankylosis can result, as in this case in the fourth metatarsophalangeal joint.*

is not frequent, especially when effective chemotherapy is instituted at an early stage. However, bony ankylosis is occasionally encountered following pyogenic processes (Fig. 60–48) and, rarely, following tuberculosis.

Degenerative Joint Disease. Significant destruction of articular cartilage from joint sepsis can lead to incongruity of apposing articular surfaces and, later, to changes of secondary degenerative joint disease. The resulting radiographic findings consisting of joint space narrowing, sclerosis, and osteophytosis may be difficult to differentiate from primary degenerative joint disease, although concentric loss of interosseous space and bony erosions are helpful indicators of preexisting articular disease.

Modifications and Difficulties in Diagnosis

Antibiotic Modified Septic Arthritis. Inadequate or inappropriate administration of antibiotics can modify articular infection. Clinical manifestations can be masked, appearing relatively late in the course of the disease, and radiographic changes may be less dramatic, less extensive, and much delayed. Furthermore, radiographic improvement following control of the infection lags behind the amelioration of clinical signs.

Preexisting Articular Abnormality. When infection is superimposed on a previous articular disorder such as rheumatoid arthritis or osteoarthritis, the roentgenographic abnormalities can be hidden or changed by the underlying disease process. In the septic rheumatoid joint, for example, the findings of soft tissue swelling, joint space narrowing, and osseous destruction related to the suppurative process are difficult to differentiate from those of rheumatoid arthritis[209] (see Chapter 26). In this clinical situation, progressive effusion and rapid acceleration of joint destruction should be viewed cautiously as the findings may indicate that worsening clinical manifestations are related not to the rheumatoid process itself but rather to a superimposed infection.

Differential Diagnosis

General Features. Any destructive monoarticular process should be regarded as infection until proved otherwise. Although numerous disorders such as pigmented villonodular synovitis, idiopathic synovial osteochondromatosis, juvenile chronic arthritis, and even adult-onset rheumatoid arthritis can be associated with monoarticular changes, infection has to be considered the prime diagnostic possibility until appropriate aspiration and culture document its absence. This is particularly true when the joint process is associated with loss of interosseous space, poorly defined or "fuzzy" osseous margins, and a sizable effusion. In patients with pyogenic infection, the articular destruction can be very rapid, with complete loss of joint space and large destructive osseous foci appearing within a period of 1 to 3 weeks; in individuals with tuberculosis or fungal disease, the articular abnormalities appear more slowly and may be associated with extensive periarticular osteoporosis. Diagnostic difficulty arises when the septic process involves more than one joint or when septic arthritis appears during the course of another articular disorder.

Of all the radiographic parameters of infection, it is the poorly defined nature of the bony destruction that is most characteristic. Osseous erosions or cysts in gout, rheumatoid arthritis, seronegative spondyloarthropathies, osteoarthritis, pigmented villonodular synovitis, idiopathic synovial osteochondromatosis, hemophilia, and calcium pyrophosphate dihydrate crystal deposition disease are more sharply marginated. Furthermore, concentric loss of interosseous space is typical in infection. A similar pattern of joint space loss accompanies rheumatoid arthritis, the seronegative spondyloarthropathies, calcium pyrophosphate dihydrate crystal deposition disease, chondrolysis, and chondral atrophy, but asymmetric diminution of the articular lumen, as noted in osteoarthritis, and relative preservation of articular space, as seen in gout, pigmented villonodular synovitis, idiopathic synovial osteochondromatosis, and hemophilia, are rare in pyogenic infection (although late loss of joint space can be encountered in tuberculosis and fungal disorders).

Osseous erosions at the marginal areas of synovial articulations are frequent in processes associated with significant synovial inflammation, such as sepsis, rheumatoid arthritis, and the seronegative spondyloarthropathies. They may also be observed in gout and, less commonly, in pigmented villonodular synovitis and idiopathic synovial osteochondromatosis. Centrally located erosions and cysts are seen in many disorders, including septic arthritis. Similarly, periarticular osteoporosis can be encountered in rheumatoid arthritis, Reiter's syndrome, juvenile chronic arthritis, hemophilia, and nonpyogenic suppurative processes, such as tuberculosis or fungal disease.

Intra-articular bony ankylosis can represent the end stage of septic arthritis, the seronegative spondyloarthropathies, and, in some locations, rheumatoid arthritis and juvenile chronic arthritis.

Specific Joint Involvement. Any articulation can be the site of an infectious process. The joint selection is influenced by the age of the patient and the specific clinical situation. In children and infants, the articulations of the appendicular skeleton, especially the knee and the hip, are commonly affected in hematogenous infections; in children and adults, the articulations of the axial skeleton, particularly the sacroiliac joint and those in the spine, are not uncommonly involved. These patterns of distribution are frequently modified when infection relates to a nonhematogenous process; any articulation can be affected following soft tissue suppuration, penetrating injury, or surgery. Furthermore, joint selection in septic arthritis is influenced by other factors. In the drug abuser, the sacroiliac, sternoclavicular, and acromioclavicular joints and the spine are common sites of involvement. In the individual with rheumatoid arthritis, any articulation affected by the primary disease process represents a potential site of infection. In the diabetic patient with infection, articulations of the foot are commonly altered. Because of this variability, the distribution of infectious processes overlaps that of other disorders.

SOFT TISSUE INFECTION

Routes of Contamination

Infection of soft tissue structures commonly results from direct contamination following trauma. Any process that disrupts the skin surface can potentially lead to secondary infection, particularly in the individual with a debilitating illness (e.g., diabetes) (Fig. 60–49) or one who is being treated with immunosuppressive agents; furthermore, nonpenetrating trauma can lead to soft tissue infection, although the exact mechanism for this complication is not entirely clear. Hematogenous spread is less important in soft tissue contamination than in osteomyelitis and septic arthritis.

Radiographic-Pathologic Correlation

Swelling with obliteration of adjacent tissue planes is characteristic of soft tissue infection. Radiolucent streaks within the contaminated area can relate to collections of air derived from the adjacent skin surface or gas formation by various bacteria[169-174, 210-212] (Fig. 60–50) (see Chapter 62). Erosion of bone owing to pressure from an adjacent soft tissue mass is much more frequent when the mass is neoplastic rather than infectious in etiology (Fig. 60–51). When osseous abnormalities appear following soft tissue contamination, infective periostitis, osteitis, or osteomyelitis is usually present (Fig. 60–52). Occasionally, periostitis of the underlying bone may represent irritation rather than true suppuration (Fig. 60–53).

A well-defined soft tissue mass is less typical of infection than of neoplasm. The edema of an infectious process usually leads to infiltration of surrounding soft tissues rather than displacement, but radiographic differentiation between infiltration and displacement of tissue planes can be exceedingly difficult. Furthermore, reaction of the soft tissue to an adjacent infection can produce pseudoneoplastic masses, which are difficult to differentiate from tumors on clinical, radiographic, and pathologic examination.[213, 214]

Complications

Although there are several complications of soft tissue infection, the most important in terms of the musculoskeletal structures is contamination of underlying osseous and articular structures. This complication has been amply discussed earlier in this chapter.

Specific Entities

Septic Subcutaneous Bursitis. There are numerous subcutaneous bursae in the human body.[215, 301] Afflictions of these structures have led to such well-known terms as "housemaid's knee" (prepatellar bursitis), "miner's elbow" (olecranon bursitis), and "weaver's bottom" (ischial bursitis). In addition, bursal swelling is often apparent in rheumatoid arthritis and gout, as well as following trauma (Fig. 60–54).

Septic bursitis is less well recognized. In most cases, bursal infection localizes to the olecranon and the prepatellar and, less frequently, the subdeltoid regions[216-220, 301, 302, 323] (Fig. 60–55). A history of recent injury, occupational trauma, or puncture (e.g., steroid administration) is frequently, although not invariably, present. Clinically detectable skin breakage and bacteriologically evident isolates of *Staphylococcus aureus* in the absence of bacteremia suggest that direct penetration by skin pathogens accounts for many cases of bursal infection. Other agents, which are less typically implicated, are *Streptococcus pneumoniae*,[216] *Mycobacterium marinum*,[217] and *Sporothrix schenckii*.[22, 220, 222] Septic subcutaneous bursitis due to hematogenous spread is very rare.[219, 221] This fact may be related to a blood supply that is less exuberant than that of the intra-articular synovial membrane, although the laboratory findings of infected bursal fluid are similar to those of septic joint fluid.[219] In some cases, the bursal reaction to infection is less intense than that of the joint.[286]

Septic bursitis is not usually associated with infectious arthritis.[322] Erosion and proliferation of subjacent bone (e.g., ulna, patella, humerus) indicate complicating infective periostitis, osteitis, and osteomyelitis. The radiographic and clinical (redness, warmth, tenderness, soft tissue swelling) findings may be misinterpreted as those of gout or rheuma-

Text continued on page 2111

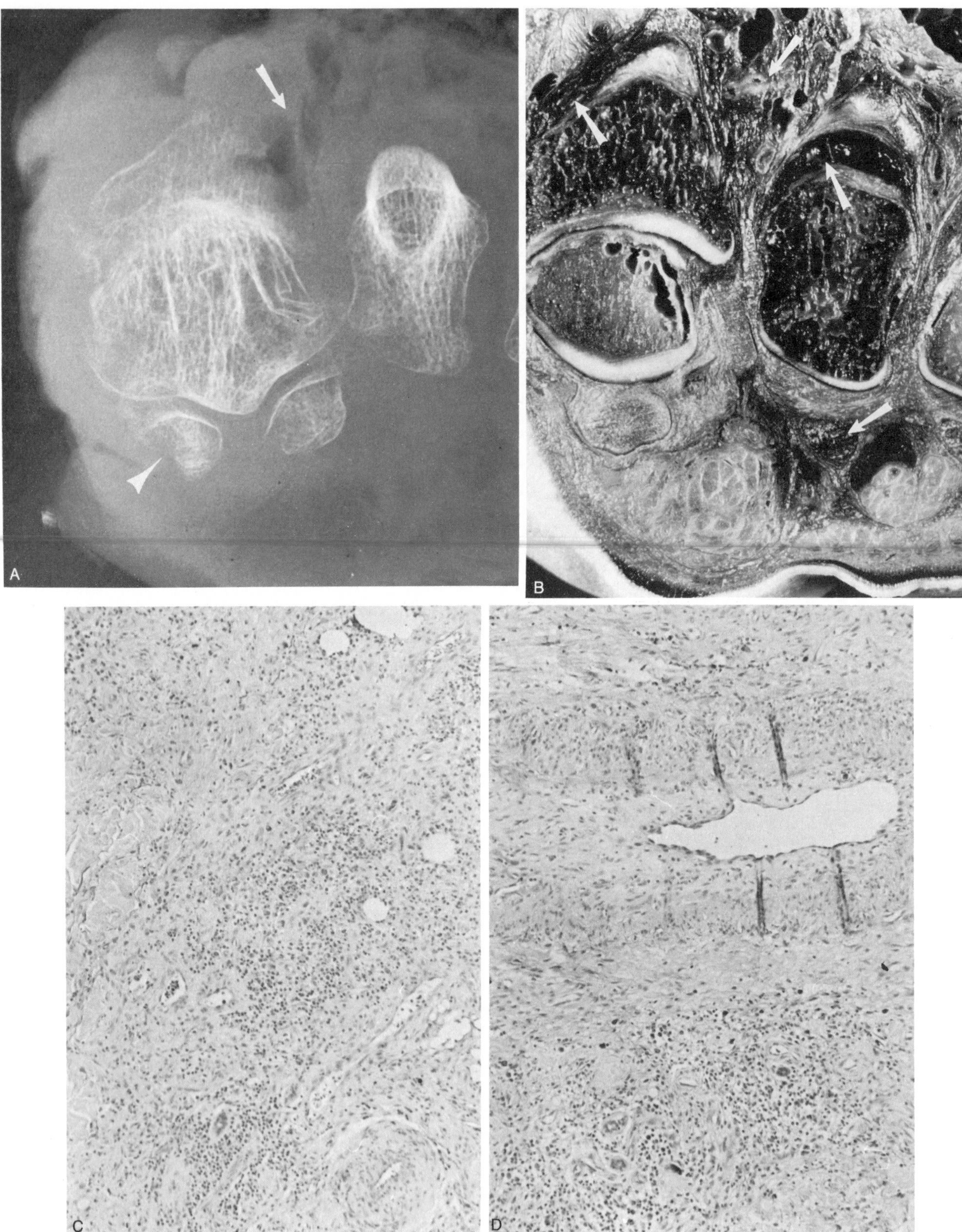

Figure 60–49. Soft tissue infection: Diabetes mellitus.

A, B A radiograph and photograph of a coronal section through the first metatarsophalangeal joint in a diabetic patient with soft tissue ulceration and infection reveal necrotic soft tissues with radiolucent streaks (arrows), soft tissue ulceration, and osseous involvement (arrowhead).

C, D Photomicrographs (140×) of a soft tissue infection in a diabetic patient indicate acute inflammatory cellular infiltration and severe intimal sclerosis.

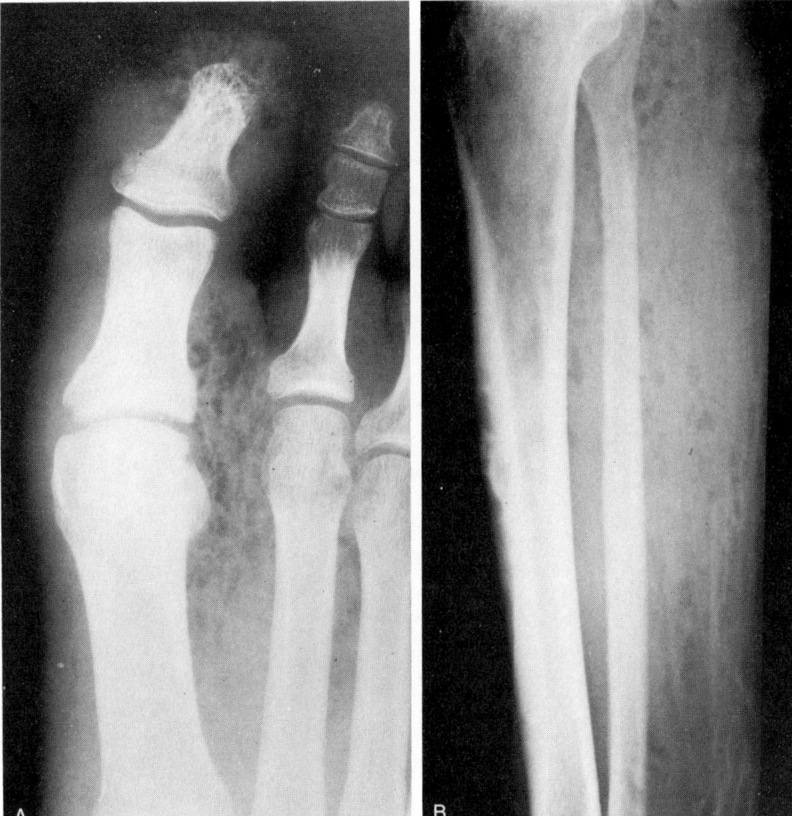

Figure 60–50. *Soft tissue infection: Gas formation. Two examples of* Escherichia coli *infection in diabetes mellitus. Note the "bubbly" radiolucent collections in the foot and lower leg.*

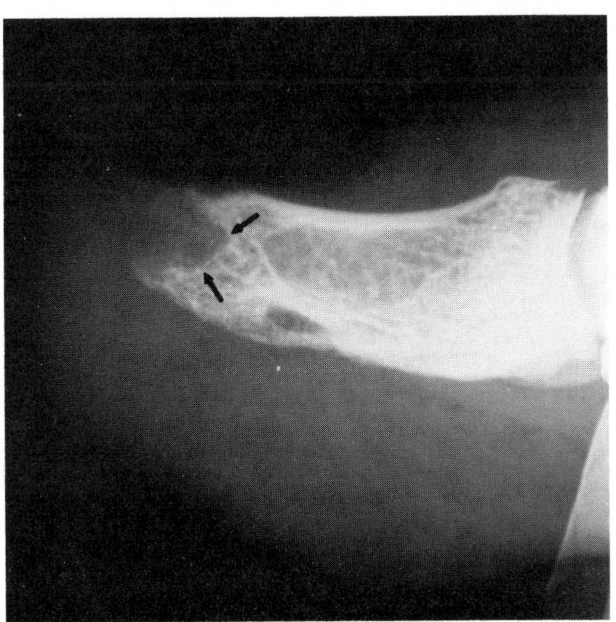

Figure 60–51. *Soft tissue infection: Osseous erosion. This 55 year old woman developed a chronic bacterial infection of the great toe, which was associated with osseous involvement. Note the erosion of the terminal tuft (arrows). Most frequently such abnormalities reflect contamination of the underlying bone rather than pressure erosion.*

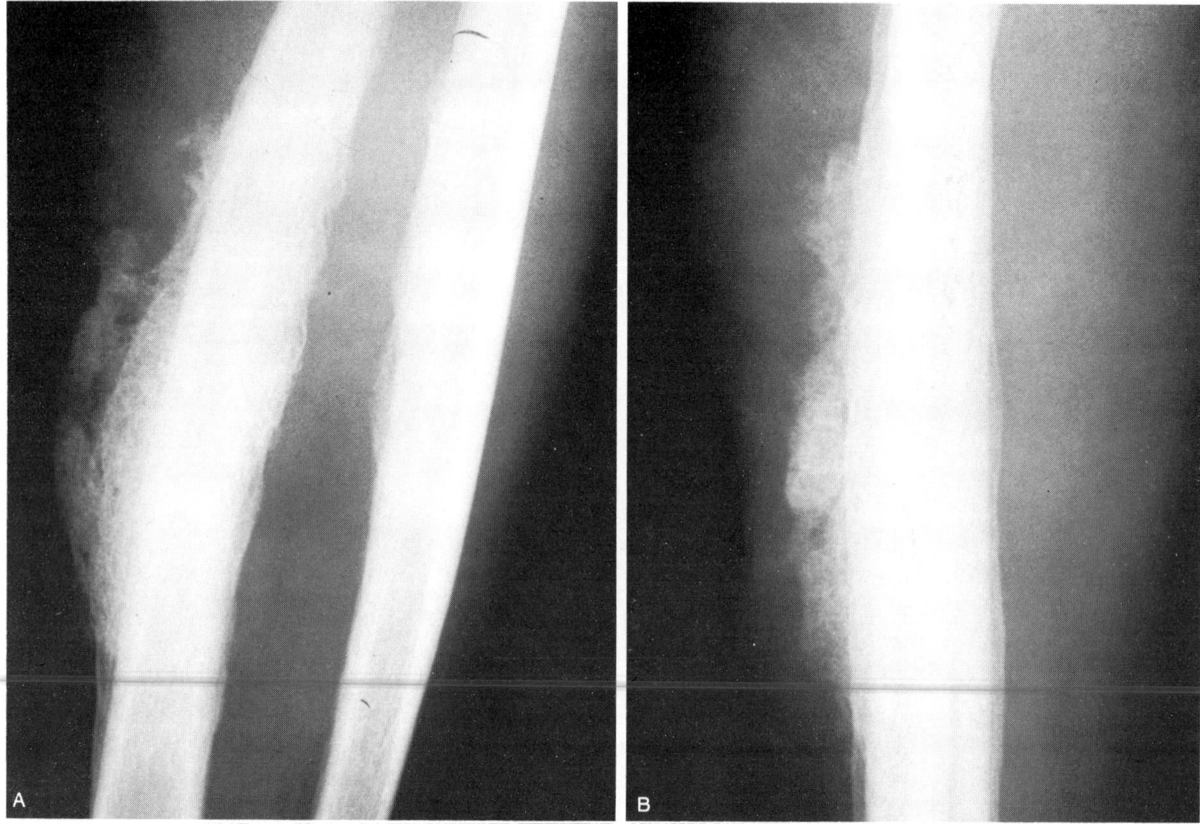

Figure 60–52. *Soft tissue infection: Infective periostitis and osteitis. A chronic soft tissue ulceration and bacterial infection of the forearm have led to contamination of the underlying periosteum and cortex, with exuberant new bone formation. The marrow does not appear to be involved on radiographic examination.*

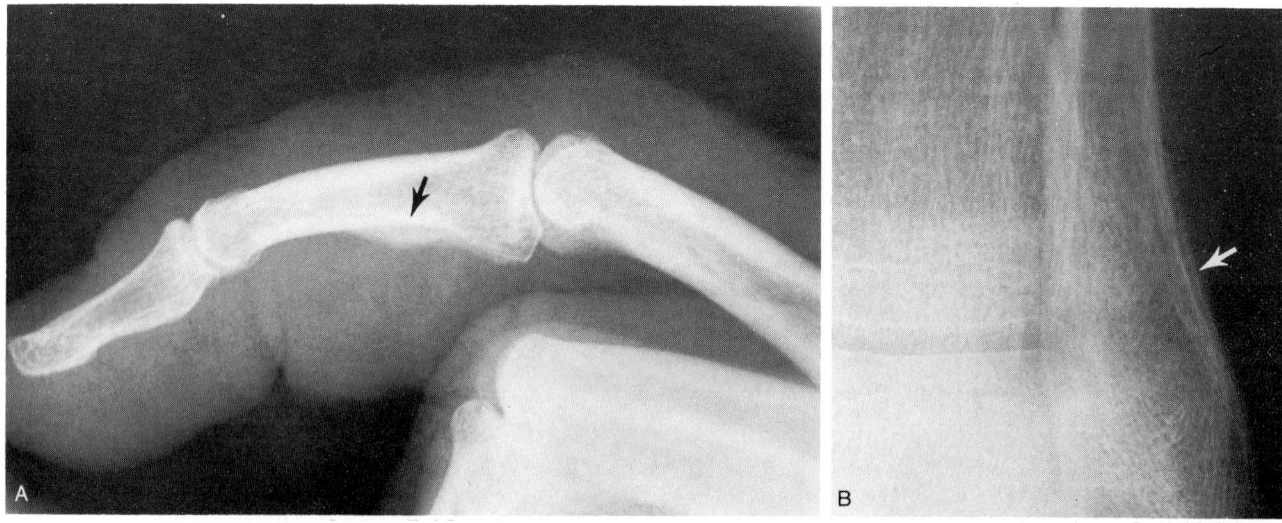

Figure 60–53. *Soft tissue infection: Periosteal irritation.*

A *A chronic infective tenosynovitis has produced irritation of the underlying phalangeal bone with periostitis (arrow). Note the soft tissue swelling and semiflexion of the digit.*

B *A chronic soft tissue ulceration and infection have led to noninfective periostitis of the underlying fibula (arrow).*

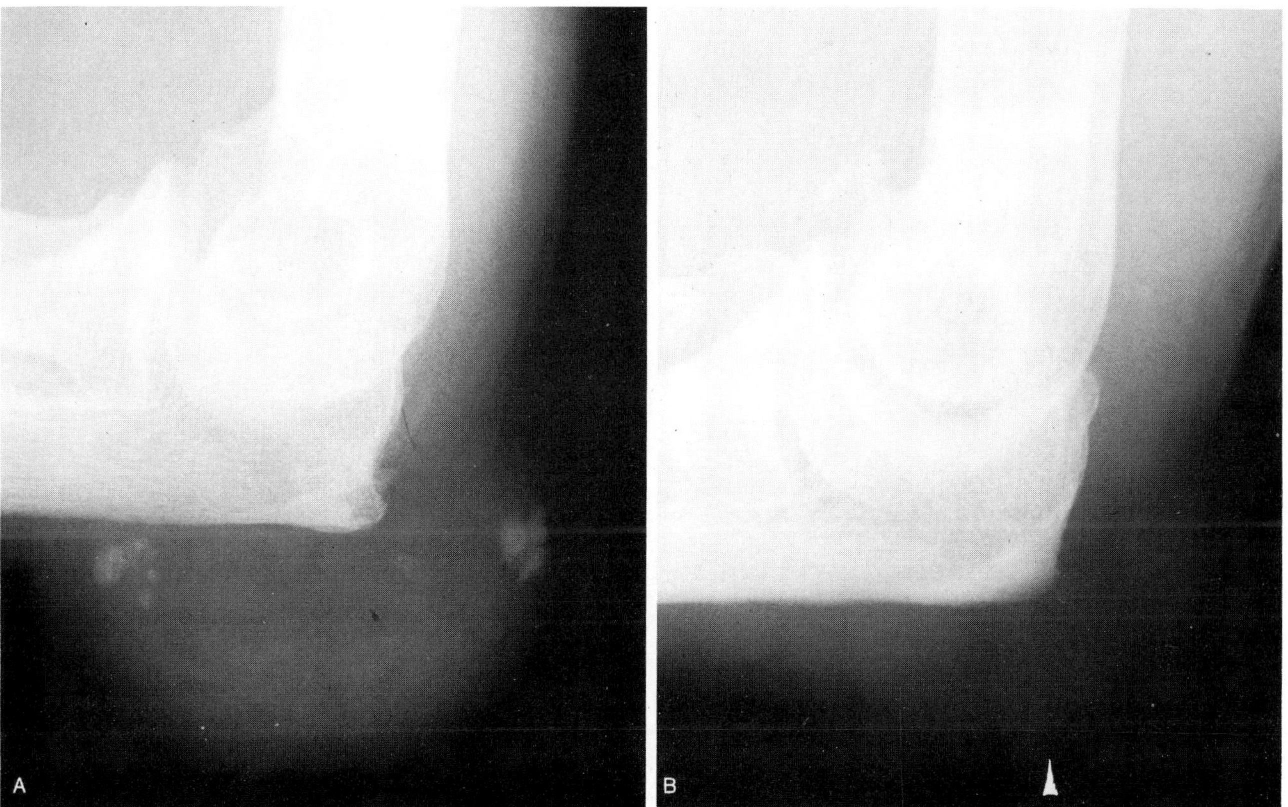

Figure 60–54. *Posttraumatic bursitis.*

A *Observe soft tissue swelling with calcification and ossification about the olecranon area related to repetitive trauma. No microorganisms were identified.*

B *Dialysis elbow. This 51 year old patient with chronic renal failure, on hemodialysis, developed olecranon bursitis due to prolonged contact of the elbow and table during the dialysis procedure. Soft tissue swelling is evident (arrowhead). No microorganisms were found.*

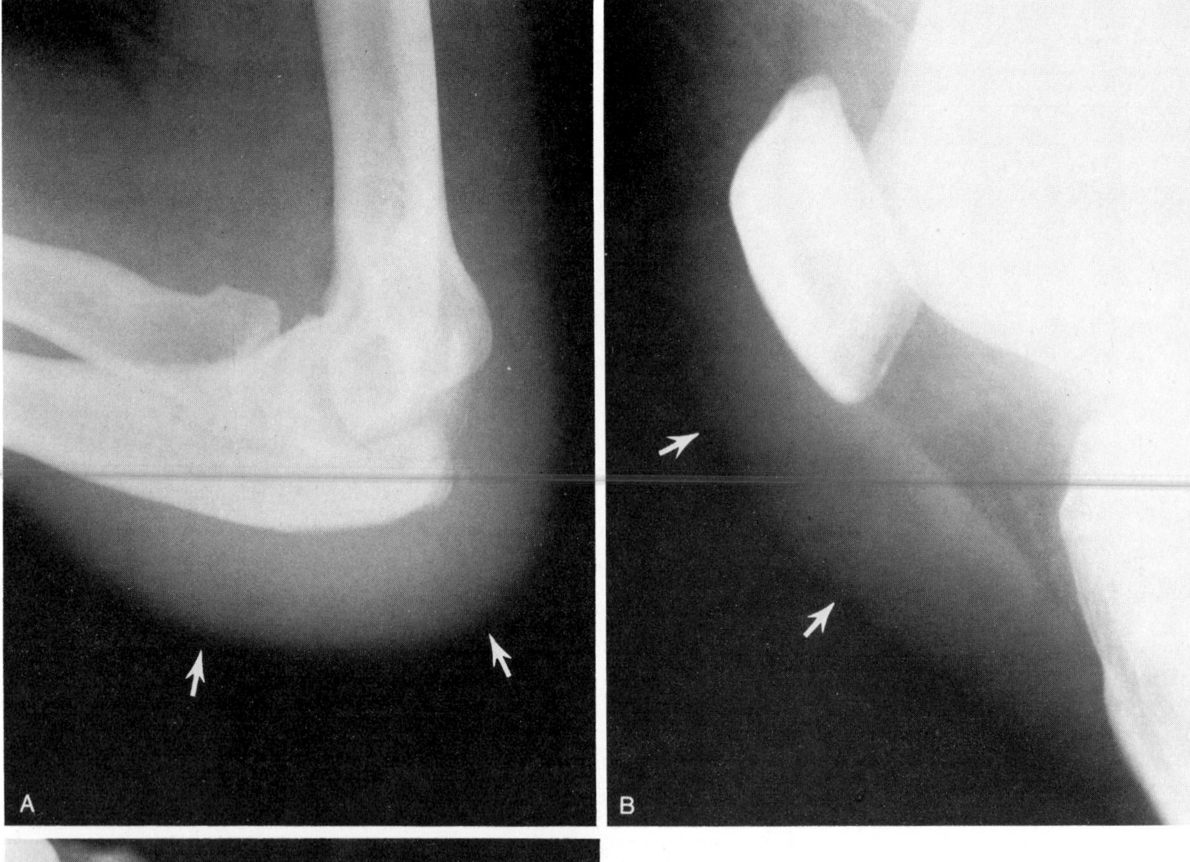

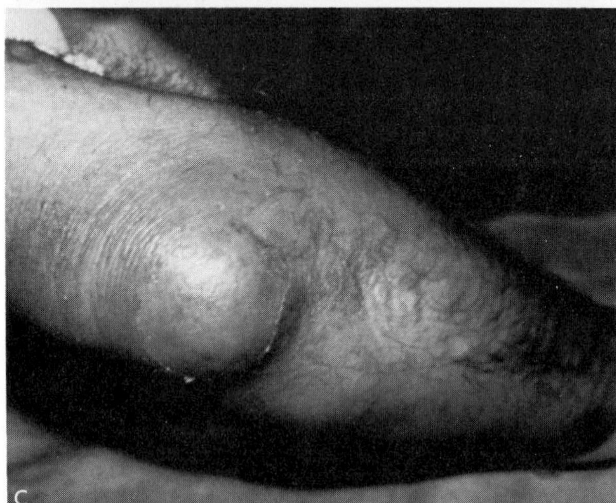

Figure 60–55. Septic bursitis.

A *Olecranon bursitis. Note olecranon swelling (arrows) and soft tissue edema due to* Staphylococcus aureus. *Previous surgery and trauma are the causes of the adjacent bony abnormalities.*

B *Prepatellar bursitis. This 28 year old carpenter who had worked on his knees for prolonged periods of time developed tender swelling in front of the knee (arrows). Inflammatory fluid which was culture positive for* Staphylococcus aureus *was recovered from the bursa.*

C *Olecranon bursitis. A clinical photograph demonstrates local skin changes over the olecranon.*

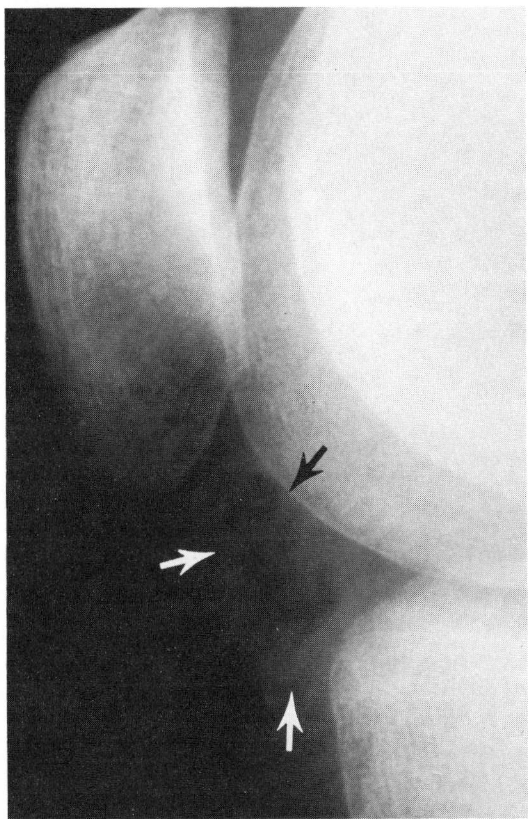

Figure 60–56. Infected intra-articular fat pad. An infection of Hoffa's fat pad in this 21 year old man had resulted in radiolucent collections and soft tissue swelling (arrows). Although staphylococcus was recovered from the area, the joint fluid was sterile, as the infection was intracapsular but extrasynovial.

toid arthritis. As these latter conditions can coexist with infection,[223] appropriate clinical and laboratory tests should be undertaken to exclude their presence. Since a sympathetic sterile effusion of a neighboring joint can be associated with septic bursitis,[302] the detection of joint fluid by radiographic techniques does not necessarily imply that a septic arthritis is present.

Septic Periarticular Bursitis. Infection of bursae that are located about articulations (e.g., popliteal) is usually related to extension of an infective process within the joint (Fig. 60–56). Rarely, primary infection of a synovial cyst can occur, although the neighboring articulations are soon contaminated.

Septic Tenosynovitis. Inflammation of the synovial lining of tendon sheaths is a common finding in various rheumatologic conditions, especially rheumatoid arthritis. Septic processes originating from a distant or local focus or following trauma can also lead to tenosynovitis. Various bacteria, mycobacteria, fungal agents, or protozoa may be implicated.[224-227, 301, 321] Soft tissue swelling and surface resorption and erosion of underlying bony structures may be evident. Appropriate microbiologic studies confirm the infective etiology of the lesion. Osteomyelitis of adjacent sesamoid bones can sometimes be identified.[303]

Granulomatous tenosynovitis may accompany sarcoidosis, beryllium exposure, or blackthorn inflammation.[304, 305]

Lymphadenitis. Lymphadenitis, usually with an accompanying cellulitis, can complicate streptococcal or staphylococcal infections. Although many sites can be involved, acute epitrochlear lymphadenitis about the elbow can produce clinical and radiologic findings that simulate osteomyelitis.[228] Nodular or diffuse soft tissue swelling and underlying periostitis can be encountered.

SPECIFIC SITUATIONS

There are a variety of situations and systemic disorders that are associated with an increased incidence of bone, joint, and soft tissue infection. Examples, such as sickle cell anemia, diabetes mellitus, rheumatoid arthritis, crystal-induced arthropathy, myeloproliferative disorders, systemic lupus erythematosus, endogenous and exogenous hypercortisolism, and hypo- and agammaglobulinemia, are discussed elsewhere in the book. A few additional situations that predispose to musculoskeletal infection are noted here.

Chronic Granulomatous Disease of Childhood

This disorder is a hereditary condition, usually transmitted as an X-linked recessive trait, which occurs in male children,[247-250, 280] although a similar syndrome has been identified in female and male children without a family history of disease.[251] The syndrome is characterized by purulent granulomatous and eczematoid skin lesions, granulomatous lymphadenitis with suppuration, hepatosplenomegaly, recurrent and persistent pneumonias, and chronic osteomyelitis (25 to 35 per cent); it is frequently fatal (40 per cent). A defect has been noted in the ability of the polymorphonuclear leukocytes and monocytes to adequately destroy certain pathogenetic organisms.[250, 252, 253] Thus, although the leukocytes can phagocytize bacteria normally, they are incapable of killing them, especially certain strains of relatively low virulence such as *Staphylococcus epidermidis*, *Staphylococcus aureus*, species of Enterobacteriaceae, *Serratia marcescans*, and certain fungi. Affected children demonstrate a normal spectrum of immunoglobulins, a normal ability to develop and express a hypersensitivity response, and normal complement and complement component levels.[254, 255]

There are certain clinical and radiologic peculiarities that characterize the osteomyelitis of chronic granulomatous disease of childhood[256]:

1. The disease lacks the usual early clinical signs and symptoms of osteomyelitis so that initial radiographs frequently reveal considerable bony involvement.
2. The causative organisms are usually of low virulence.
3. The most frequent site of involvement is the small bones of the hands and the feet.
4. The radiographic abnormalities are characterized by extensive osseous destruction with minimal reactive sclerosis.
5. The osteomyelitis may develop in new areas despite continuous therapy.
6. The osteomyelitis eventually responds to long-term antibiotic therapy so that operative intervention is rarely necessary.

The radiographic features related to the osteomyelitis of chronic granulomatous disease are not diagnostic. The predilection for the small bones of the hands and feet, the presence of extensive osteolysis, and the absence of significant bony sclerosis are helpful clues, although similar abnormalities can accompany tuberculous dactylitis. The changes may also simulate those of primary hypogammaglobulinemia and other immunodeficiency states.[257] In chronic granulomatous disease, the progression of the osseous alterations with the development of new areas of involvement, even during continuous antibiotic therapy, reflects the immunologic incompetence of the patient, although the eventual appearance of complete healing suggests that the immunologic mechanisms are ultimately capable of destroying the relatively indolent organisms that are causing the osteomyelitis.[256]

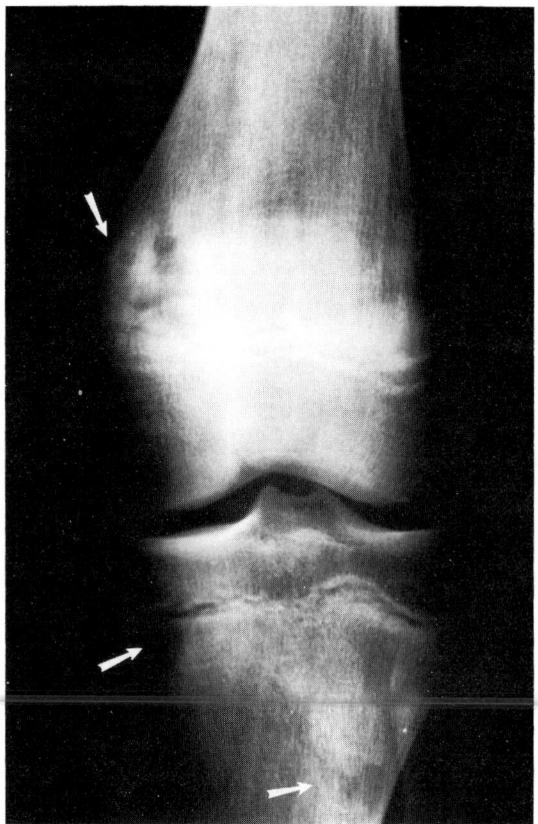

Figure 60–57. *Chronic symmetric plasma cell osteomyelitis. This 12 year old girl presented with right knee pain. Radiographs revealed bilateral and symmetric abnormalities of both knees. The metaphyseal irregularities characterized by both lysis and sclerosis (arrows) are consistent with this diagnosis. Plasma cells are typically recovered on biopsy. (Courtesy of Dr. P. Vanderstoup, St. Cloud, Minnesota.)*

Chronic Symmetric Plasma Cell Osteomyelitis

This is a variety of subacute and chronic osteomyelitis of unknown etiology that occurs in childhood and that frequently reveals multiple and symmetric alterations.[258-261, 306] The usual age of onset of the disease is 5 to 10 years, although infants may also be affected. Pain, tenderness, and swelling are common initial clinical manifestations. The metaphyses of the bones of the lower extremity and the medial ends of the clavicles are particularly vulnerable, although other osseous sites, including those in the upper extremity, can be altered (Fig. 60–57). Laboratory analysis is generally nonspecific, and cultures of the blood or of the bone following biopsy may be nonrewarding. Occasionally organisms, including pneumococci, are recovered. There is no evidence of reduced cellular or humoral immunity. Histologic evaluation is reported to be relatively specific, characterized by the predominance of plasma cells in the center of the osteolytic foci.[258, 262] However, other reports indicate that plasma cell accumulation is not always present[306] and that early osteomyelitic foci are associated with the accumulation of polymorphonuclear leukocytes, whereas chronic lesions are accompanied by lymphocyte and histiocyte infiltration.[307] Although the long-term prognosis is good, the condition may run a protracted course.

The peculiar features of this variety of osteomyelitis include a protracted clinical course with exacerbations and remissions, a striking degree of symmetric bone involvement, a predilection for the metaphyseal regions of the lower extremity, common involvement of the clavicle, difficulty in implicating specific organisms from blood or bone, and histologic evidence of plasma cells. The radiographic features may simulate those of other types of osteomyelitis, chronic granulomatous disease of childhood, infantile cortical hyperostosis, vitamin D–resistant rickets, or bone infarction. In addition, selective hyperostosis of the clavicle, as noted in this condition, may also be seen in two additional disorders. Osteitis condensans of the medial end of the bone has been reported, especially in young women[284] (see Chapter 54). Sternoclavicular hyperostosis of unknown etiology with painful swelling of the sternum, clavicles, and upper ribs has also been described.[285] Men and women are both affected, and the usual age of onset is in the fifth and sixth decades of life. In some of the patients, unilateral or bilateral subclavian vein occlusion can be seen. Hyperostotic spongiosa trabeculae are noted on histologic examination, but microorganisms are not recovered. This syndrome, termed sternocostoclavicular hyperostosis, is discussed further in Chapter 81.

Osteomyelitis and Septic Arthritis in Drug Abusers

An increased frequency of infectious disease has been noted in drug abusers.[263, 264, 308, 309] The mechanisms for this association are not entirely known. Although it appears that leukocyte function is altered in these individuals, this possibility has not been firmly established. In laboratory analyses, morphine has inhibited migration of polymorphonuclear leukocytes in animals[265] and has reduced phagocytic power of neutrophils in humans[266]; however, other experiments have indicated little effect of narcotics on bacterial destruction by polymorphonuclear leukocytes.[267] Utilization of contaminated narcotics or needles, colonization of the skin during previous hospitalizations, and alterations of the bacterial flora by pretreatment with antibiotics are three other potential mechanisms that may explain an increased incidence of infection in drug abusers.[277, 278]

Hematogenous osteomyelitis and septic arthritis in drug users are characterized by unusual localization and organisms. Although staphylococcal infection may be seen, Pseudomonas,[268-272] Klebsiella,[272] and Serratia[273, 274] are commonly implicated. Other organisms include Enterobacter, Streptococcus, Candida, and Mycobacteria. Furthermore, the axial skeleton is frequently affected, especially the spine, the sacroiliac joint, and the sternoclavicular articulation, with less common involvement of the acromioclavicular joint, the hip, the pubic symphysis, the ribs, and the ischial tuberosities[268-276] (Fig. 60–58). Alteration of the bones in the appendicular skeleton is less typical.

Osteomyelitis and Septic Arthritis in Lymphedema

A report has appeared recently of two elderly patients with lymphedema who developed beta-hemolytic streptococcal infection of the knee.[279] In these individuals, synovitis persisted for months despite the presence of adequate levels of antibiotics in the synovial fluid. Because lymphatic vessels normally drain synovial fluid from the joint, their obstruction may have interrupted normal egress of the intra-articular organisms and aided in retrograde passage of microorganisms from the site of cellulitis into the joint.

OTHER DIAGNOSTIC MODALITIES

Magnification Radiography

Optical and radiographic magnification techniques can be helpful in evaluating patients with infectious disorders. The early alterations of osteomyelitis, infective osteitis or periostitis, and septic arthritis may be readily apparent on magnification studies when conventional radiographs are equivocal or negative. The detection of small osteolytic foci in osteomyelitis, minor disruption of the subchondral bone plate in infectious arthritis, and slight periosteal proliferation in infective osteitis, periostitis, or osteomyelitis may be possible with this modality (Fig. 60–59). We have utilized magnification techniques routinely with good success in the evaluation of the feet of diabetic patients (Fig. 60–60) and in the differentiation of active versus inactive chronic osteomyelitis (Fig. 60–61). Magnification radiography may show definite bony disruption, indicating infection, in the diabetic individual in whom osseous structures are obscured on routine radiography by the presence of soft tissue gas or calcification. In chronic osteomyelitis, the documentation of ill-defined periosteal bone formation with magnification techniques implies existence of active chronic osteomyelitis at a time when the changes may be obscured on conventional radiographs by the subperiosteal alterations of the chronic infection itself.

Tomography

The major role of tomography in infectious disorders is the detection of sequestra in a patient with chronic osteomyelitis, as these pieces of necrotic bone can be obscured by the surrounding osseous abnormalities on routine radiography. With tomography, they become readily apparent, surrounded by radiolucent granulation tissue. As the presence of pieces of sequestered bone suggests activity of the infectious process, their detection is important to the orthopedic surgeon and guides the choice of therapy. Occasionally, tomographic examination will outline definite destruction of the subchondral bone plate, indicating the likely presence of septic arthri-

Text continued on page 2119

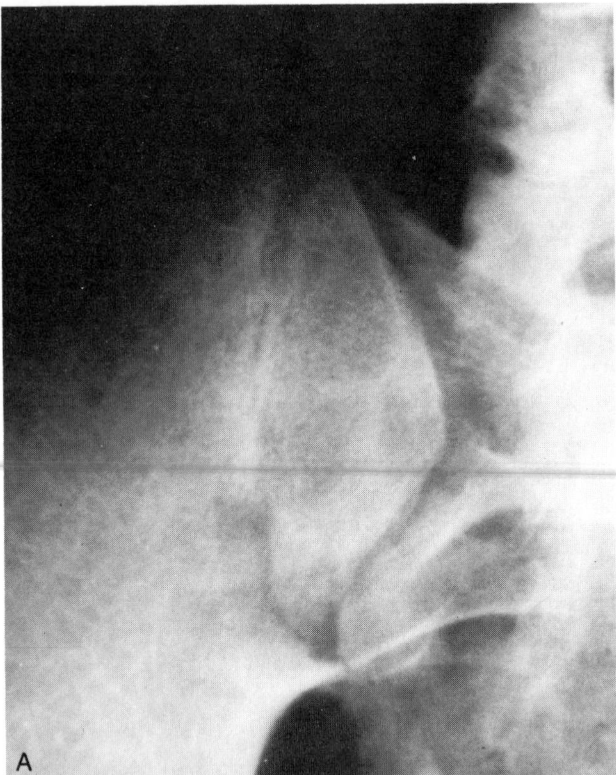

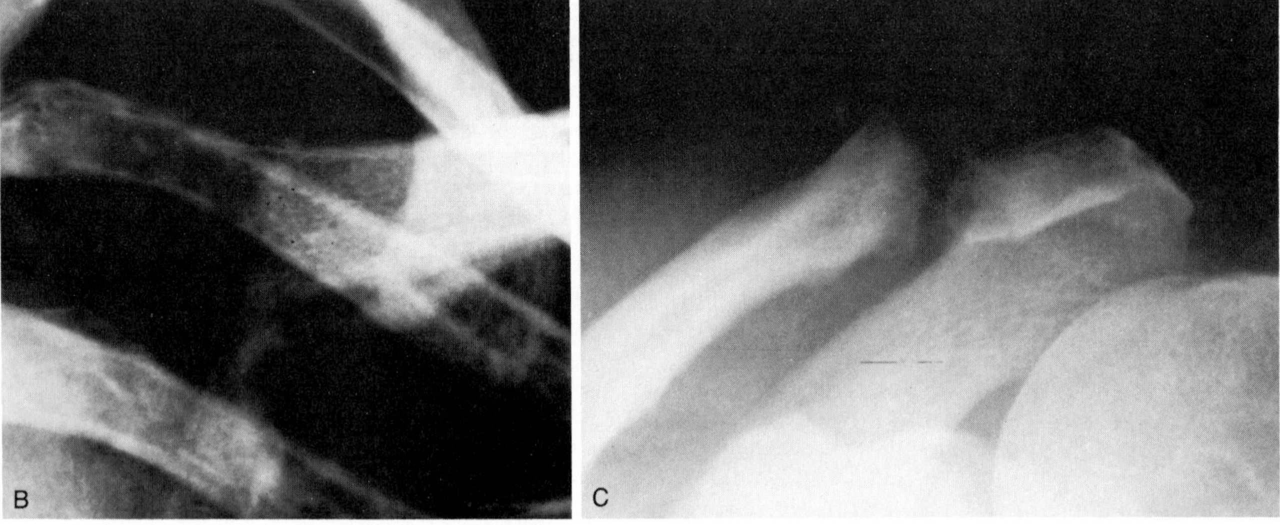

Figure 60–58. *Hematogenous osteomyelitis and septic arthritis in the drug abuser. In these individuals, common sites of involvement are the sacroiliac joint* **(A)** *and the sternoclavicular* **(B)** *and acromioclavicular* **(C)** *articulations, as well as the spine. Atypical organisms are frequently recovered.*

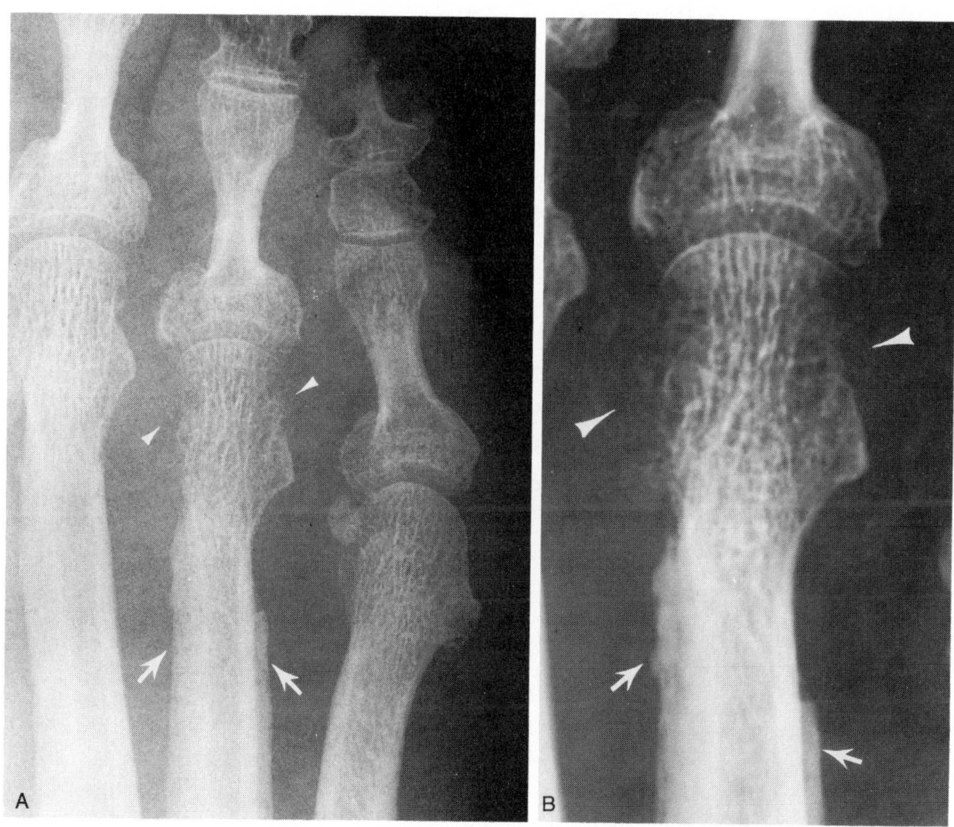

Figure 60–59. *Osteomyelitis and septic arthritis: Role of magnification radiography. Although the radiographic changes of infection, including periostitis (arrows) and osseous destruction (arrowheads), are apparent on the routine radiograph* **(A)**, *they are more obvious with magnification techniques* **(B)**.

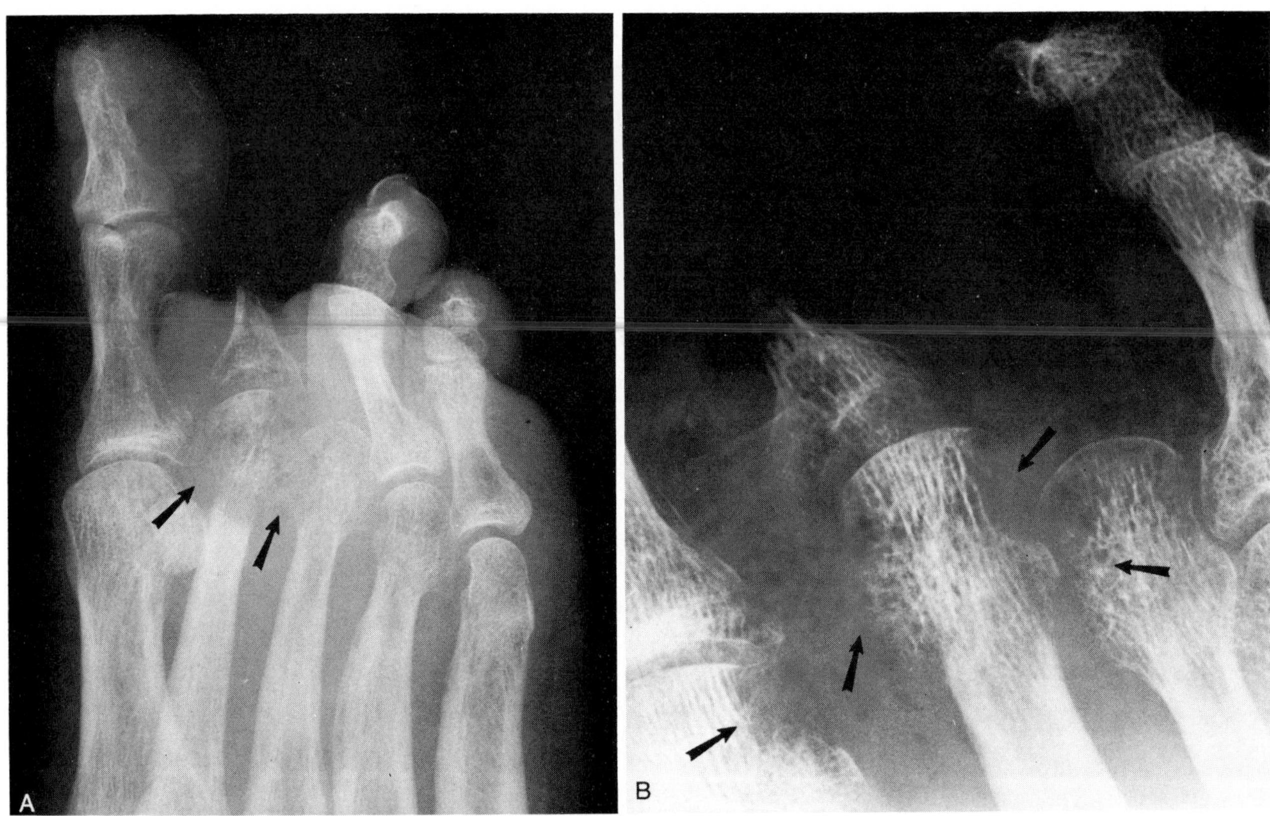

Figure 60–60. *Infection in the diabetic foot: Role of magnification radiography. This diabetic patient had a soft tissue infection with involvement of the second and third toes that required phalangectomy. The possibility of recurrent bony infection was raised.*

A *The initial film indicates apparent erosion of the second and third metatarsal heads (arrows), although the findings are obscured by the overlying soft tissues containing air. Note that the tip of the resected proximal phalanx of the second toe is not covered by soft tissue.*

B *A magnification film reveals obvious erosions of the first, second, and third metatarsal heads (arrows).*

Illustration continued on the opposite page

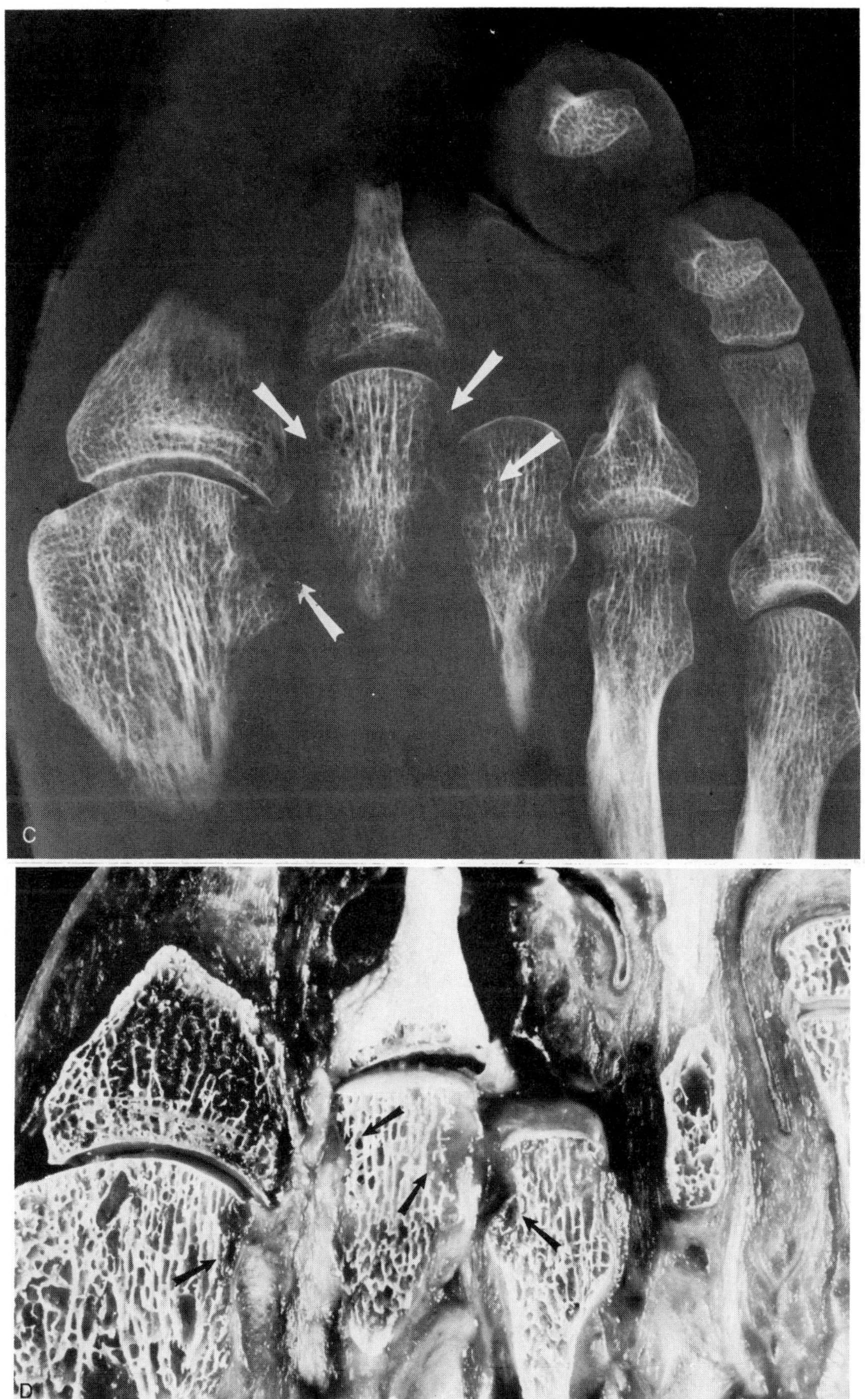

Figure 60–60. Continued

C, D *A radiograph and photograph of a transverse section of the resected foot indicate the sites of osseous erosion (arrows).*

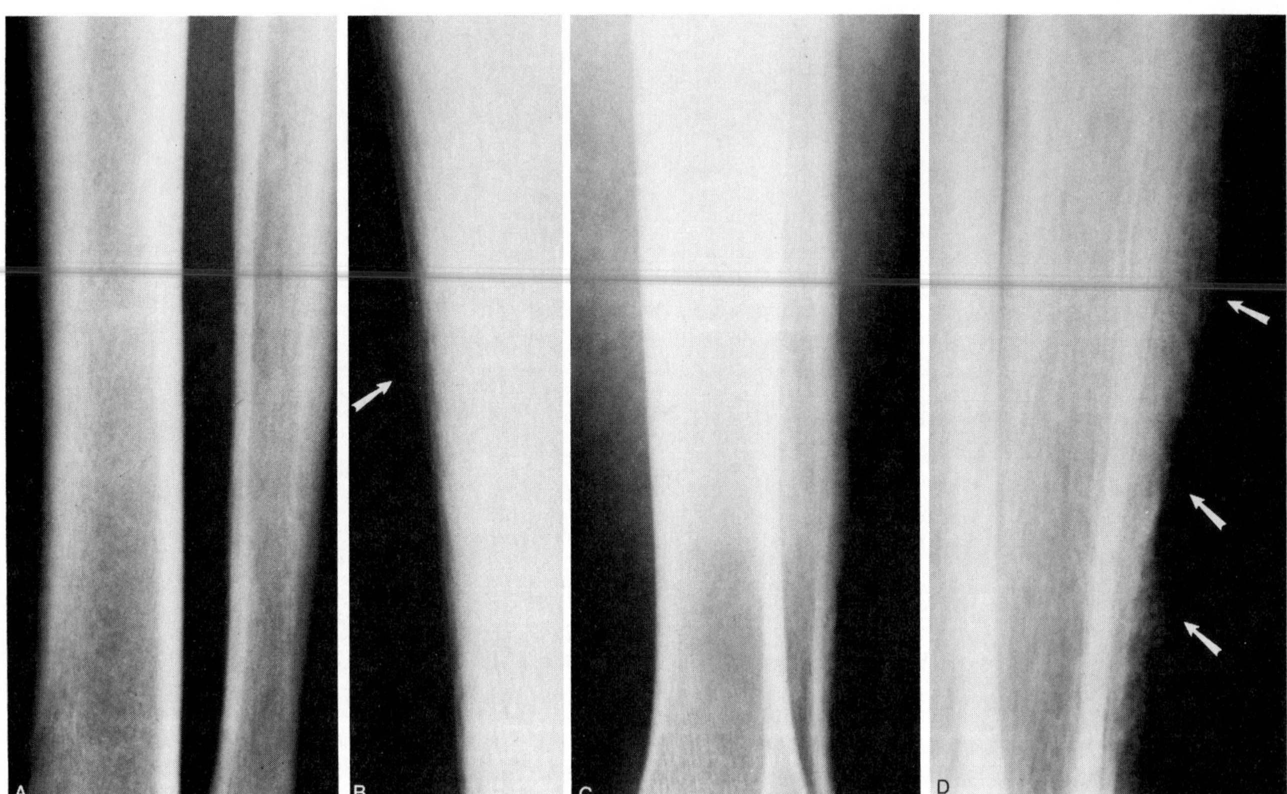

Figure 60–61. *Active versus inactive chronic osteomyelitis: Role of magnification radiography. Two examples in which magnification radiography outlines ill-defined periosteal proliferation (arrows) documenting the presence of active chronic osteomyelitis. The plain films are also shown for comparison.*

tis rather than simple osteoporosis (which usually produces a thin but otherwise intact plate).

Fistulography

Opacification of a fistulous tract can produce important information that influences the choice of therapy.[310, 320] A small catheter can be placed securely within a cutaneous opening or a Foley catheter can be placed against the opening with the balloon inflated and pressed tightly against the skin to prevent or diminish leakage. Retrograde injection of contrast material will define the course and extent of the fistula and its possible communication with an underlying bone or joint (Fig. 60–62). Although septicemia has been recorded following fistulography,[311] this is indeed a rare occurrence.

Arthrography

The principal reason for performing a joint puncture in the clinical setting of infection is to obtain fluid for bacteriologic examination. However, following removal of the joint contents, contrast opacification of the articulation will outline the extent of the synovial inflammation and the presence of capsular, tendinous, and soft tissue injury (Fig. 60–63). This is especially helpful in those joints such as the hip and the glenohumeral articulation that are relatively inaccessible to direct clinical examination because of their deep location.[312] In performing this procedure, the arthrographer should first attempt to recover some joint fluid by moving the needle about the articulation. If this fails, nonbacteriostatic saline solution should be injected and then aspirated and sent to the laboratory. These techniques should be employed prior to the injection of contrast material.

Radionuclide Examination

Although the utilization of scintigraphy in the evaluation of musculoskeletal infections is discussed elsewhere (see Chapter 17), a few comments are appropriate here. The role of this examination in

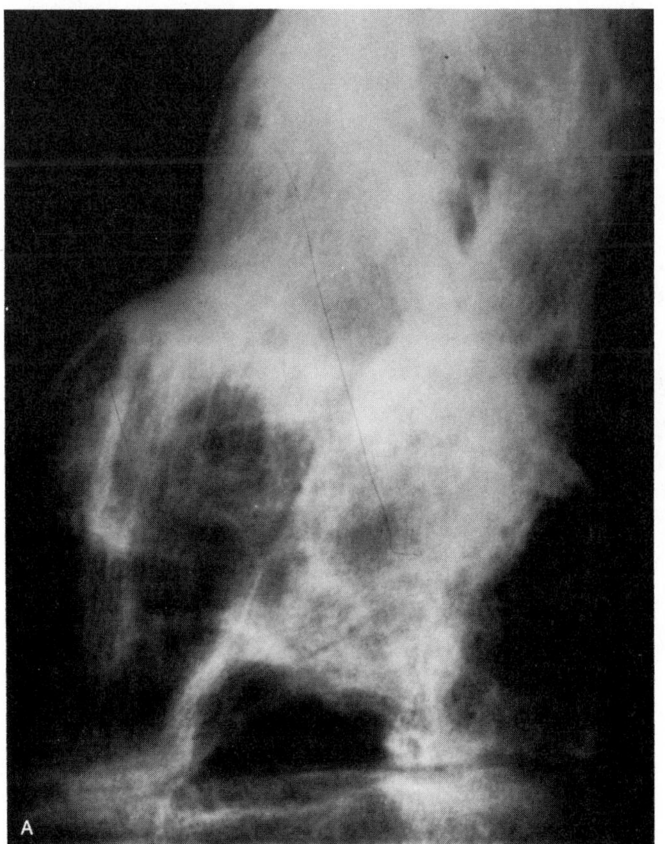

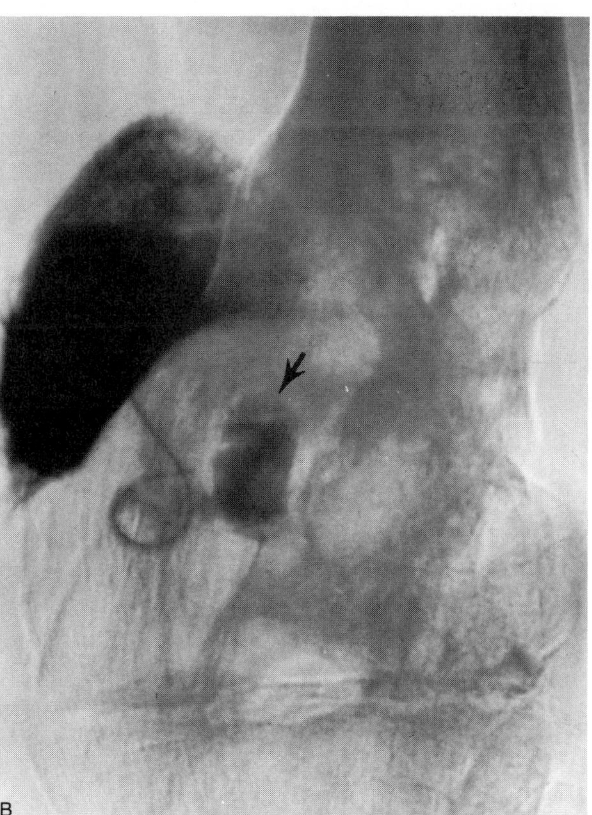

Figure 60–62. *Chronic osteomyelitis: Role of fistulography.*

A *The initial film demonstrates the radiographic features of chronic osteomyelitis of the distal femur.*

B *Subtraction film obtained during retrograde opacification of a fistulous tract confirms the communication with an abscess in the bone (arrow).*

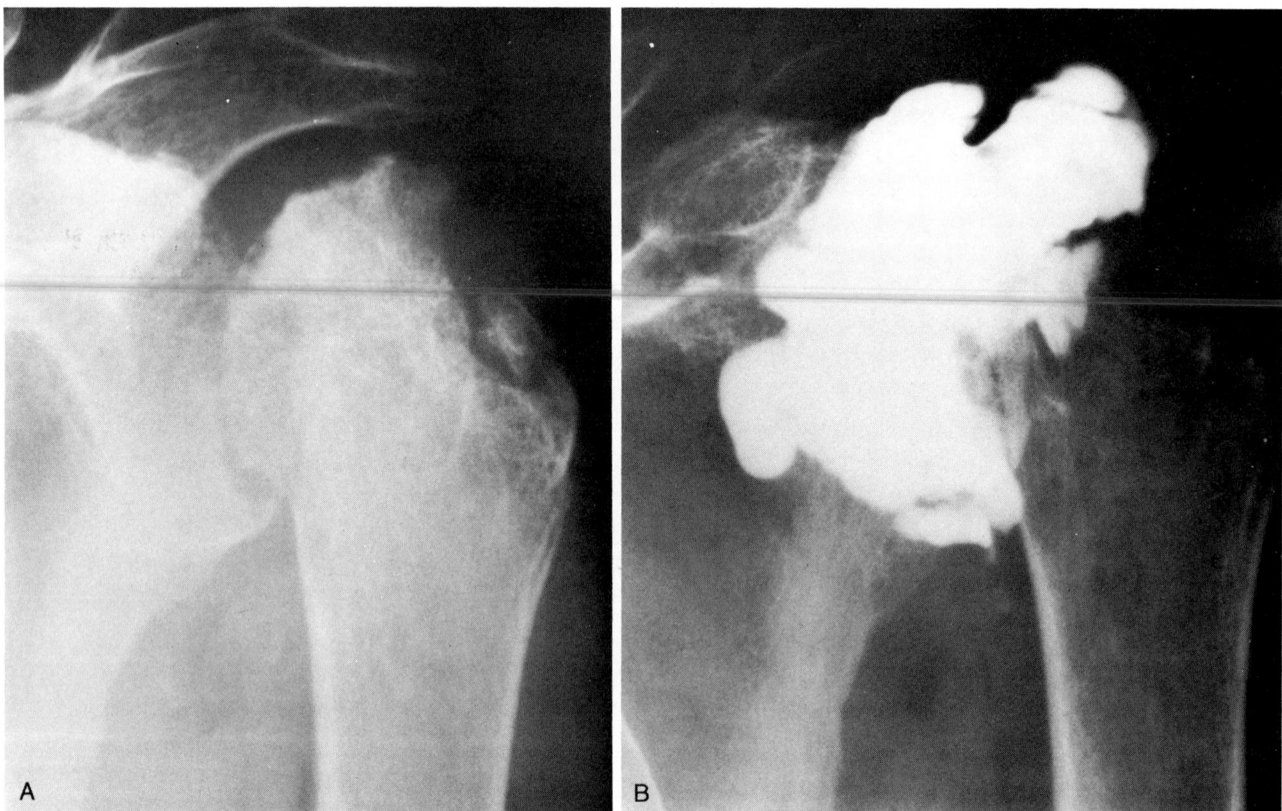

Figure 60–63. *Septic arthritis: Role of arthrography.*

A, B *The initial shoulder film in this patient who developed glenohumeral joint infection following trauma indicates the severity of the cartilaginous and osseous destruction, principally of the humeral head. Arthrography reveals the degree of synovial irregularity of the joint and the presence of "outpockets" or diverticula.*

Illustration continued on the opposite page

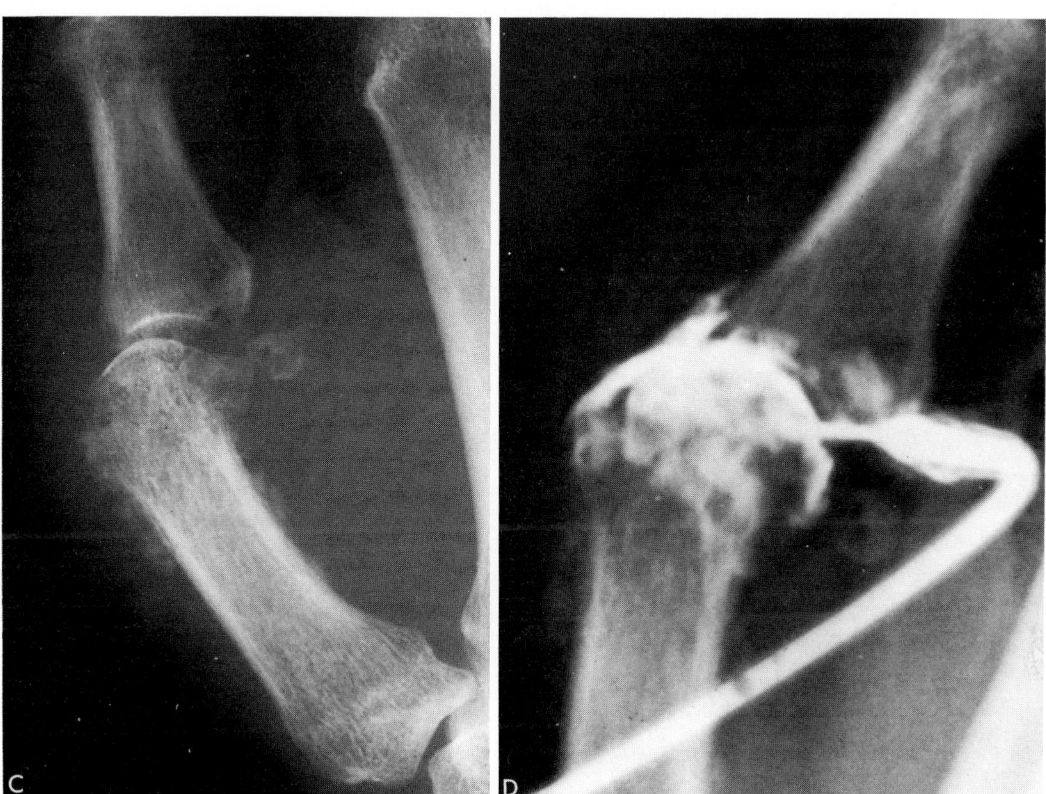

Figure 60–63. Continued

C, D *The initial film* **(C)** *demonstrates osteomyelitis of the first metacarpal and septic arthritis with marginal erosions of the metacarpal and proximal phalanx at the metacarpophalangeal joint. Osteolysis of the sesamoid is also seen. Arthrography* **(D)** *confirmed the presence of staphylococci in the joint and demonstrated considerable cartilage destruction and synovial irregularity.*

Illustration continued on the following page

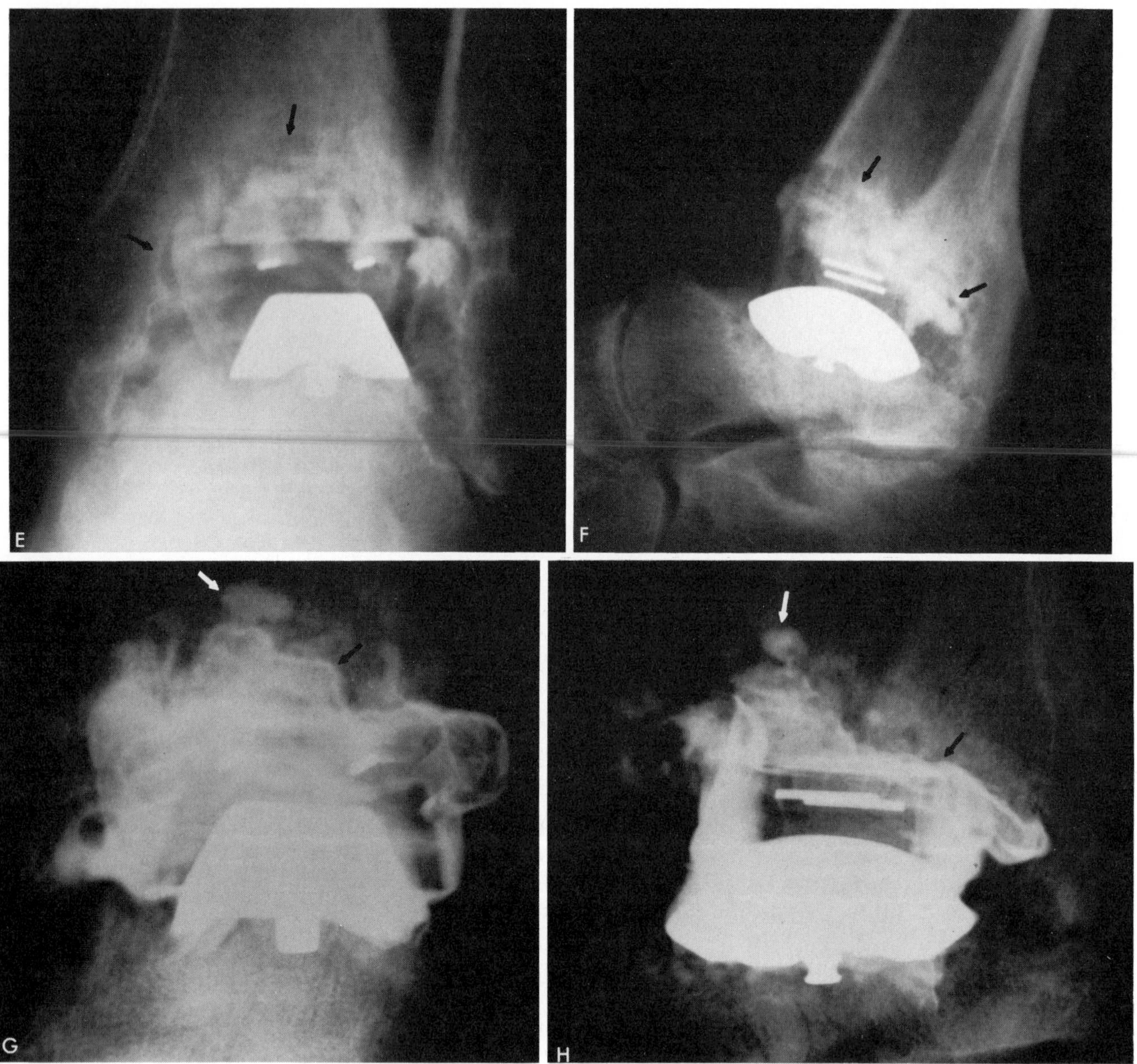

Figure 60–63. Continued

E–H *In this patient, who had had an ankle arthroplasty, initial radiographs* **(E, F)** *reveal lucent shadows between the radiopaque cement and the tibia (arrows). After joint aspiration and removal of fluid, which later confirmed the presence of infection, contrast injection* **(G, H)** *provided evidence that the tibial component was "loose." Note the contrast material between the cement and bone (arrows).*

the evaluation of bone,[229-237] joint,[238-240] and soft tissue[239, 240] infectious processes is firmly established (Fig. 60–64). Technetium phosphate bone scans will become abnormal within hours to days of the onset of bone infection and days to weeks before the disease becomes manifest on conventional radiographs. The scintigraphic abnormality may initially be evident as a photodeficient area ("cold" spot) but, within a few days, increased accumulation of the radioisotope ("hot" spot) is typical. The bone scan can also be utilized to follow the infected patient and his response to treatment, although several weeks may be required before the scan returns to an entirely normal appearance. Occasional difficulty in interpreting the bone scan in younger patients arises from differentiating normal and abnormal activity in the metaphyseal region.[315, 316] Utilization of gallium scans in this situation, although associated with less radionuclide accumulation, may allow more accurate interpretation of the metaphyseal activity. The accumulation of gallium in inflamed areas is believed to be related to the exudation of in vivo labeled serum proteins and the accumulation of in vivo labeled leukocytes, primarily neutrophils.[241, 242] Leukocytes are rich in lactoferrin, and gallium, which accumulates in leukocytes, is primarily bound to lactoferrin. Thus leukocytic uptake of gallium may explain, at least in part, augmented activity at sites of skeletal infection on gallium scans. However, similar accumulation of gallium in patients without circulating leukocytes indicates that other factors are also important.[313] It has been suggested that lactoferrin binding may be a second important mechanism explaining gallium accumulation in inflammatory foci. The lactoferrin contained in leukocytes is excreted at sites of inflammation, and the discharged lactoferrin may adhere to receptor sites in tissue macrophages. It is also possible that infective organisms themselves may take up gallium, perhaps due to siderophore production by the microorganisms.

The rationale regarding the use of gallium as an adjunct to technetium phosphates in evaluating inflammatory lesions of bone is based upon several considerations.[317, 318] As technetium accumulation is related to the integrity of the vascular tree, increased intramedullary pressure accompanying osteomyelitis can partially prevent augmented blood flow and prevent significant accumulation of the radionuclide.[314] Gallium, being less dependent upon the vascular flow, might still localize at the site of infection. Thus, in the presence of a clinical suspicion of bone or joint infection and a negative bone scan, a gallium study could be useful. Unfortunately, as gallium accumulation occurs also with soft tissue infection, differentiation of cellulitis and osteomyelitis is usually not possible with this agent, although utilization of good

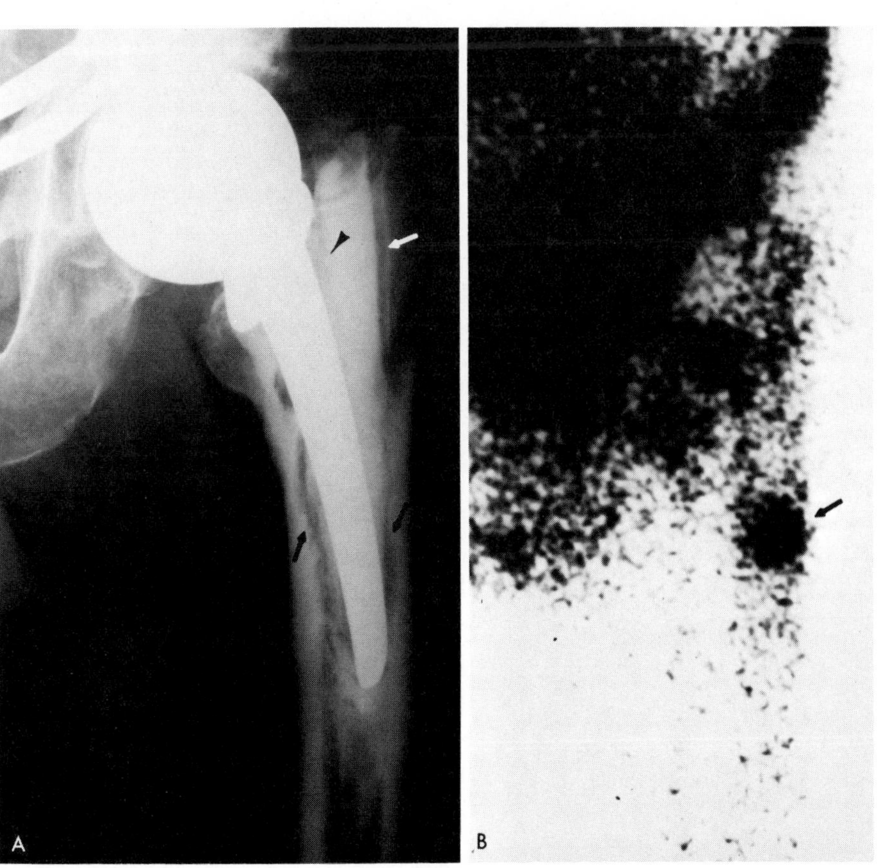

Figure 60–64. *Postoperative infection: Role of radionuclide examination (technetium phosphate studies).*

A, B *This patient had persistent pain following an arthroplasty of the hip. Exaggerated radiolucent areas between the radiopaque cement and bone (arrows,* **A***) and between the cement and metal (arrowhead) are seen. The prosthesis has "sunk" into the femur and its stem is applied to a partially eroded femoral cortex. The scan reveals focal areas of abnormal accumulation of radionuclide (arrow,* **B***).*

Illustration continued on the following page

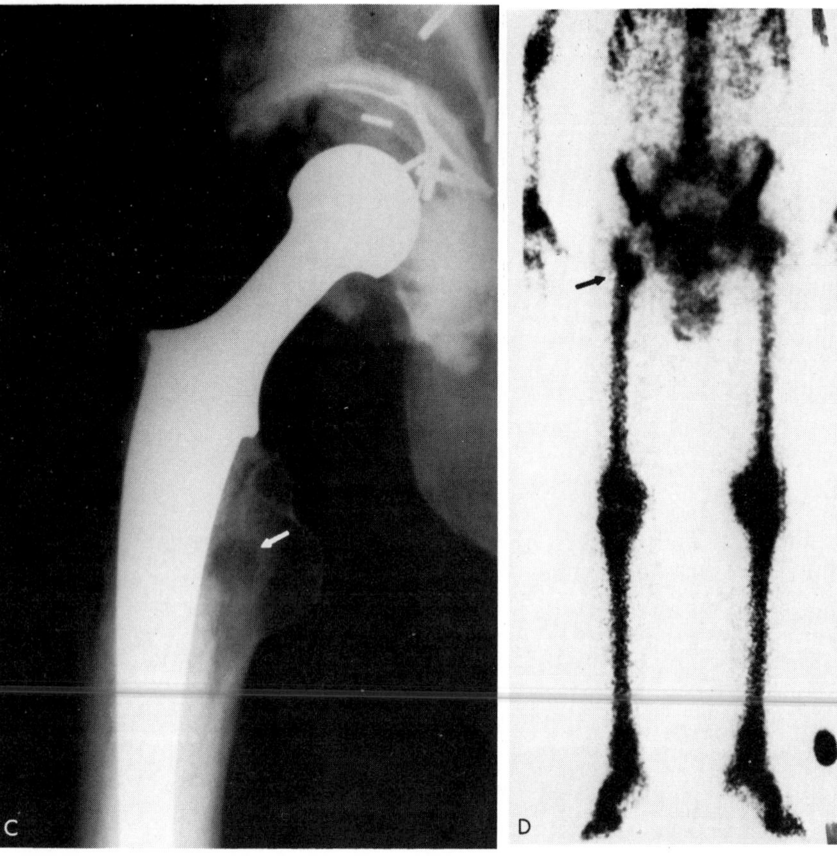

Figure 60–64. Continued
C, D *In this patient with a total hip arthroplasty, a localized abscess is identified on the radiograph and scintigraph (arrow).*

image quality may allow some differentiation of bone, joint, and soft tissue uptake.[317]

A gallium scan can be obtained in conjunction with a technetium scan in the same patient, and the information that is obtained may be even more useful than that of either examination alone (Table 60–7). Following administration of technetium agents, scans can be obtained within a few hours, documenting the presence of an inflammatory process; optimal scanning with gallium may necessitate a delay of 10 to 24 hours. Gallium scans may reveal abnormal accumulation in patients with active osteomyelitis when technetium scans reveal decreased activity ("cold" lesions) or perhaps normal activity (transition period between "cold" and "hot" lesions). Furthermore, gallium accumulation appears to correlate more closely with activity in cases of osteomyelitis than does technetium, and it may be superior in determining the response of acute osteomyelitis and chronic osteomyelitis to various therapeutic regimens. Increased accumulation of gallium in sites of cellulitis can be helpful in establishing the presence of soft tissue infection; initial technetium accumulation also occurs in cases of cellulitis, but its activity diminishes rapidly, thus affording a mechanism for differentiating between cellulitis and osteomyelitis,

Table 60–7
RADIONUCLIDE EVALUATION OF OSSEOUS AND SOFT TISSUE INFECTION

Agent	Cellulitis	Acute Osteomyelitis	Chronic Osteomyelitis
Technetium phosphates	Early scans show increased uptake; later scans are normal	Early and late scans show increased uptake (scans in early acute osteomyelitis may reveal "cold" spots)	Scans may remain positive even in inactive disease
Gallium	Increased uptake	Increased uptake	Increased uptake in areas of active disease

the latter situation associated with persistent increased radionuclide accumulation.[243, 244] Initial abnormal technetium activity also persists in patients with septic arthritis.[233]

Bone marrow imaging with technetium sulfur-colloid has been used experimentally to evaluate osteomyelitis.[236] Decrease in accumulation of the radioactive agent that is observed in osteomyelitis but not in septic arthritis may reflect obstruction to blood flow in small arteries supplying the bone and bone marrow and influx of inflammatory cells into the affected area. A similar pattern of decreased activity can be noted following technetium sulfur-colloid injection in patients with sickle cell anemia, presumably related to bone infarction.[245]

Computed Tomography

This modality may also have a role in the diagnosis of infections in bone and soft tissue[246] (see Chapter 12). Increased density of the medullary canal may be evident, related to edema or vascular congestion. Cortical destruction, periosteal proliferation, and soft tissue extension can be delineated at a time when conventional radiographs may be entirely normal. Computed tomographic evaluation of the spine may allow accurate delineation of inflammatory disease of the paravertebral musculature.[319]

SUMMARY

A thorough understanding of regional anatomy is fundamental to the accurate interpretation of clinical, radiologic, and pathologic characteristics of infections of bone, joint, and soft tissue. In most individuals with such infections, a specific mechanism of contamination can be recognized; infection may be derived from hematogenous seeding, spread from a contiguous source, direct implantation, or operative contamination. The roentgenographic findings of osteomyelitis (including abscess, involucrum, sequestration), septic arthritis (including joint space loss, marginal and central osseous erosions), and soft tissue suppuration (including swelling, radiolucent streaks, and periostitis) are generally delayed for a variable period following the clinical onset of infection. Other diagnostic modalities, including scintigraphy, allow accurate diagnosis at an earlier stage of the process.

REFERENCES

1. Nelaton A: Elements de pathologie chirurgicale. Paris, Germer-Bailliere, 1844–1859.
2. Jaffe HL: Metabolic, Degenerative, and Inflammatory Diseases of Bones and Joints. Philadelphia, Lea & Febiger, 1972.
3. Waldvogel FA, Medoff G, Swartz MN: Osteomyelitis: A review of clinical features, therapeutic considerations and unusual aspects. Part I. N Engl J Med *282*:198, 1970.
4. Garre C.: Über besondere Formen und Folgezustande der akuten infektiosen Osteomyelitis. Bruns Beitr Klin Chir *10*:241, 1893.
5. Thoma, KH, Goldman HM: Oral Pathology. 5th Ed. St Louis, CV Mosby Co, 1960, p 719.
6. Trueta J: Studies of the Development and Decay of the Human Frame. Philadelphia, WB Saunders Co, 1968, p 254.
7. Kahn DS, Pritzker KPH: The pathophysiology of bone infection. Clin Orthop Rel Res *96*:12, 1973.
8. Atcheson SG, Ward JR: Acute hematogenous osteomyelitis progressing to septic synovitis and eventual pyarthrosis. Arthritis Rheum *21*:968, 1978.
9. Capitanio MA, Kirkpatrick JA: Early roentgen observations in acute osteomyelitis. Am J Roentgenol *108*:488, 1970.
10. Nixon GW: Hematogenous osteomyelitis of metaphyseal-equivalent locations. Am J Roentgenol *130*:123, 1978.
11. Lindberg L, Lidgren L: Bone and joint infections. International Orthopaedics (SICOT) *1*:191, 1977.
12. Ferguson AB Jr: Osteomyelitis in children. Clin Orthop Rel Res *96*:51, 1973.
13. Mollan RAB, Piggot J: Acute osteomyelitis in children. J Bone Joint Surg *59B*:2, 1977.
14. Troger J, Eibner D, Otte G, Weitzel D: Diagnose und differentialdiagnose der akuten hämatogen osteomyelitis des Sauglings. Radiologe *19*:99, 1979.
15. Edwards MS, Baker CJ, Wagner ML, Taber LH, Barrett FF: An etiologic shift in infantile osteomyelitis: the emergence of the group B streptococcus. J Pediatr *93*:578, 1978.
16. Brill PW, Winchester P, Krauss AN, Symchych P: Osteomyelitis in a neonatal intensive care unit. Radiology *131*:83, 1979.
17. Butt WP: The radiology of infection. Clin Orthop Rel Res *96*:20, 1973.
18. Trueta J: The three types of acute hematogenous osteomyelitis. A clinical and vascular study. J Bone Joint Surg *41B*:671, 1959.
19. Winters JL, Cahen I: Acute hematogenous osteomyelitis: A review of sixty-six cases. J Bone Joint Surg *42A*:691, 1960.
20. Shandling B: Acute hematogenous osteomyelitis: A review of 300 cases treated during 1952–1959. S Afr Med J *34*:520, 1960.
21. Weissberg ED, Smith AL, Smith DH: Clinical features of neonatal osteomyelitis. Pediatrics *53*:505, 1974.
22. Green WT: Osteomyelitis in infancy. JAMA *105*:1835, 1935.
23. Ogden JA, Lister G: The pathology of neonatal osteomyelitis. Pediatrics *55*:474, 1975.
24. Dich VQ, Nelson JD, Haltalin KC: Osteomyelitis in infants and children. A review of 163 cases. Am J Dis Child *129*:1273, 1975.
25. Clarke AM: Neonatal osteomyelitis: A disease different from osteomyelitis of older children. Med J Aust *1*:237, 1958.
26. Lim MQ, Gresham EL, Franklin EA Jr, Leake RD: Osteomyelitis as a complication of umbilical artery catheterization. Am J Dis Child *131*:142, 1977.
27. Krauss AN, Albert RF, Kannan MM: Contamination of umbilical catheters in the newborn infant. J Pediatr *77*:965, 1970.
28. Simmons PB, Harris LE, Bianco AJ Jr: Complications of exchange transfusion. Report of two cases of septic arthritis and osteomyelitis. Mayo Clin Proc *48*:190, 1973.
29. Cohen LS, Fekety FR Jr, Cluff LE: Studies of the epidemiology of staphylococcal infection. VI. Infections in the surgical patient. Ann Surg *159*:321, 1964.
30. Davis LA: Antibiotic modified osteomyelitis. Am J Roentgenol *103*:608, 1968.
31. Blanche DW: Osteomyelitis in infants. J Bone Joint Surg *34A*:71, 1952.
32. Warwick R, Williams PL (Eds): Gray's Anatomy. 35th British Ed. Philadelphia, WB Saunders Co, 1973, pp 220, 406.
33. Crock HV: The Blood Supply of the Lower Limb Bones in Man. London, E&S Livingstone Ltd, 1967, p 29.
34. Gardner E: Blood and nerve supply of joints. Stanford Med Bull *11*:203, 1953.
35. Tachdjian MO: Pediatric Orthopedics. Philadelphia, WB Saunders Co, 1972, p 352.
36. Trueta J: Acute hematogenous osteomyelitis: Its pathology and treatment. Bull Hosp Joint Dis *14*:5, 1953.
37. Trueta J: Acute hematogenous osteomyelitis: Its pathology and treatment. Bull NY Acad Med *35*:25, 1959.
38. Trueta J: The normal vascular anatomy of the human femoral head during growth. J Bone Joint Surg *39B*:358, 1957.
39. Hobo T: Zur Pathogenese der akuten haematogenen Osteomyelitis mit

Berucksichtighg der Vitalfarbungslehre. Acta Sch Med Univ Kioto *4*:1, 1921.
40. Koch J: Untersuchungen über die Lokalisation der Bakterien: Das Verhalten des Knochenmarkes und die Veranderungen der Knochen, insbesondere der Epiphysen bei Infektionskrankheiten. Z Hyg Infektionskr *69*:436, 1911.
41. Morrey BF, Bianco AJ, Rhodes KH: Hematogenous osteomyelitis at uncommon sites in children. Mayo Clin Proc *53*:707, 1978.
42. Brookes M: The Blood Supply of Bone. London, Butterworths, 1971.
43. Wilensky AO: Osteomyelitis: Its pathogenesis. Symptomatology and Treatment. New York, Macmillan Co, 1934, p 114.
44. Green M, Nyhan WL Jr, Fousek MD: Acute hematogenous osteomyelitis.. Pediatrics *17*:368, 1956.
45. Gilmour WN: Acute haematogenous osteomyelitis. J Bone Joint Surg *44B*:841, 1962.
46. Moyson FR, Brombart JC, Wittek FR: Ostéomyélite de l'enfant. Signes radiologiques précoces. J Belge Radiol *55*:645, 1972.
47. Bretagne M-C, Jolly, A, Mouton J-N, Metaizeau J-P, Beau A, Treheux A: Mémoires originaux. Ostéomyélite pseudo-sacromateuse de l'enfant. J Radiol Electrol Med Nucl *58*:1, 1977.
48. Jorup S, Kjellberg SR: Early diagnosis of acute septic osteomyelitis, periostitis and arthritis, and its importance in treatment. Acta Radiol *30*:316, 1948.
49. Griffin PP: Bone and joint infections in children. Pediatr Clin North Am *14*:533, 1967.
50. Brodie BC: An account of some cases of chronic abscess of the tibia. Trans Med Chir Soc. *17*:238, 1832.
51. Brodie BC: Pathological and Surgical Observations of the Diseases of the Joint. 4th Ed. London, Longman, 1836, p 298.
52. Brickner WM: The treatment of chronic bone abscesses by simple evacuation through a small drill hole. Its application in non-sterile abscesses. J Bone Joint Surg *5*:492, 1923.
53. Henderson MS, Simon ME: Brodie's abscess. Arch Surg *9*:504, 1924.
54. Brailsford JF: Brodie's abscess and its differential diagnosis. Br Med J *2*:119, 1938.
55. Harris NH, Kirkaldy-Willis WH: Primary subacute pyogenic osteomyelitis. J Bone Joint Surg *47B*:526, 1965.
56. Kandel SN, Mankin HJ: Pyogenic abscess of the long bones in children. Clin Orthop Rel Res *96*:108, 1973.
57. Gledhill RB: Subacute osteomyelitis in children. Clin Orthop Rel Res *96*:57, 1973.
58. Cabanela ME, Sim FH, Beabout JW, Dahlin DC: Osteomyelitis appearing as neoplasms. A diagnostic problem. Arch Surg *109*:68, 1974.
59. Weston WT: Case report 44. Skel Radiol *2*:125, 1977.
60. Waldvogel FA, Medoff G, Swartz MN: Osteomyelitis: A review of clinical features, therapeutic considerations and unusual aspects. Part 2. N Engl J Med *282*:260, 1970.
61. VanNiekerk JP de V: Hand infections: Management and results based on a new classification: A study of more than 1000 cases. S Afr Med J *40*:316, 1966.
62. Kinnman JEG, Lee HS: Chronic osteomyelitis of the mandible: Clinical study of thirteen cases. Oral Surg *25*:6, 1968.
63. Blumenfeld RJ, Skolnik EM: Intracranial complications of sinus disease. Trans Am Acad Ophthal Otolaryngol *70*:899, 1966.
64. Francis DP, Holmes MA, Brandon G: *Pasteurella multocida* infections after domestic animal bites and scratches. JAMA *233*:42, 1975.
65. Hooper G: Tooth fragment in a metacarpophalangeal joint. Hand *10*:215, 1978.
66. Lavine LS, Isenberg HD, Rubins W, Berkman JI: Unusual osteomyelitis following superficial dog bites. Clin Orthop Rel Res *98*:251, 1974.
67. Chusid MJ, Jacobs WM, Sty JR: Pseudomonas arthritis following puncture wounds of the foot. J Pediatr *94*:429, 1979.
68. Miller EH, Semian DW: Gram-negative osteomyelitis following puncture wounds of the foot. J Bone Joint Surg *57A*:535, 1975.
69. Tscherne H, Trentz O: Gelenkinfektionen nach perforierenden wunden, punktionen und injektioner. Langenbecks Arch Chir *334*:521, 1973.
70. Brand RA, Black H: Pseudomonas osteomyelitis following puncture wounds in children. J Bone Joint Surg *56A*:1637, 1974.
71. Swischuk LE, Jorgenson F, Jorgenson A, Caper D: Wooden splinter induced "pseudotumors" and "osteomyelitis-like lesions" of bone and soft tissue. Am J Roentgenol *122*:176, 1974.
72. Manny J, Haruzi I, Yosipovitch Z: Osteomyelitis of the clavicle following subclavian vein catheterization. Arch Surg *106*:342, 1973.
73. Lilien LD, Harris VJ, Ramamurthy RS, Pildes RS: Neonatal osteomyelitis of the calcaneus: Complication of heel puncture. J Pediatrics *88*:478, 1976.
74. Koch SL: Osteomyelitis of the bones of the hand. Surg Gynecol Obstet *64*:1, 1937.
75. Whitehouse WM, Smith WS: Osteomyelitis of the feet. Semin Roentgenol *5*:367, 1970.
76. Suydam MJ, Mikity VG: Cellulitis with underlying inflammatory periostitis of the mandible. Am J Roentgenol *106*:133, 1969.
77. Martel W, Abell MR: Radiologic evaluation of soft tissue tumors. A retrospective study. Cancer *32*:352, 1973.
78. Resnick D: Osteomyelitis and septic arthritis complicating hand injuries and infections: Pathogenesis of roentgenographic abnormalities. J Can Assoc Radiol *27*:21, 1976.
79. Resnick D: The roentgenographic anatomy of the tendon sheaths of the hand and wrist: Tenography. Am J Roentgenol *124*:44, 1975.
80. Lampe EW: Surgical anatomy of the hand with special reference to infections and trauma. Clin Symp *21*:66, 1969.
81. Kanavel A: Infections of the Hand. A Guide to the Surgcal Treatment of Acute and Chronic Suppurative Processes in the Fingers, Hand, and Forearm. 7th Ed. Philadelphia, Lea & Febiger, 1939.
82. Boyes JH: Bunnell's Surgery of the Hand. 5th Ed. Philadelphia, JB Lippincott, 1970.
83. Flynn JE: Clinical and anatomical investigations of deep fascial space infections of the hand. Am J Surg *55*:467, 1942.
84. Carter SJ, Mersheimer WL: Infections of the hand. Orthop Clin North Am *1*:455, 1970.
85. Robins RHC: Infections of the hand. A review based on 1000 consecutive cases. J Bone Joint Surg *34B*:567, 1952.
86. Macey HB: Paronychia and bone felon. Am J Surg *50*:553, 1940.
87. Daniel DM: The acutely swollen hand in the drug user. Arch Surg *107*:548, 1973.
88. Neviaser RJ, Butterfield WC, Wiehe DR: The puffy hand of drug addiction. A study of the pathogenesis. J Bone Joint Surg *54A*:629, 1972.
89. Whitaker LA, Graham WP III: Management of hand infections in the narcotic addict. Plast Reconstr Surg *52*:384, 1973.
90. Ellenberg M: Diabetic foot. NY State J Med *73*:2778, 1973.
91. Levin M, O'Neal LW: The Diabetic Foot. St Louis, CV Mosby, 1973.
92. Meade JW, Mueller CB: Major infections of the foot. Med Times *96*:154, 1968.
93. Godinsky M: A study of the fascial spaces of the foot and their bearing on infections. Surg Gynecol Obstet *49*:737, 1929.
94. Kamel R, Sakla FB: Anatomical compartments of the sole of the human foot. Anat Rec *140*:57, 1961.
95. Martin BF: Observations on the muscles and tendons of the medial aspect of the sole of the foot. J Anat *98*:437, 1964.
96. Rao VR, Kini MG: Infections of the foot — an anatomical and experimental study of the fascial spaces and tendon sheaths with clinical correlations of certain types of infections of the foot. Indian Med Res Memoirs *37*:1, 1957.
97. Feingold ML, Resnick D, Niwayama G, Garetto L: The plantar compartments of the foot: A roentgen approach. I. Experimental observations. Invest Radiol *12*:281, 1977.
98. Johanson PH: Pseudomonas infections of the foot following puncture wounds. JAMA *204*:262, 1968.
99. Hagler DJ: Pseudomonas osteomyelitis: Puncture wounds of the feet. Pediatrics *48*:672, 1971.
100. Minnefor AB, Olson MI, Carver DH: Pseudomonas osteomyelitis following puncture wounds of the foot. Pediatrics *47*:598, 1971.
101. Waldvogel FA, Medoff G, Swartz MN: Osteomyelitis: A review of clinical features, therapeutic considerations and unusual aspects. Part 3. N Engl J Med *282*:316, 1970.
102. Lipscomb H, Dobson HL, Greene JA: Infection in the diabetic. South Med J *52*:16, 1959.
103. Spring M, Kahn S: Nonclostridial gas infection in the diabetic. Review of the literature and report of three cases. Arch Intern Med *88*:373, 1951.
104. Wills MR, Reece MW: Non-clostridial infections in diabetes mellitus. Br Med J *2*:566, 1960.
105. Warren S, LeCompte PM, Legg MA: The Pathology of Diabetes Mellitus. 4th Ed. Philadelphia, Lea & Febiger, 1966, p 167.
106. Deutsch SD: Non-clostridial gas infection of a fracture in a diabetic. A case report. J Bone Joint Surg *57A*:1009, 1975.
107. Boyce FF: Human bites. An analysis of 90 (chiefly delayed and late) cases from Charity Hospital of Louisiana at New Orleans. South Med J *35*:631, 1942.
108. Farmer CB, Mann RJ: Human bite infections of the hand. South Med J *59*:515, 1966.
109. Lowry TM: Infected human bites. Analysis of treatment and results in twenty-eight cases. Surg Clin North Am *21*:565, 1941.
110. Miller H, Winfield JM: Human bites of the hand. Surg Gynecol Obstet *74*:153, 1942.
111. Chuinard RG, D'Ambrosia R: Human bite infections of the hand. J Bone Joint Surg *59A*:416, 1977.
112. Mason ML, Koch SL: Human bite infections of the hand with a study of the routes of extension of infection from the dorsum of the hand. Surg Gynecol Obstet *51*:591, 1930.
113. Tindall JP, Harrison CM: *Pasteurella multocida* infections following animal injuries, especially cat bites. Arch Dermatol *105*:412, 1972.
114. Lee MLH, Buhr AJ: Dog bites and local infection with *Pasteurella septica*. Br Med J *1*:169, 1960.

115. Hubbert WT, Rosen MN: *Pasteurella multocida* infection due to animal bite. Am J Public Health *60*:1103, 1970.
116. Carithers HA: Mammalian bites of children: A problem in accident prevention. Am J Dis Child *95*:150, 1958.
117. Smith JE: Studies on *Pasteurella septica*. The occurrence in the nose and tonsils of dogs. J Comp Pathol *65*:239, 1955.
118. Owen CR, Buker EO, Bell JF, Jellison WL: *Pasteurella multocida* in animals' mouths. Rocky Mountain Med J *65*:45, 1968.
119. Stevens DB: Postoperative orthopaedic infections. A Study of etiological mechanisms. J Bone Joint Surg *46A*:96, 1964.
120. Harris WH: Sinking prostheses. Surg Gynecol Obstet *123*:1297, 1966.
121. Petty W, Bryan RS, Coventry MB, Peterson LFA: Infection after total knee arthroplasty. Orthop Clin North Am *6*:1005, 1975.
122. Kaushal SP, Galante JO, McKenna R, Bachmann F: Complication following total knee replacement. Clin Orthop Rel Res *121*:181, 1976.
123. Patterson FP, Brown CS: Complications of total hip replacement arthroplasty. Orthop Clin North Am *4*:503, 1973.
124. Bryson AF, Mandell BB: Primary closure after operative treatment of gross chronic osteomyelitis. Lancet *1*:1179, 1964.
125. Griffiths JC: Defects in long bones from severe neglected osteitis. J Bone Joint Surg *50B*:813, 1968.
126. Potter CMC: Osteomyelitis in the new-born. J Bone Joint Surg *36B*:578, 1954.
127. Smith T: On the acute arthritis of infants. St Bartholomew's Hosp Rep *10*:189, 1874.
128. Roberts PH: Disturbed epiphyseal growth at the knee after osteomyelitis in infancy. J Bone Joint Surg *52B*:692, 1970.
129. Trueta J, Amato VP: The vascular contributions to osteogenesis. III. Changes in the growth cartilage caused by experimentally induced ischaemia. J Bone Joint Surg *42B*:571, 1960.
130. Hall R McK: Regeneration of the lower femoral epiphysis. J Bone Joint Surg *36B*:116, 1954.
131. Lloyd-Roberts GC: Suppurative arthritis of infancy. Some observations upon prognosis and management. J Bone Joint Surg *42B*:706, 1960.
132. Sedlin ED, Fleming JL: Epidermoid carcinoma arising in the chronic osteomyelitis foci. J Bone Joint Surg *45A*:827, 1963.
133. Johnston RM, Miles JS: Sarcomas arising from chronic osteomyelitic sinuses. A report of two cases. J Bone Joint Surg *55A*:162, 1973.
134. Dränert K, Rüter A, Burri C, Willenegger H: Fistelmalignome bei chronischer Osteomyelitis. Arch Orthop Unfallchir *84*:199, 1976.
135. Henderson MS, Swart HA: Chronic osteomyelitis associated with malignancy. J Bone Joint Surg *18*:56, 1936.
136. Fitzgerald RH, Brewer NS, Dahlin DC: Squamous-cell carcinoma complicating chronic osteomyelitis. J Bone Joint Surg *58A*:1146, 1976.
137. Bereston ES, Ney C: Squamous cell carcinoma arising in a chronic osteomyelitic sinus tract with metastasis. Arch Surg *43*:257, 1941.
138. Lidgren L: Neoplasia in chronic fistulating osteitis. Acta Orthop Scand *44*:152, 1973.
139. Waugh W: Fibrosarcoma occurring in chronic bone sinus. J Bone Joint Surg *34B*:642, 1952.
140. Akbarnia BA, Wirth CR, Colman N: Fibrosarcoma arising from chronic osteomyelitis. Case report and review of the literature. J Bone Joint Surg *58A*:123, 1976.
141. Buxton SD: Malignant change in sinuses resulting from osteomyelitis. Med Press *232*:45, 1954.
142. Dal Monte A: Neoplasie in processi osteomielitici. Chir Organi Mov *38*:252, 1953.
143. Heilmann D: Plasmozytom auf dem Boden einer chronischen Osteomyelitis bei gleichzeitiger Ostitis deformans Paget. München Med Wochenschr *99*:1586, 1957.
144. Cruickshank AH, McConnell EM, Miller DG: Malignancy in scars, chronic ulcers, and sinuses. J Clin Pathol *16*:573, 1963.
145. Dahlin DC: Secondary amyloidosis. Ann Intern Med *31*:105, 1949.
146. Briggs GW: Amyloidosis. Ann Intern Med *55*:943, 1961.
147. Cohen AS: Amyloidosis. N Engl J Med *277*:522, 1967.
148. Curtiss PH Jr: The pathophysiology of joint infections. Clin Orthop Rel Res *96*:129, 1973.
149. Barnhart MI, Riddle JM, Bluhm GB, Quintana C: Fibrin promotion and lysis in arthritic joints. Ann Rheum Dis *26*:206, 1967.
150. Harris ED, Cohen GL, Krane SM: Synovial collagenase: Its presence in culture from joint disease of diverse etiology. Arthritis Rheum *12*:92, 1969.
151. Bobechko WP, Mandell L: Immunology of cartilage in septic arthritis. Clin Orthop Rel Res *108*:84, 1975.
152. Goldenberg DL, Cohen AS: Acute infectious arthritis. A review of patients with nongonococcal joint infections (with emphasis on therapy and prognosis). Am J Med *60*:369, 1976.
153. Kauffman CA, Watanakunakorn C, Phair JP: Pneumococcal arthritis. J Rheumatol *3*:409, 1976.
154. Paterson DC: Acute suppurative arthritis in infancy and childhood. J Bone Joint Surg *52B*:474, 1970.
155. Borella L, Goobar JE, Summitt RL, Clark GM: Septic arthritis in childhood. J Pediatr *62*:742, 1963.
156. Gillespie R: Septic arthritis of childhood. Clin Orthop Rel Res *96*:152, 1973.
157. Cole WG, Elliott BG, Jensen F: The management of septic arthritis in childhood. Aust NZ J Surg *45*:178, 1975.
158. Newman JH: Review of septic arthritis throughout the antibiotic era. Ann Rheum Dis *35*:198, 1976.
159. Hallel T, Salvati EA: Septic arthritis of the hip in infancy: End result study. Clin Orthop Rel Res *132*:115, 1978.
160. Samilson RL, Bersani FA, Watkins MB: Acute suppurative arthritis in infants and children: The importance of early diagnosis and surgical drainage. Pediatrics *21*:798, 1958.
161. Ward J, Cohen AS, Bauer W: The diagnosis and therapy of acute suppurative arthritis. Arthritis Rheum *3*:522, 1960.
162. Guiraudon C: Problèmes diagnostiques posés à l'histologiste par les monoarthrites infectieuses. Rev Rhum Mal Osteoartic *39*:787, 1972.
163. Phemister DB: Changes in the articular surfaces in tuberculosis and in pyogenic infections of joints. Am J Roentgenol *12*:1, 1924.
164. Butt WP: Radiology of the infected joint. Clin Orthop Rel Res *96*:136, 1973.
165. Shawker TH, Dennis JM: Periarticular calcifications in pyogenic arthritis. Am J Roentgenol *113*:650, 1971.
166. Kluge RM, Schmidt MC, Barth WF: Pneumococcal arthritis and joint calcification (Abstr). Arthritis Rheum *14*:394, 1971.
167. Bardenheimer JA, Morgan HC, Stamp WG: Treatment and sequelae of experimentally produced septic arthritis. Surg Gynecol Obstet *122*:249, 1966.
168. Clark RL, Cuttino JT Jr, Anderle SK, Cromartie WJ, Schwab JH: Radiologic analysis of arthritis in rats after systemic injection of streptococcal cell walls. Arthritis Rheum *22*:25, 1979.
169. Miller JM, Engle RL Jr: Metastatic suppurative arthritis with subcutaneous emphysema caused by *Escherichia coli*. Am J Med *10*:241, 1951.
170. McNae J: An unusual case of *Clostridium welchii* infection. J Bone Joint Surg *48B*:512, 1966.
171. Torg JS, Lammot TR III: Septic arthritis of the knee due to *Clostridium welchii*. Report of two cases. J Bone Joint Surg *50A*:1233, 1968.
172. Bliznak J, Ramsey J: Emphysematous septic arthritis due to *Escherichia coli*. J Bone Joint Surg *58A*:138, 1976.
173. Ziment I, Davis A, Finegold SM: Joint infection by anaerobic bacteria: A case report and review of the literature. Arthritis Rheum *12*:627, 1969.
174. Meredith HC, Rittenberg GM: Pneumoarthropathy: An unusual radiographic sign of gram negative septic arthritis. Radiology *128*:642, 1978.
175. Morganstern S, Seery W, Borshuk S, Cole AT: Septic arthritis secondary to vesico-acetabular fistula: a case report. J Urol *116*:116, 1976.
176. Chacha PB: Suppurative arthritis of the hip joints in infancy. A persistent diagnostic problem and possible complication of femoral venipuncture. J Bone Joint Surg *53A*:538, 1971.
177. Asnes RS, Arendar GM: Septic arthritis of the hip: A complication of femoral venipuncture. Pediatrics *38*:837, 1966.
178. Samilson RL, Bersani FA, Watkins MB: Acute suppurative arthritis in infants and children. The importance of early diagnoses and surgical drainage. Pediatrics *21*:798, 1958.
179. Morrey BF, Bianco AJ, Rhodes KH: Suppurative arthritis of the hip in children. J Bone Joint Surg *58A*:388, 1976.
180. Glassberg GB, Ozonoff MB: Arthrographic findings in septic arthritis of the hip in infants. Radiology *128*:151, 1978.
181. Eyre-Brook AL: Septic arthritis of the hip and osteomyelitis of the upper end of the femur in infants. J Bone Joint Surg *42B*:11, 1960.
182. Obletz BE: Suppurative arthritis of the hip joint in infants. Clin Orthop Rel Res *22*:27, 1962.
183. Obletz BE: Acute suppurative arthritis of the hip in the neonatal period. J Bone Joint Surg *42A*:23, 1960.
184. Stetson JW, DePonte RJ, Southwick WO: Acute septic arthritis of the hip in children. Clin Orthop Rel Res *56*:105, 1968.
185. Kaye JJ: Bacterial infections of the hips in infancy and childhood. Curr Probl Radiol *3*:17, 1973.
186. Smith T: On the acute arthritis of infants. St Bartholomew's Hosp Rep *10*:189, 1874.
187. Howard PJ: Sepsis in normal and premature infants with localization in the hip joint. Pediatrics *20*:279, 1957.
188. White H: Roentgen findings of acute infectious disease of the hip in infants and children. Clin Orthop Rel Res *22*:34, 1962.
189. Hefke HW, Turner VC: The obturator sign as the earliest roentgenographic sign in the diagnosis of septic arthritis and tuberculosis of the hip. J Bone Joint Surg *24*:857, 1942.
190. Guerra J, Armbuster T, Resnick D, Goergen TG, Feingold ML, Niwayama G, Danzig LA: The adult hip: An anatomic study. Part II: The soft tissue landmarks. Radiology *128*:11, 1978.
191. Chont LK: Roentgen sign of early suppurative arthritis of the hip in infancy. Radiology *38*:708, 1942.
192. Phemister DB: Changes in the articular surfaces in tuberculosis and in pyogenic infections of joints. Am J Roentgenol *12*:1, 1924.
193. Siffert RS: The effect of juxta-epiphyseal pyogenic infection on epiphyseal growth. Clin Orthop Rel Res *10*:131, 1957.

194. McWhorter GL: Operation on the neck of the femur following acute symptoms in a case of osteochondritis deformans juvenilis coxae (Perthes' disease). Surg Gynecol Obstet *38*:632, 1924.
195. Kemp HBS, Lloyd-Roberts GC: Avascular necrosis of the capital epiphysis following osteomyelitis of the proximal femoral metaphysis. J Bone Joint Surg *56B*:688, 1974.
196. Tachdjian MO, Grana L: Response of the hip joint to increased intra-articular hydrostatic pressure. Clin Orthop Rel Res *61*:199, 1968.
197. Kemp HBS: Perthes' disease. An experimental and clinical study. Ann R Coll Surg *52*:18, 1973.
198. Goldenberg DL, Brandt KD, Cathcart ES, Cohen AS: Acute arthritis caused by gram-negative bacilli: A clinical characterization. Medicine *53*:197, 1974.
199. Burton DS, Schurman DJ: Hematogenous infection in bilateral total hip arthroplasty. J Bone Joint Surg *57A*:1004, 1975.
200. Cruess RL, Bickel WS, von Kessler KLC: Infections in total hips secondary to a primary source elsewhere. Clin Orthop Rel Res *106*:99, 1975.
201. Mallory TH: Sepsis in total hip replacement following pneumococcal pneumonia. J Bone Joint Surg *55A*:1753, 1973.
202. Ahlberg A, Carlsson AS, Lindberg L: Hematogenous infection in total joint replacement. Clin Orthop Rel Res *137*:69, 1978.
203. Carlsson AS, Lidgren L, Lindberg L: Prophylactic antibiotics against early and late, deep infections after total hip replacements. Acta Orthop Scand *48*:405, 1977.
204. Good CJ, Jones MA: Posterior rupture of the knee joint in septic arthritis: Case report. Br J Surg *61*:553, 1974.
205. Stewart IM, Swinson DR, Hardinge K: Pyogenic arthritis presenting as a ruptured popliteal cyst. Ann Rheum Dis *38*:181, 1979.
206. Shapiro RF, Resnick D, Castles JJ, D'Ambrosia R, Lipscomb PR, Niwayama G: Fistulization of rheumatoid joints: A spectrum of identifiable syndromes. Ann Rheum Dis *34*:489, 1975.
207. Master R, Weisman MH, Armbuster TG, Slivka J, Resnick D, Goergen TG: Septic arthritis of the glenohumeral joint. Arthritis Rheum *20*:1500, 1977.
208. Armbuster T, Slivka J, Resnick D, Goergen TG, Weisman M, Master R: Extra-articular manifestations of septic arthritis of the glenohumeral joint. Am J Roentgenol *129*:667, 1977.
209. Resnick D: Pyarthrosis complicating rheumatoid arthritis: Report of 5 patients and a review of the literature. Radiology *114*:581, 1975.
210. Altemeier WA: Diagnosis, classification and general management of gas-producing infection, particularly those produced by *Clostridium perfringens*. *In* IW Brown Jr, BG Cox (Eds): Proceedings of the Third International Conference on Hyperbaric Medicine. Duke University, Durham, North Carolina, 1965. Washington DC National Academy of Sciences–National Research Council, 1966, p 481.
211. Bornstein DL, Weinberg AN, Swartz MN, Kunz LJ: Anaerobic infections — review of current experience. Medicine *43*:207, 1964.
212, Fee NF, Dobranski A, Bisla RS: Gas gangrene complicating open forearm fractures. Report of five cases. J Bone Joint Surg *59A*:135, 1977.
213. Angervall L, Stener B, Stener I, Ahren C: Pseudomalignant osseous tumor of soft tissue. J Bone Joint Surg *51B*:654, 1969.
214. Fu FH, Scranton PE Jr: Pseudosarcomatous proliferation of soft tissue secondary to bacterial infection. Orthopedics *1*:474, 1978.
215. Bywaters EGL: The bursae of the body. Ann Rheum Dis *24*:215, 1965.
216. Marchildon A, Slonim RR, Brown HE Jr, Howell DS: Primary septic bursitis. J Fla Med Assoc *50*:139, 1963.
217. Winter FE, Runyon EH: Prepatellar bursitis caused by mycobacterium marinum: Case report, classification, and review of the literature. J Bone Joint Surg *47A*:375, 1965.
218. Ho G Jr, Tice AD, Kaplan SR: Septic bursitis in the prepatellar and olecranon bursae. An analysis of 25 cases. Ann Intern Med *89*:21, 1978.
219. Canoso JJ, Sheckman PR: Septic subcutaneous bursitis. Report of sixteen cases. J Rheumatol *6*:96, 1979.
220. Thompson GR, Manshady BM, Weiss JJ: Septic bursitis. JAMA *240*:2280, 1978.
221. Garcia-Kutzbach A, Masi AT: Acute infectious agent arthritis (IAA): A detailed comparison of proved gonococcal and other blood-borne bacterial arthritis. J Rheumatol *1*:93, 1974.
222. Levinsky WJ: Sporotrichial arthritis. Report of a case mimicking gout. Arch Intern Med *129*:118, 1972.
223. McConville JH, Pototsky RS, Calia FM, Pachas WN: Septic and crystalline joint disease: A simultaneous occurrence. JAMA *231*:841, 1975.
224. Stratton CW, Phelps DB, Reller LB: Tuberculoid tenosynovitis and carpal tunnel syndrome caused by *Mycobacterium szulgai*. Am J Med *65*:349, 1978.
225. Danzig LA, Fierer J: Coccidioidomycosis of the extensor tenosynovium of the wrist. A case report. Clin Orthop Rel Res *129*:245, 1977.
226. Iverson RE, Vistnes LM: Coccidioidomycosis tenosynovitis in the hand. J Bone Joint Surg *55A*:413, 1973.
227. Vass M, Kulmann L, Csoka, R, Magyar, E: Polytenosynovitis caused by *Toxoplasma gondii*. J Bone Joint Surg *59B*:229, 1977.
228. Currarino G: Acute epitrochlear lymphadenitis. Pediatr Radiol *6*:160, 1977.
229. Letts RM, Sutherland JB: Technetium bone scanning as an aid in the diagnosis of atypical acute osteomyelitis in children. Surg Gynecol Obstet *140*:899, 1975.
230. Handmaker H, Leonards R: The bone scan in inflammatory osseous disease. Semin Nucl Med *6*:95, 1976.
231. Teates CD, Williamson BRJ: "Hot and cold" bone lesion in acute osteomyelitis. Am J Roentgenol *129*:517, 1977.
232. Garnett ES, Cockshott WP, Jacobs J: Classical acute osteomyelitis with a negative bone scan. Br J Radiol *50*:757, 1977.
233. Majd M: Radionuclide imaging in early detection of childhood osteomyelitis and its differentiation from cellulitis and bone infarction. Ann Radiol *20*:9, 1977.
234. Treves S, Khettry J, Broker FH, Wilkinson RH, Watts H: Osteomyelitis: Early scintigraphic detection in children. Pediatrics *57*:173, 1976.
235. Kolyvas E, Rosenthall, L, Ahronheim GA, Lisbona R, Marks MI: Serial ^{67}Ga-citrate imaging during treatment of acute osteomyelitis in childhood. Clin Nucl Med *3*:461, 1978.
236. Feigin DS, Strauss HW, James AE Jr: The bone marrow scan in experimental osteomyelitis. Skel Radiol *1*:103, 1976.
237. Smith PW, Petersen RJ, Ferlic RM: Gallium scan in sternal osteomyelitis. Am J Roentgenol *132*:840, 1979.
238. Lisbona R, Rosenthall L: Observations on the sequential use of ^{99m}Tc-phosphate complex and ^{67}Ga imaging in osteomyelitis, cellulitis and septic arthritis. Radiology *123*:123, 1977.
239. Atcheson SG, Coleman RE, Ward JR: Septic arthritis mimicking cellulitis: Distinction using radionuclide bone imaging. Clin Nucl Med *4*:79, 1979.
240. Lisbona R, Rosenthall L: Radionuclide imaging of septic joints and their differentiation from periarticular osteomyelitis and cellulitis in pediatrics. Clin Nucl Med *2*:337, 1977.
241. Hayes RL, Nelson B, Swartzendruber DC, Brown DH, Carlton JE, Byrd BL: Studies of the intra-cellular deposition of ^{67}Ga (Abstr). J Nucl Med *12*:364, 1971.
242. Swartzendruber DC, Nelson B, Hayes RL: Gallium-67 localization in lysosomal-like granules of leukemic and nonleukemic murine tissues. J Natl Cancer Inst *46*:941, 1971.
243. Gilday DL, Paul DJ: The differentiation of osteomyelitis and cellulitis in children using a combined blood pool and bone scan (Abstr). J Nucl Med *15*:494, 1974.
244. Gilday DL, Paul DJ, Paterson J: Diagnosis of osteomyelitis in children by combined blood pool and bone imaging. Radiology *117*:331, 1975.
245. Alavi A, Bond JP, Kuhl DE, Creech RH: Scan detection of bone marrow infarcts in sickle cell disorders. J Nucl Med *15*:1003, 1974.
246. Kuhn JP, Berger PE: Computed tomographic diagnosis of osteomyelitis. Radiology *130*:503, 1979.
247. Good RA, Quie PG, Windhorst DB, Page AR, Rodey GE, White J, Wolfson JJ, Holmes BB: Fatal (chronic) granulomatous disease of childhood: A hereditary defect of leukocyte function. Semin Hematol *5*:215, 1968.
248. Berendes H, Bridges RA, Good RA: A fatal granulomatosis of childhood. The clinical studies of a new syndrome. Minn Med *40*:309, 1957.
249. Landing BH, Shirkey HS: A syndrome of recurrent infection and infiltration of viscera by pigmented lipid histiocytes. Pediatrics *20*:431, 1957.
250. Holmes B, Quie PG, Windhorst DB, Good RA: Fatal granulomatous disease of childhood: An inborn abnormality of phagocytic function. Lancet *1*:1225, 1966.
251. Quie PG, Kaplan EL, Page AR, Gruskay FL, Malawista SE: Defective polymorphonuclear-leukocyte function and chronic granulomatous disease in two female children. N Engl J Med *278*:976, 1968.
252. Holmes B, Page AR, Windhorst DB, Quie PG, White JG, Good RA: The metabolic pattern and phagocytic function of leukocytes from children with chronic granulomatous disease. Ann NY Acad Sci *155*:888, 1968.
253. Quie PG, White JG, Holmes B, Good RA: In vitro bactericidal capacity of human polymorphonuclear leukocytes: Diminished activity in chronic granulomatous disease of childhood. J Clin Invest *46*:668, 1967.
254. Bridges RA, Berendes H, Good RA: A fatal granulomatous disease of childhood. Am J Dis Child *97*:387, 1959.
255. Carson MJ, Chadwick DL, Brubaker CA, Cleland RS, Landing BH: Thirteen boys with progressive septic granulomatosis. Pediatrics *35*:405, 1965.

256. Wolfson JJ, Kane WJ, Laxdal SD, Good RA, Quie PG: Bone findings in chronic granulomatous disease of childhood. A genetic abnormality of leukocyte function. J Bone Joint Surg *51A*:1573, 1969.
257. Renton P, Webster ADB: Case report 70. Skel Radiol *3*:131, 1978.
258. Giedion A, Holthusen W, Masel LF, Vischer D: Subacute and chronic symmetrical osteomyelitis. Ann Radiol *15*:329, 1972.
259. Probst FP: Chronic multifocal cleido-metaphyseal osteomyelitis of childhood. Report of a case. Acta Radiol (Diagn) *17*:531, 1976.
260. Gustavson K-H, Wilbrand HF: Chronic symmetric osteomyelitis. Report of a case. Acta Radiol *15*:551, 1974.
261. Willert H-G, Enderle A: Multifocale, symmetrische, chronische osteomyelitis. Acta Orthop Unfallchir *89*:109, 1977.
262. Exner GU: Die plasmacelluläre Osteomyelitis. Langenbecks Arch Chir *326*:165, 1970.
263. Louria DB, Hensle T, Rose J: The major medical complications of heroin addiction. Ann Intern Med *67*:1, 1967.
264. Cherubin CE: The medical sequelae of narcotic addiction. Ann Intern Med *67*:23, 1967.
265. Krueger H, Eddy NB, Sumwalt M: The Pharmacology of the Opium Alkaloids. Part I. Washington DC Government Printing Office, 1941, p 426.
266. Arkin A: The influence of strychnin, caffein, chloral, antipyrin, cholesterol, and lactic acid on phagocytosis. J Infect Dis *13*:408, 1913.
267. Nickerson DS, Williams RC, Boxmeyer M, Quie PG: Increased opsonic capacity of serum in chronic heroin addiction. Ann Intern Med *72*:671, 1970.
268. Goldwin RH, Chow AW, Edwards JE Jr, Louie JS, Guze LB: Sternoarticular septic arthritis in heroin users. N Engl J Med *289*:616, 1973.
269. Salahuddin NI, Madhavan T, Fisher EJ, Cox F, Quinn EL, Eyler WR: Pseudomonas osteomyelitis. Radiologic features. Radiology *109*:41, 1973.
270. Gifford DB, Patzakis M, Ivler D, Swezey RL: Septic arthritis due to pseudomonas in heroin addicts. J Bone Joint Surg *57A*:631, 1975.
271. Wiesseman GJ, Wood VE, Kroll LL: Pseudomonas vertebral osteomyelitis in heroin addicts. Report of five cases. J Bone Joint Surg *55A*:1416, 1973.
272. Kido D, Bryan D, Halpern M: Hematogenous osteomyelitis in drug addicts. Am J Roentgenol *118*:356, 1973.
273. Ross GN, Baraff LJ, Quismorio FP: Serratia arthritis in heroin users. J Bone Joint Surg *57A*:1158, 1975.
274. Donovan TL, Chapman MW, Harrington KD, Nagel DA: Serratia arthritis. Report of seven cases. J Bone Joint Surg *58A*:1009, 1976.
275. Holzman RS, Bishko F: Osteomyelitis in heroin addicts. Ann Intern Med *75*:693, 1971.
276. Lewis R, Gorbach S, Altner P: Spinal pseudomonas chondro-osteomyelitis in heroin users. N Engl J Med *286*:1303, 1972.
277. Tuazon CU, Sheagren JN: Increased rate of carriage of *Staphylococcus aureus* among narcotic addicts. J Infect Dis *129*:725, 1974.
278. Tuazon CU, Hill R, Sheagren JN: Microbiologic study of street heroin and injection paraphernalia. J Infect Dis *129*:327, 1974.
279. Scott JE, Harrison DH: Septic arthritis in association with primary lymphoedema. Acta Orthop Scand *47*:676, 1976.
280. Kirkpatrick JA, Capitanio MA, Pereira RM: Immunologic abnormalities: Roentgen observations. Radiol Clin North Am *10*:245, 1972.
281. Miller WB, Murphy WA, Gilula LA: Brodie abscess: Reappraisal. Radiology *132*:15, 1979.
282. Fowles JV, Lehoux J, Zlitni M, Kassab MT, Nolan B: Tibial defect due to acute haematogenous osteomyelitis. Treatment and results in twenty-one children. J Bone Joint Surg *61B*:77, 1979.
283. Terho P, Viikari J, Makela P, Toivanen A: Ruptured bilateral synovial cysts in presumed gonococcal arthritis. Sex Trans Dis *4*:100, 1977.
284. Brower AC, Sweet DE, Keats TE: Condensing osteitis of the clavicle: A new entity. Am J Roentgenol *121*:17, 1974.
285. Kohler H, Uehlinger E, Kutzner J, West TB: Sternocostoclavicular hyperostosis: Painful swelling of the sternum, clavicles, and upper ribs. Ann Intern Med *87*:192, 1977.
286. Canoso JJ, Yood RA: Reaction of superficial bursae in response to specific disease stimuli. Arthritis Rheum *22*:1361, 1979.
287. Rabe WC, Angelillo JC, Leipert DW: Chronic sclerosing osteomyelitis: Treatment considerations in an atypical case. Oral Surg *49*:117, 1980.
288. Memon IA, Jacobs NM, Yeh TF, Lilien LD: Group B streptococcal osteomyelitis and septic arthritis. Its occurrence in infants less than 2 months old. Am J Dis Child *133*:921, 1979.
289. Chilton SJ, Aftimos SF, White PR: Diffuse skeletal involvement of streptococcal osteomyelitis in a neonate. Radiology *134*:390, 1980.
290. Trias A, Fery A: Cortical circulation of long bones. J Bone Joint Surg *61A*:1052, 1979.
291. Petersen S, Knudsen FU, Andersen EA, Egeblad M: Acute haematogenous osteomyelitis and septic arthritis in childhood. A 10-year review and follow-up. Acta Orthop Scand *51*:451, 1980.
292. Green NE, Bruno J III: Pseudomonas infections of the foot after puncture wounds. South Med J *73*:146, 1980.
293. Peeples E, Boswick JA Jr, Scott FA: Wounds of the hand contaminated by human or animal saliva. J Trauma *20*:383, 1980.
294. Pinckney LE, Kennedy LA: Fractures of the infant skull caused by animal bites. Am J Roentgenol *135*:197, 1980.
295. Pinckney LE, Currarino G, Highgenboten CL: Osteomyelitis of the cervical spine following dental extraction. Radiology *135*:335, 1980.
296. Sharp JT, Lidsky MD, Duffy J, Duncan MW: Infectious arthritis. Arch Intern Med *139*:1125, 1979.
297. Cooke CP III, Levinsohn EM, Baker BE: Septic hip in pelvic fractures with urologic injury. Clin Orthop Rel Res *147*:253, 1980.
298. Hayden CK Jr, Swischuk LE: Paraarticular soft-tissue changes in infections and trauma of the lower extremity in children. Am J Roentgenol *134*:307, 1980.
299. Wood BP: The vanishing epiphyseal ossification center: A sequel to septic arthritis of childhood. Radiology *134*:387, 1980.
300. Wofsy D: Culture negative septic arthritis and bacterial endocarditis. Diagnosis by synovial biopsy. Arthritis Rheum *23*:605, 1980.
301. Bywaters EGL: Lesions of bursae, tendons, and tendon sheaths. Clinics Rheum Dis *5*:883, 1979.
302. Ho G Jr, Tice AD: Comparison of nonseptic and septic bursitis. Arch Intern Med *139*:1269, 1979.
303. Brock JG, Meredith HC: Case report 102. Skel Radiol *4*:236, 1979.
304. Nicholl EDV, Foster EA: Granulomatous tenosynovitis due to beryllium. J Bone Joint Surg *42A*:1087, 1966.
305. Kelly JJ: Blackthorn inflammation. J Bone Joint Surg *48B*:474, 1966.
306. Solheim LF, Paus B, Liverud K, Stoen E: Chronic recurrent multifocal osteomyelitis. Acta Orthop Scand *51*:37, 1980.
307. Bjorkstén B: Histopathological aspects of chronic recurrent multifocal osteomyelitis. J Bone Joint Surg *62B*:376, 1980.
308. Yarchoan R, Davies SF, Fried J, Mahowald ML: Isolated *Candida parapsilos* arthritis in a heroin addict. J Rheumatol *6*:447, 1979.
309. Roca RP, Yoshikawa TT: Primary skeletal infections in heroin users. Clin Orthop Rel Res *144*:238, 1979.
310. Metges PJ, Silici R, Kleitz C, Delahaye RP, Mine J, Pailler JL: La fistulographie. A propos de 126 éxamens. J Radiol *61*:57, 1980.
311. Halpern AA, Hasson N, Javier M: Septicemia following sinogram. Clin Orthop Rel Res *145*:187, 1979.
312. Gelberman RH, Menon J, Austerlitz MS, Weisman MH: Pyogenic arthritis of the shoulder in adults. J Bone Joint Surg *62A*:550, 1980.
313. Hofer P: Gallium: Mechanisms. J Nucl Med *21*:282, 1980.
314. Hofer P: Gallium and infection. J Nucl Med *21*:484, 1980.
315. Gilday DL: Problems in the scintigraphic detection of osteomyelitis. Radiology *135*:791, 1980.
316. Sullivan DC, Rosenfield NS, Ogden J, Gottschalk A: Problems in the scintigraphic detection of osteomyelitis in children. Radiology *135*:731, 1980.
317. Handmaker H: Acute hematogenous osteomyelitis: Has the bone scan betrayed us? Radiology *135*:787, 1980.
318. Murray IPC: Bone scanning in the child and young adult. Skel Radiol *5*:65, 1980.
319. Ralls PW, Boswell W, Henderson R, Rogers W, Boger D, Halls J: CT of inflammatory disease of the psoas muscle. Am J Roentgenol *134*:767, 1980.
320. Sequeira FW, Smith WL: Seldinger sinography. Radiology *137*:238, 1980.
321. Atdjian M, Granda JL, Ingberg HO, Kaplan BL: Systemic sporotrichosis polytenosynovitis with median and ulnar nerve entrapment. JAMA *243*:1841, 1980.
322. Viggiano DA, Garrett JC, Clayton ML: Septic arthritis presenting as olecranon bursitis in patients with rheumatoid arthritis. J Bone Joint Surg *62A*:1011, 1980.
323. Ahbel DE, Alexander AH, Kleine ML, Lichtman DM: Prothecal olecranon bursitis. J Bone Joint Surg *62A*:835, 1980.
324. Dias L, Tachdjian MO, Schroeder KE: Premature closure of the triradiate cartilage. J Bone Joint Surg *62B*:46, 1980.
325. Carandell M, Roig D, Benasco C: Plant thorn synovitis. J Rheumatol *7*:567, 1980.

OSTEOMYELITIS, SEPTIC ARTHRITIS, AND SOFT TISSUE INFECTION: THE AXIAL SKELETON

by Donald Resnick, M.D., and Gen Niwayama, M.D.

61

The distribution of osteomyelitis and septic arthritis is dramatically influenced by the age of the patient, the specific causative organism, and the presence or absence of any underlying disorder or situation. In the child and the infant, frequent involvement of the bones and the joints of the appendicular skeleton is evident, whereas in the adult, localization of infection to the osseous and articular structures of the vertebral column is common. Pyogenic organisms can affect axial or extra-axial sites, and are commonly implicated in hematogenous osteomyelitis of the tubular bones in children and infants. Tuberculous organisms can also select appendicular or axial skeletal sites, although the occurrence of tuberculous spondylitis is especially well known. In specific circumstances, infection may also show predilection for specific musculoskeletal locations. Examples of such predilection include osteomyelitis and septic arthritis of the spine and the sacroiliac and sternoclavicular articulations in the drug addict, of the foot in the diabetic patient, of the diaphyses of tubular bones in individuals with sickle cell anemia, and of altered articular sites in various arthritides.

Chapter 60 has described in detail the mechanism and the pathogenesis of bone and joint infection in various age groups and situations and has emphasized alterations of the appendicular skeleton. This chapter will delineate the radiographic and pathologic characteristics of infection in important axial skeletal locations, especially the spine and the sacroiliac articulation.

SPINAL INFECTIONS

Routes of Contamination

Hematogenous Spread of Infection. Organisms may reach the vertebrae in several fashions.[1,2] Hematogenous spread via arterial and venous routes (Batson's paravertebral venous system) can result in lodgment of organisms in the bone marrow of the vertebrae.[3-8] The basic arrangement of the nutrient vessels is similar in the cervical, the thoracic, and the lumbar spine; a vertebral, intercostal, or a lumbar artery lying closely apposed to the vertebral body supplies minute vessels to the nearby bone, which penetrate the cortex and ramify within the marrow.[9] In addition, at each intervertebral foramen, a posterior spinal branch enters the vertebral canal and divides into an ascending and a descending branch, which anastomose with similar branches from the segments above and below and from the other side, creating an arterial network on the dorsal or posterior surface of each vertebral body.[9] Three or four nutrient arteries are derived from this network and enter the vertebral body through a large dorsal, centrally placed nutrient foramen.

The venous drainage of the vertebral body is tree-like in configuration. Minute tributaries drain from the peripheral portion of the vertebral body to its center, the blood being collected by a large valveless venous channel that emerges from the central dorsal nutrient foramen and drains into an extensive loose plexus lining the vertebral canal.[9] The branching tributaries of the vertebral body are connected by channels that perforate the cortex and enter veins lying on the lateral and anterior surfaces of the vertebrae. This represents the paraspinal and spinal venous plexus of Batson. Within the vertebral body, the ramification of blood vessels at the subchondral superior and inferior limits is reminiscent of the vascular arrangement in the childhood metaphysis and adulthood epiphysis of tubular bones.

This vascular arrangement allows two direct routes for the hematogenous spread of infection: via the nutrient arteries and via the paravertebral venous system. Although the contribution of each system to cases of spinal osteomyelitis is a matter of debate, it is attractive to implicate the valveless venous plexus, whose direction and extent of flow are dramatically influenced by changes in abdominal pressure, in the frequent spread of infection (and neoplasm) to the spine from pelvic sources[10] (Fig. 61–1). Urinary tract infections or surgery,[11-17] rectosigmoid disease and enteric fistulae[18,19] and septic abortion or post-

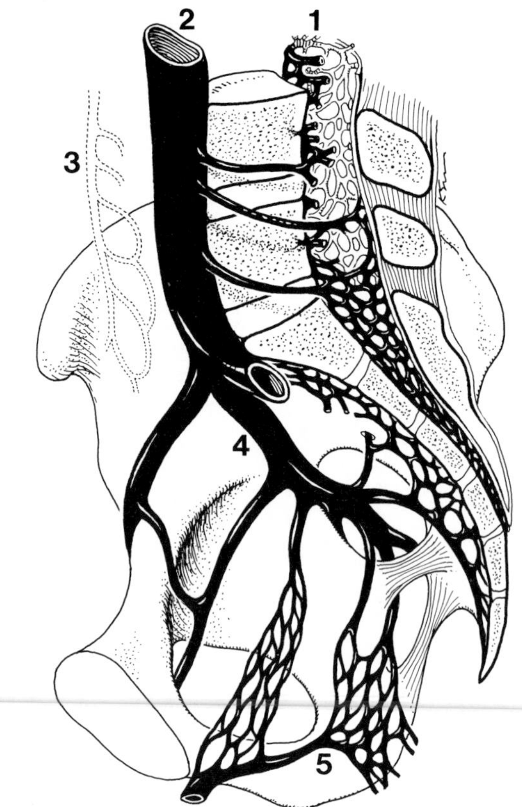

Figure 61–1. Anatomic considerations: Batson's paravertebral venous system. This valveless plexiform set of veins lies outside the thoracoabdominal cavity, anastomosing with the cavitary veins at each segmental level. Thus, communication exists between the pelvic and vertebral venous system, femoral and iliac veins, inferior vena cava and superior vena cava, as well as other important venous structures. 1, Paravertebral venous plexus; 2, inferior vena cava; 3, inferior mesenteric vein; 4, internal iliac vein; 5, pelvic plexus. (After Vider M, et al: Cancer 40:67, 1977.)

partum infection[20] are well recognized pelvic precursors of vertebral osteomyelitis (Fig. 61–2). Although experimental evidence can be found documenting the spread of malignant disease from the pelvic veins into the vertebral bodies through the paravertebral plexus,[21] the evidence is less decisive in cases of infectious diseases,[22,23] suggesting to some investigators[9] that the role of Batson's plexus in the dissemination of infectious disease has been greatly exaggerated. In addition, the common localization of early foci of osteomyelitis in the subchondral region of the vertebral body, an area richly supplied by nutrient arterioles, emphasizes that arterial rather than venous pathways may be more important in hematogenous osteomyelitis of the spine, a concept that is further underscored by the distribution of infection along the route of the ascending and descending nutrient branches of the posterior spinal arteries, the presence of prodromal findings consistent with septicemia in cases with vertebral osteomyelitis, and the absence of pathologic documentation of a spreading extradural thrombophlebitis in

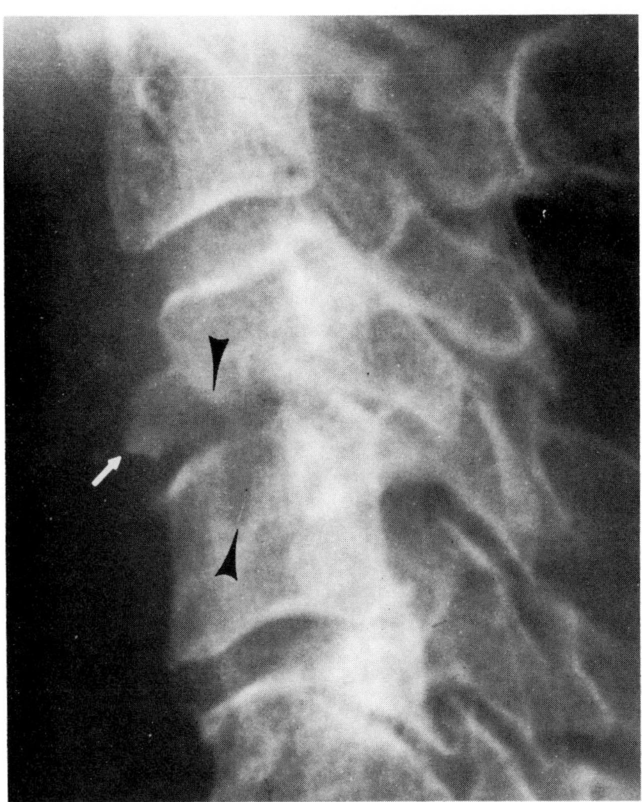

Figure 61–2. Spinal infection: Hematogenous spread. This 54 year old diabetic man developed emphysematous pyelonephritis and cystitis with septicemia and progressive neck pain (causative microorganism is Escherichia coli). Note the destructive foci in the third and fourth cervical vertebrae (arrowheads) and loss in height of the intervening intervertebral disc space. The anteriorly located ledge of bone (arrow) may represent a preexisting osteophyte that is now infected. Soft tissue swelling is also evident along the anterior aspect of the spine.

these cases.[9] Thus, in many examples of pelvic and extrapelvic infection complicated by spinal contamination, the arterial hematogenous route may be the real pathway of sepsis.

The role of hematogenous spread of infection directly into the intervertebral disc has stimulated great interest. It has been suggested that in children below the age of 18 to 20 years, vascular channels perforate the vertebral end-plate,[24] allowing organisms in the bloodstream to have direct access to the intervertebral disc.[25] This concent has led to the popular terms of "discitis,"[26] spondylarthritis,[26-28] intervertebral disc space infection[29-31] or inflammation,[32, 33] benign osteomyelitis of the spine, nonspecific spondylitis,[34, 35] and pyogenic vertebral osteomyelitis[36] that are applied to such infection.[37] A similar occurrence in adults[38] has been attributed to a persistent discal blood supply[39] or to a supply that has been reinstated by vascular invasion of degenerating discal tissue. Because of the great interest in "discitis" that has been sparked by a most heated debate, this condition is discussed separately in a later portion of the chapter.

Spread from a Contiguous Source of Infection. Vertebral or intervertebral discal infection can result from contamination by an adjacent soft tissue suppurative focus[40] (Fig. 61–3). This mechanism is not common, as many paravertebral abscesses dissect away from the spine along normal and abnormal soft tissue planes. Even in those cases in which bone or cartilage involvement follows soft tissue infection, it is extremely difficult to eliminate the possibility that osteomyelitis or discal infection does not result from hematogenous or lymphatic seeding. Tuberculous and fungal infection can, however, extend from the spine to the neighboring tissue, dissect along the subligamentous areas for a considerable distance, and then reenter the vertebral body or intervertebral disc. In cases of osteomyelitis and discal infection resulting from contamination due to a contiguous suppurative focus, soft tissue abnormalities are followed by sequential invasion of the periosteum, cortex, and marrow of the vertebrae or of the ligaments, anulus fibrosus, and nucleus pulposus of the intervertebral disc.

Direct Implantation of Infection. Organisms can be implanted directly into the intervertebral disc (and far less commonly the vertebra) during attempted punctures of the spinal canal, paravertebral and peridural tissues, or aorta[41] or in penetrating injuries. Usually the intervertebral disc is the initial site of infection, especially in cases of misguided puncture, and the vertebra becomes contaminated as a secondary event. Following inadvertent administration of a paravertebral anesthetic into the intervertebral disc, discal narrowing can occasionally represent not an infection but, perhaps, a chemical destruction of tissue.[42]

Postoperative Infection. The more frequent and aggressive spinal operations that are currently undertaken have led to an increase in postoperative infection of the spinal column. Laminectomy, diskectomy, instrumentation, and fusion can each be complicated by osteomyelitis or discal infection[43-46] (Fig. 61–4). The localization of osseous or articular contamination depends upon the precipitating surgical event; infection may involve the vertebral body, the posterior elements, the intervertebral disc, or even the spinal canal (see Chapter 14) in any region of the vertebral column.

Clinical Abnormalities

The clinical abnormalities of spinal infection depend upon the site and extent of involvement and the specific organisms that are implicated. Most of the following observations concern pyogenic infections of the spine.[1, 2, 47-58, 103]

With increasing interest and the development of more sophisticated diagnostic techniques, the re-

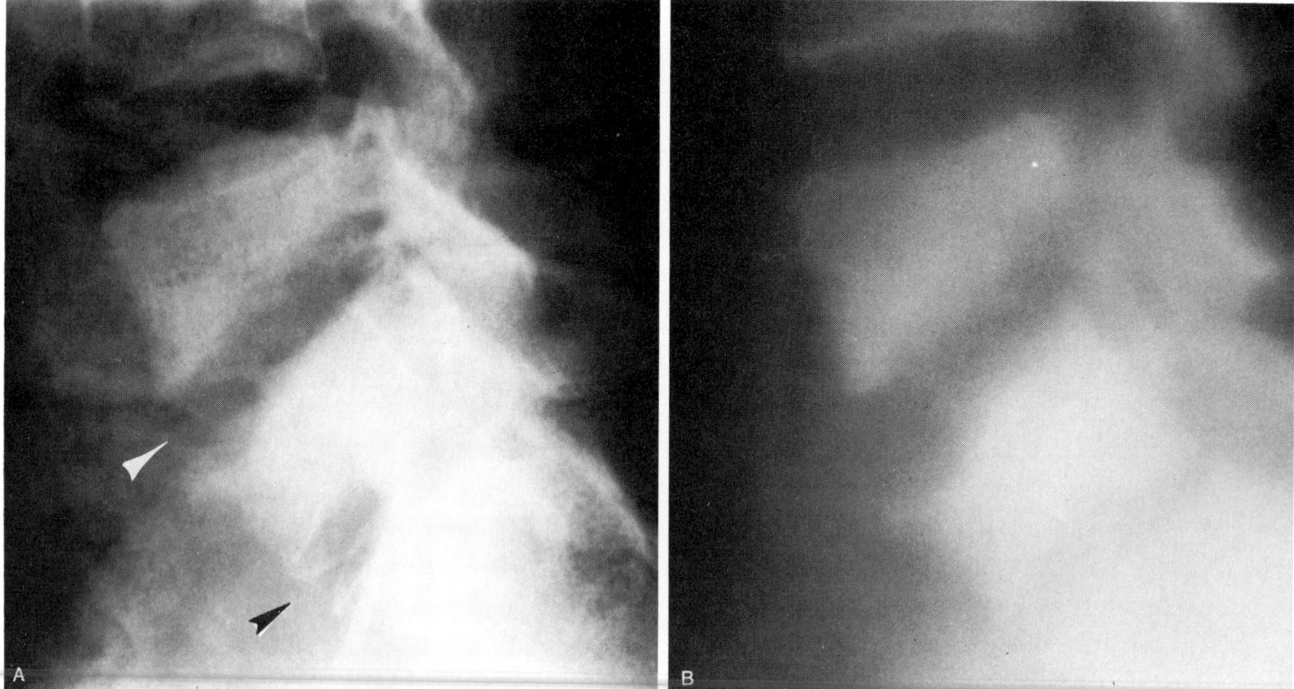

Figure 61–3. *Spinal infection: Spread from a contiguous contaminated source versus hematogenous spread. A 30 year old man developed a buttock abscess complicated by peripelvic abscess formation and osteomyelitis (causative microorganisms were mixed gram-positive and gram-negative bacteria).*

A *An initial radiograph reveals considerable destruction of the fourth and fifth lumbar vertebral bodies and, possibly, the superior surface of the sacrum with involvement of two intervening disc spaces (arrowheads).*

B *On a lateral tomogram, the osseous destruction and surrounding sclerosis are readily apparent.*

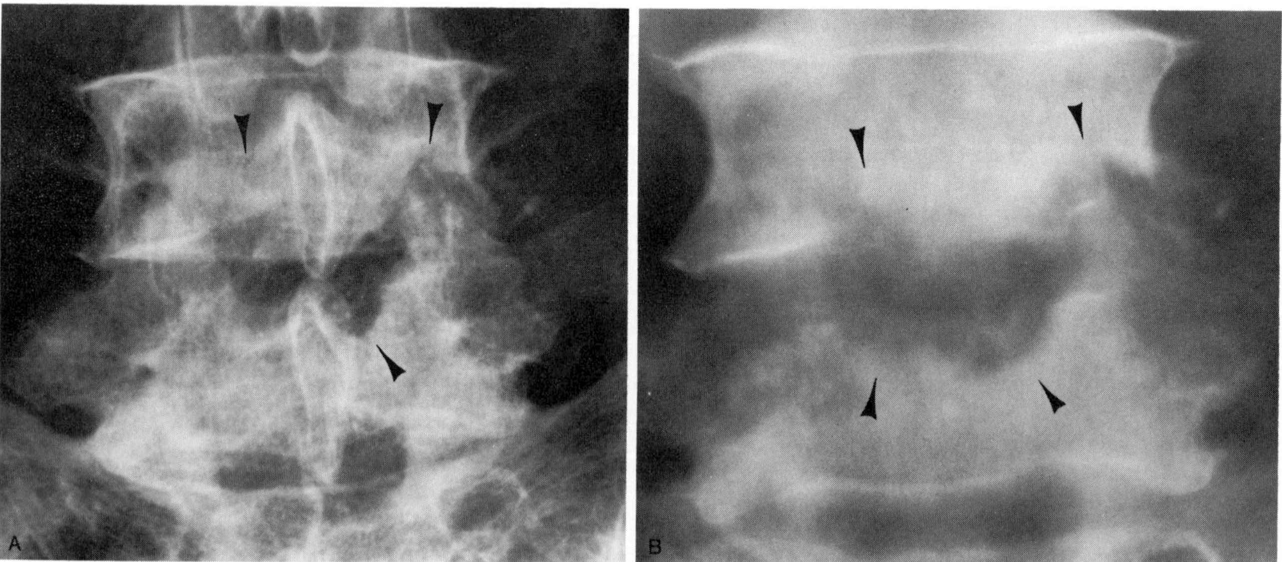

Figure 61–4. *Spinal infection: Postoperative contamination. This 71 year old man developed the onset of back and gluteal pain following a recent laminectomy. A subsequent biopsy demonstrated necrotic osseous and fibrous tissue with acute and chronic inflammatory cellular infiltration.*

A *An anteroposterior radiograph delineates destruction of apposing margins of the fourth and fifth lumbar vertebrae (arrowheads) with narrowing of the intervening disc space.*

B *Frontal tomography confirms the extent of the vertebral destruction with surrounding sclerosis (arrowheads).*

ported incidence of osteomyelitis and disc space infection (together these will be termed infective spondylitis) has risen dramatically. Initially it was suggested that infective spondylitis represented less than 1 per cent of all cases of osteomyelitis[59]; now it appears that 2 to 4 per cent is a more accurate estimation.[2, 6, 47, 60] This incidence rises rapidly in patients with pelvic infection and in those who are debilitated or who have other predisposing factors. Men are more commonly affected than women by a ratio of 1.5 to 3:1. The highest incidence of septic spondylitis occurs in the fifth and sixth decades of life, although infants, children, and elderly individuals are also affected.[53, 55, 61-63] The lumbar spine is the most typical site of involvement, followed by the thoracic spine, with sacral and cervical abnormalities about equal in frequency.[64] The usual location of infection in the vertebra is the vertebral body.[2, 54] However, alterations in the posterior elements and in unusual sites such as the odontoid process are certainly encountered.[2, 65-68]

A history of recent primary infection (urinary tract, respiratory, or skin infection), instrumentation (catheterization, cystoscopy), and diagnostic or surgical procedure (myelography, discography, bowel, urinary, or back operations) is common.[47] The most frequently encountered (80 to 90 per cent) pyogenic organism is *Staphylococcus aureus*, although other gram-positive (Streptococcus, Pneumococcus) and, less typically, gram-negative (*Escherichia coli*, Pseudomonas, Klebsiella, and Salmonella) agents may be implicated. Nonpyogenic organisms accounting for infective spondylitis include tuberculosis, syphilis, and various fungi.[1]

Clinical manifestations vary with the virulence of the organisms and the nature of the host resistance. General findings include fever, malaise, anorexia, and weight loss. Back pain is a common initial local manifestation and may be intermittent or constant, exacerbated by motion and throbbing at rest. It may have a radicular distribution. Spinal tenderness and rigidity may also be observed. With accompanying soft tissue abscess formation, hip contracture can occur (psoas muscle irritation).[2] Paraplegia, which can be reversible with appropriate antibiotic therapy, is evident in less than 1 per cent of cases.[47]

The erythrocyte sedimentation rate is almost universally elevated. Evaluation of the peripheral blood can reveal a normal or elevated leukocyte count. Appropriate culture of the blood can identify the causative organism in some cases, although more drastic methods, such as needle biopsy or aspiration, may be necessary.

Clinical diagnosis may be especially difficult in three situations[47]: Following surgical removal of a herniated intervertebral disc, the postoperative manifestations may mask the symptoms and signs of infection; in young children, absence of local manifestations can be misleading; and in the drug abuser, extraspinal abnormalities may overshadow the vertebral alterations.

Radiographic–Pathologic Correlation

Early Abnormalities. Hematogenous spread of infection frequently leads to a focus in the anterior subchondral regions of the vertebral body adjacent to the intervertebral disc (Fig. 61–5). Extension to the ventral surface of the vertebra can be associated with infection of the adjacent longitudinal ligaments[1] but more typically, discal perforation soon ensues. At this stage, radiographs may be entirely normal. Soon (1 to 3 weeks), however, a decrease in height of the intervertebral disc is accompanied by loss of normal definition of the subchondral bone plate and enlarging destructive foci within the neighboring vertebral body (Fig. 61–6). The combination of rapid loss of intervertebral disc

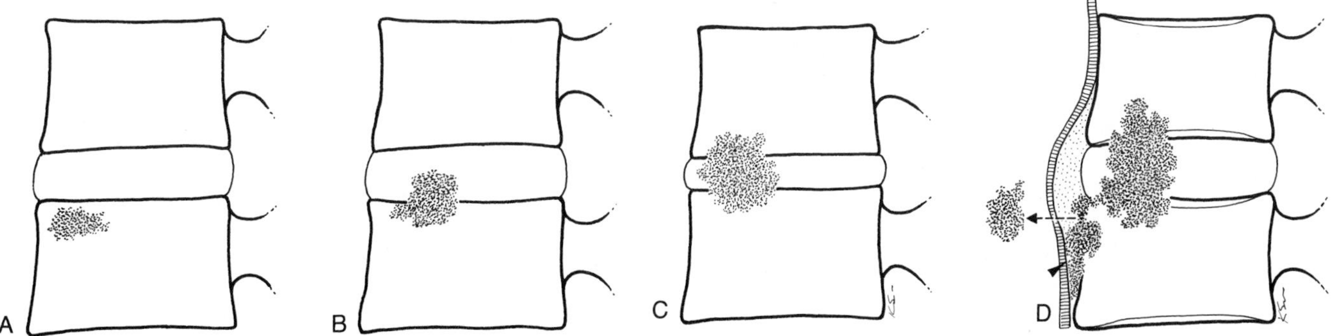

Figure 61–5. *Spinal infection: Sequential stages.*

A *An anterior subchondral focus in the vertebral body is typical.*

B *Infection may then perforate the vertebral surface, reaching the intervertebral disc space.*

C *With further spread of infection, contamination of the adjacent vertebral body and narrowing of the intervertebral disc space are recognizable.*

D *With continued dissemination, infection may spread in a subligamentous fashion, eroding the anterior surface of the vertebral body (arrowhead), or perforating the anterior ligamentous structures (arrow).*

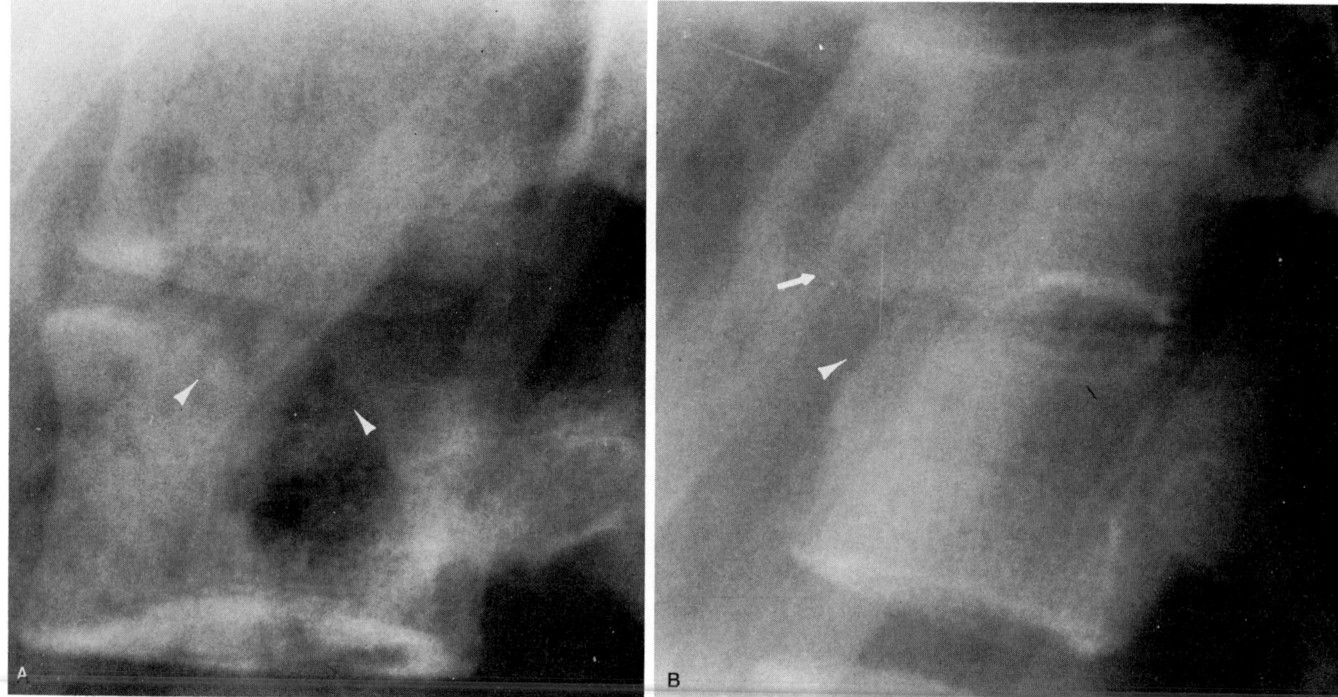

Figure 61–6. *Spinal infection: Early radiographic abnormalities.*

A *Observe loss of definition of the superior aspect of a lumbar vertebral body (arrowheads) with narrowing of the adjacent intervertebral disc space. This appearance (in a middle-aged man with pyogenic infection) conforms to the stage in Figure 61–5***B.**

B *Note the osseous destruction of the anterior aspect of the first lumbar vertebral body (arrowhead) and considerable narrowing of the intervertebral disc space. The adjacent vertebral body is osteoporotic and its anteroinferior cortex is indistinct (arrow). This appearance (in a young male drug addict with pyogenic infection) corresponds to the stage in Figure 61–5***C.**

height and adjacent lysis of bone is most suggestive of an infectious process. With further spread of infection, progressive destruction of the vertebral body and the intervertebral disc becomes evident, and the process soon contaminates the adjacent vertebra.[50] Such involvement of two contiguous vertebral bodies is almost uniformly associated with transdiscal infection and is rarely the result of multicentric involvement.[47] In a series of 150 patients with infective spondylitis, approximately two thirds had infection limited to the disc space and two vertebral bodies, 23 per cent had changes at more than one level, and in less than 1 per cent the changes were isolated to a single intervertebral disc and a single vertebral body.[50]

Later Abnormalities. After a variable period (10 to 12 weeks), regenerative changes appear in the bone with sclerosis or eburnation[50] (Fig. 61–7). The osteosclerotic response is variable in severity, and has been used in the past as a helpful sign in differentiating pyogenic from tuberculous infection.[69] Although such sclerosis is indeed common in pyogenic (nontuberculous) spondylitis,[54] it may also be evident in tuberculosis, particularly in black patients.[70, 71] Furthermore, some individuals with pyogenic spinal infection do not reveal significant eburnation, particularly when symptoms and signs have not been of long duration, so that utilizing the presence or absence of bony sclerosis as a foolproof way of differentiating tuberculous and nontuberculous spondylitis can lead to an erroneous diagnosis. More helpful in this differentiation is a combination of findings that strongly indicates tuberculous spondylitis, including the presence of a slowly progressive vertebral process with preservation of intervertebral discs, large and calcified soft tissue abscesses, and the absence of severe bony eburnation.

Soft tissue extension of infection can be observed in approximately 20 per cent of cases of pyogenic spondylitis.[47] In the lumbar spine, such extension can lead to obliteration or displacement of the psoas margin; in the thoracic spine, a paraspinal mass can be encountered; and in the cervical spine, retropharyngeal swelling can lead to displacement and obliteration of adjacent prevertebral fat planes[25, 50, 54] (Fig. 61–8).

With early and proper treatment, reconstitution can result, with production of a radiodense (ivory) vertebra, a relatively intact or ankylosed intervertebral disc, and surrounding osteophytosis[50, 72-74] (Fig. 61–9). Without such treatment, complete bony lysis and collapse, discal obliteration, deviation and deformity of the vertebral column (Fig. 61–10), and massive soft tissue abscesses which ascend or de-

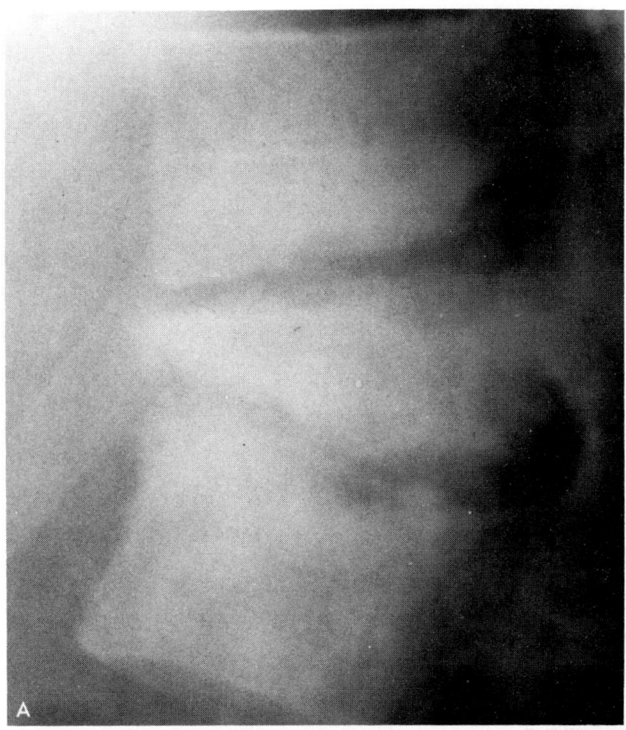

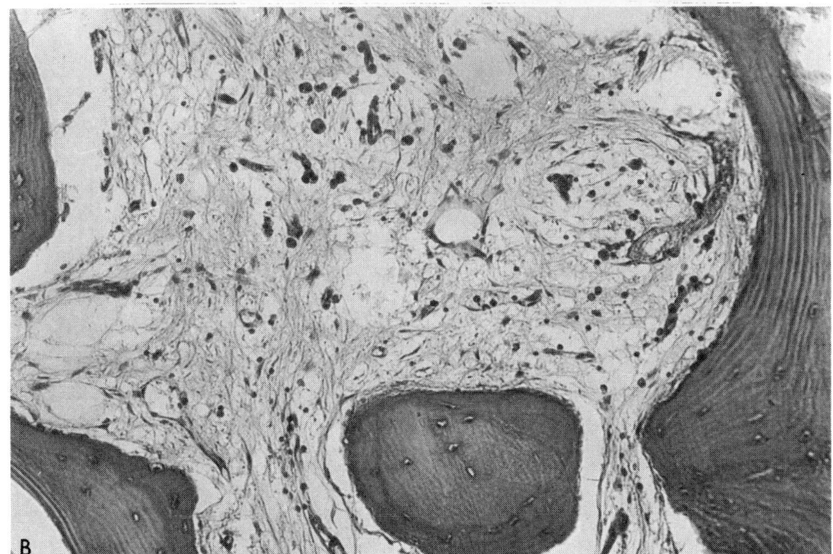

Figure 61–7. *Spinal infection: Later radiographic abnormalities.*

A *Involvement of several vertebrae is evident. Note the destruction and collapse of bone with reactive sclerosis and narrowing of two intervertebral disc spaces. Observe the poorly defined or "fuzzy" discovertebral junctions (pyogenic infection).*

B *A photomicrograph (225×) reveals that the normal cellular elements of the bone marrow have been replaced by vascular adipose and fibrous tissue. Mononuclear cells are evident, and the trabeculae are hypertrophic.*

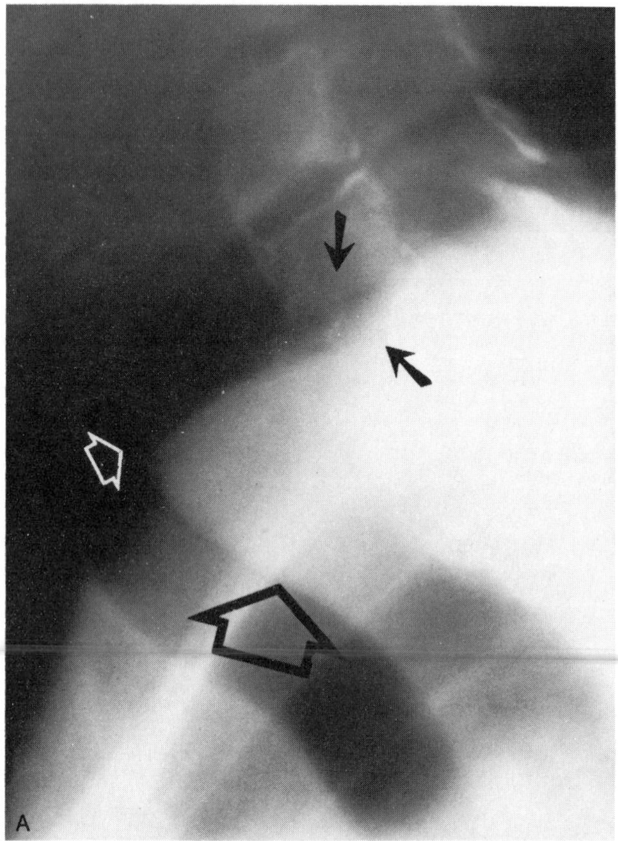

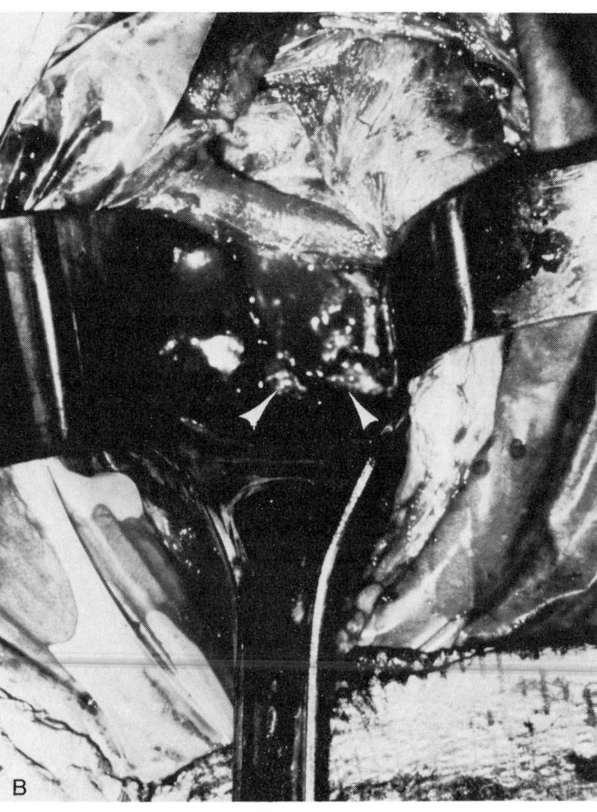

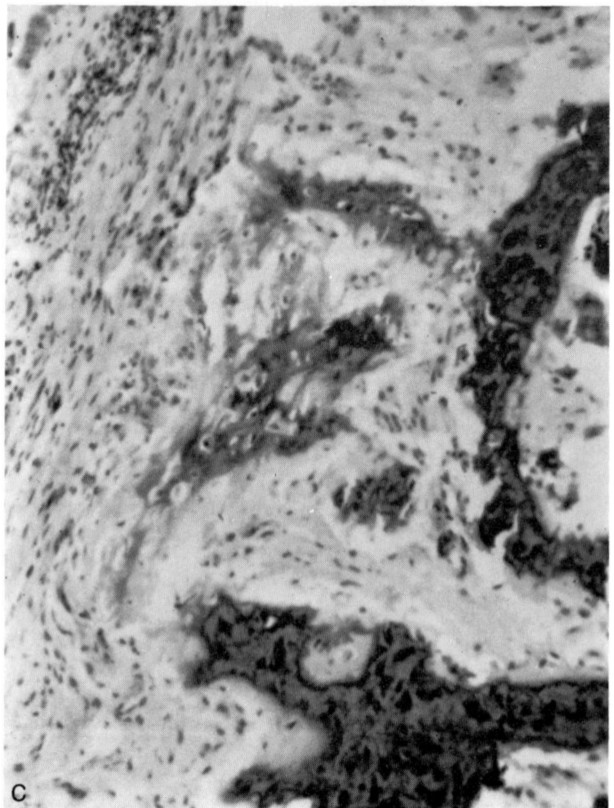

Figure 61–8. *Spinal infection: Soft tissue extension. A 49 year old man developed gram negative septicemia following genitourinary tract infection and surgery.*

A *A lateral radiograph of the neck indicates the vertebral and discal infection at the C6-C7 level (arrows) with an anterior soft tissue mass that is displacing the tracheal air column (open arrows).*

B *An operative photograph following evacuation of an anterior abscess confirms the destruction of the underlying vertebral column (arrowheads).*

C *Histologic evaluation documents the presence of necrotic bone and inflammatory cellular infiltration.*

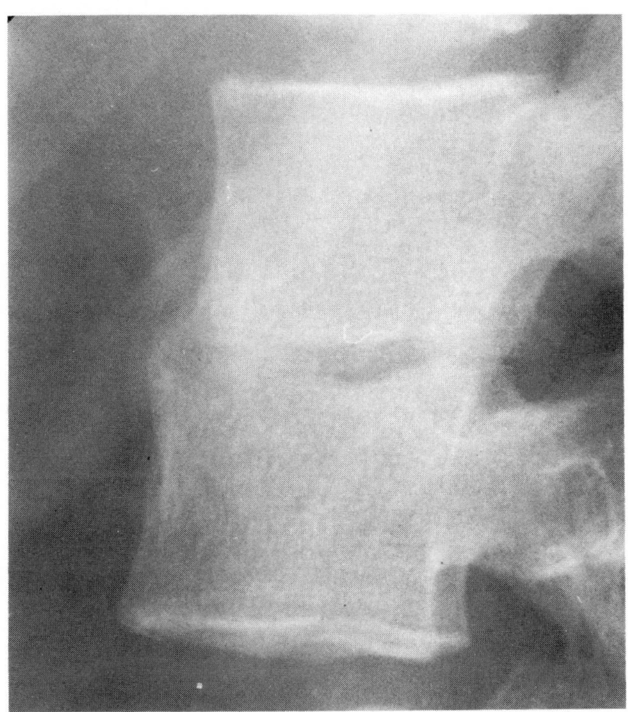

Figure 61–9. *Spinal infection: Bony fusion. Following a pyogenic infection, partial (or complete) bony ankylosis can result. Such bony fusion can also accompany trauma or congenital disorders, although the lack of hypoplasia of the vertebral bodies suggests that the process did not occur prior to the cessation of growth.*

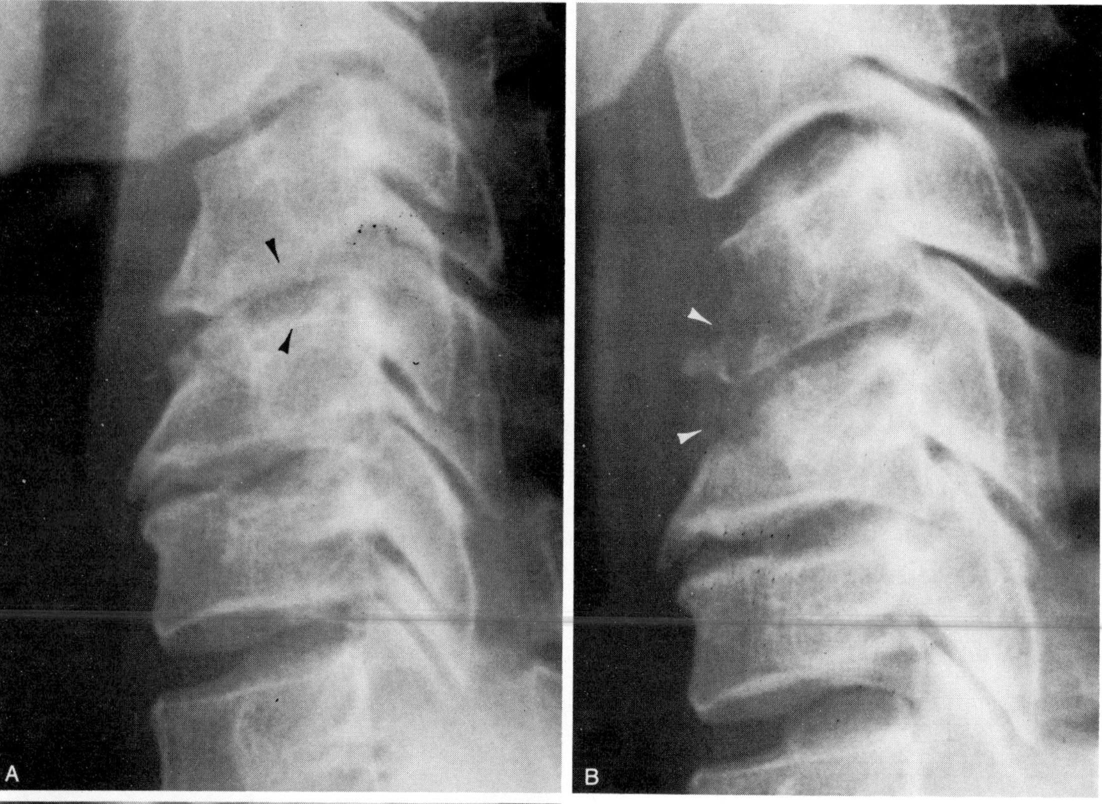

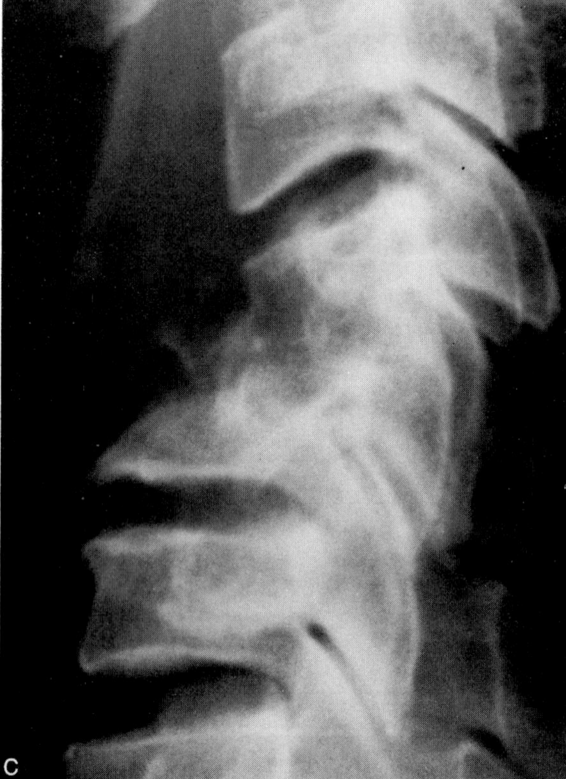

Figure 61–10. *Spinal infection: Residual deformity. A 41 year old man developed Klebsiella spondylitis in the cervical region.*

A *Initial radiograph reveals minimal bony indistinctness and destruction (arrowheads) at the C4-C5 level. Considerable degenerative disease of the intervertebral discs has resulted in disc space narrowing and osteophytes at multiple sites.*

B *Three weeks later, note the collapse and fragmentation of the superior aspect of the fifth cervical vertebral body and lysis of the inferior aspect of the fourth cervical vertebral body (arrowheads). Soft tissue swelling is evident.*

C *Two weeks after* **B,** *angulation and subluxation are apparent. Soft tissue swelling is again seen.*

scend along the spine, extending here and there into the bone or disc ("migrating" osteomyelitis),[1] can appear.

Special Types of Spinal Infection

Intervertebral Disc Infection ("Discitis"). Most infections of the intervertebral disc occur as an extension of vertebral osteomyelitis or as a direct inoculation during diagnostic or surgical procedures. However, in children, a hematogenous route to the disc still exists, which may persist until the age of 20 or 30 years[24, 75] and, according to some investigators, even in the elderly.[39] Thus, certainly in children, hematogenous contamination of the discal tissue is possible.[28-37, 76-79] Although organisms are not always isolated in cases of childhood discitis, a bacterial etiology is most frequently proposed; however, some investigators believe the condition is a noninfectious inflammatory or traumatic disorder. Clinical symptoms and signs may become evident between 1 and 16 years of age, and a preexisting infectious condition (upper respiratory tract or ear infection) is usually apparent. Low grade fever, irritability, malaise, elevation of the erythrocyte sedimentation rate, and, on occasion, leukocytosis are noted in many cases. When positive, blood or bone biopsy culture most typically reveals *Staphylococcus aureus*.

Radiologic abnormalities of discitis in children are commonly delayed (several weeks), although scintigraphy may reveal increased accumulation of bone-seeking pharmaceuticals at a relatively early stage. Roentgenographic changes are most frequent in the lumbar spine followed, in descending order of frequency, by the thoracic and cervical segments. Intervertebral disc space narrowing is later accompanied by erosion of the subchondral bone plate and osseous eburnation (Fig. 61–11). Antibiotic therapy is usually administered on an empirical basis and reconstitution, although not complete, of the intervertebral disc commonly results.

The occurrence of hematogenous spread of infection to the adult intervertebral disc has also been proposed.[80] Kemp and associates[38] described 13 men and two women between the ages of 17 and 72 years who revealed findings compatible with isolated discal infection, related primarily to staphylococci. They interpreted the radiographic manifestations, which included early decrease in the vertical height of the affected intervertebral disc and subsequent sclerosis of the neighboring bone and irregularity of the vertebral plate, as indicative of discal infection with noninfectious reactive osseous response, an interpretation that was strengthened by the lack of evidence of osteomyelitis on pathologic examination. Histologic changes included inflammatory granulation tissue within the affected disc, deposition of new bone or osteoid on existing trabeculae of the vertebral body, and fibroblastic tissues within

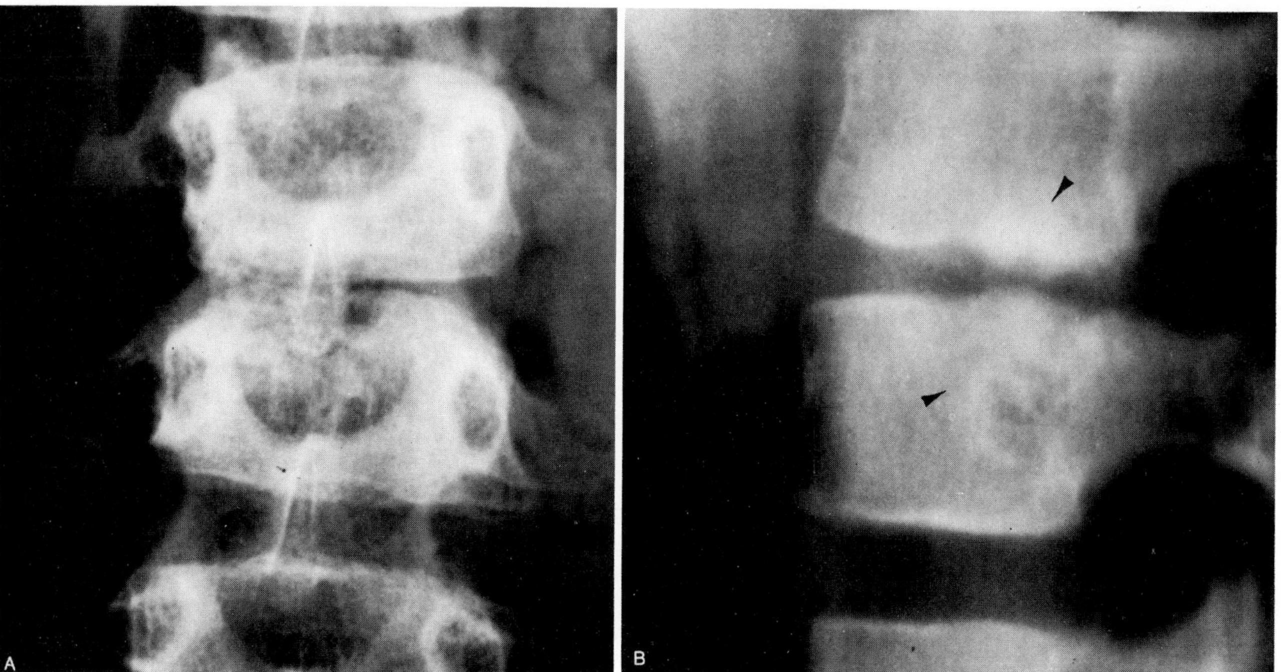

Figure 61–11. *Intervertebral disc infection: Discitis. This 6 year old girl developed symptoms and signs consistent with spinal infection. Bacteriologic studies were not helpful. Observe the narrowing of the intervertebral disc between the second and third lumbar vertebral bodies with osseous lucency and sclerosis (arrowheads). The appearance is consistent with infection. (Courtesy of Dr. L. Lurie, Chula Vista, California.)*

the intertrabecular spaces. The outcome of discitis in these patients was variable. In some, attempted repair was associated with circumferential formation of bone across the anulus; intervertebral disc fusion was not evident. Partial or complete paraplegia was observed in some of these patients.

Although the pathologic observations in this report are consistent with noninfectious bone response, it is not possible to state with certainty that some foci of infection were not present in the vertebrae. The difficulty of obtaining adequate biopsy samples and of successfully isolating organisms from the bone in documented cases of osteomyelitis is well known. Furthermore, radiologic findings in the cases reported by Kemp and co-workers are similar or identical to those in vertebral osteomyelitis. Although the concept of hematogenous infection isolated to the intervertebral disc of the adult due to persistent normal or abnormal vascular channels is indeed intriguing, further documentation of this entity is required before its existence is truly established.

Other Diagnostic Modalities

As at other sites of infection, a variety of diagnostic modalities in addition to routine radiography can be employed in cases of infective spondylitis. These include tomography, myelography, and computed tomography.[106] Especially important is the role of radionuclide studies in establishing the presence of spinal infection at a stage when radiographs are entirely normal. Technetium and gallium radiopharmaceuticals can be utilized in this regard[37, 47, 58, 76, 107, 108]; the latter agent may have a special role in the diagnosis of discitis.[81] The abnormal technetium scan may be characterized by augmented uptake in two adjacent vertebral bodies or a more diffuse pattern, reflecting reactive hyperemia[47]; in all instances, radiographic correlation must be attempted.

Differential Diagnosis

The radiographic hallmark of infective spondylitis is intervertebral disc space narrowing, frequently accompanied by lysis or sclerosis of adjacent vertebrae (Table 61–1). A similar radiographic pattern can be encountered in various articular disorders such as rheumatoid arthritis, the seronegative spondyloarthropathies, calcium pyrophosphate dihydrate crystal deposition disease, alkaptonuria, and neuroarthropathy (Fig. 61–12), but in each of these disorders, clinical and additional radiographic features usually assure accurate differential diagnosis.[82] Sarcoidosis can occasionally be associated with disc space narrowing and bone eburnation at one or more levels of the spine.

Diminution of intervertebral disc height and bony sclerosis are associated with cartilaginous node formation (Schmorl's node), which accompanies many disease processes, including traumatic, articular, and metabolic disorders.[83-85] In general, the degree of ill-definition of the subchondral bone plate is less in cases of cartilaginous nodes than in those of infection; the latter condition is characterized by "fuzzy" spiculated osseous contours. Furthermore, tomography may accurately define lucent intraosseous discal fragments in patients with cartilaginous nodes, although an intraosseous abscess can create similar lucency. Widespread cartilaginous nodes are detected in Scheuermann's disease (juvenile kyphosis), creating an appearance that should not be confused with that of infection.

Intervertebral (osteo)chondrosis also produces

Table 61–1

DIFFERENTIAL DIAGNOSIS OF DISORDERS PRODUCING DISCAL NARROWING

Disorder	Discovertebral Margin	Sclerosis	"Vacuum" Phenomena	Osteophytosis	Other Findings
Infection	Poorly defined	Variable[1]	Absent[2]	Absent	Vertebral lysis, soft tissue mass
Intervertebral osteochondrosis	Well defined	Prominent	Present	Variable	Cartilaginous nodes
Rheumatoid arthritis	Poorly or well defined with "erosions"	Variable	Absent	Absent or mild	Apophyseal joint abnormalities, subluxation
Calcium pyrophosphate dihydrate crystal deposition disease	Poorly or well defined	Prominent	Variable	Variable	Fragmentation, subluxation
Neuroarthropathy	Well defined	Prominent	Variable	Prominent	Fragmentation, subluxation, disorganization
Trauma	Well defined	Prominent	Variable	Variable	Fracture, soft tissue mass
Sarcoidosis	Poorly or well defined	Variable, may be prominent	Absent	Absent	Soft tissue mass

[1]Usually evident in pyogenic infections and in tuberculosis in the black patient.
[2]"Vacuum" phenomena may initially be evident when intervertebral osteochondrosis is also present, or, rarely, when a gas-forming microorganism is responsible for the infection.

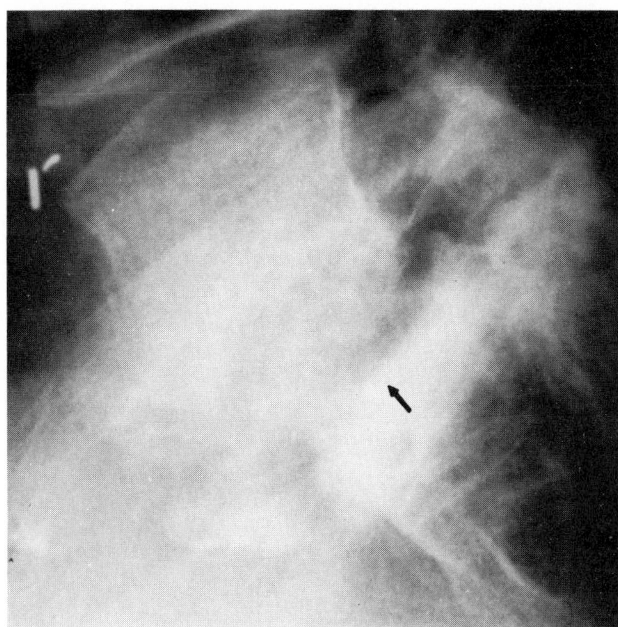

Figure 61–12. Neuroarthropathy. In this patient with tabes dorsalis, severe bony destruction and sclerosis at the lumbosacral junction are seen. The findings are similar to those in infection, although the relatively well defined nature of the superior sacral margin (arrow) is more suggestive of neuroarthropathy.

intervertebral disc space narrowing and reactive sclerosis of the neighboring bone (see Chapter 40). The resulting radiographic picture can resemble that of infective spondylitis. In intervertebral (osteo)chondrosis, the vertebral end-plates are usually smooth and well defined, although focal defects can represent sites of intravertebral discal herniation (cartilaginous nodes). Of particular diagnostic significance is the presence of one or more radiolucent collections overlying the intervertebral disc in intervertebral (osteo)chondrosis (Fig. 61–13). These "vacuum" phenomena represent gaseous collections (nitrogen) within the nucleus pulposus and are a reliable sign of discal degeneration. They are exceedingly rare in cases of discal infection, and their detection makes the diagnosis of infection very unlikely. Occasionally, however, infection that is initiated in a site of previously existing discal degeneration can be associated with a "vacuum" phenomenon. Usually, in these cases, the dissemination of infection throughout the intervertebral disc leads to disappearance of the gaseous collections (Fig. 61–14). Additionally, in rare occasions, infections with gas-forming bacteria may lead to "vacuum" phenomena.[102]

In general, primary or metastatic tumor in the spine does not lead to significant loss of intervertebral disc space; the combination of widespread lysis or sclerosis of a vertebral body and an intact adjacent intervertebral disc is much more characteristic of tumor than of infection (Fig. 61–15). However, certain neoplasms such as plasma cell myeloma and chordoma can extend across or around the intervertebral disc to involve the neighboring vertebra. Furthermore, neoplastic disruption of the subchondral bone can produce osseous weakening, allowing intraosseous discal herniation.[86] In these latter cases, some degree of disc space narrowing may accompany the bony destruction, producing a radiographic picture that simulates that of infection.

In patients with infective spondylitis involving primarily the posterior elements, bony destruction and production can simulate the findings of tumor. This is especially true when significant pedicular involvement is present.

Paraspinal masses occur in infective spondylitis and traumatic and neoplastic disorders. Intervertebral disc space ossification leading to bridging of vertebral bodies is encountered as a sequela of infective spondylitis. It may also be seen in congenital disorders and following surgery or trauma.

The accurate radiographic differentiation of pyogenic infective spondylitis from granulomatous infections (tuberculosis and fungal disorders) can be difficult. Rapid loss of intervertebral disc height, extensive sclerosis, and the absence of calcified paraspinal masses are findings that are more typical of pyogenic infection, although one or more of these signs can be encountered in some cases of tuberculous or fungal spondylitis (Fig. 61–16).

SACROILIAC JOINT INFECTIONS

Routes of Contamination

The sacroiliac joint may become infected by the hematogenous route, by contamination from a contiguous suppurative focus, by direct implantation, or following surgery (Fig. 61–17). In many instances, the exact mechanism leading to infective arthritis at this site is not clear.[87-91]

Although a hematogenous route appears likely in cases of septic sacroiliac joint disease occurring in the clinical setting of preexisting infection in a distant site (e.g., skin, pharynx), it is not certain in most patients if the primary focus is in the adjacent osseous structures or in the articulation itself.[87] The subchondral circulation of the ilium is slow, resembling the situation in the metaphysis of long bones in children. Thus, hematogenous implantation at this site is to be expected; the ilium is the most frequently infected flat bone of the body.[92, 93] From this location, extension of infection into the sacroiliac or hip joint can occur. Similarly, the association of sacroiliac joint infection with suppurative conditions of the pelvis or previous pelvic surgical procedures may indicate the importance of hematogenous spread via the paravertebral venous

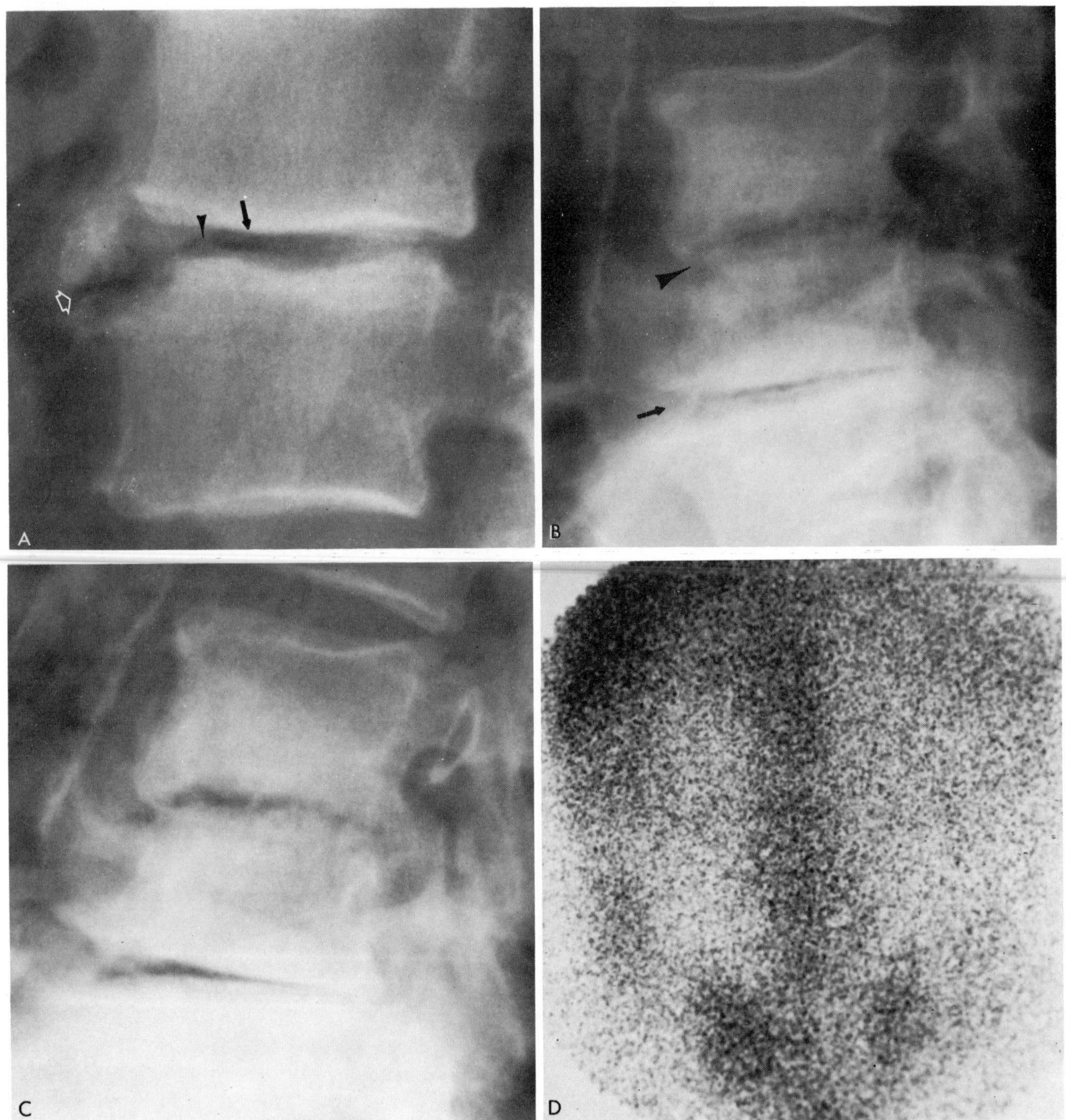

Figure 61–13. Intervertebral osteochondrosis.

A *With degeneration of the intervertebral disc, narrowing of the discal space and reactive bone formation can be seen. Note the well-defined appearance of the eburnated bone (solid arrow) and the presence of a "vacuum" phenomenon (arrowhead). The lucent zone can be traced anteriorly beneath a separated vertebral ossicle (open arrow), confirming that a "limbus" vertebra is related to anterolateral herniation of discal material.*

B–D *In this patient with back pain, an initial radiograph* **(B)** *reveals obvious intervertebral osteochondrosis at the L4-L5 vertebral level (arrow), characterized by disc space narrowing, a vacuum phenomenon, and well-defined sclerotic vertebral margins. The changes at the L3-L4 vertebral level (arrowhead) are more difficult to interpret. The vertebral bodies are irregular, and a vacuum phenomenon is not definite. On a second radiograph exposed during back extension* **(C),** *vacuum phenomena are now apparent at both vertebral levels, indicating that infection is highly unlikely. A subsequent gallium scan* **(D)** *fails to reveal augmented spinal activity and provides further documentation that infection is not present.*

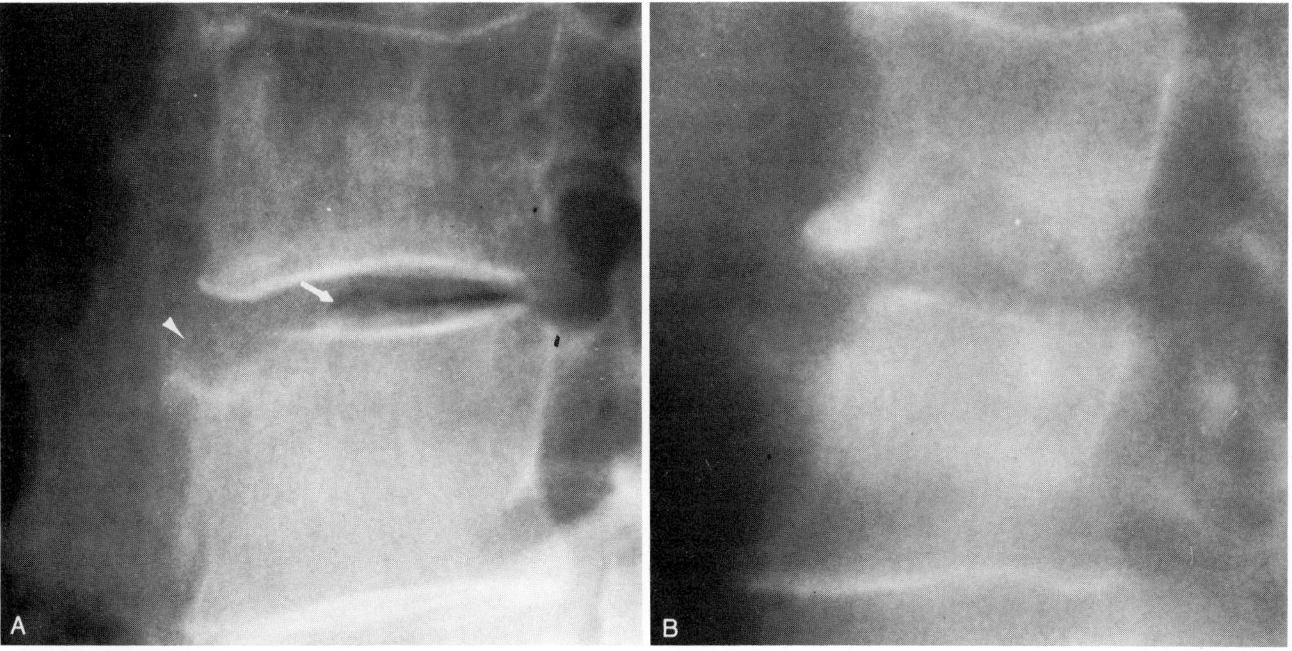

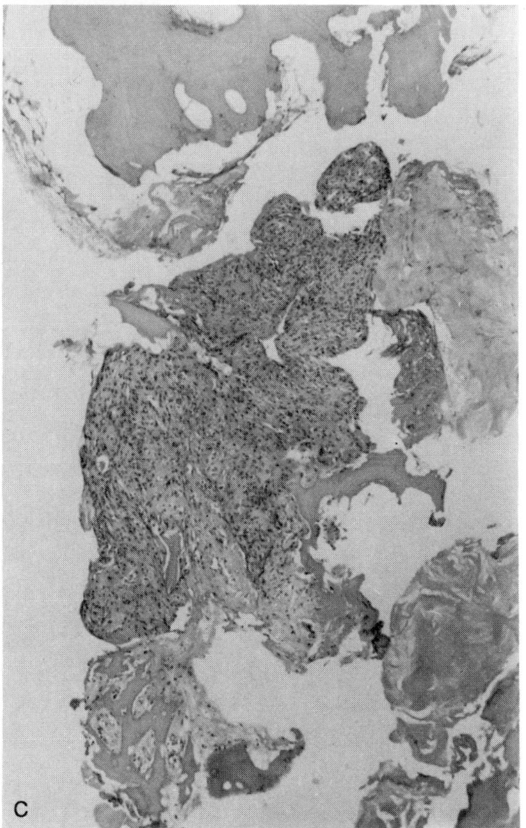

Figure 61–14. Spinal infection with disappearance of "vacuum" phenomenon. This middle-aged man developed an infective spondylitis which on histologic and laboratory examination was found to be related to brucellosis.

A An initial radiograph outlines intervertebral disc space narrowing, erosion of the anterosuperior aspect of the vertebral body (arrowhead), bony proliferation, and a "vacuum" phenomenon (arrow). Although the appearance is reminiscent of that in intervertebral osteochondrosis with cartilaginous node formation, the ill-defined nature of the destruction is more consistent with infection.

B Two weeks later, a midline lateral tomogram reveals the progressive nature of the osseous destruction and the disappearance of the "vacuum" phenomenon. At this time, the classic radiographic features of an infection are evident. The rapidity with which the abnormalities progressed in this case is consistent with brucellosis.

C Photomicrograph (86×) indicates the presence of an acute granulomatous process with destruction and necrosis of osseous trabeculae. Cultures revealed Brucella organisms.

(Courtesy of Dr. J. Usselman and Dr. V. Vint, Scripps Clinic, LaJolla, California.)

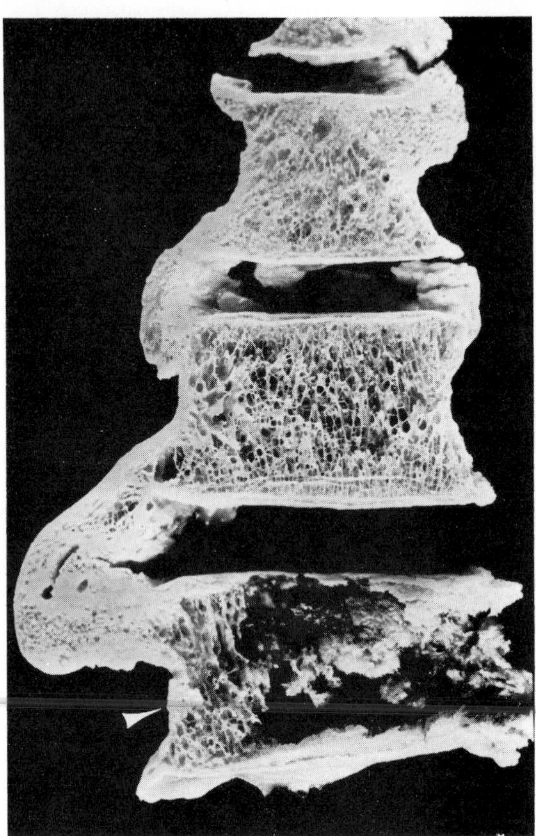

Figure 61–15. Spinal metastasis with preservation of intervertebral discs. Commonly, metastatic destruction of a vertebral body (arrowhead) is unassociated with loss of the intervertebral disc space, although, rarely, intraosseous herniation of discal material (cartilaginous nodes) into a destroyed vertebral body can lead to loss of height of the disc (see Chapter 75). In this case, a bridging osteophyte that antedated the metastatic lesion is contributing to preservation of the intervertebral disc space.

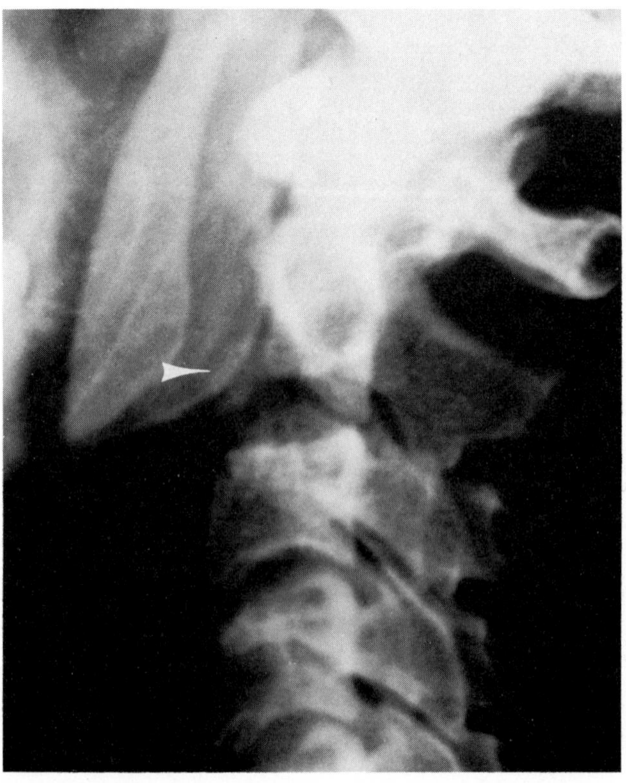

Figure 61–16. Spinal infection due to coccidioidomycosis. This adult man, living in Arizona, developed progressive neck pain. A lytic lesion of the second cervical vertebral body (arrowhead) with soft tissue swelling is evident. The absence of sclerosis and the preservation of adjacent intervertebral disc height are not uncommon in fungal or tuberculous spondylitis.

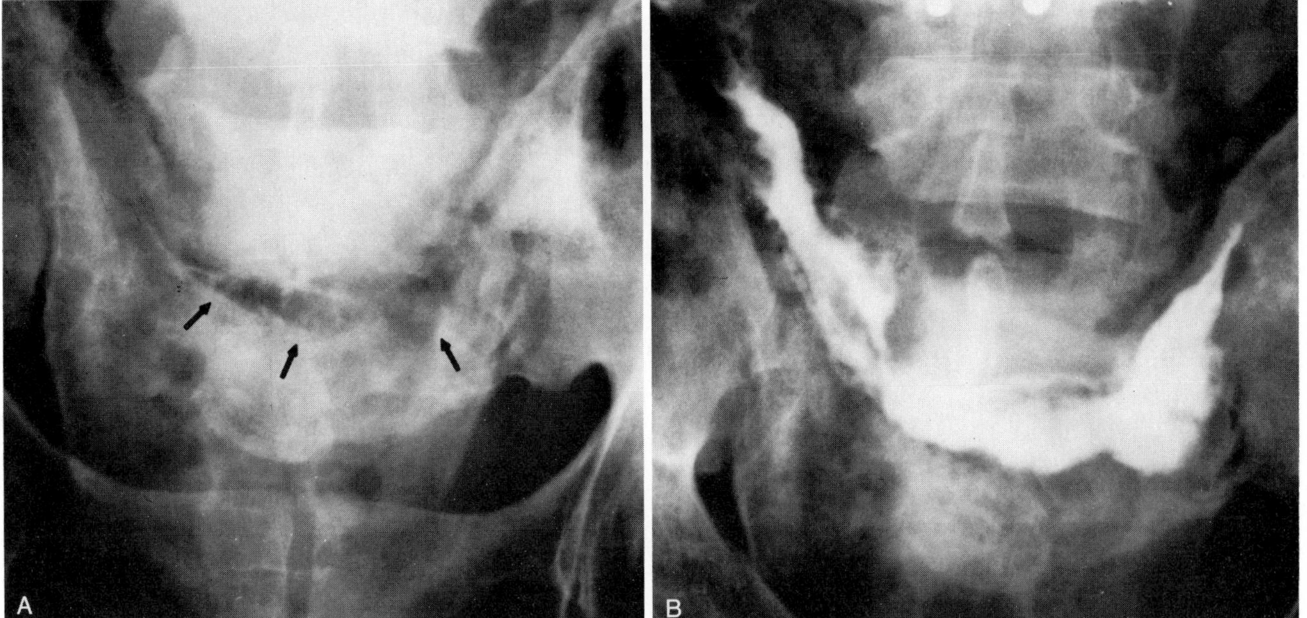

Figure 61–17. *Sacroiliac joint and sacral infection: Spread from a contiguous contaminated source. This 28 year old paralyzed man developed soft tissue infection with a fistula leading to the sacrum and sacroiliac joint.*

A *Note irregular channel-like destruction of the sacrum (arrows), with articular space widening and ill-defined bone about the left sacroiliac joint. The fifth lumbar vertebra is also affected.*

B *A fistulogram confirms the communication of the tract with the sacrum and sacroiliac joint.*

system of Batson, although, once again, the initial site of contamination (osseous or synovial) is difficult to document. The observation of a destructive process in both the iliac and the sacral aspects of the articulation in the early phases of infection suggests that direct hematogenous intra-articular contamination may be incriminated in many patients.[87]

Contamination of the sacroiliac joint or neighboring bone can occur from an adjacent infection. Pelvic abscesses can disrupt the anterior articular capsule or the periosteum and cortex of the ilium or sacrum. Thus, vaginal, uterine, ovarian, bladder, and intestinal processes can lead to iliac or sacral osteomyelitis and sacroiliac joint suppuration by contiguous contamination (as well as by hematogenous spread via Batson's plexus).[94, 95] Trauma can aggravate this situation by disrupting viscera, soft tissue, and osseous and articular structures. Abscesses following intragluteal injection of medication can lead to osteomyelitis and sacroiliac joint septic arthritis. Even infective conditions of the spine can subsequently spread beneath the spinal ligaments into the pelvis and sacroiliac articulations.[96]

Direct implantation of organisms following diagnostic or surgical procedures represents another, although uncommon, source of sacroiliac joint infection. Needle aspiration of the articulation or closed or open biopsy of the adjacent bone can be complicated by infection.

Clinical Abnormalities

Pyogenic infection of the sacroiliac articulation can lead to severe clinical manifestations, especially in children and adolescents.[104] Fever, local pain and tenderness, and a limp can be evident. Radiation of pain to the buttock, in a sciatic distribution, and even to the abdomen can be recorded. Widespread discomfort is not infrequent, perhaps reflecting the proclivity of suppurative sacroiliac joint disease to spread beyond the confines of the articulation. The discharged purulent material may follow the iliac fossa, track along the tendon of the iliopsoas muscle to the hip and toward the thigh, follow the tendons of the short external rotators to the buttock, ascend into the lumbar region or along the crest of the ilium, or penetrate the pelvic floor to be discharged through the vagina or rectum.[87]

Elevation of the erythrocyte sedimentation rate and leukocytosis are common but variable laboratory features. The identification of the causative organisms from blood culture or joint aspiration can be difficult.[105] Staphylococci, streptococci, pneumococci, Proteus, Klebsiella, Pseudomonas, Brucella, mycobacteria, and fungi can be implicated. Gram-negative bacterial agents are especially common in pyogenic arthritis of the sacroiliac joint in drug abusers.

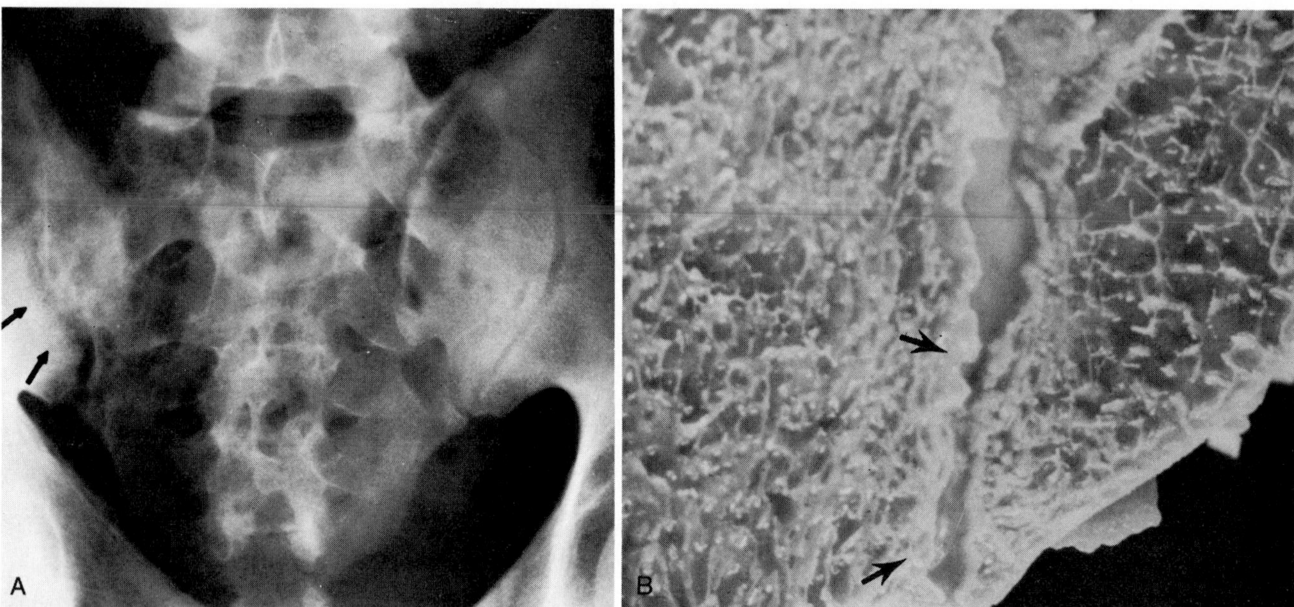

Figure 61–18. *Sacroiliac joint infection: Early abnormalities.*

A *A 35 year old male heroin addict developed Pseudomonas osteomyelitis and septic arthritis. The radiograph reveals the changes in the right sacroiliac joint, consisting of subchondral osseous erosion, ill-defined articular margins, and widening of the joint space (arrows).*

B *In the coronal section of an infected sacroiliac joint in a cadaver, observe the erosions, which predominate in the ilium (arrows).*

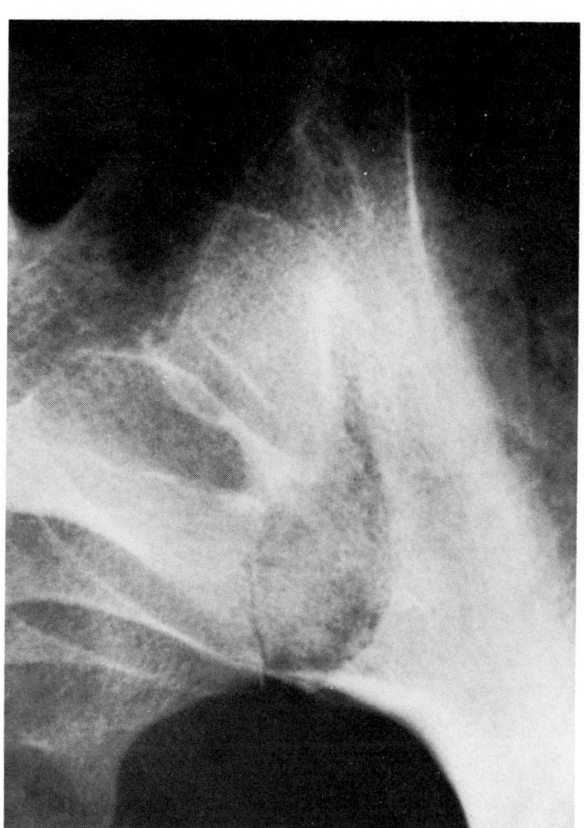

Figure 61–19. *Sacroiliac joint infection: Later abnormalities. This 28 year heroin addict presented with severe back pain. Pseudomonas was cultured from a bone biopsy. Note the articular space narrowing and osseous sclerosis about the left sacroiliac joint, especially in the ilium. Osseous fusion can ultimately result from pyogenic septic arthritis.*

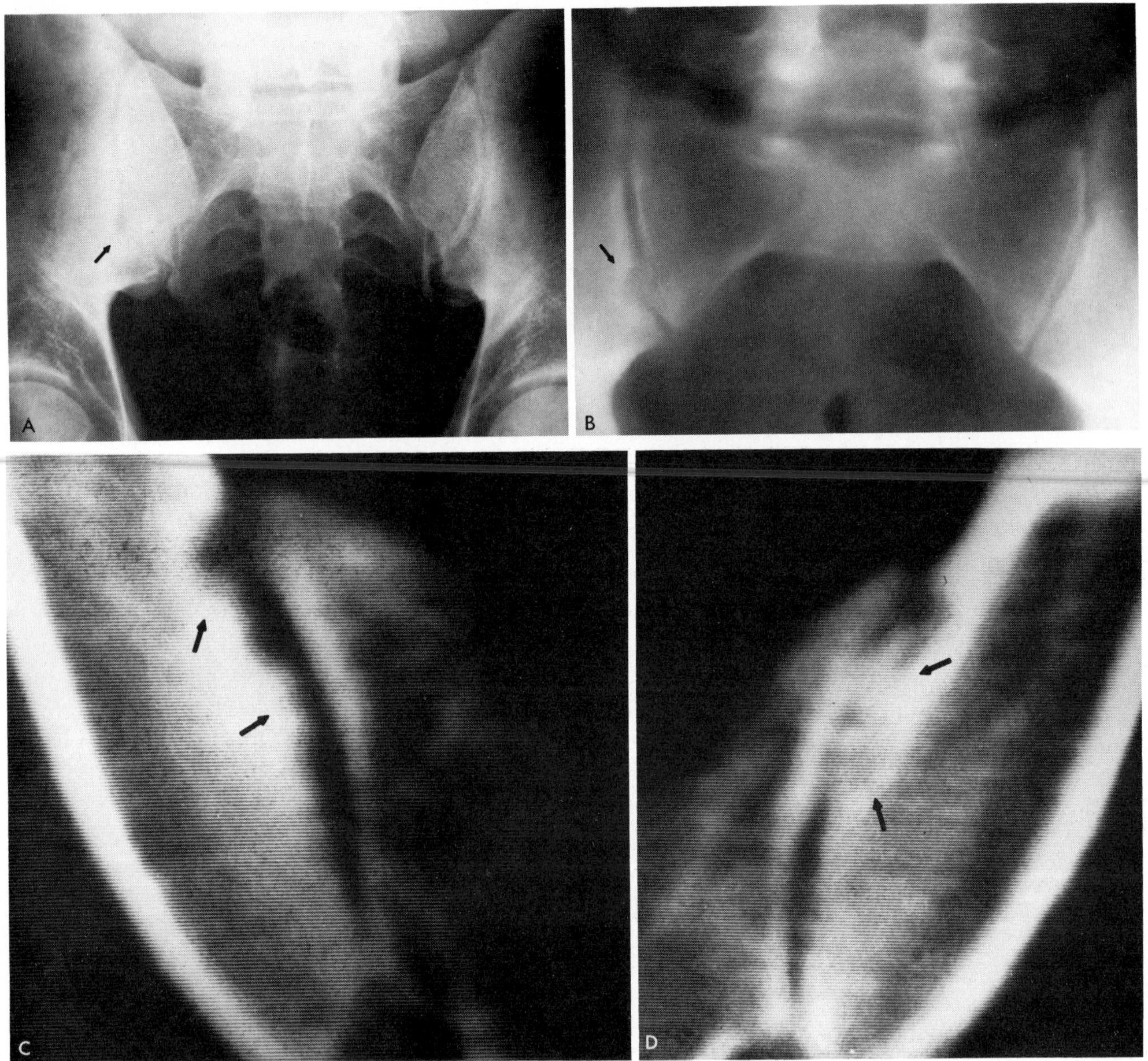

Figure 61–20. *Reiter's syndrome simulating infection.*

A *An initial radiograph reveals a definite abnormality of the right sacroiliac joint (arrow) and only equivocal changes on the opposite side.*

B *Conventional tomography indicates an iliac erosion with surrounding sclerosis on the right side (arrow) and superficial osseous irregularity about the left sacroiliac joint. Although the sacroiliac joint alterations are asymmetric in distribution, the fact that they appear to be bilateral militates against the diagnosis of infection.*

C, D *Computed tomography documents bilateral asymmetric sacroiliac joint changes with erosion and sclerosis, predominantly in the ilium (arrows).*

Radiographic–Pathologic Correlation

In almost all cases of sacroiliac joint infection, a unilateral distribution is encountered. In pyogenic arthritis, radiographic findings generally occur in 2 or 3 weeks, characterized by blurring and indistinctness of the subchondral osseous line and narrowing or widening of the interosseous space. Although these two alterations frequently coexist, their time of appearance is dictated by the initial site of contamination: If osteomyelitis precedes septic arthritis, bony abnormalities may antedate articular changes; if the joint is initially affected, cartilaginous and osseous alterations may coexist. In both situations, the most extensive findings are commonly evident about the inferoanterior aspect of the articulation. Progressive changes are accompanied by erosions, which are usually predominant on the lower ilium (Fig. 61–18). Surrounding condensation of bone is variable in incidence and degree, and it is influenced by the type and virulence of the infecting microorganism. With treatment, intra-articular osseous fusion may be encountered, ultimately leading to complete bridging of the interosseous space and disappearance of bone eburnation (Fig. 61–19).

Other Diagnostic Modalities

Tomography and radionuclide examination are two important diagnostic modalities that can be employed in patients with suspected sacroiliac joint infection. Tomograms may detect early erosive alterations when initial radiographs are normal; scintigraphy may outline increased accumulation of radionuclide at a time when findings on routine radiographs and tomograms are unimpressive.[87, 90] Abnormal unilateral uptake of isotope in the sacroiliac articulation indicates infection until proved otherwise.[111] Computed tomography can also be helpful in evaluating patients with suspected sacroiliac joint infection.

Differential Diagnosis

It is the unilateral nature of infective sacroiliac joint disease that is its most useful diagnostic feature. Bilateral symmetric or asymmetric articular changes are characteristic of ankylosing spondylitis, psoriasis, Reiter's syndrome, osteitis condensans ilii, and hyperparathyroidism (Fig. 61–20). Unilateral changes can be encountered in rheumatoid arthritis, gout, Reiter's syndrome, and psoriasis. They may also appear on the paralyzed side in hemiplegic patients (due to chondral atrophy) and on the contralateral side in patients with osteoarthritis of the hip. Unilateral sacroiliac joint disease characterized by blurring or poor definition of subchondral bone and loss of joint space is virtually diagnostic of infection.

INFECTION AT OTHER AXIAL SITES

Infection can involve almost any additional site in the axial skeleton. As elsewhere, contamination can result from hematogenous spread, spread from a contiguous source, and direct or postsurgical contamination. In the drug abuser, osteomyelitis and septic arthritis of the sternoclavicular and acromioclavicular articulations in addition to the spine and sacroiliac joint can be evident[97] (Fig. 61–21). Following urologic procedures, osteomyelitis of the symphysis pubis may be difficult to differentiate from osteitis pubis. Infection of the sternum and manubriosternal articulation can result from direct hematogenous inoculation or secondary contamination due to local injury, surgery, or diagnostic or therapeutic procedure (subclavian vein catheterization).[98-101, 109] In all cases, typical clinical and radiologic features of osteomyelitis and septic arthritis are

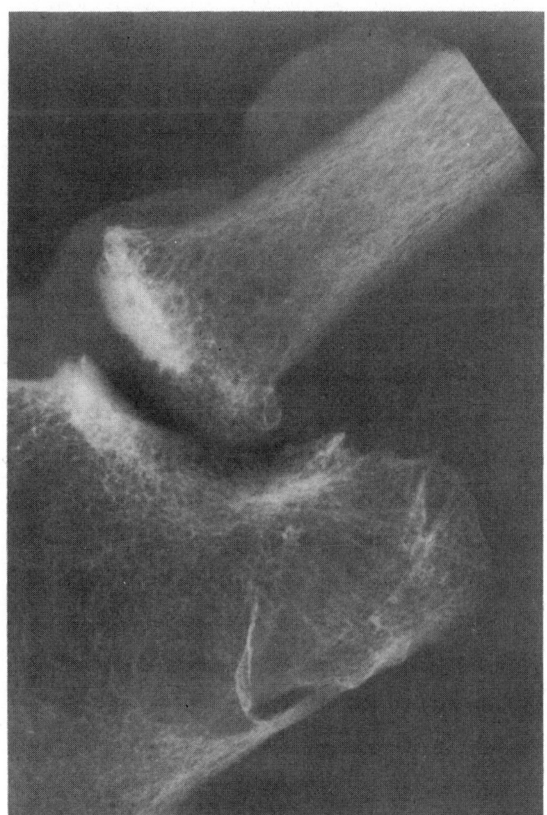

Figure 61–21. *Sternoclavicular joint infection. A coronal section through an infected sternoclavicular articulation reveals osseous destruction and reactive eburnation of both the clavicle and the sternum.*

usually apparent, allowing differentiation from other conditions.[110]

SUMMARY

The routes of contamination of the spine, the sacroiliac joint, and other axial skeletal sites are identical to those of the appendicular skeleton. In the spine, early loss of intervertebral disc space is characteristic of pyogenic infection and is associated with lysis and sclerosis of neighboring bone. These findings can simulate those of other disorders, such as rheumatoid arthritis, intervertebral (osteo)chondrosis, and conditions complicated by cartilaginous node formation. Sacroiliac joint infection is typically unilateral in distribution, a feature that allows differentiation from many other articular processes. Additional locations in the axial skeleton are not uncommonly infected in drug abusers and in patients following trauma, surgery, and diagnostic or therapeutic procedures.

REFERENCES

1. Schmorl G, Junghanns H: The Human Spine in Health and Disease. Translated by EF Besemann. 2nd Ed. New York, Grune & Stratton, 1971, p 307.
2. Hodgson AR: Infectious disease of the spine. *In* RH Rothman, FA Simeone (Eds): The Spine. Philadelphia, WB Saunders Co, 1975, p 567.
3. Batson OV: The function of the vertebral veins and their role in the spread of metastases. Ann Surg *112*:138, 1940.
4. Batson OV: The vertebral vein system. Am J Roentgenol *78*:195, 1957.
5. Harris RS, Jones DM: The arterial supply to the adult cervical vertebral bodies. J Bone Joint Surg *38B*:922, 1956.
6. Wilensky AO: Osteomyelitis of the vertebrae. Ann Surg *89*:561, 1929.
7. Willis TA: Nutrient arteries of the vertebral bodies. J Bone Joint Surg *31A*:538, 1949.
8. Ferguson WR: Some observations on the circulation in foetal and infant spines. J Bone Joint Surg *32A*:640, 1950.
9. Wiley AM, Trueta J: The vascular anatomy of the spine and its relationship to pyogenic vertebral osteomyelitis. J Bone Joint Surg *41B*:796, 1959.
10. Carson HW: Acute osteomyelitis of the spine. Br J Surg *18*:400, 1930.
11. Turner, P: Acute infective osteomyelitis of the spine. Br J Surg *26*:71, 1938.
12. Henriques CQ: Osteomyelitis as a complication in urology with special reference to the paravertebral venous plexus. Br J Surg *46*:19, 1958.
13. Henson SW Jr, Coventry MB: Osteomyelitis of the vertebrae as a result of infection of the urinary tract. Surg Gynecol Obstet *102*:207, 1956.
14. Leigh TF, Kelly RP, Weens HS: Spinal osteomyelitis associated with urinary tract infections. Radiology *65*:334, 1955.
15. Liming RW, Youngs FJ: Metastatic vertebral osteomyelitis following prostatic surgery. Radiology *67*:92, 1956.
16. De Feo E: Osteomyelitis of the spine following prostatic surgery. Radiology *62*:396, 1954.
17. Alderman EJ, Duff J: Osteomyelitis of cervical vertebra as a complication of urinary tract disease. JAMA *148*:283, 1952.
18. O'Leary JM, Lipscomb PR, Dixon CF: Enteric fistula associated with osteomyelitis of the hip and spinal column. Ann Surg *140*:897, 1954.
19. Lame EL: Vertebral osteomyelitis following operation on the urinary tract or sigmoid. Am J Roetngenol *75*:938, 1956.
20. Sherman M, Schneider GT: Vertebral osteomyelitis complicating postabortal and postpartum infection. South Med J *48*:333, 1955.
21. Coman DR, deLong RP: The role of the vertebral venous system in the metastasis of cancer to the spinal column. Cancer *4*:610, 1951.
22. Collis JL: The aetiology of cerebral abscess as a complication of thoracic disease. J Thorac Surg *13*:445, 1944.
23. Barrington FJF, Wright HD: Bacteriaemia following operations on the urethra. J Pathol Bacteriol *33*:871, 1930.
24. Coventry MB, Ghormley RK, Kernohan JW: The intervertebral disc: Its microscopic anatomy and pathology. J Bone Joint Surg *27A*:105, 1945.
25. Stauffer RN: Pyogenic vertebral osteomyelitis. Orthop Clin North Am *6*:1015, 1975.
26. Alexander CJ: The aetiology of juvenile spondylarthritis (discitis). Clin Radiol *21*:178, 1970.
27. Moes CAF: Spondylarthritis in childhood. Am J Roentgenol *91*:578, 1964.
28. Saenger EL: Spondylarthritis in children. Am J Roentgenol *64*:20, 1950.
29. Boston HC Jr, Bianco AJ Jr, Rhodes KH: Disc space infections in children. Orthop Clin North Am *6*:953, 1975.
30. Lascari AD, Graham MH, MacQueen JC: Intervertebral disk infection in children. J Pediatr. *70*:751, 1967.
31. Milone FP, Bianco AJ Jr, Ivins JC: Infections of the intervertebral disk in children. JAMA *181*:1029. 1962.
32. Spiegel PG, Kengla KW, Isaacson AS, Wilson JC Jr: Intervertebral disc-space inflammation in children. J Bone Joint Surg *54A*:284, 1972.
33. Smith RF, Taylor TKF: Inflammatory lesions of intervertebral discs in children. J Bone Joint Surg *49A*:1508, 1967.
34. Dupont A, Andersen H: Nonspecific spondylitis in childhood. Acta Paediatr *45*:361, 1956.
35. Jamison RC, Heimlich EM, Miethke JC, O'Loughlin BJ: Non-specific spondylitis of infants and children. Radiology *77*:355, 1961.
36. Bonfiglio M, Lange TA, Kim YM: Pyogenic vertebral osteomyelitis. Disk space infections. Clin Orthop Rel Res *96*:234, 1973.
37. Wenger DR, Bobechko WP, Gilday DL: The spectrum of intervertebral disc-space infection in children. J Bone Joint Surg *60A*:100, 1978.
38. Kemp HBS, Jackson JW, Jeremiah JD, Hall AJ: Pyogenic infections occurring primarily in intervertebral discs. J Bone Joint Surg *55B*:698, 1973.
39. Smith NR: The intervertebral discs. Br J Surg *18*:358, 1931.
40. Gordon EJ: Infection of disc space secondary to fistula from pelvic abscess. South Med J *70*:114, 1977.
41. Buetti VC, Lüdi H: Spondylitis nach Paravertebralanästhesie. Helv Chir Acta *25*:261, 1958.
42. Rohr H: Die angeborenen knöcherenen Fehlbildungen in der Occipito-Cervikal-Gegend und ihre Behandlung. Zbl Neurochir *16*:276, 1956.
43. McLaurin RL: Spinal suppuration. Clin Neurosurg *14*:314, 1966.
44. Keon-Cohen BT: Epidural abscess simulating disc hernia. J Bone Joint Surg *50B*:128, 1968.
45. Sullivan CR, Bickel WH, Svien HJ: Infection of the vertebral interspaces after operations on intervertebral disks. JAMA *166*:1973, 1958.
46. Stern WE, Balch RE: Surgical aspects of nonspecific inflammatory and suppurative disease of the vertebral column. Am J Surg *112*:314, 1966.
47. Goldman AB, Freiberger RH: Localized infectious and neuropathic diseases. Semin Roentgenol *14*:19, 1979.
48. Ross PM, Fleming JL: Vertebral body osteomyelitis. Spectrum and natural history. A retrospective analysis of 37 cases. Clin Orthop Rel Res *118*:190, 1976.
49. Musher DM, Thorsteinsson SB, Minuth JN, Luchi RJ: Vertebral osteomyelitis. Still a diagnostic pitfall. Arch Intern Med *136*:105, 1976.
50. Malawski SK: Pyogenic infection of the spine. International Orthopedics (SICOT) *1*:125, 1977.
51. Collert S: Osteomyelitis of the spine. Acta Orthop Scand *48*:283, 1977.
52. Chari PR: Haematogenous pyogenic osteomyelitis of the spine: A study of 17 cases. Aust N Z J Surg *42*:381, 1973.
53. Bolivar R, Kohl S, Pickering LK: Vertebral osteomyelitis in children: Report of four cases. Pediatrics *62*:549, 1978.
54. Griffiths HED, Jones DM: Pyogenic infection of the spine. A review of twenty-eight cases. J Bone Joint Surg *53B*:383, 1971.
55. Berant M, Shrem M: Vertebral osteomyelitis in a young infant. Clin Pediatr *13*:677, 1974.
56. Fredrickson B, Yuan H, Olans R: Management and outcome of pyogenic vertebral osteomyelitis. Clin Orthop Rel Res *131*:160, 1978.
57. Wedge JH, Oryschak AF, Robertson DE, Kirkaldy-Willis WH: Atypical manifestations of spinal infections. Clin Orthop Rel Res *123*:155, 1977.
58. Partio E, Hatanpaa S, Rokkanen P: Pyogenic spondylitis. Acta Orthop Scand *49*:165, 1978.
59. Hahn O: *In* Wilensky AO: Osteomyelitis of the vertebrae. Ann Surg *89*:561, 1929.

60. Kulowski J: Pyogenic osteomyelitis of the spine. An analysis and discussion of 102 cases. J Bone Joint Surg *18*:343, 1936.
61. Bremner AE, Neligan GA: Benign form of acute osteitis of the spine in young children. Br Med J *1*:856, 1953.
62. Finch PG: Staphylococcal osteomyelitis of the spine in a baby aged three weeks. Lancet *2*:134, 1947.
63. Epremian BE, Perez LA: Imaging strategy in osteomyelitis. Clin Nucl Med *2*:218, 1977.
64. Garcia A Jr, Grantham SA: Haematogenous pyogenic vertebral osteomyelitis. J Bone Joint Surg *42A*:429, 1960.
65. Shehadi WH: Primary pyogenic osteomyelitis of the articular processes of the vertebra. J Bone Joint Surg *21*:969, 1939.
66. Leach RE, Goldstein H, Younger D: Osteomyelitis of the odontoid process. J Bone Joint Surg *49A*:369, 1967.
67. Selvaggi G: Wirbelsäulenosteomyelitis. Zentr Org Ges Chir *63*:622, 1933.
68. Chinaglia A: Die akute Osteomyelitis der Wirbelsäule. Zentr Org Ges Chird *83*:342, 1937.
69. Richards AJ: Non-tuberculous pyogenic osteomyelitis of the spine. J Can Assoc Radiol *11*:45, 1960.
70. Allen EH, Cosgrove D, Millard FJC: The radiological changes in infections of the spine and their diagnostic value. Clin Radiol *29*:31, 1978.
71. Jacobs P: Osteo-articular tuberculosis in coloured immigrants: A radiological study. Clin Radiol *15*:59, 1964.
72. Waisbren BA: Pyogenic osteomyelitis and arthritis of the spine treated with combinations of antibiotics and gamma globulin. J Bone Joint Surg *42A*:414, 1960.
73. Dini P: Le spondiliti infectiose. Arch Putti Chir Organ Nov *16*:117, 1962.
74. Weber R: Considérations sur l'ostéomyélite vertébrale. Rev Chir Orthop *51*:273, 1965.
75. Mineiro JD: Coluna vertebral humana: Alguns aspectos da sua estrutura e vascularizacao. Lisboa, Dissertacao de Doutoramento, 1965.
76. Fischer GW, Popich GA, Sullivan DE, Mayfield G, Mazat BA, Patterson PH: Diskitis: A prospective diagnostic analysis. Pediatrics *62*:543, 1978.
77. Rocco HD, Eyring EJ: Intervertebral disk infections in children. Am J Dis Child *123*:448, 1972.
78. Doyle JR: Narrowing of the intervertebral disc space in children. J Bone Joint Surg *42*:1191, 1960.
79. Mathews SS, Wiltse LL, Karbelnig MJ: A destructive lesion involving the intervertebral disc in children. Clin Orthop Rel Res *9*:162, 1957.
80. Ghormley RK, Bickel WH, Dickson DD: A study of acute infectious lesions of the intervertebral disks. South Med J *33*:347, 1940.
81. Norris S, Ehrlich MG, Keim DE, Guiterman H, McKusick KA: Early diagnosis of disk-space infection using Gallium-67. J Nucl Med *19*:384, 1978.
82. Patton JT: Differential diagnosis of inflammatory spondylitis. Skel Radiol *1*:77, 1976.
83. Resnick D, Niwayama G: Intravertebral disc herniations: Cartilaginous nodes. Radiology *126*:57, 1978.
84. Williams JL, Moller GA, O'Rourke TL: Pseudoinfections of the intervertebral disk and adjacent vertebrae. Am J Roentgenol *103*:611, 1968.
85. Sauser D, Goldman AB, Kaye JJ: Discogenic vertebral sclerosis. J Can Assoc Radiol *29*:44, 1978.
86. Resnick D, Niwayama G: Intervertebral disc abnormalities associated with vertebral metastasis: Observations in patients and cadavers with prostate cancer. Invest Radiol *13*:182, 1978.
87. Coy JT III, Wolf CR, Brower TD, Winter WG Jr: Pyogenic arthritis of the sacroiliac joint. Long term follow-up. J Bone Joint Surg *58A*:845, 1976.
88. Avila L Jr: Primary pyogenic infection of the sacroiliac articulation. A new approach to the joint. Report of 7 cases. J Bone Joint Surg *23*:922, 1941.
89. L'Episcopo JB: Suppurative arthritis of the sacroiliac joint. Ann Surg *104*:289, 1936.
90. Ailsby RL, Staheli LT: Pyogenic infections of the sacroiliac joint in children. Radioisotope bone scanning as a diagnostic tool. Clin Orthop Rel Res *100*:96, 1974.
91. Delbarre F, Rondier J, Delrieu F, Evrard J, Cayla J, Menkes CJ, Amor B: Pyogenic infection of the sacro-iliac joint. Report of thirteen cases. J Bone Joint Surg *57A*:819, 1975.
92. Young F: Acute osteomyelitis of the ilium. Surg Gynecol Obstet *58*:986, 1934.
93. Morgan A, Yates AK: The diagnosis of acute osteomyelitis of the pelvis. Postgrad Med J *42*:74, 1966.
94. Ghahremani GG: Osteomyelitis of the ilium in patients with Crohn's disease. Am J Roentgenol *118*:364, 1973.
95. Goldstein MJ, Nasr K, Singer HC, Anderson JG: Osteomyelitis complicating regional enteritis. Gut *10*:264, 1969.
96. Oppenheimer A: Paravertebral abscesses associated with Strumpell-Marie disease. J Bone Joint Surg *25*:90, 1943.
97. Goldin RH, Chow A, Edwards JE Jr, Louie JS, Guze LB: Sterno-articular septic arthritis in heroin users. N Engl J Med *289*:616, 1973.
98. Biesecker GL, Aaron BL, Mullen JT: Primary sternal osteomyelitis. Chest *63*:236, 1973.
99. Wray TM, Bryant RE, Killen DA: Sternal osteomyelitis and costochondritis after median sternotomy. J Thorac Cardiovasc Surg *65*:227, 1973.
100. Lee HY, Kerstein MD: Osteomyelitis and septic arthritis, a complication of subclavian venous catheterization. N Engl J Med *285*:1179, 1971.
101. Glushakow AS, Carlson D, DePalma AF: Pyarthrosis of the manubriosternal joint. Clin Orthop Rel Res *114*:214, 1976.
102. Pate D, Katz A: Clostridia discitis: A case report. Arthritis Rheum *22*:1039, 1979.
103. Digby JM, Kersley JB: Pyogenic nontuberculous spinal infection. An analysis of thirty cases. J Bone Joint Surg *61B*:47, 1979.
104. Beaupre A, Carroll N: The three syndromes of iliac osteomyelitis in children. J Bone Joint Surg *61A*:1087, 1979.
105. Miskew DB, Block RA, Witt PF: Aspiration of infected sacro-iliac joints. J Bone Joint Surg *61A*:1071, 1979.
106. Ralls PW, Boswell W, Henderson R, Rogers W, Boger D, Halls J: CT of inflammatory disease of the psoas muscle. Am J Roentgenol *134*:767, 1980.
107. Murray IPC: Bone scanning in the child and young adult. Skel Radiol *5*:65, 1980.
108. Norris S, Ehrlich MG, McKusick K: Early diagnosis of disk space infection with ^{67}Ga in an experimental model. Clin Orthop Rel Res *144*:293, 1979.
109. Mittapalli MR: Value of bone scan in primary sternal osteomyelitis. South Med J *72*:1603, 1979.
110. Borgmeier PJ, Kalovidouris AE: Septic arthritis of the sternomanubrial joint due to Pseudomonas pseudomallei. Arthritis Rheum *23*:1057, 1980.
111. Gordon G, Kabins SA: Pyogenic sacroiliitis. Am J Med *69*:50, 1980.

OSTEOMYELITIS, SEPTIC ARTHRITIS, AND SOFT TISSUE INFECTION: THE ORGANISMS

by Donald Resnick, M.D., and Gen Niwayama, M.D.

62

The discussions of mechanisms, situations, and sites of musculoskeletal infection given in Chapters 60 and 61 leave one major area still to be covered. To correct this deficiency, consideration will now be directed toward the specific microorganisms themselves. Although the skeleton can react in only a limited number of ways, certain characteristics of its response to a particular infectious agent may differ, at least subtly, from the changes that are encountered in the presence of a different agent. Thus, certain organisms produce rapid and destructive osseous or articular disease, whereas others are associated with a more indolent process. Furthermore, some agents show predilection for certain anatomic regions of the skeleton, whereas other agents produce changes at different sites. What follows is a survey of some of the organisms that can infect the musculoskeletal system, with emphasis given to a few of the more important disorders.

BACTERIAL INFECTION

Gram-Positive Cocci

Staphylococcal Infection. Staphylococci are responsible for the majority of cases of acute osteomyelitis[1] and nongonococcal infectious arthritis.[561, 562] Estimates of the incidence of one or another strain of staphylococcus (*S. aureus* is most typical) in pyogenic osteomyelitis can reach 80 to 90 per cent. Staphylococcal osteomyelitis is primarily a disease of children under the age of 12 to 13 years, particularly boys. In cases of hematogenous spread of infection to bone, a history of a septic process at a distant site, such as the skin, the respiratory tract, or the genitourinary system,[2] and of local trauma is frequent; localization of the infection to the metaphysis of tubular bones of children is typical, although virtually any extra-axial or axial skeletal site may be affected. Brodie's abscesses may be seen (Fig. 62–1). Staphylococci are responsible also for many of the deep infections that occur after bone or joint surgery,[3-5] the foot infections in diabetic individuals, and the osseous, articular, and soft tissue suppurative processes that follow penetrating or open wounds (Fig. 62–1).

The clinical and radiologic features of musculoskeletal infections due to staphylococci were discussed in Chapters 60 and 61.

Streptococcal Infection. Streptococcal organisms, particularly beta-hemolytic streptococci, can cause osteomyelitis. In infants, hemolytic streptococcal agents were a frequent cause of osteomyelitis prior to 1940[6] and have recently been recognized as an important etiologic factor in neonatal or infantile osteomyelitis.[7-11, 520, 529, 530] The clinical manifestations of streptococcal bone infection may be mild even in the presence of significant radiologic alterations, a feature that is evident in other types of infantile osteomyelitis as well. Typically, the disease is discovered in the first few weeks of life.[10] Infection of a single bone is most frequent, and predilection for humeral involvement has been noted by some investigators. Lytic lesions with mild or absent sclerosis and periostitis can be seen. Following recovery of the organism from the blood or elsewhere, antibiotic therapy usually leads to rapid healing.

The joints may be infected by streptococcal organisms either by extension from a neighboring site of osteomyelitis or cellulitis or directly,[12] although the prevalence of such articular infection appears to be declining. Residual joint damage is infrequent if appropriate antibiotic treatment is instituted without significant delay.

Anaerobic streptococci can contaminate soft tissue wounds and fractures, producing a crepitant myositis that resembles clostridial gas gangrene. Osteomyelitis and septic arthritis due to streptococcal infection can follow human bites.[13]

Pneumococcal Infection. Pneumococcal arthritis is not frequent.[14-16] A recent report of 12 patients with this disease emphasized the prominence of underlying conditions (alcoholism, hypogammaglobulinemia), preexisting joint alterations (rheumatoid arthritis, osteoarthritis), and coexistent pneumococcal infection (meningitis, endocarditis).[17] Children or adults may be affected, and the knee appears to be the most commonly involved site. Soft tissue swelling, joint space narrowing, osseous erosions, periostitis, and periarticular calcification are encountered[18] (Fig. 62–2). Antibiotic therapy usually produces a favorable response with return of normal joint function.

Gram-Negative Cocci

Meningococcal Infection. Meningococcal arthritis is not a common condition.[19-22, 521] Three forms are recognized: an acute transient polyarthritis associated with marked pain and tenderness occurring simultaneously with a petechial rash, and perhaps related to intra-articular hemorrhage; a purulent arthritis involving one or more joints, often the knee, occurring after the fifth day of illness; and arthritis following serum therapy, a variety that is not seen currently.[23, 24] The incidence of purulent arthritis in cases of meningococcal infection is 5 to 10 per cent.[22] It may arise during septicemia or as the infection is being controlled with chemotherapy.[25] Rapid resolution of the joint disease is typical, although occasionally a protracted course with radiologic evidence of cartilaginous and osseous destruction is evident.[26, 27]

Gonococcal Infection

Clinical Abnormalities. The incidence of gonococcal arthritis is rising. Although the reasons for

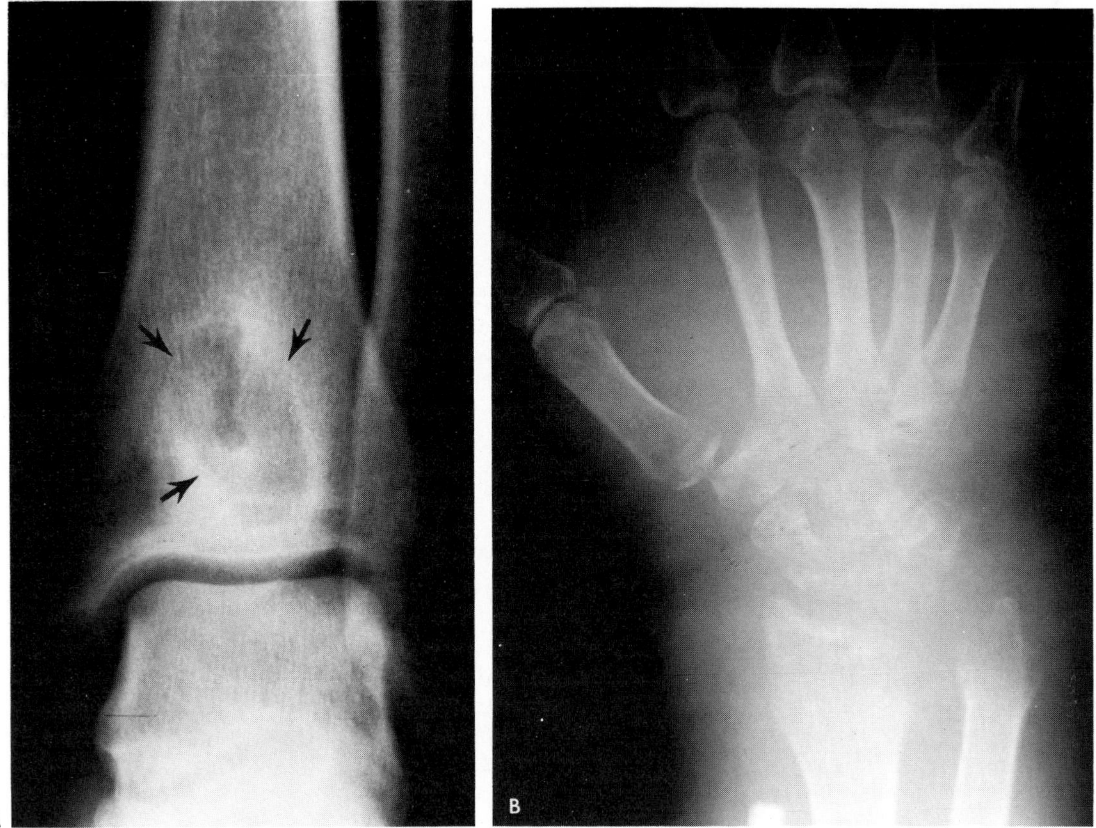

Figure 62–1. *Staphylococcal osteomyelitis and septic arthritis.*

A *A well-defined lucent lesion surrounded by a sclerotic margin at the end of the tubular bone (arrows) is typical of a Brodie's abscess.*

B *In this 43 year old woman, massive soft tissue swelling of the hand and wrist is associated with osteolysis of multiple carpal bones, radius, and ulna. Widening of the radiocarpal and inferior radioulnar joints is evident. Fistulae were apparent clinically, and culture confirmed the presence of* Staphylococcus aureus. *In this case, osteomyelitis and septic arthritis have resulted from a neglected overlying soft tissue infection.*

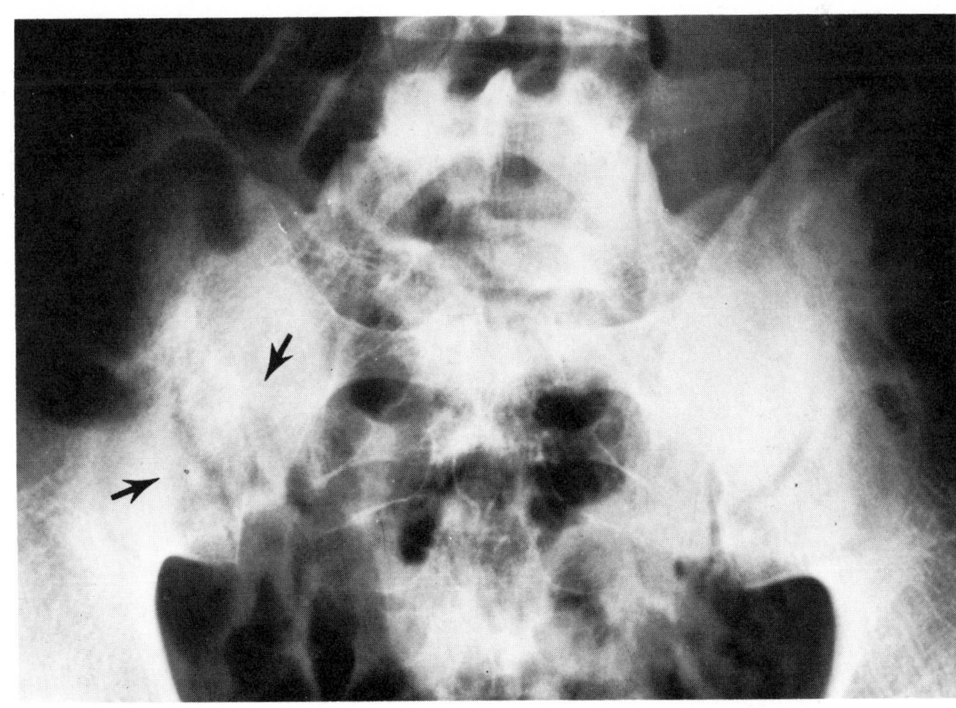

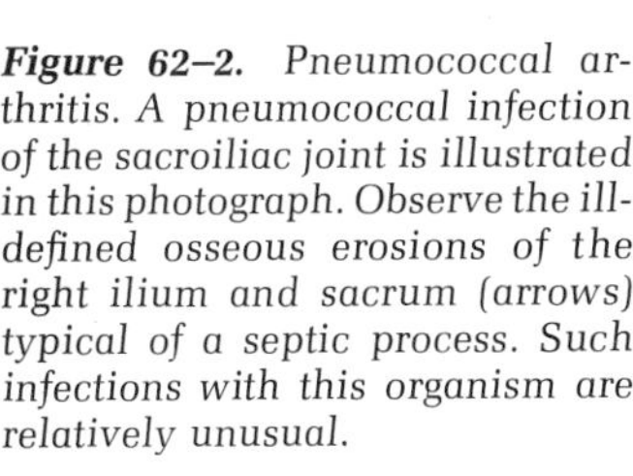

Figure 62–2. *Pneumococcal arthritis. A pneumococcal infection of the sacroiliac joint is illustrated in this photograph. Observe the ill-defined osseous erosions of the right ilium and sacrum (arrows) typical of a septic process. Such infections with this organism are relatively unusual.*

this rise are not entirely clear, there is evidence to suggest that there has been an increasing resistance of the gonococcus to antibiotics over the last few decades. The role of changing sexual mores in the resurgence of gonococcal arthritis in recent years is controversial. Although gonorrhea is more frequent in women than in men, the disease may become evident in homosexual men. It is also encountered during pregnancy and following gonococcal vulvovaginitis in children and in the neonate.[23, 28-36] It is clear that as an infant passes through the birth canal, any of its orifices may act as a portal of entry for the gonococcus; susceptible sites include the conjunctiva and the anogenital, oropharyngeal, and umbilical orifices.[34] The articular disease may have an insidious onset, with fleeting arthralgias, or a sudden onset with fever and red, hot, swollen and tender joint(s). Polyarticular findings are frequent, although the infection tends to localize in one or two joints. The affected articulations, in decreasing order of frequency, are the knee, the ankle, the wrist, and the joints of the shoulder, foot, and spine (Fig. 62–3). The articulations of the lower extremity are much more commonly involved than those of the upper extremity. In approximately 50 per cent of cases, tenosynovitis, particularly on the dorsal aspect of the fingers, is evident. Other clinical manifestations include skin rash[37] and, rarely, suppurative myositis.[38]

Recently, several stages of this articular disease have been recognized.[35] In patients with a positive blood culture or typical skin rash, clinical findings appear earlier in the disease course than in patients with positive joint culture without organisms recoverable from the blood. Dissemination of the microorganisms from the primary site of infection via the bloodstream leads to a typical and frequently toxic syndrome consisting of fever, chills, skin lesions, and polyarthritis. During this stage of the illness (1 to 3 days) aspiration of joint contents is frequently unrewarding, and polyarthritis is evanescent. By the fourth to sixth day, articular manifestations dominate the clinical picture and involve one or a few joints that commonly contain fluid from which the microorganisms can be cultured.[35, 39]

Pathologic Abnormalities. A reliable diagnosis of gonococcal arthritis depends upon recovery of the bacteria from the blood, the synovial tissue, the synovial fluid, the genitourinary tract, or the skin. This is accomplished in 50 to 60 per cent of suspected cases. The synovial fluid is an exudate that can be frankly purulent or straw-colored. The appearance of the synovial membrane is typical of that of pyogenic articular processes.[40] Initially, infiltration of the membrane with polymorphonuclear leukocytes, lymphocytes, and plasma cells is identified. With progression, the synovial lining may be destroyed and the inner surface of the articular capsule is

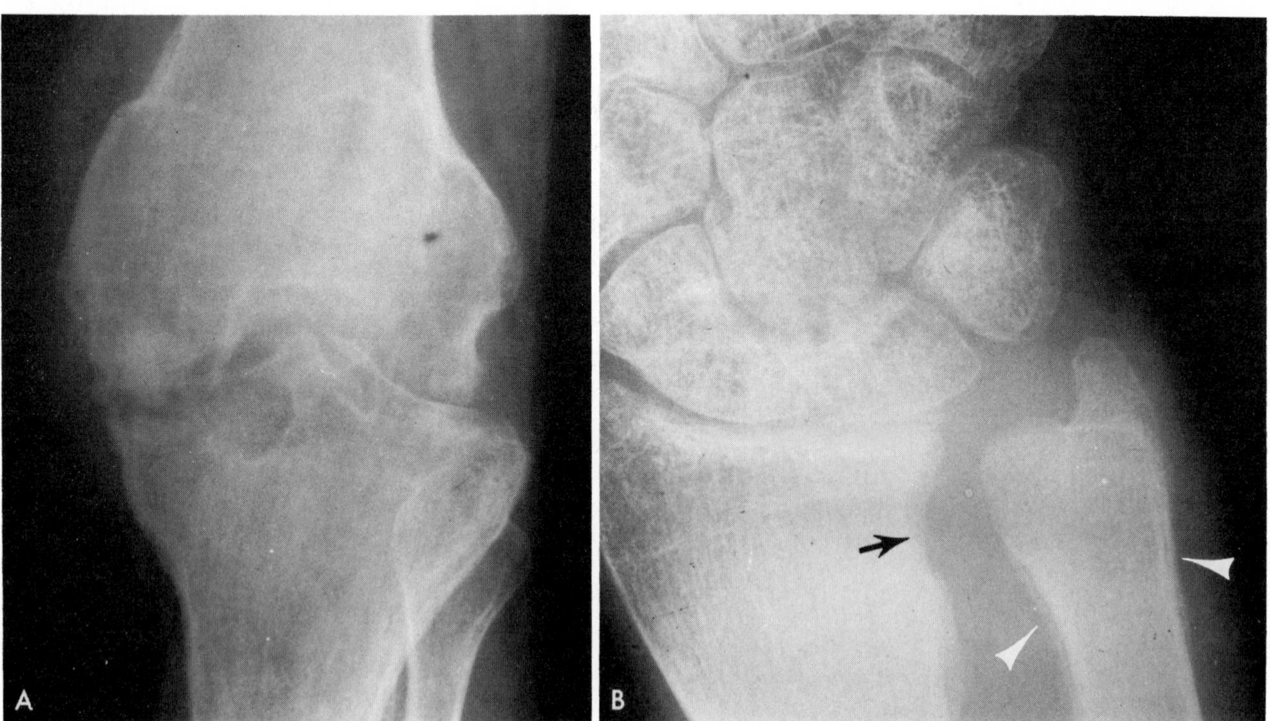

Figure 62–3. *Gonococcal arthritis.*

A *Knee. Observe joint space loss, poorly defined marginal and central osseous erosions, and soft tissue swelling. The lack of osteoporosis is impressive. Bony proliferation is evident along the distal medial femur.*

B *Inferior radioulnar joint. Note massive soft tissue swelling about the distal ulna, scalloped osseous erosions (arrow), and periostitis (arrowheads). Carpal osteoporosis is seen.*

covered with granulation tissue containing polymorphonuclear leukocytes, macrophages, and plasma cells.[1] The articular cartilage and subchondral bone may become involved in later stages of joint infection or in early stages when hematogenous implantation has produced a primary osteomyelitis.[36, 41, 42]

Radiologic Abnormalities. When antibiotic treatment is instituted at an early stage, the only significant radiographic features are soft tissue swelling and osteoporosis. If appropriate treatment is delayed, more prominent roentgenographic findings are encountered, including joint space narrowing, marginal and central osseous erosions, lytic destruction of adjacent metaphyses and epiphyses, and periostitis (Fig. 62–3). Healing can be associated with intra-articular osseous fusion. These features are identical to those accompanying other pyogenic infections. The appearance of abnormalities at multiple joints and tenosynovitis are helpful clues to a specific diagnosis of gonococcal infection.[43]

Pathogenesis. The pathogenesis of the various inflammatory lesions in disseminated gonococcemia is controversial. Numerous theories have been proposed to explain the cutaneous and articular manifestations of the disease. Although attempts at demonstrating *Neisseria gonorrhoeae* by culture and smear of the skin lesions are rarely successful,[44] identification of typical organisms with the utilization of immunofluorescent staining techniques of the involved cutaneous tissue[45] underscores the current explanation of the skin lesions, which is that they represent embolization of gonococcal organisms to cutaneous vessels.[46] Recently, circulating immune complexes have been detected in the migratory polyarthralgic phase of gonococcal arthritis.[47] Other evidence supporting[48, 49, 531] and negating[46] the role of immune complexes and gonococcal antigen in the pathogenesis of disseminated gonococcal disease is available. At this writing, the exact mechanism by which gonococcal organisms or their products affect skin and joint is not known.

Differential Diagnosis. The accurate differentiation of gonococcal joint disease and that related to other pyogenic organisms on the basis of roentgenographic findings is usually not possible; this differentiation depends upon the interpretation of the roentgenographic abnormalities in light of the clinical findings. Furthermore, differentiating the radiographic features of gonococcal pyarthrosis and Reiter's syndrome can be extremely difficult; clinical differentiation is complicated by the presence of skin rash, urethral discharge, and articular abnormalities in both conditions. Gonococcal arthritis and Reiter's syndrome both produce soft tissue swelling, osteoporosis, joint space narrowing, osseous erosion, and periostitis in one or more articulations, particularly in the lower extremity. Involvement of the joints of the foot, the calcaneus, the spine, and the sacroiliac articulation; the presence of poorly defined periosteal proliferation about the involved joints; and the absence of fuzzy or frayed central osseous margins are helpful in accurately diagnosing Reiter's syndrome.

Enteric Gram-Negative Bacilli

COLIFORM BACTERIAL INFECTION. The coliform bacteria are gram-negative bacilli that normally inhabit the human intestinal tract. The best-known organisms in this group are *Escherichia coli* and *Aerobacter aerogenes*. Articular and osseous infections with these agents (and the other gram-negative bacilli that are discussed below) are rare except in the drug abuser, the individual with preexisting joint disease, and the patient with a chronic debilitating disorder.[50] The usual mechanism of articular infection is hematogenous, although direct inoculation following a diagnostic or therapeutic procedure or injury can be implicated in some patients. Monoarticular involvement, especially of the knee, is generally associated with a poor therapeutic response. No specific radiographic features are evident, although emphysematous septic arthritis has been noted in patients with *E. coli* infection.[51, 52]

PROTEUS INFECTION. *Proteus mirabilis* infection of a joint is rarely observed.[50] The clinical situation is similar to that which is observed with coliform bacterial infection. Urinary tract abnormalities may coexist. Monoarticular involvement of the knee or another articulation is typical.

PSEUDOMONAS INFECTION. Serious infection with this organism is almost invariably associated with diminished resistance of the host or damage to local tissues (Fig. 62–4). Premature infants, children with congenital anomalies, drug abusers, patients with myeloproliferative disorders or those receiving immunosuppressive agents, and geriatric patients with debilitating diseases are individuals who may develop osteomyelitis or septic arthritis due to *Pseudomonas aeruginosa*.[50, 53-56] Hematogenous spread of infection is common in drug addicts; Pseudomonas infection commonly localizes in the axial skeleton, affecting the spine and the sacroiliac, sternoclavicular, and acromioclavicular articulations. The peculiar proclivity of drug abusers to develop Pseudomonas osteomyelitis and septic arthritis and the common localization of such disease within the central skeleton are interesting but unexplained observations.

Pseudomonas contamination of bone and joint can result also from spread of infection in an adjacent focus or from direct inoculation. Pseudomonas osteomyelitis is a recognized complication of puncture wounds,[57-60, 532] although Proteus, *E. Coli*, and other agents may also be implicated in this clinical situation.[59] Other types of trauma and surgery can lead to Pseudomonas involvement of osseous and articular structures. No specific radiographic features characterize skeletal involvement with this organism.

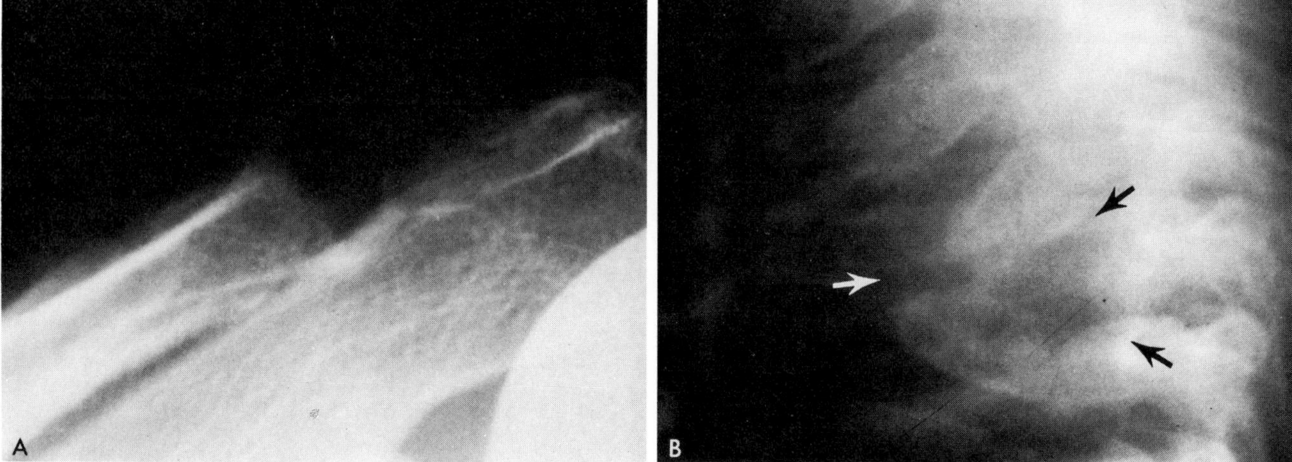

Figure 62–4. Pseudomonas osteomyelitis and septic arthritis.

A *In this drug abuser, osteomyelitis of the distal clavicle and septic arthritis of the acromioclavicular joint with osseous destruction and periostitis were related to Pseudomonas infection. Infection with this organism and in this location is not infrequent in the drug abuser.*

B *This 11 month old girl, one of twins, developed fever, back tenderness, and deformity. Aspiration and culture revealed Pseudomonas. Observe the destruction of several vertebral bodies and intervertebral discs (arrows). It is not certain whether all of the bony changes were related to infection or whether anomalies existed prior to sepsis.*

KLEBSIELLA INFECTION. Rarely, *Klebsiella pneumoniae* (or *K. friedländeri*) results in osteomyelitis and septic arthritis in a host with diminished resistance.[50]

SALMONELLA INFECTION. *Salmonella typhi* produces a systemic infection, typhoid fever. Before the advent of antibiotics, bone infection was encountered in approximately 1 per cent of patients with typhoid fever[61]; more recently, such cases have indeed become rare.[62-68] Involvement can occur in extraspinal or spinal locations (Fig. 62–5*A*). In the latter site, the radiographic picture resembles that in tuberculosis. The similarity is accentuated by histologic findings revealing an inflammatory process with or without caseating necrosis.[63, 67]

Other Salmonella organisms can involve bone and joint.[69, 70, 533] Salmonella arthritis is not common, predominates in infants and young children, and may be the initial or major manifestation of infection. It is usually monarticular, most frequently affecting the knee, the glenohumeral joint, and the hip.[23] Swelling, pain, tenderness, and limitation of articular motion may be evident.[69]

An association exists between Salmonella infection and sickle cell anemia or other hemoglobinopathies,[71-73] as well as leukemia (Fig. 62–5*B, C*), lymphoma, bartonellosis, cirrhosis of the liver, and systemic lupus erythematosus.[67] In patients with sickle cell disease, infection with *S. choleraesuis, S. paratyphi,* or *S. typhimurium* is most typical.[74] The basis for the unusual propensity of these individuals to develop Salmonella infection is not known. It has been postulated that multiple bowel infarcts allow the organisms to leave the colon and enter the bloodstream, and that Salmonella organisms are well suited for survival in areas of medullary bone infarction.[74] In fact, Salmonella osteomyelitis frequently originates in the medullary cavity of a tubular bone, although epiphyses and other osseous structures can occasionally be affected.[75] However, Salmonella spondylitis is reported to be rare.[1] In tubular bones, salmonella infection may be characterized by a symmetric distribution, a combination of lysis and sclerosis, and periostitis, findings that are difficult to differentiate from infarction alone. In addition to suppurative arthritis and osteomyelitis, a nonbacterial polyarthritis may be observed 1 to 2 weeks after infection with *S. typhimurium.*[76, 77] Its clinical manifestations resemble those of rheumatic fever.[23] A relationship between this variety of postinfectious polyarthritis and Reiter's syndrome, spondylitis, and the presence of HLA B27 antigen has been noted.[23, 78]

A Salmonella subspecies, *Salmonella arizonae (Arizona hinshawii)* bacillus, is also capable of producing osteomyelitis, especially in association with sickle cell disease.[96-98]

SHIGELLA INFECTION. Two to three weeks after acute bacillary dysentery, a noninfectious polyarthritis showing predilection for the knees, the elbows, the wrists, or the fingers can be evident, which simulates rheumatic fever and which may be associated with Reiter's syndrome and the HLA B27 antigen.[23, 78]

YERSINIA ENTEROCOLITICA INFECTION. Two types of bone or joint affliction can occur in association with infection with this organism. A nonsuppurative, self-limited polyarthritis, especially of the

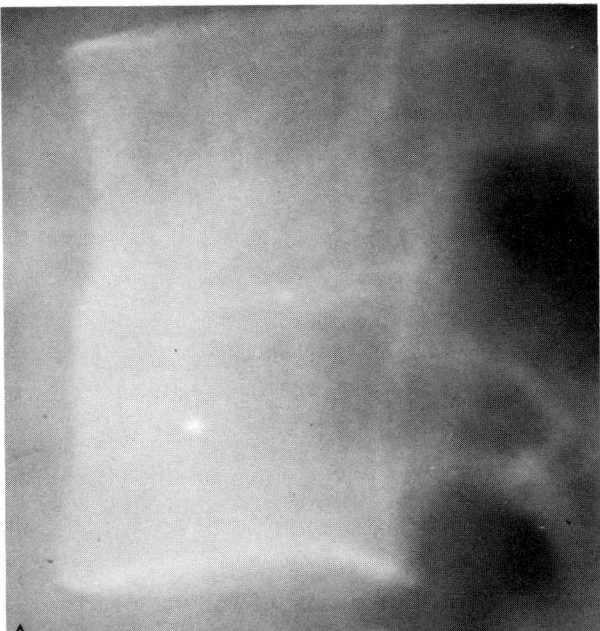

Figure 62–5. *Salmonella spondylitis and septic arthritis.*

A Salmonella typhi *infection led to vertebral and intervertebral discal involvement in this individual. The bony ankylosis of the vertebral bodies represents the end result of this infection.*

B, C *Salmonella arthritis in a child with leukemia. The plain film* **(B)** *reveals osteoporosis, subchondral radiolucent lines, and an effusion with slight lateral displacement of the femoral head. A bone scan* **(C)** *shows subtle increased activity in the right hip (arrows). Aspiration confirmed the diagnosis.*

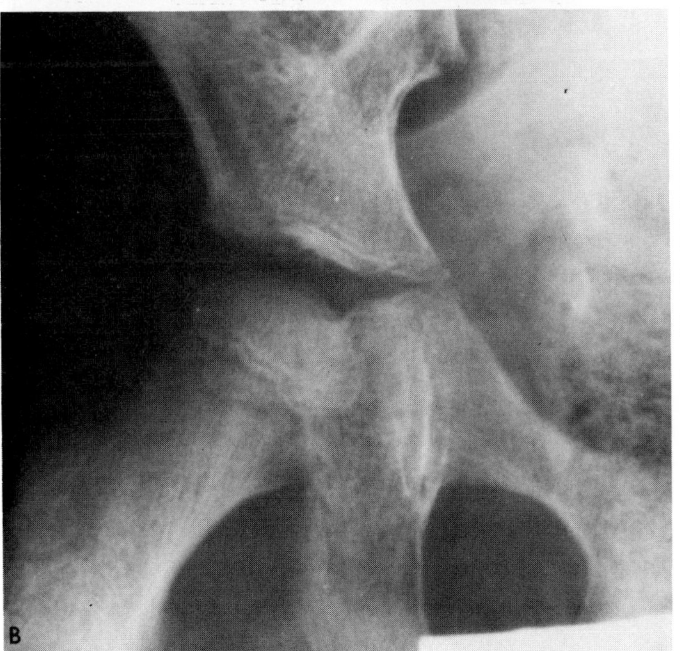

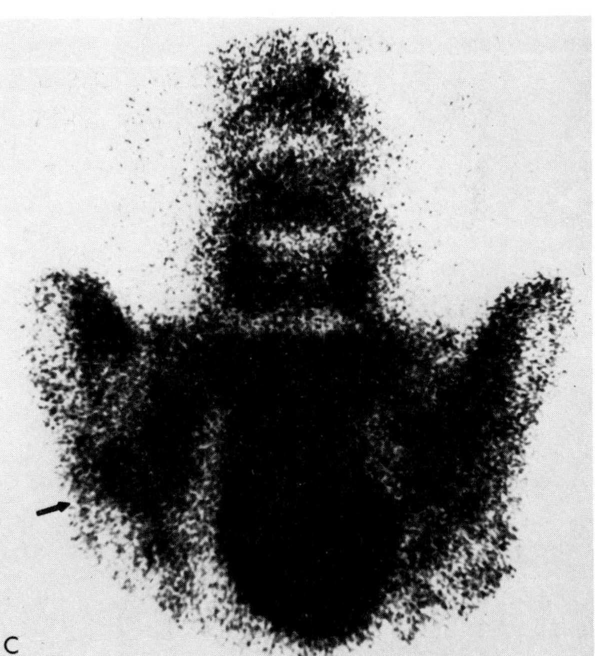

knees and the ankles, can appear approximately 3 weeks after the onset of the illness.[23, 79, 80] This articular manifestation may be complicated by sacroiliitis and the presence of the HLA B27 antigen. The second type of affliction relates to the presence of *Y. enterocolitica* septicemia, particularly in patients with underlying abnormalities (hemoglobinopathies, leukemia, diabetes, alcoholism). Septic arthritis or osteomyelitis may appear in this setting.[81-84]

Other Gram-Negative Bacilli

Hemophilus Infection. Acute septic arthritis due to *Hemophilus influenzae* has been recorded.[85-93, 522, 534] It is more frequent in children, particularly between the ages of 7 months and 4 years, than in adults (Fig. 62–6). In adult patients, alcoholism, diabetes, the nephrotic syndrome, or agammaglobulinemia may be present.[90, 94] Hematogenous spread is the usual mechanism of joint infection. Single or multiple articulations may be affected, with the knee and the ankle being the most frequent sites of involvement. Less commonly, localization in joints of the hand and the foot is apparent; a case of infection of the first metatarsophalangeal joint resembling gout has been noted.[93] Vertebral osteomyelitis caused by this organism has also been reported.[95] A relationship of hemophilus pyarthrosis and trauma has been suggested; in this regard, it is of interest that the majority of cases have affected the right side of the body (the dominant side?). Hemophilus tenosynovitis has also been described.[535, 563]

Brucella Infection. Brucellosis (undulant fever) can result from human infection with one of a variety of organisms, including *Brucella abortus, Brucella melitensis,* and *Brucella suis.*[99, 100] The disease, which is endemic in the Midwest of the United States, is transmitted to humans from lower animals such as the goat, the cow, and the hog through the ingestion of milk or milk products containing viable bacteria or through contact of skin with infected tissues or secretions. The disease is very rarely transmitted from one human to another. The invading organisms localize in tissues of the reticuloendothelial system, such as the liver, the spleen, the lymph nodes, and the bone marrow. Following an incubation period, which varies from 7 to 21 days (or

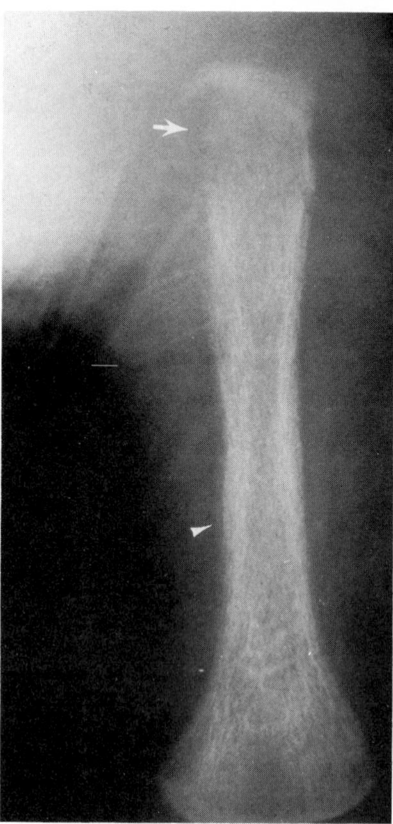

Figure 62–6. *Hemophilus osteomyelitis and septic arthritis. This infant developed osteomyelitis of the proximal metaphysis and diaphysis of the humerus with glenohumeral joint involvement due to Hemophilus. Observe metaphyseal erosion (arrow), permeative bone destruction, and periostitis (arrowhead).*

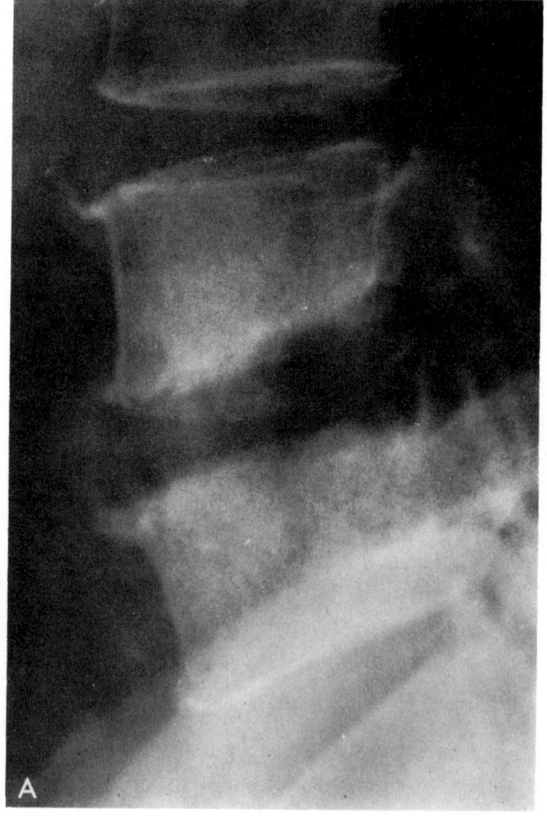

Figure 62–7. *Brucellar spondylitis.*

A *Lumbar spine involvement is characterized by irregular destruction of the osseous surfaces of two adjacent vertebrae with reactive sclerosis.*

Illustration continued on the opposite page

longer), fever, headaches, weakness, sweats, myalgia, and arthralgia become apparent.

Involvement of joints, bones, and bursae is relatively uncommon, although an inflammatory process in any one of these sites in a farmer or meathandler should arouse suspicion of brucellosis.[101] The arthritis is usually monarticular, with the hip joint being most frequently involved.[23] Alterations of bursae may be especially characteristic, with common inflammation in the prepatellar region.[101, 102] Other bursae, including that of the subdeltoid area, may also be involved.[103]

Osteomyelitis of long or flat bones may be encountered; it is frequently chronic in nature, and the osseous tissues may be secondarily invaded by staphylococci.[101] Brucellar spondylitis typically affects the lumbar spine and is associated with an acute clinical onset and rapid progression of radiologic findings (Fig. 62–7). Abnormalities include destruction of vertebrae and intervertebral discs, sclerosis, paravertebral abscess formation, and healing with intraosseous fusion and osteophytosis.[74, 101, 104-106] These radiographic abnormalities resemble those in other types of pyogenic or tuberculous spondylitis. Osteoporosis and paraspinal calcification may be somewhat less common in brucellosis than in tuberculosis.[107]

The diagnosis of brucellosis is frequently difficult to establish.[23] Culture of the organisms from a joint or bursa provides an absolute diagnosis; a rising serum agglutination titer in conjunction with developing spinal or extraspinal clinical and radio-

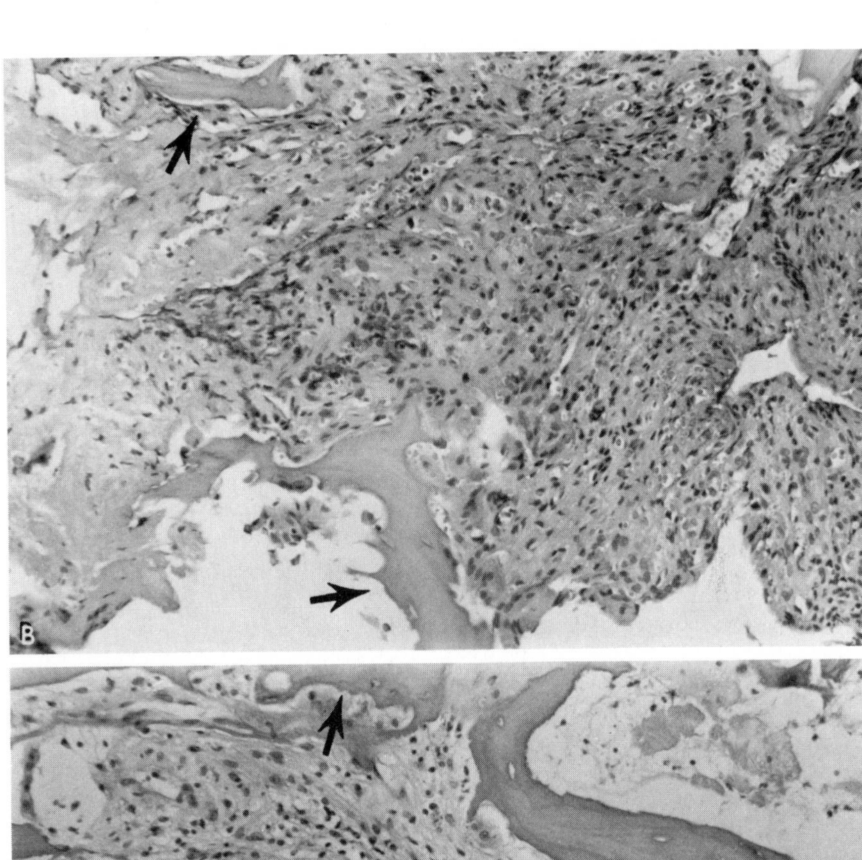

Figure 62–7. Continued

B *A photomicrograph (50×) in a different patient with brucellar spondylitis reveals necrotic osseous trabeculae (arrows) surrounded by active chronic inflammatory cells (predominantly lymphocytes and polymorphonuclear leukocytes), cellular debris, and fibroblastic cells with stromal fibrosis.*

C *In another photomicrograph (50×), osseous trabeculae show complete or incomplete necrosis (arrows). The intervening stroma reveals active chronic inflammation with polymorphonuclear leukocytes, lymphocytes, cellular debris, fibrinous exudate, and fibrosis.*

graphic findings allows a confident diagnosis. Skin tests are of little diagnostic value. Histologic examination of the synovial membrane shows granulomatous tissue, cellular infiltration with large or small mononuclear cells, and granuloma formation.[108] A granulomatous osteomyelitis may be evident on bone biopsy (Fig. 62–7).

SERRATIA INFECTION. *Serratia marcescens* can cause infection of the musculoskeletal system, especially in individuals with underlying disorders such as diabetes mellitus, systemic lupus erythematosus, and rheumatoid arthritis, or following trauma, osteonecrosis, or drug abuse.[50, 109-113, 536] The usual pathway for articular infection with this organism is the bloodstream. Radiographic features of septic arthritis include soft tissue swelling, osteoporosis, and osseous destruction and are entirely nonspecific.

AEROMONAS INFECTION. *Aeromonas hydrophilia* is an aerobic gram-negative rod found in water and stools from some individuals. Although rarely a pathogen, it can cause infection in patients with neoplasm or chronic liver disease.[114, 115] Following initiation of septic arthritis resulting from hematogenous spread of infection, the patients respond poorly to therapy.

Other Bacteria

CORYNEBACTERIUM (DIPHTHEROID) INFECTION. Diphtheroid bacteria belong to the genus Corynebacterium and are part of the normal flora of the skin, mucous membranes, and gastrointestinal tract.[116] Although these bacteria are identified in 1 to 30 per cent of all blood cultures[117] and in 3 per cent of surgical specimens obtained at total hip arthroplasty,[118] they are usually regarded as contaminants. Rarely, diphtheroid bacteria can cause septic arthritis or osteomyelitis.[116, 119, 120] In these circumstances, a preexisting condition or disease is usually evident, or previous surgery has been accomplished.

CLOSTRIDIAL INFECTION

Gas Gangrene. Wounds that are contaminated by gas gangrene may contain a mixture of clostridial organisms, including *C. tetani, C. perfringens, C. welchii, C. septicum,* and *C. novyi.* These organisms are anaerobic and are capable of producing extensive tissue destruction with gas formation at the site of invasion. Soft tissue contamination with gas gangrene develops in devitalized tissues in which arterial blood supply has been compromised. Edema, necrotizing myositis, vascular thrombosis, cellular infiltration, and interstitial gas bubbles are evident.

Clinical manifestations of clostridial myonecrosis may become evident within 6 to 8 hours of injury, and include severe pain and an edematous, pulseless, and gangrenous limb. Crepitation with detection of gas in the soft tissue is apparent in the later stages of the disease. Systemic manifestations include prostration, a normal or slightly elevated temperature, anorexia, and ultimately, circulatory collapse, coma, and death.[537]

Clinical manifestations of clostridial cellulitis are less striking. This condition relates to infection of skin and subcutaneous tissue with subsequent necrosis. The underlying skeletal muscle is not affected. Local pain and crepitus can be detected, but systemic manifestations are absent or mild.

On radiographs, radiolucent collections may appear within the subcutaneous or muscular tissues (Fig. 62–8). In the former location, they produce linear or net-like lucent areas that can extend both proximally and distally. Gas in the muscular tissues may produce circular collections of varying size.

Arthritis. *Clostridium perfringens* (or rarely *C. bifermentans*) can be introduced into an articulation by contamination from a penetrating injury or, rarely, by hematogenous spread from its normal site of residence in the gastrointestinal tract.[121-126] Diabetes mellitus and plasma cell myeloma have been present in some patients with this infection. Monoarticular disease, particularly of the knee, is typical. Synovial edema and inflammation and cartilaginous destruction can be evident, perhaps related to the effect of

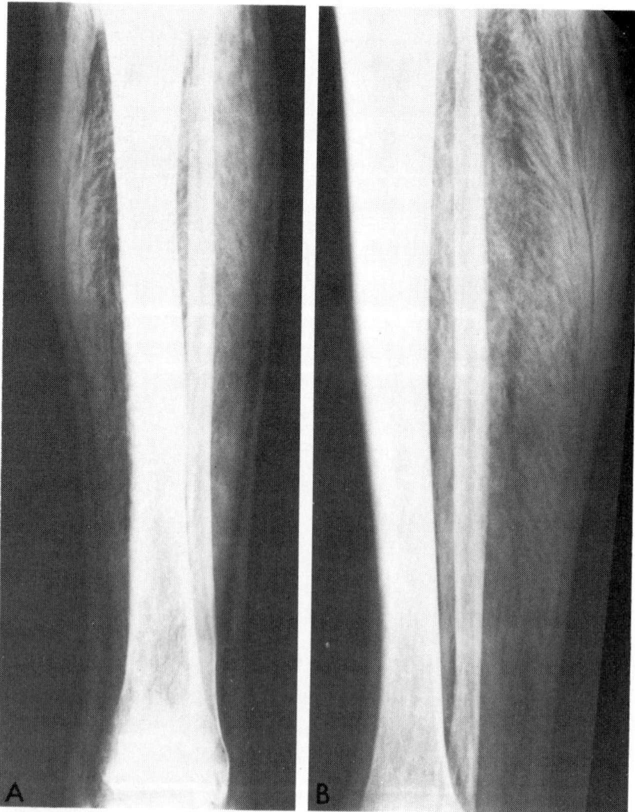

Figure 62–8. *Clostridial soft tissue infection. Linear and circular collections of gas in the subcutaneous and muscular tissues reflect the presence of clostridial myositis and cellulitis.*

the highly toxic enzymes produced by these bacteria.[125, 127] In addition to joint space narrowing and osseous defects, radiographs may delineate gas in the adjacent soft tissues or articulation itself.

Mycobacteria

TUBERCULOUS INFECTION

Incidence and Pattern. The incidence of tuberculosis has changed dramatically since the advent of appropriate chemotherapy for this disease.[128, 523] Even when pulmonary tuberculosis was a common and largely uncontrolled disorder, musculoskeletal involvement was not very frequent, the approximate incidence being 10 cases per 10,000 subjects.[1, 129, 130] In the 1940's and 1950's, osseous involvement occurred in approximately 3 to 5 per cent of tuberculous patients, although in individuals with extrapulmonary tuberculosis, the incidence of skeletal abnormalities was approximately 30 per cent.[1] These statistics varied with the country under consideration, the prevalence of the disease being greater in impoverished, undernourished, and overcrowded areas. Currently, the frequency of tuberculosis in general, and skeletal tuberculosis in particular, has diminished, although the utilization of modern therapeutic techniques, including BCG vaccination, has produced examples of iatrogenic infection (see discussion later in this chapter).

Furthermore, the pattern of osteoarticular tuberculosis has changed over the years.[23] Initially, the disease was usually encountered in children and young adults; currently, patients of all ages are affected. Individuals with underlying disorders, drug abusers, and immigrants are not infrequent hosts for this disease.[131-133] In the past, there have been two modes of infection: inhalation and ingestion.[134] The latter mechanism was more common for the bovine tubercle bacillus, *Mycobacterium bovis*, and was responsible for approximately 20 per cent of all cases of bone and joint tuberculosis, especially in children.[135] This mechanism of infection has been largely eradicated, although *Mycobacterium tuberculosis* remains an important source of the musculoskeletal alterations. Although such alterations are considered to result from hematogenous infection secondary to tuberculosis at a distant site, rarely there is no apparent primary lesion.[136]

Tuberculous spondylitis has been the most typical form of the disease. However, in recent years, articular changes in extraspinal sites, such as the hip, the knee, the wrist, and the elbow, have been more prominent.[134] Tuberculous dactylitis, multiple sites of involvement, and tendon sheath abnormalities are also commonly encountered.

Clinical Abnormalities. Skeletal tuberculosis can affect individuals of all ages, although it is rare in the first year of life. There is no significant predilection for either sex. The vertebral column, the hip, and the knee are the most frequent sites of involvement. The articulations of the lower extremity are more commonly affected than are those of the upper extremity.

The presenting symptoms and signs of the disease vary considerably.[1, 134] Tuberculous arthritis can lead to pain, swelling, weakness, muscle wasting, a draining sinus, and other manifestations, which may be present for 1 to 2 years prior to diagnosis. A history of local trauma may be obtained in 30 to 50 per cent of cases. Tuberculous spondylitis presents clinically with the insidious onset of back pain, stiffness, local tenderness, and possibly fever. Neurologic abnormalities may also be apparent. The mortality rate of tuberculous spondylitis, previously reported as 26 to 30 per cent,[1] has decreased in recent years but is still relatively high. This form of tuberculosis is most clearly associated with pulmonary disease. Tuberculous dactylitis usually presents as painless swelling of the hand or the foot. Tuberculous tenosynovitis and bursitis can produce soft tissue swelling and tenderness in the ulnar or radial bursa, the fingers, and the toes.[137]

A positive skin test for tuberculosis is of little help in the diagnosis of this disease, although a negative skin test usually excludes the diagnosis. A negative chest roentgenogram in the adult patient does not exclude the possibility of skeletal tuberculosis. In a child, such a roentgenogram makes tuberculosis an unlikely cause of bony abnormalities. The disorder is confirmed by the demonstration of the tubercle bacilli in smear or culture; this may require aspiration of joint contents or biopsy of the synovial membrane in cases of tuberculous arthritis and closed or open biopsy of bone in cases of tuberculous osteomyelitis.[23, 138]

Pathogenesis. It is generally accepted that skeletal involvement in tuberculosis occurs mainly by the hematogenous route. The localization to metaphyseal segments of long bones is noted in this disease as in hematogenously derived pyogenic osteomyelitis, perhaps related to tuberculous infarcts from emboli within the nutrient vessels[181] or to an obliterative endarteritis.[182]

Hematogenous seeding of the skeleton may arise from a primary infection of the lung, particularly in children, or at a later date, from a quiescent primary site or an extraosseous focus. With healing of the primary complex, there is a tendency toward resolution of skeletal foci, most healing without residua.[77] Occasionally, reactivation of bone and joint tuberculosis is evident. This phenomenon may occur following decreased local resistance (e.g., trauma, debilitation)[183] and is especially frequent in the hip.[134]

The incidence of associated visceral disease in patients with skeletal tuberculosis varies with the age of the patient and the method of tissue analysis (clinical, surgical, radiographic, pathologic).[177] Pulmonary involvement may be evident in 50 per cent of cases, is more frequent in children, and on radiographs may appear either active or inactive; urogenital lesions may coexist with skeletal involvement in 20 to 45 per cent of cases.[182-186]

General Pathologic Considerations. Although the specific response to tuberculosis is influenced by the anatomic structure of the skeletal part that is affected, some general characteristics can be noted.[1] The typical response of the tissue is the formation of tubercles that are sharply demarcated from the surrounding tissue (Fig. 62–9). Around a central zone are clusters of epithelioid cells with elongated vesicular nuclei. In the central part of the tubercle are multinucleated giant cells, whereas at the periphery of the tubercle is a mantle of lymphocytes.

Central caseating necrosis is characteristic of these tubercles, incited by the tuberculin produced by the bacilli.[1] During the progression of necrosis, the epithelioid cells degenerate and become grouped into an amorphous mass. Peripheral growth of the tubercle relates to the influx of new mononuclear cells, which mature into the epithelioid cells, a process that continues so long as neighboring viable tubercle bacilli are present. A prominent role of degenerating bacilli in tubercle formation is also probable.

Healing of lesions is associated with the production of hyaline fibrous nodules. Encapsulation of large caseous foci may ultimately lead to tubercle

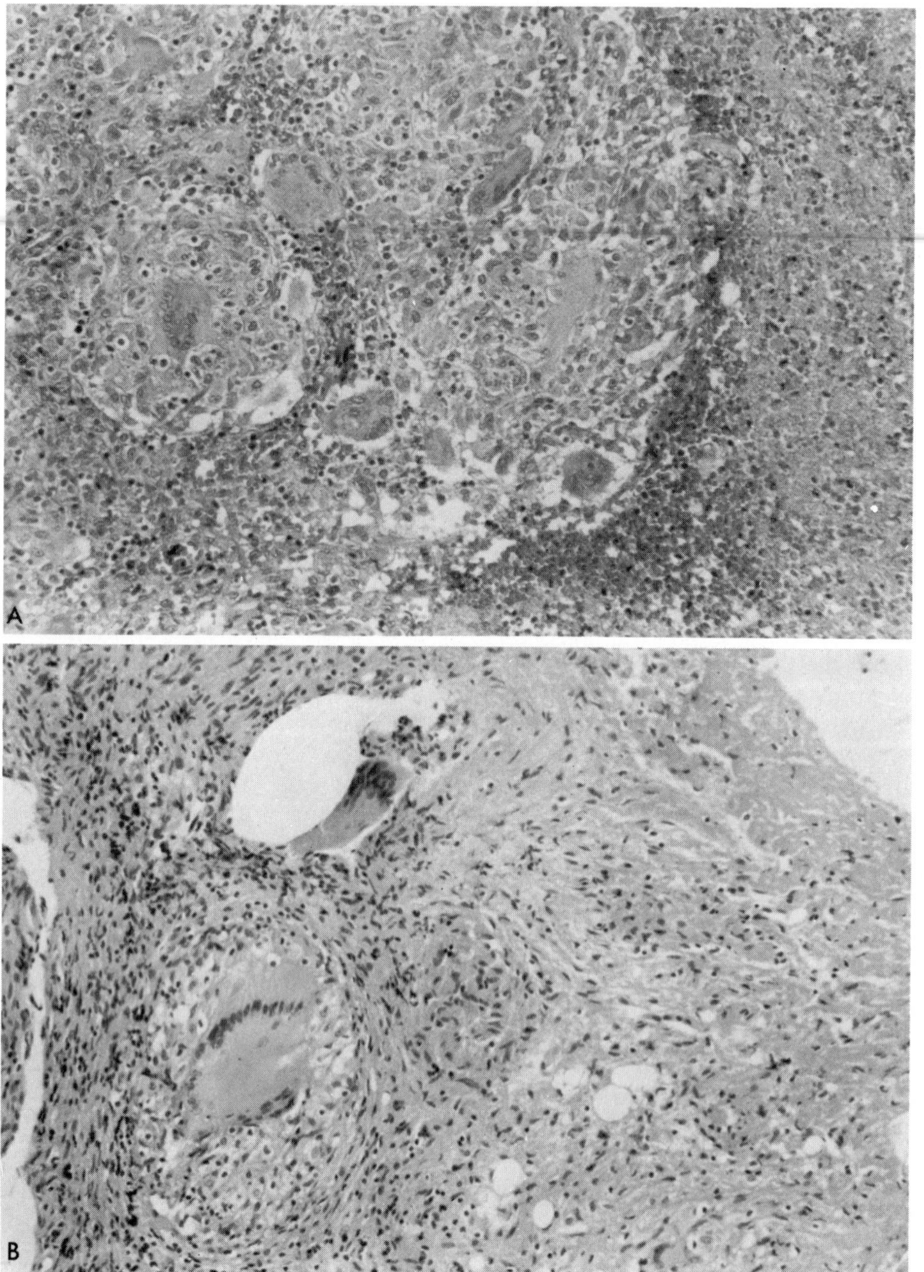

Figure 62–9. *Tuberculosis: Tubercle formation.*

A *The typical response of bone to tuberculous infection is illustrated. Note that the marrow space is completely replaced by granulomatous lesions, which consist of epithelioid cells, multinucleated giant cells (Langhans type), and lymphocytes (200×).*

B *Another example of this response to tuberculous infection. Again, a granulomatous lesion consisting of giant cells and epithelioid cells is evident. Some repair by fibroblastic cells can be noted (200×).*

replacement with a connective tissue scar. Calcification and ossification of caseating lesions may also be encountered.

Tuberculous Spondylitis

History. Tuberculous spondylitis is a disease of antiquity, having been described in a mummy from the time of 3000 BC[139, 515] and in the writings of Hippocrates (450 BC).[140] The first full account of the disease belongs to Pott in 1779.[141]

Incidence and Distribution. It is currently estimated that the vertebral column is affected in 25 to 60 per cent of cases of skeletal tuberculosis.[1, 142] The first lumbar vertebra is most commonly affected and the incidence of involvement decreases equally as one proceeds in either direction from this level.[142] The disease is relatively infrequent in the cervical and sacral segments of the vertebral column, although sacroiliac joint tuberculosis is not rare. Typically, more than one vertebra is affected, and it is not unusual to observe that as many as five or ten are altered.[1] Involved vertebrae can be located in one segment of the spine, suggesting that the disease began in a single focus and spread to neighboring vertebrae by violating the intervertebral disc. However, separate foci of tuberculosis can be detected in 1 to 4 per cent of cases.[143] With regard to its location within the vertebra, the vertebral body is more commonly involved than the posterior elements, although these latter structures may be initially or predominantly affected in some individuals[144, 145] (Fig. 62–10). In the vertebral body, an anterior predilection is striking. In a radiographic study, Westermark and Forssman[146] noted that 82 per cent of early spinal tuberculosis began in the anterior portion of the vertebral body and only 18 per cent originated in the posterior portion.

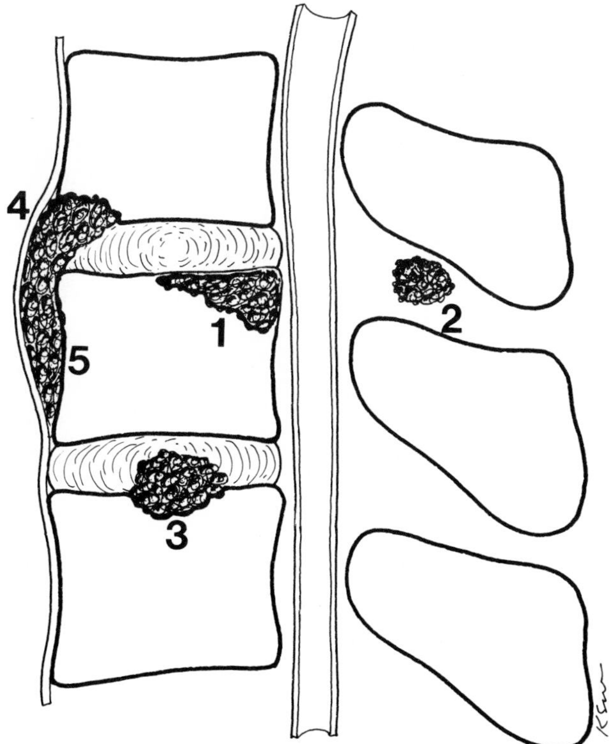

Figure 62–10. *Tuberculous spondylitis: Sites of involvement. Tuberculous lesions can localize in the vertebral body (1) or, more rarely, the posterior osseous or ligamentous structures (2). Extension to the intervertebral disc (3) or prevertebral tissues (4) is not infrequent. Subligamentous spread (5) can lead to erosion of the anterior vertebral surface.*

Men are affected slightly more frequently than women. Tuberculous spondylitis can occur in children or in adults.

Etiology and Pathogenesis. It is generally accepted that tuberculous spondylitis results from hematogenous spread of infection. A debate has existed whether the primary vascular pathway is supplied by the arterial route or the paravertebral venous plexus of Batson. It is Hodgson's belief that the latter vascular system is more important in the dissemination of tuberculosis to the spine,[142] a belief that is based upon several observations: the unusual predilection for spinal tuberculosis to involve the thoracolumbar junction; the higher incidence of spinal involvement in tuberculosis than in pyogenic osteomyelitis, in which the arterial tree appears important in vertebral contamination; the failure to produce spinal tuberculosis experimentally by injecting the bacilli locally into the vertebrae or into the left ventricle of the heart[147]; the similarity in the distribution of spinal tuberculosis and pyogenic infectious spondylitis following urologic procedures, in which Batson's plexus may be an important pathway[148]; and the production of tuberculous spinal lesions by injecting the bacilli into the abdominal or pelvic organs. Although these findings implicate the venous plexus in the spread of tuberculosis to the vertebral column, they are not incontrovertible, and a final judgment must await additional experimental or anatomic studies.

Radiographic-Pathologic Correlation. The radiographic and pathologic features of tuberculous spondylitis have been exhaustively described.[1, 47, 134, 142, 143, 149-154]

DISCOVERTEBRAL LESION. In most cases, tuberculous spondylitis begins as an infectious focus in the anterior aspect of the vertebral body adjacent to the subchondral bone plate (Fig. 62–11). Enlargement and caseation of the lesion lead to an identifiable radiographic abnormality in approximately 2 to 5 months.[155] During this time, infection may spread to the adjacent intervertebral discs. This may occur if the bacilli extend beneath the anterior longitudinal ligament or posterior longitudinal ligament to violate the peripheral discal tissue; if the organisms penetrate the subchondral bone plate and overlying cartilaginous end-plate to enter the intervertebral disc; or if an intraosseous lesion weakens the vertebral body to such a degree that it produces a discal

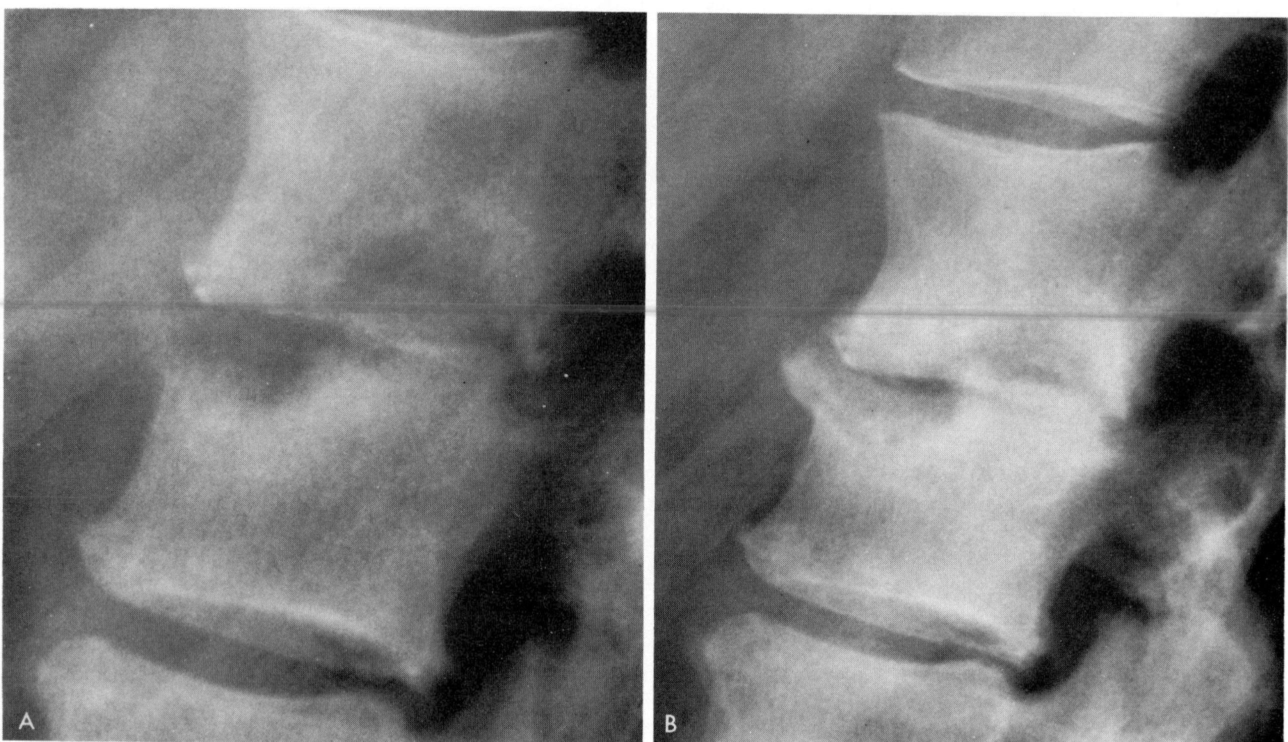

Figure 62–11. Tuberculous spondylitis: Discovertebral lesion.

A *The initial radiograph reveals subchondral destruction of two vertebral bodies with mild surrounding eburnation and loss of intervertebral disc height. The appearance is identical to that in pyogenic spondylitis.*

B *Several months later, osseous response is evident. Note the increased sclerosis. Osteophytosis and improved definition of the osseous margins can be seen.*

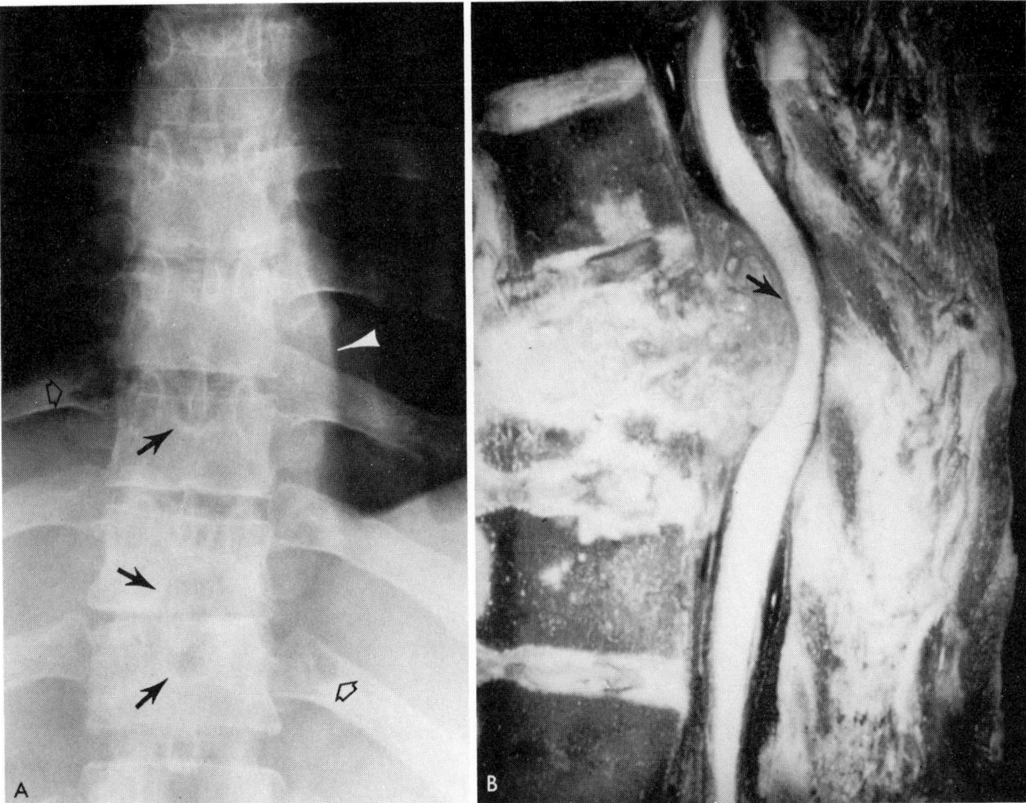

Figure 62–12. *Tuberculous spondylitis: Paraspinal abscess.*

A *Tuberculous spondylitis, resulting in vertebral and discal destruction (solid arrows), has been complicated by paraspinal swelling (arrowhead). Rib involvement is also seen (open arrows).*

B *Tuberculous spondylitis, producing vertebral and discal destruction, is associated with posterior extension, causing encroachment on the spinal cord (arrow). (Courtesy of The Arthritis Foundation.)*

herniation (cartilaginous node), contamination of invading discal tissue, and subsequent spread through the defect into the intervertebral disc. Any or all of these events can lead to decrease in height of the disc space. The combination of vertebral body and discal destruction in tuberculosis is similar to that occurring in pyogenic spondylitis, although the tuberculous process is usually not rapidly progressive. Only rarely does vertebral body tuberculosis extend into the pedicles, laminae, or transverse or spinous processes.

Once infection has reached the intervertebral disc, the loose structure of the nucleus pulposus allows its further dissemination. Extension into neighboring vertebral bodies and intervertebral discs may subsequently become evident, and eventually, long segments of the spine can be affected.

Paraspinal Extension. Extension of tuberculosis from vertebral and discal sites to the adjacent ligaments and soft tissues is frequent. This extension usually occurs anterolaterally; rarely, it is observed posteriorly in the peridural space (Fig. 62–12).[539] Once infection has been established in the paraspinal tissues, it may remain localized or extend for a considerable distance. With enlargement, the paravertebral abscesses can strip the periosteal coverings of the vertebral bodies, rendering them avascular and producing osteonecrosis.[142] Subligamentous extension of a tuberculous abscess can allow osseous and discal invasion at distant sites. The osseous changes may be subtle, including mild contour irregularity (gouge defects) and sparing of the intervertebral discs.

Burrowing abscesses can extend for extraordinary distances before perforating an internal viscus or the body surface. The direction and extent of burrowing are influenced by the site of spinal infection, the anatomy of the adjacent soft tissues, and the effect of gravity. In the lumbar region, pus collecting beneath the fascia of the psoas muscle produces a psoas abscess, which can extend into the groin and the thigh. Among the organs and tissues that have been penetrated by paravertebral abscesses are the esophagus, the bronchus, the lung, the mediastinum, the liver, the kidney, the intestine, the urinary bladder, the rectum, the vagina, and the aorta; the most frequently involved organ is the lung.[156, 157] Other body structures that have been violated by burrowing abscesses of tuberculosis are the abdominal wall, thigh, buttocks, and back.

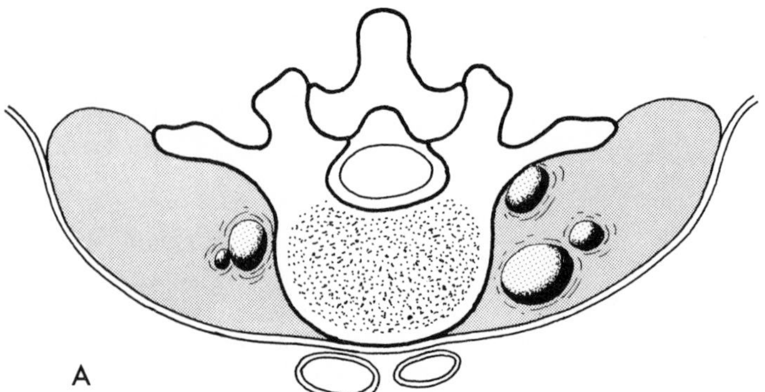

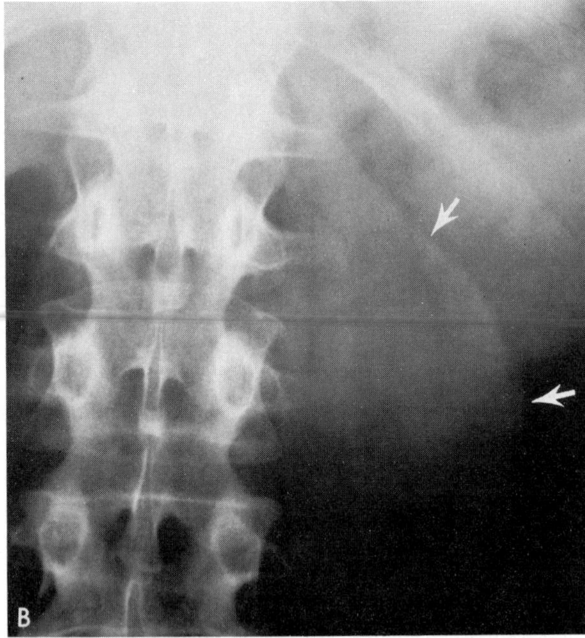

Figure 62–13. *Tuberculous spondylitis: Psoas abscess.*

A *The typical appearance of bilateral and fusiform psoas abscesses is illustrated in a cross-sectional drawing through a lumbar vertebral body.*

B *A large left noncalcified psoas abscess (arrows) can be seen.*

Illustration continued on the opposite page

Abscess formation in tuberculosis can produce soft tissue swelling on radiographs that appears out of proportion to the degree of osseous and discal destruction (Fig. 62–12). The swelling is commonly bilateral and fusiform in configuration, associated with scalloping of the anterior and lateral aspects of the vertebral bodies. Psoas abscesses are usually easy to identify and may contain calcification (Fig. 62–13). Nontuberculous psoas abscesses rarely calcify. Tuberculous abscesses of the psoas muscle calcify in two distinct patterns: faint amorphous deposits, which may become quite dense with progressive healing; and "teardrop"-shaped calcification.[152] In either situation, the calcification appears in the paraspinal area between L1 and L5.

Although psoas abscess formation can complicate 5 per cent of cases of tuberculous spondylitis, abscesses may also appear in nontuberculous conditions. Examples include inflammatory intestinal disorders (diverticulitis, appendicitis, Crohn's disease, perinephric abscess), postpartum or postoperative infections, bowel neoplasm with necrosis, and trauma with secondary infection.[152, 158-160] Implicated organisms in these cases include staphylococcus and gram-negative agents.

Posterior Element Lesions. Occasionally, the posterior elements may be the initial spinal site of tuberculosis (Fig. 62–14). In these instances, radiographic findings include pedicular or laminal destruction, erosion of the posterior cortex of the vertebral body and adjacent ribs, a large paraspinal mass, and relative sparing of the intervertebral discs.[47, 145, 538] Single or multiple levels may be affected. With involvement of the pedicles, paraplegia is frequent owing to granulomatous extension into the spinal canal. During the reparative phase, the pedicles may be reconstituted. Differential diagnosis of tuberculous spondylitis of the posterior elements includes other infections and neoplasms.

Other Spinal Lesions

Solitary Vertebral Involvement. Rarely, tuberculosis leads to isolated involvement of a single vertebral body.[47] In adults, osseous destruction will resemble that which is evident in tumors or with cartilagi-

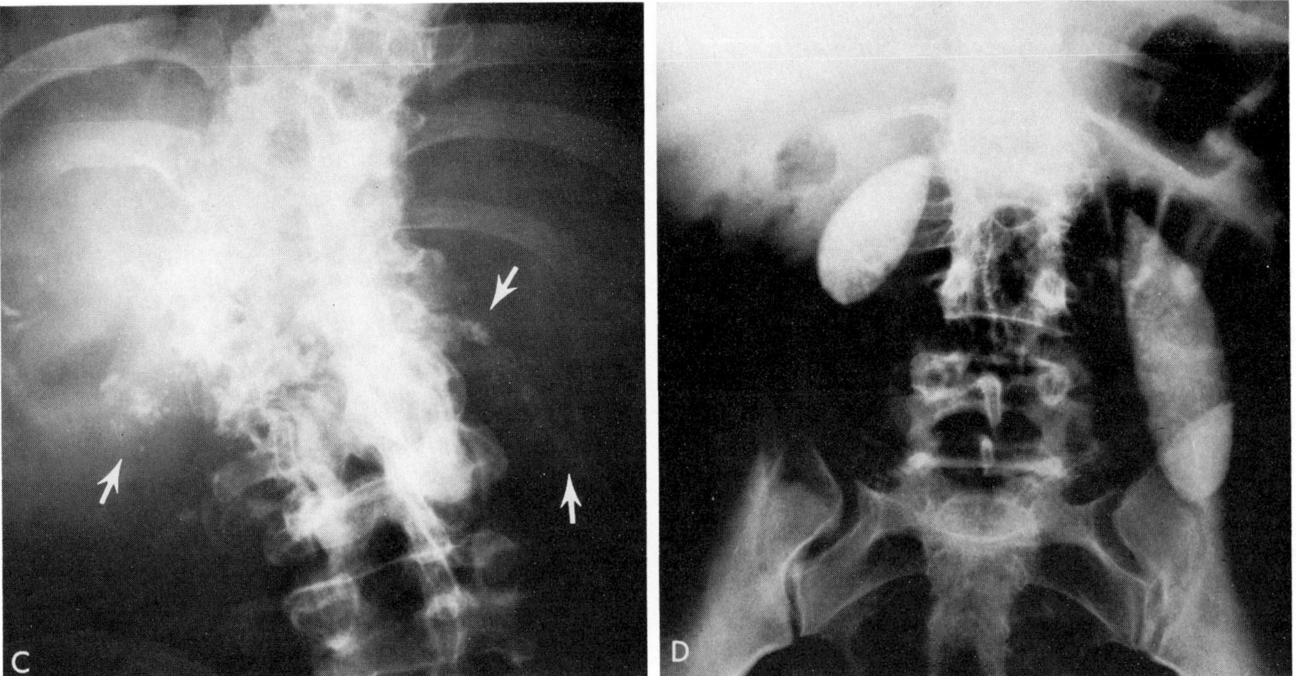

Figure 62–13. Continued
C *In this example of bilateral psoas abscesses associated with severe kyphoscoliosis of the spine, note popcorn-like calcification (arrows).*
D *Diffusely calcified psoas abscesses are noted in association with spinal abnormalities.*

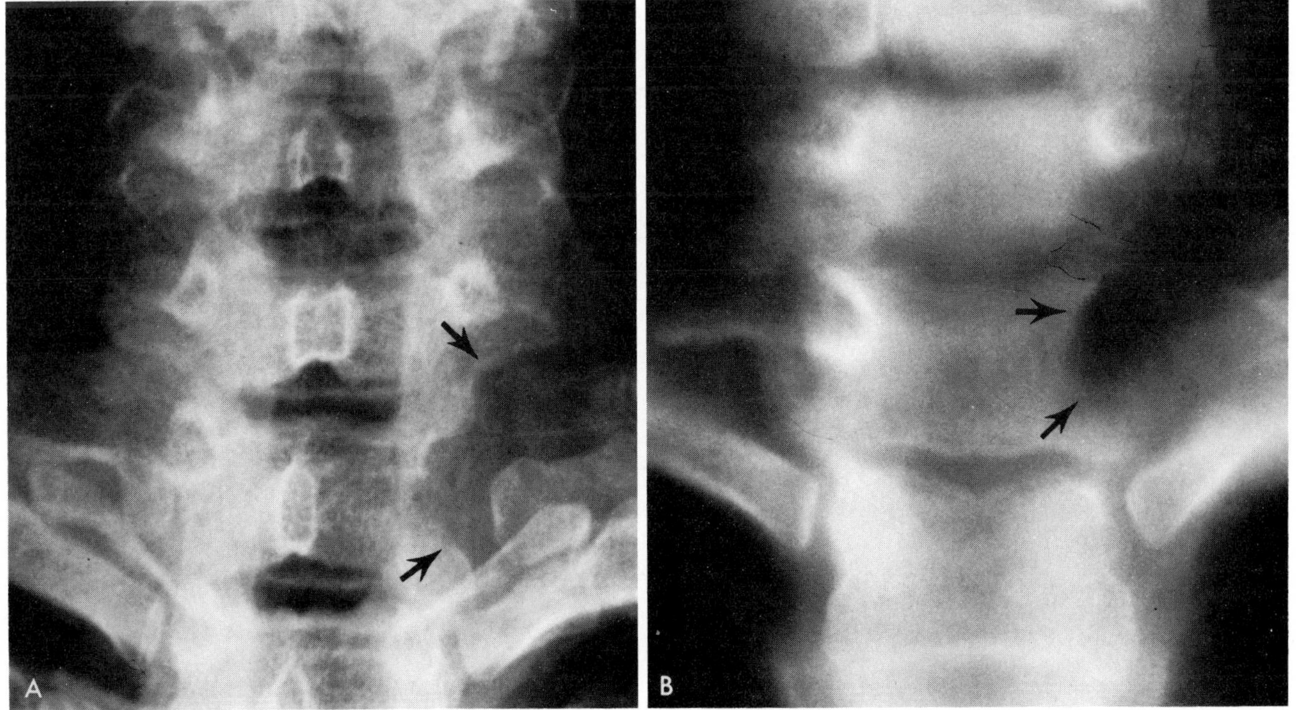

Figure 62–14. Tuberculous spondylitis: Posterior element lesions.
A *Observe destruction of the left pedicle and lateral mass of the seventh cervical vertebra (arrows).*
B *The abnormalities are better delineated on anteroposterior tomography (arrows).*

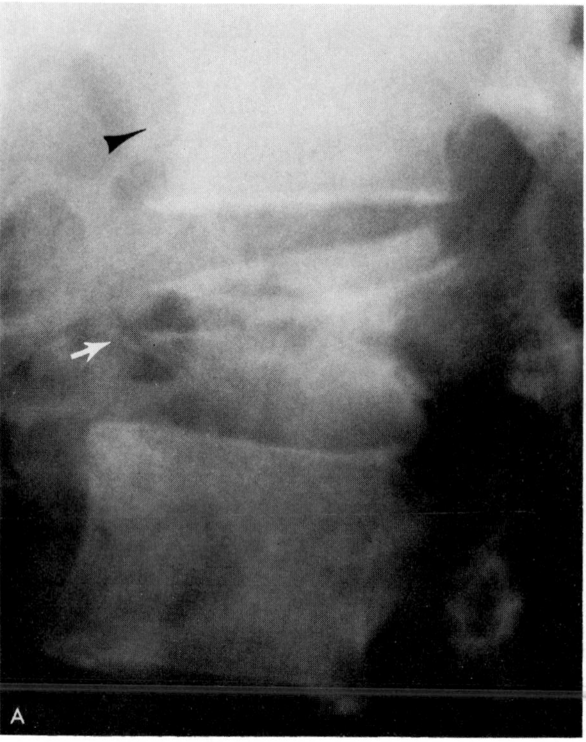
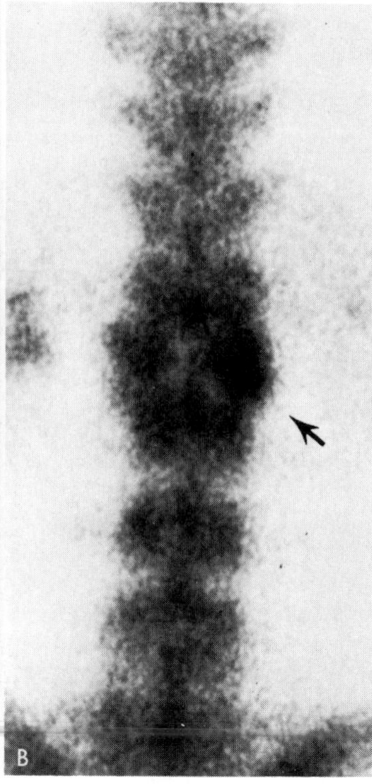

Figure 62–15. Tuberculous spondylitis: Solitary vertebral involvement.

A *A collapsed vertebral body (arrow) represents the site of tuberculous involvement in this adult patient. Note anterior scalloping of the vertebral body above this level (arrowhead), indicating subligamentous spread of infection.*

B *A technetium bone scan reveals increased accumulation of isotope in several vertebrae in this region (arrow) and right renal obstructive uropathy.*

nous node formation (Fig. 62–15).[538] In children, vertebra plana can appear, simulating the appearance of eosinophilic granuloma.

Vertebra Within a Vertebra. The appearance of "growth arrest lines" within single or multiple vertebrae in patients with tuberculosis has been noted by O'Brien.[161] These are analogous to those lines within bones of the appendicular skeleton that accompany chronic illnesses in children.

Kyphosis. Collapse of partially destroyed vertebral bodies during the course of tuberculous spondylitis can lead to severe deformities. Typically, an angulated posterior projection appears at the site of maximum spinal involvement, leading to tuberculous kyphosis or gibbus deformity. The degree of angulation varies with the site and extent of vertebral disease; angulation is more acute in the thoracic spine than in the cervical or lumbar region, and it is more severe when only one or two vertebrae are affected.[1] Despite the striking nature of the deformity, the diameter of the spinal canal may not be significantly altered. Radiography indicates destroyed vertebral bodies in the area of angulation and, in some cases of thoracic kyphosis, a remarkable increase in height of the vertebral bodies in the lordotic lumbar area.[143] Such "long" vertebrae are found only in those cases in which the growth of the vertebral bodies had not ceased at the time the disease affected the thoracic spine; they are also observed in other conditions associated with spinal deformity. A variety of operative techniques have been advocated in the treatment of tuberculous kyphosis.[162]

Scoliosis. Although not so frequent as kyphosis, lateral deviation of the spine can occur in tuberculous spondylitis.[142, 163] This accompanies asymmetric or unilateral destruction of vertebral bodies and intervertebral discs and is virtually confined to the lower thoracic and lumbar vertebrae.

Bony Ankylosis of Vertebral Bodies. Healing in tuberculous spondylitis can be associated with osseous fusion of vertebral bodies. This manifestation, which is also evident in congenital block vertebrae and following trauma or other infectious diseases, leads to partial or complete obliteration of the intervening intervertebral disc (Fig. 62–16). Not uncommonly, four to eight vertebrae are coalesced into a large osseous mass, particularly in areas of angular spinal deformity.

Ivory Vertebrae. Increased radiodensity of the vertebral body in tuberculosis can lead to an ivory vertebra.[164] This phenomenon is usually evident in the lumbar region in association with healing of the disease. At surgery, the involved vertebrae are hard; histologic examination indicates revascularization and reossification, apparently indicating a healing response to osteonecrosis.[142]

Differential Diagnosis. The differential diagnosis of tuberculous spondylitis includes a wide variety of other infectious disorders of the spine. Differentiation of tuberculous and pyogenic vertebral osteomyelitis can be extremely difficult. Clinical data that favor a diagnosis of tuberculosis are an insidious onset of symptoms, a typical tuberculous pulmonary infiltrate, the late onset of paraplegia following back pain

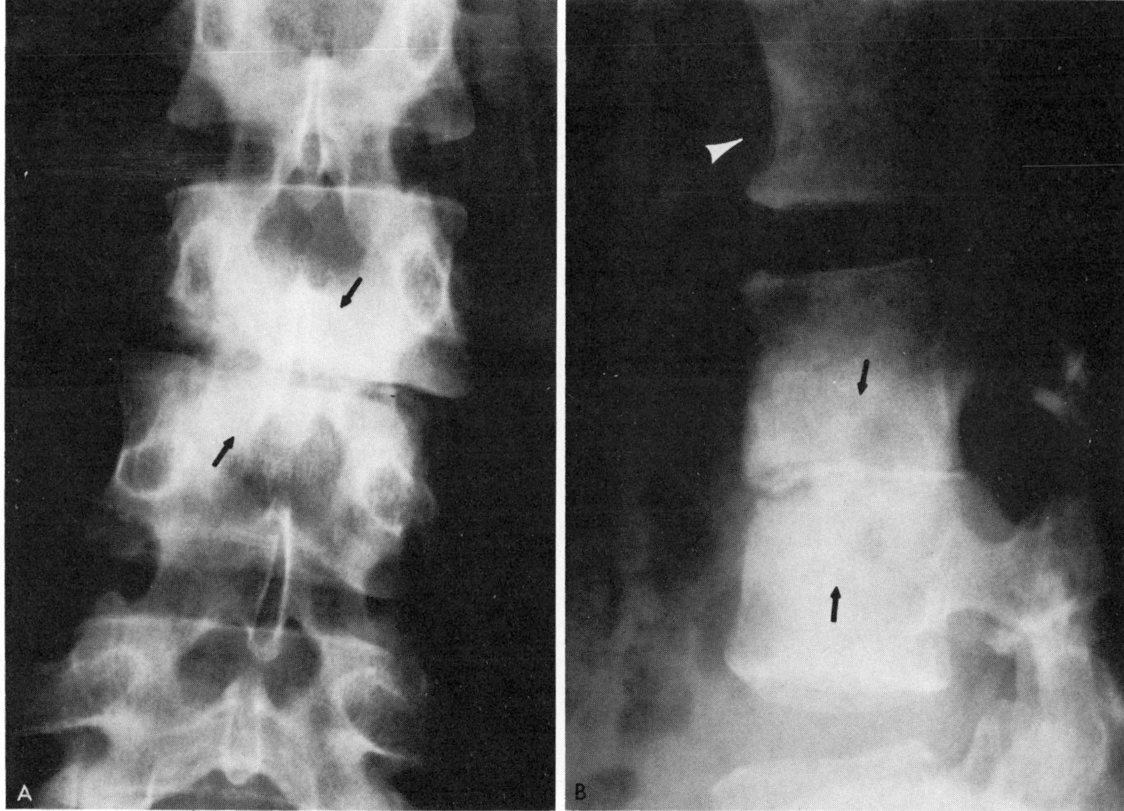

Figure 62–16. *Tuberculous spondylitis: Discal obliteration and reactive sclerosis. In this individual, discal obliteration, which subsequently led to partial bony ankylosis, and reactive sclerosis are evident (arrows). The appearance is similar to that in pyogenic spondylitis. Note anterior scalloping of an additional vertebral body (arrowhead).*

of many months' duration, and a normal erythrocyte sedimentation rate.[47] Radiographic features favoring tuberculosis are involvement of one or more segments of the spine, a delay in destruction of intervertebral discs, a large and calcified paravertebral mass, and absence of sclerosis. None of the radiographic findings is pathognomonic of tuberculosis. Furthermore, reactive bony eburnation, which is common in pyogenic osteomyelitis, is also encountered in tuberculosis, particularly in colored races[153] (Fig. 62–16).

Tuberculous spondylitis may simulate tumor. Intervertebral disc space destruction is more characteristic of infectious lesions of the spine, although it is occasionally evident in neoplastic disorders. Scalloping of the anterior surface of the vertebral bodies, evident in tuberculosis with subligamentous spread, can also be seen with paravertebral lymphadenopathy due to metastasis, myeloma, or lymphoma. Sarcoidosis can produce multifocal lesions of vertebrae and intervertebral discs with paraspinal masses, findings identical to those of tuberculosis.

Tuberculous Osteomyelitis

Incidence and Distribution. Tuberculous osteomyelitis can remain localized to bone or involve adjacent articulations. In general, tuberculosis confined to bone is relatively infrequent; occasionally, however, a tuberculous focus in one or more osseous structures is not associated with tuberculous arthritis. Virtually any bone can be affected, including the pelvis, the phalanges and metacarpals (tuberculous dactylitis), the long bones, the ribs, the sternum, the skull, the patella, and the carpal and tarsal regions.[133, 134, 165-169, 542, 543, 564]

In the long tubular bones, tuberculosis usually originates in one of the epiphyses and soon spreads into the neighboring joint (Fig. 62–17). In fact, tuberculous osteomyelitis originating in the shaft of a long bone represents less than 1 per cent of all cases of the disease,[1] although in Chinese patients, the incidence is somewhat greater.[170] Metaphyseal foci in the child can occasionally violate the growth plate (Fig. 62–17).

Radiographic-Pathologic Correlation. The pathologic process is initiated by tubercle formation in the marrow with secondary infection of the trabeculae[1] (Fig. 62–18). These trabeculae are resorbed as the focus of infection enlarges and as tuberculous granulation tissue insinuates itself between the bands of spongy trabecular bone. Caseous necrosis may be prominent or limited. In the latter situation, circumscribed lytic lesions of bone may be evident, termed

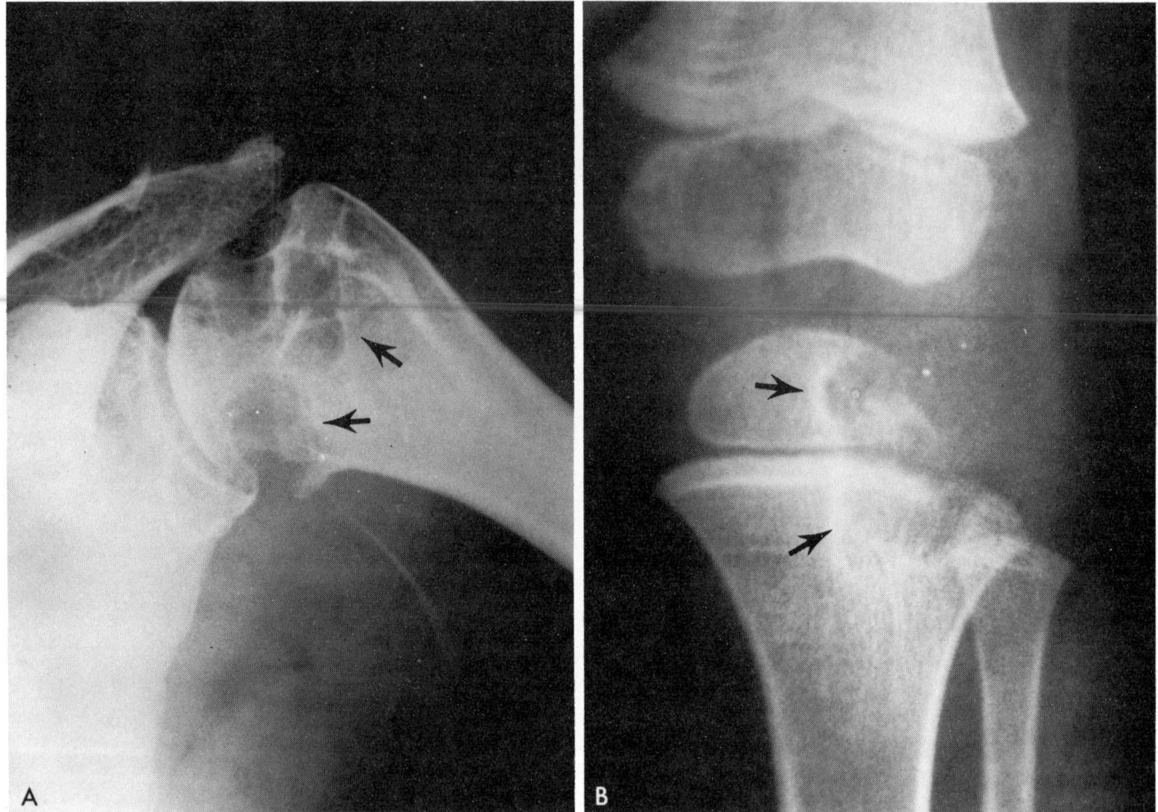

Figure 62–17. *Tuberculous osteomyelitis: Radiographic abnormalities.*

A *In this patient, an initial epiphyseal lesion (arrows) subsequently involved the glenohumeral articulation. The lesions are well circumscribed, and the glenoid and acromion are also affected.*

B *Observe the violation of the growth plate with adjacent metaphyseal and epiphyseal alterations (arrows).*

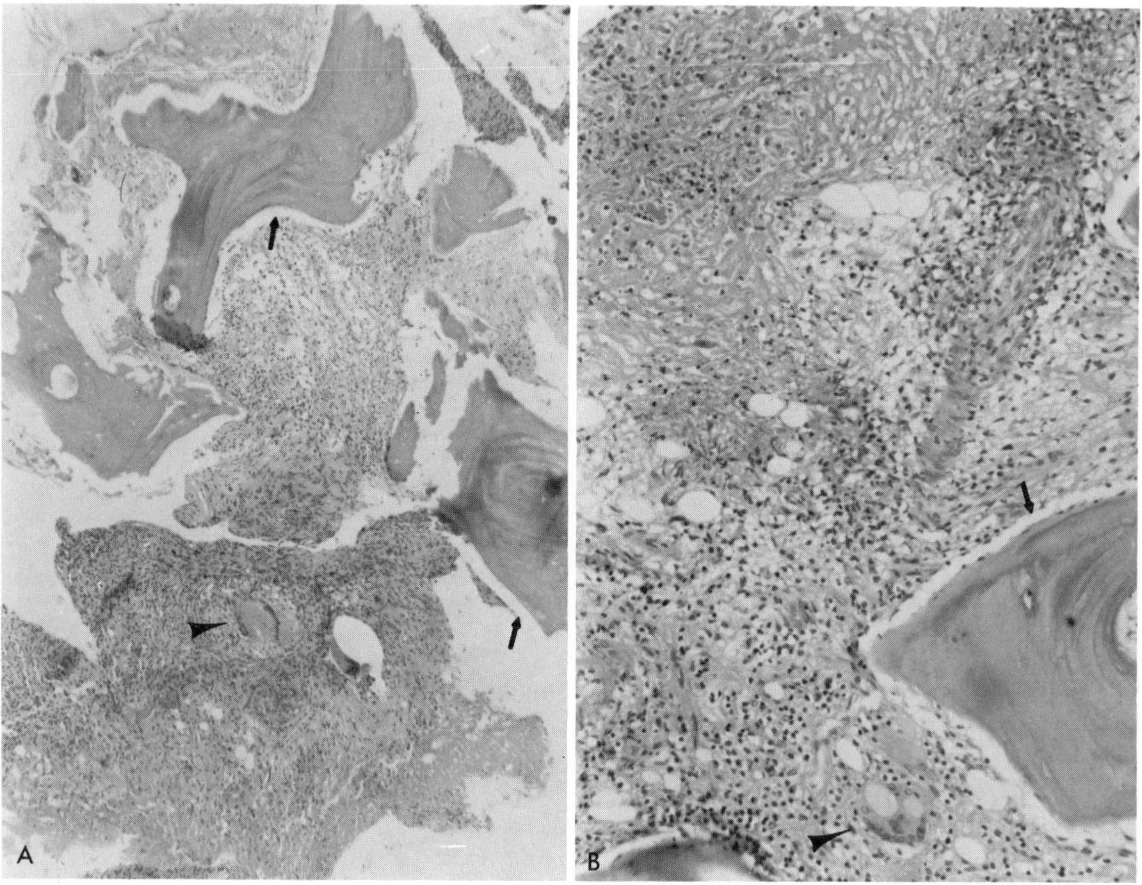

Figure 62–18. *Tuberculous osteomyelitis: Pathologic abnormalities. Photomicrographs (80×, 200×) outline eroded and necrotic trabeculae (arrows), blood vessels with surrounding cellular inflammation, and giant cells (arrowhead).*

"cystic" tuberculosis (see later discussion). With caseation and liquefaction, an abscess cavity is created containing pus and small granules of bone — "bone sand."[1] About the abscess are zones of marrow-containing granulation tissue, connective tissue with cellular elements (lymphocytes, polymorphonuclear leukocytes), and sclerotic trabeculae.

On radiographs, foci of osteolysis are accompanied by varying amounts of eburnation and periostitis. Sequestrum formation can be encountered as a spicule of increased radiodensity within the zone of destruction. The initial roentgenographic appearance in tuberculous osteomyelitis is similar to that in other types of osteomyelitis and even in aggressive neoplasm. Differentiation of tuberculous from pyogenic infection on the basis of increased osteoporosis and decreased eburnation is not feasible in most cases.

Special Types of Tuberculous Osteomyelitis

"CYSTIC" TUBERCULOSIS. A rare variety of tuberculosis is associated with disseminated lesions of the axial and the extra-axial skeleton.[165] This variety has been associated with considerable confusion regarding terminology because of a report in 1920 by Jüngling of osteitis tuberculosa multiplex cystoides, or multiple tuberculous skeletal lesions.[171] Even though it was subsequently realized that Jüngling was describing sarcoidosis rather than tuberculosis,[172] the term osteitis tuberculosa multiplex cystoides is still occasionally employed to describe cystic tuberculosis of bone.[173]

Cystic lesions of one or multiple bones in tuberculosis are much more frequently encountered in children than in adults (Fig. 62–19). In children, these lesions usually affect the peripheral skeleton, may be symmetric in distribution, are of variable size, and are generally unaccompanied by sclerosis.[165] In adults, the skull, the shoulder and pelvic girdles, and the axial skeleton are involved. In this latter age group, the lesions are small and oval, lying in the long axis of the bone, and possess well-defined margins with sclerosis.[165] It is this differing appearance in children and in adults that has led some investigators to term the juvenile lesions pseudocystic tuberculosis of bone, and the adult lesions disseminated bone tuberculosis.[174]

The prognosis of this variety of tuberculosis is good. Lesions may resolve spontaneously with low morbidity or mortality.

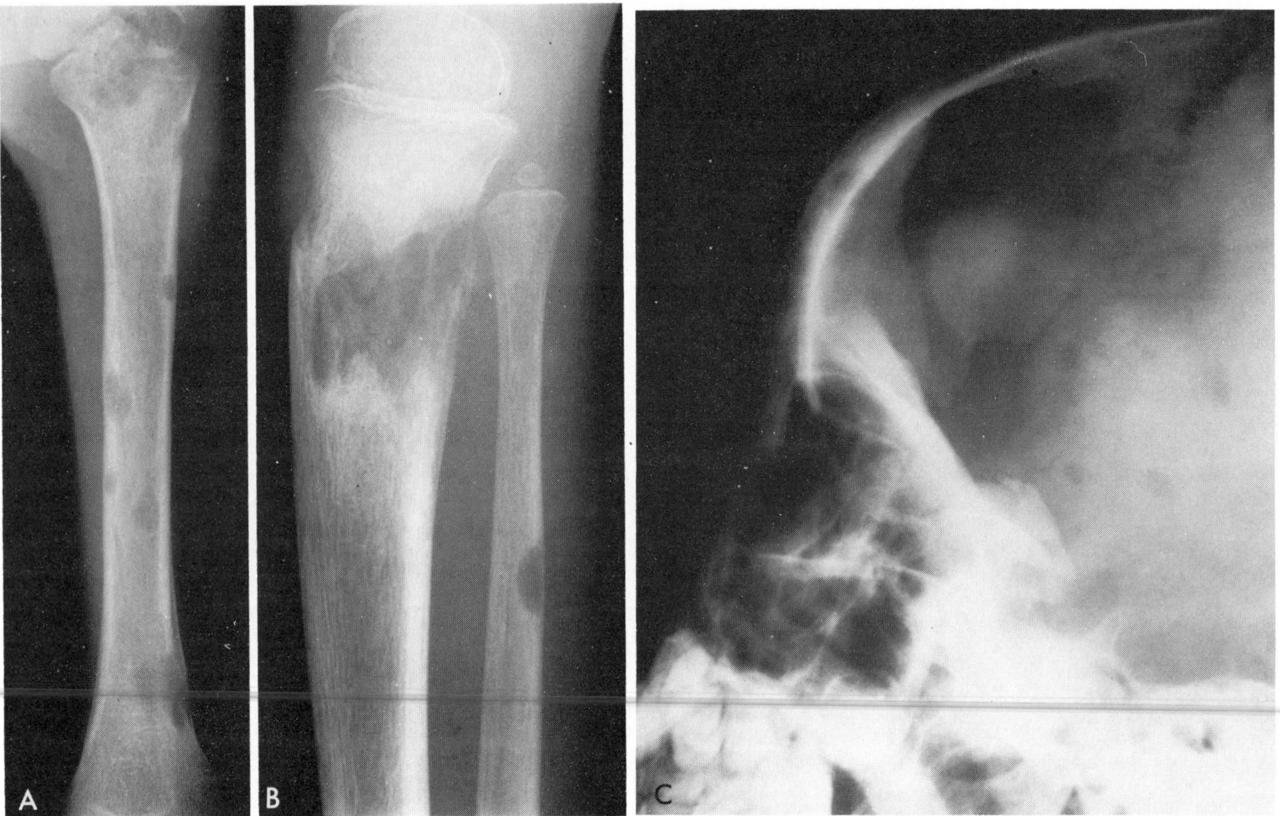

Figure 62–19. *Cystic tuberculosis. This 5 year old girl presented with axillary lymph node enlargement approximately 9 months before these films were taken. Aspiration and culture documented tuberculosis. Widespread and symmetric abnormalities were present.*

A *Note the well-defined lytic lesions of the medullary and cortical areas of the metaphysis and diaphysis of the humerus. The proximal epiphysis is also affected. Sclerosis is absent, although periostitis can be seen.*

B *Similar lesions are present in the tibia and fibula. Some of these are central, whereas others are eccentric or peripheral in location.*

C *Small and large radiolucent foci are detected in the cranium, simulating the appearance of histiocytosis.*

The radiographic characteristics of cystic tuberculosis, which include well-defined osseous lesions with or without surrounding sclerosis,[175, 176] resemble those of eosinophilic granuloma, sarcoidosis, cystic angiomatosis, plasma cell myeloma, fungal infections, metastases, and other conditions.

TUBERCULOUS DACTYLITIS. Tuberculous involvement of the short tubular bones of the hands and feet is termed tuberculous dactylitis. This form of tuberculosis is especially frequent in children, although it is also well described in adult individuals.[177] In infants and young children, the reported incidence of dactylitis in cases of tuberculosis has ranged from 0.5 to 14 per cent.[178, 179] The condition decreases in frequency after the age of 5 years and becomes rare after the age of 10 years. It then reappears in the adult.[177, 180] Although involvement of one bone of the hand or the foot is common, multiple osseous foci can be identified in 25 to 35 per cent of cases.[182, 183] Multiplicity is especially characteristic of childhood dactylitis.

Soft tissue swelling is usually the initial manifestation and can be quite extensive. Mild or exuberant periostitis of phalanges, metacarpals, or metatarsals may be evident (Fig. 62–20). Expansion of the bone with cystic quality is termed spina ventosa and is especially common in childhood. Diaphyseal destruction with extension into the epiphysis may be associated with sequestration, sinus tracts, and growth disturbance as well as brachydactyly.

These roentgenologic features appear with differing frequency in the child versus the adult.[177] In childhood dactylitis, multiplicity of sites, expansion of bone, periostitis, sequestration, fistulae, and positive chest roentgenograms are more common than in adulthood dactylitis.

The spina ventosa variety of dactylitis has received a great deal of attention. The term is derived from *spina*, meaning a spine-like projection, and *ventosa*, meaning puffed full of air,[177] and was initially applied to osseous enlargement, particularly of the diaphyses, due to marrow infiltration with tuberculous granulation tissue. Although overwhelmingly associated with tuberculous dactylitis (phalanges, metacarpals, metatarsals), a similar appearance can be evident in the radius, ulna, and humerus.[187, 188] In

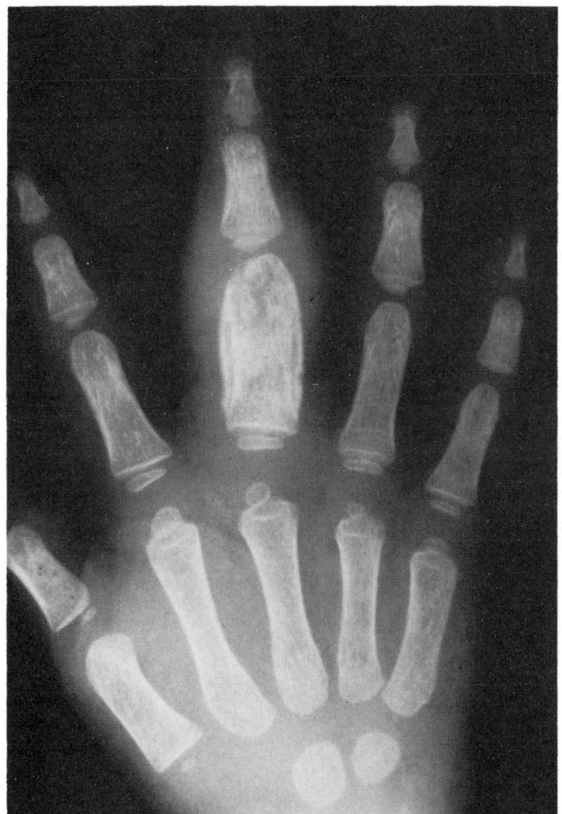

Figure 62–20. Tuberculous dactylitis. Radiographic findings in this child include soft tissue swelling of multiple digits, lytic lesions of several middle and proximal phalanges and metacarpals, and exuberant periostitis and enlargement of the proximal phalanx of the third finger.

the hands and feet, prognosis for normal function in this cystic variety of the disease is quite good.

Tuberculous dactylitis can be imitated by other conditions. Other infectious disorders of pyogenic or fungal etiology may present with similar manifestations. Syphilitic dactylitis in infants and children produces bilateral and symmetric involvement; in this disease, periostitis is more exuberant, and soft tissue swelling is less prominent than in tuberculous dactylitis.[177] Fibrous dysplasia, hyperparathyroidism, leukemia, and sickle cell anemia may produce phalangeal, metacarpal, and metatarsal changes, although characteristic roentgenographic alterations at other sites allow accurate diagnosis of these conditions.

Differential Diagnosis. Differentiation of tuberculous osteomyelitis and pyogenic osteomyelitis is difficult. Osteoporosis, bone lysis and sclerosis, and periostitis are evident in both conditions. Acute pyogenic osteomyelitis has a more rapid course and less frequently extends to the neighboring joint than tuberculous osteomyelitis. The latter condition is associated with radiographic findings that are virtually identical to those of fungal skeletal infections.

Tuberculous Arthritis

General Features. Tuberculous arthritis most typically affects large joints such as the knee and the hip, although any articular site can be involved.[134] Monoarticular disease is the rule.[189] The majority of joint lesions are secondary to adjacent osteomyelitis, although primary involvement of the synovial membrane does occur, especially in the knee.[190, 191] Most patients are middle-aged or elderly, and many have underlying disorders or have received intra-articular injections of steroids.[134] Tuberculous joint disease may persist with chronic pain and only minimal signs of inflammation. Delay in diagnosis is frequent[192]; correct diagnosis requires an awareness of the role of mycobacteria in joint disease and the utilization of synovial fluid and tissue for culture and histologic studies. The fluid is characterized by high white blood cell count, low glucose levels, and poor mucin clot formation.[193] As similar findings may be encountered in the synovial fluid in rheumatoid arthritis, culture and biopsy are frequently necessary. Synovial biopsies can be expected to reveal the histologic findings of tuberculosis in approximately 90 per cent of cases; similarly, synovial biopsies are positive on culture in about 90 per cent of cases. Culture of the synovial fluid alone is positive in approximately 80 per cent of individuals.

Pathologic Abnormalities

SYNOVIAL MEMBRANE ABNORMALITIES. Inflammatory changes in the synovial membrane are usually more marked if the infection follows the penetration of a caseous bone focus into the joint space rather than if it starts de novo in the membrane itself.[1] An enlarging joint effusion and inflammatory thickening of the periarticular connective tissue and fat contribute to soft tissue swelling. The synovial membrane thickens and is covered with heavy layers of fibrin. On microscopic examination, richly vascular tuberculous granulation tissue is found to contain necrotic and fibrin-like materal, caseous areas, and collections of leukocytes and mononuclear phagocytes. Epithelioid cells and epithelioid tubercles are frequently evident in areas of caseation. Discolored areas related to blood pigment can be observed in the synovial membrane and subsynovial connective tissue. In long-standing cases, the synovial membrane may contain pedunculated knobby masses of fibrinoid material and small rice bodies.

CARTILAGINOUS AND OSSEOUS ABNORMALITIES. The granulation tissue spreads insidiously onto the free surface of the cartilage[1] (Fig. 62–21*A*). On the basis of vascular and phagocytic processes, portions of the cartilage are eroded. The erosive process is not evenly distributed. Rather, focal areas of cartilaginous destruction may be intermixed with areas of relatively normal-appearing chondral elements. Furthermore, in certain articulations, such as the knee, contact of apposing cartilaginous surfaces

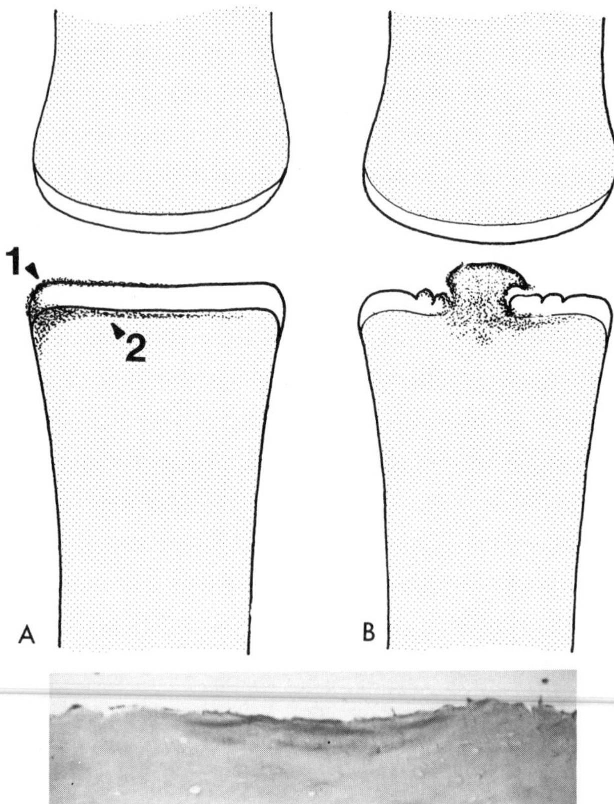

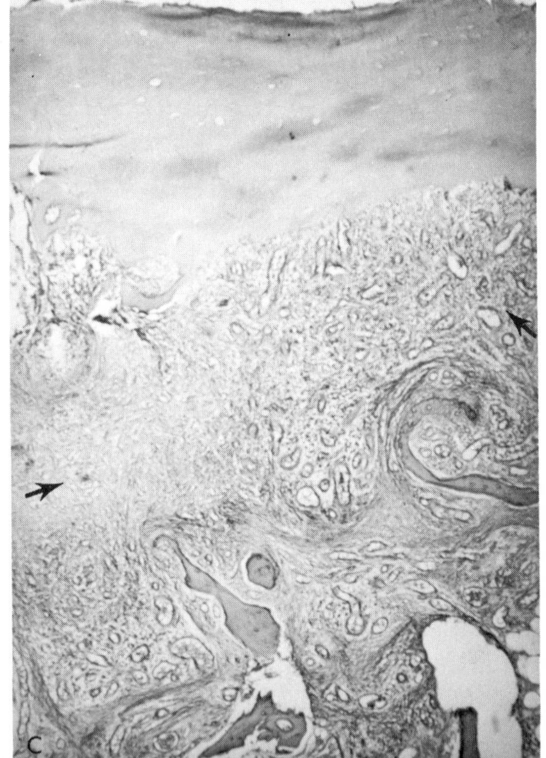

Figure 62–21. Tuberculous arthritis: Pathologic abnormalities.

A *Granulation tissue may extend onto the free surface of the cartilage (1) or between cartilage and bone (2).*

B *Subchondral trabecular granulation tissue can mushroom through gaps in the cartilage, extending into the articular cavity.*

C *A photomicrograph reveals subchondral extension of pannus (arrows), separating the cartilaginous surface and subchondral bone. (Courtesy of Dr. German Steiner, Hospital for Joint Diseases, New York, New York.)*

with resultant compression and motion slows down or prevents the advance of granulation tissue.[194]

Granulation tissue also insinuates itself between the cartilage and subchondral bone,[1] especially in articulations (e.g., hip, ankle) in which the articular cartilages are in close contact (Fig. 62–21C). This tissue originates at the peripheral margin of the chondral surface and advances beneath it, loosening and separating the cartilaginous tissue as it proceeds. The detached cartilage may become necrotic, the osseous surface can be exposed, and destruction of the subchondral bone plate and trabeculae can ensue. Occasionally, mounds of subchondral tuberculous granulation tissue may mushroom through gaps in the cartilage, extending into the articular cavity (Fig. 62–21B).

Osseous erosion may be especially marked at the periphery of the articulation. Wedge-shaped necrotic foci can become evident on either side of the joint, creating "kissing" sequestrae.

Radiographic Abnormalities. A triad of radiographic findings (Phemister's triad) is characteristic of tuberculous arthritis: juxta-articular osteoporosis, peripherally located osseous erosions, and gradual narrowing of the interosseous space (Figs. 62–22 to 62–27). Initially, soft tissue swelling and osteoporosis may dominate the radiographic picture, findings that are also evident in other infectious diseases and rheumatoid arthritis. The degree of osteoporosis can be extensive and, when severe, may resemble the abnormalities of the reflex sympathetic dystrophy syndrome or transient regional osteoporosis. The infectious etiology of the process may be obscured until osseous and cartilaginous destruction becomes evident.

Marginal erosions are especially characteristic of tuberculosis in "tight" or weight-bearing articulations, such as the hip, the knee, and the ankle. They produce corner defects simulating the erosions of other synovial processes, such as rheumatoid arthritis. The combination of regional osteoporosis, marginal erosions, and relative preservation of joint space is highly suggestive of tuberculous arthritis. In rheumatoid arthritis, early loss of articular space is more typical.

Subchondral osseous erosions are also encountered in tuberculous arthritis. They appear as ill-defined gaps in the subchondral bone plate and subjacent trabeculae that may be apparent at a stage when the articular space is well preserved.

The rapidity of joint space loss in tuberculosis is highly variable. In some patients, diminution in this space is a late finding, occurring after marginal and central erosions of large size have appeared. In other individuals, loss of interosseous space can be appreciated at a time when only small marginal osseous defects are apparent.

Bony proliferation is generally not so exuberant in tuberculous arthritis as it is in pyogenic arthritis. Subchondral eburnation is encountered, however, in

Text continued on page 2183

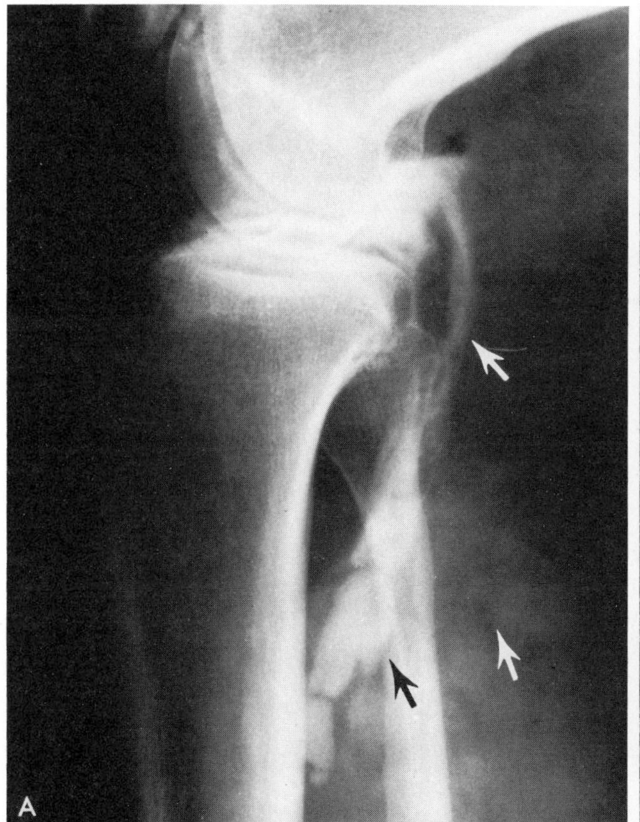

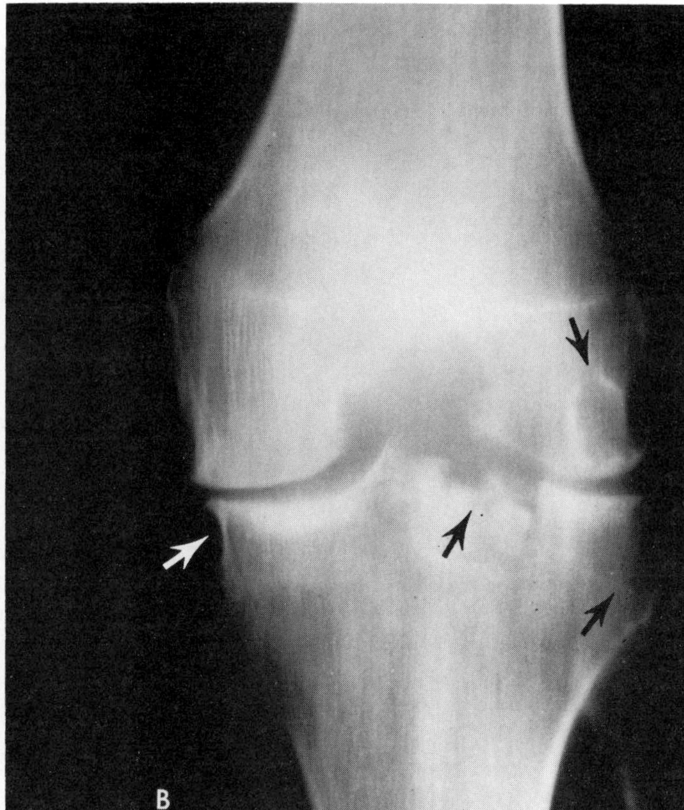

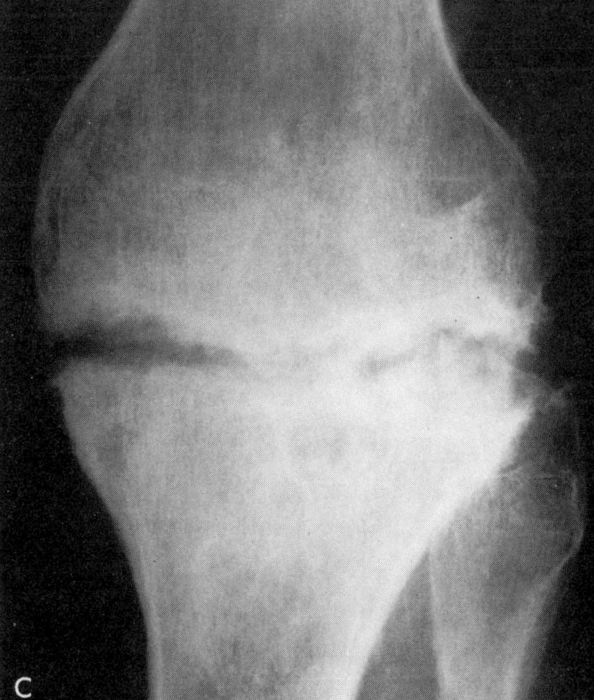

Figure 62–22. *Tuberculous arthritis: Knee.*

A *This patient presented with soft tissue swelling and a mass behind the knee. Arthrography following aspiration of the joint contents delineates a synovial (popliteal) cyst (arrows). Tuberculous organisms were later isolated.*

B *On a tomogram in another patient, typical marginal and central osseous erosions (arrows) accompany tuberculous arthritis. Osteoporosis is not prominent.*

C *In a different individual, ill-defined osseous destruction of the entire joint surface is apparent following a chronic tuberculous infection.*

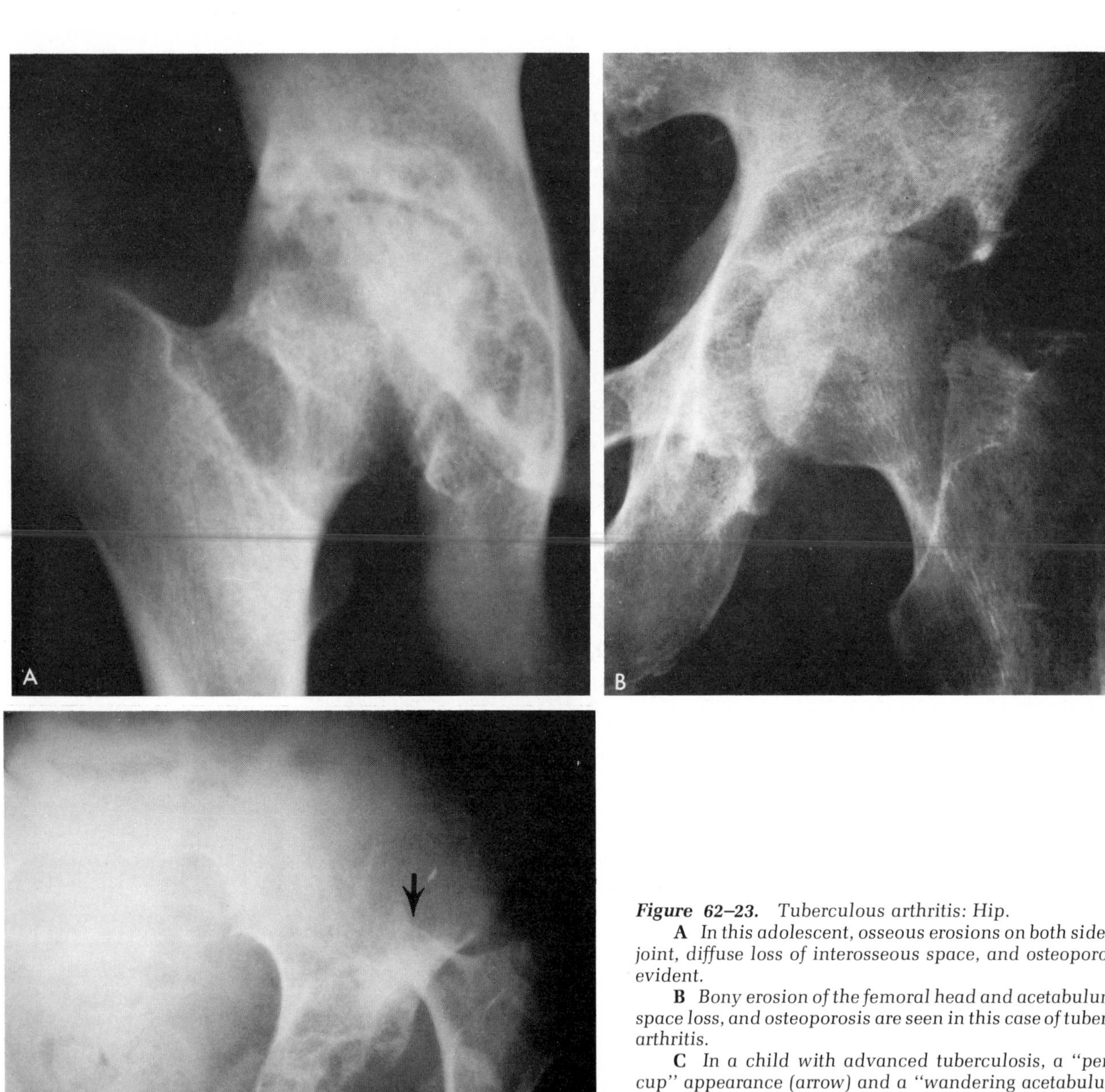

Figure 62–23. *Tuberculous arthritis: Hip.*

A *In this adolescent, osseous erosions on both sides of the joint, diffuse loss of interosseous space, and osteoporosis are evident.*

B *Bony erosion of the femoral head and acetabulum, joint space loss, and osteoporosis are seen in this case of tuberculous arthritis.*

C *In a child with advanced tuberculosis, a "pencil-in-cup" appearance (arrow) and a "wandering acetabulum" are the radiographic findings.*

*(**A, C,** Courtesy of Dr. J. Kaye, Vanderbilt University, Nashville, Tennessee)*

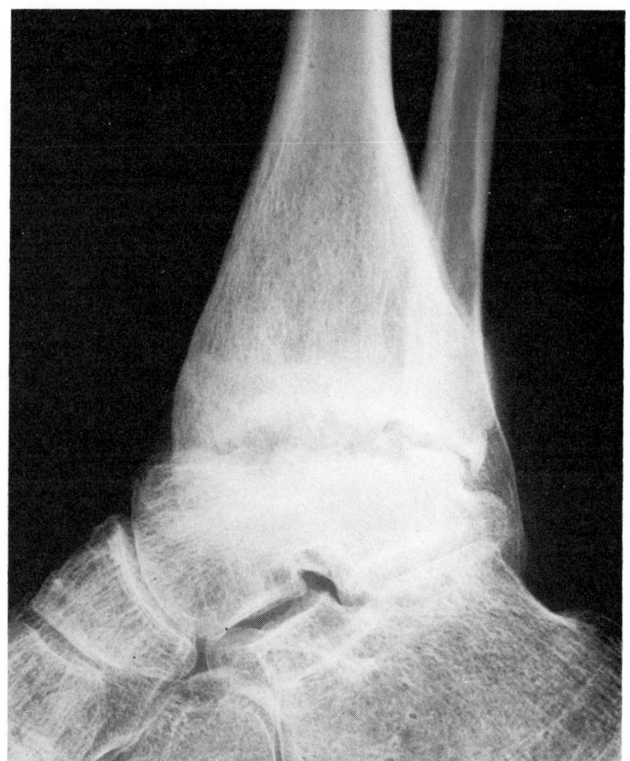

Figure 62–24. Tuberculous arthritis: Ankle. Observe poorly defined osseous erosion of the tibia and talus with reactive eburnation. Periostitis and enlargement of the distal tibial surface are noted.

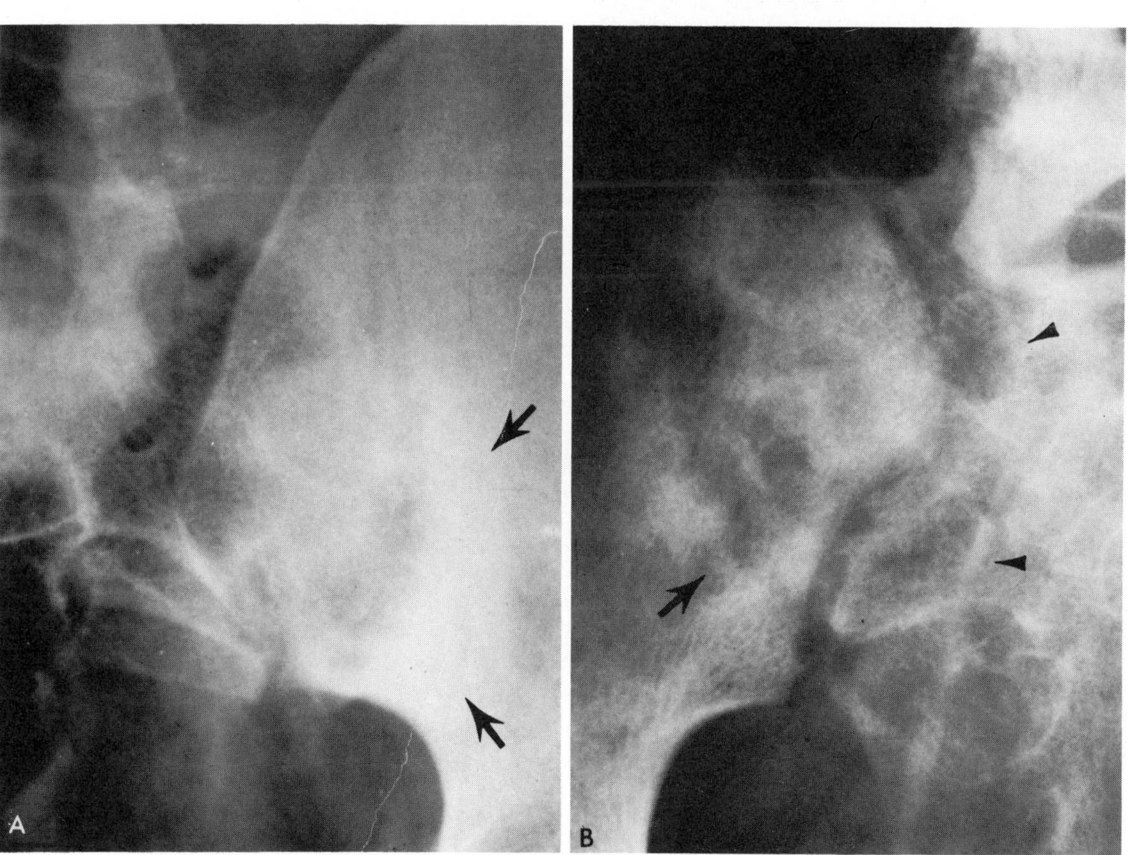

Figure 62–25. Tuberculous arthritis: Sacroiliac joint.

A *The left sacroiliac joint is abnormal. Note erosion and sclerosis, predominantly of the ilium (arrows). The appearance is identical to that of pyogenic arthritis.*

B *In another patient, changes about the right sacroiliac joint include ill-defined subchondral margins and osteoporosis (arrow). Note the displacement of the right ureter (arrowheads) during this intravenous pyelogram.*

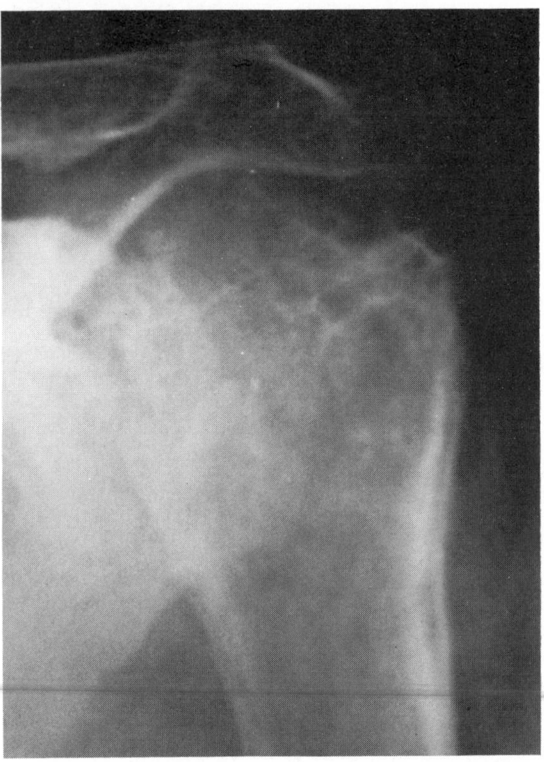

Figure 62–26. Tuberculous arthritis: Glenohumeral joint. Radiographic findings include widespread destruction of the humeral head and glenoid process, periostitis, and osteoporosis. The joint space is poorly evaluated. The tapered distal clavicle may be evidence of spread of infection to the acromioclavicular joint.

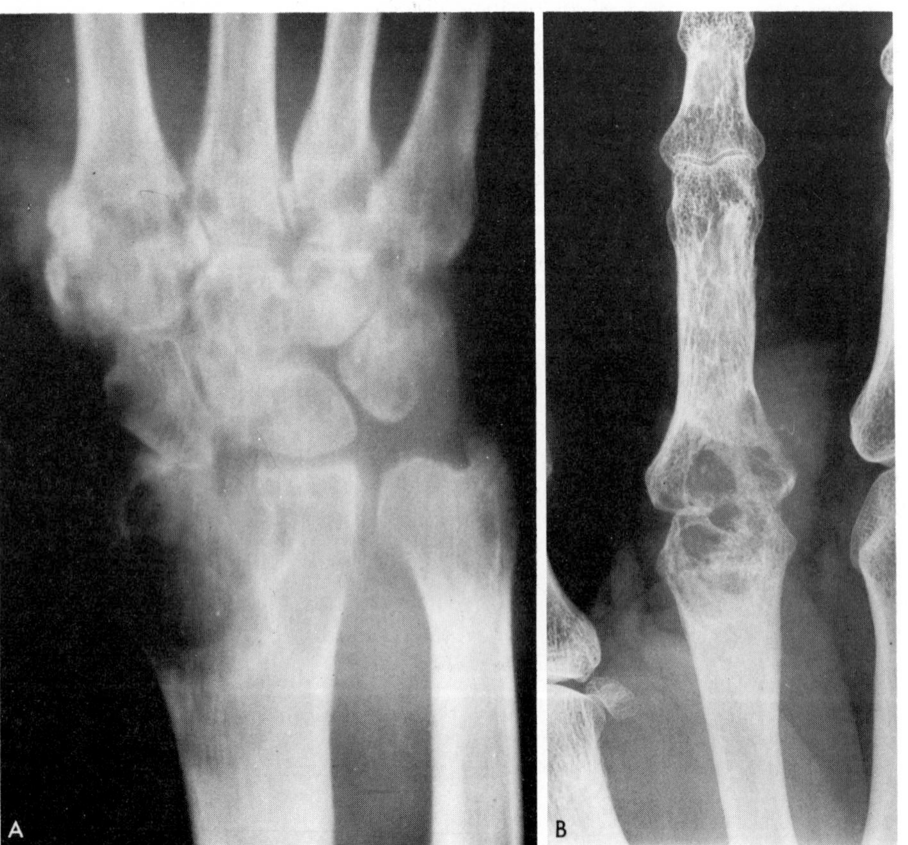

Figure 62–27. Tuberculous arthritis: Wrist and hand.

A Abnormalities include soft tissue swelling, osteoporosis, small and large osseous erosions throughout the carpus, metacarpals, and radius, and joint space narrowing.

B In a different patient, observe obliteration of the second metacarpophalangeal joint with adjacent cystic lesions. Reactive sclerosis is not apparent.

some patients with tuberculosis, particularly blacks. Similarly, periostitis can be evident, although its incidence and extent are not so great in tuberculosis as in pyogenic infection. In both tuberculosis and pyogenic processes, the periostitis is linear in nature, paralleling the osseous contour; interrupted or perpendicular varieties of periostitis as seen in neoplasms are highly unusual.

Sequestered pieces of bone appear as dense, triangular collections at the edges of the articulation. Rarely, large portions of the adjacent bone may become sequestered.[177] Fistulae can develop, and small bony fragments may be extruded.[195]

The eventual result in tuberculous arthritis is usually fibrous ankylosis of the joint. Bony ankylosis is occasionally seen, but this sequela is more frequent in pyogenic arthritis.

Differential Diagnosis. The diagnosis of tuberculous arthritis is generally not difficult when classic radiographic features appear in typical locations, such as the knee, the hip, the wrist, or the elbow.[134, 191, 194, 196-198] With unusual features or in atypical locations, the diagnosis can be more troublesome.[199] The appearance of periarticular osteoporosis, marginal erosions, and absent or mild joint space narrowing is most helpful in the accurate diagnosis of this disease. In rheumatoid arthritis, osteoporosis and marginal erosions are accompanied by early and significant loss of articular space. In gout, osteoporosis is mild or absent, although marginal erosions and preservation of interosseous space can be observed. In regional osteoporosis, marginal osseous defects are not evident, and the joint space is maintained.

A monoarticular process must be regarded as infection until proved otherwise. Although it may be difficult to define the nature of the infective agent (e.g., pyogenic, tuberculous, fungal), slow progression of disease, significant osteoporosis, and mild sclerosis are more prominent in tuberculosis and fungal disease than in pyarthrosis (Table 62–1). However, accurate diagnosis mandates synovial fluid aspiration or synovial membrane biopsy. Other monoarticular processes, such as pigmented villonodular synovitis and idiopathic synovial osteochondromatosis, can also simulate tuberculosis. In pigmented villonodular synovitis, a nodular soft tissue mass, preservation of joint space, and absence of osteoporosis are typical; in idiopathic synovial osteochondromatosis, calcified and ossified intra-articular bodies are commonly evident.

Table 62–1
COMPARISON OF TUBERCULOUS AND PYOGENIC ARTHRITIS

	Tuberculous Arthritis	Pyogenic Arthritis
Soft tissue swelling	+	+
Osteoporosis	+	±
Joint space loss	Late	Early
Marginal erosions	+	+
Bony proliferation (sclerosis, periostitis)	±	+
Bony ankylosis	±	+
Slow progression	+	–

+ = Common; ± = infrequent; – = rare or absent.

Tuberculous Bursitis and Tenosynovitis. The synovial membrane of bursae and tendon sheaths may be involved in tuberculosis. Typical sites include the radial and ulnar bursae of the hand, the flexor tendon sheaths of the fingers, and the subacromial (subdeltoid) and subgluteal bursae.[200-202] Soft tissue swelling and osteoporosis may be observed. In the region of the greater trochanter, osseous destruction can be encountered, and the hip joint may become secondarily infected,[203] particularly following surgical intervention.[204] In any bursal location, dystrophic calcification may appear; this is especially characteristic about the hip and elbow.[205]

BCG VACCINATION–INDUCED INFECTION. BCG (bacille Calmette-Guérin) is a vaccine of an attenuated bovine tubercle bacillus that has been used for immunization against tuberculosis. Although complications are unusual, generalized BCG infection[206, 207, 540] and bone and joint infection[208-219] have been identified following vaccination. The former complication is almost invariably fatal and is especially common in patients with immunologic deficiency. The latter complication results from hematogenous spread of the BCG infection to the skeleton, is not usually associated with immunologic disorders, and has a favorable prognosis.

It has been estimated that 1 in 5000 to 80,000 vaccinated children will develop bone or joint infection.[216] BCG osteomyelitis involves boys and girls between the ages of 5 months and 6 years. It usually affects the metaphyses and the epiphyses of the tubular bones or the small bones of the hands and the feet. Spinal involvement is uncommon. Solitary lesions predominate and are characterized by well-defined lytic foci with only minor degrees of sclerosis or periostitis. Small sequestra may be identified. Extension of the process from the metaphysis to the epiphysis is not uncommon.

The histologic characteristics of BCG osteomyelitis resemble those of tuberculosis, although severe plasma cell infiltration is less common in the former condition. A confident diagnosis requires the growth of the BCG strain in culture, although the difficulty in cultivating BCG is noteworthy.

ATYPICAL MYCOBACTERIAL INFECTION. Acid-fast bacteria that are morphologically similar to tubercle bacilli were long regarded as important in clinical medicine only because they might be mistaken for *M. tuberculosis* (or *M. leprae*) on histologic examination. It is now recognized that many of these bacteria are pathogenic for humans.[220] Although skin and pulmonary disease are the most recognized clinical manifestations of infection with these organisms, bone and joint alterations may also be noted. Mycobacterial osteomyelitis and arthritis can complicate connective tissue disorders and can be evident in patients with impaired resistance. The mechanisms of the musculoskeletal alterations include hematogenous spread and contamination following injury or surgery.

The atypical mycobacteria are frequently classified as follows: group I — photochromogens (*M. kansasii*); group II — scotochromogens (*M. scrofulaceum*); group III — nonchromogens (Battey type); and group IV — rapid growers (*M. fortuitum*).[221] Infection by organisms in any of these groups can lead to osteomyelitis, septic arthritis, tenosynovitis (with carpal tunnel syndrome), and bursitis.[222-229, 516, 524, 528, 541]

Although radiologic characteristics for each of these groups have not been well delineated, certain general observations include the following traits: Multiple lesions predominate over solitary lesions; metaphyses and diaphyses of long bones are commonly affected; discrete lytic areas may contain sclerotic margins; osteoporosis may not be so striking as in tuberculous infection; and articular disease can simulate tuberculosis or rheumatoid arthritis.

Pathologically, granulomatous lesions with or without caseation are typical. The diagnosis is established by culture of the synovial fluid or synovial membrane.

LEPROSY (HANSEN'S DISEASE; M. LEPRAE INFECTION)

General Features. Leprosy is an infectious disease caused by *Mycobacterium leprae*. Despite its infrequent occurrence in the United States, it is not uncommon in areas of Africa, South America, and the Orient. Leprosy is characterized by a lengthy incubation period and a chronic course with involvement of the skin, the mucous membranes, and the peripheral nervous system. It is the involvement of peripheral nerves that is especially characteristic of *M. leprae* infection.

The lesions of leprosy have been divided into four principal types according to their microscopic appearance[230]:

Lepromatous Type. Bacilli are numerous but there is very litle cellular reaction. Widespread cutaneous lesions consisting of nodules, macules, papules, and diffuse infiltration are symmetrically distributed. "Leprae cells," representing macrophages containing fat droplets and many bacilli, are distinctive.

Tuberculoid Type. Bacilli are less numerous but are capable of exciting a severe granulomatous reaction similar to that which is observed in tuberculosis or sarcoidosis. Asymmetrically distributed skin macules are evident.

Dimorphous Type. An uncommon variety in which microscopic features of both the lepromatous and tuberculoid types are seen.

Indeterminate Type. In perivascular and perineural areas, a few bacilli stimulate a slight cellular reaction whose pathologic features are not prominent enough to allow classification into tuberculoid or lepromatous types.

The clinical manifestations vary among these types of leprosy. In general, the tuberculoid type of disease is less progressive than the lepromatous type. In tuberculoid leprosy, the skin and nerves are principally affected, whereas in lepromatous leprosy, a more acute and generalized process may be evident.

Clinical Abnormalities. Although a history of prolonged contact with the bacilli is typical, the exact mode of transmission of this disease is not clear. It appears probable that the infection enters the body through the skin or mucous membranes, especially the nasal mucosa. The organisms are disseminated via the bloodstream and the lymphatics and localize in the skin, the nerves, and, in advanced cases, many of the viscera. The incubation period has been estimated to be 3 to 6 years. Men are more commonly affected than women. The disease may begin at any age, although leprosy is commonly manifest prior to 20 years of age. Prodromal symptoms and signs include malaise, fever, drowsiness, rhinitis, and profuse sweating. Skin manifestations differ in the lepromatous and tuberculoid types. Lymphadenopathy is seen in all types of leprosy, although it is most striking in the lepromatous variety.

In patients with prominent neurologic findings (neural variety of disease) lepromatous granulation tissue appears in and around the nerves, leading to tenderness and thickening of these structures, numbness, and tingling. Pruritus, anesthesia, or hyperesthesia may be evident, especially in the hands and the feet. Muscle atrophy and contractions appear, and eventually extensive multilation and secondary infection are noted.

Laboratory abnormalities may include a positive lepromin skin test (in tuberculoid leprosy), an elevated erythrocyte sedimentation rate, and a positive serologic test for syphilis (20 to 40 per cent of cases). The diagnosis is established by demonstration of the bacilli in typical histologic lesions.

Musculoskeletal Abnormalities. The musculoskeletal abnormalities include (1) those directly related to presence of the bacilli, in which granulomatous lesions appear in the osseous tissue (direct or specific effects); and (2) those that indirectly involve the skeleton due to neural abnormalities (indirect or nonspecific effects).[1, 231]

Leprous Periostitis, Osteitis, and Osteomyelitis. The incidence of direct involvement of the skeleton in leprosy is low, varying from 3 to 5 per cent among hospitalized patients.[232] The changes are usually confined to the small bones of the face, the hands, and the feet.[231] In these cases, osseous involvement is usually due to extension of the infection from overlying dermal or mucosal areas; initially the periosteum is contaminated (leprous periostitis), and subsequently the subjacent cortex, spongiosa, and marrow (leprous osteitis and osteomyelitis) become involved. Less commonly, hematogenous spread of infection to the bone can occur, leading to intramedullary foci.[1] In this situation, skeletal sites in addition to those of the face, the hand, and the foot can be altered, including the tubular bones of the extremities and the ribs.

Pathologically, intraosseous lesions are characterized by granulomatous tissue reactions that lead to trabecular destruction. The lesions are usually evident in the epiphysis and metaphysis of the tubular bones, although direct involvement of the medullary canal can also occur.[233] Progression of disease is generally slow, although the cortex and the periosteum can be violated. Periostitis and reactive sclerosis are usually not prominent in this disease. Of interest, marrow aspiration in cases of leprosy may reveal striking histiocytosis.[514]

In the face, nasal destruction is most characteristic.[234] Destruction of the alveolar process and anterior nasal spine of the maxilla appears to be related to direct lepromatous contamination of the bone as well as secondary infection.[235]

In the hands and the feet, the metaphyses of phalanges are particularly vulnerable; metacarpal and metatarsal involvement is less frequent[231] (Fig. 62–28). Soft tissue swelling, osteoporosis, endosteal thinning, enlargement of the nutrient foramina, and osseous destruction with a cystic or honeycombed appearance are evident. Pathologic fractures and epiphyseal collapse may appear. With healing, radiographs reveal increasing definition of the involved bone, although residual deformity with subluxation and malalignment can occur.

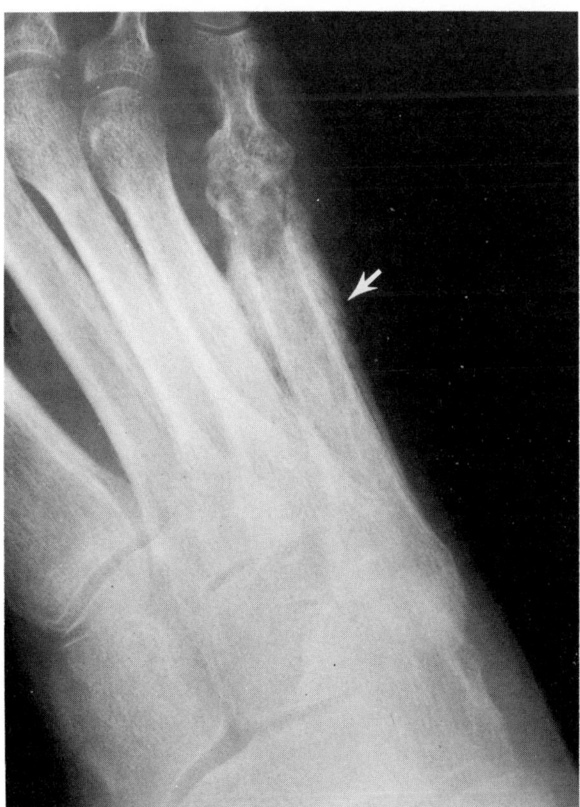

Figure 62–28. *Leprous osteomyelitis and septic arthritis. Note destruction of the metatarsal with exuberant periostitis (arrow). The fifth metatarsophalangeal joint is obliterated. The soft tissues are abnormal owing to adjacent infection.*

In the tubular bones, symmetric periostitis of the tibia, the fibula, and the distal ulna may be noted (Fig. 62–29). Intractable pain and tenderness may develop and microscopic examination usually reveals subperiosteal infiltration with *Mycobacterium leprae*.[236] The constellation of erythematous skin lesions, pain, and periostitis involving the lower extremity has been called "red leg" and has been attributed to immunologic factors present during the reactive phase of the disease.[231] The radiographs reveal periosteal proliferation reminiscent of that in hypertrophic osteoarthropathy, a similarity that is accentuated by abnormal symmetric accumulation of bone-seeking pharmaceuticals on radionuclide examination.[237]

Leprous Arthritis. Specific leprous arthritis is rare.[238] Pain and swelling with massive joint effusion are evident in the ankle, the knee, the wrist, the finger, and the elbow in order of descending frequency.[1] Joint involvement results from intra-articular extension of an osseous or periarticular infective focus or, less commonly, from hematogenous contamination of the synovial membrane. The detection of acid-fast bacilli in joint fluid is occasionally accomplished.[239, 240]

Neuropathic Musculoskeletal Lesions. The skeletal abnormalities occurring on a neurologic basis are much more frequent and severe than those produced by direct leprous infiltration of the bone.[1, 231] These changes may be evident in 20 to 70 per cent of patients in a sanatorium[232, 241, 242] They result from denervation, producing sensory or motor impairment, or both. Repeated injuries and secondary infections subsequently lead to considerable osseous and articular destruction. The bones of the hands and the feet are especially susceptible to this form of leprosy.

In leprosy, disuse of an extremity is related to the intense pain of acute leprous neuritis, the application of a cast for injury, inactivity associated with severe finger and toe contractures,[231] or a combination of these. Osteoporosis may appear, which can be complicated by fracture and deformity.

Cessation of function due to motor denervation can be associated with the absorption of cancellous bone and the development of concentric bone atrophy.[231] The result is a tapered appearance to the end of the bone, termed the "licked candy stick" (Fig. 62–30). In the foot, progressive resorption of the metatarsals and proximal phalanges occurs. In the hand and the foot, distal phalangeal resorption is also encountered, which may eventually result in loss of many of the phalanges, especially when the process is complicated by secondary infection. Although all insensitive digits can be altered, the index and long fingers

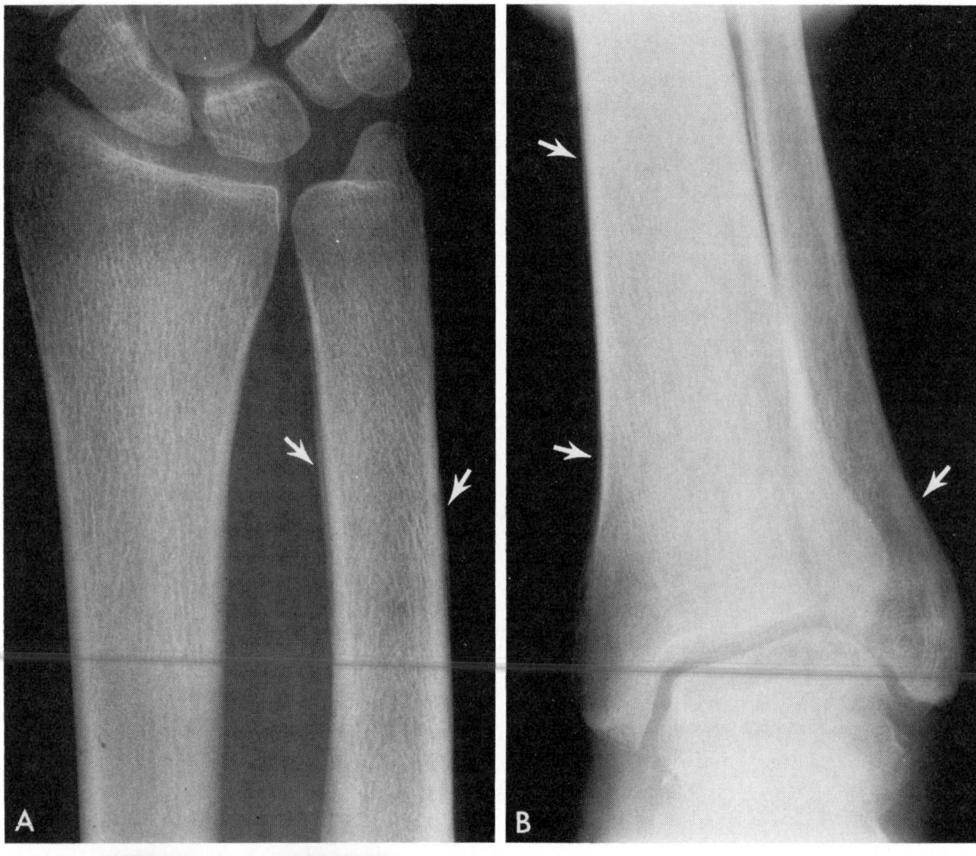

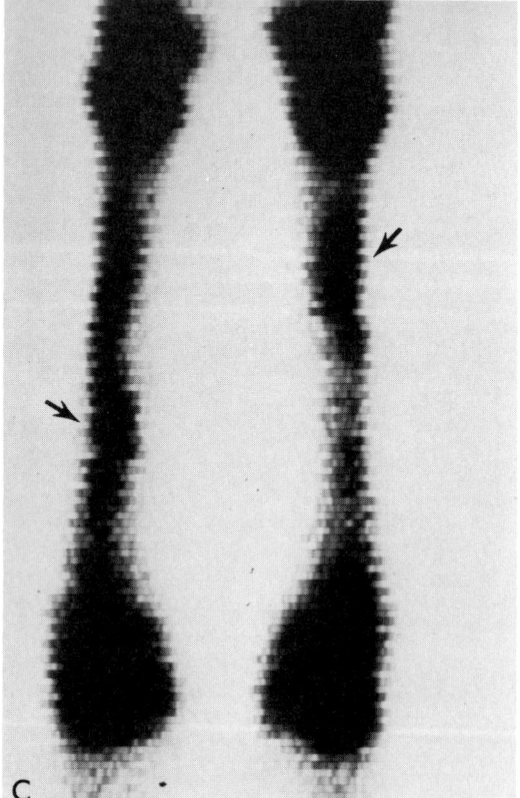

Figure 62–29. *Leprous periostitis: "Red leg." A 43 year old man presented with a 5 year history of arm and leg weakness, hypoesthesia, skin ulcerations, and rash. The lateral portions of his eyebrows had fallen out, and he had previously been treated for leprosy. A biopsy of the involved skin revealed subcutaneous infiltration with large numbers of polymorphonuclear leukocytes, histiocyte-like cells with foamy cytoplasm, and multinucleated giant cells. Special stains showed abundant acid-fast bacilli.*

A, B *Radiographs reveal periostitis of the distal ulna, tibia, and fibula (arrows). The opposite side was similarly affected.*

C *A ^{99m}Tc-pyrophosphate bone scan shows increased uptake over the knees and the ankles as well as in both tibiae and fibulae (arrows).*

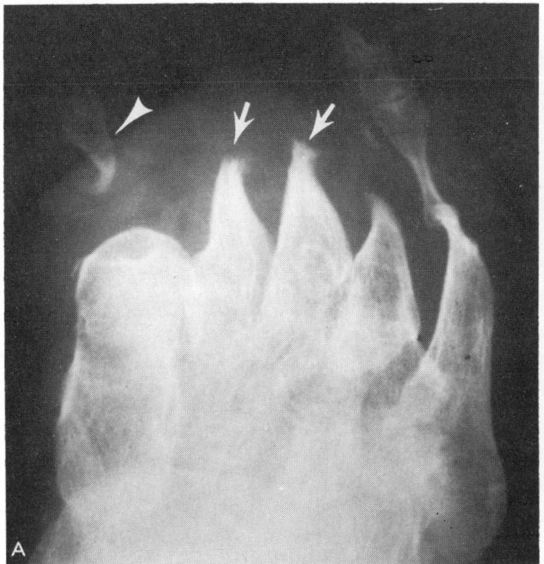
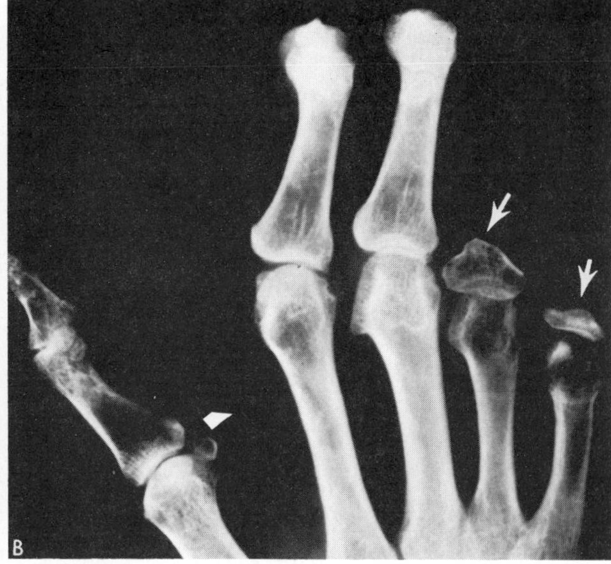

Figure 62–30. *Leprosy: Neuropathic lesions. Examples of concentric bony atrophy in the foot and the hand illustrate the tapered osseous surfaces (arrows) with isolation of distal bony fragments (arrowhead).*

are usually first affected, and seldom are all the digits equally involved.[231, 243]

Tarsal disintegration is not infrequent,[243-245, 513] attributable to sensory and motor dysfunction, trauma, and secondary infection. Changes are initiated within the medial arch, the lateral arch, the talus, and the calcaneus.[231] Osteolysis, osteosclerosis, fragmentation, and progressive resorption can be encountered (Fig. 62–31). In extreme cases, dissolution of the midfoot results in separation of the forefoot and the hindfoot, and the tibia is driven downward, becoming weight-bearing.

Figure 62–31. *Leprosy: Neuropathic lesions. Fragmentation and collapse of the talar, tibial, and calcaneal surfaces can be seen. The appearance is similar to that in tabes dorsalis.*

The histologic characteristics of involved joints in leprous patients with neurologic deficit are similar to those in other neuroarthropathies.[1] Serous effusion, villous proliferation of the synovial membrane, erosion and proliferation of cartilage, sclerosis and eburnation of bone, fragmentation, and exostoses are apparent.

The radiographic appearance of neuroarthropathy in leprosy resembles that in syphilis, diabetes, congenital insensitivity to pain, and syringomyelia. It may also simulate changes in psoriatic arthritis, collagen vascular disorders such as scleroderma, and thermal injuries.

Secondary Infection. Because of the anesthesia resulting from the neural lesions, the leper is prone to suffer injuries. Ulceration followed by secondary infection and pyogenic osteomyelitis is common in the anesthetic feet.[246] Bone destruction, florid periosteal reaction, and sequestration can appear. Septic arthritis is also seen. Differentiating the effects of pyogenic osteomyelitis and arthritis from leprous osteomyelitis or neuroarthropathy is extremely difficult.

Vascular Lesions. The incidence, nature, and importance of vascular lesions in leprosy are debated. Some investigators believe that such lesions are very common in the hand and the foot and may be delineated by arteriography, during which occlusion, narrowing, tortuosity, dilatation, irregularity, and incomplete filling of vessels can be noted.[247] Others suggest that bone absorption occurs because of interference to the mechanism controlling vasoregulation due to involvement of the nerves in the vascular reflex arch[248, 249]; in this regard, narrowing of the lumen of

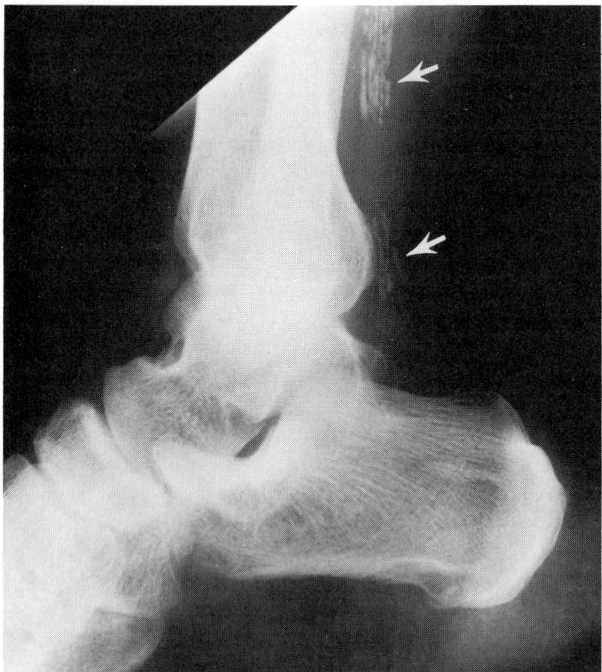

Figure 62–32. Leprosy: Calcification of nerves. The linear radiodense regions (arrows) represent calcification of nerves. This finding, although rare, is suggestive of the diagnosis of leprosy but must be distinguished from vascular calcification. (Courtesy of Dr. M. Dalinka, University of Pennsylvania, Philadelphia, Pennsylvania.)

medium-sized and small arterioles has been noted in cases with and without bone resorption.[232, 246]

Soft Tissue Calcification. Rarely, linear calcification of involved nerves can be seen on radiographs[250] (Fig. 62–32). Similarly, abscess formation within the nerve, especially in the ulnar nerve, can be associated with calcification.[251, 252]

Spirochetes

SYPHILIS

General Features. Syphilis is a chronic systemic infectious disease caused by *Treponema pallidum*, a slender spirochete with regular, evenly spaced spirals. Although the incidence and prevalence of the disorder have decreased since World War II, a recent resurgence of syphilitic infection has been noted. Syphilis is transmitted by direct and intimate contact with moist infectious lesions of the skin and mucous membranes. Thus, infection is spread during sexual contact, although less commonly the disease may be contracted during biting or kissing. The appearance of the disorder traceable to any one of these mechanisms is termed *acquired syphilis*. In addition, the fetus may be infected by transmission of the organism through the placenta; this is termed *congenital syphilis*.

Once the spirochete has violated the epithelium, it enters lymphatics and reaches the regional lymph nodes in a period of hours.[253] Subsequently, the treponema may enter the bloodstream and the ensuing spirochetemia, which can occur before the primary lesion appears at the inoculation site, allows dissemination of infection throughout the body.

Approximately 3 to 6 weeks after the organism has entered the body, a primary lesion, the *chancre*, develops at the site of inoculation. This lesion is a skin ulceration that heals spontaneously. About 6 weeks later, a generalized skin eruption known as *secondary syphilis* develops.[253] In this stage of the disease, systemic manifestations are frequent. Following healing of both primary and secondary manifestations, the patient may be without symptoms and signs for a protracted period of time, a stage termed *latent syphilis*, although progressive inflammatory alterations may be occurring slowly in many of the organ systems. Cardiovascular syphilis or neurosyphilis may become manifest 10 to 30 years later, although some individuals (approximately 50 per cent) never develop tertiary manifestations of syphilis and show no signs of the disease at autopsy.[253] In those patients with significant later alterations, large destructive lesions or *gummas* can be evident in almost any organ of the body, particularly the skin and the bones.

Congenital Syphilis

Incidence and Pathogenesis. Although earlier studies indicated that congenital syphilis might occur in 2 to 5 per cent of infants,[254] modern techniques designed to improve the recognition of this disease in pregnant women have led to an impressive reduction in the number of cases of congenital syphilis.[255] The disorder originates from transplacental migration of the treponema and invasion of the perichondrium, periosteum, cartilage, bone marrow, and sites of active endochondral ossification, especially in the metaphyseal regions of tubular bones.[1] The spirochetes inhibit osteogenesis and lead to degeneration of osteoblasts.

The fetus that is heavily infiltrated with spirochetes may abort or die shortly after birth. Others survive, developing the stigmata of congenital syphilis. Early and late lesions may be identified in these infants.

Early Osseous Lesions. In the fetus, the neonate, and the very young infant, bony abnormalities include (1) osteochondritis; (2) diaphyseal osteomyelitis (osteitis); (3) periostitis; and (4) miscellaneous changes. These have been well summarized by Jaffe,[1] and many of his observations with regard to congenital as well as acquired syphilis are included in the following pages.

1. *Syphilitic osteochondritis* usually results in symmetric involvement of sites of endochondral ossification.[256] The epiphyseal-metaphyseal junction of tubular bones, the costochondral regions, and, in

severe cases, the flat and short tubular bones and the centers of ossification of the sternum and vertebrae are affected.[1] In the growing metaphyses of the long bones, particularly about the knee, the shoulder, and the wrist, widening of the provisional calcification zone, serrations, and adjacent osseous irregularity are seen, which on histologic evaluation are found to result from a disturbance of endochondral ossification (Fig. 62–33). Radiographs outline broad horizontal radiolucent bands reminiscent of those that are identified in leukemia or metastasis from neuroblastoma.

If the process continues, metaphyseal irregularities appear (Fig. 62–34). Biopsy outlines granulation tissue within the metaphysis, which may be localized to one segment or involve the entire width of the bone, extending into the epiphysis and adjacent diaphysis. Histologically, the granulation tissue consists initially of vascular connective tissue and later of cellular infiltrations (lymphoid cells, polymorphonuclear leukocytes) and necrosis, presumably induced by the toxic effects of degenerating spirochetes.[1] On radiographs, irregular erosive lesions appear along the contour of the bone at the metaphyseal–growth plate junction. The medial surface of the proximal tibial shaft is a particularly characteristic site of erosion, a finding that is termed Wimberger's sign. These metaphyseal alterations, which may progress to osseous fragmentation, simulating the changes of scurvy, appear to be a true inflammatory change related to the spirochetes themselves.[257]

Epiphyseal separation can result from the metaphyseal destruction induced by the granulation tissue. It is usually evident in older fetuses, neonates, and infants up to the age of 3 months, and shows predilection for multiple sites in the long tubular bones, particularly in the upper extremity.[1, 258, 259] The metaphyseal line of cleavage leads to partial or complete separation of the epiphysis.

The lesions of osteochondritis generally heal quickly with specific therapy; healing is evident within 2 weeks and may be complete within 2 months.[260] Osteoblasts reappear, and new bone is deposited at the cartilaginous growth plates. Granulation tissue disappears, and normal growth ensues. Growth retardation and osseous deformity are unusual.

2. *Diaphyseal osteomyelitis (osteitis)* can appear in infants with congenital syphilis who have not received therapy or in whom treatment has been inadequate or inappropriate. Granulation tissue in the metaphysis may extend into the diaphysis, inducing infective foci of variable size (Fig. 62–34). Osteolytic lesions with surrounding bony eburnation and overlying periostitis can be encountered on radiographs of involved tubular bones. Although multiple bones are usually affected, alterations in a single tubular bone,[261] in the bones of one extremity,[544] or in nontubular bones[262] can be detected.

3. *Periostitis* is a less frequent manifestation of congenital syphilis than is osteochondritis.[1] It may result from several different processes.[263] Diffuse, widespread, symmetric, and profound periosteal proliferation can relate to its infiltration by syphilitic granulation tissue (Fig. 62–34). This variety of periostitis is observed in infants more frequently than in fetuses, and it can be associated with diaphyseal osteomyelitis. The long tubular bones and, less commonly, the flat bones are affected. Treatment produces a complete but slow resolution of the changes.

Reparative (reactive) periostitis is a second variety of periosteal response that may be noted about healing foci of osteochondritis or following epiphyseal slipping. It originates during the treatment of syphilis and represents "callus" formation rather than a response to syphilitic infiltration of the periosteum. Radiographic differentiation of infective and reparative periostitis can be difficult.

4. *Miscellaneous musculoskeletal changes* can occasionally be identified early in the course of congenital syphilis. Gummas have been reported in tubular and flat bones, although their occurrence in congenital syphilis is a rare phenomenon. Intra-articular effusions may complicate epiphyseal destruction or separation, and the joint fluid may reveal a strongly positive test for syphilis.[1]

Late Osseous Lesions. The early manifestations of congenital syphilis generally regress or disappear in the first few years of life, even in the absence of adequate therapy. However, exacerbation of disease may appear in the young child or adolescent (5 to 20 years of age). Although the evolving skeletal lesions occurring late in the course of congenital syphilis may rarely resemble those of early congenital syphilis (osteochondritis, osteomyelitis, periostitis), they more typically resemble the changes observed in acquired syphilis (see later discussion).[1] Osteomyelitis and periostitis in late congenital syphilis can involve the tubular bones, particularly the upper two-thirds of the tibial shafts, the flat bones, and even the cranium[264] (Fig. 62–35). In these sites, reactivation of spirochetes that have remained dormant for years may occur.

Gummatous or nongummatous osteomyelitis or periostitis results in diffuse hyperostosis of the involved bone. Endosteal bony proliferation produces encroachment on the medullary cavity, whereas periosteal bony proliferation creates an enlarged, undulating, and dense osseous contour.[1] In the tibia, a typical saber shin may be encountered, with anterior bending of the bone. Its radiographic appearance may resemble that of Paget's disease, although the syphilitic hyperostosis may not extend to the epiphysis. Lucent defects within areas of hyperostosis can represent gummas.

Abnormalities of the skull and mandible include destruction of the nasal bones, calvarial gumma, and

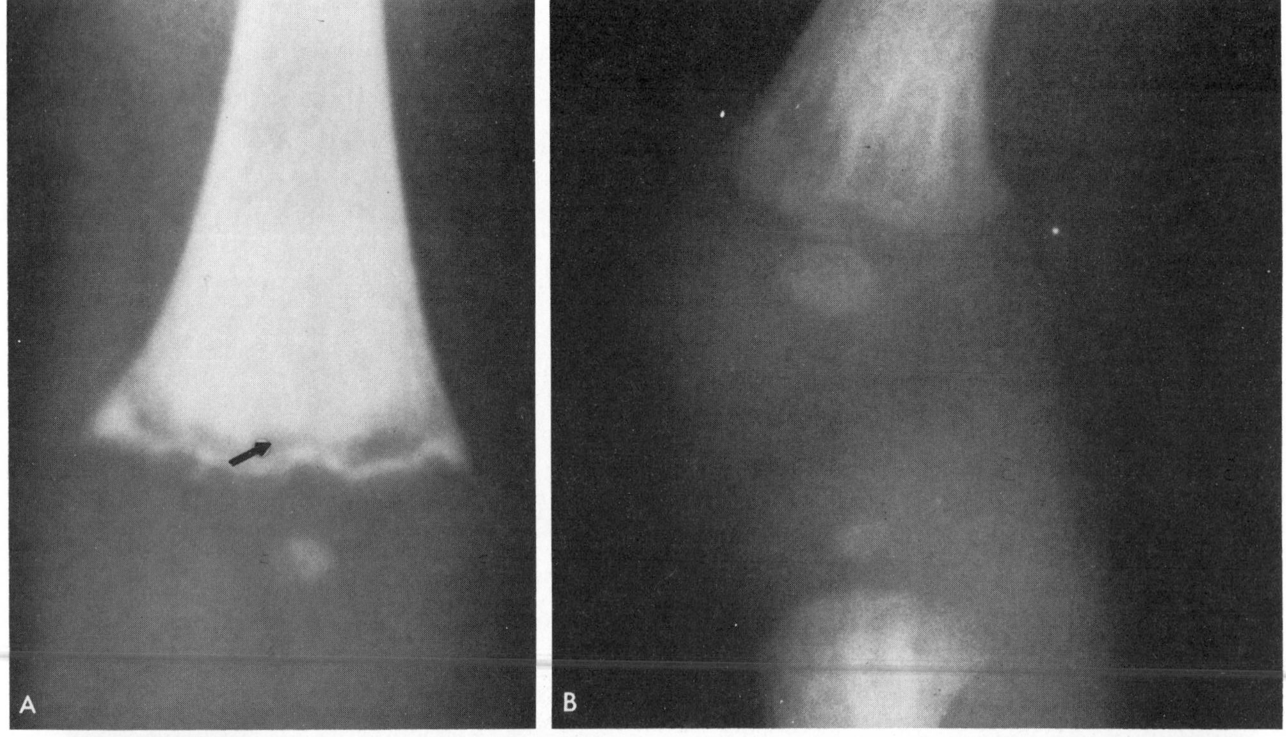

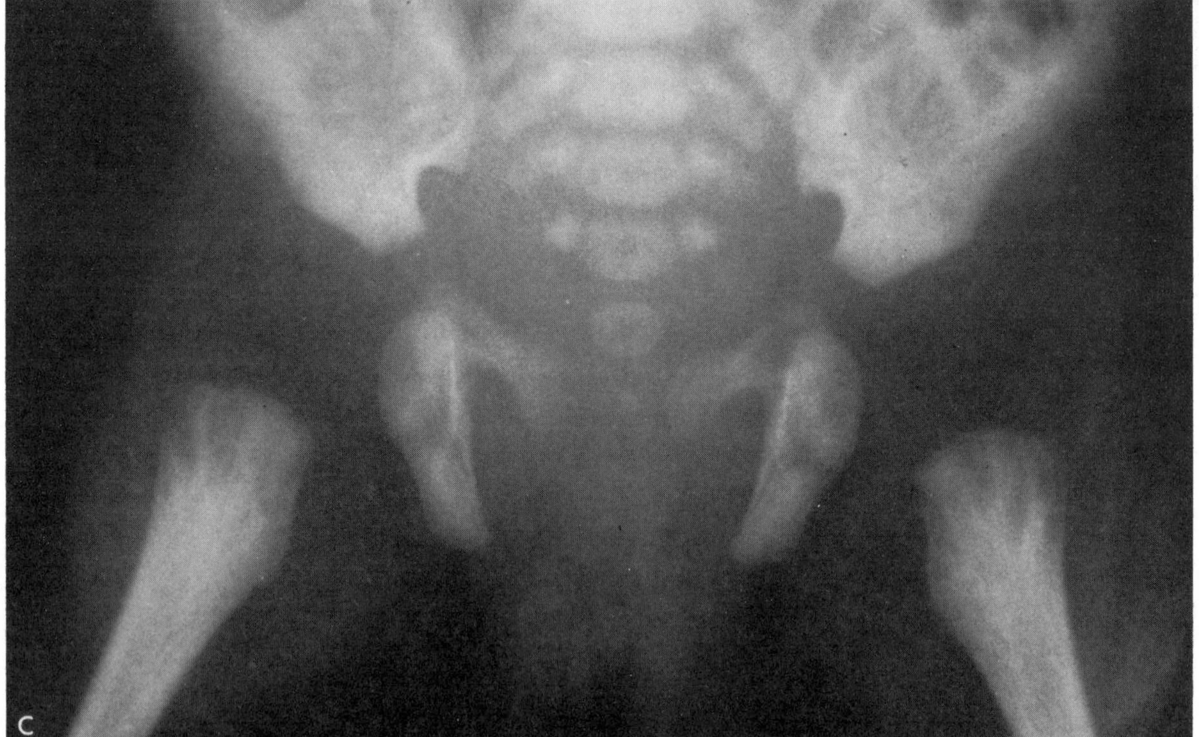

Figure 62–33. *Congenital syphilis: Osteochondritis.*

A *This 3 week old infant reveals a lucent band in the metaphysis (arrow) due to a disturbance in endochondral ossification. The appearance is similar to that in leukemia or neuroblastoma.*

B, C *In another infant with syphilis, a "celery stalk" appearance with alternating longitudinal lucent and sclerotic bands owing to abnormality of endochondral ossification resembles the changes in rubella.*

*(**B, C,** Courtesy of Dr. D. Edwards, University of California, San Diego, California.)*

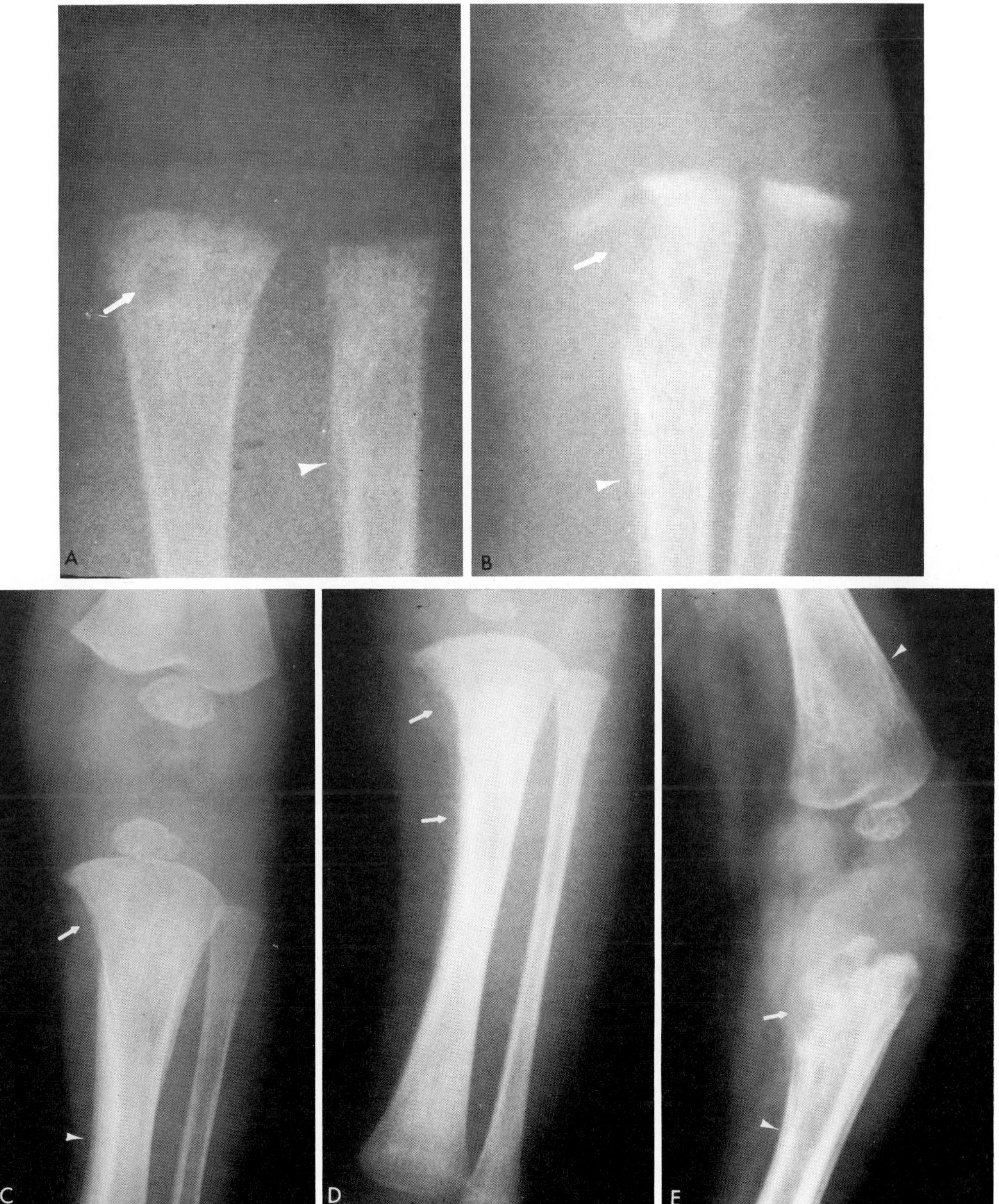

Figure 62–34. *Congenital syphilis: Osteochondritis and osteomyelitis.*

A, B *In two different infants, the progression of metaphyseal changes in the wrist can be identified. Initially* **(A),** *ill-defined lucent foci (arrow) are associated with periosteal proliferation (arrowhead). Later findings* **(B)** *include soft tissue swelling, large and destructive lesions (arrow), and more exuberant periosteal proliferation (arrowhead).*

C–E *In three different infants, the tibial alterations are well shown. Initially* **(C),** *defects in the medial tibial metaphysis (arrow) are characteristic, frequently associated with periostitis (arrowhead). Subsequently* **(D),** *the degree of osseous destruction may be more exaggerated (arrows). The predilection for the medial tibial metaphysis is again noteworthy. Eventually* **(E),** *osseous collapse can be seen (arrow). Observe the periostitis of tibia and femur (arrowheads).*

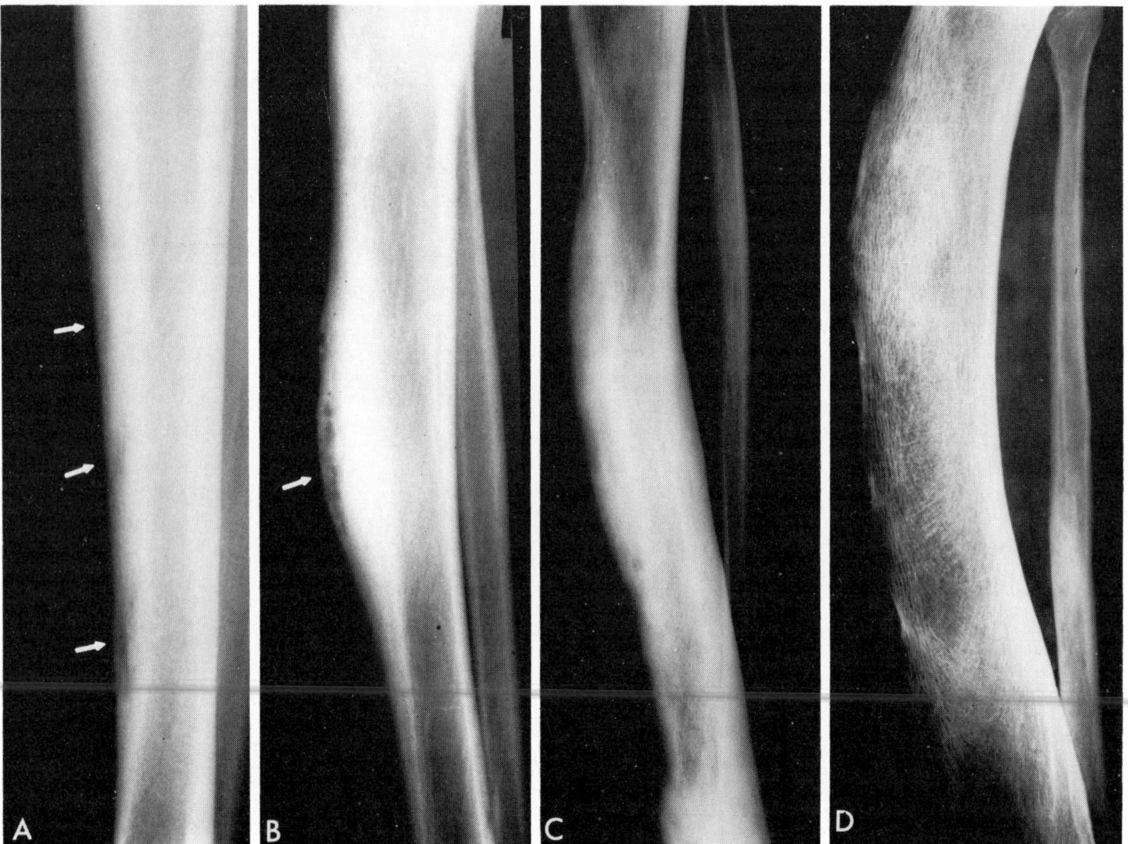

Figure 62–35. Congenital syphilis: Late osseous changes.

A Observe radiolucent foci within the anterior cortex of the tibia (arrows) with periostitis and endosteal proliferation.

B In a second patient, localized hyperostosis about a syphilitic lesion on the anterior surface of the tibia (arrow) can be observed.

C More exuberant hyperostosis of both the tibia and the fibula has resulted in bowed and prominent osseous surfaces. The changes are somewhat reminiscent of those in Paget's disease.

D A typical saber shin deformity of the tibia is associated with anterior bowing of the bone. The fibula is also involved.

Hutchinson's teeth, characterized by peg-shaped, notched, and hypoplastic dental structures.[265] The dental changes, which do not regress with antibiotic treatment, may be related to a direct action of the spirochetes on the tooth germ, a syphilic process of the mandible or the maxilla, or a metabolic effect.[1] Spirochetes are occasionally recovered from the neighboring bone.[266]

Jaffe[1] has also emphasized the late appearance of dactylitis in congenital syphilis, with periosteal proliferation and osseous expansion largely confined to the phalanges of the fingers and, less commonly, the toes.

In older syphilitic children, bilateral painless effusions, especially of the knee, have been termed Clutton's joints.[267]

Acquired Syphilis

Incidence. The incidence of osseous lesions during the course of acquired syphilis has decreased dramatically owing to improvement in diagnosis and treatment of this disease. When present, the bony and articular manifestations usually appear in the latent or tertiary phase of syphilis; similar manifestations in the early phases of the disorder are extremely unusual. In 1942, Reynolds and Wasserman[268] reviewed the cases of approximately 10,000 patients with early acquired syphilis that had accumulated over a 21 year period and were able to document only 15 cases (0.15 per cent) of destructive osseous lesions, although others have noted that the incidence may be as high as 8 to 20 per cent of these patients,[269] especially if periostitis and destructive osseous foci are both considered in the determination.

Early Acquired Syphilis

PATHOGENESIS. A spirochetemia appearing 1 to 3 months after the documentation of a primary lesion can lead to dissemination of organisms throughout the body.[270] The spirochetes can reach the deeper vascular areas of the periosteum with resulting perivascular inflammatory infiltrates and subsequent formation of highly cellular granulation tissue.[271] This tissue can extend into the haversian canals and medullary space of the involved bone(s). Conversely, initial contamination of the medullary space can lead to involvement of the cortex and the periosteum.[272, 273] Endothelial proliferation and endarteritis obliterans can develop, and infectious osteochondritis, periostitis, osteitis, or osteomyelitis may appear.

CLINICAL ABNORMALITIES. In the primary stage of syphilis, transitory, boring bone pain can be prominent, especially in febrile patients, in the tibia, humerus, and cranium, unassociated with radiographic or pathologic changes.[1] In the secondary stage, pain, soft tissue swelling, fever, and tenderness can be detected, particularly in the superficial bones, such as the frontal region of the calvarium, the anterior surfaces of the tibia, the sternum, and the ribs.[274, 275] The symptoms and signs of periostitis can vary substantially in severity and are characteristically worse at night.[274] They may resolve completely during appropriate antibiotic treatment.

RADIOGRAPHIC AND PATHOLOGIC ABNORMALITIES

Proliferative Periostitis. A proliferative periostitis is the most common osseous lesion in early acquired syphilis.[274, 276] It may be especially prominent in the tibia, the skull, the ribs, and the sternum, although other bones, such as the clavicle, the femur, the fibula, and the osseous structures of the hand and the foot, can be affected. Periosteal inflammation is associated with new bone formation, which can become extensive, leading to considerable thickening of the cortex. Although periosteal proliferation is generally laminated or solid, it can occur perpendicular to the underlying bone, simulating the appearance of an osteogenic sarcoma.[276-278] Bilateral tibial or clavicular periostitis in the adult is frequently syphilitic in origin.

Infective Osteitis and Osteomyelitis. Destructive bone lesions occur much less commonly than periostitis in early syphilis.[268-270, 279] These lesions relate to osteomyelitis and infective osteitis (as well as septic arthritis) (Fig. 62–36). Involvement of the skull is particularly characteristic,[269, 279] having been noted in nearly 9 per cent of 80 consecutive patients with secondary syphilis,[280] although any tubular and flat bone can be affected. Clinical manifestations related to skull involvement include headache and localized tumefactions. At this site, irregular areas of bone lysis are observed with a "motheaten" or permeative pattern of destruction, periostitis, and minimal or absent sclerosis. Usually, the outer table is more frequently and more significantly altered than the diploë or the inner table. Frontal, parietal, and nasopalatine areas are most often affected.[268] In the long tubular bones, osteolytic foci, cortical sequestration, periostitis, and epiphyseal separation can be noted. Syphilitic arthritis may be a complicating feature, especially of the sternoclavicular articulation (see discussion later in this chapter).

Late Acquired Syphilis

PATHOGENESIS. Osseous lesions occurring during the later stages of acquired syphilis can be related to gummatous or nongummatous inflammation.[1] Gummas within the medullary cavity, cortex, or periosteum do not usually become evident until years or decades after the acquisition of the disease.[1] Superficial bones are more commonly affected, a localization that is frequently attributed to recurrent low-grade trauma or irritation.

GUMMATOUS OSSEOUS LESIONS. A gumma represents a discrete or confluent area of variable size containing caseous necrotic material. These areas of necrosis are generally related to the effects of the toxic products of spirochetal degeneration, although the organisms themselves are usually not demonstrable within the lesions. On microscopic examination, syphilic granulation tissue within the gumma contains dense infiltration with lymphoid cells and engorged capillaries.[1] With the appearance of central caseation and peripherally located lymphoid, epithelioid, and Langhans' giant cells, the lesion resembles a tubercle. The adjacent osseous tissue undergoes necrosis. Resorption of cortical bone due to the inflammatory reaction about a gumma is frequently termed "caries sicca."[1] If the necrotic osseous area enlarges and becomes detached from the adjacent tissue, the term "caries necrotica" is utilized. The sequestered piece of cortex may become displaced into the gumma itself and may be recognized on radiographic and pathologic examination. Typically, however, cortical sequestration in syphilis is limited in extent and is not identifiable on roentgenographic evaluation. With healing, encapsulation of the caseous area by fibrous tissue is followed by gradual resorption of the caseous matter due to leukocytic and histiocytic activity.[1] Eventually a dense connective tissue scar replaces the original lesion.

The radiographic features are characterized by lytic and sclerotic areas of bone, which may reach considerable size (Fig. 62–36).[1, 281, 282] Adjacent periostitis is frequent, and, when large, the lesions may be associated with a pathologic fracture.[281]

NONGUMMATOUS OSSEOUS LESIONS. Nongummatous syphilitic periostitis, osteitis, or osteomyelitis can occur independently or in conjunction with gummas in the bone marrow.[1] Inflammation of the periosteum is associated with intimal thickening of medium-sized arteries and accumulation of lymphoid cells. Exuberant subperiosteal bone formation may follow, which may eventually merge with the underlying bone. Nongummatous syphilitic osteomyelitis is usually limited in extent, and is associated with infiltration of the marrow spaces with vascular and cellular connective tissue. Adjacent trabeculae become atrophic.

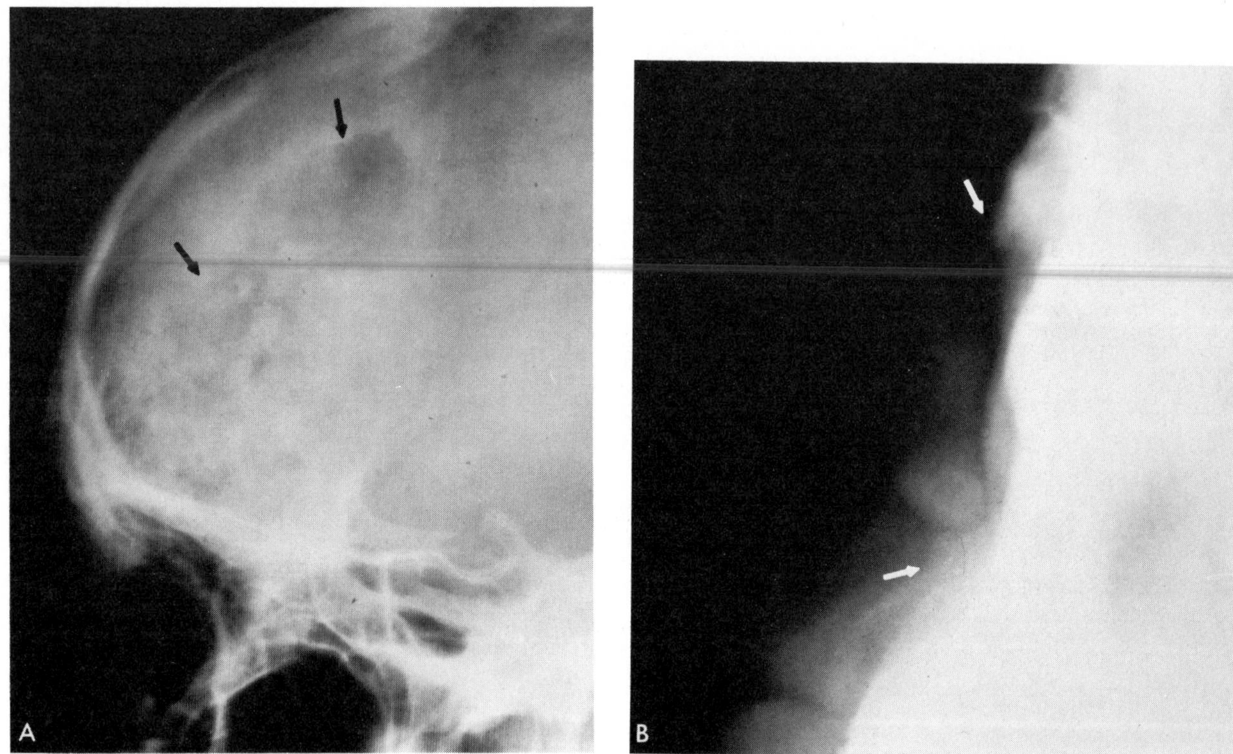

Figure 62–36. *Acquired syphilis: Osteitis, osteomyelitis, and periostitis.*

A *Lytic lesions of the frontal region of the skull (arrows) are accompanied by reactive sclerosis.*

B *Observe nasal bone destruction (arrows) associated with soft tissue deformity on this lateral radiograph of the face.*

Illustration continued on the opposite page

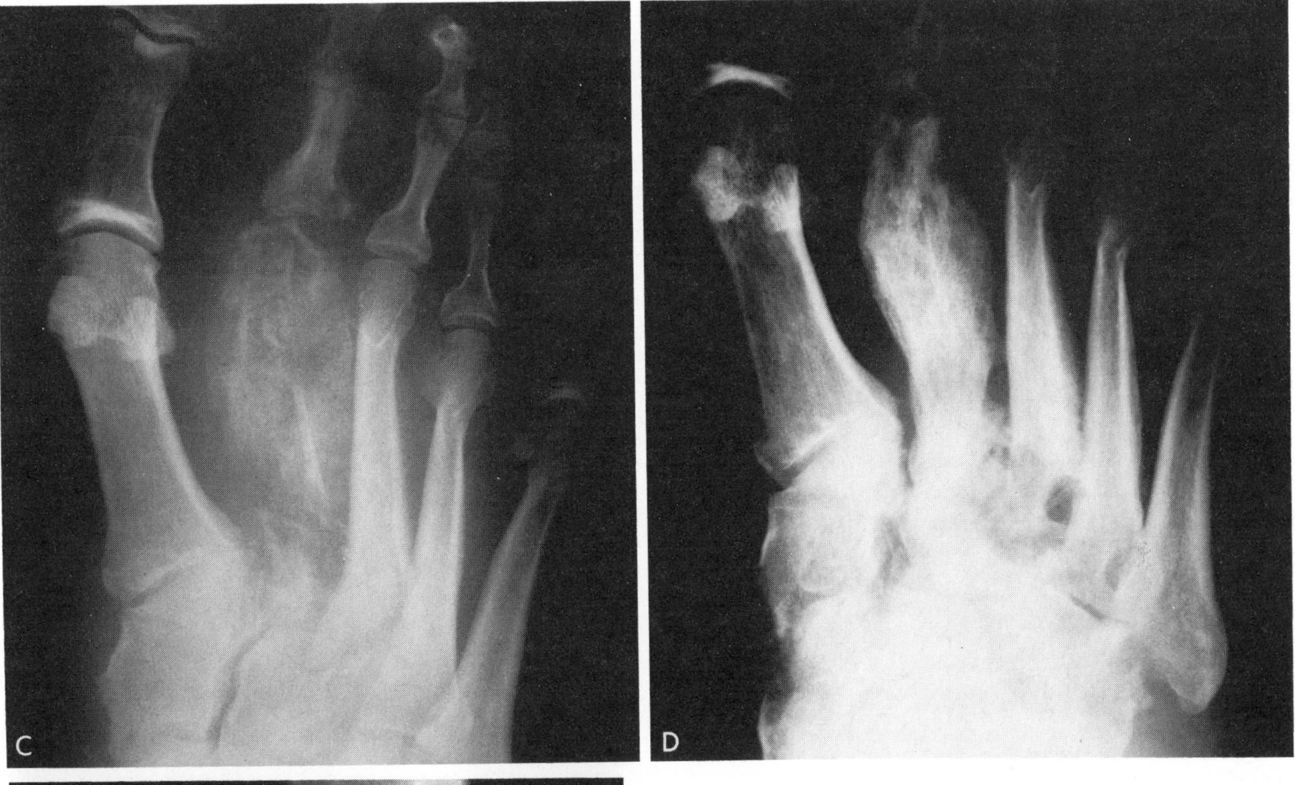

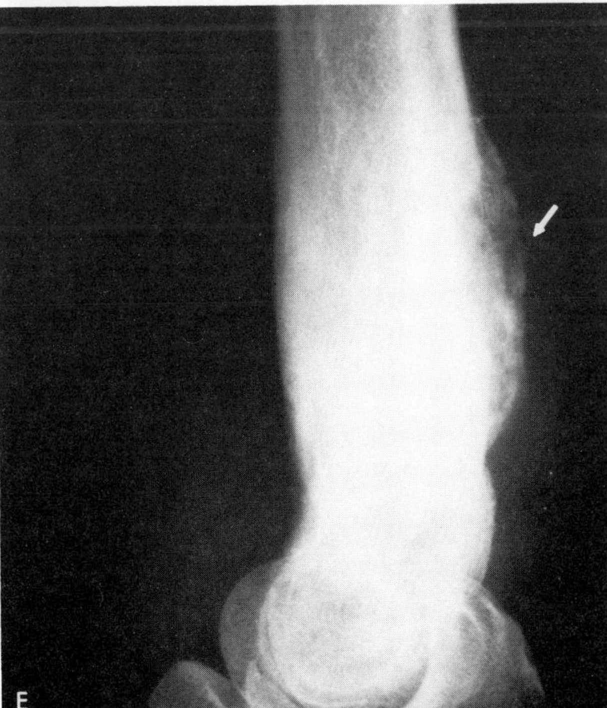

Figure 62–36. Continued

C, D *Films obtained 4 months apart illustrate initial osteolysis of metatarsals and phalanges associated with soft tissue swelling, periostitis, pathologic fracture, and articular involvement. Subsequently, exuberant new bone formation is evident in many of the metatarsal and tarsal bones.*

E *Note extreme bony proliferation of the distal humerus with soft tissue swelling (arrow) due to a gummatous lesion.*

The radiographic evaluation of nongummatous osseous lesions reveals destructive and productive bony changes associated with periostitis. Differentiation of these findings from those associated with gummas is better left to the pathologist.

DISTRIBUTION. Gummatous and nongummatous skeletal lesions can be delineated in many sites. Involvement of the cranial vault, nasal bones, maxilla, mandible, tubular bones of the appendicular skeleton, spine, and pelvis have all been noted (Fig. 62–36). The degree of periosteal proliferation can become extreme and, in tubular bones, can lead to gross enlargement of osseous tissue. The resultant radiographic and pathologic features resemble those in the late stages of congenital syphilis, including the saber shin deformity. According to Jaffe,[1] the saber shin deformity of acquired syphilis is usually related to pseudobowing of the tibia, in which the vertical direction of the marrow cavity is unchanged and the outer diameter of the bone is enlarged owing to periosteal proliferation; the saber shin deformity of congenital syphilis is associated with real bowing of the bone. Dactylitis, which is not infrequent in congenital syphilis, is less typical of acquired disease. When present in acquired syphilis, gummatous periostitis is the usual cause; in congenital syphilis gummatous osteomyelitis is typically implicated in the pathogenesis of dactylitis.

Articular Involvement

General Abnormalities. The incidence of articular involvement in syphilis is low. Joint abnormalities may occur in either congenital or acquired forms of the disease. In congenital syphilis, articular changes predominate in the late phases of the disorder; in acquired syphilis, joint manifestations appear in the tertiary or, less frequently, the secondary stage of the disorder.

The distribution of articular abnormalities varies with the age of the patient, the type of syphilitic infection, and the pathogenesis of the lesions (see later discussion). Joint effusions associated with pain and tenderness, which may be infectious or noninfectious in etiology, are commonly bilateral in distribution and most typically affect the knee. Infectious syphilitic arthritis can occur in any axial or extra-axial site, although sternoclavicular joint localization may have diagnostic importance.[565]

Pathogenesis. Joint disease appearing during the course of congenital or acquired syphilis can relate to a variety of mechanisms[1]:

1. *Spread from a contiguous source of infection.* In either congenital or acquired disease, syphilitic inflammation of periarticular bone can be complicated by joint involvement. This is usually associated with extension of an intraosseous gumma, followed by active articular inflammation resulting from the degenerating gummatous material. The inflammatory process within the joint is usually not gummatous.[283]

2. *Direct involvement of the synovial membrane.* In either congenital or acquired syphilis the luetic process can originate in the synovial or parasynovial tissues. Although the articular findings in these cases are related primarily to infection, it is frequently difficult to identify spirochetes in the synovial membrane or synovial fluid. However, electron microscopy may reveal treponema-like bodies in the synovial membrane in areas of considerable tissue necrosis.[284] Immunofluorescent antitreponemal antibody techniques can also lead to identification of spirochetes within synovial fluid.[285] Rarely, capsular thickening and synovial hypertrophy have been associated with true gummas within the synovial membrane.[286] The rapid resolution of articular symptoms after treatment with penicillin in some patients with synovitis also supports an infectious etiology.

3. *Sympathetic effusions.* In many cases of syphilis with synovitis, organisms are not identified in the articular cavity.[287, 288] In some of these cases, sympathetic effusion may relate to periosteal irritation from a neighboring intraosseous focus. In others, no adjacent bony abnormality is evident. Clinical symptoms and signs of arthralgia or arthritis may be present in the knees, hips, shoulders, and, less frequently, the joints of the fingers.[274, 288, 289] In congenital syphilis, painless intra-articular collections of fluid, especially in the knees, are termed Clutton's joints.

4. *Neuroarthropathy.* Neurosyphilis can be associated with neuroarthropathy, with fragmentation and dissolution of one or more joints of the axial and appendicular skeleton. This complication is discussed elsewhere (see Chapter 70).

Radiographic and Pathologic Abnormalities. In cases of noninfectious arthralgia or arthritis, radiographic and pathologic features may be lacking. A joint effusion may be detected, but the fluid may rapidly disappear. Osteoporosis may be evident.

Syphilitic infectious arthritis is associated with an effusion and capsular distention. The synovial membrane may become hypertrophied, with cellular infiltration. Synovial inflammation with pannus can lead to cartilaginous and osseous destruction. On radiographs, osteoporosis, joint space narrowing, bony destruction, sclerosis, and intra-articular osseous fusion can be encountered, findings that are similar to those occurring in other infectious arthritides (Fig. 62–36*C*, *D*).

YAWS. Yaws represents an infectious disorder caused by *Treponema pertenue*, an organism that is morphologically indistinguishable from *Treponema pallidum*, the cause of syphilis. Yaws occurs in tropical climates and is prevalent in Africa, South America, the South Pacific islands, and the West Indies. It is generally acquired before puberty during contact with open lesions containing the spirochetes. The transmission of the disease is rarely associated with sexual contact.

Within a period of weeks following inoculation, a granulomatous primary lesion appears, usually on

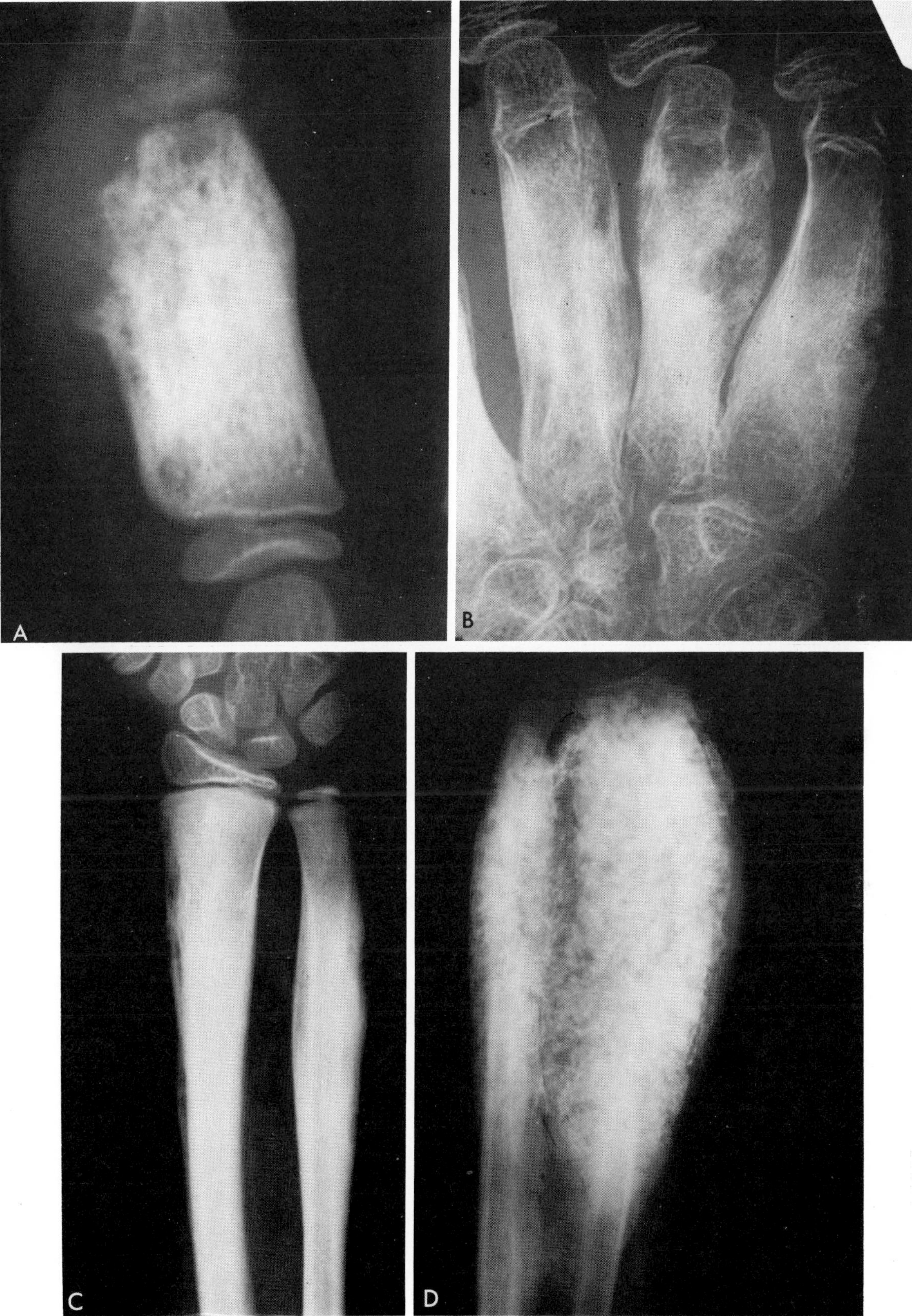

Figure 62–37. *Yaws.*

A, B *Dactylitis is characterized by lytic lesions surrounded by florid periosteal proliferation. Note the enlarged and sclerotic osseous contours.*

C, D *Osteitis and osteomyelitis produce a similar radiographic appearance at other sites, in these views the radius and ulna.*

*(**B, D,** Courtesy of Dr. W. Peter Cockshott, McMaster University, Hamilton, Ontario.)*

the legs. Approximately 1 to 3 months later, a generalized papular skin eruption occurs on the extremities, buttocks, neck, and face. After several years, late destructive lesions may become evident in the cutaneous and osseous tissues.

The tubular bones of the extremities, including those of the hands and feet, the pelvis, the skull, and the facial bones, may become the sites of periostitis or osteitis. Lucent lesions in the cortex or spongiosa are accompanied by florid periosteal bone formation (Fig. 62–37). Saber shin deformities (as in syphilis), dactylitis, and nasal destruction may be encountered. Proliferative exostoses in the maxillary bones are termed goundou. Localized expansile lesions in the epiphyses of tubular bones may simulate neoplasms.[290] Destructive changes in the fingers and toes can lead to a doigts en lorgnette appearance, in which extensive shortening and telescoping of the digits are observed.[291] In these cases, the findings may resemble leprosy or psoriatic arthritis. In yaws, however, the distal phalanges are usually spared.[292] In children, similar destructive changes of the phalangeal diaphyses can lead to growth disturbances with short, deformed fingers.[293] Bowing of the long tubular bones of the extremities with concentric atrophy and extensive joint deformities with bony ankylosis have also been recorded.

The radiographic changes in the skeleton in patients with yaws are similar to those of syphilis. A correct diagnosis is established by the isolation of *T. pertenue* from skin lesions. Both yaws and syphilis produce a positive Wassermann reaction.

Bejel. This infectious disease caused by a spirochete indistinguishable from *Treponema pallidum* is prevalent in the Middle East. Its manifestations include skin ulcerations on the lips and mouth, osteitis, and periostitis. Destruction of facial bones, including the nose, may be detected.

Miscellaneous Organisms

Tropical Ulcer. Tropical ulcers are seen in patients of all ages from Central and East Africa.[294] The initial lesions are painful and tense swellings with a serosanguineous discharge, which appear on the anterolateral aspect of the distal portions of the lower limbs and spread rapidly.[295] As the ulcer erodes muscles and tendons, it may reach the underlying bone. The favorite target area is the middle third of the tibia; fibular involvement is less frequent and, when present, is most common in the distal third of the shaft. Periostitis leads to broad-based excrescences resembling osteomas (Fig. 62–38).[295, 296] Cortical sequestra can appear, which are extruded from the body via the skin ulceration. In the medullary canal, osteoporosis[294] and bulbous expansion[295] of neighboring bone can be evident. In chronic cases, deformities appear, which consist of elongation and bowing of the osseous structures. Flexion deformities of the knee and talipes equinovarus and calcaneovalgus deformities of the foot are typical.[295] Gas gangrene and tetanus may complicate long-standing cases.[294] In approximately 25 per cent of cases, malignant degeneration leading to epidermoid carcinomas of the involved skin can produce destruction of subjacent cortical and medullary tissue,[297] with pathologic fractures. This complication appears in patients with chronic skin ulcerations (greater than 10 years in duration) and most typically involves the tibia.

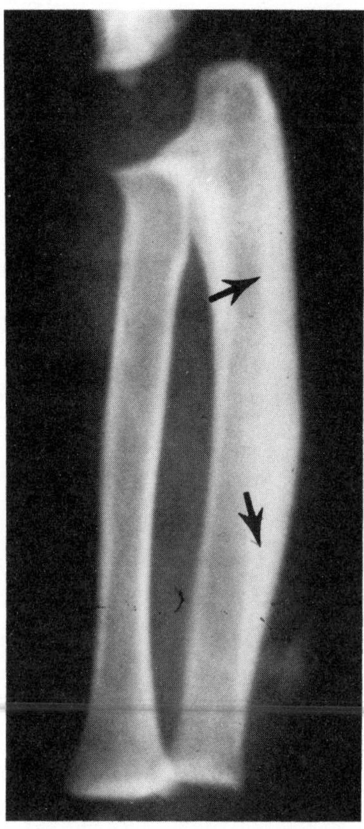

Figure 62–38. *Buruli ulcer. This is a type of chronic ulceration that may appear in the tropics. It is due to* Mycobacterium ulcerans *and can lead to exuberant periostitis (arrows). (Courtesy of Dr. W. Peter Cockshott, McMaster University, Hamilton, Ontario.)*

The etiology of tropical ulcer appears to be multifactorial. Trauma is common, and cultures of the lesion frequently isolate Vincent's types of fusiform bacilli and spirochetes.[298, 299] Staphylococcus is also frequently present.[295] An additional factor in the development of the ulcer may include malnutrition.[300]

Leptospirosis. Leptospira can produce a group of disorders that are characterized by fever, myalgia, and arthralgia.[301] Reports of arthritis are indeed rare.[302]

Rat Bite Fever. Following a bite from a rat or, less commonly, a mouse, squirrel, dog, or cat, a febrile illness can be observed that is associated with a rash and arthritis.[303] Additional clinical findings include erythema about the inoculation site and monoarticular pain, swelling, and tenderness. *Spirillum minor* or *Actinomyces muris* may be isolated on blood culture.

FUNGAL INFECTION

Actinomycosis

General Features. Actinomycosis is a noncontagious suppurative infection that is caused by anaerobic organisms that are normally found in the mouth. *Actinomyces israelii* and *Actinomyces bovis* appear to be the specific causative agents. Actinomycosis may develop in debilitated individuals or in devitalized tissues. The infections are especially frequent in the face and the neck, a fact that is probably explained by the prevalence of these organisms within the oral and nasal cavities. Pulmonary and gastrointestinal infections are also well known. From infective foci in the face, lung, or bowel, hematogenous dissemination of organisms can lead to contamination of subcutaneous tissues, liver, spleen, kidneys, brain, bones and joints.

Musculoskeletal Abnormalities. Most typically, the skeleton becomes contaminated from an adjacent infected soft tissue focus; less commonly, hematogenous seeding of osseous or articular tissues occurs. The mandible, the flat bones of the axial skeleton (pelvis, ribs, spine), and the major articulations of the appendicular skeleton are most commonly affected[107]: Mandibular and maxillary bone involvement may follow extraction of a tooth[304]; actinomycosis of the bones of the hands can

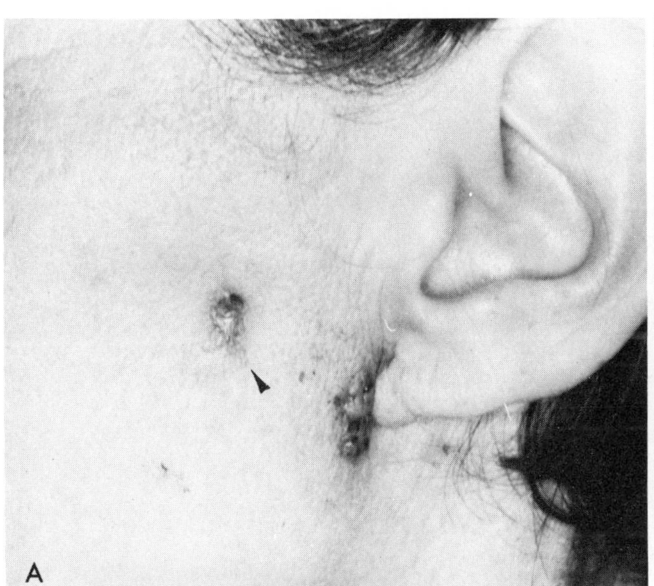

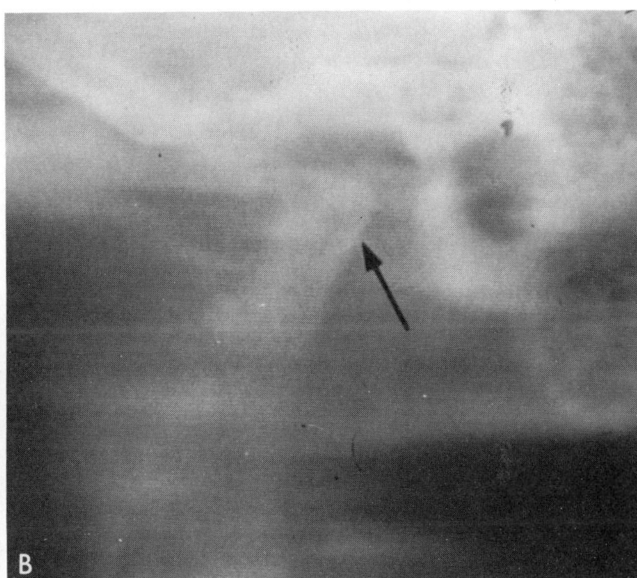

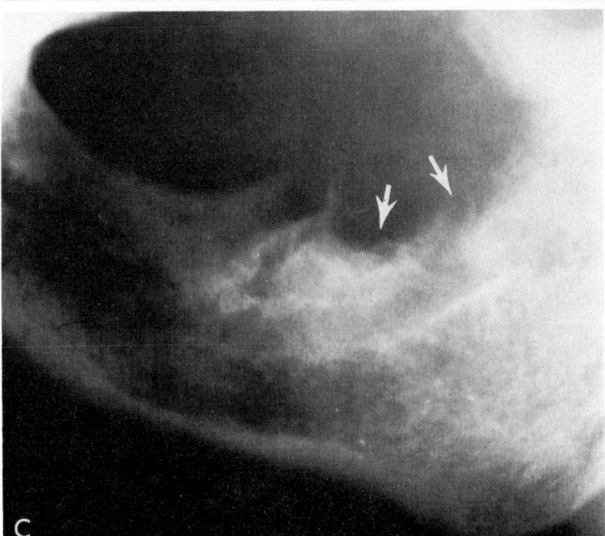

Figure 62–39. *Actinomycosis.*

A, B *A clinical photograph and radiograph of a patient with actinomycosis involving the mandible and temporomandibular joint reveal a fistulous tract (arrowhead) and erosion and sclerosis of the mandibular condyle (arrow). (Courtesy of Dr. R. Smith, University of California, San Francisco, California.)*

C *In another patient, actinomycosis has led to erosion and sclerosis of a segment of the mandible (arrows).*

Illustration continued on the following page

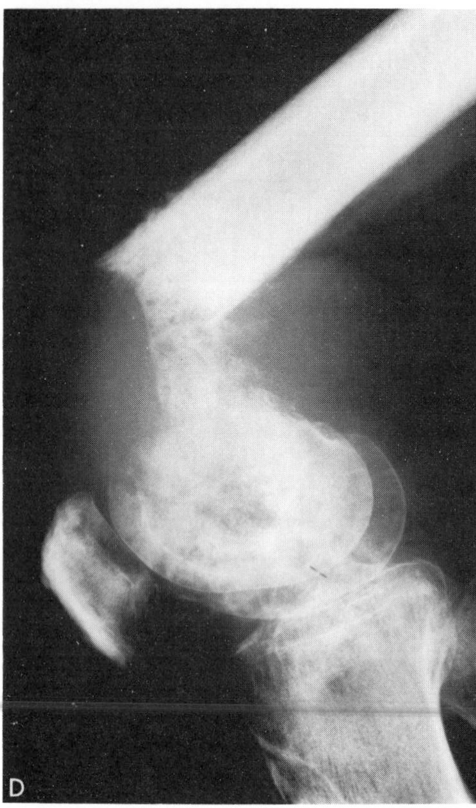

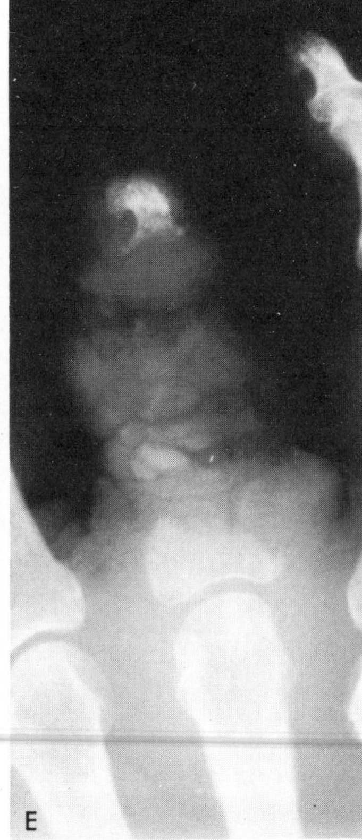

Figure 62–39. Continued

D *A neglected infection of the distal femur has resulted in a moth-eaten appearance of bone destruction, periostitis, soft tissue swelling, and a pathologic fracture.*

E *In this diabetic patient with gout and actinomycosis of the digit, observe dissolution of portions of the proximal and distal phalanges and of the entire middle phalanx. Note the accordion-like appearance of the skin due to telescoping of the digit. (Courtesy of Dr. R. Taketa, Bauer Hospital, Long Beach, California.)*

occur after a human bite[305]; solitary lesions of the tubular bones of the extremities, the ribs, the pelvis, and the spine may result either from extension of adjacent soft tissue foci or from hematogenous infection.[306-308]

Osseous involvement is characterized by a combination of lysis and sclerosis (Fig. 62–39). In the ribs, the degree of bony proliferation may be extensive, and the combination of severe osseous eburnation, cutaneous fistulae, and pleuritis is suggestive of actinomycosis. In the vertebral column, infection can originate from adjacent mediastinal or retroperitoneal foci. Several vertebrae are commonly affected, demonstrating lytic defects with surrounding sclerosis, and the intervening intervertebral discs may be spared.[309, 310] The posterior elements are often affected, including the spinous and transverse processes, laminae, and pedicles. Involvement of thoracic vertebrae is almost always associated with changes in the neighboring ribs.[311] Paravertebral abscesses may appear, but they are usually smaller than those in tuberculosis and do not calcify.[107] Additionally, collapse of the vertebrae and angulation of the spine are less frequent in actinomycosis than in tuberculosis.[1] In the mandible, a mixed lytic and sclerotic response predominates.[306]

Pathologic examination confirms the presence of a granulomatous infection with abscess formation from which actinomycotic organisms may be recovered.

Cryptococcosis (Torulosis)

General Features. This serious disease, which has a worldwide distribution, is caused by *Cryptococcus neoformans,* an organism that demonstrates unusual predilection for the central nervous system. This fungus can be recovered from the soil, pigeon droppings, fruit, and human intestinal tract and skin. Endogenous or exogenous sources may be important in the pathogenesis of this disease in humans. Once they reach the body and proliferate, cryptococci can be detected in the brain, the meninges, the lungs, other viscera, and the bones and joints. Neurologic manifestations of the disease predominate and include dizziness, ataxia, diplopia, headache, and convulsions. Many patients die within a few months.

The development of Cryptococcus infection in patients with compromised defense mechanisms is well known. Thus, the disease may be seen in association with leukemia, lymphoma, Hodgkin's disease, sarcoidosis, tuberculosis, and diabetes mellitus as well as in individuals receiving steroid medications.[312] It has been reported that the granulomatous reaction to Cryptococcus infection is similar to that of sarcoid lesions, and differentiation between the two disorders may be exceedingly difficult.[313]

Musculoskeletal Abnormalities. Osseous involvement is a manifestation of disseminated cryptococcosis, appearing in 5 to 10 per cent of such cases.[314] Occasionally, an injury may allow direct implantation of organisms into the bone. The most commonly involved skeletal sites are the spine, the pelvis, the ribs, the skull, the tibia, and the knees, in descending order of frequency.[315] Bony prominences may be affected, a peculiarity that is also evident in other fungal disorders, such as coccidioidomycosis. Single or multiple osseous foci are associated with soft tissue swelling and pain.

Radiographic features of bony involvement are not specific.[315-319] Osteolytic lesions predominate, with discrete margins, mild surrounding sclerosis, and little or no periosteal reaction (Fig. 62–40). Such findings can accompany other fungal disorders, tuberculosis, metastatic disease, and plasma cell myeloma, although the limited nature of the periostitis is more typical of cryptococcosis than of other fungal disorders.

Histologic evaluation of an osseous focus reveals granulomatous tissue containing multinucleated giant cells, histiocytes, and lymphocytes. There is a striking paucity of cellular reaction and an absence of suppuration and necrosis.[306] Cryptococcal organisms can be identified in the biopsy material.

Arthritis related to cryptococcosis is almost invariably the result of intra-articular extension of organisms from an adjacent osseous focus.[320, 321] Soft tissue swelling, effusion, and cartilaginous and bony destruction are observed in these cases. The knee is the most common site of involvement, although more than one articulation can be affected.[545] Microscopic evaluation of the synovial tissue reveals acute and chronic inflammation with granulomas and giant cells.

Rarely, extradural cryptococcal granulomas in the cervical, thoracic, or lumbar spine can lead to myelopathy or a cauda equina syndrome.[322-325] In these cases, initial radiographs may reveal osseous destruction of the spine and paravertebral swelling, and a myelogram can outline extrinsic compression of the spinal cord.

North American Blastomycosis

General Features. This fungal disease is produced by *Blastomyces dermatitidis*. In the United States, its incidence is highest in the Ohio and

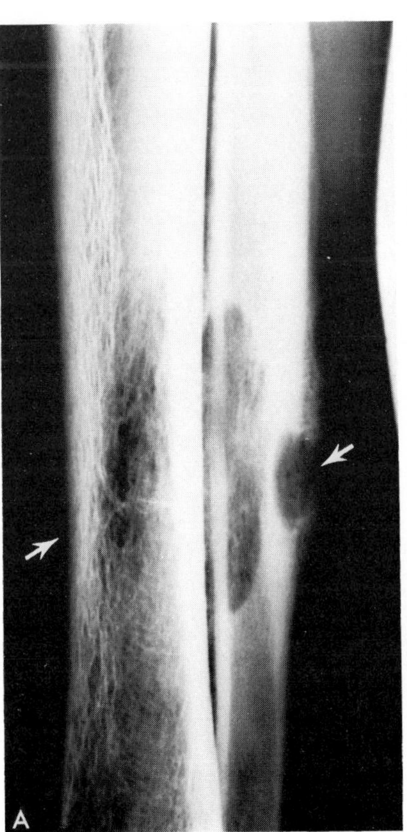

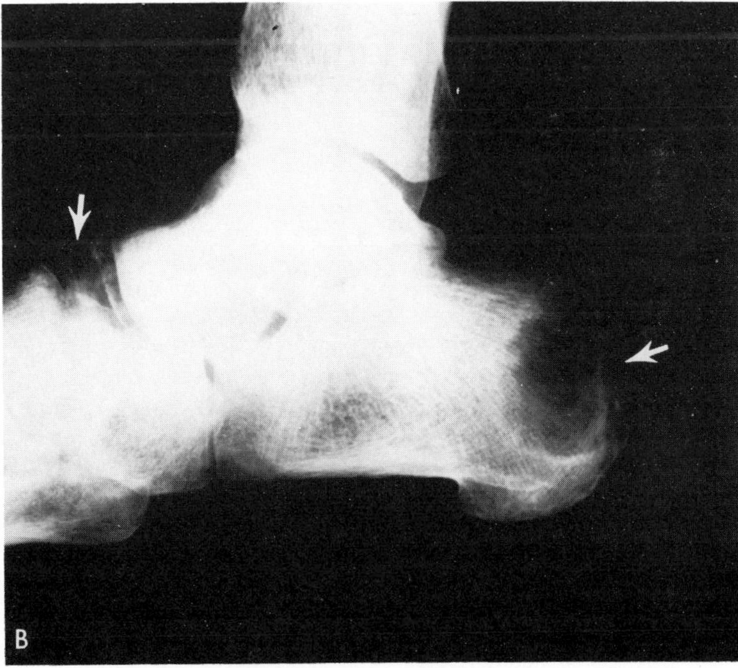

Figure 62–40. *Cryptococcosis (torulosis). Discrete osteolytic foci with surrounding sclerosis and, in some places, periosteal reaction are seen (arrows). This involvement of bony protuberances such as the calcaneus is not unexpected in this disease. The resulting appearance simulates that of other fungal diseases, especially coccidioidomycosis, as well as neoplastic disorders.*

Mississippi River valleys and in the Middle Atlantic states. The skin appears to be the portal of entry in most cases, infections commonly following cutaneous injuries. The respiratory tract may represent a second site of entry of organisms. In the skin, cutaneous abscesses develop beneath the epidermis and are surrounded by a granulomatous reaction. Similar lesions may be encountered in the lungs. Infection can subsequently spread to other viscera, lymph nodes, and bones. The disease can be noted in men and women of all ages; it predominates in individuals between the ages of 20 and 50 years.[1]

Musculoskeletal Abnormalities. The bones may be altered in as many as 50 per cent of patients with disseminated disease.[326] Skeletal changes can occur from hematogenous seeding or by direct extension from overlying cutaneous lesions. One or several osseous sites can be affected, especially the vertebrae, the ribs, the tibia, and the carpus and tarsus[1] (Fig. 62–41). No portion of the skeleton is immune.[107]

The radiologic features of blastomycotic osteomyelitis are not specific.[327-331] In the carpal and tarsal areas, cystic foci or diffuse, "moth-eaten" bony destruction can be seen, associated with osteoporosis and periostitis. In the tubular bones of the extremities, eccentric saucer-shaped erosions may be detected beneath cutaneous abscesses, or areas of focal or diffuse osteomyelitis in the subchondral regions of the epiphysis or the metaphysis can be encountered. The lesions frequently possess sclerotic margins and are surrounded by periostitis. Extension from the infected foci to soft tissues or articulations is not unusual. Draining sinuses and cortical sequestration may appear in neglected cases. In the spine, blastomycosis resembles tuberculosis[310]; a thoracolumbar predilection, anterior vertebral erosion with extension into adjacent ligamentous and soft tissue structures, osseous collapse, paraspinal masses, alteration of posterior elements, and intervertebral disc space destruction are common in both diseases. It has been noted that paravertebral abscesses of blastomycosis may erode the neighboring ribs, a finding that is unusual in tuberculosis.[329] In the flat bones such as the pelvis and sternum, extensive erosion can lead to disappearance of large osseous segments. Skull involvement consists of lysis and sclerosis.[330] Rarely, blastomycosis leads to dactylytis, producing cystic or diffuse osseous destruction, findings that are reminiscent of tuberculosis.[328]

Articular involvement is usually related to extension from an adjacent site of osteomyelitis. Rarely, however, joint destruction can occur in the absence of osseous disease.[332] In these cases,

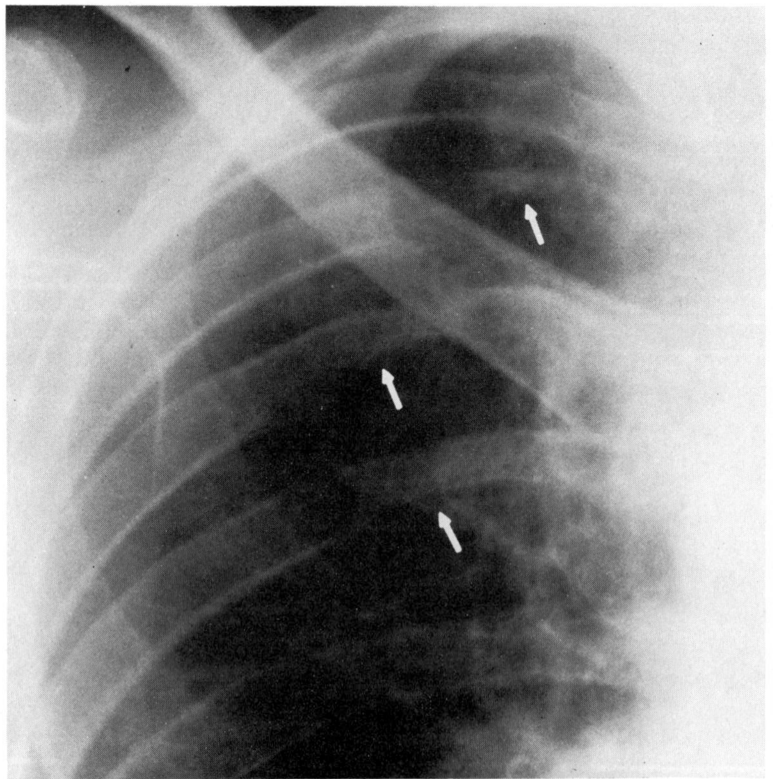

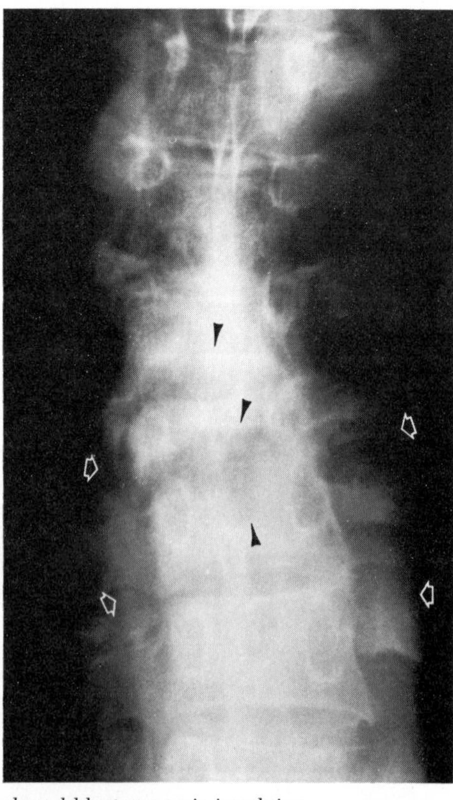

Figure 62–41. *North American blastomycosis. This patient developed blastomycosis involving lung and bone. Note osteolysis of the inferior aspects of multiple ribs (solid arrows) and vertebral body and intervertebral disc destruction (arrowheads) accompanied by a paravertebral mass (open arrows). (Courtesy of Dr. A. Brower, The Uniformed Services University for Health Sciences, Bethesda, Maryland.)*

monoarthritis predominates, especially in the knee or the ankle. Synovium, ligaments, and surrounding soft tissues are destroyed, subluxation is frequent, and the diagnosis is established by the recovery of typical organisms in the synovial fluid. Clinical or radiographic evidence of pulmonary disease aids in the correct evaluation of the joint disease.[546] Similarly, cutaneous abnormalities are also evident in most patients, creating an important "pulmonary-cutaneous-arthritic" triad.[546]

South American Blastomycosis

This fungal disorder, caused by the organism *Blastomyces brasiliensis*, occurs only in South America. The infective agents invade the pharynx and from there spread locally or are disseminated throughout the body. Nasopharyngeal ulceration and local lymphadenopathy may antedate clinical findings in other locations. Hematogenous spread of infection to the lungs, liver, spleen, other abdominal viscera, and bones can occur. In general, the features of musculoskeletal involvement are similar to those in North American blastomycosis.

Coccidioidomycosis

General Features. Coccidioidomycosis results from inhalation of the fungus *Coccidioides immitis* in endemic areas of the Southwestern portion of the United States, in Mexico, and in some regions of South America. The fungus, which is an inhabitant of soil, is disseminated in dust. Following inhalation, the organisms lodge in the terminal bronchioles and alveoli of the lungs where an inflammatory reaction may ensue. In some individuals, disseminated disease may develop with spread of infection to the liver, spleen, lymph nodes, skin, kidney, meninges, pericardium, and bones, as well as other sites. Men and women are affected equally, although the disseminated form is more common in men. Clinical manifestations vary in accordance with the distribution of the lesions, and in cases of wide dissemination, the mortality rate is quite high.

Musculoskeletal Abnormalities. Although an acute, self-limited arthritis ("desert rheumatism" with pain, swelling, and tenderness) may develop in approximately 33 per cent of cases of coccidioidomycosis,[333] only 10 to 20 per cent of patients develop granulomatous lesions in the bones and the joints. Osseous involvement can be confined to a single bone,[334] although many series note a high incidence of multiple, symmetrically distributed bony foci.[335] Involvement of the spine, the ribs, and the pelvis predominates, although any bone can be affected.[335-341] Symptoms and signs can be prominent, even in the initial phases of the disease, and consist of pain, swelling, and draining abscesses.

Radiographs frequently reveal multiple osseous lesions in the metaphyses of long tubular bones and in bony prominences (patella, tibial tuberosity, calcaneus, ulnar olecranon) (Fig. 62–42). In the bones of the hands and the feet, diaphyseal alterations are

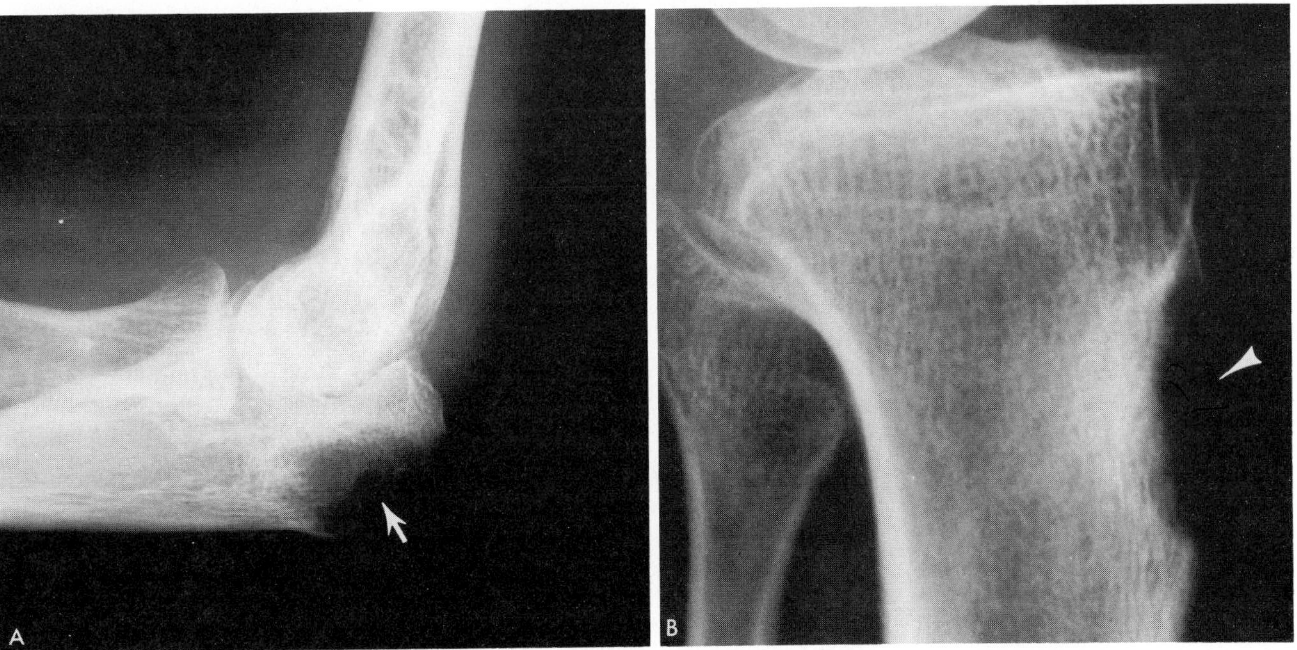

Figure 62–42. *Coccidioidomycosis: Osteomyelitis (appendicular skeleton).*
A, B *Involvement of bony protuberances such as the ulnar olecranon (arrow) and tibial tuberosity (arrowhead) is frequent. Discrete lesions with surrounding sclerosis are evident.*
Illustration continued on the following page

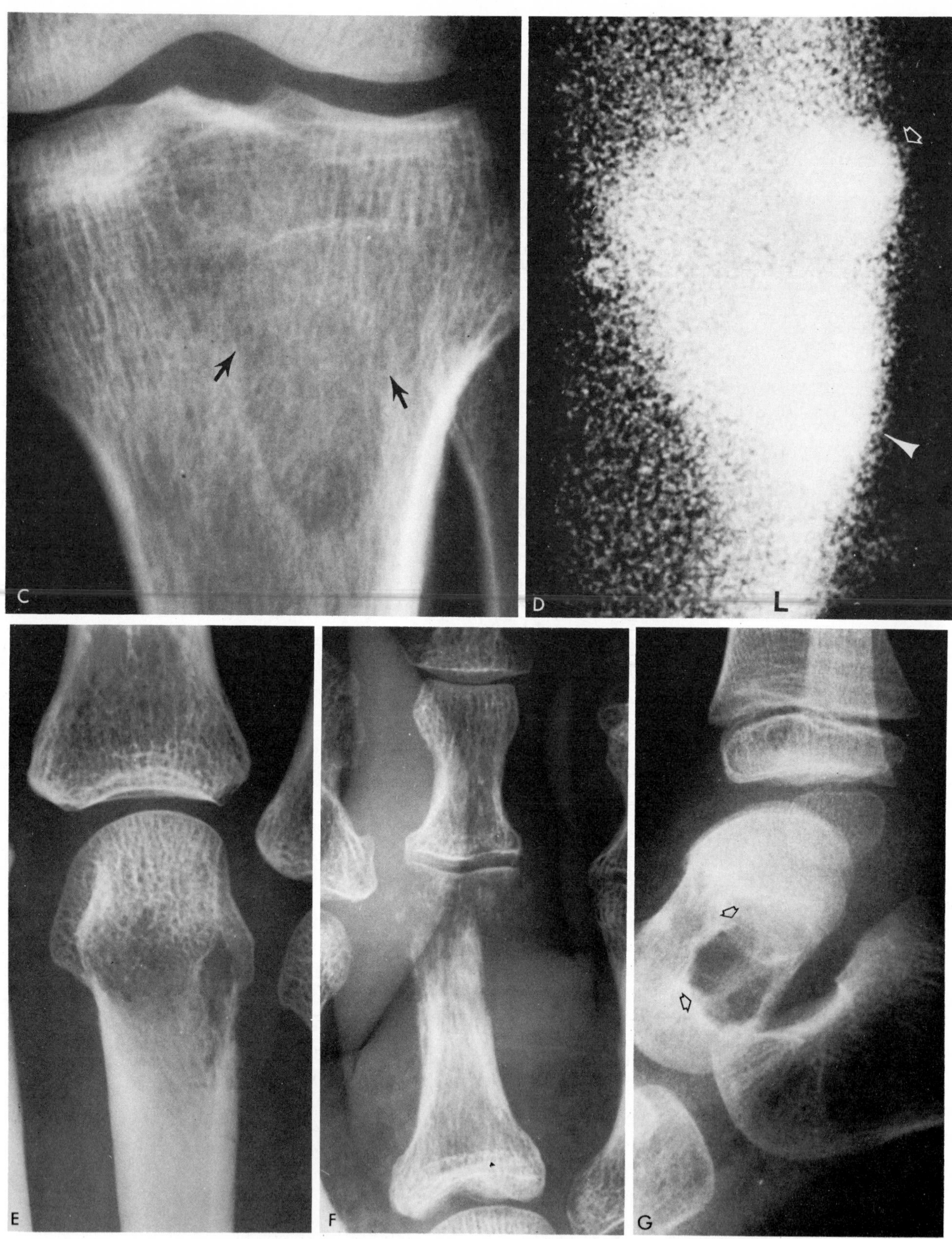

Figure 62–42. Continued

C, D *Note the osteolytic lesion of the proximal tibia (arrows), which is associated with increased accumulation of technetium pyrophosphate on radionuclide examination (arrowhead). The patella (open arrow) also reveals increased uptake of pharmaceutical agent, although an osseous lesion in this area was not evident.*

(**B–D,** From Armbuster TG, et al: J Nucl Med 18:450, 1977.)

E, F *In this patient, osteolytic foci of the metacarpal head and proximal phalanx of the toe reveal ill-defined or moth-eaten bone destruction and are associated with periostitis and soft tissue swelling. The joints appear normal, and a pathologic fracture through the phalangeal lesion is evident.*

G *In a child, a "cystic" lesion of the talus (arrows) is associated with considerable soft tissue swelling.*

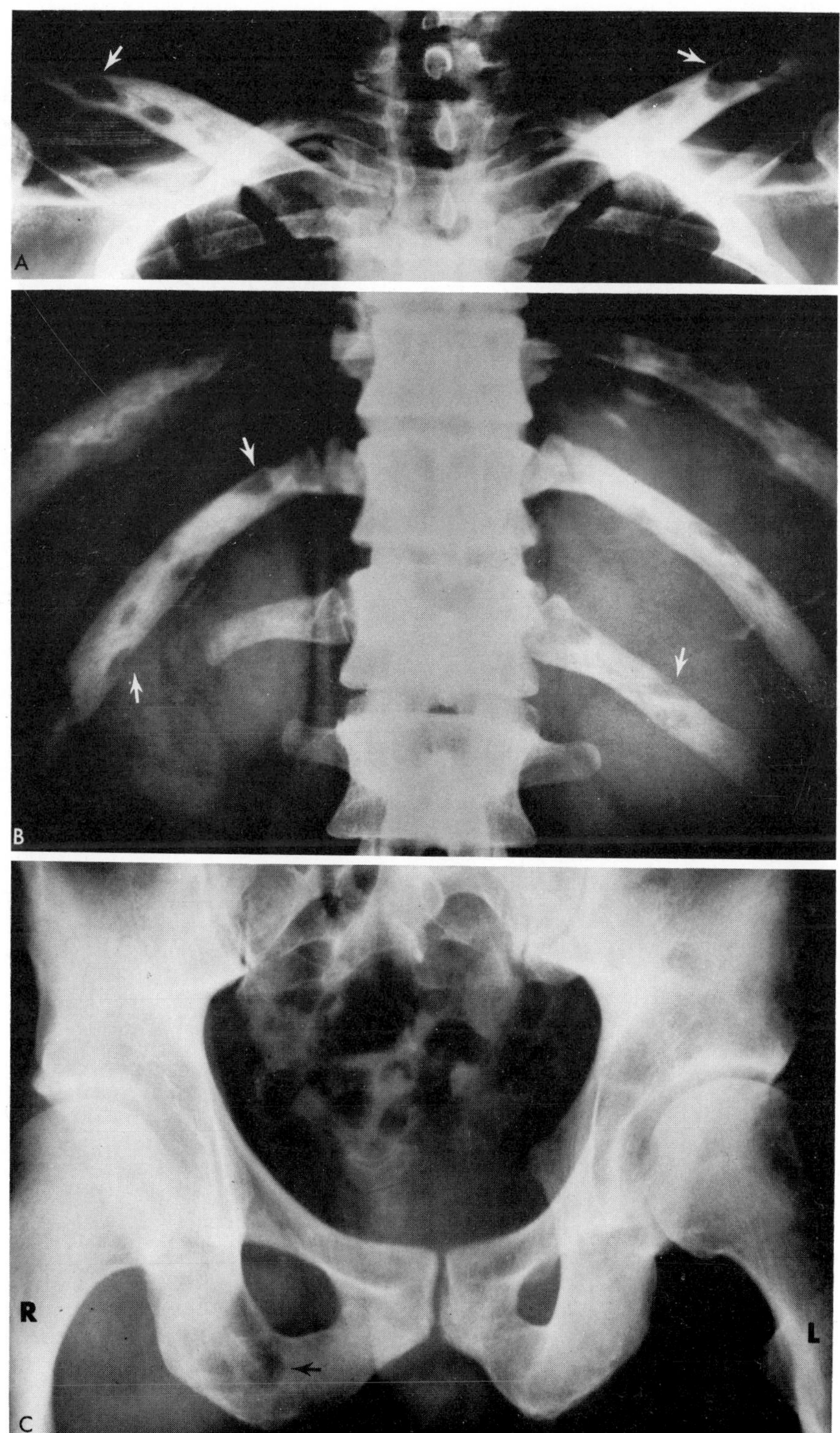

Figure 62–43. *Coccidioidomycosis: Osteomyelitis (axial skeleton). This 33 year old man presented with fever and pulmonary infiltrate. The diagnosis of disseminated coccidioidomycosis was established by skin biopsy, bone marrow and cerebral spinal fluid examination, and positive serologic test results.*

A–C *Radiography outlines lytic lesions with surrounding sclerosis involving ribs, clavicles, and pelvis (arrows).*

Illustration continued on the following page

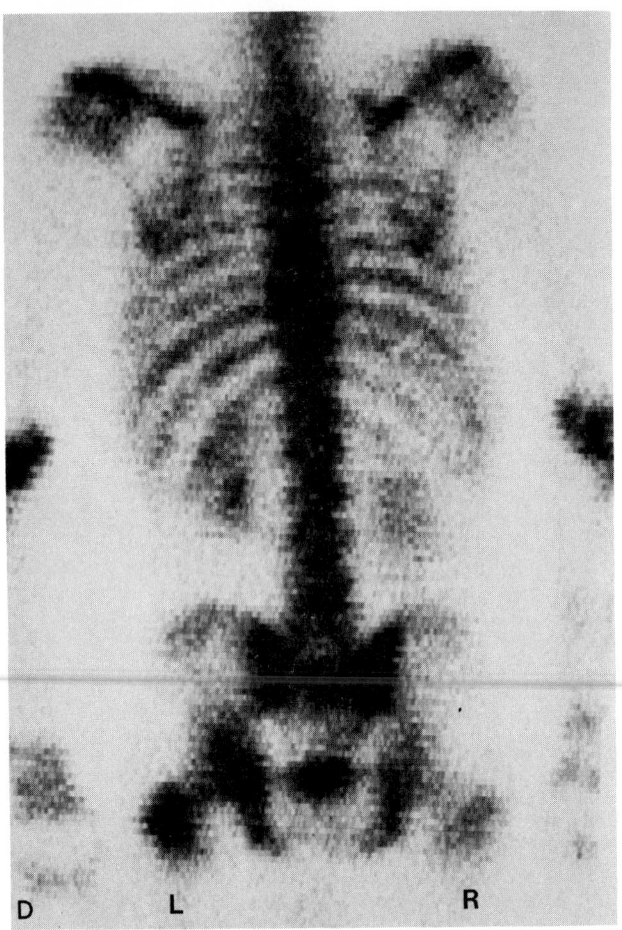

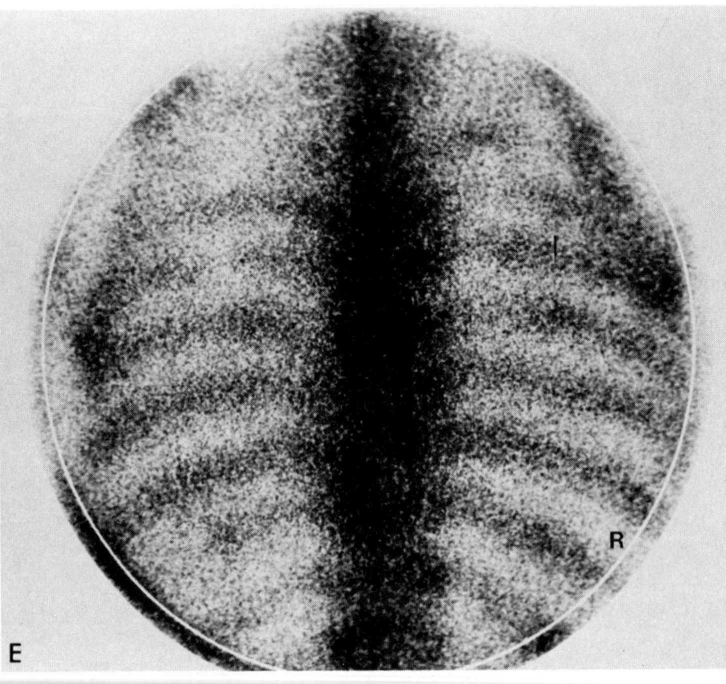

Figure 62–43. Continued
D, E *Bone scan with technetium pyrophosphate reveals several areas of increased activity, although the findings are less striking than on corresponding radiographs. On close inspection, a mottled appearance of the ribs due to diffuse osseous involvement can be seen.*
(From Armbuster, TG, et al: J Nucl Med 18:450, 1977.)

also common. Well demarcated lytic foci of the spongiosa are typical. Periostitis can be seen, but bony sclerosis and sequestration are unusual. Lesions involving the ribs are typically marginal in location and can be associated with prominent extrapleural masses[335] (Fig. 62–43). In the spine, abnormalities of one or more vertebral bodies with paraspinal masses and contiguous rib changes are typical (Fig. 62–44). There is relative sparing of the intervertebral discs, and vertebral collapse and fistulous tracts are uncommon and late manifestations. Rarely, significant vertebral sclerosis in coccidioidomycosis may simulate the changes that accompany neoplasm (metastatic disease from prostate carcinoma).[338, 547]

Joint involvement is most common in the ankle and the knee (Figs. 62–45 and 62–46), although other articulations of the appendicular and axial skeleton may be the site of an infective arthritis[342-346, 548] (Fig. 62–47). In general, articular changes result from extension of an osteomyelitic focus, although, rarely, direct hematogenous implantation of the organisms into a joint can occur. Monoarticular involvement is most typical. Synovial inflammation and cartilaginous and osseous erosion lead to radiographic findings (osteoporosis, effusion, joint space narrowing, bony destruction) similar to those in other granulomatous articular infections. In other cases, a sterile migratory polyarthritis without radiographic changes may be representative of a hypersensitivity syndrome.[548]

Coccidioidal bursitis and tenosynovitis of the hand and wrist have been reported.[347-349]

Biopsy of skeletal or articular foci in this disease reveals granulomatous lesions similar to those of tuberculosis[1]; monocytes, giant and epithelial cells, necrosis, and caseation are identified[306] (Fig. 62–48). Accurate differentiation of coccidioidomycosis and tuberculosis requires isolation of the causative agent.

Histoplasmosis

GENERAL FEATURES. Histoplasmosis is caused by the dimorphic fungus *Histoplasma capsulatum*, which is present in many areas of the United States. A similar organism, *Histoplasma capsulatum* var. *duboisii*, can also lead to disease, especially in Africa. The disorder results from exposure to soil containing the spores of this fungus. The portal of entry is usually the respiratory tract, although the gastrointestinal system may be an additional portal in some individuals. Diffuse disease can result, and the fungus proliferates most extensively in cells of

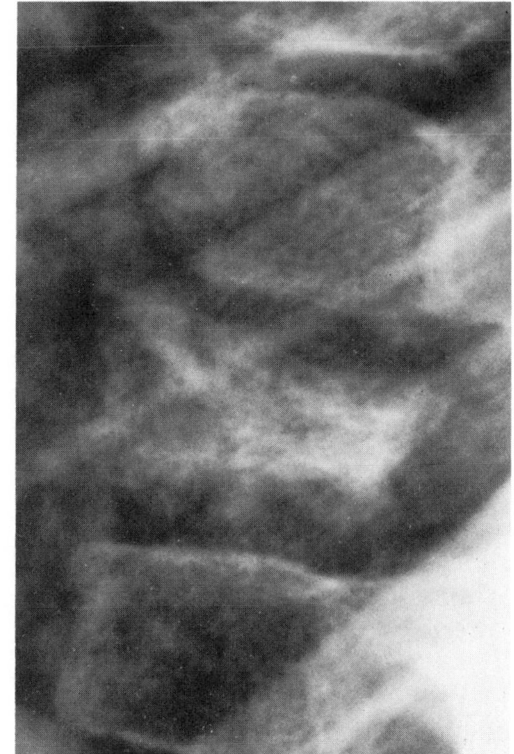

Figure 62–44. Coccidioidomycosis: Spondylitis. In this child, partial collapse of a thoracic vertebral body is accompanied by sclerosis but is unassociated with intervertebral disc space narrowing. Adjacent vertebral bodies were also abnormal.

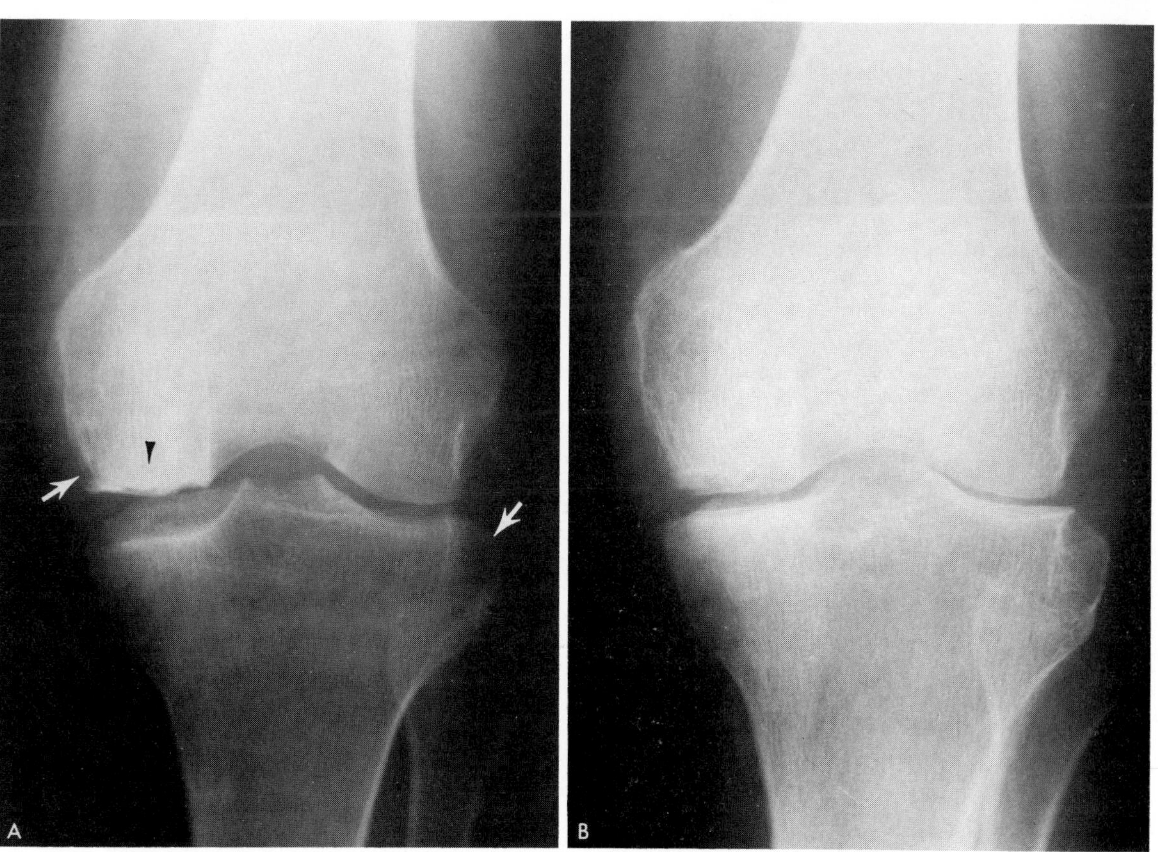

Figure 62–45. Coccidioidomycosis: Septic arthritis. This 49 year old man developed disseminated coccidioidomycosis with involvement of the right knee. Synovial biopsy and culture confirmed septic arthritis due to the fungus.

A *An initial film reveals soft tissue swelling, marginal osseous erosions (arrows), and flattening with sclerosis of the medial femoral condyle (arrowhead). The latter findings resemble those in spontaneous aseptic necrosis of the knee.*

B *One month later, further loss of joint space is evident.*

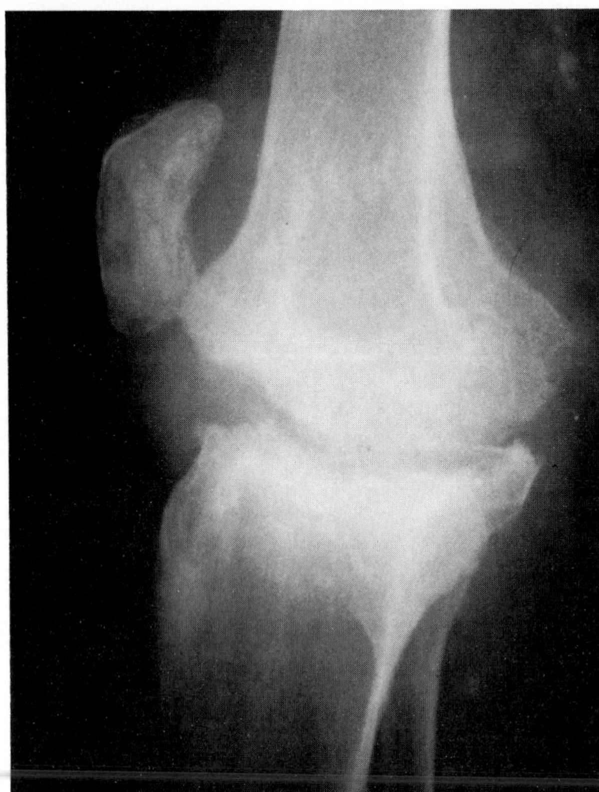

Figure 62–46. Coccidioidomycosis: Septic arthritis. *In a different patient, more extensive articular destruction of the knee is apparent. Note the degree of reactive sclerosis and the large joint effusion.*

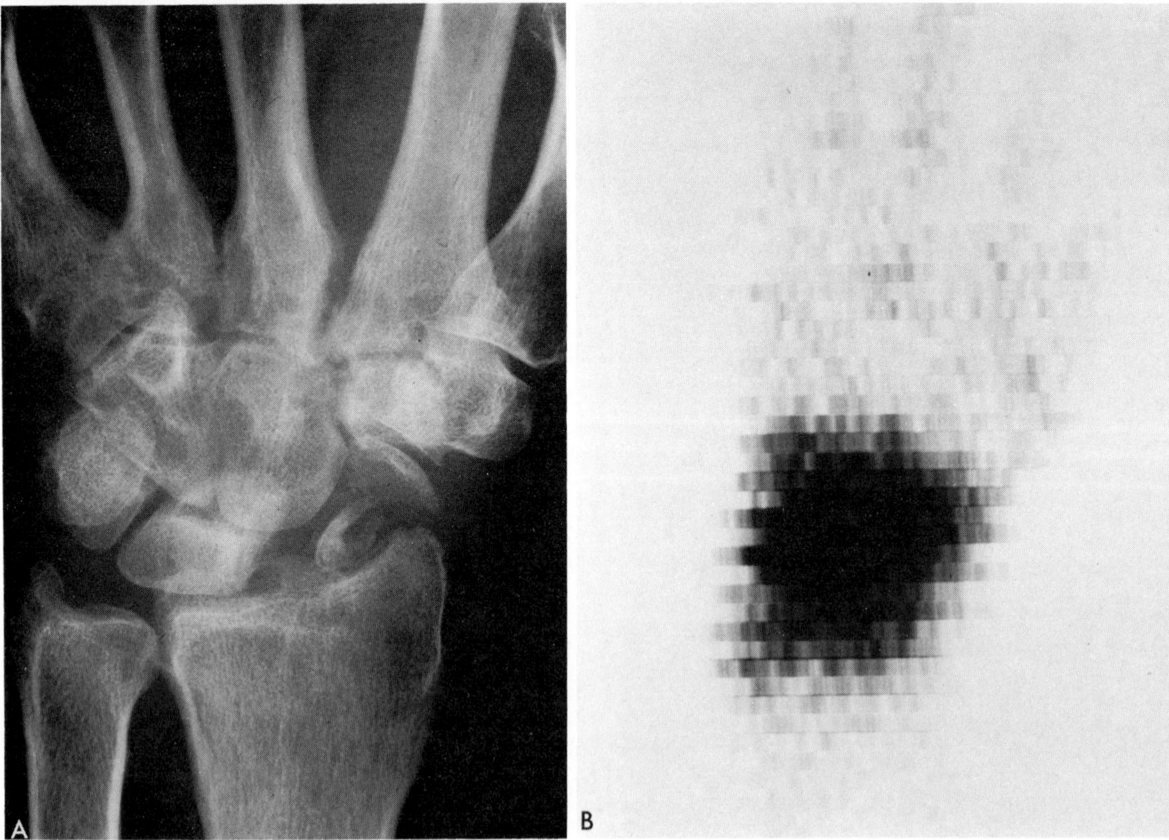

Figure 62–47. Coccidioidomycosis: Septic arthritis. *This 41 year old man presented with arthritis of the right wrist and left fifth metatarsophalangeal joint. Subsequent right wrist synovectomy and resection of the left fifth metatarsal head revealed spherules of* Coccidioides immitis.

A *The radiograph delineates destructive changes of the scaphoid, ulna, and other carpal and metacarpal bones. Narrowing of the radiocarpal, midcarpal, and common carpometacarpal articulations is evident.*

B *A radionuclide examination with technetium pyrophosphate delineates increased tracer uptake in the wrist.*

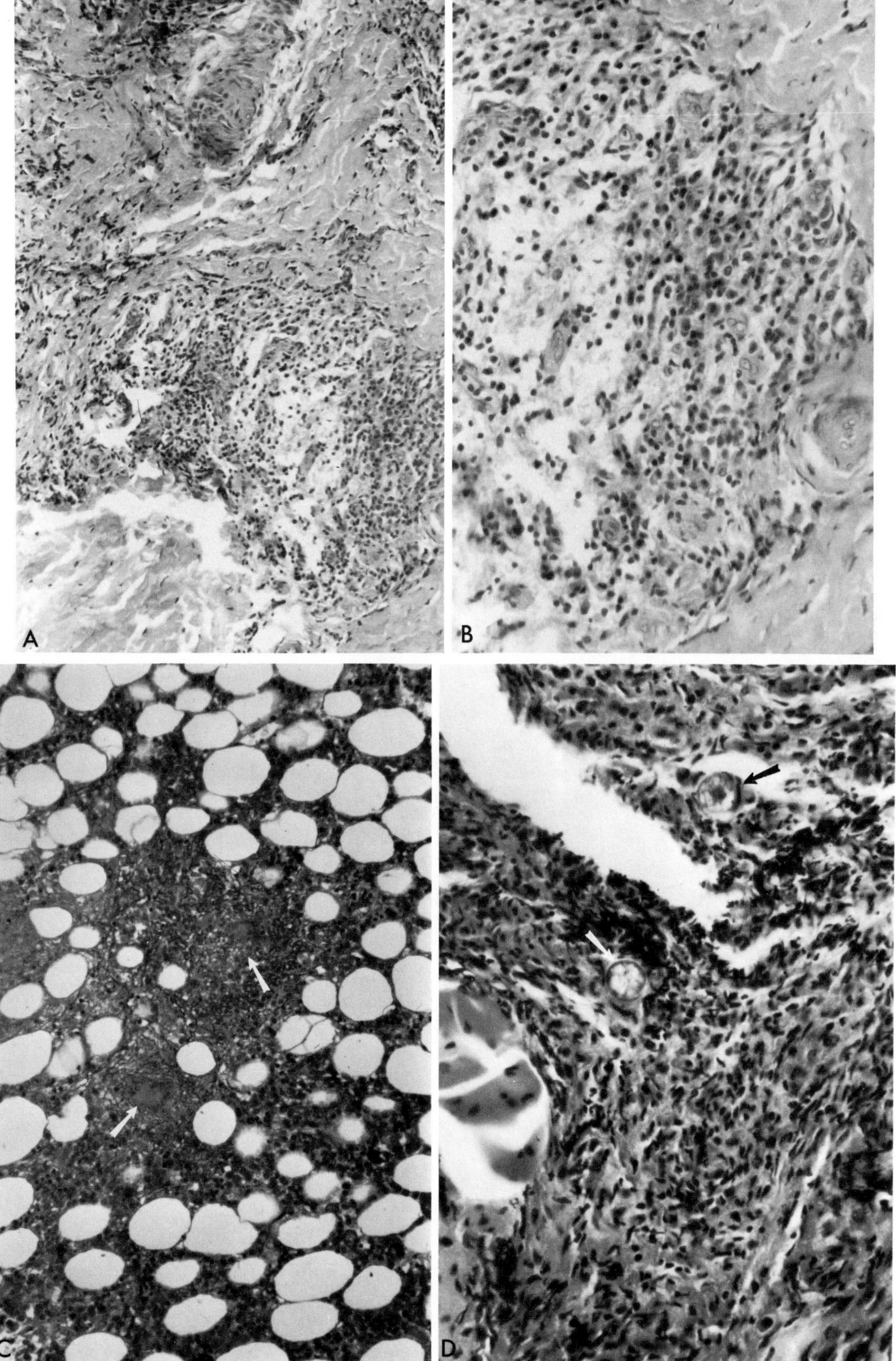

Figure 62–48. *Coccidioidomycosis: Pathologic abnormalities.*

A, B *Photomicrographs (200×, 400×) of involved parasynovial tissue show diffuse infiltration with inflammatory cells (lymphoid and plasmacytoid cells). Although microorganisms are not identified in these areas, they were apparent at other locations.*

C *Photomicrograph of bone marrow shows a granulomatous inflammatory lesion with multinuclear giant cells (arrows).*

D *In the marrow, observe coccidioidal granulomas (arrows) among acute inflammatory cells, cellular debris, and epithelioid cells.*

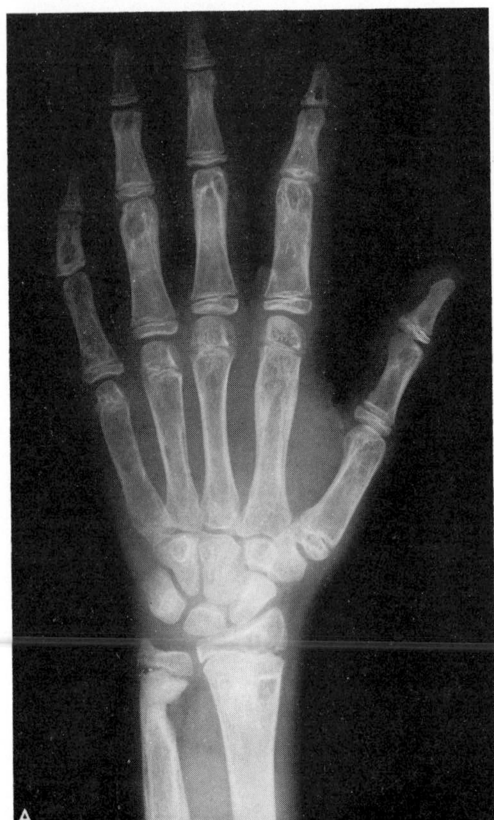

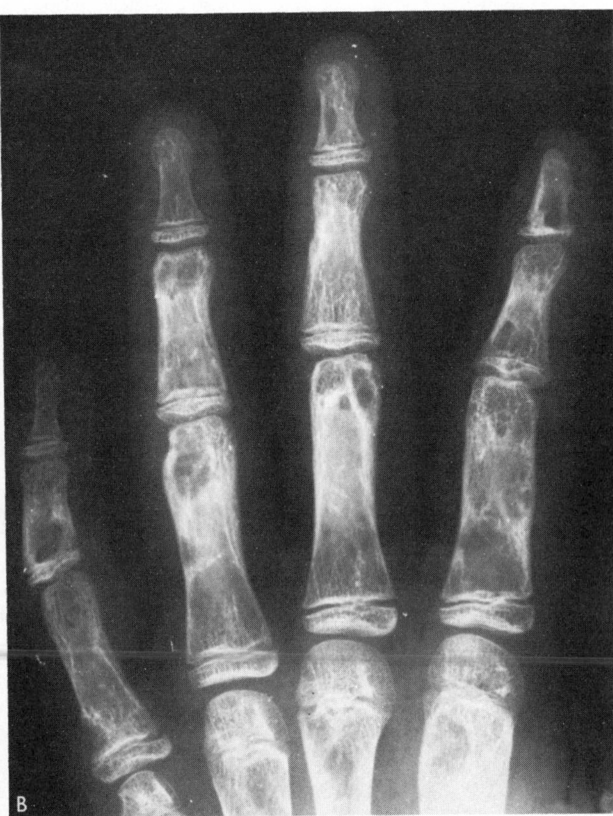

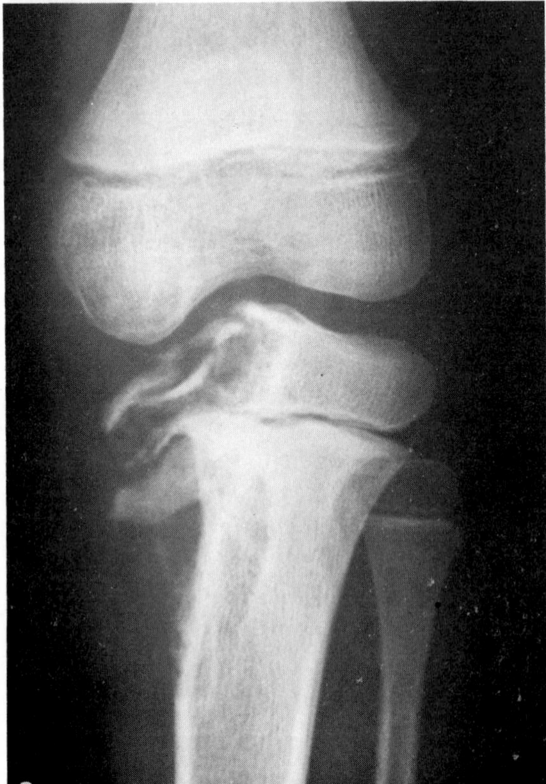

Figure 62–49. Histoplasma capsulatum var. duboisii osteomyelitis.

A, B *Radiographs of the left hand reveal cystic lesions of the radius, ulna, metacarpals, and phalanges. In many areas, they are well marginated and surrounded by reactive bone formation and mature periostitis.*

C *Extensive lesions of the tibial epiphysis and metaphysis have produced collapse of the articular surface, with sclerosis and mild periostitis. The extension across the growth cartilage is not unusual in fungal infections.*

Illustration continued on the opposite page

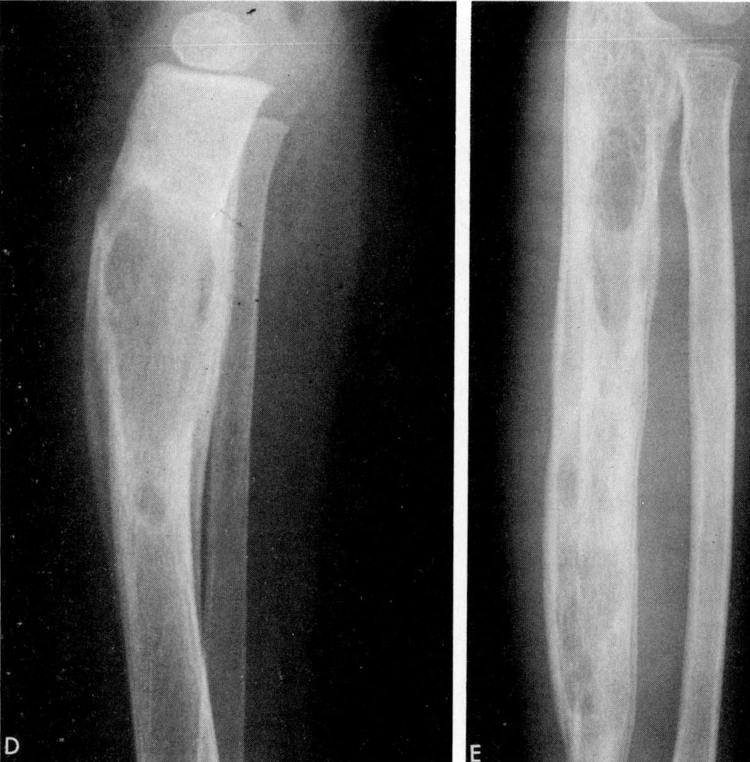

Figure 62–49. Continued

D, E *Diaphyseal involvement of the tibia and ulna is characterized by lytic lesions and exuberant periostitis.*

(**B,** *From Cockshott WP, Lucas AO: Q J Med 33:223, 1964.*)

the reticuloendothelial system. Involvement of the brain, lymph nodes, spleen, adrenal gland, lung, bowel, and bone marrow is most typical.

MUSCULOSKELETAL ABNORMALITIES. Skeletal involvement may occur in association with *H. capsulatum* or, more frequently, *H. duboisii*, infection. In histoplasmosis due to *H. capsulatum*, the pelvis, the skull, the ribs, and the small tubular bones are most typically affected[350]; children may be more commonly involved than adults.[350-353] In this variety of histoplasmosis, joint alterations have also been noted, leading to clinical (pain, swelling), radiologic (osteoporosis, joint space narrowing, erosion), and pathologic (granulation tissue with phagocytic cells) findings similar to those of tuberculosis.[353, 354, 549] In histoplasmosis due to *H. duboisii*, granulomatous ulcerating and papular lesions of the skin can be associated with osseous and articular changes in as many as 80 per cent of patients.[355] Multiple bony foci predominate in the flat bones (skull, rib, pelvis, sternum), although the spine and tubular bones can also be affected (Fig. 62–49). Cystic lytic areas are most typical.

Sporotrichosis

GENERAL FEATURES. This chronic fungal disease is caused by *Sporothrix schenckii* and is characterized by suppurating nodular lesions of the skin and the subcutaneous tissues.[356] The fungus resides as a saphrophyte on vegetation and can invade the human body through a wound of the skin; the disease is not uncommon following cutaneous puncture with thorns and is a recognized occupational hazard of florists and farmers. Human disease has also resulted from animal contact, apparently following bites of rats, mice, gophers, and parrots.[306] Following inoculation, the organisms spread locally, producing nodular lesions of the lymphatic channels. Rarely, disseminated disease can evolve, perhaps by a gastrointestinal or respiratory portal of entry. In the disseminated form of sporotrichosis, bone and joint changes may appear in 80 per cent of cases, and death can occur rapidly.

MUSCULOSKELETAL ABNORMALITIES. Osseous and articular involvement can occur from hematogenous dissemination of infection or from extension of a contaminated cutaneous or subcutaneous focus.[357-364] Localization in one or more joints is especially characteristic, with predilection for the knee, the wrist and hand, the ankle, the elbow, and the metacarpophalangeal joints. Soft tissue swelling, effusion, joint space loss, and irregularity, poor definition, and destruction of subchondral bony margins are seen (Fig. 62–50). Osteophytes may or may not be evident. Synovial biopsy reveals granulomatous inflammation, and synovial fluid or synovial tissue culture can outline the characteristic organisms.[363] Tendon and tendon sheath involvement and fistulization have been recorded.[365, 366, 566]

Bone changes may take several forms. Eccentric erosions beneath subcutaneous lesions (especially in

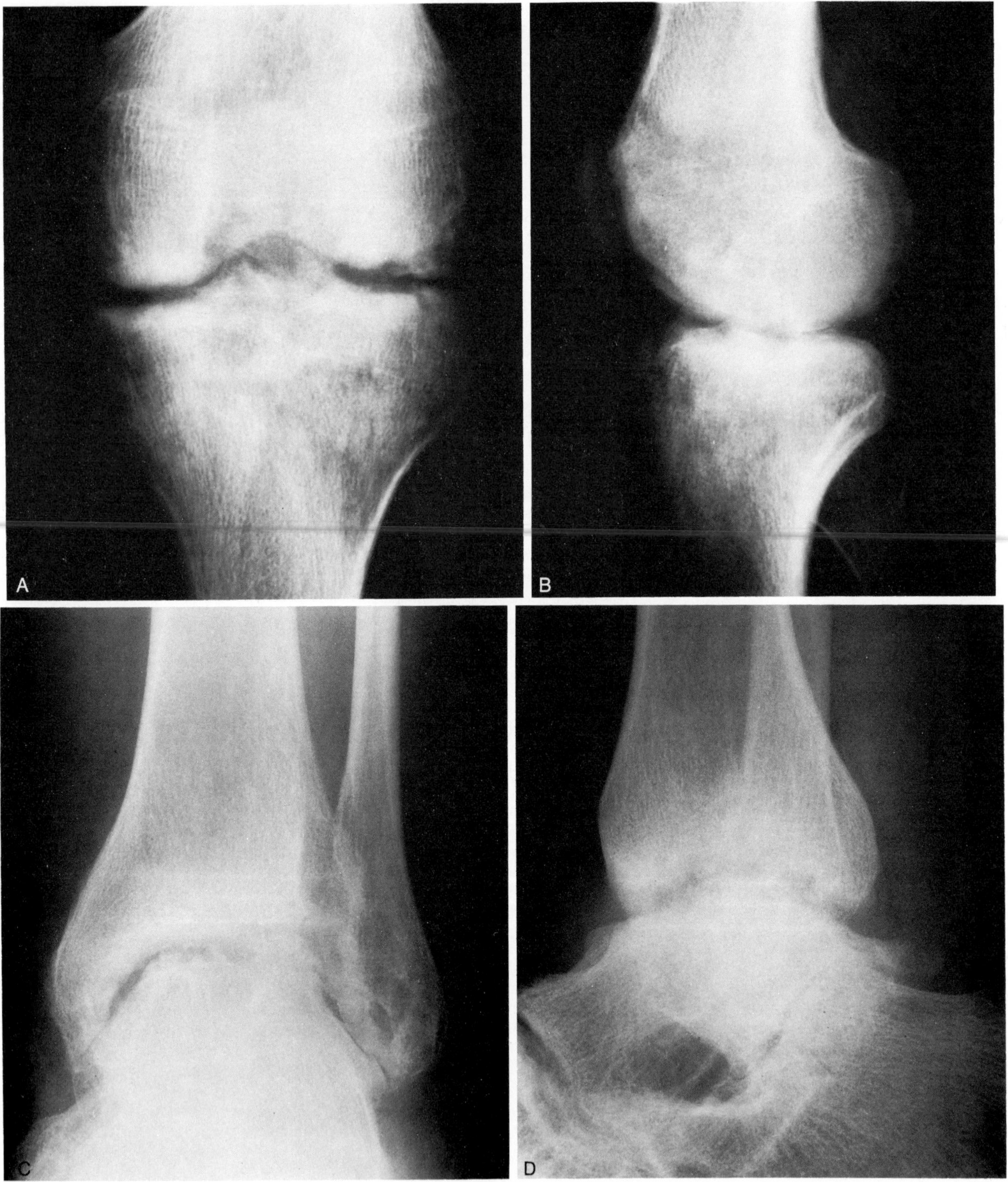

Figure 62–50. *Sporotrichosis: Septic arthritis.* ***A–F,*** *Examples of knee, ankle, and elbow involvement. The findings in each case are similar, consisting of soft tissue swelling, joint space loss, and irregularity and poor definition of subchondral bone, with marginal and central osseous erosions. The changes are identical to those in other forms of septic arthritis. Joint involvement is not infrequent in this disorder, and osteoporosis may or may not be present. Note the involvement of the posterior subtalar joint in conjunction with ankle disease, reflecting the communication of these two articulations. (Courtesy of Dr. A. Brower, The Uniformed Services University for Health Sciences, Bethesda, Maryland).*

Illustration continued on the opposite page

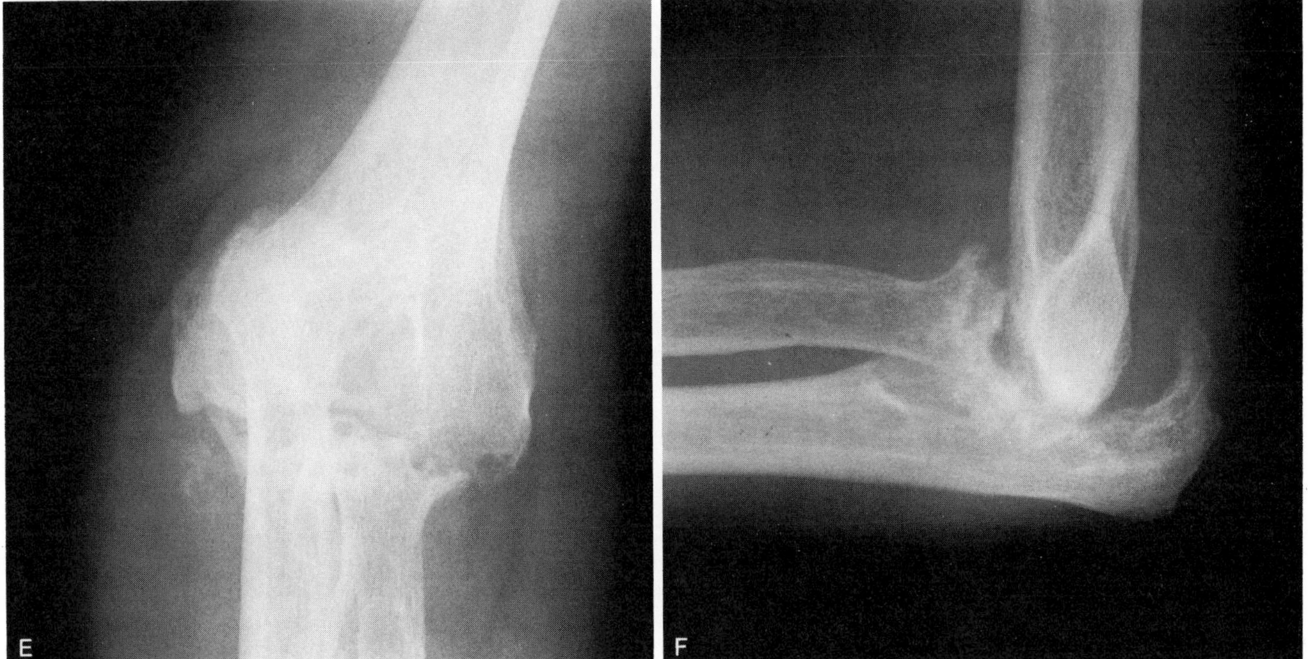

Figure 62–50. Continued

the tibia) can be encountered but are more typical of blastomycosis. Conversely, single or multiple lytic areas in bone can appear, related to hematogenous spread directly to osseous tissue or to synovium with extension into the neighboring bone.

The radiographic features of osseous and articular involvement in sporotrichosis simulate those of tuberculosis, other fungal disorders, or pigmented villonodular synovitis. Although osteoporosis may not be apparent in some individuals, perhaps allowing differentiation from tuberculosis, this is not a constant characteristic, limiting its usefulness as a diagnostic sign. Involvement of the small joints of the hands and feet appears to be more characteristic of this fungal disease than of the others.[360] Similarly, direct spread to joints without involvement of bone is more typical of sporotrichosis. Appropriate culture with isolation of *S. schenckii* allows precise diagnosis.

Candidiasis (Moniliasis)

General Features. Moniliasis is an infection caused by *Candida albicans.* This organism resides normally on the mucous membranes. In debilitated children or adults, a mucocutaneous infection consisting of white patches with subjacent inflammation appears on the buccal mucosa. Rarely, a widespread infection can follow, leading to pneumonia and hematogenous contamination of multiple viscera, including the kidney, brain, thyroid, adrenal glands, pancreas, liver, myocardium, and endocardium.

Musculoskeletal Abnormalities. Candida infection of the musculoskeletal system occurs when the host resistance is depressed, perhaps related to prolonged corticosteroid, immunosuppressive, or antibiotic therapy. Drug addicts are not uncommonly affected. In the newborn, candidiasis may be associated with prematurity, respiratory distress syndrome, parenteral feeding, and umbilical catheterization.[552] Parenteral hyperalimentation fluids with their high concentration of glucose may predispose to Candida infection. Osteomyelitis or septic arthritis can occur with this organism.

Bone involvement in cases of disseminated candidiasis is relatively rare, being evident in fewer than 1 to 2 per cent of such cases.[367, 368] When present, such osseous involvement can result from direct hematogenous seeding of the bone, hematogenous involvement of a joint with spread to the periarticular bone, or extension from an overlying soft tissue abscess.[368-371] Although *Candida albicans* is frequently implicated, other organisms, such as *Candida guilliermondi,*[372] *Candida tropicalis,*[373] *Candida parapsilosis,*[551] *Candida krusei,* and *Candida stellatoidea*[53] may be responsible for the infection. Infants, children, or adults can be affected. Osteomyelitis in any age group can occur in one or more sites, including the tubular bones of the extremities, flat bones such as the pelvis, sternum, and scapula, the ribs, and the spine.[550]

Septic arthritis is also observed in candidiasis.[373-380] Patients of all ages are affected, from the neonate to the elderly individual. As in the case of Candida osteomyelitis, debilitation and underlying disorders (carcinoma, leukemia, rheumatoid arthritis, systemic lupus erythematosus, renal failure) are frequent in Candida arthritis. Clinical findings include fever, soft tissue swelling, pain, tenderness, and restricted motion. Monoarticular disease is slightly more frequent than polyarticular disease. Typically, infection predominates in large weight-bearing articulations; the knee is the most common site of involvement. The pathogenesis of articular infection can relate to hematogenous contamination of the synovium or extension from an adjacent infected osseous or soft tissue structure. Osteomyelitis is evident in 70 to 85 per cent of patients with Candida arthritis. The frequency of spread of organisms from joint to adjacent bone has been confirmed in experimental *C. albicans* arthritis[381] and differs from the situation in some other fungal diseases, such as coccidioidomycosis in which osteomyelitis usually precedes arthritis.[335] *Candida albicans* is the most typical implicated organism (approximately 80 per cent) in cases of Candida arthritis. Radiographic findings include soft tissue swelling, joint space narrowing, irregularity of subchondral bone, and more widespread changes of osteomyelitis (Fig. 62–51). In patients undergoing surgery, a thickened synovial membrane with nonspecific mononuclear cellular infiltration can be observed. Granulomas are not usually apparent. The diagnosis is confirmed by aspiration of synovial fluid or biopsy of synovial membrane with isolation of Candida.

Mucormycosis

Mucormycosis is a rare, serious, and commonly fatal infection due to several types of fungus (Rhizopus, Mucor) in the class Phycomycetes. It appears in

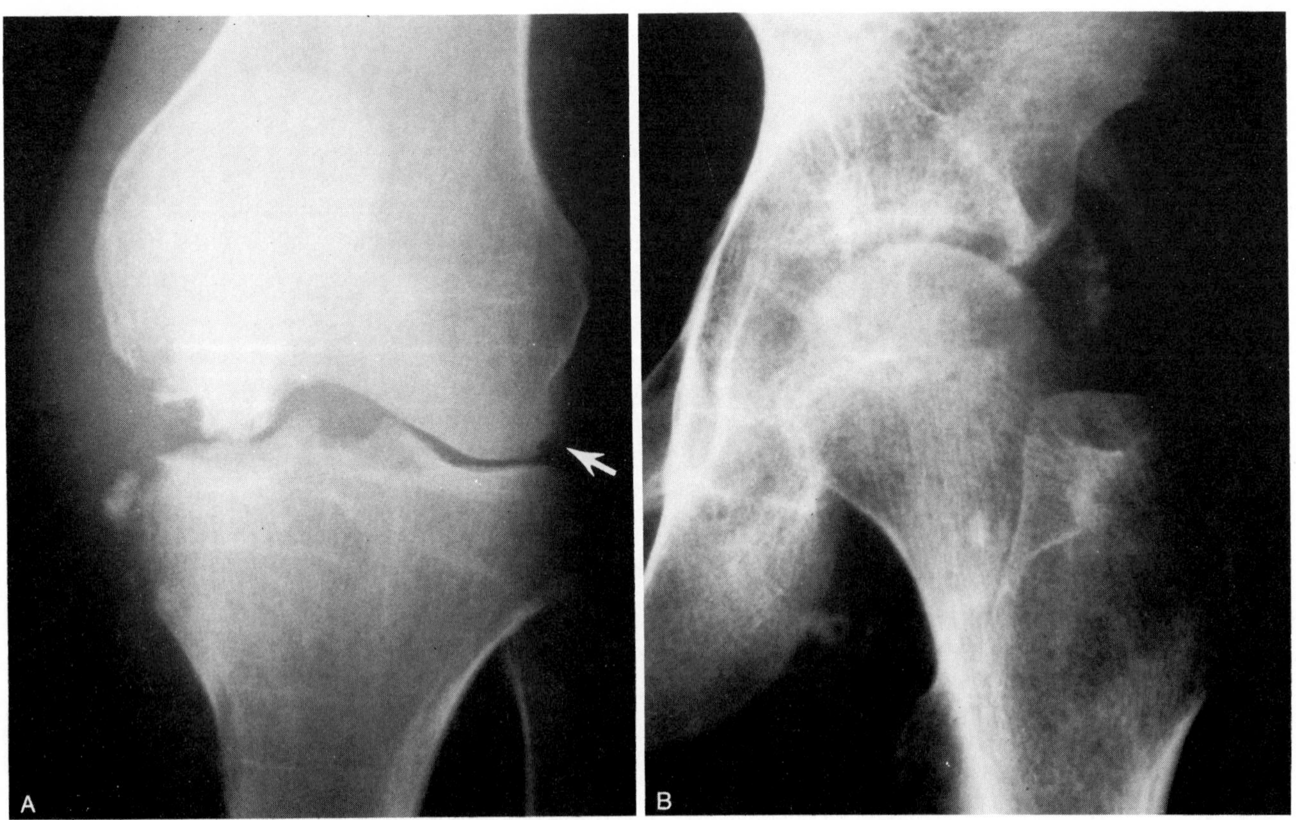

Figure 62–51. *Candidiasis: Septic arthritis.*

A *Observe massive soft tissue swelling, marginal osseous erosions (arrow), bony collapse and fragmentation, and joint space narrowing.*

B *In a different patient, loss of joint space and osteoporosis are seen. Para-articular ossification is also noted.*

association with debilitating illnesses, particularly diabetes mellitus, uremia with acidosis, lymphoma or leukemia, and extensive burns, as well as following massive corticosteroid therapy. The usual portal of entry of the fungus appears to be the paranasal sinuses, from which site infection can extend along the invaded vessels to reach the retroorbital tissues and cerebrum. In the brain, arterial and venous thrombosis leads to multiple infarcts, and hematogenous spread of mucormycosis produces infective foci, especially in the lungs and intestines. These latter sites can also be contaminated following inhalation or ingestion of fungus. The clinical varieties of mucormycosis are frequently termed rhinocerebral, pulmonary, alimentary, or disseminated.[567]

Osseous abnormalities are generally confined to the skull and the face (Fig. 62–52). Sinusitis can be complicated by destruction of the adjacent bony walls as a manifestation of infection or vascular invasion with necrosis.[382-384, 525] Bony alterations predominate about the maxillary and ethmoid sinuses; however, the frontal and sphenoid regions may also be affected.[385] Although localized osteolysis predominates, more extensive dissolution of some of the facial structures may ensue. In chronic cases, osteosclerosis is also evident. The differential diagnosis includes other varieties of osteomyelitis and neoplasm. The accurate diagnosis of mucormycosis is established by biopsy of involved tissue and demonstration of the distinctive hyphae.

A case of osteomyelitis of the proximal femur related to the fungus Rhizopus has recently been described.[399]

Aspergillosis

Aspergillus is a normal harmless inhabitant of the upper respiratory tract. Uncommonly, in patients with low resistance or in those who have received an overwhelming inoculum, a chronic localized pulmonary infection may result due to inhalation of massive numbers of spores from mycelia growing on grain. Primary infection of the ear, the nasal sinuses or the orbit may also occur. The usual organism is *A. fumigatus*.

Spinal involvement can rarely be evident, due to contiguous spread from a pulmonary focus. The thoracic spine is most typically affected,[386-388] and the radiographic features, which include osseous and intervertebral disc space destruction and paraspinal masses, resemble those of tuberculosis.[47] Similarly, extension of infection into the orbital bones and ribs can also be encountered.[389] Rarely, the tubular bones of the extremities can be affected.[386, 390, 391] In these cases a typical osteomyelitis is evident.

Maduromycosis (Mycetoma)

This chronic granulomatous fungal disease affects the feet (Madura foot) (Fig. 62–53). It may be observed throughout the world, but is especially prevalent in India. In the United States, the most frequent cause of Madura foot is *Monosporium apiospermum*, although Aspergillus, Penicillium, Mad-

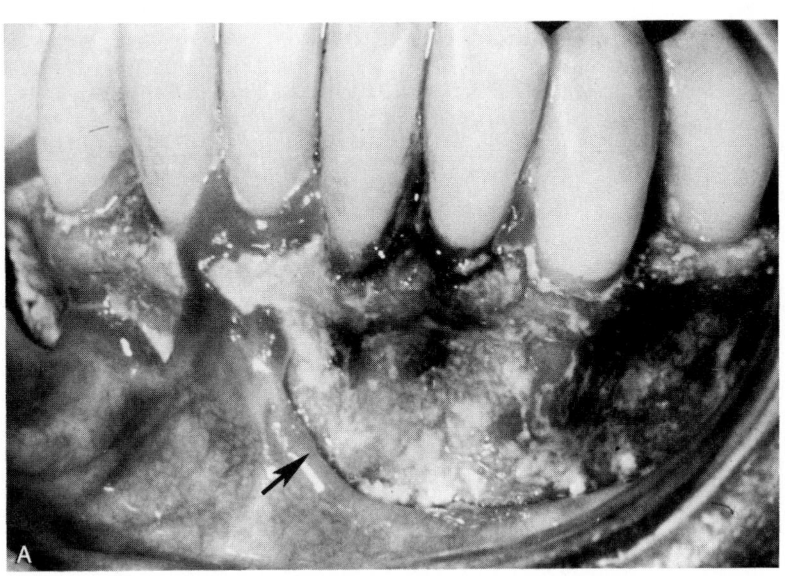

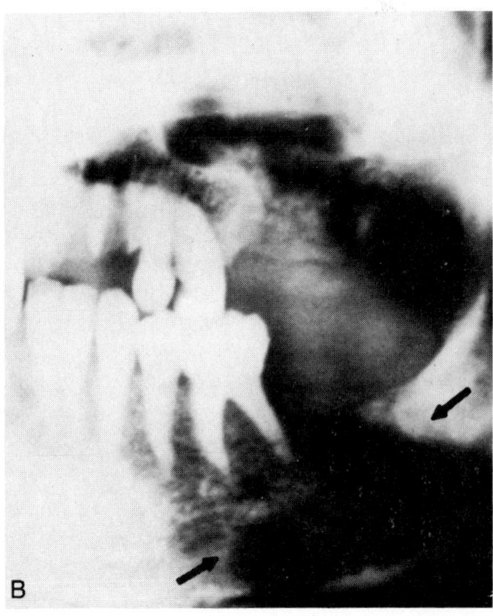

Figure 62–52. *Mucormycosis: Osteomyelitis.*

A *Observe the destructive lesion involving the left side of the mandible (arrow).*

B *A radiograph outlines lysis extending to the angle of the jaw (arrows). (Courtesy of Dr. R. Smith, University of California, San Francisco, California.)*

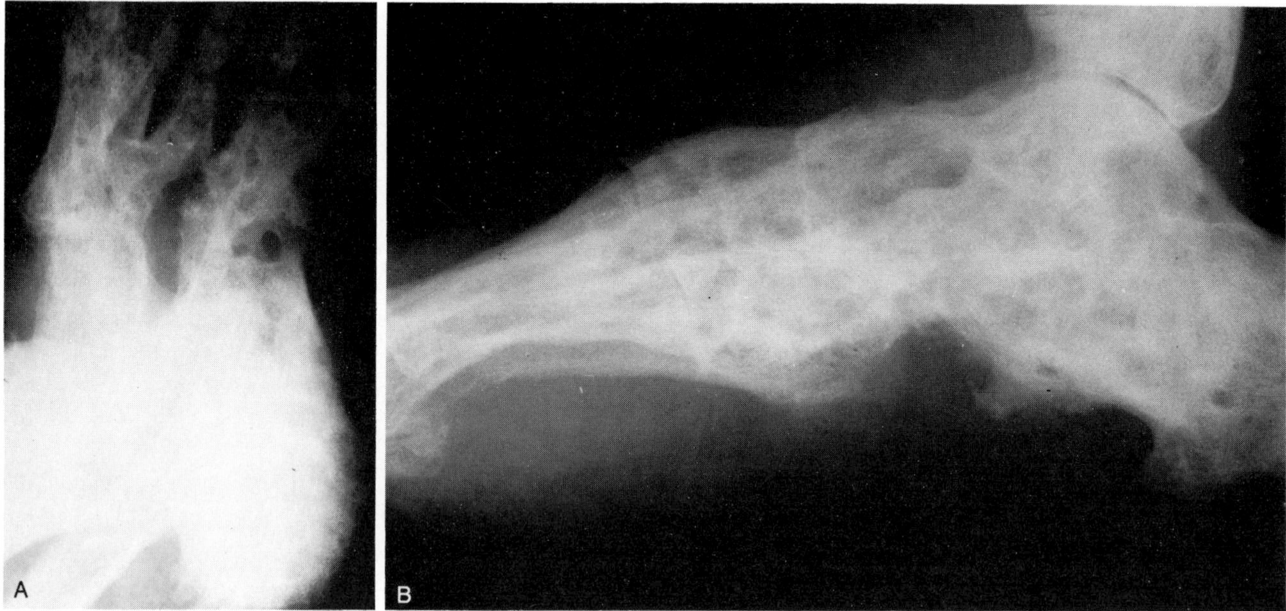

Figure 62–53. Maduromycosis: Madura foot. Oblique and lateral radiographs delineate the osseous and articular effects of chronic involvement of the foot. Bony destruction and widespread intra-articular osseous fusion can be noted.

urella, Cephalosporium, and Phialophora can produce this disease. Outside the United States, Nocardia species (*N. brasiliensis, N. madurae*) may be implicated (Fig. 62–54).

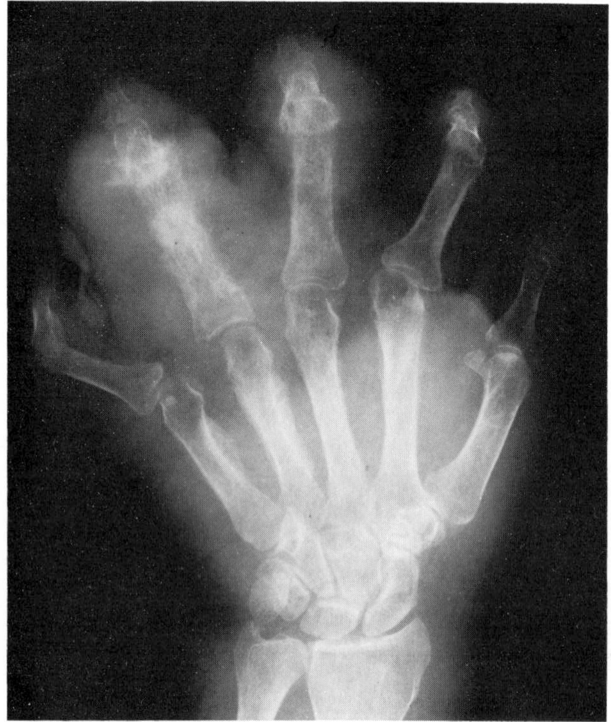

Figure 62–54. Nocardia brasiliensis: Osteomyelitis. Extensive soft tissue swelling and osseous and articular destruction with osteoporosis and periostitis have produced a deformed hand. (Courtesy of Dr. W. Peter Cockshott, McMaster University, Hamilton, Ontario.)

The infection of the foot (and less commonly the hand, arm, or leg) results from posttraumatic soft tissue invasion of organisms that are normal inhabitants of soil.[392-397] Following soft tissue contamination, the organisms may penetrate the underlying muscles, tendons, bones, and joints. Fistulae from the infected osseous tissues are common.

The course of maduromycosis is usually progressive. Initially, soft tissue swelling is seen. Over a period of months to years, a swollen, deformed, and necrotic foot appears. Dissemination of infection may occur via lymphatic channels, and death may result from secondary bacterial infection.

The radiographic findings vary with the virulence of the invading organism.[398] In some cases, single or multiple localized osseous defects are evident, whereas in others, extensive soft tissue and bony disruption occurs, with associated periostitis and sclerosis. Intra-articular osseous fusion may appear. These latter roentgenographic features can simulate other types of osteomyelitis, neuroarthropathy, and neoplasm.[107]

VIRAL INFECTION

Rubella Infection (German Measles)

This is a contagious disease of viral etiology. Although rubella is generally a benign disorder in the adult, maternal infection in the first half of pregnancy can lead to serious skeletal and nonskeletal alterations in the fetus.

Postnatal Rubella Infection. In the adult patient (especially women), rubella arthritis may occur within a few days of the skin rash.[400-402, 554] Persistent or migratory articular findings are most common in the small joints of the hands and wrists, the knees, and the ankles; in addition, the carpal tunnel syndrome may be evident. Synovial fluid aspiration can reveal mononuclear pleocytosis.

After live, attenuated rubella virus became available for active immunization, episodes of acute arthritis were noted in children injected with the virus.[403, 404] The incidence of this complication is apparently dependent upon the type of vaccination utilized. The knee is most typically affected, although the articulations of the hands and wrists may also be involved.

Recovery of the wild or attenuated rubella virus has been accomplished following natural rubella infection[405] and vaccination,[406] respectively. Histologically, a nonspecific synovitis is noted. The erythrocyte sedimentation rate may be elevated, and transiently positive results of latex fixation may occur.[407]

A chronic arthropathy has also been associated with rubella vaccination.[408] In this arthropathy, recurrent episodes of knee stiffness ("catcher's crouch syndrome") may be characterized by hypertrophy of the synovial membrane with protrusion into the intercondylar notch.

A recent report has indicated that rubella antibody levels are elevated not only in rubella vaccine arthritis but also in a significant proportion of individuals (approximately 33 per cent) with juvenile chronic arthritis, suggesting a possible role of rubella virus infection in this disease.[409] A similar laboratory finding in adult-onset Still's disease has also been noted.[553]

Intrauterine Rubella Infection. Radiographically evident osseous lesions due to intrauterine rubella infection were first reported in 1965[410, 411] and have been further documented since that time.[412-415] The roentgenographic features consist of metaphyseal lesions in long bones characterized by symmetry, linear areas of radiolucency, and increased bone density, producing a longitudinally oriented striated pattern ("celery-stalk" appearance) and the absence of periostitis, features that can disappear completely if the child recovers from the intrauterine viral infection or persist with increasing density of the juxtaepiphyseal region if the infection continues (Fig. 62–55). With healing, beak-like exostoses can be noted at the metaphyses. Histologic examination reveals variation in the thickness of the zone of mature cartilage cells adjacent to the epiphyseal line, multiple poorly calcified fragments of acellular cartilage, and osteoid.[416] Metaphyseal trabeculae may be reduced in number, and calcified bone and osteoid about the cartilaginous areas may be reduced in amount. Although positive cultures

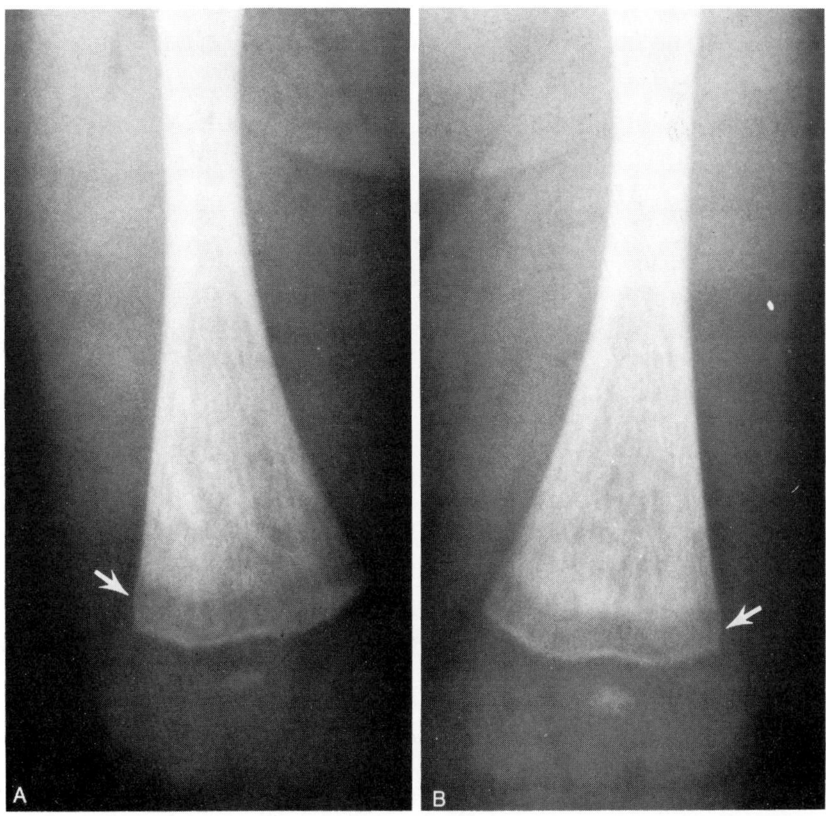

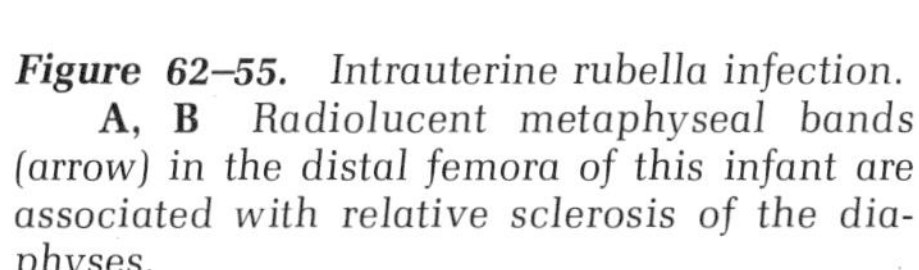

Figure 62–55. *Intrauterine rubella infection.*
A, B *Radiolucent metaphyseal bands (arrow) in the distal femora of this infant are associated with relative sclerosis of the diaphyses.*
Illustration continued on the following page

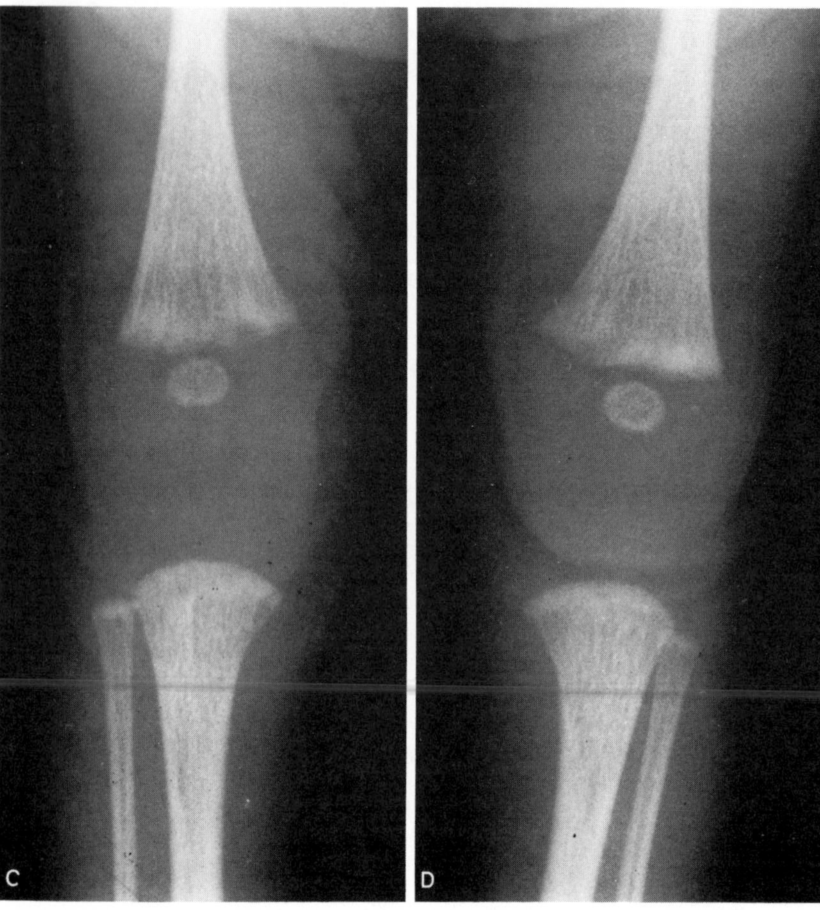

Figure 62–55. Continued

C, D *In a different infant, longitudinal striations have produced the characteristic "celery stalk" appearance. Periostitis is absent.*

for rubella can be obtained from the bone marrow, histologic evidence of osteomyelitis is generally lacking; scattered periosteal mononuclear cellular infiltration[417] and abundant plasma cellular response in the metaphyses, epiphyses, and subperiosteal locations[413] have occasionally been noted.

It is generally believed that the metaphyseal and diaphyseal lesions of rubella are related to alterations in bone formation. In a comprehensive study of the histologic characteristics of the osseous abnormalities, Reed[417] suggested that the metaphyseal radiolucent streaks in this disease were a manifestation of osteoporosis resulting from an insult to bone maturation due to the viremia. Whalen and coworkers[415] observed a delay in diaphyseal modeling in transplacental rubella, although normal modeling could be achieved within 2 months, coincident with the correction of the metaphyseal alterations. In an investigation of rabbits that were congenitally infected with rubella virus, London and colleagues[418] concluded that a direct viral action on chondrocytes was responsible for growth retardation.

These osseous alterations, which may occur in as many as 45 per cent of cases[411] of intrauterine rubella, can simulate those that are noted in other viral disorders (see discussion later in this chapter). They are usually transient in nature, disappearing after several weeks, although persistent and progressive changes can appear, and they may even lead to pathologic fracture.[419]

Cytomegalic Inclusion Disease

Intrauterine infection related to cytomegalic inclusion disease can lead to intracranial calcifications and rubella-like abnormalities of the skeleton[420-423] (Fig. 62–56). Metaphyseal osteopenia, irregularity of the growth plate, and a striated pattern parallel to the long axis of the bone characterized by alternating lucent and sclerotic bands are noted. Spontaneous pathologic fractures have also been observed in infants with cytomegalic inclusion disease.[424, 555] The metaphyseal changes are usually evident in the first few days of life and then disappear completely within a period of days to weeks. They are generally attributed to a disturbance in endochondral bone formation rather than to osteomyelitis, and these changes can be confused with findings not only of intrauterine rubella but also of erythroblastosis fetalis,[425] congenital syphilis, and hypophosphatasia. Similar alterations may be expected in other intrauterine viral infections and in premature infants of mothers with severe cyanotic cardiac abnormalities.[426]

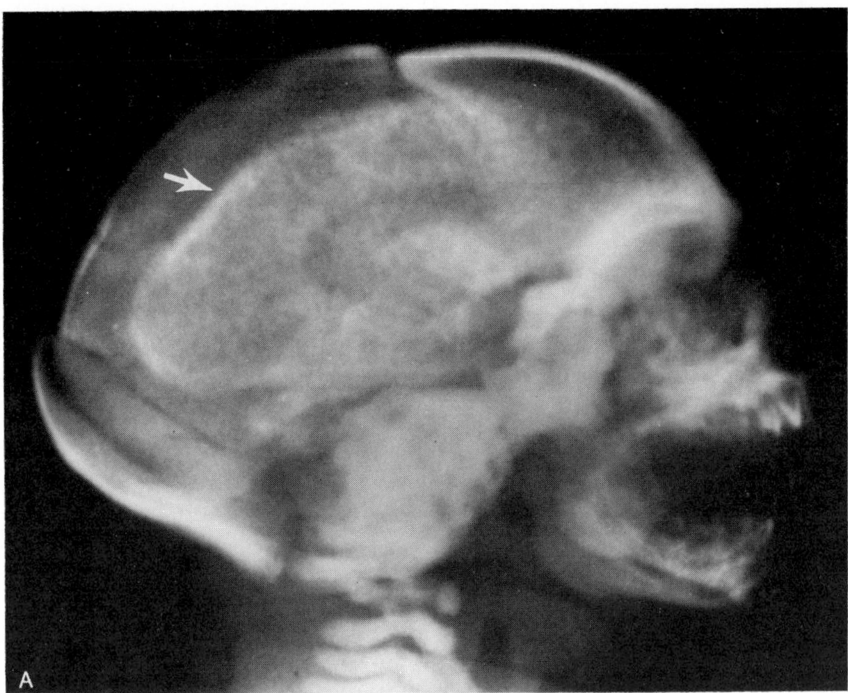

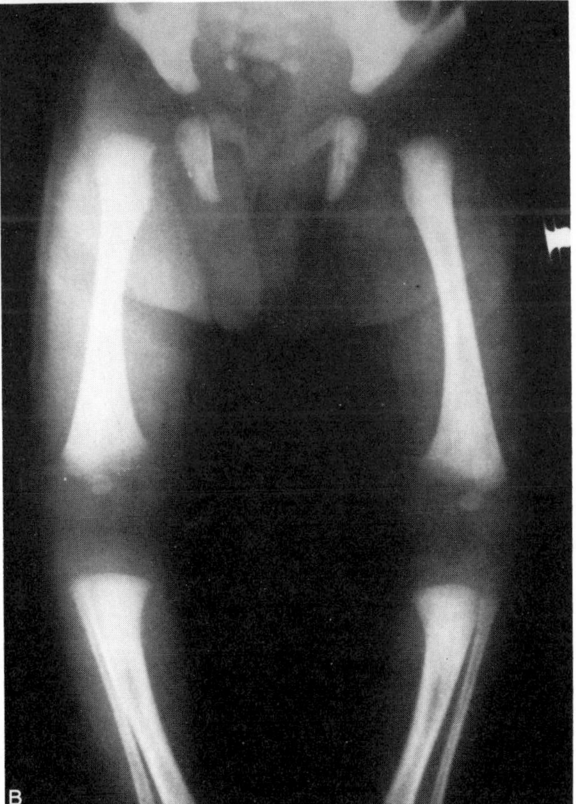

Figure 62–56. *Cytomegalic inclusion disease.*

A *This disease can be accompanied by focal cerebral necrosis and calcification. The calcific deposits are usually bilateral and symmetric in distribution, within the walls of dilated lateral ventricles (arrow).*

B *Metaphyseal changes consist of irregularity of the growth plate and osseous fragmentation, most evident in the distal femora.*

(Courtesy of Dr. F. N. Silverman, Stanford University, Palo Alto, California.)

Varicella (Chickenpox)

Varicella is a common benign disorder, usually evident in children, in which skeletal alterations are rarely encountered.[416, 556] Two fatal cases of varicella with bone marrow involvement have been recorded by Cheatham and associates[427]; in one child, irradiation and chemotherapy had been utilized for control of metastatic neuroblastoma, and in the second, steroid administration had been used for treatment of acute rheumatic fever. In both cases, the virus was isolated and serologic studies were positive. Similar examples of bone marrow lesions occurring in association with varicella in patients with malignant tumors undergoing active treatment were noted by Feldman and co-workers.[428]

Articular inflammation of the knee in varicella was reported by Ward and Bishop[429] in a 5 year old girl. Although the virus was not isolated from the joint, the fact that the arthritis subsided simultaneously with the chickenpox and that other family members developed varicella justifies the assumption that the infection was the cause of the articular abnormalities. Synovial fluid aspiration in another girl with varicella and arthritis revealed large mononuclear cells, a finding that has been observed in other virus-related arthritides.[557]

Varicella gangrenosa requiring amputation of the lower extremities has also been recorded.[430]

Mumps

Arthritis is a well recognized manifestation of this viral disease, occurring in approximately 0.5 per cent of cases.[23] This complication is usually seen in young adult men, approximately 10 to 14 days following the parotitis. A migratory polyarthralgia or polyarthritis affects predominantly the large joints, although those of the hands and the feet can also be involved.

Variola (Smallpox)

Osteomyelitis and septic arthritis are well-known complications of smallpox. The term osteomyelitis variolosa was originated by Chiari[431] in a description of nonsuppurative lesions in the bone marrow of patients who died of smallpox during the Prague epidemic of 1891–1892. Since that report, numerous further descriptions of musculoskeletal alterations in this viral disease have appeared.[432-440] There does not appear to be a relationship between the severity of the infection and the incidence or severity of the osteomyelitis or septic arthritis.[441] Infection may originate in the bone, in the joint, or in both; most typically, osseous and articular changes occur together. Symmetric involvement is frequent, and articular infection reveals an unusual affinity for the elbow (80 per cent of patients).[432, 526] This affinity may be related to the common occurrence of physiologic stresses in this articulation, which possesses a great range of motion, stresses that can lead to hyperemia and vascular seeding of the joint by the organisms.[433] However, whether or not osteomyelitis variolosa is caused directly by the virus remains controversial. The similarity of the behavior of the lesions to those accompanying other viral disorders, the presence of elementary variola inclusion bodies in the fluid of affected joints, and the demonstration of necrotic foci associated with the smallpox virus in the bone marrow in victims of the disease suggest that true infection of bone can take place.

Three types of bone and joint lesions have been described[433]:

1. A necrotic, nonsuppurative osteomyelitis, probably due to the smallpox virus itself, commonly involves the diaphyses of long tubular bones, leading to epiphyseal contamination, with destruction and deformity.
2. A suppurative arthritis related to contamination of the joint is probably due to secondary infection of a pustule.
3. A nonsuppurative arthritis may appear 1 to 4 weeks after the initial infection. Polyarticular and symmetric abnormalities are common, characterized by pain, swelling, and restriction of motion, and may be followed by secondary infection of the joint and articular deformities.

During the acute stage of osteomyelitis variolosa, findings simulate those of pyogenic osteomyelitis. Tubular bones are commonly involved; changes in the spine, the pelvis, and the skull are less typical. Juxtametaphyseal osteoporosis and destruction, epiphyseal extension, periostitis, involucrum formation, and articular contamination are seen. The elbow (Fig. 62–57), the glenohumeral joint, the knee, the hip, and the small joints of the hand, wrist and foot can be altered (Fig. 62–58).

During the later stages of the disease, joint function and bone growth are commonly affected (Fig. 62–58). In articulations, osseous destruction with or without "loose bodies," bony or fibrous ankylosis, subluxation, and secondary osteoarthritis can be encountered; in the bones, cessation or retardation of growth can be evident.

On pathologic examination, foci of necrosis may be detected throughout the marrow of the tubular bones. These focal lesions can become evident as early as 2 days and as late as 2 months after the appearance of the skin lesions. Damage to epiphyseal cartilage and premature fusion of the epiphyses account for the limb deformities that characterize this disease.

Although radiographic characteristics of osseous and articular involvement in smallpox simulate those of pyogenic infection, certain differences

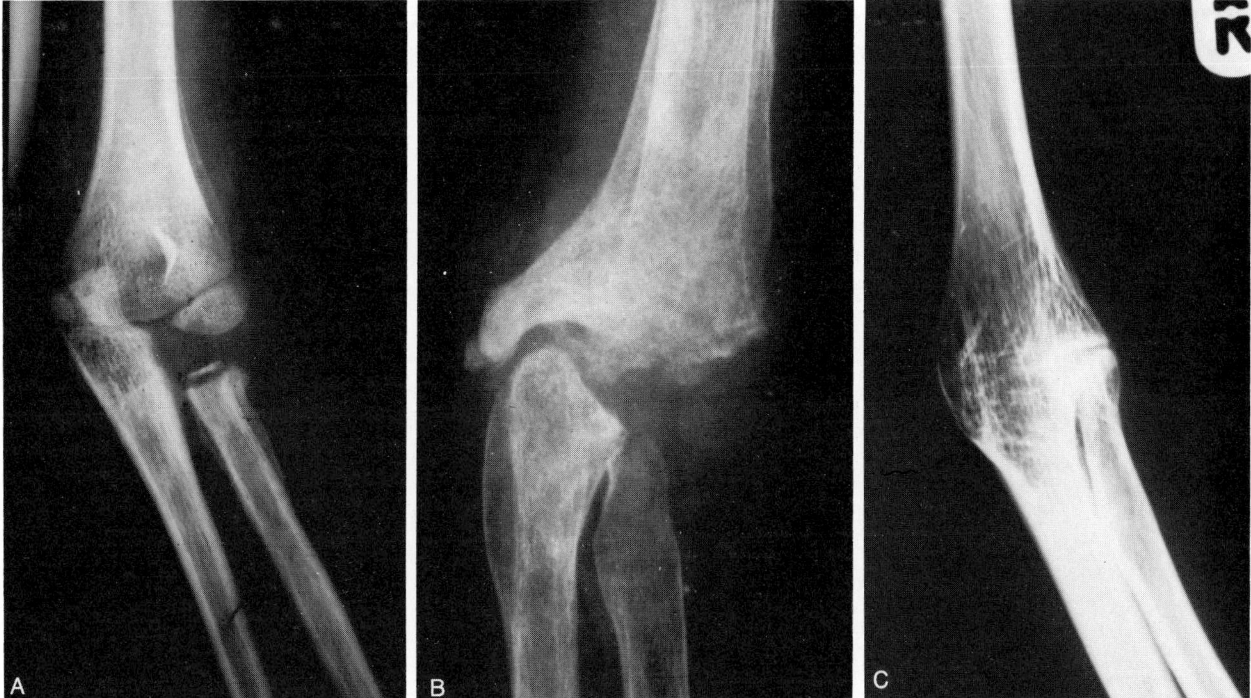

Figure 62–57. *Variola osteomyelitis and septic arthritis: Elbow involvement. Stages in the process of bone and joint disease are illustrated in three different patients. Initial findings* **(A)** *include destructive foci with periostitis. Subsequently* **(B,C)** *irregularity of articular surfaces and intra-articular osseous fusion can be seen. (Courtesy of Dr. W. Peter Cockshott, McMaster University, Hamilton, Ontario.)*

can be seen. Symmetric changes, epiphyseal extension and destruction, predilection for the elbow, extensive osteoperiostitis of diaphyses of tubular bones, and peculiar deformities suggest the diagnosis of osteomyelitis variolosa (Fig. 62–59). The low incidence of spinal involvement and the lack of response of the osseous lesions to antibiotics are also noteworthy. The musculoskeletal abnormalities of smallpox can resemble findings in tuberculosis, leprosy, chronic granulomatous disease of childhood, juvenile chronic arthritis, and bone dysplasias.

Vaccinia

Although a viremia may occur following vaccination for smallpox, osseous and articular complications are indeed unusual. However, examples of bone[442-445] and joint[446] alterations have been recorded. With osseous involvement, periostitis and hyperostosis coupled with soft tissue swelling or nodules can lead to an erroneous radiographic diagnosis of infantile cortical hyperostosis (Caffey's disease),[442, 443] although biopsy may lead to recovery of the vaccinia virus[442, 444, 445]; in some instances of vaccinia, bony lysis and involucrum formation are consistent with the radiographic findings of osteomyelitis[444] (Fig. 62–60), whereas in others, metaphyseal irregularity may represent a virus-related growth disturbance.[447] With articular involvement, aspiration of joint contents can lead to recovery of the vaccinia virus.[446]

Infectious Mononucleosis

This disorder apparently results from infection with the Epstein-Barr virus.[448] Reports of articular involvement with pain, soft tissue swelling, and elevation of the erythrocyte sedimentation rate simulating rheumatic fever or juvenile chronic arthritis have appeared,[449, 450] and biopsies of affected joints can reveal features of a subacute synovitis.[23] A patient with infectious mononucleosis has demonstrated periostitis of the ulnae and tibiae that was associated with pain and tenderness.[451] In this latter case, attempts at isolating bacterial or viral agents were unrewarding, although the individual demonstrated hyperglobulinemia.[416] The combination of periostitis and dysproteinemia has been noted in other patients.[452]

Other Viral or Viral-like Diseases

During the prodromal phase of *acute hepatitis,* a transient migratory arthritis, especially of the joints of the hands, can be evident[519] (see Chapter 32).

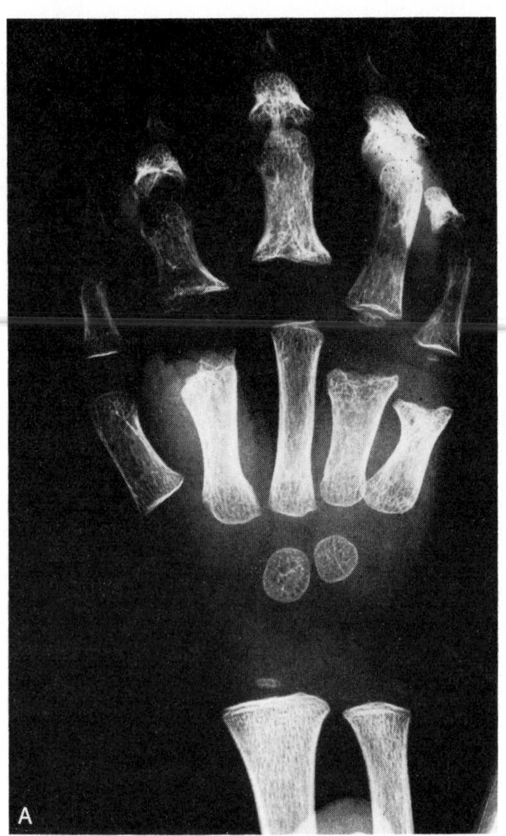

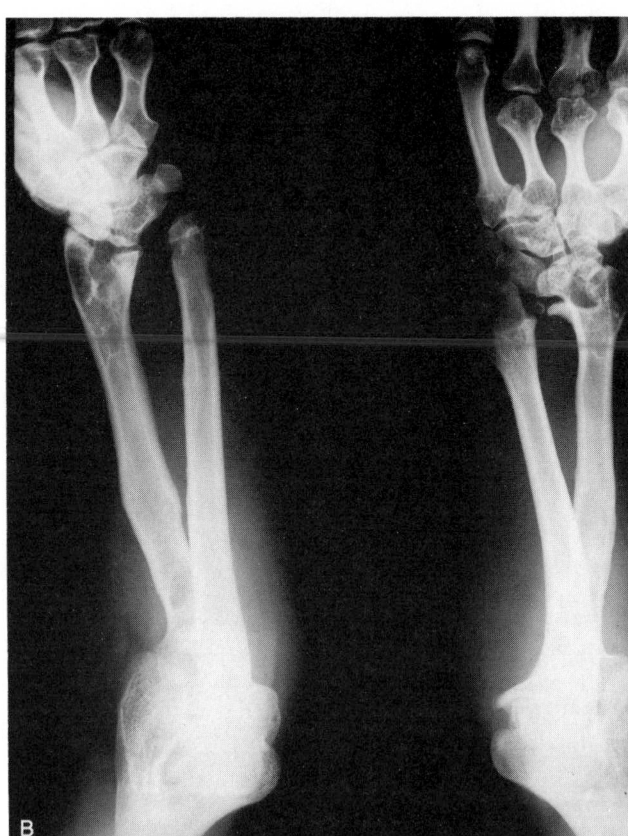

Figure 62–58. *Variola osteomyelitis and septic arthritis: Hand and wrist involvement.*

A *During the acute and subacute stages, observe epiphyseal destruction and growth deformities.*

B *In a different patient, elbow and wrist involvement has produced disturbance in bone growth. Note the shortened and deformed metacarpals.*

(Courtesy of Dr. W. Peter Cockshott, McMaster University, Hamilton, Ontario.)

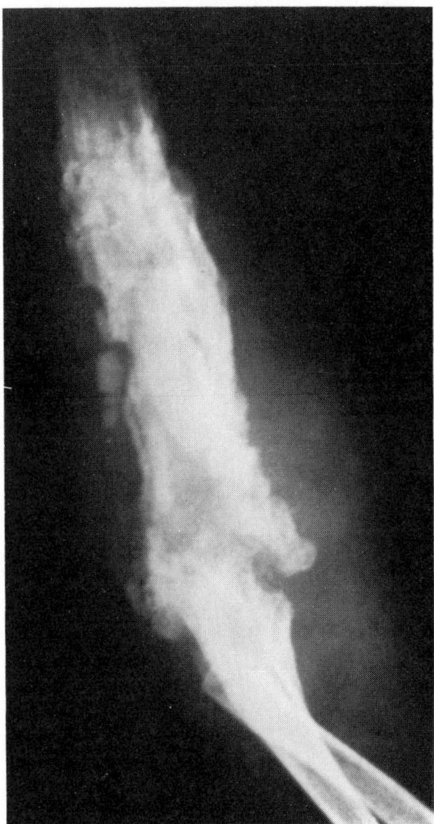

Figure 62–59. *Variola osteomyelitis. In the late phases of the disease, extreme destruction can be seen. Here, in the humeral shaft, bizarre lysis and sclerosis, fragmentation, and soft tissue swelling can be noted.*

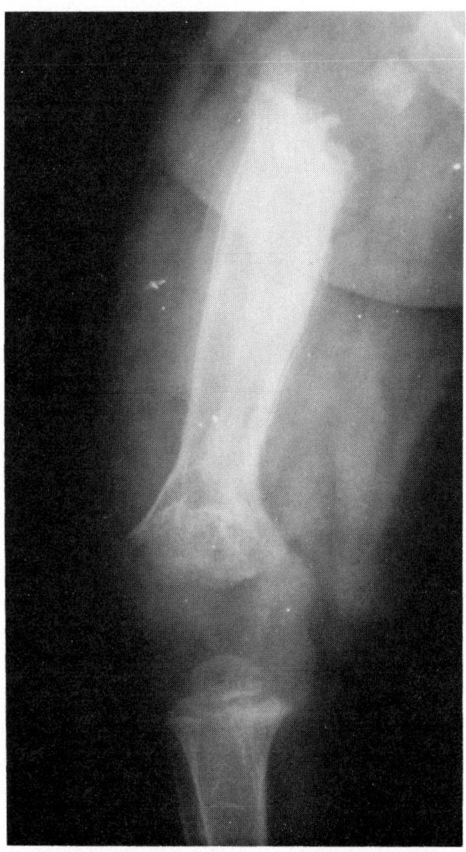

Figure 62–60. *Vaccinial osteomyelitis. Expansion of the femoral shaft, periostitis, and metaphyseal irregularities are the roentgenographic findings. (Courtesy of Dr. W. Peter Cockshott, McMaster University, Hamilton, Ontario.)*

Arthritic manifestations may also occur during *influenza,*[453] *echovirus* infections,[518] in the African disorders of *chikungunya*[558] and *O'Nyong-Nyong,*[559] and in the Australian disorder *epidemic polyarthritis.*[23] In a newborn infant with *coxsackievirus* infection, hip contractures have been noted, perhaps related to the infectious disease.[454] Although *lymphogranuloma venereum* is not a viral disorder, the infective agent is an intracellular parasite that produces intracytoplasmic "elementary bodies" that resemble the inclusion bodies of virus-infected cells.[416] In this disease, polyarthritis, principally of the knees, the ankles, and the wrists, can lead to acute or chronic symptoms and signs.[455] Joint effusions are usually sterile, and results of the Frei skin test are always positive. Osseous lesions in lymphogranuloma venereum are noted in adult patients and may relate to dissemination of the organisms via the bloodstream,[456] a contention that is supported by the isolation of the infective agent from the bone lesion.

Cat-scratch fever is a disorder of unknown etiology, possibly viral, which is characterized by local lymphadenitis within 1 or 2 weeks after being scratched by a cat.[458] Findings include soft tissue masses, erythema nodosum, and bony lesions. Osteolytic foci, when present in a child with cat-scratch fever, can resemble the lesions of eosinophilic granuloma; biopsy may reveal a granulomatous process with central necrosis and cellular infiltration.[459, 460]

RICKETTSIAL INFECTION

Although a variety of microorganisms of the family Rickettsiaceae can cause diseases in man, osseous and articular abnormalities are lacking or represent a very minor feature. In some patients, diffuse small vessel vasculitis can lead to thrombus formation, with complete or partial obliteration of the vascular lumen. These changes, which are most marked in Rocky Mountain spotted fever, are evident in many organ systems, but are especially prominent in the lung, the heart, and the brain. Occasionally, soft tissue necrosis can result in loss of cutaneous tissues in the phalanges that may be evident on roentgenograms.[461] Bony necrosis may also be recognized.

PROTOZOAN INFECTION

Toxoplasmosis

This infectious disorder is caused by an intracellular protozoan parasite, *Toxoplasma gondii*. Human infections with Toxoplasma may be either congenital or acquired.

The congenital variety of toxoplasmosis can be severe. An infant may be stillborn at term or be born prematurely with active infection characterized by fever, rash, hepatosplenomegaly, mental retardation, chorioretinitis, and convulsions, which may lead to death in 10 to 20 per cent of cases. Osseous lesions are unusual,[462] although metaphyseal alterations in tubular bones may simulate those of rubella, cytomegalic inclusion disease, or syphilis. Cerebral calcification can be evident.

The acquired variety of the disease can occur at any age and may display variable manifestations. These include rash, lymphadenopathy, ocular changes, and widespread vascular alterations. Myalgias and myositis can accompany acquired toxoplasmosis.[463] Unilateral or bilateral arthritis with articular and periarticular swelling, and tenosynovitis, especially about the ankle and the wrist, can also be apparent.[464-466] Radiographically evident osteoporosis, soft tissue swelling and osseous cystic lesions, and histologically evident synovial inflammation with granulomatous tissue, round cell infiltration, and necrosis have been described.[466]

Leishmaniasis

This disorder, produced by protozoa of the genus Leishmania, is transmitted by the bite of a sandfly, and has a widespread geographic distribution. Osseous lesions may result from extension of skin and soft tissue infection or, rarely, from hematogenous dissemination.[457]

Amebiasis

Extraintestinal manifestations of amebiasis include urticaria, neuralgia, and arthralgia. Polyarthritis coincident with enteric involvement has also been recorded.[495]

INFECTION PRODUCED BY WORMS

Hookworm Disease

This disease is produced by *Ancylostoma duodenale* or *Necator americanus*. Anemia and its complications are the major clinical manifestations of this disorder. Musculoskeletal abnormalities are indeed rare. Articular inflammation with swelling of the ankles has been described in a 7 year old boy,[467] although the exact relationship of the joint manifestations to hookworm disease was not established. O'Connor and associates[468] observed an 8 year old boy who developed a poorly defined lytic lesion of the posterior part of the talus. Stool examination documented the presence of the adult form of *Necator americanus*, and surgery with examination of the osseous lesion revealed granulation tissue with foreign body giant cells surrounding partially calcified hookworm larvae. These investigators speculated that a preexisting bony abnormality is necessary to initiate the worm's invasion of the osseous tissue.

Loiasis

This disease is prevalent in West and Central Africa, and is produced by the filaria *Loa loa* (African eye worm). Infective larvae are deposited in the victim's skin following the bite of the mango fly.[469] The larvae burrow into the deeper subcutaneous tissue, where they mature to adult worms over a period of 6 months or longer. Localized areas of allergic inflammation in the subcutaneous tissue, particularly in the forearm, produce Calabar swellings, named after the Nigerian town in which the disease is rampant. The dead worms cause abscesses or undergo calcification, or both.[470-472] Calcific deposits in the subcutaneous tissues may be fine, coiled, lace-like, and filamentous (calcification of the worm), or thicker, bead-like and lobulated (calcification of the fibrous capsule surrounding the worm).[469]

Onchocerciasis

This form of filariasis is produced by *Onchocerca volvulus* and is transmitted by flies. It is prevalent in Africa and Central and South America. Cutaneous nodules on the head and trunk consisting of adult worms and microfilariae are seen. Soft tissue calcifications, similar to those in loiasis, may be detected.[469, 473]

Filariasis

Filariasis is produced by the adult worms of the species *Wuchereria bancrofti* or *Brugia malayi*, which locate in the lymphatic and soft tissues of the human body. The disease is predominant in tropical areas of Asia, Africa, South America, Australia, and the South Pacific islands. After prolonged and repeated attacks, filariasis can lead to massive lymphedema or elephantiasis, especially of the legs and the scrotum. Lymphatic obstruction may relate to lymphangitis, a granulomatous reaction about dead worms, an allergic antigen-antibody reaction produced by the death of the parasite, or secondary bacterial infection.[469] Cutaneous and subcutaneous lymphedema and fibrous hyperplasia are seen. On radiographs, an affected limb is greatly enlarged, with soft tissue thickening, blurring of subcutaneous fat planes, and a linear striated pattern. Osseous changes are not apparent, although Reeder[292] observed irregular tuftal erosion of phalanges in the foot in one patient. Lymphangiography reveals an increase in the number of tiny lymphatic channels that have a tortuous, looping course, dermal backflow, and an increase in the size of lymph nodes that may resemble the changes in Hodgkin's disease.[474] Soft tissue calcification of *W. bancrofti* has been noted[475, 476]; elongated radiodense shadows in the subcutaneous tissue represent calcified dead encysted filariae.

Dracunculosis (Guinea Worm Disease)

The guinea worm, *Dracunculus medinensis*, can cause human disease, particularly in parts of Africa, the Middle East, South America, India, and Pakistan. The disorder is contracted when the larvae in contaminated water are ingested by a flea and are, in turn, swallowed in the drinking water by humans.[469] The larvae eventually enter the circulation and mature within the human subcutaneous tissues. Although the male worm is relatively small (2 to 3 cm in length), the female worm may reach 120 cm in length. When the female parasites die, they may calcify, producing long, curled radiodense shadows in the lower extremities and hands (Fig. 62–61*A*), and less commonly, the perineum and abdominal and chest wall[477-479]; the deposits may become fragmented because of the action of adjacent musculature. Calcification of male worms is rarely seen.[409] Of interest, Khajavi[477] noted malignant disease in 15 of 83 patients with calcifications due to infestation with guinea worms; bladder carcinoma was the most frequent neoplasm encountered. This investigator suggested that such infection might lead to secondary tumor in a way similar to that in schistosomiasis.

If a migratory guinea worm dies adjacent to an articulation, severe cellular reaction can apparently lead to joint effusion and secondary bacterial infection.[480] Calcification about the damaged articulation may also be evident (Fig. 62–61*B*,*C*).

Trichinosis

Following ingestion of infected beef, a human may develop trichinosis due to the intestinal nematode *Trichinella spiralis*. Calcification of the cysts of the parasite is commonly detected on microscopic examination but is rarely, if ever, noted on radiographic evaluation.[473]

Cysticercosis

The relationship between humans and the pork tapeworm, *Taenia solium*, is twofold: Humans are the only definitive host of the adult tapeworm, the parasite inhabiting the intestine; and humans may serve as an intermediate host (the usual intermediate host is the hog), harboring the larval stage, *Cysticercus cellulosae*. In this latter case, deposits of the larval form of the tapeworm may appear in subcutaneous and muscular tissues and in a variety of viscera, including the heart, brain, lung, liver, and eye. When the larvae die, a foreign body reaction may ensue, leading to considerable tissue response. Necrosis may occur, followed, over a period of years, by caseation and calcification.[481]

On radiographs, linear or oval elongated calcifications appear in the soft tissues and musculature; these may reach 23 mm in length.[473, 481, 482] The long axis of the calcified cysts lies in the plane of the surrounding muscle bundles[469] (Fig. 62–62).

Echinococcosis

This disorder is produced principally by the larval stage of *Echinococcus granulosus* and is most prevalent in sheep- and cattle-raising areas of North and South Africa, South America, Central Europe, Australia, and Canada; less commonly, *Echinococcus multilocularis* is the causative agent, especially in Alaska and Eurasia. In humans, *E. granulosus* is contracted by ingestion of the eggs, which are contained in the feces of the dog (sheep dog). Following ingestion, the embryos escape from the eggs, traverse the intestinal mucosa, and are disseminated via venous and lymphatic channels. Cysts may develop in various viscera, particularly the liver and the lungs.

Bone lesions are reported in 1 to 2 per cent of cases of echinococcosis.[483] Over a long period of time, osseous foci may present with pain and deformity, particularly in the 30 to 60 year old age group. Hydatid disease of bone is rarely seen in childhood. Osseous involvement is almost invariably related to primary infection and is not the result of extension from a neighboring soft tissue lesion. Although hematogenous seeding of the skeleton in echinococcosis can conceivably occur in any site, one bone, a few adjacent bones, or one skeletal region is usually affected; when several adjacent bones are involved, skeletal contamination has generally resulted from direct invasion of one or more bones from another skeletal site (e.g., pelvis to femur; vertebra to rib).[1] Echinococcal joint disease

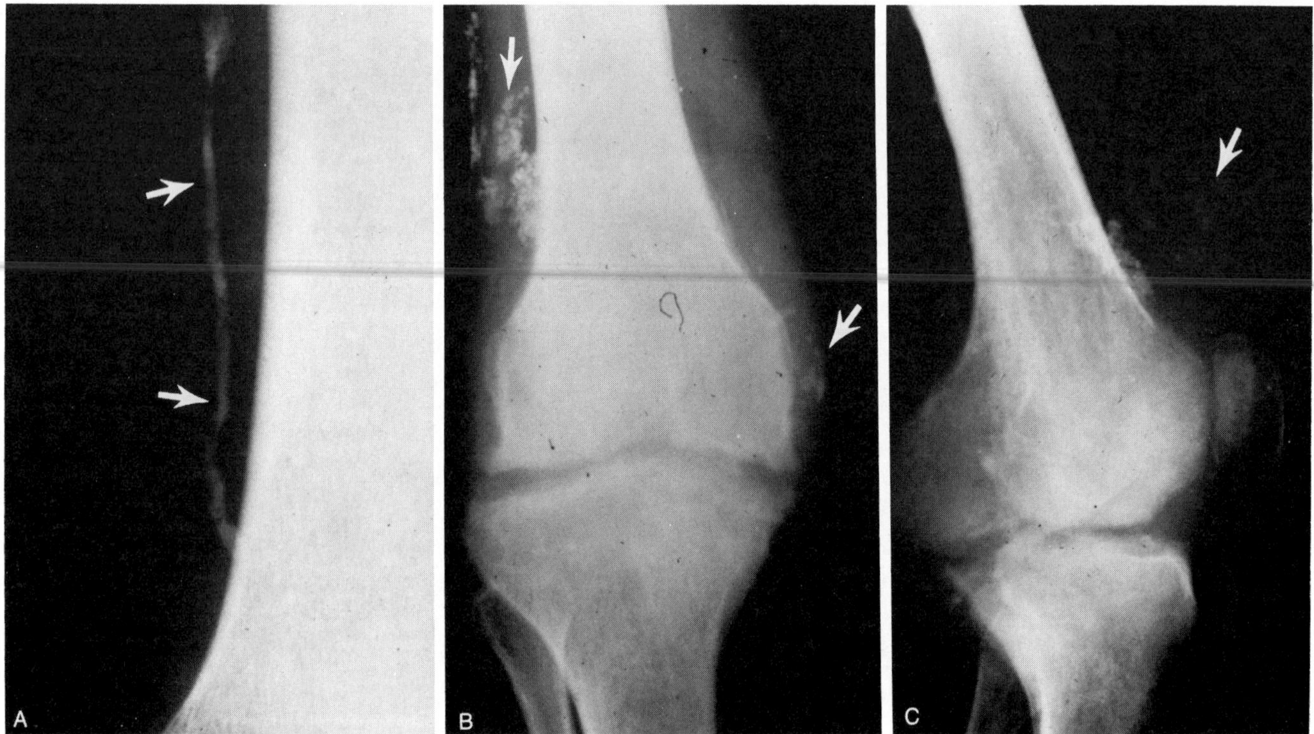

Figure 62–61. *Dracunculosis (guinea worm disease).*

A *Observe the long linear calcification (arrows) adjacent to the lower tibia due to the presence of a dying female worm.*

B, C *Guinea worm arthritis can be associated with soft tissue calcification (arrows) and swelling as well as secondary bacterial infection with osseous and cartilaginous destruction.*

*(**B, C,** Courtesy of Dr. W. Peter Cockshott, McMaster University, Hamilton, Ontario.)*

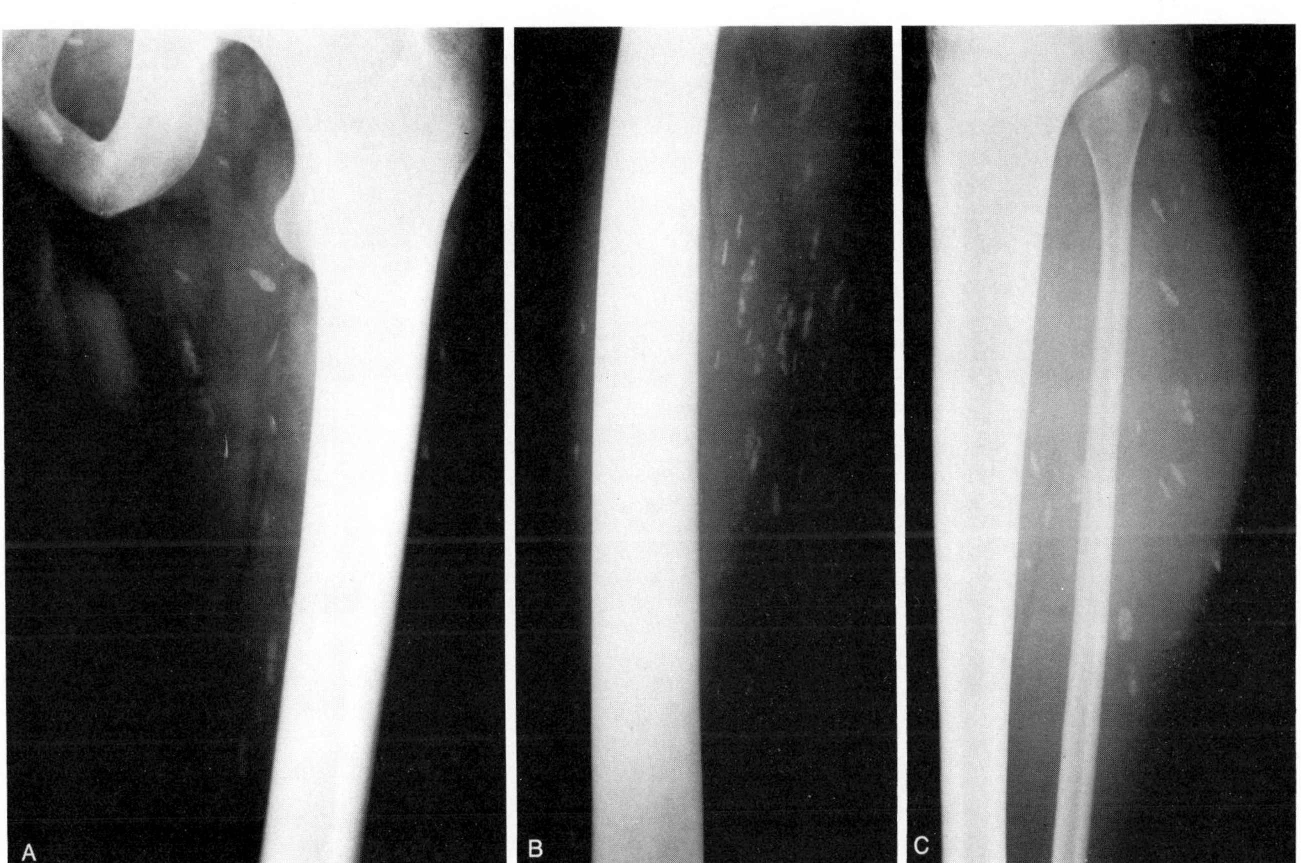

Figure 62–62. *Cysticercosis. The typical appearance of soft tissue calcification in this disorder consists of elongated linear or oval dense lesions oriented in the plane of the surrounding muscle bundles.*

without a focus of bone involvement is exceedingly rare. On the basis of available reports, the vertebral column, the pelvis, the long bones, and the skull are most commonly involved.[484-493] Rib and costochondral abnormalities can occur as an isolated phenomenon, in association with vertebral lesions, or as a result of erosion from adjacent pleural cysts.[491, 560]

Intraosseous foci of hydatid echinococcosis predominate in the spongiosa and consist of minute, separate, thin-walled cysts.[1, 492] These cysts expand at the expense of surrounding trabeculae and, in some instances, reach considerable size. Connective tissue proliferation in the marrow is accompanied by cellular infiltration, hemosiderin pigmentation, and cholesterol crystal deposition.[1] As the cysts enlarge, cortical thinning and expansion, pathologic fracture, and soft tissue extension can ensue. Periosteal bone formation is unusual. Soft tissue cysts proliferate, become delineated by a thick fibrous membrane, and may contain seropurulent fluid and detritus.[1]

Radiographs can reveal single or multiple expansile cystic osteolytic lesions containing trabeculae (Fig. 62–63). These may be associated with cortical violation and soft tissue mass formation, with calcification. The radiographic characteristics are similar to those of fibrous dysplasia, plasmacytoma, giant cell tumor, cartilaginous neoplasms (enchondroma, chondrosarcoma, chondromyxoid fibroma), skeletal metastases (especially from a tumor of the kidney or thyroid), a brown tumor of hyperparathyroidism, angiosarcoma, or a hemophilic pseudotumor. Accurate diagnosis may be aided in some individuals by eosinophilia (25 to 35 per cent of cases), a positive complement fixation test, a positive reaction to intradermal injection of hydatid fluid, and a positive indirect hemagglutination test.[494] Needle biopsy of the lesions may lead to further dissemination of infection.[491]

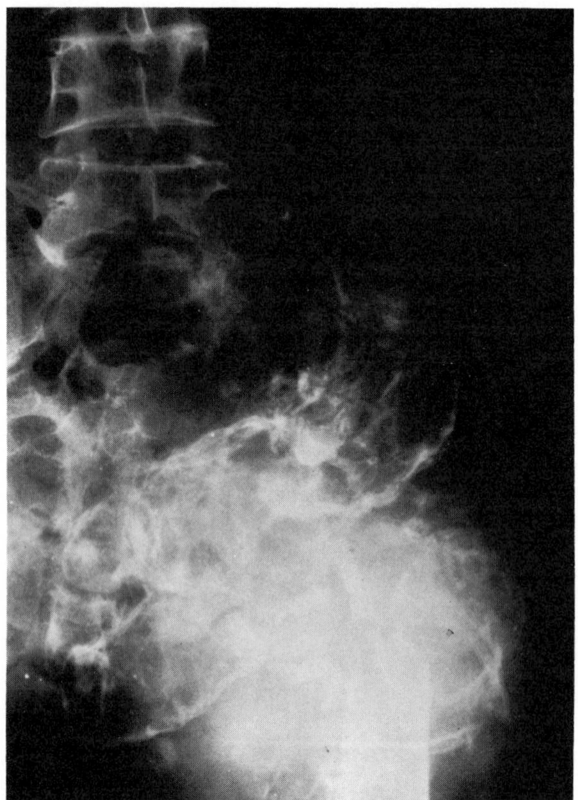

Figure 62–63. *Echinococcosis. The expansile, "bubbly" lytic lesions of the pelvis, sacrum, and proximal femur are associated with deformity, osseous fragmentation, and soft tissue swelling.*

Complications of osseous involvement in echinococcosis include pathologic fracture, secondary infection, especially with staphylococci,[492] rupture into the spinal canal with neural problems, including paraplegia, transarticular extension with osseous collapse and deformity, intrapelvic extension with compression of bladder, vagina, uterus, or colon,[490] and cranial lesions with involvement of the dura and arachnoid membranes, leading to meningitis.

Other Diseases Produced by Worms

Paragonimiasis, caused by the trematode *Paragonimus westermani,* can lead to alterations of the lung, liver, brain, mesentery, and skeletal muscle. Rarely, calcification is encountered.[473]

Schistosomiasis, due to *Schistosoma hematobium,* can produce bladder and ureteral calcification in chronic cases.

ADDITIONAL DISORDERS OF POSSIBLE INFECTIOUS ETIOLOGY

There are many other musculoskeletal disorders in which an infectious etiology is supected. Some of these, including sarcoidosis, Behçet's syndrome, and infantile cortical hyperostosis, are discussed elsewhere. Additional examples are indicated below.

Ainhum

Ainhum (dactylolysis spontanea) is a self-limited dermatologic disorder that is characteristically found in African blacks or their descendants, although rarely it is reported in other races.[496-499] In West Africa, it may be seen in 2 per cent of individuals[469]; ainhum is occasionally encountered in patients in the United States.[499] Most typically, the fifth toe on one or both feet is affected, although other toes (especially the fourth) and even the fingers can be involved.[500] Although both young and elderly men and women can be afflicted, most patients are men in the fourth and fifth decades of life.[501] A deep soft tissue groove appears[499] corresponding to a hyperkeratotic band within the epidermis,[496] asso-

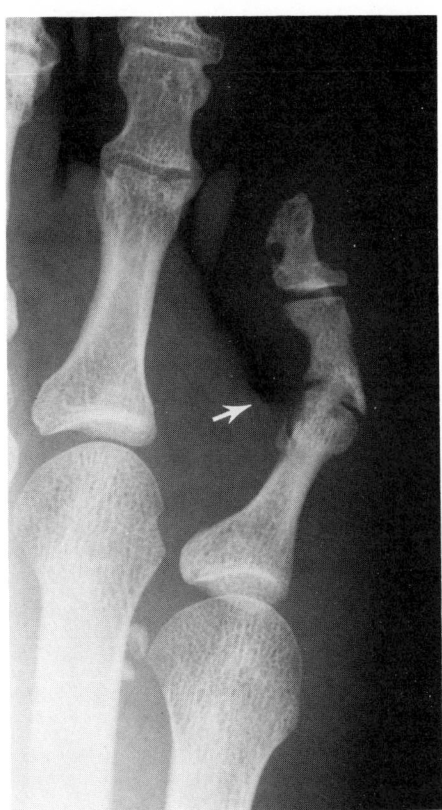

Figure 62–64. *Ainhum. Note the soft tissue groove (arrow) and the osseous resorption, especially on the medial aspect of the proximal and middle phalanges of the fifth toe. Periostitis is absent.*

ciated with dermal fibrosis.[497] The groove is evident initially along the medial aspect of the fifth toe and progressively deepens and encircles the toe. Ulceration and inflammation coexist. Digital swelling or lymphedema[496] and adjacent osseous resorption are encountered. Bony resorption begins on the medial aspect of the distal portion of the proximal phalanx or the middle phalanx of the fifth toe[499] (Fig. 62–64). Periostitis is generally absent. With further narrowing, the bone may fracture. As more bone is resorbed, including most of the middle phalanx, severe digital angulation and autoamputation are seen. The entire process may occur over a period of months or decades.

The etiology of ainhum is not clear.[499] Traumatic and infectious factors appear most likely. Although the vasculature of the involved toe is usually normal,[496] plethysmography may indicate a local increase in blood flow.[502]

Tietze's Syndrome

Tietze's syndrome, the costosternal syndrome, and costochondritis are terms that are used to describe pain, tenderness, and swelling at the costosternal articulations.[503, 504] It is a common condition, perhaps occurring in as many as 10 per cent of patients who are seen with chest pain.[503] "Epidemics" of the disease have also been noted.[505] Tietze's syndrome is benign and self-limiting. Typically, painful swelling and tenderness to local palpation of one or more costosternal junctions are observed in a patient in the second to fourth decades of life.[506] Respiratory symptoms and signs may also be apparent, and patients may reveal a distant focus of bacterial or viral infection or a recent history of thoracic surgery. Although the second costochondral junction is most commonly involved, any such junction can be affected, and xiphisternal costochondritis has also been noted.[507]

Radiographs are not commonly revealing, although soft tissue swelling, calcification, and periostitis are rarely encountered.[507] Increased activity may be demonstrated on bone scans.[508] The histopathology may be entirely unremarkable, although increased vascularity[509-511] and degeneration or proliferation of cartilage[506, 510] can be seen.[504]

The etiology is unknown. The history of a previous or coexistent viral or bacterial infection and the detection of pus within the mass suggest an infectious agent.

Lyme Arthritis

A newly recognized inflammatory articular condition is termed Lyme arthritis after the town in Connecticut in which it was first described.[512, 517, 527] Mono- or oligoarticular arthritis of large joints, especially the knee, is associated with inflammatory synovial fluid and hypertrophy, vascular proliferation, and cellular infiltration on synovial biopsy.[568] Permanent joint deformities do not occur. Although the etiology of Lyme arthritis is not known, it may be infectious in nature, based upon a geographic clustering of cases and the presence of a cutaneous lesion at the onset of the arthritis. The vector appears to be an ixodid tick.[527]

SUMMARY

Osseous, articular, and soft tissue structures may become involved in many infectious disorders. Bacteria, mycobacteria, spirochetes, fungi, viruses, rickettsiae, protozoa, and worms are all capable of affecting the musculoskeletal system. In many instances, radiographic features, although typical of an infection, do not allow diagnosis of a specific causative agent; in some cases, the distribution and the morphology of the lesions are sufficiently characteristic to suggest a single infectious process. In all cases, the roentgenograms must be interpreted in conjunction with clinical and pathologic manifestations.

REFERENCES

1. Jaffe HL: Metabolic, Degenerative and Inflammatory Diseases of Bones and Joints. Philadelphia, Lea & Febiger, 1972.
2. Felman AH, Shulman ST: Staphylococcal osteomyelitis, sepsis and pulmonary disease. Radiology *117*:649, 1975.
3. Amstutz HC: Complications of total hip replacement. Clin Orthop Rel Res *72*:123, 1970.
4. Salvati, EA, Wilson PD Jr: Long-term results of femoral head replacement. J Bone Joint Surg *55A*:516, 1973.
5. Schonholtz GJ, Borgia CA, Blair JD: Wound sepsis in orthopaedic surgery. J Bone Joint Surg *44A*:1548, 1962.
6. Green WT, Shannon JG: Osteomyelitis of infants. Arch Surg *32*:462, 1936.
7. Howard JB, McCracken GH Jr: The spectrum of group B streptococcal infections in infancy. Am J Dis Child *128*:815, 1974.
8. Hutto JH, Ayoub EM: Streptococcal osteomyelitis and arthritis in a neonate. Am J Dis Child *129*:1449, 1975.
9. Edwards MS, Baker CJ, Wagner ML, Taber LH, Barrett FF: An etiologic shift in infantile osteomyelitis: The emergence of the group B streptococcus. J Pediatr *93*:578, 1978.
10. McCook TA, Felman AH, Ayoub E: Streptococcal skeletal infections: Observations in four infants. Am J Roentgenol *130*:465, 1978.
11. Siskind B, Galliquez P, Wald ER: Group B beta-hemolytic streptococcal osteomyelitis/purulent arthritis in neonates: Report of three cases. J Pediatr *87*:659, 1975.
12. Newman JH: Review of septic arthritis throughout the antibiotic era. Ann Rheum Dis *35*:198, 1976.
13. Raff MJ, Melo JC: Anaerobic osteomyelitis. Medicine *57*:83, 1978.
14. Kluge R, Schmidt M, Barth WF: Pneumococcal arthritis. Ann Rheum Dis *32*:21, 1973.
15. Argen RJ: Suppurative pneumococcic arthritis. NY State J Med *64*:2573, 1964.
16. Torres J, Rathbun HK, Greenough WB III: Pneumococcal arthritis: Report of a case and review of the literature. Johns Hopkins Med J *132*:234, 1973.
17. Kauffman CA, Watanakunakorn C, Phair JP: Pneumococcal arthritis. J Rheumatol *3*:409, 1976.
18. Shawker TH, Dennis JM: Peri-articular calcifications in pyogenic arthritis. Am J Roentgenol *113*:650, 1971.
19. Pinals RS, Ropes MW: Meningococcal arthritis. Arthritis Rheum *7*:241, 1964.
20. Cattell J: Meningococcal meningitis with purulent arthritis. N Eng J Med *229*:49, 1943.
21. Bass M, Nothman G: Multiple purulent arthritis due to meningococcus in very early infancy. J Mt Sinai Hosp *12*:60, 1945.
22. Congeni B, Weiner DS: Meningococcal arthritis in children. Orthopedics *1*:477, 1978.
23. Ansell BM: Infective arthritis. *In* JT Scott (Ed): Copeman's Textbook of the Rheumatic Diseases. 5th Ed. Edinburgh, Churchill Livingstone, 1978, p 808.
24. Schein AJ: Articular manifestations of meningococcic infections. Arch Intern Med *62*:963, 1938.
25. Eichner HL, Dell JJ: Meningococcal arthritis. Arthritis Rheum *13*:272, 1970.
26. Hammerschlag MR, Baker CJ: Meningococcal osteomyelitis: Report of 2 cases associated with septic arthritis. J Pediatr *88*:519, 1976.
27. Koppes GM, Arnett FC: Group Y meningococcal arthritis: Case report. Milit Med *140*:861, 1975.
28. Sponzilli EE, Calabro JJ: Gonococcal arthritis in the newborn. JAMA *177*:919, 1961.
29. Graber WJ, Sanford JP, Ziff M: Sex incidence of gonococcal arthritis. Arthritis Rheum *3*:309, 1960.
30. Harris JRW, McCann JS, Mahony JDH: Gonococcal arthritis — a common rarity. Br J Vener Dis *49*:42, 1973.
31. Brown D: Gonococcal arthritis in pregnancy. South Med J *66*:693, 1973.
32. Fam A, McGillivray D, Stein J, Little H: Gonococcal arthritis: A report of six cases. Can Med Assoc J *108*:319, 1973.
33. Lightfoot RW Jr, Gotschlich EC: Gonococcal disease. Am J Med *56*:347, 1974.
34. Kohen DP: Neonatal gonococcal arthritis: Three cases and review of the literature. Pediatrics *53*:436, 1974.
35. Gelfand SH, Masi AT, Garcia-Kutzbach A: Spectrum of gonococcal arthritis: Evidence for sequential stages and clinical subgroups. J Rheumatol *2*:83, 1975.
36. Angevine CD, Hall CB, Jacox RF: A case of gonococcal osteomyelitis. A complication of gonococcal arthritis. Am J Dis Child *130*:1013, 1976.
37. Ackerman AB, Miller RC, Shapiro L: Gonococcemia and its cutaneous manifestations. Arch Dermatol *91*:227, 1965.
38. Linner JH: Suppurative myositis and purulent arthritis complicating acute gonorrhea; report of a case. JAMA *123*:757, 1943.
39. Handsfield HH, Weisner PJ, Holmes KK: Treatment of the gonococcal arthritis-dermatitis syndrome. Ann Intern Med *84*:661, 1976.
40. Ghormley RK, Deacon AE: Synovial membranes in various types of arthritis: study by differential stains. Am J Roentgenol *35*:740, 1936.
41. Cooperman MB: End results of gonorrheal arthritis: A review of 70 cases. Am J Surg *5*:241, 1928.
42. Cooperman MB: Gonococcus arthritis in infancy. Am J Dis Child *33*:932, 1927.
43. Garcia-Kutzbach A, Masi AT: Acute infectious agent arthritis (IAA): A detailed comparison of proved gonococcal and other blood-borne bacterial arthritis. J Rheumatol *1*:93, 1974.
44. Kahn G, Danielsson D: Septic gonococcal dermatitis. Arch Dermatol *99*:421, 1969.
45. Barr J, Danielsson D: Septic gonococcal dermatitis. Br Med J *1*:482, 1971.
46. Ludivico CL, Myers AR: Survey for immune complexes in disseminated gonococcal arthritis-dermatitis syndrome. Arthritis Rheum *22*:19, 1979.
47. Goldman J, Thompson S III, Jacobs N, Casey HL, Daugharty H, Wilson CH: Detection of circulating immune complexes using platelet aggregation in patients with disseminated gonococcal infection. Arthritis Rheum *18*:402, 1975.
48. Layfer LF, Parciany RK, Trenholme GM: Diagnosis of gonococcal arthritis by counterimmunoelectrophoresis: Detection of antigen and antibody in serum and synovial fluid. Arthritis Rheum *21*:572, 1978.
49. Walker LC, Ahlin TD, Tung KSK, Williams RC Jr: Circulating immune complexes in disseminated gonorrheal infection. Ann Intern Med *89*:28, 1978.
50. Goldenberg DL, Brandt KD, Cathcart ES, Cohen AS: Acute arthritis caused by gram-negative bacilli: A clinical characterization. Medicine *53*:197, 1974.
51. Miller JM, Engle RL Jr: Metastatic suppurative arthritis with subcutaneous emphysema caused by *Escherichia coli*. Am J Med *10*:241, 1951.
52. Bliznak J, Ramsey J: Emphysematous septic arthritis due to *Escherichia coli*. J Bone Joint Surg *58A*:138, 1976.
53. Holzman RS, Bishko F: Osteomyelitis in heroin addicts. Ann Intern Med *75*:693, 1971.
54. Lewis R, Gorbach S, Altner P: Spinal Pseudomonas chondro-osteomyelitis in heroin users. N Engl J Med *286*:1303, 1972.
55. Grieco MH: Pseudomonas arthritis and osteomyelitis. J Bone Joint Surg *54A*:1693, 1972.
56. Mandal AK, Fiala M, Oparah SS, Thadepalli H: Osteolytic lesion indicating pseudomonas sternal osteomyelitis. Arch Surg *111*:776, 1976.
57. Brand RA, Black H: Pseudomonas osteomyelitis following puncture wounds in children. J Bone Joint Surg *56A*:1637, 1974.
58. Chusid MJ, Jacobs WM, Sty JR: Pseudomonas arthritis following puncture wounds of the foot. J Pediatr *94*:429, 1979.
59. Miller EH, Semian DW: Gram-negative osteomyelitis following puncture wounds of the foot. J Bone Joint Surg *57A*:535, 1975.
60. Gordon SL, Evans C, Greer RB III: Pseudomonas osteomyelitis of the metatarsal sesamoid of the great toe. Clin Orthop Rel Res *99*:188, 1974.
61. Murphy JB: Bone and joint diseases in relation to typhoid fever. Surg Gynecol Obstet *23*:119, 1916.
62. Chari PR, Choudary HR, Dutt KP, Naidu ML: Typhoid osteomyelitis: Report of a case. Aust NZ J Surg *41*:174, 1971.
63. Groll A, Smith J: A case of disseminated typhoid osteitis. S Afr Med J *39*:417, 1965.
64. Mansoor IA: Typhoid osteomyelitis of the calcaneus due to direct inoculation. A case report. J Bone Joint Surg *49A*:732, 1967.
65. Miller GAH, Ridley M, Medd WE: Typhoid osteomyelitis of the spine. Br Med J *1*:1068, 1963.
66. Mnaýmneh W: Salmonella spondylitis. Report of 2 cases. Clin Orthop Rel Res *126*:235, 1977.
67. Porat S, Brezis M, Kopolovic J: *Salmonella typhi* osteomyelitis long after a fracture. J Bone Joint Surg *59A*:687, 1977.
68. Schweitzer G, Hoosen GM, Dunbar JM: *Salmonella typhi* spondylitis, an unusual presentation. S Afr Med J *45*:126, 1971.
69. David JR, Black RL: Salmonella arthritis. Medicine *39*:385, 1960.
70. Gordon HS, Hoffman SJ, Schultz A, Lomberg F: Serous arthritis of the knee joint. Report of a case caused by *Salmonella typhosa* and *Salmonella montevideo* in a child. JAMA *141*:460, 1949.
71. Hook EW, Campbell CG, Weens HS, Cooper GR: Salmonella osteomyelitis in patients with sickle cell anemia. N Engl J Med *257*;403, 1957.
72. Engh CA, Hughes JL, Abrams RC, Bowerman JW: Osteomyelitis in the patient with sickle-cell disease. Diagnosis and management. J Bone Joint Surg *53A*:1, 1971.

73. Specht EE: Hemoglobinopathic salmonella osteomyelitis. Orthopedic aspects. Clin Orthop Rel Res *79*:110, 1971.
74. Curtiss PH Jr: Some uncommon forms of osteomyelitis. Clin Orthop Rel Res *96*:84, 1973.
75. Charosky CB, Marcove RC: *Salmonella paratyphi* osteomyelitis. Report of a case simulating a giant cell tumor. Clin Orthop Rel Res *99*:190, 1974.
76. Berlof FE: Arthritis and intestinal infection. Acta Rheumatol Scand *9*:141, 1963.
77. Vartiainen J, Hurri L: Arthritis due to *Salmonella typhimurium*. Report of 12 cases of migratory arthritis in association with *Salmonella typhimurium* infection. Acta Med Scand *175*:771, 1964.
78. Aho K, Ahvonen P, Lassus A, Sairanen E, Sievers K, Tiilikainen A: HL-A 27 in reactive arthritis following infection. Ann Rheum Dis *34*:29, 1975.
79. Aho K, Ahvonen P, Lassus A, Sievers K, Tiilikainen A: HL-A 27 in reactive arthritis: A study of Yersinia arthritis and Reiter's disease. Arthritis Rheum *17*:521, 1974.
80. Jacobs JC: *Yersinia enterocolitica* arthritis. Pediatrics *55*:236, 1975.
81. Blum D, Viart P, Dachy A: Septicemie à *Yersinia enterocolitica* chez deux enfants atteints de thalassemie majeure. Arch Fr Pediatr *27*:445, 1970.
82. Mollaret HH: L'infection humaine à *Yersinia enterocolitica* en 1970, à la lumière de 642 cas récents, Aspects cliniques et perspectives épidémiologiques. Pathol Biol *19*:189, 1971.
83. Sebes JI, Mabry EH, Rabinowitz JG: Lung abscess and osteomyelitis of rib due to *Yersinia enterocolitica*. Chest *69*:546, 1976.
84. Thirumoorthi MC, Dajani AS: *Yersinia enterocolitica* osteomyelitis in a child. Am J Dis Child *132*:578, 1978.
85. Dyer RF, Romansky MJ, Holmes JR: Hemophilus pyarthrosis in an adult. Arch Intern Med *102*:580, 1958.
86. Hoaglund FT, Lord GP: *Hemophilus influenzae* septic arthritis in adults. Two case reports with review of previous cases. Arch Intern Med *119*:648, 1967.
87. Weaver JB, Sherwood L: Hematogenous pyarthrosis due to bacillus *Haemophilus influenzae* and *Corynebacterium xerosis*. Surgery *4*:908, 1938.
88. Wall JJ, Hunt DD: Acute hematogenous pyarthrosis caused by *Hemophilus influenzae*. J Bone Joint Surg *50A*:1657, 1968.
89. Patterson RL Jr, Levine DB: *Hemophilus influenzae* pyarthrosis in an adult. J Bone Joint Surg *47A*:1250, 1965.
90. Raff MJ, Dannaher CL: *Hemophilus influenzae* septic arthritis in adults. Report of a case and review of the literature. J Bone Joint Surg *56A*:408, 1974.
91. Norden CW, Sellers TF: *Hemophilus influenzae* pyarthrosis in an adult. JAMA *189*:694, 1964.
92. Krauss DS, Aronson MD, Gump DW, Newcombe DS: *Hemophilus influenzae* septic arthritis, a mimicker of gonococcal arthritis. Arthritis Rheum *17*:267, 1974.
93. McClatchey WM: Pseudopodagra from *Hemophilus influenzae* in an adult. Arthritis Rheum *22*:681, 1979.
94. Merselis JG Jr, Sellers TF Jr, Johnson JE III, Hook EW: *Hemophilus influenzae* meningitis in adults. Arch Intern Med *110*:837, 1962.
95. Oill PA, Chow AW, Flood TP, Guze LB: Adult *Haemophilus influenzae* type B vertebral osteomyelitis. A case report and review of the literature. Clin Orthop Rel Res *136*:253, 1978.
96. Hruby MA, Honig GR, Lolekha S., Gotoff SP: *Arizona hinshawii* osteomyelitis in sickle cell anemia. Am J Dis Child *125*:867, 1973.
97. Smilack JD, Goldberg MA: Bone and joint infection with *Arizona hinshawii*. Report of a case and review of the literature. Am J Med Sci *270*:503, 1975.
98. Ogden JA, Light TR: Pediatric osteomyelitis: II. *Arizona hinshawii* osteomyelitis. Clin Orthop Rel Res *139*:110, 1979.
99. Buchanan TM, Sulzer CR, Frix MK, Feldman RA: Brucellosis in the United States, 1960–1972. An abattoir-associated disease. Part I. Clinical features and therapy. Medicine *53*:403, 1974.
100. Buchanan TM, Faber LC, Feldman RA: Brucellosis in the United States, 1960–1972. An abattoir-associated disease. Part II. Diagnostic aspects. Medicine *53*:415, 1974.
101. Kelly PJ, Martin WJ, Schirger A, Weed LA: Brucellosis of the bones and joints. Experience with 36 patients. JAMA *174*:347, 1960.
102. Johnson EW, Weed LA: Brucellar bursitis. J Bone Joint Surg *36A*:133, 1954.
103. Kennedy JC: Notes on a case of chronic synovitis or bursitis due to organism of Mediterranean fever. J R Army Med Corps *2*:178, 1904.
104. Zammit F: Undulant fever spondylitis. Brit J Radiol *31*:683, 1958.
105. Papathanassiou BT, Papachristou G, Hartofilakidis-Garofalidis G: Brucellar spondylitis. Report of 6 cases. Acta Orthop Scand *43*:384, 1972.
106. Pritchard DJ: Granulomatous infections of bones and joints. Orthop Clin North Am *6*:1029, 1975.
107. Jacobson HG: Abnormalities of the Skeleton. Radiological Notes. Parts I and II. Chicago, Radiological Society of North America, 1973.
108. Rotes-Querol J: Osteo-articular sites of brucellosis. Ann Rheum Dis *16*:63, 1957.
109. Atlas E, Belding ME: *Serratia marcescens* arthritis requiring amputation. JAMA *204*:167, 1968.
110. Rogala EJ, Cruess RL: Multiple pyogenic arthritis due to *Serratia marcescens* following renal homotransplantation. Report of a case. J Bone Joint Surg *54A*:1283, 1972.
111. Martin CM, Merrill RH, Barrett O Jr: Arthritis due to Serratia. J Bone Joint Surg *52A*:1450, 1970.
112. Yosowitz GM: Serratia arthritis of the hip. Clin Orthop Rel Res *85*:122, 1972.
113. Dorwart BB, Abrutyn E, Schumacher HR: Serratia arthritis. Medical eradication of infection in a patient with rheumatoid arthritis. JAMA *225*:1642, 1973.
114. Dean HM, Post RM: Fatal infection with *Aeromonas hydrophila* in a patient with acute myelogenous leukemia. Ann Intern Med *66*:1117, 1967
115. Chmel H, Armstrong D: Acute arthritis caused by *Aeromonas hydrophila*. Clinical and therapeutic aspects. Arthritis Rheum *19*:169, 1976.
116. Morrey BF, Fitzgerald RH, Kelly PJ, Dobyns JH, Washington JA II: Diphtheroid osteomyelitis. J Bone Joint Surg *59A*:527, 1977.
117. Johnson WD, Kaye D: Serious infections caused by diphtheroids. Ann NY Acad Sci *174*:568, 1970.
118. Fitzgerald RH Jr, Peterson LFA, Washington JA II, Van Scoy RE, Coventry MB: Bacterial colonization of wounds and sepsis in total hip arthroplasty. J Bone Joint Surg *55A*:1242, 1973.
119. Tomlinson AJ: Human pathogenetic coryneform bacteria: Their differentiation and significance in public health today. J Appl Bacteriol *29*:131, 1966.
120. Kaplan K, Weinstein L: Diphtheroid infections of man. Ann Intern Med *70*:919, 1969.
121. Torg JS, Lammot TR III: Septic arthritis of the knee due to *Clostridium welchii*. Report of two cases. J Bone Joint Surg *50A*:1233, 1968.
122. Lovell WW: Infection of the knee joint by *Clostridium welchii*. J Bone Joint Surg *28*:398, 1946.
123. Korn JA, Gilbert MS, Siffert RS, Jacobson JH: *Clostridium welchii* arthritis. Case report. J Bone Joint Surg *57A*:555, 1975.
124. Nolan B, Leers W-D, Schatzker J: Septic arthritis of the knee due to *Clostridium bifermentans*. Report of a case. J Bone Joint Surg *54A*:1275, 1972.
125. Schiller M, Donnelly PJ, Melo JC, Raff MJ: *Clostridium perfringens* septic arthritis. Report of a case and review of the literature. Clin Orthop Rel Res *139*:92, 1979.
126. Schlenker JD, Vega G, Heiple KG: Clostridium pyoarthritis of the shoulder associated with multiple myeloma. Clin Orthop Rel Res *88*:89, 1972.
127. Curtiss PH, Klein L: Destruction of articular cartilage in septic arthritis. I. In vitro studies. J Bone Joint Surg *45A*:797, 1963.
128. Evans ES: Changing patterns in skeletal and articular tuberculosis. Proc R Soc Med *50*:571, 1957.
129. DeQuervain F, Hunziker H: Die Statistik der chirurgischen Tuberkulosen in Basel fur das Jahr 1913. Cor-B1 Schweiz Arzte *49*:761, 1919.
130. Johansson S: Über die Knochen- und Gelenktuberkulose im Kindesalter. Jena, Gustav Fischer, 1926.
131. Cherubin CE: The medical sequelae of narcotic addiction. Ann Intern Med *67*:23, 1967.
132. Jaffe RB, Koschman EB: Intravenous drug abuse: Pulmonary, cardiac, and vascular complications. Am J Roentgenol *109*:107, 1970.
133. Firooznia H, Seliger G, Abrams RM, Valensi V, Shamoun J: Disseminated extrapulmonary tuberculosis in association with heroin addiction. Radiology *109*:291, 1973.
134. Enarson DA, Fujii M, Nakielna EM, Grzybowski S: Bone and joint tuberculosis: A continuing problem. Can Med Assoc J *120*:139, 1979.
135. Myers JA: Tuberculosis Among Children and Adults. 3rd ed. Springfield, Ill, Charles C Thomas, 1951, p 215.
136. Griffiths DH: Orthopaedic tuberculosis. Br J Hosp Med *14*:158, 1975.
137. Pimon LH, Waugh W: Tuberculous tenosynovitis. J Bone Joint Surg *39B*:91, 1957.
138. Mills TJ, Owen R, Strach EH: Early diagnosis of bone and joint tuberculosis in children. Lancet *2*:57, 1956.
139. Smith EG, Davison WR: Egyptian Mummies. London, G Allen & Unwin, 1924, p. 157.
140. Hippocrates: The Genuine Works of Hippocrates. Translated by F Adams. London, The Sydenham Society, 1849.
141. Pott P: Remarks on that kind of palsy of the lower limbs which is frequently found to accompany a curvature of the spine. London, J Johnson, 1779.
142. Hodgson AR: Infectious disease of the spine. *In* RH Rothman, FA Simeone (Eds): *The Spine*. Philadelphia, WB Saunders Co, 1975, p 567.
143. Schmorl G, Junghans H: The Human Spine in Health and Disease. 2nd Amer Ed. Translated by EF Besemann. New York, Grune & Stratton, 1971.

144. Jacobs P: Osteo-articular tuberculosis in coloured immigrants: A radiological study. Clin Radiol *15*:59, 1964.
145. Bell D, Cockshott WP: Tuberculosis of the vertebral pedicles. Radiology *99*:43, 1971.
146. Westermark N, Forssman G: The roentgen diagnosis of tuberculous spondylitis. Acta Radiol *19*:207, 1938.
147. Blacklock JWS: Injury as an aetiological factor in tuberculosis. Proc R Soc Med *50*:61, 1957.
148. Heniques CQ: Osteomyelitis as a complication in urology with special reference to the paravertebral venous plexus. Br J Surg *46*:19, 1958.
149. Tuli SM: Tuberculosis of the craniovertebral region. Clin Orthop Rel Res *104*:209, 1974.
150. Martin NS: Tuberculosis of the spine. A study of the results of treatment during the last twenty-five years. J Bone Joint Surg *52B*:613, 1970.
151. Bailey HL, Gabriel M, Hodgson AR, Shin JS: Tuberculosis of the spine in children. J Bone Joint Surg *54A*:1633, 1972.
152. Graves VB, Schrieber MH: Tuberculous psoas muscle abscess. J Can Assoc Radiol *24*:268, 1973.
153. Goldblatt M, Cremin BJ: Osteo-articular tuberculosis: Its presentation in coloured races. Clin Radiol *29*:669, 1978.
154. Paus B: Tumour, tuberculosis, and osteomyelitis of the spine. Acta Orthop Scand *44*:372, 1973.
155. Hellstadius A: Tuberculous necrosis of the entire vertebral body with negative x-ray findings. Acta Orthop Scand *16*:163, 1946.
156. Boeminghaus H: Senkungsabszesse. Dtsch Med Wochenschr *59*:1559, 1933.
157. Fang HSY, Ong GB, Hodgson AR: Anterior spinal fusion. The operative approaches. Clin Orthop Rel Res *35*:16, 1964.
158. Kyle J: Psoas abscess in Crohn's disease. Gastroenterology *61*:149, 1971.
159. Tordoir BM: Spasm of and abscess formation in psoas muscle caused by renal calculus. J Urol *66*:638, 1951.
160. Zadek I: Acute nontuberculous psoas abscess. J Bone Joint Surg *32A*:433, 1950.
161. O'Brien JP: The manifestation of arrested bone growth. The appearance of a vertebra within a vertebra. J Bone Joint Surg *51A*:1376, 1969.
162. Yau ACMC, Hsu LCS, O'Brien JP, Hodgson AR: Tuberculous kyphosis. Correction with spinal osteotomy, halo-pelvic distraction, and anterior and posterior fusion. J Bone Joint Surg *56A*:1419, 1974.
163. Lovett RW: Lateral deviation of the spine as a diagnostic symptom in Pott's disease. Trans Am Orthop Assoc *3*:182, 1890.
164. Cleveland M, Bosworth DM: The pathology of tuberculosis of the spine. J Bone Joint Surg *24*:527, 1942.
165. O'Connor BT, Steel WM, Sanders R: Disseminated bone tuberculosis. J Bone Joint Surg *52A*:537, 1970.
166. Alexander GH, Mansuy MM: Disseminated bone tuberculosis (so-called multiple cystic tuberculosis). Radiology *55*:839, 1950.
167. Wolstein D, Rabinowitz JG, Twersky J: Tuberculosis of the rib. J Can Assoc Radiol *25*:307, 1974.
168. Scoggin CH, Schwarz MI, Dixon BW, Durrance JR: Tuberculosis of the skull. Arch Intern Med *136*:1154, 1976.
169. Hartofilakidis-Garofalidis G: Cystic tuberculosis of the patella. Report of three cases. J Bone Joint Surg *51A*:582, 1969.
170. Hsieh CK, Miltner LJ, Chang CP: Tuberculosis of the shaft of the large long bones of the extremities. J Bone Joint Surg *16*:545, 1934.
171. Jüngling O: Ostitis tuberculosa multiplex cystica—eine eigenartige Form der Knochentuberkulose. Fortschr Geb Roentgenstr Nuklearmed *27*:375, 1920.
172. Ellis FA: Jungling's "ostitis tuberculosa multiplex cystoides" is not cystic tuberculosis osteitis. Acta Med Scand *104*:221, 1940.
173. Girdwood W: Multiple cystic tuberculosis of bone (Jüngling's disease). Report of a case. J Bone Joint Surg *35B*:285, 1953.
174. Komins C: Multiple cystic tuberculosis; review and revised nomenclature. Br J Radiol *25*:1, 1952.
175. Edeiken J, De Palma Af, Moskowitz H, Smythe V: "Cystic" tuberculosis of bone. Clin Orthop Rel Res *28*:163, 1963.
176. Karlén A: On cystic tuberculosis of bone. Acta Orthop Scand *31*:163, 1961.
177. Feldman F, Auerbach R, Johnston A: Tuberculous dactylitis in the adult. Am J Roentgenol *112*:460, 1971.
178. Hardy JB, Hartmann JR: Tuberculosis dactylitis in childhood. Prognosis. J Pediatr *30*:146, 1947.
179. Herzfeld G, Tod MC: Tuberculous dactylitis in infancy. Arch Dis Child *1*:295, 1926.
180. Robins RH: Tuberculosis of the wrist and hand. Br J Surg *54*:211, 1967.
181. König F: Die Tuberkulose der Menschlichen Gelenke Sowie der Brustwand und des Schadels. Berlin, August Hirschwald, 1906.
182. Auerbach O: Tuberculosis of skeletal system. Bull Seaview Hosp *6*:117, 1941.
183. Poppel MH, Lawrence LR, Jacobson HG, Stein J: Skeletal tuberculosis: Roentgenographic survey with reconsideration of diagnostic criteria. Am J Roentgenol *70*:936, 1953.
184. Reisner D: Relations between extrapulmonary and pulmonary tuberculosis. Am Rev Tuberc *30*:375, 1934.
185. Auerbach O, Stemmerman MG: Roentgen interpretation of pathology in Pott's disease. Am J Roentgenol *52*:57, 1944.
186. Mann KJ: Lung lesions in skeletal tuberculosis: Review of 500 cases. Lancet *2*:744, 1946.
187. Steinbach HL: Infections of bone. Semin Roentgenol *1*:337, 1966.
188. Poznanski AK: The Hand in Radiologic Diagnosis. Philadelphia, WB Saunders Co, 1974.
189. Berney S, Goldstein M, Bishko F: Clinical and diagnostic features of tuberculous arthritis. Am J Med *53*:36, 1972.
190. Murray RC: Tuberculosis of the knee; follow-up investigation of old cases. Br Med J *2*:10, 1940.
191. Rose GK: Tuberculosis of the knee joint. Br J Clin Pract *13*:241, 1959.
192. Wolfgang GL: Tuberculous joint infection. Clin Orthop Rel Res *136*:275, 1978.
193. Wallace R, Cohen AS: Tuberculous arthritis. A report on two cases with review of biopsy and synovial fluid findings. Am J Med *61*:277, 1976.
194. Phemister DB, Hatcher CH: Correlation of pathological and roentgenological findings in the diagnosis of tuberculous arthritis. Am J Roentgenol *29*:736, 1933.
195. Stenstrom B: Über Phalangentuberkulose bei alteren Individuen. Acta Radiol *16*:471, 1935.
196. Polo G DeV, Coradin CC: Tuberculosis of the hip: Treatment with closed irrigation and suction using streptomycin. Clin Orthop Rel Res *110*:154, 1975.
197. Flatman JG: Hip disease with referred pain to the knee. JAMA *234*:967, 1975.
198. Brashear HR, Winfield HG: Tuberculosis of the wrist: a report of ten cases. South Med J *68*:1345, 1975.
199. Davis JA, Bluestone R: Case report 84. Skel Radiol *4*:41, 1979.
200. David-Chausse J, Dehais J, Bullier R, Chabellard JP: Les ostéo-arthrites et synovites tuberculeuses a foyers multiples. A propos de 10 observations. Revue Rhum *45*:463, 1978.
201. Mayers LB: Carpal tunnel syndrome secondary to tuberculosis. Arch Neurol *10*:426, 1964.
202. Klofkorn RW, Steigerwald JC: Carpal tunnel syndrome as the initial manifestation of tuberculosis. Amer J Med *60*:583, 1976.
203. Meyerding HW, Mrox RJ: Tuberculosis of the greater trochanter. JAMA *101*:1308, 1933.
204. McNeur JC, Pritchard AE: Tuberculosis of the greater trochanter. J Bone Joint Surg *37B*:246, 1955.
205. Sharma SV, Varma BP, Khanna S: Dystrophic calcification in tubercular lesions of bursae. Acta Orthop Scand *49*:445, 1978.
206. Thrap-Meyer H: Generalized BCG infection in man. I. Clinical report. Acta Tuberc Scandinav *29*:173, 1954.
207. Waaler E, Oeding P: Generalized BCG infection in man. III. Autopsy findings. Acta Tuberc Scandinav *29*:188, 1954.
208. Morbak A: Osteomyelitis ulnae after BCG vaccination. Nordisk Medicin *52*:1482, 1954.
209. Imerslund O, Jonsen T: Lupus vulgaris and multiple bone lesions caused by BCG. Acta Tuberc Scandinav *30*:116, 1955.
210. Haraldsson S: Osteitis tuberculosa fistulosa following vaccination with BCG stain. Acta Orth Scandinav *29*:121, 1959.
211. Felländer M: Tuberculous osteitis following BCG vaccination. Acta Orthop Scandinav *33*:116, 1963.
212. Foucard T, Hjelmstedt A: BCG-osteomyelitis and -osteoarthritis as a complication following BCG vaccination. Acta Orthop Scandinav *42*:142, 1971.
213. Bang J, Engbaek HC, Nielsen E: Osteomyelitis following BCG vaccination. Acta Tuberc Scand *39*:203, 1960.
214. Eng J, Aaneland T: BCG osteitis in a child: a bacteriological investigation. Scand J Resp Dis *47*:182, 1966.
215. Virtanen S, Lindgren I: Osteomyelitis of the femur caused by BCG. Acta Tuberc Scand *41*:260, 1962.
216. Bergdahl S, Felländer M, Robertson B: BCG osteomyelitis. Experience in the Stockholm region over the years 1961–1974. J Bone Joint Surg *58B*: 212, 1976.
217. Mortensson W, Eklöf O, Jorulf H: Radiologic aspects of BCG-osteomyelitis in infants and children. Acta Radiol (Diag) *17*:845, 1976.
218. Torklus DV: Bovine tuberkulöse Osteomyelitis nach BCH-Impfung. Z Orthop *115*:249, 1977.
219. Kallesoe O, Jespersen A: Metastatic osteomyelitis following BCG vaccination. Acta Orthop Scand *49*:134, 1978.
220. Chapman JS: The ecology of the atypical mycobacteria. Arch Environ Health *22*:41, 1971.
221. Runyon EH: Anonymous mycobacteria in pulmonary disease. Med Clin N Am *43*:273, 1959.
222. Omar MM: Case report 26. Skel Radiol *1*:245, 1977.
223. Danigelis JA, Long RE: Anonymous mycobacterial osteomyelitis. A case report of a six-year old child. Radiology *93*:353, 1969.
224. Cheatum DE, Hudman V, Jones SR: Chronic arthritis due to mycobac-

terium intracellulare. Sacroiliac, knee, and carpal tunnel involvement in a young man and response to chemotherapy. Arth Rheum *19*:777, 1976.
225. Dorff GJ, Frerichs L, Zabransky RJ, Jacobs P, Spankus JD: Musculoskeletal infections due to mycobacterium kansasii. Clin Orth Rel Res *136*:244, 1978.
226. Halpern AA, Nagel DA: Mycobacterium fortuitum infections: a review with two illustrative cases. Clin Orth Rel Res *136*:247, 1978.
227. Girard DE, Bagby GC Jr, Walsh JR: Destructive polyarthritis secondary to myobacterium kansasii. Arth Rheum *16*:665, 1973.
228. Stratton CW, Phelps DB, Reller LB: Tuberculoid tenosynovitis and carpal tunnel syndrome caused by mycobacterium szulgai. Amer J Med *65*: 349, 1978.
229. Ellis W: Multiple bone lesions caused by avian-battey mycobacteria. Report of a case. J Bone Joint Surg *56B*:323, 1974.
230. Binford CH: Leprosy—a model in geographic pathology. Internat Path *7*:6, 1966.
231. Enna CD, Jacobson RR, Rausch RO: Bone changes in leprosy: a correlation of clinical and radiographic features. Radiology *100*:295, 1971.
232. Paterson DE, Rad M: Bone changes in leprosy, their incidence, progress, prevention, and arrest. Int J Leprosy *29*:393, 1961.
233. Sawtschenko J: Zur Frage Über die Veränderungen der Knochen beim Aussatze (Osteitis et Osteomyelitis leprosa). Beitr Path Anat *9*:241, 1890.
234. Moller-Christensen V, Bakke SN, Melsom RS, Waaler AE: Changes in anterior nasal spine and alveolar process of maxillary bone in leprosy. Int J Lepr *20*:335, 1952.
235. Job CK, Karat S, Karat ABA: Pathological study of nasal deformity in lepromatous leprosy. Lepr India *40*:42, 1968.
236. Karat S, Karat ABA, Foster R: Radiological changes in the bones of the limbs in leprosy. Lepr Rev *39*:147, 1968.
237. Goergen TG, Resnick D, Lomonaco A, O'Dell CW Jr: Radionuclide bone scan abnormalities in leprosy: Case reports. J Nucl Med *17*:788, 1976.
238. Hirschberg M, Biehler R: Lepra der Knochen. Dermatol Ztschr *16*:415, 1909.
239. Louie JS, Koransky JR, Cohen AH: Lepra cells in synovial fluid of a patient with erythema nodosum leprosum. N Engl J Med *289*:1410, 1973.
240. Karat ABA, Karat S, Job CK, Furness MA: Acute exudative arthritis in leprosy: Rheumatoid arthritis–like syndrome in association with erythema nodosum leprosum. Br Med J *3*:770, 1967.
241. Faget GH, Mayoral A: Bone changes in leprosy: A clinical and roentgenological study of 505 cases. Radiology *42*:1, 1944.
242. Esguerra-Gomez G, Acosta E: Bone and joint lesions in leprosy: A radiologic study. Radiology *50*:619, 1948.
243. Wastie ML: Radiological changes in serial x-rays of the foot and tarsus in leprosy. Clin Radiol *26*:285, 1975.
244. Harris JR, Brand PW: Patterns of disintegration of the tarsus in the anaesthetic foot. J Bone Joint Surg *48B*:4, 1966.
245. Warren G: Tarsal bone disintegration in leprosy. J Bone Joint Surg *53B*:688, 1971.
246. Skinsnes OK, Sakurai I, Aquino TI: Pathogenesis of extremity deformity in leprosy. Int J Lepr *40*:375, 1972.
247. Wahi PL, Kaur S, Vadwa MB, Sodhi JS, Chakravarti RN: Peripheral arteriographic studies in leprosy. Clin Radiol *27*:365, 1976.
248. Lechat MF: Bone lesions in leprosy. Int J Lepr *30*:125, 1962.
249. Barnetson J: Pathogenesis of bone changes in neural leprosy. Int J Lepr *19*:297, 1951.
250. Trapnell DH: Calcification of nerves in leprosy. Br J Radiol *38*:796, 1965.
251. Ellis BP: Calcification of the ulnar nerve in leprosy. Lepr Rev *46*:297, 1975.
252. Lichtman DM, Swafford AW, Kerr DM: Calcified abscess in the ulnar nerve in a patient with leprosy. A case report. J Bone Joint Surg *61A*:620, 1979.
253. Heyman A: Syphilis *In* TR Harrison, et al (Eds): Principles of Internal Medicine. 4th Ed. New York, McGraw-Hill Book Co, 1962, p 1068.
254. Herxheimer G: Die pathologische Anatomie der angeborenen Syphilis. Allgemeime Gesichtspunkte. Verh Dtsch Ges Pathol *23*:144, 1928.
255. McCord JR: Syphilis and pregnancy. A clinical study of 2150 cases. JAMA *105*:89, 1935.
256. Cremin BJ, Fisher RM: The lesions of congenital syphilis. Br J Radiol *43*:333, 1970.
257. Schneider P: Über die Organveränderungen bei der angeborenen Fruhsyphilis. Verh Dtsch Ges Pathol *23*:177, 1928.
258. McLean S: The roentgenographic and pathologic aspects of congenital osseous syphilis. Am J Dis Child *41*:130, 1931.
259. McLean S: The correlation of the roentgenographic and pathologic aspects of congenital osseous syphilis with particular reference to the first months of life. Am J Dis Child *41*:363, 1931.
260. Levin EJ: Healing in congenital osseous syphilis. Am J Roentgenol *110*:591, 1970.
261. Chipps BE, Swischuk LE, Voelter WW: Single bone involvement in congenital syphilis. Pediatr Radiol *5*:50, 1976.
262. Lilien LD, Harris VJ, Pildes RS: Congenital syphilitic osteitis of scapulae and ribs. Pediatr Radiol *6*:183, 1977.
263. Fraenkel E: Die kongenitale Knochensyphilis im Röntgenbilde. Fortschr Geb Roentgenstr Nuklearmed, Suppl 26, 1911.
264. Pendergrass EP, Gilman RL, Castleton KB: Bone lesions in tardive heredosyphilis. Am J Roentgenol *24*:234, 1930.
265. Hutchinson J: Syphilis. London, Cassell & Co, 1887.
266. Bauer WH: Tooth buds and jaws in patients with congenital syphilis. Correlation between distribution of *Treponema pallidum* and tissue reaction. Am J Pathol *20*:297, 1944.
267. Clutton HH: Symmetrical synovitis of the knee in hereditary syphilis. Lancet *1*:391, 1886.
268. Reynolds FW, Wasserman H: Destructive osseous lesions in early syphilis. Arch Intern Med *69*:263, 1942.
269. Bauer MF, Caravati CM: Osteolytic lesions in early syphilis. Br J Vener Dis *43*:175, 1967.
270. Ehrlich I, Kricun ME: Radiographic findings in early acquired syphilis: Case report and critical review. Am J Roentgenol *127*:789, 1976.
271. Ungerman AH, Vicary WH, Eldridge WW: Luetic osteitis simulating malignant disease. Am J Roentgenol *40*:224, 1938.
272. Truog CP: Bone lesions in acquired syphilis. Radiology *40*:1, 1943.
273. Speed JS, Boyd HB: Bone syphilis. South Med J *29*:371, 1936.
274. Wile UJ, Senear FE: A study of the involvement of the bones and joints in early syphilis. Am J Med Sci *152*:689, 1916.
275. Roy RB, Laird SM: Acute periostitis in early acquired syphilis. Br J Vener Dis *49*:555, 1973.
276. Metcalfe JW: Syphilitic osteoperiostitis — skull, ribs, and phalanges. Report of a case. US Nav Med Bull *49*:528, 1949.
277. Sante LR: Radiographic manifestations of syphilitic diseases of bone. Am J Syph *12*:510, 1928.
278. Skapinker S, Minnaar D: Syphilitic diseases of the long bones in the Bantu. J Bone Joint Surg *33B*:578, 1951.
279. Dismukes WE, Delgado DG, Mallernee SV, Myers TC: Destructive bone disease in early syphilis. JAMA *236*:2646, 1976.
280. Thompson RG, Preston RH: Lesions of the skull in secondary syphilis. Am J Syph *36*:332, 1952.
281. Burrows HJ: Pathological fracture of the humerus complicating late secondary syphilis. Br J Surg *24*:452, 1937.
282. Johns D: Syphilitic disorders of the spine. Report of two cases. J Bone Joint Surg *52B*:724, 1970.
283. Gangolphe M: Contribution à l'étude des localisations articulaires de la syphilis tertiare. De l'osteoarthrite syphilitique. Ann Dermatol Syphiligr *6*:449, 1885.
284. Reginato AJ, Schumacher HR, Jimenez S, Maurer K: Synovitis in secondary syphilis. Clinical, light, and electron microscopic studies. Arthritis Rheum *22*:170, 1979.
285. Smith JL, Israel CW, McCrary JA, Harner RE: Recovery of *Treponema pallidum* from aqueous humor removed at cataract surgery in man by passive transfer to rabbit testis. Am J Ophthalmol *65*:242, 1968.
286. Borchard: Ueber luetische Gelenkentzundungen. Dtsch Ztschr Chir *61*:110, 1901.
287. Kling DH: Syphilitic arthritis with effusion. Am J Med Sci *183*:538, 1932.
288. Gerster JC, Weintraub A, Vischer TL, Fallet GH: Secondary syphilis revealed by rheumatic complaints. J Rheumatol *4*:197, 1977.
289. Kahn MF, Baillet F, Amouroux J, DeSeze S: Le rhumatisme inflammatoire subaigu de la syphilis secondaire. A propos de quatre observations. Rev Rhum Mal Osteoartic *37*:431, 1970.
290. Cockshott WP, Davies AGM: Tumoral gummatous yaws. J Bone Joint Surg *42B*:785, 1960.
291. Jones BS: Doigt en lorgnette and concentric bone atrophy associated with healed yaws osteitis. Report of two cases. J Bone Joint Surg *54B*:341, 1972.
292. Reeder MM: Tropical diseases of the foot. Semin Roentgenol *5*:378, 1970.
293. Riseborough AW, Joske RA, Vaughan BF: Hand deformities due to yaws in Western Australian aborigines. Clin Radiol *12*:109, 1961.
294. Ngu VA: Medicine in tropics: Tropical ulcers. Br Med J *1*:283, 1967.
295. Kolawole TM, Bohrer SP: Ulcer osteoma — bone response to tropical ulcer. Am J Roentgenol *109*:611, 1970.
296. Brown JS, Middlemiss JH: Bone changes in tropical ulcer. Br J Radiol *29*:213, 1956.
297. Lodwick GS: Reactive response to local injury in bone. Radiol Clin North Am *2*:209, 1964.
298. Adamson PB: Tropical ulcer in British Somaliland. J Trop Med Hyg *52*:68, 1949.
299. Smith EC: Note on bacteriology of tropical ulcers. W Afr Med J *4*:68, 1931.
300. Thompson IG: Pathogenesis of tropical ulcer amongst Hausas of Northern Nigeria. Trans R Soc Trop Med Hyg *50*:485, 1956.

301. Edwards GA: Clinical characteristics of leptospirosis. Am J Med *27*:4, 1959.
302. Sutliff WD, Shepard R, Dunham WB: Acute *Leptospira pomona* arthritis and myocarditis. Ann Intern Med *39*:134, 1952.
303. Brown T McP, Nunemaker JC: Rat-bite fever. A review of the American cases with re-evaluation of etiology; report of cases. Bull Johns Hopkins Hosp *70*:201, 1942.
304. Nathan MH, Radman WP, Barton HL: Osseous actinomycosis of the head and neck. Am J Roentgenol *87*:1048, 1962.
305. Rhangos WC, Chick EW: Mycotic infections of bone. South Med J *57*:664, 1964.
306. Pritchard DJ: Granulomatous infections of bones and joints. Orthop Clin North Am *6*:1029, 1975.
307. Martinelli B, Tagliapietra EA: Actinomycosis of the arm. Bull Hosp J Dis *31*:31, 1970.
308. Simpson WM, McIntosh CA: Actinomycosis of the vertebrae (actinomycotic Pott's disease). Arch Surg *14*:1166, 1927.
309. Cope, VZ: Actinomycosis of bone with special reference to infection of the vertebral column. J Bone Joint Surg *33B*:205, 1951.
310. Baylin GJ, Wear JM: Blastomycosis and actinomycosis of spine. Am J Roentgenol *69*:395, 1953.
311. Young WB: Actinomycosis with involvement of the vertebral column. Clin Radiol *11*:175, 1960.
312. Collins VP, Gellhorn A, Trimble JR: The coincidence of cryptococcosis and disease of the reticulo-endothelial and lymphatic systems. Cancer *4*:883, 1951.
313. Shields LH: Disseminated cryptococcosis producing a sarcoid type reaction. The report of a case treated with amphotericin B. Arch Intern Med *104*:763, 1959.
314. Littman ML: Cryptococcosis (torulosis). Am J Med *27*:976, 1959.
315. Chleboun J, Nade S: Skeletal cryptococcosis. J Bone Joint Surg *59A*:509, 1977.
316. Woolfitt R, Park H-M, Greene M: Localized cryptococcal osteomyelitis. Radiology *120*:290, 1976.
317. Meredith HC, John JF Jr, Rogers CI, Gooneratne N, Kreutner A Jr: Case report 89. Skel Radiol *4*:53, 1979.
318. Tchang FKM, Gilardi GL: Osteomyelitis due to *Torulopsis inconspicua*. Report of a case. J Bone Joint Surg *55A*:1739, 1973.
319. Bryan CS: Vertebral osteomyelitis due to *Cryptococcus neoformans*. Case report. J Bone Joint Surg *59A*:275, 1977.
320. Levinson DJ, Silcox DC, Rippon JW, Thomsen S: Septic arthritis due to nonencapsulated *Cryptococcus neoformans* with coexisting sarcoidosis. Arthritis Rheum *17*:1037, 1974.
321. Chand K, Lall KS: Cryptococcosis (torulosis, European blastomycosis) of the knee joint. A case report with review of the literature. Acta Orthop Scand *47*:432, 1976.
322. Ley A, Jacas R, Oliveras C: Torula granuloma of the cervical spinal cord. J Neurosurg *8*:327, 1951.
323. Rao SB, Rao KS, Dinakar I: Spinal extradural cryptococcal granuloma. A case report. Neurol India *18*:192, 1970.
324. Ramamurthi B, Anguli VC: Intramedullary cryptococcic granuloma of the spinal cord. J Neurosurg *11*:622, 1954.
325. Litvinoff J, Nelson M: Extradural lumbar cryptococcosis. Case report. J Neurosurg *49*:921, 1978.
326. Cherniss EI, Waisbren BA: North American blastomycosis: A clinical study of 40 cases. Ann Intern Med *44*:105, 1956.
327. Riegler HF, Goldstein LA, Betts RF: Blastomycosis osteomyelitis. Clin Orthop Rel Res *100*:225, 1974.
328. Gelman MI, Everts CS; Blastomycotic dactylitis. Radiology *107*:331, 1973.
329. Gehweiler JA, Capp MP, Chick EW: Observations on the roentgen patterns in blastomycosis of bone. A review of cases from the blastomycosis study of the Veterans Administration and Duke University Medical Center. Am J Roentgenol *108*:497, 1970.
330. Gill JA, Gerald B: Blastomycosis in childhood. Radiology *91*:965, 1968.
331. Joyce PF, Sundarim M, Burdge RE, Riaz MA: A rare clinical presentation of blastomycosis. Skel Radiol *2*:239, 1978.
332. Sanders LL: Blastomycosis arthritis. Arthritis Rheum *10*:91, 1967.
333. Dickson EC, Gifford MA: Coccidioides infection (coccidioidomycosis): Primary type of infection. Arch Intern Med *62*:853, 1938.
334. Conaty JP, Biddle M, McKeever FM: Osseous coccidioidal granuloma. J Bone Joint Surg *41A*:1109, 1959.
335. Dalinka MK, Dinnenberg S, Greendyke WH, Hopkins R: Roentgenographic features of osseous coccidioidomycosis and differential diagnosis. J Bone Joint Surg *53A*:1157, 1971.
336. Wesselius LJ, Brooks RJ, Gall EP: Vertebral coccidioidomycosis presenting as Pott's disease. JAMA *238*:1397, 1977.
337. Santos GH, Cook WA: Vertebral coccidioidomycosis. Unusual polymorphic disease. NY State J Med *72*:2784, 1972.
338. Eller JL, Siebert PE: Sclerotic vertebral bodies: An unusual manifestation of disseminated coccidioidomycosis. Radiology *93*:1099, 1969.
339. Cortner JW, Schwartzmann JR: Bone lesions in disseminated coccidioidomycosis. Ariz Med *14*:401, 1957.
340. Bisla RS, Taber TH Jr: Coccidioidomycosis of bone and joints. Clin Orthop Rel Res *121*:196, 1976.
341. Armbruster TG, Goergen TG, Resnick D, Catanzaro A: Utility of bone scanning in disseminated coccidioidomycosis: Case report. J Nucl Med *18*:450, 1977.
342. Rettig AC, Evanski PM, Waugh TR, Prietto CA: Primary coccidioidal synovitis of the knee. A report of four cases and review of the literature. Clin Orthop Rel Res *132*:187, 1978.
343. Pankovich AM, Jevtic MM: Coccidioidal infection of the hip. A case report. J Bone Joint Surg *55A*:1525, 1973.
344. Greenman R, Becker J, Campbell G, Remington J: Coccidioidal synovitis of the knee. Arch Intern Med *135*:526, 1975.
345. Pollock S, Morris J, Murray W: Coccidioidal synovitis of the knee. J Bone Joint Surg *49A*:1397, 1967.
346. Haug WA, Merrifield RC: Coccidioidal villous synovitis. Am J Clin Pathol *31*:165, 1959.
347. Iverson RE, Vistnes LM: Coccidioidomycosis tenosynovitis in the hand. J Bone Joint Surg *55A*:413, 1973.
348. Danzig LA, Fierer J: Coccidioidomycosis of the extensor tenosynovium of the wrist. A case report. Clin Orthop Rel Res *129*:245, 1977.
349. Winter WG, Larson RK, Honeggar MM, Jacobsen DT, Pappagianis D, Huntington RW: Coccidioidal arthritis and its treatment — 1975. J Bone Joint Surg *57A*:1152, 1976.
350. Klingberg WG: Generalized histoplasmosis in infants and children. Review of ten cases, one with apparent recovery. J Pediatr *36*:728, 1950.
351. Lunn HF: A case of histoplasmosis of bone in East Africa. J Trop Med Hyg *63*:175, 1960.
352. Allen JH Jr: Bone involvement with disseminated histoplasmosis. Am J Roentgenol *82*:250, 1959.
353. Key JA, Large AM: Histoplasmosis of the knee. J Bone Joint Surg *24*:281, 1942.
354. Omer GE Jr, Lockwood RS, Travis LO: Histoplasmosis involving the carpal joint. A case report. J Bone Joint Surg *45A*:1699, 1963.
355. Cockshott WP, Lucas AO: Histoplasmosis duboisii. Q J Med *33*:223, 1964.
356. Forester HR: Sporotrichosis: An occupational dermatosis. JAMA *87*:1605, 1926.
357. Mikkelsen WM, Brandt RL, Harrell ER: Sporotrichosis: A report of 12 cases, including two with skeletal involvement. Ann Intern Med *47*:435, 1957.
358. Altner PC, Turner RR: Sporotrichosis of bones and joints. Review of the literature and report of six cases. Clin Orthop Rel Res *68*:138, 1970.
359. Lurie HI: Five unusual cases of sporotrichosis from South Africa showing lesions in muscles, bones, and viscera. Br J Surg *50*:585, 1963.
360. Winter TQ, Pearson KD: Systemic sporothrixosis. Radiology *104*:579, 1972.
361. Comstock C, Wolson AH: Roentgenology of sporotrichosis. Am J Roentgenol *125*:651, 1975.
362. Serstock DS, Zinneman HH: Pulmonary and articular sporotrichosis. Report of two cases. JAMA *233*:1291, 1975.
363. Crout JE, Brewer NS, Tompkins RB: Sporotrichosis arthritis. Clinical features in seven patients. Ann Intern Med *86*:294, 1977.
364. Satterwhite TK, Kageler MV, Conklin RH, Portnoy BL, DuPont HL: Disseminated sporotrichosis. JAMA *240*:771, 1978.
365. Dehaven KE, Wilde AH, O'Duffy JD: Sporotrichosis arthritis and tenosynovitis. Report of a case cured by synovectomy and amphotericin B. J Bone Joint Surg *54A*:874, 1972.
366. Kedes LH, Siemienski J, Braude AI: The syndrome of the alcoholic rose gardener. Sporotrichosis of the radial tendon sheath. Report of a case cured with amphotericin B. Ann Intern Med *61*:1139, 1964.
367. Louria DB, Stiff DP, Bennett B: Disseminated moniliasis in the adult. Medicine *41*:307, 1962.
368. Edwards JE Jr, Turkel SB, Elder HA, Rand RW, Guze LB: Hematogenous candida osteomyelitis. Am J Med *59*:89, 1975.
369. Connor CL: Monilia from osteomyelitis. J infect Dis *43*:108, 1928.
370. Hirschmann JV, Everett ED: Candida vertebral osteomyelitis. Case report and review of the literature. J Bone Joint Surg *58A*:573, 1976.
371. Noble HB, Lyne ED: Candida osteomyelitis and arthritis from hyperalimentation therapy. Case report. J Bone Joint Surg *56A*:825, 1974.
372. O'Connell CJ, Cherry AV, Zoll JG: Osteomyelitis of cervical spine: *Candida guilliermondi*. Ann Intern Med *79*:748, 1973.
373. Svirsky-Fein S, Langer L, Milbauer B, Khermosh O, Rubinstein E: Neonatal osteomyelitis caused by *Candida tropicalis*. Report of two cases and review of the literature. J Bone Joint Surg *61A*:455, 1979.
374. Noyes FR, McCabe JD, Fekety FR: Acute candida arthritis. Report of a case and use of amphotericin B. J Bone Joint Surg *55A*:169, 1973.
375. Fitzgerald E, Lloyd-Still J, Gordon SL: Candida arthritis. A case report and review of the literature. Clin Orthop Rel Res *106*:143, 1975.
376. Smilack JD, Gentry LO: Candida costochondral osteomyelitis. Report of a case and review of the literature. J Bone Joint Surg *58A*:888, 1976.

377. Bayer AS, Guze LB: Fungal arthritis. I. Candida arthritis: Diagnostic and prognostic implications and therapeutic considerations. Semin Arthritis Rheum *8*:142, 1978.
378. Lachman RS, Yamauchi T, Klein J: Neonatal systemic candidiases and arthritis. Radiology *105*:631, 1972.
379. Murray HW, Fialk MA, Roberts RB: Candida arthritis—a manifestation of disseminated candidiasis. Am J Med *60*:587, 1976.
380. Adler S, Randall J, Plotkin SA: Candida osteomyelitis and arthritis in a neonate. Am J Dis Child *123*:595, 1972.
381. Hollingsworth JW, Carr J: Experimental candidal arthritis in the rabbit. Sabouraudia *11*:56, 1973.
382. Green WH, Goldberg HI, Wohl GT: Mucormycosis infection of the craniofacial structures. Am J Roentgenol *101*:802, 1967.
383. Straatsma BR, Zimmerman LE, Gass JDM: Phycomycosis. A clinicopathologic study of fifty-one cases. Lab Invest *11*:963, 1962.
384. Addlestone RB, Baylin GJ: Rhinocerebral mucormycosis. Radiology *115*:113, 1975.
385. Kaufman RS, Stone G: Osteomyelitis of frontal bone secondary to mucormycosis. NY State J Med *73*:1325, 1973.
386. Grossman M: Aspergillosis of bone. Br J Radiol *48*:57, 1975.
387. Seres JL, Ono H, Benner EJ: Aspergillosis presenting as spinal cord compression. Case report. J Neurosurg *36*:221, 1972.
388. Seligsohn R, Rippon JW, Lerner SA: *Aspergillus terreus* osteomyelitis. Arch Intern Med *137*:918, 1977.
389. Green WR, Font RL, Zimmerman LE: Aspergillosis of the orbit. Report of ten cases and review of the literature. Arch Ophthalmol *82*:302, 1969.
390. Casscells SW: Aspergillus osteomyelitis of the tibia. A case report. J Bone Joint Surg *60A*:994, 1978.
391. Omar MM, Brown J: Case report 81. Skel Radiol *3*:250, 1979.
392. Josefiak EJ, Kokiko GV: Mycetoma of the hand. Arch Pathol *67*:55, 1959.
393. Cockshott WP, Rankin AM: Medical treatment of mycetoma. Lancet *2*:1112, 1960.
394. Symmers D, Sporer A: Maduromycosis of the hand. Arch Pathol *37*:309, 1944.
395. Hogshead HP, Stein GH: Mycetoma due to *Nocardia brasiliensis*. J Bone Joint Surg *52A*:1229, 1970.
396. Kulowski J, Stovall S: Maduramycosis of tibia in a native American. JAMA *135*:429, 1947.
397. Majid MA, Mathias PF, Seth HN, Thirumalachar MJ: Primary mycetoma of the patella. J Bone Joint Surg *46A*:1283, 1964.
398. Cockshott WP: Radiological patterns of the deep mycoses. *In* GEW Wolstenholme, R Porter (Eds): Ciba Foundation Symposium on Systemic Mycoses. London, J & A Churchill Ltd, 1968, p 113.
399. Moore PH Jr, McKinney RG, Mettler FA Jr: Radiographic and radionuclide findings in Rhizopus osteomyelitis. Radiology *127*:665, 1978.
400. Chambers RJ, Bywaters EGL: Rubella synovitis. Ann Rheum Dis *22*:263, 1963.
401. Lee PR: Arthritis and rubella. Br Med J *2*:925, 1962.
402. Lee PR, Barnett AF, Scholer JF, Bryner S, Clark WH: Rubella arthritis: Study of 20 cases. Calif Med *93*:125, 1960.
403. Spruance SL, Klock LE Jr, Bailey A, Ward JR, Smith CB: Recurrent joint symptoms in children vaccinated with HPV-77 DK-12 rubella vaccine. J Pediatr *80*:413, 1972.
404. Thompson GR, Ferreyra A, Brackett RG: Acute arthritis complicating rubella vaccination. Arthritis Rheum *14*:19, 1971.
405. Hildebrandt HM, Maassab HF: Rubella synovitis in a one year old patient. N Engl J Med *274*:1428, 1966.
406. Ogra PL, Herd JK: Arthritis associated with induced rubella infection. J Immunol *107*:810, 1971.
407. Johnson RE, Hall AP: Rubella arthritis: Report of cases studied by latex tests. N Engl J Med *258*:743, 1958.
408. Spruance SL, Metcalf R, Smith CB, Griffiths MM, Ward JR: Chronic arthropathy associated with rubella vaccination. Arthritis Rheum *20*:741, 1977.
409. Ogra PL, Ogra SS, Chiba Y, Dzierba JL, Herd JK: Rubella virus infection in juvenile rheumatoid arthritis. Lancet *1*:1157, 1975.
410. Randolph AJ, Yow MD, Phillips CA, Desmond MM, Blattner RJ, Melnick JL: Transplancental rubella infection in newly born infants. JAMA *191*:843, 1965.
411. Rudolph AJ, Singleton EB, Rosenberg HS, Singer DB, Phillips CA: Osseous manifestations of the congenital rubella syndrome. Am J Dis Child *110*:428, 1965.
412. Peters ER, Davis RL: Congenital rubella syndrome. Cerebral mineralization and subperiosteal new bone formation as expressions of this disorder. Clin Pediatr *5*:743, 1966.
413. Sekeles E, Ornoy A: Osseous manifestations of gestational rubella in young human fetuses. Am J Obstet Gynecol *122*:307, 1975.
414. Rabinowitz JG, Wolf BS, Greenberg EI, Rausen AR: Osseous changes in rubella embryopathy (congenital rubella syndrome). Radiology *85*:494, 1965.
415. Whalen JP, Winchester P, Krook L, O'Donohue N, Dische R, Nunez E: Neonatal transplacental rubella syndrome. Its effect on normal maturation of the diaphysis. Am J Roentgenol *121*:166, 1974.
416. Silverman FN: Virus diseases of bone. Do they exist? Am J Roentgenol *126*:677, 1976.
417. Reed GB Jr: Rubella bone lesions. J Pediatr *74*:208, 1969.
418. London WT, Fucillo DA, Anderson B, Sever JL: Concentration of rubella virus antigen in chondrocytes of congenitally infected rabbits. Nature *226*:172, 1970.
419. Sacks R, Habermann ET: Pathological fracture in congenital rubella. A case report. J Bone Joint Surg *59A*:557, 1977.
420. Sacrez R, Fruhling L, Korn R, Juif J-G, Francfort C, Geiger R: Trois observations de maladie des inclusions cytomegaliques. Arch Fr Pediatr *17*:129, 1960.
421. Graham CB, Thal A, Wassum CS: Rubella-like bone changes in congenital cytomegalic inclusion disease. Radiology *94*:39, 1970.
422. Merten DF, Gooding CA: Skeletal manifestations of congenital cytomegalic inclusion disease. Radiology *95*:333, 1970.
423. McCandless AE, Davis C, Hall EG: Bone changes in congenital cytomegalic inclusion disease. Arch Dis Child *50*:160, 1975.
424. Kopelman AE, Halsted CC, Minnefor AB: Osteomalacia and spontaneous fractures in twins with congenital cytomegalic inclusion disease. J Pediatr *81*:101, 1972.
425. Ritvo M, Schauffer IA, Krosnick G: Clinical and roentgen manifestations of erythroblastosis fetalis. Am J Roentgenol *61*:291, 1949.
426. Black-Schaffer B: Fetal nanosomia and bone athrepsia in newborn of women with severe cyanotic cardiovascular anomaly. Am J Obstet Gynecol *59*:656, 1950.
427. Cheatham WJ, Weller TH, Dolan TF Jr, Dower JC: Varicella: Report of two fatal cases with necropsy, virus isolation and serologic studies. Am J Pathol *32*:1015, 1956.
428. Feldman S, Hughes WT, Daniel CB: Varicella in children with cancer: Seventy-seven cases. Pediatrics *56*:388, 1975.
429. Ward JR, Bishop B: Varicella arthritis. JAMA *212*:1954, 1970.
430. Bogumill GP: Bilateral above-the-knee amputations: A complication of chickenpox. J Bone Joint Surg *47A*:371, 1965.
431. Chiari H: Über osteomyelitis variolosa. Beitr Z Pathol Anat Allg Pathol *13*:13, 1893.
432. Cockshott P, MacGregor M: The national history of osteomyelitis variolosa. J Fac Radiol *10*:57, 1959.
433. Cockshott P, MacGregor M: Osteomyelitis variolosa. Q J Med *27*:369, 1958.
434. Gupta SK, Srivastava TP: Roentgen features of skeletal involvement in small pox. Australas Radiol *17*:205, 1973.
435. Nathan PA, Trung NB: Osteomyelitis variolosa. Report of a case. J Bone Joint Surg *56A*:1525, 1974.
436. Bertcher RW: Osteomyelitis variolosa. Am J Roentgenol *76*:1149, 1956.
437. Eeckels R, Vincent J, Seynhaeve V: Bone lesions due to smallpox. Arch Dis Child *39*:591, 1964.
438. Margolis HS, Subbarao K, Pitt MJ, Boyer J: Case report 58. Skel Radiol *2*:261, 1978.
439. Davidson JC, Palmer PES: Osteomyelitis variolosa. J Bone Joint Surg *45B*:687, 1963.
440. Srivastava AN: Orthopaedic complications of smallpox. J Bone Joint Surg *48B*:183, 1966.
441. Bery K, Chawla S: Radiological features in smallpox osteomyelitis. (A review of six cases.) Indian J Radiol *23*:11, 1969.
442. Cochran W, Connolly JH, Thompson ID: Bone involvement after vaccination against smallpox. Br Med J *2*:285, 1963.
443. Delano PJ, Butler CD: Etiology of infantile cortical hyperostosis. Am J Roentgenol *58*:633, 1947.
444. Sewall S: Vaccinia osteomyelitis; report of a case with isolation of the vaccinia virus. Bull Hosp J Dis *10*:59, 1949.
445. Barbero GJ, Gray A, Scott TF, Kempe CH: Vaccinia gangrenosa treated with hyperimmune vaccinal gamma globulin. Pediatrics *16*:609, 1955.
446. Silby HM, Farber R, O'Connell CJ, Ascher J, Marine EJ: Acute monoarticular arthritis after vaccination. Report of a case with isolation of vaccina virus from synovial fluid. Ann Intern Med *62*:347, 1965.
447. Elliott WD: Vaccinial osteomyelitis. Lancet *2*:1053, 1959.
448. Tamir D, Benderly A, Levy J, Ben-Porath E, Vonsover A: Infectious mononucleosis and Epstein-Barr virus in childhood. Pediatrics *53*:330, 1974.
449. Adenbonojo FO: Monoarticular arthritis: Unusual manifestation of infectious mononucleosis. Clin Pediatr *11*:549, 1972.
450. Wechsler HF, Rosenblum AH, Sills CT: Infectious mononucleosis; report of epidemic in army post. Ann Intern Med *25*:113, 1946.
451. Burrows FG: Transient periosteal reaction in illness diagnosed as infectious mononucleosis. Radiology *98*:291, 1971.
452. Goldbloom RB, Stein PB, Eisen A, McSheffrey JB, Brown BS, Wigglesworth FW: Idiopathic periosteal hyperostosis with dysproteinemia: New clinical entity. N Engl J Med *274*:873, 1966.

453. Price GE, Ford DK, Gofton JP, Robinson HS: An outbreak of "infectious" polyarthritis in a Haida Indian family. Arthritis Rheum *6*:633, 1963.
454. Greudenberg E, Roulet F, Nicole R: Kongenital Infektion mit Coxsackie-virus. Ann Pediatr *178*:150, 1952.
455. Dawson MH, Boots RL: Arthritis associated with lymphogranuloma venereum. JAMA *113*:1162, 1939.
456. Wright LT, Logan M: Osseous changes associated with lymphogranuloma venereum. Arch Surg *39*:108, 1939.
457. Kirkpatrick DJ: Donovanosis (granuloma inguinale): A rare cause of osteolytic bone lesions. Clin Radiol *21*:101, 1970.
458. Warwick WJ: Cat-scratch syndrome, many diseases or one disease? Progr Med Virol *9*:256, 1967.
459. Collipp PJ, Koch R: Cat-scratch fever associated with an osteolytic lesion. N Engl J Med *260*:278, 1959.
460. Adams WC, Hindman SM: Cat-scratch disease associated with an osteolytic lesion. J Pediatr *44*:665, 1954.
461. Lees RF, Harrison RB, Williamson BRJ, Schaffer HA Jr: Radiographic findings in Rocky Mountain spotted fever. Radiology *129*:17, 1978.
462. Milgram JW: Osseous changes in congenital toxoplasmosis. Arch Pathol *97*:150, 1974.
463. Chandar K, Mair HJ, Mair NS: Case of toxoplasma polymyositis. Br Med J *1*:158, 1968.
464. Thiers H, Coudert J, Romagny G, Garin JP: Deux observations posant le problème d'une localization synoviale de l'infection toxoplasmique. Rev Rhum Mal Osteoartic *18*:548, 1951.
465. Ippolito A, Giacovazzo M, Badalamneti G, Spagna G: Toxoplasmosi acquisita e artrite reumatoide. G Mal Infett Parassit *20*:955, 1968.
466. Vass M, Kullmann L, Csoka R, Magyar E: Polytenosynovitis caused by *Toxoplasma gondii*. J Bone Joint Surg *59B*:229, 1977.
467. VanMeter BF: Hookworm arthritis (report of a case). Kentucky Med J *12*:429, 1914.
468. O'Connor RL, Luedke DC, Harkess JW: Hookworm lesion of bone. J Bone Joint Surg *53A*:362, 1971.
469. Reeder MM: Tropical diseases of the soft tissue. Semin Roentgenol *8*:47, 1973.
470. Greig EDW: Notes on cases of Calabar swellings with radiological observations. J Trop Med Hyg *43*:19, 1940.
471. Johnstone RDC: Loiasis. Lancet *1*:250, 1947.
472. Williams I: Calcification in loiasis. J Fac Radiol *6*:142, 1954.
473. Samuel E: Roentgenology of parasitic calcification. Am J Roentgenol *63*:512, 1950.
474. Montangerand Y, Atlan D, Laluque P, Fillaudeau G: Lymphographic aspects of Filarian adenopathy. J Radiol Electr Med Nucl *50*:135, 1969.
475. O'Connor FW, Golden R, Auchincloss H: Roentgen demonstration of calcified *Filaria bancrofti* in human tissues. Am J Roentgenol *23*:494, 1930.
476. Christopherson JB: Radioscopical diagnosis of filariasis. Br Med J *1*:808, 1929.
477. Khajavi A: Guinea worm calcification: A report of 83 cases. Clin Radiol *19*:433, 1968.
478. Brocklebank JA: Calcification in the guinea worm. Br J Radiol *17*:163, 1944.
479. Cohen G: The radiological demonstration of *Dracunculus medinensis*. S Afr Med J *33*:1094, 1959.
480. Sivaramappa M, Reddy CRRM, Sita Devi C, Reddy AC, Reddy PK, Murthy DP: Acute guinea worm synovitis of the knee joint. J Bone Joint Surg *51A*:1324, 1969.
481. Brailsford JF: *Cysticerus cellulosae:* Its radiographic detection in the musculature and central nervous system. Br J Radiol *14*:79, 1941.
482. Keats TE: Cysticercosis: A demonstration of its roentgen manifestations. Mo Med *58*:457, 1961.
483. Alldred AJ, Nisbet NW: Hydatid disease of bone in Australia. J Bone Joint Surg *46B*:260, 1964.
484. Pasquali E: Sulla localizzazione ossea dell'echinococco. Chir Organi Mov *15*:355, 1930.
485. Duran H, Ferrandez L, Gomez-Castresana F, Lopez-Duran L, Mata P, Brandau D, Sanchez-Barba A: Osseous hydatidosis. J Bone Joint Surg *60A*:685, 1978.
486. Hooper J, McLean I: Hydatid disease of the femur. Report of a case. J Bone Joint Surg *59A*:974, 1977.
487. Gharbi HA, Cheikh MB, Hamaza R, Jeddi M, Hamza B, Jedidi H, Bendridi MF: Les localisations rares de l'hydatidose chez l'enfant. Ann Radiol *20*:151, 1977.
488. Booz MK: The management of hydatid disease of bone and joint. J Bone Joint Surg *54B*:698, 1972.
489. Teymoorian GA, Bagheri F: Hydatid cyst of the skull: Report of four cases. Radiology *118*:97, 1976.
490. Mnaymneh W, Yacoubian V, Bikhazi K: Hydatidosis of the pelvic girdle — treatment by partial pelvectomy. A case report. J Bone Joint Surg *59A*:538, 1977.
491. Bonakdarpour A, Zadeh YFA, Maghssoudi H, Shariat S, Levy W: Costal echinococcosis. Report of six cases and review of the literature. Am J Roentgenol *118*:371, 1973.
492. Hutchison WF, Thompson WB, Derian PS: Osseous hydatid (echinococcus) disease. JAMA *182*:81, 1962.
493. Stewart GR, Loewenthal J: Vertebral hydatidosis. Aust NZ J Surg *36*:175, 1967.
494. Garabedian GA, Matossian RM, Djanian AY: An indirect hemagglutination test for hydatid disease. J Immunol *78*:269, 1957.
495. Rappaport EM, Rossien AX, Rosenblum LA: Arthritis due to intestinal amebiasis. Ann Intern Med *34*:1224, 1951.
496. Cole GT: Ainhum: Account of fifty-four patients with special reference to etiology and treatment. J Bone Joint Surg *47B*:43, 1965.
497. Auckland G, Ball J, Griffiths D: Ainhum. J Bone Joint Surg *39B*:513, 1957.
498. Browne SG: Ainhum: Clinical and etiological study of 83 cases. Ann Trop Med *55*:314, 1961.
499. Fetterman LE, Hardy R, Lehrer H: The clinico-roentgenologic features of Ainhum. Am J Roentgenol *100*:512, 1967.
500. Earle KV: Ainhum of the fingers: Case from Sierra Leone. Trans R Soc Trop Med Hyg *52*:570, 1958.
501. Spinzig EW: Ainhum: Its occurrence in the United States with report of three cases. Am J Roentgenol *42*:246, 1939.
502. Burch GE, Hale AR: Plethysmographic study of a toe of a patient with Ainhum. Arch Intern Med *100*:113, 1957.
503. Wolf E, Stern S: Costosternal syndrome. Arch Intern Med *136*:189, 1976.
504. Cameron HU, Fornasier VL: Tietze's disease. J Clin Pathol *27*:960, 1974.
505. Gill GV: Epidemic of Tietze's syndrome. Br Med J *2*:499, 1977.
506. Tietze A: Ueber eine eigenartige Haufung von Fallet mit Dystrophie der Rippenknorpel. Berl Klin Wschr *58*:829, 1921.
507. Jelenko C III: Tietze's syndrome at the xiphisternal joint. South Med J *67*:818, 1974.
508. Sain AK: Bone scan in Tietze's syndrome. Clin Nucl Med *3*:470, 1978.
509. Gill AM, Jones RA, Pollak L: Tietze's disease. Br Med J *2*:155, 1942.
510. Leger L, Moinnereau R: Tuméfaction douloureuse de la jonction chondro-costal (syndrom de Tietze). Presse Med *58*:336, 1950.
511. Geddes AK: Tietze's syndrome. Can Med Assoc J *53*:571, 1945.
512. Steere AC, Malawista SE, Hardin JA, Ruddy S, Askenase PW, Andiman WA: Erythema chronicum migrans and Lyme arthritis. The enlarging clinical spectrum. Ann Intern Med *86*:685, 1977.
513. Harverson G, Warren AG: Tarsal bone disintegration in leprosy. Clin Radiol *30*:317, 1979.
514. Lawrence C, Schreiber AJ: Leprosy's footprints in bone-marrow histiocytes. N Engl J Med *300*:834, 1979.
515. Zimmerman MR: Pulmonary and osseous tuberculosis in an Egyptian mummy. Bull NY Acad Med *55*:604, 1979.
516. Khermosh O, Weintroub S, Topilsky M, Baratz M: *Mycobacterium abscessus (M. chelonei)* infection of the knee joint. Report of two cases following intra-articular injection of corticosteroids. Clin Orth Rel Res *140*:162, 1979.
517. Steere AC, Gibofsky A, Patarroyo ME, Winchester RJ, Hardin JA, Malawista SE: Chronic Lyme arthritis. Clinical and immunogenetic differentiation from rheumatoid arthritis. Ann Intern Med *90*:896, 1979.
518. Blotzer JW, Myers AR: Echo virus–associated polyarthritis. Report of a case with synovial fluid and synovial histologic characterization. Arthritis Rheum *21*:978, 1978.
519. Hyer FH, Gottlieb NL: Rheumatic disorders associated with viral infection. Semin Arthritis Rheum *8*:17, 1978.
520. Ancona RJ, McAuliffe J, Thompson TR, Speert DP, Ferrieri P: Group B streptococcal sepsis with osteomyelitis and arthritis. Its occurrence with acute heart failure. Am J Dis Child *133*:919, 1979.
521. Fam AG, Tenenbaum J, Stein JL: Clinical forms of meningococcal arthritis: A study of five cases. J Rheumatol *6*:567, 1979.
522. Leek JC, Robbins DL: Infectious arthritis due to *Hemophilus influenzae*. J Rheumatol *6*:432, 1979.
523. Chapman M, Murray RO, Stoker DJ: Tuberculosis of the bones and joints. Semin Roentgenol *14*:266, 1979.
524. Zvetina JR, Foster J, Reyes CV: *Mycobacterium kansasii* infection of the elbow joint. A case report. J Bone Joint Surg *61A*:1099, 1979.
525. Henriquez M, Levy R, Raja RM, Kramer MS, Rosenbaum JL: Mucormycosis in a renal transplant recipient with successful outcome. JAMA *242*:1397, 1979.
526. Lentz MW, Noyes FR: Osseous deformity from osteomyelitis variolosa. A case report. Clin Orthop Rel Res *143*:155, 1979.
527. Hardin JA, Steere AC, Malawista SE: Immune complexes snd the evolution of Lyme arthritis. Dissemination and localization of abnormal C1q binding activity. N Engl J Med *301*:1358, 1979.
528. Halla JT, Gould JS, Hardin JG: Chronic tenosynovial hand infection from *Mycobacterium terrae*. Arthritis Rheum *22*:1386, 1979.

529. Memon IA, Jacobs NM, Yeh TF, Lilien LD: Group B streptococcal osteomyelitis and septic arthritis. Am J Dis Child *133*:921, 1979.
530. Chilton SJ, Aftimos SF, White PR: Diffuse skeletal involvement of streptococcal osteomyelitis in a neonate. Radiology *134*:390, 1980.
531. Rosenthal L, Olhagen B, Ek S: Aseptic arthritis after gonorrhea. Ann Rheum Dis *39*:141, 1980.
532. Green NE, Bruno J III: Pseudomonas infections of the foot after puncture wounds. South Med J *73*:146, 1980.
533. Gray RG, Poppo MJ: *Salmonella hartford* septic arthritis. J Rheumatol *7*:422, 1980.
534. Rumans LW, Allen MS: *Haemophilus influenzae* septic arthritis in adults. Am J Med Sci *279*:67, 1980.
535. Bansal S, Magnussen CR, Napodano RJ: *Haemophilus influenzae* tenosynovitis. Ann Rheum Dis *38*:561, 1979.
536. Thomas JM, Lowes JA, Tabaqchali S: *Serratia marcescens* in mixed aerobic infections of bone. J Bone Joint Surg *62B*:389, 1980.
537. Seradge H, Anderson MG: Clostridial myonecrosis following intra-articular steroid injection. Clin Orthop Rel Res *147*:207, 1980.
538. Rahman NU: Atypical forms of spinal tuberculosis. J Bone Joint Surg *62B*:162, 1980.
539. Postacchini F, Montanaro A: Tuberculous epidural granuloma simulating a herniated lumbar disk: A report of a case. Clin Orthop Rel Res *148*:182, 1980.
540. Perelman R, Danis F, Nathanson M, Lafay F, Garcia J, Fischer A: A propos d'un cas de "bécégite" généralisée mortelle sans déficit immunitaire apparent. Sem Hôp Paris *56*:480, 1980.
541. Lakhanpal VP, Tuli SM, Singh H, Sen PC: *Mycobacterium kansasii* and osteoarticular lesions. Acta Orthop Scand *51*:471, 1980.
542. Brown TS, Franklyn PP, Marikkar MSK: Tuberculosis of the skull vault. Clin Radiol *31*:313, 1980.
543. Meck JM, Colettis E, Parrot R, LeGal J: Aspects radiologiques de l'ostéite tuberculeuse chez l'africain immigré. Ann Radiol *22*:634, 1979.
544. Dzebolo NN: Congenital syphilis: An unusual presentation. Radiology *136*:372, 1980.
545. Bayer, AS, Choi C, Tillman DB, Guze LB: Fungal arthritis. V. Cryptococcal and histoplasmal arthritis. Semin Arthritis Rheum *9*:218, 1980.
546. Bayer AS, Scott VJ, Guze LB: Fungal arthritis. IV. Blastomycotic arthritis. Semin Arthritis Rheum *9*:145, 1980.
547. McGahan JP, Graves DS, Palmer PES: Coccidioidal spondylitis. Usual and unusual radiographic manifestations. Radiology *136*:5, 1980.
548. Bayer AS, Guze LB: Fungal arthritis. II. Coccidioidal synovitis. Clinical diagnostic, therapeutic, and prognostic considerations. Semin Arthritis Rheum *8*:200, 1979.
549. Rosenthal J, Brandt K, Wheat LJ, Slama TG: Rheumatologic manifestations of histoplasmosis (Abstr). Arthritis Rheum *23*:738, 1980.
550. Shaikh BS, Appelbaum PC, Aber RC: Vertebral disc space infection and osteomyelitis due to *Candida albicans* in a patient with acute myelomonocytic leukemia. Cancer *45*:1025, 1980.
551. Yarchoan R, Davies SF, Fried J, Mahowald ML: Isolated *Candida parapsilosis* arthritis in a heroin addict. J Rheumatol *6*:447, 1979.
552. Yousefzadeh DK, Jackson JH: Neonatal and infantile candidal arthritis with or without osteomyelitis: A clinical and radiographical review of 21 cases. Skel Radiol *5*:77, 1980.
553. Huang SHK, DeCoteau WE: Adult-onset Still's disease: An unusual presentation of rubella infection. Can Med Assoc J *122*:1275, 1980.
554. Bayer AS: Arthritis related to rubella. Postgrad Med *67*:131, 1980.
555. Smith RK, Specht EE: Osseous lesions and pathologic fractures in congenital cytomegalic inclusion disease: Report of a case. Clin Orthop Rel Res *144*:280, 1979.
556. Dickey LE: Possible varicella lesion of the humerus: A case report. Clin Orthop Rel Res *148*:237, 1980.
557. Pasqual-Gomez E: Identification of large mononuclear cells in varicella arthritis. Arthritis Rheum *23*:519, 1980.
558. Kennedy AC, Fleming J, Solomon L: Chikungunya viral arthropathy: a clinical description. J Rheumatol *7*:231, 1980.
559. Haddow AJ, Davies CW, Walker AJ: O'nyong nyong fever: An epidemic virus in East Africa. Trans R Soc Trop Med Hyg *54*:517, 1960.
560. Saksouk FA: Extrapleural extraosseous costal echinococcosis. Br J Radiol *52*:918, 1979.
561. Rosenthal J, Bole GG, Robinson WD: Acute nongonococcal infectious arthritis. Arthritis Rheum *23*:889, 1980.
562. Manshady BM, Thompson GR, Weiss JJ: Septic arthritis in a general hospital 1966–1977. J Rheumatol *7*:523, 1980.
563. Leek JC, Robbins DL: *Haemophilus influenzae* tenosynovitis. Ann Rheum Dis *39*:530, 1980.
564. Albeniz FE, Martin RG, Del Rio AA: Osteomielitis tuberculosa de localización diafisaria. Radiologia *21*:455, 1979.
565. Taillandier J, Manigand G, Fixy P, Sebag A: Le rhumatisme inflammatoire de la syphilis secondaire. Sem Hôp Paris *56*:979, 1980.
566. Atdjian M, Granda JL, Ingberg HO, Kaplan BL: Systemic sporotrichosis polytenosynovitis with median and ulnar nerve entrapment. JAMA *243*:1841, 1980.
567. Lehrer RI, Howard DH, Sypherd PS, Edwards JE, Segal GP, Winston DJ: Mucormycosis. Ann Intern Med *93*:93, 1980.
568. Steere AC, Brinckerhoff CE, Miller DJ, Drinkler H, Harris ED Jr, Malawista SE: Elevated levels of collagenase and prostaglandin E2 from synovium associated with erosion of cartilage and bone in a patient with chronic Lyme arthritis. Arthritis Rheum *23*:591, 1980.

SECTION XIV

TRAUMATIC, IATROGENIC, AND NEUROGENIC DISEASES

PHYSICAL INJURY

by Donald Resnick, M.D., and Gen Niwayama, M.D.

63

No other facet of musculoskeletal disease occupies a more fundamental or important role than that related to physical abuse. The evaluation of the complications of trauma is an integral part of orthopedic surgery, a large part of the practice of emergency room medicine, and the most common indication for skeletal roentgenograms. Complete textbooks are devoted to a discussion of the consequences of such trauma both in the child and in the adult.

Physical injury contributes to a wide variety of alterations in the bones, the joints, and the soft tissues. In addition to fractures, dislocations, subluxations, and capsular, tendinous, and ligamentous tears, trauma can affect the growth plate of the immature skeleton as well as the hyaline cartilaginous and fibrocartilaginous articular structures. Further complications of trauma include the reflex sympathetic dystrophy syndrome (see Chapter 48), osteolysis (see Chapter 82), osteonecrosis (see Chapter 77), many of the osteochondroses (see Chapter 78), neuroarthropathy (see Chapter 70), infection (see Chapters 60 to 62), and heterotopic bone formation (see Chapter 85). Trauma has also been implicated in the development of certain neoplasms, such as aneurysmal bone cysts (Fig. 63–1). Non-mechanical trauma to the musculoskeletal system can result from thermal and electrical injury (see Chapter 64), irradiation (see Chapter 65), and chemical substances (see Chapters 66 to 68).

This chapter presents an overview of the subject of physical trauma. Emphasis is placed upon the consequences of injuries to joints and certain conditions whose radiographic manifestations simulate

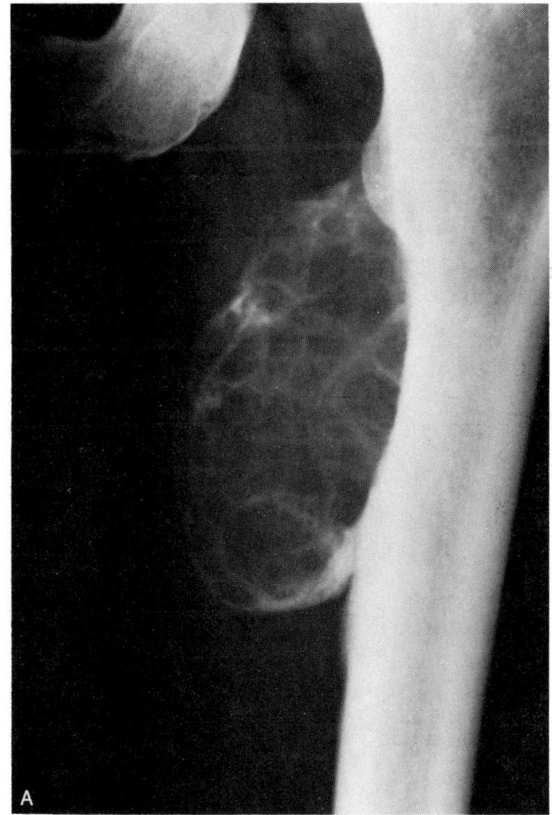

Figure 63–1. *Aneurysmal bone cyst. This patient gradually developed a soft tissue mass following an injury.*

A *A radiograph reveals an eccentric lesion of the proximal femur containing a rim of calcification and a trabecular pattern. Note the scalloping of the external surface of the cortex.*

Illustration continued on the following page

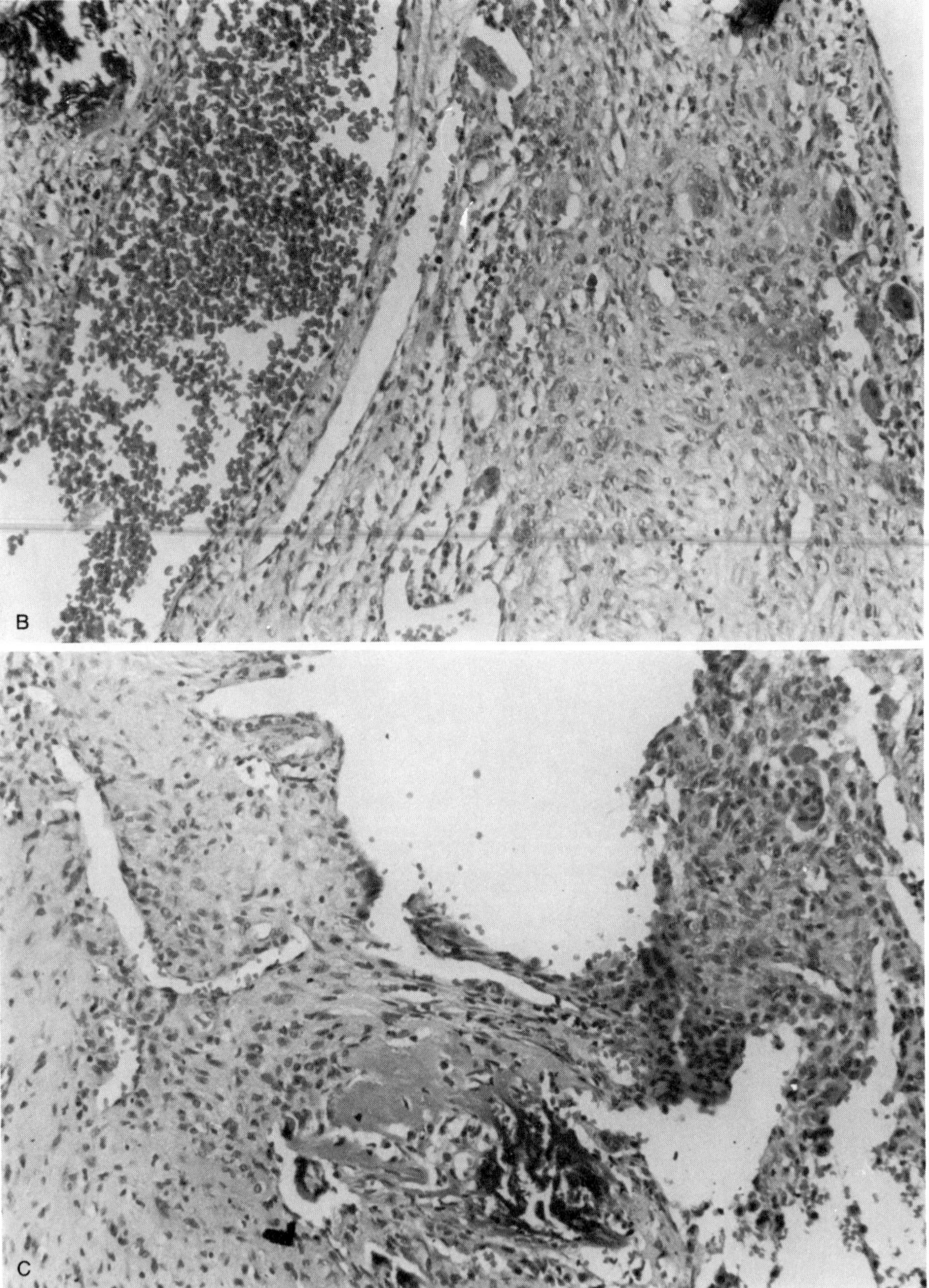

Figure 63–1. Continued

B *A photomicrograph (170×) demonstrates granulation tissue and flattened cells lining a blood space, with multinucleated giant cells.*

C *Note the granulation tissue lining a blood space, occasional multinucleated giant cells, and a focal calcium deposit (170×).*

those associated with non-traumatic skeletal disorders. Although a detailed discussion of fractures is not included, some attention is directed to specific types of fractures and those associated with joint dislocation and subluxation.

AVAILABLE DIAGNOSTIC MODALITIES

Plain film radiographic examination is well suited for the evaluation of most skeletal injuries. However, obtaining an adequate radiologic examination in emergency room patients can be extremely difficult.[1] These patients are frequently uncooperative because of pain and restricted motion, and their consciousness may be altered. Despite these difficulties, it is imperative that both the technologist and the radiologist be patient and thorough. Immediate review of the roentgenograms must be accomplished while the patient is still in the radiology department so that inadequate or suboptimal films can be identified and repeat roentgenograms can be obtained without delay. When the individual's condition limits maneuverability, alternate projections can be substituted for more standard views (see Chapter 7). Fluoroscopy can be a useful adjunct to the initial radiographic examination, as the patient can be conveniently turned to the proper obliquity to visualize a possible abnormality.

In the evaluation of trauma in children, a debate has existed regarding the necessity of obtaining comparison radiographs of the opposite extremity. Although this practice has been generally advocated in available textbooks,[2-4] a survey of members of the Society for Pediatric Radiology indicated that less than 30 per cent of these individuals routinely utilized comparison views and that the additional roentgenograms provided important information in less than 5 per cent of cases.[5] McCauley and associates,[6] in a review of 300 cases of childhood injury, noted that when pediatric radiologists were initially interpreting the films, comparison roentgenograms were rarely indicated. These investigators concluded that comparison views should be obtained selectively, not routinely, if the diagnosis is in doubt. Most typically, such a situation arises in the evaluation of Salter-Harris type 1 growth plate injuries and hip trauma. Radiographs of the opposite side may also be helpful in the assessment of bowing fractures and injuries about the elbow.

Specialized radiographic techniques such as tomography and magnification radiography are generally not necessary for proper diagnosis in cases of skeletal trauma. Occasionally, such techniques can identify subtle fracture lines when initial radiographs are normal, but routine utilization of these modalities is not indicated. When the clinical suspicion of a bone infraction is great, the patient can be treated as if a definite fracture has been identified, even when initial roentgenograms are normal. Radiographs obtained two or three weeks later may identify callus formation, substantiating the presence of a fracture.

Xeroradiography (see Chapter 11) and low KV radiography (see Chapter 10) can be helpful in the evaluation of trauma, especially when a soft tissue injury is suspected. Stereoradiography, too, may be of aid.

Radionuclide examination[523] (see Chapter 17) and computed tomography (see Chapter 12) can also be useful in the diagnosis of skeletal trauma. The role of scintigraphy is perhaps best exemplified in the evaluation of fatigue fractures (see later discussion), whereas that of computed tomography is most strongly established in the appraisal of spinal and pelvic fractures.[582-584] Scintigraphy may also be useful in detecting subtle acute fractures when radiographs are normal (e.g., in the carpal bones) or in excluding fractures in the presence of significant clinical findings,[578-580] and can be used to evaluate the healing response.[581] Difficulty arises in determining the age of a fracture by scintigraphy because of considerable variability in radionuclide activity in the posttraumatic period. In general, activity diminishes steadily following the fracture and eventually returns to normal levels. The minimal time required for the scan to return to normal following fracture appears to be about 5 to 6 months and in 90 per cent of cases the scan is normal by 2 years following the injury.[585]

FRACTURES

General Principles

Following a fracture, a remarkable series of events occurs that leads to osseous healing in the majority of cases.[7-12] Initially, there is bleeding from the damaged ends of the bones and from the neighboring soft tissues. Formation of a hematoma within the medullary canal, between the fracture ends, and beneath the elevated periosteum is followed by clot formation. Interruption of blood vessels produces osteocytic death, and the necrotic material induces an intense, acute inflammatory response. Vasodilatation, exudation of plasma and leukocytes, and infiltration of polymorphonuclear leukocytes, histiocytes, and mast cells are identified.

A reparative phase begins with organization of the fracture hematoma and invasion by fibrovascular tissue, which replaces the clot and lays down the collagen fibers and the matrix, which will later become mineralized to form the woven bone of the provisional or primary callus.[12] Participation of cells in the periosteum, endosteum, and granulation tissue can be recognized in the healing process, although the site of cellular activity and the amount of new bone that is formed are variable and influenced by the nature of the bone that is affected. Callus rapidly envelops the bone ends, producing increasing stability at the fracture site. In some areas, particularly at the periphery of the callus, cartilage appears and is converted to bone by the process of endochondral ossification.

During the process of repair, a remodeling phase can also be identified which is associated with resorption of unnecessary segments of the callus and proliferation of trabeculae along lines of stress. The exact location of osteoblastic and osteoclastic activity is apparently mediated by electrical mechanisms.[7] The fate of the dead bone at the fracture site is influenced by mechanical factors. It may be resorbed, or incorporated into the bony mass, providing osseous continuity and stability.

The three phases of fracture healing — inflammatory, reparative, and remodeling — overlap, and cellular activity at a fracture site, which can be outlined utilizing radioisotopic studies, persists long after the radiographic changes appear static[7]; for example, it has been estimated that increased activity is present at the site of a tibial fracture for a period of 6 to 9 years. Many local factors can modify the healing process: the degree of trauma (retarded healing is expected in fractures associated with extensive osseous and soft tissue injury); the degree of bone loss (retarded healing occurs when the bone loss is substantial); the type of bone involved (cancellous bone unites rapidly at sites of osseous contact, whereas cortical bone may unite with or without extensive external callus, depending upon the degree of apposition of the fragments); the extent of immobilization (improper immobilization may lead to delayed union or nonunion); the presence of infection (retarded bone healing occurs when infection is present); the presence of an underlying pathologic process (neoplastic, metabolic, and other disorders delay the healing process); utilization of radiation therapy (irradiated bone unites at a slower rate); the presence of extensive osteonecrosis (avascular bone impedes fracture healing); and the occurrence of intra-articular extension (fibrinolysins in the synovial fluid may destroy the initial clot, producing a delay in fracture union).[7] Systemic factors such as the age of the patient (healing is more rapid in the immature skeleton) and the presence of certain hormones (corticosteroids inhibit fracture healing) can also be influential in fracture repair.

Special Types of Fractures

Pathologic Fractures. A pathologic fracture is one in which the bone is disrupted at a site of preexisting abnormality, frequently by a stress that would not have fractured a normal bone. Any process that structurally weakens the osseous tissue, particularly if it involves cortical bone, can result in a pathologic fracture. The most common underlying abnormalities are tumors and osteoporosis, although infectious, articular, and metabolic processes can all present in this fashion. The term "insufficiency fracture" has been utilized to describe disruption occurring at sites of nontumorous lesions.[13] Large and aggressive lesions are more likely to produce pathologic fractures than small nonaggressive processes.

The radiographic distinction between a pathologic and a nonpathologic fracture is not always easy. This differentiation is not difficult when a fracture line traverses a large area of osseous destruction or when the adjacent or distant bones are riddled with additional lesions (Fig. 63–2). When a smaller lesion is present, the fracture itself may obscure the area of lysis or sclerosis, especially in the presence of displacement at the fracture site. The absence of a history of trauma or fracture pain and the presence of symptoms and signs of preexisting abnormality such as angular deformity, painless swelling, or generalized bone pain are clinical aids to the diagnosis of a pathologic fracture. The roentgenographic diagnosis is substantiated by the presence of bone destruction, altered architecture or

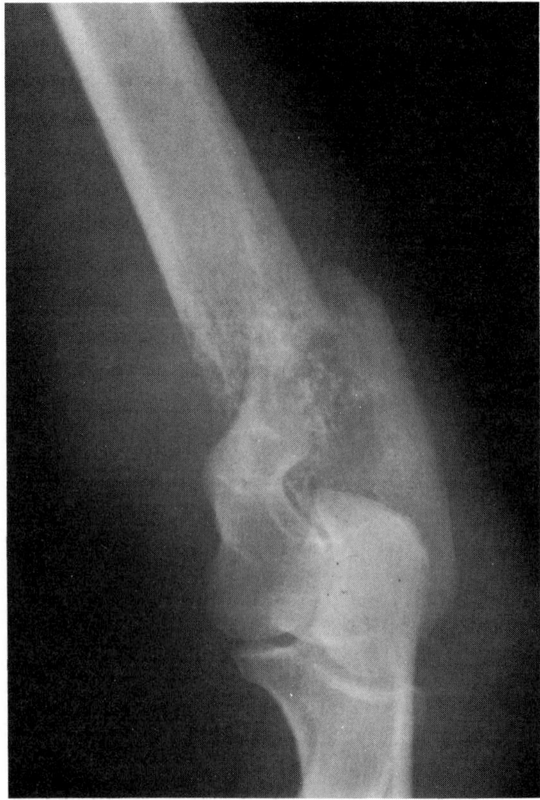

Figure 63–2. *Pathologic fracture. A transverse fracture line through a metastatic focus from bronchogenic carcinoma can be detected in the distal humerus. Note the osteolysis, cortical irregularity, and soft tissue swelling.*

density, and deformity. A transverse fracture line and an inability to mentally reconstruct the entire bone by "piecing together" the fracture fragments are additional radiographic clues. Diagnostic difficulty may be encountered in the patient who presents with a nonpathologic fracture that is days to weeks old, as resorption, osteolysis, or rotation about the fracture site may create the illusion of an underlying lesion. This is especially true with fractures of the femoral neck, pubic rami, and distal clavicle (see Chapter 82).

STRESS FRACTURES. Stress fractures can occur in normal or abnormal bone that is subjected to repeated cyclic loading, with the load being less than that which causes acute fracture of bone.[14-18] Two types of stress fractures can be recognized: a *fatigue fracture*, resulting from the application of abnormal stress or torque to a bone with normal elastic resistance; and an *insufficiency fracture*, occurring when normal stress is placed on a bone with deficient elastic resistance. Both fatigue and insufficiency fractures can occur in the same individual if an abnormal stress is placed upon an abnormal bone. Fatigue fractures frequently share the following features: the activity is new or different for the individual; the activity is strenuous; and the activity is repeated with a frequency that ultimately produces symptoms and signs.[13, 14] Typical examples are the fatigue fractures that occur in the metatarsals of military recruits ("march" fractures),[16, 17, 19-21] and in the lower extremities in athletes, joggers, and dancers,[22-24] although other strenuous activities can produce similar infractions at these and additional sites.[25-34, 588] The causes of insufficiency fractures are diverse[14] and include rheumatoid arthritis,[35-37] osteoporosis,[38] Paget's disease,[13] osteomalacia or rickets,[39] hyperparathyroidism,[13] renal osteodystrophy, osteogenesis imperfecta,[13] osteopetrosis,[13] fibrous dysplasia,[13] and irradiation[13] (Fig. 63–3). Fatigue and insufficiency fractures are not infrequent following certain surgical procedures that result in altered stress or an imbalance of muscular force on normal or abnormal bones. Common examples are noted in the metatarsals following bunion surgery,[40, 41] in the lower extremities following arthrodesis or arthroplasty,[36] in the pubic rami following hip[540, 587] or knee[541] surgery, and in the clavicles following radical neck dissection[42] (Fig. 63–4).

Although the roentgenogram plays an essential role in the diagnosis of stress fractures (see following discussion), it is the radionuclide examination that provides not only a means of early detection,[43-45, 531-535] but also a visual account of the biochemical properties of bone that are fundamental to the pathogenesis of stress fractures. Roub and others[15] have provided an excellent summary of these properties (Fig. 63–5). When a bone is stressed, osteonal remodeling or osteonization takes place in which resorption of circumferential lamellar bone and its subsequent replacement by dense osteonal bone are identified.[46, 47] Because of this process, there exists a vulnerable period following a stressful occurrence in

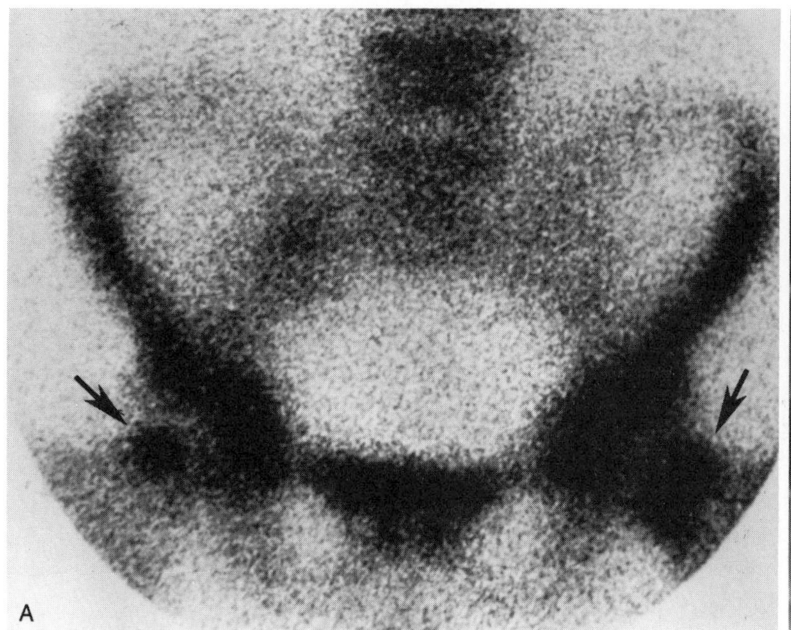

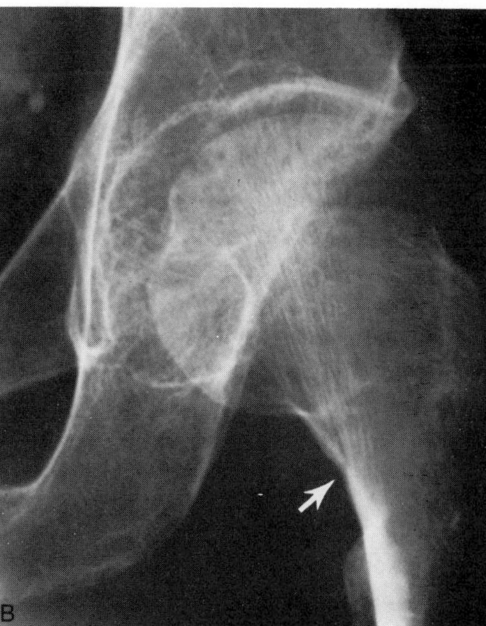

Figure 63–3. *Insufficiency fractures: Rheumatoid arthritis and osteoporosis. This patient with long-standing rheumatoid arthritis, being treated with corticosteroids, developed spontaneous bilateral hip pain.*

A *A scan of the pelvis utilizing technetium pyrophosphate delineates increased accumulation of radionuclide in both femoral necks (arrows), more marked on the left side.*

B *A radiograph of the left hip delineates the site of the stress fracture (arrow). A similar roentgenographic abnormalitiy was present on the opposite side.*

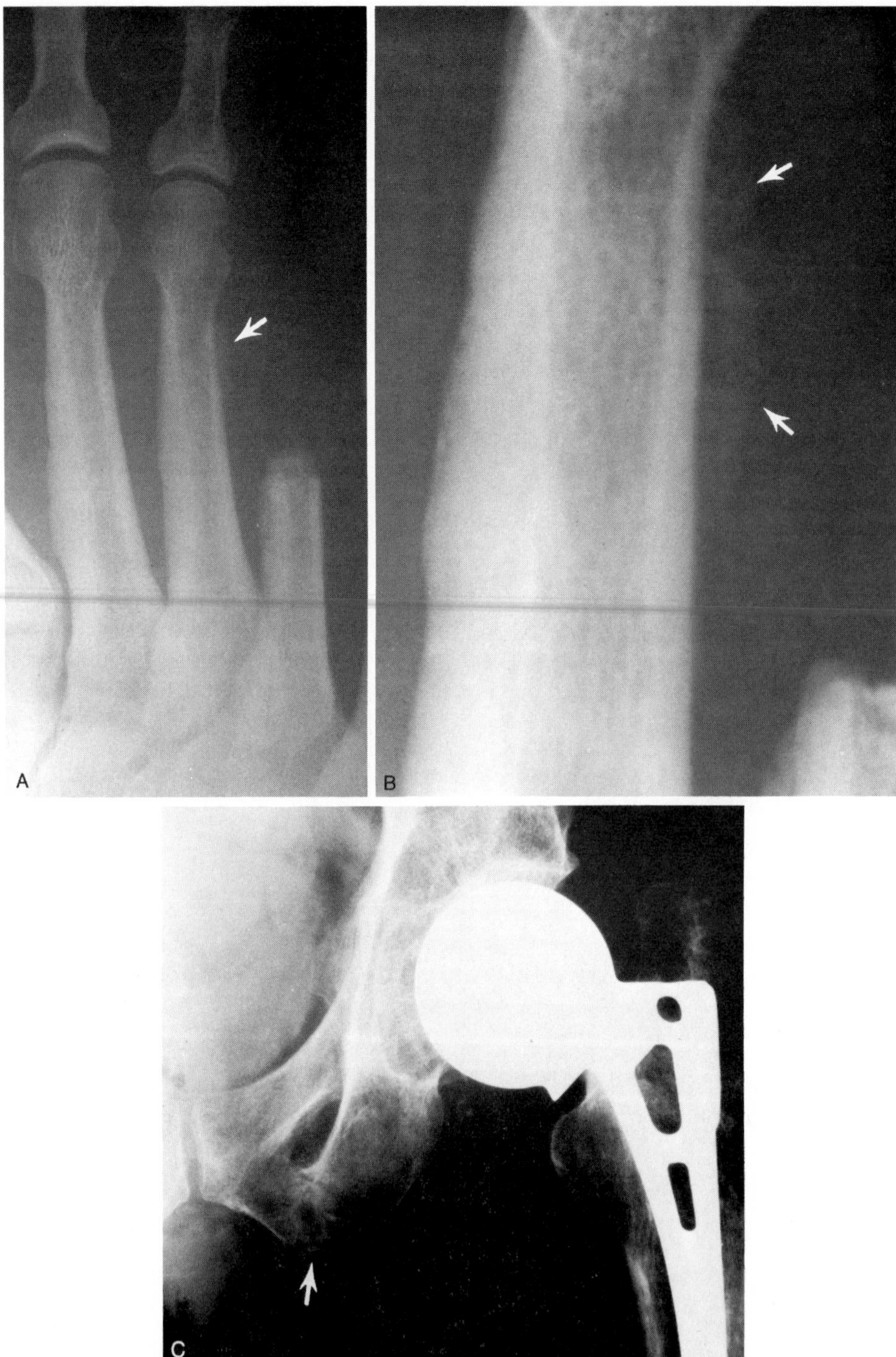

Figure 63–4. *Fatigue fractures — following surgical procedures.*

A, B *This diabetic patient developed osteomyelitis that required surgical resection of the fourth and fifth digits of the foot. Subsequently, activity-related foot pain occurred, which was due to a stress fracture of the shaft of the third metatarsal (arrows), characterized by periostitis, which is best delineated on a magnification roentgenogram* **(B).** *No evidence of infection was apparent.*

C *Increasing hip pain in this patient following hip surgery was related not to loosening or infection of the prosthesis but to a fatigue fracture of the inferior pubic ramus (arrow).*

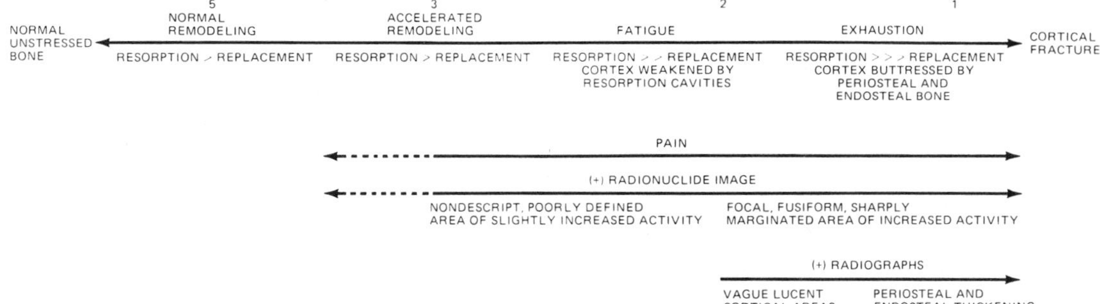

Figure 63–5. *Stress reaction in bone. A comparison of the histologic, clinical, scintigraphic, and radiologic responses. (From Roub LW, et al: Radiology 132:431, 1979.)*

which the cortical bone is less capable of withstanding further stress and in which the foci of osseous resorption may be transformed into sites of microfracture. This complication is especially likely to occur when unusual and unaccustomed activity leads to increased tone and strength of a muscle in a relatively short period of time while the increased strength of the bone lags behind.[14] The stress fracture begins as a small cortical crack, which progresses as the stress continues or becomes more exaggerated[48, 49]; such progression is characterized by the appearance of subcortical infraction in front of the advancing main crack in the bone.[50] If the stress is eliminated, the sequence is interrupted or slowed so that new bone formation "catches up" to the increased demand, and a state of increased bone strength is then reached. Increasing physical activity under controlled circumstances can produce osseous hypertrophy without evidence of microfracture. Exercise programs of the professional athlete are designed to allow the bone to compensate for the exaggerated muscular stresses that are encountered; bony hypertrophy is well recognized in the lower extremities of long distance runners and ballet dancers[24] as well as in the upper extremities of baseball pitchers and tennis players.[51, 52] This is radiologic evidence of Wolff's law at work.[53]

The biochemical properties of bone that have been outlined have their scintigraphic counterparts.[15] The stressed and "painful" bone undergoing accelerated remodeling produces an abnormal radionuclide image in which nondescript, poorly defined areas of increased accumulation of bone-seeking pharmaceuticals are observed in the absence of ra-

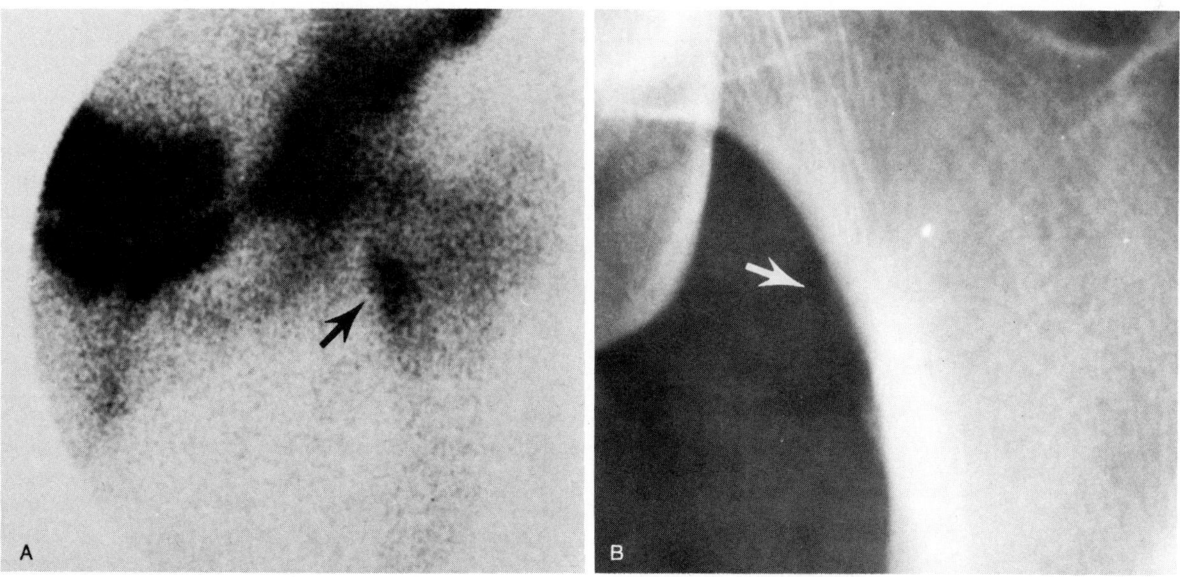

Figure 63–6. *Stress fractures: Radionuclide abnormalities. An athletic young woman developed persistent hip pain aggravated by activity.*

A *A radionuclide examination reveals a focal, sharply marginated area of increased activity in the femoral neck (arrow).*

B *A radiograph of the hip delineates a minimal amount of indistinct new bone formation along the medial aspect of the femoral neck (arrow).*

diographic findings. Appropriate modification of the physical activity may allow osseous "healing" without the appearance of cortical infraction. If the strenuous activity continues, the painful bone may reveal focal fusiform, sharply marginated areas of increased radionuclide activity that can be associated with radiolucent cortical areas and periosteal and endosteal thickening on the roentgenogram, and a diagnosis of a true stress factor is substantiated (Fig. 63–6). Thus, a stress fracture appears to represent one end of the spectrum of bony response to stress.

The clinical findings of stress fractures are characteristic. Activity-related pain that is relieved by rest is typical. Localized tenderness and soft tissue swelling can also be observed. Almost any bone in the body can be affected, and the specific site of involvement is influenced by the type of physical activity that is being undertaken. The bones in the lower extremity are more frequently affected than those in the upper extremity. More than one site can be involved simultaneously, and symmetric changes are not unusual.

The radiographic abnormalities are influenced by the location of the fracture and the interval between the time of injury and that of the roentgenographic examination. Certain features are more characteristic of stress fractures in the diaphysis of a tubular bone, whereas others are encountered in stress fractures in the end of a tubular bone (e.g., the tibial plateau) or in areas that are predominantly cancellous bone (e.g., the tarsus). In a diaphysis, a linear cortical radiolucent area is frequently associated with periosteal and endosteal cortical thickening (Fig. 63–7). The degree of bone formation can be extreme, obscuring the radiolucent defect within the cortex. Magnification radiography and tomography can outline the linear or band-like nature of the radiolucent area and the disruption of the osseous surface, findings that can then be differentiated from those of an osteoid osteoma (circular or elliptical cortical radiolucent area with or without calcification in an area of sclerosis) and an abscess (circular or oval radiolucent area without calcification with surrounding sclerosis). In an epiphyseal location or in a cancellous area, focal sclerosis representing condensation of trabeculae is the typical finding, and periostitis is not prominent (Fig. 63–8). With healing at either site, the sclerosis may become more diffuse, and eventually it and the fracture line can disappear. Biochemical principles can be applied to

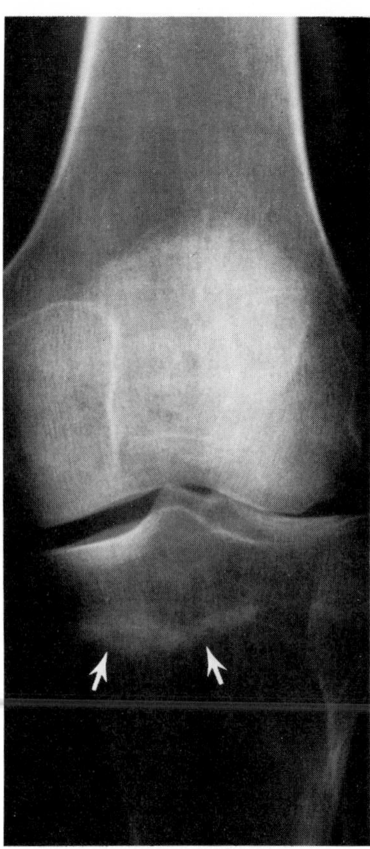

Figure 63–8. *Stress fractures: Radiographic abnormalities in epiphyses. Band-like focal sclerosis (arrows) is typical of a stress fracture in the proximal tibia.*

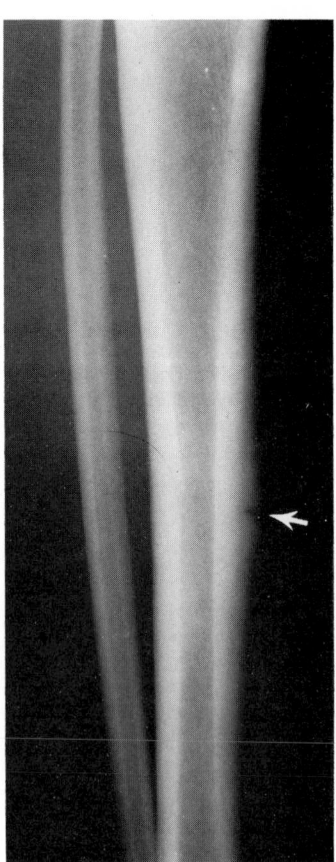

Figure 63–7. *Stress fractures: Radiographic abnormalities in diaphyses. A horizontally oriented, linear cortical lucent area with surrounding periosteal proliferation (arrow) is typical of a stress fracture of the diaphysis of the tibia.*

the explanation of stress fractures in various sites of the body.[14] A few specific examples are included in Table 63–1.

1. *Calcaneal stress fracture.* Fatigue fracture of the calcaneus is not uncommon in military recruits,[54, 55] and insufficiency fractures in this site can accompany rheumatoid arthritis, neurologic disorders, as well as other diseases[56] (Fig. 63–9). The failure of bone is related to the antagonistic action of the Achilles and plantar tendons and is accentuated when osteoporosis or spastic muscular tension is present. Less commonly, other tarsal bones reveal stress fractures.[542]

2. *Fibular stress fracture.* In the act of running, the calf musculature is active in flexion and extension of the ankle and in closer approximation of the tibia and fibula. The magnitude of the muscular activity is influenced by the type of ground surface, increasing in the presence of hard turf. Changing muscular stresses can result in the "runner's fracture."[14, 38] Jumping can also produce fibular stress fractures; classically, the proximal portion of the bone is affected in jumping, whereas the distal portion may be altered in running.[536]

3. *Tibial stress fracture.* Stress fracture of the proximal diaphysis of the tibia can occur during running,[57] particularly in children,[58, 60] and stress fracture of the middle and distal tibial diaphysis can take place during long-distance running, marching, and ballet dancing[24, 28, 57, 59, 61] (Fig. 63–10).

4. *Femoral stress fracture.* Stress fracture of the shaft or neck of the femur can result from numerous activities, including long-distance running, ballet dancing, and marching[25, 28, 30, 62-65] (Fig. 63–10). Although both adults and children can be affected, stress fractures of the femoral neck are rare in children with open capital epiphyseal growth plates.[25, 66] In this area, Devas[67] has described two types of stress fracture: a transverse type, more frequent in older patients, appearing as a small radiolucent area in the superior aspect of the femoral neck and becoming displaced in some situations; and a compression type, more common in younger patients, appearing as a haze of callus in the inferior aspect of the neck, and being stable in most cases.

5. *Metatarsal stress fracture.* The metatarsals are a very frequent site of stress fracture, which may accompany marching, ballet dancing, prolonged standing, and surgical resection of adjacent metatarsals[16, 17, 19-21, 40, 537] (Fig. 63–11). The middle and distal portions of the shafts of the second and third metatarsals are most often affected,[68] but any metatarsal, including the first, may be involved. In the latter location, it is the base of the bone that is altered, and periostitis, a frequent finding at other metatarsal sites, is relatively uncommon.

6. *Upper extremity stress fracture.* These fractures are far less frequent than stress fractures in the bones of the lower extremity. Typical sites include the ribs in golfers and tennis players,[27] the coracoid process of the scapula in trapshooters,[26] the ulnae of patients using wheelchairs,[69] the hook of the hamate in tennis players, golfers, and baseball players,[70, 71] the olecranon process in baseball pitchers and javelin throwers,[72] the phalangeal tufts in guitar players,[34] and the inferior edge of the glenoid fossa in baseball pitchers.[73] Radial stress fractures are also recorded.[538, 539]

7. *Stress fracture of the neural arch of the vertebra (spondylolysis).* Spondylolysis represents a defect in the pars interarticularis of the vertebra. It may or may not be associated with a slippage of one vertebral body onto the adjacent one, the slippage being termed spondylolisthesis. Spondylolysis is most frequently observed in the lumbar region of the spine, although reports of cervical spondylolysis are

Table 63–1

LOCATION OF STRESS FRACTURE BY ACTIVITY*

Location	Activity
Sesamoids of metatarsals	Prolonged standing
Metatarsal shaft	Marching; stamping on ground; prolonged standing; ballet; postoperative bunionectomy
Navicular	Stamping on ground; marching; long distance running
Calcaneus	Jumping; parachuting; prolonged standing; recent immobilization
Tibia—Mid and distal shaft	Long distance running
Proximal shaft (children)	Running
Fibula—Distal shaft	Long distance running
Proximal shaft	Jumping; parachuting
Patella	Hurdling
Femur—Shaft	Ballet; long distance running
Neck	Ballet; marching; long distance running; gymnastics
Pelvis—Obturator ring	Stooping; bowling; gymnastics
Lumbar vertebra (pars interarticularis)	Ballet; lifting heavy objects; scrubbing floors
Lower cervical, upper thoracic spinous process	Clay shoveling
Ribs	Carrying heavy pack; golf; coughing
Clavicle	Postoperative radical neck
Coracoid of scapula	Trap shooting
Humerus—Distal shaft	Throwing a ball
Ulna—Coronoid	Pitching a ball
Shaft	Pitchfork work; propelling wheelchair
Hook of hamate	Holding golf club, tennis racquet, baseball bat

*Modified from Daffner RH: Skel Radiol 2:221, 1978.

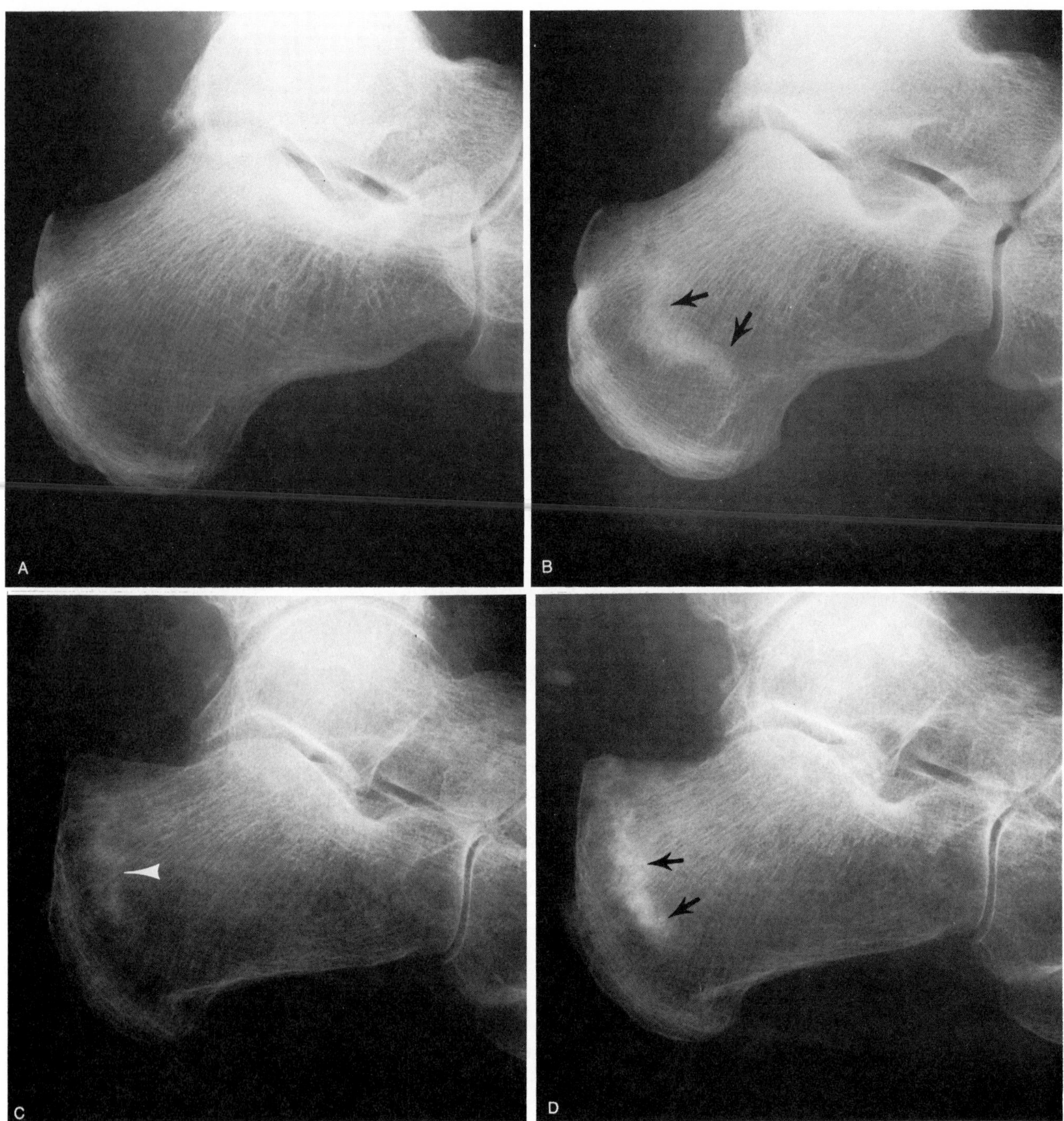

Figure 63–9. *Calcaneal stress fractures in two patients.*

A, B *Examinations obtained 2 months apart reveal an initially normal radiograph, and subsequently, a meandering vertically oriented sclerotic line (arrows). This illustrates the typical location and appearance of a stress fracture in this bone.*

C, D *In a different patient, radiographs obtained several weeks apart delineate an initially ill-defined area of sclerosis (arrowhead), which, on subsequent examination, becomes better delineated (arrows).*

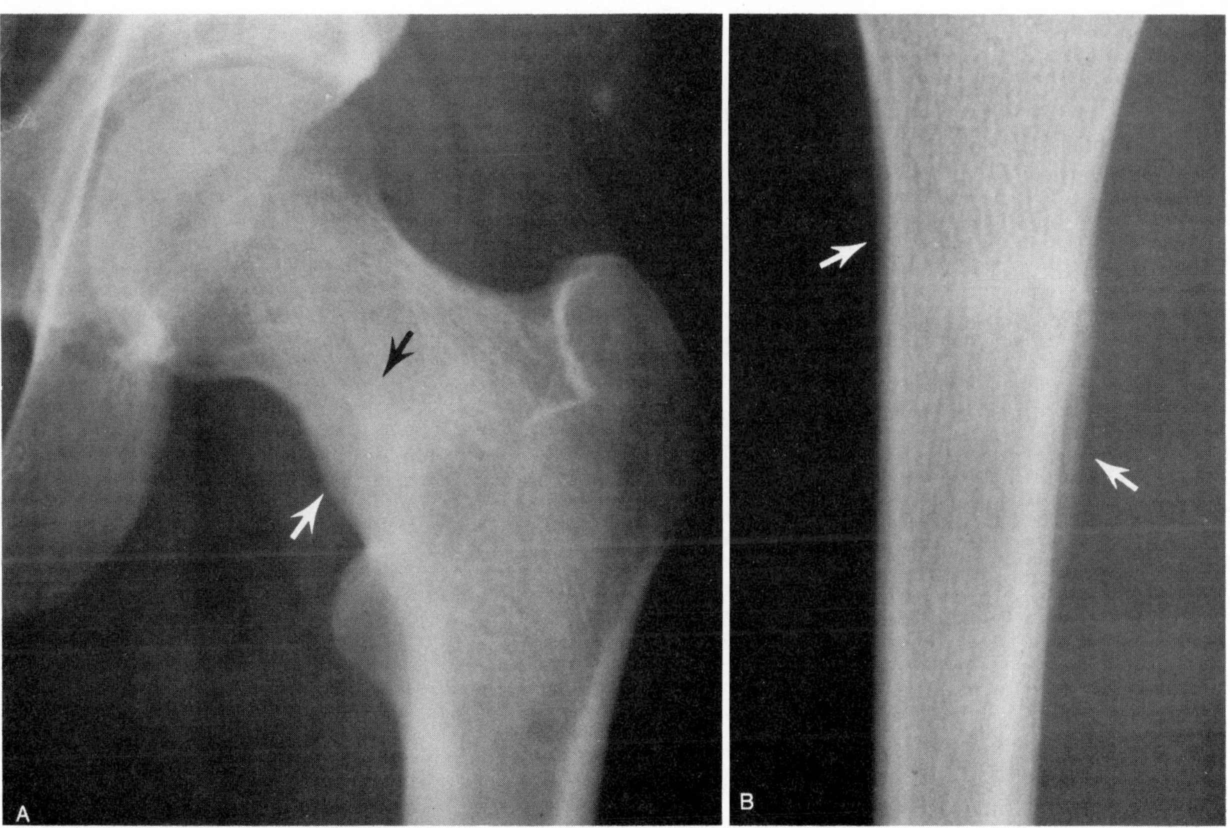

Figure 63–10. *Femoral and tibial stress fractures.*

A *In the femoral neck, observe buttressing and sclerosis (arrows).*

B *In the proximal tibial shaft, periostitis and sclerosis (arrows) are the radiographic abnormalities.*

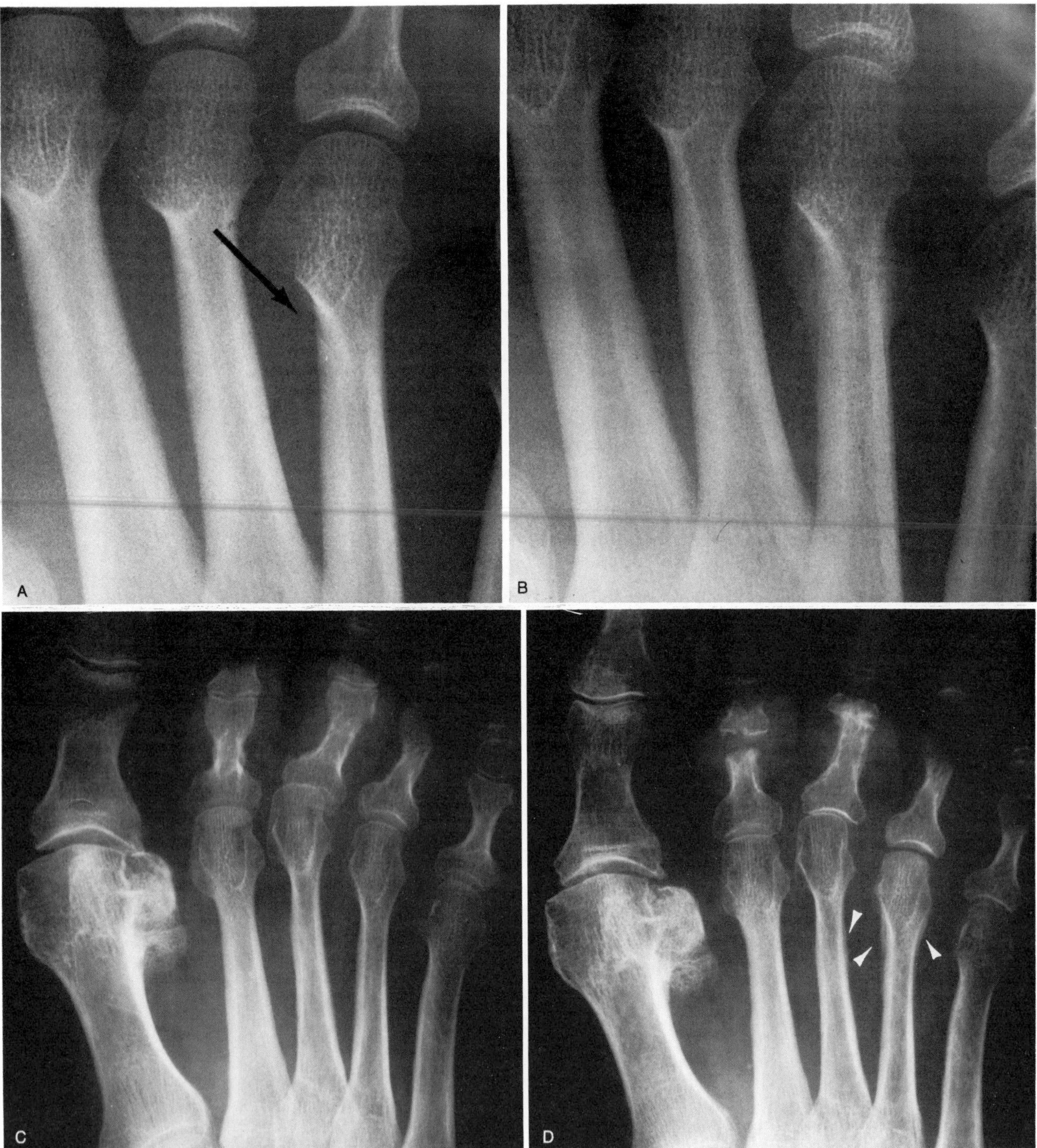

Figure 63–11. *Metatarsal stress fractures.*

A, B *In a military recruit, the initial radiograph delineates an oblique linear radiolucent line through the distal shaft of the fourth metatarsal (arrow). Several weeks later* **(B),** *considerable new bone formation can be seen.*

C, D *In a different patient, resection of the distal portions of the proximal phalanges of the second and third toes is followed by stress periostitis of the shafts of the third and fourth metatarsals (arrowheads).*

numerous (these cervical abnormalities may have a different pathogenesis).[74-78] The fifth lumbar vertebra is most commonly affected (approximately 67 per cent), and the incidence of spondylolysis diminishes as one proceeds cephalad in the lumbar region (L4: 15 to 30 per cent; L3:1 to 2 per cent). Symptoms and signs may be absent, although back and radicular pain, tenderness, gait abnormality, and neurologic deficits can be observed.

The considerable attention that has been focused upon defects in the neural arch of the lumbar vertebrae is not surprising in view of the overall incidence of spondylolysis in the general population. It has been estimated that 3 to 7 per cent of vertebral columns reveal at least one area of spondylolysis.[79-81] This incidence may be greater in Japanese subjects,[82] Eskimos,[83] and in whites than in blacks.[81, 84] Most series demonstrate a male predominance, with the ratio of affected men to affected women ranging from 2:1 to 4:1.[81, 85, 86] Typically, spondylolysis is discovered in childhood or early adulthood, and the incidence of the abnormality does not increase after the age of 20 years.[81] Radiologic and anatomic studies confirm the rarity of pars defects in infants,[87, 88] although documented cases of spondylolysis in infants between the ages of 3 and 8 months have appeared.[84, 89] The incidence of these defects rises precipitously between the ages of 5 and 7 years.[90]

The etiology of lumbar spondylolysis has long been debated. Conflicting opinions have related the osseous defects to congenital or traumatic factors, although the current consensus strongly supports an acquired traumatic lesion originating sometime between infancy and early adult life.[84, 91-98] It is the *type* of fracture — fatigue versus acute — that is not clear. It seems probable that spondylolysis results most frequently from a fatigue fracture occurring after repeated trauma rather than from an acute fracture following a single traumatic episode,[84, 99] although an acute pathogenesis is supported by some observers.[100] The pars interarticularis appears to be the vulnerable point when repetitive stresses act upon the vertebral arch.[94, 589] Yet, there are differences between spondylolysis and other types of fatigue fractures: it frequently develops at an earlier age than other fatigue fractures; there is an hereditary predisposition; the fluffy periosteal callus formation that is commonly noted at sites of other stress fractures is rarely observed in spondylolysis; it develops following minor trauma; and the defect in the pars interarticularis commonly persists.[84] These differences are not uniformly present. For example, some patients do recall a single traumatic event that initiated the back complaints. Furthermore, callus and healing with disappearance of the defect can be noted in some cases,[84, 96, 101-103] although fibrous union and a pseudarthrosis can be detected on histologic examination of the defect in others.[102]

Genetic influences are important in this condition. Spondylolysis "families" can be discovered in which over 25 per cent of individuals demonstrate a defect in the pars interarticularis.[88, 524] Furthermore, there is an increased incidence of nearby congenital anomalies of the spine, such as transitional vertebrae and spina bifida. However, these findings may indicate not that the defect itself is inherited, but rather that there is a genetic influence on the strength of the bone of the pars interarticularis that predisposes certain individuals to stress fracture. Local dysplastic osseous changes have not been demonstrated histologically, and it is possible that the genetic influences in some cases are being confused with environmental and occupational factors, e.g., the occurrence of spondylolysis in the athletic child of athletic parents.[79]

The experimental production of spondylolysis also supports a traumatic rather than a genetic origin. Lamy and associates[100] produced fractures through the pars interarticularis of approximately 35 per cent of cadaveric lumbar vertebrae that were stressed in flexion, whereas Cyron and co-workers[93] were able to create spondylolytic-type fractures in lumbar vertebrae by creating strains in extension. The fractures commenced in the anterolateral cortical layers of the pars, an area of relatively thick bone.[96, 104] These studies and others underscore the importance of trauma in the pathogenesis of spondylolysis.

It is possible that either a single traumatic episode or repeated trauma can result in spondylolysis; thus acute fractures or stress fractures can conceivably produce the same roentgenographic findings. Using this assumption, Wiltse and colleagues[110] have classified lumbar spondylolysis and spondylolisthesis into five types:

Type I: Dysplastic with associated congenital abnormality of the upper sacrum and the arch of the lumbar vertebra.

Type II: Isthmic with a defect in the pars interarticularis that may be: (a) a fatigue fracture, (b) an elongated but intact pars, or (c) an acute fracture.

Type III: Degenerative due to long-standing intersegmental instability.

Type IV: Traumatic due to fractures in areas of the posterior elements other than the pars interarticularis.

Type V: Pathologic due to generalized or localized bone disease.

Radiographic alterations of spondylolysis are diagnostic[97, 105, 106] (Figs. 63–12 and 63–13). The spine has a "Scotty dog" appearance on oblique projections. A unilateral or bilateral radiolucent area through the neck of the "Scotty dog" is well demonstrated. Reactive sclerosis about the radiolucent band may be seen, although true callus is unusual. Slippage or spondylolisthesis may be encountered in some cases, a phenomenon that is more obvious if roentgenograms are obtained with the patient in a standing position[107, 543] or under stress with 30

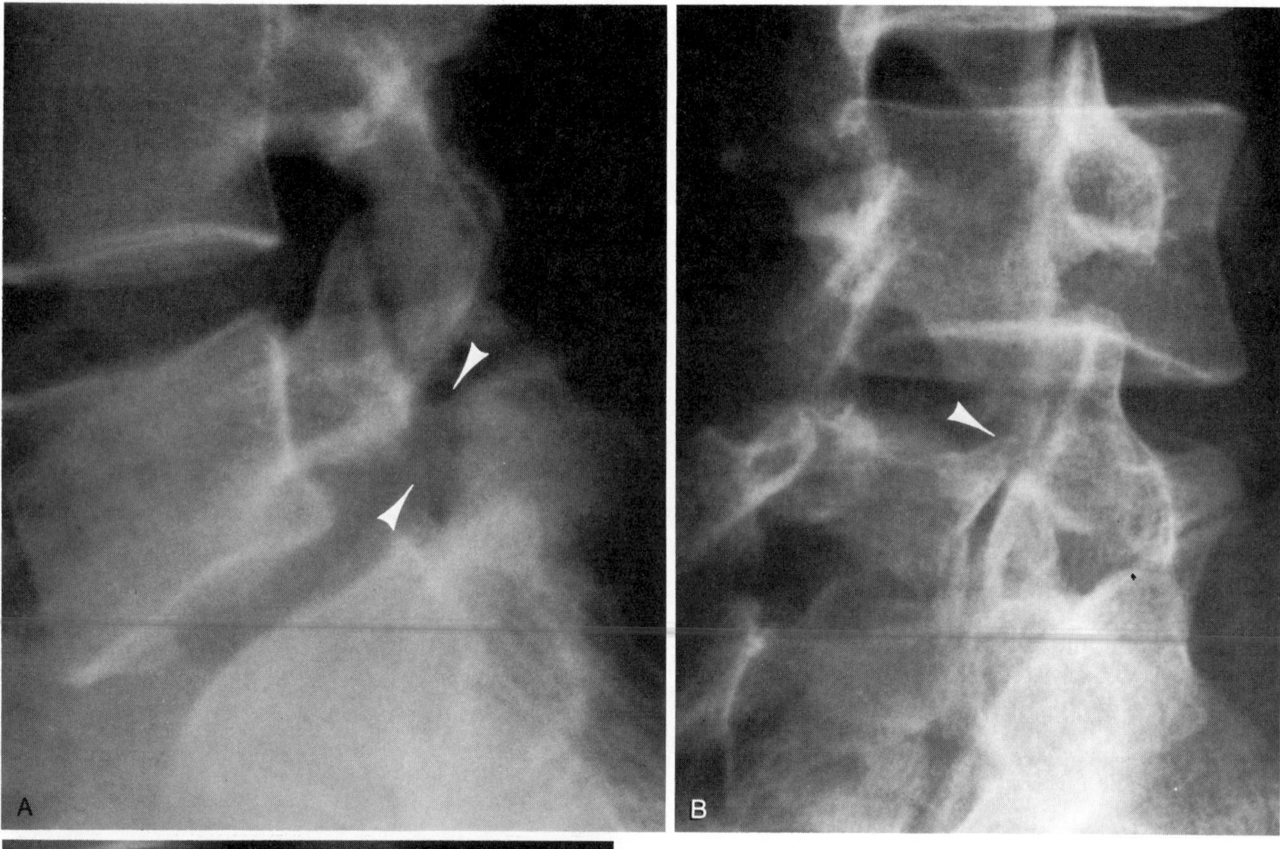

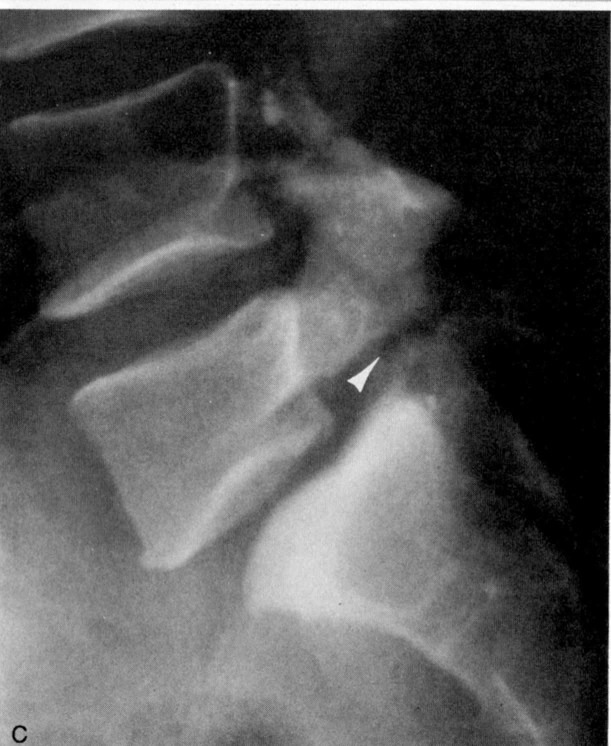

Figure 63–12. *Spondylolysis in adults.*

A, B *Lateral and left posterior oblique projections reveal a defect through the pars interarticularis (arrowheads). The spine has a "Scotty dog" appearance on oblique views. The resulting lucent lesion has produced a break in the "neck" of the "Scotty dog" on the oblique projection. A Grade I spondylolisthesis of L5 on S1 can be noted on the lateral radiograph.*

C *In a different patient, a more exaggerated spondylolisthesis of L5 on S1 is associated with a spondylolysis (arrowhead), intervertebral disc space narrowing, and reactive sclerosis of the sacrum. A myelogram had been performed.*

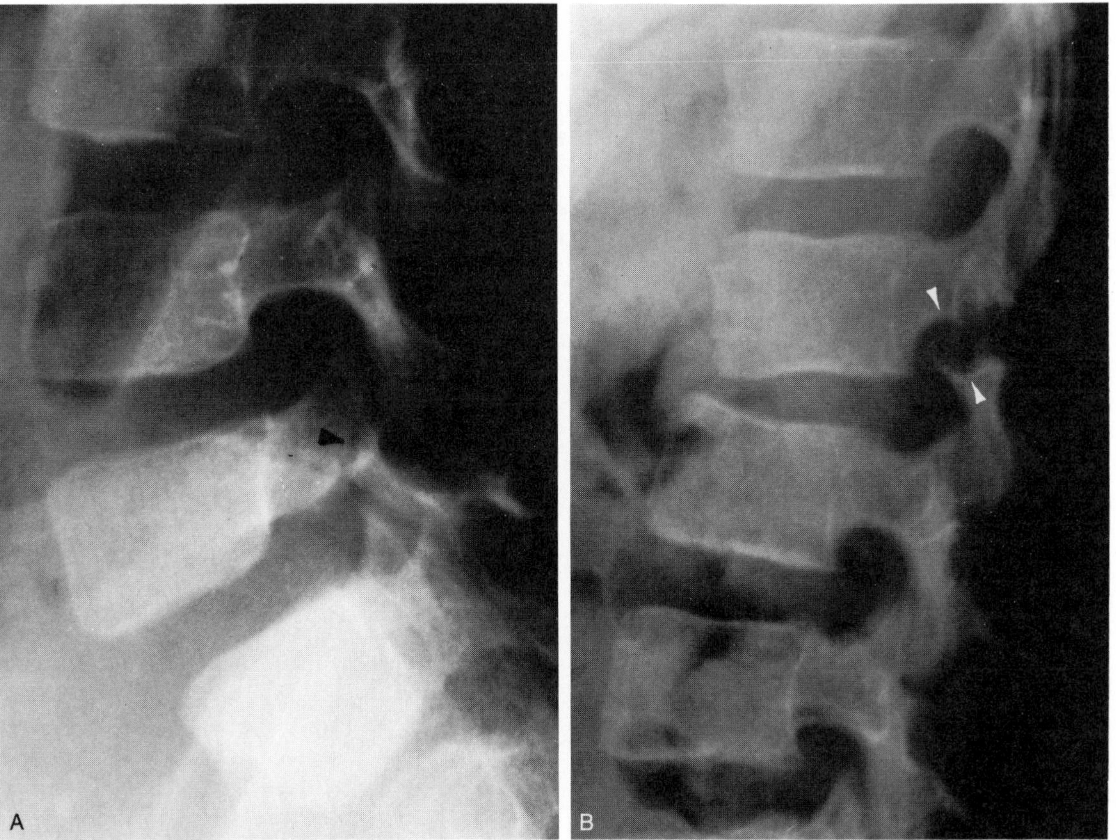

Figure 63–13. *Spondylolysis in children.*

A *A 5 year old boy reveals a fracture (arrowhead) through the pars interarticularis of L5 with spondylolisthesis.*

B *A 9 year old boy demonstrates traumatic spondylolysis of L1 (arrowheads) with spondylolisthesis and spinal angulation.*

pounds of weight on the shoulders. In cases of unilateral spondylolysis, hypertrophy and reactive sclerosis of the contralateral pedicle and lamina may be detected as a physiologic response to the presence of an unstable neural arch[108] (Fig. 63–14). Differentiation of the sclerotic bone from that which occurs in an osteoid osteoma must be accomplished, as excision of an eburnated pedicle associated with contralateral spondylolysis will create painful instability. Additional radiographic abnormalities detected on frontal projections[544] and on flexion and extension films[545] in cases of spondylolysis with or without spondylolisthesis aid in differential diagnosis.

Scintigraphy can be a helpful diagnostic modality in obscure cases of low back pain in which a definite pars interarticularis defect cannot be verified. Increased uptake of bone-seeking pharmaceuticals may indicate increasing stress in the pars with or without a definite fracture.[109]

Greenstick, Torus, and Bowing Fractures. In the immature skeleton, fractures that do not completely penetrate the entire shaft of a bone are not infrequent. The main types of incomplete fractures, in addition to stress fractures, are greenstick, torus, and bowing fractures.

A *greenstick fracture* is one that perforates one cortex and ramifies within the medullary bone.[111] The name is derived from the resemblance of these fractures to a young branch of a tree, which, when broken, is disrupted on its outer surface but remains intact on its inner surface. Greenstick fractures are commonly converted to complete fractures because of the exaggeration of the deformity as the bone continues to grow. Typical locations of greenstick fractures are the proximal metaphysis or diaphysis of the tibia and the middle third of the radius and ulna.

A *torus fracture* results from an injury insufficient in force to create a complete discontinuity of bone but sufficient to produce a buckling of the cortex[111] (Fig. 63–15). Torus fractures are common in metaphyseal regions and in patients with osteoporosis. Significant clinical abnormalities may accompany these fractures, and the radiographs may be interpreted as normal, unless subtle bulging of the cortex is identified. Oblique and lateral roentgeno-

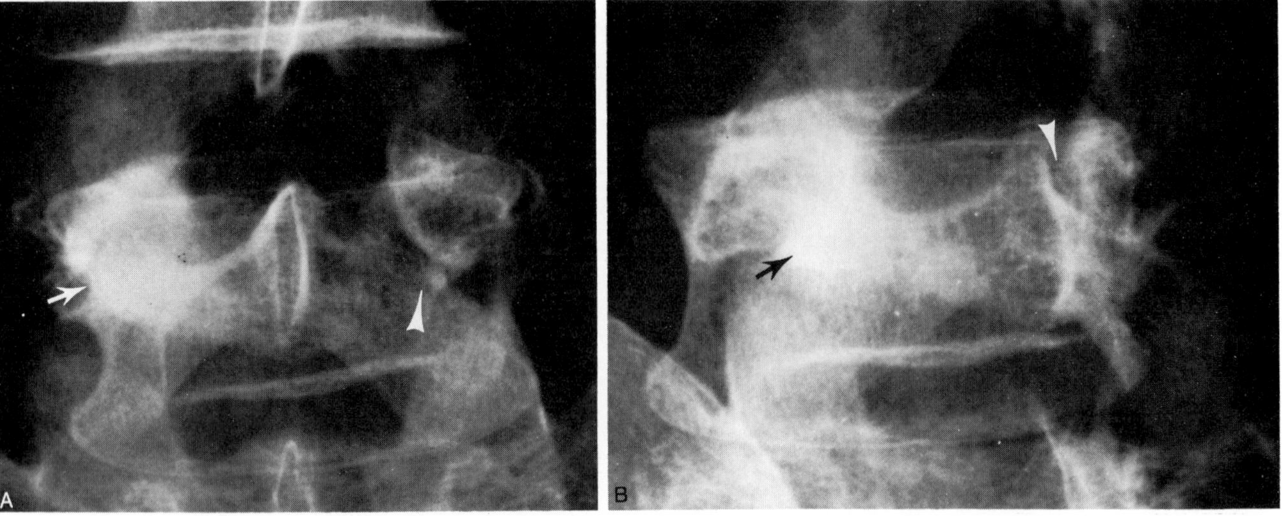

Figure 63–14. Unilateral spondylolysis with bony hypertrophy and reactive sclerosis of the contralateral pedicle. A left spondylolysis (arrowhead) of L5 is associated with eburnation on the opposite side (arrow).

grams are commonly more helpful than frontal projections. Follow-up examination confirms the presence of a torus fracture and may reveal transverse bands of increased radiodensity, indicating osseous impaction.

Bowing fractures are a plastic response, usually to longitudinal stress in a bone.[112-122] They are virtually confined to children and are most typically apparent in the radius and the ulna, although their presence in adults[119] and involvement of other areas such as the fibula and femur[119-122, 546] are encountered.

Experimental data have indicated specific patterns of bony deformation related to longitudinal compression forces[48, 53] (Fig. 63–16). An initial zone

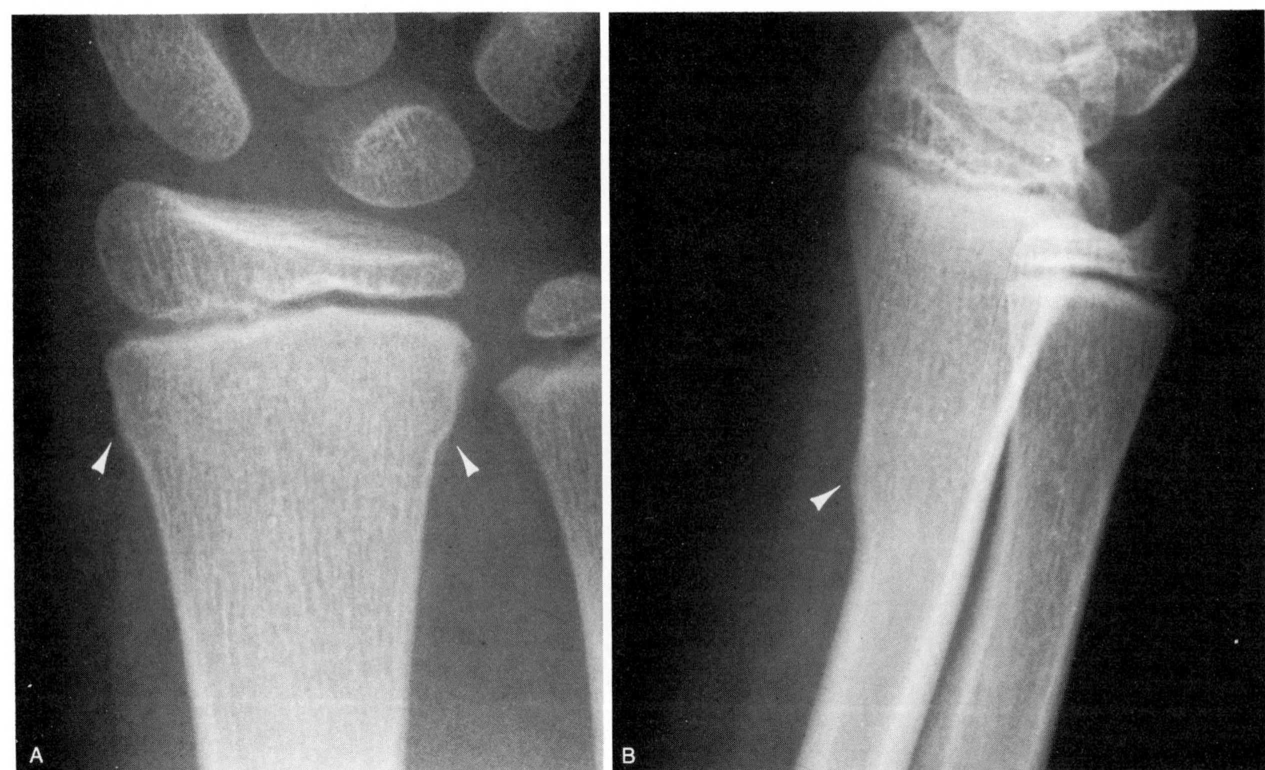

Figure 63–15. Torus fractures. Two examples of torus fractures of the distal radius in children. Note the buckling of the cortex (arrowheads).

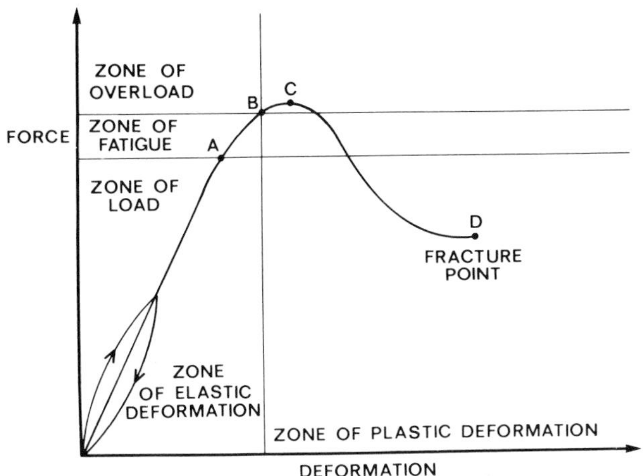

Figure 63–16. *Graphic relationship of bony deformation (bowing) and force (longitudinal compression), after Chamay and Tschantz.*[49, 53] *The linear response in the zone of elastic deformation and the weakening of bone in the zone of plastic deformation are demonstrated. (From Borden S IV: Roentgen recognition of acute plastic bowing of the forearm in children. Am J Roentgenol 135:524, 1975. Copyright 1975, American Roentgen Ray Society.)*

of elastic deformation of bone is characterized by bowing that disappears with release of the offending force. With greater force, plastic deformation occurs, which results in permanent bowing of the bone. Still further increase in stress will lead to fracture. Histologic analysis of the bowed bone will reveal cortical fatigue lines and microfractures. These experimental results can be applied to the analysis of bowing fractures in humans. The deforming force is usually longitudinal without a shear component, particularly with regard to bowing fractures of the radius or ulna, although a direct blow can lead to bowing fracture of the fibula; the deforming force must be greater than the maximal strength of the bone (approximately 100 to 150 per cent of body weight); and the duration of the force must be shorter than the time necessary to reach the point of fracture.[116] Commonly, bowing is identified in one of two neighboring bones (e.g., radius and ulna; fibula and tibia), and a fracture of the adjacent bone is evident. The latter fracture is usually diaphyseal in location and may allow dispersion of enough of the stress to prevent a similar fracture of the bowed bone. Similarly, dislocation of one bone can be associated with bowing of the adjacent one; an example of this is a dislocation of the radial head in association with a bowed ulna. Bowing may also involve one bone without an abnormality of an adjacent one or may affect both bones simultaneously.

Roentgenographic analysis of bowing deformities reveals lateral or anteroposterior bending of the affected bone (Fig. 63–17). The abnormality may be subtle, necessitating comparison radiographs of the opposite side for correct diagnosis. Sequential radiographs of a plastic bowing deformity usually reveal no evidence of periostitis, although thickening of the involved cortex may be detected. Scintigraphy may identify increased uptake of bone-seeking pharmaceuticals even when radiographs are only equivocal. A bowed bone remains bowed, resists attempts at reduction, holds an adjacent fracture in angulation, and prevents relocation of an adjacent dislocation.[116] The force necessary to reduce a plastic deformity is equivalent in magnitude to that required to create it.

The principles that govern the appearance of bowed fractures in children can be applied to these lesions in other clinical settings.[116] In the adult, the range of plastic deformation is narrower than in the child or adolescent, although a longitudinal force of the correct magnitude and duration can create a bowed bone. Similar deformities may appear in pathologic bone, as in fibrous dysplasia, Paget's disease, and osteogenesis imperfecta.

TRANSCHONDRAL FRACTURES (OSTEOCHONDRITIS DISSECANS). Osteochondritis dissecans indicates fragmentation and possible separation of a portion of the articular surface. The clinical manifestations are variable, related to the specific site of involvement. The age of onset varies from childhood to middle age, but an adolescent onset is most frequent. Patients may be entirely asymptomatic; however, pain aggravated by movement, limitation of

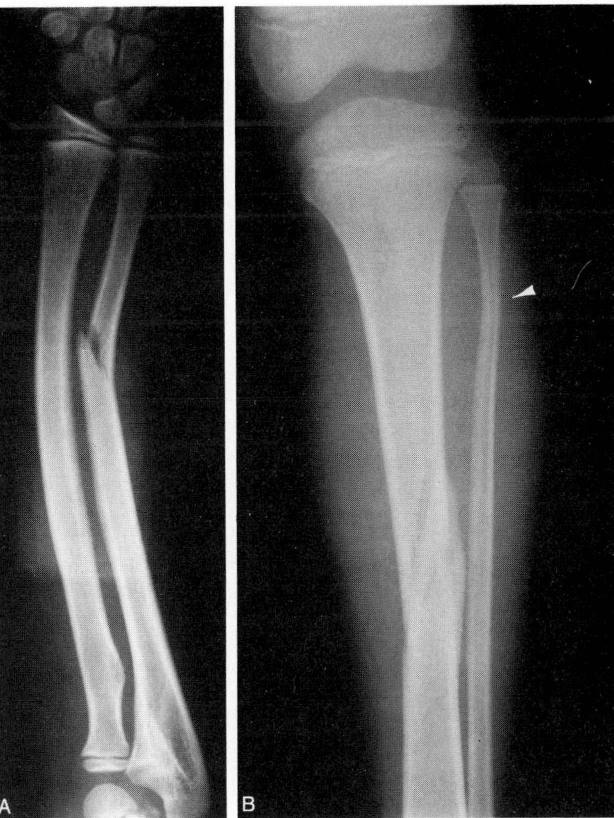

Figure 63–17. *Bowing deformities of bone.*

A *Note the bowing of the radius associated with a fracture of the adjacent ulna.*

B *Observe subtle bowing of the proximal fibula (arrowhead) associated with a tibial fracture.*

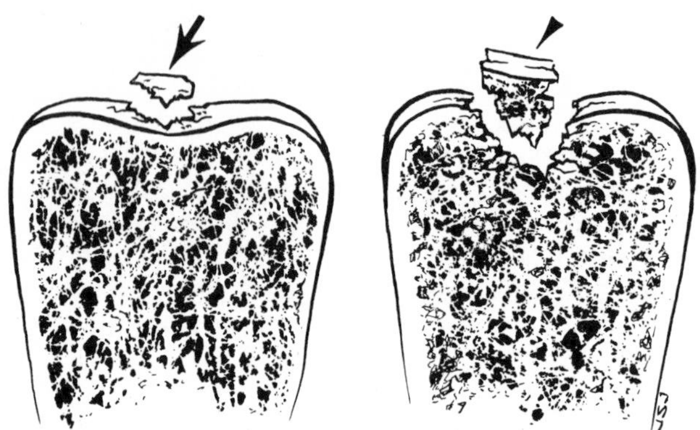

Figure 63–18. Transchondral fractures (osteochondritis dissecans): Components of fragments. Fragments can consist of cartilage alone (arrow) or both cartilage and bone (arrowhead).

motion, clicking, locking, and swelling may be apparent. Single or multiple sites can be affected. Although the role of trauma is undeniable in most locations, a familial history has been evident in some cases, especially in osteochondritis of the knee,[123-126, 547] and an autosomal dominant mode of inheritance has been suggested.[127, 142] Major alterations associated with familial osteochondritis are short stature, endocrine dysfunction, and tibia vara,[142] and it is possible that a separate variety of osteochondritis dissecans occurs in the juvenile patient owing to irregularities of ossification.

Osteochondral fractures are the result of shearing, rotatory, or tangentially aligned impaction forces.[128] Because of the insensitivity of subchondral bone, with the absence of recognizable symptoms and signs in many cases, it is not always possible to define the exact time and mechanism of the injury. Acute injuries can produce fragments consisting of cartilage alone (chondral fractures) or cartilage and underlying bone (osteochondral fractures)[128-130] (Fig. 63–18). In general, the fracture line parallels the joint surface, and it is the depth of the lesion that defines the cartilaginous and osseous components of the fragment. Obviously, a purely cartilaginous fragment creates no direct radiographic abnormalities, whereas one containing calcified cartilage and bone becomes apparent owing to a varying degree of radiodensity. Secondary roentgenographic signs consisting of soft tissue swelling and a joint effusion can be apparent with either chondral or chondro-osseous fragments. Arthrography may be utilized to define the nature and location of the fracture more accurately; defects in the cartilaginous surface, contrast filling of an osseous excavation, and intra-articular chondral and osseous bodies may be recognized (see Chapter 15).

Following the injury, the detached portion of the articular surface can remain in situ, be slightly displaced, or become "loose" within the joint cavity (Figs. 63–19 and 63–20). In many cases, the osteocartilaginous fragments attach to the synovial lining at a distant site and become reabsorbed. If a fragment maintains some attachment to its site of origin, it can undergo revascularization, and new bone formation and radiographically evident growth and trabeculation can be seen. Free chondral or osteochondral fragments can undergo (a) proliferation of new layers of cartilage and bone, (b) resorption due to surface osteoclasis, or (c) degenerative calcification of cartilage in both the original cartilage and the cartilage of the layers that have formed about the initial nidus or fragment.[128] These histologic findings have radiographic counterparts; "loose" bodies may become more visible with time owing to proliferation of new cartilage and bone or secondary degenerative calcification, or both. With the proliferation of new cartilage

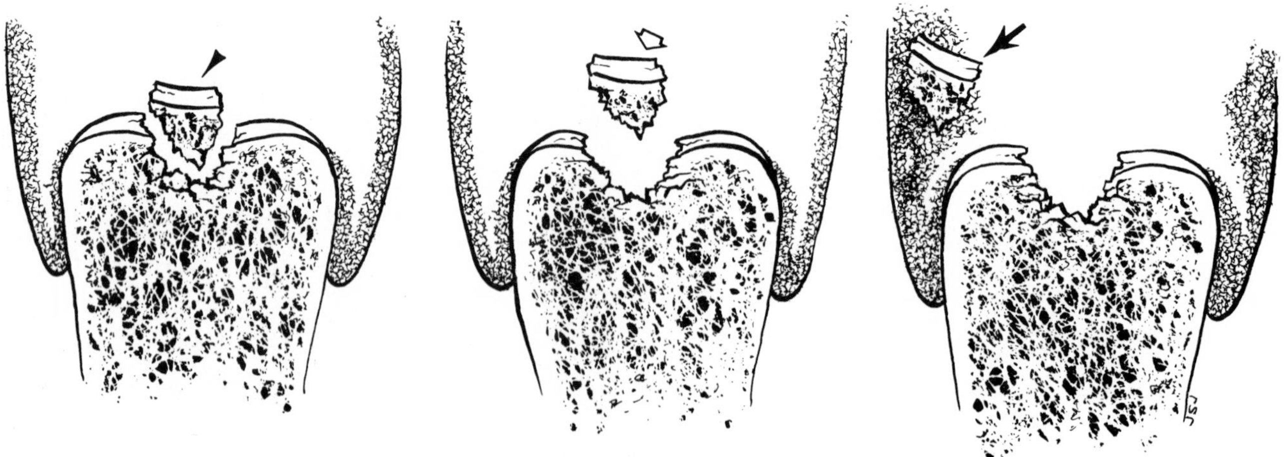

Figure 63–19. Transchondral fractures (osteochondritis dissecans): Fate of fragments. Chondral or osteochondral fragments can remain in situ (arrowhead), be slightly displaced or "loose" in the articular cavity (open arrow), or become embedded at a distant synovial site, evoking a local inflammatory reaction (solid arrow).

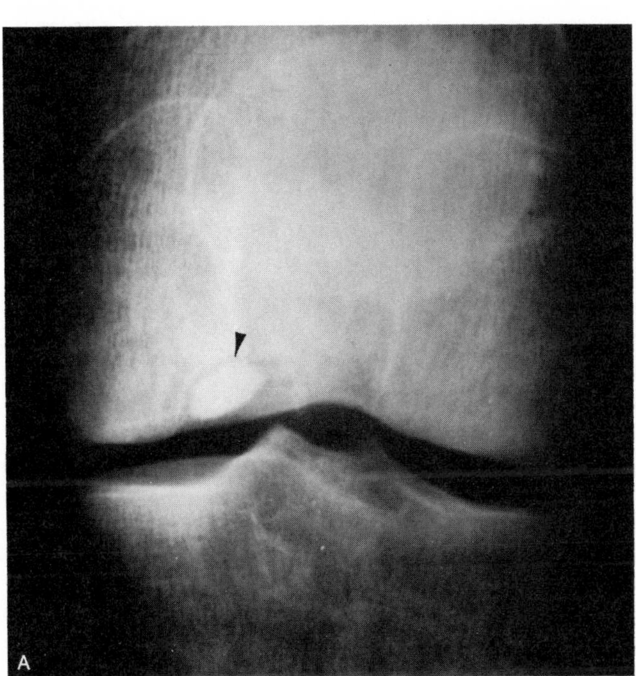

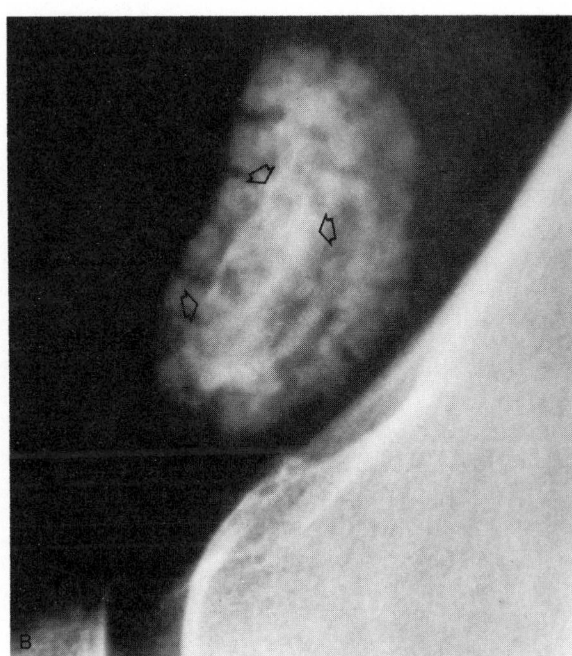

Figure 63–20. *Transchondral fractures (osteochondritis dissecans): Fate of fragments.*

A *Fragment remaining in situ: Note the osseous dense area (arrowhead) indicating a fragment that remains in its bed in the medial femoral condyle.*

B *"Loose" body with proliferation of new cartilage. Note the layered appearance as calcification has occurred about the original nidus (open arrows) in the suprapatellar pouch.*

Illustration continued on the following page

and bone, a laminated appearance is identified, whereas with secondary degenerative calcification, a more or less homogeneous increase in radiodensity is seen.

The identification of "loose" osteocartilaginous bodies or those attached to the synovial lining on roentgenographic examination should stimulate a search for their site of origin. A rather small defect in the articular surface may be the only evidence of the initial fracture location, even in the presence of multiple and large intra-articular bodies. Special views and tomograms may be required for identification of the fracture site. Such identification is important, as single or multiple chondral or osseous bodies can accompany a variety of other conditions, including idiopathic synovial osteochondromatosis and articular disorders such as neuroarthropathy, crystal-induced arthropathy, degenerative joint disease, and osteonecrosis. In idiopathic synovial osteochondromatosis, radiographic clues include the presence of multiple opaque areas of approximately equal size scattered throughout the articular cavity,

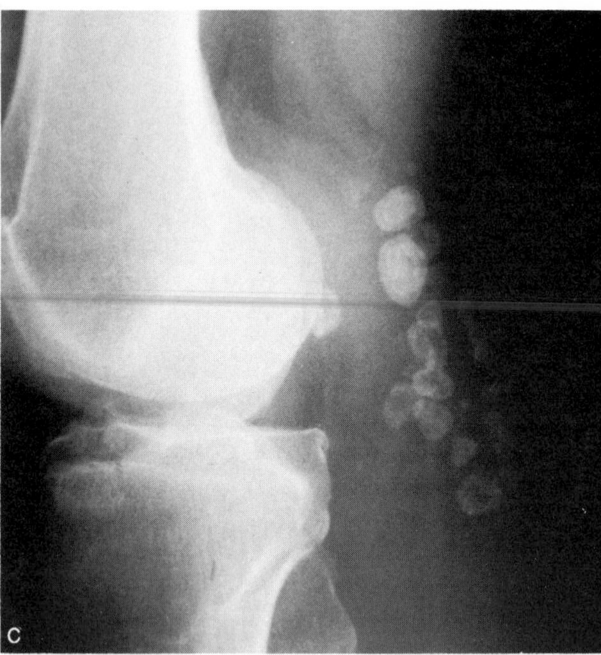

Figure 63–20. Continued

C *Migration of fragments to a distant location. In this situation, intra-articular bodies have passed into a communicating synovial (popliteal) cyst.*

D, E *Reattachment of fragments to synovial membrane with resorption. Radiographs obtained several months apart reveal resorption of synovium-embedded fragments (arrow).*

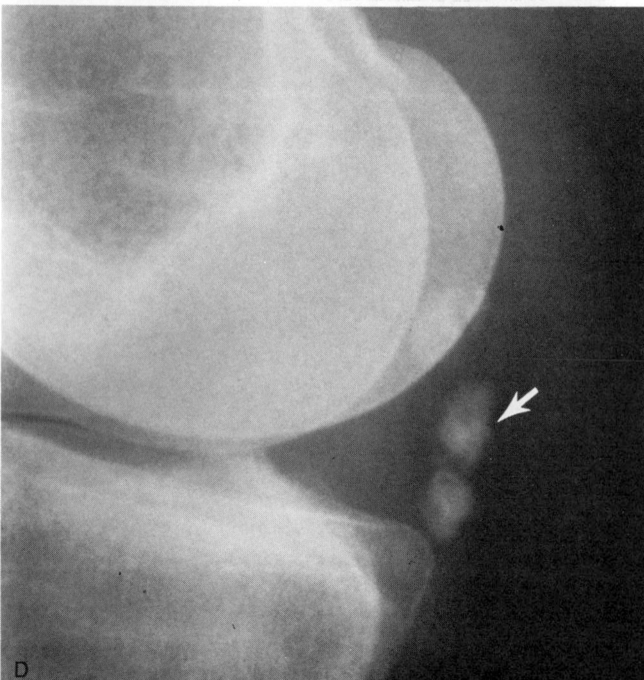

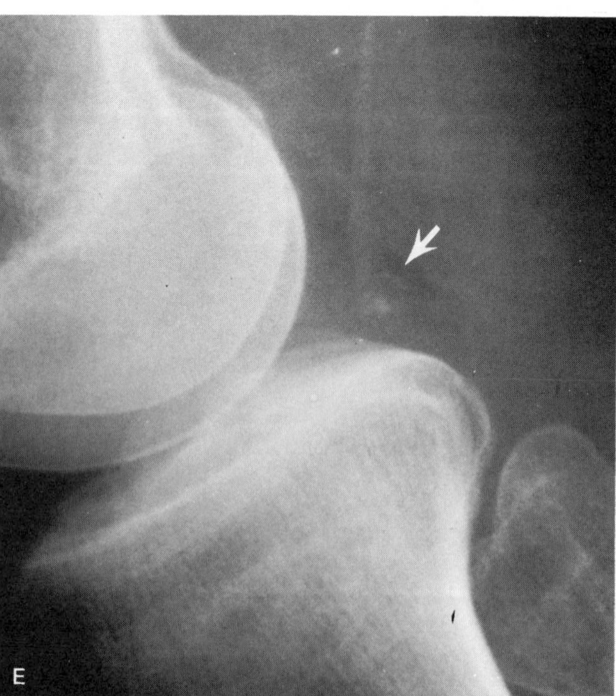

confined to one segment of the joint, or even within a synovial cyst, and the absence of evidence of an underlying articular disorder or trauma (Fig. 63–21). The diagnosis of idiopathic synovial osteochondromatosis is substantiated by the pathologist, who frequently notes metaplasia of synovial lining cells into cartilage and bone.

Femoral Condyles. The most typical location of osteochondritis dissecans is the condylar surfaces of the distal femur.[131-141] Men are affected more frequently than women, and the average age at onset of symptoms and signs is 15 to 20 years, although the age range is highly variable. Unilateral changes predominate over bilateral changes in a ratio of approximately 3:1. A significant history of knee trauma can be elicited in about 50 per cent of cases. Pain and swelling may be prominent. The possible locations of the osteochondral defect have been

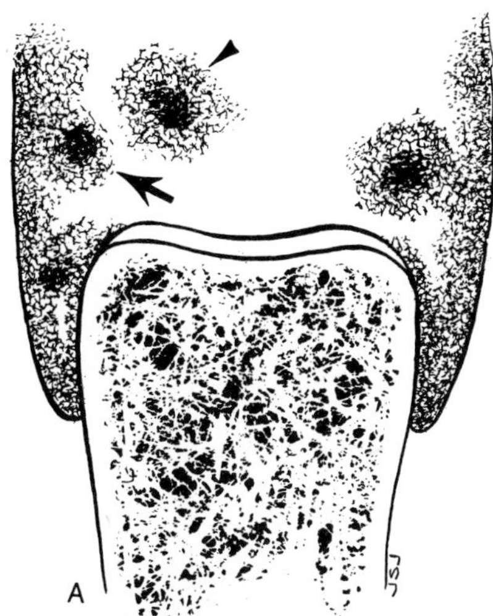

Figure 63–21. *Idiopathic synovial osteochondromatosis.*

A *In this condition, metaplasia of synovial lining cells into cartilage and bone is identified. The resulting nidi can remain in the synovial membrane (arrow) or become displaced into the articular cavity (arrowhead).*

B, C *This 67 year old woman developed progressive pain and swelling in the elbow over a 6 month period. The radiograph* **(B)** *outlines irregular ossification in the joint (solid arrows) with displacement of the anterior fat pad (arrowhead) and minor osseous erosion (open arrow) and osteophytic lipping. The arthrogram* **(C)** *identifies multiple radiolucent filling defects (arrows). The diagnosis was confirmed histologically.*

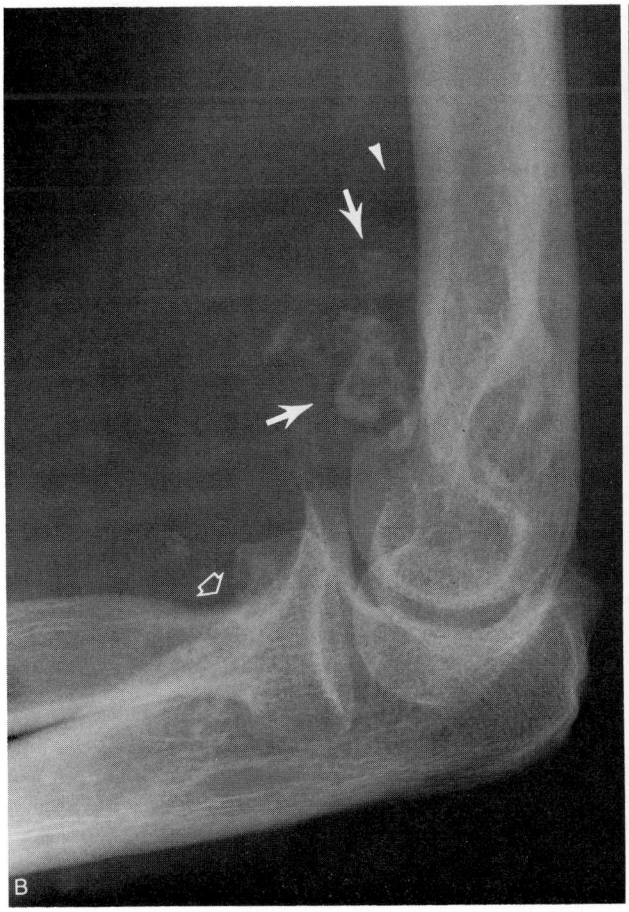

B

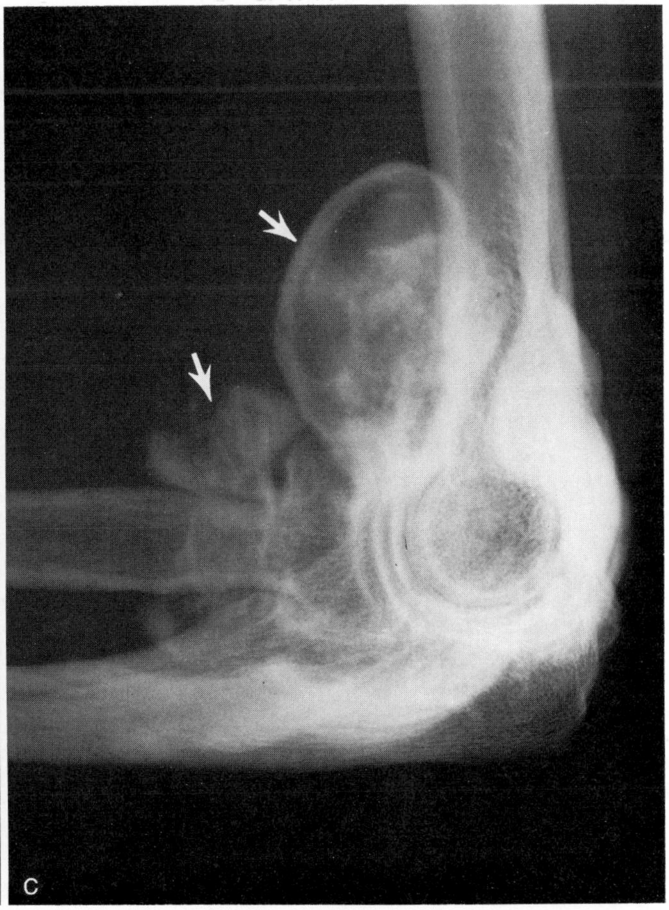

C

summarized by Aichroth,[131] who, in an analysis of over 100 patients, determined that the medial condyle was affected in approximately 85 per cent of cases and the lateral condyle in 15 per cent of cases. A classic defect on the inner (lateral) aspect of the medial femoral condyle occurred in 69 per cent of cases, whereas an extended classic or inferocentral medial condylar lesion was evident in 6 per cent and 10 per cent of cases, respectively (Figs. 63–22 and 63–23). Other investigators have detected a somewhat higher incidence of lateral condylar lesions, in the order of magnitude of approximately 30 per cent.[136, 137, 150]

The pathogenesis of osteochondritis dissecans of the femoral condyles is not agreed upon.[143] That bone necrosis may be recognized on histologic evaluation of some of the lesions is undeniable. Rather, it is the cause of the osteonecrosis and the role of trauma that have been debated. Milgram's observations that some of the fragments originating from the joint surface in this disease contain articular cartilage alone, with no

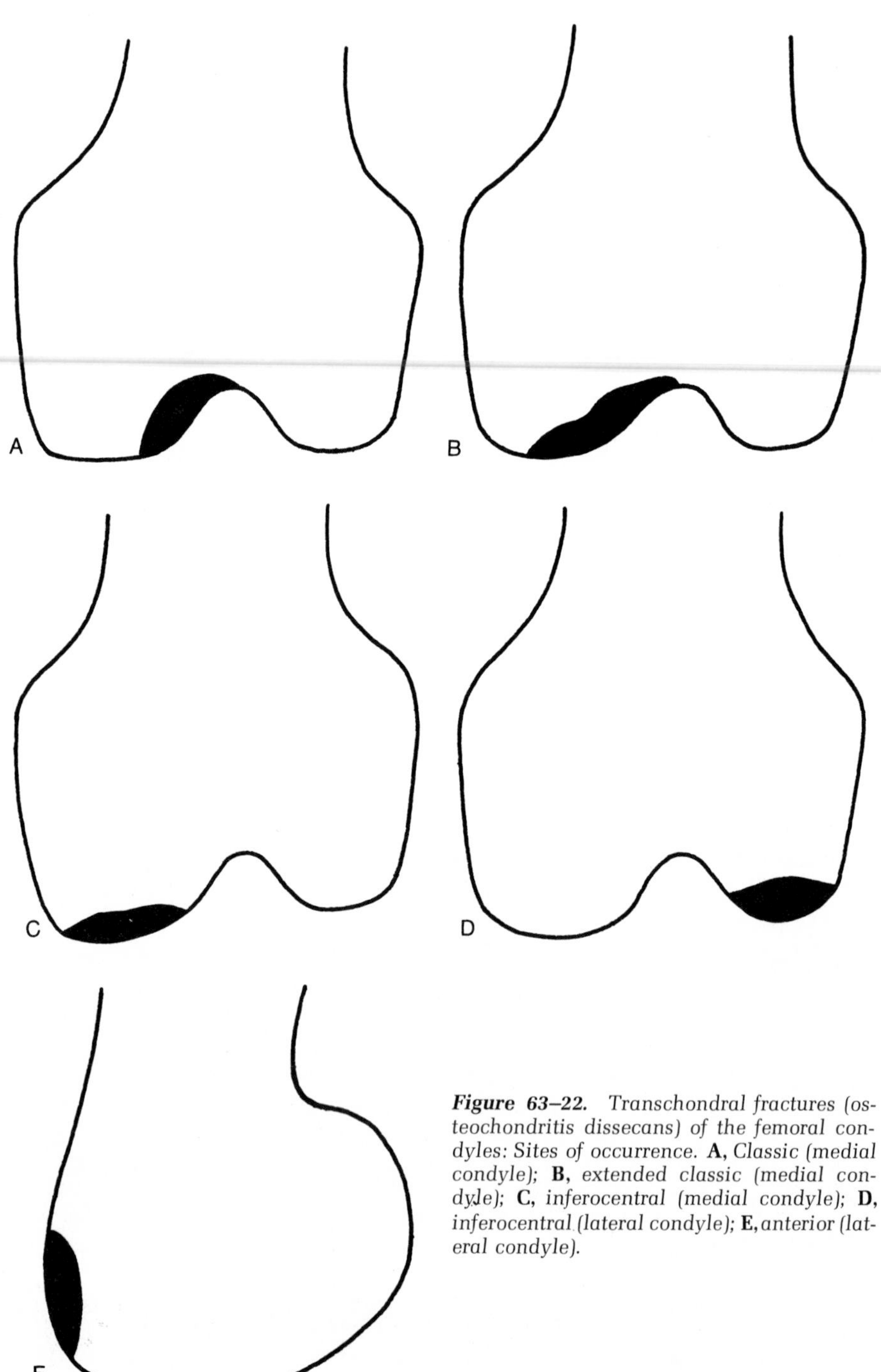

Figure 63–22. *Transchondral fractures (osteochondritis dissecans) of the femoral condyles: Sites of occurrence.* **A,** *Classic (medial condyle);* **B,** *extended classic (medial condyle);* **C,** *inferocentral (medial condyle);* **D,** *inferocentral (lateral condyle);* **E,** *anterior (lateral condyle).*

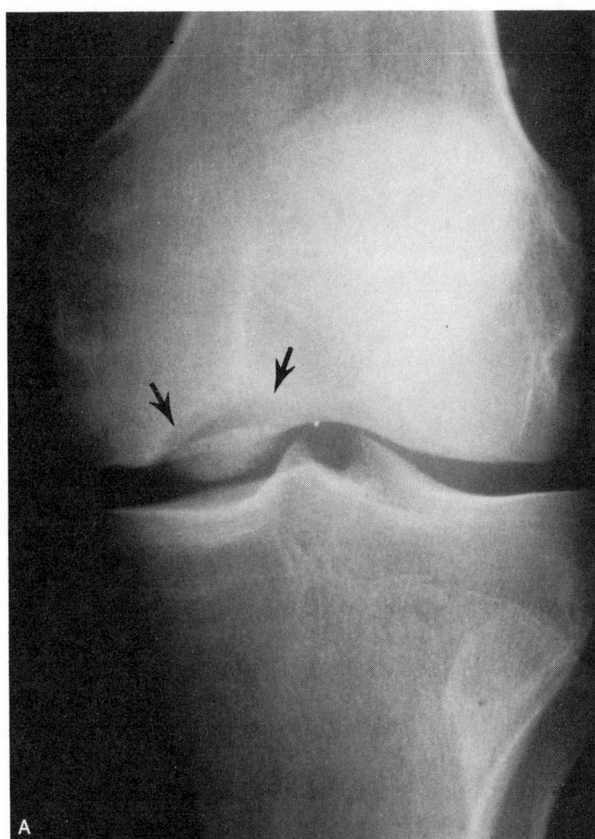

Figure 63–23. Transchondral fractures (osteochondritis dissecans) of the femoral condyles: Sites of occurrence.

A Extended classic defect of medial condyle (arrows).

B, C Inferocentral lesion of lateral condyle (arrow).

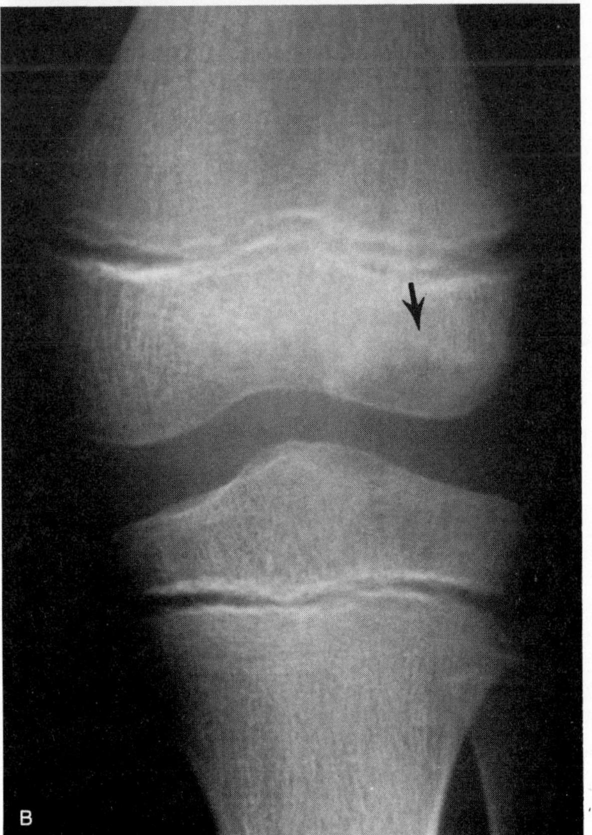

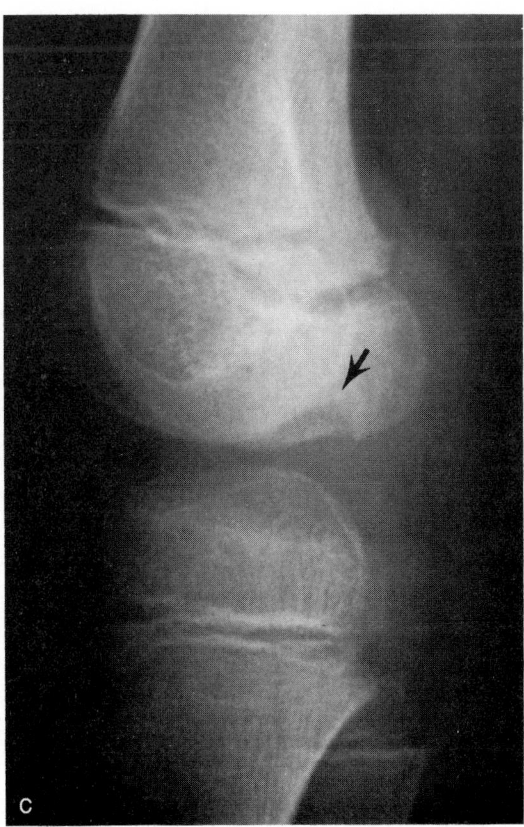

evidence of necrotic subchondral bone,[132] an observation also confirmed by other investigators,[135, 144, 145] would support a primary traumatic etiology. Even fragments with osseous components can reveal evidence of bone marrow viability.[132, 144, 146] Furthermore, examination of specimens of bone at the femoral origin of the fragments has not shown evidence of bone infarction.[132, 145, 147] These pathologic observations appear to underscore the importance of trauma in initiating this condition. The mechanism of the traumatic event is not clear but may be related to rotatory forces acting on the fixed weight-bearing knee. Shearing forces, direct blows, and ligamentous avulsions could produce osteochondral fragments.[138, 148, 149] The trauma may be major or minor, and the relative insensitivity of cancellous bone would account for the absence of acute symptoms and signs in some patients.[132, 144] The presence and degree of displacement of the chondral or osteochondral fragment can apparently vary; some bodies may be immediately torn free, whereas others remain attached and undergo remodeling owing to retained blood supply from adjacent soft tissue structures.[132] Subsequent trauma could lead to progressive disruption, and motion may induce the formation of cartilaginous callus in the cleft within the subchondral bone.

The roentgenographic characteristics of osteochondritis dissecans in situ of the femoral condyles have been well summarized by Milgram.[132] Rarely, in acute cases, a linear radiolucent fracture line in the subchondral bone may be observed. More commonly, a small osseous lesion may be separated from the normal or sclerotic base of the femoral defect by a radiolucent crescentic zone. Fragmentation and collapse of the partially separated body can be recognized. Disruption and displacement of the osteochondral fragment produce a loose or synovium-embedded intra-articular osseous body (Fig. 63–24). The site of origin on the femur may be gradually remodeled, although a slightly flattened or irregular articular surface can frequently be detected for decades. Secondary degenerative joint disease has been described in long-term follow-up examinations of those patients with osteochondritis dissecans of the knee who have had the first manifestation of the disorder following the closure of the growth plate[136]; the pattern of degenerative joint disease in these individuals has been described as atypical in that it begins about 10 years earlier in life than does usual osteoarthritis of the knee, more commonly involves the three compartments of the knee, and is frequently associated with "loose bodies." In some of the reported cases of degenerative joint disease following osteochondritis dissecans, the initial lesion may have represented spontaneous osteonecrosis of the knee (see Chapter 77).

The major differential diagnosis of the radio-

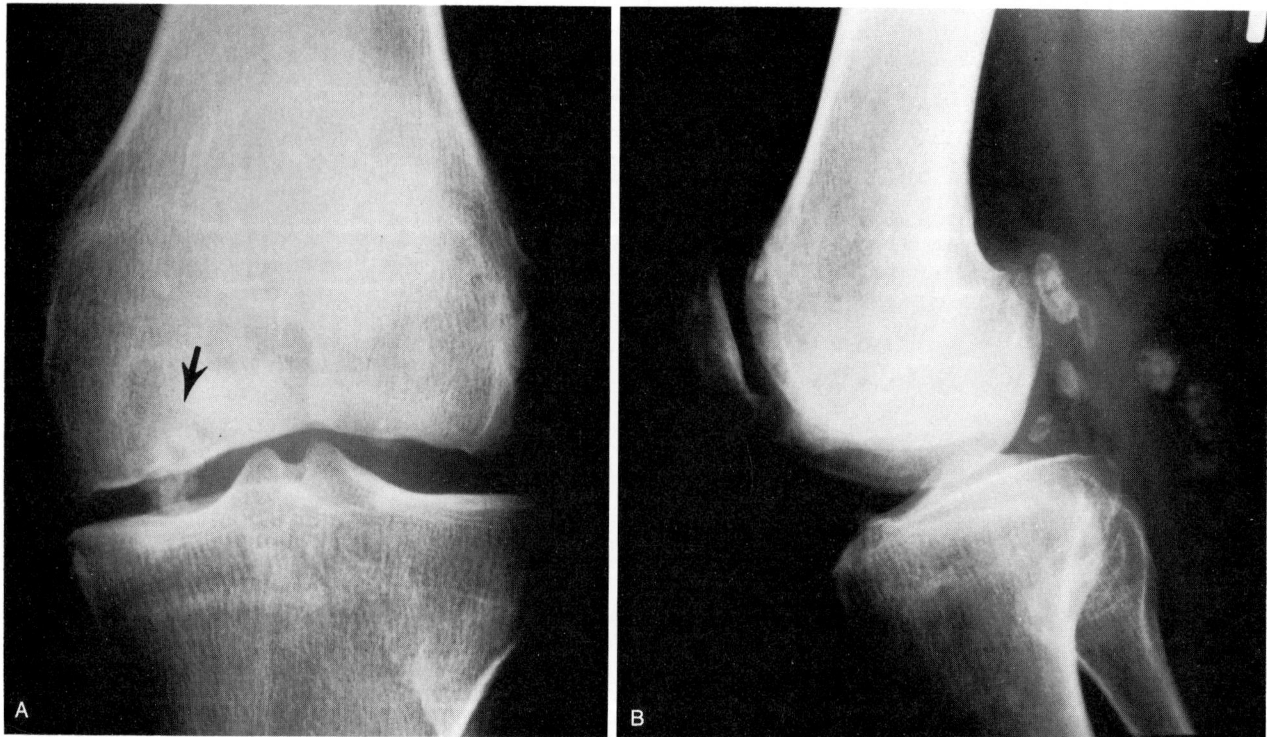

Figure 63–24. *Transchondral fractures (osteochondritis dissecans) of the femoral condyles. Note the healed defect in the medial femoral condyle (arrow), osseous bodies in the joint and in a popliteal cyst, and secondary degenerative joint disease.*

graphic features of condylar osteochondritis dissecans is spontaneous osteonecrosis of the knee. This lesion occurs in older individuals, is associated with the sudden onset of clinical manifestations, and almost invariably involves the weight-bearing portion of the medial femoral condyle. It appears to represent a true osteonecrosis, although the cause of the necrosis is not certain. Osteochondritis dissecans of the knee must also be differentiated from the fragmentation that may accompany neuroarthropathy and from the normal grooves that appear on the medial and lateral femoral condyles on lateral roentgenograms (see Chapter 3).

Patella. In comparison with osteochondritis dissecans of the femoral condyles, that of the patella is rare.[151-155, 548] Unilateral involvement predominates. Men are affected more frequently than women, and the age of clinical onset is usually between 15 and 20 years. The typical site of the lesion is the medial facet of the patella. Involvement of the lateral facet occurs in approximately 30 per cent of cases, and the most medial or "odd" facet is generally spared. The middle or lower portion of the bone is almost universally affected, whereas the superior portion is uninvolved.

The etiology of the lesion appears to be traumatic, although support for primary ischemic necrosis does exist[156] despite the rich blood supply to the subchondral patellar bone.[157] Although a history of an injury may not be elicited, it is well recognized that the articular surface is repeatedly exposed to trauma, and a tangential shearing force may be responsible for the lesion. Historically, patients frequently note pain, originating when the knee was flexed under load, supporting the concept of a shearing fracture. An association with ligamentous laxity and lateral patellar subluxation also supports this concept of a traumatic etiology.[155] The lesions are optimally identified on lateral and axial radiographs, appearing as osseous defects near the convexity between the condylar articular surfaces of the patella (Fig. 63–25). Single or multiple intra-articular osseous bodies may also be recognized. Arthrography can identify the chondral component of the injury.

The major differential diagnoses are chondromalacia patellae, dorsal defect of the patella, and osteochondral fractures related to direct injury or recurrent dislocation. Chondromalacia patellae is usually confined to the cartilaginous layer of the bone. Radiographs may be entirely normal, although local subchondral sclerosis and detached flakes of calcified cartilage have been recognized. The dorsal defect of the patella is a benign lesion associated with a round and lytic defect with well-defined margins in the superolateral aspect of the bone[158, 159] (Fig. 63–26). Arthrography reveals intact cartilage in almost all cases.[525] This defect occurs in both sexes, may be bilateral, and is unassociated with symptoms and signs.

Dislocation of the patella is associated with an osteochondral fracture at the medial side of the patella and, less frequently, at the lateral margin of the lateral femoral condyle[160-164] (Fig. 63–27). Although this diagnosis may be facilitated by seeing the patient when the patella is dislocated, the patella may reduce itself spontaneously, and the patient may not volunteer an appropriate history. Thus, identification of the typical fractures is important in the accurate diagnosis of this condition. The radiographic abnormalities are characteristic, appearing on axial views of the patella. The findings relate both to true fracture of the patella and femur and to calcification and ossification of adjacent hematomas.[164] The cause of the patellar and femoral fractures relates to the contraction of the quadriceps muscle during relocation, driving the patella into the lateral femoral condyle.[128]

Although tumors and infection may also affect the patella (Fig. 63–28), the resulting radiographic picture does not resemble that of osteochondritis dissecans.

Talus. Osteochondral fractures are also recognized in the talar dome.[165-169, 526, 549-551] The middle third of the lateral border of the talus and the posterior third of the medial border are the two most common sites of injury, and they are involved with approximately equal frequency.[165] Men are affected more often than women, and the patients are usually in the second to fourth decades of life. Clinical and experimental evidence confirms the etiology of trauma in the production of these lesions, although the exact mechanism of injury has not been agreed upon.[165, 170, 171] The lateral talar lesion appears to relate to an inversion injury of the ankle[165] (Fig. 63–29). As the foot is inverted, the lateral border of the talar dome is compressed against the fibula. Further inversion ruptures the lateral collateral ligament and results in an avulsion of a small piece of the dome. This osteochondral fragment may remain in place or be displaced by continued inversion. If the injury is mild and the lateral ligament remains intact, clinical manifestations may be relatively mild; more severe injury with ligamentous tear is associated with pain and swelling. The medial talar dome lesion may be related to plantar flexion of the foot with inversion, followed by rotation of the tibia on the talus[165] (Fig. 63–30). This combination of forces produces compression of the talus, while the collateral ligaments remain intact. Greater force causes the posteroinferior lip of the tibia to ride medially across the everted medial margin of the talus, producing an osteochondral fragment that may remain in situ or become partially or completely displaced. The same force can injure portions of the deltoid and lateral collateral ligaments. The medial talar fracture is frequently cup-shaped, deeper, and larger than the lateral talar lesion, which may be shallow and wafer-shaped.[549]

Carefully obtained radiographs can usually delineate the site of injury. Anteroposterior, lateral, internal, and external oblique projections should be

Text continued on page 2272

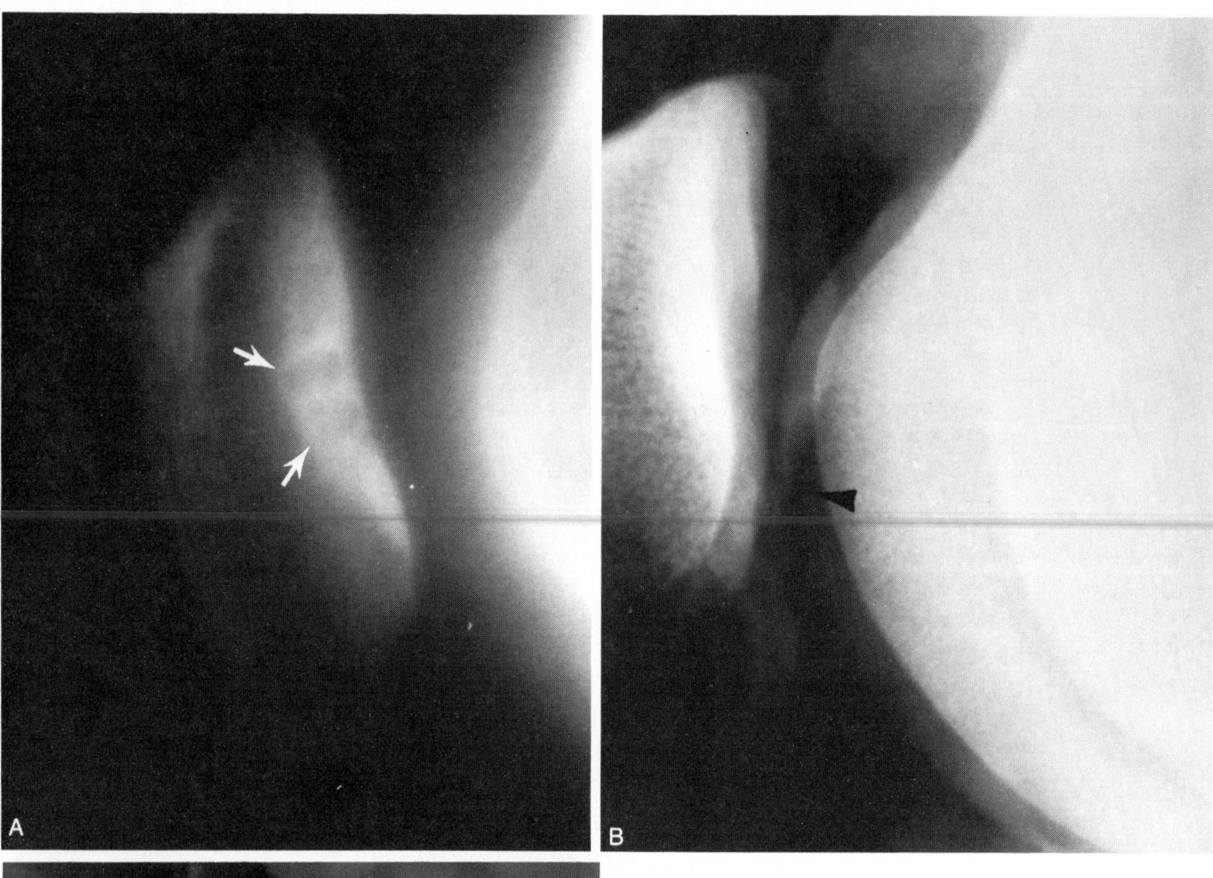

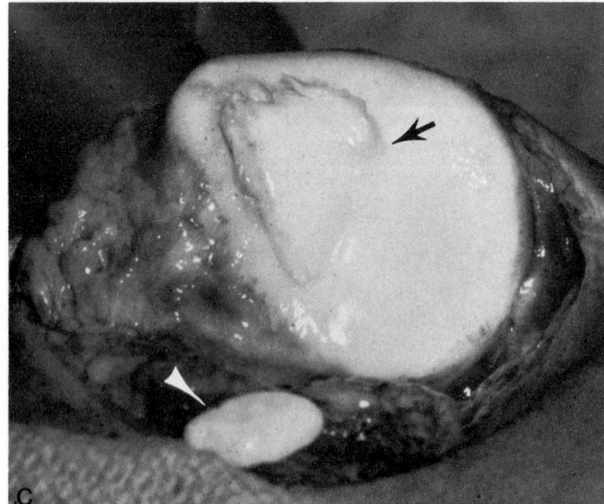

Figure 63–25. *Transchondral fractures (osteochondritis dissecans) of the patella.*

A *A lateral tomogram identifies the site of injury, appearing as a cystic area with surrounding sclerosis (arrows).*

B *In a different patient, arthrography outlines a chondral defect (arrowhead) on the lower surface of the patella.*

C *An operative photograph outlines a fracture site of the patella (arrow) with a button-like fragment (arrowhead). (**C**, Courtesy of Dr. R. Convery, University Hospital, University of California, San Diego, California.)*

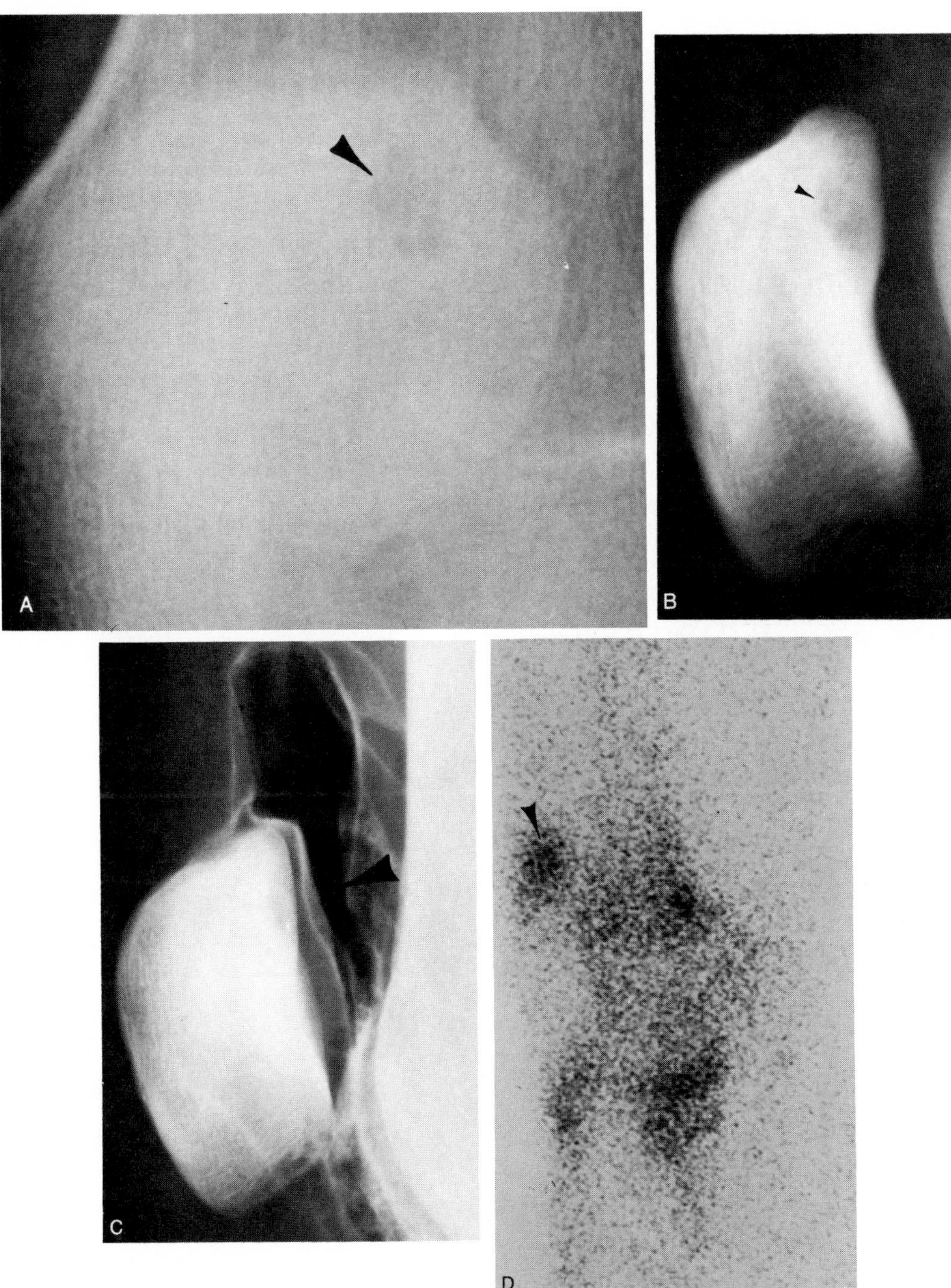

Figure 63–26. *Dorsal defect of the patella (DDP).*

A, B *Anteroposterior and lateral views of the patella identify a well-circumscribed lytic lesion (arrowhead) in the superolateral aspect of the patella, bordering on the subchondral bone.*

C *In a different patient with a DDP, an arthrogram reveals intact patellar cartilage with slight thinning of the chondral surface over the upper pole (arrowhead), a normal finding.*

D *In a symptomatic 18 year old patient with a DDP, a lateral view of a bone scan following injection of technetium pyrophosphate shows diffuse increased patellar activity (arrowhead). Normal growth plate activity is also noted.*

Illustration continued on the following page

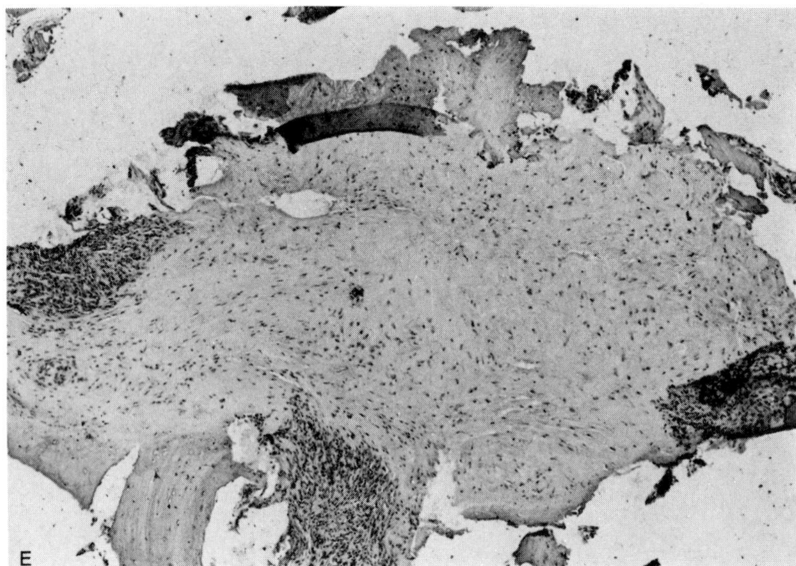

Figure 63–26. Continued

E *The histology of a DDP consists of dense fibrous tissue separating spicules of viable bone. Collections of lymphocytes are present (240×).*

(From Goergen TG et al: Radiology 130:333, 1979.)

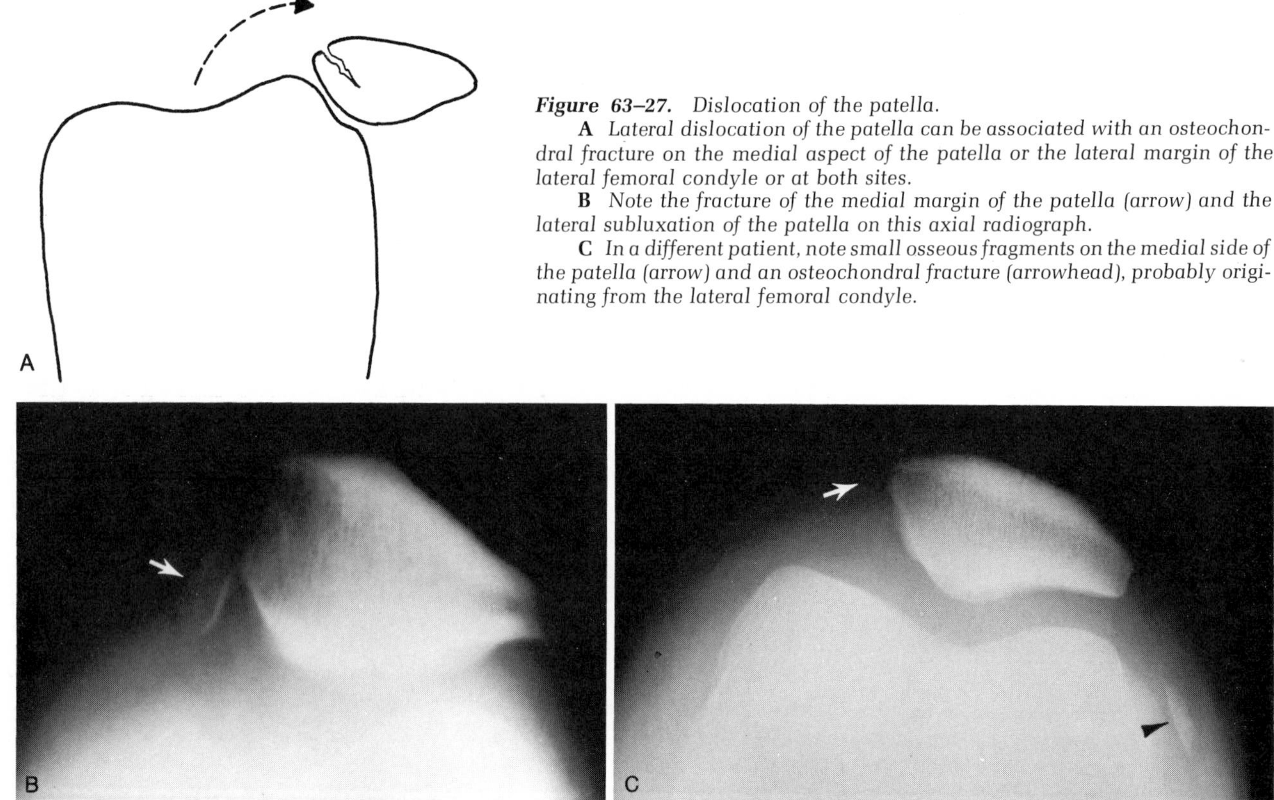

Figure 63–27. *Dislocation of the patella.*

A *Lateral dislocation of the patella can be associated with an osteochondral fracture on the medial aspect of the patella or the lateral margin of the lateral femoral condyle or at both sites.*

B *Note the fracture of the medial margin of the patella (arrow) and the lateral subluxation of the patella on this axial radiograph.*

C *In a different patient, note small osseous fragments on the medial side of the patella (arrow) and an osteochondral fracture (arrowhead), probably originating from the lateral femoral condyle.*

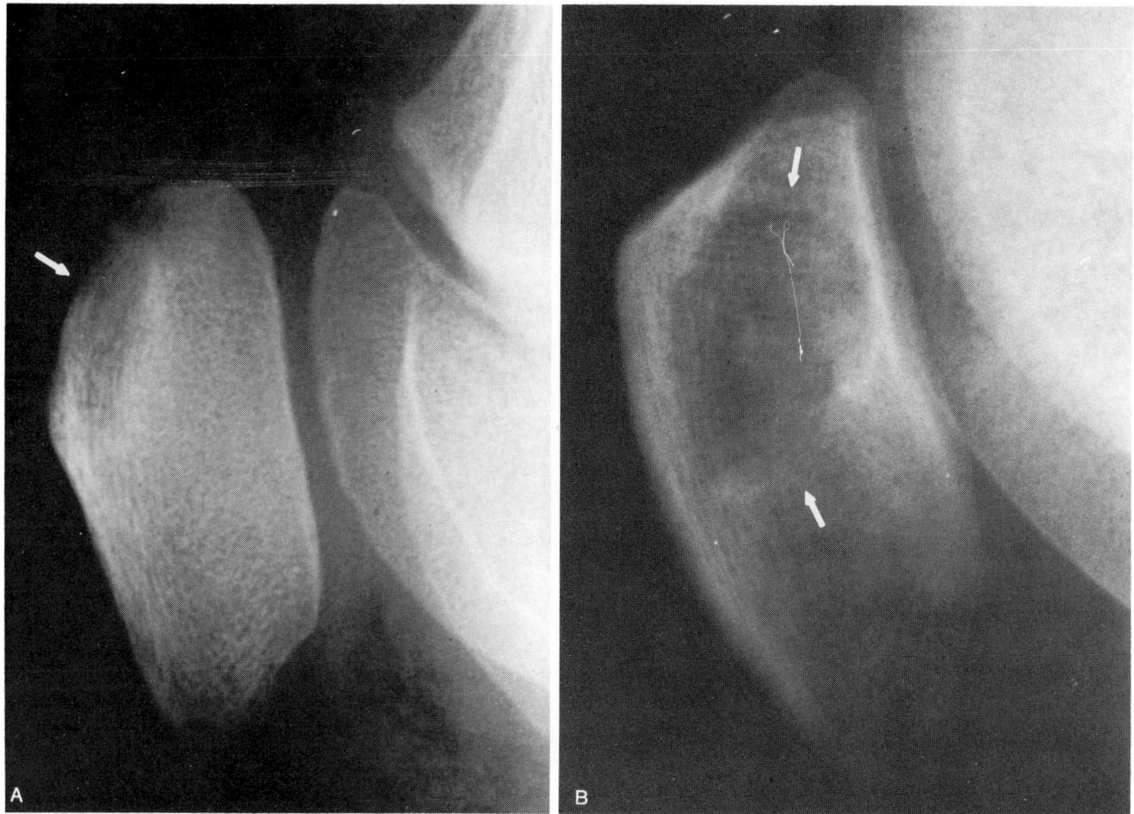

Figure 63–28. Other patellar lesions.

A Osteomyelitis. A lateral view of the patella in this 7 year old boy reveals a lytic lesion with ill-defined margins on the anterior surface of the bone (arrow).

B Chondroblastoma. In this 19 year old man, the large, lytic, well-circumscribed lesion is a chondroblastoma (arrows).

(From Goergen TG, et al: Radiology 130:333, 1979.)

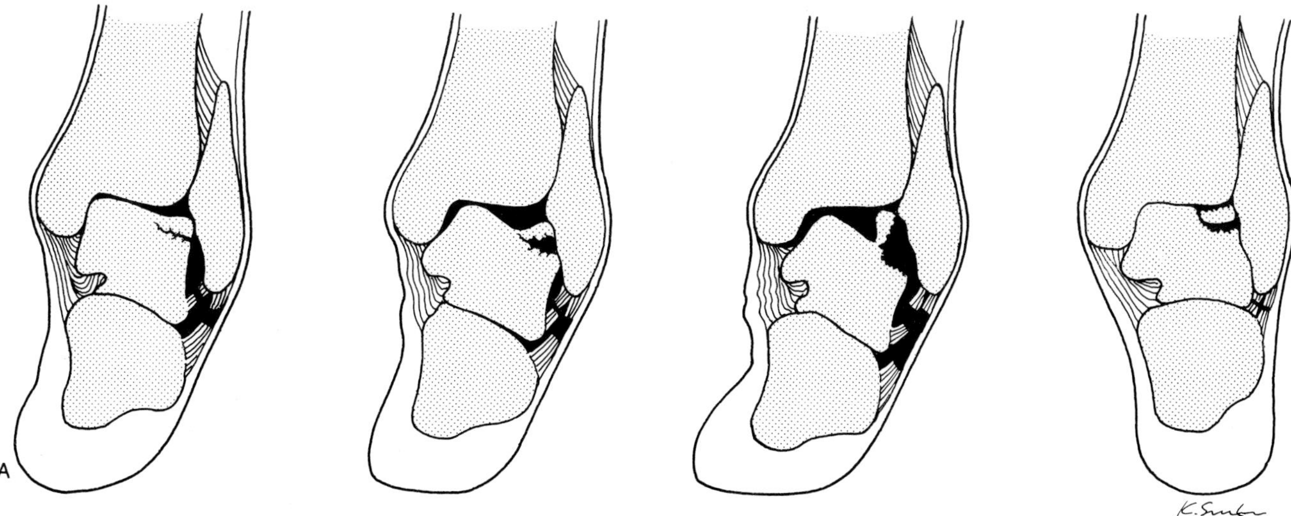

Figure 63–29. Transchondral fractures (osteochondritis dissecans) of the talus: Lateral lesion.

A As the foot is inverted, the lateral border of the talar dome is compressed against the face of the fibula. Although initially the adjacent ligaments may remain intact, further inversion can produce rupture of these ligaments, with avulsion of the osteochondral fragment. This fragment can remain in situ or be displaced. (**A**, After Berndt AL, Harty M: J Bone Joint Surg 41A:988, 1959.)

Illustration continued on the following page

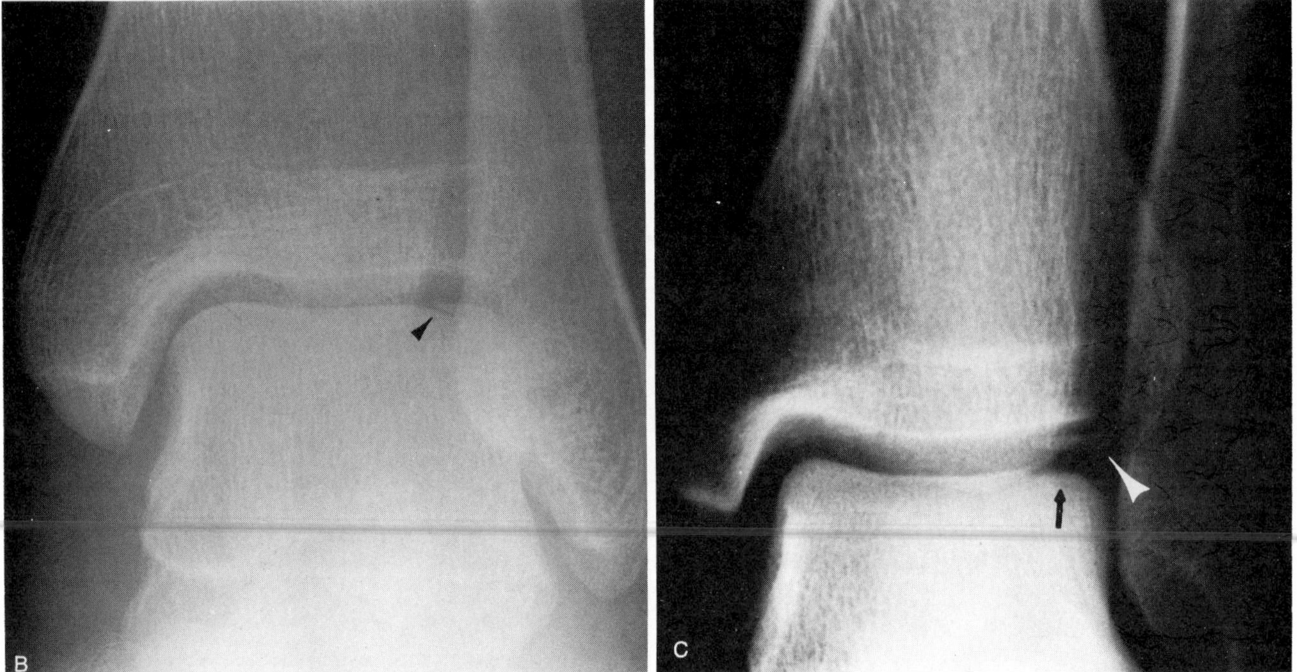

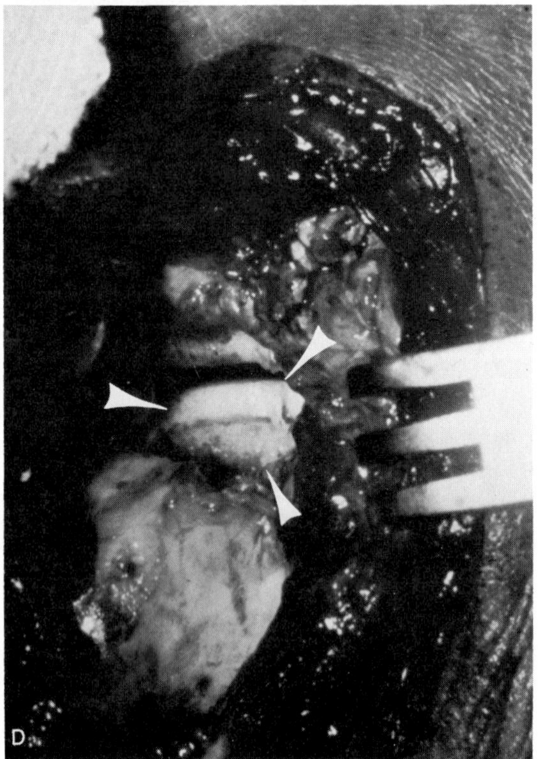

Figure 63–29. Continued

B, C *Two examples of the lateral talar transchondral fracture. In* **B** *note the oblique fracture line (arrowhead) and in* **C** *observe the displaced fragment (arrowhead) and irregular talar surface (arrow).*

D *An intraoperative photograph of such a lesion reveals a slightly displaced osteochondral fragment (arrowheads).*

A

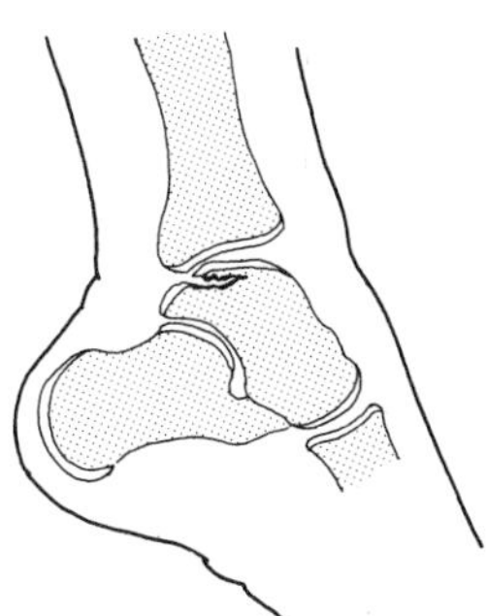

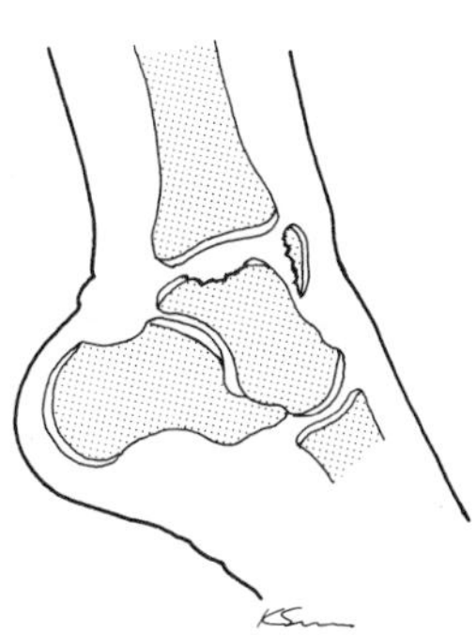

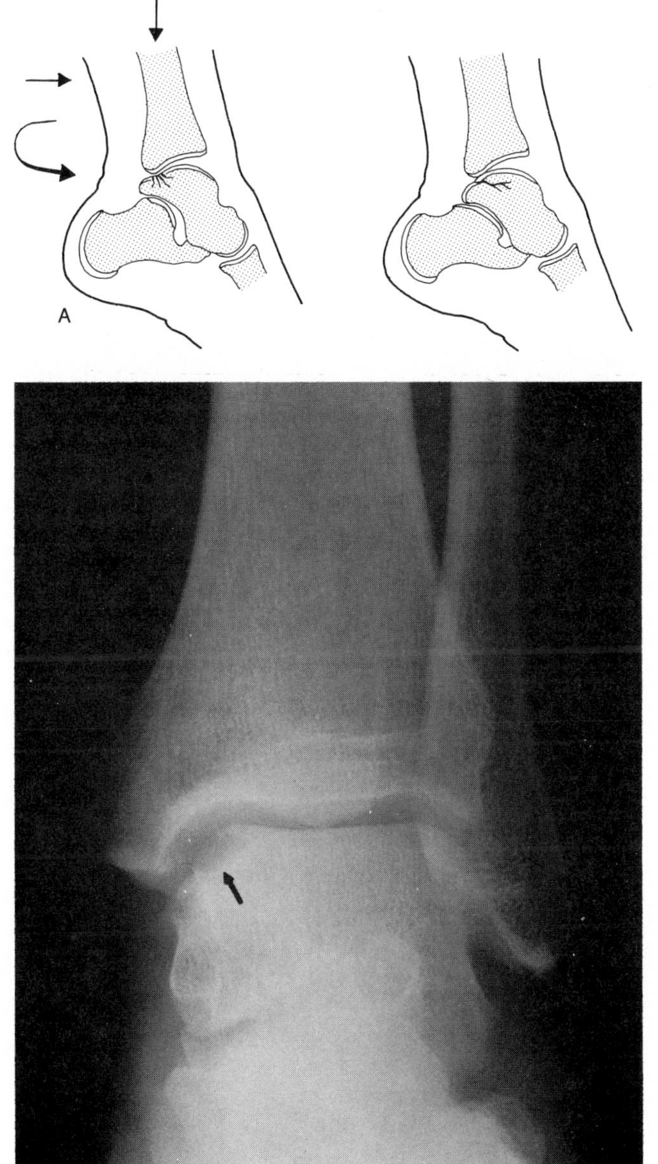

Figure 63–30. *Transchondral fractures (osteochondritis dissecans) of the talus: Medial lesion.*

A *Plantar flexion of the foot, inversion, and rotation produce a small area of talar compression. Greater forces lead to "gouging out" of an osteochondral fragment owing to the presence of the adjacent tibia. This fragment may remain in situ or become displaced. (***A,** *After Berndt AL, Harty, M: J Bone Joint Surg 41A:988, 1959).*

B *In this patient, note the lucent lesion of the medial talar dome (arrow), the site of an osteochondral fragment.*

obtained. These views may be supplemented with radiographs taken with the ankle in stress and with varying degrees of plantar and dorsiflexion of the ankle, and with fluoroscopy and tomography.[166, 168, 169] The osseous defects may be quite subtle, consisting of slight irregularity of the articular surface, shallow excavations with or without adjacent sclerosis, and small "flake" fracture fragments. Frequently, they appear larger on lateral radiographs and tomograms. Arthrography and arthrotomography are indicated in some cases to delineate the fracture site better, to define the condition of the overlying chondral coat, and to detect intra-articular osseous and cartilaginous bodies. Precise identification of the location and the extent of injury are important in the determination of the need for surgery and the specific surgical approach that must be utilized.

Other Sites. Posttraumatic osteochondral fractures, "osteochondritis dissecans," and necrosis can be identified at other sites (see Chapter 78), including the elbow[172-175, 552] and the wrist.[176] In fact, osteochondral fractures can accompany a variety of joint dislocations, a typical example of which is the Hill-Sachs deformity that complicates anterior dislocation of the humeral head (see discussion that follows).

DISLOCATIONS

General Principles

A dislocation results when there is complete loss of contact between two osseous surfaces that normally articulate. A subluxation represents a partial loss of this contact. Subluxations and dislocations are usually caused by physical trauma, although they may also occur when congenital or acquired conditions produce muscular imbalance (e.g., congenital dislocation of the hip, neurologic disorders) or when articular disorders produce incongruities of the joint surface and instability (e.g., rheumatoid arthritis). Many dislocations and subluxations due to trauma are associated with fractures of the neighboring bone.[177] Although the radiographic diagnosis of a dislocation or subluxation is not difficult when the bones remain malaligned following the injury, spontaneous reduction can occur. In these cases, characteristic fractures in periarticular bone can confirm the presence of a previous dislocation. Typical examples of such fractures are the Hill-Sachs lesion of the humeral head following an anterior dislocation of the glenohumeral joint, and the medial patellar fracture following lateral dislocation of the patella. Furthermore, these fractures may dispose the joint to future dislocations.

Accurate roentgenographic diagnosis of subluxations and dislocations requires that films be obtained in more than a single projection. Ideally, at least two projections oriented at right angles to each other should be utilized, and, frequently, supplementary radiographs may be necessary. Roentgenograms exposed during stress or weight-bearing (e.g., for the acromioclavicular joint) and comparison views of the uninvolved side (e.g., for the child's elbow joint) can be useful.

Special Types of Dislocations or Subluxations

GLENOHUMERAL JOINT DISLOCATION. The glenohumeral joint is relatively unstable. The glenoid cavity has an articular surface that is approximately one third as large as that of the humeral head, and the stability of the articulation is provided in large part by surrounding capsular and ligamentous structures.[178] Because of these anatomic characteristics and the frequency of injury to the shoulder region, dislocations of this joint occur often. These dislocations can be classified into anterior, posterior, superior, and inferior types. Anterior dislocation is, by far, the most frequent, representing over 95 per cent of such injuries (Fig. 63–31). This type of dislocation is associated with a compression fracture on the posterolateral aspect of the humeral head that is produced by impaction of the humerus against the anterior rim of the glenoid fossa. This osseous defect of the humerus has been recognized for a century,[179] although the report of Hill and Sachs in 1940[180] of the humeral lesion was the first review of the subject in the English language. Because of this, the osseous defect is frequently termed the Hill-Sachs lesion.

This lesion is observed in many cases of anterior dislocation of the glenohumeral joint. It is frequently larger in those cases that are dislocated for a considerable period of time, those that are recurrent, and those in which the direction of dislocation is anteroinferior rather than purely anterior.[181] The reported incidence of the lesion has varied considerably. Hill and Sachs detected it in 27 per cent of 119 cases of acute anterior dislocation and in 74 per cent of 15 cases of recurrent anterior dislocation.[180] Other investigators have noted the Hill-Sachs defect in 50 to 100 per cent of cases of recurrent dislocations.[182-187] Much of this variation is related to the difference in the roentgenographic technique utilized to investigate patients with glenohumeral joint dislocation.[181, 188] In fact, many different radiographic projections have been described in this clinical setting (see Chapter 7). Films obtained in various degrees of internal rotation are mandatory, as such rotation of the humerus will produce a tangential view of the osseous lesion (Figs. 63–31 and 63–32). Fluoroscopy can also be helpful in equivocal cases. The role of computed tomography has not yet been defined. The

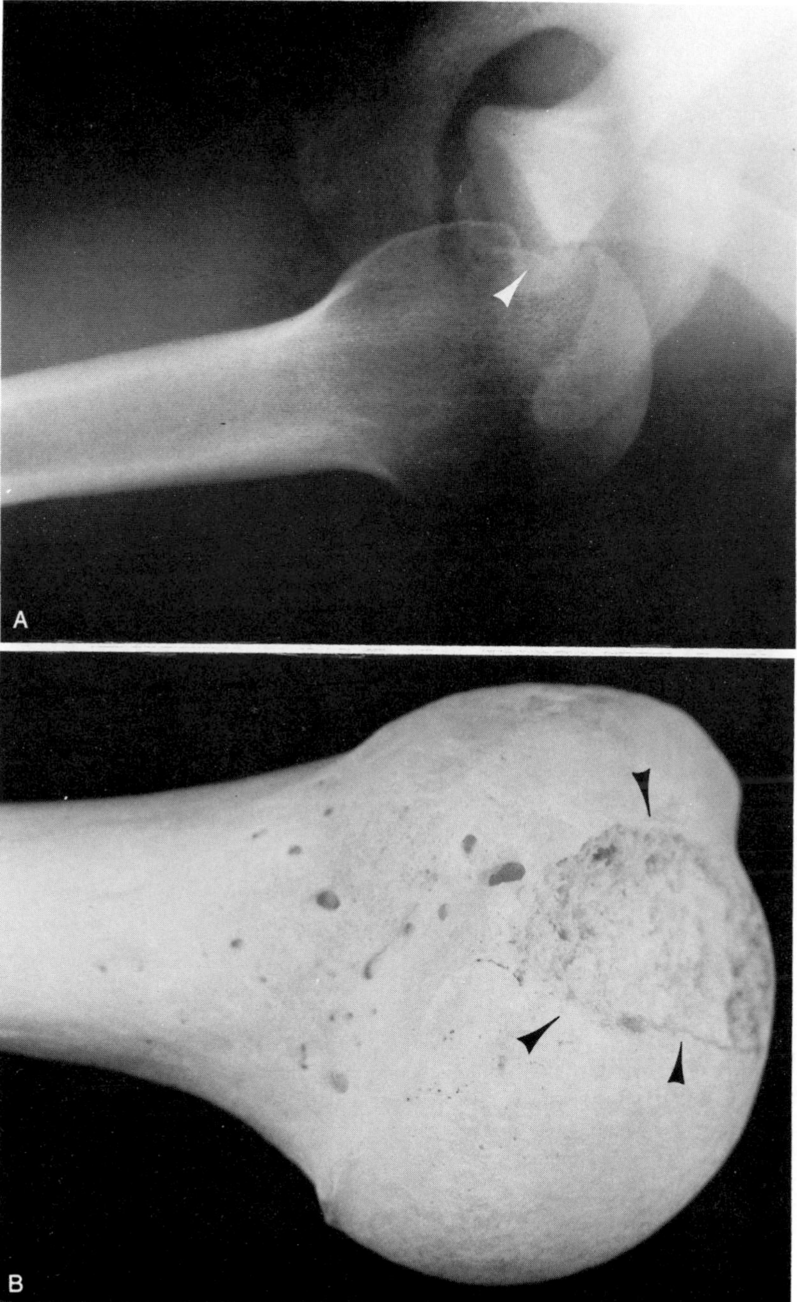

Figure 63–31. *Glenohumeral joint: Anterior dislocation —Hill-Sachs lesion.*

A *An axillary radiograph reveals an anterior dislocation of the humeral head. Note the impaction of the anterior glenoid process and the posterolateral aspect of the humeral head, producing a Hill-Sachs lesion (arrowhead). Although the dislocation is well shown on this radiograph, axillary projections are difficult to obtain while the humeral head is still displaced.*

B *A photograph of the posterior surface of the humeral head demonstrates the characteristics of a Hill-Sachs lesion (arrowheads).*

Illustration continued on the following page

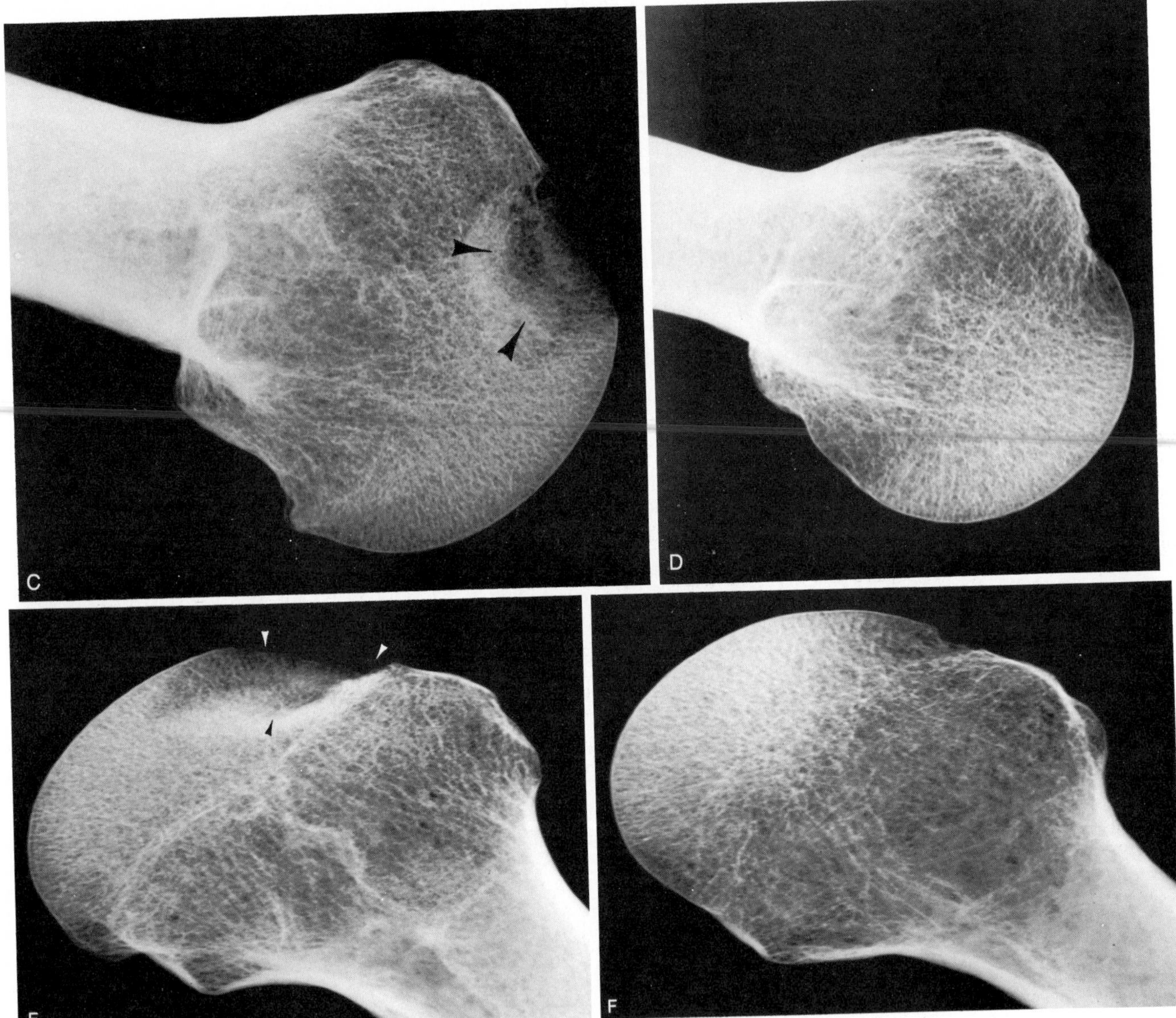

Figure 63–31. Continued
C, D *"Notch" views of a humeral head with a Hill-Sachs lesion (arrowheads)* **(C)** *and a normal humeral head* **(D).**
E, F *"Modified Didiee" views of a humeral head with a Hill-Sachs lesion (arrowheads)* **(E)** *and a normal humeral head* **(F).**

Illustration continued on the opposite page

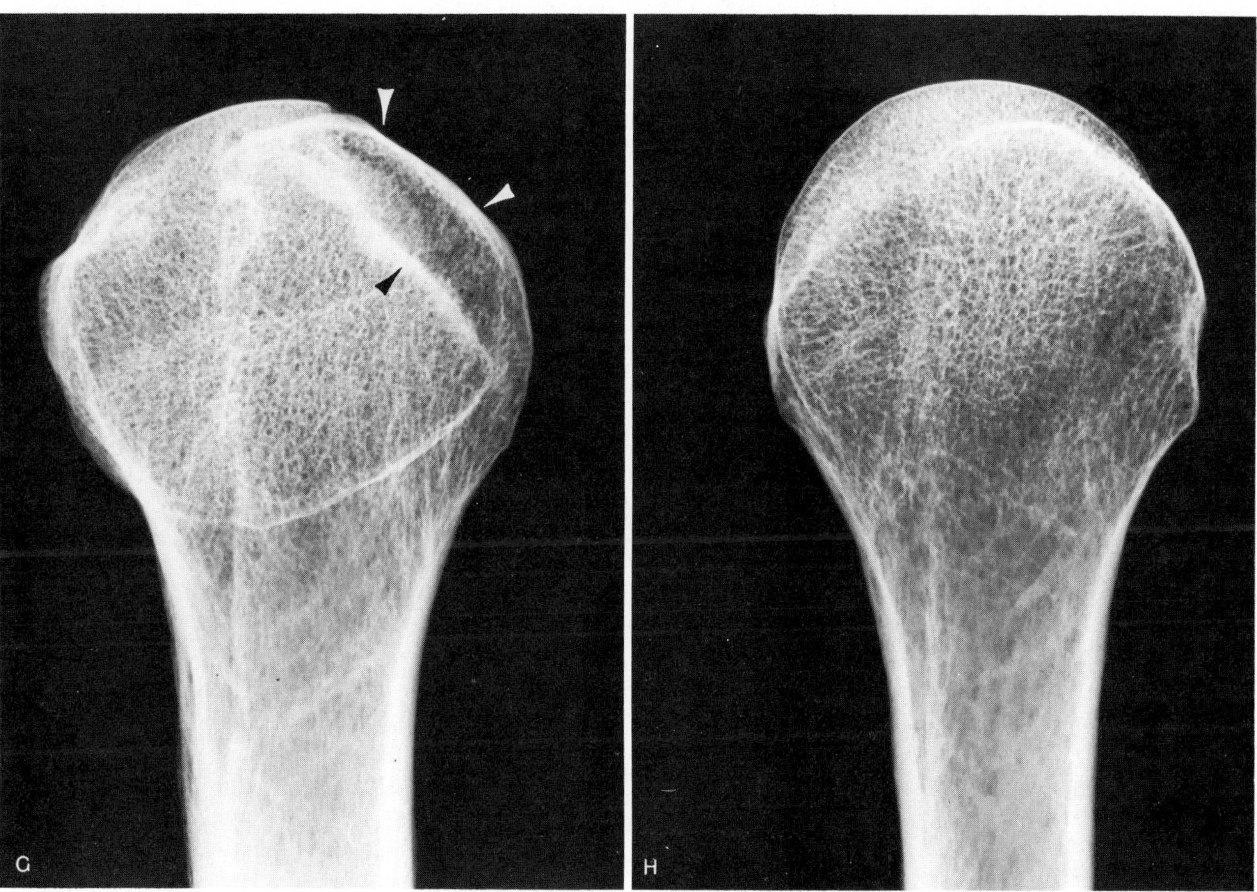

Figure 63–31. Continued

G, H *Internal rotation views of a humeral head with a Hill-Sachs lesion (arrowheads)* **(G)** *and a normal humeral head* **(H)**.

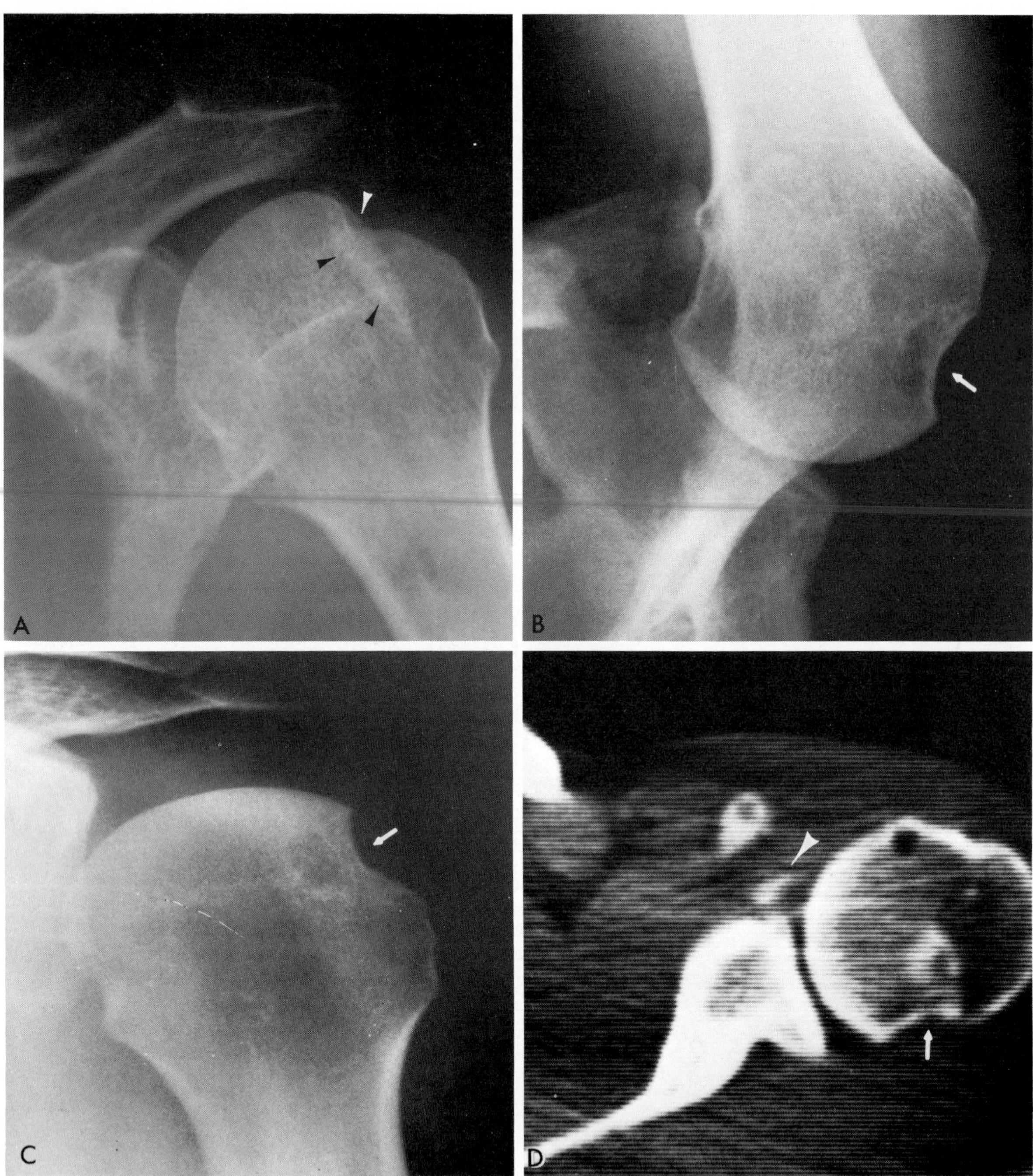

Figure 63–32. *Glenohumeral joint: Anterior dislocation —Hill-Sachs lesion.*

A *In a patient with a previous anterior dislocation, the internal rotation view reveals the extent of the Hill-Sachs lesion (arrowheads).*

B–D *In a different patient, a large Hill-Sachs lesion is evident on both the "notch"* **(B)** *and "Didiee"* **(C)** *views (arrow). Note its presence on the computed tomogram* **(D)** *(arrow) in association with fragmentation of the anterior glenoid rim (arrowhead).*

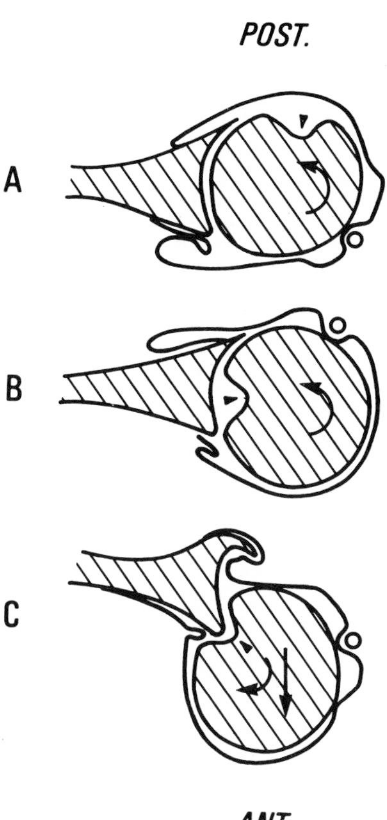

Figure 63–33. Hill-Sachs lesion: Propensity for recurrent dislocation. In a patient with a Hill-Sachs lesion (arrowhead), external rotation **(B)** may allow the lesion to engage the glenoid process so that during subsequent internal rotation **(C)**, the humeral head is levered out of the glenoid fossa, producing an anterior dislocation. (**A**, Neutral position.) (Courtesy of Dr. G. Greenway, Dallas, Texas).

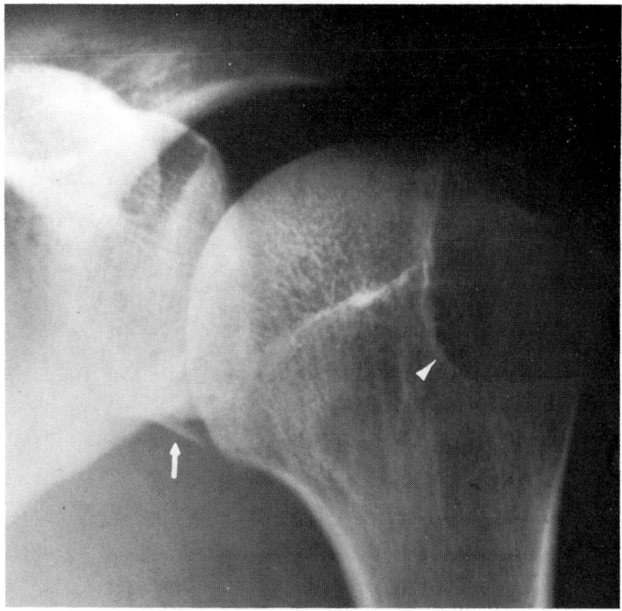

Figure 63–34. Glenohumeral joint: Anterior dislocation — Bankart lesion. In addition to the Hill-Sachs lesion (arrowhead), note the fragmentation of the glenoid rim (arrow).

radiographic detection of a Hill-Sachs lesion is important, as it delineates the nature of a shoulder injury that may be clinically obscure, implies a propensity for recurrent dislocation, and influences the necessity for and choice of a surgical procedure (Fig. 63–33).

A second fracture accompanying anterior dislocation of the humeral head involves the glenoid fossa and is called the Bankart lesion[189] (Fig. 63–34). When osseous fragmentation of the anterior glenoid rim occurs, the abnormality may be apparent on plain film radiographs in frontal or axillary projections, or both.[190] Although large osseous fractures of the glenoid are occasionally apparent,[191] the fracture may include only the cartilaginous surface of the bone, and an arthrogram may be necessary to detect the changes (see Chapter 15). Double contrast arthrography (air and contrast media) utilizing the axillary projection is especially helpful in delineating the cartilaginous Bankart lesion. This technique also identifies the large anterior recesses of the glenohumeral joint that are produced by single or recurrent dislocation.

Posterior dislocation of the glenohumeral joint is rare, constituting approximately 2 to 4 per cent of all shoulder dislocations. Over 50 per cent of these cases are unrecognized on initial evaluation, despite the presence of a history of trauma, pain, swelling, and limitation of motion. The diagnosis of adhesive capsulitis ("frozen shoulder") is often suggested in such cases.[192, 193] Many cases of posterior dislocation result from convulsions, and in these instances, bilateral dislocations may be evident.[200, 553] Physical examination reveals a posteriorly displaced humeral head that is held in internal rotation.[194] Absence of external rotation and limitation of abduction are present in virtually all cases of posterior dislocation. Associated injuries include stretching of the posterior capsule, fracture of the posterior aspect of the glenoid rim, an avulsion fracture of the lesser tuberosity of the humerus, and a stretched or detached subscapularis tendon.

Radiographs are diagnostic; the routine examination must include a lateral view of the scapula or an axillary view of the shoulder, or both, and additional projections may also be helpful.[195] On an anteroposterior radiograph, posterior dislocation of the humeral head distorts the normal elliptical radiodense area created by the overlapping of the head and the glenoid fossa (Fig. 63–35). An empty or vacant glenoid cavity is a second radiographic sign of dislocation in this projection; the posteror displacement of the humeral head may create a space between the anterior rim of the glenoid and the humeral head that is frequently greater than 6 mm.[196] Thirdly, the normal parallel pattern of the articular surfaces of the glenoid concavity and the humeral head convexity is lost. Additional roentgenographic signs of posterior dislocation on frontal radiographs

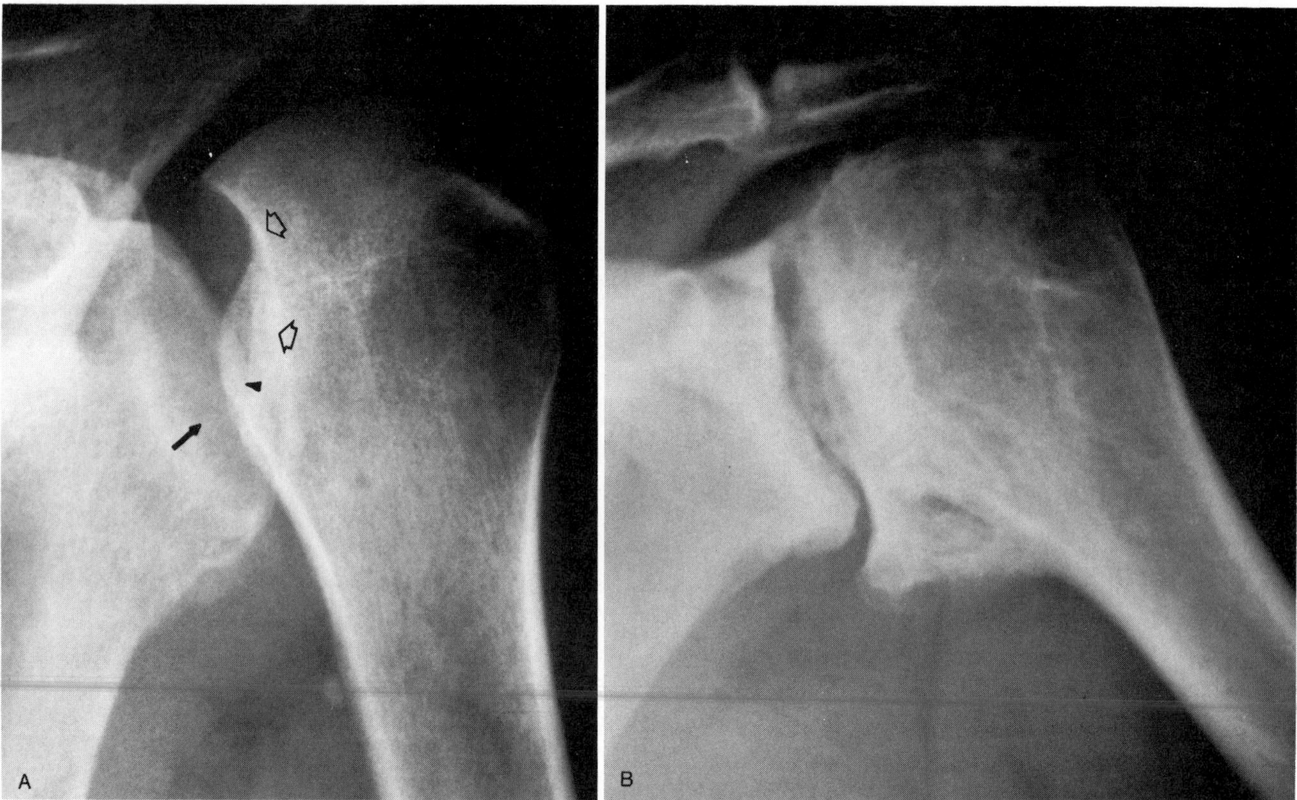

Figure 63–35. *Glenohumeral joint: Posterior dislocation.*

A *An anteroposterior roentgenogram in a patient with a posterior glenohumeral joint dislocation. Findings include distortion of the normal elliptical radiodense region created by overlying of the humeral head and glenoid fossa (arrowhead), a "vacant" glenoid cavity (solid arrow), loss of parallelism between the articular surfaces of the glenoid cavity and humeral head, internal rotation of the humerus, and an impaction fracture (open arrows). An osseous fragment adjacent to the medial proximal diaphysis of the humerus is also identified.*

B *Recurrent posterior dislocations of the glenohumeral joint have led to secondary degenerative joint disease with articular space narrowing, deformity, sclerosis, and bizarre osteophytosis.*

include a fixed position of internal rotation of the humerus, and a second cortical line, the "trough" line, parallel and lateral to the subchondral articular surface of the humeral head.[197] This line represents the margin of a trough-like impaction fracture of the head created when this structure contacts the posterior glenoid rim during the dislocation.[198] As such, it is analogous to the Hill-Sachs lesion that is seen in association with anterior glenohumeral joint dislocation and is quite diagnostic of a posterior dislocation. However, the medially located lesser tuberosity that appears during marked internal rotation in the normal shoulder should not be misintrepreted as a trough or as a site of impaction fracture.

A tangential view of the glenoid normally demonstrates no overlapping of the humeral head and glenoid rim.[199] In patients with posterior glenohumeral joint dislocation, the humeral head is displaced medially and abnormal overlapping may be seen. An axillary or lateral scapular projection directly delineates the posterior position of the humeral head with respect to the glenoid.

Superior dislocation of the glenohumeral joint is rare. An extreme forward and upward force on the adducted arm can produce extensive damage to the rotator cuff, capsule, biceps tendon, and surrounding musculature, and fracture of the acromion, clavicle, coracoid process, or humeral tuberosities. Inferior dislocation of the glenohumeral joint (luxatio erecta) is also rare.[201, 202] Following this injury, the superior aspect of the articular surface of the humeral head is directed inferiorly and does not contact the inferior glenoid rim.

In addition to traumatic glenohumeral joint dislocation, voluntary subluxation or dislocation may be encountered.[203, 204] In these cases, spontaneous displacements of the humeral head occur anteriorly or, more frequently, posteriorly. Although it has been proposed that generalized ligamentous laxity may be responsible for this phenomenon[205] and that some patients may also reveal genu valgus and weak arches, widespread abnormalities are generally not evident in patients with voluntary dislocation of the glenohumeral joint.[204]

A special type of inferior displacement of the humeral head is termed the "drooping shoulder"[206-208]

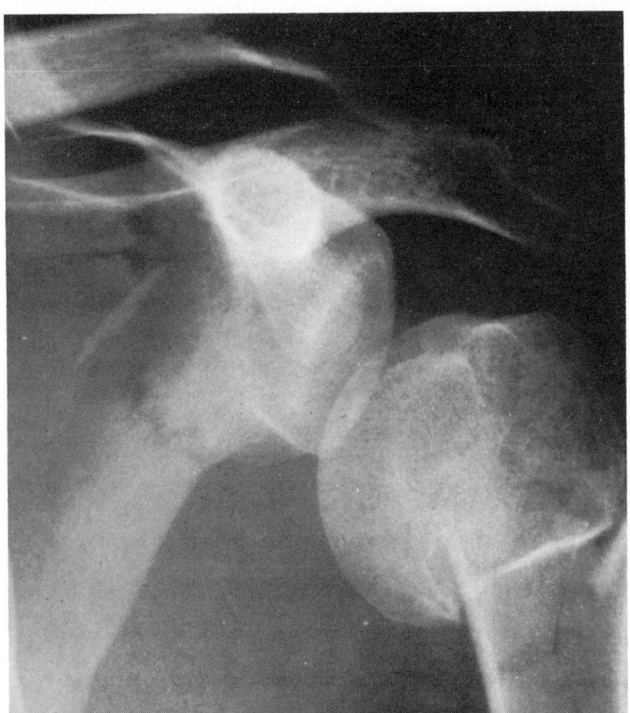

Figure 63–36. Glenohumeral joint: "Drooping shoulder." A fracture of the surgical neck of the humerus is associated with inferior subluxation of the head with respect to the glenoid cavity. Observe an associated scapular fracture.

(Fig. 63–36). It can be associated with uncomplicated fractures of the surgical neck of the humerus. The pathogenesis of the displacement is not clear, although relaxation or stretching of the supporting musculature, detachment of the capsule, and hemarthrosis have each been proposed as possible mechanisms. The appearance of a similar displacement in patients with neurologic injuries of the brachial plexus, especially those involving the axillary nerve, supports the view that muscular alterations produce the subluxation, whereas the detection of a "drooping shoulder" in patients with various articular disorders may indicate that joint effusion can also lead to inferior displacement of the humeral head. Recognition of this condition will eliminate erroneous diagnosis of fracture-dislocation of the proximal humerus, and conservative therapy will lead to disappearance of the "drooping shoulder" over a period of weeks.

Acromioclavicular Joint Dislocation. Subluxation or dislocation of the acromioclavicular joint is a common injury.[209-211] The injury, which can result from direct or indirect forces, has been classified into three types.[212, 213] Type I consists of intra-articular damage to the acromioclavicular joint without ligamentous instability either of the joint capsule or of the coracoclavicular ligaments. Thus, the joint remains stable. Type II is subluxation of the acromioclavicular joint with disruption of the capsule. The coracoclavicular ligaments remain intact. Type III consists of acromioclavicular joint dislocation with disruption of the coracoclavicular and acromioclavicular ligaments. This produces an unstable clavicle. Occasionally, the coracoclavicular ligaments remain intact, and an avulsion fracture or epiphyseal separation of the coracoid process is evident.[214-216]

Type I injuries are diagnosed clinically rather than roentgenographically, although there may be soft tissue swelling and minimal widening of the acromioclavicular joint. The radiographic diagnosis of Type II and Type III injuries is based upon the detection of displacement of the distal clavicle with relation to the acromion and upon the degree of displacement that is evident (Fig. 63–37). Special roentgenograms may be required, including an angulated frontal projection[217] and films obtained with weight held in the hand (stress radiographs). The stress radiograph should include both shoulders so that comparison between the uninvolved and involved joints is facilitated. A difference of 3 to 4 mm in the distance between the superior aspect of the coracoid process and the inferior aspect of the clavicle in the two shoulders indicates an acromioclavicular subluxation or dislocation in which the injured distal clavicle moves superiorly. A complete coracoclavicular ligament disruption is suggested by an increase of the coracoclavicular distance by 40 to 50 per cent.[218] In cases of acromioclavicular joint dislocation, follow-up roentgenograms may reveal calcification and ossification of the coracoclavicular ligament[208, 219, 220] (Fig. 63–37).

Sternoclavicular Joint Dislocation. Sternoclavicular joint injuries are rare compared with those of the glenohumeral or acromioclavicular joints. Anterior dislocations predominate over posterior (retrosternal) dislocations, although the seriousness of posterior dislocations has resulted in many reports of this injury.[221, 222] Almost all cases of sternoclavicular subluxation and dislocation are traumatic, although congenital[223] and spontaneous[224] displacements have been recorded. Radiographic analysis is facilitated by a variety of special projections (see Chapter 7) and may be supplemented with conventional or computed tomography in some instances.[225, 554] In the more common anterior sternoclavicular joint dislocation, the medial end of the clavicle is displaced anteriorly or anterosuperiorly to the anterior margin of the manubrium. In posterior sternoclavicular joint dislocation, the medial end of the clavicle is displaced posteriorly or posterosuperiorly with respect to the posterior margin of the manubrium.[226] Prompt recognition of the latter injury is required because the displaced clavicle may impinge on the trachea, the esophagus, the great vessels, or the major nerves in the superior mediastinum, leading to vascular compromise, cough, dysphagia, and dyspnea. Death may ensue in unrecognized or severe injuries.[227]

An additional injury of the medial end of the clavicle is an epiphyseal fracture or separation. The growth plate at this site is among the last to become

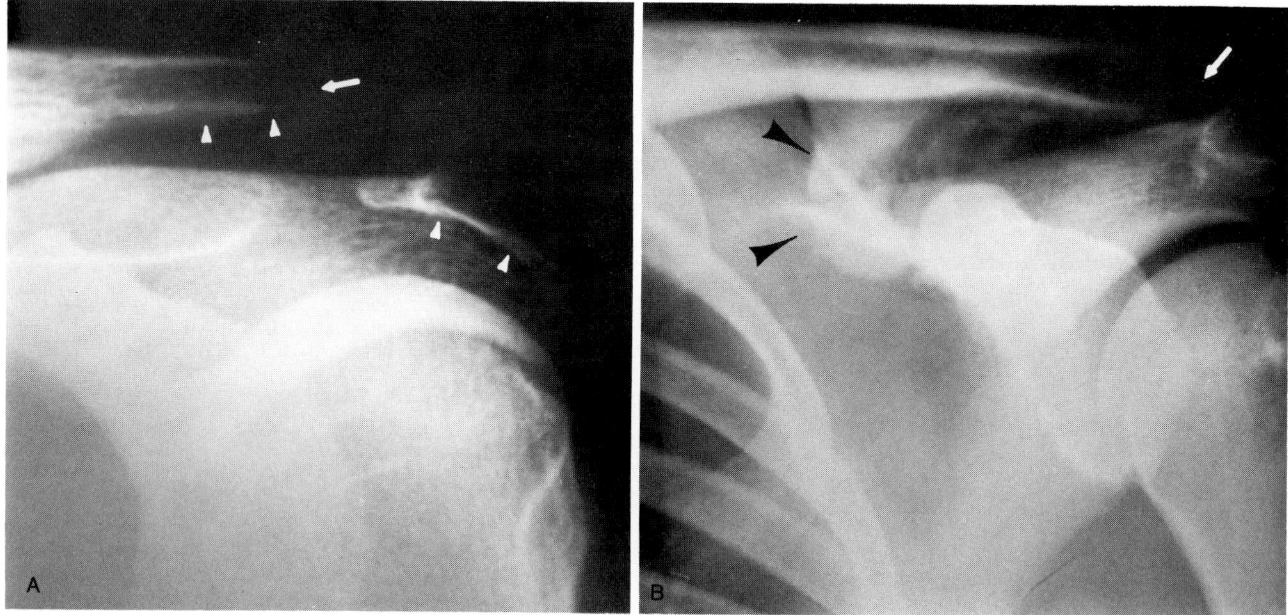

Figure 63–37. Acromioclavicular joint dislocation.
A A Grade III dislocation has resulted in superior displacement of the clavicle (arrow) with respect to the acromion. Note that the inferior margin of the clavicle no longer is aligned with the inferior margin of the acromion (arrowheads).
B Follow-up roentgenograms in patients with acromioclavicular joint dislocations (arrow) may reveal ossification of the coracoclavicular ligament (arrowheads).

obliterated during skeletal maturation, disappearing at approximately 25 years of age. Various types of injuries to the growth plate can occur.[228] Before the medial clavicular epiphysis ossifies at the age of about 18 years, it is extremely difficult to differentiate between a dislocation of the sternoclavicular joint and a fracture through the growth plate.

Elbow Dislocation. Dislocation of the elbow is a relatively frequent injury, especially in the immature skeleton.[229] The classification of such injuries is based upon the direction of displacement and the presence of radial or ulnar dislocation. In cases of dislocation involving both the radius and the ulna, a posterior dislocation is most frequent (approximately 80 to 90 per cent of all elbow dislocations), as these two bones are displaced in a posterior direction in relation to the distal humerus.[230, 231] In adults, this injury may be complicated by fracture of the coronoid process of the ulna or the radial head, and in children and adolescents, the medial epicondylar ossification center is frequently avulsed and may become entrapped during reduction.[229] Entrapment of the medial nerve in the elbow joint after closed reduction of a posterior dislocation of the elbow with fracture of the medial epicondyle can produce a depression in the cortex on the ulnar side of the distal humeral metaphysis.[232]

Medial and lateral dislocations of the elbow are not common.[233] Anterior dislocation is also unusual.[234] Rarely, elbow dislocations may be recurrent.[235] The cause of this last injury varies, but a residual defect in the articular surface of the trochlea, attenuation of the collateral ligaments, failure of union of the coronoid process, or anterior capsular stripping may be observed.

Isolated dislocation of the ulna at the elbow is unusual. Similarly, isolated radial head dislocation without an associated fracture in the ulna is rare in adults. In the child, traumatic dislocation of the radial head must be differentiated from congenital dislocaton of this bone[236, 237] or dislocation associated with hereditary onycho-osteodysplasia (nail-patella syndrome).[238] Because of the rarity of isolated traumatic dislocation of the radial head,[239] all such cases should be extensively investigated for an associated fracture of the ulna.

The combination of an ulnar fracture and radial head dislocation is termed a Monteggia fracture-dislocation[240-242] (Fig. 63–38). Various types of Monteggia fracture-dislocations are recognized: Type I — fracture of the middle or upper third of the ulna with anterior dislocation of the radial head and anterior angulation of the ulna; Type II — fracture of the middle or upper third of the ulna with posterior dislocation of the radial head and posterior angulation of the ulna; Type III — fracture of the ulna just distal to the coronoid process with lateral dislocation of the radial head; and Type IV — fracture of the upper or middle third of the ulna with anterior dislocation of the radial head and fracture of the upper third of the radius below the bicipital tuberosity.[243] Type I injuries are most frequent (approxi-

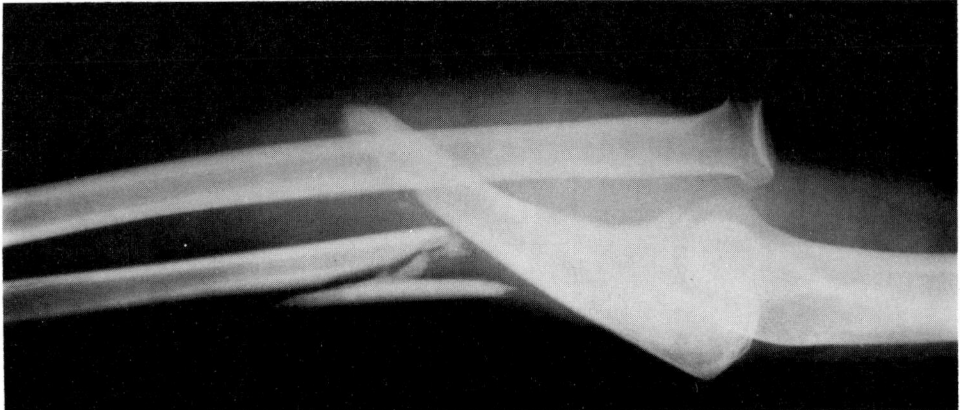

Figure 63–38. Monteggia fracture-dislocation (Type I). Note the fracture of the upper one third of the ulna with anterior angulation at the fracture site and anterior dislocation of the radial head.

mately 65 per cent), followed by Type II (approximately 18 per cent), Type III (approximately 16 per cent), and Type IV (approximately 1 per cent).[240] As the Monteggia fracture-dislocation is common and easily overlooked, multiple views of the elbow should be obtained in all patients who demonstrate fractures of the proximal half of the ulna. A line drawn through the radial shaft and radial head should align with the capitulum in any projection.[244]

In infants and young children, separation of the entire distal humeral epiphysis may be confused with elbow dislocation.[245, 246] The correct diagnosis of this injury rests upon two observations: a normal relationship between the capitulum and radius; and medial displacement of the radius and ulna with respect to the humerus.

Complications of elbow dislocations include heterotopic calcification and ossification,[247, 248] and neural and vascular injury.[231, 249]

Wrist Dislocation. The bones about the wrist are commonly injured. Various fractures, each with its own eponym, may be encountered, including Colles' fracture (fracture of the distal radius with posterior displacement), Smith's fracture (fracture of the distal radius with anterior displacement), Barton's fracture (dorsal rim fracture of the distal radius), and Hutchinson's fracture (radial styloid fracture). Dislocation of the radiocarpal joint is very uncommon. When present, the dorsally dislocating carpus frequently fractures the dorsal rim of the distal radius. More typical dislocations, subluxations, or malalignments about the wrist involve the distal ulna and carpal bones.

Although isolated dislocations of the inferior radioulnar joint are infrequently seen,[250-252] dislocation or subluxation of this articulation may occur in association with a fracture of the radius. This combination of findings is termed a Galeazzi fracture-dislocation[250, 253-255] (Fig. 63–39). Classically, the shaft of the radius is fractured in this injury; fractures of the distal end of the radius, which may be associated with dislocation of the ulnar head, and of the radial neck and head, which may be associated with a dislocation of the inferior radioulnar joint, are not regarded as Galeazzi fracture-dislocations. Most commonly, the fracture occurs at the junction of the middle and distal thirds of the radius and has a short oblique or transverse configuration. The distal radial fragment is displaced in an ulnar direction. Usually, the dislocation of the ulnar head is readily apparent, although, in some cases, ulnar head subluxation may be more apparent on clinical evaluation. In equivocal cases, arthrography of the radiocarpal joint can be helpful in establishing an injury to the distal ulna or surrounding structures.[256] Disruption of the inferior radioulnar joint requires injury to the triangular fibrocartilage, the major stabilizing structure of the distal ulna. Thus, contrast opacification of the radiocarpal joint will be associated with filling of the inferior radioulnar joint due to perforation of the intervening triangular fibrocartilage.[255, 257] Fracture of the ulnar head or styloid process may also be identified. Dislocation of the ulna usually occurs in a distal, dorsal, and medial direction; volar dislocation is less frequent.

In the carpal bones, fractures predominate, although several characteristic dislocations or subluxations may be observed with or without associated fractures. Recognition of these injuries on the roentgenogram requires a knowledge of the normal osseous alignment of the wrist (see Chapter 3). On lateral roentgenograms, alterations in the normal relationship of the radius, lunate, scaphoid, and capitate can be classified as dorsiflexion carpal instability (in which the lunate is tilted dorsally and the scapholunate angle is greater than 70 degrees), and palmar flexion instability (in which the lunate is tilted in a palmar direction and the scapholunate angle is decreased below the normal value of approximately 47 degrees).[258-262, 555-557]

Posttraumatic instability of the carpus relates to the fact that the scaphoid is a mechanical link that stabilizes the intercarpal joint during wrist motion. Injury to the wrist may disrupt this stability, leading to zigzag collapse deformities of the articulation.[258] Dorsiflexion instability occurs commonly after scaphoid fracture with scapholunate dissociation,

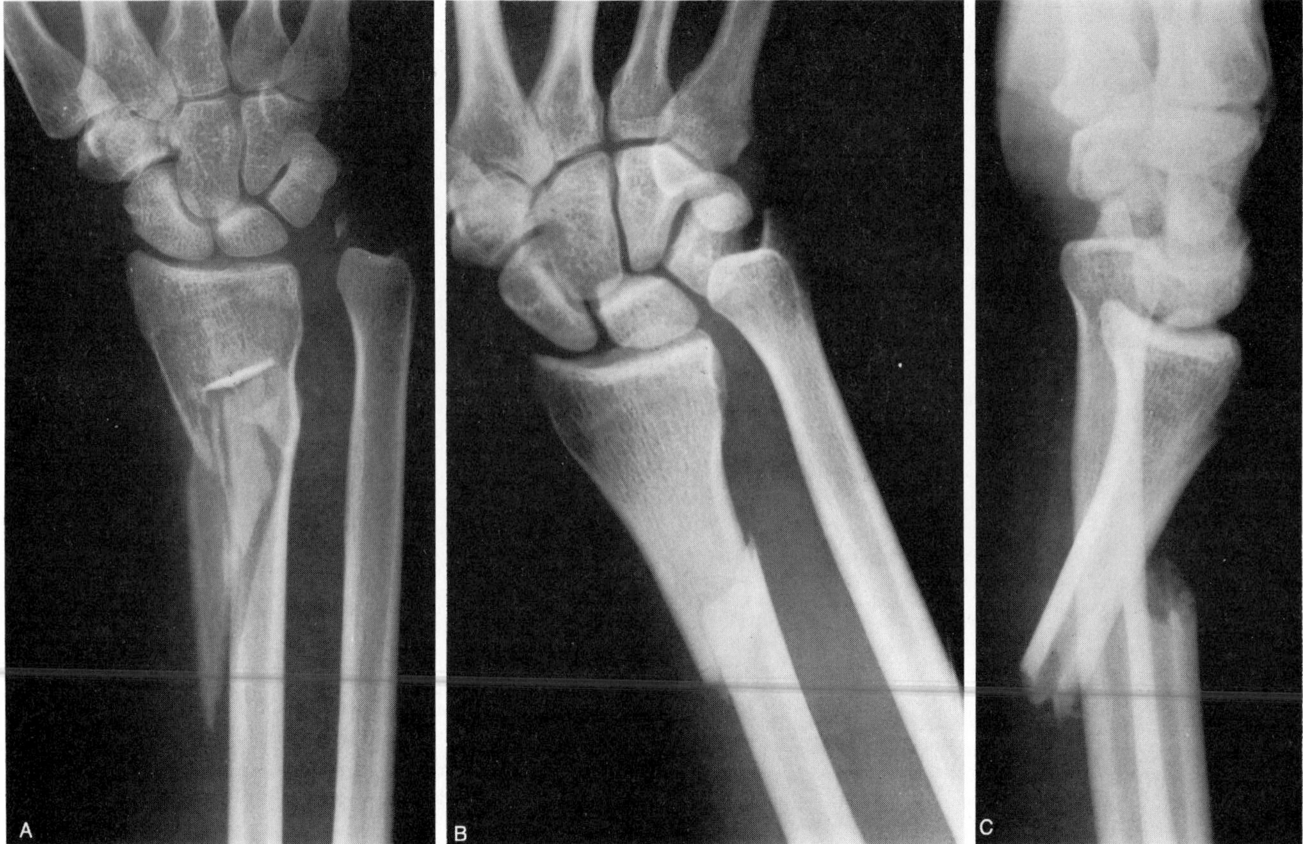

Figure 63–39. *Galeazzi fracture-dislocation.*

A *Observe an oblique fracture of the distal portion of the radial diaphysis, a fracture of the ulnar styloid, and dorsomedial dislocation of the ulna.*

B, C *In a different patient, a transverse radial fracture is associated with significant overlapping, shortening, and angulation as well as a volar dislocation of the distal ulna.*

whereas palmar flexion instability is less frequently seen following scaphoid fracture. Similar patterns of carpal instability can be identified in various articular disorders, including rheumatoid arthritis and calcium pyrophosphate dihydrate crystal deposition disease.[263] Patients with traumatically induced carpal ligament instability may have pain, snapping, crepitus, swelling, tenderness, limited range of motion, and decreased strength. Diagnosis of the alignment deformity requires special views, including posteroanterior projections in neutral, ulnar, and radial deviation, an anteroposterior projection with tightly clenched fist, and oblique and lateral projections.[259] Fluoroscopic monitoring can also be useful in detecting transient subluxations in the wrist.[558]

Dissociated scapholunate movements may accompany tears of the ventral radiocarpal ligaments and scapholunate interosseous ligament complex. This may occur as a complication of lunate or perilunate dislocation, rheumatoid arthritis, and other articular diseases, and as an isolated injury. Scapholunate dissociation (rotatory subluxation of the scaphoid) is suggested when the distance between the scaphoid and lunate is 2 mm or wider and can be unequivocally diagnosed when this distance is 4 mm or wider[259] (Fig. 63–40). This finding implies that an abnormality exists in the scapholunate interosseous ligament. When the scaphoid is also tilted in a palmar direction, a ventral radiocarpal ligament tear is also present. Rotatory subluxation of the scaphoid is associated with roentgenographic findings in addition to widening of the scapholunate space (Terry-Thomas sign) and palmar tilting of the scaphoid.[264-268] These findings include, on the posteroanterior view, a "ring" produced by the cortex of the distal pole of the scaphoid and a foreshortened scaphoid. Radiographs exposed during radial deviation of the wrist may accentuate the gap or space between the scaphoid and the lunate,[264] although a false-positive "ring" sign may also be seen with the wrist in this position. Wrist arthrography can substantiate the diagnosis of rotatory subluxation of the scaphoid by revealing communication between the radiocarpal and midcarpal compartments. However, this communication is frequent in older patients owing to small perforations or tears of the interosseous ligaments between the bones of the proximal carpal row, so caution must be applied to the inter-

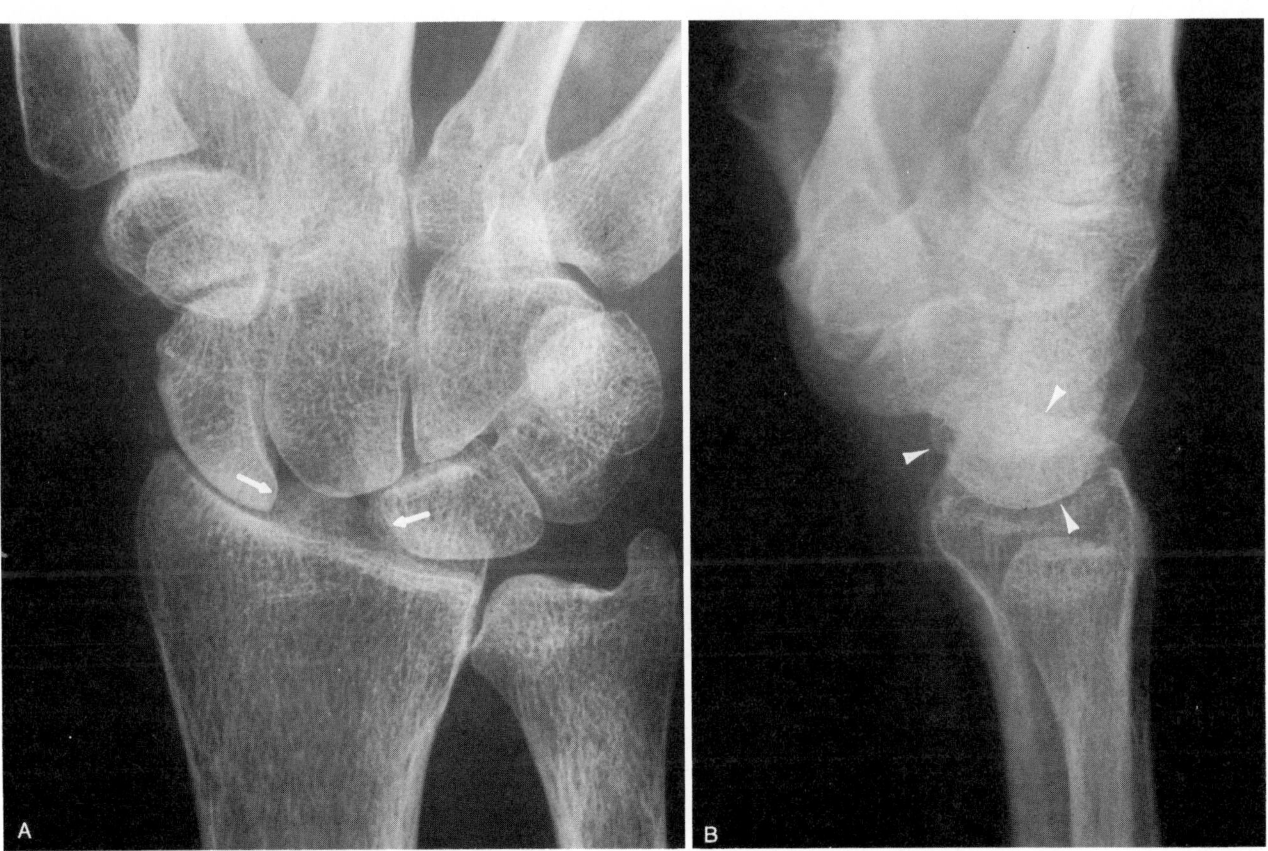

Figure 63–40. *Scapholunate dissociation (rotary subluxation of the scaphoid).*

A, B *Observe the gap or widening in the scapholunate space (arrows) on the posteroanterior roentgenogram, and dorsiflexion of the lunate (arrowheads) on the lateral roentgenogram. The radiocarpal and midcarpal joints are narrowed. A small fracture of the volar surface of the lunate is seen.*

Illustration continued on the following page

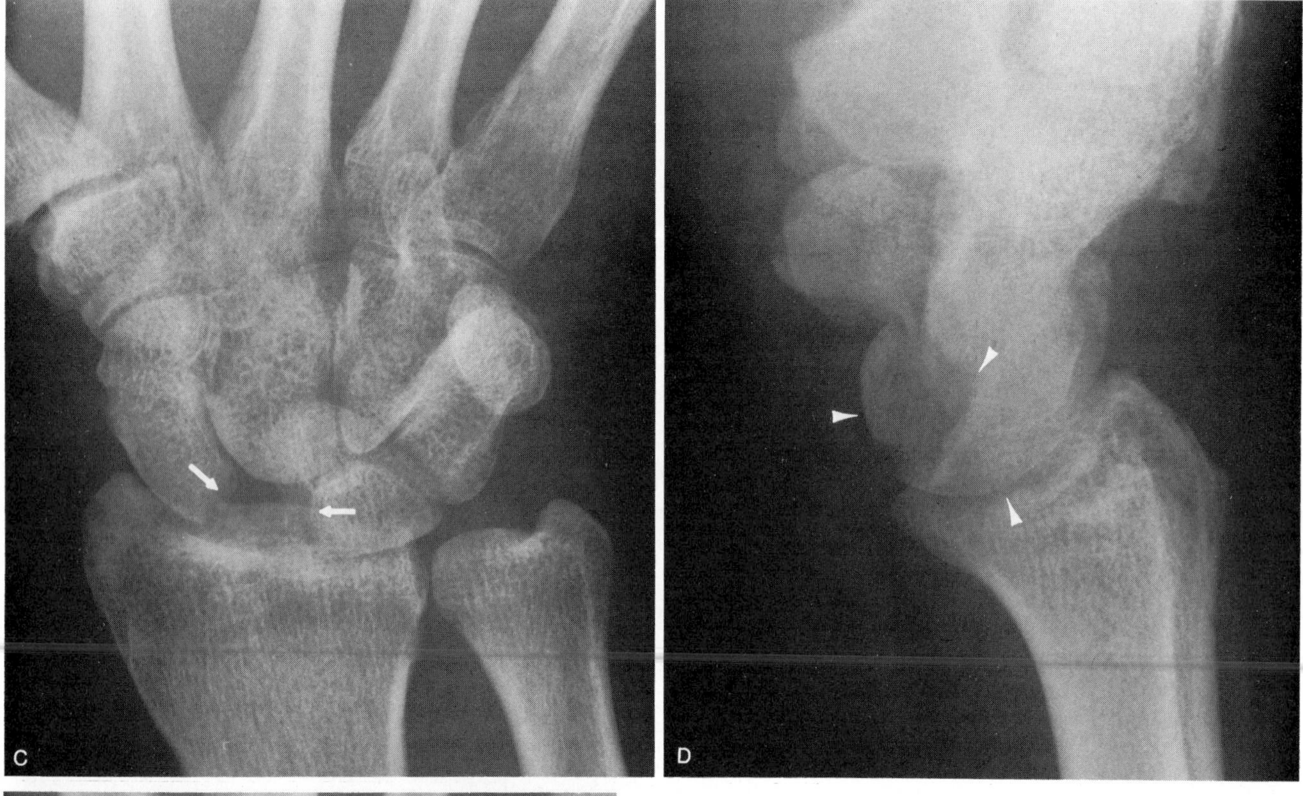

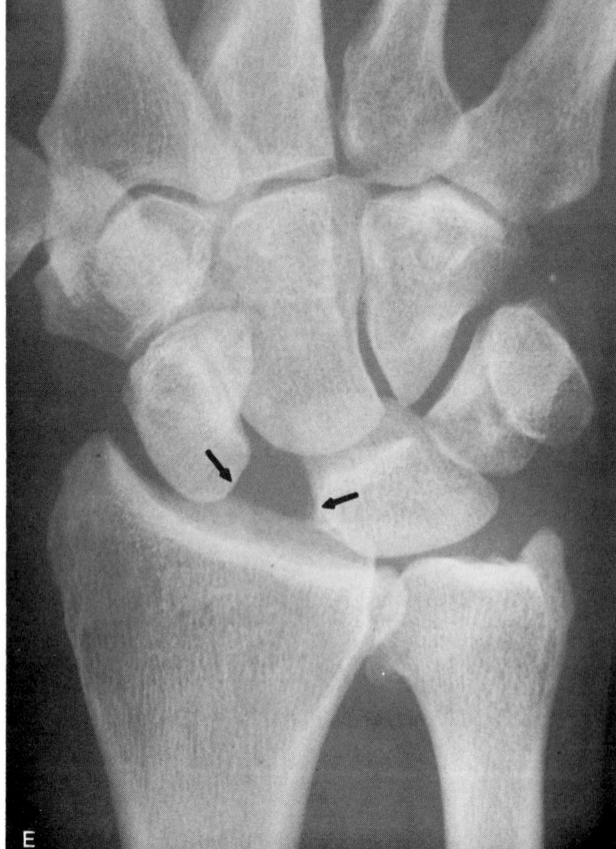

Figure 63–40. Continued

C, D *Similar findings are observed in a different patient with scapholunate dissociation (arrows) and dorsiflexion instability (arrowheads).*

E *In a third patient, findings include widening of the scapholunate distance (arrows) and a foreshortened scaphoid.*

pretation of the arthrographic findings. Degenerative joint disease of the radiocarpal and midcarpal compartments may complicate this condition.

Virtually any of the carpal bones may be dislocated following an injury. Because the lunate and the proximal scaphoid are protected to some extent by the distal radius, a common pattern of injury is a perilunate or transscaphoid perilunate dislocation (Fig. 63–41). In a perilunate dislocation, the lunate remains aligned with the distal radius, and the other carpal bones dislocate, usually dorsally, although on rare occasions in a volar direction.[269] When the wrist is hyperextended, the dorsal cortex of the distal radial articular surface fixes the lunate in place and apposes the scaphoid waist. A fall on the hyperextended hand, producing an abnormal force through the radius, can produce a fracture of the scaphoid,[270] and, with sufficient stress, a dislocation of the carpus occurs. The distal fragment may move with the distal carpal row and the proximal fragment may move with the proximal carpal row. With continued hyperextension force, the capitate may force the lunate ventrally, thus converting the perilunate dislocation into a lunate dislocation in which the lunate is displaced in a palmar direction and the capitate appears to be aligned with the distal radius[271, 272] (Fig. 63–41*D*). Variations in the classic patterns of dislocation and associated fractures are common, dependent upon the exact position of the wrist at the time of injury.[559] Transscaphoid, transcapitate, and transtriquetral fracture-dislocations are encountered, and the radial and ulnar styloid processes may also be affected. Proper radiographic interpretation requires multiple projections, including frontal, lateral, and oblique views. Difficulty in interpretation arises when a fragment is displaced for a considerable distance or when a fracture fragment rotates (e.g., the proximal end of the capitate)[270] so that its site of origin is obscure. The radiographic approach to carpal injuries is well summarized by Gilula.[260]

Metacarpophalangeal and Interphalangeal Joint Dislocation. Dislocation of a metacarpophalangeal joint (excluding the thumb) results from a fall on the outstretched hand that forces the joint into hyperextension. The volar plate is disrupted, allowing dorsal displacement of the base of the proximal phalanx.[273] Radiographs may reveal a widened joint space, indicating interposition of the volar plate within the joint. An adjacent sesamoid can also become displaced into the joint space.[274]

Dislocation of the proximal interphalangeal joint can occur in a posterior or, more rarely, anterior direction. Posterior dislocation results from a hyperextension injury. Ligamentous and volar plate

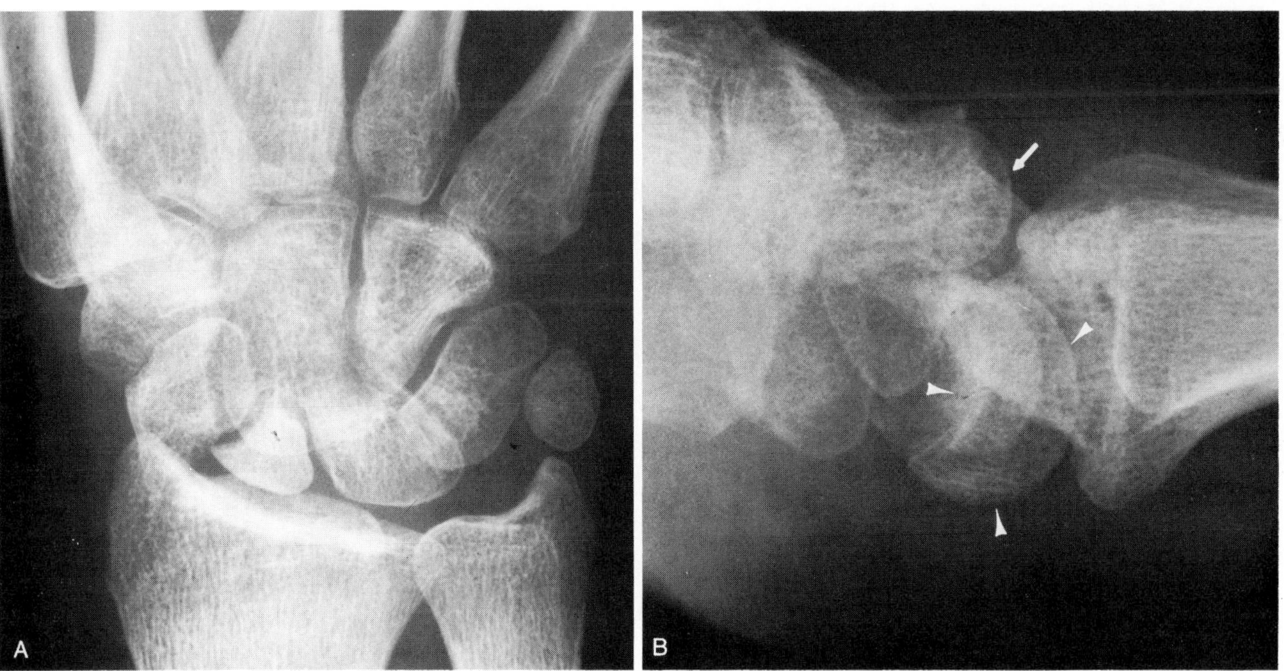

Figure 63–41. *Perilunate and lunate dislocations.*

A, B *Transscaphoid perilunate dislocation. Findings include a fracture of the scaphoid with osteonecrosis of the proximal pole and a perilunate dislocation characterized by a lunate bone (arrowheads) aligned with the distal radius as well as dorsal displacement of the capitate (arrow) and the rest of the carpus.*

Illustration continued on the following page

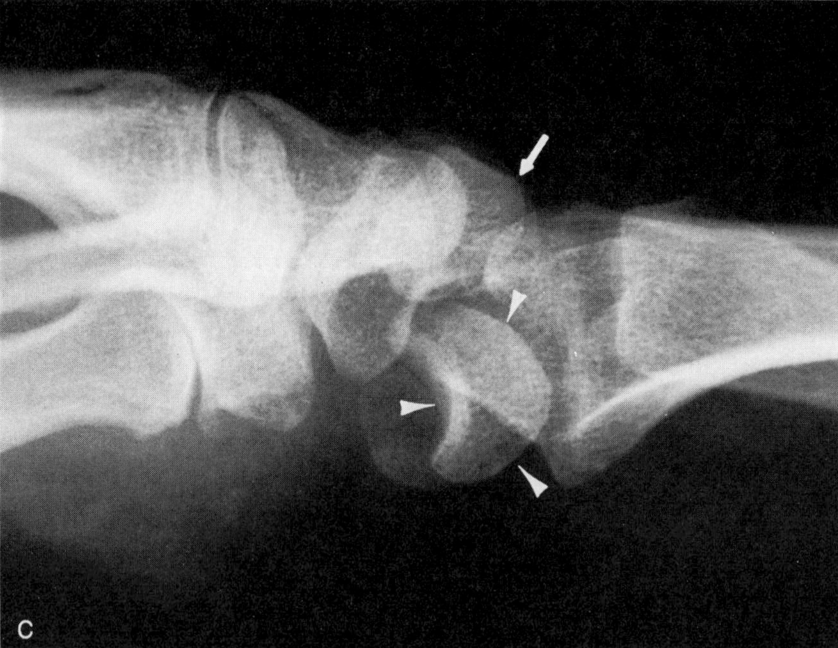

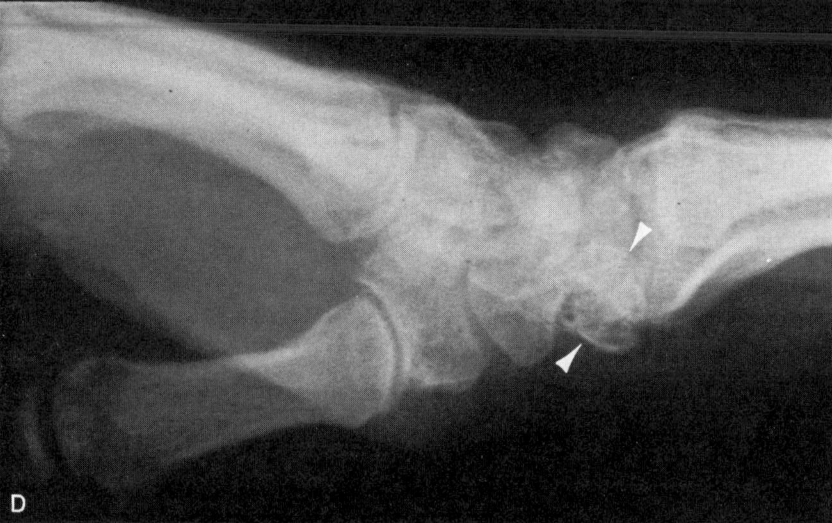

Figure 63–41. Continued
C *Perilunate dislocation. Observe the alignment of the lunate (arrowheads) with the distal radius and dorsal displacement of the capitate (arrow) and the rest of the carpal bones.*
D *Lunate dislocation. In this case, the lunate is displaced in a volar direction (arrowheads) and the capitate and other carpal bones are aligned with the distal radius.*

disruption is a frequent associated finding[275, 276] (Fig. 63–42). Radiographs reveal the abnormal position of the phalanx and, in many cases, small avulsed fragments of bone. Posterior dislocation of a distal interphalangeal joint can also be encountered.

A Bennett's fracture-dislocation is a relatively common intra-articular injury that occurs at the base of the first metacarpal[277, 278] (Fig. 63–43*A*). Following an axial blow to a partially flexed first metacarpal, an oblique fracture line separates the major portion of the bone from a small fragment of the volar lip. The base of the metacarpal is pulled dorsally and radially. The Bennett's fracture represents only one of several different fracture patterns that occur at the base of the thumb and should not be confused with a second intra-articular fracture, the Rolando's fracture, in which a Y- or T-shaped comminuted fracture line is evident (Fig. 63–43*B*).

Dislocations and collateral ligament injuries of the first metacarpophalangeal joint are important complications of trauma. Although several types of injuries can be identified, that related to a sudden valgus stress applied to the metacarpophalangeal joint of the thumb, the gamekeeper's thumb, has received the most attention.[279-283] Initially described as an occupational hazard in English gamewardens, who, in killing rabbits by twisting their necks, sustained repeated stresses about the first metacarpophalangeal joint, the injury is now recognized to occur in various settings, including skiing[284] (Fig. 63–44). Attenuation or disruption of the ligamentous apparatus along the ulnar aspect of the thumb is

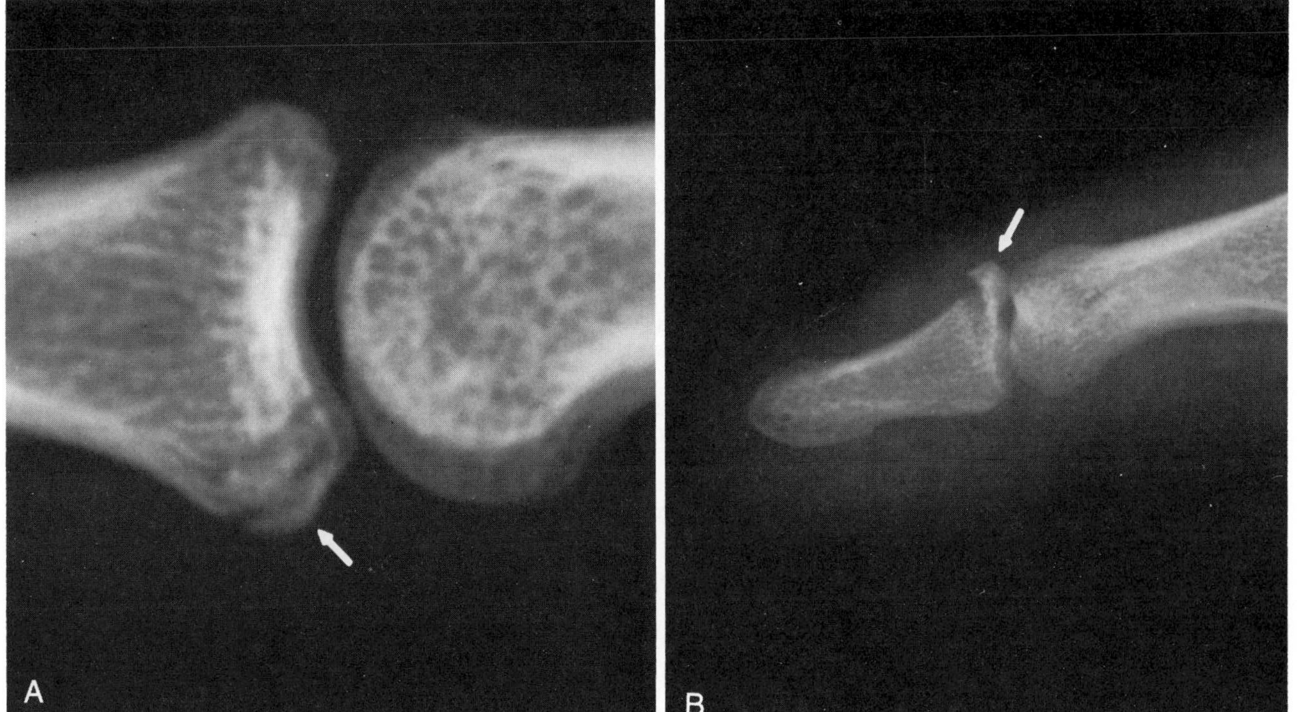

Figure 63–42. *Interphalangeal joint injuries.*

A, B *Small avulsion fractures (arrow) of the proximal interphalangeal or distal interphalangeal joint can result from traction on the volar plate* **(A)** *or extensor tendons* **(B).** *Dislocations may also be evident.*

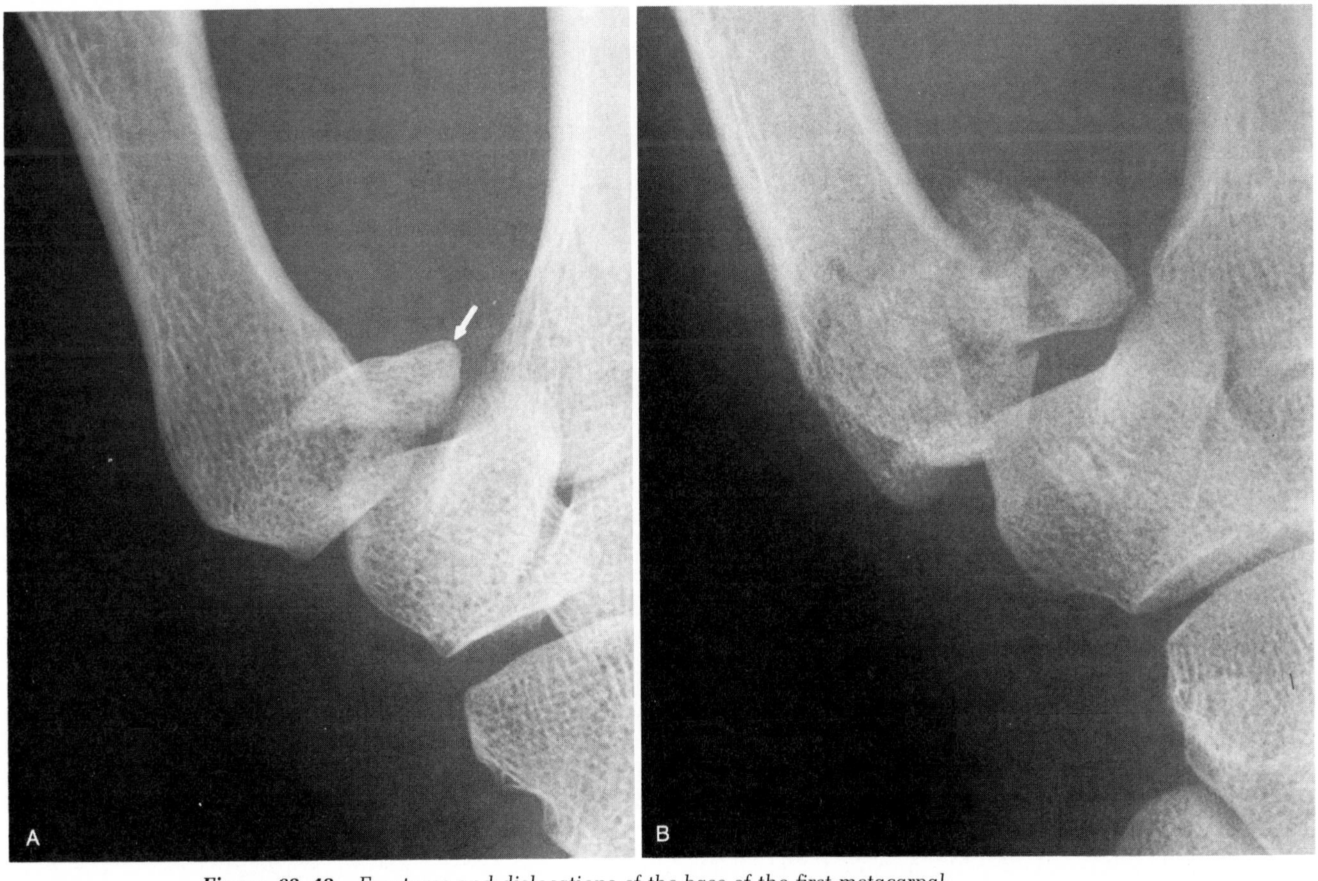

Figure 63–43. *Fractures and dislocations of the base of the first metacarpal.*

A *Bennett's fracture-dislocation. Observe the typical oblique fracture of the volar lip of the first metacarpal (arrow).*

B *Rolando's fracture. A comminuted fracture of the metacarpal base is evident.*

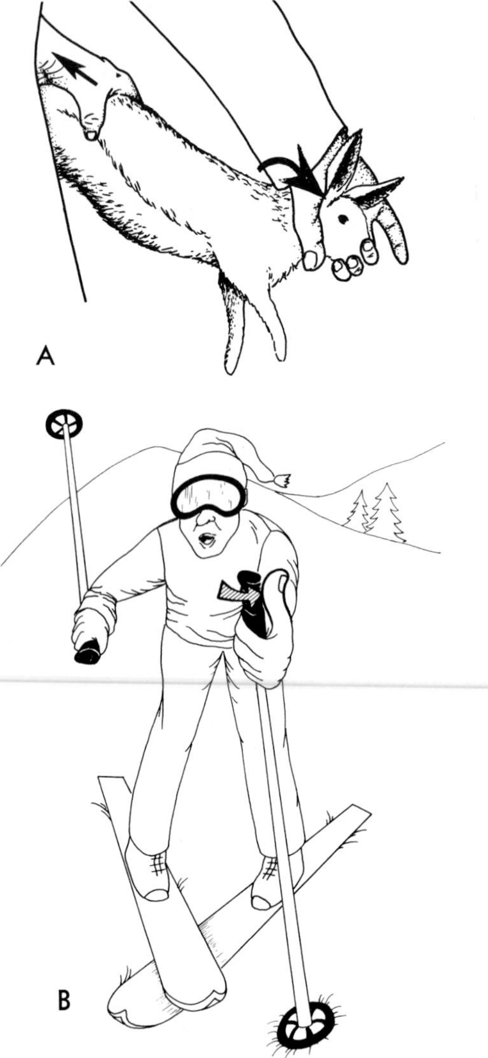

Figure 63–44. Gamekeeper's thumb: Mechanism of injury.

A *Classic mechanism of injury. To kill a wounded rabbit, a gamekeeper extends rabbit's neck and applies traction. Although a strong pull in the direction of the arrow would normally exert pressure only in the cleft between the first and second fingers, a loose grip produces strain along the ulnar aspect of the thumb (curved arrow), stretching the ulnar collateral ligament.*

B *More modern mechanism of injury. Incorrect implantation of a ski pole produces abduction and extension of thumb (arrow) as momentum carries skier downhill. This creates stress on the ulnar aspect of the first metacarpophalangeal joint, with injury to the ulnar collateral ligament.*

(From Resnick D, Danzig LA: Am J Roentgenol 126:1046, 1976. Copyright 1976, American Roentgen Ray Society.)

seen, which may be associated with pain, swelling, tenderness, edema, and pinch instability (Fig. 63–45). Initial radiographs can be negative, although small avulsed fragments from the base of the proximal phalanx can be delineated in some instances (Fig. 63–46). These fragments may be displaced proximally and rotated from 45 degrees to 90 degrees. Roentgenograms obtained with radial stress applied to the first metacarpophalangeal joint can reveal subluxation, and arthrography may outline leakage of contrast material from the ulnar aspect of the articulation and an abnormal folded position of the ulnar collateral ligament[285, 286] (see Chapter 15).

Hip Dislocation. Dislocation of the femoral head with or without an acetabular fracture is an injury that usually follows considerable trauma and that may be associated with significant injury elsewhere in the body. Dislocations are classified as anterior, posterior, and central in type.

Anterior dislocation of the hip is due to forced abduction.[287] It is a rather rare type of dislocation, representing 5 to 10 per cent of all hip dislocations. On radiographs, the abnormal position of the femoral head is readily apparent, and associated femoral head fractures may be identified.[288] A characteristic depression or flattening of the posterosuperior and lateral portion of the femoral head can be seen[560, 591] (Fig. 63–47). Rarely, anterior dislocation of the hip may be recurrent.[289, 290]

Posterior dislocation of the hip is more common (approximately 80 to 85 per cent of all hip dislocations) and may result from a "dashboard injury" in which the flexed knee strikes the dashboard during a head-on automobile collision.[287, 291-295] The leg is shortened, internally rotated, and adducted. Associated problems include knee trauma, femoral head or shaft fractures, and sciatic nerve injury. The frequent occurrence of posterior acetabular rim fractures following posterior dislocation of the hip requires careful analysis of routine radiographs and utilization of oblique and lateral projections[296-298] (see Chapter 3) (Fig. 63–47). A persistently widened hip joint may indicate abnormally placed fragments or significant acetabular injury. Tomography can be used to identify small osseous fragments, deformity of the femoral head, and the extent of damage to the posterior acetabular rim. Additional complications of this injury are periarticular soft tissue calcification and ossification, acetabular labrum tears, osteonecrosis of the femoral head, and secondary degenerative joint disease.[299-302] Osteonecrosis may complicate as many as 25 per cent of posterior hip dislocations, especially when the injury is associated with a delay in diagnosis and treatment and a fracture of the posterior acetabular margin.

Central acetabular fracture-dislocation usually results from a force applied to the lateral side of the trochanter and pelvis, with the stress applied through the femoral head. Various patterns of acetabular fracture complicate this injury, and hemorrhage into the pelvis may also be observed. Secondary degenerative joint disease is not infrequent.

Traumatic dislocation of the hip is usually encountered in adults, although children and infants can also be affected.[303-306, 527, 561] In the younger age group, dislocation is almost always posterior in type, and in the infant, traumatic displacement must be differentiated from congenital dislocation of the hip.

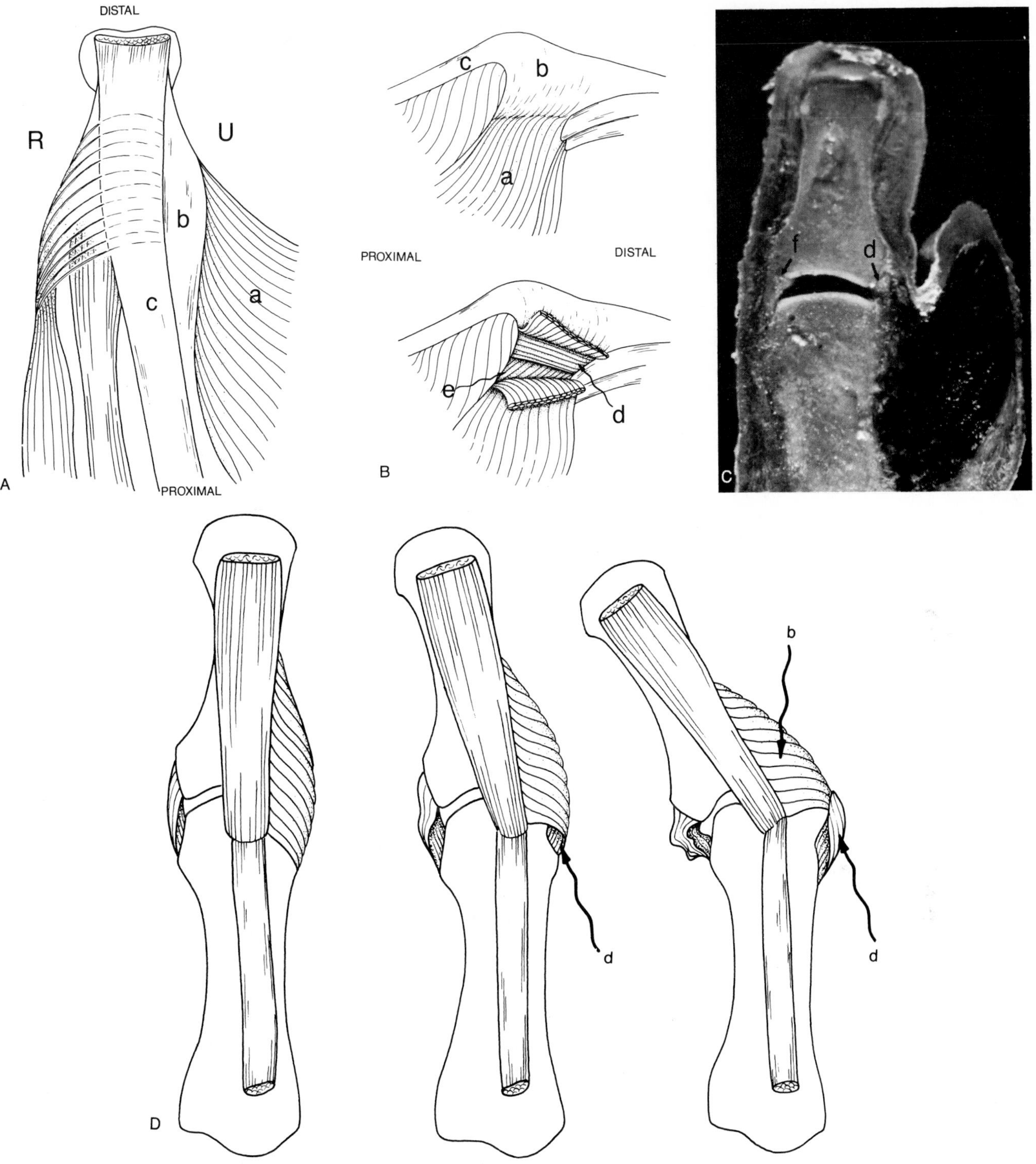

Figure 63–45. *Gamekeeper's thumb: Mechanism of injury. Anatomy of ligaments of metacarpophalangeal joint of thumb.*

A *Dorsal aspect showing radial* (R) *and* (U) *sides of metacarpophalangeal joint. Tendon of extensor pollicis longus* (c) *passes over the metacarpophalangeal joint, running from proximal to distal aspect of digit. The adductor pollicis* (a) *inserts in part on the proximal phalanx, some of its fibers fusing with a portion of the dorsal aponeurosis, termed the adductor aponeurosis* (b).

B *Ulnar aspect showing adductor pollicis* (a), *adductor aponeurosis* (b), *and tendon of the extensor pollicis longus* (c). *In lower drawing, the adductor pollicis has been incised and opened, exposing the ulnar collateral* (d) *and accessory collateral* (e) *ligaments.*

C *Coronal section of first metacarpophalangeal joint. Note position of ulnar* (d) *and radial* (f) *collateral ligaments.*

D *Dorsal aspect of first metacarpophalangeal joint following rupture of ulnar collateral ligament. With time, torn ligament* (d) *can protrude from the proximal edge of the adductor aponeurosis* (b), *the latter preventing its return.*

(From Danzig LA: Am J Roentgenol 126:1046, 1976. Copyright 1976, American Roentgen Ray Society.)

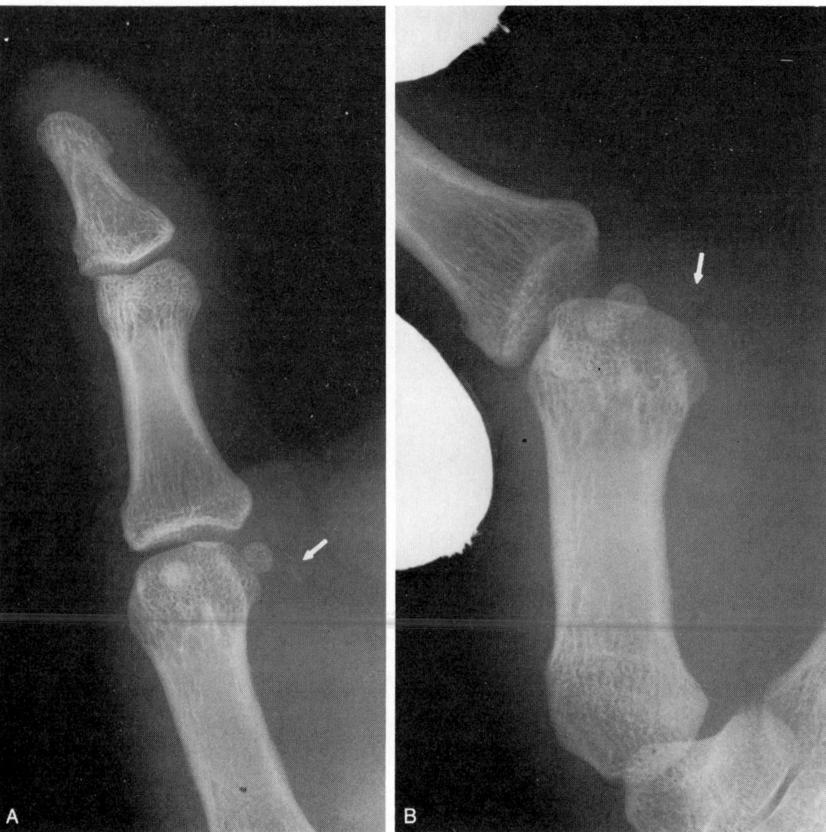

Figure 63–46. *Gamekeeper's thumb.*

A *An initial radiograph outlines small osseous fragments adjacent to the first metacarpophalangeal joint (arrow).*

B *A radiograph obtained during radial stress reveals subluxation of the phalanx on the metacarpal. The fracture fragments are again identified (arrow).*

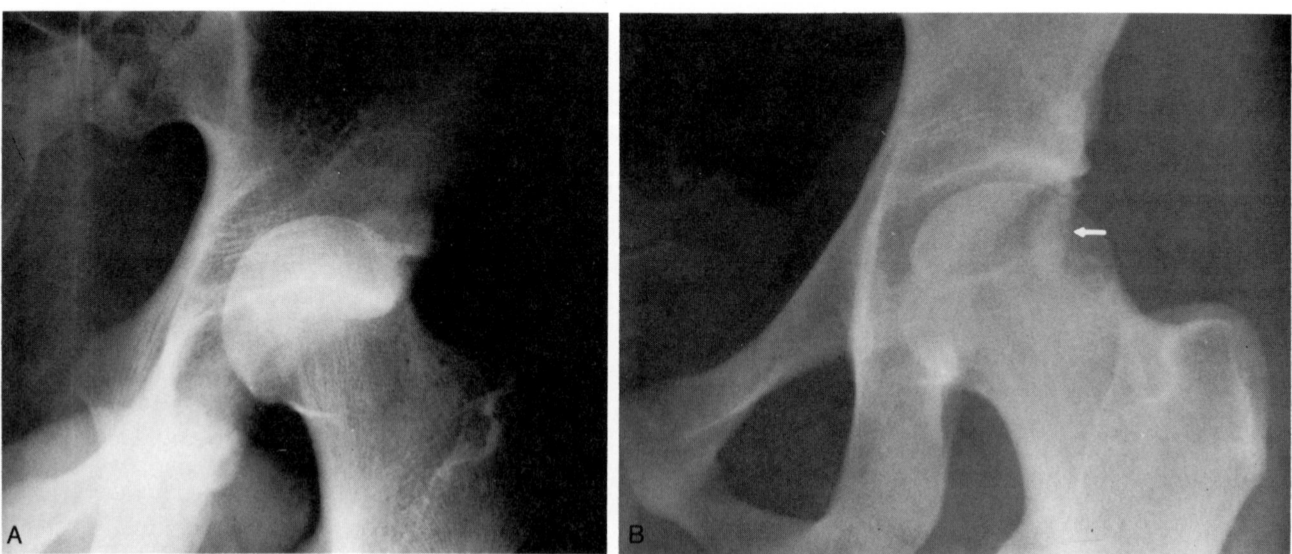

Figure 63–47. *Hip dislocation.*

A, B *Posterior dislocation. The initial oblique radiograph reveals a posterosuperior dislocation of the femoral head. Following reduction, note the large osseous fragment of the posterior acetabular rim (arrow).*

Illustration continued on the opposite page

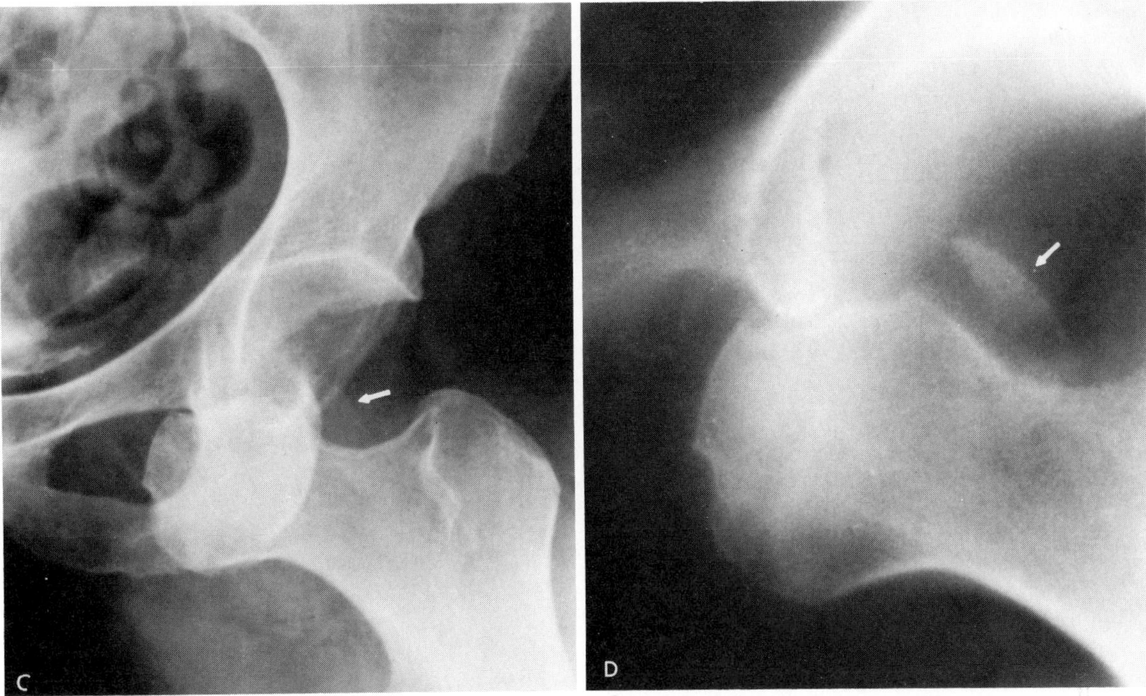

Figure 63–47. Continued
C, D *Anterior dislocation. Plain film and tomogram reveal inferomedial position of the dislocated femoral head and a fracture fragment of the lateral portion of the head (arrow).*

Knee Dislocation. This is a rare but serious injury due to the neurovascular insult that may result from popliteal artery and peroneal nerve damage.[307-310] Anterior, posterior, lateral, medial, and rotatory types of dislocation are recognized. Anterior dislocation is the most common type (30 to 50 per cent of all knee dislocations), apparently resulting from hyperextension of the knee with tearing of the posterior capsule and cruciate ligament. The adjacent popliteal artery may be stretched, leading to thrombosis or laceration. Peroneal nerve damage is most likely to occur in patients with posterolateral dislocation. Following any type of dislocation, capsular, cruciate, and ligamentous injury can be seen.

Radiographic diagnosis is not difficult, although multiple views are required to detect associated osteochondral and fibular head fractures as well as avulsion injuries of the tibial spines. Arteriography should be employed to delineate the status of the popliteal artery in patients in whom operative intervention is being contemplated owing to vascular symptoms and signs.

Patellar Dislocation. Traumatic dislocation of the patella can be produced by a direct blow or an exaggerated contraction of the quadriceps mechanism. Abnormalities predisposing to displacement may include an abnormally high patella (patella alta), deficient height of the lateral femoral condyle, shallowness of the patellofemoral groove, genu valgum or recurvatum, lateral insertion of the patellar tendon, muscular weakness, and excessive tibial torsion.[311, 312] Lateral dislocation predominates, although rare patterns of displacement include vertical (superior), intercondylar, and intra-articular dislocation.[313-316] Recurrent dislocation and osteochondral fractures of the medial patellar facet and lateral femoral condyle are common[160-164, 317-319] (Fig. 63–27). Analysis of patients with recurrent dislocation or subluxation of the patella frequently requires special axial projections[593] (see Chapter 7).

Proximal Tibiofibular Joint Dislocation. Although rare, proximal tibiofibular joint dislocation may be seen in parachuting, hang-gliding, sky-diving, and horseback riding injuries. Anterior or, less frequently, posterior dislocation of the fibular head can be noted.[320, 321] Peroneal nerve injury can appear following a posterior dislocation of this joint. Rarely, a superior dislocation can be seen, which is associated with injury to the interosseous membrane and superior dislocation of the lateral malleolus.

Radiographic findings associated with dislocation of the proximal tibiofibular joint may be subtle. As the fibular head is displaced anteriorly, it also moves laterally. This anterolateral movement can be better appreciated when comparison radiographs of the uninvolved side are available or when the relationship of the fibular head to the osseous groove on the posterolateral aspect of the tibia is carefully analyzed (see Chapter 3). Oblique roentgenograms may reveal complete separation of the tibia and the fibula. In cases of posterior dislocation, the fibular head is displaced medially, overlapped in large part by the tibia on anteroposterior roentgenograms.

Subluxation of the proximal tibiofibular joint refers to excessive and symptomatic movement without frank dislocation.[322-324] This is a self-limited condition of youth with decreasing symptoms as the patient approaches skeletal maturity, although persistent symptoms and signs may require surgical intervention.

Ankle Dislocation. Subluxations and dislocations of the ankle, particularly those in a medial or lateral direction, are commonly associated with fracture of the adjacent malleolar surfaces. Displacements due to extensive ligamentous and capsular injury without fracture can occur in an anterior or posterior direction. Posterior dislocation is more frequent than anterior dislocation, and either may be associated with fracture of the tibial surface. The diagnosis of the specific type of fracture-dislocation is usually easily accomplished by routine radiography; asymmetry of the ankle joint is best delineated on mortise views obtained in 10 degrees of internal rotation.[325] Such assessment is important, as even minor degrees of displacement of the talus with respect to the tibia can result in secondary degenerative joint disease.[326] Arthrography can be utilized to demonstrate the presence and site of ligamentous injury, although the examination must be accomplished shortly after the traumatic insult (see Chapter 15).

Tarsal Dislocation. Subluxation, dislocation, and fracture-dislocation are common injuries in the midfoot and hindfoot.[327-329] Of particular interest is the Lisfranc's fracture-dislocation of the tarsometatarsal joints[330-333] (Fig. 63–48). Normally, the heads of the metatarsals are joined by transverse ligaments.[332] Similarly, the bases of the metatarsals reveal ligamentous connections, except between the base of the first and that of the second metatarsal. An oblique ligament extends between the medial cuneiform and the second metatarsal base, anchoring the base of this metatarsal. This metatarsal is also stabilized because of its recessed position between the cuneiforms.

Injuries of the tarsometatarsal joints can result from direct or, more commonly, indirect trauma. In the latter situation, violent abduction of the forefoot can lead to lateral displacement of the four lateral metatarsals with or without a fracture at the base of the second metatarsal and cuboid bone (Fig. 63–48). Accompanying dorsal displacement is more frequent than plantar displacement, a predilection that is explained, at least in part, by the relatively wide configuration of the dorsal surface of the base of the second metatarsal.[331] The first metatarsal may dislocate in the same direction or in the opposite direction of the other metatarsals, depending upon the precise vectors of the force.[334, 335]

Radiographic examination usually identifies the dislocation and accompanying fractures, although the findings may be subtle. Proper recognition of abnormal alignment in the tarsometatarsal joints requires knowledge of normal radiographic anatomy.[331] A consistent relationship in the normal foot is the alignment of the medial edge of the base of the second metatarsal with the medial edge of the second cuneiform on the frontal and oblique views of the foot. A small space or gap between the bases of the first and second metatarsals does not, by itself, represent a definite sign of dislocation; rather, disruption of the alignment of the second metatarsal and second cuneiform with a step-off between the bones is more diagnostic of an injury. The normal alignment of the bases of the fourth and fifth metatarsals with the cuboid and that of the base of the first metatarsal with the medial cuneiform are more variable.

Metatarsophalangeal and Interphalangeal Joint Dislocation. Dislocations at the metatarsophalangeal joints can occur in any direction, related to the mechanism of injury. The first metatarsophalangeal joint is commonly affected.[336] Similarly, patterns of dislocation of interphalangeal joints in the foot are variable. The interphalangeal joint of the hallux is most typically affected. Pseudodislocation of the proximal interphalangeal joint of the fifth toe following trauma has been related to accumulation of joint fluid or soft tissue injury.[337]

Pelvic Dislocation. The sacroiliac joint is extremely stable owing to the strong ligaments that surround it. Rarely, isolated fractures or separations of the articulation can occur, producing a single break in the pelvic ring.[338] Much more frequently, sacroiliac joint disruption is accompanied by a fracture through the relatively weak anterior portion of the ring, resulting in a double break of the pelvic ring. One type of injury producing disruption of the pelvic ring in two places consists of an anterior abnormality characterized by pubic fractures or symphyseal separation and a posterior abnormality consisting of a sacroiliac joint dislocation or fracture of the neighboring bone, usually the ilium. This injury is termed a Malgaigne fracture. In most instances, identifying the sites of fracture or dislocation is easy, although subtle cases are encountered.[339] Asymmetry in the configuration and width of the two sacroiliac articulations and a minor step-off at the symphysis pubis may be the only radiographic clues to a significant pelvic injury.

In all cases of pelvic fracture and dislocation, a search for associated injuries of neighboring soft tissues and viscera must be accomplished.

Spinal Dislocation. Fracture-dislocation of the spine can occur at any level in the lumbar, thoracic, or cervical segments. In most instances, prominent clinical manifestations, which may include neurologic deficit, and radiologic abnormalities assure prompt and accurate diagnosis. Vertebral displacements are commonly accompanied by characteristic fractures, which vary in accordance with the mechanism of injury. In some cases, significant ligamentous injuries are unassociated with obvious radiographic changes on routine examination, although carefully monitored flexion and extension

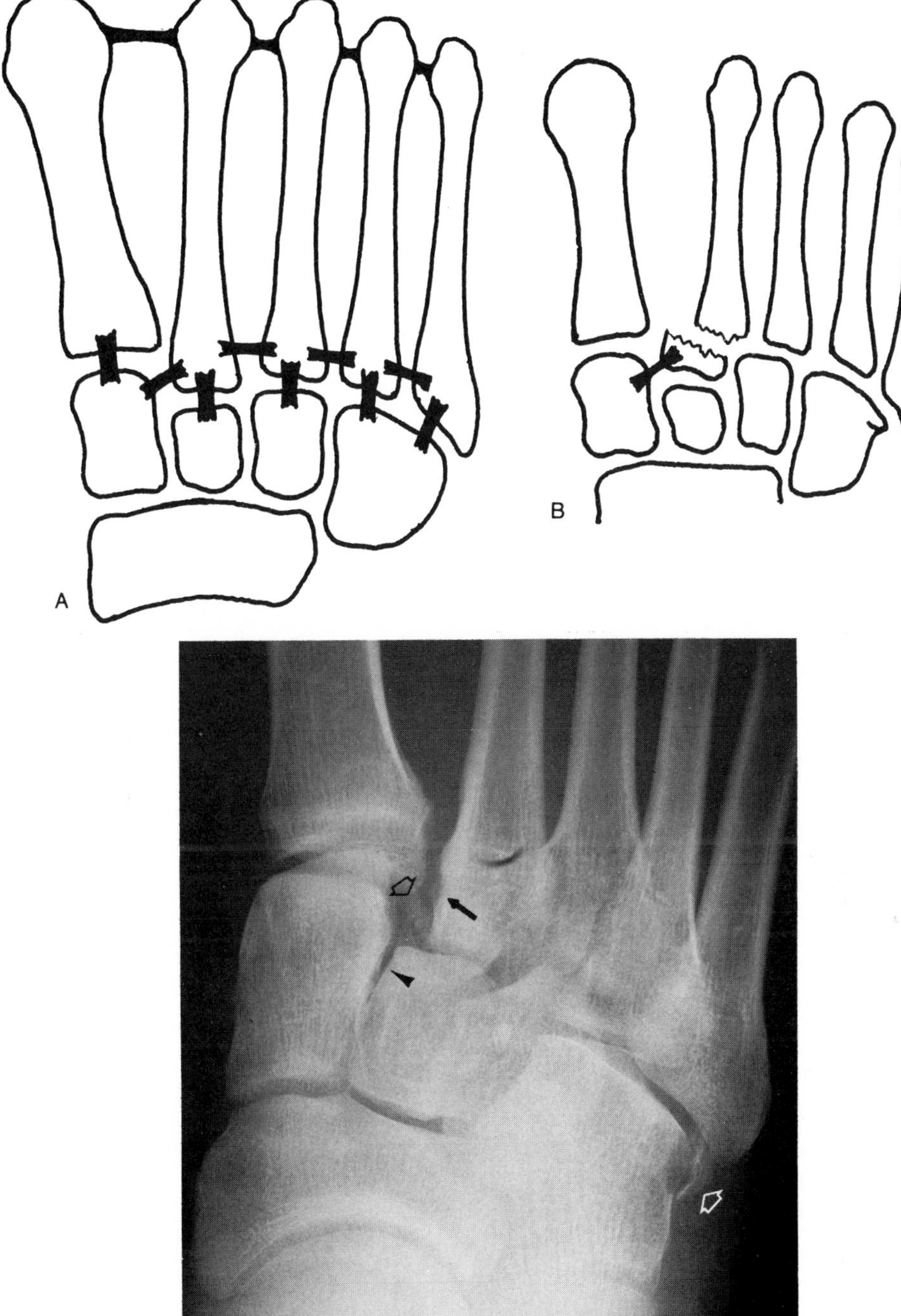

Figure 63–48. *Lisfranc's fracture-dislocation of tarsometatarsal joints.*

A *Normal ligamentous anatomy (see text).*

B *Lateral dislocation of the second through fifth metatarsals may be associated with fractures of the base of the second metatarsal and cuboid.*

C *In this patient, note subtle displacement of the second through fifth metatarsal bases. The medial edge of the second metatarsal base (solid arrow) is not aligned with the medial edge of the second cuneiform (arrowhead). Fractures of the base of the second metatarsal and cuboid are evident (open arrows).*

(From Wiley JJ: J Bone Joint Surg 53B:474, 1971.)

studies can reveal the presence and degree of spinal instability.

Because of the frequency of abnormalities of the atlanto-axial articulations in arthritis, a brief discussion of several traumatic alterations at this site follows.

Atlanto-axial Rotary Fixation. The principal motion that occurs at the atlanto-axial articulations is rotation, although some degree of lateral translation, flexion-extension, and vertical approximation also appears at this level. It has been estimated that approximately 50 degrees of all rotatory cervical motion takes place at the atlanto-axial junction.[340]

Self-limited and completely reversible rotation at the atlanto-axial junction can accompany a variety of processes.[341] Such atlanto-axial rotary displacement is especially frequent in children with torticollis and may follow trivial trauma or upper respiratory tract infection or may occur on a spontaneous basis. Occasionally, the abnormal displacement persists and the condition is termed rotary fixation.[342, 343] Rotary fixation may occur as an isolated injury or in combination with a transverse ligament rupture or fracture of the atlas or the axis, or both. The patient presents with the head tilted to one side and rotated to the opposite side with slight flexion. Subsequently, the abnormal position of the head may appear to lessen in severity owing to compensation in the lower cervical spine. If accompanied by ligamentous deficiency and fracture with atlanto-axial instability, atlanto-axial rotary fixation can rarely lead to neurologic deficit, vascular compromise, and death.[341]

The correct diagnosis can be established on a carefully performed radiographic examination. In a *normal* subject, an anteroposterior roentgenogram (open-mouth projection) reveals symmetrically placed articular masses of the atlas and the axis, with the odontoid process located midway between the masses[342] (Fig. 63–49). A radiograph obtained with 10 to 15 degrees of rotation of the head to the right side shows anteromedial rotation and upward shifting of the left atlantal articular mass with an apparent medial approximation to the odontoid. The right atlantal articular mass moves posteromedially and inferiorly, and its profile narrows with concomitant widening of the profile of the left atlantal articular mass. The upward slide of the left atlantal articular mass may provide a slight widening of the left lateral atlanto-axial joint space, whereas the downward slide of the right atlantal articular mass may lead to narrowing of the right lateral atlanto-axial joint space. In the normal situation, rotation of the head to the opposite side produces the converse of all of these radiographic changes.

In patients with atlanto-axial rotary fixation, a persistent asymmetry of the odontoid process in its relationship to the articular masses of the atlas is seen that is not corrected by changes in head position (Fig. 63–50). Documentation of this abnormal situation is provided by a radiographic study that includes five open-mouth views of the odontoid process: anteroposterior (AP) view in neutral position; AP views with the head tilted 10 degrees to either side; and AP views with the head rotated 10 degrees to either side. Normally, the relative position of the odontoid process and lateral masses of the atlas will vary among these views; in the presence of atlanto-axial rotary fixation, no change in alignment is apparent. Cineradiography, laminography, and computed tomography can be utilized to detect these changes in selected cases.[344] If rotary fixation is complicated by rupture or attenuation of the transverse ligament of the atlas, the distance between the atlas and the dens will be increased on lateral radiographs obtained during neck flexion.

The exact pathogenesis of this lesion is not clear.

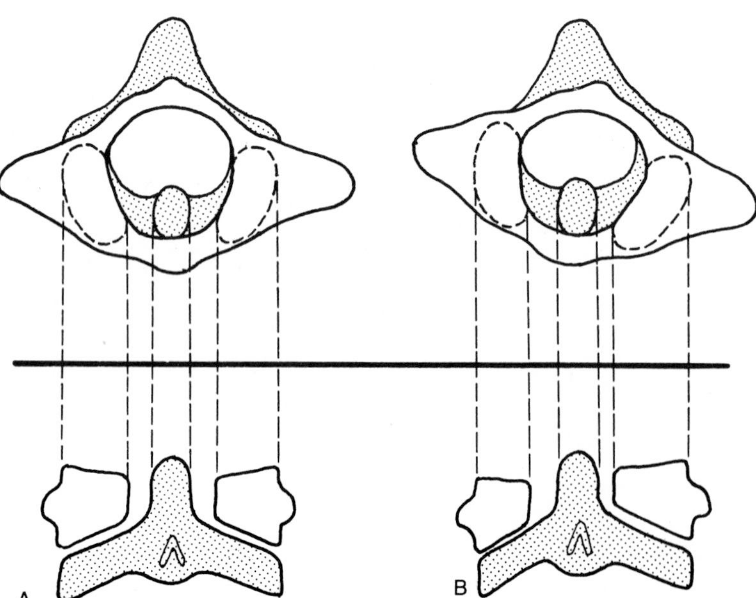

Figure 63–49. *Atlanto-axial joint in neutral position* **(A)** *and on rotation to the right side* **(B)**, *viewed from above (on top) and from the frontal plane (on bottom).*

A *In neutral position, the odontoid process is located midway between the lateral masses of the atlas. The lateral atlanto-axial joints are symmetric in appearance.*

B *With rotation, anteromedial rotation and upward shift of the left atlantal articular mass are associated with its medial approximation to the odontoid process. The right atlantal articular mass moves inferiorly and posteromedially, and it possesses a narrow profile. The left lateral atlanto-axial joint is widened, and the right is narrowed. Persistence of the findings is consistent with atlanto-axial rotary fixation.*

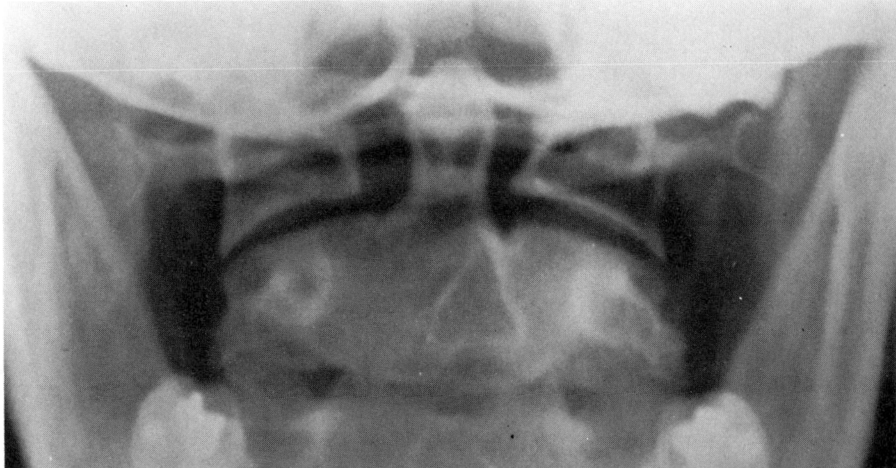

Figure 63–50. Atlanto-axial rotary fixation. In this patient, persistent alignment changes identical to those described in Figure 63–49**B** are seen.

It may result from tear and invagination of capsular ligaments about the lateral atlanto-axial joints.[345] This invagination might lead to pain and muscle spasm in the initial stages of the disorder. Rupture of one or both alar ligaments,[346] hyperemia with ligament laxity,[347] and muscle contraction due to inflammation[348] are other suggested etiologies.

Atlanto-axial Subluxation/Dislocation. Traumatic subluxation of the atlas and the axis is almost always accompanied by a fracture of the odontoid process.[349] Isolated atlanto-axial subluxation (without fracture) indicates abnormality of the transverse ligament that may be related to trauma, inflammation, or congenital anomaly; underlying inflammatory disease processes include rheumatoid arthritis, juvenile chronic arthritis, ankylosing spondylitis, pharyngitis, and tonsillitis, processes that presumably lead to ligament laxity due to hyperemia.[354] With isolated atlanto-axial subluxation, the atlas almost always slides anteriorly, increasing the distance between the anterior arch of the atlas and the dens[350]; rarely, posterior displacement of the atlas with respect to the axis can occur without fracture of the odontoid process.[351, 352] An abnormal distance between the atlas and the dens following anterior atlanto-axial subluxation is best detected on carefully obtained lateral radiographs during neck flexion. This distance in normal individuals varies with age; it may reach 2.5 to 3.0 mm in adults and 3.5 to 4.5 mm in children.[353] In normal children, minor subluxations may also appear at other cervical levels, particularly between the second and third cervical vertebrae.

Isolated traumatic anterior atlanto-axial subluxation is associated with tear or disruption of the transverse ligament.[355] Congenital anomalies of regional bones (e.g., the odontoid process) or ligaments (e.g., the transverse ligament) increase the individual's susceptibility to traumatic subluxation.

Fracture of the odontoid process with atlanto-axial subluxation can result from either a hyperflexion or hyperextension injury[356] (Fig. 63–51). In hyperflexion injuries, the dens is displaced anteriorly with the atlas; in hyperextension injuries, it is displaced posteriorly. Considerable instability following either injury can be outlined during radiographic examination performed in the lateral projection during neck flexion and extension. Fractures of the odontoid process may be complicated by nonunion; the incidence of this complication is dependent upon the age of the patient, the type and location of the fracture, and the method of treatment.[357-360] Osteolysis following fracture can produce a separate ossicle above the base of the odontoid[361-364] (Figs. 63–52 and 63–53). This ossicle resembles an os odontoideum, which has generally been considered a developmental anomaly

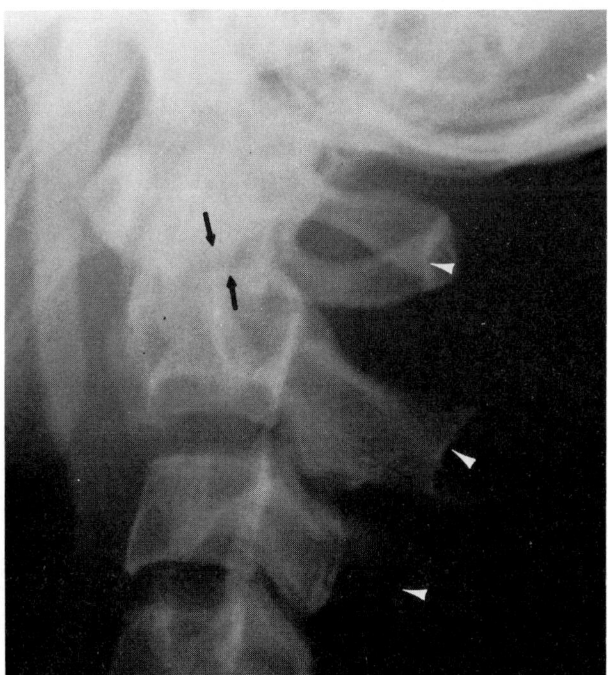

Figure 63–51. Odontoid fracture with atlanto-axial subluxation. Note the odontoid fracture (arrows) with anterior displacement of the atlas and odontoid with respect to the remainder of the axis. Note the "malalignment" of the spinolaminar lines (arrowheads), indicating the degree of subluxation.

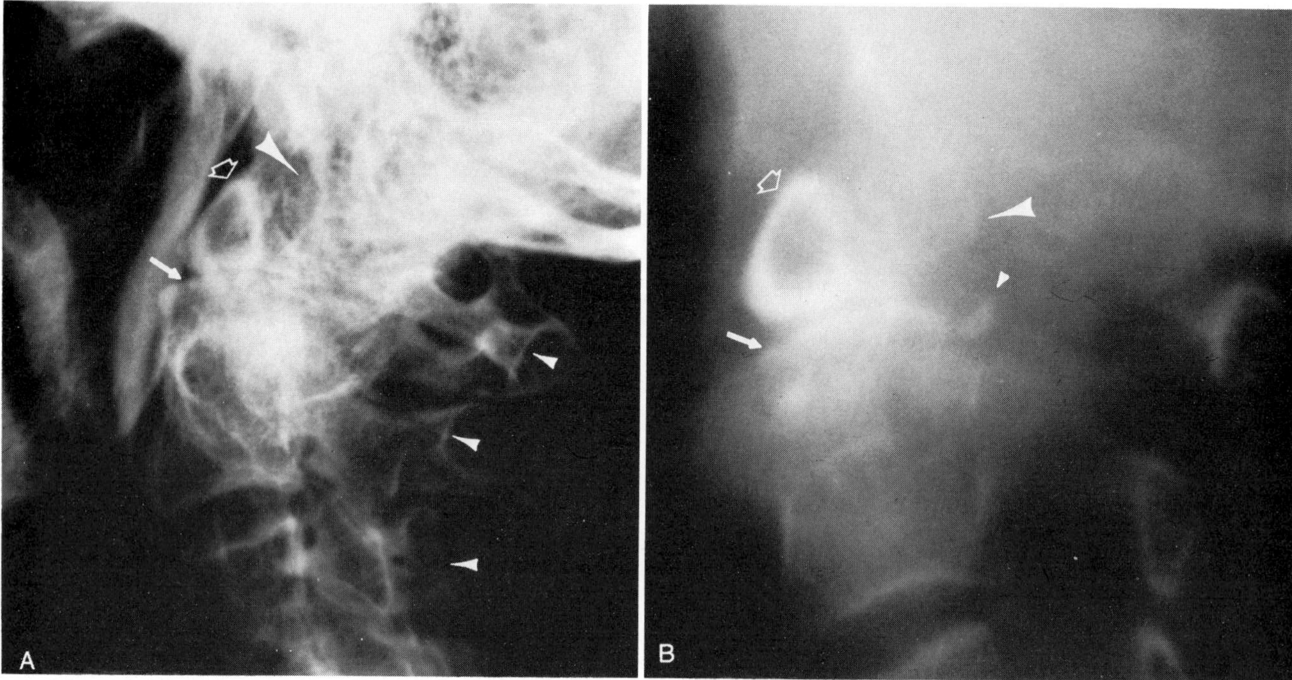

Figure 63–52. Nonunion of an odontoid fracture with separate ossicle. Following an injury many years before, this patient developed persistent neck pain.

A A lateral radiograph reveals amputation of the axis (solid arrow) without identification of an odontoid process. The anterior arch of the atlas (open arrow) is displaced posteriorly with respect to the axis, as evidenced by the alignment of the spinolaminar lines (small arrowheads). A separate bony fragment is seen (large arrowhead).

B A midline tomogram reveals the abnormal position of the anterior arch of the atlas (open arrow) and the axis (solid arrow), the separate ossific dense area (large arrowhead), and a small fracture of the axis (small arrowhead). Flexion-extension tomograms indicated considerable movement at the atlanto-axial junction with abnormal contact between the arch of the atlas and the amputated axis, accounting for the sclerotic bony margins.

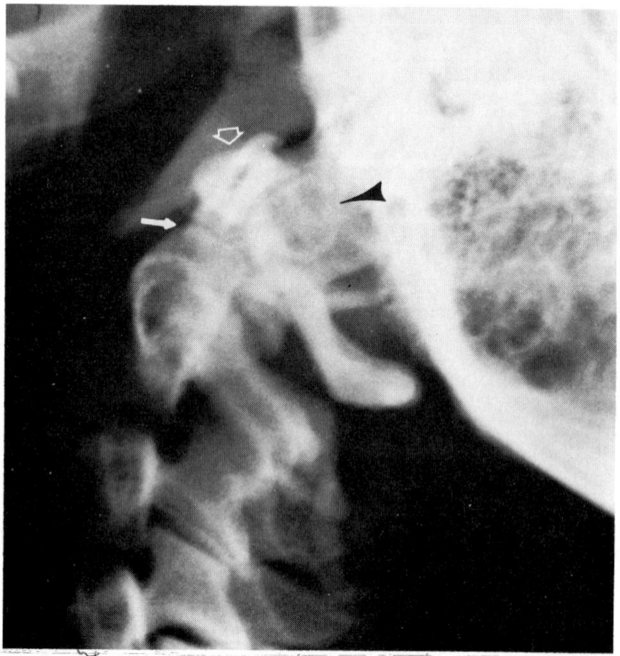

Figure 63–53. Nonunion of an odontoid fracture with separate ossicle. The findings are similar to those in Figure 63–52, including an amputated axis (solid arrow), posterior displacement of the anterior arch of the atlas (open arrow), and a separate ossific dense area (arrowhead).

of the axis. The appearance of a separate odontoid tip following fracture or even acute ligamentous injury[365, 562, 563] suggests that at least some instances of os odontoideum are acquired rather than congenital in etiology. The possibility that posttraumatic resorption of a portion of the odontoid process relates to vascular insufficiency and osteonecrosis has been suggested, and, in fact, osteonecrosis of the proximal end of the dens has been noted in association with halo-pelvic distraction.[366]

Fractures of the odontoid process must be differentiated from pseudofractures due to Mach bands, an optical illusion that leads to the appearance of a radiolucent line across the base of the dens.[367]

TRAUMA TO SYNOVIAL JOINTS

Traumatic Synovitis and Hemarthrosis

Following a blow or abnormal stress, joint swelling and pain may develop. A joint effusion appearing within the first few hours following trauma is usually related to a hemarthrosis; nonbloody effusions usually appear 12 to 24 hours after in-

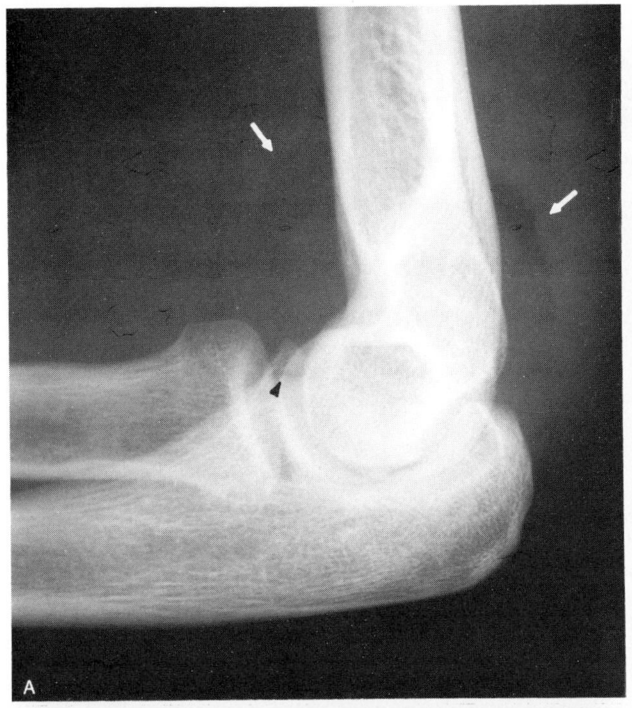

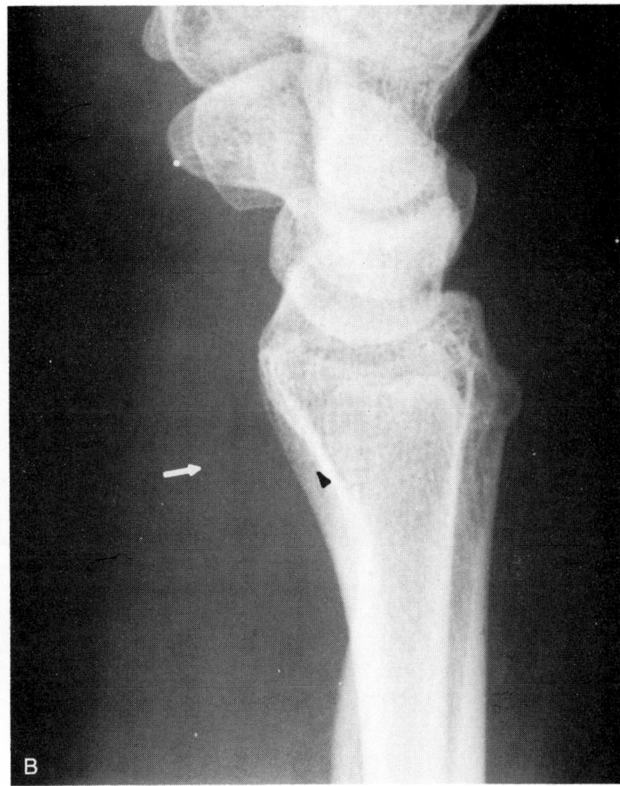

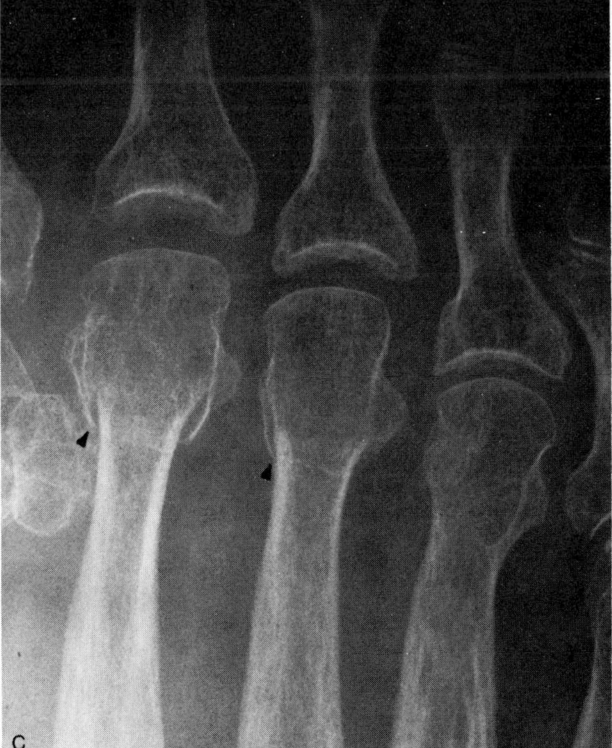

Figure 63–54. *Traumatic synovitis, hemarthrosis, and soft tissue edema.*

A *Displacement of the anterior and posterior fat pads (arrows) about the elbow following trauma usually indicates intra-articular fluid or blood. Note the fracture of the coronoid process of the ulna (arrowhead).*

B *Obliteration of the fat plane about the pronator quadratus muscle (arrow) is associated with a subtle fracture (arrowhead).*

C *Widening of the second and third metatarsophalangeal joints accompanies fractures of the metatarsal heads (arrowheads) and may be related to synovitis, hemarthrosis, or osseous shortening.*

jury.[368, 369] Pain and, occasionally, fever may be apparent in cases of hemarthrosis, and in all such cases, occult fractures or ligamentous injury must be excluded by careful clinical and radiologic examination.[564] Hemarthrosis may also be associated with hemophilia, pigmented villonodular synovitis, neuropathic arthropathy, and intra-articular tumors in addition to injuries.

Bloody or nonbloody effusions following trauma are associated with radiographic findings that are related to displacement of intra-articular fat pads and edema of extra-articular fat planes. Typical examples of these findings are widening of the suprapatellar pouch in cases of knee trauma; ventral and posterior displacement of the fat pads about the distal humerus (Fig. 63–54*A*) and distortion of the fat planes overlying the supinator muscle in cases of elbow trauma; displacement and obliteration of the fat plane overlying the pronator quadratus muscle (Fig. 63–54*B*) and about the carpal scaphoid in cases of wrist trauma; and "bulging" of the "capsular" fat in cases of hip trauma in children.[370-374] In general, the displacement and distortion of many of these fat planes indicate only the presence of fluid or mass in the joint and may be evident in a variety of articular processes; however, in the clinical setting of trauma, detection of these changes should encourage a thorough search for a subtle fracture or subluxation. Similarly, widening of the articular space due to accumulation of fluid can follow intra-articular trauma[375] (Fig. 63–54*C*), but may also be observed in other articular conditions. Chronic accumulation of blood in the joint, as in cases of hemophilia and pigmented villonodular synovitis, may lead to hemosiderin deposition in the synovial membrane and increased radiodensity of the distended joint.

Careful evaluation of synovial fluid in some joints may document the presence of "wear particles" consisting of chondral fragments and debris.[586] Their presence in a traumatized joint, such as the knee, may indicate damage to the fibrocartilaginous meniscus. The particles are more readily identified in the absence of a hemarthrosis as they may be obscured by abundant erythrocytes in the synovial fluid.

Lipohemarthrosis

Bloody synovial fluid containing fat droplets can be noted grossly and microscopically following trauma to a joint.[376-378] The discovery of intra-articular fat, when combined with bone marrow spicules, is reliable evidence of an intra-articular fracture, the fat being released from the marrow following cortical violation. Frequently, however, a hemorrhagic effusion containing fat may be observed in patients without fracture, probably related to significant cartilaginous or ligamentous injury.[379-381] As fat is also present in the synovium, it is possible that damage to the synovium alone can release fat into the synovial fluid.[381] The amount of fat in the synovial fluid is directly proportional to the severity of the joint injury.[379] Although fat globules are occasionally seen in many other types of effusion, their accumulation is much greater in cases of trauma. Following trauma, synovitis with synovial fluid leukocytosis may result as a response to intra-articular lipid droplets and may be associated with intracellular (leukocytes) accumulation of the lipids due to phagocytosis.[381]

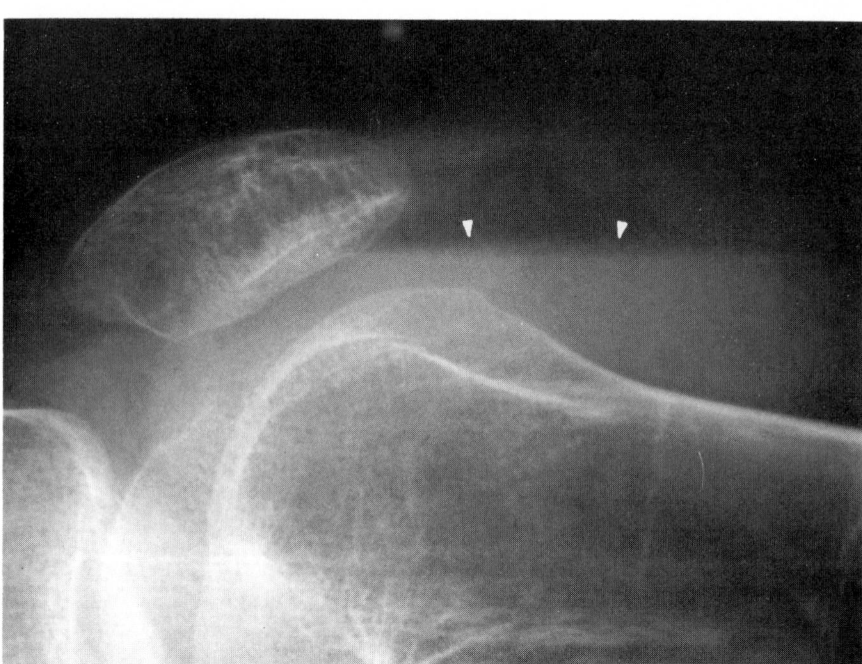

Figure 63–55. *Lipohemarthrosis. On a cross-table lateral radiograph, a straight radiodense fluid line (arrowheads) at a fat-blood interface can be a helpful clue to an underlying yet subtle fracture.*

Radiographic examination utilizing horizontal beam technique may demonstrate a fat-blood fluid level following injury to the joint[377, 380, 382-387] (Fig. 63–55). Most commonly, this finding is seen in a knee or a shoulder, although it may also be noted in other articulations, including the elbow.[388] In the knee, subtle tibial plateau fractures may be the source of the fat, requiring careful radiography and tomography for detection,[389-391] although fat may also originate from fibular, femoral, or patellar fractures as well as soft tissue injury to cartilage, ligaments, fat pads, or synovium.[565] Small amounts of fat and blood in this joint may not be sufficient to produce a fat-blood fluid level on cross-table radiography, although large amounts will reveal a typical radiopaque straight line at the interface of the fat above and the blood below. Occasionally, routine lateral knee films taken without horizontal beam technique in patients with significant intra-articular fat will allow visualization of the capsule as a water-dense linear structure outlined on both sides by fat.[392]

In the shoulder and the elbow, fat-blood fluid levels can accompany fractures, dislocations, and, perhaps, injuries to the synovium or surrounding soft tissue structures.[383, 385, 388]

TRAUMA TO SYMPHYSES

Traumatic insult to symphyses, including the symphysis pubis, manubriosternal joint, and intervertebral disc, is not infrequent. Subluxation or dislocation of the symphysis pubis leads to a single break in the pelvic ring and is commonly combined with a second injury with pelvic disruption such as a fracture of the ilium or sacrum or a diastasis of the sacroiliac joint. Minor degrees of instability in this location may be discovered during radiographic examination performed with the patient standing first on one leg, then on the other. Exaggerated movement at the articulation indicates violation of its integrity, although, under normal circumstances, some motion at the symphysis pubis may be observed, especially in pregnant women (see Chapter 54). Subluxation or dislocation of the manubriosternal joint usually indicates significant trauma, and may be seen after automobile accidents in which the chest strikes the steering wheel.

Violation of the intervertebral disc may be combined with fractures of the vertebral bodies and posterior elements, leading to spinal instability. One example of an injury that can lead to disruption of both the intervertebral disc (and surrounding bone) and the posterior spinal structures is the "seat-belt" fracture (Fig. 63–56). During an automobile accident, the trunk flexes over the seat belt. A horizontal fracture of a vertebral body (Chance fracture) or tearing of the intervertebral disc can be combined with laminal and spinous process fractures or ligamentous tear.

Trauma to the discovertebral junction can result from obvious or occult injury. In either situation, violation of the cartilaginous end-plate and subchondral bone plate of the vertebral body may allow intraosseous herniation of discal material (cartilaginous or Schmorl's nodes)[393-396] (Figs. 63–57 and 63–58). Cartilaginous nodes may appear in acute injuries in which excessive axial loading of the spine occurs. This can result in obvious compression fracture of the vertebral body or subtle injury at the

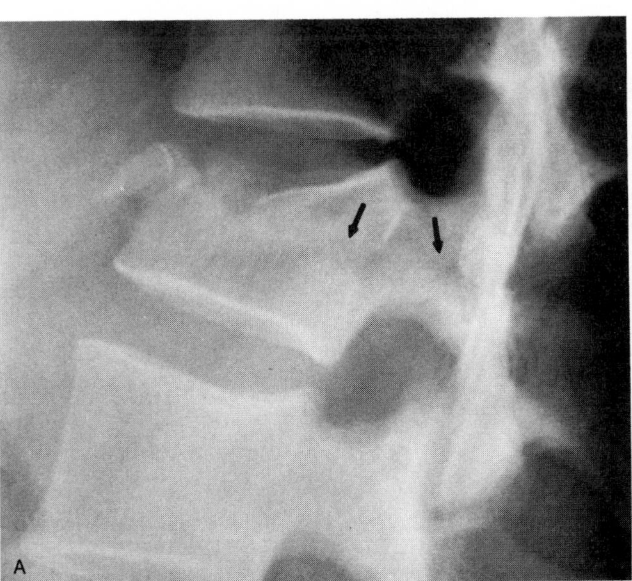

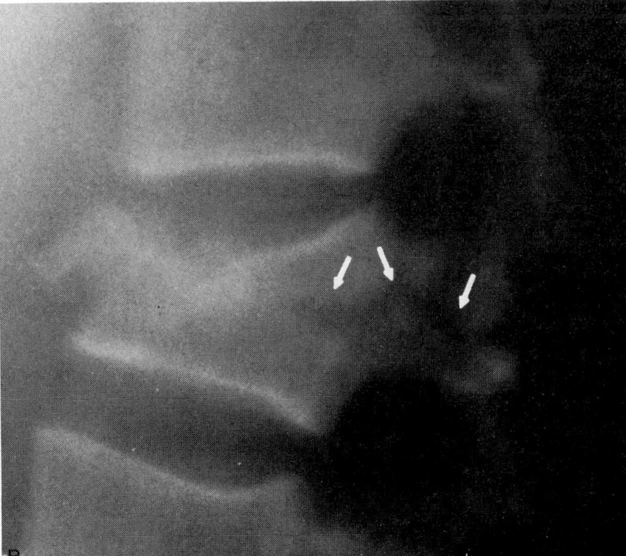

Figure 63–56. *"Seat-belt" fracture. Following an automobile accident, a transverse fracture of an upper lumbar vertebra is sometimes associated with a transverse fracture through the pedicles and laminae (arrows).*

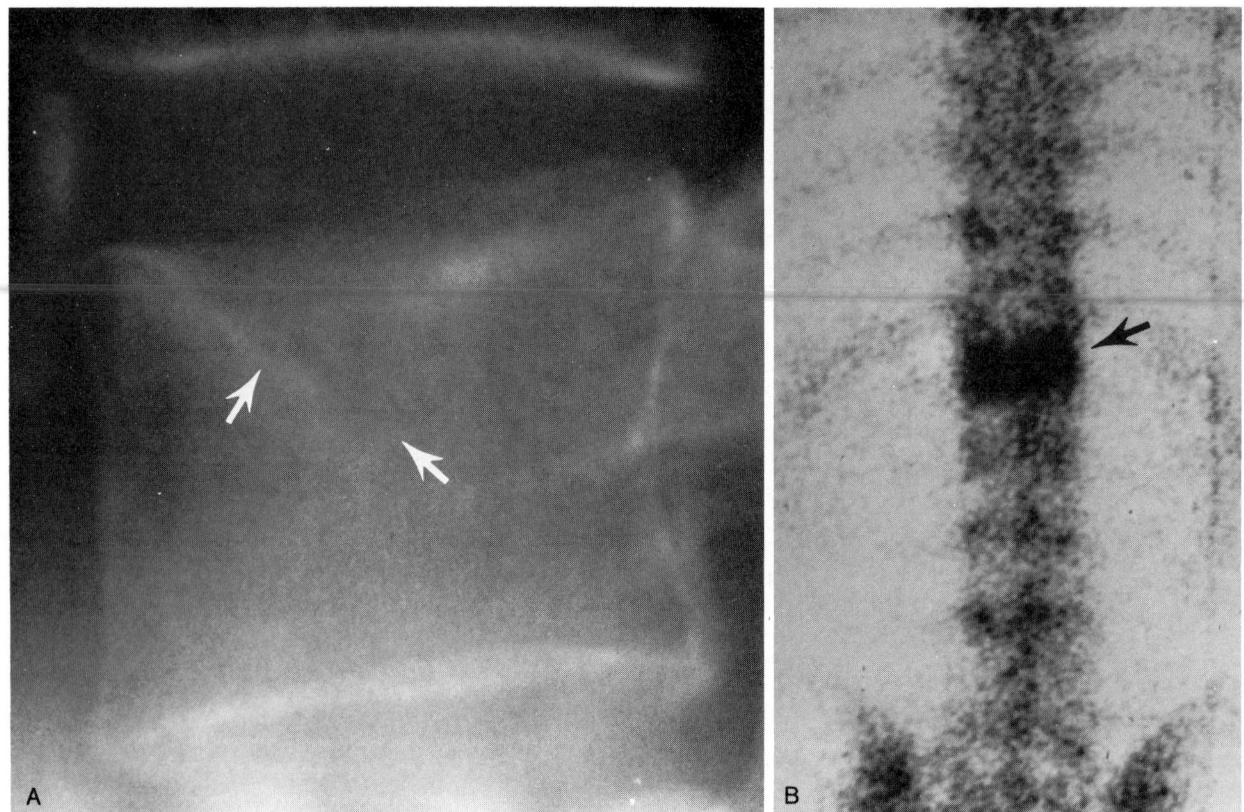

Figure 63–57. *Discovertebral trauma. Acute compression fracture.*

A *Following an injury with axial loading of the spine, intraosseous herniation of discal material (cartilaginous node) (arrows) can be seen.*

B *A radionuclide study with technetium pyrophosphate reveals increased accumulation of isotope at the site of injury (arrow).*

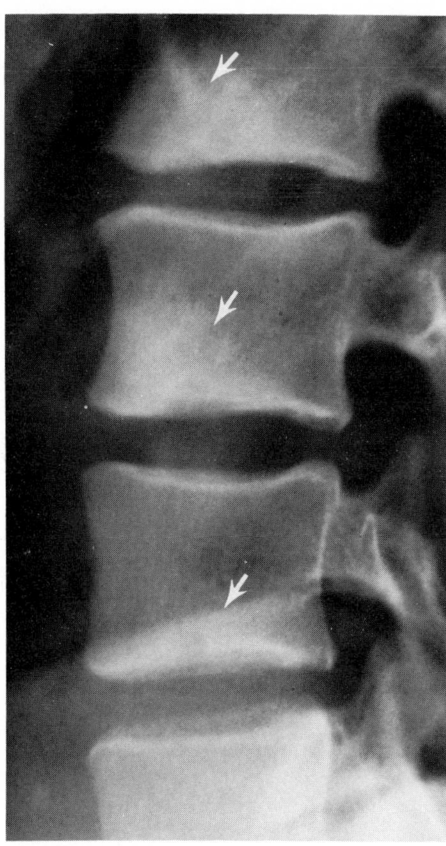

Figure 63–58. Discovertebral trauma: Occult injury. The reactive sclerosis of the inferior surfaces of multiple lumbar vertebrae (arrows) represents the sequelae of intraosseous discal herniations (cartilaginous nodes).

discovertebral junction. With axial loading, there is an increase in nuclear pressure. Fracture of the cancellous bone of the vertebral body and disruption of the cartilaginous end-plate allow discal material to enter the vertebral body. Typically, the cranial disc protrudes into the vertebra, although both cranial and caudal discs may be involved. In the latter instance, the invading cranial and caudal discal tissue may split the vertebral body, producing a bursting fracture of the vertebra. This sequence of events requires the presence of a relatively normal nucleus pulposus; compression injuries in patients with intervertebral osteochondrosis (see Chapter 40) produce uniform flattening of the vertebral body.[397]

The intravertebral discal material may be associated with surrounding osseous compression and reactive bone formation. Radiographs reveal one or more radiolucent areas, with bony sclerosis in the vertebral body that may be combined with intervertebral disc space loss. The roentgenographic appearance may simulate that of infection or tumor.

Another type of injury of the discovertebral junction occurs at the site of attachment of the anulus fibrosus to the rim of the vertebral body. At this site, fibrous extensions of the anulus (Sharpey's fibers) are firmly attached to the vertebral rim. In the developing skeleton, this union is far more solid than that between the cartilage in the vertebral rim and the ossified portion of the vertebral body.[398] Thus, in the young patient, prolapse of the contiguous intervertebral disc can lead to displacement of the ossified portion of the vertebral rim owing to separation of the osteocartilaginous junction between the rim and the remaining vertebral body. In the mature skeleton, osseous union between the rim and vertebral body occurs, producing a much stronger connection. Even in the adult, however, injury can lead to osseous avulsion at the site of attachment of Sharpey's fibers. Hyperextension injury to the cervical spine can be associated with a small bony flake at this site.

TRAUMA TO SYNCHONDROSES (GROWTH PLATES)

Mechanisms and Classification

The growth plate of the immature skeleton is especially vulnerable to injury; approximately 6 to 15 per cent of fractures of the tubular bones in children under the age of 16 years involve the growth plate and neighboring bone.[399-404] Forces that produce ligamentous tear or joint dislocation in the adult may lead to growth plate injury in the child and adolescent, as the joint capsule and ligamentous structures are approximately two to five times stronger than the cartilaginous plate.[405] Four types of stress may produce growth plate injury; shearing or avulsive forces account for approximately 80 per cent of injuries, and splitting or compressive stresses account for the remainder.[402] Sites that are most typically affected are the distal tibial, fibular, ulnar, and radial growth plates and the proximal humeral growth plate. Subtle clinical findings may follow the traumatic insult; pain, swelling, tenderness, and limitation of motion may be encountered. Identification of the abnormality of the growth plate on the roentgenogram may also be difficult. The irregular band-like radiolucency of the normal cartilaginous plate can obscure minor degrees of separation or diastasis. Well-coned roentgenograms and multiple projections are mandatory, and tomograms may also be necessary. Early diagnosis and treatment can prevent significant growth disturbance and deformity.

Of the various regions of the growth plate, it is the hypertrophic zone that is most vulnerable to shearing and avulsive injuries. The germinal cells are usually spared, and growth will continue as long as there has been no interference with the blood supply.[406] The vulnerability of the blood supply varies with the specific region of the body that is traumatized. In certain locations, such as the proximal femur, the growth plate is situated intra-articularly, and the vascular supply to the epiphysis is closely applied to the periphery of the plate, increasing its susceptibility to injury.[402] In these areas and others, growth disturbance can ensue, and the degree of deformity is dependent upon the potential for future growth of the undamaged segment of the growth cartilage.[403] The younger the patient, the longer the period of growth and the greater the potential for future deformity. Once a deformity has appeared, its progression may be stimulated by abnormal mechanical forces.

The vulnerability of the hypertrophic zone of the growth plate to shearing injury appears to be influenced by the rate of growth.[404, 407] An increase in the thickness of this zone during periods of rapid growth may promote epiphyseal separations. However, other factors also influence the susceptibility of the growth plate to shearing forces.[404] Furthermore, compression forces produce failure of the metaphysis rather than the growth plate in most instances. This may be observed in the normal skeleton as well as in certain pathologic states such as scurvy.[408] Metaphyseal failure is more common at the sites at which the metaphysis is not protected from compression stress; one example is the vertebral endplate, where a compression fracture can produce a cartilaginous node. Metaphyseal fragility is also accentuated by any condition associated with osseous weakening, be it related to the osteoclastosis of hyperparathyroidism or the hypervascularity of the normal growth spurt.

Avulsion injury to the growth plate is commonly observed at sites of apophyses. Examples include the lesser trochanter, the medial epicondyle of the distal humerus, and the base of the fifth metatarsal.[404] At some sites, notably the calcaneus, the iliac crest, and the vertebral body, irregularity of the metaphysis provides some degree of protection against avulsion injury.[409] At any site, the age of appearance of the injury is dependent upon the time of appearance and fusion of the apophysis. The avulsed cartilage may continue to demonstrate osteogenesis, producing small or large bony ossicles.[410, 411]

A splitting injury of the growth plate produces a fracture that crosses the entire epiphyseal complex, perpendicular to the growth plate. With healing, callus formation may take place across the plate, anchoring the epiphysis to the metaphysis.[401] Cessation of growth occurs at this focus, and as the remainder of the epiphyseal complex continues to grow, angular deformity may ensue.

Following an injury to the growth plate, repair is quickly initiated, unless an injury to the germinal layer of the cartilage or to the vascular supply of the epiphysis has occurred.[402] Initially, there is a transient increase in the thickness of the growth plate, which reaches a peak in approximately 10 days. Fibrin appears within the line of cleavage; the cartilage cells continue to grow, and the epiphyseal plate thickens as the cellular columns lengthen.[401] In about three weeks, dissolution and resorption of fibrin are observed and normal growth resumes.[406]

Although there are several proposed classification systems of growth plate injuries, that of Salter and Harris is most widely accepted.[406] This system separates the lesions according to their radiographic appearance (Fig. 63–59).

Type I (6 per cent). This represents a pure epiphyseal separation, with the fracture isolated to the growth plate itself (Fig. 63–60*A*). A shearing or avulsion force causes a cleavage through the zone of hypertrophic cells. This type of injury has a favorable prognosis and becomes apparent at a relatively young age, at a time when the growth plate is wide; it is especially frequent under the age of 5 years and as a result of birth injury.[412] The proximal humerus and femur and distal humerus are the most commonly affected sites. Radiographic recognition of this injury is not difficult when the growth plate is wide and when the epiphysis remains displaced. In many instances, however, spontaneous reduction of the separation takes place, and the roentgenographic diagnosis is more difficult. Helpful signs are soft tissue swelling and minimal widening or irregularity of the growth plate.

Type II (75 per cent). This most common type of growth plate injury results from a shearing or avulsion force that splits the growth plate for a variable distance before entering the metaphyseal bone, separating a small fragment of the bone, the "corner sign" (Fig. 63–60*B*). The periosteum on the side of the metaphyseal fracture remains intact, but that on the opposite side is disrupted in conjunction with growth plate separation. Because of the intact periosteum, the fracture fragment is usually easily reduced, and the eventual prognosis is generally favorable. The usual age of injury is 10 to 16 years, and the common sites of involvement are the distal radius, distal tibia, distal fibula, distal femur, and ulna, in order of decreasing frequency. The predilection is for areas with large ossification centers.

Type III (8 per cent). In this variety of injury, the fracture line extends vertically through the epiphysis and growth plate to the hypertrophic zone, and then horizontally across the growth plate itself, usually on one side or the other (Fig. 63–60C). Type III injuries are especially common in children between the ages of 10 and 15 years and in the distal tibia, with less frequent involvement of the proximal tibia and distal femur. Radiography usually allows prompt recognition of the fracture, although multiple projections and stress views are sometimes necessary. Displacement is generally minimal, and if care is exercised in the reduction of the fracture, growth arrest and deformities are rare. If reduction is not complete, the gap in the growth plate may become replaced with bone.[403]

Type IV (10 per cent). A vertically oriented

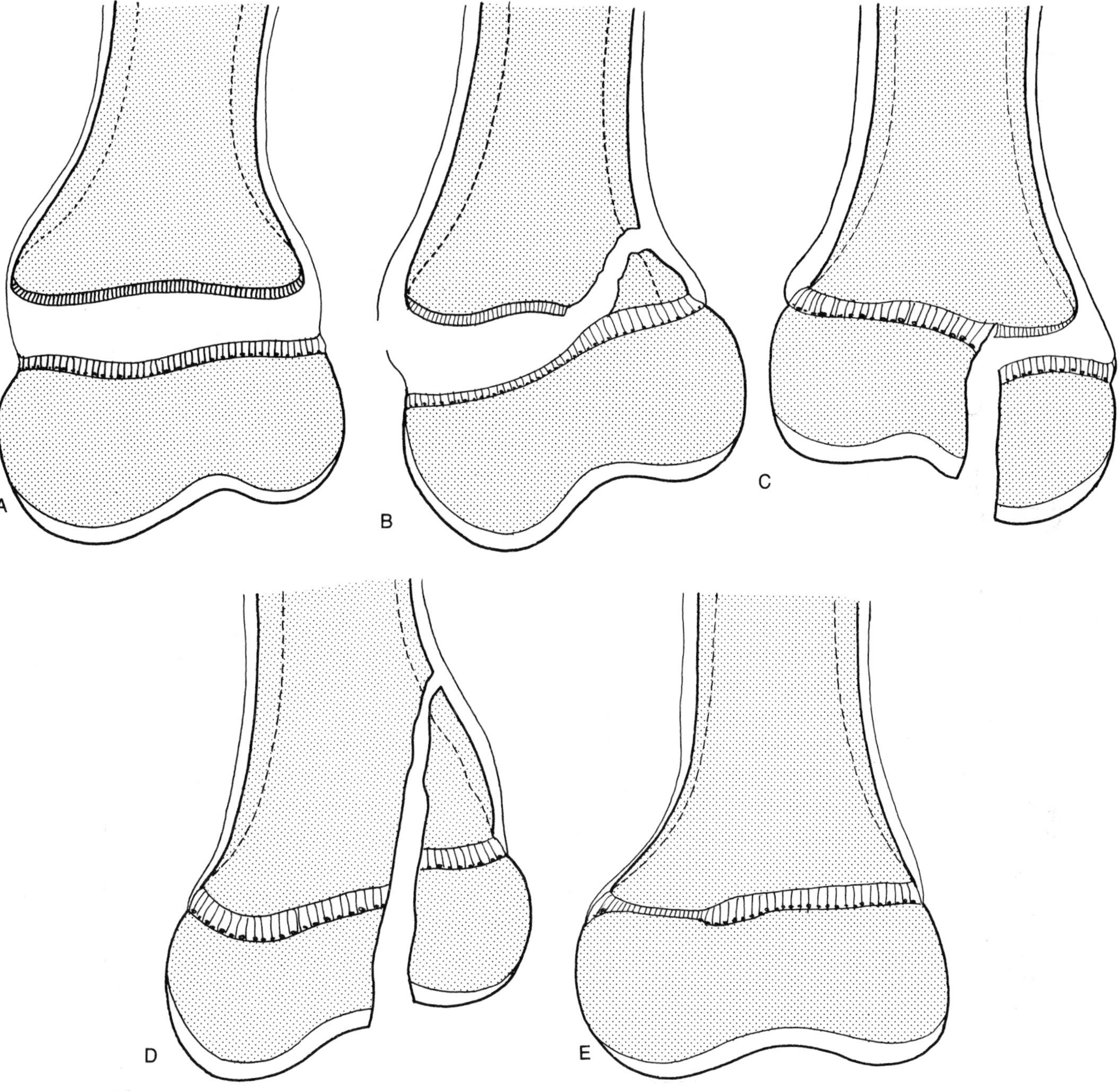

Figure 63–59. *Growth plate injuries: Classification system.*

A *Type I: A split in the growth plate occurs through the zone of hypertrophic cells. The periosteum is intact.*

B *Type II: The growth plate is split and the fracture enters the metaphyseal bone, creating a triangular fragment. The periosteum about the fragment is intact, whereas that on the opposite side may be torn.*

C *Type III: A vertical fracture line extends through the epiphysis to enter the growth plate. It then extends transversely across the hypertrophic zone of the plate.*

D *Type IV: A fracture extends across the epiphysis, growth plate, and metaphysis. Note the incongruity of the articular surface and the violation of the germinal cells of the growth plate.*

E *Type V: Compression of a portion of the growth plate may be unassociated with immediate radiographic abnormalities.*

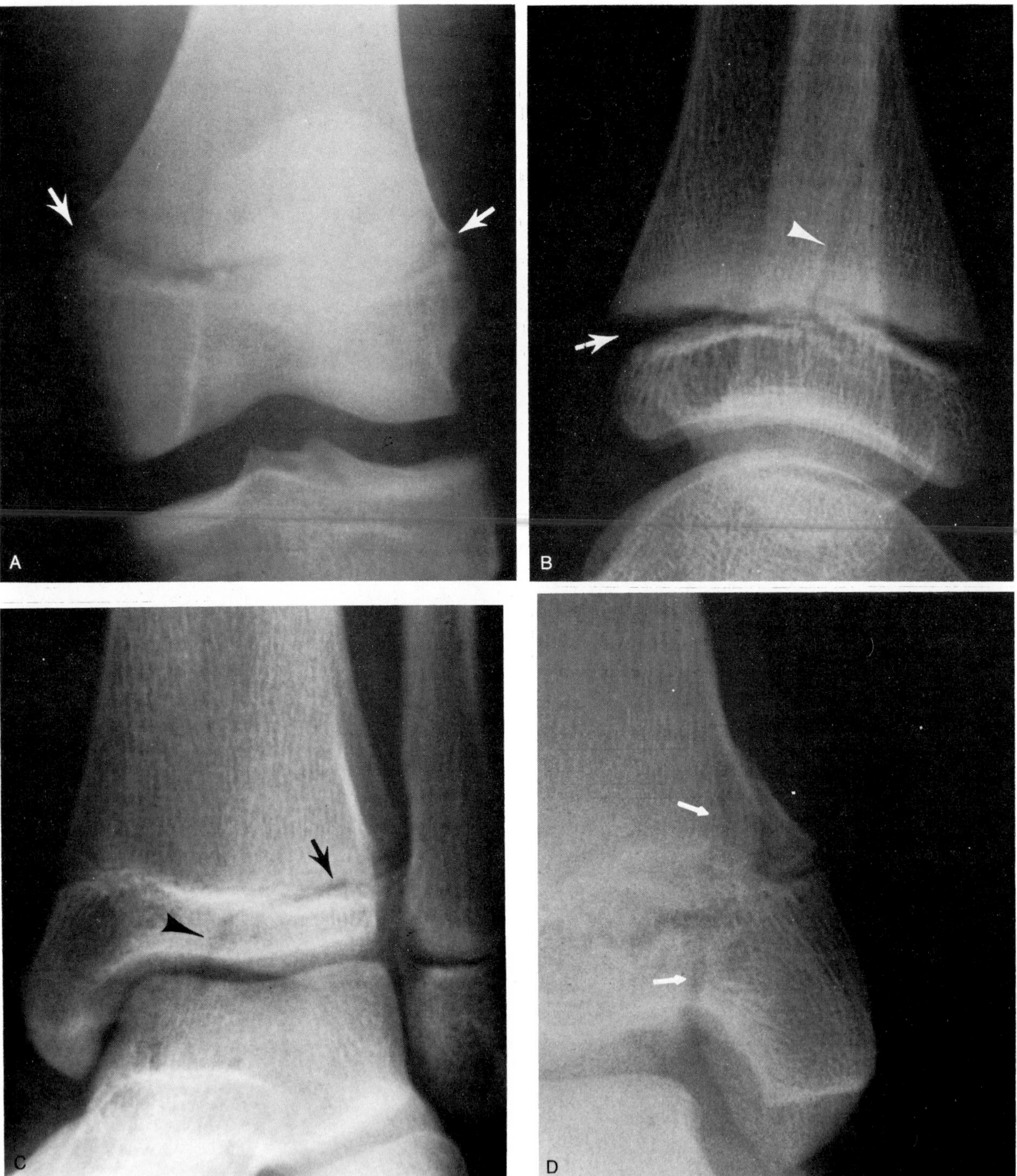

Figure 63–60. *Growth plate injuries: Different types of fractures.*

A *Type I: Note the widening (arrows) of the growth plate of the distal femur.*

B *Type II: Observe the widening of the growth plate (arrow) and the metaphyseal fracture (arrowhead).*

C *Type III: The epiphyseal fracture line (arrowhead) and growth plate violation (arrow) can be recognized.*

D *Type IV: Observe the fracture line extending vertically through the epiphysis and metaphysis (arrows).*

splitting force can produce a fracture that extends across the epiphysis, the growth plate, and the metaphysis, producing a fragment that consists of a portion of both the epiphysis and the metaphysis (Fig. 63–60*D*). This injury is most frequently encountered in the distal humerus and the distal tibia. The radiographic diagnosis is facilitated by the presence of considerable metaphyseal and epiphyseal bone within the fragment; however, in younger children in whom the epiphysis is unossified or only partially ossified, the injury may be mistaken for a Type II growth plate fracture. This is an important distinction, as the prognosis in Type II and Type IV injuries is different. The former injury is easily reduced and is associated with a good prognosis, whereas the latter injury may require open reduction and careful realignment so that growth arrest and joint deformity are not encountered at a later date.

Type V (1 per cent). A crushing or compressive injury to the end of a tubular bone can lead to this rare type of growth plate fracture. Injury to the vascular supply in the germinal cells of the plate occurs without any immediate radiographic signs; there is no irregularity or widening of the growth plate. Subsequent roentgenographic examination may indicate focal areas of diminished or absent bony growth, which, in the presence of normal development in adjacent areas, can lead to angular deformity. Premature osseous fusion of the injured portion of the plate may be identified. This injury is more prominent in older children and adolescents, particularly those between the ages of 12 and 16 years. The distal femoral and distal tibial physes are more typically affected.

Ozonoff[402] has emphasized two additional types of injury to the growth plate or neighboring bone, or both.

Type VI. An injury to the perichondrium can produce reactive bone formation external to the growth plate. The resultant osseous bridge may act as a barrier to growth of the adjacent portion of the plate so that progressive osseous angulation may appear. This rare injury may follow a glancing blow or burn.

Type VII. This relatively common type of injury is associated with epiphyseal alterations in the absence of involvement of the growth plate or metaphysis. Transchondral fractures (osteochondritis dissecans) are examples of Type VII injuries. The fragment may be purely cartilaginous in nature or may consist of both cartilage and bone. Complications include irregularity of the articular surface with secondary degenerative joint disease, and intra-articular osteocartilaginous bodies.

Approximately 25 to 30 per cent of patients with growth plate injuries develop some degree of growth deformity, and in 10 per cent of individuals, this deformity is quite significant.[402] The prognosis is related to the age of the patient, the anatomy of the vascular supply to the region, the type of injury, and the immediacy and adequacy of the reduction. In general, the younger the patient at the time of injury, the poorer the prognosis for residual deformity. Types I, II, and III injuries have a relatively good prognosis, whereas Type IV injuries carry a guarded prognosis, and Types V and VI injuries, a poor prognosis. Late sequelae include growth impairment, premature growth plate fusion, epiphyseal malposition and rotation, and osteonecrosis.[402]

Specific Injuries

SLIPPED CAPITAL FEMORAL EPIPHYSIS. Slippage of the capital femoral epiphysis is a well-recognized occurrence in children and adolescents. It is most typically observed between the ages of 10 and 17 years in boys and 8 and 15 years in girls, with the average age of onset being 13 or 14 years in boys and 11 or 12 years in girls.[413-419] Rarely, a slipped epiphysis occurs in a younger child or neonate who has had severe trauma[420-423, 566] or another disorder such as malnutrition, congenital dislocation of the hip, or tuberculosis,[417, 424] and in an older adolescent or adult with delayed skeletal maturation.[415, 416, 424-426] Boys are more frequently affected than girls, although the ratio of male to female cases varies from one series to another. The incidence of slipped capital femoral epiphysis is greater in black patients than in whites,[424, 427, 428] and is especially high in overweight children.[417, 418] The occurrence of slipped capital femoral epiphysis in tall, thin children is unusual. The left side is affected almost twice as frequently as the right side in male patients, whereas among female patients, both hips are affected with equal frequency. About 20 to 25 per cent of patients with slipped capital femoral epiphysis have bilateral involvement,[416, 417] an occurrence that is more frequent in girls.

A variety of contributing factors have been emphasized in the pathogenesis of slipped capital femoral epiphysis.

1. *Trauma.* Although trauma is an important precipitating event in slipped epiphyses in infants and young children, it appears to have only a minor contributing role in older individuals. Less than 50 per cent of patients have a history of significant injury.

2. *Adolescent Growth Spurt.* The association of slipped capital femoral epiphysis with the adolescent growth spurt is well recognized. Experimental observations in animals have indicated that a minimal amount of shearing stress is necessary to displace the epiphysis when the growth plate is relatively wide, as during periods of rapid growth.[429] The vulnerability of the growth plate during this period is further accentuated by its change in configuration from a horizontal to an oblique plane, increasing the shearing stresses.[417] A higher incidence of this disorder in boys than in girls may be related

to a greater and longer growth spurt in the former.[430]

3. *Hormonal Influences.* The relationship of slipped capital femoral epiphysis to periods of rapid growth has led to speculation regarding the influence of various hormones in the pathogenesis of this condition.[417, 592] Experimental observations have indicated that a deficit of sex hormones relative to growth hormone can produce a widening of the growth plate and a reduction of the shearing force necessary to displace the epiphysis[429, 431, 567]; a delay in skeletal maturation, which is associated with a higher incidence of slipped capital femoral epiphysis, may accentuate this imbalance between growth and sex hormonal levels by lengthening the period of vulnerability because of the late closure of the growth plate. Despite these observations, however, there is no clear evidence that levels of growth hormone are abnormal in patients with slipped capital femoral epiphysis.

4. *Weight and Activity*: One of the most striking characteristics of patients with this condition is a tendency to be overweight. Obesity increases the shearing stress on the growth plate and can lead to slippage even during usual activity. The propensity for epiphyseal slippage appears to be greater in physically active adolescents than in those who are less active, probably related to their exposure to greater shearing forces during strenuous activity.[432]

The stresses about the hip that are most likely to produce growth plate shear are those of abduction and external rotation.[402] With the exception of the adductor group, the musculature about this articulation inserts laterally into the region below the greater trochanter and thus pulls the femoral shaft laterally and anteriorly in external rotation. The femoral head seated in the acetabulum is located in a posterior and medial direction with respect to the remainder of the femur. Although a posteromedioinferior "slippage" of the capital femoral epiphysis is typical,[433] other directions in which the epiphysis can "move" are anteriorly[434] and superiorly or valgus.[435, 436] Histologic studies following slippage have indicated a fracture or cleft through the hypertrophic cells of the growth plate, widening of the growth plate, formation of cartilage clusters and bars divided by longitudinally arranged eosinophilic septae, and islands of unorganized cartilage dispersed irregularly in the proximal metaphysis.[437-439] Mickelson and co-workers[439] observed a change in composition of cartilage matrix in the distal region of the growth plate that might predispose that region to slippage.

The radiographic analysis is essential to the diagnosis of slipped capital femoral epiphysis.[402, 440-443] Both anteroposterior and "frog-leg" or lateral projections are mandatory; abnormalities on the frontal projection alone may be quite subtle, even in the presence of significant epiphyseal displacement. Comparison roentgenograms of the opposite side

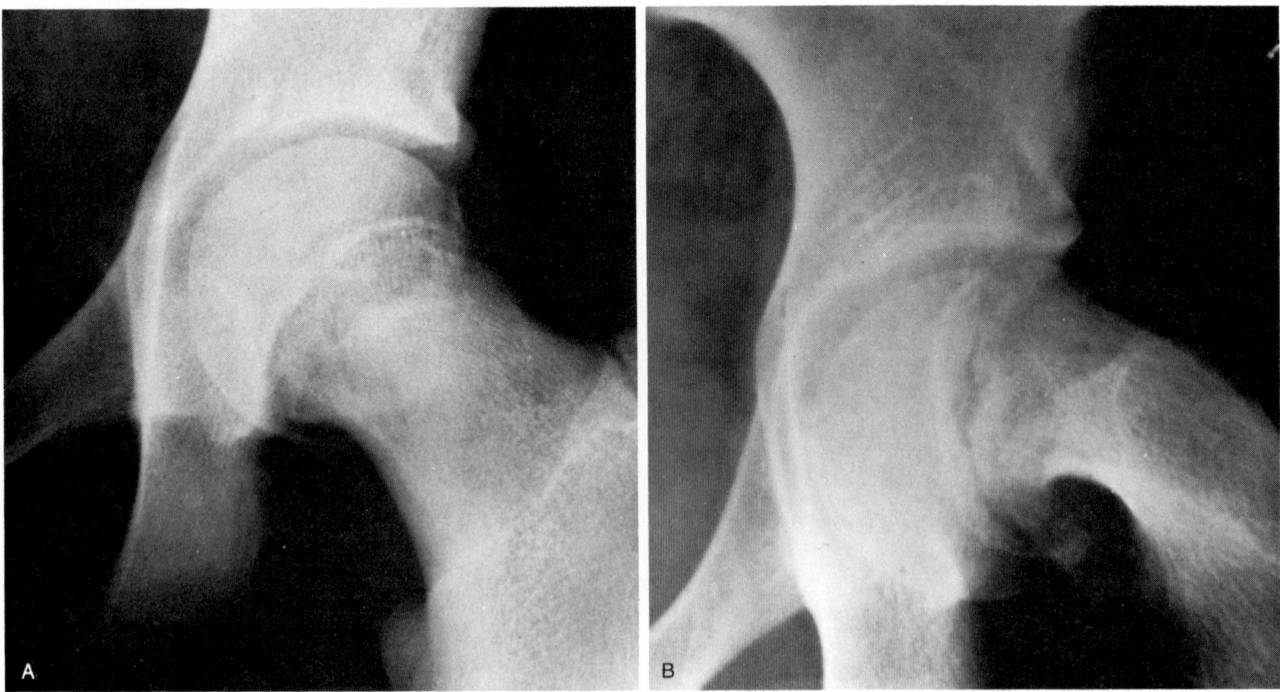

Figure 63–61. *Slipped capital femoral epiphysis: Radiographic abnormalities.*

A *Anteroposterior view. Subtle findings include mild osteoporosis of the proximal femur and an indistinct metaphyseal margin.*

B *"Frog-leg" view. The degree of posterior slippage is readily apparent. Note the widened growth plate.*

can be very useful. In acute or subacute stages of this disorder, several roentgenographic signs may be apparent. On the anteroposterior view, osteoporosis of both the femoral head and neck is common (Fig. 63–61*A*). The margin of the metaphysis may appear blurred or indistinct, and the growth plate may appear increased in width. The epiphyseal height is frequently reduced. A tangential line along the lateral border of the femoral neck may fail to intersect any of the epiphysis or may cross only a small portion of it. The metaphysis may appear to be displaced from the acetabulum so that no overlap exists between the medial third of the metaphysis and the posterior margin of the acetabulum.[444] On the lateral or "frog-leg" view, the degree of epiphyseal displacement is usually quite easy to ascertain (Fig. 63–61*B*). The anterior or posterior margins of the epiphysis and metaphysis fail to correspond to each other.[402] The degree of slippage can be estimated by dividing the amount of displacement by the total width of the metaphysis.

In chronic stages of slipped capital femoral epiphysis, reactive bone formation appears along the medial and posterior portions of the femoral neck, a "buttressing" phenomenon that is similar to that which occurs in degenerative joint disease.[402] Premature fusion of the growth plate may result in femoral shortening.

Sequelae of slipped capital femoral epiphysis include severe varus deformity, shortening and broadening of the femoral neck, osteonecrosis, chondrolysis, and degenerative joint disease. Osteonecrosis has been described in 6 to 15 per cent of patients with this disorder[402, 445-448] (Fig. 63–62*A*). This complication results from an insult to the precarious blood supply to the proximal femur and is accentuated after acute severe slippage, closed or delayed manipulation, open reduction, and a femoral neck osteotomy. Clinical findings include persistent or exacerbated pain after treatment of the slippage. Chondrolysis may be observed in as many as 40 per cent of patients with epiphyseal slippage, is more frequent in black than in white patients and in individuals with severe slippage, usually occurs within one year of the slippage, may be evident in untreated or treated individuals, and may appear in

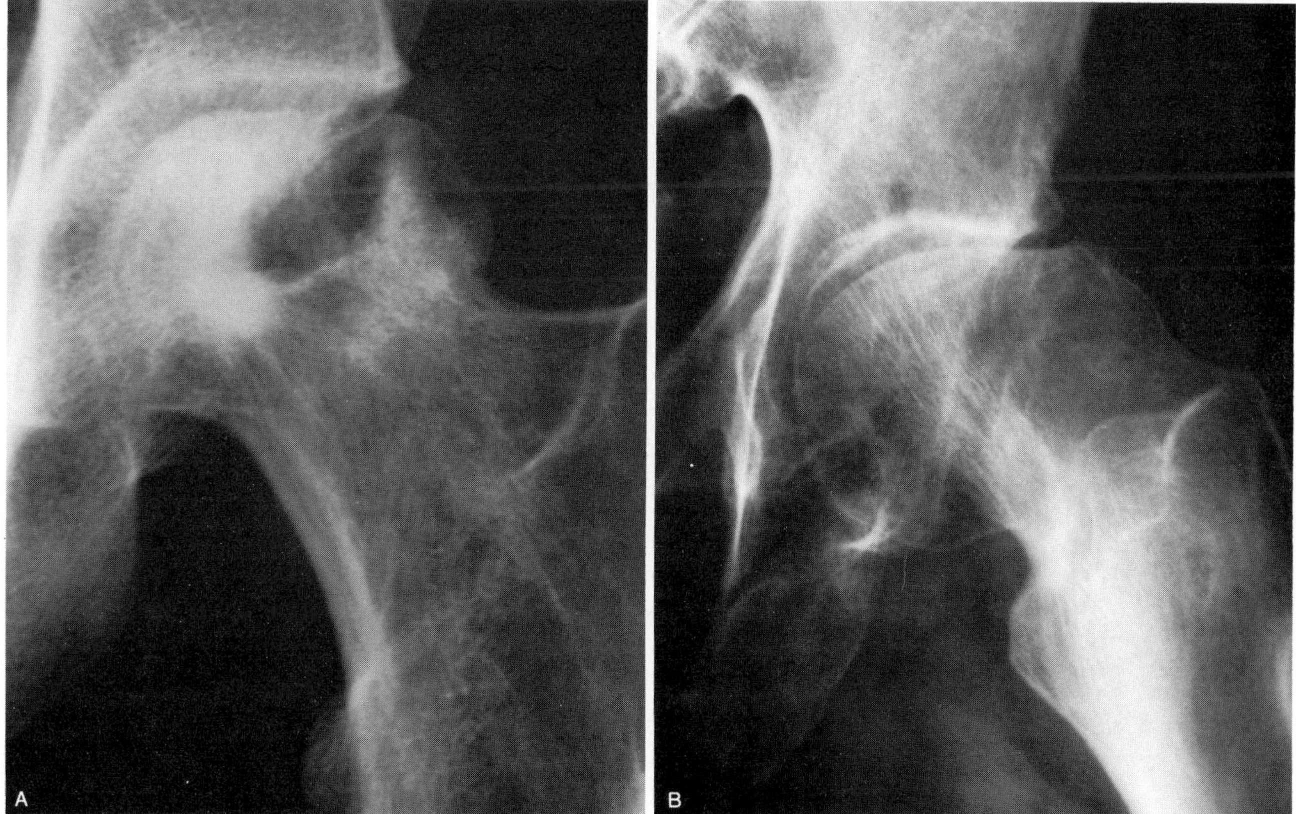

Figure 63–62. *Slipped capital femoral epiphysis: Sequelae.*

A *Osteonecrosis. Note the collapsed and fragmented epiphysis with irregular articular margin. Buttressing of the femoral neck is prominent.*

B *Degenerative joint disease. Observe the malalignment of the femoral head and neck indicating the presence of a previous epiphysiolysis. The joint space is narrowed superiorly, and buttressing of the medial portion of the femoral neck is observed. The absence of a curvilinear radiodense line on the medial aspect of the femoral head distinguishes this appearance from that seen in the "tilt deformity" of osteoarthritis.*

conjunction with osteonecrosis[402, 449-452] (see Chapter 82). Radiographs outline osteoporosis, concentric narrowing of the interosseous space, and eburnation and osteophytosis of apposing osseous margins. Some recovery in the joint space may be seen after a period of months in approximately one third of individuals.[449, 453] Degenerative joint disease following a slipped capital femoral epiphysis can produce a narrowed interosseous space associated with typical displacement of the femoral head (Fig. 63–62*B*). This appearance should not be confused with the "tilt deformity" of the femoral head that is common in patients with osteoarthritis who have not had a previous epiphysiolysis (see chapter 39).

GROWTH PLATE INJURIES ABOUT THE KNEE. Growth plate trauma in the distal femur may be related, in many cases, to birth, athletic, or automobile injury[454-458] (Fig. 63–60*A*). Examples include the "wagon-wheel" fracture resulting when children catch their legs between the spokes of wagon or bicycle wheels[456] and the "clipping injury" of adolescent football players.[458] Type II and Type III Salter-Harris injuries are especially common. The prognosis is guarded in many instances because of the possible sequelae of shortening and angulation.

Injury to the proximal tibial physis is relatively rare,[459, 460, 528] as the collateral ligaments attach distal to the growth plate, the medial on the tibial shaft and the lateral on the fibula.[401] Any type of Salter-Harris injury can be encountered, and stress roentgenograms are frequently required for accurate diagnosis.[460]

GROWTH PLATE INJURIES ABOUT THE ELBOW. The accurate diagnosis of elbow injury in the immature skeleton is complicated by the presence of multiple ossification centers.[229, 402] Although comparison views of the opposite elbow may be helpful, there is some degree of asymmetry that can occur in the normal individual. Thus, it is necessary to know the time and the pattern of ossification of the various epiphyseal centers (Fig. 63–63). At birth, the entire distal humerus is cartilaginous, and there are no centers of ossification. The first distal humeral ossification center to appear is the capitulum, which ossifies during the first year of life. The medial epicondyle appears at approximately 5 to 7 years of age, followed by the trochlea at ages 9 to 10 years and, finally, by the lateral epicondyle at ages 9 to 13 years.[292] These centers fuse with the shaft between the ages of 14 and 16 years, except for the medial epicondyle, which may not fuse until 18 or 19 years of age. The ossification center of the radial head appears at ages 3 to 6 years, and the olecranon center of the ulna appears at ages 6 to 10 years. An acronym that may be utilized as an aid in remembering the sequence of appearance of some of these ossification centers is CRIT: C—capitulum, R—radial head, I—internal or medial epicondyle, T—trochlea.[461]

Normally, the distal humeral metaphysis and capitulum are anteverted about 140 degrees relative to the shaft of the humerus. A line that is drawn along the anterior cortex of the humerus on the lateral radiograph, the anterior humeral line, should intersect the middle third of the capitellar ossification center.[462] In the presence of supracondylar fractures of the humerus, the most common fracture of the elbow in children, posterior displacement or angulation of the distal fragment will allow the anterior humeral line to pass anterior to the capitulum.

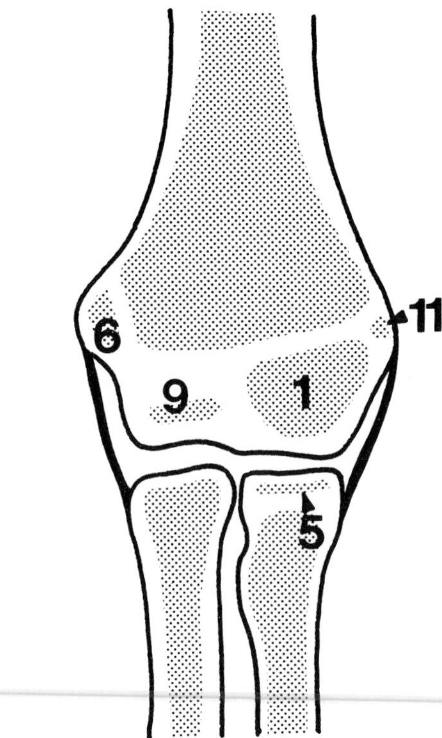

Figure 63–63. *Normal pattern of ossification about the elbow. Numbers indicate approximate age in years at which the center ossifies (see text).*

Many types of epiphyseal injuries affect the child's elbow.[590] A fracture of the lateral condyle is frequent and represents a Salter-Harris Type IV injury. The fracture line splits the epiphysis and separates a portion of the adjacent metaphysis and the capitulum. Because the extensors of the forearm are attached to the fragment, it is commonly displaced posteriorly and inferiorly by muscle traction.[229] Separation of the medial epicondyle ossification center is the result of stress placed on the flexor pronator tendon that attaches to this site. It represents approximately 10 percent of all elbow injuries and leads to a transverse fracture or inferior displacement of the epicondyle.[463] In some instances, the epicondyle may become entrapped within the joint[570] (Fig. 63–64). In this situation, the displaced epicondylar ossification center can simulate a normal trochlear center, and the diagnosis may be missed; however, the appearance of a "trochlear" center without a medial epicondylar center is inconsistent with the normal sequence of ossification about the distal humerus, a fact that facilitates proper diagnosis of the injury in some

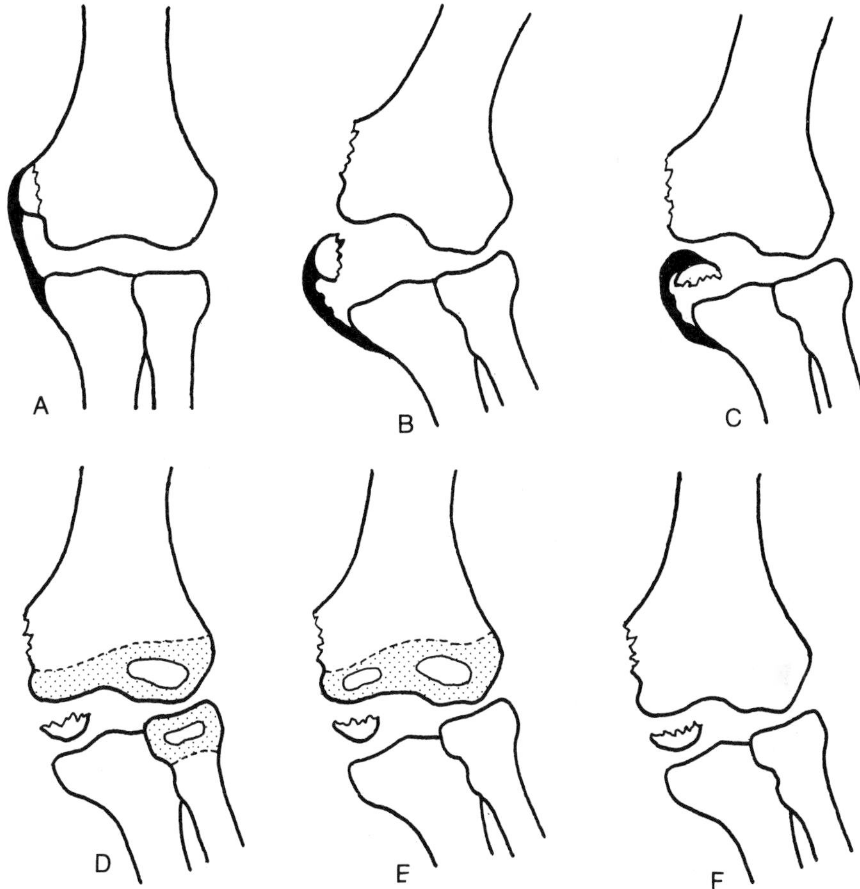

Figure 63–64. *Injuries of the medial epicondyle of the humerus.*

A *The initial site of fracture is indicated.*

B, C *Following a valgus stress with temporary opening of the medial aspect of the elbow joint, the epicondyle is avulsed, and it may be drawn into the joint by traction from its attached flexor pronator muscle group and the ulnar collateral ligament. When the force is relieved, the joint closes, entrapping the medial epicondyle.*

D–F *The radiographic appearance depends upon the age of the patient at which the injury occurs. When entrapment takes place before ossification of the trochlear center* **(D)**, *the entrapped medial epicondyle may be mistaken for a "normal" trochlea. If the entrapment occurs at a slightly older age* **(E)**, *the medial epicondyle is usually visualized between the trochlea and the coronoid process of the ulna in the anteroposterior projection. If it lies slightly posterior to the trochlea, identification may be possible only on the lateral view. In the older adolescent* **(F)**, *the entrapped epicondyle is located between the coronoid process of the ulna and the site of fusion between the trochlea and distal humeral metaphysis.*

(From Chessare JW, et al: Am J Roentgenol 129:49, 1977. Copyright 1977, American Roentgen Ray Society.)

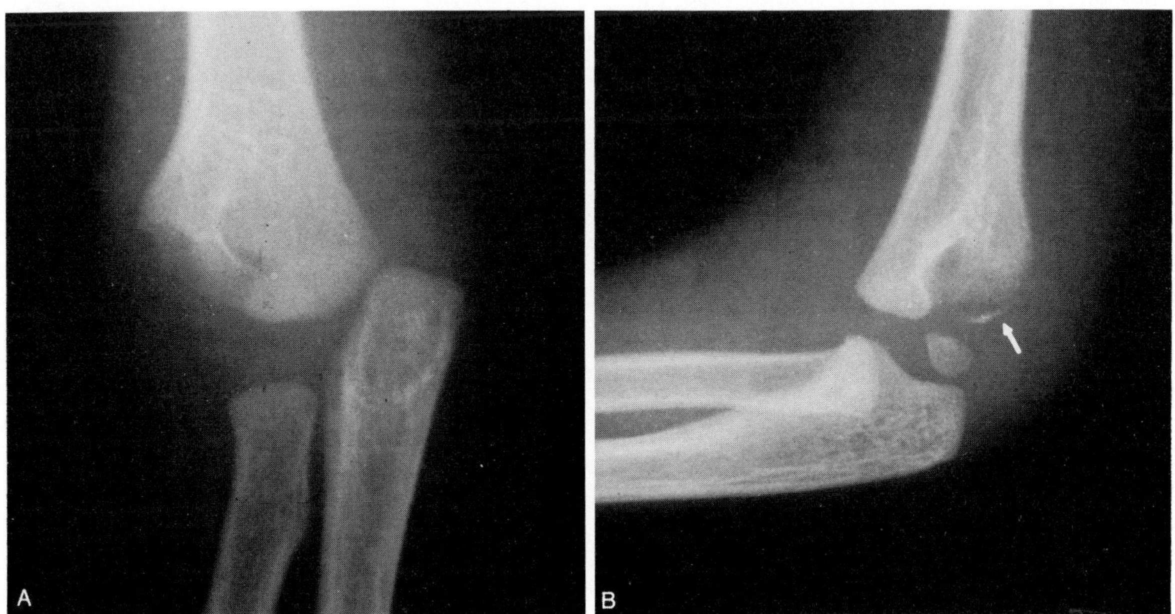

Figure 63–65. *Growth plate injury of the distal humerus. Although the anteroposterior radiograph* **(A)** *appears to delineate a dislocation of the elbow with medial displacement of the ulna and the radius, the lateral radiograph* **(B)** *identifies the metaphyseal ossific flake (arrow) and the normal alignment of the radius and capitulum, indicating that a separation of the distal humeral growth plate has occurred.*

patients. The posterior location of the ossific focus on the lateral projection of the elbow is another useful sign.

Separation with or without fracture of the entire distal humeral epiphysis may be mistaken for a fracture of the lateral humeral condyle or a dislocation of the elbow[464, 568, 569] (Fig. 63–65).

OTHER GROWTH PLATE INJURIES. Similar injuries may appear about the wrist, shoulder, ankle, hands, and feet, and even the bones of the axial skeleton.[465-470] These have been well summarized by Rogers.[401]

TRAUMA TO SUPPORTING STRUCTURES, SYNDESMOSES, AND ENTHESES

Tendon and Ligament Injury and Healing

In an intact musculotendinous system, complete with its bony attachment, the muscle belly itself is the weakest point; in a tendon-bone preparation, the bone-tendon junction is the weakest point.[7, 471] The ultimate strength of such a system is dependent upon many factors, including the rate of loading. Tendons derive their nutrition from a mesotenon that brings a vascular network in an arcade comparable to that in the mesentery of the gut.[7] A tendon deprived of blood supply degenerates and dies. Following injury, tendon healing is related to fibroblastic infiltration from surrounding soft tissues.[472, 473] Proliferating connective tissue penetrates between the ends of sutured tendons and deposits collagen fibers that reveal progressive orientation, finally forming tendon fibers identical to those in normal tendons.[7, 571] An effective healing process requires close approximation of the ends of the divided tendon; complete tendon ruptures leading to separation of tendon ends will not heal unless they are closely applied to each other so that collagenous tissue from the periphery can proliferate and penetrate the injured areas. Similarly, healing of ligaments is encouraged by direct apposition of the divided surfaces; collagenation about closely applied or sutured pieces of ligament can result in repair and restoration of a relatively normal ligamentous apparatus.[474, 475]

Tendon tears or ruptures can appear at virtually any site in the body. Typical examples are injuries of the tendons in the hands and feet and of the patellar, triceps, peroneal, quadriceps, rotator cuff, and Achilles tendons[476-479, 529] (Fig. 63–66). In most cases, significant trauma initiates the tendon injury, although spontaneous ruptures have been documented,[572] especially in patients with rheumatoid arthritis and systemic lupus erythematosus and in those receiving local corticosteroid injection (see Chapters 26, 27, 33, and 66). Radiographic diagnosis of a purely soft tissue injury can be difficult, although soft tissue swelling, changes in tendon contour, and bony displacement may be detected. Additional diagnostic modalities such as xeroradiography, low KV radiography, and arthrography can be helpful (see Chapters 10, 11, and 15).

Ligament tears or ruptures are also widely distributed and are particularly noteworthy about the wrist, ankle, elbow, and knee.[480-482, 573, 574] In these cases, plain film radiography may require supplementation with stress radiography and arthrography. Stress roentgenograms are especially helpful in the investigation of ligamentous injuries of the knee[483-487] and the ankle[488-490]; application of force during radiography can outline displacement or tilting of the apposing articular surfaces. Difficulty in interpretation of stress radiographs relates to incomplete or inappropriate force application and to mild displacement that may occur in normal individuals. Arthrography, as in the ankle, the knee, and the articulations of the hand (e.g., the first metacarpophalangeal joint), following ligamentous injury may indicate abnormal leakage or extravasation of contrast media. Similarly,

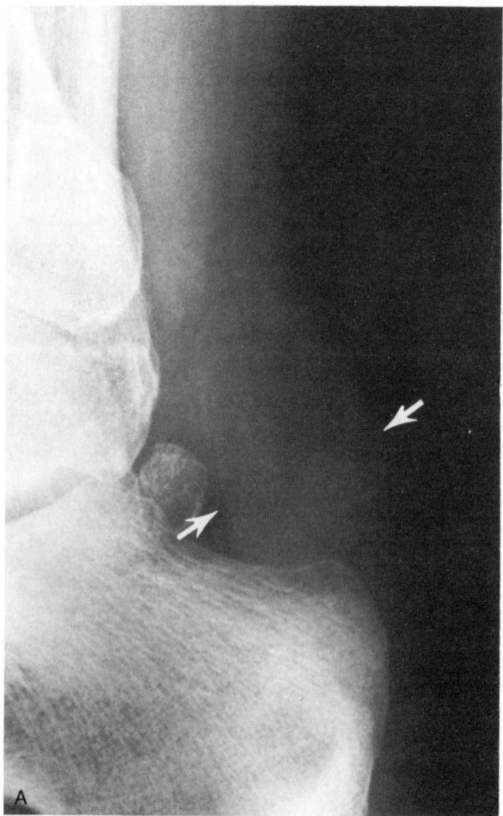

Figure 63–66. *Tendon and ligament injuries.*

A *Achilles tendon rupture. Observe the soft tissue swelling (arrows) and indistinctness of the tendon outline. The pre-achilles fat pad has been obscured.*

Illustration continued on the opposite page

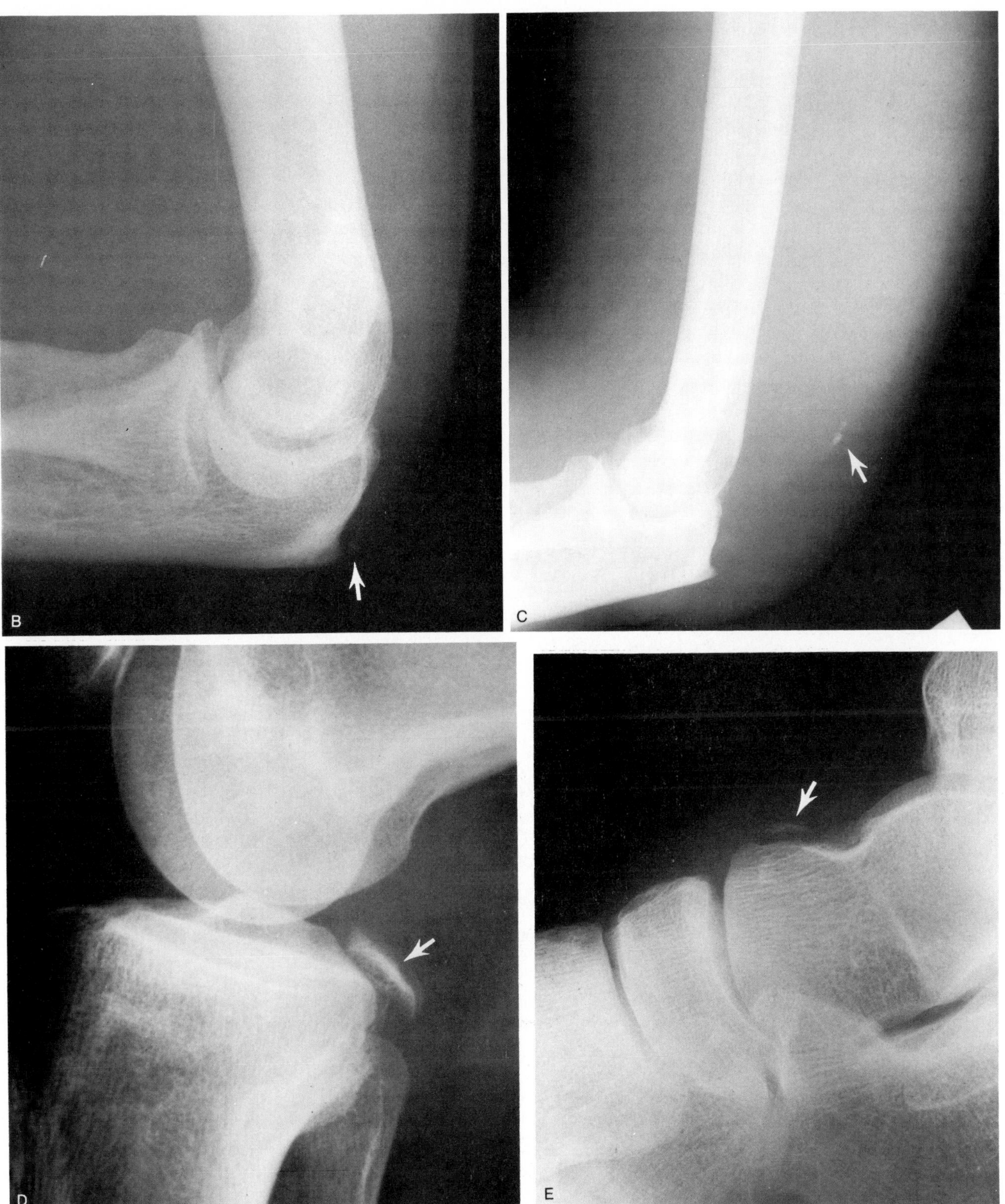

Figure 63–66. Continued

B, C *Triceps tendon avulsion. The initial radiograph* **(B),** *obtained prior to trauma, indicates a small outgrowth (arrow) at the site of attachment of the tendon to the ulnar olecranon. Following injury* **(C),** *note massive soft tissue swelling and avulsion of the fragment (arrow).*

D *Cruciate ligament avulsion. Observe the posterior bony fragment (arrow), resulting from an old posterior cruciate injury.*

E *Talonavicular ligament avulsion. Observe the small osseous dense area (arrow).*

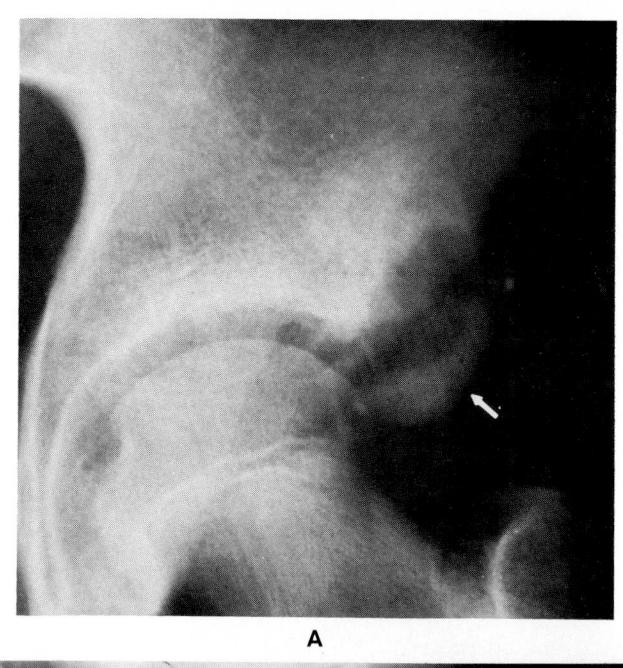

A

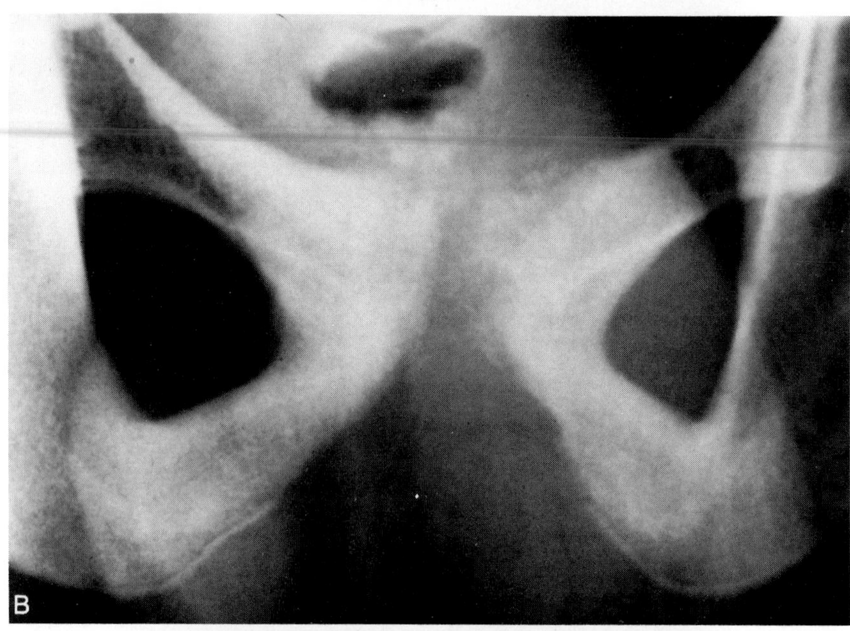

B

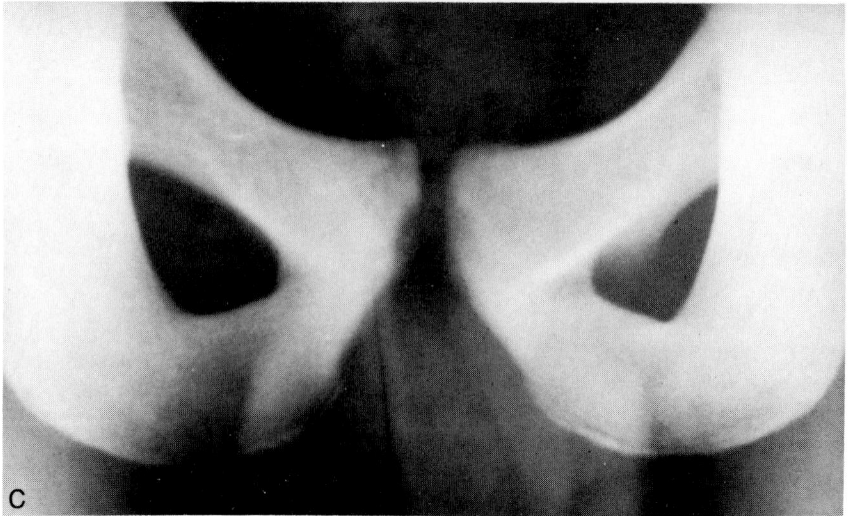

C

Figure 63–67. *See legend on opposite page*

contrast opacification of tendon sheaths (tenography) or tendons themselves (tendinography) may reveal abnormal patterns in patients with tendon or ligament tears.[575]

Avulsion Injuries

Abnormal stress on ligaments and tendons may lead to characteristic avulsions at their site of attachment to bone. For example, avulsion of a portion of the calcaneus, the patella, or the ulnar olecranon may accompany exaggerated pull of the Achilles, quadriceps, or triceps tendon, respectively (Fig. 63–66). Avulsion may also accompany cruciate ligament injuries and spinal trauma (e.g., clay shoveler's fracture of the spinous processes of the lower cervical and upper thoracic vertebrae.)[530] Cartilaginous or cartilaginous and bony fragments may be avulsed. The size of the avulsed fragment is quite variable; in the adult, only small osseous flecks may be pulled from the parent bone, whereas in the child or adoles-

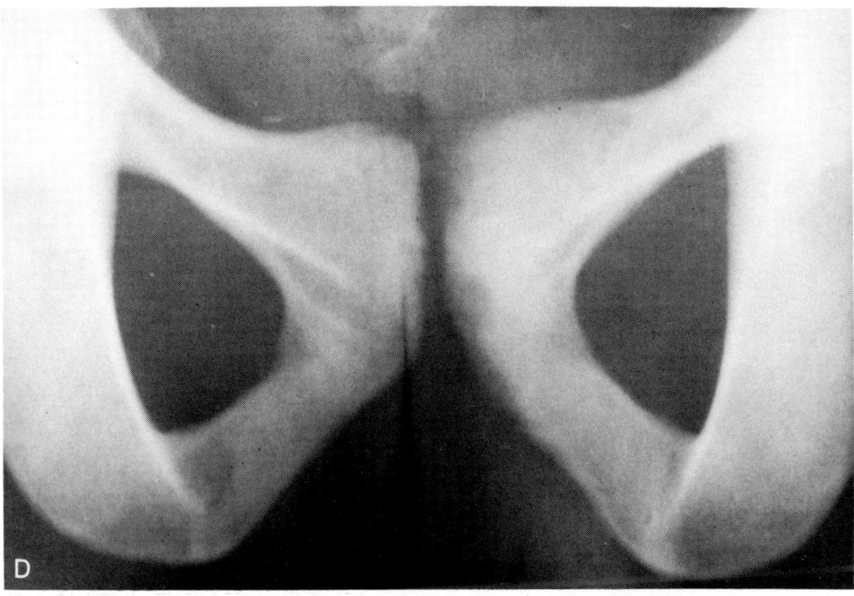

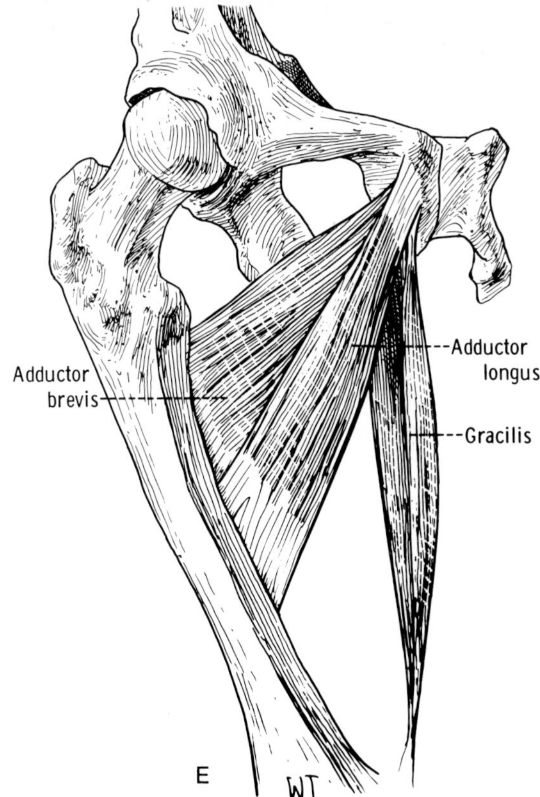

Figure 63–67. *Avulsion injuries of the pelvis.*

A *Anterior inferior iliac spine. The avulsed fragment (arrow) is related to stress at the origin of the rectus femoris muscle.*

B–E *Symphysis pubis and inferior pubic ramus. Examples of the type of osseous irregularity that may result from avulsion injuries due to stress in the adductor brevis, adductor longus, and gracilis muscles.*

*(**B–E**, From Schneider R, et al: Radiology 120:567, 1976.)*

cent, an entire apophysis may undergo avulsion. The degree of displacement of the fragment is also variable.

There are several avulsion injuries about the pelvis and the hips in young athletes that have characteristic radiographic features.[491] These include (a) avulsion injuries of the anterior superior iliac spine, which occur in sprinters as the result of stress at the origin of the tensor fasciae femoris or the sartorius muscle; (b) avulsion injuries of the anterior inferior iliac spine and of a groove just above the superior aspect of the acetabular rim, which relate to stress at the origins of the straight and reflected heads of the rectus femoris (Fig. 63–67*A*); (c) avulsion injuries of the apophysis of the lesser trochanter due to stress of the psoas major during strenuous hip flexion; (d) avulsion injuries of the apophysis of the ischial tuberosity due to violent contraction of the hamstring muscles, often occurring in hurdlers; (e) avulsion injuries of the greater trochanter of the femur produced by gluteal muscle contraction; (f) avulsion of the apophysis of the iliac crest due to severe contraction of the abdominal muscles associated with abrupt directional change during running; and (g) avulsion injuries near the symphysis pubis related to adductor muscle (adductor longus, adductor brevis, gracilis) insertion sites[491-495] (Fig. 63–67*B* to *E*). Clinical findings accompanying these avulsion injuries include local pain, tenderness, and swelling. Radiographs reveal irregularity at the site of avulsion and displaced pieces of bone of variable size. Follow-up roentgenograms may reveal considerable new bone formation or healing with incorporation of the fragment into the parent bone, which, in some cases, is associated with bizarre skeletal overgrowth or deformity simulating neoplasm.

Rotator Cuff Tear

The rotator cuff, composed of the teres minor, infraspinatus, supraspinatus, and subscapularis muscles, is a common site of abnormality. Acute or chronic tears of this structure may be encountered[496-498] (Fig. 63–68). Traumatically induced tears can be associated with pain and full passive range of motion. The presence of inflammation or degeneration of the cuff accentuates its vulnerability to rupture. The torn tendon retracts and becomes ineffective in its normal action as an antagonist to the upward pull of the deltoid muscle. This loss of function in combination with a decrease in the soft tissue mass between humerus and acromion allows the humeral head to become juxtaposed to the undersurface of the acromion process. This superior displacement, however, is not constant, so that it is important to recognize additional radiographic manifestations that accompany rotator cuff injuries.[496, 499, 500] The incidence of these manifestations is greater in cases of chronic rotator cuff tears than in acute injury (Fig. 63–69).

1. *Narrowing of the acromiohumeral head space.* This interosseous space may measure less than the lower limit of normal, 0.7 cm.[499, 501] The narrowing should be evident in both internal and external rotation roentgenograms, as some diminution of the humeroacromial space can be seen in external rotation projections in normal individuals.

2. *Reversal of the normal inferior acromial convexity.* Elevation of the humeral head leads to closer apposition of the humerus and the acromion and repeated traumatic insult to the acromion. Straightening and concavity of the undersurface of the acromion may then become evident. This finding must be evident on both internal rotation and external rotation projections, as a pseudoconcavity can be seen in normal individuals on a single view owing to the anatomic characteristics of the acromion process.

3. *Cystic lesions and sclerosis of the acromion and humeral head.* Small cystic lesions surrounded by a thin rim of sclerosis can be noted along the inferior aspect of the acromion. Similarly, cysts appear within the greater tuberosity in areas of bony sclerosis and contour irregularity. These latter cystic lesions may develop by the process of synovial intrusion in which synovial fluid is forced into the subchondral bone because of repeated stress.[502] The loss of soft tissue and the elevation of the humeral head may allow abutment of the acromion and greater tuberosity in full abduction. Notching of the superior aspect of the humeral neck may also be seen.[500]

Several limitations of these radiographic findings as diagnostic aids in rotator cuff tear must be noted. Acute tears of the rotator cuff in younger patients may be unaccompanied by significant roentgenographic changes; the diagnosis in these individuals is better established by arthrography in which contrast material extends from the glenohumeral joint into the subacromial (subdeltoid) bursa. Second, apparent elevation of the humeral head with "malalignment" of the humerus and glenoid and "narrowing" of the humeroacromial space can be an artifact of the x-ray technique related to incident beam angulation. Third, severe degeneration and atrophy of the rotator cuff without tear can lead to many of the same abnormalities that are noted in association with chronic tears of the rotator cuff. Finally, many of the radiographic changes can also appear in patients with other disorders, particularly those with "frozen" shoulders.

Rotator cuff atrophy and tear can complicate a variety of articular diseases, such as rheumatoid arthritis, ankylosing spondylitis, and septic arthritis. In these processes, synovial inflammation may lead to erosion of the undersurface of the cuff and subsequent disruption. Radiographs reveal the typical roentgenographic signs that are listed above and, additionally, changes of the glenohumeral joint consistent with the underlying disease (e.g., joint space narrowing, osseous erosion). In rotator cuff disrup-

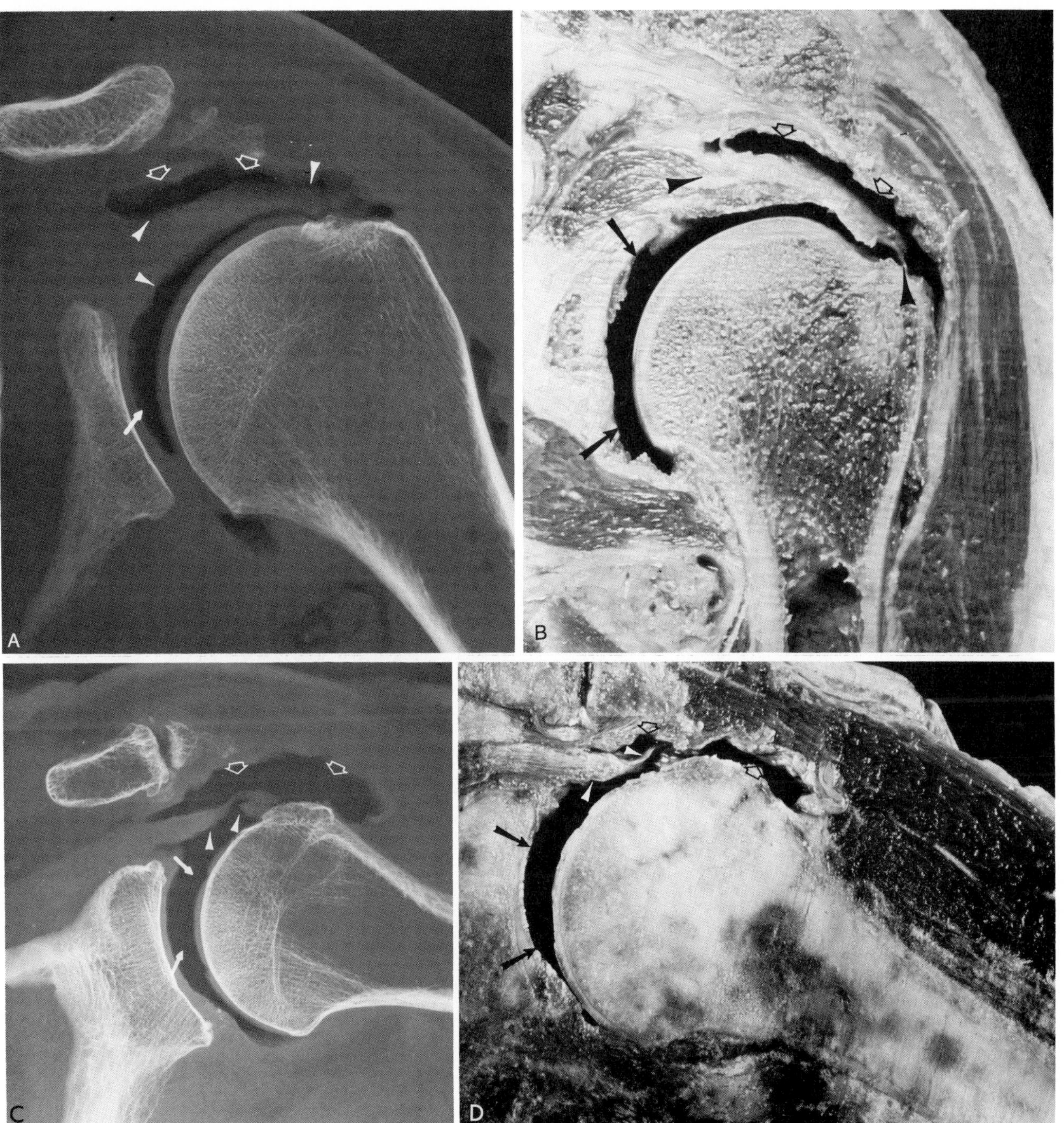

Figure 63–68. *Rotator cuff tears: Radiographic-pathologic correlation. These coronal sections were prepared following air arthrography of the glenohumeral joint in cadavers of elderly persons.*

A, B *On a corresponding sectional radiograph and photograph, note the irregular and torn rotator cuff (arrowheads), allowing communication of the glenohumeral joint (solid arrows) and subacromial (subdeltoid) bursa (open arrows).*

C, D *In a different cadaver, note the irregular rotator cuff (arrowheads) with communication of the glenohumeral joint (solid arrows) and subacromial (subdeltoid) bursa (open arrows). The articular cartilage is eroded.*

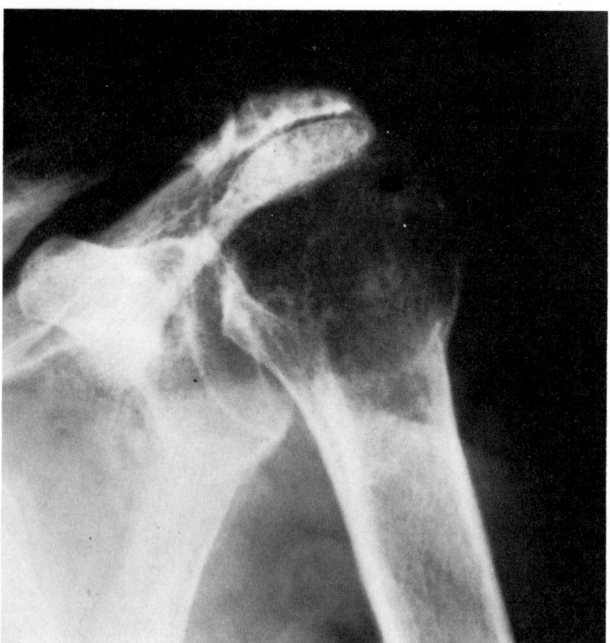

Figure 63–69. Rotator cuff tears: Radiographic abnormalities. This patient with a chronic rotator cuff tear reveals elevation of the humeral head with respect to the glenoid, contact of the humeral head and the acromion, concavity of the inferior surface of the acromion, and sclerosis and cyst formation on apposing surfaces of acromion and humeral head.

tion uncomplicated by the presence of an underlying disorder, the glenohumeral joint may appear surprisingly normal, although secondary degenerative joint disease can develop later.

Diastasis

The term diastasis implies a separation of normally joined bony elements; it is frequently applied to injuries of the ligaments that extend between the lower tibia and the lower fibula.[503] Complete or partial diastasis can appear, depending upon the extent of damage to the tibiofibular and interosseous ligaments. Radiographs may reveal abnormal separation of the tibia and fibula in which the space (la ligne claire) between the medial cortex of the fibula and the posterior edge of the peroneal groove is greater than 5.5 mm in the anteroposterior roentgenogram.[504] Fractures of the neighboring bones may also be evident.

TRAUMATIC ABUSE OF CHILDREN (THE BATTERED CHILD SYNDROME)

A great deal of attention has recently been directed toward the problem of deliberate child abuse.[505-516, 576] It has been estimated that as many as 25,000 incidents are reported each year in the United States.[402] Boys and girls are affected in equal numbers, and most children are younger than 6 years of age, with 25 per cent of the children being under the age of 2 years. Radiographic abnormalities can be detected in 50 to 70 per cent of cases. Although these abnormalities may involve multiple systems in the body, it is the skeletal alterations that have received a great deal of emphasis.

Traumatic insult to the child's skeleton can produce elevation of the periosteal membrane, which is loosely attached to the diaphysis of tubular bones. The vascularity of the osteogenic layer of the periosteum is responsible for the appearance of a subperiosteal hematoma. Although the resultant periostitis is a delayed roentgenographic finding (Fig. 63–70*A*), the firm attachment of the periosteal membrane to the metaphyses of the tubular bones can lead to an immediate radiographic abnormality — single or multiple metaphyseal bone fragments (Fig. 63–70*B*,*C*). Reactive bone formation with sclerosis can be a prominent change associated with periostitis and metaphyseal fracture.

The proper work-up of a child suspected of receiving physical abuse includes a radiographic survey of all of the long bones, the pelvis, the spine, the ribs, and the skull.[402] Scintigraphy with bone-

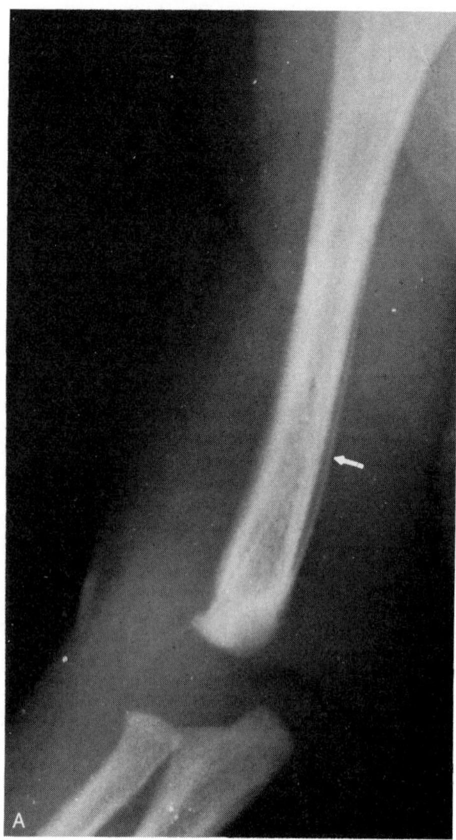

Figure 63–70. Battered child syndrome.

A Periostitis (arrow) is a delayed radiographic sign of trauma.

Illustration continued on the opposite page

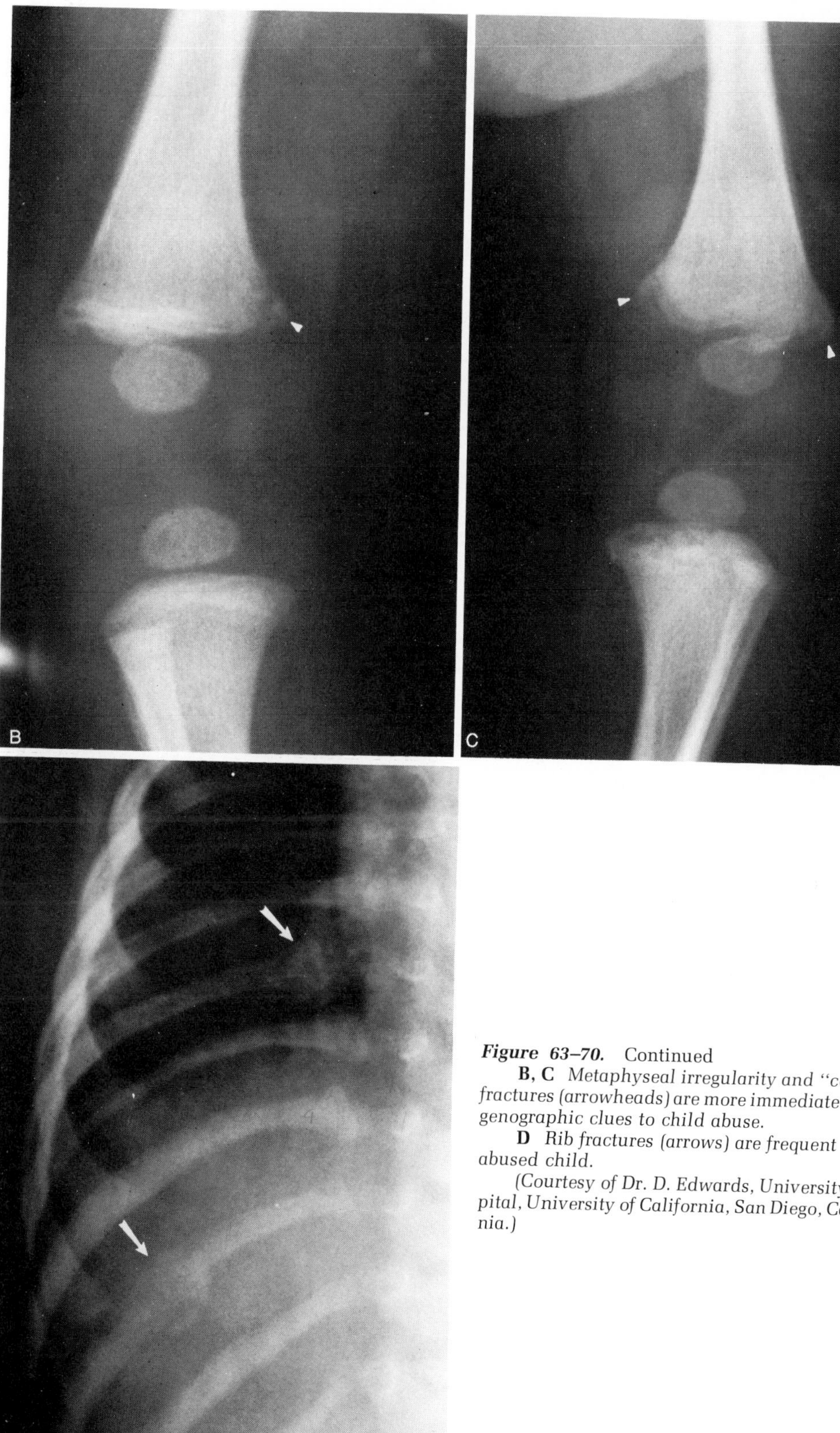

Figure 63–70. Continued

B, C *Metaphyseal irregularity and "corner" fractures (arrowheads) are more immediate roentgenographic clues to child abuse.*

D *Rib fractures (arrows) are frequent in the abused child.*

(Courtesy of Dr. D. Edwards, University Hospital, University of California, San Diego, California.)

seeking pharmaceuticals may also be a useful adjunct to the roentgenographic examination,[517, 518] although false-negative radionuclide studies have been noted.[519] Roentgenographic findings include single or multiple fractures, especially in the ribs (Fig. 63–70*D*), but also involving, in order of descending frequency, the humerus, the femur, the tibia, and the skull. Diaphyseal or metaphyseal fractures can be seen in various stages of healing. The metaphyseal infractions may be quite subtle, requiring multiple projections for adequate visualization. "Unusual" fractures such as those of the sternum, the lateral aspect of the clavicle, the scapula, and the vertebral bodies should arouse suspicion of battering. Injury of the spinal cord may accompany vertebral trauma.

Subperiosteal bone formation may be apparent in a period of 7 to 14 days following the injury. It varies in appearance from focal, thin periosteal deposits to massive bone formation. Periostitis with intramedullary foci of necrosis may also represent the sequela of traumatically induced pancreatitis in the battered child.[508] Late skeletal findings include metaphyseal cupping, growth disturbances, subluxation, and diaphyseal widening due to subperiosteal apposition.

Extraosseous alterations may include cutaneous lesions, malnutrition with decrease in subcutaneous fat, pulmonary contusion and laceration with pneumothorax, gastrointestinal hemorrhage with mass formation and obstruction, pancreatitis, mucosal alterations in the mouth and palate, ocular lesions such as retinal detachment, and intracranial and subdural hematomas.

The accurate diagnosis of the battered child syndrome is facilitated by radiographic changes that include multiple and unusual fractures in different stages of healing, metaphyseal infractions, and subperiosteal hemorrhage with periostitis. Disorders that must be differentiated from this syndrome are the normal periostitis of infancy, osteogenesis imperfecta, congenital insensitivity to pain, and infantile cortical hyperostosis. Metaphyseal avulsion fractures may also accompany abnormal copper metabolism in the kinky hair syndrome (Menkes' syndrome).[520-522] Metaphyseal changes in a variety of other congenital disorders may resemble those in the battered child syndrome.[577]

SUMMARY

In addition to such complications as the reflex sympathetic dystrophy syndrome, osteolysis, osteonecrosis, many of the osteochondroses, neuroarthropathy, heterotopic bone formation, and infection, physical trauma may lead to a variety of radiographic abnormalities. Special types of injuries include pathologic, stress, greenstick, torus, bowing, and transchondral fractures and osseous infractions accompanying subluxations and dislocations. Trauma to synovial joints may lead to synovitis, hemarthrosis, and lipohemarthrosis; trauma to symphyses may result in intraosseous cartilaginous herniations (cartilaginous nodes); trauma to synchondroses may cause variable patterns of growth plate injury; and trauma to supporting structures, syndesmoses, and entheses may lead to tendinous and ligamentous laceration and disruption, avulsion, and diastasis. Characteristic skeletal abnormalities also appear in the abused or battered child.

REFERENCES

1. Resnick D: Skeletal aches and pains. Radiol Clin North Am *16*:37, 1978.
2. Caffey J: Pediatric X-Ray Diagnosis. 5th Ed. Chicago, Year Book Medical Publishers, 1967.
3. Poznanski AK: Practical Approaches to Pediatric Radiology. Chicago, Year Book Medical Publishers, 1976.
4. Rang M: Children's Fractures. Philadelphia, JB Lippincott, 1974.
5. Merten D: Comparison radiographs in extremity injuries of childhood: Current application in radiological practice. Radiology *126*:209, 1978.
6. McCauley RGK, Schwartz AM, Leonidas JC, Darling DB, Bankoff MS, Swan CS II: Comparison views in extremity injury in children: An efficacy study. Radiology *131*:95, 1979.
7. Cruess RL, Dumont J: Healing of bone, tendon and ligament. *In* Rockwood CA Jr, Green DP (Eds.): Fractures. Philadelphia, JB Lippincott, 1975, p 97.
8. Mulholland MC, Pritchard JJ: The fracture gap (Abstr). J Anat *93*:590, 1959.
9. McClements, P, Templeton RW, Pritchard JJ: Repair of a bone gap (Abstr). J Anat *95*:616, 1961.
10. Ham AW: A histological study of the early phases of bone repair. J Bone Joint Surg *12*:827, 1930.
11. Lindholm R, Lindholm S, Liukko P, Paasimaki J, Isokaanta S, Rossi R, Autio E, Tamminen E: The mast cell as a component of callus in healing fractures. J Bone Joint Surg *51B*:148, 1969.
12. McKibbin B: The biology of fracture healing in long bones. J Bone Joint Surg *60B*:150, 1978.
13. Pentecost RL, Murray R, Brindley HH: Fatigue, insufficiency and pathologic fractures. JAMA *187*:1001, 1964.
14. Daffner RH: Stress fractures: Current concepts. Skel Radiol *2*:221, 1978.
15. Roub LW, Gumerman LW, Hanley EN Jr, Clark MW, Goodman M, Herbert DL: Bone stress: A radionuclide imaging perspective. Radiology *132*:431, 1979.
16. Wilson ES Jr, Katz FN: Stress fractures. An analysis of 250 consecutive cases. Radiology *92*:481, 1969.
17. Savoca CJ: Stress fractures. A classification of the earliest radiographic signs. Radiology *100*:519, 1974.
18. Gilbert RS, Johnson HA: Stress fractures in military recruits — review of twelve years' experience. Milit Med *131*:716, 1966.
19. Zatzkin HR: Trauma to the foot. Semin Roentgenol *5*:419, 1970.
20. Protzman RR, Griffis CG: Stress fracture in men and women undergoing military training. J Bone Joint Surg *59A*:825, 1977.

21. Levy JM: Stress fractures of the first metatarsal. Am J Roentgenol *130*:679, 1978.
22. Newberg AH, Kalisher L: Case report: An unusual stress fracture in a jogger. J Trauma *18*:816, 1978.
23. Miller EH, Schneider HJ, Bronson JL, McLain D: A new consideration in athletic injuries. The classical ballet dancer. Clin Orthop Rel Res *111*:181, 1975.
24. Schneider HJ, King AY, Bronson JL, Miller EH: Stress injuries and developmental change of lower extremities in ballet dancers. Radiology *113*:627, 1974.
25. Miller F, Wenger DR: Femoral neck stress fracture in a hyperactive child. A case report. J Bone Joint Surg *61A*:435, 1979.
26. Sandrock AR: Another sports fatigue fracture. Stress fracture of the coracoid process of the scapula. Radiology *117*:274, 1975.
27. Rasad S: Golfer's fractures of the ribs. Report of 3 cases. Am J Roentgenol *120*:901, 1974.
28. Hallel T, Amit S, Segal D: Fatigue fractures of tibial and femoral shaft in soldiers. Clin Orthop Rel Res *118*:35, 1976.
29. Cohen HR, Becker MH, Genieser NB: Fatigue fracture in Hare Krishna converts. New group at risk. NY State J Med *74*:1998, 1974.
30. Provost RA, Morris JM: Fatigue fracture of the femoral shaft. J Bone Joint Surg *51A*:487, 1969.
31. Brower AC, Neff JR, Tillema DA: An unusual scapular stress fracture. Am J Roentgenol *129*:519, 1977.
32. Engber WD: Stress fractures of the medial tibial plateau. J Bone Joint Surg *59A*:767, 1977.
33. Lecestre P, Benoit J, Dabos N, Ramadier JO: Les fractures de fatigue. A propos de 8 cas. Rev Chir Orthop *63*:815, 1977.
34. Young RS, Bryk D, Ratner H: Selective phalangeal tuft fractures in a guitar player. Br J Radiol *50*:147, 1977.
35. Rappoport AS, Sosman JL, Weissman BN: Spontaneous fractures of the olecranon process in rheumatoid arthritis. Radiology *119*:83, 1976.
36. Schneider R, Kaye JJ: Insufficiency and stress fractures of the long bones occurring in patients with rheumatoid arthritis. Radiology *116*:595, 1975.
37. Miller B, Markheim HR, Towbin MN: Multiple stress fractures in rheumatoid arthritis. J Bone Joint Surg *49A*:1408, 1967.
38. Devas M: Stress Fractures. London, Churchill Livingstone, 1975.
39. Milkman LA: Pseudofractures (hunger osteopathy, late rickets, osteomalacia). Report of a case. Am J Roentgenol *24*:29, 1930.
40. Ford LT, Gilula LA: Stress fractures of the middle metatarsals following the Keller operation. J Bone Joint Surg *59A*:117, 1977.
41. Michetti ML: March fracture following a McBride bunionectomy. A case report. J Am Podiatry Assoc *60*:286, 1970.
42. Cummings CW, First R: Stress fracture of the clavicle after a radical neck dissection. Case report. Plast Reconstr Surg *55*:366, 1975.
43. Prather JL, Nusynowitz ML, Snowdy HA, Hughes AD, McCartney WH, Bagg RJ: Scintigraphic findings in stress fractures. J Bone Joint Surg *59A*:869, 1977.
44. Geslien GE, Thrall JH, Espinosa JL, Older RA: Early detection of stress fractures using ^{99m}Tc-polyphosphate. Radiology *121*:683, 1976.
45. Wilcox JR Jr, Moniot AL, Green JP: Bone scanning in the evaluation of exercise-related stress injuries. Radiology *123*:699, 1977.
46. Sweet DE, Allman RM: Stress fracture. RPC of the month from the AFIP. Radiology *99*:687, 1971.
47. Johnson LC: Morphologic analysis in pathology: The kinetics of disease and general biology of bone. *In* Frost HH (Ed): Bone Biodynamics. Henry Ford Hospital International Symposium. Boston, Little, Brown and Co., 1964, p 607.
48. Brooks DB, Burstein AH, Frankel VH: The biomechanics of torsional fractures: The stress concentration of a drill hole. J Bone Joint Surg *52A*:507, 1970.
49. Chamay A: Mechanical and morphological aspects of experimental overload and fatigue in bone. J Biomech *3*:263, 1970.
50. Wright TM, Hayes WC: The fracture mechanics of fatigue crack propagation in compact bone. J Biomed Mater Res *10*:637, 1976.
51. Jones HH, Priest JD, Hayes WC, Tichenor CC, Nagel DD: Humeral hypertrophy in response to exercise. J Bone Joint Surg *59A*:204, 1977.
52. Torg JS, Pollack H, Sweterlitsch P: The effect of competitive pitching on the shoulders and elbows of preadolescent baseball pitchers. Pediatrics *49*:267, 1972.
53. Chamay A, Tschantz P: Mechanical influence in bone remodeling. Experimental research on Wolff's law. J Biomech *5*:173, 1972.
54. Winfield AC, Dennis JM: Stress fractures of the calcaneus. Radiology *72*:415, 1959.
55. Hullinger CW: Insufficiency fracture of the calcaneus similar to march fracture of the metatarsal. J Bone Joint Surg *26*:751, 1944.
56. Stein RE, Stelling FH: Stress fracture of the calcaneus in a child with cerebral palsy. J Bone Joint Surg *59A*:131, 1977.
57. Orava S, Puranen J, Ala-Ketola L: Stress fractures caused by physical exercise. Acta Orthop Scand *49*:19, 1978.
58. Devas M: Stress fractures in children. J Bone Joint Surg *45B*:528, 1963.
59. Singer M, Maudsley RH: Fatigue fractures of the lower tibia: A report of five cases. J Bone Joint Surg *36B*:647, 1954.
60. Pilgaard S, Poulsen JO, Christensen JH: Stress fractures. Acta Orthop Scand *47*:167, 1976.
61. Burrows HJ: Fatigue infraction of the middle of the tibia in ballet dancers. J Bone Joint Surg *38B*:83, 1956.
62. Levin DC, Blazina ME, Levine E: Fatigue fractures of the shaft of the femur: Simulation of malignant tumor. Radiology *89*:883, 1967.
63. Devas MB: Stress fractures of the femoral neck. J Bone Joint Surg *47B*:728, 1965.
64. Haggert GE, Eberle HJ: Bilateral stress fractures of the neck of the femur. A case report. Lahey Clin Bull *10*:15, 1956.
65. Branch HE: March fractures of the femur. J Bone Joint Surg *26*:387, 1944.
66. Wolfgang GL: Stress fracture of the femoral neck in a patient with open capital femoral epiphyses. A case report. J Bone Joint Surg *59A*:680, 1977.
67. Devas MB: Compression stress fractures in man and the greyhound. J Bone Joint Surg *43B*:540, 1961.
68. Delahaye RP, Doury P, Pattin S, Metges PJ, Mine J: Les fractures des métatarsiens. Rev Rhum Mal Osteoartic *43*:707, 1976.
69. Evans DL: Fatigue fracture of the ulna. J Bone Joint Surg *37B*:618, 1955.
70. Stark HH, Jobe FW, Boyes JH, Ashworth CR: Fracture of the hook of the hamate in athletes. J Bone Joint Surg *59A*:575, 1977.
71. Carter PR, Eaton RG, Littler JW: Ununited fracture of the hook of the hamate. J Bone Joint Surg *59A*:583, 1977.
72. Torg JS, Moyer RA: Non-union of a stress fracture through the olecranon epiphyseal plate observed in an adolescent baseball pitcher. J Bone Joint Surg *59A*:264, 1977.
73. Bennett GE: Shoulder and elbow lesions of the professional baseball pitcher. JAMA *117*:510, 1941.
74. Sheikholeslamzadeh S, Aalami-Harandi B, Fateh H: Spondylolisthesis of the cervical spine. Report of a case. J Bone Joint Surg *59B*:95, 1977.
75. Moseley I: Neural arch dysplasia of the sixth cervical vertebra. "Congenital cervical spondylolisthesis." Br J Radiol *49*:81, 1976.
76. Bellamy R, Lieber A, Smith SD: Congenital spondylolisthesis of the sixth cervical vertebra. Case report and description of operative findings. J Bone Joint Surg *56A*:405, 1974.
77. Charlton OP, Gehweiler JA Jr, Martinez S, Morgan CL, Daffner RH: Spondylolysis and spondylolisthesis of the cervical spine. Skel Radiol *3*:79, 1978.
78. Kosnik EJ, Johnson JC, Scoles PV, Rossel CW: Cervical spondylolisthesis. Spine *4*:203, 1979.
79. Eisenstein S: Spondylolysis. A skeletal investigation of two population groups. J Bone Joint Surg *60B*:488, 1978.
80. Willis TA: The separate neural arch. J Bone Joint Surg *13*:709, 1931.
81. Roche MB, Rowe GG: The incidence of separate neural arch and coincidental bone variations. Anat Rec *109*:233, 1951.
82. Hasebe K: Die Wirbelsäule der Japaner. Z Morphol Anthropol *15*:259, 1912.
83. Stewart TD: The age incidence of neural-arch defects in Alaskan natives, considered from the standpoint of etiology. J Bone Joint Surg *35A*:937, 1953.
84. Wiltse LL, Widell EH Jr, Jackson DW: Fatigue fracture: The basic lesion in isthmic spondylolisthesis. J Bone Joint Surg *57A*:17, 1975.
85. Meyerding AW: Low backache and sciatic pain associated with spondylolisthesis and protruded intervertebral disc: Incidence, significance, and treatment. J Bone Joint Surg *23*:461, 1941.
86. Nathan H: Spondylolysis. J Bone Joint Surg *41A*:303, 1959.
87. Batts M Jr: The etiology of spondylolisthesis. J Bone Joint Surg *21*:879, 1939.
88. Wiltse LL: The etiology of spondylolisthesis. J Bone Joint Surg *44A*:539, 1962.
89. Borkow SE, Kleiger B: Spondylolisthesis in the newborn. A case report. Clin Orthop Rel Res *81*:73, 1971.
90. Baker DR, McHollick W: Spondyloschisis and spondylolisthesis in children. J Bone Joint Surg *38A*:933, 1956.
91. Farfan HF, Osteria V, Lamy C: The mechanical etiology of spondylosis and spondylolisthesis. Clin Orthop Rel Res *117*:40, 1976.
92. Hadley LA: Stress fracture with spondylolysis. Am J Roentgenol *90*:1258, 1963.
93. Cyron BM, Hutton WC, Troup JDG: Spondylolytic fracture. J Bone Joint Surg *58B*:462, 1976.
94. Cyron BM, Hutton WC: The fatigue strength of the lumbar neural arch in spondylolysis. J Bone Joint Surg *60B*:234, 1978.
95. Cyron BM, Hutton WC: Variations in the amount and distribution of cortical bone across the partes interarticularis of L5. A predisposing factor in spondylolysis? Spine *4*:163, 1979.

96. Krenz J, Troup JDG: The structure of the pars interarticularis of the lower lumbar vertebrae and its relation to the etiology of spondylolysis, with a report of a healing fracture in the neural arch of a fourth lumbar vertebra. J Bone Joint Surg *55B*:735, 1973.
97. Fullenlove TM, Wilson JG: Traumatic defects of the pars interarticularis of the lumbar vertebrae. Am J Roentgenol *122*:634, 1974.
98. Rowe GG, Roches MB: The etiology of separate neural arch. J Bone Joint Surg *35A*:102, 1953.
99. Pfeil E: Experimentelle Untrsuchungen zur Frage der Entstehung der Spondylolyse. Z Orthop *109*:231, 1971.
100. Lamy C, Eng B, Bazergui A, Kraus H, Farfan HF: The strength of the neural arch and the etiology of spondylolysis. Orthop Clin North Am *6*:215, 1975.
101. Murray RO, Colwill MR: Stress fractures of the pars interarticularis. Proc R Soc Med *61*:555, 1968.
102. Zippel H, Runge H: Pathologische Anatomie und Pathogenese von Spondylolyse und Spondylolisthesis im Kindesalter. Z Orthop *114*:189, 1976.
103. Rabushka SE, Apfelbach H, Love L: Spontaneous healing of spondylolsis of the fifth lumbar vertebra. Case report. Clin Orthop Rel Res *93*:256, 1973.
104. Troup JDG: The etiology of spondylolysis. Orthop Clin North Am *8*:57, 1977.
105. Leger J-L, Bouchard R, Maltais R: Étude radiologique de 305 cas de spondylolyse avec ou sans spondylolisthesis. J Can Assoc Radiol *30*:86, 1979.
106. Epstein BS, Epstein JA, Jones MD: Lumbar spondylolisthesis with isthmic defects. Radiol Clin North Am *15*:261, 1977.
107. Lowe RW, Hayes TD, Kaye J, Bagg RJ, Luekens CA Jr: Standing roentgenograms in spondylolisthesis. Clin Orthop Rel Res *117*:80, 1976.
108. Sherman FC, Wilkinson RH, Hall JE: Reactive sclerosis of a pedicle and spondylolysis in the lumbar spine. J Bone Joint Surg *59A*:49, 1977.
109. Jackson DW, Wiltse LL, Cirincione RJ: Spondylolysis in the female gymnast. Clin Orthop Rel Res *117*:68, 1976.
110. Wiltse LL, Newman PH, Macnab I: Classification of spondylolysis and spondylolisthesis. Clin Orthop Rel Res *117*:23, 1976.
111. Silverman FN: Problems in pediatric fractures. Semin Roentgenol *13*:167, 1978.
112. Naga AH, Broadrick GL: Traumatic bowing of the radius and ulna in children. NC Med J *38*:452, 1977.
113. Crowe JE, Swischuk LE: Acute bowing fractures of the forearm in children: A frequently missed injury. Am J Roentgenol *128*:981, 1977.
114. Rydholm U, Nilsson JE: Traumatic bowing of the forearm. A case report. Clin Orthop Rel Res *139*:121, 1979.
115. Borden S IV: Traumatic bowing of the forearm in children. J Bone Joint Surg *56A*:611, 1974.
116. Borden S IV: Roentgen recognition of acute plastic bowing of the forearm in children. Am J Roentgenol *125*:524, 1975.
117. Manoli A II: Traumatic fibular bowing with tibial fracture: Report of two cases. Orthopedics *1*:145, 1978.
118. Voumard C, Lopez J, Queloz J, Landry M: Les fractures plastiques de l'avant-bras chez l'enfant. Ann Radiol *21*:551, 1978.
119. Cook GC, Bjelland JC: Acute bowing fracture of the fibula in an adult. Radiology *131*:637, 1979.
120. Martin W III, Riddervold HO: Acute plastic bowing fractures of the fibula. Radiology *131*:639, 1979.
121. Cail WS, Keats TE, Sussman MD: Plastic bowing fracture of the femur in a child. Am J Roentgenol *130*:780, 1978.
122. Stenström R, Gripenberg L, Bergius A-R: Traumatic bowing of forearm and lower leg in children. Acta Radiol [Diagn] (Stockh) *19*:243, 1978.
123. Pick M: Familial osteochondritis dissecans. J Bone Joint Surg *37B*:142, 1955.
124. Stougaard J: Familial occurrence of osteochondritis dissecans. J Bone Joint Surg *46B*:542, 1964.
125. Stougaard J: The hereditary factor in osteochondritis dissecans. J Bone Joint Surg *43B*:256, 1961.
126. Hanley W, McKusick VA, Barranco FT: Osteochondritis dissecans with associated malformations in two brothers: A review of familial aspects. J Bone Joint Surg *49A*:925, 1967.
127. Robinson RP, Franck WA, Carey EJ Jr, Goldberg EB: Familial polyarticular osteochondritis dissecans masquerading as juvenile rheumatoid arthritis. J Rheumatol *5*:2, 1978.
128. Milgram JW, Rogers LF, Miller JW: Osteochondral fractures: mechanisms of injury and fate of fragments. Am J Roentgenol *130*:651, 1978.
129. Milgram JW: The classification of loose bodies in human joints. Clin Orthop Rel Res *124*:282, 1977.
130. Milgram JW: The development of loose bodies in human joints. Clin Orthop Rel Res *124*:292, 1977.
131. Aichroth P: Osteochondritis dissecans of the knee. A clinical study. J Bone Joint Surg *53B*:440, 1971.
132. Milgram JW: Radiological and pathological manifestations of osteochondritis dissecans of the distal femur. A study of 50 cases. Radiology *126*:305, 1978.
133. Linden B, Telhag H: Osteochondritis dissecans. A histologic and autoradiograph study in man. Acta Orthop Scand *48*:682, 1977.
134. Lipscomb PR Jr, Lipscomb PR Sr, Bryan RS: Osteochondritis dissecans of the knee with loose fragments. Treatment by replacement and fixation with readily removed pins. J Bone Joint Surg *60A*:235, 1978.
135. Chiroff RT, Cooke CP: Osteochondritis dissecans: A histologic and microradiographic analysis of surgically excised lesions. J Trauma *15*:689, 1975.
136. Linden B: Osteochondritis dissecans of the femoral condyles. A long-term follow-up study. J Bone Joint Surg *59A*:769, 1977.
137. Linden B: The incidence of osteochondritis dissecans in the condyles of the femur. Acta Orthop Scand *47*:664, 1976.
138. Aichroth P: Osteochondral fractures and their relationship to osteochondritis dissecans of the knee. An experimental study in animals. J Bone Joint Surg *53B*:448, 1971.
139. Matthewson MH, Dandy DJ: Osteochondral fractures of the lateral femoral condyle. A result of indirect violence to the knee. J Bone Joint Surg *60B*:199, 1978.
140. Mollan RAB: Osteochondritis dissecans of the knee. A case report of an unusual lesion on the lateral femoral condyle. Acta Orthop Scand *48*:517, 1977.
141. Mansat CH, Mansat M, Duroureau L, Metton G: Ostéochondrite disséquante du genou. Rev Rhum Mal Osteoartic *45*:177, 1978.
142. Mubarak SJ, Carroll NC: Familial osteochondritis dissecans of the knee. Clin Orthop Rel Res *140*:131, 1979.
143. Nagura S: The so-called osteochondritis dissecans of Konig. Clin Orthop Rel Res *18*:100, 1960.
144. Phemister DB: The causes of and changes in loose bodies arising from the articular surface of the joint. J Bone Joint Surg *6*:278, 1924.
145. Fisher AGT: A study of loose bodies composed of cartilage or of cartilage and bone occurring in joints, with special reference to their pathology and etiology. Br J Surg *8*:493, 1921.
146. Fairbank HAT: Osteochondritis dissecans. Br J Surg *21*:67, 1933.
147. Campbell CJ, Ranawat CS: Osteochondritis dissecans: The question of etiology. J Trauma *6*:201, 1966.
148. Rosenberg NJ: Osteochondral fractures of the lateral femoral condyle. J Bone Joint Surg *46A*:1013, 1964.
149. Kennedy JC, Grainger RW, McGraw RW: Osteochondral fractures of the femoral condyles. J Bone Joint Surg *48B*:436, 1966.
150. Dexel M, Doerig M: Osteochondrosis dissecans, 10-und mehrjahresergebnisse. a) Spatresultate nach konservativer und operativer behandlung der Osteochondrosis dissecans ain Kniegelenk. Orthopade *8*:120, 1979.
151. Pantazopoulos T, Exarchou E: Osteochondritis dissecans of the patella. Report of four cases. J Bone Joint Surg *53A*:1205, 1971.
152. Rombold C: Osteochondritis dissecans of the patella. J Bone Joint Surg *18*:230, 1936.
153. Rideout DF, Davis S, Navani SV: Osteochondritis dissecans patellae. Br J Radiol *39*:673, 1966.
154. Kleinberg S: Bilateral osteochondritis dissecans of the patella. J Bone Joint Surg *31A*:185, 1949.
155. Edwards DH, Bentley, G: Osteochondritis dissecans patellae. J Bone Joint Surg *59B*:58, 1977.
156. Smillie IS: Osteochondritis Dissecans. Edinburgh, E & S Livingstone Ltd, 1960.
157. Scapinelli R: Blood supply of the human patella. J Bone Joint Surg *49B*:563, 1967.
158. Haswell DM, Berne AS, Graham CB: The dorsal defect of the patella. Pediatr Radiol *4*:238, 1976.
159. Goergen, TG, Resnick D, Greenway G, Saltzstein SL: Dorsal defect of the patella (DDP): A characteristic radiographic lesion. Radiology *130*:333, 1979.
160. Milgram JE: Tangential osteochondral fracture of the patella. J Bone Joint Surg *25*:271, 1943.
161. Morscher E: Cartilage-bone lesions of the knee joint following injury. Reconstr Surg Traumatol *12*:2, 1971.
162. Ahstrom JP: Osteochondral fracture in the knee joint associated with hypermobility and dislocation of the patella. J Bone Joint Surg *47A*:1491, 1965.
163. Frandsen PA, Kristensen H: Osteochondral fracture associated with dislocation of the patella: Another mechanism of injury. J Trauma *19*:195, 1979.
164. McDougall A, Brown JD: Radiological sign of recurrent dislocation of the patella. J Bone Joint Surg *50B*:841, 1968.
165. Berndt AL, Harty M: Transchondral fracture (osteochondritis dissecans) of the talus. J Bone Joint Surg *41A*:988, 1959.
166. Smith GR, Winquist RA, Allan TNK, Northrop CH: Subtle transchondral fractures of the talar dome: A radiological perspective. Radiology *124*:667, 1977.

167. Scharling M: Osteochondritis dissecans of the talus. Acta Orthop Scand *49*:89, 1978.
168. Yvars MF: Osteochondral fractures of the dome of the talus. Clin Orthop Rel Res *114*:185, 1976.
169. Newberg AH: Osteochondral fractures of the dome of the talus. Br J Radiol *52*:105, 1979.
170. DeGinder WL: Osteochondritis dissecans of the talus. Radiology *65*:590, 1955.
171. Roden S, Tillegard P, Unander-Scharin, L: Osteochondritis dissecans and similar lesions of the talus. Report of fifty-five cases with special reference to etiology and treatment. Acta Orthop Scand *23*:51, 1953.
172. Roberts N, Hughes R: Osteochondritis dissecans of the elbow joint: A clinical study. J Bone Joint Surg *32B*:348, 1950.
173. Woodward AH, Bianco AJ Jr: Osteochondritis dissecans of the elbow. Clin Orthop Rel Res *110*:35, 1975.
174. Lerner HH, Watkins MB, Resnick B: Osteochondritis dissecans of the supratrochlear septum of the humerus. Am J Roentgenol *55*:717, 1946.
175. Martel W, Abell MR: Case report 46. Skel Radiol *2*:173, 1978.
176. Meves H, Schneider-Sickert F: Gibt es eine Osteochondrosis dissecans am Kahnbein der Hand? Z Orthop *113*:424, 1975.
177. Perkins G: The ruminations of an orthopaedic surgeon. London, Butterworths, 1970.
178. Saha AK: Dynamic stability of the glenohumeral joint. Acta Orthop Scand *42*:491, 1971.
179. Joessel D: Ueber die recidive der humerusluxationen. Dtsch Z Chir *13*:167, 1880.
180. Hill HA, Sachs MD: The grooved defect of the humeral head. A frequently unrecognized complication of dislocations of the shoulder joint. Radiology *35*:690, 1940.
181. Hermodsson I: Röntgenologische studien über die traumatischen und habituellen Schultergelenkverrenkungen nach vorn und nach unten. Acta Radiol (Suppl) *20*:1, 1934.
182. Symeonides PP: The significance of the subscapularis muscle in the pathogenesis of recurrent anterior dislocation of the shoulder. J Bone Joint Surg *54B*:476, 1972.
183. Eyre-Brook AL: Recurrent dislocation of the shoulder. Physiotherapy *57*:7, 1971.
184. Rowe CR: Prognosis in dislocations of the shoulder. J Bone Joint Surg *38A*:957, 1956.
185. Brav EA: Recurrent dislocation of the shoulder. Ten years' experience with Putti-Platt reconstruction procedure. Am J Surg *100*:423, 1960.
186. Palmar I, Widen A: The bone-block method for recurrent dislocation of the shoulder joint. J Bone Joint Surg *30B*:53, 1948.
187. Adams JC: Recurrent dislocations of the shoulder. J Bone Joint Surg *30B*:26, 1948.
188. Hall RH, Isaac F, Booth CR: Dislocations of the shoulder with special reference to accompanying small fractures. J Bone Joint Surg *41A*:489, 1959.
189. Bankart ASB: Recurrent or habitual dislocation of the shoulder joint. Br Med J *2*:1132, 1923.
190. Pavlov H, Freiberger RH: Fractures and dislocations about the shoulder. Semin Roentgenol *13*:85, 1978.
191. Aston JW Jr, Gregory CF: Dislocation of the shoulder with significant fracture of the glenoid. J Bone Joint Surg *55A*:1531, 1973.
192. Hill NA, McLaughlin HL: Locked posterior dislocation simulating a "frozen shoulder." J Trauma *3*:225, 1963.
193. McLaughlin HL: Posterior dislocation of the shoulder. J Bone Joint Surg *34A*:584, 1952.
194. Dimon JH III: Posterior dislocation and posterior fracture-dislocation of the shoulder. A report of 25 cases. South Med J *60*:661, 1967.
195. Bloom MH, Obata WG: Diagnosis of posterior dislocation of the shoulder with use of Velpeau axillary and angle-up roentgenographic views. J Bone Joint Surg *49A*:943, 1967.
196. Arndt JH, Sears AD: Posterior dislocation of the shoulder. Am J Roentgenol *94*:639, 1965.
197. Cisternino SJ, Rogers LF, Stufflebam BC, Kruglik GD: The trough line: A radiographic sign of posterior shoulder dislocation. Am J Roentgenol *130*:951, 1978.
198. Bernageau J, Patte D: Diagnostic radiologique des luxations postérieures de l'épaule. Rev Chir Orthop *65*:101, 1979.
199. Slikva J, Resnick D: An improved radiographic view of the glenohumeral joint. J Can Assoc Radiol *30*:83, 1979.
200. Shaw JL: Bilateral posterior fracture-dislocation of the shoulder and other trauma caused by convulsive seizures. J Bone Joint Surg *53A*:1437, 1971.
201. Lynn FS: Erect dislocation of the shoulder. Surg Gynecol Obstet *39*:51, 1921.
202. Laskin RS, Sedlin ED: Luxatio erecta in infancy. Clin Orthop Rel Res *80*:126, 1971.
203. Rowe CR, Pierce DS, Clark JG: Voluntary dislocation of the shoulder. J Bone Joint Surg *55A*:445, 1973.
204. Braunstein EM, Martel W: Voluntary glenohumeral dislocation. Am J Roentgenol *129*:911, 1977.
205. Howorth MB: Generalized relaxation of the ligaments. Clin Orthop Rel Res *30*:133, 1963.
206. Cotton F: Subluxation of the shoulder downward. Boston Med Surg J *185*:405, 1921.
207. Hammond R: Relaxation of the shoulder following bone injury. J Bone Joint Surg *5*:712, 1923.
208. Laskin RS, Schreiber S: Inferior subluxation of the humeral head: The drooping shoulder. Radiology *98*:585, 1971.
209. Uhrist MR: Complete dislocations of the acromioclavicular joint. The nature of the traumatic lesion and effective methods of treatment with an analysis of 41 cases. J Bone Joint Surg *28*:813, 1946.
210. Powers JA, Bach PJ: Acromioclavicular separations. Closed or open treatment? Clin Orthop Rel Res *104*:213, 1974.
211. Weaver JK, Dunn HK: Treatment of acromioclavicular injuries, especially complete acromioclavicular separation. J Bone Joint Surg *54A*:1187, 1972.
212. Allman FL Jr: Fractures and ligamentous injuries of the clavicle and its articulation. J Bone Joint Surg *49A*:774, 1967.
213. Zlotsky NA, Ballard A: Acromioclavicular injuries in athletes. J Bone Joint Surg *48A*:1224, 1966.
214. Montgomery SP, Loyd RD: Avulsion fracture of the coracoid epiphysis with acromioclavicular separation. Report of two cases in adolescents and review of the literature. J Bone Joint Surg *59A*:963, 1977.
215. Protass JJ, Stampfli FV, Osmer JC: Coracoid process fracture diagnosis in acromioclavicular separation. Radiology *116*:61, 1975.
216. Smith DM: Coracoid fracture associated with acromioclavicular dislocation. A case report. Clin Orthop Rel Res *108*:165, 1975.
217. Zanca P: Shoulder pain: Involvement of the acromioclavicular joint. Analysis of 1000 cases. Am J Roentgenol *112*:493, 1971.
218. Bearden JM, Hughston JC, Whatley GS: Acromioclavicular dislocation: Method of treatment. J Sports Med Phys Fitness *1*:5, 1973.
219. Millbourn E: On injuries to the acromioclavicular joint. Treatment and results. Acta Orthop Scand *19*:349, 1950.
220. Arner O, Sandahl U, Ohrling H: Dislocation of the acromioclavicular joint — review of the literature and report of 56 cases. Acta Chir Scand *113*:140, 1957.
221. Nettles JL, Linscheid R: Sternoclavicular dislocations. J Trauma *8*:158, 1968.
222. Tyer HDD, Sturrock WDS, Callow FM: Retrosternal dislocation of the clavicle. J Bone Joint Surg *45B*:132, 1963.
223. Newlin NS: Congenital retrosternal subluxation of the clavicle simulating an intrathoracic mass. Am J Roentgenol *130*:1184, 1978.
224. Sadr B, Swann M: Spontaneous dislocation of the sternoclavicular joint. Acta Orthop Scand *50*:269, 1979.
225. Levinsohn EM, Bunnell WP, Yuan HA: Computed tomography in the diagnosis of dislocations of the sternoclavicular joint. Clin Orthop Rel Res *140*:12, 1979.
226. Lee FA, Gwinn JL: Retrosternal dislocation of the clavicle. Radiology *110*:631, 1974.
227. McKenzie JM: Retrosternal dislocation of the clavicle: A report of two cases. J Bone Joint Surg *45B*:138, 1963.
228. Brooks AL, Henning GD: Injury to the proximal clavicular epiphysis. J Bone Joint Surg *54A*:1347, 1972.
229. Rogers LF: Fractures and dislocations of the elbow. Semin Roentgenol *13*:97, 1978.
230. Kini MG: Dislocation of the elbow and its complications. J Bone Joint Surg *22*:107, 1940.
231. Linscheid RL, Wheeler DK: Elbow dislocations. JAMA *194*:1171, 1965.
232. Matev I: A radiological sign of entrapment of the median nerve in the elbow joint after posterior dislocation. A report of two cases. J Bone Joint Surg *58B*:353, 1976.
233. Exarchou EJ: Lateral dislocation of the elbow. Acta Orthop Scand *48*:161, 1977.
234. Cohn I: Fractures of the elbow. Am J Surg *55*:210, 1942.
235. Symeonides PP, Paschaloglou C, Stavrou Z, Pangalides TH: Recurrent dislocation of the elbow. Report of three cases. J Bone Joint Surg *57A*:1084, 1975.
236. Caravias D: Some observations on congenital dislocation of the head of the radius. J Bone Joint Surg *39B*:86, 1957.
237. White J: Congenital dislocation of the head of the radius. Br J Surg *30*:377, 1942.
238. Elliott KA, Elliott GB, Kindrachuk WH: The radial subluxation-fingernail defect-absent patella syndrome. Am J Roentgenol *87*:1067, 1962.
239. Wiley JJ, Pegington J, Horwich JP: Traumatic dislocation of the radius at the elbow. J Bone Joint Surg *56B*:501, 1974.
240. Bruce HE, Harvey JP Jr, Wilson JC Jr: Monteggia fractures. J Bone Joint Surg *56A*:1563, 1974.

241. Peiro A, Andres F, Fernandez-Esteve F: Acute Monteggia lesions in children. J Bone Joint Surg *59A*:92, 1977.
242. Giustra PE, Killoran PJ, Furman RS, Root JA: The missed Monteggia fracture. Radiology *110*:45, 1974.
243. Bado JL: The Monteggia Lesion. Springfield, Illinois, Charles C Thomas, 1962.
244. Storen G: Traumatic dislocation of the radial head as an isolated lesion in children: Report of one case with special regard to roentgen diagnosis. Acta Chir Scand *116*:144, 1959.
245. Rogers LF, Rockwood CA Jr: Separation of the entire distal humeral epiphysis. Radiology *106*:393, 1973.
246. Mizuno, K, Hirohata K, Kashiwagi D: Fracture-separation of the distal humeral epiphysis in young children. J Bone Joint Surg *61A*:570, 1979.
247. Loomis LK: Reduction and after-treatment of posterior dislocation of the elbow. Am J Surg *63*:56, 1944.
248. Thompson HC III, Garcia A: Myositis ossificans (aftermath of elbow injuries). Clin Orthop Rel Res *50*:129, 1967.
249. Kerin R: Elbow dislocation and its association with vascular disruption. J Bone Joint Surg *51A*:756, 1969.
250. Hughston JC: Fracture of the distal radial shaft. Mistakes in management. J Bone Joint Surg *39A*:249, 1957.
251. Heiple KG, Freehafer AA, Van't Hof A: Isolated traumatic dislocation of the distal end of the ulna or distal radio-ulnar joint. J Bone Joint Surg *44A*:1387, 1962.
252. Snook GA, Chrisman D, Wilson TC, Wietsma RD: Subluxation of the distal radio-ulnar joint by hyperpronation. J Bone Joint Surg *51A*:1315, 1969.
253. Wong PCN: Galeazzi fracture-dislocations in Singapore 1960–1964. Incidence and results of treatment. Singapore Med J *8*:186, 1967.
254. Reckling FW, Cordell LD: Unstable fracture-dislocations of the forearm. The Monteggia and Galeazzi lesions. Arch Surg *96*:999, 1968.
255. Mikic ZD: Galeazzi fracture-dislocations. J Bone Joint Surg *57A*:1071, 1975.
256. Rienau G, Gay R, Martinez C, Mansat C, Mansat M: Lesions de l'articulation radio-cubitale inférieure dans les traumatismes de l'avant-bras et du poignet. Intérêt de l'arthrographie. Rev Chir Orthop *57*(Suppl 1):253, 1971.
257. Resnick D: Arthrography in the evaluation of arthritic disorders of the wrist. Radiology *113*:331–340, 1974.
258. Linscheid RL, Dobyns JH, Beabout JW, Bryan RS: Traumatic instability of the wrist. Diagnosis, classification, and pathomechanics. J Bone Joint Surg *54A*:1612, 1972.
259. Gilula LA, Weeks PM: Post-traumatic ligamentous instabilities of the wrist. Radiology *129*:641, 1978.
260. Gilula LA: Carpal injuries: Analytic approach and case exercises. Am J Roentgenol *133*:503, 1979.
261. Meyrueis JP, Cameli M, Jan P: Instabilité du carpe. Diagnostic et formes cliniques. Ann Chir *32*:555, 1978.
262. Sebald JR, Dobyns JH, Linscheid RL: The natural history of collapse deformities of the wrist. Clin Orthop Rel Res *104*:140, 1974.
263. Resnick D, Niwayama G: Carpal instability in rheumatoid arthritis and calcium pyrophosphate deposition disease. Pathogenesis and roentgen appearance. Ann Rheum Dis *36*:311–318, 1977.
264. Hudson TM, Caragol WJ, Kaye JJ: Isolated rotatory subluxation of the carpal navicular. Am J Roentgenol *126*:601, 1976.
265. Boyes JG: Subluxation of the carpal navicular bone. South Med J *69*:141, 1976.
266. Frankel VH: The Terry-Thomas sign. Letter to Editor. Clin Orthop Rel Res *129*:321, 1977.
267. Howard FM, Fahey T, Wojcik E; Rotatory subluxation of the navicular. Clin Orthop Rel Res *104*:134, 1974.
268. Crittenden JJ, Jones DM, Santarelli AG: Bilateral rotational dislocation of the carpal navicular. Case report. Radiology *94*:629, 1970.
269. Pournaras J, Kappas A: Volar perilunar dislocation. A case report. J Bone Joint Surg *61A*:625, 1979.
270. Stein F, Siegel MW: Naviculocapitate fracture syndrome. A case report — new thoughts on the mechanism of injury. J Bone Joint Surg *51A*:391, 1969.
271. MacAusland WR: Perilunar dislocation of the carpal bones and dislocation of the lunate bone. Surg Gynecol Obstet *79*:256, 1944.
272. Dunn AW: Fractures and dislocations of the carpus. Surg Clin North Am *52*:1513, 1972.
273. Kaplan EB: Dorsal dislocation of the metacarpophalangeal joint of the index finger. J Bone Joint Surg *39A*:1081, 1957.
274. Sweterlitsch PR, Torg JS, Pollack H: Entrapment of a sesamoid in the index metacarpophalangeal joint: Report of two cases. J Bone Joint Surg *51A*:995, 1969.
275. Moberg E: Fractures and ligamentous injuries of the thumb and fingers. Surg Clin North Am *40*:297, 1960.
276. Nance EP Jr, Kaye JJ, Milek MA: Volar plate fractures. Radiology *133*:61, 1979.
277. Green DP, O'Brien ET: Fractures of the thumb metacarpal. South Med J *65*:807, 1972.
278. Griffiths JC: Fractures at the base of the first metacarpal bone. J Bone Joint Surg *46B*:712, 1964.
279. Neviaser RJ, Wilson JN, Lievano A: Rupture of the ulnar collateral ligament of the thumb (gamekeeper's thumb). Correction by dynamic repair. J Bone Joint Surg *53A*:1357, 1971.
280. Coonrad RW, Goldner JL: A study of the pathological findings and treatment in soft-tissue injury of the thumb metacarpophalangeal joint with a clinical study of the normal range of motion in one thousand thumbs and a study of post mortem findings of ligamentous structures in relation to function. J Bone Joint Surg *50A*:439, 1968.
281. Campbell CS: Gamekeeper's thumb. J Bone Joint Surg *37B*:148, 1955.
282. Stener B: Displacement of the ruptured ulnar collateral ligament of the metacarpophalangeal joint of the thumb. A clinical and anatomical study. J Bone Joint Surg *44B*:869, 1962.
283. Sakellarides HT, DeWeese JW: Instability of the metacarpophalangeal joint of the thumb. Reconstruction of the collateral ligaments using the extensor pollicis brevis tendon. J Bone Joint Surg *58A*:106, 1976.
284. Schultz RJ, Fox JM: Gamekeeper's thumb: Result of skiing injuries. NY State J Med *73*:2329, 1973.
285. Linscheid RL: Arthrography of the metacarpophalangeal joint. Clin Orthop Rel Res *103*:91, 1974.
286. Resnick D, Danzig LA: Arthrographic evaluation of injuries of the first metacarpophalangeal joint: Gamekeeper's thumb. Am J Roentgenol *126*:1046, 1976.
287. Epstein HC: Traumatic dislocations of the hip. Clin Orthop Rel Res *92*:116, 1973.
288. Scham SM, Fry LR: Traumatic anterior dislocation of the hip with fracture of the femoral head. Clin Orthop Rel Res *62*:133, 1969.
289. Dall D, Macnab I, Gross A: Recurrent anterior dislocation of the hip. J Bone Joint Surg *52A*:574, 1970.
290. Haddad RJ Jr, Drez D: Voluntary recurrent anterior dislocation of the hip. A case report. J Bone Joint Surg *56A*:419, 1974.
291. Larson CB: Fracture dislocations of the hip. Clin Orthop Rel Res *92*:147, 1973.
292. Whitehouse GH: Radiological aspects of posterior dislocation of the hip. Clin Radiol *29*:431, 1978.
293. Canale ST, Manugian AH: Irreducible traumatic dislocations of the hip. J Bone Joint Surg *61A*:7, 1979.
294. Epstein HC: Posterior fracture-dislocations of the hip; long-term follow-up. J Bone Joint Surg *56A*:1103, 1974.
295. Smith GR, Loop JW: Radiologic classification of posterior dislocations of the hip: Refinement and pitfalls. Radiology *119*:569, 1976.
296. Armbuster TG, Guerra, J, Resnick D, Goergen TG, Feingold ML, Niwayama G, Danzig LA: The adult hip: An anatomic study. Part I. The bony landmarks. Radiology *128*:1–10, 1978.
297. Quackenbush D, DiDonato R, Butler D: A modified lateral projection for anterior and posterior lips of the acetabulum. Radiology *125*:536, 1977.
298. Judet R, Judet J, Letournel E: Fracture of the acetabulum: Classification and surgical approaches for open reduction. J Bone Joint Surg *46A*:1615, 1964.
299. Proctor H: Dislocations of the hip joint (excluding "central" dislocation) and their complications. Injury *5*:1, 1973.
300. Paterson I: The torn acetabular labrum. A block to reduction of a dislocated hip. J Bone Joint Surg *39B*:306, 1957.
301. Dameron TB Jr: Bucket-handle tear of acetabular labrum accompanying posterior dislocation of the hip. J Bone Joint Surg *41A*:131, 1959.
302. Connolly JF: Acetabular labrum entrapment associated with a femoral-head fracture-dislocation. A case report. J Bone Joint Surg *56A*:1735, 1974.
303. Hovelius L: Traumatic dislocation of the hip in children. Report of two cases. Acta Orthop Scand *45*:746, 1974.
304. Hammelbo T: Traumatic hip dislocation in childhood. A report of three cases. Acta Orthop Scand *47*:546, 1976.
305. Schlonsky J, Miller PR: Traumatic hip dislocations in children. J Bone Joint Surg *55A*:1057, 1973.
306. Gaul RW: Recurrent traumatic dislocation of the hip in children. Clin Orthop Rel Res *90*:107, 1973.
307. Kennedy JC: Complete dislocation of the knee joint. J Bone Joint Surg *45A*:889, 1963.
308. Reckling FW, Peltier LF: Acute knee dislocations and their complications. J Trauma *9*:181, 1969.
309. Meyers MH, Harvey JR Jr: Traumatic dislocation of the knee joint. A study of eighteen cases. J Bone Joint Surg *53A*:16, 1971.
310. Taylor AR, Arden GP, Rainey HA: Traumatic dislocation of the knee. A report of forty-three cases with special reference to conservative treatment. J Bone Joint Surg *54B*:96, 1972.
311. Brattstrom H: Shape of the intercondylar groove normally and in recurrent dislocation of the patella. Acta Orthop Scand (Suppl) *68*:5, 1964.

312. Brattstrom H: Patella alta in non-dislocating knee joints. Acta Orthop Scand *41*:578, 1970.
313. Frangakis EK: Intra-articular dislocation of the patella. A case report. J Bone Joint Surg *56A*:423, 1974.
314. Allen FJ: Intercondylar dislocation of the patella. South Afr Med J *18*:66, 1944.
315. Deaderick C: Case of rupture of quadriceps femoris tendon with dislocation of the patella beneath the intercondyloid groove of the femur. Ann Surg *11*:102, 1890.
316. Feneley RCL: Inter-articular dislocation of the patella. Report of a case. J Bone Joint Surg *50B*:653, 1968.
317. Freiberger RH, Kotzen LM: Fracture of the medial margin of the patella, a finding diagnostic of lateral dislocation. Radiology *88*:902, 1967.
318. Rorabeck CH, Bobechko WP: Acute dislocation of the patella with osteochondral fracture. A review of eighteen cases. J Bone Joint Surg *58B*:237, 1976.
319. Jacobsen K, Metz P: Occult traumatic dislocation of the patella. J Trauma *16*:829, 1976.
320. Ogden JA: Dislocation of the proximal fibula. Radiology *105*:547, 1972.
321. Parkes JC II, Zelko RR: Isolated acute dislocation of the proximal tibiofibular joint. Case report. J Bone Joint Surg *55A*:177, 1973.
322. Ogden JA: Subluxation and dislocation of the proximal tibiofibular joint. J Bone Joint Surg *56A*:145, 1974.
323. Baciu CC, Tudor A, Olaru I: Recurrent luxation of the superior tibiofibular joint in the adult. Acta Orthop Scand *45*:772, 1974.
324. Sijbrandij S: Instability of the proximal tibio-fibular joint. Acta Orthop Scand *49*:621, 1978.
325. Goergen TG, Danzig LA, Resnick D, Owen CA: Roentgenographic evaluation of the tibiotalar joint. J Bone Joint Surg *59A*:874, 1977.
326. Ramsey PL, Hamilton W: Changes in tibiotalar area of contact caused by lateral talar shift. J Bone Joint Surg *58A*:356, 1976.
327. Main BJ, Jowett RL: Injuries of the midtarsal joint. J Bone Joint Surg *57B*:89, 1975.
328. Dewar FP, Evans DC: Occult fracture-subluxation of the midtarsal joint. J Bone Joint Surg *50B*:386, 1968.
329. Brantigan JW, Pedegana LR, Lippert FG: Instability of the subtalar joint. Diagnosis by stress tomography in three cases. J Bone Joint Surg *59A*:321, 1977.
330. Cassebaum WH: Lisfranc-fracture-dislocations. Clin Orthop Rel Res *30*:116, 1963.
331. Foster SC, Foster RR: Lisfranc's tarsometatarsal fracture-dislocation. Radiology *120*:79, 1976.
332. Wiley JJ: The mechanism of tarso-metatarsal joint injuries. J Bone Joint Surg *53B*:474, 1971.
333. Wilson DW: Injuries of the tarso-metatarsal joints. Etiology, classification and results of treatment. J Bone Joint Surg *54B*:677, 1972.
334. Ashhurst APC: Divergent dislocation of the metatarsus. Ann Surg *83*:132, 1926.
335. Aitken AP, Poulson D: Dislocations of the tarsometatarsal joint. J Bone Joint Surg *45A*:246, 1963.
336. Salamon PB, Gelberman RH, Huffer JM: Dorsal dislocation of the metatarsophalangeal joint of the great toe. A case report. J Bone Joint Surg *56A*:1073, 1974.
337. Howland WJ: Pseudo-dislocation of the proximal interphalangeal joint of the fifth toe. Am J Roentgenol *103*:653, 1968.
338. Watson-Jones R: Dislocations and fracture-dislocations of the pelvis. Br J Surg *25*:773, 1938.
339. Langloh ND, Johnson EW Jr, Jackson CB: Traumatic sacro-iliac disruptions. J Trauma *12*:931, 1972.
340. Fielding JW: Cineroentgenography of the normal cervical spine. J Bone Joint Surg *39A*:1280, 1957.
341. Fielding JW, Hawkins RJ, Hensinger RN, Francis WR: Atlantoaxial rotary deformities. Orthop Clin North Am *9*:955, 1978.
342. Wortzman G, Dewar FP: Rotary fixation of the atlantoaxial joint: Rotational atlantoaxial subluxation. Radiology *90*:479, 1968.
343. Fielding JW, Hawkins RJ: Atlanto-axial rotatory fixation. (Fixed rotatory subluxation of the atlanto-axial joint). J Bone Joint Surg *59A*:37, 1977.
344. Fielding JW, Stillwell WT, Chynn KY, Spyropoulos EC: Use of computed tomography for the diagnosis of atlanto-axial rotatory fixation. A case report. J Bone Joint Surg *60A*:1102, 1978.
345. Coutts MB: Atlanto-epistropheal subluxations. Arch Surg *29*:297, 1934.
346. Fiorani-Gallotta G, Luzzatti G: Sublussazione laterale e sublussazione rotatoria dell'atlanta. Arch Ortop *70*:467, 1957.
347. Watson-Jones R: Spontaneous hyperaemic dislocation of the atlas. Proc R Soc Med *25*:586, 1932.
348. Hess JH, Bronstein IP, Abelson SM: Atlanto-axial dislocation unassociated with trauma and secondary to inflammatory foci of the neck. Am J Dis Child *49*:1137, 1935.
349. Garber JN: Abnormalities of the atlas and axis vertebrae — congenital and traumatic. J Bone Joint Surg *46A*:1782, 1964.
350. Jackson H: The diagnosis of minimal atlanto-axial subluxation. Br J Radiol *23*:672, 1950.
351. Sassard WR, Heinig CF, Pitts WR: Posterior atlanto-axial dislocation without fracture. Case report with successful conservative treatment. J Bone Joint Surg *56A*:625, 1974.
352. Patzakis MJ, Knopf A, Elfering M, Hoffer M, Harvey JP Jr: Posterior dislocation of the atlas on the axis; a case report. J Bone Joint Surg *56A*:1260, 1974.
353. Cattell HS, Filtzer DL: Pseudosubluxation and other normal variations in the cervical spine in children. A study of one hundred and sixty children. J Bone Joint Surg *47A*:1295, 1965.
354. Marar BC, Balachandran N: Non-traumatic atlanto-axial dislocation in children. Clin Orthop Rel Res *92*:220, 1973.
355. Fielding JW, Cochran GVB, Lawsing JF III, Hohl M: Tears of the transverse ligament of the atlas. A clinical and biochemical study. J Bone Joint Surg *56A*:1683, 1974.
356. Shapiro R, Youngberg AS, Rothman SLG: The differential diagnosis of traumatic lesions of the occipito-atlanto-axial segment. Radiol Clin North Am *11*:505, 1973.
357. Anderson LD, D'Alonzo RT: Fractures of the odontoid process of the axis. J Bone Joint Surg *56A*:1663, 1974.
358. Sherk HH, Nicholson JT, Chung SMK: Fractures of the odontoid process in young children. J Bone Joint Surg *60A*:921, 1978.
359. Schatzker J, Rorabeck CH, Waddell JP: Fractures of the dens (odontoid process). An analysis of thirty-seven cases. J Bone Joint Surg *53B*:392, 1971.
360. Schatzker J, Rorabeck CH, Waddell JP: Non-union of the odontoid process. An experimental investigation. Clin Orthop Rel Res *108*:127, 1975.
361. Fielding JW, Griffin PP: Os odontoideum: An acquired lesion. J Bone Joint Surg *56A*:187, 1974.
362. Freiberger RH, Wilson PD Jr, Nicholas JA: Acquired absence of the odontoid process. A case report. J Bone Joint Surg *47A*:1231, 1965.
363. Hawkins RJ, Fielding JW, Thompson WJ: Os odontoideum: Congenital or acquired. J Bone Joint Surg *58A*:413, 1976.
364. Stillwell WT, Fielding JW: Acquired os odontoideum. A case report. Clin Orthop Rel Res *135*:71, 1978.
365. Ricciardi JE, Kaufer H, Louis DS: Acquired os odontoideum following acute ligament injury. Report of a case. J Bone Joint Surg *58A*:410, 1976.
366. Tredwell SJ, O'Brien JP: Avascular necrosis of the proximal end of the dens. J Bone Joint Surg *57A*:332, 1975.
367. Daffner RH: Pseudofracture of the dens: Mach bands. Am J Roentgenol *128*:607, 1977.
368. Davie B: The significance and treatment of haemarthrosis of the knee following trauma. Med J Aust *1*:1355, 1969.
369. Wilkinson A: Traumatic haemarthrosis of the knee. Lancet *2*:13, 1965.
370. MacEwan DW: Changes due to trauma in the fat plane overlying the pronator quadratus muscle: A radiologic sign. Radiology *82*:879, 1964.
371. Rogers SL, MacEwan DW: Changes due to trauma in the fat plane overlying the supinator muscle: A radiologic sign. Radiology *92*:954, 1969.
372. Bledsoe RC, Izenstark JL: Displacement of fat pads in disease and injury of the elbow: A new radiographic sign. Radiology *73*:717, 1959.
373. Bohrer SP: The fat pad sign following elbow trauma. Its usefulness and reliability in suspecting "invisible fractures." Clin Radiol *21*:90, 1970.
374. Hunter RD: Swollen elbow following trauma. JAMA *230*:1573, 1974.
375. Weston WJ: Joint space widening with intracapsular fractures in joints of the fingers and toes of children. Australas Radiol *15*:367, 1971.
376. Lawrence C, Seife B: Bone marrow in joint fluid: A clue to fracture. Ann Intern Med *74*:740, 1971.
377. Kling DH: Fat in traumatic effusions of the knee joint. Am J Surg *6*:71, 1929.
378. Berk RN: Liquid fat in the knee joint after trauma. N Engl J Med *277*:1411, 1967.
379. Gregg JR, Nixon JE, DiStefano V: Neutral fat globules in traumatized knees. Clin Orthop Rel Res *132*:219, 1978.
380. Holmagren BS: Flussiges fett in kniegelenk nach trauma. Acta Radiol *23*:131, 1942.
381. Graham J, Goldman JA: Fat droplets and synovial fluid leukocytes in traumatic arthritis. Arthritis Rheum *21*:76, 1978.
382. Peirce CB, Eaglesham DC: Traumatic lipohemarthrosis of the knee. Radiology *39*:655, 1942.
383. Saxton HM: Lipohaemarthrosis. Br J Radiol *35*:122, 1962.
384. Nelson SW: Some important diagnostic and technical fundamentals in radiology of trauma, with particular emphasis on skeletal trauma. Radiol Clin North Am *4*:241, 1966.
385. Arger PH, Oberkircher PE, Miller WT: Lipohemarthrosis. Am J Roentgenol *121*:97, 1974.

386. Feldman F, Ellis K, Green WM: The fat embolism syndrome. Radiology *114*:535, 1975.
387. Schwegler N, Hug I: Fettflussigkeitsspiegel bei Tibiakopf-Impressionsfraktur. Fortschr Geb Roentgenstr Nuklearmed *122*:301, 1975.
388. Yousefzadeh DK, Jackson JH Jr: Lipohemarthrosis of the elbow joint. Radiology *128*:643, 1978.
389. Newberg AH, Greenstein R: Radiographic evaluation of tibial plateau fractures. Radiology *126*:319, 1978.
390. Fagerberg S: Tomographic analysis of depressed fractures within the knee joint, and of injuries to the cruciate ligaments. Acta Orthop Scand *27*:219, 1958.
391. Chuinard EG: Fractures of the condyles of the tibia. Clin Orthop Rel Res *37*:115, 1964.
392. Sacks BA, Rosenthal DI, Hall FM: Capsular visualization in lipohemarthrosis of the knee. Radiology *122*:31, 1977.
393. Resnick D, Niwayama G: Intravertebral disk herniations: cartilaginous (Schmorl's) nodes. Radiology *126*:57, 1978.
394. Hilton RC, Ball J, Benn RT: Vertebral end-plate lesions (Schmorl's nodes) in the dorsolumbar spine. Ann Rheum Dis *35*:127, 1976.
395. Martel W, Seeger JF, Wicks JD, Washburn RL: Traumatic lesions of the discovertebral junction in the lumbar spine. Am J Roentgenol *127*:457, 1976.
396. Williams JL, Moller GA, O'Rourke TL: Pseudoinfections of the intervertebral disc and adjacent vertebrae. Am J Roentgenol *103*:611, 1968.
397. Roaf R: A study of the mechanics of spinal injuries. J Bone Joint Surg *42B*:810, 1960.
398. Keller RH: Traumatic displacement of the cartilaginous vertebral rim: A sign of intervertebral disc prolapse. Radiology *110*:21, 1974.
399. Sakakida K: Clinical observations on the epiphyseal separation of long bones. Pacif Med Surg *73*:108, 1965.
400. Larson RL, McMahon RO: The epiphyses and the childhood athlete. JAMA *196*:607, 1966.
401. Rogers LF: The radiography of epiphyseal injuries. Radiology *96*:289, 1970.
402. Ozonoff MB: Pediatric Orthopedic Radiology. Philadelphia, W. B. Saunders Company, 1979.
403. Siffert RS: The effect of trauma to the epiphysis and growth plate. Skel Radiol *2*:21, 1977.
404. Alexander CJ: Effect of growth rate on the strength of the growth plate-shaft junction. Skel Radiol *1*:67, 1976.
405. Harsha WN: Effects of trauma upon epiphyses. Clin Orthop Rel Res *10*:140, 1957.
406. Salter RB, Harris WR: Injuries involving the epiphyseal plate. J Bone Joint Surg *45A*:587, 1963.
407. Salter RB, Harris WR: Injuries of the growth plate. *In* M Rang (Ed): The Growth Plate and Its Disorders. London, E & S Livingstone, 1969, p 132.
408. Park EA, Guild HG, Jackson D, Bond M: The recognition of scurvy with especial reference to the early x-ray changes. Arch Dis Child *10*:265, 1935.
409. Alexander CJ: The etiology of juvenile spondyloarthritis (discitis). Clin Radiol *21*:178, 1970.
410. Berry JM: Fracture of the tuberosity of the ischium due to muscular action. JAMA *59*:1450, 1912.
411. Stayton CA: Ischial epiphysiolysis. Am J Roentgenol *76*:1161, 1956.
412. Haliburton RA, Barber JR, Fraser RL: Pseudodislocation: An unusual birth injury. Can J Surg *10*:455, 1967.
413. Howorth MB: Slipping of the upper femoral epiphysis. Surg Gynecol Obstet *73*:723, 1941.
414. Burrows HJ: Slipped upper femoral epiphysis. J Bone Joint Surg *39B*:641, 1957.
415. Jerre T: A study in slipped upper femoral epiphysis. Acta Orthop Scand (Suppl) *6*:1, 1950.
416. Sorensen KH: Slipped upper femoral epiphysis, clinical study on aetiology. Acta Orthop Scand *39*:499, 1968.
417. Kelsey JL: Epidemiology of slipped capital femoral epiphysis: A review of the literature. Pediatrics *51*:1042, 1973.
418. Kelsey JL, Acheson RM, Keggi KJ: The body build of patients with slipped capital femoral epiphysis. Am J Dis Child *124*:276, 1972.
419. Ninomiya S, Nagasaka Y, Tagawa H: Slipped capital femoral epiphysis. A study of 68 cases in the eastern half area of Japan. Clin Orthop Rel Res *119*:172, 1976.
420. Towbin R, Crawford AH: Neonatal traumatic proximal femoral epiphysiolysis. Pediatrics *63*:456, 1979.
421. Milgram JW, Lyne ED: Epiphysiolysis of the proximal femur in very young children. Clin Orthop Rel Res *110*:146, 1975.
422. Lindseth RE, Rosene HA: Traumatic separation of the upper femoral epiphysis in a newborn infant. J Bone Joint Surg *53A*:1641, 1971.
423. Ogden JA, Gossling HR, Southwick WO: Slipped capital femoral epiphysis following ipsilateral femoral fracture. Clin Orthop Rel Res *110*:167, 1975.
424. Kelsey JL, Keggi KJ, Southwick WO: The incidence and distribution of slipped capital femoral epiphysis in Connecticut and Southwestern United States. J Bone Joint Surg *52A*:1203, 1970.
425. Moore RD: Aseptic necrosis of the capital femoral epiphysis following adolescent epiphyseolysis. Surg Gynecol Obstet *80*:199, 1945.
426. Al-Aswad BI, Weinger JM, Schneider AB: Slipped capital femoral epiphysis in a 35 year old man. A case report. Clin Orthop Rel Res *134*:131, 1978.
427. Henrikson B: The incidence of slipped capital femoral epiphysis. Acta Orthop Scand *40*:365, 1969.
428. Bishop JO, Oley TJ, Stephenson CT, Tullos HS: Slipped capital femoral epiphysis. A study of 50 cases in Black children. Clin Orthop Rel Res *135*:93, 1978.
429. Morscher E: Strength and morphology of growth cartilage under hormonal influence of puberty. Reconstr Surg Traumatol *10*:3, 1968.
430. Hillman JW, Hunter WA Jr, Barrow JA III: Experimental epiphysiolysis in rats. Surg Forum *8*:566, 1957.
431. Harris WR: The endocrine basis for slipping of the upper femoral epiphysis. An experimental study. J Bone Joint Surg *32B*:5, 1950.
432. Murray RO, Duncan C: Athletic activity in adolescence as an etiological factor in degenerative hip disease. J Bone Joint Surg *53B*:406, 1971.
433. Howorth B: History of slipping of the capital femoral epiphysis. Clin Orthop Rel Res *48*:11, 1966.
434. Kampner SL, Wissinger HA: Anterior slipping of the capital femoral epiphysis. Report of a case. J Bone Joint Surg *54A*:1531, 1972.
435. Finch AD, Roberts WM: Epiphyseal coxa valga. J Bone Joint Surg *28*:869, 1946.
436. Skinner SR, Berkheimer GA: Valgus slip of the capital femoral epiphysis. Clin Orthop Rel Res *135*:90, 1978.
437. LaCroix P, Verbrugge J: Slipping of the upper femoral epiphysis. A pathological study. J Bone Joint Surg *33A*:371, 1951.
438. Ponseti IV, McClintock R: The pathology of slipping of the upper femoral epiphysis. J Bone Joint Surg *38A*:71, 1956.
439. Mickelson MR, Ponseti IV, Cooper RR, Maynard JA: The ultrastructure of the growth plate in slipped capital femoral epiphysis. J Bone Joint Surg *59A*:1076, 1977.
440. Loyd RD, Evans JP: Acute slipped capital femoral epiphysis. South Med J *68*:857, 1975.
441. Bloomberg TJ, Nuttall J, Stoker DJ: Radiology in early slipped femoral capital epiphysis. Clin Radiol *29*:657, 1978.
442. Aadalen RJ, Weiner DS, Hoyt W, Herndon CH: Acute slipped capital femoral epiphysis. J Bone Joint Surg *56A*:1473, 1974.
443. Scham SM: The triangular sign in the early diagnosis of slipped capital femoral epiphysis. Clin Orthop Rel Res *103*:16, 1974.
444. Jacobs P: A note on the diagnosis of early adolescent coxa vara (slipped epiphysis). Br J Radiol *35*:619, 1962.
445. Mickelson MR, El-Khoury GY, Cass JR, Case KJ: Aseptic necrosis following slipped capital femoral epiphysis. Skel Radiol *4*:129, 1979.
446. Dalinka MK, Alavi A, Forsted DH: Aseptic (ischemic) necrosis of the femoral head. JAMA *238*:1059, 1977.
447. Lowe HG: Avascular necrosis after slipping of the upper femoral epiphysis. Bone Joint Surg *43B*:688, 1961.
448. Hall JE: The results of treatment of slipped femoral epiphysis. J Bone Joint Surg *39B*:659, 1957.
449. Lowe HG: Necrosis of articular cartilage after slipping of the capital femoral epiphysis. Report of six cases with recovery. J Bone Joint Surg *52B*:108, 1970.
450. Gage JR, Sundberg AB, Nolan DR, Sletten RG, Winter RB: Complications after cuneiform osteotomy for moderately or severely slipped capital femoral epiphysis. J Bone Joint Surg *60A*:157, 1978.
451. Cruess RL: The pathology of acute necrosis of cartilage in slipping of the capital femoral epiphysis. A report of two cases with pathological sections. J Bone Joint Surg *45A*:1013, 1963.
452. Tillema DA, Golding JSR: Chondrolysis following slipped capital femoral epiphysis in Jamaica. J Bone Joint Surg *53A*:1528, 1971.
453. Hartman JT, Gates DJ: Recovery from cartilage necrosis following slipped capital femoral epiphysis. A seven year study of 166 cases. Orthop Rev *1*:33, 1972.
454. Larson RL: Epiphyseal injuries in the adolescent athlete. Orthop Clin North Am *4*:839, 1973.
455. Smith L: A concealed injury to the knee. J Bone Joint Surg *44A*:1659, 1962.
456. Cassebaum WH, Patterson AH: Fractures of the distal femoral epiphysis. Clin Orthop Rel Res *41*:79, 1965.
457. Stephens DC, Louis DS: Traumatic separation of the distal femoral epiphyseal cartilage plate. J Bone Joint Surg *56A*:1383, 1974.
458. Rogers LF, Jones S, Davis AR, Dietz G: "Clipping injury" fracture of the epiphysis in the adolescent football player: An occult lesion of the knee. Am J Roentgenol *121*:69, 1974.
459. Aitken AP, Ingersoll RE: Fractures of the proximal tibial epiphyseal cartilage. J Bone Joint Surg *38A*:787, 1956.
460. Shelton WR, Canale ST: Fractures of the tibia through the proximal tibial epiphyseal cartilage. J Bone Joint Surg *61A*:167, 1979.
461. Poznanski A: Personal communication, 1979.
462. Rogers LF, Malave S Jr, White H, Tachdjian MO: Plastic bowing, torus

and greenstick supracondylar fractures of the humerus: Radiographic clues to obscure fractures of the elbow in children. Radiology *128*:145, 1978.
463. Chessare JW, Rogers LF, White H, Tachdjian MO: Injuries of the medial epicondylar ossification center of the humerus. Am J Roentgenol *129*:49, 1979.
464. Mizuno K, Hirohata K, Kashiwagi D: Fracture-separation of the distal humeral epiphysis in young children. J Bone Joint Surg *61A*:570, 1979.
465. Aitken AP: The end results of the fractured distal radial epiphysis. J Bone Joint Surg *17*:302, 1935.
466. Holland CT: A radiological note on injuries to distal epiphyses on the radius and ulna. Proc R Soc Med *22*:695, 1929.
467. Aitken AP: The end results of the fractured distal tibial epiphysis. J Bone Joint Surg *18*:685, 1936.
468. Kleiger B, Barton J: Epiphyseal ankle fractures. Bull Hosp Joint Dis *25*:240, 1964.
469. Dameron TB Jr, Reibel DB: Fractures involving the proximal humeral epiphyseal plate. J Bone Joint Surg *51A*:289, 1969.
470. Godshall RW, Hansen CA: Incomplete avulsion of a portion of the iliac epiphysis. An injury of young athletes. J Bone Joint Surg *55A*:1301, 1973.
471. Welsh RP, MacNab I, Riley V: Biomechanical studies of rabbit tendon. Clin Orthop Rel Res *81*:171, 1971.
472. Peacock EE: Biological principles in the healing of long tendons. Surg Clin North Am *45*:461, 1965.
473. Peacock EE: A study of the circulation in normal tendons and healing grafts. Ann Surg *149*:415, 1959.
474. Clayton ML, Weir GL Jr: Experimental investigations of ligamentous healing. Am J Surg *98*:373, 1959.
475. Tipton CM, Schild RJ, Flatt AE: Measurement of ligamentous strength in rat knees. J Bone Joint Surg *49A*:63, 1967.
476. Mornet J, Doliveux P: La maladie des tendons d'achille et sa complication: La rupture. Rev Rhum Mal Osteoartic *40*:607, 1973.
477. Reveno PM, Kittleson AC: Spontaneous Achilles tendon rupture. Radiology *93*:1341, 1969.
478. Margles SW, Lewis MM: Bilateral spontaneous concurrent rupture of the patellar tendon without apparent associated systemic disease: A case report. Clin Orthop Rel Res *136*:186, 1978.
479. Newberg A, Wales L: Radiographic diagnosis of quadriceps tendon rupture. Radiology *125*:367, 1977.
480. Staples OS: Ruptures of the fibular collateral ligaments of the ankle. Result study of immediate surgical treatment. J Bone Joint Surg *57A*:101, 1975.
481. Moore TM, Meyers HM, Harvey JP Jr: Collateral ligament laxity of the knee. Long-term comparison between plateau fractures and normal. J Bone Joint Surg *58A*:594, 1976.
482. Liljedahl S-O, Lindvall N, Wetterfors J: Early diagnosis and treatment of acute ruptures of the anterior cruciate ligament. A clinical and arthrographic study of forty-eight cases. J Bone Joint Surg *47A*:1503, 1965.
483. Jacobsen K: Demonstration of rotatory instability in injured knees by stress radiography. Acta Orthop Scand *49*:195, 1978.
484. Jacobsen K: Stress radiographic measurements of post-traumatic knee instability. A clinical study. Acta Orthop Scand *48*:301, 1977.
485. Jacobsen K: Stress radiographical measurement of the anteroposterior, medial and lateral stability of the knee joint. Acta Orthop Scand *47*:335, 1976.
486. Sylvin LE: A more exact measurement of the sagittal stability of the knee joint. Acta Orthop Scand *46*:1008, 1975.
487. Kennedy JC, Fowler PJ: Medial and anterior instability of the knee. J Bone Joint Surg *53A*:1257, 1971.
488. Freeman MAR: Instability of the foot after injuries to the lateral ligament of the ankle. J Bone Joint Surg *47B*:669, 1965.
489. Rubin G, Witten M: The talar tilt angle and the fibular collateral ligaments. J Bone Joint Surg *42A*:311, 1960.
490. Johannsen A: Radiological diagnosis of lateral ligament lesion of the ankle. A comparison between talar tilt and anterior drawer sign. Acta Orthop Scand *49*:295, 1978.
491. Schneider R, Kaye JJ, Ghelman B: Adductor avulsive injuries near the symphysis pubis. Radiology *120*:567, 1976.
492. Stayton CA: Ischial epiphysiolysis. Am J Roentgenol *76*:1161, 1956.
493. Symeonides P: Isolated traumatic rupture of the adductor longus muscle of the thigh. Clin Orthop Rel Res *88*:64, 1972.
494. Ellis R, Greene A: Ischial apophyseolysis. Radiology *87*:646, 1966.
495. Krahl H, Rompe G: Ermüdungsbruch der pars symphysica des Schambeines. Beitrag zur Differentialdiagnose der Uberlastungsschaaden am vordern Beckenring. Z Orthop *111*:216, 1973.
496. Cotton RE, Rideout DF: Tears of the humeral rotator cuff: A radiological and pathological necropsy study. J Bone Joint Surg *46B*:314, 1964.
497. McLaughlin HL: Rupture of the rotator cuff. J Bone Joint Surg *44A*:979, 1962.
498. Wolfgang GL: Surgical repair of tears of the rotator cuff of the shoulder. J Bone Joint Surg *56A*:14, 1974.
499. Kotzen LM: Roentgen diagnosis of rotator cuff tear. Report of 48 surgically proven cases. Am J Roentgenol *112*:507, 1971.
500. DeSmet AA, Ting YM: Diagnosis of rotator cuff tear on routine radiographs. J Can Assoc Radiol *28*:54, 1977.
501. Golding FC: The shoulder — the forgotten joint. Br J Radiol *35*:149, 1962.
502. Golding C: Radiology and orthopedic surgery. J Bone Joint Surg *48B*:320, 1966.
503. Wilson FC: Fractures and dislocations of the ankle. *In* Rockwood CA and Green DP (Eds): Fractures. Philadelphia, JB Lippincott Co, 1975, p. 1361.
504. Husfeldt E: Significance of roentgenography of ankle joint in oblique projection in malleolar fractures. Hospitalstid *80*:788, 1937.
505. Kogutt MS, Swischuk LE, Fagan CJ: Patterns of injury and significance of uncommon fractures in the battered child syndrome. Am J Roentgenol *121*:143, 1974.
506. Spackman TJ: Pediatric trauma: Medical abuse of infants. Radiol Clin North Am *11*:633, 1973.
507. Akbarnia B, Torg JS, Kirkpatrick J, Sussman S: Manifestations of the battered-child syndrome. J Bone Joint Surg *56A*:1159, 1974.
508. Slovis TL, Berdon WE, Haller JO, Baker DH, Rosen L: Pancreatitis and the battered child syndrome. Report of 2 cases with skeletal involvement. Am J Roentgenol *125*:456, 1975.
509. Hiller HG: Battered or not — a reappraisal of metaphyseal fragility. Am J Roentgenol *114*:241, 1972.
510. Silverman FN: Unrecognized trauma in infants, the battered child syndrome, and the syndrome of Ambroise Tardieu. Radiology *104*:337, 1972.
511. Caffey J: Some traumatic lesions in growing bones other than fractures and dislocations: Clinical and radiological features. Br J Radiol *30*:225, 1957.
512. O'Neill JA Jr, Meacham WF, Griffin PP, Sawyers JL: Patterns of injury in the battered child syndrome. J Trauma *13*:332, 1973.
513. Tröger J: Das misshandelte Kind. Radiologe *18*:233, 1978.
514. Swischuk LE: Spine and spinal cord trauma in the battered child syndrome. Radiology *92*:733, 1969.
515. Faure C, Steadman C, Lalande G, Al Moudares N, Marsault C, Bennett J: La vertèbre vagabonde. Ann Radiol *22*:96, 1979.
516. Cullen JC: Spinal lesions in battered babies. J Bone Joint Surg *57B*:364, 1975.
517. Fordham EW, Ramachandran PC: Radionuclide scanning of osseous trauma. Semin Nucl Med *4*:411, 1974.
518. Marty R, Denney JD, McKamey MR, Rowley MJ: Bone trauma and related benign disease: Assessment by bone scanning. Semin Nucl Med *6*:107, 1976.
519. DeSmet AA, Kuhns LR, Kaufman RA, Holt JF: Bony sclerosis and the battered child. Skel Radiol *2*:39, 1977.
520. Wesenberg RL, Gwinn JL, Barnes GR Jr: Radiological findings in the kinky-hair syndrome. Radiology *92*:500, 1969.
521. Menkes JH: Kinky hair disease. Pediatrics *50*:181, 1972.
522. Adams PC, Strand RD, Bresnan MJ, Lucky AW: Kinky hair syndrome: Serial study of radiological findings with emphasis on the similarity to the battered child syndrome. Radiology *112*:401, 1974.
523. Rosenthall L, Hill RO, Chuang S: Observation on the use of ^{99m}Tc phosphate imaging in peripheral bone trauma. Radiology *119*:637, 1976.
524. Shahriaree H, Sajadi K, Rooholamini SA: A family with spondylolisthesis. J Bone Joint Surg *61A*:1256, 1979.
525. Hunter LY, Hensinger RN: Dorsal defect of the patella with cartilaginous involvement. A case report. Clin Orthop Rel Res *143*:131, 1979.
526. Yuan HA, Cady RB, DeRosa C: Osteochondritis dissecans of the talus associated with subchondral cysts. Report of three cases. J Bone Joint Surg *61A*:1249, 1979.
527. Barquet A: Traumatic hip dislocation in childhood. A report of 26 cases and a review of the literature. Acta Orthop Scand *50*:549, 1979.
528. Burkhart SS, Peterson HA: Fractures of the proximal tibial epiphysis. J Bone Joint Surg *61A*:996, 1979.
529. Kamali M: Bilateral traumatic rupture of the infrapatellar tendon. Clin Orthop Rel Res *142*:131, 1979.
530. Torisu T: Avulsion fracture of the tibial attachment of the posterior cruciate ligament. Indications and results of delayed repair. Clin Orthop Rel Res *143*:107, 1979.
531. Mills GQ, Marymont JH III, Murphy DA: Bone scan utilization in the differential diagnosis of exercise-induced lower extremity pain. Clin Orthop Rel Res *149*:207, 1980.
532. Meurman KOA, Elfving S: Stress fractures in soldiers: A multifocal bone disorder. Radiology *134*:483, 1980.
533. Spencer RP, Levinson ED, Baldwin RD, Sziklas JJ, Witek JT, Rosenberg R: Diverse bone scan abnormalities in "shin splits." J Nucl Med *20*:1271, 1979.
534. Saunders AJS, Sayed TF, Hilson AJW, Maisey MN, Grahame R: Stress lesions of the lower leg and foot. Clin Radiol *30*:649, 1979.

535. Norfray JF, Schlachter L, Kernahan T Jr, Arenson DJ, Smith SD, Roth IE, Schlefman BS: Early confirmation of stress fractures in joggers. JAMA *243*:1647, 1980.
536. Symeonides PP: High stress fractures of the fibula. J Bone Joint Surg *62B*: 192, 1980.
537. Drez D Jr, Young JC, Johnston RD, Parker WD: Metatarsal stress fractures. Am J Sports Med *8*:123, 1980.
538. Weigl K, Amrami B: Occupational stress fracture in an unusual location: Report of a case in the distal end of the shaft of the radius. Clin Orthop Rel Res *147*:222, 1980.
539. Farquharson-Roberts MA, Fulford PC: Stress fracture of the radius. J Bone Joint Surg *62B*:194, 1980.
540. Oh I, Hardacre JA: Fatigue fracture of the inferior pubic ramus following total hip replacement for congenital hip dislocation. Clin Orthop Rel Res *147*:154, 1980.
541. Torisu T: Fatigue fracture of the pelvis after total knee replacements: Report of a case. Clin Orthop Rel Res *149*:216, 1980.
542. Meurman KOA, Elfving S: Stress fracture of the cuneiform bones. Br J Radiol *53*:157, 1980.
543. Leger JL, Bouchard R, Maltais R: Etude radiologique de 305 cas de spondylolyse avec ou sans spondylolisthesis. J Can Assoc Radiol *30*:86, 1979.
544. Ravichandran G: A radiologic sign in spondylolisthesis. Am J Roentgenol *134*:113, 1980.
545. Penning L, Blickman JR: Instability in lumbar spondylolisthesis: A radiologic study of several concepts. Am J Roentgenol *134*:293, 1980.
546. Tetiz CC, Carter DR, Frankel VH: Problems associated with tibial fractures with intact fibulae. J Bone Joint Surg *62A*:770, 1980.
547. Auld CD, Chesney RB: Familial osteochondritis dissecans and carpal tunnel syndrome. Acta Orthop Scand *50*:727, 1979.
548. Orava S, Weitz H, Holopainen O: Osteochondritis dissecans patellae. Z Orthop *117*:906, 1979.
549. Canale ST, Belding RH: Osteochondral lesions of the talus. J Bone Joint Surg *62A*:97, 1980.
550. McCullough CH, Venugopal V: Osteochondritis dissecans of the talus: The natural history. Clin Orthop Rel Res *144*:264, 1979.
551. Alexander AH, Lightman DM: Surgical treatment of transchondral talar-dome fractures (osteochondritis dissecans). J Bone Joint Surg *62A*: 646, 1980.
552. Lindholm TS, Osterman K, Vankka E: Osteochondritis dissecans of elbow, ankle and hip: A comparison survey. Clin Orthop Rel Res *148*:245, 1980.
553. Vastamaki M, Solonen KA: Posterior dislocation and fracture-dislocation of the shoulder. Acta Orthop Scand *51*:479, 1980.
554. Lourie JA: Tomography in the diagnosis of posterior dislocation of the sterno-clavicular joint. Acta Orthop Scand *51*:579, 1980.
555. Gerard FM: Post-traumatic carpal instability in a young child. A case report. J Bone Joint Surg *62A*:131, 1980.
556. Taleisnik J: Post-traumatic carpal instability. Clin Orthop Rel Res *149*:73, 1980.
557. Hockley B: Carpal instability and carpal injuries. Aust Radiol *23*:158, 1979.
558. Protas JM, Jackson WT: Evaluating carpal instabilities with fluoroscopy. Am J Roentgenol *135*:137, 1980.
559. Myfield JK, Kilcoyne RK: Carpal dislocations: Pathomechanics and progressive perilunar instability. J Hand Surg *5*:226, 1980.
560. Dussault RG, Beauregard G, Fauteaux P, Laurin C, Boisjoly A: Femoral head defect following anterior hip dislocation. Radiology *135*:627, 1980.
561. Pettersson H, Theander G, Danielsson L: Voluntary habitual dislocation of the hip in children. Acta Radiol (Diag) *21*:303, 1980.
562. Fielding JW, Hensinger RN, Hawkins RJ: Os odontoideum. J Bone Joint Surg *62A*:376, 1980.
563. Hukuda S, Ota H, Okabe N, Tazima K: Traumatic atlantoaxial dislocation causing os odontoideum in infants. Spine *5*:207, 1980.
564. Noyes FR, Bassett RW, Grood ES, Butler DL: Arthroscopy in acute traumatic hemarthrosis of the knee. J Bone Joint Surg *62A*:687, 1980.
565. Train JS, Hermann G: Lipohemarthrosis: Its occurrence with occult cortical fracture of the knee. Orthopedics *3*:416, 1980.
566. Wojtowycz M, Starshak RJ, Sty JR: Neonatal proximal femoral epiphysiolysis. Radiology *136*:647, 1980.
567. Oka M, Miki T, Hama H, Yamamuro T: The mechanical strength of the growth plate under the influence of sex hormones. Clin Orthop Rel Res *145*:264, 1979.
568. DeLee JC, Williams KE, Rogers LF, Rockwood CA: Fracture-separation of the distal humeral epiphysis. J Bone Joint Surg *62A*:46, 1980.
569. Holda ME, Manoli A II, LaMont RL: Epiphyseal separation of the distal end of the humerus with medial displacement. J Bone Joint Surg *62A*:52, 1980.
570. Tayob AA, Shively RA: Bilateral elbow dislocations with intra-articular displacement of the medial epicondyles. J Trauma *20*:332, 1980.
571. Minns RJ, Steven FS: Local denaturation of collagen fibres during the mechanical rupture of collagenous fibrous tissue. Ann Rheum Dis *39*:164, 1980.
572. Stern RE, Harwin SF: Spontaneous and simultaneous rupture of both quadriceps tendons. Clin Orthop Rel Res *147*:188, 1980.
573. Van de Berg A, Collard A: Diagnosis of the disorders of the knee ligaments. A radiological measurement of laxity. J Belge Radiol *62*:49, 1979.
574. Seligson D, Gassman J, Pope M: Ankle instability: Evaluation of the lateral ligaments. Am J Sports Med *8*:39, 1980.
575. Grevsten S, Eriksson K: Tendinography for diagnosing injuries of tendons and ligaments. Acta Radiol (Diag) *20*:447, 1979.
576. Barrett IR, Kozlowski K: The battered child syndrome. Aust Radiol *23*: 72, 1979.
577. Horan FT, Beighton PH: Infantile metaphysial dysplasia or "battered babies"? J Bone Joint Surg *62B*:243, 1980.
578. Jorgensen TM, Andresen JH, Thommesen P, Hansen HH: Scanning and radiology of the carpal scaphoid bone. Acta Orthop Scand *50*:663, 1979.
579. Jung H, Schlenkhoff D, Barry BA, Arlt B: Die Knochenszintigraphie mit ^{99m}Technetium-phosphat-komplexen in der Diagnostik von Frakturen spongioser Knochen. Unfallheilkunde *83*:103, 1980.
580. Murray IPC: Bone scanning in the child and young adult. Skel Radiol *5*:65, 1980.
581. Hughes S: Radionuclides in orthopaedic surgery. J Bone Joint Surg *62B*: 4, 1980.
582. O'Callaghan JPO: CT of facet distraction in flexion injuries of the thoracolumbar spine: The "naked" facet. Am J Roentgenol *134*:563, 1980.
583. Shirkhoda A, Brashear HR, Staab EV: Computed tomography of acetabular fractures. Radiology *134*:683, 1980.
584. Faerber EN, Wolpert SM, Scott M, Belkin SC, Carter BL: Computed tomography of spinal fractures. J Comput Assist Tomogr *3*:657, 1979.
585. Matin P: The appearance of bone scans following fractures, including immediate and long-term studies. J Nucl Med *20*:1227, 1979.
586. Sedgwick WG, Gilula LA, Lesker PA, Whiteside LA: Wear particles: Their value in knee arthrography. Radiology *136*:11, 1980.
587. Resnick D, Guerra J Jr: Stress fractures of the inferior pubic ramus following hip surgery. Radiology *137*:335, 1980.
588. Meuerman KOA: Stress fracture of the pubic arch in military recruits. Br J Radiol *53*:521, 1980.
589. Schulitz K-P, Niethard FU: Strain on the interarticular stress distribution. Arch Orthop Traumatol *96*:197, 1980.
590. Fowles JV, Kassab MT: Displaced fractures of the medial humeral condyle in children. J Bone Joint Surg *62A*:1159, 1980.
591. DeLee JC, Evans JA, Thomas J: Anterior dislocation of the hip and associated femoral head fractures. J Bone Joint Surg *62A*:960, 1980.
592. Jayakumar S: Slipped capital femoral epiphysis with hypothyroidism treated by nonoperative method. Clin Orthop Rel Res *151*:179, 1980.
593. Newberg AH, Seligson D: The patellofemoral joint: 30°, 60°, and 90° views. Radiology *137*:57, 1980.

64

THERMAL AND ELECTRICAL INJURIES

by Donald Resnick, M.D.

Exposure of the human body to extremes in temperature or to electricity can lead to significant abnormality. Osseous and articular structures may participate in the body's response to such insult, and the changes that are induced may be irreparable. Chapter 64 summarizes musculoskeletal manifestations of thermal and electrical injury.

FROSTBITE

Terminology and General Abnormalities

Local damage can follow nonfreezing (immersion foot) and freezing (frostbite) injuries.[1] *Immersion foot* is related to prolonged exposure to low but not freezing temperatures in combination with persistent dampness.[2] Typical examples of immersion foot occur in soldiers (trench foot) and in survivors of shipwrecks. Contributory to the tissue injury in this entity are prolonged exposure to cold and dampness, immobility and dependency of the extremities, semistarvation, dehydration, and exhaustion. Singly or in combination, these factors lead to hypoxic injury in response to decreased blood flow to the affected body part. Plasma escapes through the injured capillary wall, producing edema, which further compromises the integrity of the vascular supply to nerve and muscle tissue. The resulting clinical manifestations pass through three distinct stages: an ischemic stage of hours to days in which cold, pulseless, and anesthetic extremities are seen; a hyperemic stage lasting 1 to 12 weeks in which a bounding, pulsatile circulation is associated with tissue swelling, blistering, and weeping; and a posthyperemic recovery phase, with restoration of normal vascular tones, skin color, and temperature. Although gangrene and necrosis of skin are frequent in the hyperemic stage, and induration and fibrosis of subcutaneous tissue with limitation of joint motion may be seen for several years following the injury, complete recovery in immersion foot is common.

Frostbite differs from immersion foot in that blood vessels are severely or irreparably injured, the circulation of blood ceases, and the vascular beds within the frozen tissue are occluded by thrombi and cellular aggregation.[3] Frostbite results from exposure to cold air that is usually at a temperature below −13° C (8° F). Once the freezing process has been initiated, it progresses rapidly, and superficially located tissue, such as that in the ears, nose, and digits, is increasingly damaged by the formation of tiny crystals of ice. The involved cutaneous areas are firm or hard, white, and numb. In part, the cutaneous injury consists of a separation of the epidermal-dermal interface.[3]

Musculoskeletal Abnormalities

Pathogenesis. The development and progression of frostbite injuries are directly related to abnormality in circulation.[4-8] During the period of exposure, vascular spasm in the involved extremities is evident. With warming or thawing of the injured parts, vasodilatation leads to increased permeability of the vascular wall, transudation of fluid, perivascular edema, and intravascular stasis, with agglutination of erythrocytes and deposition of fibrin. In this latter stage, vasoconstriction may persist in less damaged areas.

Angiography can be utilized to assess these

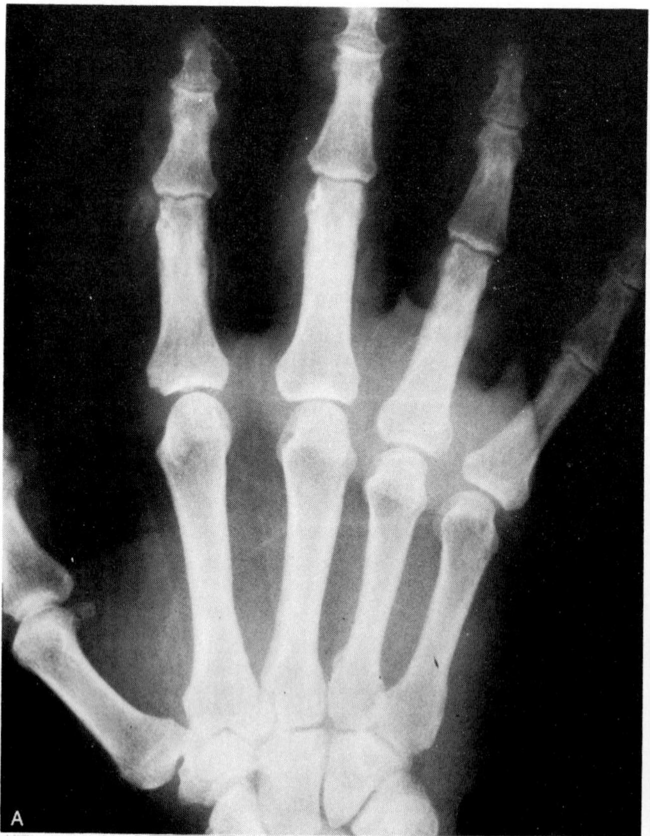

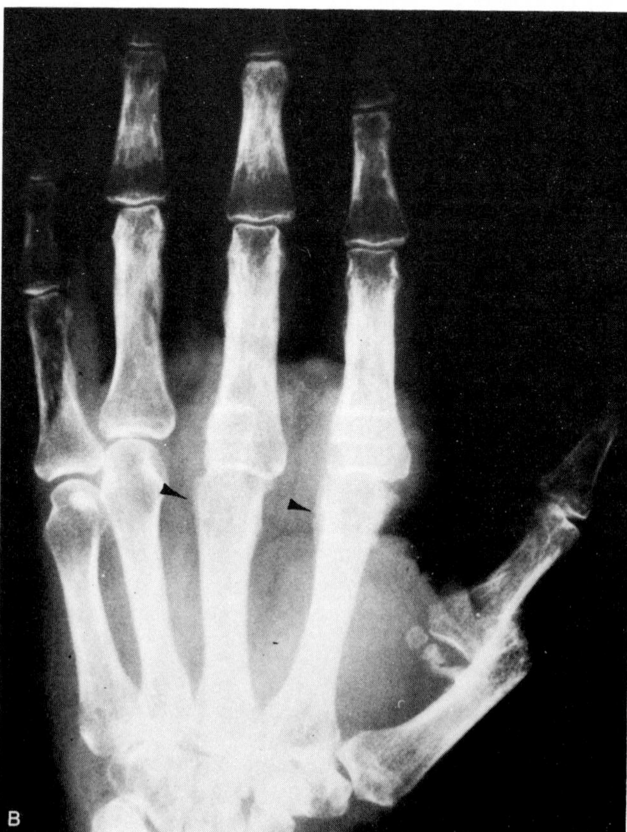

Figure 64–1. *Frostbite: Early changes.*

A *Observe soft tissue swelling, especially of the second through fifth digits. Osteoporosis and small cystic lucent areas are also evident.*

B *At a somewhat later stage in another patient, note soft tissue swelling, osteoporosis, periostitis (arrowheads), osteolysis, and subluxation of metacarpophalangeal articulations. (**B**, Courtesy of Dr. M. Dalinka, University of Pennsylvania, Philadelphia, Pennsylvania.)*

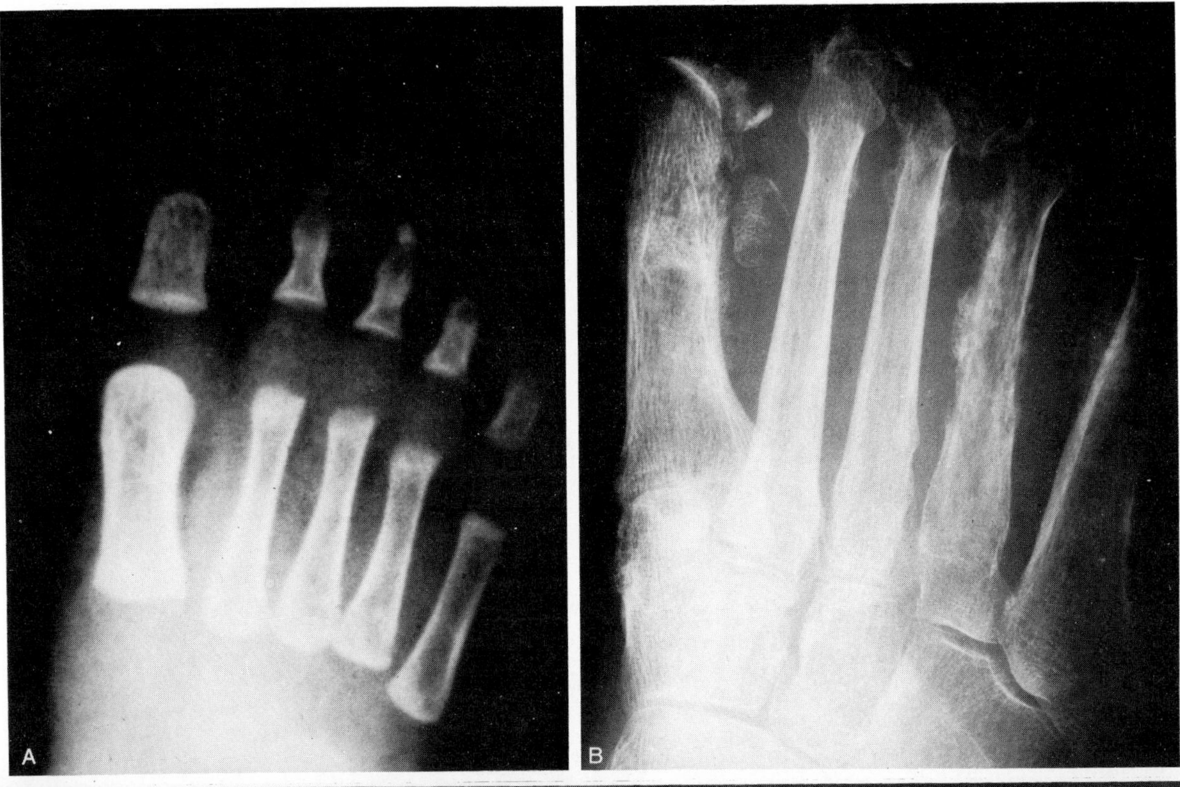

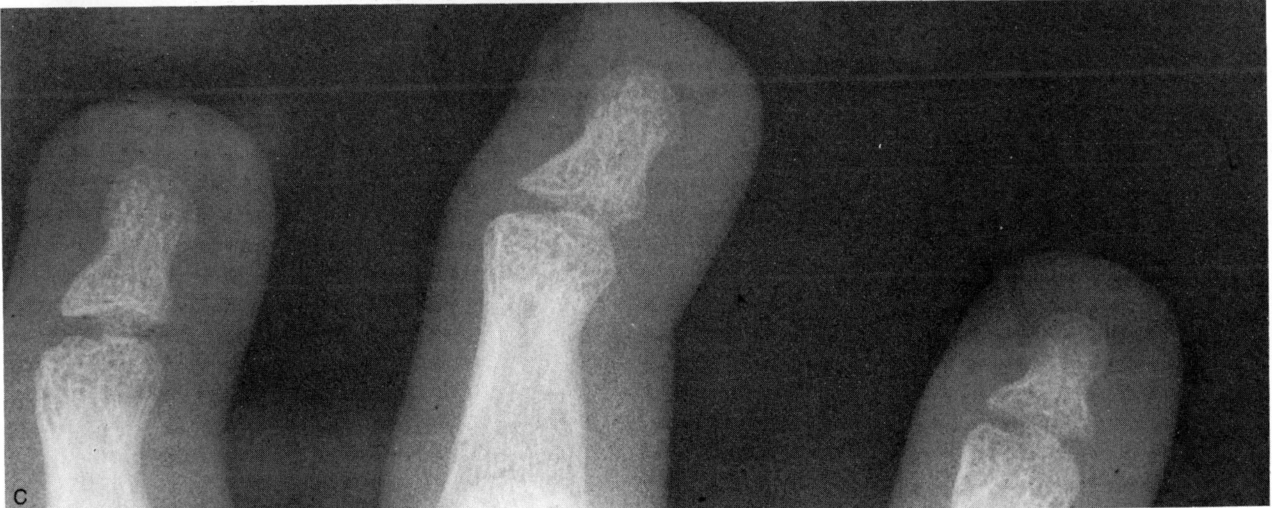

Figure 64–2. Frostbite: Late changes.

A *This baby was left as a newborn on a doorstep in subzero weather. At the time this radiograph was taken, the child's chronologic age was 11 months, although the skeletal bone age is markedly retarded. Also note amputation of multiple phalanges in the toes.* (**A,** *Courtesy of Dr. R. Fellow, Fairbanks Memorial Hospital, Fairbanks, Alaska.*)

B *This 75 year old man had a previous history of severe frostbite involving the hands and the feet. Recently he had developed soft tissue swelling and infection in the lower extremity. The changes on this roentgenogram, which include soft tissue swelling, acro-osteolysis, and ill-defined destruction of the metatarsals with periostitis, can be attributed to frostbite or infection, or both.*

C *Epiphyseal destruction and disappearance can occur following frostbite in children.* (**C,** *Courtesy of Dr. M. Dalinka, University of Pennsylvania, Philadelphia, Pennsylvania.*)

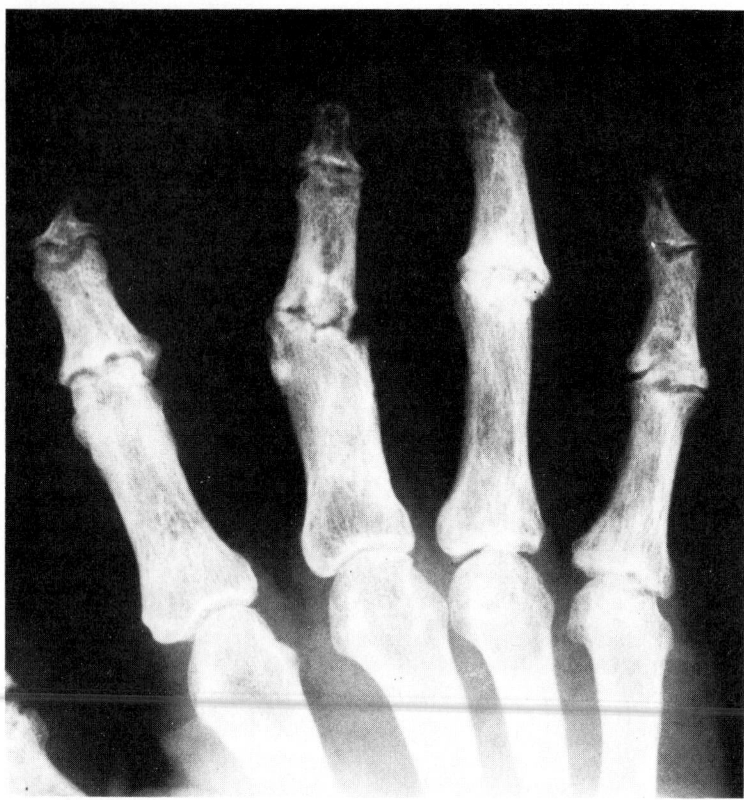

Figure 64–3. Frostbite: Interphalangeal joint abnormalities. In addition to acro-osteolysis, osseous and cartilaginous destruction is evident in the proximal interphalangeal, distal interphalangeal, and, to a lesser extent, metacarpophalangeal articulations. Subchondral erosion and collapse, sclerosis, osteophytosis, and joint space narrowing with or without intra-articular bony ankylosis simulate the findings of inflammatory (erosive) osteoarthritis. (Courtesy of Dr. M. Dalinka, University of Pennsylvania, Philadelphia, Pennsylvania.)

vascular changes.[9-12] Varying degrees of vasospasm as well as vascular stenosis and occlusion can be identified. Proliferation of collateral vessels involving both arterial and venous components occurs in the recovery phase.[5, 13] Transcatheter administration of sympathetic blocking agents may have a role in the treatment of vasospasm complicating frostbite.[9]

Radiographic Abnormalities. Bony and articular manifestations of frostbite are apparently related to cellular injury and necrosis from the freezing process itself or from the vascular insufficiency it produces.[14] Findings are most marked in the hands and the feet, and their severity depends on the length of exposure and the prevailing temperature.

Initially, no abnormality may be apparent. Early radiographic manifestations include soft tissue swelling and loss of tissue, especially at the tips of the digits; osteoporosis and periostitis may occur at a slightly later stage (Fig. 64–1). In the hand, the findings predominate in the four ulnar digits; sparing of the thumb is characteristic although not invariable, and can be attributed to clenching of the fist with the thumb clasped in the palm during the exposure to cold.

Late skeletal manifestations are variable (Fig. 64–2). In children, epiphyseal abnormalities are frequent.[14-20] The epiphyseal injuries involve primarily the distal phalanges, although other phalangeal epiphyses and, rarely, metacarpal (or metatarsal) epiphyses can be affected. Fragmentation, destruction, and disappearance of epiphyseal centers are seen. Premature epiphyseal fusion is also noted, resulting in brachydactyly. Metaphyseal irregularities consist of expansion and coarse trabeculation. Secondary infection of bone or joint can develop. Injury to articular cartilage can lead to an arthritis that is symptomatic and disabling.[63] Chondrocyte injury may relate to vascular changes or direct effect of the depressed temperature.

Interphalangeal joint abnormalities may eventually simulate those of osteoarthritis[16, 21-23] (Fig. 64–3). Unilateral or bilateral changes with joint space narrowing, sclerosis, osteophytosis, and soft tissue hypertrophy are seen. Juxta-articular punched-out cystic defects may also be observed.[22] Deformity and deviation can result from uneven digital involvement.[20] Tuftal resorption of terminal phalanges can be traced to loss of overlying soft tissue structures. Unilateral changes and the presence of subchondral cysts may aid in differentiating frostbite arthritis from osteoarthritis.[63, 64] Acute bouts of interphalangeal arthritis occurring years after the exposure to cold temperatures have been described.[64]

Frostbite injury of the ears can become manifest as calcification and ossification of the pinna.[24, 25] Cartilage calcification at this site following cold injury must be differentiated from that due to mechanical trauma, hyperparathyroidism, calcium pyrophosphate dihydrate crystal deposition disease, gout, Addison's disease, alkaptonuria, and acromegaly.[25]

Other Diagnostic Modalities

The role of arteriography in the diagnosis and treatment of frostbite has been noted above. In addition, scintiscanning with bone-seeking pharmaceuticals can be utilized to assess the viability of involved osseous tissue.[26] The uptake of radionuclide in the region of frostbite is dependent upon the integrity of the vascular tree; absence of such uptake indicates bone that lacks vascular perfusion, providing useful information to the surgeon.

Differential Diagnosis

The normal occurrence of sclerosis of one or more epiphyses ("ivory" epiphyses) should not be misinterpreted as evidence of epiphyseal necrosis following frostbite. Thiemann disease (epiphyseal acrodysplasia) is a poorly defined condition occurring predominantly in men in their late teens, in which swelling of the fingers is associated with epiphyseal irregularity, sclerosis, and fragmentation, particularly of the proximal and middle phalanges.[27-29] Although a dominant inheritance has been noted in some patients with Thiemann disease, its exact etiology is unknown. The distribution of epiphyseal abnormalities (changes predominate in proximal and middle phalanges, especially in the third finger, with sparing of the distal phalanges) differs from that in frostbite. Rarely, Volkmann's ischemia can apparently be associated with epiphyseal growth arrest.[15]

Ungual tuftal resorption can occur in a variety of conditions other than frostbite, including collagen vascular disease, epidermolysis bullosa, neuroarthropathy, hyperparathyroidism, and psoriatic arthritis. In these conditions, the thumb is frequently affected, and other, more diagnostic findings are generally present.

THERMAL BURNS

General Abnormalities

Thermal injury results in coagulative tissue necrosis.[30] An inflammatory response is evoked, with subsequent changes in cellular structure and configuration.[31] The thickness of burn injury is related to the magnitude of the heat exposure. A second degree burn implies that coagulative necrosis involves only the epidermis and part of the dermis, and that there are elements available for epithelial regeneration; a third degree burn implies death of tissue to such an extent that epithelial regeneration cannot occur.[32] In both second and third degree burns, massive outpouring of protein-rich fluid is due to both endothelial capillary damage and interference with normal lymphatic absorption. Secondary bacterial invasion is frequent, and may contribute to ischemic necrosis of tissue by the presence of perivascular infiltration and arterial thrombosis.

Musculoskeletal Abnormalities

Thermal burns can produce significant skeletal and soft tissue abnormalities. Such abnormalities are generally more frequent and severe in children than in adults, perhaps related to a more exuberant response of the immature skeleton to injury.[33] The changes may involve the bone, the joint, or the periarticular tissue; the pathogenesis of many of the findings is not clear.[33-38]

The incidence of radiographic changes following burns is dependent upon the severity of the thermal injury and the method of radiographic examination. Schiele and associates[39] observed osteoporosis in 34 per cent and heterotopic calcification and ossification in 23 per cent of 70 patients with upper extremity burns.

RADIOGRAPHIC ABNORMALITIES. Early radiographic alterations include soft tissue loss, osteoporosis, and periostitis; late alterations include articular and periarticular changes and growth disturbances.

Soft Tissue Loss. Necrosis of soft tissue following a burn produces a decrease in its outline on radiographic examination. This finding can occur during the acute stage or in chronic stages subsequent to further loss of skin and subcutaneous structures.

Osteoporosis. Osteoporosis is the most frequent bony response to thermal burns[33-35] (Fig. 64–4). It may be localized to the burned area or more generalized in distribution. The pathogenesis of such osteoporosis probably includes immobilization and disuse, a reflex vasomotor response, or a metabolic reaction to tissue destruction. Osteoporosis is more extensive in cases of severe burn or long immobilization.

In the burned region, localized hyperemia can produce osteoporosis, which, depending upon the distribution of the burn, can be unilateral or bilateral in appearance, although symmetric changes are somewhat unusual. Osteoporosis can appear within a period of weeks to months following injury, and with increased mobilization of the patients during the recovery phase, the finding may diminish or disappear completely.

Periostitis. Generally, periosteal bone formation appears within a period of months following the injury in those bones that underlie areas of severe burn[33] (Fig. 64–4). It represents a local response to periosteal irritation and in tubular bones produces

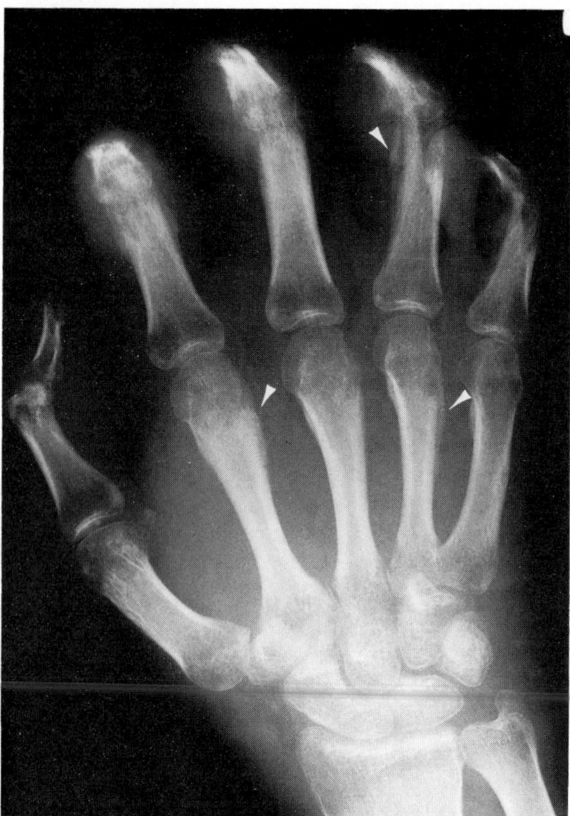

Figure 64–4. Thermal burn: Early changes. The early radiographic findings in this patient who had burned his hand include diffuse soft tissue swelling, soft tissue and bony loss of the digits, severe periarticular osteoporosis, and periostitis, especially of the phalanges and metacarpals (arrowheads).

diaphyseal and metaphyseal changes that are similar to those in hypertrophic osteoarthropathy.

Osteophytosis. Periarticular osseous excrescences that attach to the underlying bone are more frequent in adults than children. Although they cannot always be clearly differentiated from soft tissue calcification and ossification, these outgrowths may contain recognizable trabeculae and appear to arise from the subjacent bone. They are most prevalent about the elbow, where they appear at the articular margins of the olecranon or coronoid process (Fig. 64–5). They lie in the planes of ligaments and correspond histologically to new bone formation in a fibrous connective tissue stroma.[33] Osteophytes are invariably associated with adjacent burns of the soft tissue and are a response to the thermal injury itself or to the stress of nearby atrophic ligaments. Their course is variable; they may gradually decrease in size or progress, leading to complete osseous bridging of the articulation.[62]

Periarticular Calcification and Ossification. The appearance of irregular periarticular calcification is not infrequent within one or more months following thermal injury. The deposits create ill-defined and flocculent radiodense areas that are separate from the underlying bone. They are most commonly found about the elbow, near the radial head, or along the anterior and posterior surfaces of the distal humerus.[39] Calcification can remain unchanged in extent or become incorporated into enlarging areas of soft tissue ossification.

Periarticular ossification is most commonly encountered about the hip, the elbow, and the glenohumeral joint (Fig. 64–5). Such ossification usually becomes evident in the second or third months following injury,[33] although it may occasionally occur as early as the fourth or fifth week.[39] The relationships among heterotopic bone formation, periarticular calcification, and osteophytosis are not clear, although all three abnormalities may represent various stages of the same process and frequently occur at the same location. Heterotopic ossification is intimately associated with the surrounding musculature, although it does not appear to replace the muscle tissue. The bony ridges commonly attach to the adjacent osseous structure. When extensive, ossification is accompanied by a decrease in joint mobility.

The pathogenesis of heterotopic calcification and ossification following burns is unknown. Although the deposits may be prominent in proximity to the area of burn, calcification and bone formation can also be observed in the contralateral unburned extremity.[33, 40] Thus, superimposed mechanical trauma, immobility, and vascular alterations may be important in the development of periarticular calcific and ossific deposits following burns (as well as following neurologic injury). In this regard, Schiele and colleagues[39] were unable to detect a correlation between the occurrence of heterotopic ossification and either the per cent total body surface burned or the average extent of third degree burns, suggesting that factors other than the burn itself were important in the appearance of periarticular radiodense shadows.

Acromutilation. Acromutilation with partial or complete loss of phalanges can be a prominent finding when the hand or the foot is burned[36, 39] (Fig. 64–6). Adjacent soft tissue loss is typical.

Abnormalities in Bone Growth. Increased bone growth can be seen in children who are burned, presumably as a result of hyperemia. Even in adults, a similar phenomenon has been observed.[33]

Articular Abnormalities. Progressive destruction of one or more joints with eventual fibrous or bony ankylosis can be evident following thermal burns.[33, 39, 41-42] Destruction may appear within a period of a few weeks, and ankylosis may appear within a few months. These changes can occur either close to the initial site of injury or at a remote site. The elbow, the hip, the ankle, and the articulations of the hand are most typically affected (Fig. 64–7).

Initially, fusiform soft tissue swelling and osteoporosis can be observed about the involved articulation. Progressive loss of interosseous space and

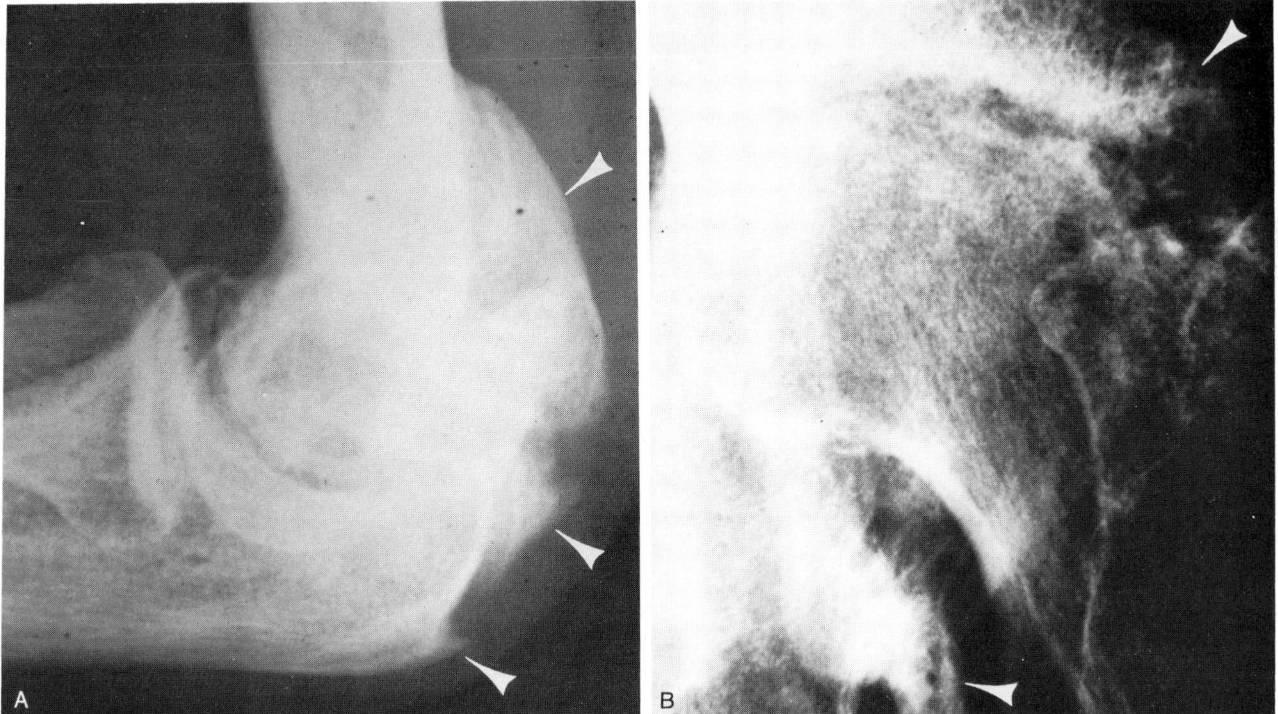

Figure 64–5. *Thermal burn: Osteophytes, soft tissue calcification, and ossification.*
A *Several months following a thermal burn, local ossification (arrowheads) appears along the posterior surface of the humerus and ulna.*
B *In the hip of another patient, observe osseous excrescences (arrowheads) in the acetabulum and intra-articular cartilaginous and bony destruction with reactive sclerosis.*

subchondral irregularity are seen. Eventually, intra-articular osseous fusion may result.

Thermal injury, mechanical trauma, infection, neuroarthropathy, and immobilization have all been considered as possible factors in the pathogenesis of these articular changes. The fact that joint alterations can occur in areas that are not burned indicates that agents other than the thermal injury itself must be implicated in their pathogenesis. Although minor or significant mechanical trauma may occur during positioning or movement of the burn patient, and can even lead to fracture, subluxation, and dislocation, this factor does not appear to be responsible for many of the articular manifestations of burns. Bacteremia with hematogenous dissemination of infection to bones and joints may account for some of the destructive articular changes,[33, 39, 43] although the lack of substantial pathologic evidence of joint sepsis and the poor correlation between the degree of sepsis and the amount of articular destruction are noteworthy. Nerve injury leading to neuroarthropathy does not appear to be a significant factor in these joint manifestations.

Chondral lysis and atrophy following immobilization due to interference with normal pathways of cartilaginous nutrients may be a prominent cause of the joint space loss and ankylosis that accompany thermal burns.[42] Indeed, immobilization and compression of joint surfaces have been found experimentally to cause acute necrosis of cartilage.[44-46] Closely applied cartilaginous surfaces can be associated with chondrocyte death and chondral degen-

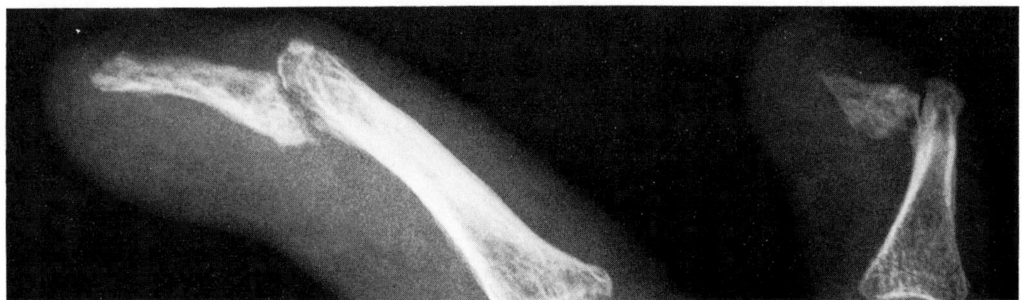

Figure 64–6. *Thermal burn: Acromutilation. Observe the terminal phalangeal destruction of two burned digits. Joint destruction and subluxation are also evident.*

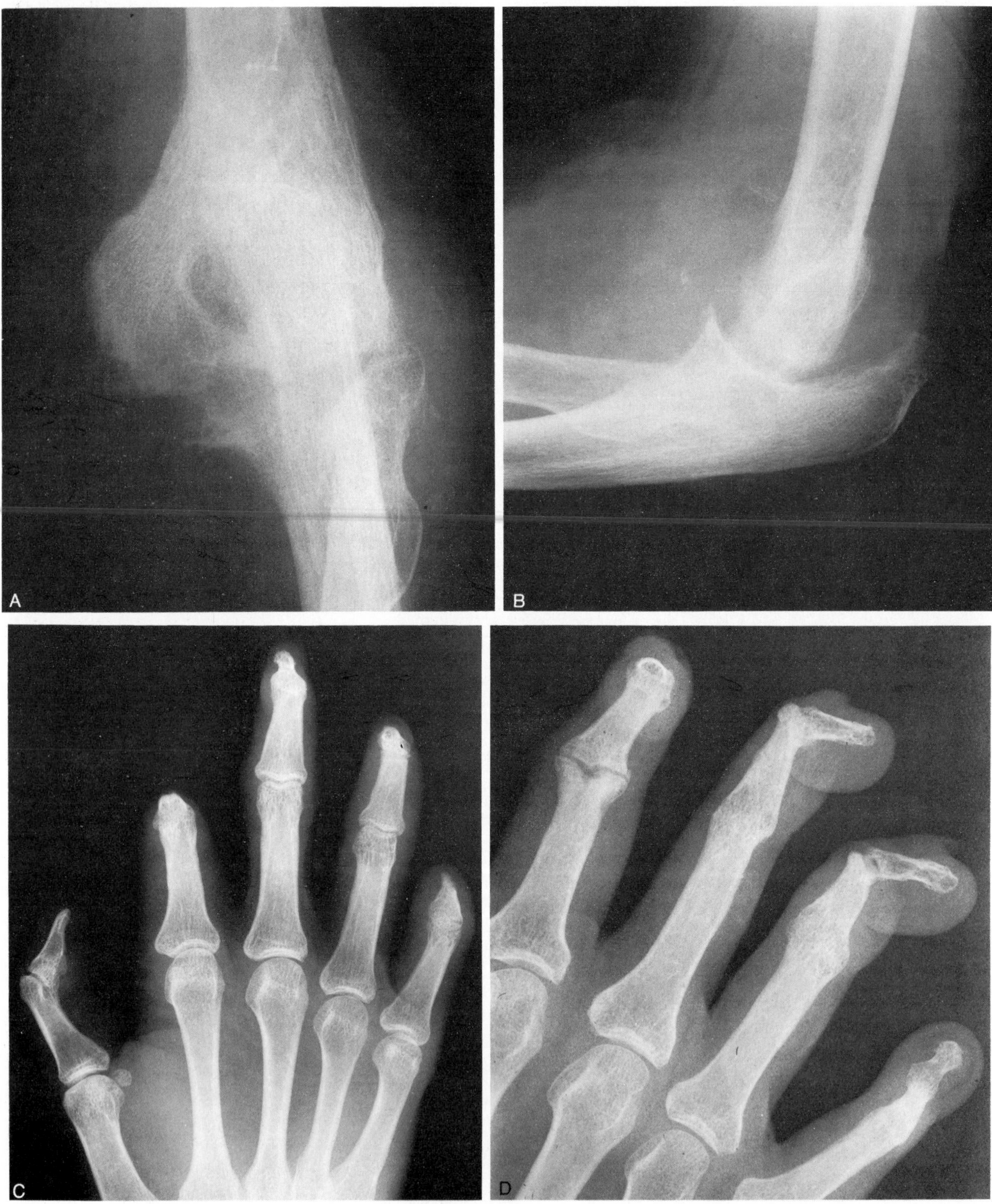

Figure 64–7. *Thermal burn: Articular abnormalities.*

A, B *This 54 year old man developed destructive changes of the elbow following severe burns. Findings, which include osteoporosis, soft tissue swelling, an effusion, and osteolysis and fragmentation of the humerus, radius, and ulna, simulate those of infection or neuroarthropathy.*

C, D *Two examples of articular and osseous changes following burns of the hand. Note osteolysis with deformity of phalanges and intra-articular osseous fusion.*

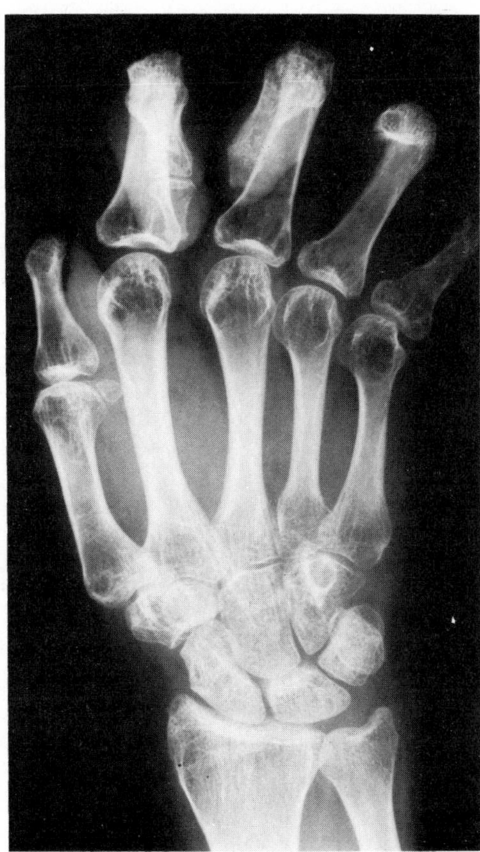

Figure 64–8. Thermal burn: Contractures. Flexion contractures of the digits, osteolysis, and osteoporosis represent the sequelae of a burn that had occurred many years previously.

eration, whereas unapposed cartilage may remain relatively viable. During immobilization of burn patients, the intimacy of the articular surfaces and the stasis of the synovial fluid may produce chondrolysis.[42] A similar phenomenon may accompany paralysis or immobilization for treatment of slipped capital femoral epiphyses[47, 48] or scoliosis.[49]

Contractures. Contractures due to soft tissue and muscular changes in the burn patient are frequent, especially about the elbow and the hand.[32,50] Joint malalignment, subluxation, and dislocation as well as disuse osteoporosis may be evident (Fig. 64–8).

Differential Diagnosis

The radiographic features of osteoporosis, periarticular calcification and ossification, joint space loss, intra-articular bony ankylosis, and contracture that are encountered in burn patients may also be seen following paralysis (or immobilization). Heterotopic ossification in these situations is identical; it may occur in the area of the thermal injury or neurologic defect, although it may also be noted in remote locations, suggesting that common factors may be operational. Accurate differential diagnosis is often dependent upon appropriate clinical history.

In some patients with thermal burns, articular abnormalities resemble those in pyogenic arthritis and may reflect an accompanying bacteremia with septic embolization.

Phalangeal tuftal resorption or destruction following burns must be differentiated from similar changes occurring in association with frostbite, collagen vascular disorders, and articular diseases.

ELECTRICAL BURNS

General Abnormalities

Electricity can produce severe injury or death. The extent of bodily harm is dependent upon the type of electricity, the voltage, the water content of tissues, and the points of entry and exit of the charge.[51, 52] Alternating currents produce tetanization of muscles and sweating; direct currents produce electrolytic changes in the tissues.[53] Alternating currents are estimated to be approximately four to five times more dangerous than direct currents; fatal electrocution can be produced by exposure to household circuits of 115 volts at 60 cycles.[53]

The pathway of the current influences the body's response to injury. Electrical injury associated with a relatively short route from a point of entry in an arm to a point of exit in a finger is associated with less tissue damage than an injury in which the electricity enters the head and exits at the foot. The duration of contact is also crucial. With alternating currents, muscular contraction following injury may prevent the individual's releasing the source of electricity, leading to more prolonged and severe tissue damage. Furthermore, the electrical conductivity of tissues influences their susceptibility to injury from electricity. Structures with a high water content, such as the vascular tree, the muscles, and the perspiring skin, are good conductors, whereas the bones are tissues of high resistance.

Electrical energy is converted to heat in traversing the skin.[53] Resulting burns are accentuated by vascular spasm, leading to electrical necrosis. Death from low voltage electrical injury (below 200 volts) is usually due to ventricular fibrillation; death related to high voltage electricity (greater than 1000 volts) is due to inhibition of the respiratory center in the brain.[54]

Musculoskeletal Abnormalities

Severe injury induced by electricity is much more common in adults than in children because of

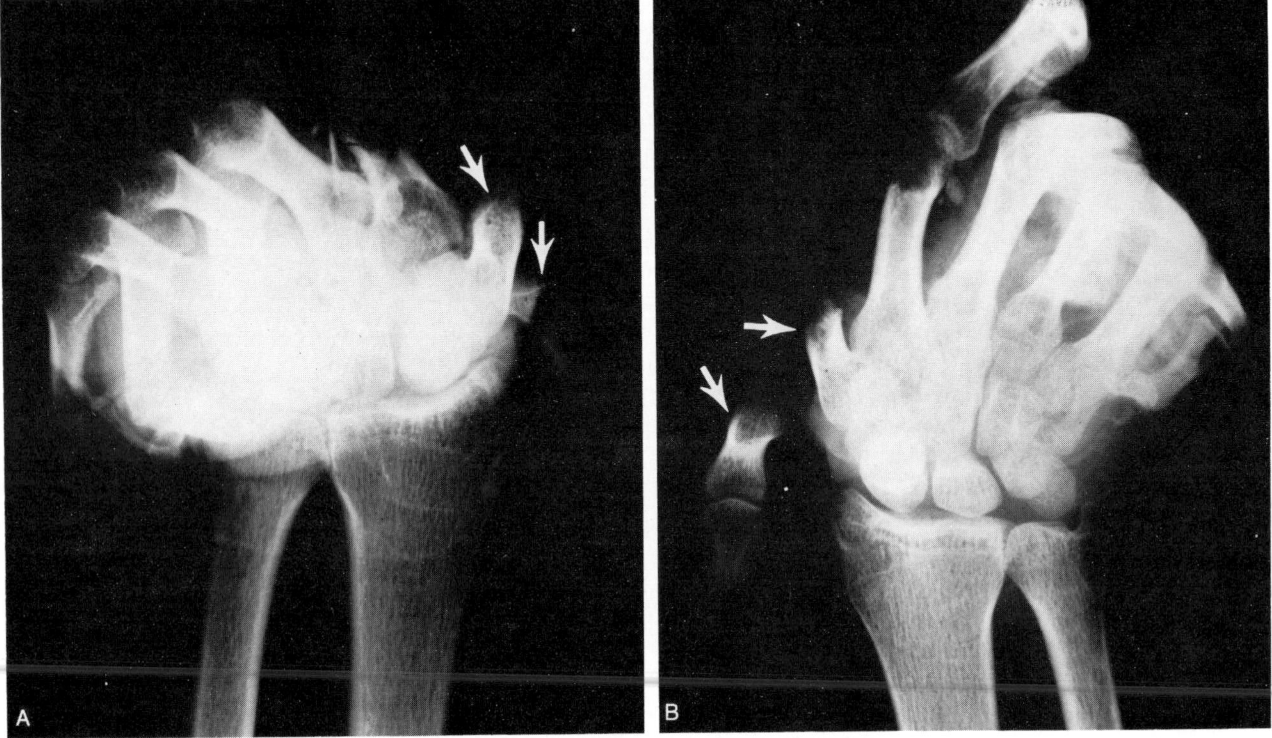

Figure 64–9. *Electrical burn. This man developed changes after touching a high tension wire.*
A, B *The severe alterations in both hands resulted from sustained grasping of the wire. They include contracture, soft tissue injury, subluxation, dislocation, and fracture (arrows).*

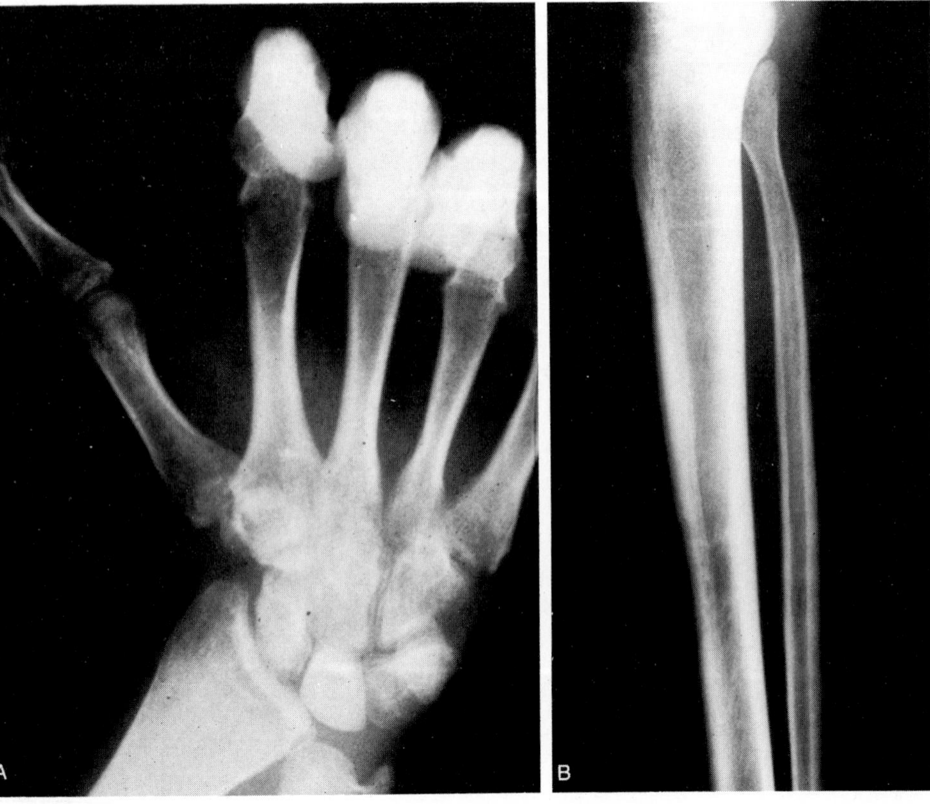

Figure 64–10. Electrical burn. *A 21 year old man came into contact with a high tension wire, resulting in a severe injury to both hands (entrance wounds) and to the pretibial regions (exit wounds).*

A *A radiograph of a hand reveals contractures of multiple digits and periarticular osteoporosis.*

B Osteolysis *of the mid-diaphysis of the tibia reflects bony changes at the point of exit of the electric current.*

(Courtesy of Drs. J. Barry, University of California, San Diego, California, and J. Ogden, Yale University, New Haven, Connecticut.)

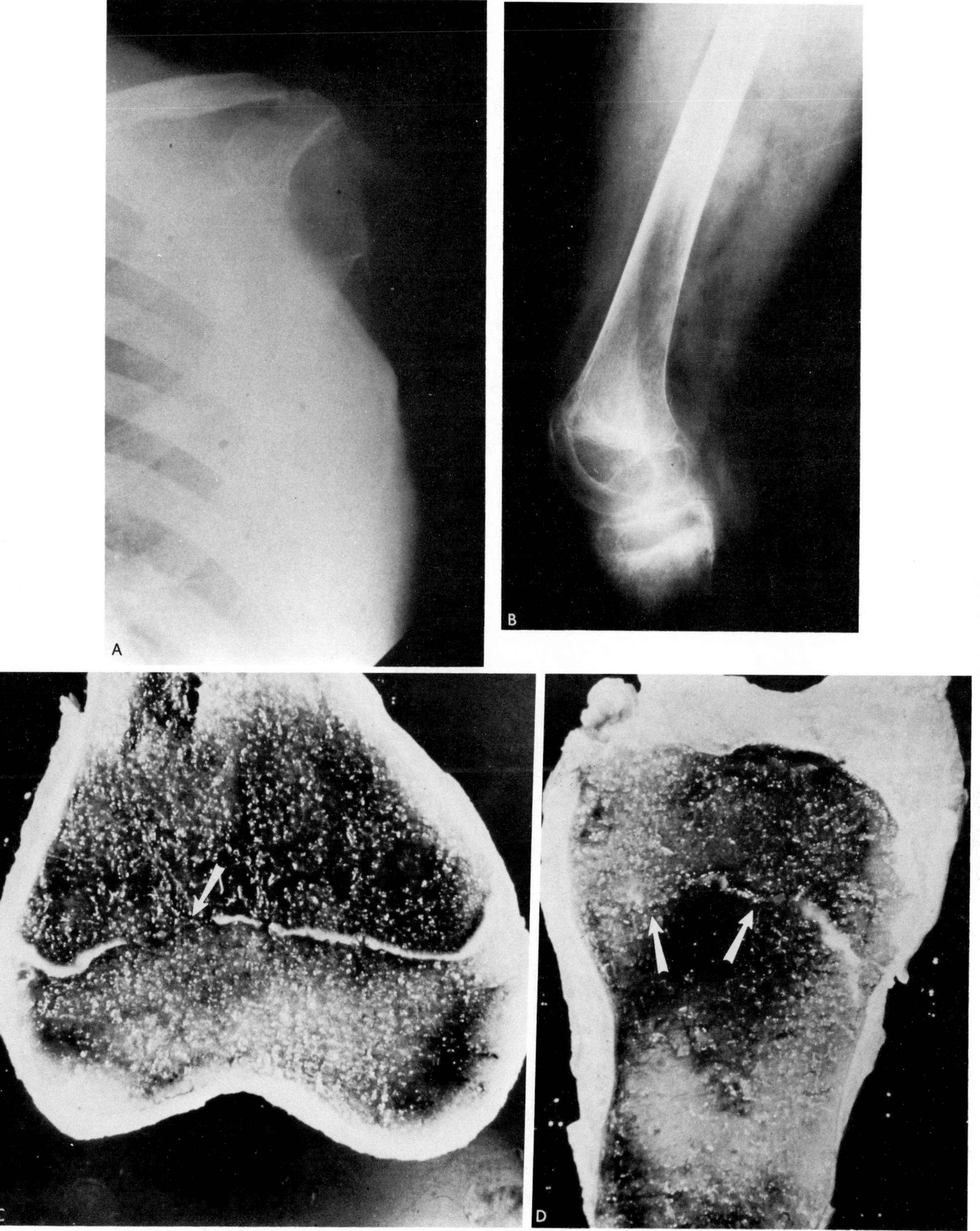

Figure 64–11. *Electrical burn. This 17 year old boy developed injuries following contact with a high tension wire. He required an immediate amputation of one leg and one arm. Subsequently, a phalangeal amputation of the opposite arm and an extension of his leg amputation were also necessary.*

A *A radiograph of the shoulder demonstrates the site of amputation, tapering of the distal clavicle, and glenoid osteoporosis.*

B *A lateral roentgenogram of the femur and knee reveals the site of amputation, osteoporosis, sclerosis, and a coarsened trabecular pattern. There is loss of joint space and irregularity of the growth plate.*

C, D *Coronal sections of the distal femur* **(C)** *and proximal tibia* **(D)** *reveal premature fusion of the growth plates (arrows), presumably an effect of the electric current itself.*

(Courtesy of Drs. J. Barry, University of California, San Diego, California, and J. Ogden, Yale University, New Haven, Connecticut.)

the increased occupational risk in the former age group. The hand, because of its grasping function, is the most commonly affected area in the body. Severe skin burns are encountered at the point of entry and exit of the electrical charge. Osseous and articular changes relate to the effects of heat, mechanical trauma from accompanying uncoordinated muscle spasm, neural and vascular tissue damage, infection, disuse or immobilization, and perhaps a specific effect of the electricity itself.[55]

Initial roentgenographic features include loss of cutaneous, subcutaneous, and osseous tissues owing to tissue charring. Other findings are soft tissue hematomas; compression fractures of the spine, dislocation of joints, and avulsions at tendinous insertions related to muscle spasm; and various fractures due to accompanying falls[56] (Fig. 64–9). Small, rounded osseous dense lesions resembling wax drippings may be attributable to melting of the bone due to the intense heat.[56] Focal tiny disruptions in bony continuity (microfractures) may also be a direct effect of the heat.[57, 58] They can possess a zig-zag contour with discrete margins and may occur anywhere along the route of electricity. Osteolysis and periostitis are also encountered[55] (Figs. 64–10 and 64–11). Epiphyseal fragmentation and osteochondral fractures may be noted.[56]

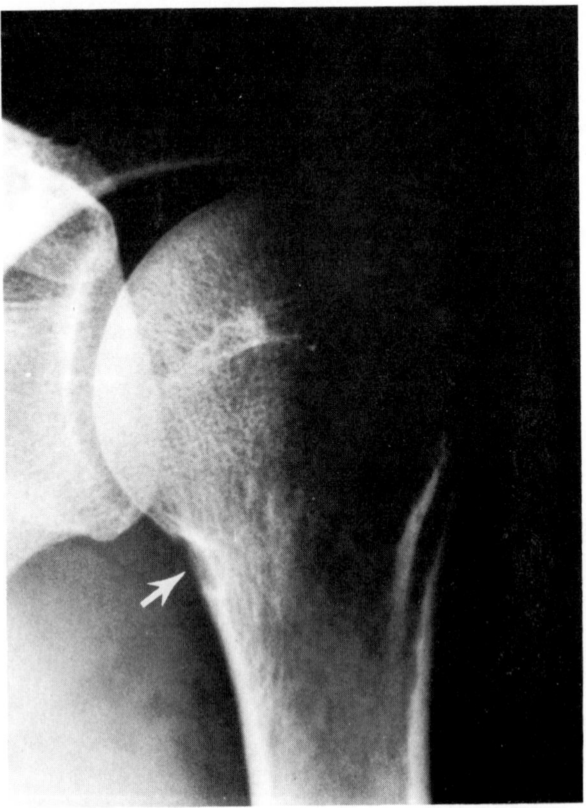

Figure 64–12. *Electrical burn. A 48 year old woman developed an electrical injury with a point of entrance in the hand and a point of exit in the shoulder. The small, eccentric, cortical lucent lesion (arrow) evident in the proximal humerus months later is consistent with bone lysis at the exit point following an electrical burn.*

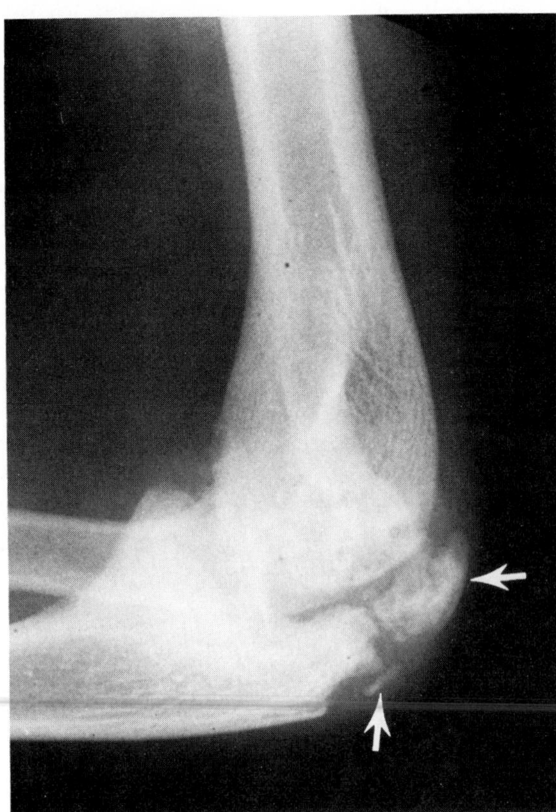

Figure 64–13. *Electrical burn. Bony fragmentation, periarticular calcification and ossification (arrows), and joint contracture occur at sites remote from an electrical burn. (Courtesy of Drs. J. Barry, University of California, San Diego, California, and J. Ogden, Yale University, New Haven, Connecticut.)*

Delayed musculoskeletal alterations, which may appear months or years later, are related predominantly to ischemia.[59] Osteonecrosis, which develops at sites distal to the entry and exit wounds, may be attributed to periosteal stripping or damage to the vascular wall with thrombosis. Medullary lucent areas in the diaphyses and metaphyses of tubular bones, endosteal resorption with medullary expansion, cystic rarefactions, cortical sequestration, and epiphyseal collapse and fragmentation can be evident (Fig. 64–12). Accelerated bone growth and premature fusion of damaged epiphyses may follow electrical injury in children (Fig. 64–11).[61] Secondary infection with osteomyelitis and septic arthritis, nonunion of pathologic fractures, neuroarthropathy, and contracture with joint subluxation or dislocation have also been described. Periarticular calcification and ossification (Fig. 64–13), and intra-articular bony ankylosis may eliminate joint motion.[55] Some of these osseous and soft tissue changes have been reproduced experimentally.[60]

Differential Diagnosis

The radiographic findings following this type of injury represent a combination of thermal, mechani-

Table 64–1

RADIOGRAPHIC FINDINGS ASSOCIATED WITH THERMAL AND ELECTRICAL INJURIES

Soft tissue swelling, loss, or contracture
Osteoporosis
Acro-osteolysis
Periostitis
Epiphyseal injury and growth disturbance
Articular abnormalities
Periarticular calcification and ossification
Osteolysis, osteosclerosis, and fracture

cal, and electrical effects on bones and joints. They are complicated by vascular and neurologic damage and secondary infection. The resulting roentgenographic picture is nonspecific; some of the radiographic abnormalities are identical to those following trauma from any cause, whereas others resemble those of septic arthritis, neuroarthropathy, osteoporosis, thermal burns, frostbite, and neurologic deficit.

SUMMARY

The radiographic features of the skeleton following thermal and electrical injuries can be varied (Table 64–1). In many cases, they are not specific and must be interpreted with knowledge of the mechanism of injury. Of particular interest are the appearance of epiphyseal abnormalities in frostbite, periarticular calcification and ossification following thermal burns, and pathologic fractures in the electrocuted individual.

REFERENCES

1. Meryman HT: Tissue freezing and local cold injury. Physiol Rev *37*:233, 1957.
2. Ungley CC: The immersion foot syndrome. Adv Surg *1*:209, 1949.
3. Brauer RW, Behnke AR: Hypothermia and cold injury. *In* TR Harrison, et al (Eds): Principles of Internal Medicine. 4th Ed. New York, McGraw-Hill Book Co, 1962, p 835.
4. Bellman S, Adams-Ray J: Vascular reactions after experimental cold injury. A microangiographic study on rabbit ears. Angiology *7*:339, 1956.
5. Hurley LA: Angioarchitectural changes associated with rapid rewarming subsequent to freezing injury. Angiology *8*:19, 1957.
6. Martinez A, Golding M, Sawyer PN, Wesolowski SA: The specific arterial lesions in mild and severe frostbite: Effect of sympathectomy. J Cardiovasc Surg *7*:495, 1966.
7. Edwards EA, Leeper RW: Frostbite: An analysis of seventy-one cases. JAMA *149*:1199, 1952.
8. Quintanilla R, Krusen FH, Essex HE: Studies on frostbite with special reference to treatment and the effect on minute blood vessels. Am J Physiol *149*:149, 1947.
9. Gralino BJ, Porter JM, Rosch J: Angiography in the diagnosis and therapy of frostbite. Radiology *119*:301, 1976.
10. Tishler J: The soft tissue and bone changes in frostbite injuries. Radiology *102*:511, 1972.
11. Smith SP, Walker WF: Arteriography in cold injury. Br J Radiol *37*:471, 1964.
12. Erikson U, Ponten B: The possible value of arteriography supplemented by a vasodilator agent in the early assessment of tissue viability in frostbite. Injury *6*:150, 1974.
13. Likhoded VI: Angiografiia v diagnostike otmorozhenii. Vestn Khir *110*:90, 1973.
14. Bigelow DR, Ritchie GW: The effects of frostbite in childhood. J Bone Joint Surg *45B*:122, 1963.
15. Bennett RB, Blount WP: Destruction of epiphyses by freezing. JAMA *105*:661, 1935.
16. Dreyfuss JR, Glimcher MJ: Epiphyseal injury following frostbite. N Engl J Med *253*:1065, 1955.
17. Florkiewicz L, Kozlowski K: Symmetrical epiphyseal destruction by frostbite. Arch Dis Child *37*:51, 1962.
18. Thelander HE: Epiphyseal destruction by frostbite. J Pediatr *36*:105, 1950.
19. Wenzl JE, Burke EC, Bianco AJ: Epiphyseal destruction from frostbite of the hands. Am J Dis Child *114*:668, 1967.
20. Selke AC Jr: Destruction of phalangeal epiphyses by frostbite. Radiology *93*:859, 1969.
21. Ellis R, Short JG, Simonds BD: Unilateral osteoarthritis of the distal interphalangeal joints following frostbite. A case report. Radiology *93*:857, 1969.
22. Blair JR, Schatzki P, Orr KD: Sequelae to cold injury in one hundred patients. A follow-up study four years after occurrence of cold injury. JAMA *163*:1203, 1957.
23. Schumacher HR Jr: Unilateral osteoarthritis of the hand. JAMA *191*:246, 1965.
24. Sessions DG, Stallings JO, Mills WJ Jr, Beal DD: Frostbite of the ear. Laryngoscope *81*:1223, 1971.
25. Yeh CW, Chan KF: Case report 87. Skel Radiol *4*:49, 1979.
26. Lisbona R, Rosenthall L: Assessment of bone viability by scintiscanning in frostbite injuries. J Trauma *16*:989, 1976.
27. Thiemann H: Juvenile epiphysenstorungen. Fortschr Geb Roentgenstr Nuklearmed *14*:79, 1909.
28. Giedion A: Acrodysplasias: cone-shaped epiphyses, peripheral dysostosis, Thiemann's disease, and acrodysostosis. Progr Pediatr Radiol *4*:325, 1973.
29. Shaw EW: Avascular necrosis of the phalanges of the hand (Thiemann's disease). JAMA *156*:711, 1954.
30. Order SE, Moncrief JA: The Burn Wound. Springfield, Ill, Charles C Thomas, 1965.
31. Foley FD: Pathology of cutaneous burns. Surg Clin North Am *50*:1201, 1970.
32. Brown HC: Current concepts of burn pathology and mechanisms of deformity in the burned hand. Orthop Clin North Am *4*:987, 1973.
33. Evans EB, Smith JR: Bone and joint changes following burns. A roentgenographic study — preliminary report. J Bone Joint Surg *41A*:785, 1959.
34. Owens N: Osteoporosis following burns. Br J Plast Surg *1*:245, 1949.
35. Colson P, Stagnara P, Houot H: L'ostéoporose chez les brûlés des membres. Lyon Chir *48*:950, 1953.
36. Rabinov D: Acromutilation of the fingers following severe burns. Radiology *77*:968, 1961.
37. Boyd BM Jr, Roberts WM, Miller GR: Peri-articular ossification following burns. South Med J *52*:1048, 1959.
38. Evans EB: Orthopaedic measures in the treatment of severe burns. J Bone Joint Surg *48A*:643, 1966.
39. Schiele HP, Hubbard RB, Bruck HM: Radiographic changes in burns of the upper extremity. Radiology *104*:13, 1972.
40. Johnson JTH: Atypical myositis ossificans. J Bone Joint Surg *39A*:189, 1957.
41. Schwartz EE, Weiss W, Plotkin R: Ankylosis of the temporomandibular joint following burn. JAMA *235*:1477, 1976.
42. Pellicci PM, Wilson PD Jr: Chondrolysis of the hips associated with severe burns. A case report. J Bone Joint Surg *61A*:592, 1979.
43. Artz CP, Reiss E: The Treatment of Burns. Philadelphia, WB Saunders Co, 1957, p 169.
44. Thaxter TH, Mann RA: Factors contributing to the degeneration of immobilized normal synovial joints in rats. J Bone Joint Surg *46A*:921, 1964.
45. Trias A: Effects of persistent pressure on the articular cartilage. An experimental study. J Bone Joint Surg *43B*:376, 1961.
46. Salter RB, Field P: The effects of continuous compression on living articular cartilage. J Bone Joint Surg *42A*:31, 1960.
47. Cruess RL: The pathology of acute necrosis of cartilage in slipping of the capital femoral epiphysis. A report of two cases with pathological sections. J Bone Joint Surg *45A*:1013, 1963.
48. Maurer RC, Larsen IJ: Acute necrosis of cartilage in slipped capital femoral epiphysis. J Bone Joint Surg *52A*:39, 1970.
49. Heppenstall RB, Marvel JP Jr, Chung SMK, Brighton CT: Chondrolysis

of the hip joint — usual and unusual presentations. J Bone Joint Surg *55A*:1308, 1973.

50. Jackson D: Acquired vertical talus due to burn contractures. A report of two cases. J Bone Joint Surg *60B*:215, 1978.
51. Maclachlan W: Electrical injuries. J Ind Hyg *16*:52, 1934.
52. Langworthy OR, Kouwenhoven WB: An experimental study of abnormalities produced in the organism by electricity. J Ind Hyg *12*:31, 1930.
53. Bennett IL Jr: Electrical injury. *In* TR Harrison, et al (Eds): Principles of Internal Medicine. 4th Ed. New York, McGraw-Hill Book Co, 1962, p 855.
54. Pearl FL: Electric shock: Presentation of cases and review of the literature. Arch Surg *27*:227, 1933.
55. Brinn LB, Moseley JE: Bone changes following electrical injury. Case report and review of literature. Am J Roentgenol *97*:682, 1966.
56. Kolar J, Vrabec R: Roentgenological bone findings after high voltage injury. Fortschr Geb Roentgenstr Nuklearmed *92*:385, 1960.
57. Jellinek S: Roentgen bone changes found in the treatment of electrical accidents. Wien Med Wochenschr *79*:543, 1929.
58. Jellinek S: Changes in electrically injured bones: Examined microscopically and by x-rays. Br J Radiol *31*:23, 1926.
59. Barber JW: Delayed bone and joint changes following electrical injury. Radiology *99*:49, 1971.
60. Granberry WM, Janes JM: The effect of electrical current on the epiphyseal cartilage: A preliminary experimental study. Proc Mayo Clin *38*:87, 1963.
61. Ogden JA, Southwick WO: Electrical injury involving the immature skeleton. J Bone Joint Surg (in press).
62. Clark GS, Naso F, Ditunno JF Jr: Marked bone spur formation in a burn amputee patient. Arch Phys Med Rehabil *61*:189, 1980.
63. Carrera GF, Kozin F, McCarty DJ: Arthritis after frostbite injury in children. Arthritis Rheum *22*:1082, 1979.
64. Glick R, Parhami N: Frostbite arthritis. J Rheumatol *6*:456, 1979.

65

RADIATION CHANGES

by Murray K. Dalinka, M.D., and John A. Bonavita, M.D.

The use of X rays in diagnosis and therapy became well established shortly after Roentgen discovered them. The deleterious effects of radiation were noted as early as 6 months following Roentgen's initial description, with the development of pigmentation, telangiectasia, fibrosis, alopecia, scarring, ulceration, and dermatitis, which are recognized as precancerous changes.[13] Radiation-induced neoplasia was described in 1902 in a 33 year old demonstrator of x-ray tubes.[37]

The harmful side effects of radiation were soon publicized in the lay press, as evidenced by an editorial in a now-defunct London newspaper:

> "We are sick of the Roentgen Ray; . . . you can see other people's bones with the naked eye, and also see through 8″ of solid wood. On the revolting indecency of this there is no need to dwell. But what we seriously put before the attention of the government . . . that it will call for legislative restriction of the severest kind. Perhaps the best thing would be for all civilized nations to combine to burn all works on the roentgen rays, to execute all discoverers, and to corner all the tungstate in the world and whelm it in the middle of the ocean."[13]

Beck[5] later described neoplasms in patients irradiated for tuberculous arthritis, and Martland and Humphries[65] implicated radium as a cause of skeletal tumors in radium dial workers. This showed that the effects of radiation were independent of their method of production and could be produced by internal or external sources.[105, 106]

RADIUM

In 1924 Blum described radium jaw, a type of osteomyelitis seen in radium dial workers.[9] Workers who painted luminous dials on watches pointed the paintbrushes with their lips and teeth, causing them to ingest luminous paint containing radium (^{226}Ra) and mesothorium (^{228}Ra). The average mixture of the isotopes was approximately 6 to 1 (mesothorium to radium) and the radiation dosage for the mixture was 10 times that of radium.[52] The fluorescence of the watch dials came from the bombardment of the zinc sulfide in the paint by the alpha particles of radium and mesothorium.[52]

Radium has a half-life of 1622 years and emits continuous radiation, mostly alpha particles with a range of 40 micrometers in tissue.[52] Mesothorium has a half-life of 6.7 years, and thorium, its major daughter product, has a half-life of 52 seconds.[52]

Radium was used therapeutically, both orally and intravenously, in the treatment of many ailments between 1910 and 1930. Parenteral and oral radium preparations were not contaminated with mesothorium, but the effects on the osseous system were identical.[46, 61]

Oral radium is deposited mainly in the outer cortex of bone, with an irregular and generalized distribution.[65] With parenteral administration, the early peak blood level leads to "flush labeling" with an unequal distribution.[46]

In 1929 Martland and Humphries described osseous neoplasms in radium dial workers.[65] Similar neoplasms were later described secondary to oral and parenteral radium administration.[61] Squamous cell carcinomas of the mastoids and paranasal sinuses have been reported in dial workers.[46] This is not surprising in view of the proximity of the epithelium to underlying bone.

Many of the deaths in radium dial workers were secondary to severe aplastic anemia. Loutit postulated that this anemia may have been aleukemic leukemia.[62] He thought that radium might have a direct effect on the bone marrow.[62]

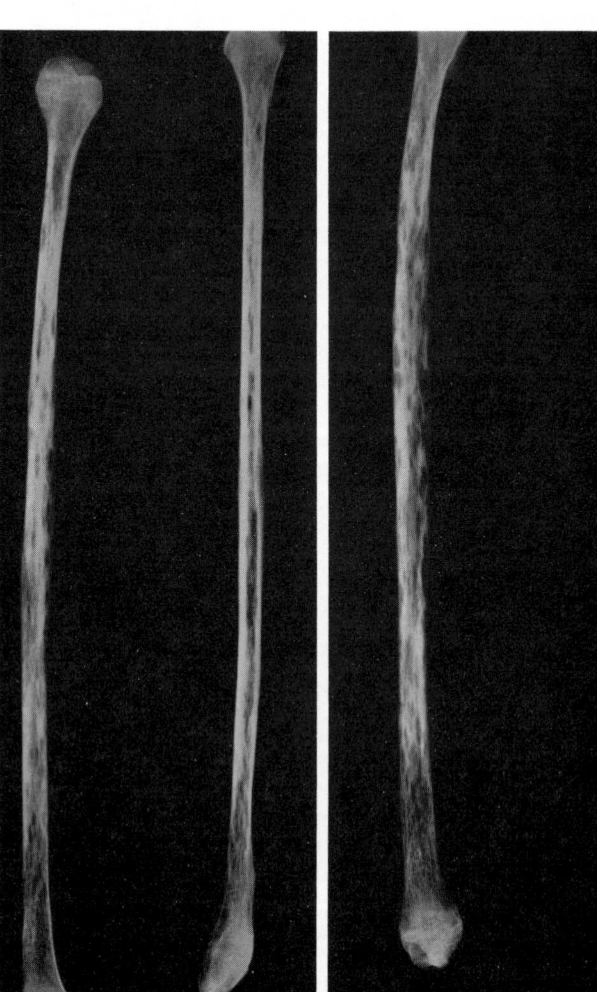

Figure 65–1. *Radiograph of specimen from radium dial worker showing both fibulae with multiple resorption cavities within the shafts. Note the well-defined lucent lesions somewhat resembling multiple myeloma.*

There is a general correlation between the bony lesions produced and the body burden of radium acquired. With a body burden of less than 0.1 microgram of ^{226}Ra, no radiographic changes occur.[47] Bone neoplasms have been reported with doses greater than 0.4 microgram of uncontaminated radium.[61] With time, there is an increase in the number and severity of osseous lesions.[46]

When large quantities of radium are deposited in bone for more than 20 years, mostly dead osteoid tissue remains. Normal bone physiology becomes erratic and large resorption cavities are formed.[47, 61] These cavities contain gelatinous material with osteoid-like matrix and appear as sharply defined bone lesions resembling multiple myeloma. They occur in the long bones (Fig. 65–1) and skull (Fig. 65–2) and increase in size with time. These areas of cortical resorption are secondary to constant alpha particle irradiation.[46]

Metaphyseal sclerosis is frequent, particularly in patients who ingest radium prior to epiphyseal closure.[46] Areas of increased density probably represent the deposition of new bone upon unresorbed bony trabeculae, a manifestation of bone ischemia secondary to vascular changes in the central arteries of the haversian canals. These density changes may simulate Paget's disease, but the bone is of normal size.[46] Large areas of aseptic necrosis indistinguishable from ischemic necrosis from other causes may be seen. Pathologic fractures can occur, and they frequently heal normally. Osteosarcomas (Fig. 65–3) and fibrosarcomas, sometimes multicentric, are seen.[46] The average latent period of these sarcomas is 23 years. Carcinomas of the paranasal sinuses and mastoids have also been reported.[46]

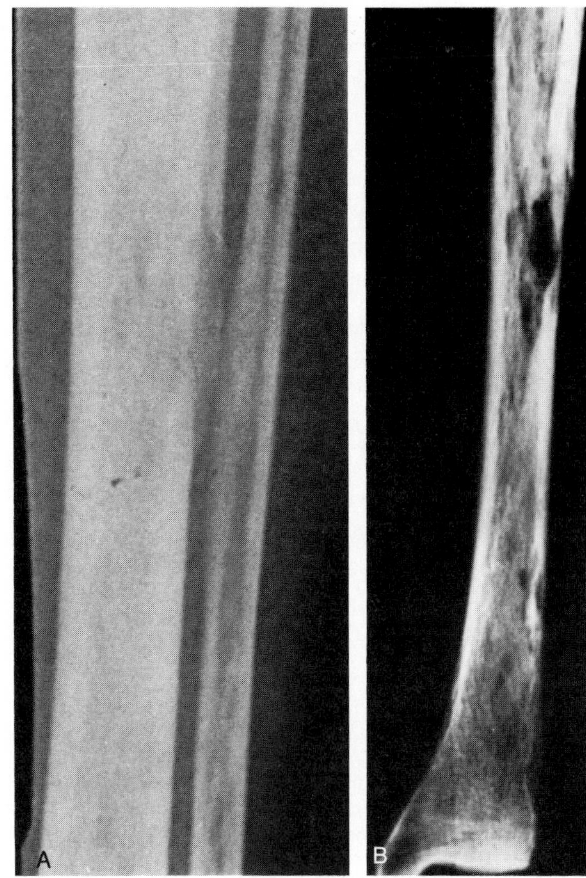

Figure 65–3. *Osteosarcoma in radium dial worker.*

A *Radiograph demonstrating a lytic lesion in tibia with poorly defined resorption cavities in the shaft.*

B *Radiograph of amputated specimen showing lytic osteosarcoma. The resorption cavities are now well visualized.*

(From Dalinka MK, et al: Semin Roentgenol 9:29, 1974.)

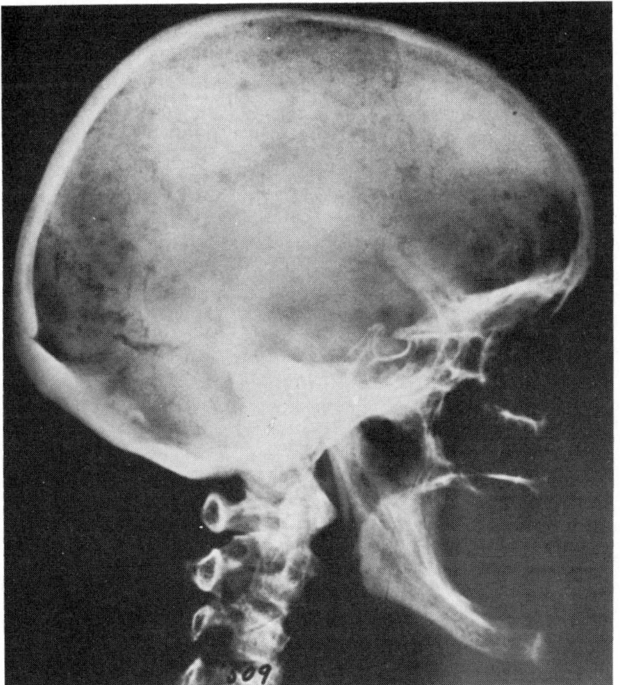

Figure 65–2. *Skull of radium dial worker demonstrating multiple small lucent areas within the calvarium, mainly in the parietal region, simulating multiple myeloma. (From Dalinka MK, et al: Semin Roentgenol 9:29, 1974.)*

THORIUM

Thorium dioxide in dextran (Thorotrast) was introduced as a contrast agent in 1928 and was widely used in the United States between 1930 and the early 1950s.[39, 53] Its clinically inert properties and high atomic number made it the agent of choice for hepatolienography, peripheral and cerebral angiography, and the opacification of body cavities.[53]

Extravasation of Thorotrast at the site of injection leads to continuous alpha particle irradiation, resulting in an expanding cicatricial mass, which invades contiguous structures, leading to tissue destruction and vascular compromise.[21, 59] In addition to these "Thorotrastomas" (i.e., Thorotrast granulomas), sarcomas, including extraskeletal chondro-

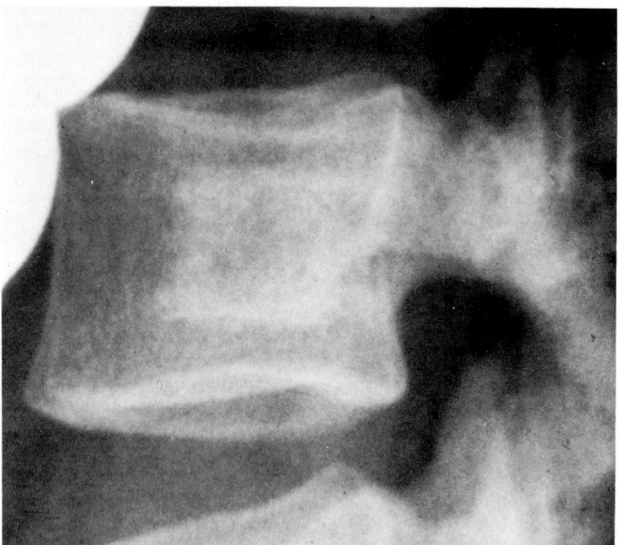

Figure 65–4. Coned-down view of lumbar vertebra showing "bone within a bone" appearance in patient injected with Thorotrast at the age of 3 years. (From Teplick JG et al: Radiology 129:657, 1978.)

sarcomas and osteosarcomas, have been described at the extravasation sites.[45, 81]

Thorotrast is a colloidal suspension that is phagocytized by the reticuloendothelial system, with 70 per cent deposited in the liver, 20 per cent in the spleen, and 1.5 to 3 per cent in the subendosteal cancellous bone.[20] It has a physical half-life of 1.4×10^{10} years and a biologic half-life of 400 years; hence, the liver, spleen, and bone marrow are subjected to continuous low-dose alpha radiation. The reticuloendothelial system and adjacent tissues are therefore at risk for radiation-induced neoplasia, particularly hemangioendothelial sarcoma of the liver.[20]

Jee and co-workers have studied the distribution of thorium and its daughter products in bone.[54] Histologic and autoradiographic studies demonstrated that most of the Thorotrast was deposited along the endosteum. The weekly bone marrow exposure of a 25 ml injection of Thorotrast was calculated at 0.3 rad.[60] Irradiation leads to thickened trabeculae and sclerosis adjacent to the endosteum, probably secondary to vascular ischemia. Diffuse osteosclerosis, bone marrow aplasia, and osteomalacia have been described by Murphy and colleagues.[71]

The injection of Thorotrast into growing children may give rise to a bone-within-bone or "ghost vertebra" appearance[102] (Fig. 65–4). The Thorotrast deposition causes constant alpha radiation and temporary growth arrest. The size of the ghost vertebra corresponds to the vertebral size at the time of injection.[102]

Sindelar and associates reviewed five patients with skeletal sarcomas following Thorotrast injection. Four patients had osteosarcomas and one had a vertebral fibrosarcoma.[94] These tumors occurred at least 16 years following administration of the contrast agent. Three of these patients demonstrated

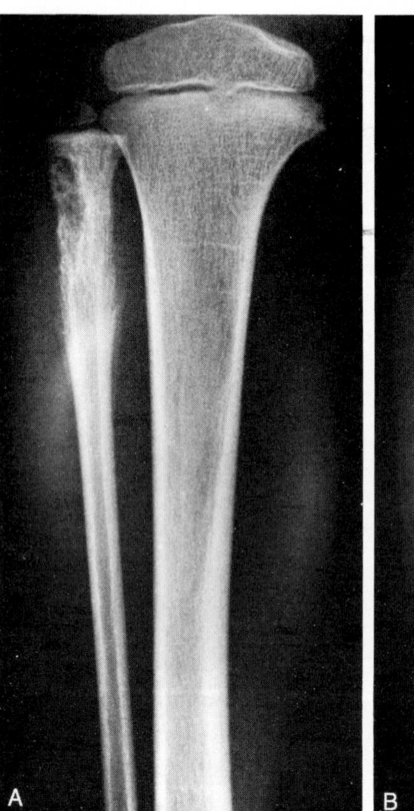

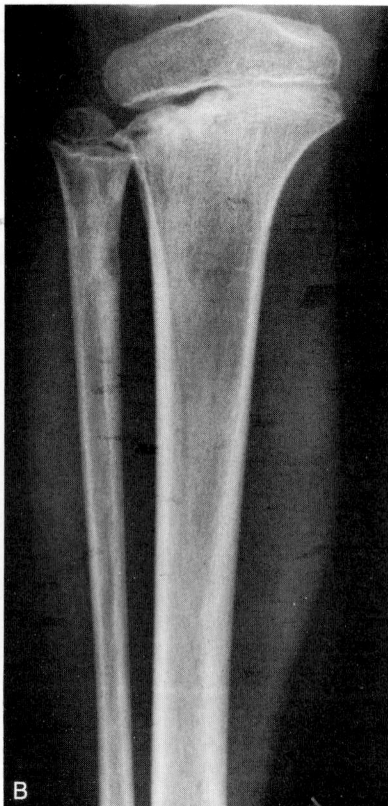

Figure 65–5. Ewing's tumor prior to and following radiation therapy.

A Ewing's tumor of proximal fibula with destructive metaphyseal and diaphyseal lesion and layered periosteal new bone formation.

B Same patient 6 months following radiation therapy. There is widening of the cartilaginous growth plate in the lateral aspect of the tibia and adjacent fibula. Note the dense metaphyseal band in the tibia.

thorium within the vicinity of the tumor on autoradiography.[94]

EFFECTS OF RADIATION THERAPY

Bone Growth

The effects of radiation on bone growth were first demonstrated in 1903, when Perthes showed that the growth of chick wings was retarded by radiation.[79] In 1906, Fösterling demonstrated gross impairment of the growth of rabbits following radiation to the upper half of the body.[35] The effects of radiation on bone growth in humans were reported in the German literature in 1929 by Hueck and Spiess[51]; Desjardins[26] and Bisgard and Hunt[8] reported similar changes in the United States.

It has been shown experimentally that the epiphysis is the area most sensitive to radiation.[22, 83, 85] Microscopic changes may occur with a dose as low as 300 rads, and decreased growth can occur with as little as 400 rads.[22] The histologic changes can be demonstrated as early as 2 to 4 days following therapy.[85] The early radiation effects are in the zone of provisional calcification, which shows a decrease in the number of chondrocytes and an abnormal columnar arrangement of the cartilage cells. There is swelling, pyknosis, and fragmentation of the chondrocytes, as well as chondrocyte degeneration with irregular, faintly stained cells.[85] With a low dose of 600 to 1200 rads, there is rapid histologic recovery. Secondary changes are limited, but some residua may remain.[100] With 1200 rads or more, the damage is increased and is maximal to the chondroblasts. Delayed changes take 6 months or longer to occur and are dose related.[85, 89] Late changes may occur secondary to vascular damage and include premature cartilage degeneration and bone marrow atrophy.[85] The dose-related changes are decreased with protraction. Growth impairment is related to the age of the animal or patient, with the effect of the given dose being greater at a younger age.

Rubin and Casarett have shown that when the entire bone is irradiated, there is decrease in overall size and diameter, simulating osteogenesis imperfecta.[85] If only the epiphysis is irradiated, there is growth deformity, with a decrease in width resembling achondroplasia.[85] Irradiation of the metaphysis leads to a bowing deformity, whereas diaphyseal irradiation causes a narrow shaft with normal cortical diameter.[85]

The effects of radiation are independent of their method of production and can be produced by internal or external sources.[105, 106] In growing bone the quality of radiation is of little significance, as cartilage is almost of water density and there is no differential absorption.[25, 82] The larger the field irradiated, the greater the effects.

Reidy and co-workers showed that there was a decrease in overall length and retardation in growth rate following epiphyseal irradiation in dogs.[83] They demonstrated that the epiphysis at the untreated end of a bone contributed more to length than the corresponding epiphysis on the opposite side.[83] Epiphyseal irradiation was utilized to decrease growth in patients with unequal leg length.[36] Frantz reported a patient with marked shortening of an extremity following treatment of a soft tissue hemangioma.[36] The treated bone had a decrease in shaft diameter, cortical thickness, and overall bone length.[36] Abnormal tubulation and premature epiphyseal fusion may also occur following radiation therapy with larger doses.[25, 27]

Widening of the growth plate has been described as early as 1 to 2 months following treatment. If mild, this returns to normal after approximately 6 months.[27] Joint space widening has also been reported 8 to 10 months following therapy[27] (Fig. 65–5). Metaphyseal irregularity and fraying

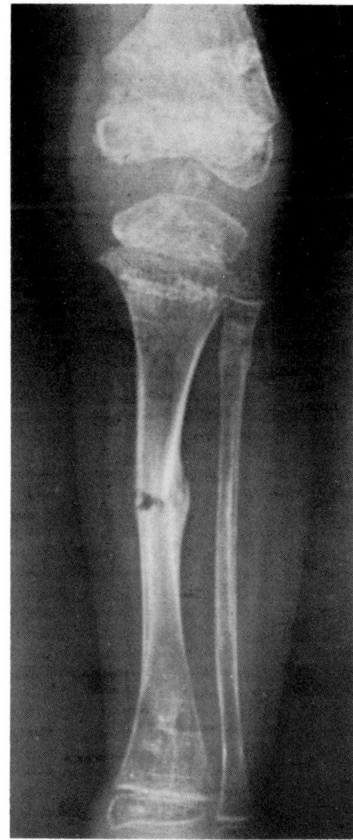

Figure 65–6. *This patient was irradiated approximately 2 years prior to this film for leukemia and knee pain. The treated field included most of the tibia as well as the knee. There is a fracture through the midshaft of the tibia with periosteal reaction about it. Periosteal reaction is also noted about the midshaft of the fibula. There is metaphyseal irregularity of the distal femur, with deformity secondary to radiation therapy. Diffuse osteopenia is also present. (Courtesy of Dr. Patricia Borns, Wilmington, Delaware.)*

may occur when the epiphyseal widening begins to heal (Fig. 65–6). Metaphyseal sclerosis may also be seen (Fig. 65–5). Patients with metaphyseal changes may develop a broad band of increased density, which may be a manifestation of repair. This can resolve, leading to normal trabeculae.[27]

In humans, the diaphysis is relatively resistant to radiation, and periosteal new bone formation is affected less than enchondral bone formation.[22] Dawson thought that growth impairment did not occur following radiation of the shaft of long bones if the epiphysis was spared.[22] The degree of sensitivity was dependent upon the bone involved.[22] Osteoporosis was a frequent and nonspecific finding.[22]

Wolf and associates[108] and Rubin and Casarett[85] have reported slipped capital femoral epiphysis as a sequel to radiation therapy (Fig. 65–7). In these patients, the femoral head was included in the field of therapy. The damaged growth plate was not able to withstand the shearing stresses of growth, leading to epiphyseal slippage.[25, 108, 115] Radiation-induced slipped epiphyses usually occur at an earlier age than the idiopathic variety.[108] Ryan and Walters[114] and others[109] believe that the chemotherapy admini-

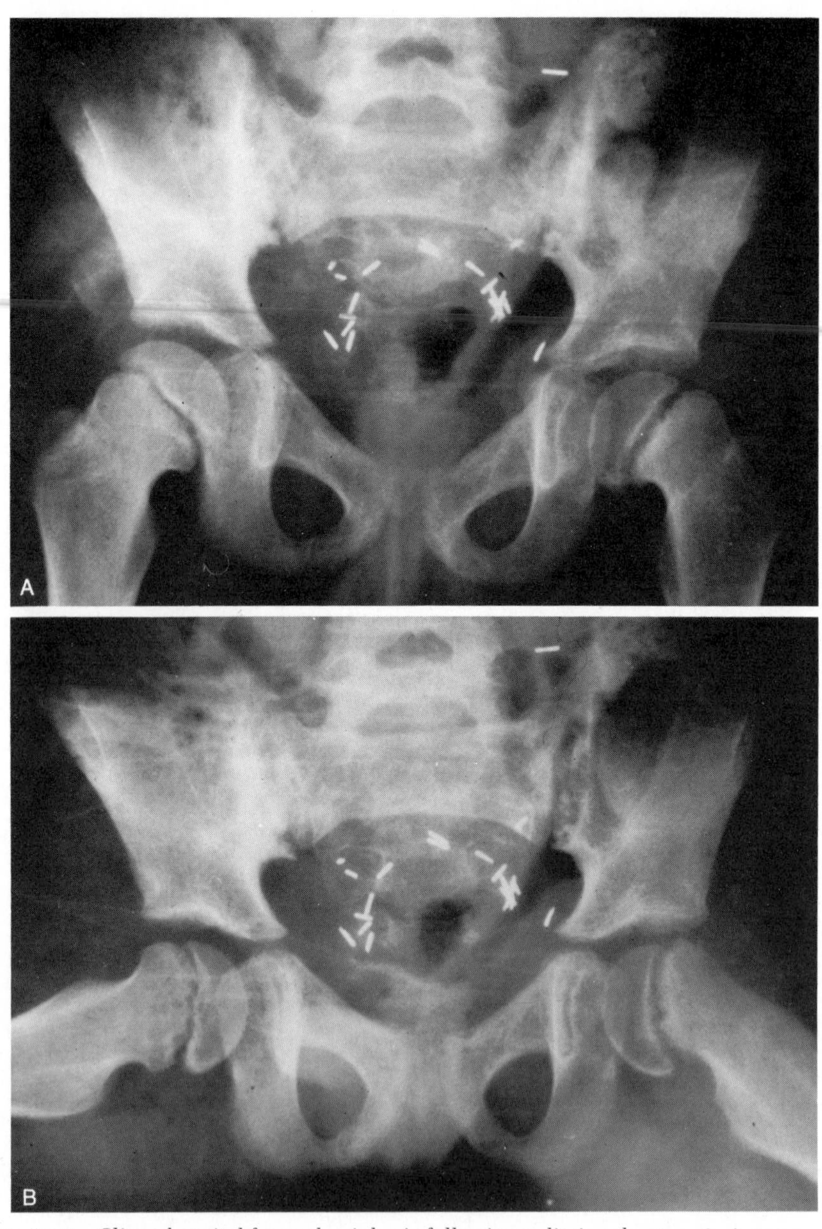

Figure 65–7. *Slipped capital femoral epiphysis following radiation therapy.* **A,** *Anteroposterior (AP) view.* **B,** *Frog-leg lateral view of the pelvis in an 8 year old child following radiation therapy for an embryonal rhabdomyosarcoma. The pelvis was treated with 5940 rads with a femoral shield added at 4500 rads. Note the slipped epiphysis on the left side. The right sacroiliac joint has sclerotic margins also secondary to the radiation therapy. (Courtesy of Dr. Arthur Newburg, Burlington, Vermont.)*

stered along with the radiation may contribute to the toxicity to the growth cartilage, leading to the slipped capital femoral epiphysis.

Rarely, changes secondary to radiation therapy in children may not be clinically manifest until adulthood. Bilateral aseptic necrosis has been reported in a 25 year old patient who was treated with 2200 rads to the pelvis at the age of 13 months.[29]

Scoliosis

Engel produced scoliosis in rabbits, dogs, and goats by implanting radium needles unilaterally in the spine.[30] There was loss of height and destruction of the adjacent bone marrow in the irradiated area. The disc cartilage was 2 to 3 times thicker on the irradiated side as it hypertrophied to compensate for the bone loss.[30]

Arkin and Simon used radon seeds and asymmetric external beam irradiation to produce scoliosis in rabbits.[2] A single dose of 1000 rads was sufficient. Histologically, the vertebra demonstrated an absence of cartilaginous columns and an irregular zone of provisional calcification. There was no gross or microscopic evidence of necrosis, inflammation, or marrow fibrosis.

Arkin and colleagues reported the first case of radiation-induced scoliosis in humans.[3] The patient developed an isolated lumbar scoliosis with uniform wedging of the vertebral bodies following therapy to the back for melanotic nevi.[3]

In 1952, Neuhauser and co-workers published a classic paper on the effects of radiation on the growing spine.[73] They described 45 patients treated for abdominal malignancies, with autopsy data for 11 patients and roentgenograms from 34 patients. The roentgenographic findings were dose related. There were no radiologic abnormalities in patients treated with less than 1000 rads. Those children receiving 1000 to 2000 rads developed changes secondary to growth arrest. These changes consisted of horizontal lines of increased density, which were parallel to the vertebral end-plates; on occasion, there was a "bone-within-bone" appearance. These abnormalities were not confined to the treatment field and hence were related to the general effect on bone growth. Irregularity and scalloping of the end-plates was confined to the irradiated area. Benign exostoses were identified in five patients (Fig. 65–8), and a mild, nonprogressive scoliosis was common (Figs. 65–9 and 65–10). The changes were more severe in patients treated prior to the age of 2 years, hence the effects of radiation were believed to be dose- and age-related.

The earliest histologic changes occur in the zone of provisional calcification. The gross aberrations are not detected until the osseous changes take place, usually at least a year following therapy.[100] Bony abnormalities may occur earlier if the patient is treated with over 3000 rads or prior to 18 months of age.[85, 87]

Neuhauser and associates thought that radiation of the entire vertebral body would eliminate the scoliosis.[73] Whitehouse and Lampe,[107] in agreement with Neuhauser and his colleagues, stated that the complications could be minimized by protracting the course of radiation with small daily doses. Vaeth and co-workers also believed that the scoliosis was mild and nonprogressive.[104] In their series, four of six women conceived following therapy, and all six had normal menses.

In many later series, scoliosis occurred despite therapy to the entire vertebral body and even megavoltage therapy.[49, 74] Rubin and co-workers[85, 87] and Katzman and associates[55] stated that the scoliosis was more severe if osseous involvement was present

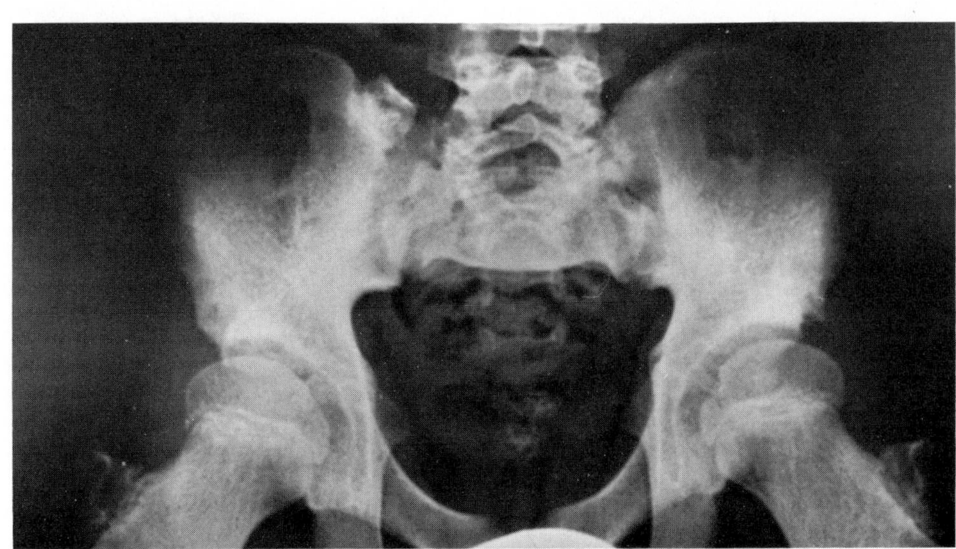

Figure 65–8. *Anteroposterior view of pelvis in patient irradiated for Wilms' tumor. Note the exostosis arising from the posterior iliac crest on the right side. (Courtesy of Dr. Patricia Borns, Wilmington, Delaware.)*

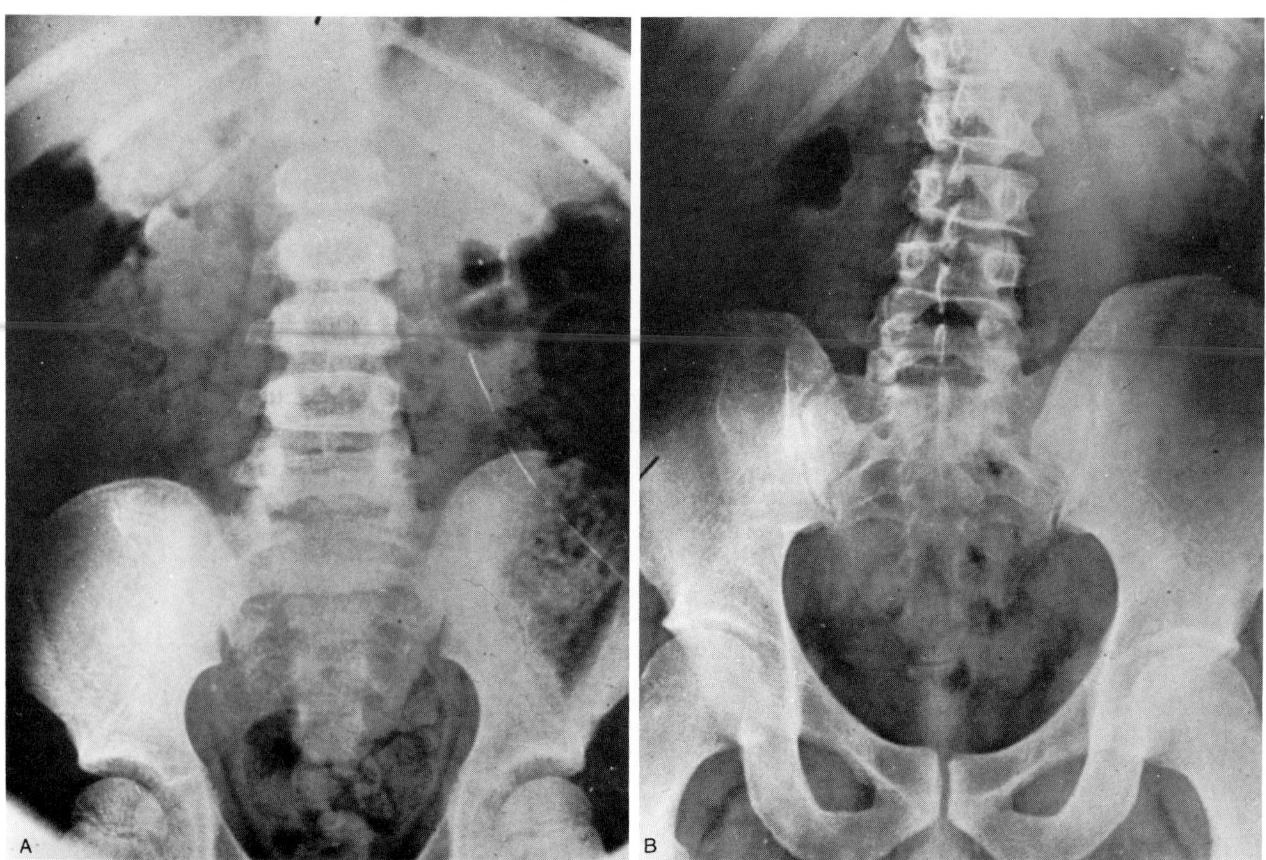

Figure 65–9. *Films of the abdomen before and after therapy for a right-sided Wilms' tumor.*

A *Normal film taken in July 1938, prior to therapy.*

B *Film taken 26 years later, demonstrating a levoscoliosis. The right sides of the vertebral bodies are decreased in height, and the pedicles are decreased in size. The right iliac crest is hypoplastic. Note that the intervertebral discs are thickened, probably representing hypertrophy because of the decrease in bony size.*

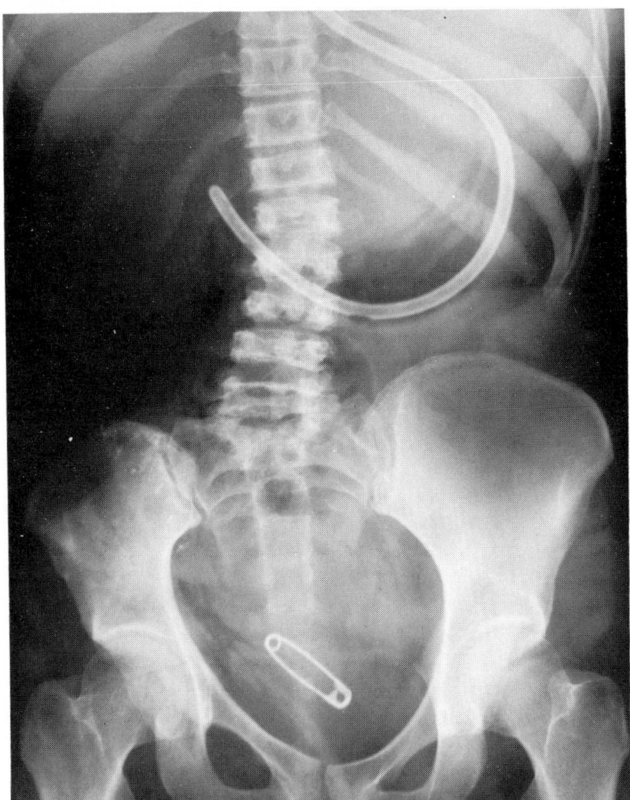

Figure 65–10. Another patient irradiated for a right-sided Wilms' tumor in childhood. Note the severe decrease in the height of the vertebral bodies and a slight scoliosis convex to the left. The ribs and iliac crest on the right side are also hypoplastic. The long tube was present because of intestinal obstruction, which was later shown to be secondary to radiation enteritis.

prior to therapy. Scoliosis is most likely secondary to a combination of factors, including "fall off" at the edge of the roentgen beam, changes in the small blood vessels, and fibrosis of the overlying soft tissues.[7, 87] The scoliosis is usually not severe enough to require orthopedic management.[112]

Riseborough and colleagues believed the scoliosis could be progressive, particularly when high doses were given to young patients.[84] The increase in scoliosis occurred during the adolescent growth spurt despite treatment with Milwaukee bracing. Surgical therapy with Harrington rods was necessary in 8 of 57 scoliotic patients. The degree of scoliosis was not proportional to the changes in the vertebral body.[84] Kyphosis occurred in 21 of 81 patients and was usually associated with scoliosis. There was an increased incidence of pseudarthrosis following surgical therapy for kyphoscoliosis.[84]

Changes in the axial growth of the vertebral bodies have also been described.[82] These usually occur following irradiation of patients less than 6 years of age or at puberty.[82] The decreased growth might be overlooked if sitting heights are not measured.[82] Children receiving more than 3500 rads show a decrease in sitting height, whereas those receiving less than 2500 rads do not.[82]

The effects of radiation on growing bone have important radiotherapeutic implications. Growth disturbances are largely independent of the quality of radiation.[25, 82] The major radiation changes occur in the fine physeal blood vessels and chondroblasts, which are both of unit density material and therefore affected equally by all types of radiation.[25, 82]

In radiotherapy, the radiation field size should be as small as possible. When treating the spine, the entire vertebral body is included. The iliac crest apophysis should be shielded if possible as it is responsible for 40 per cent of the growth of the ilium.

Radiation Necrosis

The pathologic effects of radiation are independent of their method of production. Immediate or delayed cell death, injury with recovery, arrest of cellular division, abnormal repair, or neoplasia may occur.[105, 106] These changes may be seen secondary to either internal or external sources of radiation.

Ewing used the term "radiation osteitis" to define the effects of radiation on bone.[31] He classified radiation changes into different stages, which were dose related. Abnormalities included temporary cessation of growth with recovery, periostitis, bone sclerosis with increased fragility, aseptic necrosis, and infection with osteoradionecrosis.[31]

Rubin and Casarett thought that osteonecrosis of mature bone and cartilage was secondary to a combination of irradiation, infection, and trauma, with irradiation causing a susceptibility to damage by other noxious stimuli.[86]

Howland and co-workers believed that radiation causes bone atrophy, not necrosis; secondary infection must be present for true necrosis to occur.[50, 110] The atrophy is followed by repair. Attempts at regeneration result in the deposition of new bone on the unresorbed ischemic trabeculae.[24] There is a mottled appearance with a mixture of osteoporosis, increased density, and coarse trabeculation.[24] Fractures through the osteopenic bone may heal normally, as true necrosis is absent.[10]

The osseous changes are secondary to destruction of the osteoblasts, which disappear following therapy.[50, 92] Vascular damage may contribute to the late radiation changes.[86] The bony abnormalities are dependent upon the dosage, quality of the roentgen beam, method of fractionation, length of time following therapy, specific bone or bones involved, and the superimposition of trauma or infection.[86]

Radiation changes are dose related; the larger the dose, the greater the effect. The threshold of radiation changes in bone is believed to be 3000 rads, with cell death occurring at 5000 rads.[12]

The quality of the x-ray beam determines the energy absorption and hence the radiation effect. The energy absorption in bone of 250 KV in rads is three times greater than the exposure dose in roentgens.[86] With orthovoltage, the changes are caused mainly by the photoelectric effect, which is mostly scattered radiation dependent upon the third power of the atomic number. With low kilovoltage, the greater radiation effect is therefore in bone. With supervoltage therapy, the Compton effect predominates, and it is independent of the atomic number of the tissue irradiated. The absorbed dose in bone is similar to the exposure dose.

The larger the size of the treatment field, the greater the area at risk and the higher the integral dose necessary. With supervoltage therapy, tumor dose may be reached with smaller fields, causing less damage to the surrounding structures.

Ellis derived a formula relating the total dose, number of fractions, and treatment time to a nominal single dose (NSD).[28] The empirically derived formula is as follows:

$$\underset{\text{(Total dose)}}{TD} = NSD \times \underset{\text{(Number of fractions)}}{N^{0.24}} \times \underset{\text{(Treatment time in days)}}{T^{0.11}}$$

This formula was based upon extensive clinical data and radiobiologic principles.[28] The nominal single dose (NSD) is of value in comparing different treatment regimens.[28, 56] Montague believed that the margin of tolerance was narrow and clinical trials were necessary before changes in fractionation were established.[68] Individual and geometric field variations were such that complete reliance should not be placed upon empirical formulas.[68]

The temporal relationships vary with different bones. Mandibular osteonecrosis frequently presents within a year following therapy, whereas in most other sites the latent period is longer. Minimal changes usually occur at least a year after treatment and are slowly progressive. When fractures occur in irradiated bone, other radiation changes are usually present.

Regional Effects

Mandible. Osteonecrosis is considerably more common in the mandible than in the maxilla because of its compact bone and poor blood supply.[42, 64, 75] The mandible, because of its superficial location, receives a large dose of radiation in the treatment of intraoral cancer.[19] A high complication rate is considered an acceptable risk when treating a potentially curable lesion.[40]

The incidence of osteonecrosis increases with an increasing mandibular dose. It varies with the treatment method and is least common with parallel opposing fields.[40] Osteonecrosis is more common when the tumor involves or is adjacent to bone.[6] In one series of 176 patients treated with supervoltage therapy for tonsillar lesions, 66 developed mandibular necrosis.[40] The necrosis was usually of a mild and temporary nature.[40] Mandibular necrosis may be aseptic or septic; the aseptic or simple type is usually of no consequence.[42]

There is a high incidence of poor oral hygiene, smoking, and alcoholism in patients with carcinoma of the oral cavity.[15] Considerable controversy exists regarding the role of dental extraction in radiation therapy. Grossly carious teeth should be removed prior to treatment. Teeth with periodontal disease without opposing teeth should be extracted if they are within the treatment field.[42] The extraction should take place prior to therapy so that the tooth bed can heal before irradiation begins. Salvageable teeth should be preserved.[6] Following treatment, good oral care is imperative, as radiation decreases salivary function and mandibular vascularity.[40] If teeth are removed after therapy, the trauma and bare sockets predispose to infection.

Mandibular osteonecrosis may be difficult to differentiate from tumor recurrence.[12] Recurrence and osteoradionecrosis both usually occur within a year following therapy. Pain, ulceration, bleeding, and weight loss are common to both.[86] Mandibular necrosis frequently presents as an ill-defined destructive lesion without sequestration (Fig. 65–11). The absence of a soft tissue mass helps in the differentiation of necrosis from tumor recurrence, but an inflammatory mass may be present with osteonecrosis. Cortical destruction is frequent. The necrosis is confined to the treated area. Radiation necrosis may progress slowly or heal with vigorous conservative therapy. Hyperbaric oxygenation and intraoral mandibular surgery are sometimes necessary.[63]

Shoulder. Radiation changes in the shoulder girdle following therapy for breast carcinoma have been reported in 1 to 3 per cent of patients.[24] With the advent of supervoltage therapy, the incidence and severity of these changes have decreased.[50]

Osteopenia is common following irradiation but occurs in a substantial number of patients treated by radical mastectomy alone.[58] Osteopenia is frequently associated with a coarse, disorganized trabecular pattern, which may superficially resemble Paget's disease.[66]

Rib fractures are common and may be subtle. The early finding is frequently a sharp change in alignment with or without a fracture line. The rib lesions frequently occur in the anterior or anterolateral aspects of the ribs and are usually multiple[77] (Figs. 65–12 and 65–13). Involvement of the posterior rib surfaces is also common (Fig. 65–13). The edges of the fracture fragments are frequently resorbed, and they may show sclerotic or pointed ends (Fig. 65–12). Fractures are frequently painless, and the resorption may be progressive.[19] The fractures may heal spontaneously with increased bony density.[77] Involved osseous structures frequently show other changes at the time of fracture (Fig. 65–13).

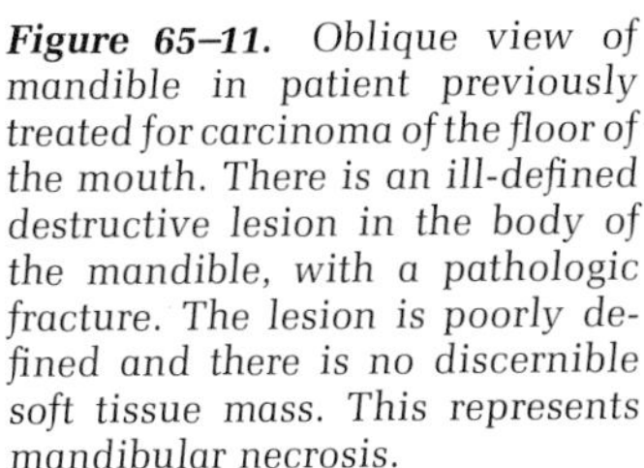

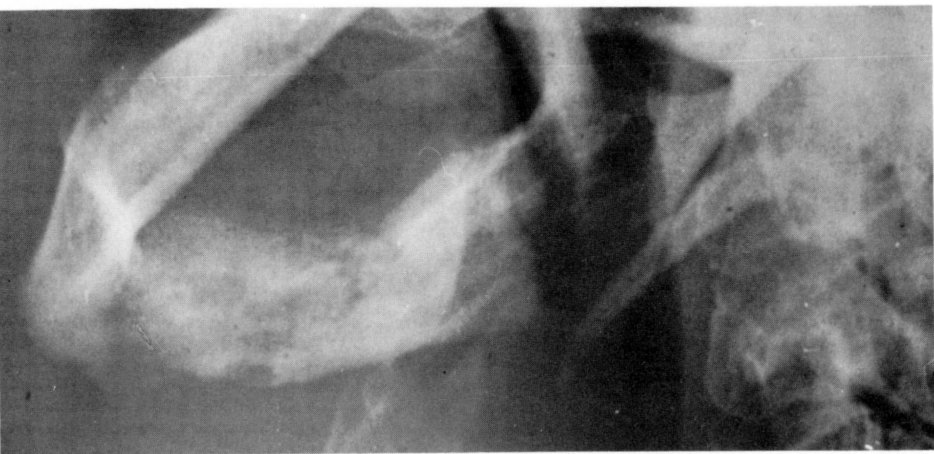

Figure 65–11. *Oblique view of mandible in patient previously treated for carcinoma of the floor of the mouth. There is an ill-defined destructive lesion in the body of the mandible, with a pathologic fracture. The lesion is poorly defined and there is no discernible soft tissue mass. This represents mandibular necrosis.*

Clavicular fractures are commonly associated with rib fractures and may also be resorbed at the edges.[12] Symptoms are usually minimal unless there is associated ulceration or infection of the skin. Slaughter stated that osseous infection may lead to rapid clavicular destruction simulating malignancy[95]; however, this may occur in the absence of infection.[12] Scapular fractures can be associated with rib and clavicular fractures, but the fragments are usually not resorbed (Fig. 65–12). Fractures about the shoulder girdle frequently progress to nonunion, as they are relatively asymptomatic and the fragments are not immobilized.[12]

Radiation necrosis of the humerus (Fig. 65–13) can be seen 7 to 10 years following therapy.[92] Associated findings in the ribs, clavicle, and scapula are frequent. DeSantos and Libshitz state that humeral necrosis is almost always symptomatic.[24] Changes may include resorption cavities, fractures, and avascular necrosis of the humeral head. Histologically there are no osteoblasts. New bone formation is absent and there are normal blood vessels, including capillaries.[92]

Pelvis. Fractures of the femoral neck following radiation therapy to the pelvis (Fig. 65–14) were

Figure 65–12. *Changes of radiation necrosis following orthovoltage therapy and radical mastectomy for carcinoma of the breast. A pathologic fracture is present in the scapula. Multiple rib fractures are present, with resorption of the edges of the second rib and a large gap in the first rib. Pathologic fractures are present in the posterior fourth and fifth ribs. Diffuse osteopenia is seen in the proximal humeral shaft. (From Dalinka MK, et al: Semin Roentgenol 9:29, 1974.)*

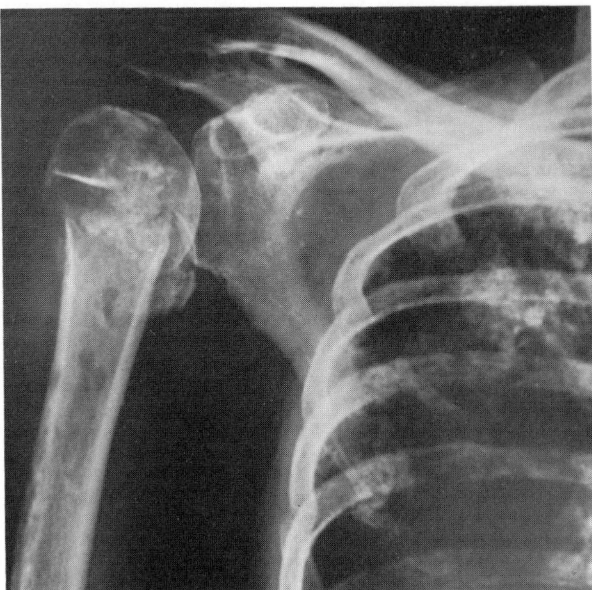

Figure 65–13. *Radiation necrosis. Examination of the shoulder 10 years following radiation for carcinoma of the breast reveals pathologic fractures of the right humerus and multiple ribs. The lucent lesions in the proximal humeral shaft are also secondary to radiation necrosis. (From Dalinka MK, et al: Semin Roentgenol 9:29, 1974.)*

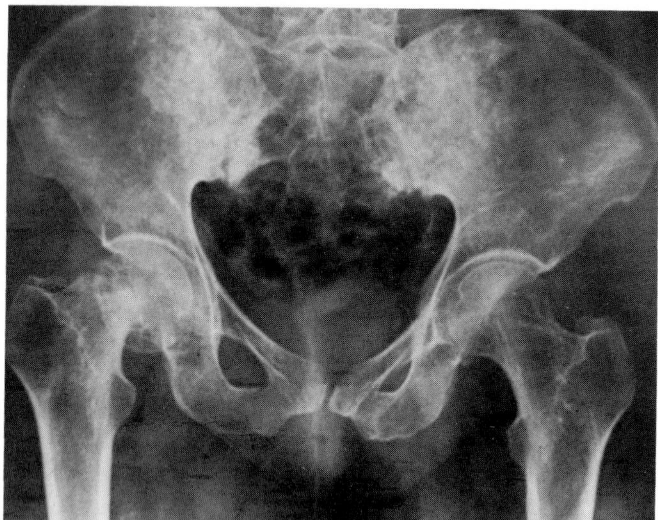

Figure 65–14. *Fracture of right femoral neck 4 years following therapy for carcinoma of the cervix. The patient was treated with 2500 rads of external radiation plus two applications of radium. There are sclerotic changes about both sacroiliac joints with adjacent calcification.*

first reported in the late 1920s in the German literature.[41] Dalby and co-workers[18] and others[10, 12, 41, 95] later reported similar findings in the United States. Patients in these series were all treated with orthovoltage therapy, and lateral fields were used in most cases except for the series by Dalby and associates.[18] Fractures occurred in approximately 2 per cent of patients treated with pelvic radiation.[10] Fractures of the femoral neck have been reported following as little as 1540 rads and as early as 5 months following therapy.[41] Sclerotic changes in the femoral neck with increased trabecular density were frequently present prior to fracture.[41] Bonfiglio thought that the fractures were stress or insufficiency fractures in osteoporotic bone.[10]

Pain, frequently in the knee or groin, commonly precedes the onset of the fractures, which are usually subcapital.[86] The average radiation dose is estimated

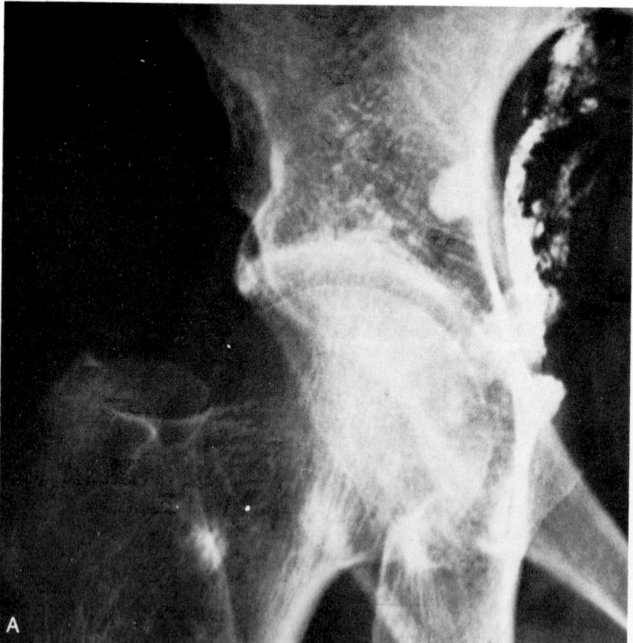

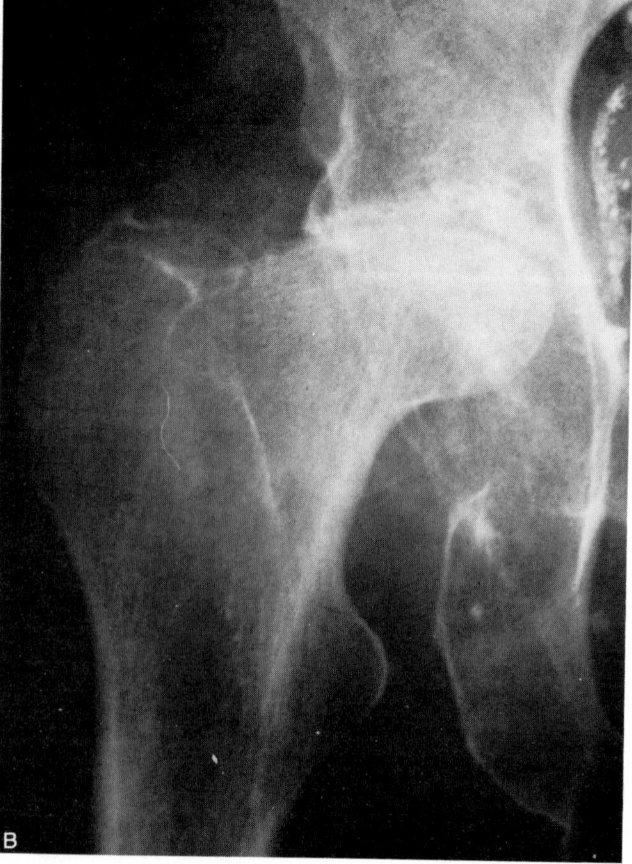

Figure 65–15. *Radiation necrosis following treatment for carcinoma of the cervix.*

A *Anteroposterior view of right hip prior to therapy shows no evidence of abnormality. Note contrast medium within lymphatic vessels from lymphangiogram.*

B *Same patient 9 months following therapy. The femoral head has collapsed and there is marked narrowing of the hip joint, with an irregular femoral head.*

at 3000 rads. Vascular damage is not sufficient to prevent repair, and fractures heal with routine treatment, with adequate callus formation.[10] Avascular necrosis may occur (Fig. 65–15) but is rare following fractures in irradiated bone.[10]

The sacroiliac joints may be wide and irregular, with sclerosis about the joint margins (Fig. 65–16). This sclerosis may extend from the region of the joint to the ilium, simulating osteitis condensans ilii.[86, 88] Fractures may radiate from the middle of the posterior superior iliac crest through the iliac wing.[86]

Occasionally soft tissue calcifications occur, and they are not associated with masses or underlying bony destruction (Fig. 65–17), which differentiates them from radiation-induced sarcoma.[24]

Changes in the pubis simulating osteitis pubis (Fig. 65–16) may occur, as may fractures about the pubic rami or ischium. These may be secondary to the high dosage of internal radiation to the anterior pelvis. Fractures can occur anywhere in the pelvis, particularly if the patient is re-treated (Fig. 65–18).

Protrusio acetabuli has been reported following radiation. This can occur following orthovoltage or supervoltage therapy. In one case, it was seen following irradiation for transitional cell carcinoma of the prostatic urethra[44] (Fig. 65–19). The mechanism of protrusion in these patients is unclear but may be related to remodeling and revascularization of weakened, previously irradiated bone.[43]

The changes secondary to pelvic irradiation have decreased markedly with increased awareness in using supervoltage therapy. Use of lateral fields in pelvic cancer has long since been abandoned.[86] The femoral neck is usually shielded during treatment; the fields for the pelvis are smaller, and re-treatment is rare.

Radiation changes are usually easy to differentiate from recurrence or spread of disease. Metastases may involve the lateral pelvic walls from direct extension or the vertebral bodies via spread to the retroperitoneal lymph nodes.[86, 88] Hematologic dissemination frequently occurs to sites outside of the treatment field and is associated with multiple lesions.[86, 88] Radiation-induced tumors occur following long latent periods and are frequently associated with soft tissue masses or characteristic osseous lesions.

STERNUM. Morris and co-workers reported sternal changes following therapy for Hodgkin's disease and compared the changes following megavoltage to those following orthovoltage therapy.[69] The incidence and severity of the changes were directly related to the dose and length of follow-up examination and were best explained by damage to the microvascular structures, similar to that seen in sickle cell disease with infarction.[69]

Mild changes consisted of osteoporosis, abnormal bony trabeculae, and localized bone necrosis with sclerosis. Moderate changes included the development of localized pectus excavatum and necro-

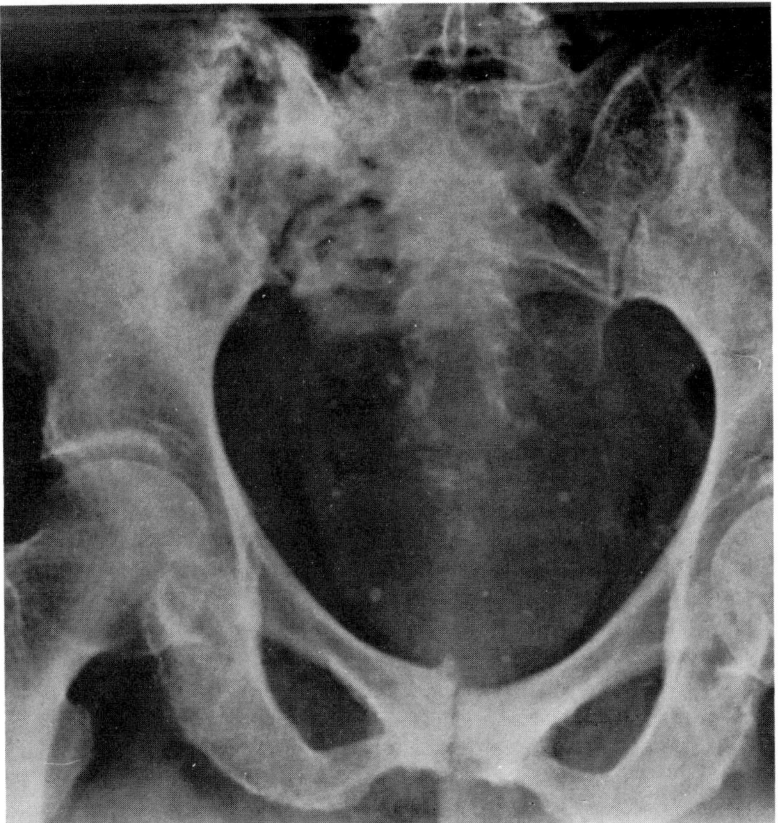

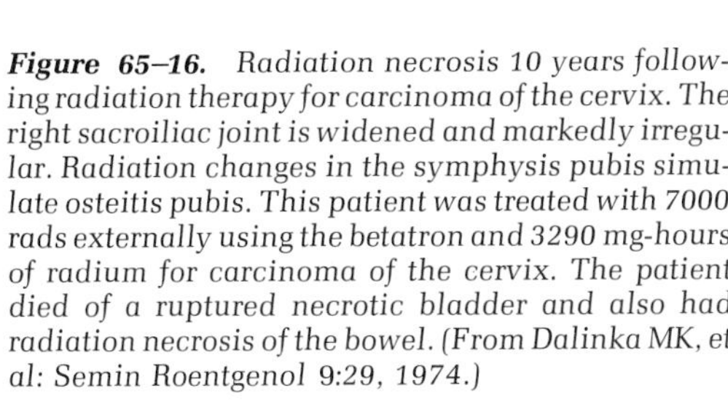

Figure 65–16. *Radiation necrosis 10 years following radiation therapy for carcinoma of the cervix. The right sacroiliac joint is widened and markedly irregular. Radiation changes in the symphysis pubis simulate osteitis pubis. This patient was treated with 7000 rads externally using the betatron and 3290 mg-hours of radium for carcinoma of the cervix. The patient died of a ruptured necrotic bladder and also had radiation necrosis of the bowel. (From Dalinka MK, et al: Semin Roentgenol 9:29, 1974.)*

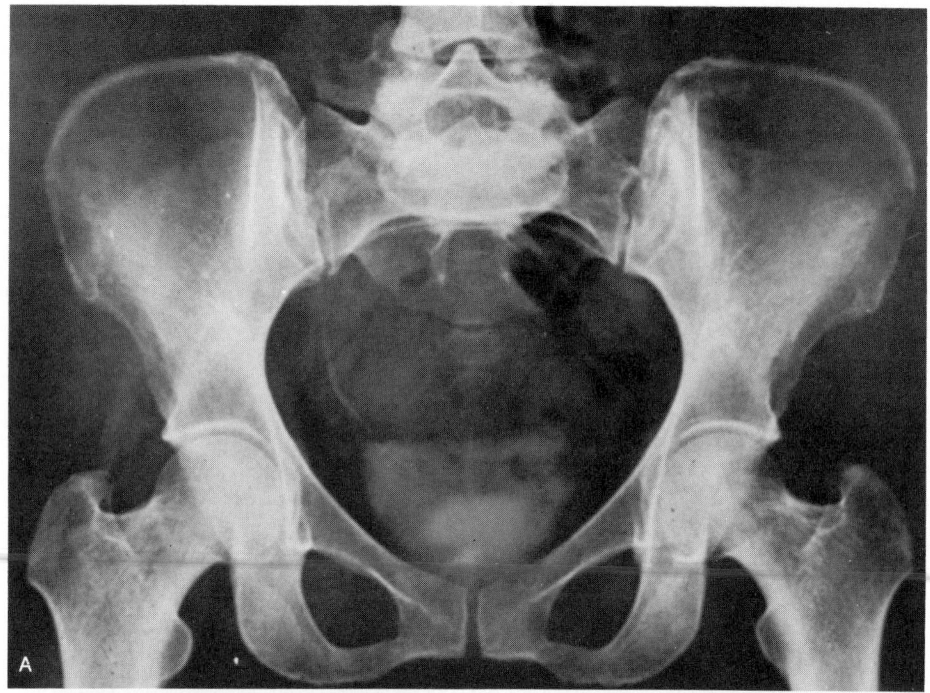

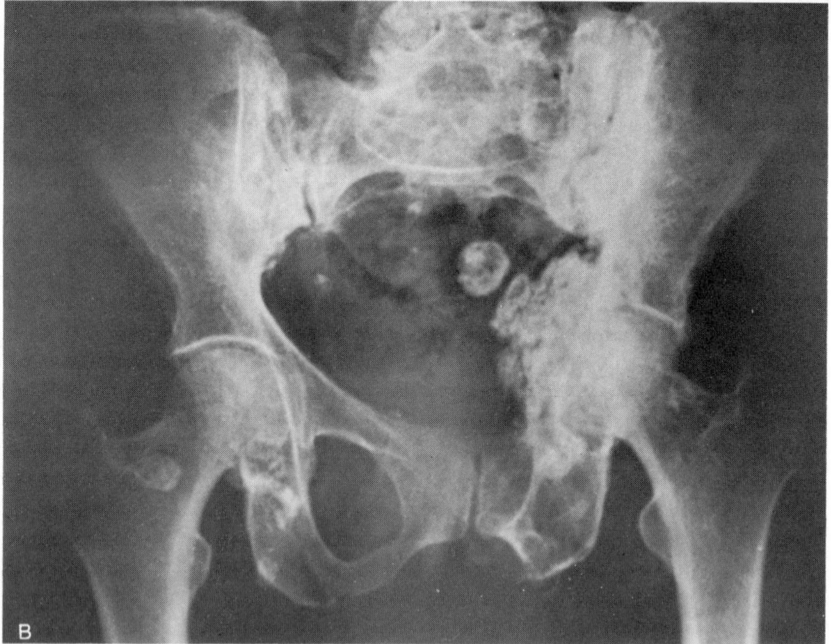

Figure 65–17. *Pelvic changes following radiation therapy.*

A *Normal film prior to therapy in 1949.*

B *Same patient 23 years following therapy, revealing extensive soft tissue calcification about the pelvis. The left hemipelvis is deformed secondary to a previous ischial fracture. Sclerosis is present about both sacroiliac joints, particularly on the left side.*

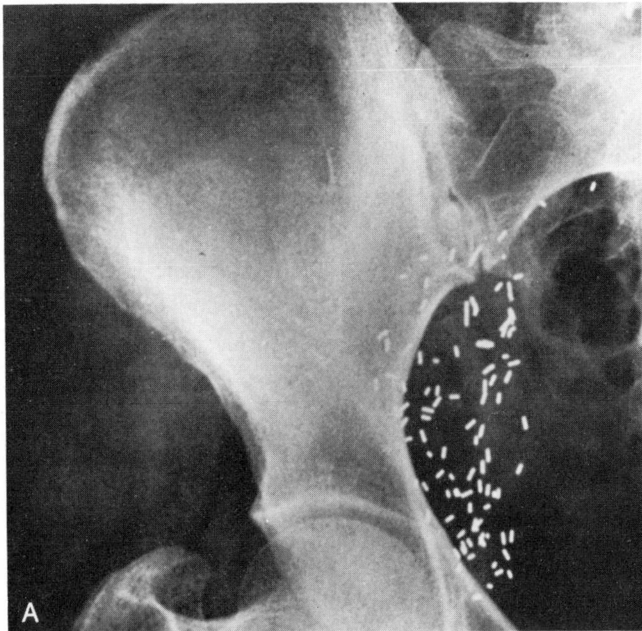

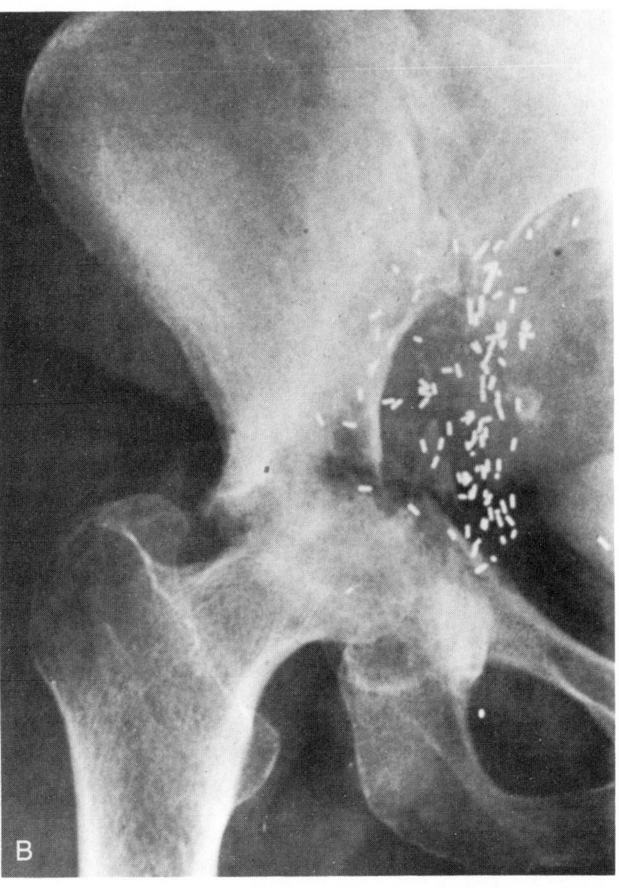

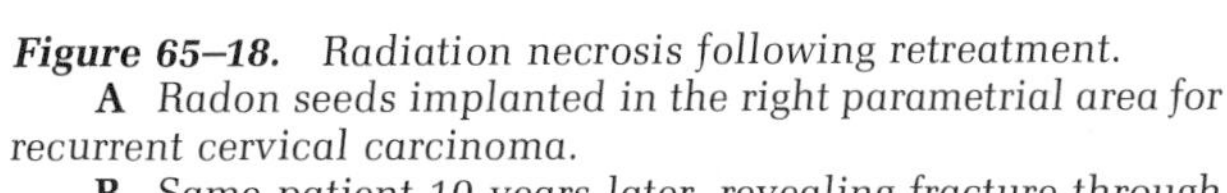

Figure 65–18. *Radiation necrosis following retreatment.*

A *Radon seeds implanted in the right parametrial area for recurrent cervical carcinoma.*

B *Same patient 10 years later, revealing fracture through the medial wall of the acetabulum with loss of the joint space and large cyst formation.*

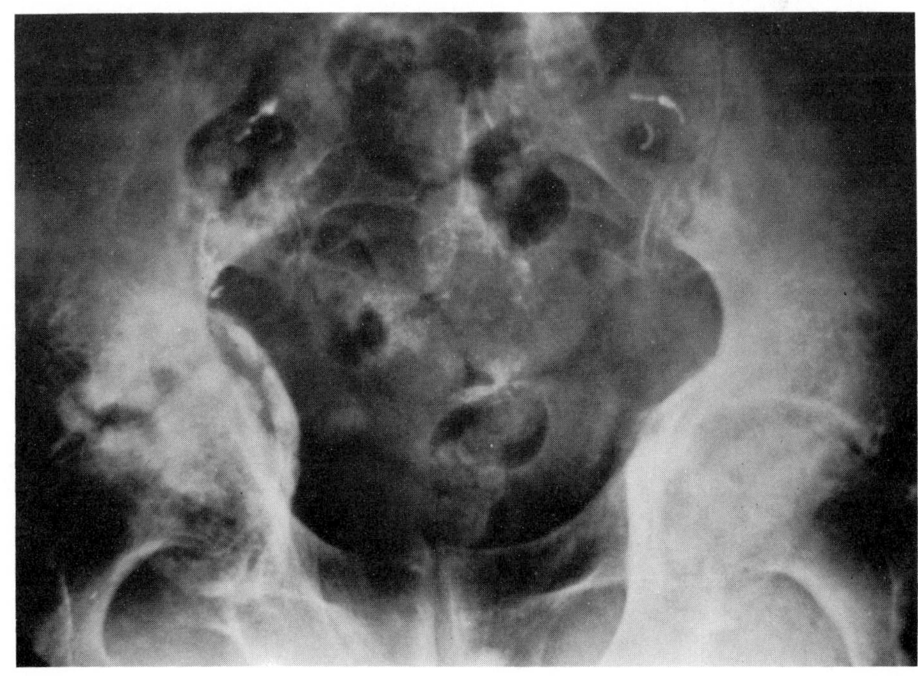

Figure 65–19. Protrusio *acetabuli following treatment of prostatic carcinoma with 7000 rads. There is a considerable degree of protrusio acetabuli on the right side with an acetabular fracture and loss of the joint space. Mild protrusio is present on the left. (From Hasselbacher P, Schumacher HR: J Rheumatol 41:189, 1977.)*

sis involving more than one sternal segment. Severe changes were defined as complete osseous necrosis of one or more sternal segments with deformity.[69] The changes were more common and more severe in those patients treated with orthovoltage therapy.[69]

Miscellaneous Sites. Radiation changes in other areas usually follow a similar pattern. Well-defined lucent shadows are sometimes identified within the field of therapy.[116] These can occur in normal bone following therapy for a soft tissue neoplasm (Figs. 65–20 and 65–21) or in bone previously treated for an osseous lesion (Fig. 65–22). Small areas of trabecular sclerosis may occur, as can larger areas of ischemic necrosis. Bragg and co-workers have described faint sclerosis in phalangeal lesions.[12]

Articular cartilage is relatively radioresistant and Dawson stated that osteoarthritis does not occur following radiotherapy.[22] Occasionally, severe cartilaginous destruction can be seen with joint space narrowing and productive osteophyte formation. This may represent secondary degenerative arthritis caused by destructive changes with collapse of the subchondral bone. However, it may be a direct effect of radiation therapy[72] (Fig. 65–15).

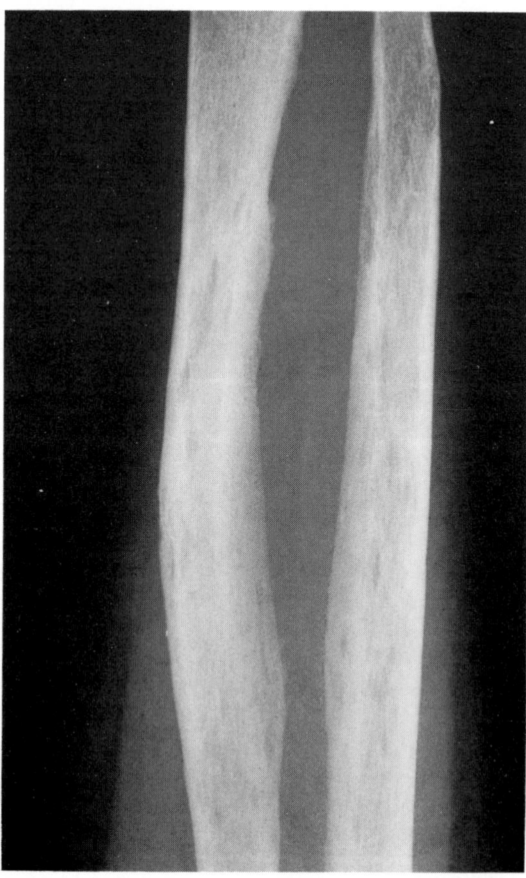

Figure 65–20. *Anteroposterior view of forearm revealing multiple lucent lesions within the shaft of the radius and ulna, representing radiation necrosis following therapy for soft tissue tumor.*

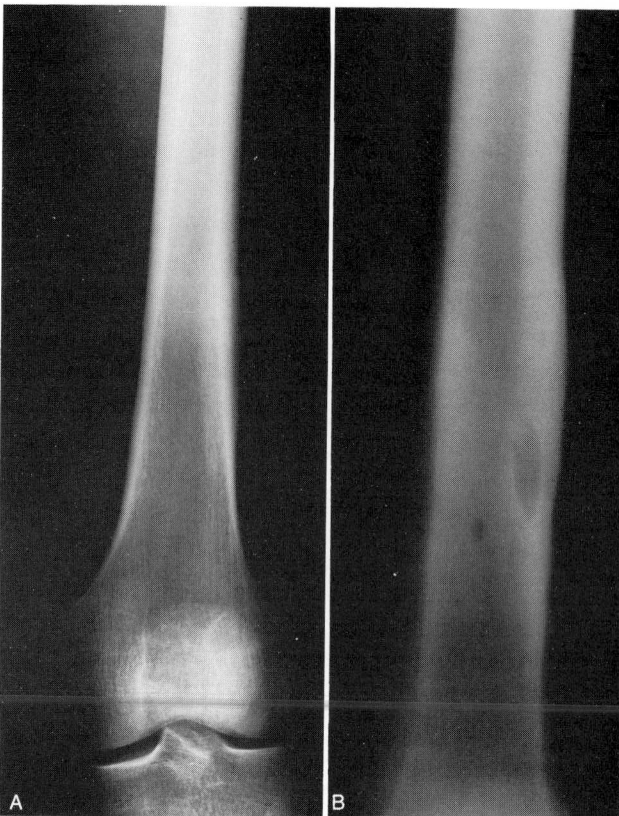

Figure 65–21. *Radiation necrosis following treatment for soft tissue liposarcoma.*

A *Normal femur.*

B *Same patient 2 years following therapy, revealing resorption cavities within the femur secondary to radiation.*

(Courtesy of Dr. Ferris Hall, Boston, Massachusetts.)

Radiation-Induced Neoplasms

Benign. Exostoses (osteochondromas) have been reported to arise in normal bone treated with radiation therapy. Osteochondromas are the only benign radiation-induced tumors reported in humans. Experimentally, enchondromas identical to those seen in Ollier's disease have been produced secondary to internal[98] or external radiation. Exostoses can be seen in any bone within the irradiated field (Figs. 65–23 and 65–24). Osteochondromas occur exclusively in children[25] and are more likely to occur if the patient has been irradiated prior to the age of 2 years. They have been reported with doses ranging from 1600 to 6425 rads,[70] although Murphy and Blount reported an exostosis in a patient who received 125 rads during the first week of life,[70] and Sanger and associates[91] reported three patients treated prior to the age of 2 years who developed osteochondromas with doses of less than 1000 rads. All five of Murphy and Blount's cases arose at the periphery of the irradiated field.[70] Radiation-induced exostoses are histologically and radiologically identical to spontaneously occurring osteochondromas, but to date there has

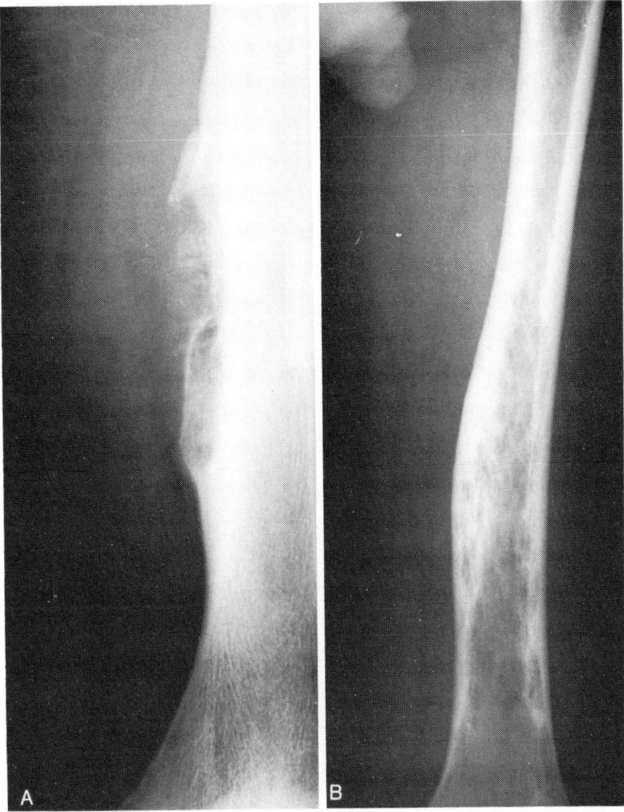

Figure 65–22. *Ewing's tumor followed by late radiation necrosis.*

A *Oblique view of femur demonstrating destructive diaphyseal lesion with saucerization, perpendicular periosteal new bone formation, and a large soft tissue mass. Codman's triangles are present at both edges of the lesion.*

B *Same patient 31 years later, revealing multiple well-defined lucent areas in the shaft of the femur secondary to radiation necrosis.*

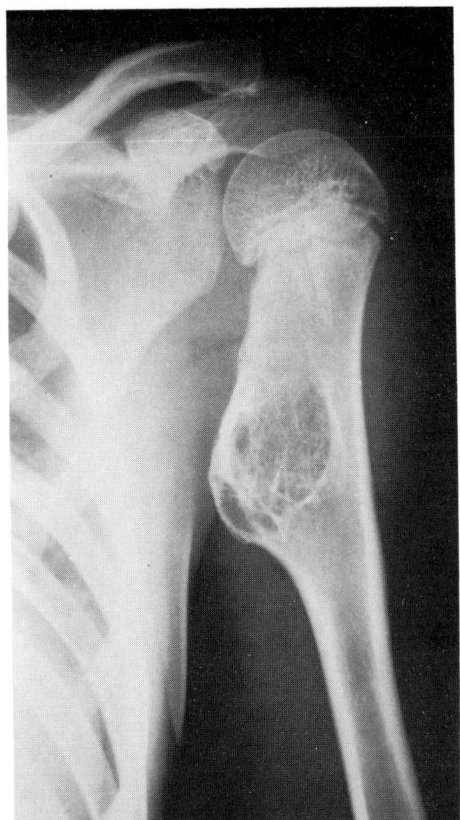

Figure 65–23. *Radiation-induced exostosis in the proximal humerus following radiation therapy. This appearance is identical to that of a spontaneously occurring osteochondroma. (Courtesy of Dr. Walter E. Berdon, Babies Hospital, New York, New York.)*

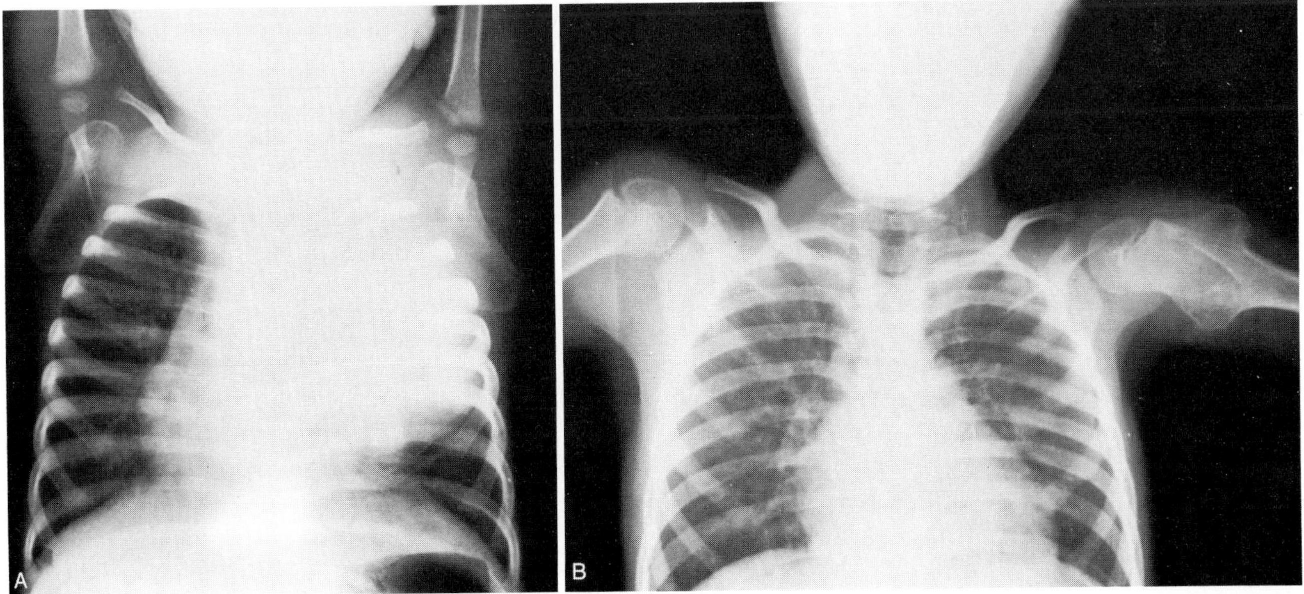

Figure 65–24. *Exostoses secondary to radiation therapy.*

A *Left posterior mediastinal neuroblastoma, which was biopsied, partially excised, and treated with 2500 rad tumor dose.*

B *Same patient 8 years later, revealing two benign exostoses.*

(From Berdon WE, et al: Am J Roentgenol 93:565, 1964. Copyright 1945, American Roentgen Ray Society.)

been no well-documented case of malignant degeneration.[89]

MALIGNANT. Radiation-induced neoplasia was first reported in 1902 by Frieben, who reported a case of squamous cell carcinoma of the skin with lymph node metastases.[37] Other early workers described cases of squamous cell carcinoma of the skin following x-ray dermatitis and continuous x-ray exposures.[13] In 1922 Beck reported three patients who developed osteogenic sarcoma following roentgen therapy for tuberculous arthritis.[5] Martland and Humphries in 1929 reported on the development of osteosarcomas in radium dial workers.[65]

In the laboratory, osteosarcomas have been produced by external radiation[11, 111] as well as by bone-seeking radionuclides.[32] Fabrikant and Smith have shown that in mice osteosclerotic changes frequently precede the development of osteosarcomas.[32]

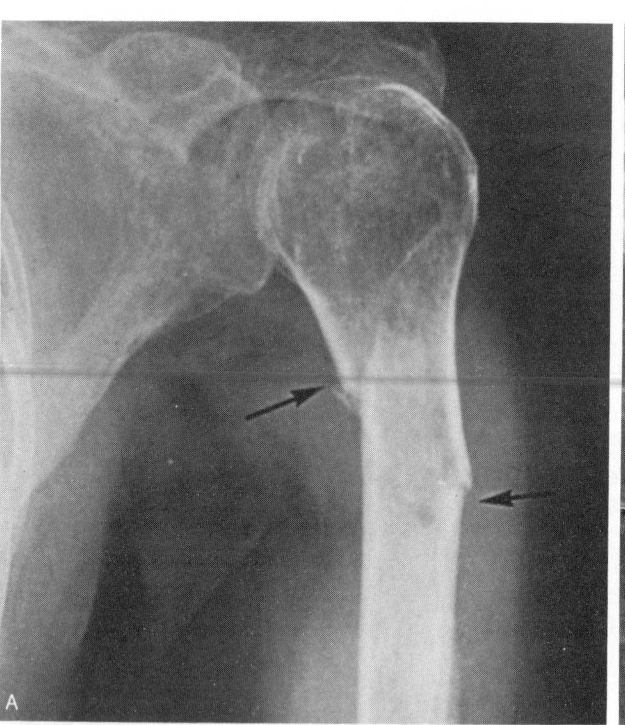

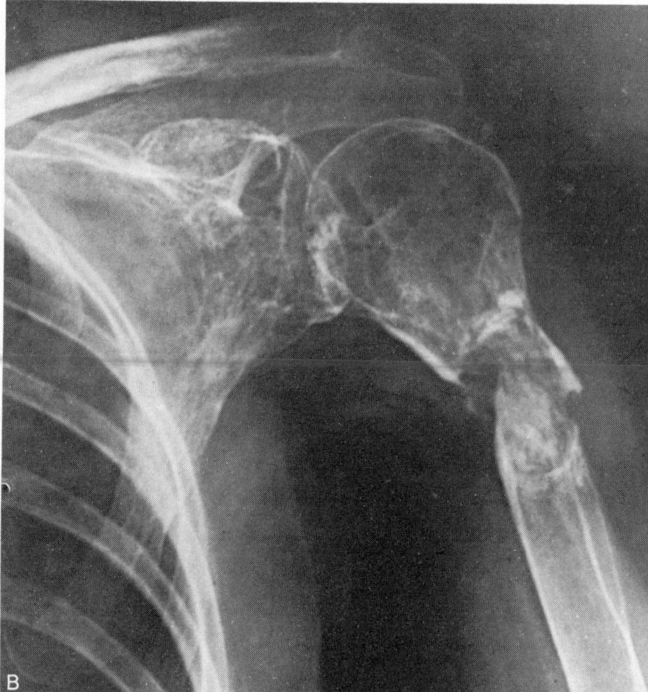

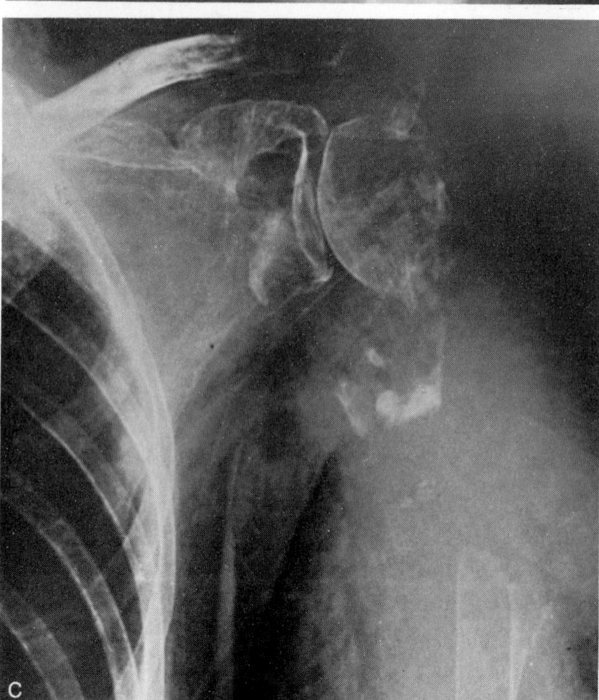

Figure 65–25. *Sarcoma arising in irradiated bone.*

A *Pathologic fracture (arrows) of proximal humerus 6 years following radiation therapy for carcinoma of the breast.*

B *Same patient 2 years later, revealing pseudoarthrosis of the humerus with radiation changes in the scapula and humerus.*

C *Same patient 6 years following* **B,** *with an undifferentiated radiation-induced sarcoma of the humerus.*

*(***A, C,** *From Dalinka MK, et al: Semin Roentgenol 9:29, 1974.)*

They produced sarcomas utilizing both alpha and beta emitters and showed that the osseous changes were independent of the method of production. The location of the tumors was mainly in the long bones with phosphorus-32, a beta emitter.[32] Tumors induced by the alpha emitters plutonium-239 and americium-211 had a more widespread distribution.[32] King and co-workers[111] believe that combined radiographic and scintigraphic techniques should be utilized for the early detection of radiation-induced osteosarcomas.

Arlen and co-workers[4] and others[67, 99, 103] have shown that radiation osteitis is frequently present adjacent to radiation-induced tumors. This was present in 50 per cent of Arlen and colleagues' cases[4] and in 10 of 11 patients in Steiner's series.[99] In humans as well as animals, bony changes usually precede the development of radiation-induced tumors (Fig. 65–25). Cruz and associates stated that these changes usually occur in the areas of intermediate radiation damage, as heavily damaged areas lack the capability to regenerate.[17]

Cahan and collaborators established the following criteria for the diagnosis of radiation-induced sarcoma[14]:

1. Microscopic or radiologic evidence of a nonmalignant condition.
2. Sarcoma must arise within the irradiated field.
3. A long latent period must be present — at least 4 years.
4. There must be histologic proof of sarcoma.

Arlen and co-workers modified these criteria slightly by stating that a malignant tumor with different histology from the primary lesion would also be acceptable as radiation induced.[4] In a series of 50 radiation-induced sarcomas, there were two osteosarcomas that arose in areas of treated round cell tumors: one Ewing's tumor and one reticulum cell sarcoma.[4]

Radiation-induced sarcomas can arise in areas of normal bone or bone treated for benign or malignant tumors.[4] Histologically a radiation-induced sarcoma is identical to a spontaneously occurring sarcoma.[57] In most series, osteosarcoma is the most common radiation-induced sarcoma,[11, 14, 101] but in some series, fibrosarcoma is the most common.[4] Chondrosarcomas have occasionally been reported[34, 78] and account for approximately 9 per cent of radiation-induced tumors.[8] Feintuch reported a patient with fibrous dysplasia, which degenerated into chondrosarcoma following radiation.[33] Unusual bone tumors with confusing histology may also occur following radiation.[16]

The evidence that radiation can induce sarcomas is overwhelming. Sarcomas have been reported with doses as low as 800 rads for the treatment of bursitis.[38] Radiation-induced sarcomas usually require a dose of at least 3000 rads in 3 weeks, with a threshold appearing at about 1000 rads.[57] In children, one would expect a higher incidence of radiation-induced tumors because of the longer potential period at risk.[103] However, the latent period does not seem to differ between children and adults.[93]

The latent period for radiation-induced tumors varies between 4 and 42 years, with an average of 11 years[67] (Fig. 65–26). These tumors have been produced by supervoltage as well as orthovoltage therapy.

Sarcomas have been produced in the skull following pituitary radiation[1, 97] and therapy for retinoblastoma.[90, 113] Sagerman and co-workers believed that the minimal risk for developing osteosarcoma was 1.5 per cent of survivors.[90] However, two of their 23 patients developed osteosarcoma outside the irradiated field, which may indicate an increased incidence of osteosarcoma in patients with retinoblastoma.[90]

The incidence of radiation-induced sarcoma has ranged from 0.1 per cent of 5 year survivors[80] to 0.2 per cent of 10 year survivors from breast carcinoma.[48, 57] In one series of 50 radiation-induced sarcomas, 35 patients had preexisting bone disease.[4] In the most recent literature, most cases of radiation-induced tumors have occurred in patients with previously normal bone.

Radiation necrosis can usually be differentiated from sarcoma arising in irradiated bone, although

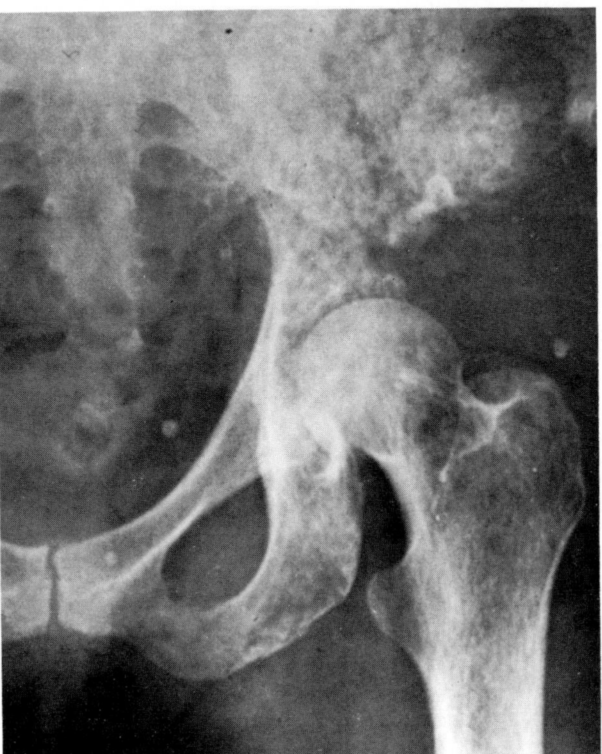

Figure 65–26. *Anteroposterior view of pelvis with osteosarcoma of left iliac wing 17 years following therapy for cervical carcinoma. (From Dalinka MK, et al: Semin Roentgenol 9:29, 1974.)*

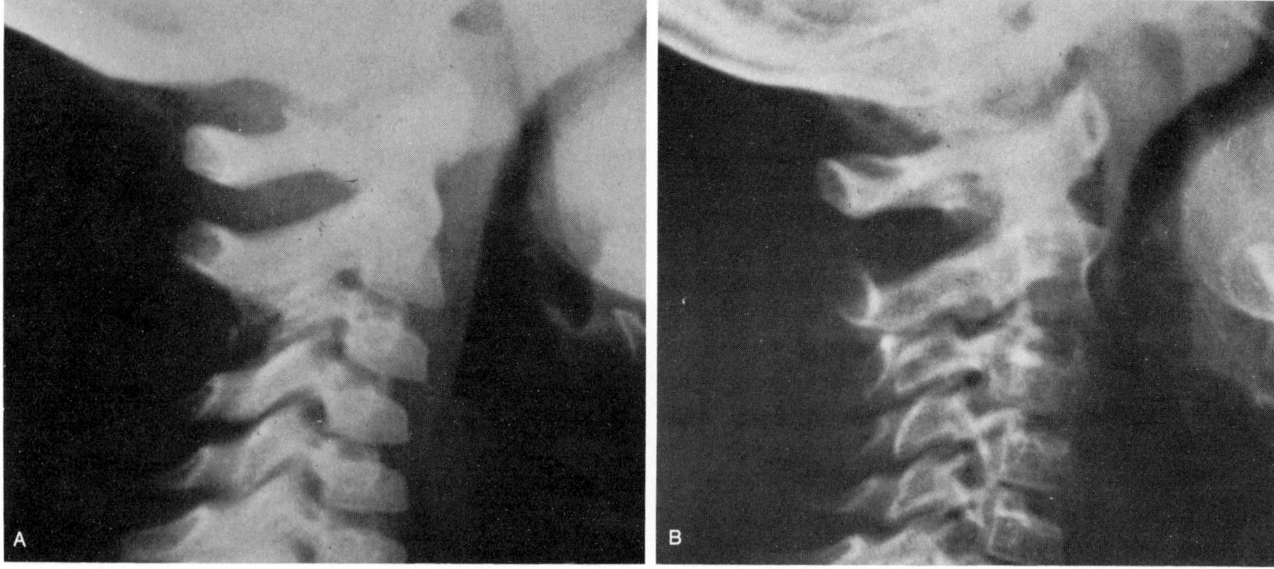

Figure 65–27. Healing of eosinophilic granuloma of spine following radiation therapy.
A There is a destructive lesion involving the spinous process and the lamina of C3.
B Same patient following 600 rads of radiation therapy, showing complete healing of the destructive osseous lesion.

occasional cases may cause difficulty. Both necrosis and sarcoma occur within the field of radiation and often have long latent periods. The presence of pain and a soft tissue mass favors the diagnosis of neoplasia, whereas their absence favors radiation necrosis. The relative lack of progression on serial roentgenograms favors the diagnosis of radiation necrosis.

Healing of Irradiated Osseous Lesions

Recognition of the inherent dangers and complications of radiation therapy has led to its more judicious use. Occasionally aggressive benign lesions in inaccessible areas, particularly the spine, are still treated by radiation. Patients with histiocytosis are frequently given low dose radiation, usually 550 to 600 rads.[96] Following therapy, the lytic lesions frequently heal and appear normal (Fig. 65–27).

Radiation and combination chemotherapy are utilized in the management of primary malignant round cell tumors of bone, particularly Ewing's tumor and lymphoma of bone. The radiation dose is usually between 5000 and 6000 rads. Radiation leads to healing of the osseous lesions (Fig. 65–5) and may convert layered periosteal reaction into thick periosteal new bone. With the large doses used in the treatment of these lesions, the changes of radiation necrosis frequently occur with long-term survival (Fig. 65–22).

Radiation is used extensively in the management of painful metastatic lesions. These patients are treated symptomatically with relatively low doses, frequently with large fractions. A favorable clinical response is often followed by sclerosis in the treated area, with partial or complete healing of the metastatic focus.

Parametrial Calcifications in Patients Treated for Cervical Carcinoma with Radioactive Gold

Deeths and Stanley found soft tissue calcification in the parametrium in 17 of 31 patients treated with colloidal gold-198 injections for cervical carcinoma.[23] In 16 of 17 cases, the calcifications were confined to the area of injection. Calcification varied in appearance from linear to globular and was sometimes associated with periosteal reactions, thought to be either reactive in nature or secondary to partial subperiosteal injection. This adjuvant therapy was used between 1950 and 1964 in conjunction with radiation and surgery; it was abandoned when supervoltage therapy became available because of its excess complications.

SUMMARY

The effects of radiation on bone occur secondary to accidental exposure (radium dial workers) as well as to diagnostic (Thorotrast) and therapeutic administration. Radiation therapy may affect bone growth, cause osseous necrosis, and induce neoplasia.

REFERENCES

1. Amine ARC, Sugar O: Suprasellar osteogenic sarcoma following radiation for pituitary adenoma: Case report. J Neurosurg *44*:88, 1976.
2. Arkin AM, Simon N: Radiation scoliosis; an experimental study. J Bone Joint Surg *32A*:396, 1950.
3. Arkin AM, Pack GT, Ransohoff NS, Simon N: Radiation induced scoliosis; a case report. J Bone Joint Surg *32A*:401, 1950.
4. Arlen M, Higinbotham NL, Huvos AG, Marcove RC, Miller T, Shah IC: Radiation induced sarcoma of bone. Cancer *28*:1087, 1971.
5. Beck A: Zur Frage des Röntgensarkoms, zugleich ein Beitrag zur Pathogenese des Sarkoms. Münch Med Wochenschr *69*:623, 1922. (Cited in Cahan WG, Woodard HQ, Higinbotham NL, Stewart FW, Coley BL: Sarcoma arising in irradiated bone: Report of eleven cases. Cancer *1*:3, 1948.)
6. Bedwinek JM, Shukovsky LJ, Fletcher GH, Daley TE: Osteonecrosis in patients treated with definitive radiotherapy for squamous cell carcinomas of the oral cavity and naso- and oropharynx. Radiology *119*:665, 1976.
7. Berdon WE, Baker DH, Boyer J: Unusual benign and malignant sequelae to childhood radiation therapy including "unilateral hyperlucent lung." Am J Roentgenol *93*:545, 1945.
8. Bisgard JD, Hunt HB: Influence of roentgen rays and radium on epiphyseal growth in long bones. Radiology *26*:56, 1936.
9. Blum T: Osteomyelitis of the mandible and maxilla. J Am Dent Assoc *11*:802, 1924.
10. Bonfiglio M: The pathology of fractures of the femoral neck following irradiation. Am J Roentgenol *70*:449, 1953.
11. Brady LW: Radiation induced sarcomas of bone. Skel Radiol *41*:72, 1979.
12. Bragg DG, Shidnia H, Chu FCH, Higinbotham NL: The clinical and radiographic aspects of radiation osteitis. Radiology *97*:103, 1970.
13. Cade S: Radiation induced cancer in man. Br J Radiol *30*:393, 1957.
14. Cahan WG, Woodard HQ, Higinbotham NL, Stewart FW, Coley B: Sarcoma arising in irradiated bone; report of 11 cases. Cancer *1*:3, 1948.
15. Cheng VST, Wang CC: Osteonecrosis of the mandible resulting from external megavoltage radiation therapy. Radiology *112*:685, 1974.
16. Cohen J, D'Angio GJ: Unusual bone tumors after roentgen therapy of children. Am J Roentgenol *86*:502, 1961.
17. Cruz MN, Coley BL, Stewart FW: Post-radiation bone sarcoma; report of eleven cases. Cancer *10*:72, 1957.
18. Dalby RG, Jacox HW, Miller NF: Fracture of the femoral neck following irradiation. Am J Obstet Gynecol *32*:50, 1936.
19. Dalinka MK, Edeiken J, Finkelstein JB: Complications of radiation therapy: Adult bone. Semin Roentgenol *9*:29, 1974.
20. da Silva Horta J: Late effects of thorotrast on the liver and spleen and their efferent lymph nodes. Ann NY Acad Sci *145*:676, 1967.
21. da Silva Horta J: Effects of colloidal thorium dioxide extravasates in the subcutaneous tissues of the cervical region in man. Ann NY Acad Sci *145*:776, 1967.
22. Dawson WB: Growth impairment following radiotherapy in childhood. Clin Radiol *19*:241, 1968.
23. Deeths TM, Stanley RJ: Parametrial calcification in cervical carcinoma patients treated with radioactive gold. Am J Roentgenol *127*:511, 1976.
24. DeSantos LA, Libshitz HI: Adult bone. *In* HI Libshitz (Ed): Diagnostic Roentgenology of Radiotherapy Change. Baltimore, Williams & Wilkins, 1979.
25. DeSantos LA, Libshitz HI: Growing bone and radiation induced neoplasia. *In* HI Libshitz (Ed): Diagnostic Roentgenology of Radiotherapy Change. Baltimore, Williams & Wilkins, 1979.
26. Desjardins AU: Osteogenic tumor: Growth injury of bone and muscular atrophy following therapeutic irradiation. Radiology *14*:296, 1930.
27. DeSmet AA, Kuhns LR, Fayos JV, Holt JF: Effects of radiation therapy on growing long bones. Am J Roentgenol *127*:935, 1976.
28. Ellis F: Dose, time and fractionation, a clinical hypothesis. Clin Radiol *20*:1, 1969.
29. El-Mahdi AM, Marks R, Thornton WN, Constable WC: Sequelae of pelvic irradiation in infancy. Radiology *110*:665, 1974.
30. Engel D: Experiments on the production of spinal deformities by radium. Am J Roentgenol *42*:217, 1939.
31. Ewing J: Radiation osteitis. Acta Radiol *6*:399, 1926.
32. Fabrikant JI, Smith CLD: Radiographic changes following the administration of bone seeking radionuclides. Br J Radiol *37*:53, 1964.
33. Feintuch TA: Chondrosarcoma arising in a cartilagenous area of previously irradiated fibrous dysplasia. Cancer *31*:877, 1973.
34. Fitzwater JE, Cabaud HE, Farr GH: Irradiation induced chondrosarcoma. A case report. J Bone Joint Surg *58A*:1037, 1976.
35. Försterling K: Über allgemeine und partielle Wachstumsstorungen nach Kurz dauernden Röntgenbestrahlungen von säugethieren. Arch Klin Chir *81*:505, 1906. (Cited in Dawson WB: Growth impairment following radiotherapy in childhood. Clin Radiol *19*:241, 1968.)
36. Frantz CH: Extreme retardation of epiphyseal growth from roentgen irradiation. A case study. Radiology *55*:720, 1950.
37. Frieben A: Cancroid des Handrückens nach langdauernder Einwirkung von Röntgenstrahlen. Fortschr Geb Rontgenstr Nuklearmed *6*:106, 1902. (Cited in Cade S: Radiation induced cancer in man. Br J Radiol *30*:393, 1967.)
38. Glicksman AS, Toker C: Osteogenic sarcoma following radiotherapy for bursitis. Mt Sinai Med *43*:163, 1976.
39. Gondos B: Late clinical and roentgen observations following Thorotrast administration. Clin Radiol *24*:195, 1973.
40. Grant BP, Fletcher GH: Analysis of complications following megavoltage therapy for squamous cell carcinomas of the tonsillar area. Am J Roentgenol *96*:28, 1966.
41. Gratzek FR, Holmstrom EG, Rigler LG: Post-irradiation bone changes. Am J Roentgenol *53*:62, 1945.
42. Guttenberg SA: Osteoradionecrosis of the jaw. Am J Surg *127*:326, 1974.
43. Hall FM, Mauch PM, Levene MB, Goldstein MA: Protrusio acetabuli following pelvic irradiation. Am J Roentgenol *132*:291, 1979.
44. Hasselbacher P, Schumacher HR: Bilateral protrusio acetabuli following pelvic irradiation. J Rheumatol *4*:189, 1977.
45. Hasson J, Hartman KS, Milikow E, Mittelman JA: Thorotrast induced extra-skeletal osteosarcoma of the cervical region. Cancer *36*:1827, 1975.
46. Hasterlik RJ, Finkel AJ: Diseases of bones and joints associated with intoxication by radioactive substances, principally radium. Med Clin North Am *49*:285, 1965.
47. Hasterlik RJ, Miller CE, Finkel AJ: Radiographic development of skeletal lesions in man many years after acquisition of radium burden. Radiology *93*:599, 1969.
48. Hatfield PM, Schulz, MD: Post irradiation sarcoma: Including five cases after x-ray therapy of breast carcinoma. Radiology *96*:593, 1970.
49. Heaston DK, Libshitz HI, Chan RC: Skeletal effects of megavoltage irradiation in survivors of Wilms' tumor. Am J Roentgenol *133*:389, 1979.
50. Howland WJ, Loeffler RK, Starchman DE, Johnson RG: Post irradiation atrophic changes of bone and related complications. Radiology *117*:677, 1975.
51. Hueck H, Spiess W: Zur Fräge der Wachstumsstorungen bei röntgenbestrahlten Knochen- und Gelenktuberkulosen. Strahlentherapie *32*:322, 1929. (Cited in DeSantos LA, Libshitz HI: Growing bone and radiation induced neoplasia. *In* HI Libshitz [Ed]: Diagnostic Roentgenology of Radiotherapy Change. Baltimore, Williams & Wilkins, 1979.)
52. Janower ML: Occupational hazard. JAMA *190*:769, 1964.
53. Janower ML, Miettinen OS, Flynn MJ: Effects of long term Thorotrast exposure. Radiology *103*:13, 1972.
54. Jee WSS, Dockum NL, Mical RS, Arnold JS, Looney WB: Distribution of thorium daughters in bone. Ann NY Acad Sci *145*:660, 1967.
55. Katzman H, Waugh T, Berdon W: Skeletal changes following irradiation of childhood tumors. J Bone Joint Surg *51A*:825, 1969.
56. Kim JH, Chu FCH, Pope RA, Woodard HQ, Bragg DB, Shidnia H: Time dose factors in radiation induced osteitis. Am J Roentgenol *120*:684, 1974.
57. Kim JH, Chu FCH, Woodard HQ, Melamed MR, Huvos A, Cantin J: Radiation induced soft tissue and bone sarcoma. Radiology *129*:501, 1978.
58. Langlands AO, Souter WA, Samuel E, Redpath AT: Radiation osteitis following irradiation for breast cancer. Clin Radiol *28*:93, 1977.
59. Levowitz BS, Hughes RE, Alford TC: Treatment of thorium dioxide granulomas of the neck. N Engl J Med *268*:340, 1963.
60. Looney WB: Investigation of the late clinical findings following Thorotrast (thorium dioxide) administration. Am J Roentgenol *83*:163, 1960.
61. Looney WB, Hasterlik RJ, Brues AM, Skirmont E: A clinical investigation of the chronic effects of radium salts administered therapeutically (1915–1931). Am J Roentgenol *73*:1006, 1955.
62. Loutit JF: Malignancy from radium. Br J Cancer *24*:195, 1970.
63. Mainous EG, Hart GB: Osteoradionecrosis of the mandible treated with hyperbaric oxygen. Arch Otolaryngol *101*:173, 1975.
64. Marciani RD, Bowden CM Jr: Osteoradionecrosis of the maxilla: Report of a case. J Oral Surg *31*:56, 1973.
65. Martland HS, Humphries RE: Osteogenic sarcoma in dial painters using luminous paint. Arch Pathol *7*:406, 1929.
66. Meyer JE: Thoracic effects of therapeutic irradiation for breast carcinoma. Am J Roentgenol *130*:877, 1978.
67. Mindell ER, Shah NK, Webster JH: Post radiation sarcoma of bone and soft tissues. Orthop Clin North Am *8*:821, 1977.
68. Montague ED: Experience with altered fractionation in radiation therapy of breast cancer. Radiology *90*:962, 1968.
69. Morris LL, Cassady JR, Jaffe N: Sternal changes following mediastinal irradiation for childhood Hodgkin's disease. Radiology *115*:701, 1975.

70. Murphy FD Jr, Blount WP: Cartilaginous exostoses following irradiation. J Bone Joint Surg *44A*:662, 1962.
71. Murphy WA, Seligman PA, Tillack T, Eichling, JO, Teitelbaum SL, Joist JH: Osteosclerosis, osteomalacia, and bone marrow aplasia; a combined late complication of Thorotrast administration. Skel Radiol *3*:234, 1979.
72. Murphy W: Personal communication, 1979.
73. Neuhauser EBD, Wittenborg MH, Berman CZ, Cohen J: Irradiation effects of roentgen therapy on the growing spine. Radiology *59*:637, 1952.
74. Oliver JH, Gluck G, Gledhill RB, Chevalier L: Musculoskeletal deformities following treatment of Wilms' tumor. Can Med Assoc J *119*:459, 1978.
75. Parker RG: Tolerance of mature bone and cartilage in clinical radiation therapy. Front Radiat Ther Oncol *6*:312, 1972.
76. Parker RG, Berry HC: Late effects of therapeutic irradiation on the skeleton and bone marrow. Cancer *37*:1162, 1976.
77. Paul LW, Pohle EA: Radiation osteitits of the ribs. Radiology *38*:543, 1942.
78. Peimer CA, Yuan HA, Sagerman RH: Post radiation chondrosarcoma, a case report. J Bone Joint Surg *58A*:1033, 1976.
79. Perthes G: Ueber den Einfluss der Roentgenstrahlen auf epitheliale Gewebe, insbesondere aus des Carcinom. Arch Klin Chir *71*:955, 1903. (Cited in Dawson WB: Growth impairment following radiotherapy in childhood. Clin Radiol *19*:241, 1968.)
80. Phillips TL, Sheline GE: Bone sarcomas following radiation therapy. Radiology *81*:992, 1963.
81. Plenge K, Kruckenmeyer K: Über ein Sarkom am Ort der Thorotrast injektion. Zentralbl. Allg Pathol *92*:255, 1954. (Cited in da Silva Horta J: Effects of colloidal thorium dioxide extravasates in the subcutaneous tissues of the cervical region in man. Ann NY Acad Sci *145*:776, 1967.)
82. Probert JC, Parker BR: The effects of radiation therapy on bone growth. Radiology *114*:155, 1975.
83. Reidy JA, Lingley JR, Gall EA, Barr JS: The effect of roentgen irradiation on epiphyseal growth. II. Experimental studies upon the dog. J Bone Joint Surg *29A*:853, 1947.
84. Riseborough EJ, Grabias SL, Burton R, Jaffe N: Skeletal alterations following irradiation for Wilms' tumor, with particular reference to scoliosis and kyphosis. J Bone Joint Surg *58A*:526, 1976.
85. Rubin P, Casarett GW: Growing cartilage and bone. *In* Clinical Radiation Pathology. Vol 2. Philadelphia, WB Saunders Co, 1968, p 518.
86. Rubin P, Casarett GW: Mature cartilage and adult bone. *In* Clinical Radiation Pathology. Vol 2. Philadelphia, WB Saunders Co, 1968, p 557.
87. Rubin P, Duthie RB, Young LW: The significance of scoliosis in postirradiated Wilms' tumor and neuroblastoma. Radiology *79*:539, 1962.
88. Rubin P, Probhasawat D: Characteristic bone lesions in post irradiated carcinoma of the cervix — metastases versus osteonecrosis. Radiology *76*:703, 1961.
89. Rutherford H, Dodd GD: Complications of radiation therapy: Growing bone. Semin Roentgenol *9*:15, 1974.
90. Sagerman RH, Cassady JR, Tretter P, Ellsworth RM: Radiation induced neoplasia following external beam therapy for children with retinoblastoma. Am J Roentgenol *105*:529, 1969.
91. Saenger EL, Silverman F, Sterling TD, Turner ME: Neoplasia following therapeutic irradiation for benign conditions in childhood. Radiology *74*:889, 1960.
92. Sengupta S, Prathap K: Radiation necrosis of the humerus. A report of three cases. Acta Radiol (Ther) *12*:313, 1973.
93. Sim FH, Cupps RE, Dahlin DC, Ivins JC: Post radiation sarcoma of bone. J Bone Joint Surg *54A*:1479, 1972.
94. Sindelar WF, Costa J, Ketcham AS: Osteosarcoma associated with Thorotrast administration. Report of two cases and literature review. Cancer *42*:2604, 1978.
95. Slaughter DP: Radiation osteitis and fractures following irradiation with report of five cases of fractured clavicle. Am J Roentgenol *48*:201, 1942.
96. Smith DG, Nesbit ME Jr, D'Angio GJ, Levitt SH: Histiocytosis X: Role of radiation therapy in management with special reference to dose levels employed. Radiology *106*:419, 1973.
97. Sparagana M, Eells RW, Stefani S, Jablokow V: Osteogenic sarcoma of the skull: A rare sequela of pituitary irradiation. Cancer *29*:1376, 1972.
98. Spiess H: Exostotische Dysplasie durch Strahlenwirkung? Dtsch Med Wochenschr *35*:1483, 1957. (Cited in Berdon WE, Baker DH, Boyer J: Unusual benign and malignant sequelae to childhood radiation therapy including "unilateral hyperlucent lung." Am J Roentgenol *93*:545, 1965.)
99. Steiner: Post radiation sarcoma of bone. Cancer *18*:603, 1965.
100. Tefft M: Irradiation effect on growing bone and cartilage. Front Radiat Ther Oncol *6*:289, 1972.
101. Tefft M, Vawter GF, Mitus A: Second primary neoplasms in children. Am J Roentgenol *103*:800, 1968.
102. Teplick JG, Head GL, Kricun ME, Haskin MD: Ghost infantile vertebrae and hemi-pelves within adult skeleton from Thorotrast administration in childhood. Radiology *129*:657, 1978.
103. Tountas AA, Fornasier VL, Harwood AR, Leung PMK: Post irradiation sarcoma of bone—a perspective. Cancer *43*:182, 1979.
104. Vaeth JM, Levitt SH, Jones MD, Holtfreter C: Effects of radiation therapy in survivors of Wilms' tumor. Radiology *79*:560, 1962.
105. Vaughan J: Bone disease induced by radiation. Int Rev Exp Pathol *1*:243, 1962.
106. Vaughan J: The effects of skeletal irradiation. Clin Orthop Rel Res *56*:283, 1968.
107. Whitehouse WM, Lampe I: Osseous damage in irradiation of renal tumors in infancy and childhood. Am J Roentgenol *70*:721, 1953.
108. Wolf EL, Berdon WE, Cassady JR, Baker DH, Freiberger R, Paviov H: Slipped femoral capital epiphysis as a sequela to childhood irradiation for malignant tumors. Radiology *125*:781, 1977.
109. Dickerman JD, Newberg AH, Moreland, MD: Slipped capital femoral epiphysis (SCFE) following pelvic irradiation for rhabdomyosarcoma. Cancer *44*:480, 1979.
110. Erglin H, Howland WJ: Postradiation atrophy of mature bone. CRC Crit Rev in Diag Imag *12*:225, 1980.
111. King MA, Casarett GW, Weber DA, Burgener FA, O'Mara RE, Wilson GA: A study of irradiated bone. III. Scintigraphic and radiographic detection of radiation-induced osteosarcomas. J Nucl Med *21*:426, 1980.
112. Mayfield JK: Postradiation spinal deformity. Orthop Clin NA *10*:829, 1979.
113. Pagani JJ, Bassett LW, Winter J, Gold RH, Brawer M: Osteogenic sarcoma after retinoblastoma radiotherapy. AJR *133*:399, 1979.
114. Ryan BR, Walters TR: Slipped capital femoral epiphysis following radiotherapy and chemotherapy. Med and Ped Oncol *6*:279, 1979.
115. Chapman JA, Deakin DP, Green JH: Slipped upper femoral epiphysis after radiotherapy. J Bone Joint Surg *62B*:337, 1980.
116. Paling MR, Herdt JR: Radiation osteitis: A problem of recognition. Radiology *137*:339, 1980.

66

DISORDERS DUE TO MEDICATIONS AND OTHER CHEMICAL AGENTS

by Donald Resnick, M.D.

Significant musculoskeletal changes can result from medications and other chemical agents. The effects of some of these agents, such as heavy metals (Chapter 68), vitamins A, C, and D (Chapter 67), phenytoin (Chapter 49), polyvinyl chloride (Chapter 82), and alcohol (Chapter 70), are discussed elsewhere. In this chapter, consideration will be given to the musculoskeletal alterations that may accompany administration of certain teratogenic drugs, corticosteroids and other anti-inflammatory agents, fluorine, dopamine, calcium gluconate, and milk-alkali. The nonspecific alterations that may result from the trauma associated with the administration process itself will not be considered, although, for example, subcutaneous injection of drugs can lead to infection, calcification, pseudomalignant soft tissue reaction, and even introduction of foreign material.[1-4]

TERATOGENIC DRUGS

It is a well-recognized fact that medications administered to the pregnant woman can affect the fetus, a fact that is becoming increasingly important, as it has been recently estimated that more than 80 per cent of expectant mothers take at least one drug during pregnancy.[5-7] Certain of the drugs act on the somatic cells of the developing organism during vulnerable periods of embryogenesis and organogenesis and are termed teratogens. The teratogenicity of a drug is dependent upon several factors, including its chemical and pharmacologic properties, the duration of its use, the modification of the drug by the mother, the access of the fetus to the drug, the developmental stage of the fetus at the time of exposure, a possible genetic susceptibility to the agent, and the effect of the drug on fetal metabolism.[8] Some substances are known to be teratogenic, whereas others are suspected of possessing this property.[9] Of particular importance are four chemicals that appear to be teratogenic to the musculoskeletal system.[10]

Thalidomide

The thalidomide disaster became evident in the reports of McBride in 1961[11] and Lenz and Knapp in 1962.[12] This drug was used to induce sleep in the pregnant woman, and when its ingestion occurred in the first trimester, particularly between days 34 and 50 following the start of the last menstrual period,[12] thalidomide exposure could produce reduction deformities of the limbs. The anomalies included dysplasia of the thumb and radial hemimelia, phocomelia, or complete four limb amelia and were associated with hypoplasia or aplasia of the external ear and canal, congenital heart defects, gastrointestinal tract atresia or stenosis, and capillary hemangioma of the face.[10] The teratogenic effect of thalidomide may be related to inhibition of the early mesodermal precursors of the anlagen of the developing parts[10] or a chemical injury to the neural crest, which inhibits migration of its cells for the sensory nerve of the appropriate segment so that the tissues normally supplied by that nerve are deficient in growth.[13, 14, 162]

Anticonvulsants

When administered to expectant mothers, anticonvulsant medications, especially phenytoin,[15-17] may lead to congenital anomalies in infants, including hypoplasia of the distal phalanges, a digitate thumb, cleft palate, and peculiar facies.[10] The teratogenic potential of the anticonvulsants is not uniformly accepted by all investigators.[18]

Alcohol

Infants born to severely and chronically alcoholic women may reveal the fetal alcohol syndrome, consisting of prenatal and postnatal growth deficiency and delayed development.[10, 19-21] Findings may include clinodactyly, camptodactyly, and congenital dislocation of the hip. An association of the fetal alcohol syndrome (as well as the fetal phenytoin syndrome) with adrenal neoplasms has been suggested.[161]

Folic Acid Antagonists

Fetal malformations have been associated with maternal exposure to folic acid antagonists, especially aminopterin, and include cranial dysplasia and foot and hand anomalies.[22]

Other Drugs

There are a number of reports that implicate other drugs as teratogens. Examples include the potential role of warfarin (Coumadin) in the development of chondrodysplasia punctata (Conradi-Hünermann disease, chondrodystrophica calcificans congenita)[23, 24] and of estrogen and progestogen in certain congenital abnormalities.[25] It is certain that additional examples of teratogenic agents will be identified in the future; in this regard, the warning of Wilson[8] should be noted: "All chemicals are capable of producing some embryotoxic effect under the right conditions of dosage, developmental stage and species selection."

CORTICOSTEROIDS AND OTHER ANTI-INFLAMMATORY AGENTS

In 1949, Hench and colleagues[26] isolated a hormone of the adrenal cortex, compound E, and reported on its beneficial properties in the treatment of rheumatoid arthritis. In the subsequent decades, the anti-inflammatory characteristics of this agent became well known, as did certain of its side effects.

The complications of cortisone therapy can become manifest in almost all systems of the body, including the skeleton (Table 66–1). Detrimental effects include osteoporosis, osteonecrosis, neuropa-

Table 66–1

MUSCULOSKELETAL ABNORMALITIES ASSOCIATED WITH CORTICOSTEROID MEDICATION

Osteoporosis
Osteonecrosis
Neuropathic-like arthropathy
Osteomyelitis (septic arthritis)
Tendinous injury or rupture
Soft tissue atrophy

thic-like articular destruction, osteomyelitis, septic arthritis, and tendinous and soft tissue injury.

Osteoporosis

The occurrence of generalized osteoporosis in patients receiving systemic corticosteroids has been noted by many observers (Chapter 48). Pathologic fractures occur that heal with extensive callus formation.[27, 28] Collapse of single or multiple vertebral bodies with condensation of bone at the superior and inferior surfaces (Fig. 66–1) and infractions of ribs are particularly characteristic and are relatively asymptomatic in these steroid-medicated patients, who lack normal protective pain responses. The contribution of osteoporosis in periarticular locations to subchondral bony collapse and disintegration has been emphasized by some investigators[29] but is not universally accepted.[30]

Assessment of the exact role of corticosteroid medication in the production of osteoporosis is difficult because many of the conditions for which the drug is utilized are themselves associated with bone loss. This is particularly true in the inflammatory arthritides, in which immobilization and disuse are additional factors leading to osteoporosis.[31] It seems probable that accelerated bone loss is associated with the use of corticosteroids in noninflammatory conditions and that it is also evident in inflammatory disorders, particularly when the patients are more than 50 years of age. In the latter situation, however, the anti-inflammatory action of the drug could decrease the bone loss associated with the inflammation, and, in some cases, the net result may be a reduction in local bone turnover.[32] Although reports have been conflicting, steroid-induced osteoporosis may be more significant in patients receiving larger cumulative doses[167] and may be uninfluenced by the exact schedule of the therapeutic regimen.[168]

Osteonecrosis

Although osteonecrosis is a recognized complication of steroid therapy, it should not be equated

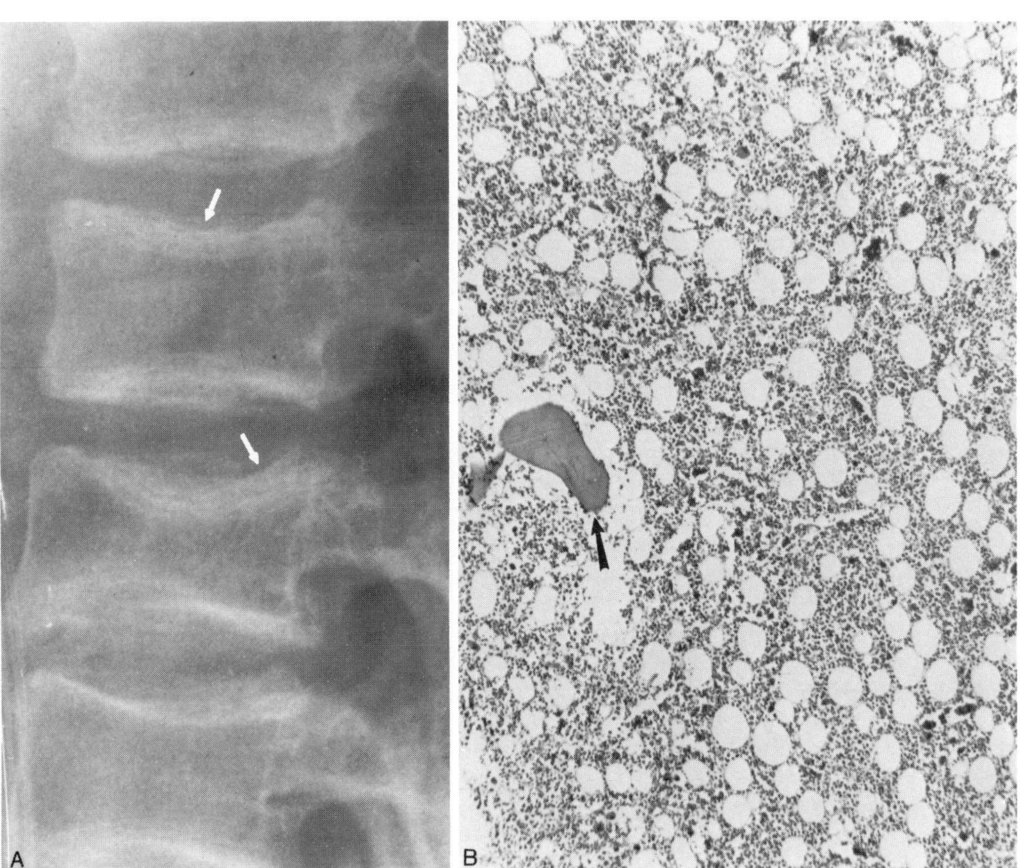

Figure 66–1. *Steroid-induced osteoporosis.*

A *A lateral radiograph of the lumbar spine reveals biconcave deformities of multiple vertebral bodies with bony condensation at the superior and inferior aspects of each vertebra (arrows). This appearance can be seen with exogenous or endogenous hypercortisolism.*

B *A photomicrograph (90×) indicates sparse bony trabeculae (arrow) surrounded by marrow.*

Illustration continued on the following page

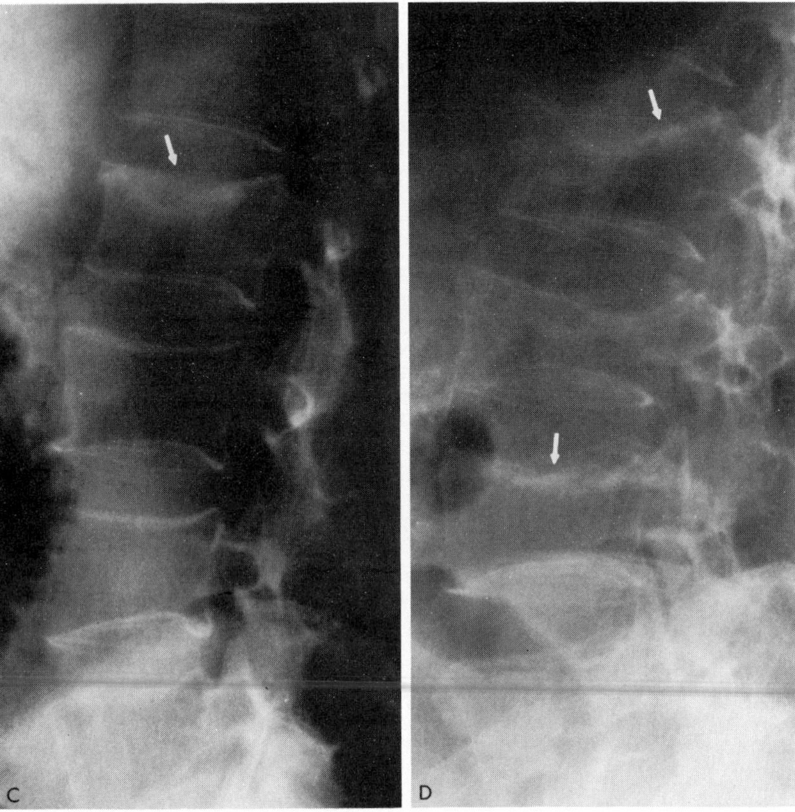

Figure 66–1. Continued

C, D *In another patient being treated with corticosteroids, radiographs of the lumbar spine exposed several months apart reveal osteoporosis, progressive collapse of vertebral bodies, and bony condensation (arrows) on the superior aspect of multiple collapsed vertebrae.*

with the term steroid arthropathy.[33] Steroid arthropathy indicates structural joint damage occurring in association with local or systemic administration of steroids; it may relate to osteoporosis and bony collapse, perhaps accelerated by the absence of pain sensation (following oral, parenteral, topical, or, most strikingly, intra-articular administration of steroids), or it may relate to osteonecrosis (following oral, parenteral, or topical administration of steroids). It is not always possible to distinguish which of the two processes is operational even on radiographic and pathologic examination, and in many cases, both may be occurring simultaneously.

Since the report of Pietrogrande and Mastromarino in 1957,[34] descriptions of steroid-induced osteonecrosis have been numerous.[27-30, 35-46] In some cases, the reports are complicated by the fact that the underlying disease for which the corticosteroids had been utilized, such as systemic lupus erythematosus,[165] may itself be capable of producing osteonecrosis, although the occurrence of bone necrosis in steroid-treated patients with conditions not associated with necrosis (asthma, tuberculosis, pemphigus, and thrombocytopenia purpura) is also well recognized.

The true incidence of steroid-induced osteonecrosis is difficult to determine because of the many variables that are included in the various studies. In patients receiving corticosteroids following renal transplantation, the incidence appears to be approximately 10 per cent;[47] this complication is probably less frequent in other conditions. In many reviews of patients with osteonecrosis, steroid medications have been implicated in 20 to 35 per cent of cases. The occurrence of steroid-induced bone necrosis appears to be directly related to the dosage level of the medication and may become prominent in many individuals after prolonged high intake.[39, 44] Other factors that may be important include the mode and the schedule of steroid administration.

The onset of symptoms and signs related to osteonecrosis usually is delayed for a period of 2 to 3 years following administration of the drug. Although it is uncommon to recognize clinical and radiographic manifestations of this complication within 6 months of the onset of the therapy, occasional examples of more acute bony necrosis are seen, and the rapidity of the radiographic and pathologic changes may be striking.[44] Single or multiple osseous sites can be affected; the femoral head, the humeral head, the distal femur, and the proximal tibia, in decreasing order of frequency, are most commonly altered. In general, although one site may be involved at the time of initial clinical presentation, there is a tendency for more widespread abnormalities to appear over a period of time. In fact, it is expected that approximately 30 to 50 per cent of patients who reveal steroid-induced osteonecrosis of one femoral head will later demonstrate changes on the contralateral side.

Radiographic and pathologic characteristics of

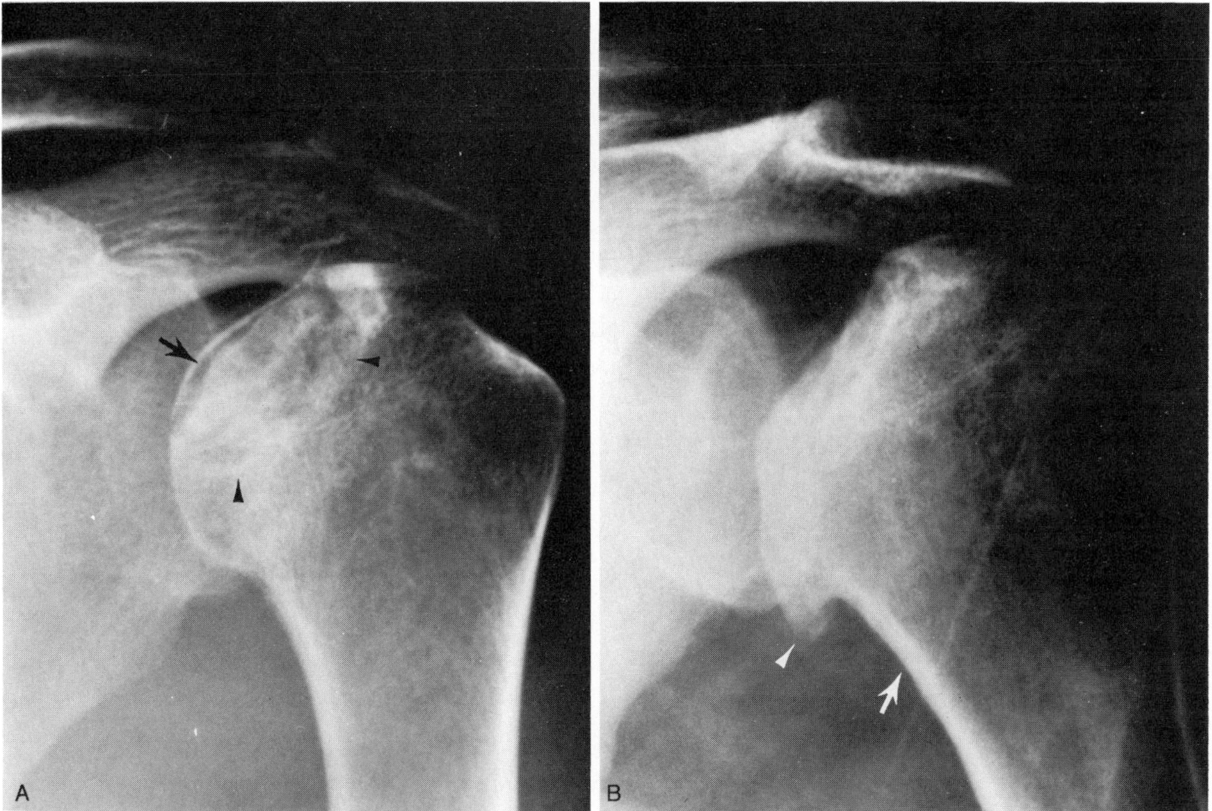

Figure 66–2. *Steroid-induced osteonecrosis: Proximal humerus.*

A *Abnormalities consist of flattening of the humeral head with a subchondral radiolucent line (crescent sign) (arrow), surrounding osteolysis and osteosclerosis (arrowheads), and relative preservation of joint space.*

B *In a more advanced case, significant collapse and fragmentation of bone with eburnation are evident. Thickening or "buttressing" of the medial humeral cortex (arrow) and osteophytosis (arrowhead) are also apparent.*

osteonecrosis due to corticosteroids are not unique, being evident in cases of bony necrosis due to other causes (Chapter 76). Osteoporosis, patchy osteosclerosis, subchondral radiolucent lines (crescent sign), osseous collapse, and fragmentation are recognized (Figs. 66–2 and 66–3). Preservation of joint space is also typical during the early stages of the process.

The pathogenesis of steroid-associated osteonecrosis is not clear (Table 66–2). Osteoporosis leading to microfractures and eventual bony collapse (mechanical factors) and vascular compromise due to compression from marrow accumulation of adjacent relatively inelastic fat cells, fat embolization, vasculitis, or hyperviscosity (vascular factors) are frequently proposed mechanisms for this complication. The mechanical theory gained support from Frost's observation that trabecular cracks can be observed in subchondral bone prior to collapse,[48] whereas the vascular theory is supported by demonstrated alterations in coagulation mechanisms and viscosity,[49, 50] by changes similar to giant cell arteritis in the soft tissues about the necrotic bone,[51] and by identification of fat globules in subchondral vessels in areas of osteonecrosis.[38, 52] The importance of intravascular fatty deposits in the production of osteonecrosis has been further popularized by Jones and his collaborators,[53-56] who emphasized the following sequence of events: corticosteroid-induced fatty liver, systemic fatty embolization, infarction of bone, and osteonecrosis. The latter hypothesis was partially confirmed by Jaffe and co-workers,[57] who detected significant intraosseous fat embolization in rabbits that were administered systemic corticosteroids, an observation that was also supported in other investigations.[43] Currently, the theory of fat embolization is most widely accepted, although an ancillary role of altered mechanical forces acting on weakened osteoporotic bone or vulnerability of vascular circulation at certain sites, such as the proximal femur, or both factors, may be important.

Additional analgesics may be associated with drug-induced arthropathy and osteonecrosis.[14, 29, 58] These medications include phenylbutazone and indomethacin. The pathogenesis of the articular abnormalities that are evident following treatment with nonsteroidal anti-inflammatory agents is presumed to be similar to that following corticosteroid administration.

Changes in the diaphyses and metaphyses of tubular bones are less frequently encountered than epiphyseal alterations in patients being treated with steroids or other anti-inflammatory agents. Wilken-

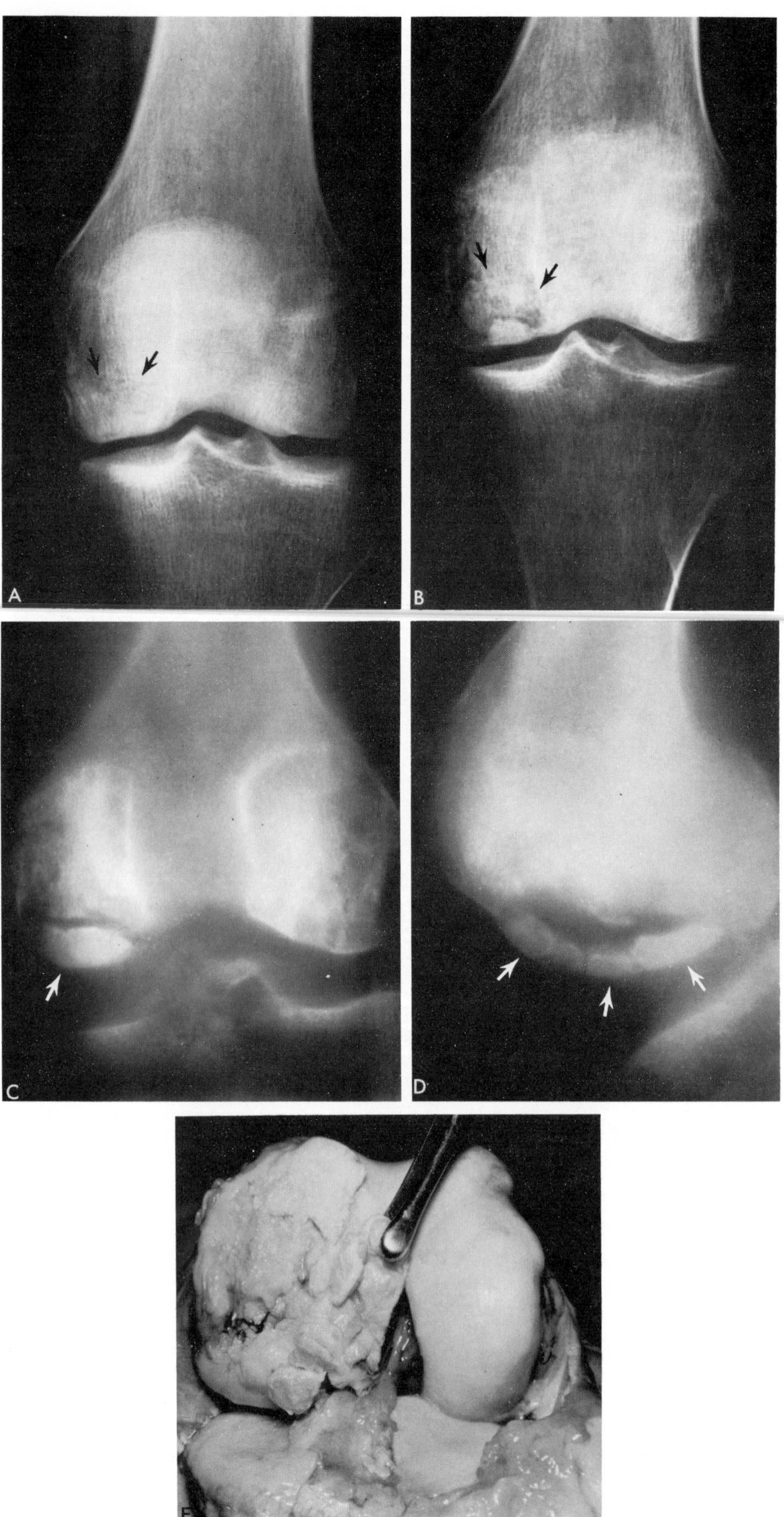

Figure 66–3. *Steroid-induced osteonecrosis: Distal femur. Progressive changes in a 1 year period are illustrated in a young patient who was treated with corticosteroids following renal transplantation. Both knees were similarly affected.*

A *An initial film indicates a subtle radiolucent line (arrows) of the medial femoral condyle, indicating definite osteonecrosis.*

B *One year later, considerable fragmentation (arrows) of the articular surface is seen.*

C, D *Frontal and lateral tomograms demonstrate the fragmentation of the osseous surface with the creation of multiple intra-articular bony pieces (arrows).*

E *An operative photograph of the distal femoral condylar surface reveals the severity of the osteocartilaginous abnormalities on the medial side. (**E,** Courtesy of Dr. R. Convery, University of California, San Diego, California.)*

Table 66–2

PATHOGENESIS OF STEROID-INDUCED OSTEONECROSIS

Theory	Possible Mechanisms
Mechanical	Osteoporosis leading to microfractures and osseous collapse
Vascular	Vascular compression from marrow accumulation of fat
	Fat embolization following steroid-induced fatty liver
	Vasculitis
	Hyperviscosity

feld and Sliwinski[59] noted osteolytic lesions of both humeri in a rheumatoid patient who was receiving corticosteroids and cyclophosphamide that on biopsy were characterized by fatty cellular infiltration and cortical thinning. This finding is consistent with the corticosteroid-induced fatty overgrowth of the bone marrow that has been observed experimentally.[60]

Osteonecrosis of vertebral bodies in association with steroid medications has recently been recognized. Radiolucent linear shadows in the subchondral bone reflect fractures of necrotic bone and are reminiscent of the radiolucent areas that appear at other sites of osteonecrosis, such as the femoral and humeral heads (Fig. 66–4).[163, 164]

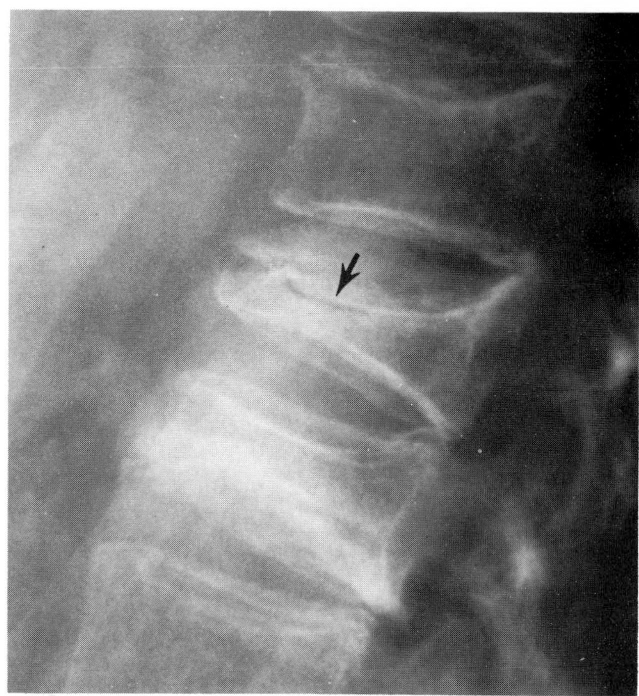

Figure 66–4. *Steroid-induced osteonecrosis: Vertebral bodies. Observe collapse of multiple osteoporotic lumbar vertebral bodies, reactive sclerosis of end-plates, and a radiolucent line or "crescent" within the bone (arrow). The latter finding differs from a "vacuum" intervertebral disc, in which the radiolucent collection is located over the disc itself.*

Neuropathic-like Articular Destruction

A neuropathic-like, rapidly progressive joint disease characterized by severe osseous and cartilaginous destruction represents one variety of steroid arthropathy that appears most typically following intra-articular injection of the drug[33, 61-64] (Table 66–3). It may be associated with osteoporosis, osteonecrosis, and an underlying articular disorder, such as rheumatoid arthritis or degenerative joint disease (Figs. 66–5 and 66–6). Although any joint can be affected, it is the hip and the knee that are most frequently involved. The rapidity of the process may be remarkable, with the transition in a short period of time from an articulation with minor alterations (perhaps due to underlying osteoarthritis or rheumatoid arthritis) to one with significant osseous collapse and fragmentation. Gouged-out areas of bony destruction have been compared to animal bites, the "bite" sign.[61]

The pathogenesis of the process is not certain. Although osteonecrosis may be an accompanying feature, it does not appear to be the initial event in this articular manifestation; joint space narrowing, contour defects and eburnation may appear before osseous collapse and fragmentation become evident.

Table 66–3

STEROID-INDUCED NEUROPATHIC-LIKE ALTERATIONS

Possible Pathogenesis	Characteristics
Neuroarthropathy due to sensory loss induced by medication	Usually evident following intra-articular administration of drug
Osteonecrosis	Predilection for the hip and the knee
	Rapid onset and progression
	Osseous defects ("bites"), collapse, and fragmentation
	Cartilaginous destruction

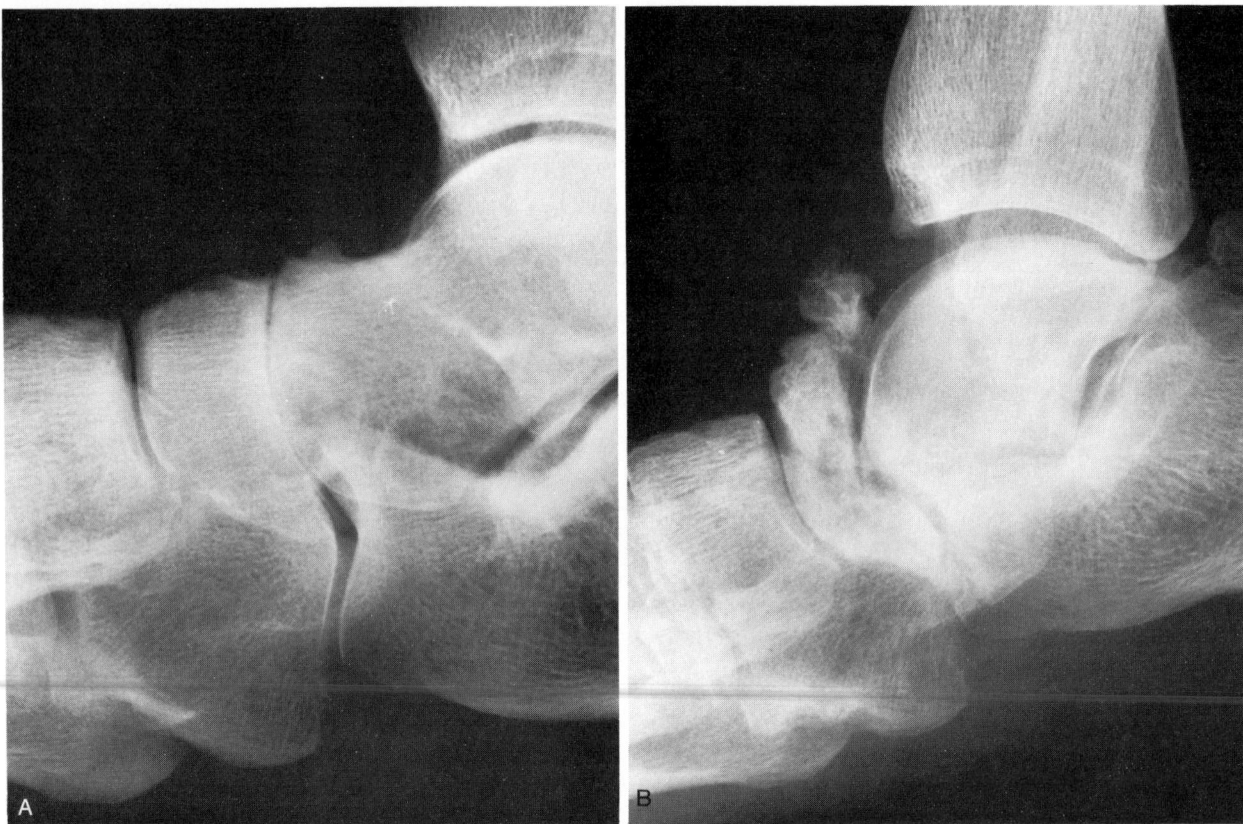

Figure 66–5. *Steroid-induced neuropathic-like arthropathy. This patient with rheumatoid arthritis had had repeated injections of corticosteroids into the talonavicular space. Radiographs obtained 2 years apart indicate progressive abnormalities. The initial film* **(A)** *demonstrates joint space narrowing, sclerosis, and subchondral cyst formation, whereas the later film* **(B)** *reveals fragmentation of the talus and navicular bone. The findings are unlike uncomplicated rheumatoid arthritis and resemble neuropathic changes.*

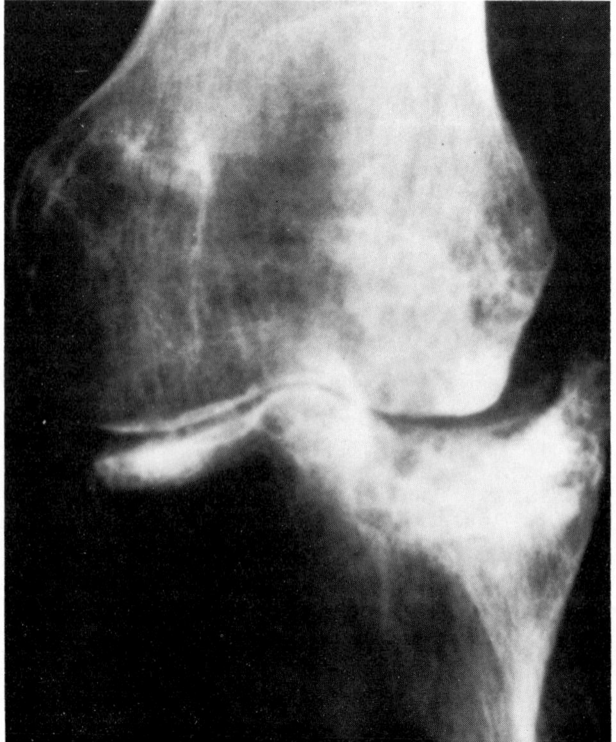

Figure 66–6. *Steroid-induced neuropathic-like arthropathy. Another patient with rheumatoid arthritis developed rapid collapse of the lateral tibial plateau following intra-articular steroid injections. The flattening and sclerosis of bone and valgus deformity may represent steroid-induced arthropathy, although the contribution of the rheumatoid process may be considerable.*

The process resembles an infection, but organisms are not recovered from the joint in most instances. The fact that there is a relative absence of pain in the presence of severe osseous and cartilaginous destruction may indicate that the analgesic effect of the steroid medication may be fundamental to the pathogenesis of the articular changes. Most probably, therefore, the joint destruction is due to a neuroarthropathy created by the steroid-induced obscuration of pain and is aggravated by the steroid-related osteoporosis of the neighboring bone. Recurrent trauma in this painless situation leads to disintegration of weakened subchondral bone and acceleration of any underlying articular disorder. Cartilaginous destruction can appear as a secondary event in a joint that reveals increasing incongruity of apposing articular surfaces, although a direct effect of the corticosteroids on the articular cartilage may also be important. Experimentally, cartilaginous fibrillation and cystic degeneration can accompany intra-articular or intramuscular steroid injection[65, 66] (Fig. 66–7). Inhibition of protein and polysaccharide synthesis by the chondrocyte can be evident.[67-69]

The ability of steroids to provoke neuropathic-like changes is not universally accepted. Gibson and colleagues[70] were unable to document significant joint changes in monkeys that were subjected to intra-articular steroid injections. They emphasized the anecdotal nature of many of the previous reports of pseudoneuropathic steroid-induced joint changes in humans[62, 64, 71, 72] and the inconsistency of the reported changes in other series,[73, 74] although these investigators did concede that the medication might have a harmful effect on cartilage already compromised by inflammatory disease,[75] especially if administered at frequent intervals.

Osteomyelitis and Septic Arthritis

Bone and joint infections can complicate steroid therapy. Septic arthritis can appear following oral, intravenous, or intra-articular administration[76-79] and can affect any articulation, particularly the knee. Single or multiple joints may be involved, and bacterial organisms, especially *Staphylococcus*

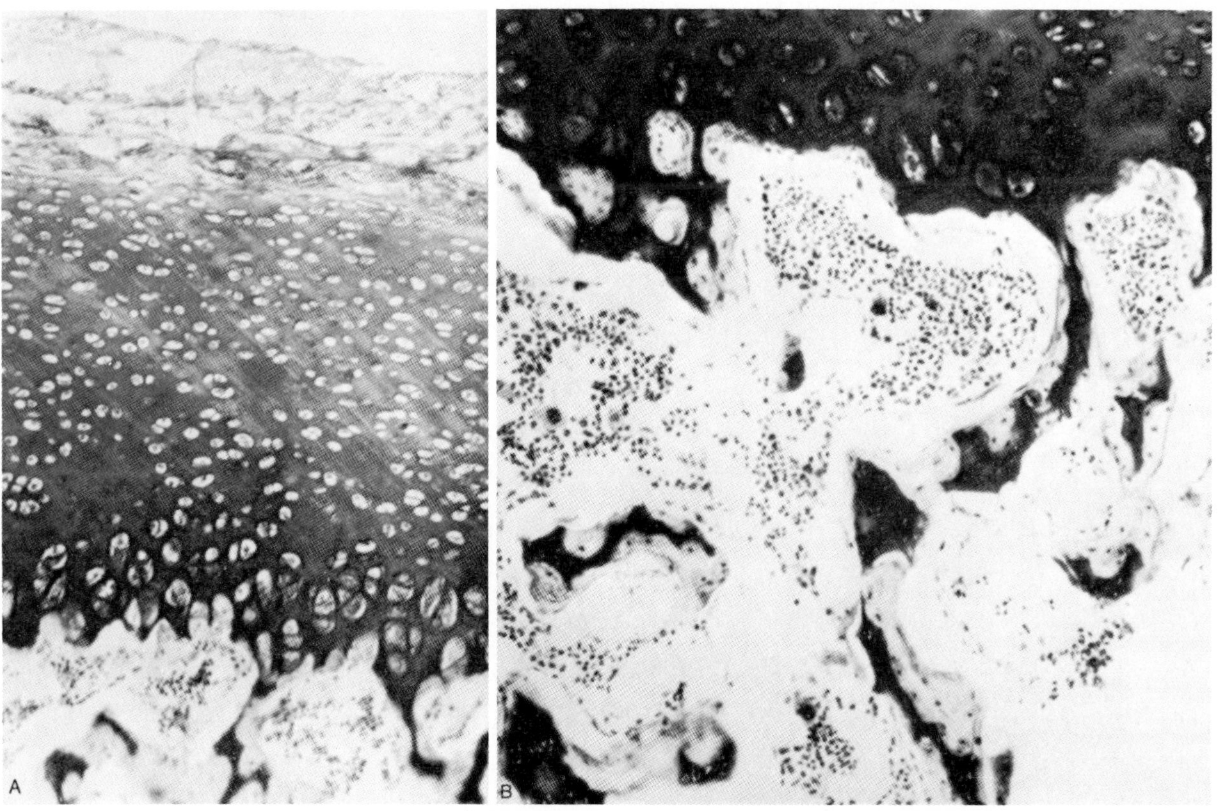

Figure 66–7. *Steroid-induced cartilaginous abnormalities. Intra-articular or intramuscular injection of corticosteroids in the rabbit may lead to significant abnormalities.*

A *After 13 daily intramuscular injections of cortisone, superficial cartilage fibrillation, a decrease in hypertrophic cells, and poor organization of subchondral trabeculae can be seen (160 ×).*

B *Twelve days after intra-articular methylprednisolone administration, the zone of hypertrophic cells is shallow, the calcified matrix is not remodeled in the normal dentate pattern, and osteoblasts are few and spindle-shaped (160×).*

(From Shaw NE, Lacey E: J Bone Joint Surg 55B:197, 1973.)

aureus, predominate. Similarly, osteomyelitis can appear alone or in conjunction with septic arthritis. The initiation and spread of infection are promoted by the medication's interference with normal host defense mechanisms; in addition, direct inoculation of joint, bone, or soft tissue can result from the usage of contaminated needles or syringes during the injection process. Rarely, nonseptic joint effusions may be identified in patients receiving steroid medications, especially those who have had renal transplantations.[169] In these cases, the synovial fluid may be colorless and contain an unusually low protein content.

Tendinous and Soft Tissue Injury

Tendinous rupture has been described in association with systemically or locally administered corticosteroids,[80-85] but it is not certain if the complication relates to the effect of steroids or the disease process for which the steroids are being utilized (Fig. 66–8). Experimental evidence suggests that steroids may induce changes in healthy tendons and that they may inhibit the healing process of unhealthy tendons. Langhoff and colleagues[86] reported the dissolution of fibrocytes and fibroblasts following injection of methylprednisolone into tendons, although Phelps and co-workers[87] were unable to confirm a change in the biochemical properties of rabbit patellar tendons following corticosteroid injection. Wrenn and associates[88] found that corticosteroid therapy partially inhibited the healing process of tendons, decreasing the amount of fibrous tissue, reducing the tendon strength, and delaying regeneration of the tendon sheath. Hydrocortisone injection into a tendon has also been associated with fatty degeneration and collagen necrosis.[89, 90] At this time, it appears likely that steroids, particularly when locally administered, accelerate degeneration and rupture of a tendon that is already the site of a pathologic process; whether or not similar complications can occur in healthy tendons following steroid administration is not certain. Locally administered steroids may also have a detrimental effect on ligaments, decreasing the strength of ligamentous attachments to bone.[166]

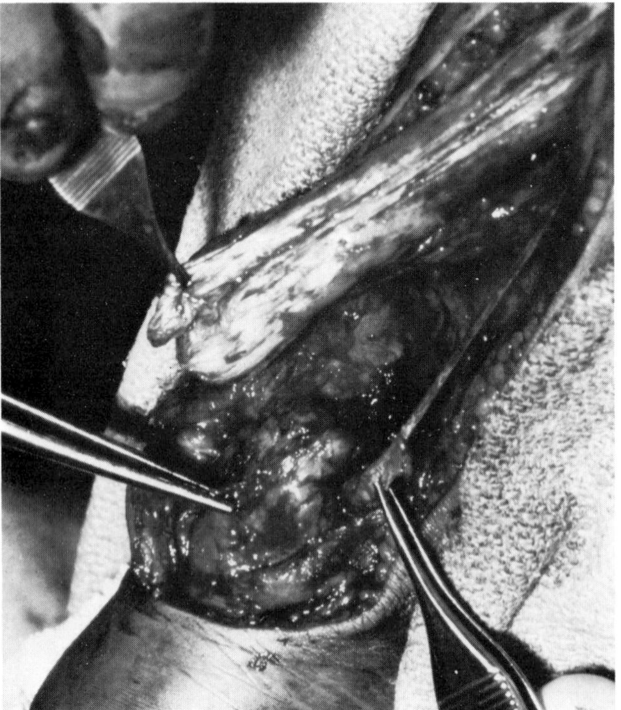

Figure 66–8. *Steroid-induced rupture of the Achilles tendon. The upper forceps holds the proximal torn end of the Achilles tendon in a patient who had received steroid injections adjacent to this tendon. (Courtesy of Dr. R. Convery, University of California, San Diego, California.)*

Atrophy of subcutaneous tissues may appear following local application of various steroid preparations, especially triamcinolone; this can occur when the medication is applied topically or when it is injected in or beneath the skin.[91-95] Rarely, intra-articular injection can lead to periarticular (perilymphatic) skin atrophy.[96] Although some recovery of the cutaneous tissue may occur after a number of years, complete restoration of the local fat is not common.

FLUORINE

Chronic fluorine intoxication, fluorosis, arises when the drinking water contains fluoride in concentrations higher than 4 parts per million (ppm)[97-100]; fluorosis occurs endemically in certain regions of the world, especially India, where it was first described in the 1930s,[101] and sporadically in almost a worldwide distribution. The entity may also appear in industrial workers who are exposed to fluorine compounds over a period of years,[171] in laboratory personnel who have inhaled fluorine vapors, in patients receiving medications containing high doses of fluorine, such as niflumic acid (a nonsteroidal anti-inflammatory agent),[173] and in individuals who habitually drink fluorine-containing wine (wine fluorosis).[114, 116] It is this well-recognized intoxication by fluoride that has generated interest and criticism in public health programs for the prevention of dental caries.[98] It is paradoxical that the cumulative effects of fluorine may be detrimental not only to the skeleton but also to the dental tissues. The investigation of Smith and Hodge[102] has revealed that although fluoride concentration in 1 ppm can reduce dental caries, a level of 2 ppm or more can lead to mottled enamel, that of 8 ppm can produce osteosclerosis in 10 per cent of individuals, and a concentration greater than 100 ppm may induce growth disturbances, kidney damage, or death.

Dental Fluorosis

Mottled enamel is an early dental sign of fluoride intoxication.[98, 103-105] The teeth appear polished and hard and contain minute opaque flecks, which may be scattered about the tooth surface (Fig. 66–9). Progression of the dental changes leads to depressions or pits of variable size and discoloration.[106] Radiographs outline hypoplasia, irregular dental roots, and periapical sclerosis and root resorption.

Skeletal Fluorosis

Radiographic Abnormalities. Involvement of the axial skeleton is characteristic[98, 99, 107-113] (Table 66–4) (Fig. 66–10). Changes are most marked in the spine, the pelvis, and the ribs. Although osteopenia can appear initially, particularly in children. osteosclerosis usually appears first. Increasing trabecular condensation eventually creates a radiodense or chalky appearance throughout the thorax, vertebral column, and pelvis with obscuration of bony architecture. The skull and tubular bones of the appendicular skeleton are relatively spared in this sclerotic process.

Vertebral osteophytosis can lead to encroachment in the spinal canal and intervertebral foramina. In the axial skeleton, hyperostosis and bony excrescences develop at sites of ligamentous attachment, especially in the iliac crests, ischial tuberosities, and inferior margins of the ribs. Calcification of paraspinal ligaments as well as sacrotuberous and iliolumbar ligaments can be noted.

In the appendicular skeleton, periosteal thickening, calcification of ligaments, and excrescences at ligamentous and muscular attachments to bone can be seen at one or more sites, particularly near the interosseous membranes of the forearm and leg, the calcaneus, the posterior surface of the femur, the tibial tuberosity, and the proximal humerus (Fig. 66–11). In some cases, the degree of periosteal bone formation can become profound and is termed periostitis deformans.[114, 115] This variety of fluorosis can lead to unilateral or bilateral cloaks of undulating periosteal bone, which may surround the humeri, femora, ulnae, radii, tibiae, fibuli, metatarsals, metacarpals, and phalanges, and is associated with cortical thickening, medullary diminution with endosteal bone formation, "invading" osteophytes that extend into tendons, fasciae, or muscles, and periarticular excrescences, especially about the hip, the knee, or the elbow. Soft tissue ossification resembling "myositis" ossificans and cartilaginous "atrophy" and "ulceration" have been noted.[115]

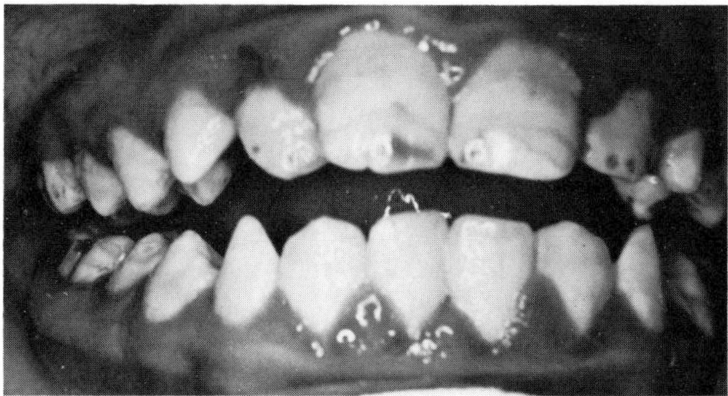

Figure 66–9. Fluorosis: Dental abnormalities. Depressions, discoloration, and opaque flecks are evident in this individual with fluorosis. (Courtesy of Dr. R. Smith, University of California, San Francisco, California.)

Table 66–4

RADIOGRAPHIC ABNORMALITIES IN FLUOROSIS

Hypoplasia and irregularity of dental structures
Osteosclerosis
Vertebral osteophytosis
Ligamentous calcification
Periostitis

Pathologic Abnormalities. Histopathologic assessments of skeletal fluorosis have been inconsistent. Although cortical thickening with narrowing of the marrow cavity, decreased bone resorption, and virtual absence of osteoclasts have been noted in some reports,[107] others have cited an increase in bone surfaces lined by osteoid and striking evidence of osseous resorption (Fig. 66–12).[117] Accelerated bone formation and resorption may occur simultaneously; irregular laying down of periosteal bone on the surface may be associated with an increased rate of resorption, as indicated by cancellization of the cortex, the presence of enlarged haversian canals (resorption tunnels), and an increased number of lacunae.[118] Tetracycline studies have indicated that subperiosteal bony deposition may create disordered or irregular lamellae,[98, 119] whereas histologic investigations have indicated an increase in resorption surfaces that correlates with plasma levels of alkaline phosphatase, bone fluoride, and the radiologic findings of coarse osseous striations.[117] It has been suggested that the concomitant increase in bone formation and osteoclastic resorption in skeletal fluorosis is caused by overactivity of parathyroid hormone,[117] a suggestion that is supported by clinical, laboratory, and radiologic data.[120] It has been recognized that fluorine can markedly influence the response of bone to parathyroid hormone and calcitonin, an action that appears to be mediated, in large part, by an effect on bone mineral.[121, 122] The fluoroapatite crystals, which are of large size, may be more stable and less reactive in surface exchange reactions,[117] increasing the resistance of bone to the actions of parathyroid hormone.[120]

Text continued on page 2378

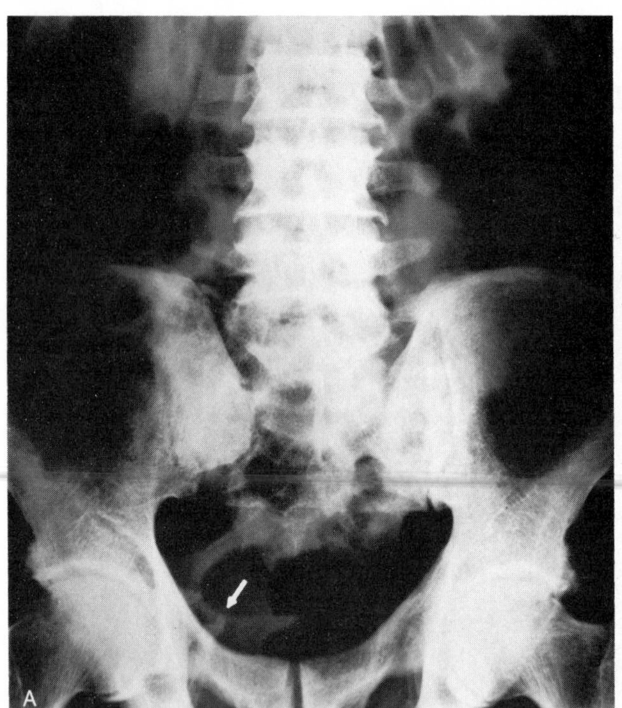

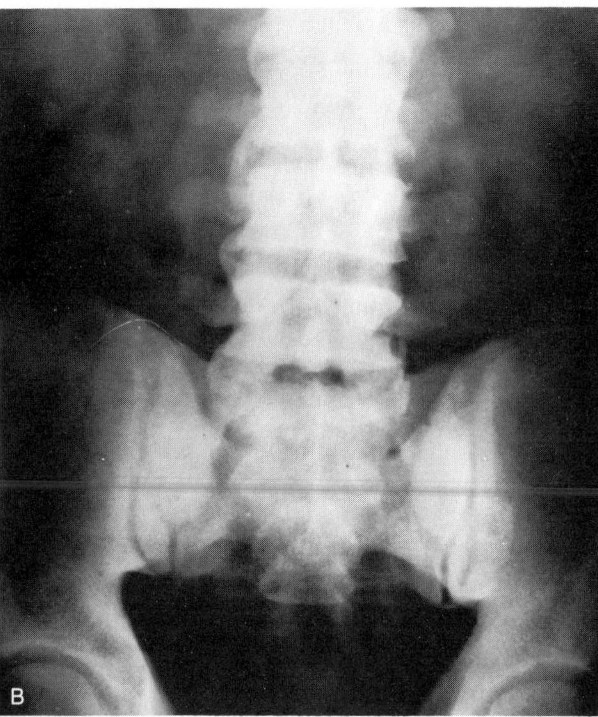

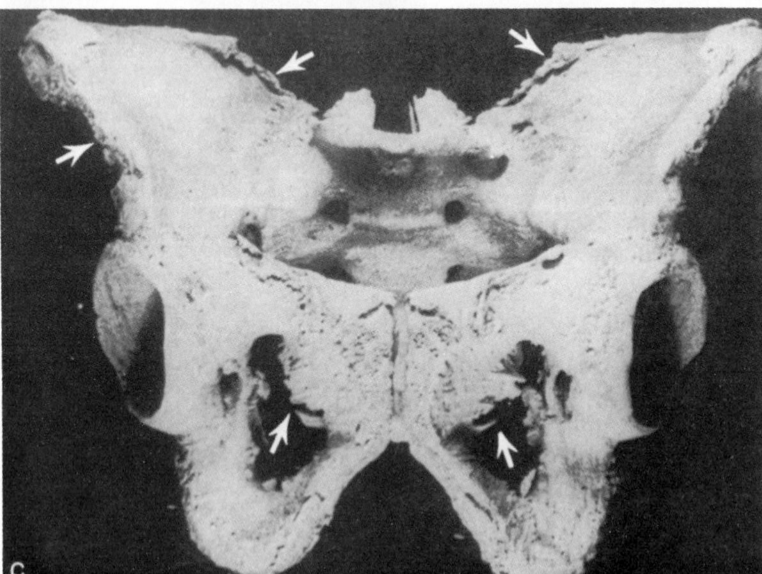

Figure 66–10. *Fluorosis: Axial skeletal abnormalities.*

A *Osteosclerosis with a coarsened trabecular pattern, vertebral osteophytosis, and sacrotuberous ligament ossification (arrow) are the observed radiographic changes.*

B *Osteosclerosis and vertebral osteophytosis are evident in a different patient with fluorosis. Note the bony eburnation about the sacroiliac joints.*

C *A macerated pelvis of a 45 year old farmer from India with fluorosis reveals proliferation at ligamentous attachments, especially about the iliac crests and the ischial and pubic rami (arrows).*

Illustration continued on the opposite page

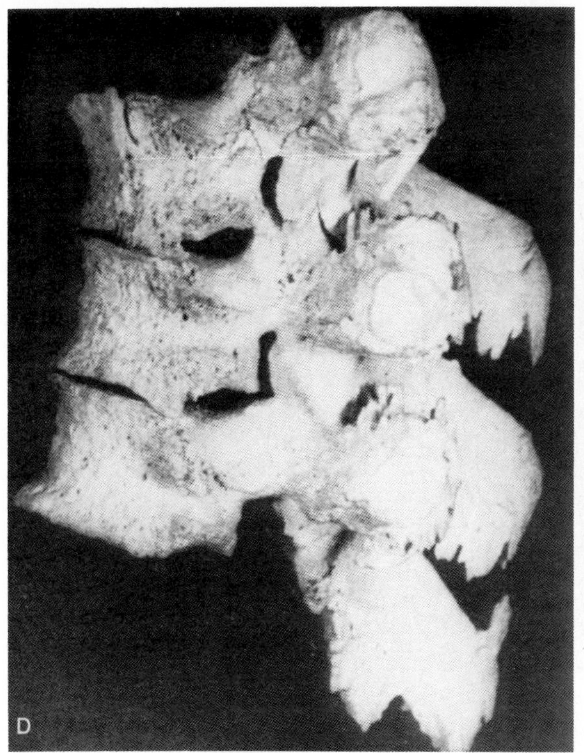

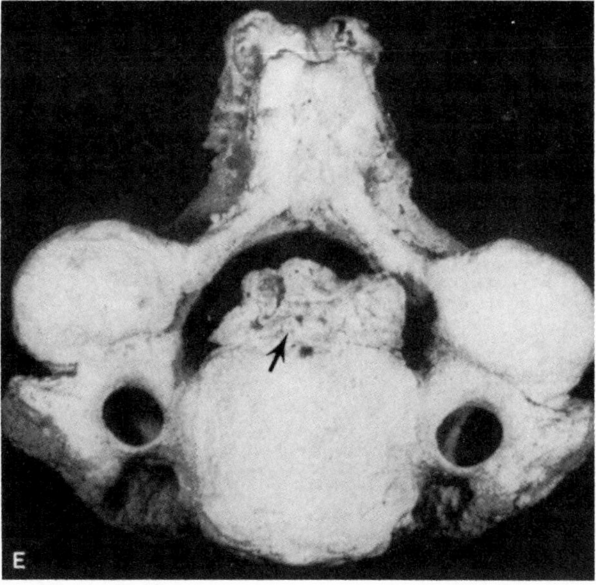

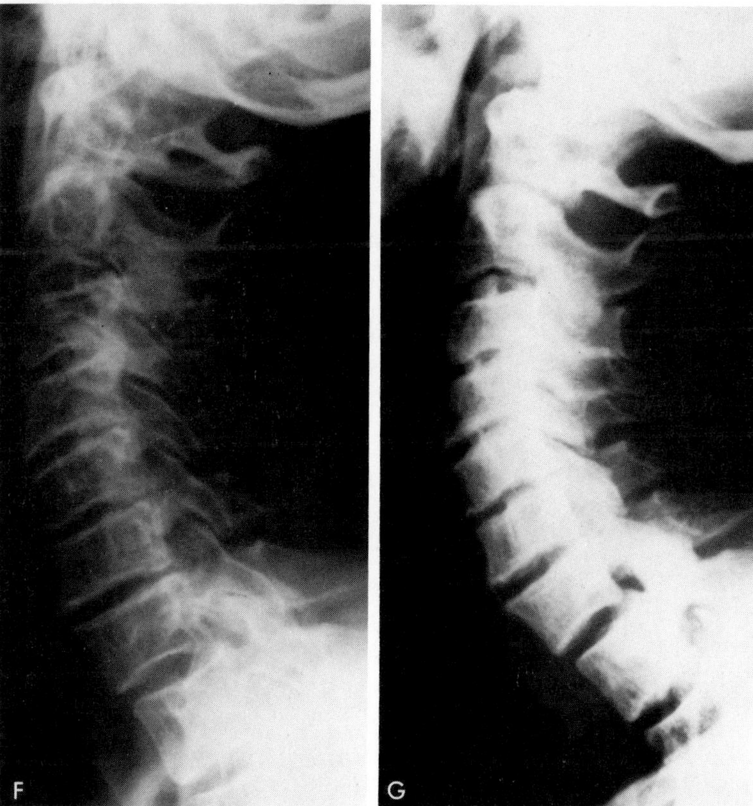

Figure 66–10. Continued

D *In the same patient as in* **C**, *note osseous fusion of the second to fourth thoracic vertebrae, narrowing of the intervertebral foramina, and osteophytes.*

E *In the same patient as in* **C** *and* **D**, *a photograph of the inferior surface of the third cervical vertebra reveals calcification and ossification of the posterior longitudinal ligament (arrow) and osseous overgrowth about the spinous processes and articular pillars.*

F, G *Lateral radiographs of the cervical spine obtained 5 years apart in a 70 year old woman receiving fluoride treatment for osteoporosis. Initially* **(F)**, *prior to treatment, osteoporosis is apparent. Subsequently* **(G)**, *note the increased radiodensity and coarsened trabecular pattern in the cervical vertebrae.*

*(***F, G**, *Courtesy of Drs. V. Vint and G. Williams, Scripps Clinic, LaJolla, California.)*

*(***C–E**, *From Singh A, et al: J Bone Joint Surg 44B:806, 1962.)*

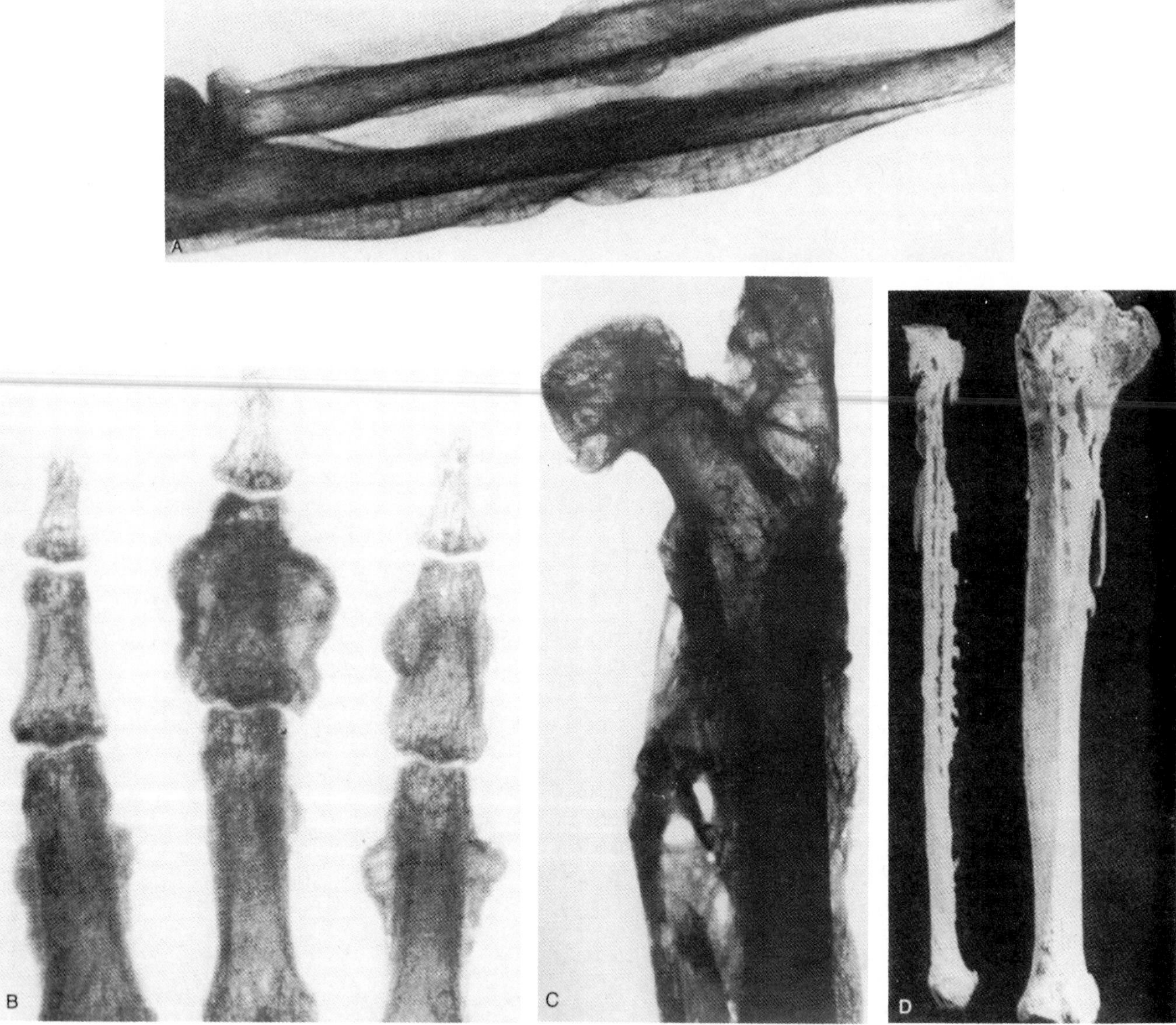

Figure 66–11. *Fluorosis: Appendicular skeletal abnormalities.*

A–C *Extensive periosteal proliferation of the radius, ulna, proximal femur, and phalanges can be noted in fluorosis. A striking appearance consisting of enlarged and undulating osseous contours is seen. (From Soriano M, Manchon F: Radiology 87:1089, 1966.)*

D *A macerated tibia and fibula from the cadaver in Figure 66–10***C** *reveal periosteal proliferation. (From Singh A, et al: J Bone Joint Surg 44B:806, 1962.)*

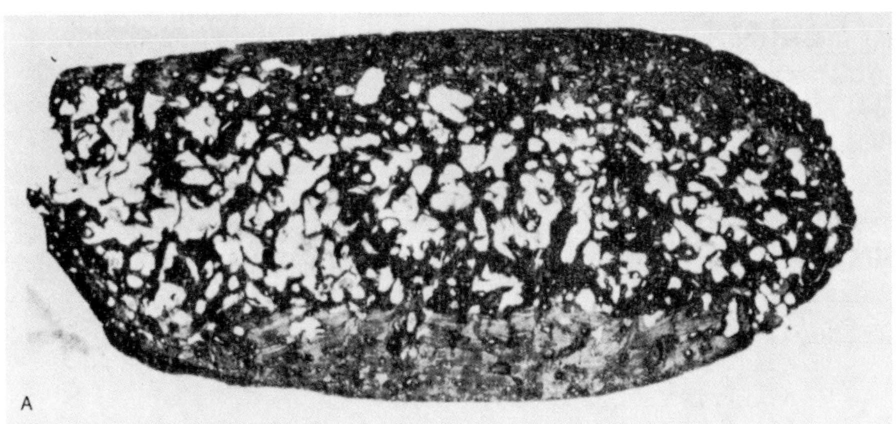

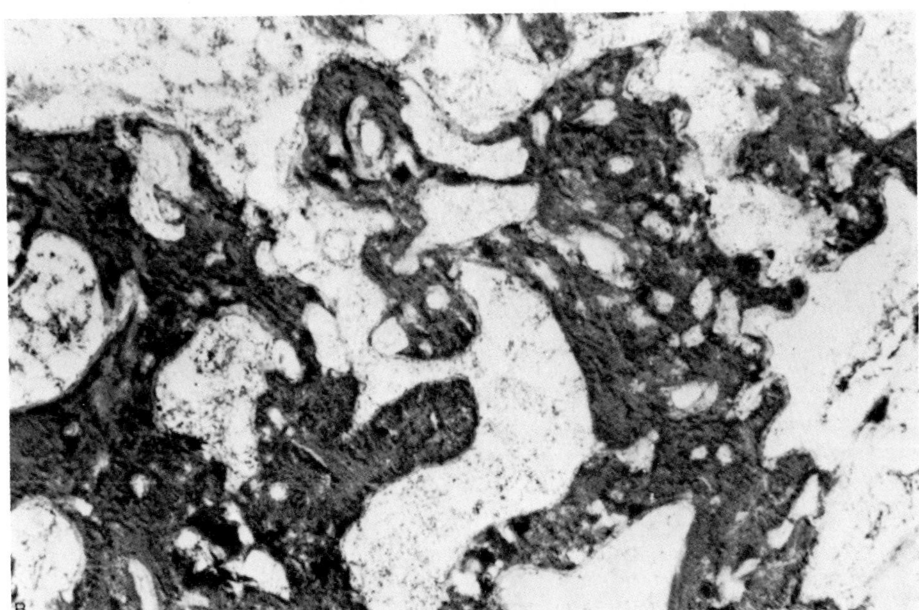

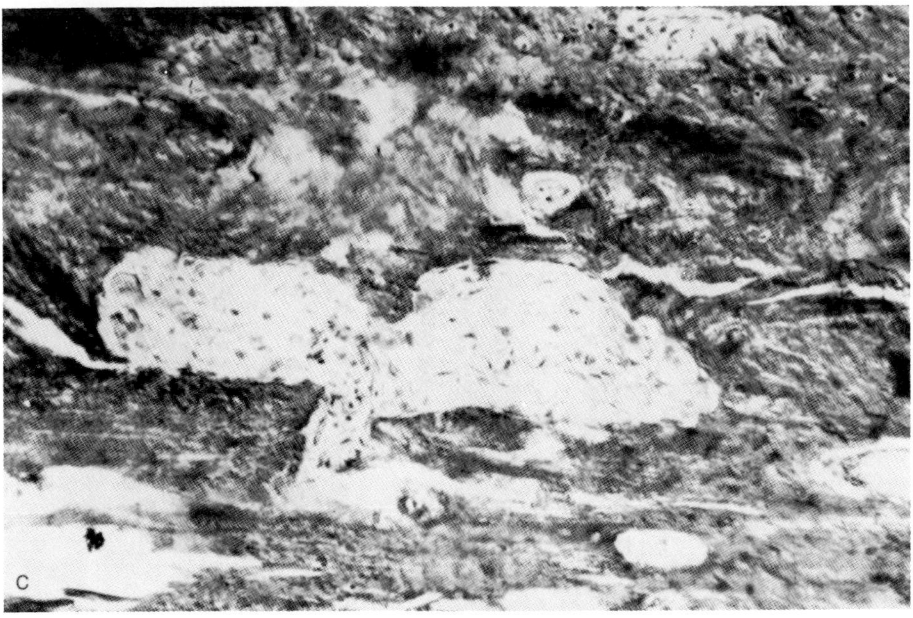

Figure 66–12. *Skeletal fluorosis: Pathologic abnormalities.*

A *A photograph of a cross section of a fluorotic rib reveals cortical thickening and prominent trabeculae in the medullary cavity.* (**A,** *From Singer L, et al: Clin Orthop Rel Res 99:303, 1974.*)

B *An iliac crest biopsy from a patient with fluorosis indicates a filigree pattern of trabecular bone, with loops and bridges of osteoid and internal resorption (50×).*

C *In another site in the same patient as in* **B,** *resorption of bone with tunneling and osteoclastosis is observed (125×).*

(**B, C,** *From Faccini JM, Teotia SPS: Calcif Tiss Res 16:45, 1974.*)

Whether this structural change is a major factor in exciting parathyroid stimulation is not known, although animal experiments indicating that an increase in circulating hormone can appear within days of fluoride administration[123] suggest that other mechanisms are also important in the production of elevated parathormone levels in association with skeletal fluorosis.

The mechanical properties of bone in fluorosis have also been studied, although not without disagreement.[172] Evans and Wood[124] discovered that certain characteristics, such as tensile strength, tensile strain, energy absorbed to failure, and modulus of elasticity, were less in fluorotic human bone specimens than in normal bone specimens, whereas other characteristics, such as compressive strength and compressive strain, were increased in the fluorotic bone. Franke and colleagues[125] observed an increase in bone strength in fluorosis, an effect that was related to an increase in the amount of osseous tissue, although methodology in this latter experiment was later challenged by Lindahl and Lindwall.[126] Chemical analysis of fluorotic bone has indicated elevated fluoride and carbonate content and reduced citrate and magnesium content.[127] The fluoride content may decrease slowly after exposure has ceased.[128]

Complications. Advanced stages of fluorosis can lead to significant and crippling abnormalities, including kyphosis, restricted spinal and chest motion, and contractures and deformities of extraspinal articulations, such as the hips and the knees.[98] A high incidence of genu valgum deformity has been cited in some reports.[129] Neurologic complications include paresthesias, muscular weakening and wasting, sensory disturbances, and paralysis.[98] Although neurologic and musculoskeletal complications are more frequently reported in adults with fluorosis, they are also evident in some children with the disease.[170]

Differential Diagnosis. The combination of findings noted on radiographs of patients with skeletal fluorosis is virtually diagnostic. Osteosclerosis, osteophytosis, and ligamentous calcification represent a useful triad of abnormalities that are evident on pelvis and spine roentgenograms. The other alterations that occur in both axial and extra-axial locations, such as periostitis and osseous excrescences at sites of tendinous and ligamentous attachment, provide additional clues to the correct diagnosis.

Osteosclerosis alone is not diagnostic of fluorosis, being evident in skeletal metastasis, myelofibrosis, mastocytosis, certain hemoglobinopathies, renal osteodystrophy, Paget's disease, congenital disorders, and other conditions. Likewise, vertebral osteophytosis or similar outgrowths can accompany many diseases, including fluorosis, spondylosis deformans, diffuse idiopathic skeletal hyperostosis, ankylosing spondylitis, the spondylitis of psoriasis, Reiter's syndrome, and inflammatory bowel disorders, acromegaly, neuroarthropathy, and alkaptonuria. Proliferative changes at ligamentous and tendinous insertions on bones are apparent not only in fluorosis but also in diffuse idiopathic skeletal hyperostosis and certain plasma cell dyscrasias. Periostitis similar to that which may be seen in fluorosis can be detected in hypertrophic osteoarthropathy, pachydermoperiostosis, and thyroid acropachy. Thus, each individual radiographic finding of skeletal fluorosis can be apparent in other disorders as well; it is the combination of findings in fluorosis that is diagnostic.

DOPAMINE AND RELATED SUBSTANCES

Dopamine is a direct-acting catecholamine that at lower doses dilates the mesenteric, renal, cerebral, and coronary vessels and at high doses has a vasoconstrictor action due to stimulation of alpha receptors.[130-132] Utilization of this drug in large amounts can be associated with ischemic necrosis and gangrene.[133-137] These complications, which may be more severe in patients with underlying vascular diseases, such as diabetes mellitus and atherosclerosis, can, in unusual circumstances, require amputation of one or more extremities[138, 139] (Fig. 66–13).

Gangrene may also occur during the course of treatment with other vasoconstrictive drugs. Ergotamine and its derivatives, such as methysergide, which have been used in the treatment of migraine headaches to reduce the vasodilatation and excessive pulsation of the branches of the external carotid artery, can lead to vasoconstriction of peripheral vessels and gangrene.[140-144] Administration of vasopressin (Pitressin) can induce gangrene and perhaps osteonecrosis (Fig. 66–14).[145] Repeated self-administered injections of epinephrine into the thighs of asthmatic individuals have eventuated in massive soft tissue calcification, perhaps attributable to capillary spasm, decreased vascularity, and pH alterations.[4, 14]

CALCIUM GLUCONATE

Intravenous administration of calcium gluconate has been utilized in the treatment of neonatal tetany and neonatal asphyxia. Subcutaneous masses of calcification at sites of recent or previous injections can appear.[146, 147] Clinical findings include erythema and bulla formation, becoming evident in a period of days, which may be followed by skin sloughing and secondary infection. Calcification can be noted within 4 or 5 days or as late as 3 weeks following injection (Fig. 66–15). It is amorphous and can be localized or distributed along fascial planes.

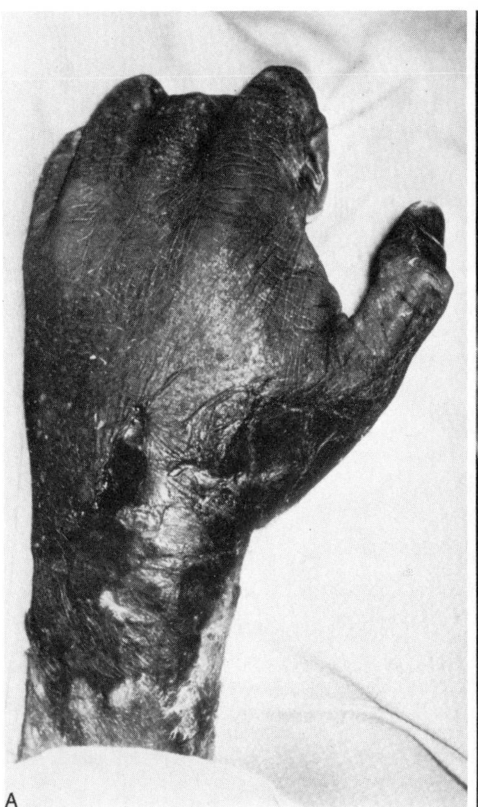

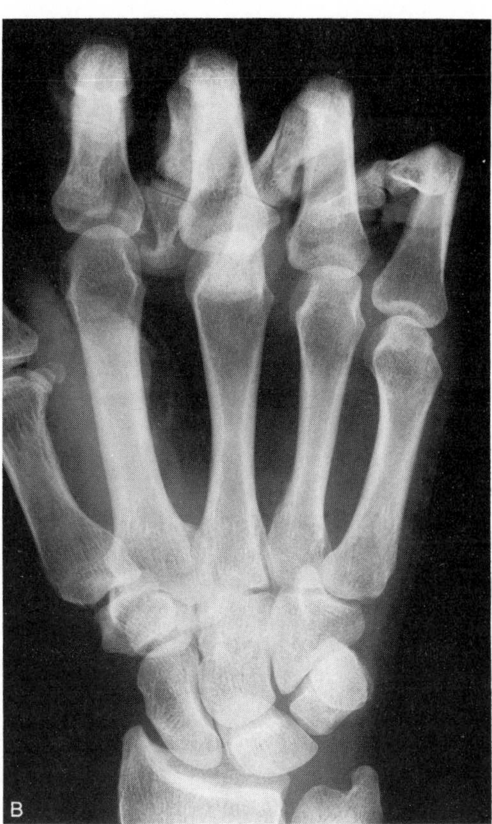

Figure 66–13. *Dopamine-induced gangrene. A 46 year old man, admitted to the hospital with severe hypotension, was given a dopamine infusion of 8 to 16 micrograms/kg/min. He developed progressive cyanosis of both hands and both feet. He required bilateral below-the-knee amputations and a unilateral below-the-elbow amputation.*

A *A photograph of the left hand indicates the severity of the necrosis.*

B *A radiograph reveals the extent of soft tissue contracture. The bones are intact.*

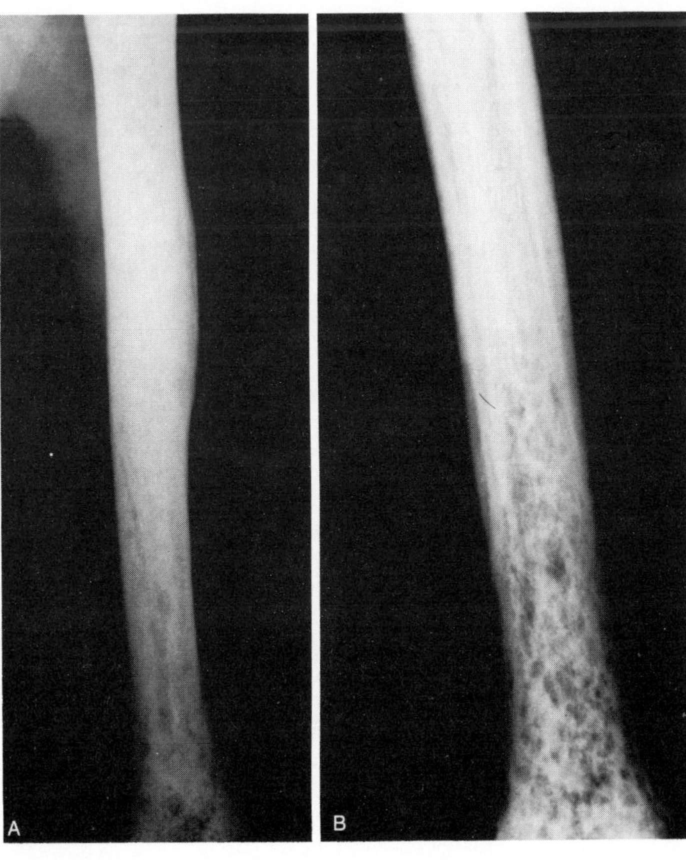

Figure 66–14. *Possible vasopressin-induced osteonecrosis. This elderly woman with carcinoma of the breast had required extensive surgery and irradiation, pituitary ablation, and vasopressin medication for over 10 years. The changes in the humeral and femoral shafts consisting of patchy sclerosis are apparently related to osteonecrosis. (Courtesy of Dr. W. Murphy, Mallinckrodt Institute, St. Louis, Missouri.)*

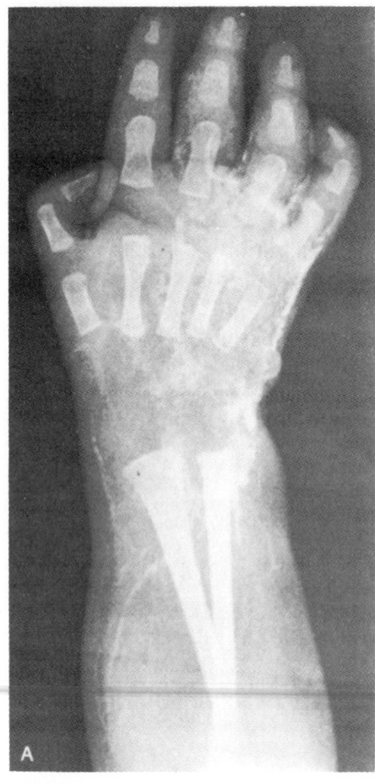

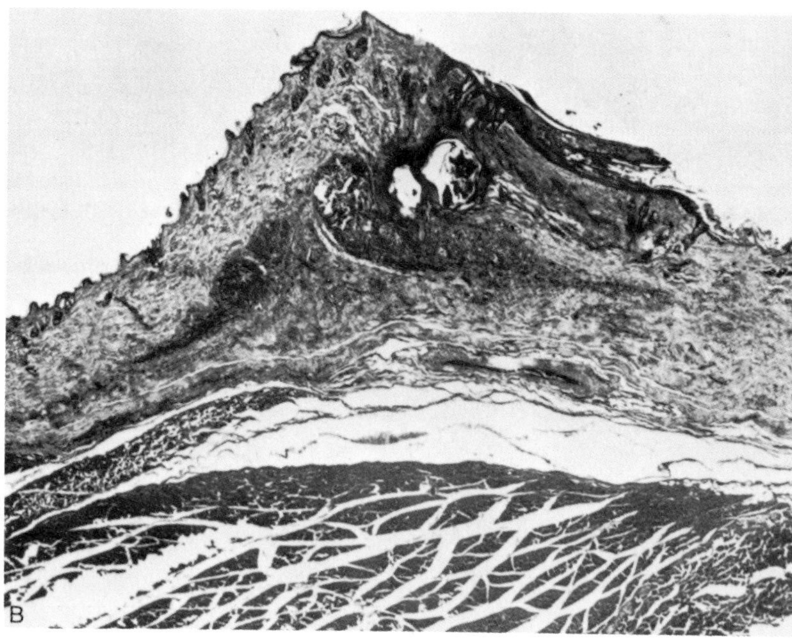

Figure 66–15. *Calcium gluconate extravasation.*

A *This 3 lb 6 ounce black infant received an infusion of calcium gluconate into a vein in the dorsum of the hand that subsequently infiltrated into the soft tissues. A radiograph taken approximately 1 week later reveals extensive linear and plate-like subcutaneous deposits with vascular calcification.*

B *A cross section of the skin, subcutaneous tissue, and muscle of a rabbit 37 days after subcutaneous injection of 4 ml calcium gluconate reveals a calcium-filled inclusion cyst in the upper dermis with adjacent calcification in fibrous tissue (9 ×).*

(From Berger PE, et al: Am J Roentgenol 121:109, 1974. Copyright 1974, American Roentgen Ray Society.)

Vascular calcification may also be apparent. With healing, clinical and radiologic manifestations may disappear. The roentgenographic changes simulate those in subcutaneous fat necrosis and hematomas following trauma.[146]

MILK-ALKALI

In 1949, Burnett and co-workers[148] observed six patients with chronic peptic ulcer disease and renal insufficiency in whom excessive intake of milk and alkali (for a few to many years) led to metastatic calcification. These patients revealed hypercalcemia without hypercalciuria or hypophosphatemia, normal serum alkaline phosphatase levels, azotemia, and mild alkalosis. Although all six individuals revealed clinical improvement following the withdrawal of milk and alkali from the diet, the calcification persisted and none survived. These investigators postulated that the following sequence of events was important: excessive intake of milk and alkali, kidney damage, fixation in urinary calcium excre-

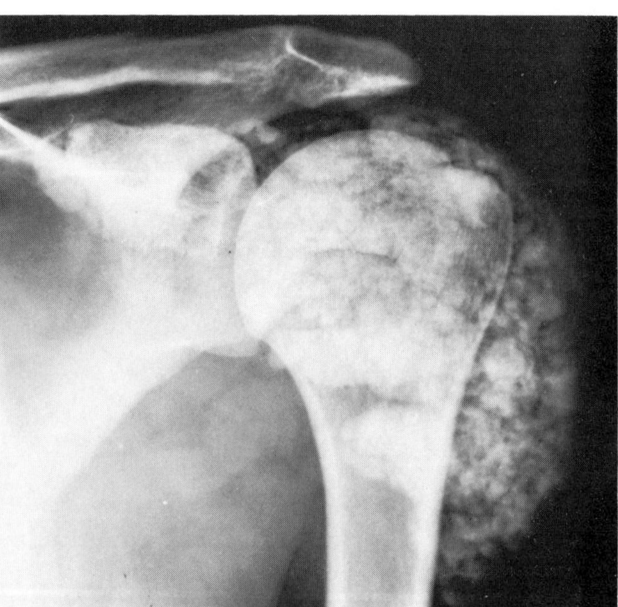

Figure 66–16. *Milk-alkali syndrome. In this patient, periarticular calcific deposits appear about the shoulder. A similar appearance can be seen in hypervitaminosis D, renal osteodystrophy, and certain collagen vascular disorders.*

tion, hypercalcemia, supersaturation of calcium phosphate, and calcinosis.

Other reports of this complication soon appeared,[149-151] and the reversibility of both clinical and radiologic findings and the importance of renal insufficiency and the simultaneous ingestion of milk and alkali were emphasized.[152] Poppel and Zeitel[153] outlined the roentgenologic manifestations of milk-drinker's syndrome; unilateral or bilateral periarticular deposits predominate, which are amorphous

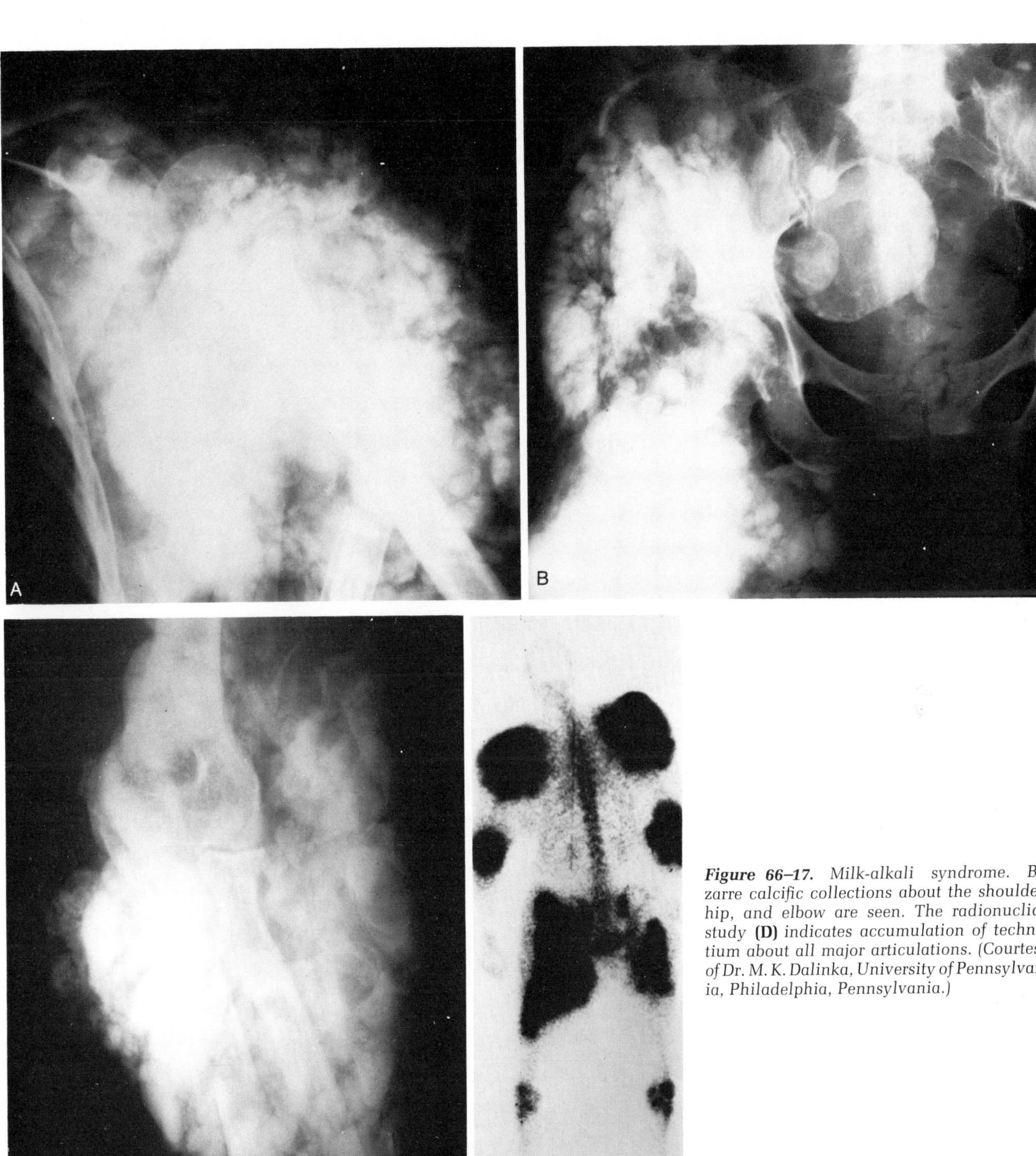

Figure 66–17. *Milk-alkali syndrome. Bizarre calcific collections about the shoulder, hip, and elbow are seen. The radionuclide study* **(D)** *indicates accumulation of technetium about all major articulations. (Courtesy of Dr. M. K. Dalinka, University of Pennsylvania, Philadelphia, Pennsylvania.)*

and vary in size from small nodules to bulky tumors (Figs. 66–16 and 66–17). Widespread calcification in blood vessels, kidneys, ligaments, and falx cerebri are also observed, and the osseous tissues are normal.[154-159]

Wenger and associates[160] summarized their experiences at the University of Chicago; 35 patients with the milk-alkali syndrome were detected in 33,000 patients who were hospitalized for the management of peptic ulcer disease. They noted that the syndrome might appear within several days to weeks after the start of therapy with calcium carbonate, milk, and cream, the interval averaging one week. The typical clinical manifestations were nausea, vomiting, anorexia, weakness, headache, and dizziness. No definite relationship with primary hyperparathyroidism was detected, although the exact mechanism could not be determined.

The differential diagnosis of periarticular calcific deposits accompanying the milk-alkali syndrome includes collagen vascular disorders, hyperparathyroidism, renal osteodystrophy, hypervitaminosis D, and tumoral calcinosis.

SUMMARY

A survey of some of the musculoskeletal manifestations associated with certain medications and chemical substances indicates that at times the therapeutic regimen may indeed be more detrimental than the disease. A variety of teratogenic drugs can lead to significant fetal anomalies. Corticosteroids and other anti-inflammatory agents can produce osteoporosis, osteonecrosis, and neuropathic-like alterations. Osteosclerosis, periostitis, osseous excrescences, ligamentous calcification, and dental abnormalities can accompany fluorosis. Injection of dopamine and related substances may lead to gangrene, requiring amputation, whereas soft tissue calcification may appear following calcium gluconate injection or milk and alkali ingestion.

REFERENCES

1. Keats TE: Post-injection calcification of the deltoid muscle. J Can Assoc Radiol *29*:165, 1978.
2. Goldman AB: Myositis ossificans circumscripta: A benign lesion with a malignant differential diagnosis. Am J Roentgenol *126*:32, 1976.
3. Imray TJ, Hiramatsu Y: Radiographic manifestations of Japanese acupuncture. Radiology *115*:625, 1975.
4. Murray RO: Radiological importance of soft tissue lesions related to skeletons. Ann R Coll Surg *54*:109, 1974.
5. Forfar JO, Nelson MM: Epidemiology of drugs taken by pregnant women: Drugs that may affect the fetus adversely. Clin Pharmacol Ther *14*:632, 1973.
6. Bleyer WA, Au WYW, Lange WA, Raisz LG: Studies on the detection of adverse drug reactions in the newborn. 1. Faetal exposure to maternal medications. JAMA *213*:2046, 1970.
7. Hill RM: Drugs ingested by pregnant women. Clin Pharmacol Ther *14*:654, 1973.
8. Wilson JG: Factors determining the teratogenicity of drugs. Ann Rev Pharmacol *14*:205, 1974.
9. Wilson JG: Present status of drugs as teratogens in man. Teratology *7*:3, 1973.
10. Harris, JM III, Pashayan HM: Teratogenesis. Orthop Clin North Am *7*:281, 1976.
11. McBride WG: Thalidomide and congenital anomalies. Lancet *2*:1358, 1961.
12. Lenz W, Knapp K: Thalidomide embryopathy. Arch Environ Health *5*:100, 1962.
13. McCredie J, McBride WG: Some congenital abnormalities: Possibly due to embryonic peripheral neuropathy. Clin Radiol *24*:204, 1973.
14. Murray RO: Iatrogenic lesions of the skeleton. Am J Roentgenol *126*:5, 1976.
15. Loughnan PM, Gold H, Vance JC: Phenytoin teratogenicity in man. Lancet *1*:70, 1973.
16. Hill RM, Verniaud WM, Horning MG, McCulley LB, Morgan NF: Infants exposed in utero to antiepileptic drugs. A prospective study. Am J Dis Child *127*:645, 1974.
17. Monson RR, Rosenberg L, Hartz SC, Shapiro S, Heinonen OP, Slone D: Diphenylhydantoin and selected congenital malformations. N Engl J Med *289*:1049, 1973.
18. Lowe CR: Congenital malformations among infants born to epileptic women. Lancet *1*:9, 1973.
19. Palmer RH, Quellette EM, Warner L, Leichtman SR: Congenital malformations in offspring of a chronic alcoholic mother. Pediatrics *53*:490, 1974.
20. Ferrier PE, Nicod I, Ferrier S: Fetal alcohol syndrome. Lancet *2*:1496, 1973.
21. Jones KL, Smith DW: Recognition of the fetal alcohol syndrome in early infancy. Lancet *2*:999, 1973.
22. Milunsky A, Graef JW, Gaynor MF: Methotrexate-induced congenital malformations. J Pediatr *72*:790, 1968.
23. Becker MH, Genieser NB, Finegold M, Miranda D, Spackman T: Chondrodysplasia punctata. Is maternal warfarin therapy a factor? Am J Dis Child *129*:356, 1975.
24. Shaul WL, Emery H, Hall JG: Chondrodysplasia punctata and maternal warfarin use during pregnancy. Am J Dis Child *129*:360, 1975.
25. Greenberg G, Inman WHW: Hormonal pregnancy tests and congenital malformations. Br Med J *2*:191, 1975.
26. Hench PS, Kendall EC, Slocumb CH, Polley HF: Effect of hormone of adrenal cortex (17-hydroxy-11-dehydro cortisone, compound E) and of pituitary adrenocorticotrophic hormone on rheumatoid arthritis: Preliminary report. Ann Rheum Dis *8*:97, 1949.
27. Murray RO: Radiological bone changes in Cushing's syndrome and steroid therapy. Br J Radiol *33*:1, 1960.
28. Murray RO: Steroids and skeleton. Radiology *77*:729, 1961.
29. Solomon L: Drug-induced arthropathy and necrosis of the femoral head. J Bone Joint Surg *55B*:246, 1973.
30. Fisher DE, Bickel WH: Corticosteroid-induced avascular necrosis. A clinical study of seventy-seven patients. J Bone Joint Surg *53A*:859, 1971.
31. Saville, PD, Kharmosh O: Osteoporosis of rheumatoid arthritis. Influence of age, sex and corticosteroids. Arthritis Rheum *10*:423, 1967.
32. Heaney RP, Walch JJ, Steffes P, Skillman TG: Periarticular bone remodelling in rheumatoid arthritis. Calcif Tissue Res *2*:Suppl 33, 1968.
33. Sweetman R: Corticosteroid arthropathy and tendon rupture. J Bone Joint Surg *51B*:397, 1969.
34. Pietrogrande V, Mastromarino R: Osteopatia da prolungata trattamento cortisonico. Ortop Traum Appar Mot *25*:791, 1957.
35. Gold EW, Fox OD, Weissfeld S, Curtiss PH: Corticosteroid-induced avascular necrosis: An experimental study in rabbits. Clin Orthop Rel Res *135*:272, 1978.
36. Cruess RL: Cortisone-induced avascular necrosis of the femoral head. J Bone Joint Surg *59B*:308, 1977.
37. Cruess RL: Steroid-induced avascular necrosis of the head of the humerus. Natural history and management. J Bone Joint Surg *58B*:313, 1976.
38. Fisher DE, Bickel WH, Holley KE: Histologic demonstration of fat emboli in aseptic necrosis associated with hypercortisonism. Mayo Clin Proc *44*:252, 1969.
39. Velayos EE, Leidholt JD, Smyth CJ, Priest R: Arthropathy associated with steroid therapy. Ann Intern Med *64*:759, 1966.
40. Smyth CJ, Leidholt JD: Steroid arthropathy of the hip. Clin Orthop Rel Res *90*:50, 1973.
41. Fisher DE: The role of fat embolism in the etiology of corticosteroid-induced avascular necrosis. Clinical and experimental results. Clin Orthop Rel Res *130*:68, 1978.
42. Cruess RL: Experience with steroid-induced avascular necrosis of the shoulder and etiologic considerations regarding osteonecrosis of the hip. Clin Orthop Rel Res *130*:86, 1978.

43. Cruess RL, Ross D, Crawshaw E: The etiology of steroid-induced avascular necrosis of bone. A laboratory and clinical study. Clin Orthop Rel Res *113*:178, 1975.
44. Heimann WG, Freiberger RH: Avascular necrosis of the femoral and humeral heads after high-dosage corticosteroid therapy. N Engl J Med *263*:672, 1960.
45. Boksenbaum M, Mendelson CG: Aseptic necrosis of the femoral head associated with steroid therapy. JAMA *184*:262, 1963.
46. Serre H, Simon L: Le role de la corticothérapie dans l'osteo-necrose primitive de la tète femorale chez l'adulte. Presse Med *69*:1995, 1961.
47. Harrington KD, Murray WR, Kountz SL, Belzer FO: Avascular necrosis of bone after renal transplantation. J Bone Joint Surg *53A*:203, 1971.
48. Frost HM: The etiodynamics of aseptic necrosis of the femoral head. *In* Proceedings of the Conference on Aseptic Necrosis of the Femoral Head. St. Louis, National Institute of Health, 1964, p 393.
49. Boettcher WG, Bonfiglio M, Hamilton HH, Sheets RF, Smith K: Non-traumatic necrosis of the femoral head. Part I. Relation of altered hemostasis to etiology. J Bone Joint Surg *52A*:312, 1970.
50. Cosgriff SW: Thromboembolic complications associated with ACTH and cortisone therapy. JAMA *147*:924, 1951.
51. Merle d'Aubigne R, Postel M, Mazabraud A, Massias P, Guerguen J: Idiopathic necrosis of the femoral head in adults. J Bone Joint Surg *47B*:612, 1965.
52. Fisher DE, Bickel WH, Holley KE, Ellefson RD: Corticosteroid-induced aseptic necrosis. II. Experimental study. Clin Orthop Rel Res *84*:200, 1972.
53. Jones JP, Engleman EP, Steinbach HL, Murray WR, Rambo O: Fat embolization as a possible mechanism producing avascular necrosis. Arthritis Rheum *8*:449, 1965.
54. Jones JP, Sakovich L: Fat embolism of bone: A roentgenographic and histological investigation with use of intra-arterial lipiodol in rabbits. J Bone Joint Surg *48A*:149, 1966.
55. Jones JP, Engleman EP: Fat embolization complicating hypercortisonism. Arthritis Rheum *8*:448, 1965.
56. Jones JP, Engleman EP, Najarian JS: Systemic fat embolism after renal homotransplantation and treatment with corticosteroids. N Engl J Med *273*:1453, 1965.
57. Jaffe WL, Epstein M, Heyman N, Mankin HJ: The effect of cortisone on femoral and humeral head in rabbits. Clin Orthop Rel Res *82*:221, 1972.
58. Arora JS: Indomethacin arthropathy of hips. Proc R Soc Med *61*:669, 1968.
59. Wilkenfeld MJ, Sliwinski AJ: Fatty lesions of both humeri in a patient on corticosteroids and cyclophosphamide. Arthritis Rheum *22*:199, 1979.
60. Sakai T, Cruess RL: Effect of cortisone on the lipids of bone matrix in the rat. Proc R Soc Exp Bio Med *124*:490, 1967.
61. Miller WT, Restifo RA: Steroid arthropathy. Radiology *86*:652, 1966.
62. Chandler GN, Jones DT, Wright V, Hartfall SJ: Charcot's arthropathy following intra-articular hydrocortisone. Br Med J *1*:952, 1959.
63. Steinberg CL, Duthe RB, Piva AE: Charcot-like arthropathy following intra-articular hydrocortisone. JAMA *181*:851, 1962.
64. Bentley G, Goodfellow JW: Disorganization of the knees following intra-articular hydrocortisone injections. J Bone Joint Surg *51B*:498, 1969.
65. Salter RB, Gross A, Hall JH: Hydrocortisone arthropathy — an experimental investigation. Can Med Assoc J *97*:374, 1967.
66. Shaw NE, Lacey E: The influence of corticosteroids on normal and papain-treated articular cartilage in the rabbit. J Bone Joint Surg *55B*:197, 1973.
67. Mankin HJ, Conger KA: The acute effects of intra-articular hydrocortisone on articular cartilage in rabbits. J Bone Jont Surg *48A*:1383, 1966.
68. Moskowitz RW, Davis W, Sammarco J, Mast W, Chase SW: Experimentally induced corticosteroid arthropathy. Arthritis Rheum *13*:236, 1970.
69. Mankin HJ, Zarins A, Jaffe WL: The effect of systemic corticosteroids on rabbit articular cartilage. Arthritis Rheum *15*:593, 1972.
70. Gibson T, Burry HC, Poswillo D, Glass J: Effect of intra-articular corticosteroid injections on primate cartilage. Ann Rheum Dis *36*:74, 1977.
71. Zachariae L: Deleterious effects of corticosteroids administered topically, in particular intra-articularly. Acta Orthop Scand *36*:127, 1965.
72. Alarcon-Segovia D, Ward LE: Marked destructive changes occurring in osteoarthritic finger joints after intra-articular injection of corticosteroids. Arthritis Rheum *9*:443, 1966.
73. Wright V, Chandler GN, Morison RAH, Hartfall SJ: Intra-articular therapy in osteoarthritis. Comparison of hydrocortisone acetate and hydrocortisone tertiary butylacetate. Ann Rheum Dis *19*:257, 1960.
74. Keagy RD, Keim HA: Intra-articular steroid therapy: Repeated use in patients with chronic arthritis. Am J Med Sci *253*:45, 1967.
75. Chandler GN, Wright V: Deleterious effect of intra-articular hydrocortisone. Lancet *2*:661, 1958.
76. Rabinowitz MS: Pyarthrosis of knee joint following intra-articular hydrocortisone. Bull Hosp J Dis *16*:158, 1955.
77. Thomet M: Le danger des injections intra-articulaires d'hydrocortisone. Praxis *46*:152, 1957.
78. Mills LC, Boylston BF, Greene JA, Moyer JH: Septic arthritis as a complication of orally given steroid therapy. JAMA *164*:1310, 1957.
79. Tondreau RL, Hodes PJ, Schmidt ER Jr: Joint infections following steroid therapy: Roentgen manifestations. Am J Roentgenol *82*:258, 1959.
80. Ismail AM, Balakrishnan R, Rajakumar MK: Rupture of patellar ligament after steroid infiltration. J Bone Jont Surg *51B*:503, 1969.
81. Melmed EP: Spontaneous bilateral rupture of the calcaneal tendon during steroid therapy. J Bone Joint Surg *47B*:104, 1965.
82. Bedi SS, Ellis W: Spontaneous rupture of the calcaneal tendon in rheumatoid arthritis after local steroid injection. Ann Rheum Dis *29*:494, 1970.
83. Morgan J, McCarty DJ: Tendon ruptures in patients with systemic lupus erythematosus treated with corticosteroids. Arthritis Rheum *17*:1033, 1974.
84. Halpern AA, Horowitz BG, Nagel DA: Tendon ruptures associated with corticosteroid therapy. West J Med *127*:378, 1977.
85. Smaill GB: Bilateral rupture of achilles tendons. Br Med J *1*:1657, 1961.
86. Langhoff J, Krahl H, Langhoff I: Mikroskopische unde submikroskopische veranderungen an kaninchensehen nach lokaler injektion von 6-methylprednisolon. Bruns Beitr Klin Chir *218*:736, 1971.
87. Phelps D, Sonstegard DA, Matthews LS: Corticosteroid injection effects on the biomechanical properties of rabbit patellar tendons. Clin Orthop Rel Res *100*:345, 1974.
88. Wrenn RN, Goldner JL, Markee JL: An experimental study of the effect of cortisone on the healing process and tensile strength of tendons. J Bone Joint Surg *36A*:588, 1954.
89. Salter RB, Murray D: Effect of hydrocortisone on musculoskeletal tissue. J Bone Joint Surg *51B*:195, 1969.
90. Balasubramaniam P, Prathrap K: The effect of injection of hydrocortisone into rabbit calcaneal tendons. J Bone Joint Surg *54B*:729, 1972.
91. Goldman L: Reactions following intralesional and sublesional injections of corticosteroids. JAMA *182*:613, 1962.
92. Fisherman EW, Feinberg AR, Feinberg SM: Local subcutaneous atrophy. JAMA *179*:971, 1962.
93. Beardwell A: Subcutaneous atrophy after local corticosteroid injection. Br Med J *3*:600, 1967.
94. Schetman D, Hambrick GW Jr, Wilson CE: Cutaneous changes following local injection of triamcinolone. Arch Dermatol *88*:820, 1963.
95. Rostron PKM, Calver RF: Subcutaneous atrophy following methylprednisolone injection in Osgood-Schlatter epiphysitis. J Bone Joint Surg *61A*:627, 1979.
96. Gottlieb NL, Penneys NS, Brown HE Jr: Periarticular perilymphatic skin atrophy after intra-articular corticosteroid injections. JAMA *240*:559, 1978.
97. Singh A, Jolly SS: Endemic fluorosis. Quart J Med *30*:357, 1961.
98. Singh A, Jolly SS, Bansal BC, Mathur CC: Endemic fluorosis. Epidemiological, clinical and biochemical study of chronic fluorine intoxication in Panjab (India). Medicine *42*:229, 1963.
99. Singh A, Dass R, Hayreh SS, Jolly SS: Skeletal changes in endemic fluorosis. J Bone Joint Surg *44B*:806, 1962.
100. Singh A, Vazirani, SJ, Jolly SS, Bansal BC: Endemic fluorisis. Postgrad Med J *38*:150, 1962.
101. Shortt HE, McRobert GR, Barnard TW, Nayar ASM: Endemic fluorosis in the madras presidency. Ind J Med Res *25*:553, 1937.
102. Smith FA, Hodge HC: Fluoride toxicity. *In* JC Muhler, MK Hine (Eds): Fluorine and Dental Health. Bloomington, Indiana University Press, 1959.
103. Dean HT: Distribution of mottled enamel in the United States. Pub Health Rep *48*:703, 1933.
104. McClure FJ, Likins RC: Fluorine in human teeth studied in relation to fluorine in the drinking water. J Dent Res *30*:172, 1951.
105. Smith MC, Lantz EM, Smith HV: The cause of mottled enamel. Science *74*:244, 1931.
106. Siddiqui AH: Fluorosis in Nalgonda district Hyderabad-Deccan. Br Med J *2*:1408, 1955.
107. Roholm K: Fluorine intoxication. A clinical hygienic study with a review of the literature and some experimental investigations. London, HK Lewis & Company, Ltd., 1937.
108. Stevenson CA, Watson AR: Fluoride osteosclerosis. Am J Roentgenol *78*:13, 1957.
109. Stevenson CA, Watson AR: Roentgenologic findings in fluoride osteosclerosis. Arch Indust Health *21*:340, 1960.
110. Linsman JF, McMurray CA: Fluoride osteosclerosis from drinking water. Radiology *40*:474, 1943.
111. Moller PF, Gudjonsson SV: Massive fluorosis of bones and ligaments. Acta Radiol *13*:269, 1932.
112. Largent EJ, Bovard PG, Heyroth FF: Roentgenographic changes and

urinary fluoride excretion among workmen engaged in the manufacture of inorganic fluorides. Am J Roentgenol *65*:42, 1951.
113. Leone NC, Stevenson CA, Hilbish TF, Sosman MC: A roentgenologic study of a human population exposed to high fluoride domestic water. Am J Roentgenol *74*:874, 1955.
114. Soriano M: Periostitis deformans (un nuevo tipo de fluorosis osea en el hombre) la fluorosis vinica. Rev Clin Esp *97*:375, 1965.
115. Soriano M, Manchon F: Radiological aspects of a new type of bone fluorosis, periostitis deformans. Radiology *87*:1089, 1966.
116. Johnson FF, Fischer LL: Report on fluorine in wine. Am J Pharm *107*:512, 1939.
117. Faccini JM, Teotia SPS: Histopathological assessment of endemic skeletal fluorosis. Calcif Tissue Res *16*:45, 1974.
118. Aggarwal ND: Structure of human fluorotic bone. J Bone Joint Surg *55A*:331, 1973.
119. Singh A, Jolly SS, Bansal BC: Skeletal fluorosis and its neurological complications. Lancet *1*:197, 1961.
120. Teotia SPS, Teotia M: Secondary hyperparathyroidism in patients with endemic skeletal fluorosis. Br Med J *1*:637, 1973.
121. Messer HH, Armstrong WD, Singer L: Fluoride, parathyroid hormone and calcitonin: Inter-relationships in bone calcium metabolism. Calcif Tissue Res *13*:217, 1973.
122. Messer HH, Armstrong WD, Singer L: Fluoride, parathyroid hormone, and calcitonin: Effects on metabolic processes involved in bone resorption. Calcif Tissue Res *13*:227, 1973.
123. Faccini JM: Fluoride and bone. Calcif Tissue Res *3*:1, 1969.
124. Evans FG, Wood JL: Mechanical properties and density of bone in a case of severe endemic fluorosis. Acta Orthop Scand *47*:489, 1976.
125. Franke J, Runge H, Grau P, Fengler F, Wanka C, Rempel H: Physical properties of fluorosis bone. Acta Orthop Scand *47*:20, 1976.
126. Lindahl O, Lindwall L: Physical properties of fluorosis bone. Critical comments. Acta Orthop Scand *49*:382, 1978.
127. Singer L, Armstrong WD, Zipkin I, Frazier PD: Chemical composition and structure of fluorotic bone. Clin Orthop Rel Res *99*:303, 1974.
128. Baud CA, Lagier R, Boivin G, Boillat MA: Value of the bone biopsy in the diagnosis of industrial fluorosis. Virchows Arch Pathol Anat Histol *380*:283, 1978.
129. Krishnamachari KAVR, Krishnaswamy K: Genu valgum and osteoporosis in an area of endemic fluorosis. Lancet *2*:877, 1973.
130. Reid PR, Thompson WL: The clinical use of dopamine in the treatment of shock. Johns Hopk Med J *137*:265, 1975.
131. Goldberg LI: Dopamine — clinical uses of an endogenous catecholamine. N Engl J Med *291*:707, 1974.
132. Stetson JB, Reading GP: Avoidance of vascular complications associated with the use of dopamine. Can Anaesth Soc J *24*:727, 1977.
133. Holzer J, Karliner JS, O'Rourke RA, Pitt W, Ross J Jr: Effectiveness of dopamine in patients with cardiogenic shock. Am J Cardiol *32*:79, 1973.
134. Boltax RS, Dineen JP, Scarpa FJ: Gangrene resulting from infiltrated dopamine solution. N Engl J Med *296*:823, 1977.
135. Buchanan N, Cane RD, Miller N: Symmetrical gangrene of the extremities associated with the use of dopamine subsequent to ergometrine administration. Intensive Care Med J *3*:55, 1977.
136. Green SI, Smith JW: Dopamine gangrene. N Engl J Med *294*:114, 1976.
137. Alexander CS, Sako Y, Mikulic E: Pedal gangrene associated with the use of dopamine. N Engl J Med *293*:591, 1975.
138. Golbranson F, Vance R, Vandell R, Lurie L: Multiple extremity amputations in hypotensive patients treated with dopamine. JAMA (in press).
139. Ebels T, Homan van der Heide JN: Dopamine-induced ischaemia. Lancet *2*:762, 1977.
140. Graham JR: Methysergide for prevention of headache. N Engl J Med *270*:67, 1964.
141. Johnson TD: Severe peripheral arterial constriction, acute ischemia of a lower extremity with use of methysergide and ergotamine. Arch Intern Med *117*:237, 1966.
142. Imrie CW: Arterial spasm associated with oral ergotamine therapy. Br J Clin Pract *27*:457, 1973.
143. Ureles A, Rob C: Acute ischemia of a limb complicating methysergide maleate therapy. JAMA *183*:1041, 1963.
144. Vaughan-Lane T: Gangrene induced by methysergide and ergotamine. A case report. J Bone Joint Surg *61B*:213, 1979.
145. Twiford TW Jr, Granmayeh M, Tucker MJ: Gangrene of the feet associated with mesenteric intra-arterial vasopressin. Am J Roentgenol *130*:558, 1978.
146. Berger PE, Heidelberger KP, Poznanski AK: Extravasation of calcium gluconate as a cause of soft tissue calcification in infancy. Am J Roentgenol *121*:109, 1974.
147. Harris V, Ramamurthy RS, Pildes RS: Late onset of subcutaneous calcifications after intravenous injections of calcium gluconate. Am J Roentgenol *123*:845, 1975.
148. Burnett CH, Commons RR, Albright F, Howard JE: Hypercalcemia without hypercalcuria or hypophosphatemia, calcinosis, and renal insufficiency. N Engl J Med *240*:787, 1949.
149. Miller JM, Freeman I, Heath WH: Calcinosis due to treatment of duodenal ulcer. JAMA *148*:198, 1952.
150. McQueen EG: "Milk poisoning" and "calcium gout." Lancet *2*:67, 1952.
151. Wermer P, Kuschner M, Riley EA: Reversible metastatic calcification associated with excessive milk and alkali intake. Am J Med *14*:108, 1953.
152. Dworetzky M: Reversible metastatic calcification (milk-drinker's syndrome). JAMA *155*:830, 1954.
153. Poppel MH, Zeitel BE: Roentgen manifestations of milk drinker's syndrome. Radiology *67*:195, 1956.
154. Snapper I, Bradley WG, Wilson VE: Metastatic calcification and nephrocalcinosis from medical treatment of peptic ulcer. Arch Intern Med *93*:807, 1954.
155. Foltz EE: Calcinosis complicating peptic ulcer therapy. Gastroenterology *27*:50, 1954.
156. Ogle JC, Harvey CM Jr: Hypercalcemia and renal impairment following milk and alkali therapy for peptic ulcer. South Med J *48*:126, 1955.
157. Scholz DA, Keating FR Jr: Milk-alkali syndrome. Review of eight cases. Arch Intern Med *95*:460, 1955.
158. Kessler E: Hypercalcemia and renal insufficiency secondary to excessive milk and alkali intake. Ann Intern Med *42*:324, 1955.
159. Rodnan G, Johnson H: Chronic renal failure in association with the excessive intake of calcium and alkali. Gastroenterology *27*:584, 1954.
160. Wenger J, Kirsner JB, Palmer WL: The milk-alkali syndrome. Hypercalcemia, alkalosis and temporary renal insufficiency during milk-antacid therapy for peptic ulcer. Am J Med *24*:161, 1958.
161. Seeler, RA, Israel JN, Royal JE, Kaye CI, Rao S, Abulaban M: Ganglioneuroblastoma and fetal hydantoin-alcohol syndromes. Pediatrics *63*:524, 1979.
162. Hamanishi C: Congenital short femur. Clinical, genetic, and epidemiological comparison of the naturally occurring condition with that caused by thalidomide. J Bone Joint Surg *62B*:307, 1980.
163. Maldague B, Noel H, Malghem J: The intravertebral vacuum cleft: A sign of ischemic vertebral collapse. Radiology *129*:23, 1978.
164. Maldague B, Malghem J, Huaux JP, Rombouts-Lindemans C, Noel H: Ischemic collapse of the vertebral body: Myth or reality. J Belge Radiol *62*:61, 1979.
165. Zizic TM, Hungerford DS, Stevens MB: Ischemic bone necrosis in systemic lupus erythematosus. I. The early diagnosis of ischemic necrosis of bone. Medicine *59*:134, 1980.
166. Oxlund H: The influence of a local injection of cortisol on the mechanical properties of tendons and ligaments and the indirect effect on skin. Acta Orthop Scand *51*:231, 1980.
167. Gluck O, Murphy W, Hahn T, Hahn B: Risk factors for steroid-induced bone loss (Abstr). Arthritis Rheum *23*:681, 1980.
168. Gluck O, Hahn T, Hahn B: Comparison of bone loss in patients receiving alternate or daily glucocorticoid therapy (Abstr). Arthritis Rheum *23*:681, 1980.
169. Weinstein J: Benign joint effusion associated with glucocorticosteroid therapy. J Rheumatology *7*:245, 1980.
170. Christie DP: The spectrum of radiographic bone changes in children with fluorosis. Radiology *136*:85, 1980.
171. Boillat MA, Garcia J, Velebit L: Radiological criteria of industrial fluorosis. Skel Radiol *5*:161, 1980.
172. Alhava EM, Olkkonen H, Kauranen P, Kari T: The effect of drinking water fluoridation on the fluoride content, strength and mineral density of human bone. Acta Orthop Scand *51*:413, 1980.
173. Meunier PJ, Courpron P, Smoller JS, Briancon D: Niflumic acid-induced skeletal fluorosis: Iatrogenic disease or therapeutic perspective for osteoporosis? Clin Orthop Rel Res *148*:304, 1980.

67

HYPERVITAMINOSIS AND HYPOVITAMINOSIS

by Donald Resnick, M.D.

Musculoskeletal manifestations accompany deficiencies and excesses of certain vitamins. A classic example of a disorder that illustrates the fundamental dependence of normal osseous development and maturation on vitamin intake is rickets, which is due to a deficiency in vitamin D or its active metabolites (Chapter 49). In addition, excessive levels of the vitamins D and A and depressed levels of the vitamins A and C can produce characteristic changes in the skeleton, which will be illustrated in the following pages.

HYPERVITAMINOSIS A

Vitamin A poisoning appears in both children and adults. Its clinical and radiologic manifestations are influenced by the acute or chronic nature of the vitamin abuse. In infants and children, short-term or long-term ingestion of excessive amounts of vitamin A are due, in many cases, to the actions of an overly concerned or enthusiastic parent and may be accompanied by significant skeletal alterations. In adults, extraskeletal changes predominate, and the affected individual can reveal prominent dermatologic aberrations in addition to anorexia and weight loss.[1-3]

Acute Poisoning

Following a massive dose of vitamin A (several hundred thousand units), acute clinical findings can develop. These were first alluded to by Kane,[4] an Arctic explorer, who in 1856 recorded transient symptoms of vertigo and headache that followed the ingestion of polar bear liver, a substance that contains a high concentration of vitamin A.[5, 6] Approximately one century later, nausea, vomiting, headache, drowsiness, and irritability were noted in adults with acute hypervitaminosis A resulting from ingestion of shark liver, also rich in this vitamin.[7] The findings of acute intoxication due to vitamin A were further delineated in 1954 by Marie and See[8] in children who developed drowsiness, vomiting, and bulging of the fontanels from accidental overdose of vitamin drops. The symptoms and signs cleared within a few days after the cessation of vitamin A intake.

Bulging of the fontanels can appear within 12 hours following vitamin ingestion, usually disappearing after 36 to 48 hours[9, 10]; the acute hydrocephalus may be attributable to an increase in production or a decrease in absorption of cerebrospinal fluid.[30] Although skull films can reveal widening of the sutures, the finding is transient, and the ocular fundi and cerebral electroencephalogram are generally normal.

Subacute and Chronic Poisoning

Chronic vitamin A poisoning was first recorded in a child in 1944 by Josephs,[11] and several years later, its association with soft tissue swellings of the extremities and roentgenographic osseous abnormalities was recognized.[12] The skeletal changes were later described in detail,[13] and a similar condition occurring in adults was noted.[14] In both age groups, anorexia and itching represent nonspecific early findings of the disorder. After a period of weeks or months, hard and tender soft tissue nodules appear in the extremities, particularly in the forearms. Additional manifestations include dry scaly skin, coarse and sparse hair, hepatosplenomegaly, and digital clubbing. An elevated serum vitamin A level is diagnostic in this clinical setting, and rapid diminution and disappearance of the symptoms and signs follow withdrawal of vitamin A intake.[9]

Radiographic signs are characteristic. They are virtually confined to children, usually appearing near the end of the first year of life, although infants and teenagers can occasionally reveal similar abnormalities. Cortical thickening of the tubular bones is a constant finding and is usually related to the areas in which soft tissue nodules are present.[9, 12, 15-18] Typically, hyperostosis is observed in the ulnae and metatarsals, producing a wavy or undulating diaphyseal contour; metaphyseal and epiphyseal segments do not participate in the cortical thickening (Fig. 67–1). The clavicles, tibiae, and fibulae are not uncommonly affected; involvement of the femora, humeri, metacarpals, and ribs is less constant, and changes in the mandible are rarely observed. Microscopic examination indicates that subperiosteal deposition of bone accounts for the increased thickening of the cortices.[9]

Additional findings may appear in the epiphyseal and metaphyseal segments of tubular bones that may lead to crippling deformities.[19-21] The distal femora are most commonly altered. Cupping, shortening, and splaying of the metaphyses, irregularity and narrowing of the cartilaginous growth plates, and hypertrophy and premature fusion of the epiphyseal ossification centers can be noted (Fig. 67–2). Although the areas of cortical hyperostosis may gradually disappear following removal of the excess vitamin A, the damage to the epiphyseal cartilage may be irreversible if the poisoning has been protracted. Flexion contractures, short stature, and leg length discrepancies may ensue. Furthermore, scoliosis and fractures have been recorded,[20] although the relationship of these findings to hypervitaminosis A is not clear.

As in cases of acute poisoning, increased intracranial pressure has been noted in association with chronic hypervitaminosis A.[6, 22, 88] In those cases in which chronic hypervitaminosis A appears in the first 6 months of life, the skull may be poorly mineralized with relatively dense sutural margins.[23] After this age, cranial findings include widening of the sutures with elongation of the head, hyperostosis in the occipital and the temporal bones, and ventricular dilatation.[24]

Certain effects of vitamin A on the skeleton have been observed in the laboratory. In weaning rats and guinea pigs, premature maturation and vascularization of the cartilaginous growth plates can be produced with excessive intake of vitamin A. Premature closure of the plates can produce early cessation of growth in these animals.[25] Furthermore, an accelerated remodeling of the transverse diameter of the tubular bones, particularly in the juxtaepiphyseal areas, can lead to osseous fracture.[26] On the basis of organ cultures, Dingle and associates[27-29] have postulated that vitamin A produces activation or release of cell proteases, which destroy extracellular cartilage matrix.[20] The simultaneous administration of cortisone to animals receiving high doses of vitamin A may prevent the cartilaginous destruction.[30]

The condition that produces skeletal changes that most resemble those of chronic hypervitaminosis A is infantile cortical hyperostosis (Caffey's disease) (Table 67–1). In vitamin A intoxication, cortical hyperostosis usually becomes manifest no earlier than the end of the first year of life (whereas infantile cortical hyperostosis may produce changes in the first 6 months of life), mandibular and facial involvement is unusual (whereas these areas are typically affected in infantile cortical hyperostosis), metatarsal alterations are frequent (whereas these bones are generally spared in infantile cortical hyperostosis),

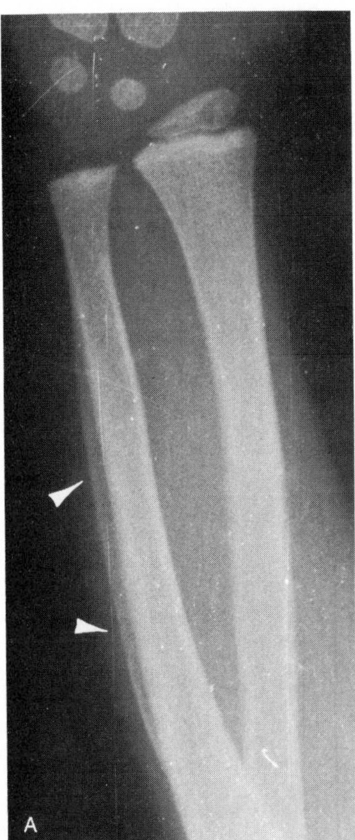

Figure 67–1. *Hypervitaminosis A: Periostitis and cortical hyperostosis.*

A *Note periosteal bone formation in the diaphysis of the ulna (arrowheads).* (**A**, *Courtesy of Dr. F. Silverman, Department of Radiology, Stanford University Medical Center, Stanford, California.*)

B, C *In a different child, periosteal proliferation is evident in the diaphyses of multiple metatarsals (arrowheads) in both feet.*

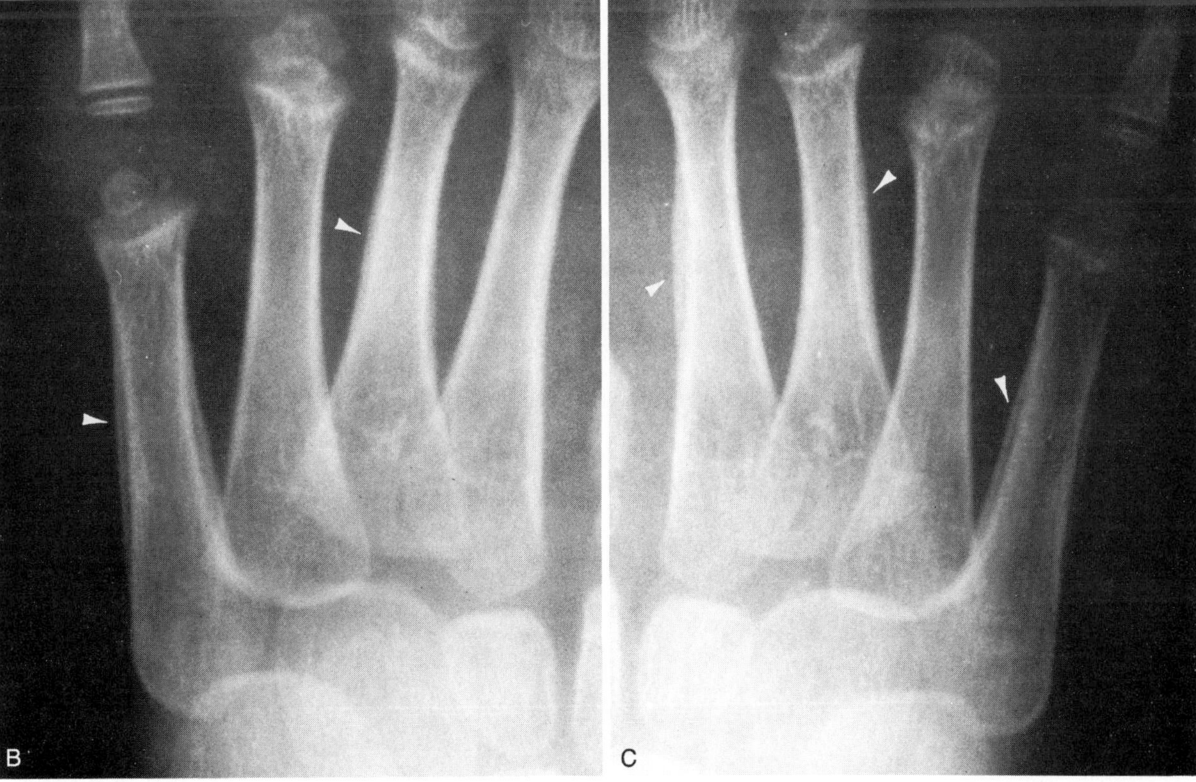

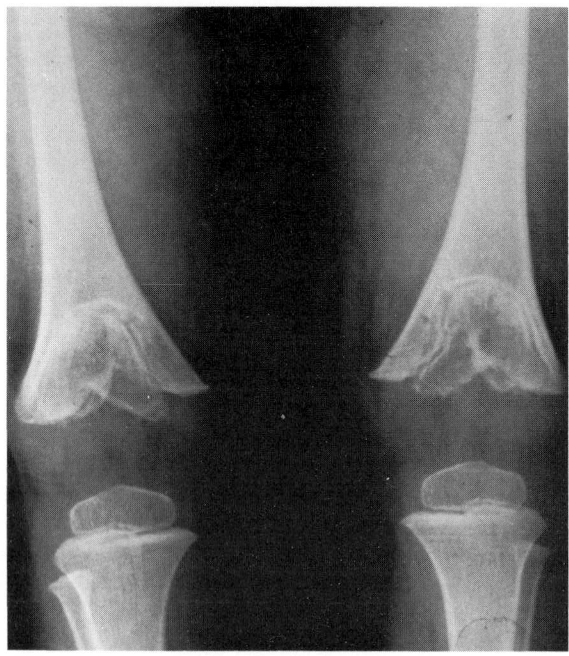

Figure 67–2. Hypervitaminosis A: Metaphyseal and epiphyseal changes. Observe the striking splaying and cupping of the distal femoral metaphyses, with narrowing of the cartilaginous growth plates and hypertrophy and invagination of the epiphyses.

and biochemical analysis of the blood reveals marked elevation of vitamin A concentration.[31]

HYPOVITAMINOSIS A

Vitamin A dietary deficiency in a pregnant woman can lead to an abortion or stillbirth of the fetus, or, in less severe cases, birth of a child who may reveal ophthalmic defects. Chronic vitamin A deficiency in infancy, childhood, or adulthood produces a variety of epithelial alterations, including dry and scaly skin, photophobia, night blindness, and dry conjunctivae; in infancy, additional manifestations include a susceptibility to infection, anemia, cranial nerve injury, and growth retardation.[33, 34] Increased intracranial pressure of unknown pathogenesis is observed in this condition,[24, 32, 34, 35] which in infants below the age of 6 months may lead to widening of the cranial sutures with bulging fontanels.[36, 37]

Additional skeletal changes in vitamin A deficiency are recognized in experimental situations.[31] In animals deprived of vitamin A, stimulation of periosteal and endosteal bone formation[38] and retardation of endochondral bone formation[39] can lead to the appearance of short and thick tubular bones and may contribute to neural damage due to the effect of osseous pressure on neurologic tissue in the bones that are encasing the nervous system.[31] Furthermore, in experimental and nonexperimental situations, vitamin A deficiency may have a dramatic effect on dental development.[40-42]

HYPOVITAMINOSIS C (SCURVY)

A long-term deficiency of dietary vitamin C (ascorbic acid) results in scurvy. This disease can be divided into those cases that develop in infancy or childhood (infantile scurvy) and those that occur in adults (adult scurvy).

Table 67–1

HYPERVITAMINOSIS A VERSUS INFANTILE CORTICAL HYPEROSTOSIS (CAFFEY'S DISEASE)

	Hypervitaminosis A	Infantile Cortical Hyperostosis
Age of onset	End of first year of life	First 6 months of life
Findings	Soft tissue nodules Periostitis and hyperostosis Metaphyseal changes Growth disturbances Increased intracranial pressure	Soft tissue nodules Periostitis and hyperostosis Growth disturbances
Sites of hyperostosis (descending order of frequency)	Ulnae Metatarsals Clavicles Tibiae Fibulae Metacarpals Other tubular bones Ribs	Mandible Clavicles Scapulae Ribs Tubular bones
Etiology	Vitamin A poisoning	Unknown; possibly a viral disease

Infantile Scurvy

Infantile scurvy occurs in babies who are administered pasteurized or boiled milk[9]; the process of heating the milk leads to disruption of vitamin C and the appearance of the disorder. Clinically apparent disease develops after deficiency of the vitamin has existed for 4 to 10 months; thus, it is exceedingly unusual to detect this disorder in infants below the age of 4 months, the manifestations generally becoming apparent at 8 to 14 months of age. However, there are reports of scurvy appearing in the first and second months of life,[43-45] although the authenticity of some of these cases is open to question.[9] Prior to the appearance of hemorrhagic tendencies, infants with scurvy can develop nonspecific findings, including a failure to thrive and digestive alterations. The onset of pale skin with petechial hemorrhages, swollen, red, and ulcerated gums, palatal petechiae, hematuria, melena, hematemesis, and secondary infections, when combined with characteristic radiographic changes and depressed levels of serum ascorbic acid, assures accurate diagnosis; this hemorrhagic tendency that is a hallmark of the disease may be related to a lack of intercellular cement substance in the endothelial layer of the capillaries. Additional clinical findings of infantile scurvy include inactivity, soft tissue swelling due to edema and hemorrhage, and costochondral tenderness and prominence.

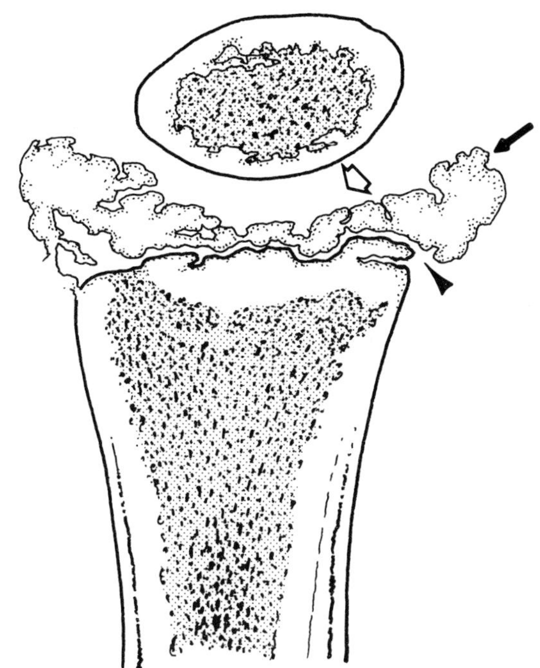

Figure 67–3. *Hypovitaminosis C (scurvy): Pathologic abnormalities. The changes in the ends of tubular bones consist of an irregular arrangement of cartilage cells in the proliferating zone of the growth plate (open arrow), a metaphyseal area containing a latticework of calcified cartilage that is free of osseous tissue (solid arrow), and a decrease in trabeculae, fracture, and detritus in the junctional area (arrowhead). Metaphyseal excrescences can develop.*

Metaphyseal Changes. Skeletal alterations are due to a depression of normal cellular activity, which is manifest in the collagen of the bony tissues.[31, 46] The activity of the osteoblast is reduced, thereby leading to a decrease in the formation of bony matrix, which is most marked in areas of active endochondral bone growth (ends of tubular bones and costochondral junctions). In the region of the cartilaginous growth plate, proliferating cartilage cells are reduced in number, modified osteoblasts are identified, and a disorganization of the growth zone is evident. An irregular arrangement of cartilage cells appears in the proliferating zone of the plate, and a small area of the adjacent metaphysis contains a trabecular latticework of calcified cartilage matrix that is strikingly free of borders of osseous tissue[31] (Fig. 67–3). A sparsity of newly formed trabeculae is evident in this junctional region, and a brittleness of trabecular structure is demonstrated. Extensive resorption of cortical and spongy bone contributes to a tendency to fracture through this zone, leading to evidence of fresh and remote hemorrhage. The abnormal marrow in the junctional area is termed "gerüstmark," and the entire zone consists of detritus ("Trümmerfeldzone").[31] Lateral extension of the heavy provisional zones of calcification in conjunction with elevation and stimulation of the adjacent periosteal membrane produces small spicules or excrescences of the metaphysis.

A roentgenogram of the end of an involved tubular bone will reveal several zones (Table 67–2) (Fig. 67–4). A radiodense line borders on the growth plate, representing the sclerotic provisional zone. On its metaphyseal side between the provisional zone of calcification and the heavy spongiosa deeper in the shaft exists a transverse band of diminished density, the "scurvy" line. Small beak-like outgrowths of the metaphysis, incomplete or complete separation of the plate from the shaft due to subepiphyseal marginal clefts and infractions ("corner" or "angle" sign), and periosteal elevation with new bone formation due to subperiosteal hemorrhage complete the distinctive radiographic picture of the metaepiphyseal regions of tubular bones (and costochondral junctions).[9] These changes are most marked in areas of active endochondral bone formation, such as the distal end of the femur, proximal and distal ends of the tibia and fibula, the distal end of the radius and ulna, the proximal end of the humerus, and the sternal ends of the ribs.

Epiphyseal Changes. In the ossification centers of the epiphyses of tubular bones and in the carpus and tarsus, similar but less marked alterations are seen. Persistence and thickening of the provisional zone of calcification produce a radiodense shell around the ossification center that is accentuated by central rarefaction owing to atrophy of the adjacent spongiosa (Wimberger's sign of scurvy).[9] These epiphyseal abnormalities, which do not include infraction or fracture, are invariably

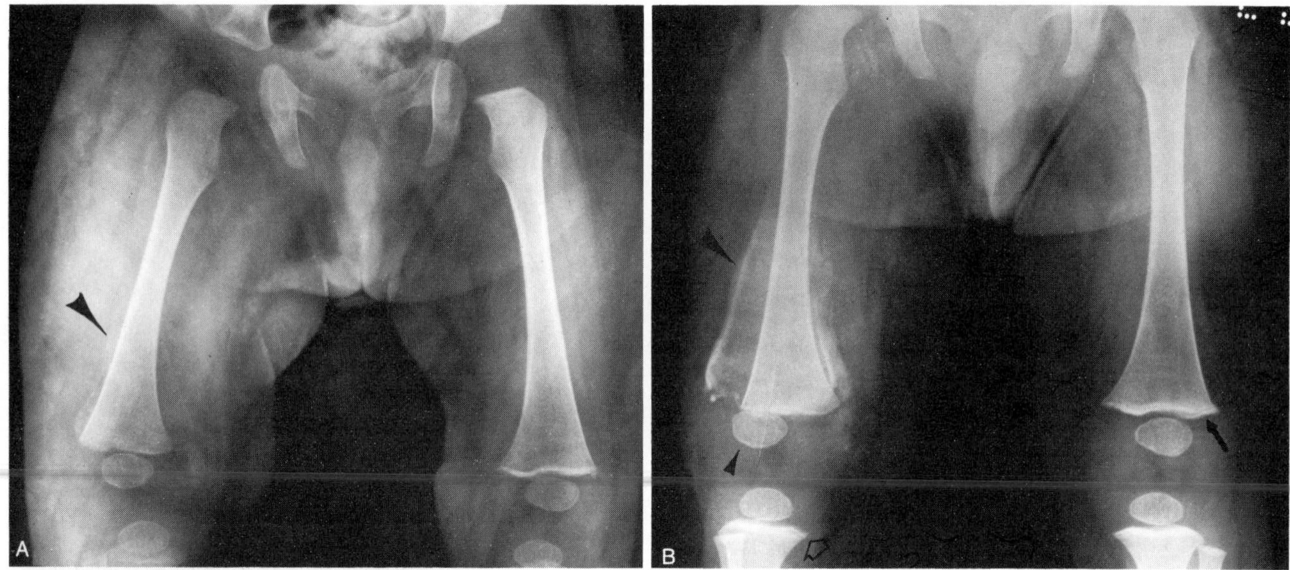

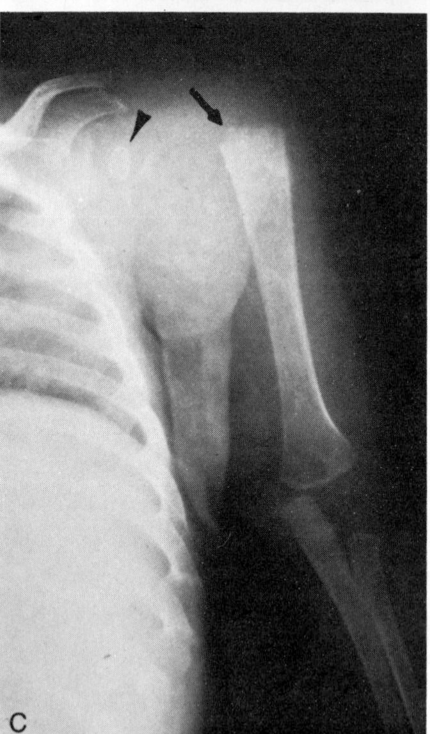

Figure 67–4. *Hypovitaminosis C (scurvy): Radiographic abnormalities.*

A, B *At the ends of tubular bones, one can note osteoporosis, a thick sclerotic metaphyseal line beneath which is a radiolucent line ("scurvy line") (solid arrow), small beak-like excrescences (open arrow), epiphyseal displacement (small arrowhead), and subperiosteal hemorrhage with periostitis (large arrowhead). (***A, B,** *Courtesy of Dr. F. Silverman, Department of Radiology, Stanford University Medical Center, Stanford, California.)*

C *In another child, observe osteoporosis, soft tissue swelling, and epiphyseal displacement (arrowhead) with metaphyseal irregularity (arrow).*

Table 67–2

HYPOVITAMINOSIS C (SCURVY): RADIOGRAPHIC-PATHOLOGIC CORRELATION

Radiographic Finding	Pathologic Finding
Transverse metaphyseal line of increased density	Prominent thickened provisional zone of calcification
Transverse metaphyseal line of decreased density ("scurvy" line)	Decrease in trabeculae and detritus in junctional area of metaphysis ("Trümmerfeldzone")
Metaphyseal excrescences or beaks	Lateral extension of the heavy provisional zone of calcification with periosteal elevation and stimulation
Subepiphyseal infractions ("corner" or "angle" sign)	Decrease and brittleness of trabeculae in junctional area with fracture and hemorrhage
Periostitis	Subperiosteal hemorrhage with elevation and stimulation of periosteum
Epiphyseal shell of increased density with central lucency (Wimberger's sign of scurvy)	Prominent thickened provisional zone of calcification with atrophy of central spongiosa

combined with the metaphyseal changes that were outlined previously.

Diaphyseal Changes. Atrophy of spongiosa in the shafts of tubular bones accounts for a nonspecific decreased radiodensity and a "ground-glass" appearance of the diaphyses. Cortical diminution is common and often severe, yet fracture of the shafts is unusual. Subperiosteal hemorrhage is most frequent in the larger tubular bones, such as the femur, the tibia, and the humerus, although similar but less extensive bleeding may appear in other sites, including the flat bones of the calvarium and shoulder girdle.[9] The degree of hemorrhage is variable and can produce focal or diffuse elevation of the periosteal membrane. The entire length of the diaphysis may be affected; epiphyseal hemorrhage is exceedingly rare. Radiographically, soft tissue masses of increased density, displacement of adjacent bones, and small or large shells of periosteal bone, particularly during the healing phase of the disease, are observed.

Articular Changes. Hemarthrosis is a rare manifestation of scurvy,[47, 48] demonstrating a predilection for the large weight-bearing articulations of the lower extremities. A bloody effusion and thickened synovial membrane with hemosiderin deposition in the macrophages of the deep connective tissue can be observed. Hemarthrosis and intrasynovial hemorrhage can be attributed to loss of the structural integrity of the collagen tissue in the synovial membrane coupled with the trauma of normal activity.[48]

Dental Changes. Cyst formation and hemorrhage in the enamel and interruptions of the lamina dura may be dental manifestations of scurvy in humans.[49, 50] In animals, dental changes in experimental vitamin C deficiency can be prominent with arrested growth and hemorrhage.[31]

Growth Disturbances. Permanent growth disturbances following scurvy are unusual despite the frequency and severity of epiphyseal separations. Central segmental metaphyseal cupping in a bilateral or unilateral distribution can lead to intrusion of the epiphysis into the exaggerated concavity of the metaphysis and apparent early fusion of the growth plate.[51, 52] This complication is not frequent, however, and the degree of limb shortening may be minimal. The pathogenesis of metaphyseal cupping is not clear, although impaired ossification in the central portion of the growth plate due to interruption of vascular supply, perhaps related to periosteal stripping, has been suggested as one possible mechanism for this alteration.[51] The change may be accentuated by osseous weakening of the neighboring metaphyseal bone.[53] Similar cupping may be observed following trauma, infection, irradiation, immobilization, and vitamin A poisoning, as well as in sickle cell anemia and hereditary bone disorders.[54]

Effects of Therapy. With treatment of the disease, roentgenographic signs may accompany healing scurvy.[55] Thickening of the cortex, increased density of the radiolucent zone of the metaphysis, transverse densities within the shaft due to burying of the thickened provisional zone of calcification, massive subperiosteal bone formation, which later merges with the underlying cortex, spontaneous shifting of the diaphysis to realign with the displaced epiphysis, and increased density of the epiphysis can all be observed.[9] Circular central radiolucent foci in the epiphyseal ossification centers corresponding to the original outline of the osteoporotic epiphyses have been noted.

Differential Diagnosis. The appearance of a radiolucent metaphyseal band in scurvy does not represent a pathognomonic finding. Other chronic illnesses, such as leukemia and neuroblastoma, can produce bony atrophy in this region. The identification of radiodense lines at the metaphysis and about the epiphysis, metaphyseal fractures, osseous beaks, epiphyseal displacements, and diaphyseal periostitis allows an accurate diagnosis of scurvy. Leukemia can lead to periostitis and diaphyseal destruction in combination with band-like metaphyseal radiolucency, but fracture and epiphyseal separation are not identified. Syphilis produces symmetric destructive foci in the metaphyses, particularly in the proximal tibia, but the distinctive findings are not confused with those of scurvy. Metaphyseal changes can also accompany rubella, cytomegalic inclusion disease, toxoplasmosis, and a variety of traumatic and dysplastic disorders.

Adult Scurvy

Currently, scurvy is rarely encountered in adults, although it may be observed in severely malnourished individuals, especially the elderly. The findings require a protracted period of vitamin deficiency for clinical expression.[49] Nonspecific weakness, anorexia, weight loss, and fatigue generally antedate the more diagnostic hemorrhagic manifestations, such as petechiae and ecchymoses of the skin, subcutaneous tissues, and gums.[56]

Hemarthrosis and bleeding at synchondroses can be observed in adult scurvy[48, 57] (Fig. 67–5). Osteoporosis is prominent in the axial skeleton, especially the spine, and in the tubular bones of the appendicular skeleton. In the vertebral column, biconcave deformities of vertebral bodies, condensation of bone at the superior and inferior vertebral margins, and central rarefaction are identical to changes of osteoporosis accompanying a wide spectrum of disorders; in the extremities, cortical thinning can be associated with mild periosteal proliferation. The cranium may also be osteoporotic in adult-onset scurvy.

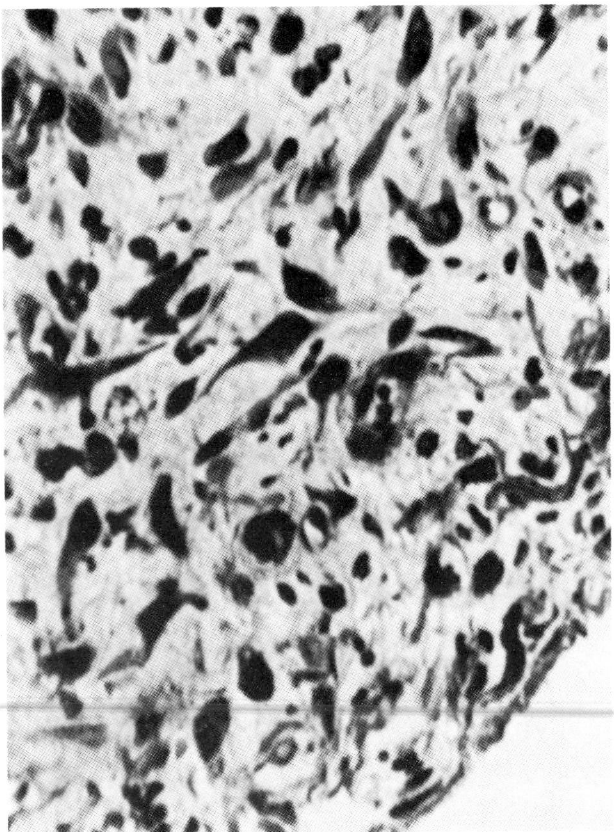

Figure 67–5. *Hypovitaminosis C (scurvy): Articular abnormalities. In a 56 year old man with scurvy, knee hemarthrosis appeared. The synovial membrane shows many elongated fibroblasts and smaller erythrocytes scattered throughout the interstitium (360×). (From Bevelaqua P, et al: JAMA 235:1874, 1976. Copyright 1976, American Medical Association.)*

HYPERVITAMINOSIS D

Excessive intake of vitamin D can be associated with clinical and radiologic manifestations in both children and adults. Initial reports noted findings of intoxication in infants and young children who had been administered excessive levels of vitamin D for the treatment of rickets and other skeletal disorders[58]; similar intoxication in adults was later identified in patients who were receiving inordinate amounts of vitamin D for the therapy of Paget's disease or rheumatoid arthritis.[31, 59, 60]

Musculoskeletal Abnormalities

Vitamin D poisoning can be acute or chronic. The level of the vitamin that is required to produce toxic symptoms and signs is extremely variable; patients with preexisting renal or gastrointestinal dysfunction are especially susceptible.[31] Acute clinical manifestations may appear within 3 to 9 days following massive doses (4 to 18 million units per day) of the vitamin and include vomiting, fever, dehydration, abdominal cramps, bone pain and tenderness, convulsions, and coma.[61] With chronic poisoning, lassitude, thirst, anorexia, and polyuria are followed by vomiting, abdominal pain, and diarrhea.[9] Laboratory analysis indicates albuminuria, hematuria, hypercalciuria, and hypercalcemia. With the onset of renal insufficiency, the levels of serum phosphorus and nonprotein nitrogen become elevated.

In infants and in children, metaphyseal bands of increased density, reflecting heavy calcifications of the matrix of the proliferating cartilage, alternating with areas of increased lucency are evident in the tubular bones.[62] Cortical thickening due to periosteal apposition[63] may be observed at certain sites, and osteoporosis and thinning of the cortices may be evident at other locations. Widespread osteosclerosis has also been noted.[64] Metastatic calcification of viscera, blood vessels, periarticular structures, muscles, laryngeal and tracheal cartilage, the falx cerebri, and the tentorium cerebelli can be noted.[63, 65, 66]

In adults, hypervitaminosis D can lead to focal or generalized osteoporosis. The bones of the appen-

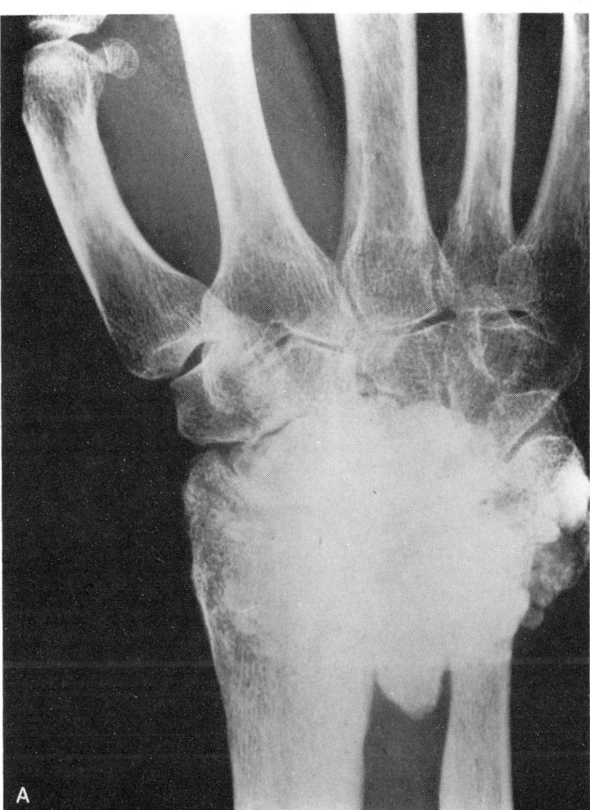

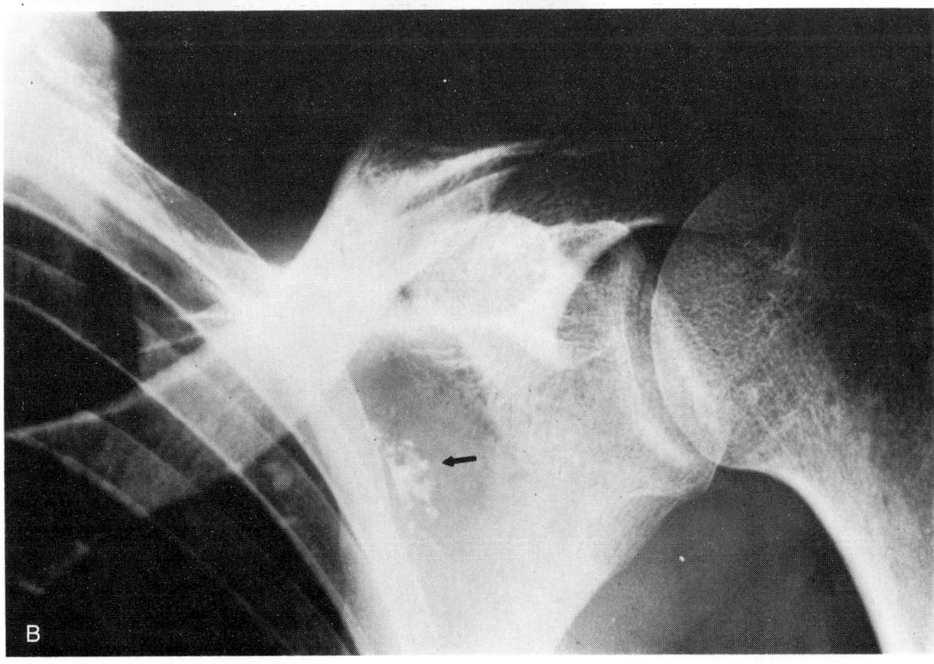

Figure 67–6. *Hypervitaminosis D: Soft tissue abnormalities.*

A *In a patient with rheumatoid arthritis who was treated with vitamin D, note massive soft tissue calcification about the wrist.*

B *In a different patient without articular disease, small calcific deposits in the soft tissue are evident (arrow).*

dicular skeleton, the spine, the pelvis, and even the skull reveal varying degrees of bone loss. Massive soft tissue calcification can become apparent, especially in patients with rheumatoid arthritis or gout being treated with excessive amounts of the vitamin, and is frequently combined with severe osteoporosis. Lobulated, smooth, amorphous masses of calcium are evident in periarticular regions, bursae, tendon sheaths, joint capsules, and intra-articular cavities[31, 67] (Fig. 67–6). On pathologic evaluation, thick white granular calcareous material, usually representing hydroxyapatite, is identified, and an inflammatory reaction in the bursal wall or adjacent soft tissues can be seen. In patients with rheumatoid arthritis or gout, calcification of soft tissue nodules or tophi is observed.

Experimentally, toxic doses of vitamin D administered to animals lead to osteoporosis, hypercalcemia, hyperphosphatemia, and metastatic calcification,[68, 69] although smaller doses cause little effect on calcium and phosphorus balance.[70] Although it is not precisely known why metastatic calcification occurs at specific sites, previous tissue degeneration does not appear to be an essential factor,[71] but local alkalinity may favor deposition of calcium phosphate.[31] Experimentally, withdrawal of the vitamin can be followed by reversion to normal serum levels and metabolic balance of calcium and phosphorus with recalcification of bone and resorption of metastatic deposits.[72]

Metastatic soft tissue calcification accompanies a variety of disorders, including hypervitaminosis D, milk-alkali syndrome, hyperparathyroidism, plasma cell myeloma, and skeletal metastasis.[73, 74] Furthermore, soft tissue calcinosis can be evident in various collagen vascular disorders, and dystrophic calcification can occur following tissue injury or devitalization from any cause. Periarticular deposits are most characteristic of hypervitaminosis D, milk-alkali syndrome, hyperparathyroidism, renal osteodystrophy, collagen vascular disorders, and tumoral calcinosis.

Chronic Idiopathic Hypercalcemia

Idiopathic infantile hypercalcemia was first described in 1952.[75, 76] The major clinical manifestations of this disorder include a peculiar facies, anorexia, hypotonia, mental and physical retardation, and vomiting. Radiographically, a generalized increase in skeletal density is observed.[77, 78] Although the exact pathogenesis of chronic idiopathic hypercalcemia is not known, the disease may relate to the excessive ingestion of vitamin D over prolonged periods by infants who are slightly sensitive to this vitamin.[79, 80]

In 1963, Black and Bonham-Carter[81] noted that infants with a facies similar to that of patients with idiopathic hypercalcemia could reveal supravalvular aortic stenosis and mental retardation (Williams' syndrome), an observation that was subsequently verified by numerous investigators. Furthermore, the vascular manifestations that were encountered in these patients were varied and included, in addition to supravalvular aortic stenosis, stenosis of the branches of the aorta, the peripheral pulmonary vessels, or carotid arteries and aortic hypoplasia.[24]

The detection of hypercalcemia and these variable vascular anomalies suggests that vitamin D excess or hypersensitivity in the expectant mother may represent a fundamental cause of congenital malformations of the cardiovascular system of the fetus. Clinical evidence supporting this concept includes the detection of elevated levels of vitamin D in the blood of some infants with idiopathic hypercalcemia, osteosclerosis, and aortic stenosis[82-86]; supporting experimental findings include the observations of Friedman and Roberts[87] in the offspring of pregnant rabbits given high doses of vitamin D. These investigators noted an elevated level of serum calcium and aortic lesions similar to supravalvular aortic stenosis in some of the newborn rabbits. In addition, disturbances in the development of the bones of the face and cranium were evident.

SUMMARY

Deficiencies and excesses of certain vitamins may have a pronounced effect on the musculoskeletal system. In addition to vitamin D deficiency leading to rickets, hypervitaminosis A and D and hypovitaminosis C (scurvy) are examples of vitamin-related disorders that affect the osseous, articular, or soft tissue structures.

REFERENCES

1. Jeghers H, Marraro H: Hypervitaminosis A: Its broadening spectrum. Am J Clin Nutr *6*:335, 1958.
2. Sulzberger MG, Lazar MP: Hypervitaminosis A. JAMA *146*:788, 1951.
3. DiBenedetto RJ: Chronic hypervitaminosis A in an adult. JAMA *201*:700, 1967.
4. Kane EK: Arctic Explorations in the Years 1853, 1854, 1855. Philadelphia, Childs & Peterson Publishers, 1856, p 392.
5. Rodahl K, Moore T: The vitamin A content and toxicity of bear and seal liver. Biochem J *37*:166, 1943.
6. Feldman MH, Schlezinger NS: Benign intracranial hypertension associated with hypervitaminosis A. Arch Neurol *22*:1, 1970.
7. Lonie TC: Excess vitamin A as a cause of food poisoning. N Z Med J *49*:680, 1950.
8. Marie J, See G: Acute hypervitaminosis A of the infant: Its clinical manifestations with benign acute hydrocephalus and pronounced bulge of the fontanel; a clinical and biologic study. Am J Dis Child *87*:731, 1954.
9. Caffey J: Pediatric X-Ray Diagnosis. 7th Ed. Chicago, Year Book Medical Publishers, 1978, p 1466.
10. Moore LA, Sykes JF: Cerebrospinal fluid pressure and vitamin A deficiency. Amer J Physiol *130*:684, 1940.
11. Josephs HW: Hypervitaminosis A and carotenemia. Am J Dis Child *67*:33, 1944.

12. Toomey JA, Morissette RA: Hypervitaminosis A. Am J Dis Child *73*:473, 1947.
13. Caffey J: Chronic poisoning due to excess of vitamin A. Description of the clinical and roentgen manifestations in seven infants and young children. Pediatrics *5*:672, 1950.
14. Sulzberger MB, Lazar MP: Hypervitaminosis A: Report of a case in an adult. JAMA *146*:788, 1951.
15. Dickey LB, Bradley EJ: Hypervitaminosis A. Stanford Med Bull *6*:345, 1948.
16. Woodard WK, Miller LJ, Legant O: Acute and chronic hypervitaminosis A in a 4 month old infant. J Pediatr *59*:260, 1961.
17. Tunell R, Pierson B: Chronic vitamin A intoxication in infants. Acta Paediatr Scand *50*:319, 1961.
18. Pickup JD: Hypervitaminosis A. Arch Dis Child *31*:229, 1956.
19. Pease CN: Focal retardation and arrestment of growth due to vitamin A intoxication. JAMA *182*:980, 1962.
20. Ruby LK, Mital MA: Skeletal deformities following chronic hypervitaminosis A. A case report. J Bone Joint Surg *56A*:1283, 1974.
21. Persson B, Tunell R, Ekengren K: Chronic vitamin A intoxication during the first half year of life; description of five cases. Acta Paediatr Scand *54*:49, 1965.
22. Grossman LA: Increased intracranial pressure: Consequence of hypervitaminosis A. South Med J *65*:916, 1972.
23. Arena, JM, Sarazen P Jr, Baylin GJ: Hypervitaminosis A: Report of an unusual case with marked craniotabes. Pediatrics *8*:788, 1951.
24. Taybi H: Vitamin deficiency and intoxication. *In* TH Newton, DG Potts (Eds): Radiology of the skull and brain. Vol 1. The Skull. St Louis, The CV Mosby Co, 1971, p 678.
25. Wolbach SB: Vitamin-A deficiency and excess in relation to skeletal growth. J Bone Joint Surg *29*:171, 1947.
26. Wolke RE, Nielsen SW: Pathogenesis of hypervitaminosis A in growing porcine bone. Lab Invest *16*:639, 1967.
27. Dingle JT, Lucy JA, Fell HB: Studies on the mode of action of excess vitamin A. 1. Effect of excess of vitamin A on the metabolism and composition of embryonic chick-limb cartilage grown in organ culture. Biochem J *79*:497, 1961.
28. Lucy JA, Dingle JT, Fell HB: Studies on the mode of action of excess vitamin A. 2. A possible role of intracellular proteases in the degradation of cartilage matrix. Biochem J *79*:500, 1961.
29. Dingle JT: Studies on the mode of action of excess vitamin A. 3. Release of a bound protease by the action of vitamin A. Biochem J *79*:509, 1961.
30. Thomas L, McCluskey RT, Li J, Weissmann G: Prevention by cortisone of the changes in cartilage induced by an excess of vitamin A in rabbits. Am J Pathol *42*:271, 1963.
31. Jaffe HL: Metabolic, Degenerative and Inflammatory Diseases of Bones and Joints. Philadelphia, Lea & Febiger, 1972, p 448.
32. Bass MH: The relation of vitamin A intake to cerebrospinal fluid pressure; a review. J Mt Sinai Hosp *24*:713, 1957.
33. Bass MH, Caplan J: Vitamin A deficiency in infancy. J Pediatr *47*:690, 1955.
34. Keating JP, Feigin RD: Increased intracranial pressure associated with probable vitamin A deficiency in cystic fibrosis. Pediatrics *46*:41, 1970.
35. Eaton HD: Chronic bovine hypo- and hypervitaminosis A and cerebrospinal fluid pressure. Am J Clin Nutr *22*:1070, 1969.
36. Cornfeld D, Cooke RE: Vitamin A deficiency: Case report; unusual manifestations in a 5½ month old baby. Pediatrics *10*:33, 1952.
37. Bass MH, Fisch GR: Increased intracranial pressure with bulging fontanel; a symptom of vitamin A deficiency in infants. Neurology *11*:1091, 1961.
38. Mellanby E: Skeletal changes affecting the nervous system produced in young dogs by diets deficient in vitamin A. J Physiol *99*:467, 1941.
39. Wolbach SB, Bessey OA: Vitamin A deficiency and the nervous system. Arch Pathol *32*:689, 1941.
40. Boyle PE: Manifestations of vitamin A deficiency in a human tooth-germ. J Dent Res *13*:39, 1933.
41. Orten AU, Burn CG, Smith AH: Effects of prolonged chronic vitamin A deficiency in the rat with special reference to odontomas. Proc Soc Exp Biol Med *36*:82, 1937.
42. Burn CG, Orten AU, Smith AH: Changes in the structure of the developing tooth in rats maintained on a diet deficient in vitamin A. Yale J Biol Med *13*:817, 1941.
43. Jackson D, Park EA: Congenital scurvy. J Pediatr *7*:741, 1935.
44. Burns RR: The unusual occurrence of scurvy in an eight week old infant. Am J Roentgenol *89*:923, 1963.
45. Dennis JM, Mercado R: Scurvy following folic acid antagonist therapy. Radiology *67*:412, 1956.
46. Wolbach SB, Howe PR: Intercellular substances in experimental scorbutus. Arch Pathol *1*:1, 1926.
47. Pirani CL, Bly CG, Sutherland K: Scorbutic arthropathy in the guinea pig. Arch Pathol *49*:710, 1950.
48. Bevelaqua FA, Hasselbacher P, Schumacher HR: Scurvy and hemarthrosis. JAMA *235*:1874, 1976.
49. Crandon JH, Lund CC, Dill DB: Experimental human scurvy. N Engl J Med *223*:353, 1940.
50. Boyle PE: The tooth germ in acute scurvy. J Dent Res *14*:172, 1934.
51. Silverman FN: Recovery from epiphyseal invagination: Sequel to an unusual complication of scurvy. J Bone Joint Surg *52A*:384, 1970.
52. Sprague PL: Epiphyseo-metaphyseal cupping following infantile scurvy. Pediatr Radiol *4*:122, 1976.
53. Siffert RS: The growth plate and its affections. J Bone Joint Surg *48A*:546, 1966.
54. Caffey J: Traumatic cupping of the metaphyses of growing bones. Am J Roentgenol *108*:451, 1970.
55. McLean S, McIntosh R: Healing in infantile scurvy as shown by x-ray. Am J Dis Child *36*:875, 1928.
56. Mitra ML: Vitamin-C deficiency in the elderly and its manifestations. J Am Geriatr Soc *18*:67, 1970.
57. Joffe N: Some radiological aspects of scurvy in the adult. Br J Radiol *34*:429, 1961.
58. Thatcher L: Hypervitaminosis-D with report of a fatal case in a child. Edinburgh Med J *38*:457, 1931.
59. Wells HG, Holley SW: Metastatic calcification in osteitis deformans. (Paget's disease of bone). Arch Pathol *34*:435, 1942.
60. Danowski TS, Winkler AW, Peters JP: Tissue calcification and renal failure produced by massive dose vitamin D therapy of arthritis. Ann Intern Med *23*:22, 1945.
61. Ruziczka O: Injuries due to overdosage of vitamin D. Wien Klin Wochenschr *64*:964, 1952.
62. Ross, SG: Vitamin D intoxication in infancy. A report of four cases. J Pediatr *41*:815, 1952.
63. Swoboda W: Die rontgensymptomatik der vitamin-D-intoxikation im kindesalter. Fortschr Geb Roentgenstr Nuklearmed *77*:534, 1952.
64. DeWind LT: Hypervitaminosis D with osteosclerosis. Arch Dis Child *36*:373, 1961.
65. Debre R: Toxic effects of overdosage of vitamin D_2 in children. Am J Dis Child *75*:787, 1948.
66. Holman CB: Roentgenologic manifestations of vitamin D intoxication. Radiology *59*:805, 1952.
67. Christensen WR, Liebman C, Sosman MC: Skeletal and peri-articular manifestations of hypervitaminosis D. Am J Roentgenol *65*:27, 1951.
68. Kreitmair H, Moll T: Hypervitaminose nach grossen dosen vitamin D. Munch Med Wochenschr *75*:1113, 1928.
69. Shohl AT, Goldblatt H, Brown HB: The pathological effects upon rats of excess irradiated ergosterol. J Clin Invest *8*:505, 1930.
70. Bauer W, Marble A, Claflin D: Studies on mode of action of irradiated ergosterol; its effect on calcium, phosphorus and nitrogen metabolism of normal individuals. J Clin Invest *11*:1, 1932.
71. Ham AW: Mechanism of calcification in the heart and aorta in hypervitaminosis D. Arch Pathol *14*:613, 1932.
72. Steck IE, Deutsch H, Reed CI, Struck HC: Further studies on intoxication with vitamin D. Ann Intern Med *10*:951, 1937.
73. Barr DP: Pathological calcification. Physiol Rev *12*:593, 1932.
74. Bauer JM, Freyberg RH: Vitamin D intoxication with metastatic calcification. JAMA *130*:1208, 1946.
75. Fanconi G, Girardet P: Chronische Hypercalcämie kombiniert mit Osteosklerose, Hyperazotämie, Minderwuchs, und kongenitalen missbildungen. Helv Paediatr Acta *7*:314, 1952.
76. Schlesinger B, Butler N, Black J: Chronische Hypercalcämie kombiniert mit Osteosklerose, hyperazotämie, Minderwuchs, und kongenitalen missbildungen. Helv Paediatr Acta *7*:335, 1952.
77. Shiers JA, Neuhauser EBD, Bowman JR: Idiopathic hypercalcemia. Am J Roentgenol *78*:19, 1957.
78. Singleton EB: The radiographic features of severe idiopathic hypercalcemia of infancy. Radiology *68*:721, 1957.
79. Forbes GB, Cafarelli C, Manning J: Vitamin D and infantile hypercalcemia. Pediatrics *42*:203, 1968.
80. Fraser D, Kidd BSL, Kooh SW, Paunier LD: A new look at infantile hypercalcemia. Pediatr Clin North Am *13*:503, 1966.
81. Black JA, Bonham-Carter RE: Association between aortic stenosis and facies of severe infantile hypercalcemia. Lancet *2*:745, 1963.
82. Garcia RE, Friedman WF, Kaback MM, Rowe RD: Idiopathic hypercalcemia and supravalvular aortic stenosis. N Engl J Med *271*:117, 1964.
83. Kurlander GJ, Petry EL, Taybi H, Lurie PR, Campbell JA: Supravalvular aortic stenosis; roentgen analysis of twenty-seven cases. Am J Roentgenol *98*:782, 1966.
84. Seelig MS: Vitamin D and cardiovascular, renal, and brain damage in infancy and childhood. Ann NY Acad Sci *147*:537, 1969.
85. Friedman WF: Vitamin D as a cause of the supravalvular aortic stenosis syndrome. Am Heart J *73*:718, 1967.
86. Manios SG, Antener I: A study of vitamin D metabolism in idiopathic hypercalcemia of infancy. Acta Paediatr Scand *55*:600, 1966.
87. Friedman WF, Roberts WC: Vitamin D and the supravalvular aortic stenosis syndrome; the transplacental effects of vitamin D on the aorta of the rabbit. Circulation *34*:77, 1966.
88. Mahoney CP, Margolis T, Knauss TA, Labbe RF: Chronic vitamin A intoxication in infants fed chicken liver. Pediatrics *65*:893, 1980.

68

HEAVY METAL POISONING

by Donald Resnick, M.D.

Poisoning with certain heavy metals can produce characteristic musculoskeletal alterations. One of the most well-recognized changes associated with ingestion, inhalation, or injection of lead or other heavy metals is the appearance of radiodense lines at the ends of tubular bones or along the contours of flat and irregular bones. These lines must be differentiated from the transverse radiodense areas that are commonly observed at some of these locations in individuals who have not been poisoned with metals. This chapter reviews initially the nature and appearance of "growth arrest" lines and subsequently the radiographic changes of the skeleton associated with heavy metal poisoning.

TRANSVERSE OR STRESS LINES (OF PARK OR HARRIS)

The appearance of opaque transverse lines that extend across the metaphyses of tubular bones is a common radiographic phenomenon[1, 2] that may be observed in children and adults (Fig. 68–1). They are

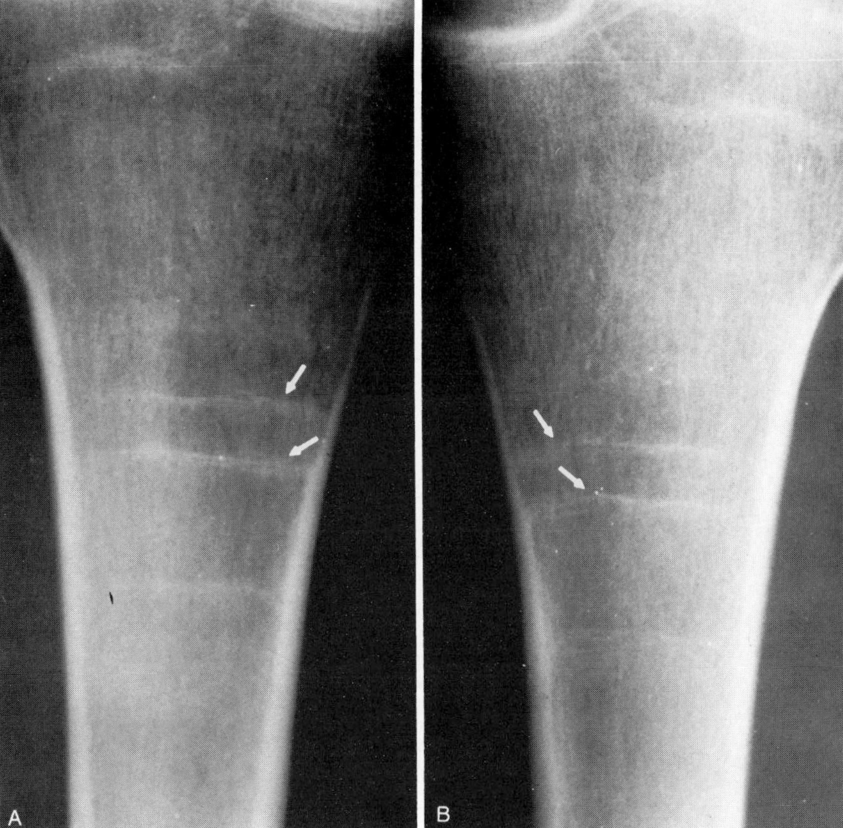

Figure 68–1. Transverse or stress lines: Appendicular skeleton. In the proximal tibiae, multiple transverse radiodense lines extend almost completely across the medullary cavity (arrows).

often referred to as Park or Harris lines (as a tribute to the contributions of these two investigators)[3-6] as well as transverse or "growth arrest" lines.[4, 7] A historical summary[8-40] of the numerous investigations of these lines, which is beautifully tabulated by Garn and colleagues[2] (Table 68–1), emphasizes that they have been recognized in both healthy and sick individuals, that similar lines have been encountered in patients who have been poisoned with a variety of heavy metals, that the lines may be utilized as a determinant of growth potential and magnitude, that they may be produced experimentally in animals restricted to specific dietary intakes, and that their exact pathogenesis is not uniformly agreed upon by all investigators. It is now generally recognized that these transverse radiodense lines can be evident at birth or during infancy and that they do not appear after growth has ceased but that, once formed, they persist into adult life. They are without local symptoms and signs. Similar lines can appear about the margins of the round and the flat bones and in both the appendicular and the axial skeletons (Fig. 68–2). The radiodense lines are more frequent and prominent as sites of rapid bone growth, such as the femora and tibiae about the knee. Although they are usually symmetric and widespread in distribution, atypical patterns are encountered.

In the tubular bones, single or multiple lines of increased density parallel the contours of the nearby provisional zones of calcification. Although the pathogenesis of the dense lines is not certain, it is the close proximity and similarity between the lines and the growth plate that have suggested that the bands are related to a disturbance of normal growth patterns. Indeed, the term "arrest" lines, which is still applied to these dense shadows, underscores the early belief that their appearance signified an arrest in normal growth. However, as shown by Park and his associates,[3, 4] they are more properly termed "recovery" lines, indicating periods of renewed or increased growth, presumably following a period of inhibited growth of the bone. The discovery of the radiodense bands suggests a previous occurrence of an episode or episodes of trauma or infection. Although this association between disease or stress and linear radiodense shadows is useful, certain limitations must be recognized:[2] The association is significant but of low order; the disease-line association is highest in the earliest age group (3 to 18 months); and, despite the fact that a new line may be encountered following episodes of trauma or disease, it may also be observed without such an episode.

Anatomically, the transverse bands consist of horizontally oriented trabeculae that partially or completely cross the medullary cavity at right angles to the normal longitudinally directed trabecular

Table 68–1

HISTORICAL SUMMARY OF PUBLISHED STUDIES ON LINES AND BANDS

Date	Author	Summary of Findings
1874	Wegner[8]	Produced transverse bands of trabeculae by administration of phosphorus to rabbits and chickens.
1877	Gies[9]	Produced transverse bands by administration of arsenic to rabbits.
1903	Ludloff[10]	Reported transverse striations in radiographs of legs of normal individuals.
1904	Lehndorff[11]	Described transverse striations in scurvy.
1918	Phemister[12]	Described radiopaque transverse bands in long bones after administration of phosphorus.
1921	Stettner[13]	Interpreted transverse lines as lines of arrested growth.
1924	Asada[14]	Reported experimental production of lines by encasing extremities in plaster.
1926	Harris[5]	Reviewed earlier literature on lines, utilized lines to demonstrate nonexistence of interstitial growth, explained their presence as manifestations of arrested growth, and discussed their formation with reference to vitamins.
1927	Eliot, Souther, and Park[15]	Concluded from histologic studies that transverse lattice formation might be regarded as temporary halting of cartilage growth but with continuation of osteoblastic activity.
1931	Harris[6]	Presented historical review, case histories and illustrations of various clinical conditions, and experimental evidence indicating that transverse stratum first appears as calcification in proliferative zone of cartilage.
1931	Park, Jackson, and Kajdi[16]	Reported radiopaque bands following lead poisoning, and suggested that lead produced more densely packed trabeculae.
1933	Park, Jackson, Goodwin, and Kajdi[17]	Discussed transverse formations in lead poisoning and distinguished these "bands" from transverse lines.
1933	Harris[18]	Presented essentially a repetition of his earlier article.[6]
1938	Sontag[19]	Reported striae in tarsal bones of 1-month-old infants, and attributed their presence to shift from prenatal to postnatal environment.
1941	Stammel[20]	Reported two individuals marked by multiple lines and bands on vertebrae, round bones, epiphyses, and phalanges, as well as major long bones and pelvis.
1941	Siegling[21]	Used radiopaque lines to determine growth loci in epiphyses of long bones.
1942	Gill and Abbott[22]	Described shifting proportions of relative growth at both ends of tibia and femur between prenatal and postnatal life in child whose mother had been administered bismuth during pregnancy.
1945	Caffey[23]	Reported lines in sites of accelerated growth, and doubted that growth retardation is essential to development of these lines.
1952	Follis and Park[24]	Distinguished between lattice formations, or zones of increased density, and transverse strata, or lines of increased density—the former being primarily a defect in resorptional activity by osteoblasts, whereas in the latter, a cessation of cartilaginous growth is primary.
1953	Park and Richter[4]	Indicated that though initiation of a transverse line is caused by cessation of cartilage growth, thickening is caused by lag of cartilage cell maturation behind resumed osteoblastic activity in recovery phase.
1955	Hewitt, Westropp, and Acheson[25]	Demonstrated statistically significant association between transverse lines in radiographs of knees and periods of illness in 650 normal children.
1956	Jones and Dean[26]	Reported that more children with kwashiorkor had transverse lines on distal radius than normal children, and followed development of these lines in serial radiographs.
1956	Dreizen, Currie, Gilley, and Spies[27]	Found transverse lines and nutritive status not to be significantly associated, although relation between resorption of lines and nutritive status was reported.
1959	Acheson[28]	Suggested that in starvation and illness, withdrawal of growth hormone is primary cause of slowing of cartilage growth.
1960	Goff[29]	Reviewed previous uses of transverse lines to elucidate relative growth, and gave additional examples of their utility.
1962	Platt and Steward[30]	Produced transverse lines in growing pigs subjected to low-protein diets.
1964	Dreizen, Spirakis, and Stone[31]	Indicated in longitudinal study of 679 children that frequency of transverse lines on distal radius reached a maximum by 5 years of age and decreased thereafter.
1964	Park[3]	Presented summary and review of work by him and his colleagues on formation and distribution of transverse lines and their distinction from bands produced by phosphorus and heavy metals.
1964	Wells[32]	Showed prevalence of transverse tibial lines in skeletal remains of children and adults.
1965	Roche[33]	Utilized transverse lines to demonstrate articular apposition at nonepiphyseal ends of metacarpals.
1966	Marshall[34]	Found presence of new transverse lines on radius to be associated with illness and inoculation and discussed their use in paleopathology.
1967	Garn and Schwager[35]	Showed persistent transverse lines on distal tibias of adults into ninth decade, with decreasing frequency after sixth decade in both sexes.
1967	Gray[36]	Observed radiopaque lines in 30 percent of 133 Egyptian mummies, and suggested ". . . a general poor state of health during adolescence in ancient Egypt."

Table 68–1

HISTORICAL SUMMARY OF PUBLISHED STUDIES ON LINES AND BANDS *(Continued)*

Date	Author	Summary of Findings
1968	Garn, Hempy, and Schwager[37]	Used transverse lines on distal tibia in longitudinal series to partition relative contribution of proximal and distal and of diaphyseal and epiphyseal growth increments.
1968	Cornwell and Littleton[38]	Identified radiopaque lines on tibia as subcortical, reaching from endosteal surface to endosteal surface, as confirmed by axial tomograms and bone sections.
1968	Schwager[39]	Reported statistically significant, low-order associations between episodes of disease and trauma in childhood and appearance of new transverse lines in succeeding period.
1968	McHenry[40]	Showed high frequency of transverse lines on distal femur in prehistoric populations, and demonstrated such lines to be manifestations of bony lattices within marrow cavity.

(From Garn SM, Silverman FN, Hertzog KP, Rohmann CG: Med Radiogr Photogr *44*:60, 1968.)

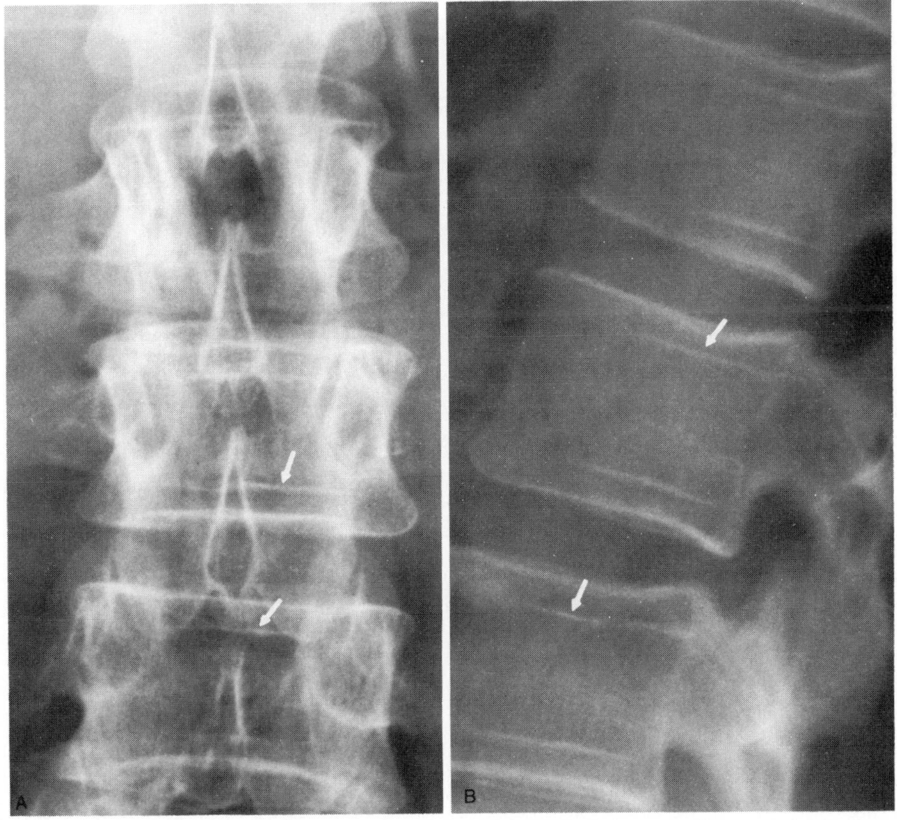

Figure 68–2. *Transverse or stress lines: Axial skeleton. In multiple vertebral bodies, observe radiodense lines paralleling the superior and inferior osseous margins (arrows), creating a "bone-within-bone" appearance.*

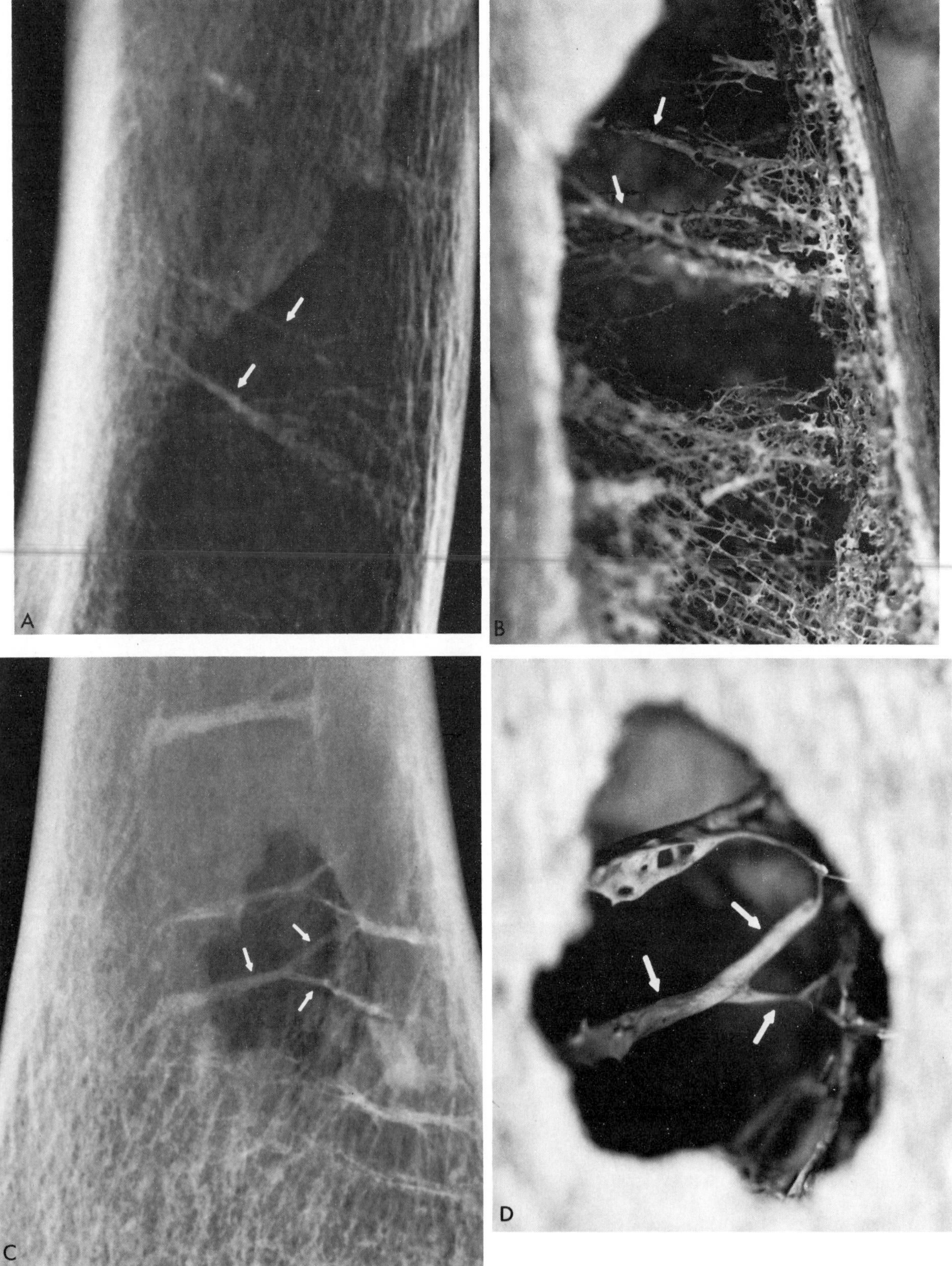

Figure 68–3. Transverse or stress lines: Anatomic correlation.

A, B On this radiograph and photograph of a sectioned femur, note that the radiodense lines are produced by bony strands within the marrow cavity (arrows). The bony projections, from 0.2 to 1.3 mm in diameter, are thick compared to the surrounding bone.

C, D In another sectioned femur, a radiograph and photograph reveal the branching strands that create the radiodense lines (arrows).

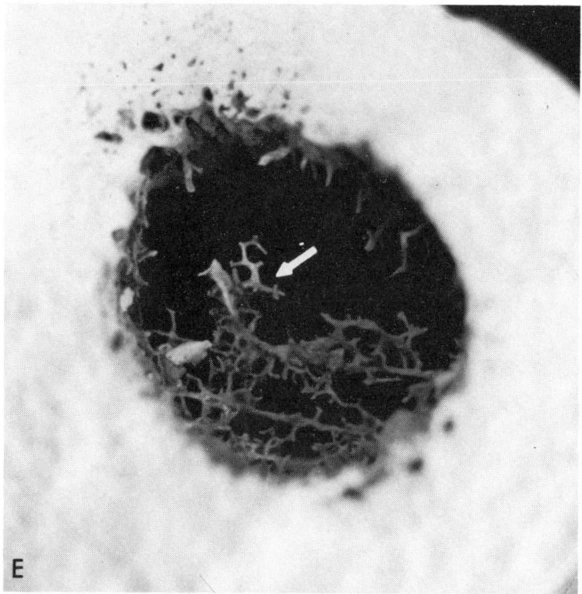

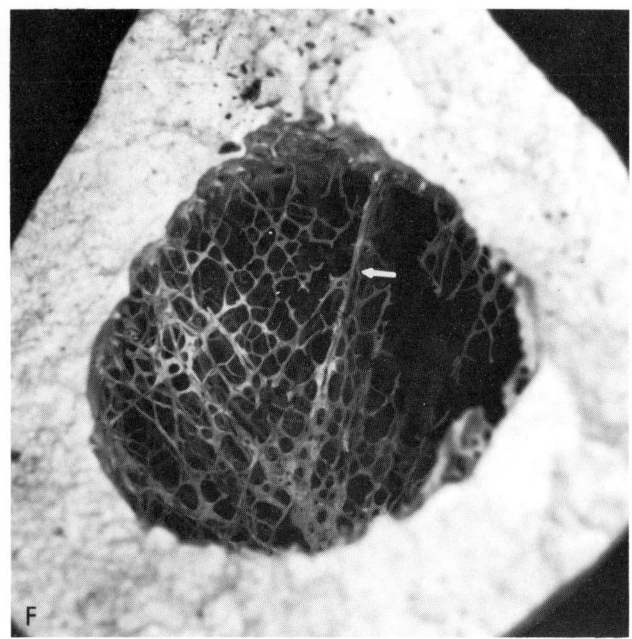

Figure 68–3. Continued

E, F *On transverse sections through two femora, the horizontally oriented lattice networks of bone within the medullary canal (arrow) are responsible for the linear radiodense areas on frontal radiographs.*

(From Medical Radiography and Photography 44:58, 1968. Published by Health Sciences Markets Division, Eastman Kodak Company, Rochester, New York. Courtesy of Dr. S. M. Garn, Dr. F. N. Silverman, K. P. Hertzog, and C. G. Rohmann.)

structures (Fig. 68–3). According to Park,[3, 4] during the initial stage of growth arrest, the osteoblasts form a very thin transverse bony template beneath the zone of proliferative cartilage. With resurgence of growth during the recovery phase, cartilaginous proliferation and increased osteoblastic activity contribute to the thickening and metaphyseal migration of the transverse line, which, at this stage, can be recognized radiographically. Thus, these radiodense areas are not "growth arrest" lines but are "postarrest," "poststress," or "recovery" lines.

LEAD POISONING

General Abnormalities

Lead poisoning results from prolonged ingestion of lead-containing materials, such as paint; inhalation of fumes from burning storage batteries or similar substances[41]; or, rarely, absorption of the material from bullets or buckshot that is contained within a serous cavity after a wound.[58-60] Lead poisoning may also appear in the fetus of a mother exposed to lead since lead may cross the placenta as early as the twelfth to fourteenth week of gestation, a process that increases throughout pregnancy.[63] Delayed dental and skeletal development, lead lines, and osteosclerosis may be evident in infants with congenital lead poisoning.

The onset of symptoms and signs following chronic lead poisoning may be abrupt. Poorly localized cramping abdominal pain, encephalopathy with convulsions, delirium, coma or death, peripheral neuritis with muscular paralysis, and mild anemia are recognized clinical manifestations of the disorder.[42, 43] Examining the urine for porphyrin is a useful screening test for establishing the diagnosis. Other chemical tests of blood and urine can also be utilized for diagnostic purposes. It has been suggested that children with reduced serum levels of 1,25-dihydroxyvitamin D may demonstrate increased intestinal absorption of lead.[64]

Musculoskeletal Abnormalities

Lead poisoning is associated with the appearance of thick transverse radiodense lines in the metaphyses of growing tubular bones.[14, 17, 44] The pathogenesis and morphology of these lead lines are different from those of the transverse or stress lines of Park and Harris. Although it has been suggested that the increased radiodensity of the metaphysis in cases of lead poisoning is due to laying down of lead within the cartilaginous matrix ("leadification"),[17] it seems more probable that deposition of calcium is the basis of the transverse lines; even though lead is deposited in the metaphysis, it is in very minute amounts relative to the content of calcium.[44] Caffey[1] terms the process chondrosclerosis and notes the

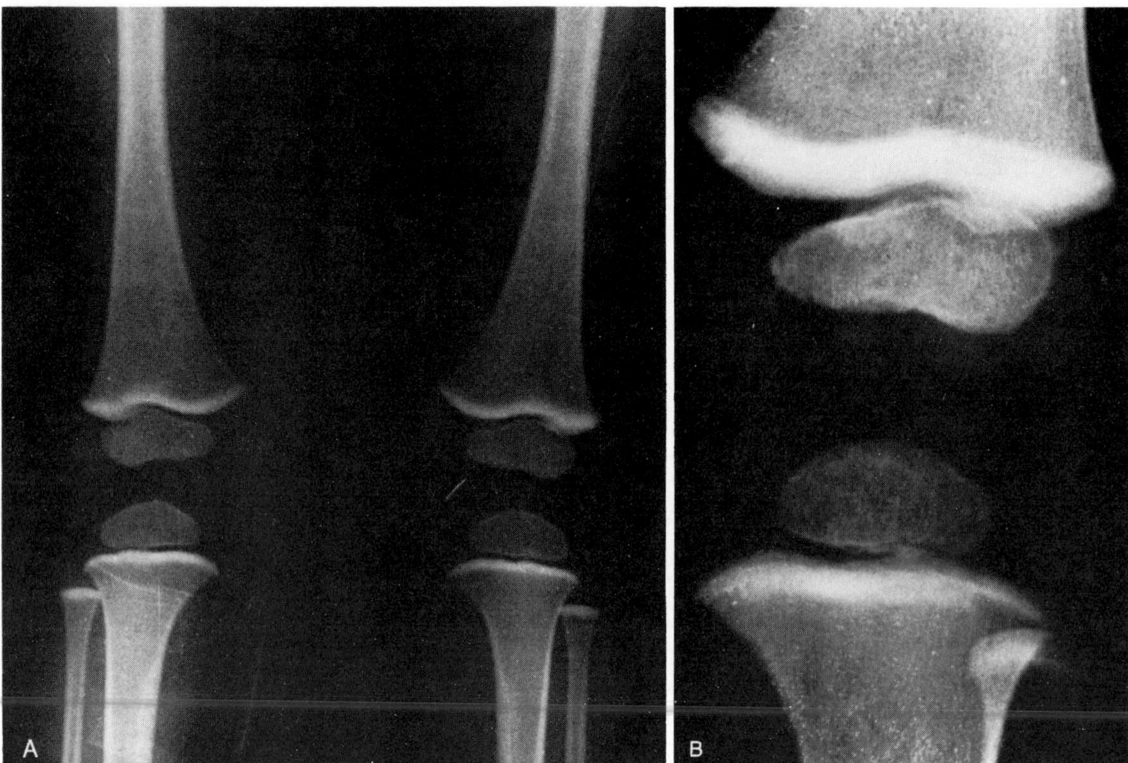

Figure 68–4. Lead poisoning: Knee.

A *In this child, observe the transverse radiodense bands of the metaphyses of femur, tibia, and fibula.* (**A,** Courtesy of Dr. F. Silverman, Department of Radiology, Stanford University Medical Center, Stanford, California.)

B *An enlargement of this region in another patient indicates radiodense bands in the metaphyses of the same bones.*

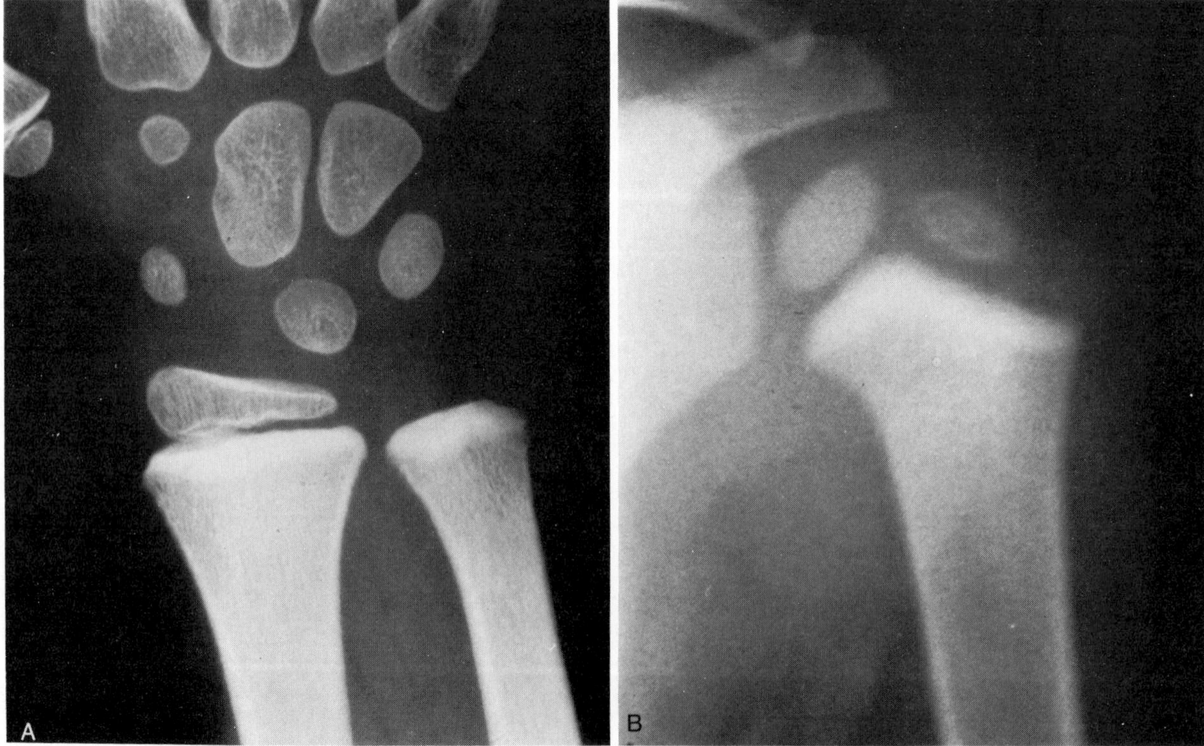

Figure 68–5. Lead poisoning: Wrist and shoulder. *In two different children, radiodense metaphyseal bands are identified in the distal radius, distal ulna, and proximal humerus.*

presence of trabeculae composed of calcified thick cartilaginous cores covered by thin sleeves of endosteal bone almost devoid of osteoblasts. The process may be initiated by oligemia of the metaphyseal segment of the cartilage plate due to a prolonged decrease in blood flow in the metaphyseal arteries.

The lead lines that are almost invariable in chronic infantile and juvenile plumbism are not an early manifestation of the process and are, therefore, of little diagnostic aid. The radiodense zones are expecially prominent in the bones about the knees (Fig. 68–4); identification of density in the proximal fibular metaphysis may be particularly helpful in establishing a radiographic diagnosis of lead poisoning, as similar changes in the distal femur and proximal tibia can be seen in apparently healthy children. Radiodense lines can also be evident at other sites, particularly in the wrist (Fig. 68–5). Single transverse bands predominate; however, multiple lines may result from several episodes of lead poisoning. Even the axial skeleton may be affected (Fig. 68–6).

An additional manifestation of plumbism is failure of normal modeling of the tubular bones, which is most prominent in the femora.[45] Widening of the metaphyses can resemble the changes in Pyle's disease and may persist for months or years before resolving spontaneously.

Lead poisoning can be associated with clinical and radiologic signs of increased intracranial pressure.[46] Mild pleocytosis and an increase in the protein content of the cerebrospinal fluid are frequent, and decompression craniotomy may be required to sustain life.[47] Widening of the cranial sutures, especially the coronal and sagittal sutures, may be evident in as many as 10 per cent of cases of chronic lead poisoning.[48]

Saturnine gout is also termed the "moonshine malady"[49] because of the appearance of the condition in moonshiners whose home-brewed liquor contained an appreciable quantity of lead.[50, 51] Saturnine gout appears to be an expression of renal injury from lead in which a tubular defect leading to uric acid retention becomes evident.

Differential Diagnosis

Radiodense lines in the metaphyses of tubular bones can be seen as a normal variant,[1] as an indication of previous stress, in heavy metal poisoning, including lead poisoning, and in the healing stages of leukemia, rickets, and scurvy (Table 68–2). Similar findings may accompany hypothyroidism, hypervitaminosis D, and transplacental infections (rubella, cytomegalic inclusion disease, herpes, toxoplasmosis, and syphilis). Metaphyseal flaring or

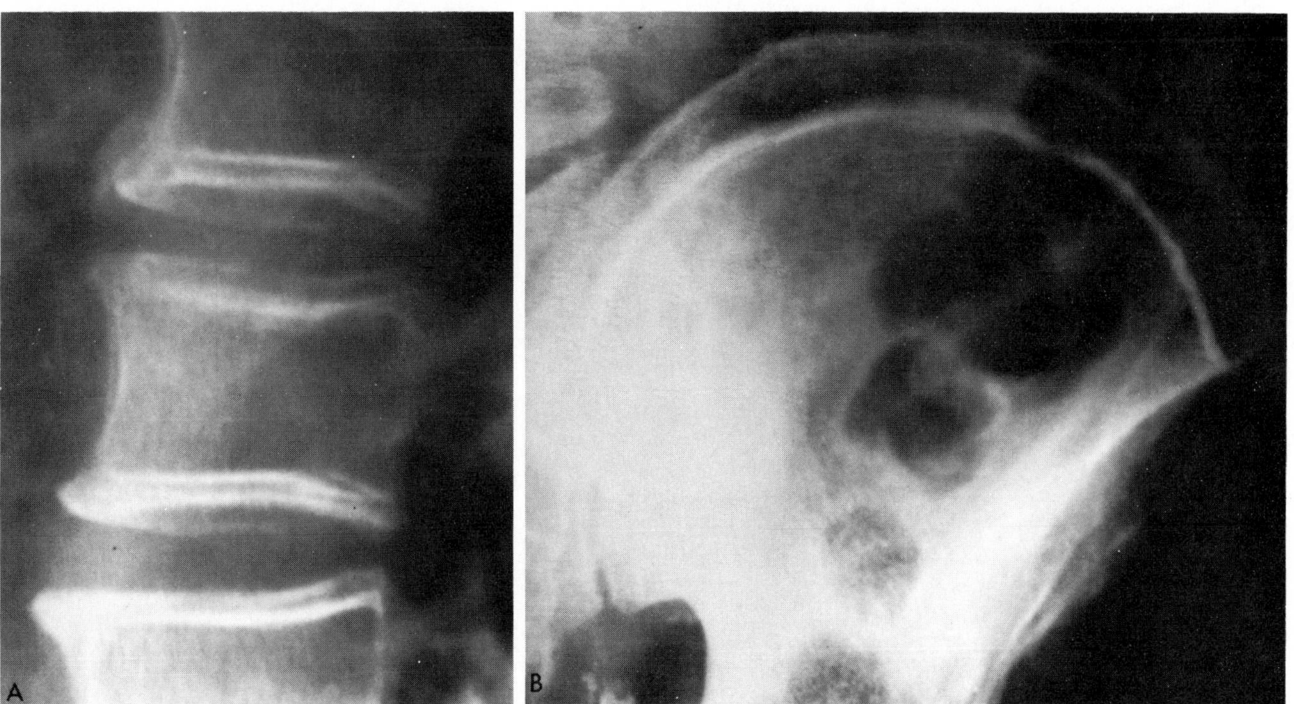

Figure 68–6. *Lead poisoning: Spine and pelvis. Radiodense lines are evident in the vertebral bodies and ilium. (Courtesy of Dr. A. Brower, Bethesda, Maryland.)*

Table 68–2
RADIODENSE METAPHYSEAL LINES

Stress lines
Heavy metal poisoning
Leukemia
Rickets
Scurvy
Hypothyroidism
Hypoparathyroidism
Hypervitaminoses
Transplacental infections

widening is seen not only in lead poisoning but also in various anemias (sickle cell anemia, thalassemia), storage disorders (Gaucher's disease, Niemann-Pick disease), congenital syndromes (Pyle's disease, multiple familial exostoses, osteopetrosis, Ollier's disease), and as a normal variant.

PHOSPHORUS POISONING

Phosphorus poisoning had previously been seen in rachitic and tuberculous children who were being treated with phosphorized cod liver oil,[52, 53] although it is rarely encountered today. It may be reproduced experimentally by feeding metallic (yellow) phosphorus to growing rats. Single or multiple deep bands of increased radiodensity are produced in the ends of growing tubular bones and within flat or irregular bones and persist for many years. The phosphorus shadow is caused by numerous and closely packed trabeculae that are composed of solid bone or small central cartilaginous cores surrounded by heavy sleeves of endosteal bone containing many osteoblasts.[1] Caffey indicates that the process is an osteosclerosis that differs from the chondrosclerosis that is evident in lead (or bismuth) poisoning and concludes that the lines result from chronic hyperemia in the metaphyseal side of the cartilaginous end-plate due to excessive blood flow in terminal metaphyseal vessels.

BISMUTH POISONING

In the pregnant woman with syphilis, injected bismuth may cross the placenta and enter the fetal circulation to be deposited in the skeleton.[54-56] Single or multiple radiodense bands or lines in the metaphyses of the tubular bones in cases of bismuth poisoning share radiographic and morphologic characteristics with those that appear in cases of lead poisoning.[57] The roentgenographic findings may resemble syphilitic osteochondritis, and differentiation of this condition from bismuth poisoning in the fetus of a syphilitic mother who has received bismuth during pregnancy can be difficult.[1] In adults, radiographic abnormalities simulating those of osteonecrosis have been described in cases of bismuth poisoning.[65]

POISONING FROM OTHER METALS

In experimental and perhaps in clinical situations, other heavy metals, such as radium, gold, mercury, and silver, may lead to metaphyseal changes.[1] In addition, metallic mercury emboli in arterial and venous circulation can appear following blood sampling utilizing mercury-sealed syringes and after accidents or suicide attempts and can lead to mercurialism, mercury abscesses, and local ischemia.[61-62, 66]

SUMMARY

In some cases of heavy metal poisoning, radiodense lines or bands may appear in the metaphyses of tubular bones and within flat or irregular bones. The resulting radiographic findings, which are most characteristically observed in lead, phosphorus, and bismuth poisoning, must be differentiated from normal variants, stress lines of Park and Harris, and changes in various metabolic, endocrine, and infectious disorders.

REFERENCES

1. Caffey J: Pediatric X-Ray Diagnosis. 7th Ed. Chicago, Year Book Medical Publishers, 1978, p 1125.
2. Garn SM, Silverman FN, Hertzog KP, Rohmann CG: Lines and bands of increased density. Their implication to growth and development. Med Radiogr Photogr *44*:58, 1968.
3. Park EA: The imprinting of nutritional disturbances on the growing bone. Pediatrics *33*:815, 1964.
4. Park EA, Richter CP: Transverse lines in bone: The mechanism of their development. Bull Johns Hopk Hosp *93*:234, 1953.
5. Harris HA: The growth of the long bones in childhood with special reference to certain bony striations of the metaphysis and to the role of the vitamins. Arch Intern Med *38*:785, 1926.
6. Harris HA: Lines of arrested growth in the long bones in childhood. Correlation of histological and radiographic appearances in clinical and experimental conditions. Br J Radiol *4*:561, 622, 1931.
7. Schwager PM: The frequency of appearance of transverse lines in the tibia in relation to chronic illnesses. Am J Phys Anthropol *29*:130, 1968.
8. Wegener G: Ueber das normale and pathologische Wachstum der Rohrenknochen. Eine dritische Untersuchung auf experimenteller und casiustischer Grundlage. Arch Pathol Anat *61*:44, 1874.

9. Gies T: Experimentelle Untersuchungen über den Einfluss des Arsens auf den Organismus. Arch Exp Pathol Pharmakol *8*:175, 1877.
10. Ludloff K: Ueber wachstum und architektur der unteren femurepiphyse und oberen tibiaepiphyse. Ein beitrag zur Röntgendiagnostik. Bruns Beitr Klin Chir *38*:64, 1903.
11. Lehndorff H: Zur kenntniss des morbus barlow. Röntgenbefund Arch Kinderheilk *38*:161, 1904.
12. Phemister DB: The effect of phosphorus on growing, normal and diseased bones. JAMA *70*:1737, 1918.
13. Stettner E: Uber die beziehungen der ossifikation des handskeletts zu alter und langenwachstum bei gesunden und kranken kindern von der gebutt bis zur pubertat. Arch Kinderheilk *68*:342, 439, 1920; *69*:27, 1921.
14. Asada T: Uber die Entstehung und pathologische bedeutung der im Röntgenbild des rohrenknochens am diaphysenende zum vorschein kommenden parallelen querlinienbildung. Mitt Med Fak Univ Kyushu Fukuoka *9*:43, 1924.
15. Eliot MM, Souther SP, Park EA: Transverse lines in x-ray plates of the long bones of children. Bull Johns Hopkins Hosp *41*:364, 1927.
16. Park EA, Jackson D, Kajdi L: Shadows produced by lead in x-ray pictures of growing skeleton. Am J Dis Child *41*:485, 1931.
17. Park EA, Jackson D, Goodwin TC, Kajdi L: X-ray shadows in growing bones produced by lead; their characteristics, cause, anatomical counterpart in bone and differentiation. J Pediatr *3*:265, 1933.
18. Harris HA: Bone Growth in Health and Disease: The Biological Principles Underlying the Clinical, Radiological and Histological Diagnosis of Perversions of Growth and Disease in the Skeleton. London, Oxford University Press, 1933, p 3.
19. Sontag LW: Evidences of disturbed prenatal and neonatal growth in bones of infants aged one month. Am J Dis Child *55*:1248, 1938.
20. Stammel CA: Multiple striae parallel to epiphyses and ring shadows around bone growth centers. Am J Roentgenol *46*:497, 1941.
21. Siegling JA: Growth of epiphyses. J Bone Joint Surg *23*:23, 1941.
22. Gill GG, Abbott LRC: A practical method of predicting the growth of the femur and tibia in the child. Arch Surg *45*:286, 1942.
23. Caffey J: Pediatric X-ray Diagnosis. A Textbook for Students and Practitioners of Pediatrics, Surgery & Radiology. Chicago, Year Book Medical Publishers, 1945, p 597.
24. Follis RH Jr, Park EA: Some observations on bone growth with particular respect to zones and transverse lines of increased density in the metaphysis. Am J Roentgenol *68*:709, 1952.
25. Hewitt D, Westropp CK, Acheson RM: Oxford child health survey: Effect of childish ailments on skeletal development. Br J Prev Soc Med *9*:179, 1955.
26. Jones PRM, Dean RFA: The effects of kwashiorkor on the development of the bones of the hand. J Trop Pediatr *2*:51, 1956.
27. Dreizen S, Currie C, Gilley EJ, Spies TD: Observations on the association between nutritive failure, skeletal maturation rate and radiopaque transverse lines in the distal end of the radius in children. Am J Roentgenol *76*:482, 1956.
28. Acheson RM: Effects of starvation, septicaemia, and chronic illness on the growth cartilage plate and metaphysis of the immature rat. J Anat *93*:123, 1959.
29. Goff CW: Surgical Treatment of Unequal Extremities. Publication 418, American Lecture Series, Monograph in the Bannerstone Division of American Lectures in Orthopaedic Surgery. Springfield, Ill. Charles C Thomas, 1960, p 3.
30. Platt BS, Steward RJC: Transverse trabeculae and osteoporosis in bones in experimental protein-calorie deficiency. Br J Nutr *16*:483, 1962.
31. Dreizen S, Spirakis CN, Stone RE: The influence of age and nutritional status on "bone scar" formation in the distal end of the growing radius. Am J Phys Anthropol *22*:295, 1964.
32. Wells C: Les lignes de Harris et les maladies anciennes. Scalpel *117*:665, 1964.
33. Roche AF: The sites of elongation of human metacarpals and metatarsals. Acta Anat *61*:193, 1965.
34. Marshall WA: Problems in relating radiopaque transverse lines in the radius to the occurrence of disease. Symp Soc Hum Biol *8*:245, 1966.
35. Garn SM, Schwager PM: Age dynamics of persistent transverse lines in the tibia. Am J Phys Anthropol *27*:375, 1967.
36. Gray PHK: Radiography of ancient Egyptian mummies. Med Radiogr Photogr *43*:34, 1967.
37. Garn SM, Hempy HO III, Schwager PM: Measurement of localized bone growth employing natural markers. Am J Phys Anthropol *28*:105, 1968.
38. Cornwell WS, Littleton JT: An investigation of transverse lines by axial tomography. Abstracted in Am J Phys Anthropol *29*:130, 1968.
39. Schwager PM: The frequency of appearance of transverse lines in the tibia in relation to childhood illnesses. Abstracted in Am J Phys Anthropol *29*:130, 1968.
40. McHenry H: Transverse lines in long bones of prehistoric California Indians. Am J Phys Anthropol *29*:1, 1968.
41. Browder AA, Joselow MM, Louria DB: The problem of lead poisoning. Medicine *52*:121, 1973.
42. Jones RR: Symptoms in early stages of industrial plumbism. JAMA *104*:195, 1935.
43. Aub JC, Fairhall LT, Minot AS, Reznikoff P: Lead poisoning. Medicine *4*:1, 1925.
44. Leone AJ Jr: On lead lines. Am J Roentgenol *103*:165, 1968.
45. Pease CN, Newton GG: Metaphyseal dysplasia due to lead poisoning in children. Radiology *79*:233, 1962.
46. Greengard J: Lead poisoning in childhood: Signs, symptoms, current therapy, clinical expression. Clin Pediatr *5*:269, 1966.
47. McLaurin RL, Nichols JB Jr: Extensive cranial decompression in the treatment of severe lead encephalopathy. Pediatrics *20*:653, 1957.
48. Freeman R: Chronic lead poisoning in children; a review of 90 children diagnosed in Sydney 1948–1967. Med J Aust *1*:640, 1970.
49. Klinenberg JR: Saturnine gout — a moonshine malady. N Engl J Med *280*:1238, 1969.
50. Emmerson BT: The clinical differentiation of lead gout from primary gout. Arthritis Rheum *11*:623, 1968.
51. Ball GV, Sorensen LB: Pathogenesis of hyperuricemia in saturnine gout. N Engl J Med *280*:1199, 1969.
52. Hess, AE, Weinstock M: The value of elementary phosphorus in rickets. Am J Dis Child *32*:483, 1926.
53. Phemister BD: The effect of phosphorus in growing normal and diseased bone. JAMA *70*:1737, 1918.
54. Heyman A: Systemic manifestations of bismuth toxicity; observations on 4 patients with pre-existent kidney disease. Am J Syph Gonorr Vener Dis *28*:721, 1944.
55. Caffey J: Changes in the growing skeleton after the administration of bismuth. Am J Dis Child *53*:56, 1937.
56. Whitridge J Jr: Changes in the long bones of newborn infants following the administration of bismuth during pregnancy. Am J Syph Gonorr Vener Dis *24*:223, 1940.
57. Russin LA, Stadler HE, Jeans PC: The bismuth lines in the long bones in relation to linear growth. J Pediatr *21*:211, 1942.
58. Leonard MH: The solution of lead of synovial fluid. Clin Orthop Rel Res *64*:255, 1969.
59. Switz DM, Elmorshidy ME, Deyerle WM: Bullets, joints, and lead intoxication. A remarkable and instructive case. Arch Intern Med *136*:939, 1976.
60. Windler EC, Smith RB, Bryan WJ, Woods GW: Lead intoxication and traumatic arthritis of the hip secondary to retained bullet fragments. A case report. J Bone Joint Surg *60A*:254, 1978.
61. Buxton JT Jr, Hewett JC, Gadsden RH, Bradham GB: Metallic mercury embolism, JAMA *193*:573, 1965.
62. Naidich TP, Bartelt D, Wheeler PS, Stern WZ: Metallic mercury emboli. Am J Roentgenol *117*:886, 1973.
63. Pearl M, Boxt LM: Radiographic findings in congenital lead poisoning. Radiology *136*:83, 1980.
64. Rosen JF, Chesney RW, Hamstra A, DeLuca HF, Mahaffey KR: Reduction in 1,25-dihydroxyvitamin D in children with increased lead absorption. N Engl J Med *302*:1128, 1980.
65. Gaucher A, Netter P, Faure G, Pourel J, Hutin MF, Burnel D: Les ostéoarthropathies "bismuthiques." Intérêt du dosage du bismuth osseux. Rev Rhum Mal Osteoartic *47*:31, 1980.
66. Krohn IT, Solof A, Mobini J, Wagner DK: Subcutaneous injection of metallic mercury. JAMA *243*:548, 1980.

69

NEUROMUSCULAR DISORDERS

by Donald Resnick, M.D.

Osseous, articular, and soft tissue changes accompany many neuromuscular disorders. Although the specific response of the musculoskeletal system is dependent to some degree on the nature of the disorder, certain general abnormalities are evident in many of the diseases. These alterations, which include osteoporosis, soft tissue atrophy or hypertrophy, growth disturbances and deformities due to altered muscular forces, growth plate and epiphyseal changes, soft tissue, bone, and joint infections, heterotopic ossification, cartilage atrophy, and synovitis, are discussed in this chapter. Neuroarthropathy, which may also accompany neurologic disorders, is described in Chapter 70.

OSTEOPOROSIS

Profound osteoporosis accompanies immobilization, disuse, or paralysis. It can affect the entire skeleton or a portion of it, according to the cause or the circumstances[1, 2] (Fig. 69–1). The pathogenesis of the osteoporosis is not clear, although the bone atrophy accompanying muscle paralysis due to conditions of the central nervous system, spinal cord, or peripheral nerves may be similar in its cause to that which follows muscular inactivity due to longstanding debilitating diseases, immobilization of a fracture, or weightlessness. It appears that immobilization causes stasis of blood flow, changes in arterial and venous blood gases with accumulation of carbon dioxide within bone, and an increase in intraosseous

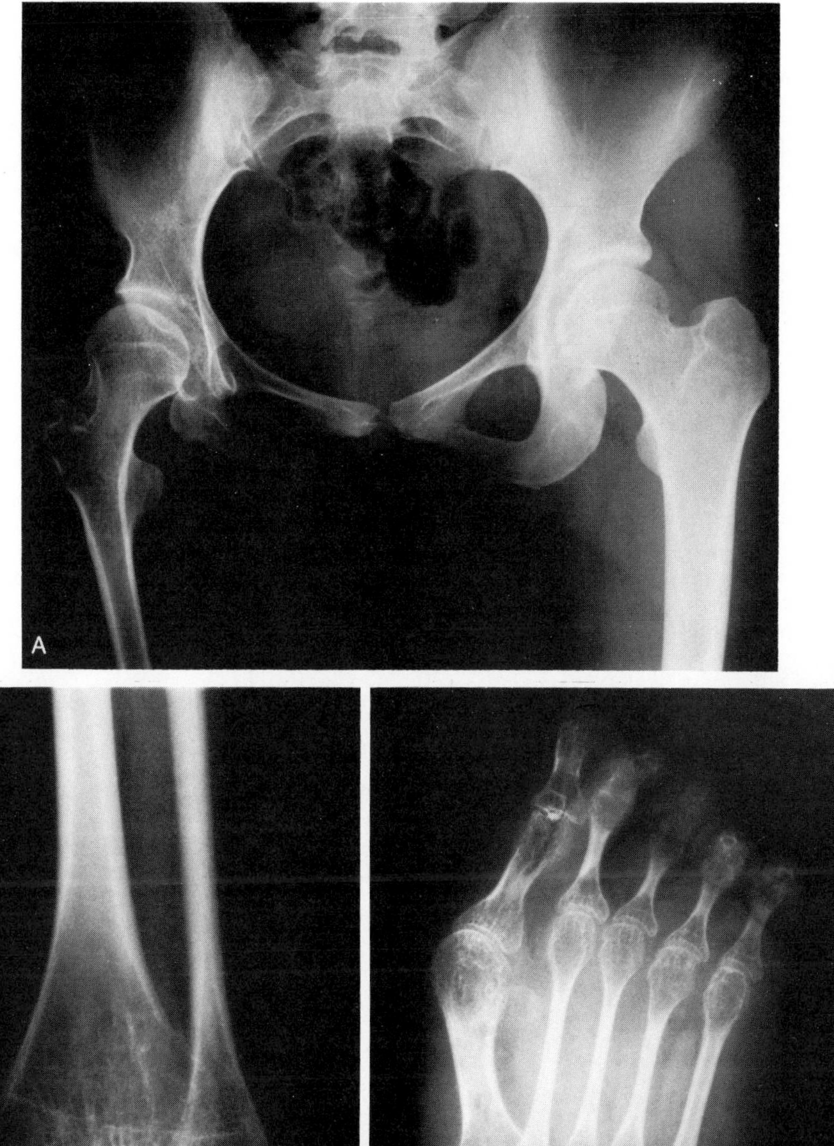

Figure 69–1. *Osteoporosis, bony underdevelopment, and soft tissue atrophy: Patients with poliomyelitis.*

A *Note osteoporosis and underdevelopment of the hemipelvis and femur on the right, paralyzed side. Coxa valga and external rotation of the femur and stress changes at the contralateral sacroiliac articulation are also noted.*

B, C *In the ankle and foot, thin or slender diaphyses, soft tissue atrophy and periarticular osteoporosis are prominent.*

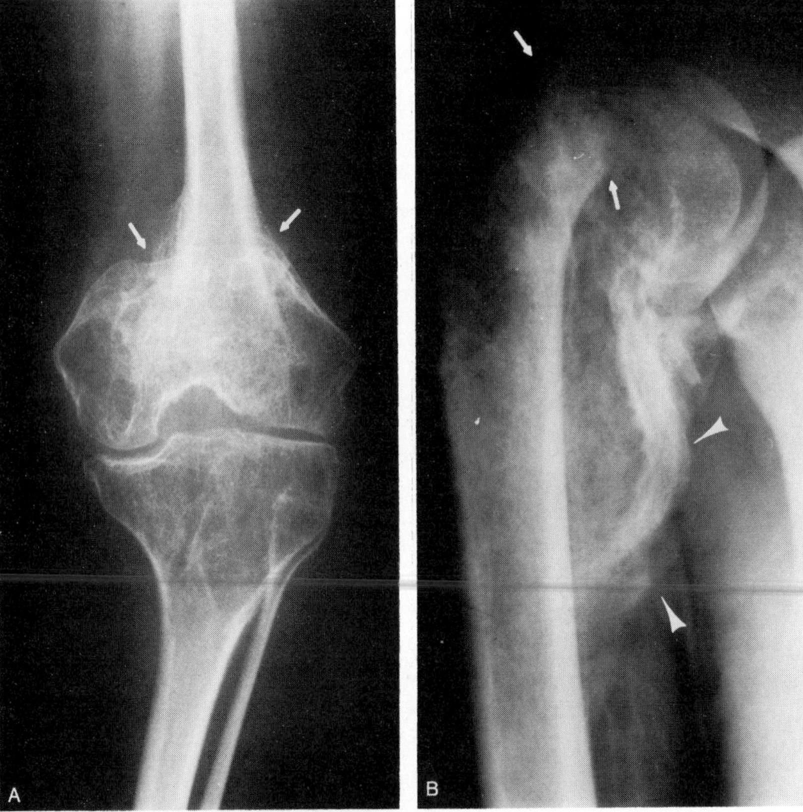

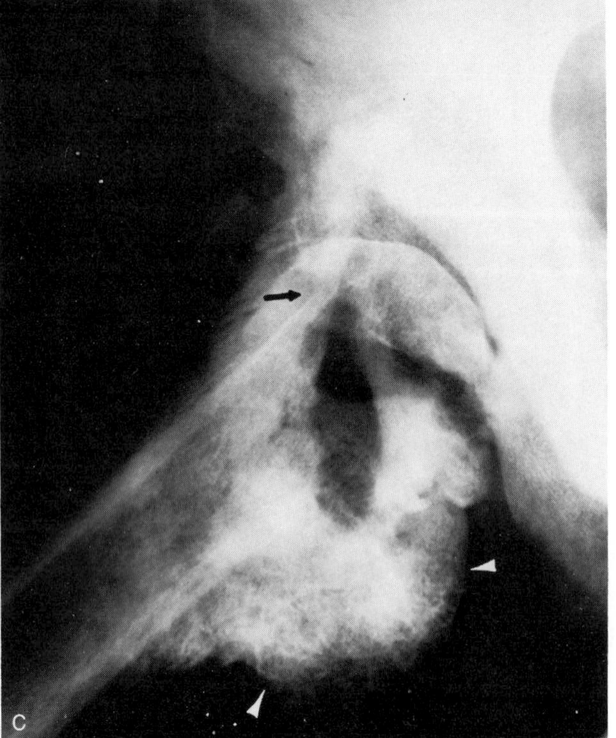

Figure 69–2. Osteoporosis and fracture.

A *In a patient with poliomyelitis, observe osteoporosis about the knee, thin tubular diaphyses, and a healed fracture of the distal femoral shaft (arrows).*

B *This 17 year old boy sustained injuries in an automobile accident, which included a fracture-dislocation of the shoulder and spinal fractures resulting in quadriplegia. Observe the displaced fracture of the proximal humerus (arrows) and excessive callus formation (arrowheads).*

C *This 51 year old quadriplegic patient developed flexion contractures of the hips. During a vigorous physical therapy session, a "snap" was audible in the right hip. A subcapital fracture (arrow) was demonstrated, which was later found to be associated with excessive callus formation (arrowheads).*

venous pressure.[3-5, 123] The alterations in bone circulation can modify cellular differentiation and function[6, 7]; initially, osteoclastic activity may be stimulated and osteoblastic activity may be reduced. Bone resorption predominates over bone formation, although subsequent osteoblastic activation allows repair of the bone resorption.[8, 9] In tubular bones, all three cortical envelopes (periosteal, intracortical or haversian, and endosteal envelopes) appear to participate in bone loss.[10] The contribution of each cortical envelope as well as trabecular bone[11] to osseous resorption and formation is influenced by the nature of the underlying disorder, the length of the observation period following immobilization or paralysis, the method of evaluation, and the integrity of certain endocrine glands.[12, 13, 117]

The radiographic counterpart of the altered cellular dynamics is osteopenia (Chapter 48). The axial and appendicular skeletons participate in this process. A generalized or localized, uniform or patchy, diffuse or periarticular decrease in spongy bone density is associated with diminution of the cortex and accentuation of stress trabeculae in the peripheral or central skeleton or both. "Spontaneous" fractures may be encountered as a result of bony atrophy and weakening aggravated by spasticity, contractures, deformities, and, in some instances, vigorous physical therapy[14-17]; excessive callus formation can appear in the healing phase,[111, 112] probably the result of continued active or passive motion at the fracture site[16, 17] (Fig. 69–2). Furthermore, focal areas of cortical resorption can develop, such as in the ribs, owing to pressure erosion from apposing bone or muscle atrophy with loss of normal mechanical stress.[18, 19, 116]

SOFT TISSUE ATROPHY AND HYPERTROPHY

Soft tissue atrophy with muscle wasting and fatty infiltration accompanies most neuromuscular disorders and can be detected on roentgenograms of the extremities[108] (Fig. 69–1). However, in Duchenne muscular dystrophy and congenital myotonia, the actual bulk of the musculature is increased.[20, 21] In the former condition, fatty infiltration of muscle is evident, and additional radiographic signs include congestive heart failure, osteoporosis, and a peculiar increased anteroposterior thickness of the diaphysis of the fibula.[22]

GROWTH DISTURBANCES AND DEFORMITIES DUE TO ALTERED MUSCULAR FORCES

Activity is essential to the normal growth and development of bones. With inactivity from any cause, muscle contraction diminishes or is lost, and, in the immature skeleton, the growth cartilage, which loses the healthy intermittent compression that everyday activity brings, is damaged. Although the specific alterations of growth may vary from one disorder to another, certain changes are common and well recognized. Inactive children who spend most of their time in a horizontal position can reveal vertebral bodies with increased vertical dimensions and narrowed intervertebral discs.[23-25] The increase in the height index (ratio of superoinferior diameter to anteroposterior diameter) is approximately proportional to the degree of inactivity; the presence of an inhibitory effect of the compressive force of weight-bearing on the potential longitudinal growth of vertebral bodies may be lost in prolonged recumbency. The similarity of the resulting radiographic appearance of the vertebral bodies in the immobilized child to that of certain animals, such as dogs, with horizontally oriented vertebral columns is of interest in this regard. The reported occurrence of increased height of vertebral bodies in young children with Down's syndrome suggests that genetic mechanisms may also affect bone development.[26]

Similarly, an increase in the neck-shaft angle of the femur, producing coxa valga, can result from muscular imbalance or a decrease in weight-bearing, particularly in very young children.[23, 24, 27-29] In severe cases, subluxation or dislocation of the hip may occur[30, 31] (Fig. 69–3). The opposite situation, coxa

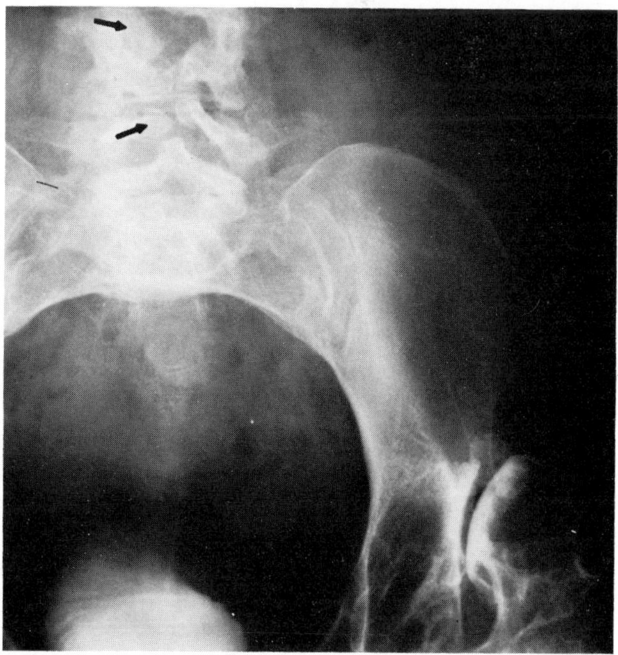

Figure 69–3. *Dislocation of the hip. In a paraplegic individual with spina bifida (arrows) and meningomyelocele, note the dislocated left femoral head, which is flattened and sclerotic. A neurogenic bladder is also apparent.*

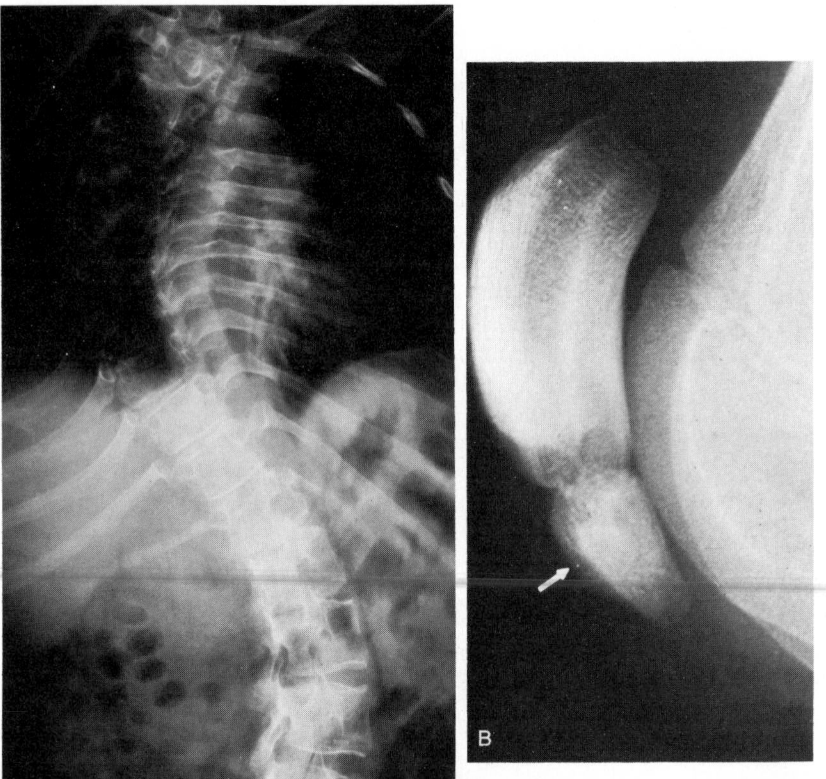

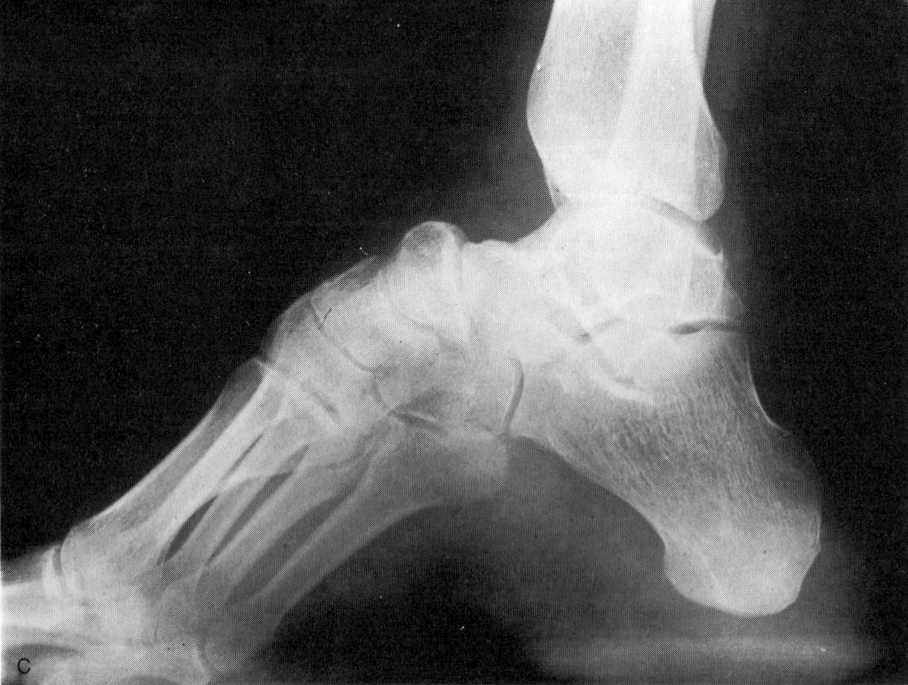

Figure 69–4. *Additional osseous effects related to altered muscular activity.*

A *Scoliosis in cerebral palsy. Note the prominent scoliotic curvatures, which were associated with considerable pelvic obliquity.*

B *Patellar fragmentation in cerebral palsy. Observe the large fragment of the inferior pole of the patella (arrow) due to altered stress in the quadriceps mechanism.*

C *Pes cavus deformity in poliomyelitis. Observe the exaggerated arch of the foot, soft tissue atrophy, and osteoporosis.*

vara, develops when the normal amount of upward muscle pull exceeds the force that can be resisted by weakened bone, such as in osteomalacia and Paget's disease.[24]

Additional examples of the effects of altered muscular activity on neighboring bone can be easily identified (Fig. 69–4). In the child with cerebral palsy, scoliosis, lordosis, and pelvic obliquity may result from unbalanced spine and hip muscle contraction and spasticity[32]; external rotation of the upper femur with a prominent lesser trochanter is due to the exaggerated pull of the iliopsoas muscle; flexion contractures of the hips and the knees with abnormal stress in the quadriceps mechanism may lead to patella alta, an elongated patellar shape, and fragmentation of the lower pole of the patella[33-36] and the tibial tuberosity.[36] An exaggerated pull of the flexor muscles of the leg relative to the extensors can produce equinus at the ankle.[37, 38] In the child with poliomyelitis or peroneal muscle atrophy, a pes cavus deformity is due to altered muscular function and stress.

GROWTH PLATE AND EPIPHYSEAL CHANGES

Premature closure of the growth plate, particularly in the metatarsals and knees, is noted in patients with poliomyelitis[39, 40] (Fig. 69–5). Currarino[41] noted evidence of premature fusion of one or more epiphyses in 9 per cent of 250 patients with polio, in all cases limited to the feet or the knees. Unilateral or bilateral changes occur, always corresponding to sites that are involved in the neurologic disease; the fourth metatarsal is most frequently affected. The altered epiphyses in the foot or the knee can be buried in the adjacent metaphyses ("ball and socket" epiphyses), and, following epiphyseal fusion, the involved bone is shortened. Although the pathogenesis of the change is not known, chronic growth plate trauma due to angular deformity and muscular and osseous weakening may be responsible for the premature epiphyseal fusion.

Epiphyseal and metaphyseal trauma is a recognized manifestation in patients with certain neurologic disorders (meningomyelocele and congenital insensitivity to pain) owing to their sensory deficiency, osteoporosis, and musculoligamentous laxity[42-49, 113, 114] (Chapter 70). Following injury, the absence of significant pain allows continued activity, and neuropathic alterations appear, characterized by metaphyseal and growth plate hemorrhage, epiphyseal displacement, widening and irregularity of the cartilaginous plate, metaphyseal and epiphyseal fragmentation, and periosteal bone formation. The appearance may simulate that of rickets or infection.

OSSEOUS, ARTICULAR, AND SOFT TISSUE INFECTION

The immobilized and debilitated patient with neuromuscular disease frequently develops generalized or localized infections. Skin breakdown over

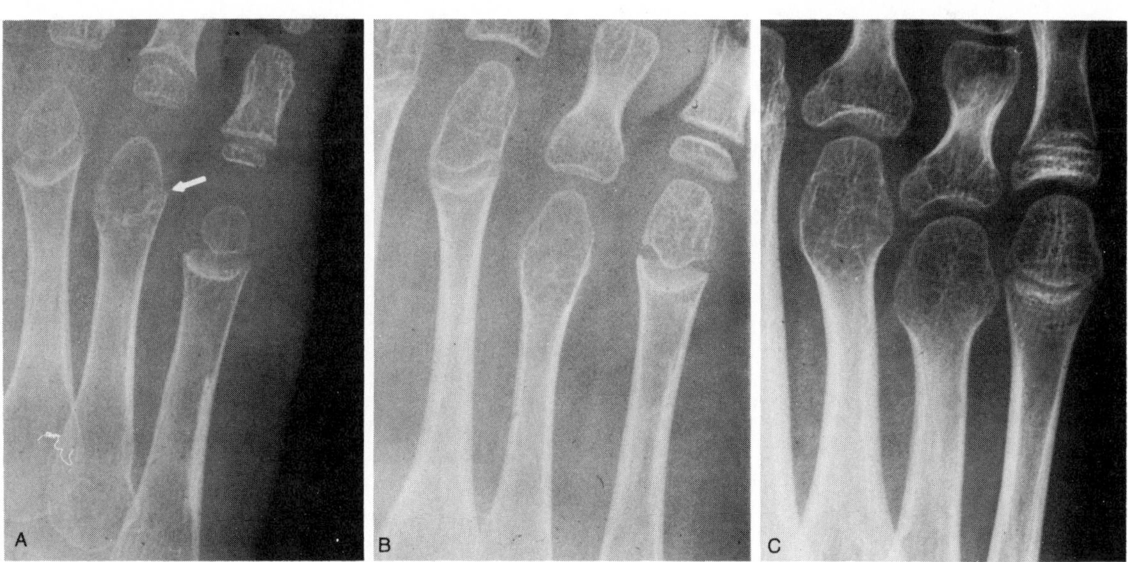

Figure 69–5. *Premature closure of the growth plate in a patient with poliomyelitis.*

A *In the initial film, the growth plate of the fourth metatarsal is partially closed (arrow), whereas those of the third and fifth metatarsals are still open. Furthermore, the fourth metatarsal is shortened and considerable osteoporosis is evident.*

B *Five years later, note the solid fusion of the fourth metatarsal epiphysis and the shortening of the digit. Observe fusion of the growth plate of the proximal phalanx of the fourth toe.*

C *At this stage, closure of the growth plate of the third metatarsal has produced shortening of this digit as well.*

pressure points is a common and frustrating problem in these individuals,[50-52] and with penetration of the subcutaneous and fascial tissue, infection may reach the underlying bones and joints. The ischial tuberosities, the femoral trochanters, the hip articulations, and other bony protuberances are most typically affected, and the characteristic radiographic findings of osteomyelitis or septic arthritis (or both) ensue (Chapter 60). The degree of osteolysis in these cases may become extreme,[53] the bone loss being aggravated by factors other than infection, such as disuse, the trauma of continual pressure, and neuropathy.

The frequency of sacroiliac joint abnormality in paralyzed individuals has been attributed, at least in part, to chronic pelvic sepsis resulting in osseous contamination. This articular manifestation is discussed later in this chapter.

HETEROTOPIC OSSIFICATION

Heterotopic new bone formation is a well-documented complication of central nervous system and spinal cord disorders.[54-59] It is most commonly reported in association with paraplegia secondary to spinal cord trauma, where it may be observed in 16 to 53 per cent of cases.[60-65] Less frequently, heterotopic ossification is evident following acute anoxia, head injury,[124] cerebrovascular accident, encephalomyelitis, poliomyelitis, multiple sclerosis, neoplastic disease, and tetanus.[58, 59, 63, 66-71] It occurs in both flaccid and spastic forms of paralysis and is more common and severe in young men.

In general, ossification appears 2 to 6 months following injury. However, it has been evident as early as 19 days after trauma.[61, 65] Single or multiple, unilateral or bilateral sites may be affected. The most typically involved areas are the hip (Fig. 69–6), the knee (Fig. 69–7), and the shoulder (Fig. 69–8); less commonly, the elbow (Fig. 69–9)[109] and the small joints of the hand and the foot are altered.[59] Although ossification is almost always seen in a paralyzed limb or limbs, this association is not constant.

The clinical manifestations are variable. Many patients have no symptoms or signs in addition to those of the primary neurologic disorder itself. Others develop pain, swelling, and restricted joint motion simulating the findings of an acute arthritis. Aspiration of articular contents may reveal clear yellow or serosanguineous synovial fluid with a meager number of erythrocytes or leukocytes.[59, 60] Additional laboratory findings may be unrewarding, although elevation of the serum alkaline phosphatase level has been observed.[72] The frequency of certain histocompatibility antigens in patients with heterotopic ossification appears to be identical to that in healthy individuals.[73]

Radiographic examination delineates initially ill-defined periarticular radiodense areas that do not contain recognizable trabeculae. The collections enlarge, merge with the underlying bone in the form of an irregular excrescence, and demonstrate trabecular architecture. Eventually, complete periarticular osseous bridging may result, associated with significant loss or absence of joint motion. In some instances, ossification develops at a distance from a joint and eventually becomes attached to the subjacent bone, forming a peculiar exostosis.

Scintigraphic examination may also be utilized to determine the evolution of this process and the maturity of the heterotopic ossification.[57, 74, 75] This determination is important, as surgical removal of immature new bone is frequently followed by recurrence of the abnormal deposits, whereas excision of mature ossification is not associated with such recurrence. Images obtained with bone-seeking pharmaceutical agents reveal an acute phase with increased radionuclide activity prior to the appearance of radiographic abnormalities, a subacute phase with a rapid increase in activity, a chronic active immature phase with a steady state of increased activity, a chronic active maturing phase with decreased activity, and a chronic mature phase with a return of the normal scan.[57] The time necessary for the bone scan to pass from one stage to the next appears to be variable, but operative intervention should not be contemplated before the activity of the radionuclide begins to diminish. Supplementing the study with a scintigraphic examination with a bone marrow–seeking agent may further document the maturity of the deposited bone; the accumulation of radionuclide in this study indicates mature marrow-containing ectopic bone.

Histologically, the maturing heterotopic ossification consists of essentially normal bone with haversian canals, osteoblasts, blood vessels, and marrow.[60, 61, 76, 77]

The cause of the ectopic bone formation is unknown.[59] Local factors, such as continuous pressure, decubitus ulceration, and trauma from vigorous therapy, have been emphasized by some investigators[122]; however, the occurrence of heterotopic ossification in areas remote from the pressure points or the decubitus ulcers and in the absence of physical manipulation has been documented. Systemic factors, such as hypoproteinemia and urinary tract infections, have also been implicated,[77] but studies have failed to confirm this.[61] The appearance of excessive callus formation around fractures in some paralyzed individuals has suggested that an exaggerated healing response or bone-forming tendency may be operational,[112] but this, too, appears unlikely.[54] A genetic predisposition to bone formation has also been postulated as a cause of ossification in these patients (as well as in those with diffuse idiopathic skeletal hyperostosis),[78] but results of histocompatibility antigen determinations have not been reward-

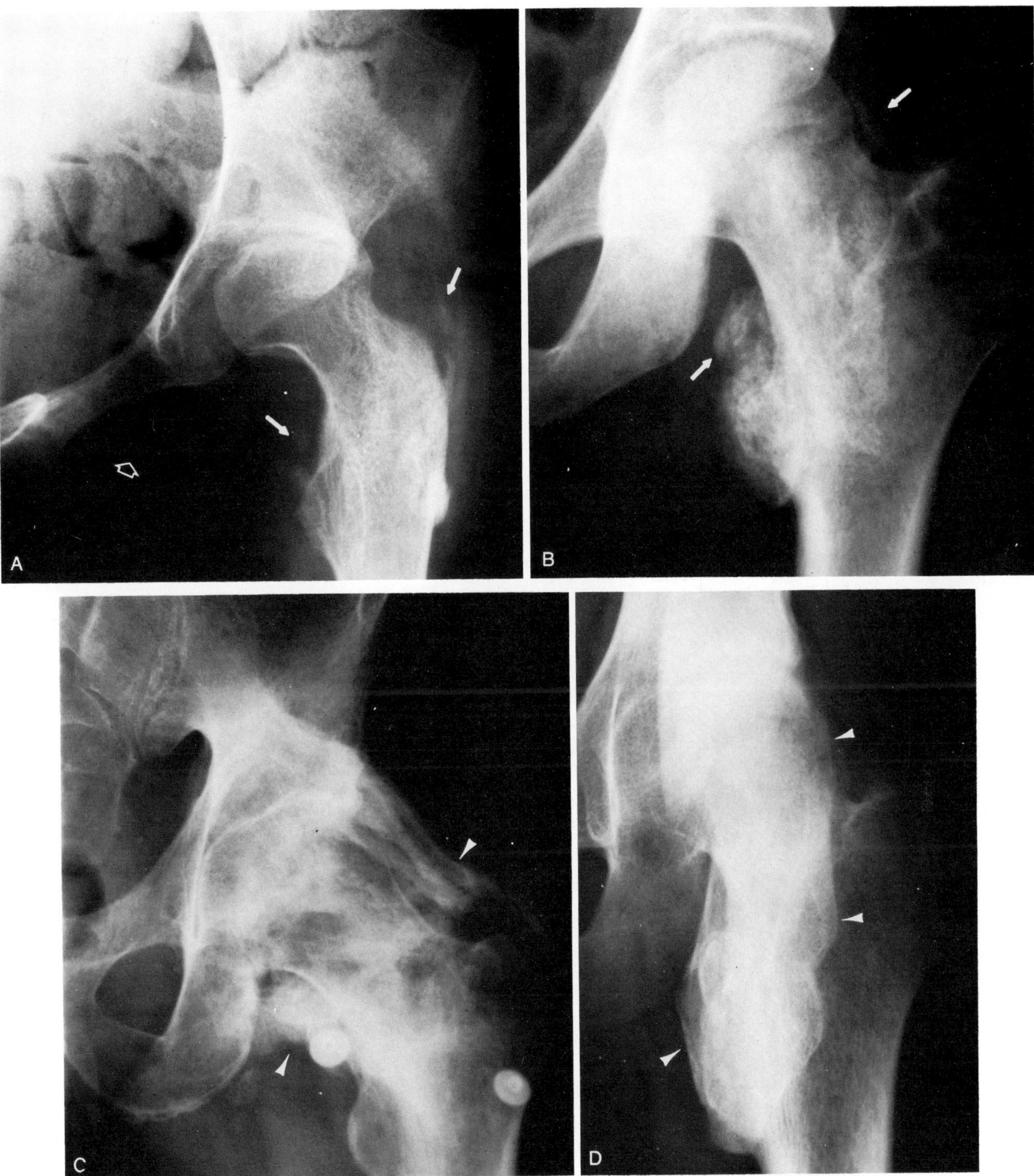

Figure 69–6. *Heterotopic ossification: The hip. Four examples of ossification of varying severity about the hip. The deposits begin as ill-defined opacities (solid arrows) and progress to radiodense lesions of considerable size possessing trabecular pattern (arrowheads). Osteoporosis of neighboring bone can be considerable. Additional findings may include articular space diminution and osteomyelitis of the ischial tuberosity that may require surgical resection (open arrow).*

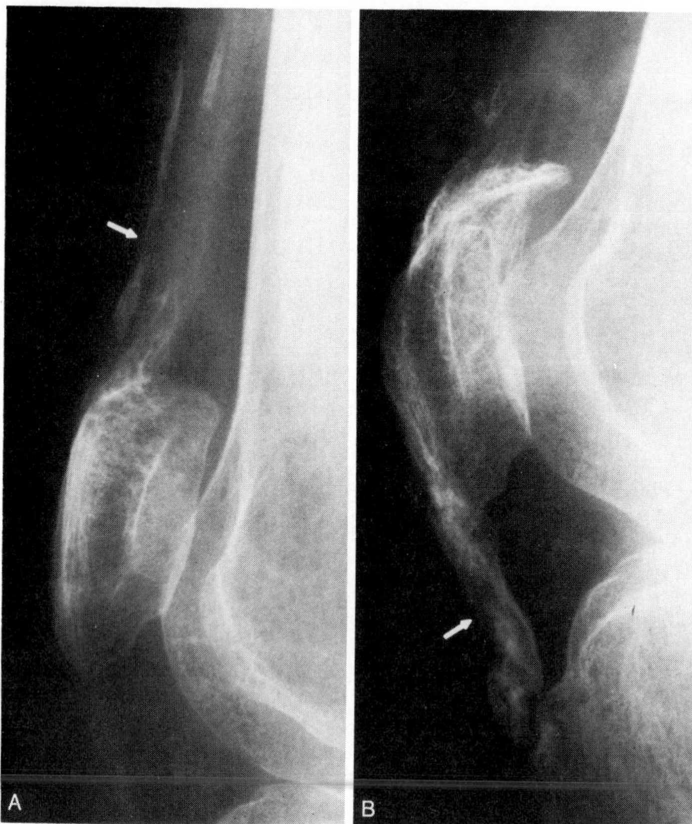

Figure 69–7. *Heterotopic ossification:* The knee. Two examples of soft tissue and tendinous ossification (arrow) about the knee. Observe the accompanying osteoporosis.

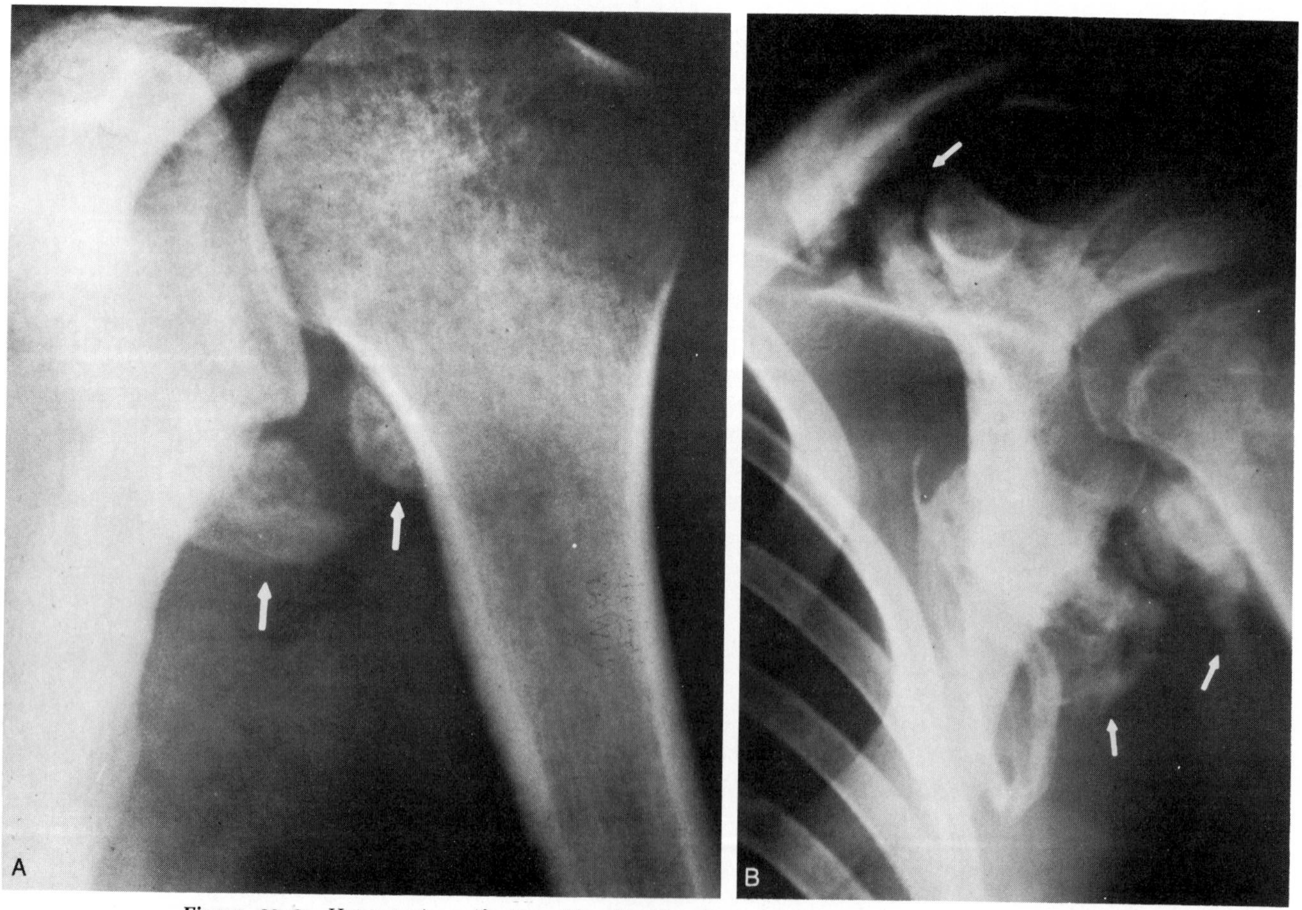

Figure 69–8. *Heterotopic ossification:* The shoulder. Deposits of varying size can also be noted about the shoulder (arrows). Again observe the associated osteoporosis.

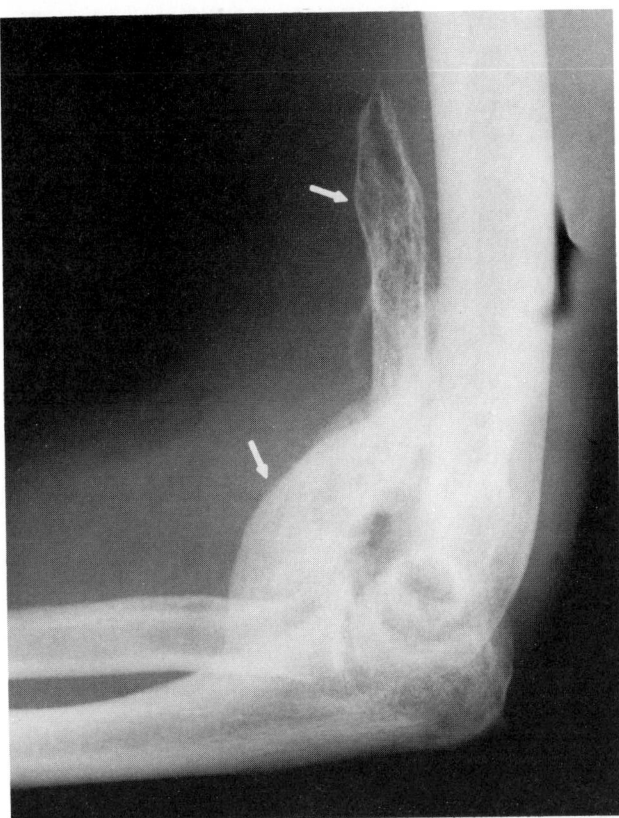

Figure 69–9. Heterotopic ossification: The elbow. Striking mature ossification (arrows) has produced "ankylosis" along the anterior aspect of the elbow.

ing.[73, 121] It has also been theorized that denervation stimulates the connective tissue to recover its embryonic osteogenic function,[79] but the exact basis for this stimulation and the variability of this response in different individuals remain unexplained.

The common factor in heterotopic ossification in neurologic disorders is immobilization. The deposition of calcium and bone may relate to vascular stasis,[125] perhaps in Batson's paravertebral plexus (which has tributaries in the appendicular skeleton as well),[80] but the exact pathogenesis of such ossification and why it is present in some individuals and absent in others remain mysteries.

Heterotopic ossification of soft tissues is not confined to patients with neuromuscular disease. Burns, mechanical trauma, and venous stasis (varicosities) can lead to similar changes. In addition, a progressive form of ossification of unknown etiology, myositis ossificans progressiva, is also recognized.

CARTILAGE ATROPHY

Articular cartilage is nourished predominantly by diffusion of synovial fluid[81-84] (Fig. 69–10). A subchondral route for nutrition of the innermost portion of the cartilaginous surface appears probable based upon data from experimental studies in animals.[85, 86] This latter process may be more prominent in the immature skeleton than in the mature skeleton owing to differences in the anatomic configuration of the junctional region between articular cartilage and subchondral bone; nutrition in the young animal may be enhanced by the presence of prominent vascular buds extending from the subchondral circulation into the cartilage mass, whereas in the older animal, mature cortical bone may separate the cartilage from the subchondral vascular spaces.[87, 118] These experimental observations may indeed have relevance to chondral nutrition in the human.[88] The diffusion into cartilage of nutrients from the synovial fluid and subchondral bone is aided by the pliability and hydrophilic characteristics of the chondral surface,[89, 90] and is dependent upon a pumping action that develops during normal activity.[91]

Immobilization leads to significant changes in cartilaginous nutrition. The production of synovial fluid is greatly curtailed.[92] In animals, progressive contracture of capsular and pericapsular structures and encroachment on the joint by intra-articular fibro-fatty connective tissue are observed.[93-96] At sites at which the articular surfaces are in contact, chondral fibrillation, erosion, and necrosis with liquefaction are identified.[94-98, 110] The subchondral bone may be thickened and invaded by proliferating primitive mesenchymal tissue from the marrow spaces, which replaces the deep layer of articular cartilage.[95, 99]

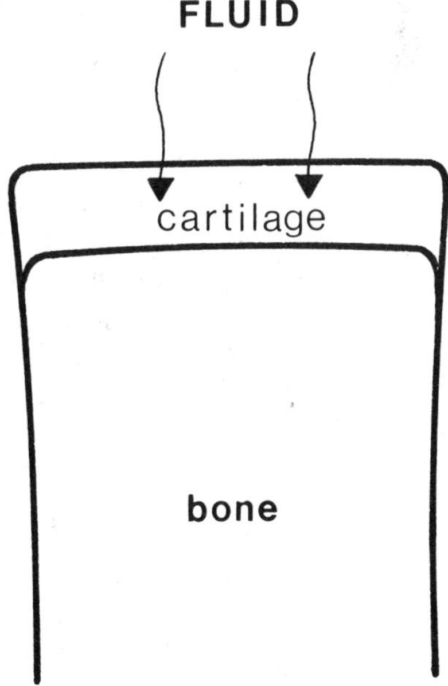

Figure 69–10. Normal cartilage nutrition. The predominant mechanism of cartilage nutrition is derived from a "pumping" action in which synovial fluid diffuses into the chondral substance. A subchondral route of nutrition is present but of less magnitude.

Repair of chondral elements may follow short periods of immobilization.[100]

Similar events may accompany immobilization of human joints.[101, 102] In the knee, prolonged immobilization is associated with proliferation of fibrofatty tissue, which subsequently envelops intra-articular ligaments and obliterates the articular lumen, and is associated with gradual resorption of peripheral cartilage[102] (Fig. 69–11). In areas of apposed articular surfaces, fibrillation and cystic defects appear within the cartilage, and a reparative effort associated with proliferation and transchondral extension of primitive mesenchymal tissue within the marrow and with endochondral ossification may result in total replacement of articular cartilage and intra-articular fibrous or bony ankylosis.[102] Both intra-articular and periarticular changes are important in the limitation of joint motion that follows long-term immobilization.[95-102]

These observations on animals and humans suggest that the chondral alterations following immobilization result from a decrease in cartilage nutrition due to the presence of an atrophic synovial membrane and the absence of normal movement with a concomitant decrease in fluid diffusion. A decrease in loading of the cartilage due to absence of contraction of muscles that span the articulation may contribute to these alterations.[119] The radiographic counterpart is a loss of interosseous (joint) space in the patient with neurologic disease (Fig. 69–12). Although this may be observed in any paralyzed body part, changes are especially characteristic in the hip, the knee, and the sacroiliac joint. Pool[91] noted significant joint space narrowing (by at least 50 per cent) of the hip articulation in 12.5 per cent of 200 patients with flaccid paralysis, in some cases within 2 years of injury; the incidence of this abnormality in spastic paralysis is probably less

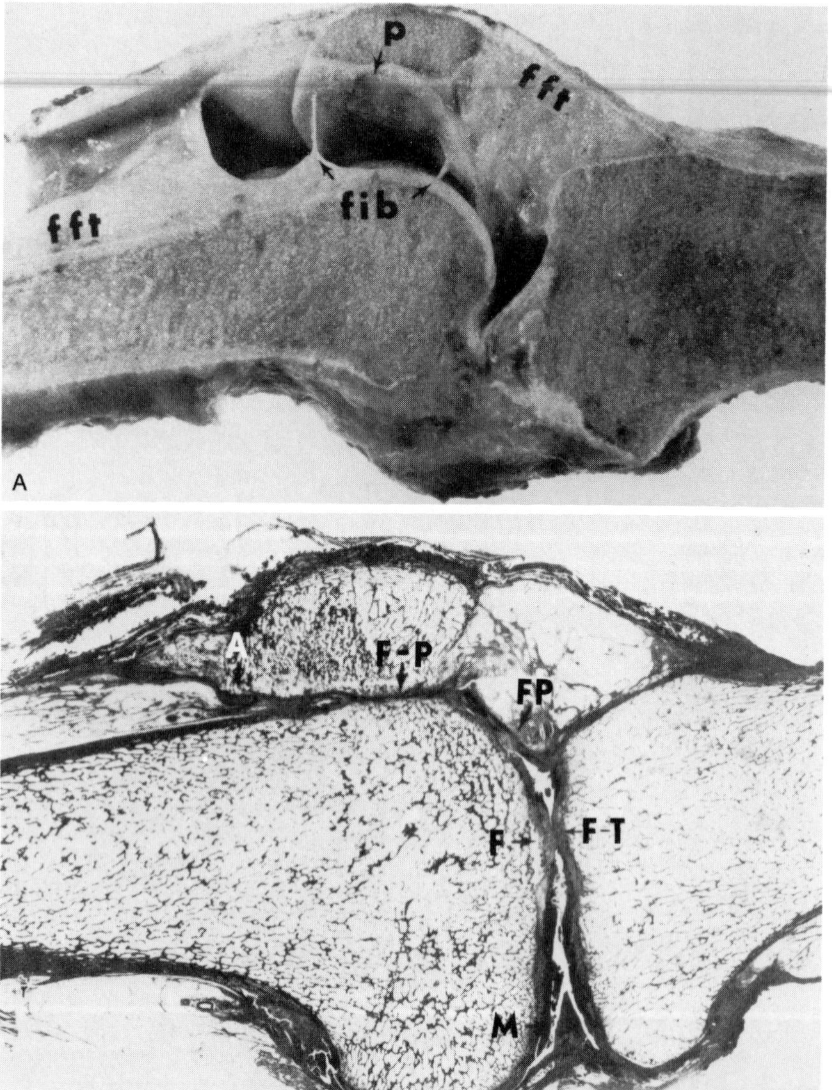

Figure 69–11. *Cartilage atrophy: Pathologic abnormalities.*

A *On a photograph of a sagittal section of an immobilized knee (period of immobilization — over 12 months), note fibrofatty tissue (fft) filling the inferior portion of the joint cavity as well as a portion of the suprapatellar pouch. Fibrous septa (fib) extend from the femoral condyle to the patella. The patellar articular cartilage (p) is irregular.*

B *On a photomicrograph (1×) of a similar sagittal section in a different patient (period of immobilization — 16 months), note osteoporosis. Replacement of the articular cartilages of the femoral condyle, patella, and tibia by fibrous connective tissue is apparent. Small islands of cartilage remain in the patella (A), the femoral condyle (F), and the tibia. Mature fibrous connective tissue, in which ossification is occurring, joins the femoral condyle and the patella (F–P), and the femoral condyle and the tibia (F–T). Obliteration of portions of the joint cavity as well as the suprapatellar pouch by fibrofatty tissue (FP) is evident.*

(From Enneking WF, Horowitz M: J Bone Joint Surg 54A:973, 1972.)

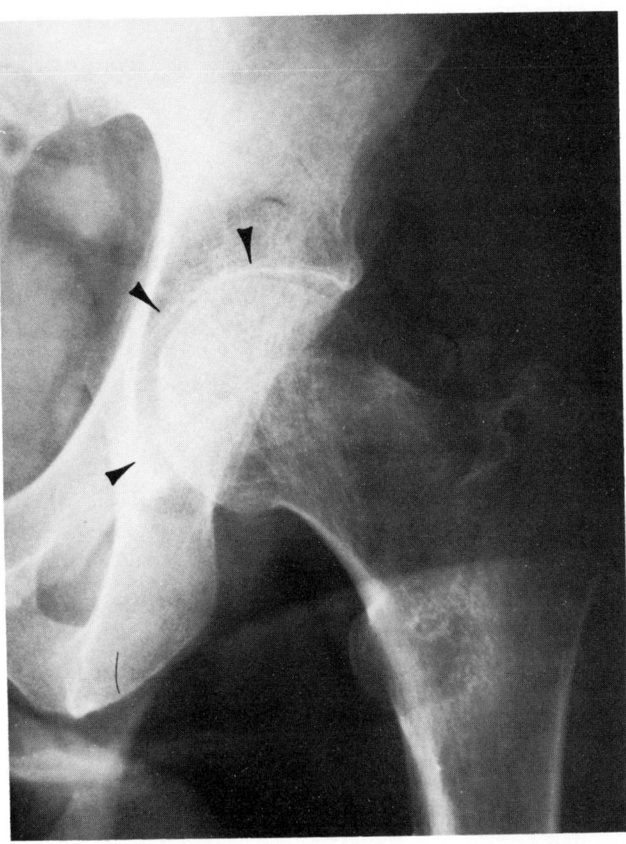

Figure 69–12. *Cartilage atrophy: Radiologic abnormalities. A typical example of symmetric loss of the joint space (arrowheads) in the hip due to cartilage atrophy resulting from paralysis is presented.*

because of the muscular tension across the articulation. Characteristically, diffuse loss of interosseous space is evident with axial migration of the femoral head, although narrowing of the superolateral aspect of the articulation may be prominent in some individuals because of associated lateral subluxation of the femoral head. Accompanying osteoporosis may be evident.

Changes may also be observed in one or both sacroiliac joints, although the interpretation of the alterations in this location has been a matter of debate (Fig. 69–13). In 1950, Abel[103] reported radiographic changes of the sacroiliac articulation in 98 of 160 patients (61 per cent) with traumatic paraplegia. The abnormalities consisted of periarticular osteoporosis and joint space narrowing, which, in some cases, progressed to intra-articular bony ankylosis. On biopsy of the sacroiliac joint in one patient, atrophic bone with vascular marrow, cartilaginous denudation, and osseous fusion were noted. This investigator cited the radiographic and histologic similarity of sacroiliac joint involvement in paraplegia to that in ankylosing spondylitis, perhaps indicating a common pathogenesis in both disorders. It was subsequently suggested that chronic genitourinary tract infection might produce the osteoarticular lesions of ankylosing spondylitis owing to dissemination of infection via the paravertebral venous plexus,[104] a mechanism that would also be operational in paralyzed individuals. In 1965, Wright and colleagues[105] studied 38 paraplegic men, noting sacroiliac joint abnormalities on radiographs of 12 (32 per cent) of these individuals. Major osseous erosion, complete bony ankylosis of the joint, or spondylitis was not evident, thus creating a roentgenographic picture that differed from that in ankylosing spondylitis. Furthermore, these investigators found that the sacroiliac joint changes were not related to the presence or severity of genital infection, leading them to postulate that sacroiliac articular alterations in paraplegia are due not to sacroiliitis or chronic infection but to damage by the severe mechanical stresses to which the pelvis is subjected acting on osteoporotic bone. The differing pathogeneses of sacroiliac joint changes in paralysis and ankylosing spondylitis were further underscored by histocompatibility antigen typing of 54 paraplegic or quadriplegic individuals, 24 of whom had abnormal radiographs of the sacroiliac articulations.[106] Although the sacroiliac joint alterations were more severe in quadriplegic than in paraplegic patients, there was no association between these alterations and any of the HLA antigens of the A and B loci in either group.

Thus, the pathogenesis of sacroiliac joint changes in paralyzed individuals remains a mystery. The findings may relate to a combination of cartilage atrophy due to immobilization and subchondral osseous collapse due to weakening and fracture of osteoporotic bone. Sacroiliac joint abnormalities may be more common in patients with high spinal levels of paraplegia than in those with low levels of paraplegia, perhaps related to more severe limitation of trunk mobility in the former individuals.[115] The abnormalities appear to be more frequent and severe in patients with paralysis of longer duration.[120] Rarely, they are combined with changes in the spine, including syndesmophytes, interspinous ossification, osteophytes, and intervertebral discal calcification.[120]

SYNOVITIS

The occurrence of soft tissue swelling about certain joints in the paralyzed patient in conjunction with heterotopic ossification has already been noted. Noninflammatory fluid is usually recovered on joint aspiration in these individuals. Occasionally, however, an acute inflammatory joint reaction can be seen in the early convalescent stage following a cerebrovascular accident, exclusively or predominantly in the paralyzed limb.[107] The arthritis may be preceded by an infection of the respiratory, urinary, or biliary tract, although the synovial fluid is sterile. The articular inflammation heals without sequelae in a few weeks and does not recur.

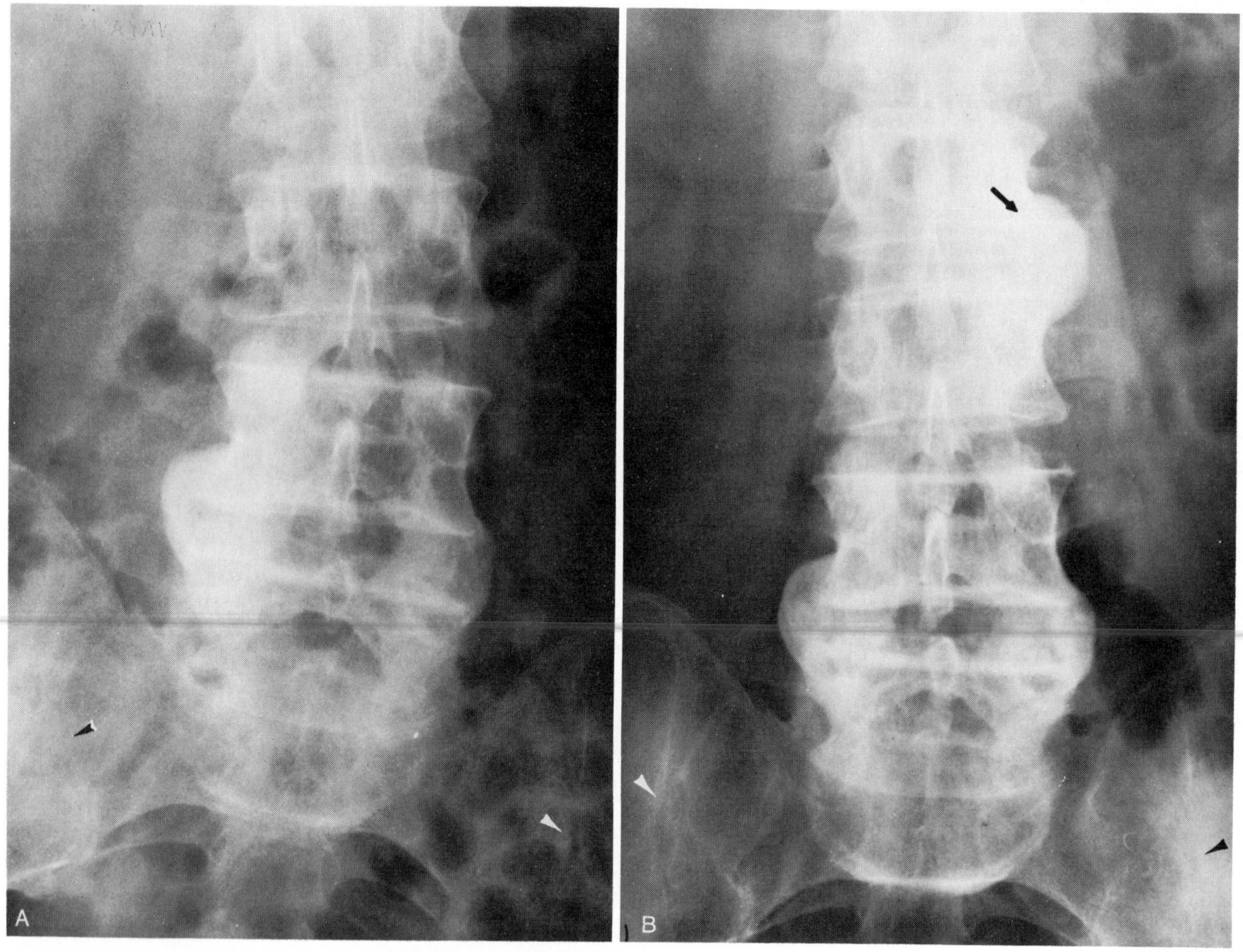

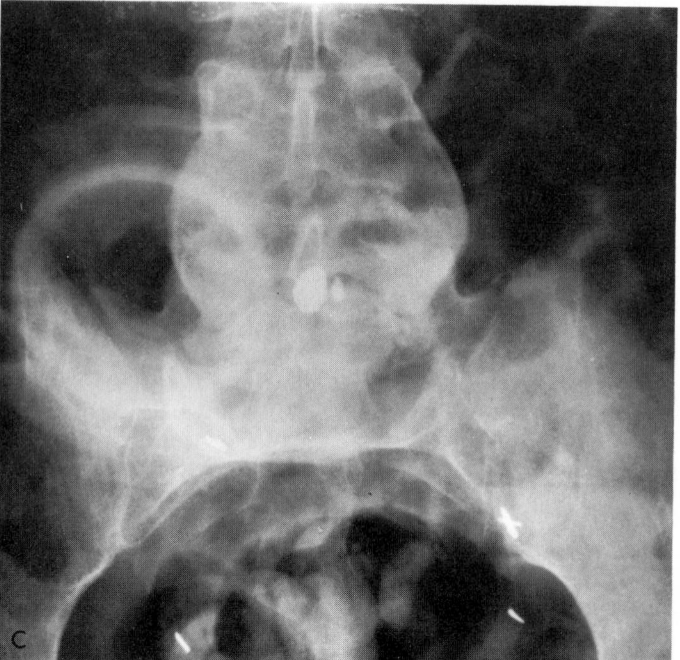

Figure 69–13. *Sacroiliac joint and spinal abnormalities.*

A, B *In this patient, who had been quadriplegic for over 5 years, two sets of radiographs obtained 2 years apart indicate loss of interosseous space in both sacroiliac joints (arrowheads) and spinal ossification. One of the vertebral outgrowths appeared during the period of paralysis (arrow). Whether these excrescences represent typical osteophytes or heterotopic bone formation is not clear.*

C *In a different patient with quadriplegia, bilateral sacroiliac joint changes consisting of narrowing of the interosseous space are combined with peculiar spinal outgrowths at the discovertebral junction that resemble syndesmophytes. Previous surgery and myelography had been accomplished.*

This clinical situation leading to arthritis in paralyzed limbs is in sharp contrast to that which is evident when rheumatoid arthritis (or other articular disorders) occurs in a hemiplegic individual (Chapter 27). In the latter case, relative sparing of the paralyzed limbs is apparent.

MISCELLANEOUS ABNORMALITIES

Significant digital clubbing may be encountered in paralyzed patients.[105] This finding is seen in patients in whom paralysis has been present for more than a year and appears to correlate with the presence of decubitus ulcers and persistent subcutaneous edema.

SUMMARY

The musculoskeletal abnormalities accompanying neuromuscular disorders include osteoporosis, soft tissue atrophy, growth disturbances, deformities, growth plate injuries, infection, heterotopic ossification, cartilage atrophy, synovitis, clubbing, and neuroarthropathy (Table 69–1). Typical radiographic changes are encountered that are easy to interpret when an adequate clinical history is provided. Although the pathogenesis of some of the findings is clear, that of heterotopic ossification and sacroiliac joint alterations is unknown.

Table 69–1

MUSCULOSKELETAL ABNORMALITIES IN PARALYSIS

Osteoporosis
Soft tissue atrophy or hypertrophy
Osseous deformities
Growth disturbances
"Stress" fragmentation of bone
Epiphyseal and metaphyseal fracture or fragmentation
Infection
Heterotopic ossification
Cartilage atrophy
Synovitis

REFERENCES

1. Albright F, Burnett CH, Cope O, Parsons W: Acute atrophy of bone (osteoporosis) simulating hyperparathyroidism. J Clin Endocrinol *1*:711, 1941.
2. Eichler J: Inaktivitätsosteoporose. Z Rheumaforsch *31*:367, 1972.
3. Little K: Bone Behavior. London, Academic Press, 1973.
4. Benassy J, Mazabraud J, Diverres JC: L'osteogenese neurogene. Rev Chir Orthop *49*:95, 1963.
5. Trueta J: The dynamics of bone circulation. *In* HM Frost (Ed): Bone Dynamics. Boston, Little, Brown and Co, 1964, p 245.
6. Dhem A: Les mecanismes des destruction du tissue osseux. Acta Orthop Belg *39*:423, 1973.
7. Andrew C, Basset L: Biophysical Principles Affecting Bone Structure. *In* GH Bourne (ed): Biochemistry and Physiology of Bone. Vol. 3. New York, Academic Press, 1971, p 584.
8. Chantraine A: Actual concept of osteoporosis in paraplegia. Paraplegia *16*:51, 1978.
9. Rasmussen H, Bordier P: The cellular basis of metabolic bone disease. N Engl J Med *289*:25, 1973.
10. Uhthoff HK, Jaworski ZFG: Bone loss in response to long-term immobilization. J Bone Joint Surg *60B*:420, 1978.
11. Griffiths HJ, Bushueff B, Zimmerman RE: Investigation of the loss of bone mineral in patients with spinal cord injury. Paraplegia *14*:207, 1976.
12. Burkhart JM, Jowsey J: Parathyroid and thyroid hormones in the development of immobilization osteoporosis. Endocrinology *81*:1053, 1967.
13. Minaire P, Meunier P, Edouard C, Bernard J, Courpron P, Bourret J: Quantitative histological data on disuse osteoporosis. Comparison with biological data. Calcif Tissue Res *17*:57, 1974.
14. Eichenholtz N: Management of long-bone fractures in paraplegic patients. J Bone Joint Surg *45A*:299, 1963.
15. McIvor WC, Samilson RL: Fractures in patients with cerebral palsy. J Bone Joint Surg *48A*:858, 1966.
16. Handelsman JE: Spontaneous fractures in spina bifida. J Bone Joint Surg *54B*:381, 1972.
17. Miller PR, Glazer DA: Spontaneous fractures in the brain-crippled, bedridden patient. Clin Orthop Rel Res *120*:138, 1976.
18. Bernstein C, Loeser WD, Manning LE: Erosive rib lesions in paralytic poliomyelitis. Radiology *70*:368, 1958.
19. Woodlief RM: Superior marginal rib defects in traumatic quadriplegia. Radiology *126*:673, 1978.
20. Litt RE, Altman DH: Significance of the muscle cylinder ratio in infancy. Am J Roentgenol *100*:80, 1967.
21. Furukawa T, Peter JB: The muscular dystrophies and related disorders. I. The muscular dystrophies. JAMA *239*:1537, 1978.
22. Harris VJ, Harris WS: Increased thickness of the fibula in Duchenne muscular dystrophy. Am J Roentgenol *98*:744, 1966.
23. Houston CS, Zaleski WA: The shape of vertebral bodies and femoral necks in relation to activity. Radiology *89*:59, 1967.
24. Houston CS: The radiologist's opportunity to teach bone dynamics. J Can Assoc Radiol *29*:232, 1978.
25. Gooding CA, Neuhauser EBD: Growth and development of the vertebral body in the presence and absence of normal stress. Am J Roentgenol *93*:388, 1965.
26. Rabinowitz JG, Moseley JE: The lateral lumbar spine in Down's syndrome: A new roentgen feature. Radiology *83*:74, 1964.
27. Stevenson FH: The osteoporosis of immobilization in recumbency. J Bone Joint Surg *34B*:256, 1952.
28. Lamb DW, Pollock GA: Hip deformities in cerebral palsy and their treatment. Dev Med Child Neurol *4*:488, 1962.
29. Baker LD, Dodelin R, Bassett FH: Pathological changes in the hip in cerebral palsy; incidence, pathogenesis, and treatment. A preliminary report. J Bone Joint Surg *44A*:1331, 1962.
30. Tachdjian MO, Minear WL: Hip dislocation in cerebral palsy. J Bone Joint Surg *38A*:1358, 1956.
31. Sharrard WJW, Allen JMH, Heaney SH, Prendiville GRG: Surgical prophylaxis of subluxation and dislocation of the hip in cerebral palsy. J Bone Joint Surg *57B*:160, 1975.
32. Samilson R, Bechard R: Scoliosis in cerebral palsy: Incidence, distribution of curve patterns, and thoughts on etiology. Curr Pract Orthop Surg *5*:183, 1973.
33. Saupe E: Beitrag zur patella bipartita. Fortschr Geb Roentgenstr Nuklearmed *28*:37, 1921.
34. Roberts WM, Adams JP: The patellar-advancement operation in cerebral palsy. J Bone Joint Surg *35A*:958, 1953.
35. Kaye JJ, Freiberger RH: Fragmentation of the lower pole of the patella in spastic lower extremities. Radiology *101*:97, 1971.
36. Rosenthal RK, Levine DB: Fragmentation of the distal pole of the patella in spastic cerebral palsy. J Bone Joint Surg *59A*:934, 1977.
37. Baker LD, Hill LM: Foot alignment in the cerebral palsy patient. J Bone Joint Surg *46A*:1, 1964.
38. Sharrard WJW, Bernstein S: Equinus deformity in cerebral palsy. A comparison between elongation of the tendocalcaneus and gastrocnemius recession. J Bone Joint Surg *54B*:272, 1972.
39. Ross D: Disturbance of longitudinal growth associated with prolonged disability of the lower extremity. J Bone Joint Surg *30A*:103, 1948.

40. Ratliff AH: The short leg in poliomyelitis. J Bone Joint Surg *41B*:56, 1959.
41. Currarino G: Premature closure of epiphyses in the metatarsals and knees: A sequel of poliomyelitis. Radiology *87*:424, 1966.
42. Edvardsen P: Physeo-epiphyseal injuries of lower extremities in myelomeningocele. Acta Orthop Scand *43*:550, 1972.
43. Gyepes MT, Newbern DH, Neuhauser EBD: Metaphyseal and physeal injuries in children with spina bifida and meningomyeloceles. Am J Roentgenol *95*:168, 1965.
44. Poznanski AK: Diagnostic clues in the growing ends of bone. J Can Assoc Radiol *29*:7, 1978.
45. Nellhaus G: Neurogenic arthropathies (Charcot's joints) in children. Clin Pediatr *14*:647, 1975.
46. Drummond RP, Rose GK: A twenty-one-year review of a case of congenital indifference to pain. J Bone Joint Surg *57B*:241, 1975.
47. Franklyn PP: Congenital indifference to pain. Ann Radiol *15*:343, 1972.
48. Gold RH, Mirra JM: Case report 45. Skel Radiol *2*:127, 1977.
49. Schneider R, Goldman AB, Bohne WHO: Neuropathic injuries to the lower extremities in children. Radiology *128*:713, 1978.
50. Shea JD: Pressure sores. Classification and management. Clin Orthop Rel Res *112*:89, 1975.
51. Enis JE, Sarmiento A: The pathophysiology and management of pressure sores. Orthop Rev *2*:25, 1973.
52. Griffith BH: Pressure sores. Mod Trends Plast Surg *2*:150, 1966.
53. Abel MS, Smith GR: The case of the disappearing pelvis. Radiology *111*:105, 1974.
54. Rosin AJ: Ectopic calcification around joints of paralysed limbs in hemiplegia, diffuse brain damage, and other neurological diseases. Ann Rheum Dis *34*:499, 1975.
55. Hsu JD, Sakimura I, Stauffer ES: Heterotopic ossification around the hip joint in spinal cord injured patients. Clin Orthop Rel Res *112*:165, 1975.
56. Wharton GW, Morgan TH: Ankylosis in the paralyzed patient. J Bone Joint Surg *52A*:105, 1970.
57. Tibone J, Sakimura I, Nickel VL, Hsu JD: Heterotopic ossification around the hip in spinal cord-injured patients. J Bone Joint Surg *60A*:769, 1978.
58. Roberts PH: Heterotopic ossification complicating paralysis of intracranial origin. J Bone Joint Surg *50B*:70, 1968.
59. Goldberg MA, Schumacher HR: Heterotopic ossification mimicking acute arthritis after neurologic catastrophies. Arch Intern Med *137*:619, 1977.
60. Nicholas JJ: Ectopic bone formation in patients with spinal cord injury. Arch Phys Med Rehabil *54*:354, 1973.
61. Hardy AG, Dickson JW: Pathological ossification in traumatic paraplegia. J Bone Joint Surg *45B*:76, 1963.
62. Furman R, Nicholas JJ, Jivoff L: Elevation of the serum alkaline phosphatase coincident with ectopic-bone formation in paraplegic patients. J Bone Joint Surg *52A*:1131, 1970.
63. Liberson M: Soft tissue calcification in cord lesions. JAMA *152*:1010, 1953.
64. Dejerine Mme, Ceillier A: Para-osteoarthropathies des paraplegiques par lesions medullairies: Etude clinique et radiographique. Ann Medecine *5*:497, 1918.
65. Abramson AS: Bone disturbances in injuries to the spinal cord and cauda equina (paraplegia): Their prevention by ambulation. J Bone Joint Surg *30A*:982, 1948.
66. Money RA: Ectopic para-articular ossification after head injury. Med J Aust *1*:125, 1972.
67. Hossack DW, King A: Neurogenic heterotopic ossification. Med J Aust *1*:326, 1967.
68. Freiberg JA: Para-articular calcification and ossification following acute anterior poliomyelitis in an adult. J Bone Joint Surg *34A*:339, 1952.
69. Storey G, Tegner WS: Paraplegic para-articular calcification. Ann Rheum Dis *14*:176, 1955.
70. Gunn DR, Young WB: Myositis ossificans as a complication of tetanus. J Bone Joint Surg *41B*:535, 1959.
71. Rosin AJ: Peri-articular calcification in a hemiplegic limb: A rare complication of a stroke. J Am Geriatr Soc *18*:916, 1970.
72. Nechwatal E: Early recognition of heterotopic calcifications by means of alkaline phosphatase. Paraplegia *11*:79, 1973.
73. Weiss S, Grosswasser Z, Ohri A, Mizrachi Y, Orgad S, Efter T, Gazit E: Histocompatibility (HLA) antigens in heterotopic ossification associated with neurological injury. J Rheumatol *6*:88, 1979.
74. Donath A, Muheim G, Rossier A: Valeurs des scintigraphies iteratives dans l'évaluation des calcifications ectopiques des paraplegiques. Radiol Clin Biol *43*:387, 1974.
75. Muheim G, Donath A, Rossier AB: Serial scintigrams in the course of ectopic bone formation in paraplegic patients. Am J Roentgenol *118*:865, 1973.
76. Miller LF, O'Neill CJ: Myositis ossificans in paraplegics. J Bone Joint Surg *31A*:283, 1949.
77. Damanski M: Heterotopic ossification in paraplegia: A clinical study. J Bone Joint Surg *43B*:286, 1961.
78. Shapiro RF, Utsinger PD, Wiesner KB, Resnick D, Bryan BL, Castles JJ: HLA-B27 and modified bone formation. Lancet *1*:230, 1976.
79. Radt P: Peri-articular ectopic ossification in hemiplegics. Geriatrics *25*:142, 1970.
80. Major P, Resnick D, Greenway G: Heterotopic ossification in paraplegia: A possible disturbance of the paravertebral venous plexus. Radiology *136*:797, 1980.
81. Brower TD, Akahoshi Y, Orlic P: The diffusion of dyes through articular cartilage in vivo. J Bone Joint Surg *44A*:456, 1962.
82. Maroudas A, Bullough P, Swanson SAV, Freeman MAR: The permeability of articular cartilage. J Bone Joint Surg *50B*:166, 1968.
83. Mankin HJ: Localization of tritiated cytidine in articular cartilage of immature and adult rabbits after intra-articular injection. Lab Invest *12*:543, 1963.
84. Bollet AJ: An essay on the biology of osteoarthritis. Arthritis Rheum *12*:152, 1969.
85. McKibbin B, Holdsworth FW: The nutrition of immature joint cartilage in the lamb. J Bone Joint Surg *48B*:793, 1966.
86. Hodge JA, McKibbin B: The nutrition of mature and immature cartilage in rabbits. An autoradiographic study. J Bone Joint Surg *51B*:140, 1969.
87. Ogata K, Whiteside LA, Lesker PA: Subchondral route for nutrition to articular cartilage in the rabbit. Measurement of diffusion with hydrogen gas in vivo. J Bone Joint Surg *60A*:905, 1978.
88. Greenwald AS, Haynes DW: A pathway for nutrients from the medullary cavity to the articular cartilage of the human femoral head. J Bone Joint Surg *51B*:747, 1979.
89. Reynolds JJ: Degradation processes in bone and cartilage. Calcif Tissue Res *4*(Suppl):52, 1970.
90. Thaxter TH, Mann RA, Anderson CE: Degeneration of immobilized knee joints in rats: Histological and autoradiographic study. J Bone Joint Surg *47A*:567, 1965.
91. Pool WH Jr: Cartilage atrophy. Radiology *112*:47, 1974.
92. Thompson RC Jr, Bassett CA: Histological observations on experimentally induced degeneration of articular cartilage. J Bone Joint Surg *52A*:435, 1970.
93. Ginsberg JM, Eyring EJ, Curtiss PH Jr: Continuous compression of rabbit articular cartilage producing loss of hydroxyproline before loss of hexosamine. J Bone Joint Surg *51A*:467, 1969.
94. Hall MC: Cartilage changes after experimental relief of contact in the knee joint of the mature rat. Clin Orthop Rel Res *64*:64, 1969.
95. Evans EB, Eggers GWN, Butler JK, Blumel J: Experimental immobilization and remobilization of rat knee joints. J Bone Joint Surg *42A*:737, 1960.
96. Akeson WH, Woo SLY, Amiel D, Coutts RD, Daniel D: The connective tissue response to immobility: Biochemical changes in peri-articular connective tissue of the immobilized rabbit knee. Clin. Orthop Rel Res *93*:356, 1973.
97. Trias A: Effect of persistent pressure on the articular cartilage. An experimental study. J Bone Joint Surg *43B*:376, 1961.
98. Salter RB, Field P: The effects of continuous compression on living articular cartilage: An experimental investigation. J Bone Joint Surg *42A*:31, 1960.
99. Finsterbush A, Friedman B: Early changes in immobilized rabbits knee joints: A light and electron microscopic study. Clin Orthop Rel Res *92*:305, 1973.
100. Finsterbush A, Friedman B: Reversibility of joint changes produced by immobilization in rabbits. Clin. Orthop Rel Res *111*:290, 1975.
101. Baker WD, Thomas TG, Kirkaldy-Willis WH: Changes in the cartilage of the posterior intervertebral joints after anterior fusion. J Bone Joint Surg *51B*:736, 1969.
102. Enneking WF, Horowitz M: The intra-articular effects of immobilization on the human knee. J Bone Joint Surg *54A*:973, 1972.
103. Abel MS: Sacroiliac joint changes in traumatic paraplegics. Radiology *55*:235, 1950.
104. Mason RM, Murray RS, Oates JK, Young AC: Prostatitis and ankylosing spondylitis. Br Med J *1*:748, 1958.
105. Wright V, Catterall RD, Cook JB: Bone and joint changes in paraplegic men. Ann Rheum Dis *24*:419, 1965.
106. Hunter T, Hildahl CR, Smith NJ, Dubo HIC, Schroeder ML: Histocompatibility antigens in paraplegic or quadriplegic patients with sacroiliac joint changes. J Rheumatol *6*:92, 1979.
107. Hermann E: Acute arthritis in hemiplegics. Scand J Rheumatol *1*:87, 1972.
108. Pálvölgyi R: Roentgenmorphological muscle changes in anterior horn cell lesions. Fortschr Geb Roentgenstr Nuklearmed *130*:338, 1979.
109. Roberts JB, Pankratz DG: The surgical treatment of heterotopic ossification at the elbow following long-term coma. J Bone Joint Surg *61A*:760, 1979.
110. Lagenskiold A, Michelsson JE, Videman T: Osteoarthritis of the knee in the rabbit produced by immobilization. Acta Orthop Scand *50*:1, 1979.

111. Heuwinkel R: Zur ätiologie und pathogenese der knochenneubildungen bei hirnverletzen und paraplegiken. I. Das lokale milieu — untersuchungen im frakturhamatom. Unfallheilkunde *82*:252, 1979.
112. Heuwinkel R, Schneider H-M: Zur ätiologie und pathogenese der knochenneubildungen bei hirnverletzen und paraplegikern. II. Histochemie der frakturnahen weichgewebe (enzymmuster im bereich der heilenden fraktur). Unfallheilkunde *82*:349, 1979.
113. Townsend PF, Cowell HR, Steg NL: Lower extremity fractures simulating infection in myelomeningocele. Clin Orthop Rel Res *144*:255, 1979.
114. Wenger DR, Jeffcoat BT, Herring JA: The guarded prognosis of physeal injury in paraplegic children. J Bone Joint Surg *62A*:241, 1980.
115. Khan MA, Kushner I, Freehafer AA: Sacroiliac joint abnormalities in paraplegics. Ann Rheum Dis *38*:317, 1979.
116. Wignall KB, Williamson BRJ: The chest x-ray in quadriplegia: A review of 119 patients. Clin Radiol *31*:81, 1980.
117. Hancock DA, Reed GW, Atkinson PJ: Bone and soft tissue changes in paraplegic patients. Paraplegia *17*:267, 1979–1980.
118. Ogata K, Whiteside LA: Barrier to material transfer at the bone-cartilage interface. Measurement with hydrogen gas in vivo. Clin Orthop Rel Res *145*:273, 1979.
119. Palmoski MJ, Colyer RA, Brandt KD: Joint motion in the absence of normal loading does not maintain normal articular cartilage. Arthritis Rheum *23*:325, 1980.
120. Bhate DV, Pizarro AJ, Seitam A, Mak EK: Axial skeletal changes in paraplegics. Radiology *133*:55, 1979.
121. Hunter T, Dubo HIC, Hildahl CR, Smith NJ, Schroeder ML: Histocompatibility antigens in patients with spinal cord injury or cerebral damage complicated by heterotopic ossification. Rheumatol Rehabil *19*:97, 1980.
122. Michelsson JE, Granroth G, Andersson LC: Myositis ossificans following forcible manipulation of the leg. J Bone Joint Surg *62A*:811, 1980.
123. Chantraine A, Van Ouwenaller C, Hachen HJ, Schinas P: Intra-medullary pressure and intra-osseous phlebography in paraplegia. Paraplegia *17*:391, 1979.
124. Garland DE, Blum CE, Waters RL: Periarticular heterotopic ossification in head-injured adults. Incidence and location. J Bone Joint Surg *62A*:1143, 1980.
125. Seigel RS: Heterotopic ossification in paraplegia. Radiology *137*:259, 1980.

70

NEURO-ARTHROPATHY

by Donald Resnick, M.D.

The report that first acknowledged the relationship of arthropathy and neural disease was that of Mitchell[1] in 1831, in which a patient with a spinal disorder ("caries of the lumbar spine") developed a peripheral joint affliction that did not respond to the "usual treatment by leeches, purgatives, and cooling diaphoretics."[2] Thirty-seven years later, in 1868, Charcot[3] described an apparent cause-and-effect relationship between primary lesions of the central nervous system and certain arthropathies, naming the condition "l'arthropathie des ataxiques." Charcot continued to study and to characterize the disorder during the next 15 years,[4-6] and although his description was virtually confined to patients with tabes dorsalis, the name "Charcot joint" has become synonymous with all articular abnormalities related to neurologic deficits, regardless of the nature of the primary disease.[7] Other terms applied to this articular disorder are neuroarthropathy and neurotrophic and neuropathic joint disease.[126]

ETIOLOGY AND PATHOGENESIS

Central (upper motor neuron) and peripheral (lower motor neuron) lesions can lead to neuroarthropathy. Included in a list of central lesions that may produce neuroarthropathy are syphilis, syringomyelia, meningomyelocele, trauma, multiple sclerosis, Charcot-Marie-Tooth syndrome, congenital vascular anomalies, and other causes of cord compression, injury, or degeneration; peripheral causes include diabetes mellitus, alcoholism, amyloidosis, infection (tuberculosis, yaws, leprosy), pernicious anemia, trauma, and intra-articular or systemic administration of steroids.[7] Additionally, congenital insensitivity to pain and dysautonomia produce similar alterations.

Despite the prominent role that neurologic disorders play in the development of neuroarthropathy, there is no uniform agreement on the pathogenesis of the articular changes. In fact, following early reports of this disorder, two fundamental theories of pathogenesis arose. The "French theory,"[8] as supported by Mitchell[1] and Charcot,[3] maintained that joint changes were the result of damage to the central nervous system trophic centers, which controlled nutrition of the bones and the joints, leading to atrophy of osseous and articular structures. This theory was immediately challenged by Volkmann, who maintained that unusual mechanical stresses about a weight-bearing joint in an ataxic individual led to recurrent subclinical trauma.[8] This latter concept was later championed by Virchow and became known as the "German theory."

Eloesser[9] in 1917, on the basis of the results of a series of experiments, supported the role of trauma in the development of neuropathic joints. He noted that cats' joints rendered anesthetic by posterior sensory nerve section remained intact, whereas those articulations that were subjected to additional damage developed neuropathic-like alterations. Furthermore, chemical analysis and in vitro stress studies of both denervated and normal bones failed to reveal any atrophy or inherent osseous weakening, "making untenable Charcot's theory that atrophic disturbance causing a wasting of the bone [was] at the root of these arthropathies," and suggesting that Charcot joints were due to "the sudden response of an anesthetic joint to. . .acute trauma."[2] The results of other investigations supported this concept[10] and demonstrated the obvious pattern of repetitive trauma resulting in intra-articular osseous fragments that arises in an anesthetic joint.[11]

Although additional theories emphasized the contributory role of lesions of the autonomic nervous system,[12] vascular insufficiency,[13] or infection[14] in the production of neuropathic joints, the current consensus supports the prominent role of misuse or abuse of insensitive joints in this arthropathy (Fig. 70–1). Loss of the protective sensations of pain and proprioception leads to relaxation of the supporting structures and chronic instability of the joint. In this setting, the daily stresses of normal movement produce injury, malalignment, and abnormal joint loading. Cumulative injury leads to progressive degeneration and disorganization of the articulation.[15]

The radiographic and pathologic features reflect the joint disorganization with excessive cartilaginous and osseous destruction. However, the appearances may vary with the specific etiology of the neurologic deficit. Productive changes are common-

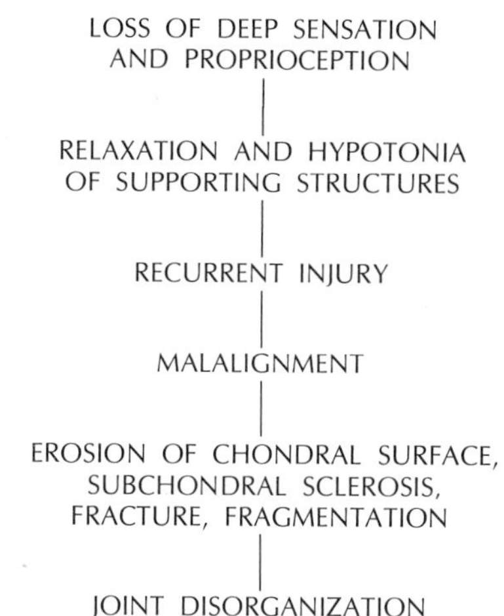

Figure 70–1. *Pathogenesis of neuroarthropathy. The probable sequential steps in the development of the joint disease are indicated.*

ly associated with central spinal cord lesions, such as trauma, tumor, or congenital malformations, and with diseases that commonly spare the sympathetic nervous system, such as tabes dorsalis and syringomyelia, whereas destructive manifestations are typically linked to peripheral nerve injuries and related to trauma, alcoholism, and diabetes, which presumably affect postganglionic nerve segments carrying sympathetic vasoconstrictive as well as sensory and motor fibers.[16] The importance in neuroarthropathy of a neurally mediated vascular reflex leading to increased osteoclastic bone resorption in hyperemic areas that are devoid of vasoconstrictive impulses has been postulated by Johnson.[17] Angiography may confirm hypervascularity,[18] although the increased blood flow may promote both lysis and sclerosis in the neuropathic joint. Associated osteonecrosis could be caused by mechanical compromise of the vascular supply produced by osseous fragmentation.[16]

Proponents of a neurovascular cause for neuroarthropathy cite the inconclusive results of Eloesser's classic experiment in cats.[125] They emphasize that osteoclastic resorption of bone due to hyperemia could explain all of the radiographic changes of this joint disease, which could be considered neurotrophic rather than neurotraumatic in nature. This mechanism is supported by histologic evidence of hypervascularity of bone, osteoclastic activity, and dilatation of haversian canals, as well as radiologic evidence of osteolysis and fracture at sites not subject to unusual trauma.[125]

GENERAL RADIOGRAPHIC AND PATHOLOGIC ABNORMALITIES

Although the pathologic and radiologic features of advanced neuroarthropathy are indeed charac-

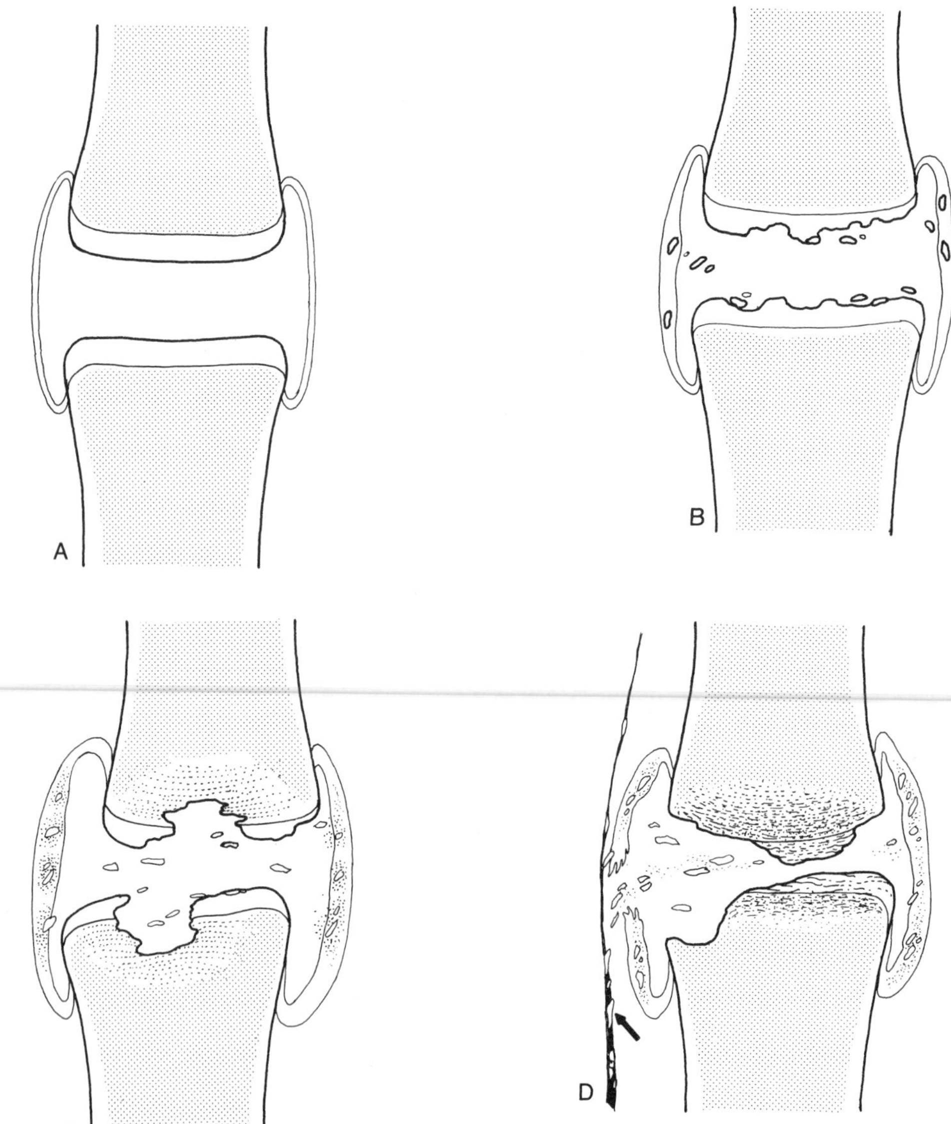

Figure 70–2. *General radiographic and pathologic abnormalities: stages of neuroarthropathy.*

A *A normal synovial articulation is illustrated.*

B *Initially, cartilaginous fibrillation and fragmentation can be observed; some of the cartilaginous debris remains attached to the chondral surface, some is displaced into the articular cavity, and some becomes embedded in the synovial membrane.*

C *Subsequently, osseous and cartilaginous destruction becomes more extensive, the embedded pieces of cartilage and bone producing local synovial irritation. Bony eburnation and subluxation are also evident.*

D *Eventually, large portions of the chondral coat are lost, sclerosis is extreme, capsular rupture can occur, and shards of bone can dissect along the soft tissue planes (arrow).*

teristic,[10, 15, 19] early features may simulate those of osteoarthritis (Fig. 70–2). Thus, cartilaginous fibrillation and erosion, subchondral trabecular thickening, and osteophytosis on pathologic examination and joint space narrowing, sclerosis, and osseous excrescences on roentgenographic examination are similar to findings in degenerative joint disease. The presence of an enlarging and persistent effusion, minimal subluxation, fracture, and fragmentation should alert the radiologist to the possibility of neuroarthropathy[20]; similarly, the finding of considerable amounts of cartilaginous and osseous debris attached to and incorporated into the synovial membrane (detritic synovitis) in a patient who is presumed to have degenerative joint disease should suggest to a pathologist that the changes may indeed represent neuropathic joint disease (Table 70–1). These early changes may show rapid progression, suggesting that microfractures exist that evolve quickly into gross fragmentation,[16, 21] and the articulation may appear to fall apart in a matter of days or weeks[22] (Fig. 70–3). The rapid nature of the evolving neuropathic process has also been verified experimentally,[9] and in clinical situations, acute subluxations or dislocations may be encountered.[23] It is the focal disruption of chondral and osseous surfaces in

Table 70–1

SOME CAUSES OF DETRITIC SYNOVITIS

Neuroarthropathy
Osteonecrosis
Calcium pyrophosphate dihydrate crystal deposition disease
Psoriatic arthritis
Osteoarthritis
Osteolysis with detritic synovitis

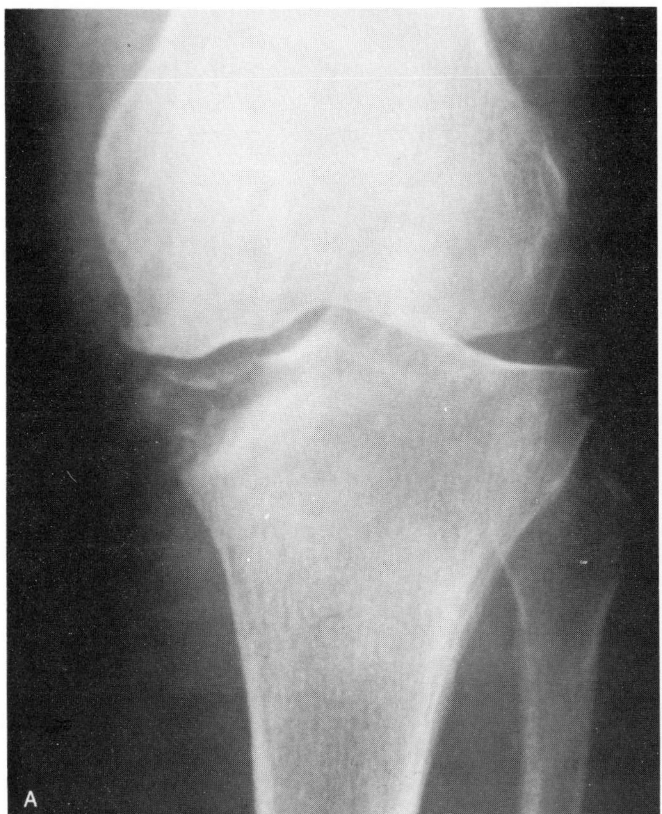

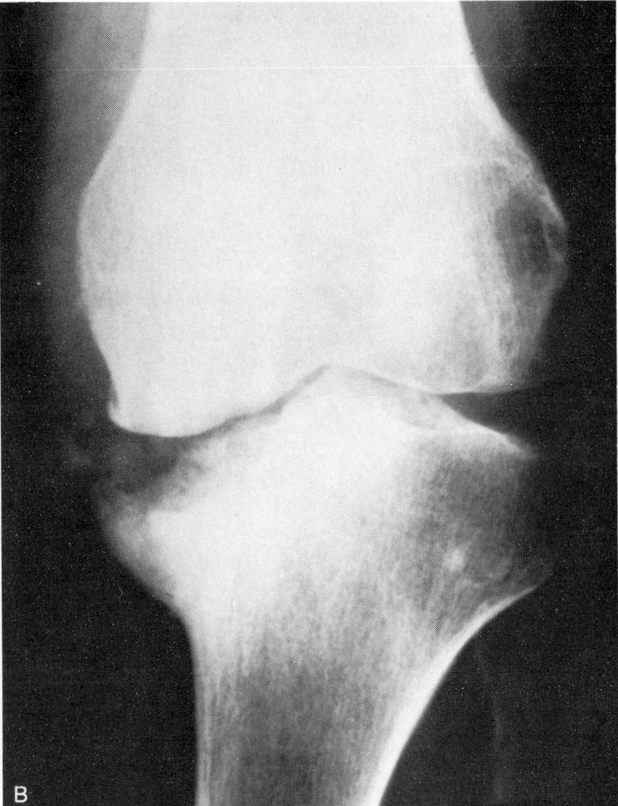

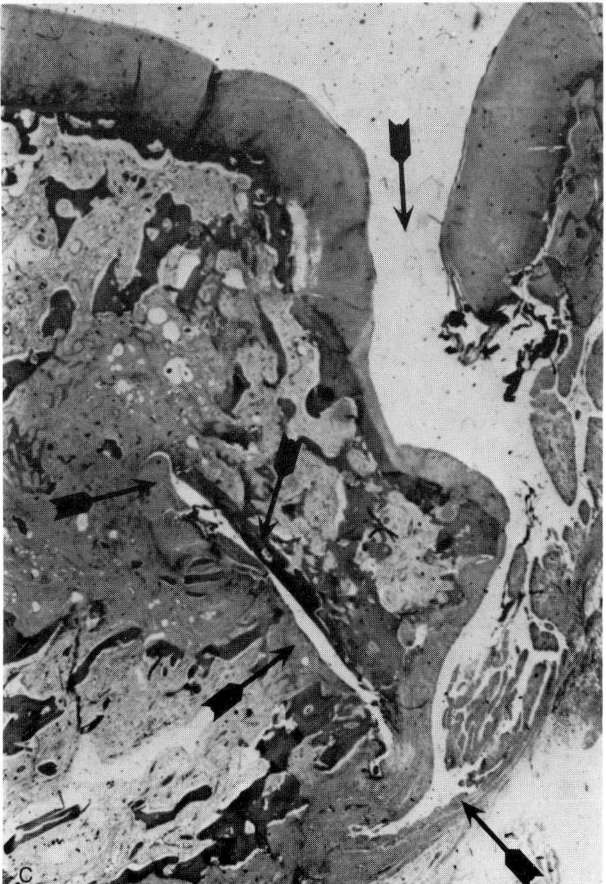

Figure 70–3. *General radiographic and pathologic abnormalities of neuroarthropathy: Rapid progression of disease.*

A, B *The appearance and progression of articular destruction can occur rapidly. Initial foci of chondral and osseous destruction can lead to fragmentation and collapse in a period of weeks. This is a patient with tabes dorsalis.*

C *This photomicrograph (3×) of the articular margin of the talus of a diabetic patient demonstrates unhealed linear microfractures, which are not visible to the naked eye or on radiographs of specimen slices (arrows). The extension of the microfracture through the subarticular bone and the cavitation at the fracture site suggest motion between adjacent surfaces. (**C,** From Feldman F, et al: Radiology 111:1, 1974.)*

the early stages of neuropathic joint disease that leads to collections of bone and cartilage debris, which are ground into the synovial and subsynovial tissues (Fig. 70–4), and that produces radiographic and pathologic clues to the nature of the articular abnormality months to years before gross fragmentation becomes evident.[24]

When an articulation is the site of more advanced abnormalities, diagnostic roentgenographic features appear, consisting of depression, absorption, and shattering of subchondral bone, osseous proliferation in the form of significant sclerosis and osteophytosis, intra-articular osseous fragments, subluxation, massive soft tissue enlargement and effusion, and fracture of neighboring bones (Fig. 70–5). On pathologic examination, the capsule is irregularly thickened by fibrous tissue and ossified, the synovial membrane is indurated with villous transformation, and considerable fluid and connective tissue adhesions are evident within the joints.[15] In the synovial membrane, fragments of cartilage and bone may reveal growth activity. In addition, diffuse metaplasia of the synovium with formation of cartilage and calcification of cartilage within the deeper layers of the membrane can be noted.[25] The embedded and metaplastic osteocartilaginous

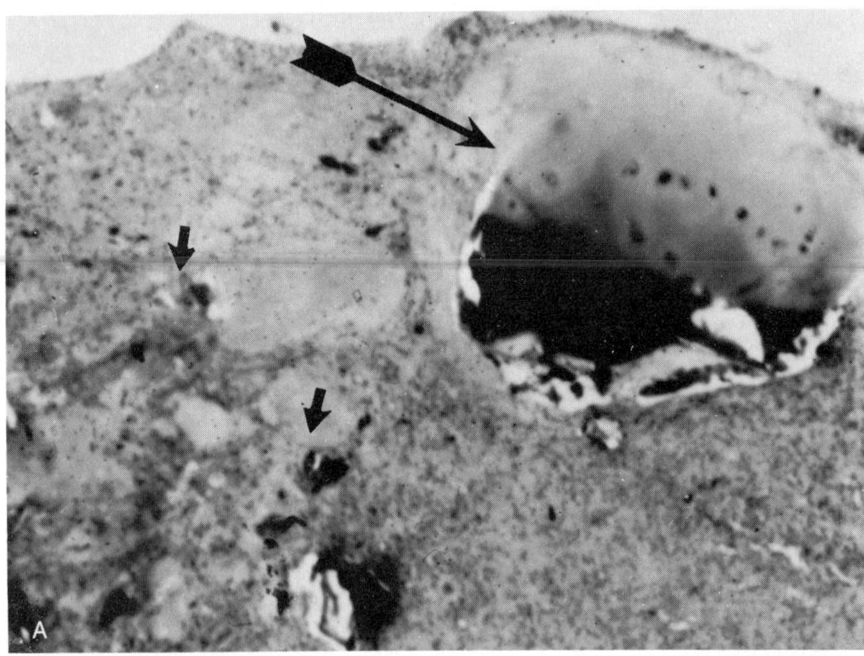

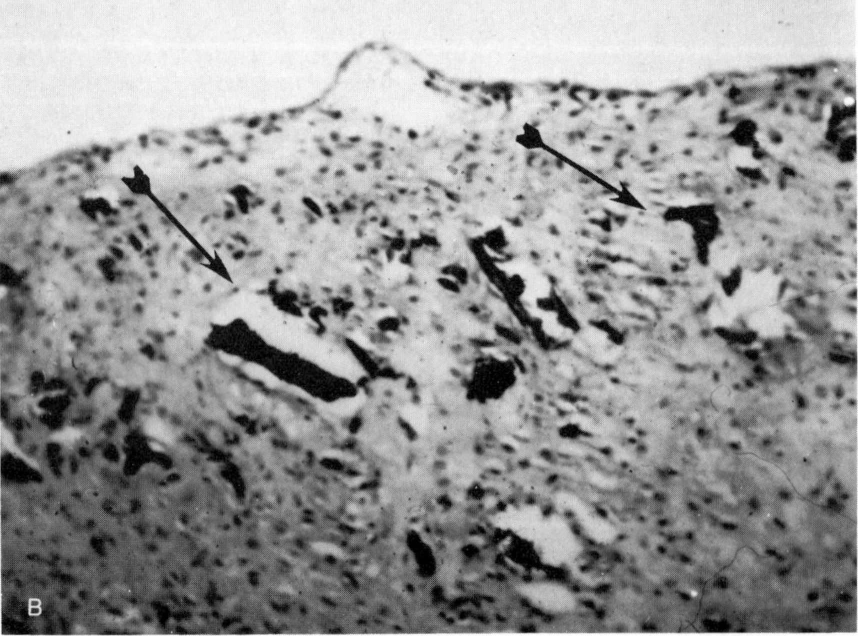

Figure 70–4. *General radiographic and pathologic abnormalities of neuroarthropathy: Detritic synovitis.*

A *Note the large fragment of recognizable articular cartilage and subchondral bone embedded within the synovium (large arrow). Other fragments of bone and cartilage are visible (small arrows) (52×).*

B *On higher magnification (160×), multiple microscopic bony spicules (arrows) are seen below the surface of the scarred synovial membrane. Note the reactive histiocytosis and young fibroblasts in the background.*

(From Feldman F, et al: Radiology 111:1, 1974.)

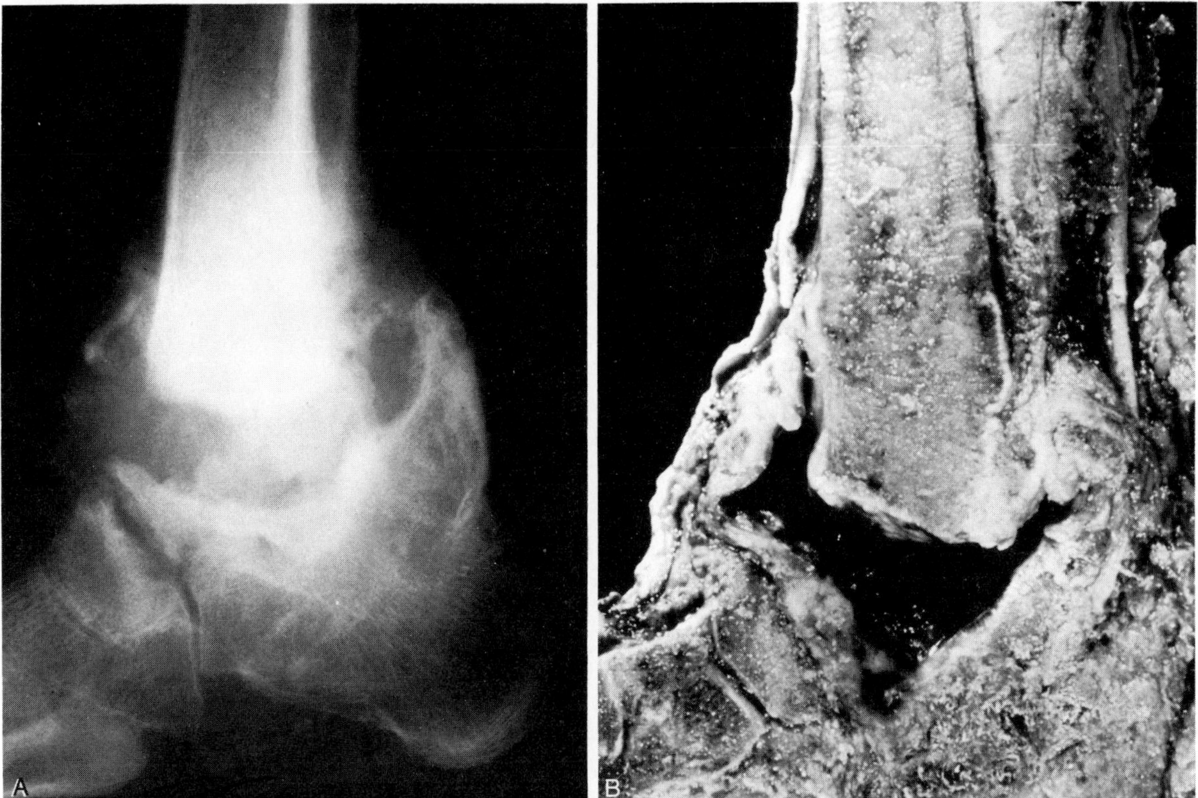

Figure 70–5. *General radiographic and pathologic abnormalities of neuroarthropathy: Advancing lesions.*

A *Note soft tissue swelling and considerable fragmentation and resorption of the talus, tibia, and fibula, with extreme sclerosis, osteophytosis, and intra-articular osseous bodies.*

B *On a sagittal section of the amputated extremity, the degree of osseous resorption and fragmentation is apparent, as are synovial and capsular hypertrophy and distention.*

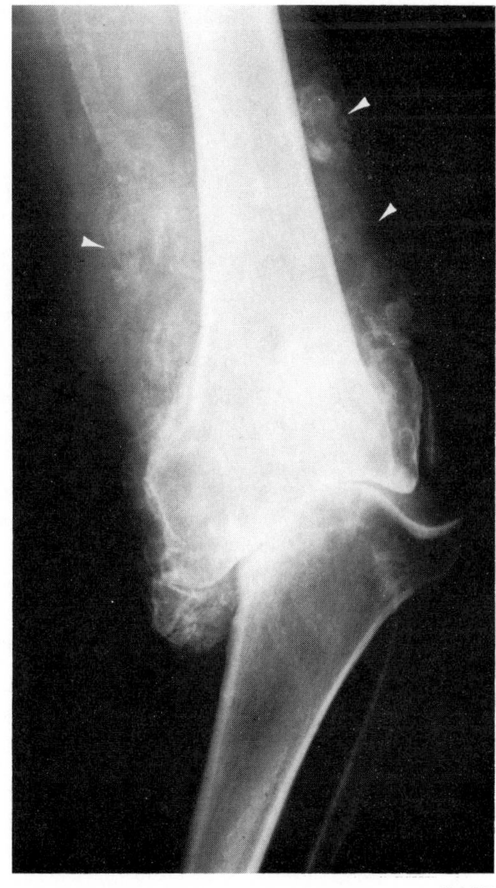

Figure 70–6. *General radiographic and pathologic abnormalities of neuroarthropathy: Migration of bony shards. In this patient with syphilis, numerous fragments of bone originating from the destroyed articular surfaces have moved into the far recesses of the joint or migrated along adjacent tissue planes (arrowheads).*

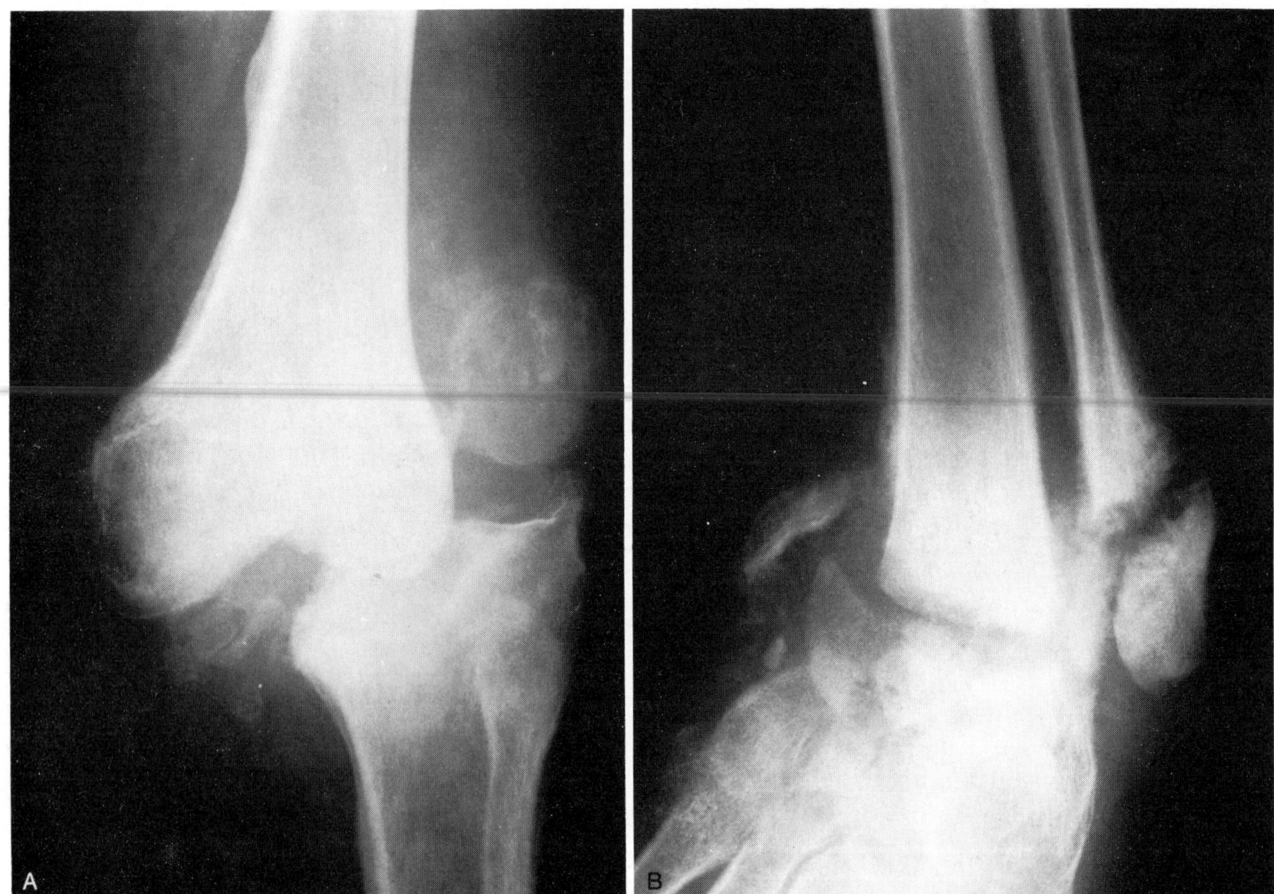

Figure 70–7. *General radiographic and pathologic abnormalities of neuroarthropathy: Fractures and subluxations.*

A *Gross disorganization of the joint in a tabetic patient is characterized by lateral subluxation of the tibia on the femur, lateral patellar dislocation, soft tissue swelling, osseous fragmentation and sclerosis, and periostitis.*

B *In a different patient with the same disease, note the angular deformity of the ankle with fragmentation, sclerosis, and fractures. Periostitis and soft tissue swelling are evident.*

C–F *This patient with diabetes mellitus developed spontaneous fractures of the distal tibia and fibula* **(C)**, *which became displaced in the following few weeks* **(D)**. *After amputation, a photograph* **(E)** *and radiograph* **(F)** *of a coronal section of the specimen indicate severe displacement and angulation. The patient had been relatively asymptomatic during this period.*

Illustration continued on the opposite page

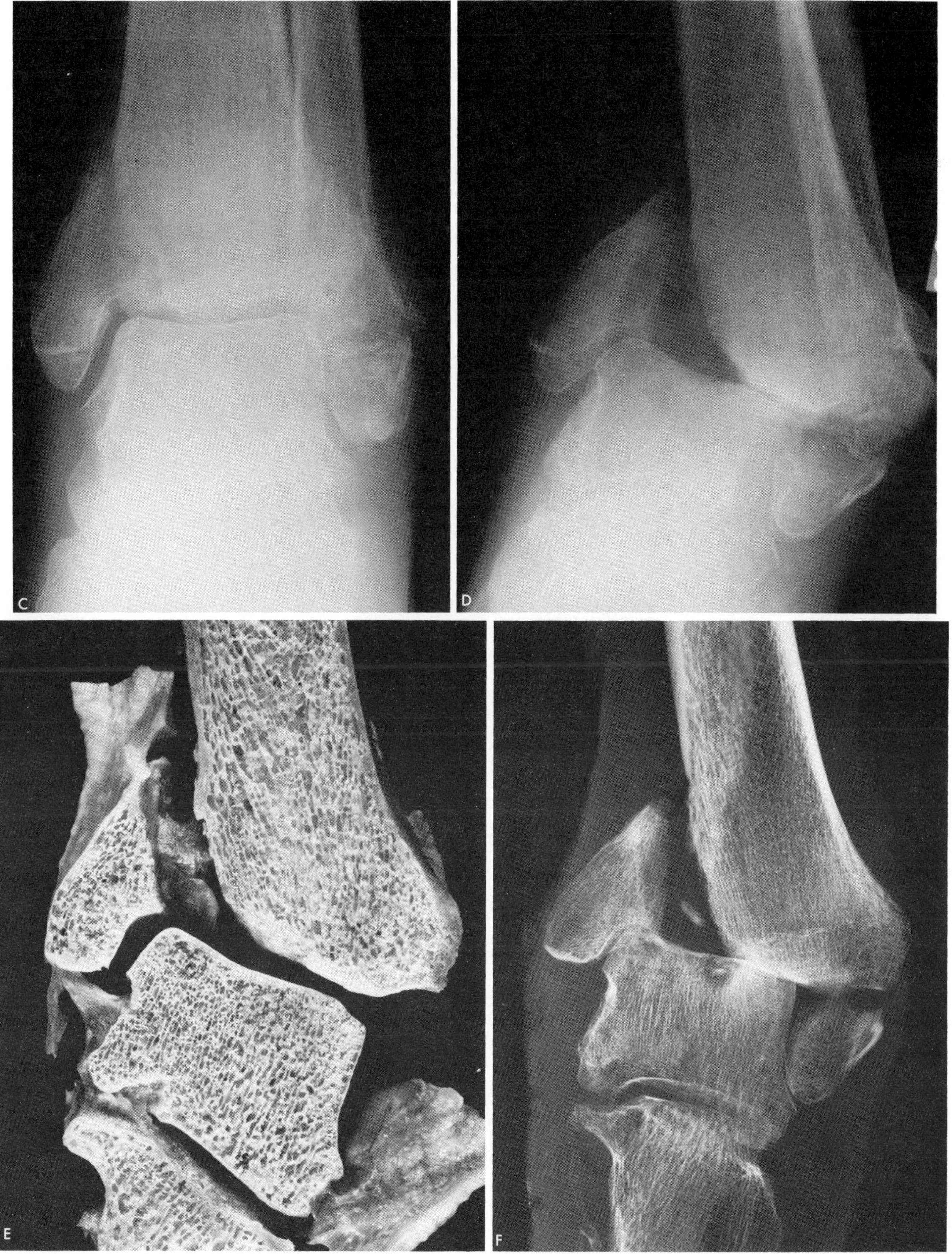

Figure 70–7. Continued

bodies in the synovium of neuropathic articulations produce radiographically detectable calcific and ossific dense lesions, which may eventually become far removed from the joint itself[26, 27] (Fig. 70–6). This latter phenomenon represents migration of bone shards into the distant recesses of an enlarging joint cavity, into a neighboring synovial cyst, or along muscle tissue planes. In some instances, the radiodense shadows later disappear.[26]

The articular ends of the bones that are contained within a neuropathic joint become devoid of cartilage, the surface being replaced by fibrous tissue or fibrocartilage.[15] The exposed subchondral bone appears eburnated and shiny, and it may be deformed, distorted, or worn away by the apposing articular surface. Marginal exostoses can reach considerable size, although others fragment and disintegrate. Malalignment with angular deformity, subluxation, or dislocation leads to increased stress on the articular bone, contributing to sclerosis and gross fractures (Fig. 70–7). Fracture lines can originate in the subchondral region and extend extra-articularly, or they may occur at a site distant from the joint — e.g., the diaphysis of a tubular bone. Fracture repair with periostitis is encountered, and the exuberant callus may merge with the endosteal sclerosis and marginal osteophytic lips; in some patients, pseudarthrosis develops at sites of fracture or, following healing, refracture occurs.

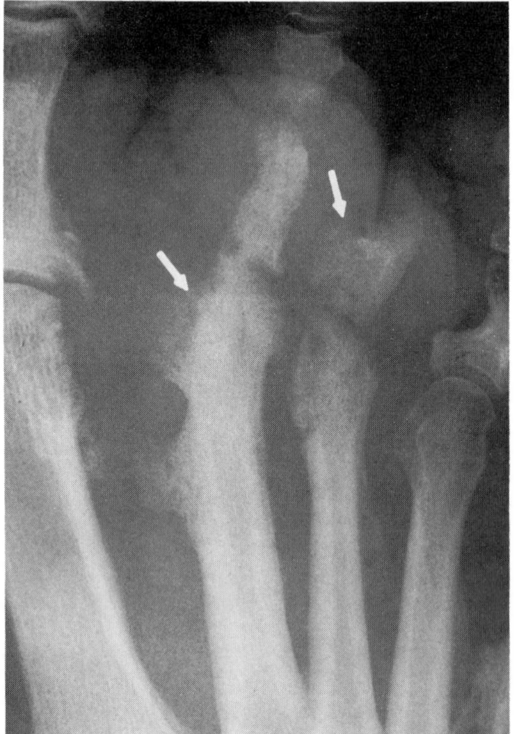

Figure 70–8. *General radiographic and pathologic abnormalities of neuroarthropathy: superimposed infection. In diabetic patients, neuroarthropathy of superficial articulations such as the metatarsophalangeal joints is frequently complicated by osteomyelitis and septic arthritis. In such instances, the ill-defined contour of the involved bones (arrows) usually allows diagnosis of both conditions.*

In long-standing neuroarthropathy, the resulting radiographic picture is that of a disorganized joint, characterized by simultaneously occurring bone resorption and formation. The degree of sclerosis, osteophytosis, and fragmentation in this articular disorder is greater than that in any other process. Yet, the bone shards and irregular articular surfaces that are produced by the considerable osseous fragmentation and collapse accompanying this disease are generally well defined and sharp. Poorly marginated, "fuzzy" bone contours, as occur in septic arthritis, are not evident unless infection has become superimposed on the neuropathic process. This latter complication, however, is not infrequent, especially in diabetic patients and in those articulations that are superficially located in the body (e.g., metatarsophalangeal joints) (Fig. 70–8).[127] Intra-articular bony fusion is an uncommon manifestation of neuroarthropathy at any site, with the exception of the spine. In fact, attempts at arthrodesis in this disease are frequently unsuccessful.

SPECIFIC DISORDERS

Although Charcot's original description of neuroarthropathy emphasized its occurrence in tabes dorsalis,[3-6] Charcot anticipated that similar abnormalities might accompany other neurologic processes, and, in fact, he described neuropathic joint changes in two nontabetic individuals with spinal injuries and hemiplegia.[2] Subsequent reports of neuroarthropathy in poliomyelitis,[28] syringomyelia,[2] peripheral nerve injuries,[29] and diabetes mellitus[30] confirmed the accuracy of this anticipation. It is now known that neuroarthropathy can accompany many disorders that lead to sensory disturbances, includ-

Table 70–2

COMMON SITES OF INVOLVEMENT IN NEUROARTHROPATHY

Disease	Sites of Involvement
Tabes dorsalis	Knee, hip, ankle, spine
Syringomyelia	Glenohumeral joint, elbow, wrist, spine
Diabetes mellitus	Metatarsophalangeal, tarsometatarsal, intertarsal joints
Alcoholism	Metatarsophalangeal, interphalangeal joints
Amyloidosis	Knee, ankle
Congenital indifference to pain	Ankle, intertarsal joints
Meningomyelocele	Ankle, intertarsal joints
Congenital sensory neuropathy/hereditary sensory radicular neuropathy	Knee, ankle, intertarsal, metatarsophalangeal, interphalangeal joints
Idiopathic	Elbow

ing the utilization of intra-articular or oral corticosteroids.[31] Although some motor function is fundamental in the pathogenesis of the articular lesions, patients with both sensory and motor loss can develop neuroarthropathy, presumably related to vigorous physical therapy.

Although the radiographic and pathologic features of neuroarthropathy are generally similar in these various disorders, certain subtle differences can be evident. Furthermore, the distribution of the articular abnormalities varies among these disorders, providing an important clue to a proper specific diagnosis (Table 70–2).

Tabes Dorsalis

It is estimated that 5 to 10 per cent of patients with tabes dorsalis will reveal neuroarthropathy.[15] The articulations of the lower extremity are affected in 60 to 75 per cent of cases; those of the upper extremity or elsewhere are involved in the remaining instances. The knee (Fig. 70–9*A*), the hip (Fig. 70–9*B*), the ankle (Fig. 70–9*C*), the shoulder, and the elbow (Fig. 70–9*D*) are altered, in descending order of frequency. Other involved sites include the joints of the forefoot, midfoot, vertebral column, and fingers, and the temporomandibular and sternoclavicular articulations.[15, 16, 32-34] Monoarticular involvement predominates but polyarticular alterations are not unusual, and bilateral symmetric changes affecting as many as eight joints may be encountered.[15]

Most typically, painless swelling, deformity, weakness, and instability represent the clinical manifestations of tabetic neuropathic joints. However, affected articulations may indeed be painful, although the mild nature of the discomfort appears relatively insignificant in the face of extensive soft tissue swelling. The soft tissue prominence results from sizable joint effusions, dissection of fluid into periarticular structures, and capsular and soft tissue hypertrophy. In some instances, patients present with evidence of a spontaneous fracture of the neighboring bone, which, when combined with significant capsular and ligamentous laxity, leads to considerable deformity or angulation. The radiographs will reveal typical features of neuroarthropathy, which, in this disease, include exuberant eburnation and fragmentation. Abnormalities in certain laboratory parameters, such as the *Treponema pallidum* Immobilization (TPI) test, the fluorescent treponemal antibody absorption (FTA-ABS) test, the Venereal Disease Research Laboratory (VDRL) test, and the Automated Reagin Test (ART), although not without false-positive and false-negative results, provide important clues to the specific diagnosis.

Axial neuroarthropathy is not uncommon in tabes[7, 16, 35-40] and may represent 20 per cent of all cases of neuropathic disease encountered in tabetic patients. It is most frequently seen in men and in the sixth and seventh decades of life, predominantly in the lumbar spine, less commonly in the thoracic spine, and rarely in the cervical spine.[7, 16, 41] One or more vertebrae can be affected. As opposed to the situation in peripheral neuropathic joint disease, axial neuroarthropathy is often symptomatic, leading to significant pain; this symptom is related to the preservation of some nerve fibers and the compression of nerve roots by intervertebral disc herniation, osteophytes, or debris.[7, 16, 42, 43] Clinical signs include abnormal spinal curvature (kyphosis or scoliosis) and motor and sensory disturbances. Rarely, paraplegia is evident.[42, 43]

Radiographic features of tabetic axial neuroarthropathy may be productive or destructive in nature.[16] In the former group, changes such as intervertebral disc space and apophyseal joint narrowing, sclerosis, and osteophytosis can simulate findings in degenerative joint disease. However, the productive alterations of neuroarthropathy are generally more exaggerated than those of degenerative joint disease, representing "osteoarthritis with a vengeance."[16] Thus, eburnation may be florid, intervertebral disc space narrowing may be complete, osteophytes can reach mammoth proportions, and apophyseal joint subluxation with neighboring bony sclerosis can be profound (Fig. 70–10). Fracture with osseous fragmentation in spinal and paraspinal locations as well as malalignment can also be evident. The resulting roentgenographic findings, when severe, are unique to this disorder, differing from the spinal manifestations of degenerative joint disease, infection, skeletal metastasis, and Paget's disease (Table 70–3).

Less commonly, osteolytic or destructive changes predominate in axial neuroarthropathy. These can appear acutely and progress rapidly, leading to significant bony dissolution in a period of weeks or months. Anterior (intervertebral discs and vertebral bodies) or posterior (apophyseal joints) structures can be more extensively affected, and the irregular destructive changes that ensue can produce osseous surfaces resembling the pieces of a jigsaw puzzle.[16] The appearance of this lytic variety of neuroarthropathy can resemble that in infection or skeletal metastasis.

Pathologic features in axial and appendicular skeletal sites of tabetic neuroarthropathy resemble those of other neuropathic disorders (Fig. 70–11). Initial "stress" or microfractures precede the more extensive destructive and productive changes. Degeneration of adjacent nerves and superimposed infection can be encountered.

Syringomyelia

It has been estimated that 20 to 25 per cent of patients with syringomyelia develop neuroarthrop-

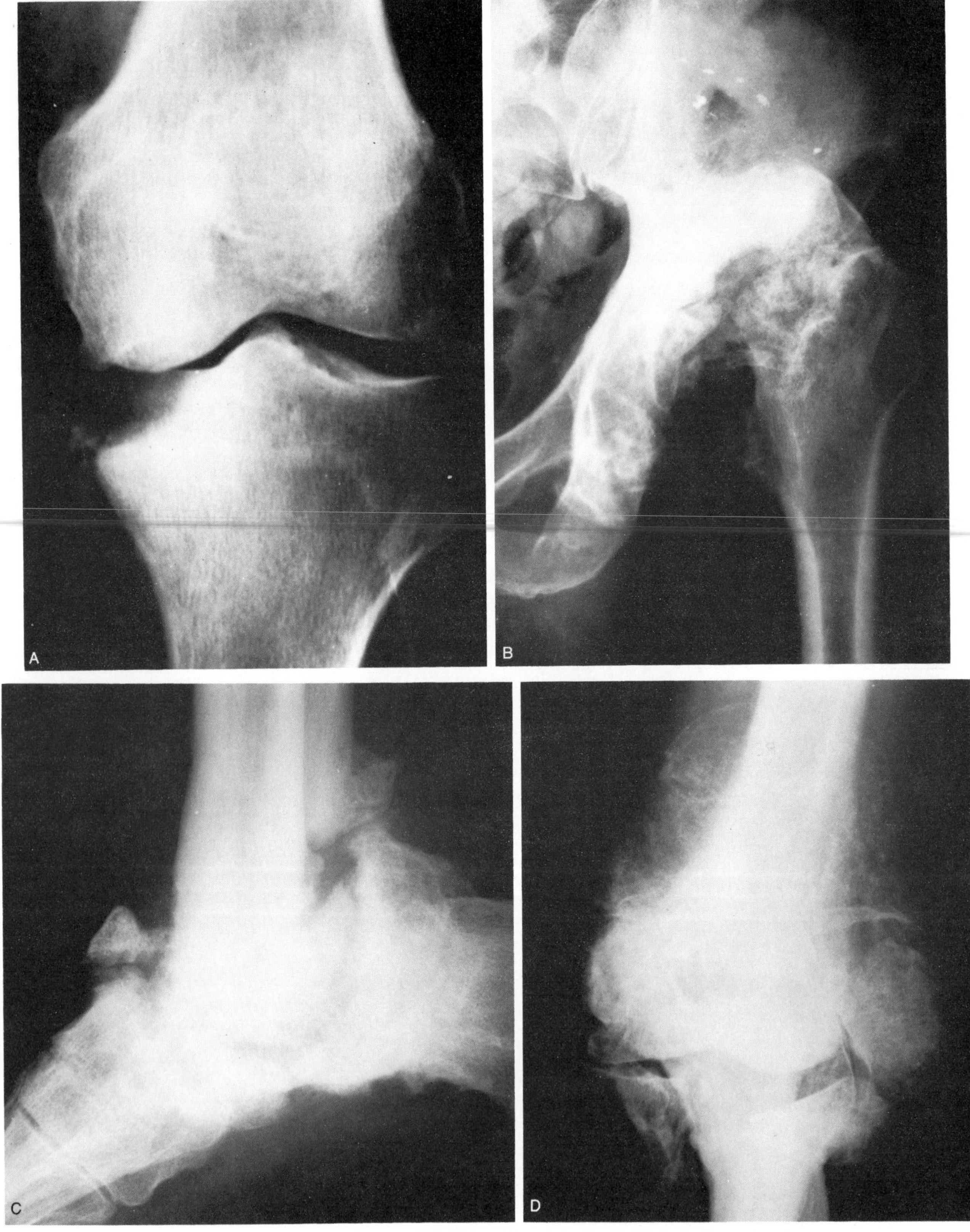

Figure 70–9. *Tabes dorsalis: Neuroarthropathy of the appendicular skeleton. Examples of neuropathic joint disease of the knee* **(A)**, *the hip* **(B)**, *the ankle* **(C)**, *and the elbow* **(D)** *are shown. In all cases, sclerosis and fragmentation are prominent, and deformities, subluxation, and dislocation may be evident.*

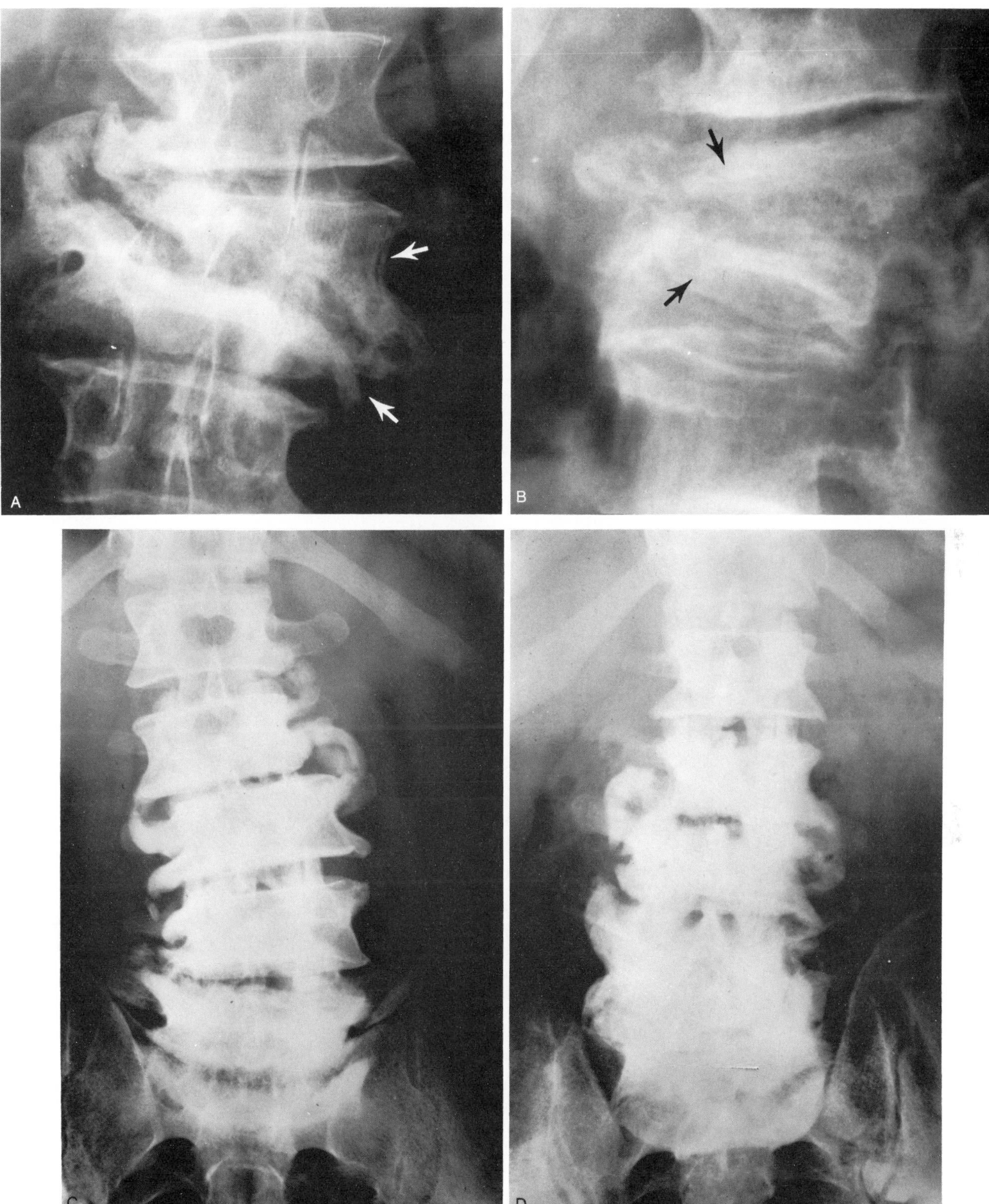

Figure 70–10. *Tabes dorsalis: Neuroarthropathy of the axial skeleton.*

A, B *Localized disease. Frontal and lateral radiographs of the lumbar spine reveal extensive disorganization involving two vertebral bodies (arrows) and the intervening intervertebral disc. Note the loss of intervertebral disc space, sclerosis, and osteophytosis. The resulting osseous contours are relatively well defined.*

C, D *Generalized disease. Two examples of widespread abnormalities in the lumbar spine consisting of loss of height of multiple intervertebral discs, extreme sclerosis, osteophytes, subluxation, and vertebral angulation are shown.*

Table 70–3

AXIAL NEUROARTHROPATHY AND ITS DIFFERENTIAL DIAGNOSIS

	Neuroarthropathy	Intervertebral Osteochondrosis	Infection	CPPD Crystal Deposition Disease[1]
Sites of involvement	One or more levels Predominates in thoracolumbar spine[2]	Frequently widespread Cervical, thoracic, or lumbar spine	Frequently one level Predominates in thoracolumbar spine	Widespread Cervical, thoracic, or lumbar spine
Intervertebral disc spaces	Narrowed or obliterated	Narrowed	Narrowed or obliterated	Calcification; narrowed
Bony sclerosis	May be extreme	Usually mild to moderate	Variable[3]	Variable[5]
Osteophytosis	May be massive	Absent or moderate in size	Usually absent	Variable
Bony fragmentation	May be extreme	Absent or minimal	Usually absent	Variable[6]
Subluxation, angulation	Common	Rare	Variable[4]	Variable
Paravertebral mass	Usually absent	Absent	Common	Absent

[1]CPPD, calcium pyrophosphate dihydrate.
[2]Influenced by the specific underlying disorder.
[3]Sclerosis more typical in pyogenic spondylitis and in black patients with tuberculous spondylitis.
[4]In tuberculosis, kyphosis may become prominent.
[5]Discal calcification may appear without sclerosis, or disc space loss may be combined with moderate or severe sclerosis.
[6]In some patients, fragmentation and deformity may be severe, especially in the cervical spine.

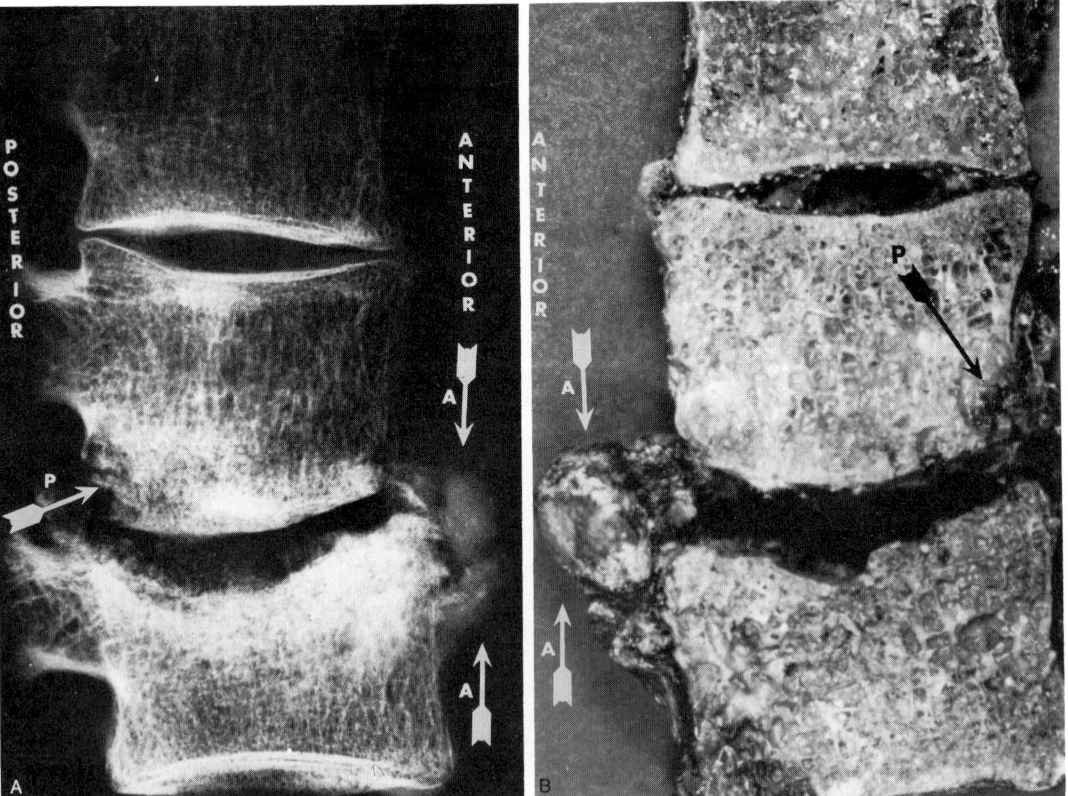

Figure 70–11. Tabes dorsalis: Neuroarthropathy of the axial skeleton. A radiograph and photograph of a sagittal section of the lumbar spine in another syphilitic patient reveal subarticular fractures, particularly evident in the lower vertebral body, which provide the pathogenesis for the radiopacity, crumbling margins, and displacement of detritus into adjacent paravertebral tissue (arrows marked A). Note the loss of bone along the posterior margin of the upper vertebra (arrows marked P). (From Feldman F, et al: Radiology 111:1, 1974.)

athy.[15, 36, 44-49] Although the radiographic and pathologic characteristics of neuropathic joint disease in syringomyelia resemble those of tabes, striking differences in the distribution of the abnormalities can be noted. Neuroarthropathy in syringomyelia is common in the joints of the upper extremity, especially the glenohumeral articulation, as well as the elbow (Fig. 70–12 *A*, *B*) and the articulations of the wrist and fingers (Fig. 70–12 *C*). Approximately 75 to 80 per cent of syringomyelia patients with neuroarthropathy demonstrate abnormalities in one or more of these sites; the remainder have changes in the articulations of the lower extremity or the spine. In the lower extremity, the knee, the ankle, and the hip are affected with approximately equal frequency; in both the upper and lower limbs, bilateral symmetric changes are not so common as in tabes.[15] Changes in the spine are

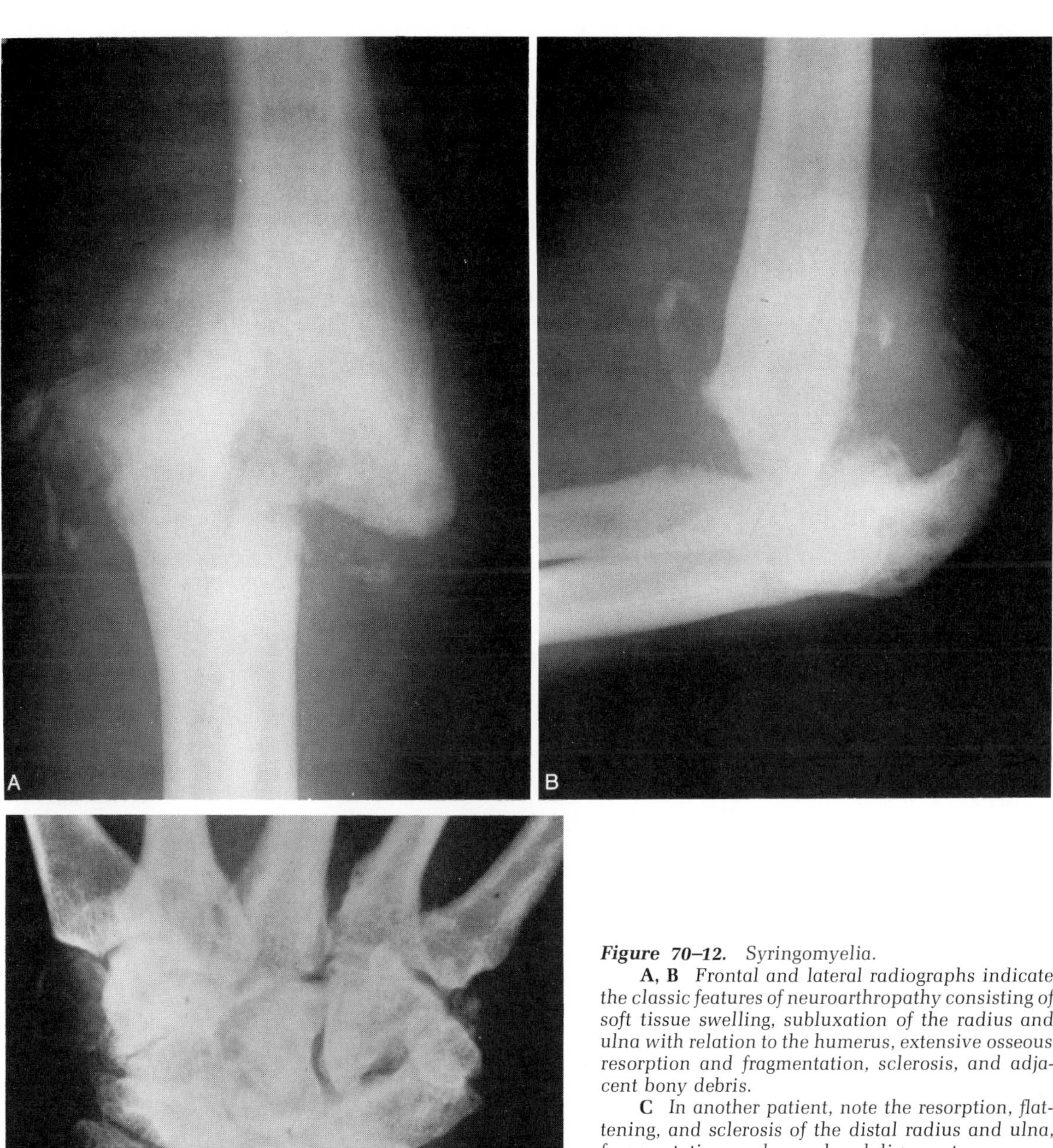

Figure 70–12. Syringomyelia.

A, B *Frontal and lateral radiographs indicate the classic features of neuroarthropathy consisting of soft tissue swelling, subluxation of the radius and ulna with relation to the humerus, extensive osseous resorption and fragmentation, sclerosis, and adjacent bony debris.*

C *In another patient, note the resorption, flattening, and sclerosis of the distal radius and ulna, fragmentation, and carpal malalignment.*

most characteristic in the cervical region, although localized alterations in the thoracic and lumbar segments are encountered.

Generally, neuroarthropathy occurs during the later phases of syringomyelia, although occasionally joint findings may be the initial or predominant manifestation of the disease. Accompanying or preceding neurologic changes due to spinal cord damage are variable and include decreased reflexes, ataxia, bladder disturbances, muscle atrophy, and spastic weakness or paralysis.[118] Myelography can demonstrate spinal cord enlargement, especially in the cervical region, and laboratory analysis can indicate increases in cerebrospinal fluid pressure and protein content.

The clinical, radiographic, and pathologic alterations of neuroarthropathy in syringomyelia are similar to those in tabes, although the incidence of spontaneous fractures of the diaphyses and metaphyses of tubular bones may be somewhat less in the former disease. Rapid and painless swelling of the affected region appears.[50] The degree of fragmentation and sclerosis of the humeral head can be striking, and these changes may be associated with fractures of neighboring bones, including the scapula, clavicle, and ribs. In the spine, productive or destructive changes can predominate, and the appearance in the initial stages of the disease can simulate degenerative joint disease.

Diabetes Mellitus

The complexity of diabetic arthropathy is well known.[30, 51-65] The first description of a typical painless "Charcot joint" in a patient with diabetes mellitus belongs to Jordan in 1936,[66] an association that was subsequently emphasized by Bailey and Root in 1947.[67] Since the latter report, countless descriptions of "neuropathic," "neuroarthropathic," "osteoarthropathic," "osteopathic," "neurogenic," and "atrophic" articular changes in this disease have appeared, and the wide variation of terms applied to the alterations reflects a continuing debate as to their pathogenesis.[30] Loss of pain and loss of proprioceptive sensation appear to be of major importance in diabetic neuroarthropathy,[68] and, in the presence of repetitive micro- or macrotrauma, initiate the changes. The role of ischemia may be important[69] despite the preservation of peripheral pulses[30, 70]; small blood vessel disease may act synergistically with other factors, such as neuropathy, trauma, or infection, to promote the osteoarticular alterations. However, adequate blood supply is a prerequisite for the occurrence of osteolysis,[63] and the prominent role of vascular insufficiency in the initiation of diabetic osteoarthropathy remains controversial.[30] That infectious processes are commonly superimposed on neuropathic changes in the diabetic patient is well recognized,[53, 71] especially in superficially located articulations. The addition of suppuration to neuroarthropathy can accentuate and accelerate the joint destruction, although recovery from the infection may be followed by remarkable reconstitution of the bony architecture.[30]

Although the exact incidence of neuropathic joint changes in diabetic individuals is not clear, this disease appears to be overtaking both syphilis and syringomyelia as the leading cause of neuroarthropathy. Sinha and co-workers[30] noted neuroarthropathic alterations in 0.15 per cent of 68,000 consecutive hospital admissions of diabetic patients, although these investigators speculated that the true incidence was greater because of the asymptomatic nature of the articular lesions. Typically, diabetic neuroarthropathy appears in a man or a woman with long-standing diabetes mellitus, generally in the fifth to seventh decades of life. Changes in younger and older patients, however, can occur.[72] The joints of the forefoot and midfoot are most commonly altered, although the ankle, the knee, the spine, and the articulations of the upper extremity, in descending order of frequency, can be affected.[52] Painless soft tissue swelling, skin ulceration, and joint deformity are encountered. Mono- or polyarticular involvement can occur; spontaneous arrest of clinical and radiographic changes at one site may be followed by the onset and progressive growth of alterations at a previously unaffected joint.[30]

Destructive or resorptive bony abnormalities can predominate, depending upon the location of the neuroarthropathy.[54] In the intertarsal or tarsometatarsal articulations, osseous fragmentation, sclerosis, and subluxation or dislocation can be prominent and the complete disintegration of one or more tarsal bones can occur rapidly.[54, 119, 120] (Figs. 70–13 to 70–15). Talar disruption and dorsolateral displacement of the metatarsals in relation to the cuneiforms and cuboid bones are characteristic, and the resulting radiographic picture may resemble that which is observed in an acute "Lisfranc's fracture-dislocation"[65] (Fig. 70–16). At the metatarsophalangeal joints, osseous resorption is frequent, leading to partial or complete disappearance of the metatarsal heads and proximal phalanges with tapering or "pencil-pointing" of phalangeal and metatarsal shafts[54, 62, 63] (Fig. 70–17). Occasionally, the bases of the proximal phalanges may broaden, forming a cup,[54] an appearance which has been termed "intrusion," "mortar and pestle," "bulbous," "pencil and cup," or "balancing pagoda."[64] With continued forefoot involvement, progressive resorption of phalanges and dorsiflexion and foreshortening of the toes appear. Concomitant ulceration of soft tissues over a bony prominence due to downward subluxation of the proximal phalangeal head leads to osteomyelitis or septic arthritis or both.

Although less frequent than changes in the forefoot or midfoot, ankle involvement can be detect-

Text continued on page 2442

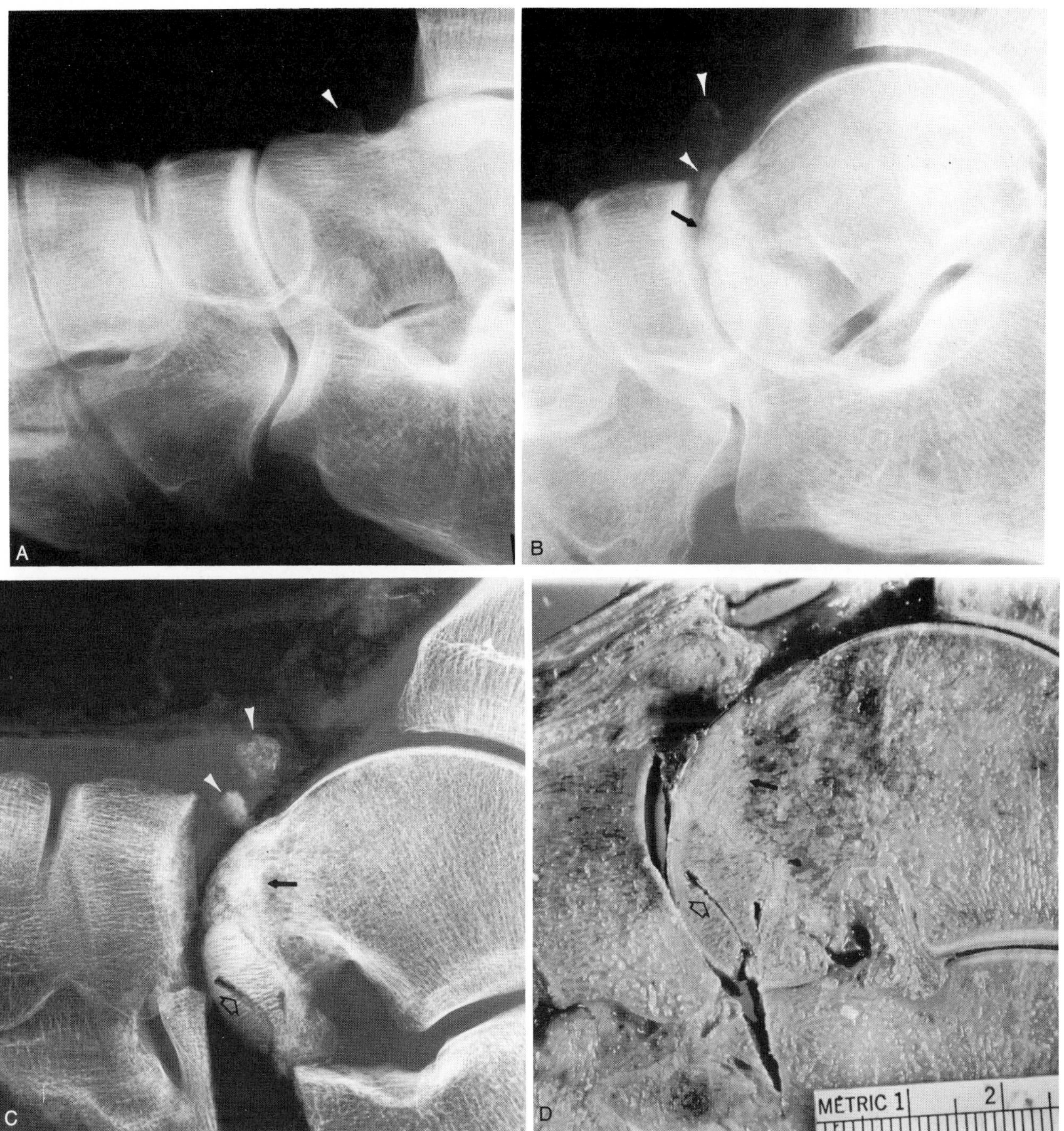

Figure 70–13. *Diabetes mellitus: Intertarsal joints. A 32 year old patient with diabetes mellitus developed neuroarthropathy without signs of infection.*

A *An initial radiograph reveals a talar bony outgrowth (arrowhead) but is otherwise unremarkable.*

B *Four months later, resorption and sclerosis of the articular surface of the distal talus (arrow) are associated with fragmentation (arrowheads) of the dorsal surface of the bone, including the previously noted outgrowth.*

C, D *A radiograph and photograph of a sagittal section of the amputated foot show the sclerosis (closed arrow) and fragmentation (arrowheads). An artifact produced by the band-saw (open arrow) is also evident.*

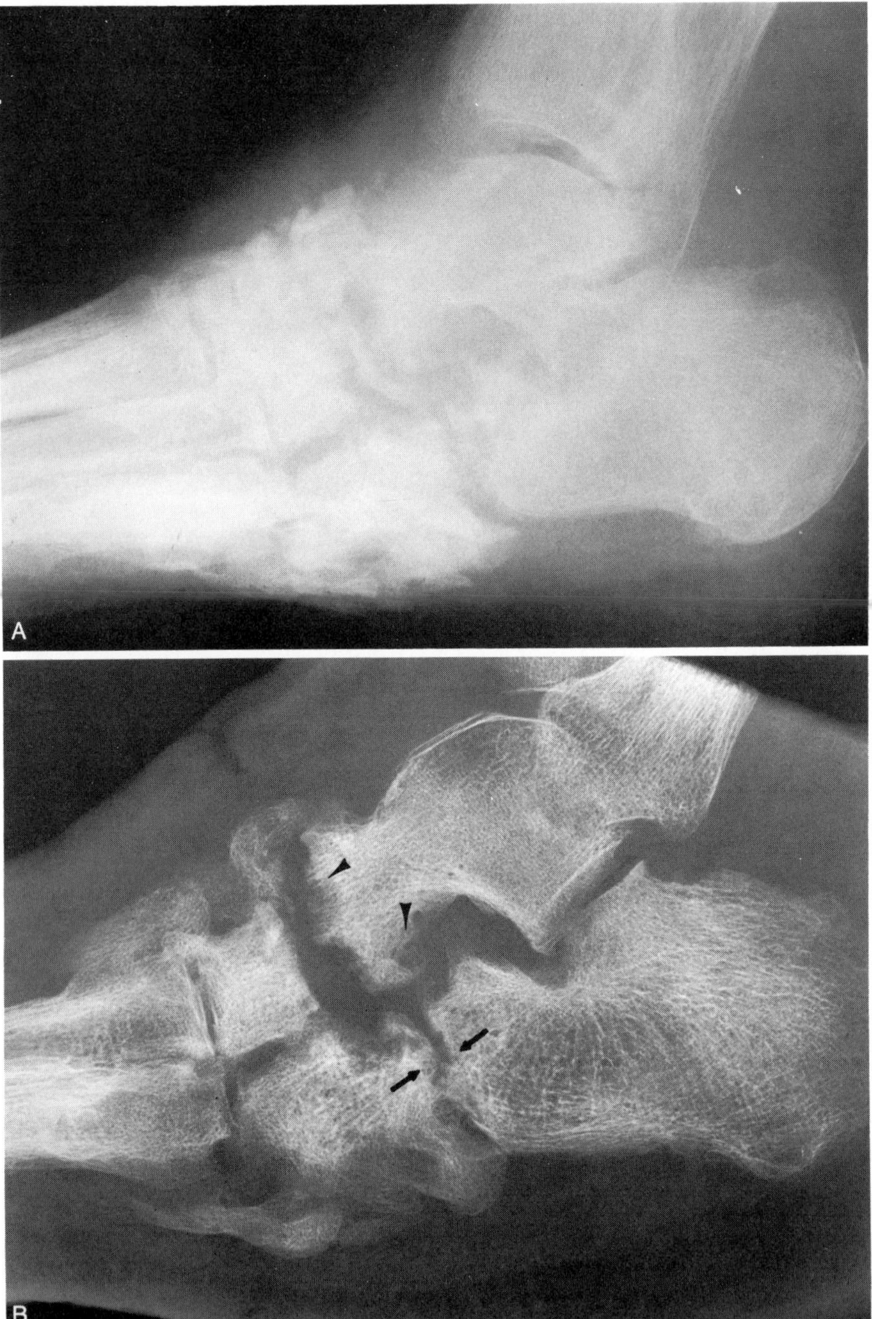

Figure 70–14. *Diabetes mellitus: Intertarsal and tarsometatarsal joints. This 55 year old patient with diabetes mellitus had signs of neuroarthropathy and infection, with soft tissue ulcerations.*

A *The radiograph reveals articular destruction throughout the midfoot. Note, in addition to eburnation, the ill-defined or fuzzy appearance to the osseous margins (compare with Figure 70–13).*

B *A lateral sagittal section of the amputated foot reveals extensive involvement of the anterior talocalcaneonavicular joint (arrowheads) and calcaneocuboid joint (arrows). The poorly marginated osseous destruction and fragmentation are evident. Most of the navicular bone has been resorbed.*

Illustration continued on the opposite page

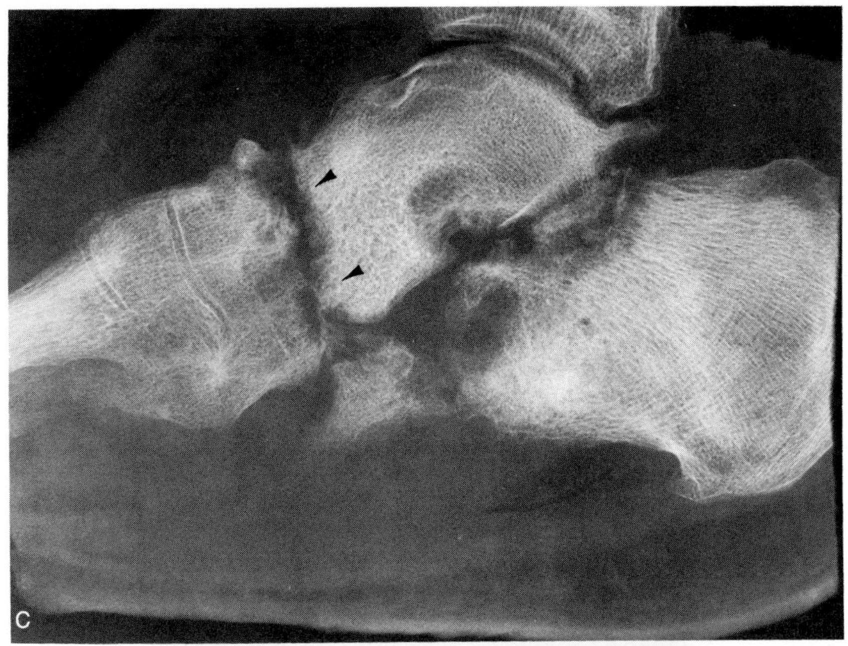

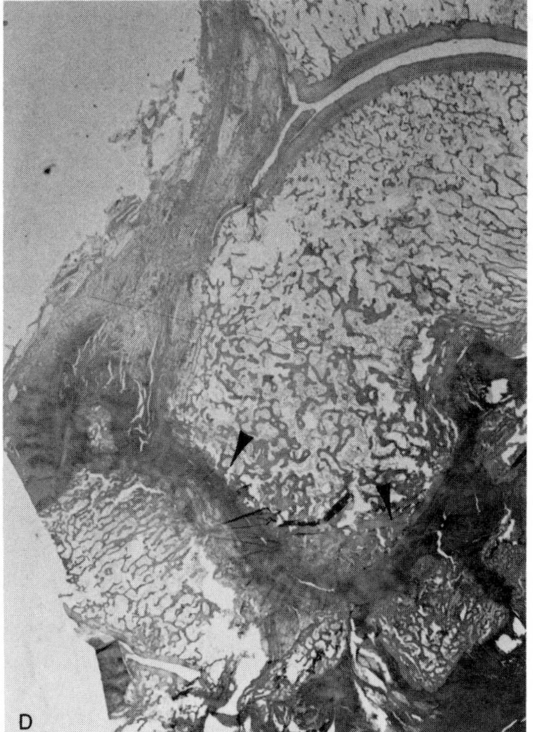

Figure 70–14. Continued

C *On a more medial sagittal section, the destruction of the talocalcaneonavicular joint (arrowheads) is again evident. Note the absence of a recognizable navicular bone and the degree of calcaneal involvement.*

D *A photomicrograph (2×) of the section in* **C** *indicates fibrous ankylosis of the talocalcaneonavicular joint (arrowheads) and subchondral sclerosis. Observe the intact articular cartilage of the ankle joint.*

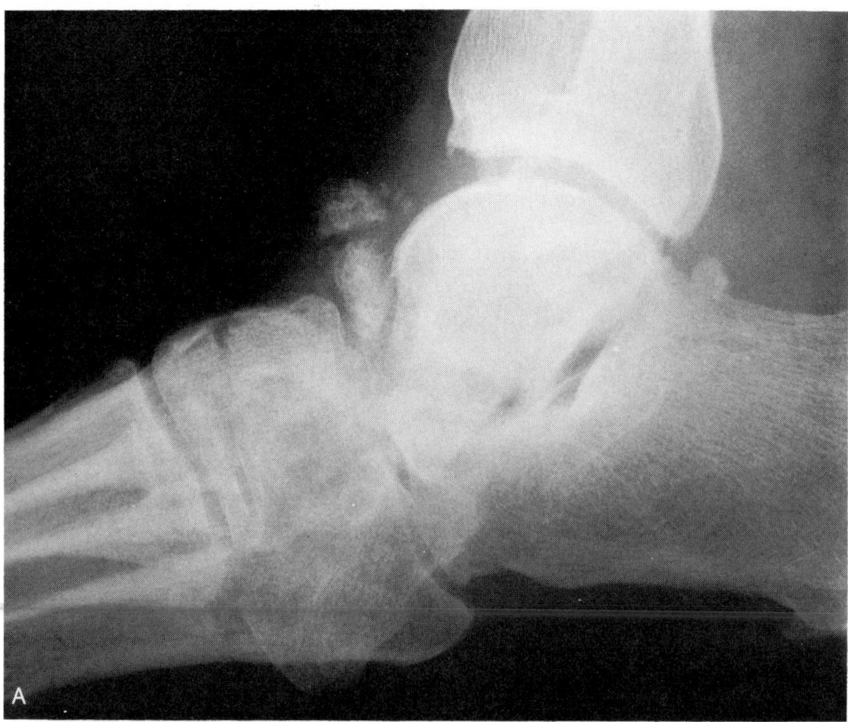

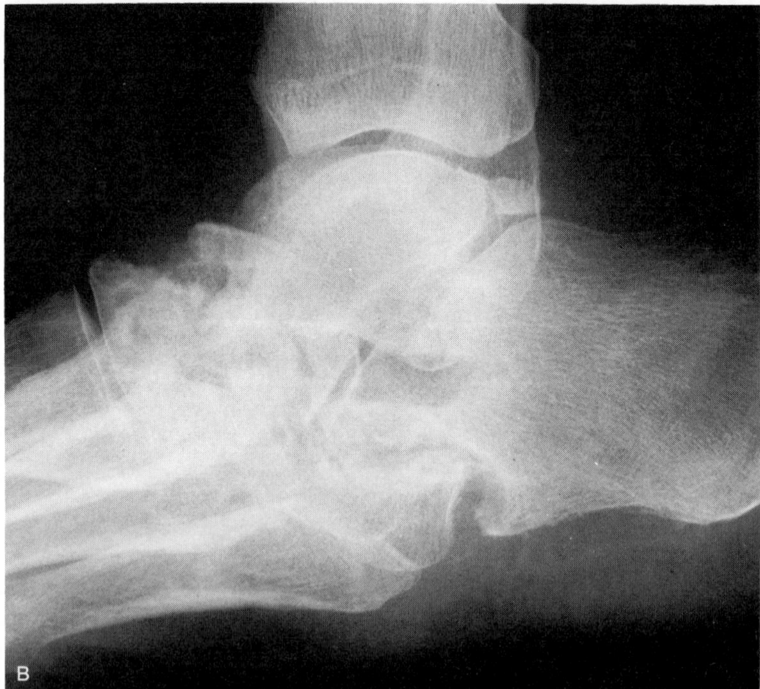

Figure 70–15. *Diabetes mellitus: Intertarsal joints.*

A *Typical fragmentation and sharply defined osseous debris characterize the involvement of the dorsal aspect of the talus and the entire navicular bone in this patient without signs of infection.*

B *In a different individual, talonavicular and calcaneocuboid areas are predominantly affected.*

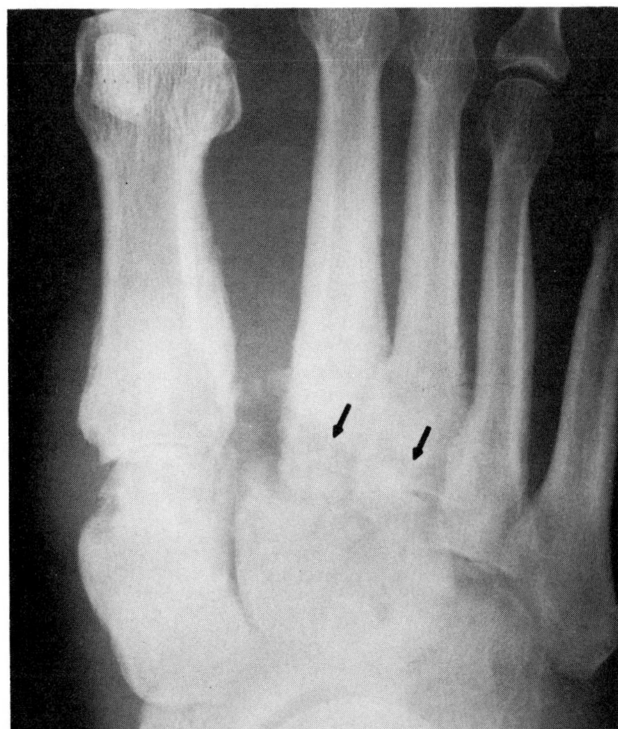

Figure 70–16. *Diabetes mellitus: Tarsometatarsal joints. Note the lateral displacement of the bases of the metatarsals (arrows) with respect to the tarsals. This finding, combined with soft tissue swelling and fragmentation, resembles a Lisfranc's fracture-dislocation.*

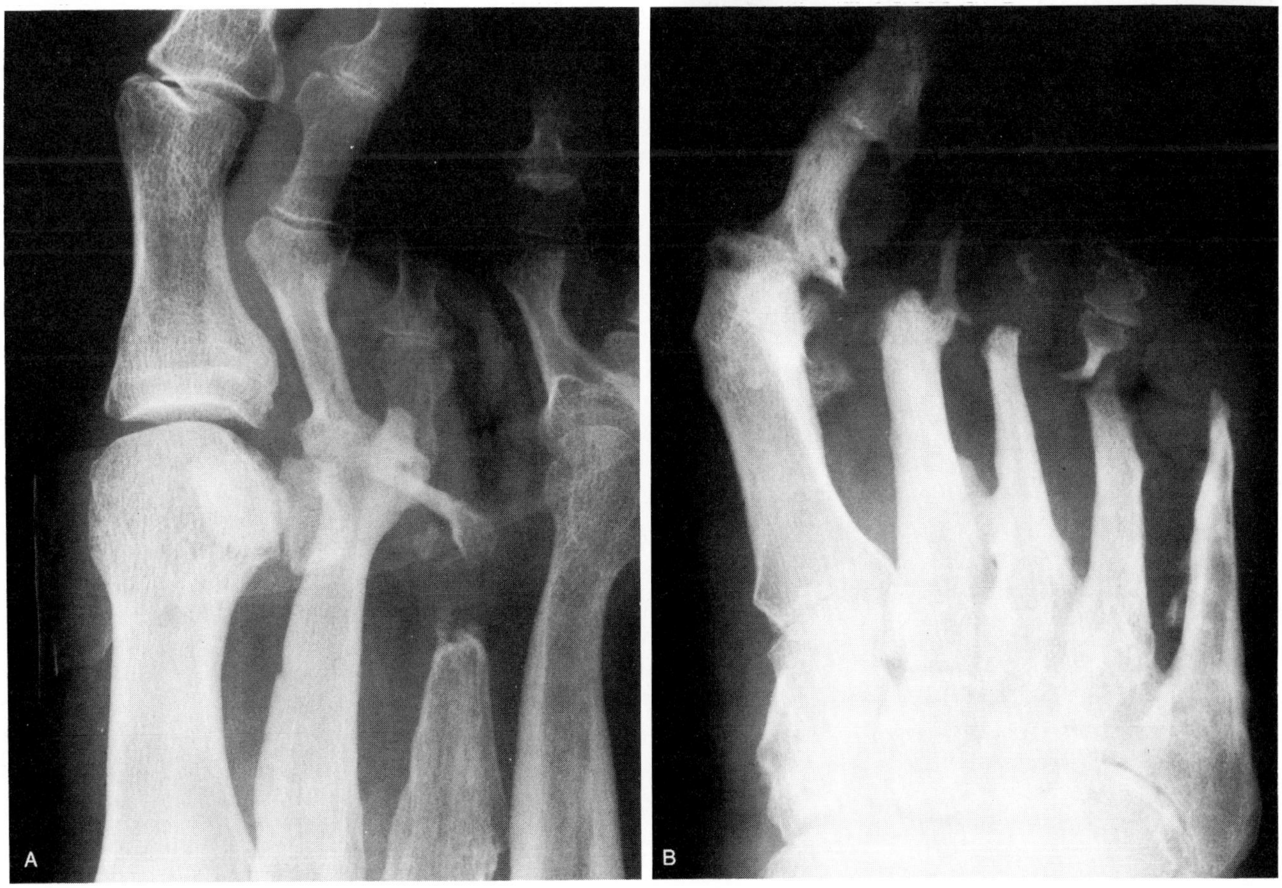

Figure 70–17. *Diabetes mellitus: Metatarsophalangeal and interphalangeal joints.*

A, B *Neuroarthropathy and infection in the forefoot of a diabetic patient can combine to produce bizarre abnormalities consisting of osteolysis of distal metatarsals and proximal phalanges, with tapering of the osseous contours. The changes can be exaggerated due to surgical removal of some of the bony fragments.*

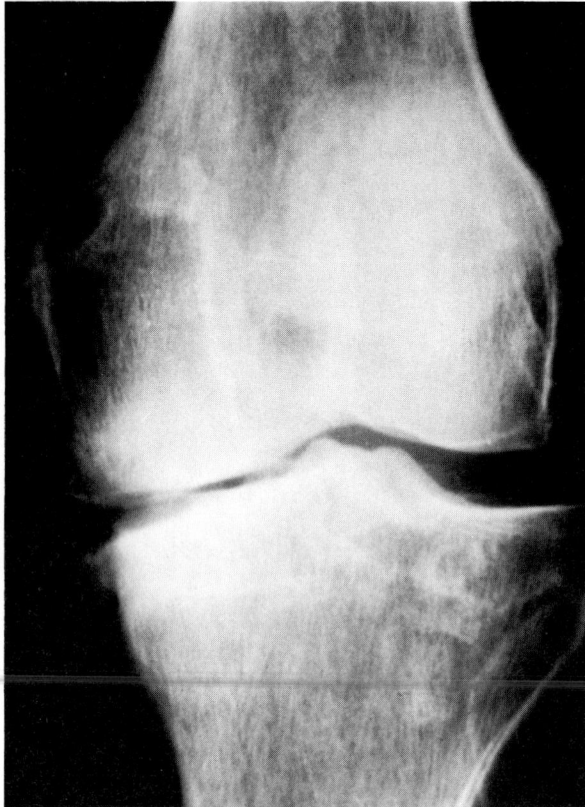

Figure 70–18. Diabetes mellitus: Knee. Neuroarthropathic abnormalities in this diabetic patient consist of sclerosis and flattening of the medial femoral condyle and tibial plateau. The changes could easily be interpreted as degenerative joint disease, although they are slightly more severe.

ed.[56, 60] A history of severe trauma is common in diabetic individuals with ankle changes,[30] and significant fragmentation, eburnation, and dislocation can be seen. Knee abnormalities are indeed rare (Fig. 70–18).

Reports of changes in the articulations of the upper extremities are limited.[59, 64] Sensory neuropathy is not infrequent in the upper limbs[73, 74] and can apparently lead to neuropathic abnormalities in the glenohumeral joint, elbow, wrist, and hand. The changes in the shoulder consist of joint space loss, humeral head deformity, subchondral lysis and sclerosis, cystic changes, and subluxation[59] (Fig. 70–19). Although fragmentation may be less frequent and prominent about the joints of the upper limbs, cases with severe bone fracture, eburnation, and dissolution are seen. Flexion contracture of the hand can accompany diabetic neuropathy. Subchondral and periarticular cystic bony changes about the shoulder and the hands are more frequent in diabetic than in nondiabetic individuals, although their relationship to neuropathic or "degenerative" disease remains speculative.[59]

Diabetic axial neuroarthropathy may be generalized or localized in distribution.[16, 75] The resulting radiographic changes, which include destruction of vertebral bodies, sclerosis, osteophytosis, fragmentation, bony ankylosis, and spinal angulation, resemble those in tabes or syringomyelia.

The pathologic aberrations accompanying neuroarthropathy in the diabetic patient are not significantly different from those in other neurologic disorders.[30, 72, 76, 77] Articular cartilage and osseous destruction with the appearance of debris in intra-articular and intrasynovial locations is typical. Alterations in the blood vessels and nerves of diabetic patients have also been recorded.[78, 79]

Alcoholism

Although peripheral neuropathy may be evident in as many as 30 per cent of alcoholic patients who are examined at a hospital,[80] reports of neuroarthropathy in these individuals are infrequent. Only a few descriptions of this articular complication in alcoholic patients had appeared[81, 82] prior to the report by Thornhill and colleagues[80] of 10 such patients with neuroarthropathy in the feet. These patients had prolonged histories of heavy alcoholic intake and revealed soft tissue ulceration, edema, increased skin pigmentation, and peripheral neuropathy, as

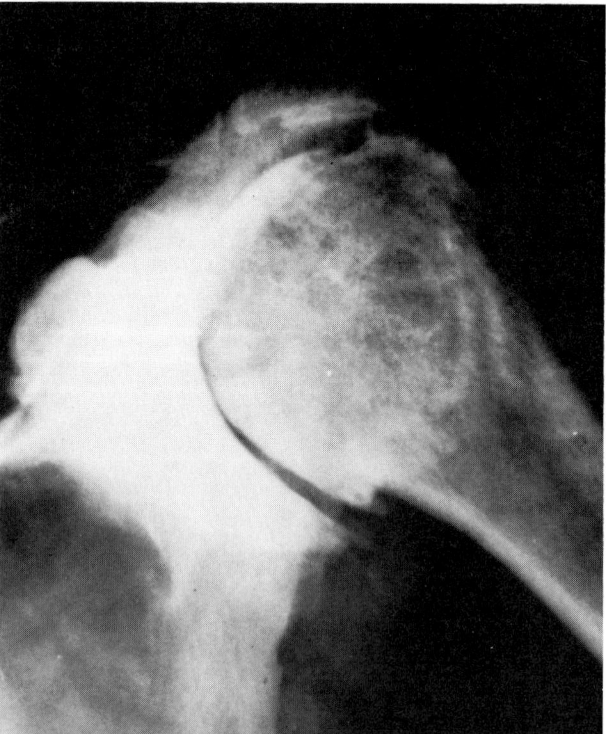

Figure 70–19. Diabetes mellitus: Glenohumeral joint. The findings include joint space narrowing, sclerosis, cyst formation, and osteophytosis. Although these changes might be misinterpreted as osteoarthritis, the history of diabetes mellitus, the presence of neurologic abnormality on clinical examination, and the degree of sclerosis on radiographic examination should suggest the correct diagnosis. Furthermore, osteoarthritis of the glenohumeral joint is unusual.

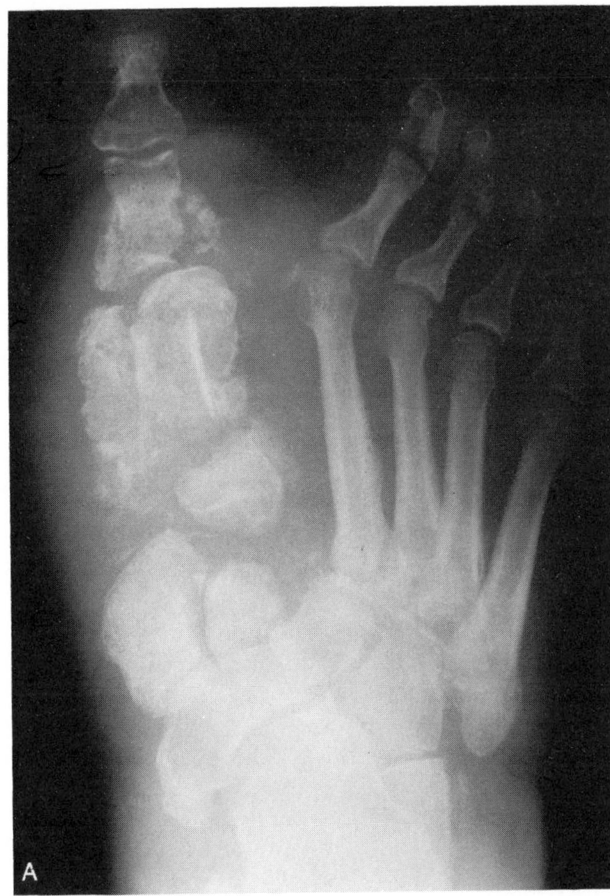

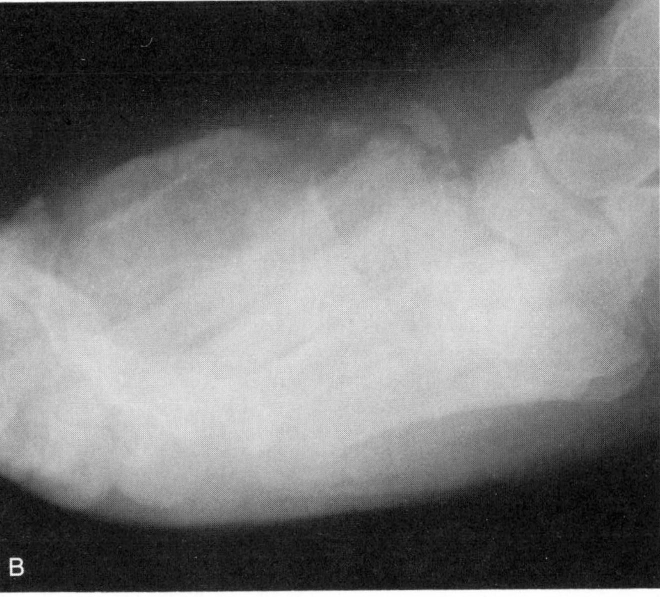

Figure 70–20. Alcoholism. This man with chronic alcoholism who had severe peripheral neuropathy developed painless swelling and subsequent infection (staphylococcal) of the foot. He was not diabetic. The radiographic findings are consistent with neuroarthropathy with or without osteomyelitis, although the extent of such changes in association with alcoholic neuropathy is indeed unusual. Observe soft tissue swelling, fracture, fragmentation, and new bone formation about the metatarsal and phalanx of the great toe, fragmentation of the cuneiforms, and lateral displacement of the metatarsal bases. The bony detritus appears remarkably well defined.

well as roentgenographic changes consistent with neuroarthropathy. The radiographic findings included soft tissue swelling, atrophy of phalangeal and metatarsal bones, osteolysis of terminal phalanges, subluxation, sclerosis, and pathologic fractures, and they were reminiscent of those accompanying diabetic neuropathic disease (Fig. 70–20). Infection was frequent (e.g., *Staphylococcus albus*), although its role in the articular disorder could not be ascertained. Furthermore, the incidence and contribution of diabetes mellitus to the clinical and radiographic features in this study were not clear.

Amyloidosis

Neuropathy, which is encountered in certain variants of amyloidosis,[83, 84] is not commonly associated with neuroarthropathy despite an impairment of sensory more than of motor function. Occasionally, patients with amyloidosis with or without additional plasma cell dyscrasias will develop neuropathic joint disease.[85, 86] The knee and the ankle appear to be the predominant sites of involvement. Vascular amyloid infiltration in nerve tissue can be demonstrated on histologic examination[86] (see Chapter 56).

Congenital Indifference to Pain

This condition was first described in 1932 by Dearborn.[87] Although pain sensation is decreased, there may be normal perception of touch and temperature and normal tendon reflexes. It is generally believed that the abnormalities lie somewhere in the cerebral cortex; the nerve endings in the skin and periosteum may be normal.[88]

The neurologic deficit can be recognized in infancy or childhood. A decreased or absent reaction to pain, scars on the tongue or finger related to burns or infections, corneal opacities resulting from unnoticed foreign bodies, and aggressive behavior may be found.[89] These clinical manifestations, coupled with progressive deformities, may lead to radiographic evaluation with demonstration of typical skeletal abnormalities[89-96] (Fig. 70–21).

Schneider and co-workers[95] have characterized the skeletal lesions in congenital indifference to pain (and related disorders) into fractures of the metaphysis and diaphysis of long bones; epiphyseal separations; neuroarthropathy; and soft tissue ulcerations. These injuries, which are often unrecognized and untreated, can lead to severe disability and are more frequent in the lower extremity than in the upper extremity. Diaphyseal and metaphyseal fractures re-

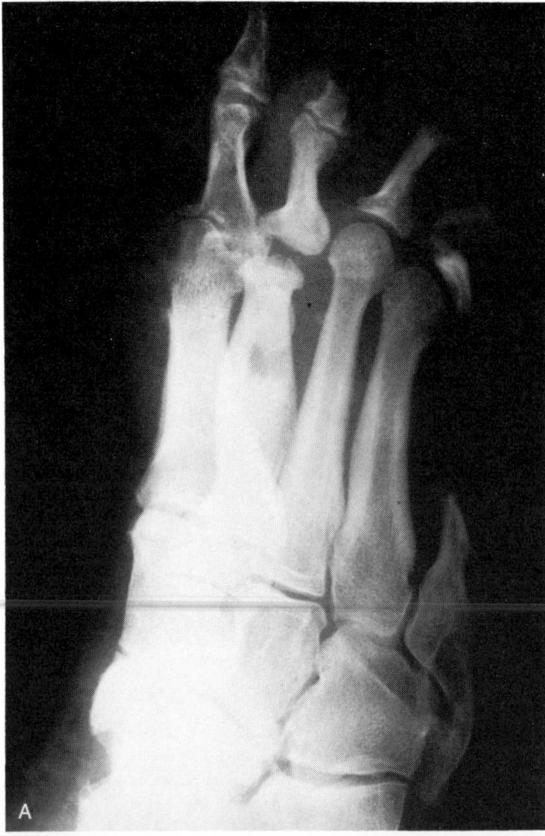

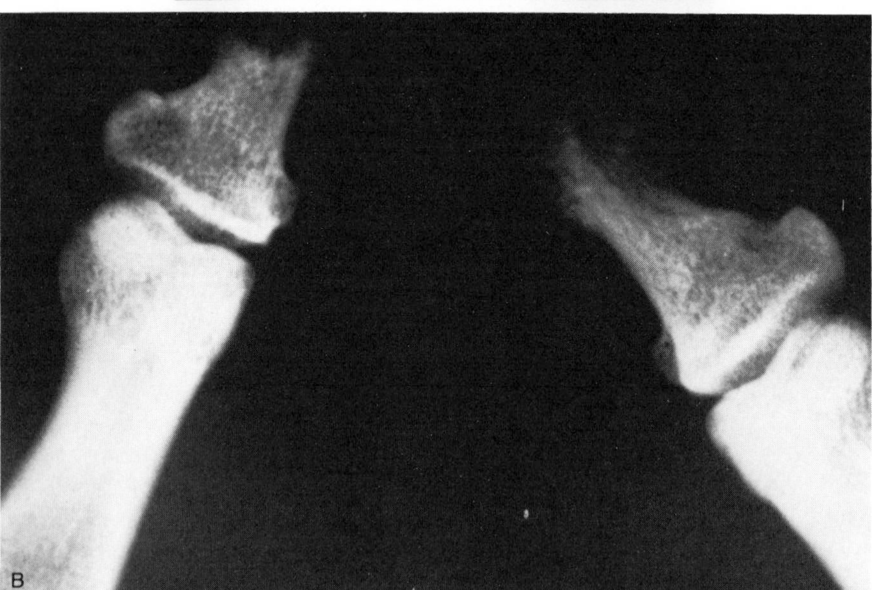

Figure 70–21. *Congenital indifference to pain.*

A, B *In this woman, observe the resorption and tapering of metatarsals and phalanges of the foot, with periostitis, sclerosis, and fragmentation, and the osteolysis of the terminal tufts of the thumbs. The changes are consistent with neuroarthropathy, although, in the lower extremity, infection is also probable. (***A, B,** *Courtesy of Dr. M. Pallayew, Montreal, Quebec.)*

Illustration continued on the opposite page

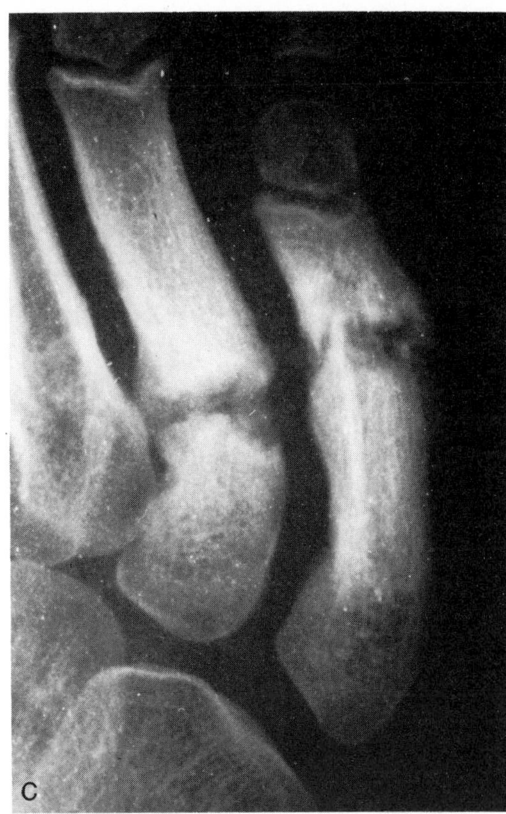

Figure 70–21. Continued
C *This 10 year old boy with congenital indifference to pain developed fractures of multiple metatarsals on both feet, which failed to heal and which were later associated with deformity.*

late to both osteoporosis and neurologic deficit; the bony fragments can heal, with abundant callus formation, although displacement with deformity or osteomyelitis can appear. Epiphyseal separations are the result of chronic trauma or stress, as the growth plate represents the weak link in the child's skeleton; widening and irregularity of the growth plate, lysis and sclerosis of the metaphysis, periostitis and callus, and variable degrees of epiphyseal displacement are recognized. Neuroarthropathy is especially common in the ankle and tarsal areas, although multiple sites can be affected; fragmentation and sclerosis can be prominent. Soft tissue ulcerations appear at the pressure areas on weight-bearing articulations or over bony prominences; the ulcers may deepen and lead to contamination of underlying bones and joints.

Many of the lesions may heal under proper supervision and treatment. However, recurrent osteomyelitis, fractures, dislocations, and progressive joint or skeletal deformity can be seen.[89, 94, 122]

Skeletal abnormalities similar to those of congenital indifference to pain are encountered in familial dysautonomia or the Riley-Day syndrome, which is characterized by autonomic dysfunction, sensory and motor disturbance, and spinal deformities [97-99, 107]; in congenital sensory neuropathy with anhidrosis, which is characterized by a probable autosomal recessive mode of inheritance, inability to detect noxious stimuli, defective intelligence, and reduced temperature and touch sensation[100, 101, 121]; and in hereditary sensory radicular neuropathy (acrodystrophic neuropathy), which is characterized by sensory neuropathy, trophic ulceration, and severe neuropathic skeletal alterations.[102-104, 117]

Meningomyelocele (Spinal Dysraphism)

Skeletal abnormalities are detected in patients with various types of spinal dysraphism.[95, 105-109] Sensory impairment resulting from spina bifida and meningomyelocele is the most frequent basis of neuropathic arthropathy in childhood, principally affecting the ankle and the tarsal articulations. In active children, changes may appear in the first 3 years of life. These changes are identical to those in congenital indifference to pain and include osteoporosis, diaphyseal and metaphyseal fractures, injuries of the growth plate, epiphyseal separations, persistent effusions, articular destruction, and soft tissue ulcerations[123, 124] (Fig. 70–22).

Other Diseases

There are numerous other causes of neuropathic skeletal alterations. These include spinal cord or peripheral nerve injury,[95, 110] myelopathy of pernicious anemia,[111] Charcot-Marie-Tooth disease,[112] arachnoiditis,[113, 114] paraplegia, familial interstitial hypertrophic polyneuropathy of Déjérine and Sottas, leprosy, and yaws. An idiopathic variety of neuroarthropathy of the elbow has also been identified[115, 116] (Fig. 70–23). Neuropathic-like changes that follow intra-articular injection of steroids were discussed in Chapter 66.

DIFFERENTIAL DIAGNOSIS

When severe, neuroarthropathy is associated with radiographic changes that are virtually pathognomonic. Bony eburnation, fracture, subluxation, and joint disorganization can be more profound in this disorder than in any other arthropathy. It is the mild and moderate stages of neuropathic joint disease that can be confused with other diseases.

In the articulations of the appendicular skeleton, joint space loss, sclerosis, and fragmentation in early stages of neuroarthropathy can resemble changes in osteoarthritis. With the progressive flattening and deformity of the articular surfaces, the production of numerous intra-articular osseous dense areas, and the appearance of increasing sclerosis and osteophytosis, the diagnosis of neuroarthrop-

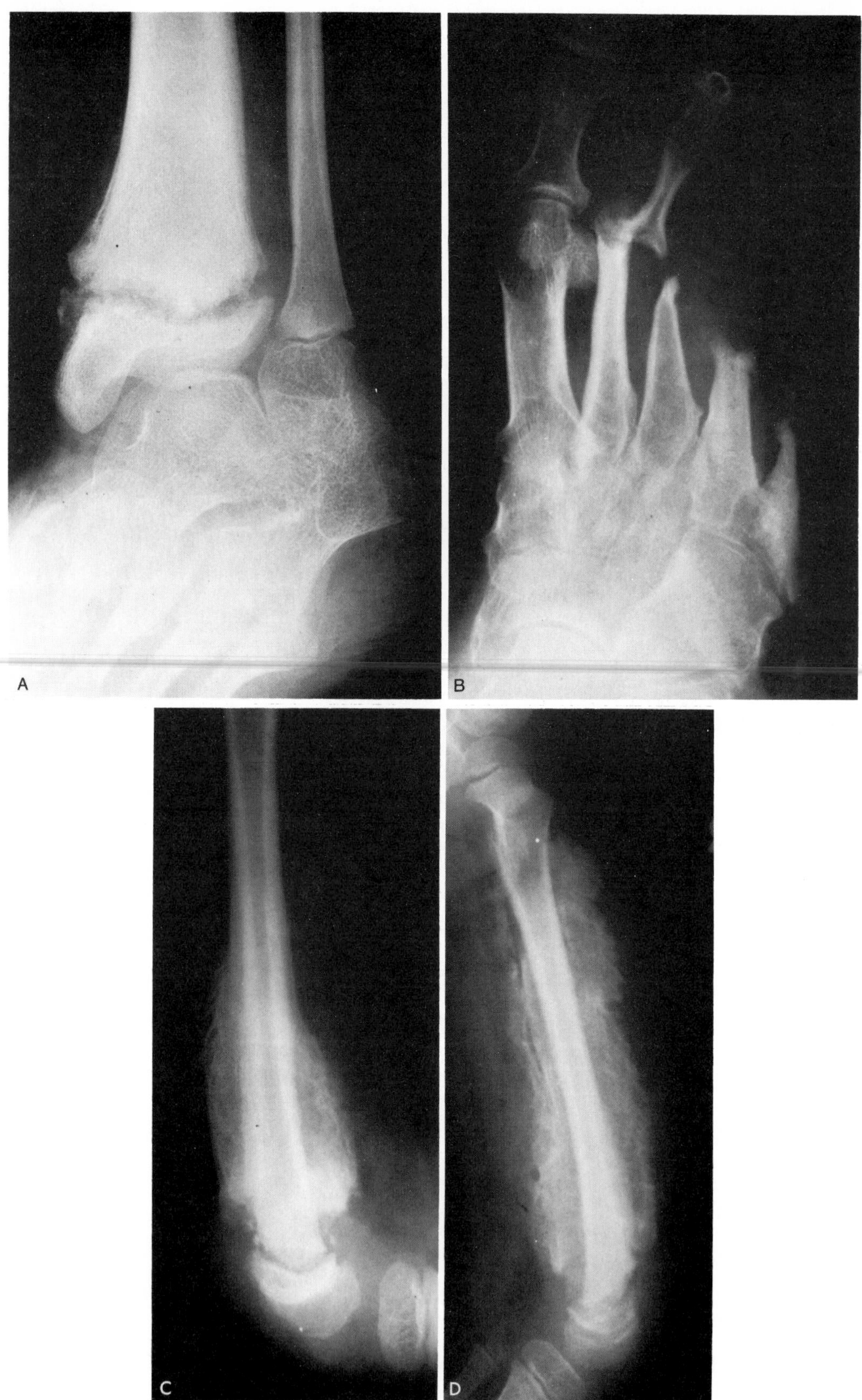

Figure 70–22. *Meningomyelocele (spinal dysraphism).*

A *In this child with a meningomyelocele, note an epiphyseal separation of the distal tibia, with a widened and irregular growth plate, sclerosis, and periostitis.*

B *In a 20 year old man with a meningomyelocele, progressive osteolysis of metatarsals and phalanges occurrred over a period of years. Some of the findings may be related to secondary infection or surgical intervention. (***B,** *Courtesy of Dr. F. Feldman, Columbia University, New York, New York.)*

C, D *Lateral radiographs of the femora in this child with a meningomyelocele reveal irregular and widened distal femoral growth plates, fracture and fragmentation, and exuberant periostitis. (Courtesy of Dr. J. E. L. Desautels, University of Calgary, Calgary, Alberta.)*

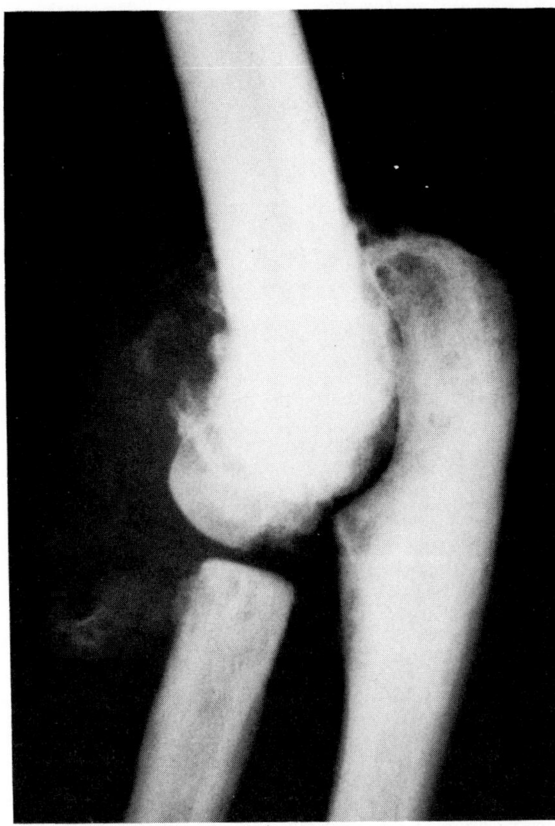

Figure 70–23. Idiopathic neuroarthropathy of the elbow. This middle-aged man developed a neurologic deficit and progressive painless elbow deformity. No underlying disease could be detected. The changes of severe sclerosis and fragmentation are consistent with neuroarthropathy. A radial head resection had been accomplished.

athy becomes more obvious. In calcium pyrophosphate dihydrate crystal deposition disease, a neuropathic-like arthropathy characterized by joint space narrowing, eburnation, and fragmentation can appear, especially in the knee, the wrist, and the metacarpophalangeal articulations; the identification of articular and periarticular calcification, the involvement of specific areas of the joint, such as the radiocarpal compartment of the wrist, the patellofemoral compartment of the knee, and the talonavicular space of the midfoot, and the variability of osteophyte formation are helpful clues to the accurate diagnosis of pyrophosphate arthropathy. However, neuroarthropathy and calcium pyrophosphate dihydrate crystal deposition disease can appear in the same individual (see Chapter 44). Bony fragmentation and collapse are also manifestations of osteonecrosis, posttraumatic osteoarthritis, intra-articular steroid arthropathy, neglected infection, and alkaptonuria. Additional clinical and radiographic manifestations in these latter disorders usually assure proper differential diagnosis.

In the articulations of the axial skeleton, early findings of neuroarthropathy, such as intervertebral disc space narrowing and vertebral sclerosis, resemble those of intervertebral osteochondrosis, infection, or alkaptonuria. With the appearance of significant fragmentation, sclerosis, and osteophytosis, the diagnosis of axial neuropathic disease is not difficult (Table 70–3).

Once the radiographic findings are interpreted as those of neuroarthropathy, the identification of the underlying disorder usually depends upon the location of the changes. Although there is considerable overlap in the distribution patterns of the various diseases, tabes typically produces changes in the hip, the knee, the ankle, and the spine; diabetes mellitus leads to alterations in the midfoot and forefoot; syringomyelia affects the articulations of the upper extremity and cervical spine; and congenital indifference to pain and meningomyelocele commonly localize in the articulations of the lower extremity. In the last two disorders, the presence of metaphyseal and growth plate destruction in the immature skeleton is especially characteristic.

SUMMARY

The effect of the deprivation of sensory feedback on the musculoskeletal system can be profound. The anesthetized articulation that is subject to continuing stress progressively deteriorates, leading to specific radiographic abnormalities. These changes, which include articular space narrowing, bony eburnation, osteophytosis, fragmentation, fracture, and subluxation, can accompany a variety of disorders but are most common in tabes dorsalis, diabetes mellitus, and syringomyelia. When severe, the resulting radiographic picture is diagnostic, although in earlier stages the findings may resemble those of osteoarthritis, calcium pyrophosphate dihydrate crystal deposition disease, osteonecrosis, or, in the spine, intervertebral osteochondrosis.

REFERENCES

1. Mitchell JK: On a new practice in acute and chronic rheumatism. Am J Med Sci *8*:55, 1831.
2. Kidd JG Jr: The Charcot joint: Some pathologic and pathogenetic considerations. South Med J *67*:597, 1974.
3. Charcot JM: Sur quelques arthropathies qui paraissent dépendre d'une lésion du cerveau ou de la moelle épinière. Arch Physiol Norm Pathol *1*:161, 1868.
4. Charcot JM: Lectures on the Diseases of the Nervous System. Vol 2. Edited and translated by S Sigerson. London, The New Sydenham Society, 1881, p 47.
5. Charcot JM: Ataxie locomotrice progressive: Arthropathie de l'épaule gauche. Resultats necropsiques. Arch Physiol Norm Pathol *2*:121, 1869.
6. Charcot JM, Joffrov A: Note sur une lésion de la substance grise de la moelle epinière observée dans un cas d'arthropathie née a l'ataxie locomotrice progressive. Arch Physiol Norm Pathol *3*:306, 1870.

7. Goldman AB, Freiberger RH: Localized infectious and neuropathic diseases. Semin Roentgenol *14*:19, 1979.
8. Delano PJ: The pathogenesis of Charcot's joint. Am J Roentgenol *56*:189, 1946.
9. Eloesser L: On the nature of neuropathic affections of the joints. Ann Surg *66*:201, 1917.
10. Potts WJ: Pathology of Charcot joints. Ann Surg *86*:596, 1927.
11. Leriche R, Brenckmann E: Recherches experimentales sur le mécanisme de formation de la chondromatose articulaire et de l'arthrite deformante. Presse Med *2*:1441, 1928.
12. Foster D, Bassett R: Neurogenic arthropathy (Charcot joint) associated with diabetic neuropathy. Arch Neurol Psychiatry *57*:173, 1947.
13. Parsons H, Norton W: The management of diabetic neuropathic joints. N Engl J Med *244*:935, 1951.
14. Hodgson J, Pugh D, Young H: Roentgenologic aspects of certain lesions of bone: Neurotropic or infectious? Radiology *50*:65, 1948.
15. Jaffe HL: Metabolic, Degenerative and Inflammatory Diseases of Bones and Joints. Philadelphia, Lea & Febiger, 1972, p 847.
16. Feldman F, Johnson AM, Walter JF: Acute axial neuroarthropathy. Radiology *111*:1, 1974.
17. Johnson LC: Discussion. Arthritis Rheum *9*:358, 1966.
18. Rabaiotti A, Rossi L, Schittone N, Gandini GE: Le alterazioni vascolari nell'arthropatia tabetica. Ann Radiol Diagn *33*:115, 1960.
19. Soto-Hall R, Halderman KO: The diagnosis of neuropathic joint disease (Charcot joint). An analysis of forty cases. JAMA *114*:2076, 1940.
20. Katz I, Rabinowitz JG, Dziadiw R: Early changes in Charcot's joints. Am J Roentgenol *86*:965, 1961.
21. Johnson JTH: Neuropathic fractures and joint injuries. Pathogenesis and rationale of prevention and treatment. J Bone Joint Surg *49A*:1, 1967.
22. Norman A, Robbins H, Milgram JE: The acute neuropathic arthropathy — a rapid severely disorganizing form of arthritis. Radiology *90*:1159, 1968.
23. Stewart A, Kettelkamp DB, Brandt KD: Acute joint dislocation — an early feature of neuropathic arthropathy. Arthritis Rheum *19*:1367, 1976.
24. Horwitz T: Bone and cartilage debris in the synovial membrane. Its significance in the early diagnosis of neuroarthropathy. J Bone Joint Surg *30A*:579, 1948.
25. Lloyd-Roberts GC: The role of capsular changes in osteoarthritis of the hip joint. J Bone Joint Surg *35B*:627, 1953.
26. Harrison RB: Charcot's joints: Two new observations. Am J Roentgenol *128*:807, 1977.
27. Forrester DM, Magre G: Migrating bone shards in dissecting Charcot joints. Am J Roentgenol *130*:1133, 1978.
28. Steindler A: The tabetic arthropathies. JAMA *96*:250, 1931.
29. Philips H, Rosenheck C: Neuro-arthropathies of peripheral nerve injury origin. JAMA *86*:169, 1926.
30. Sinha S, Munichoodappa C, Kozak GP: Neuro-arthropathy (Charcot joints) in diabetes mellitus. Medicine *51*:191, 1972.
31. Alarcon-Segovia D, Ward LE: Charcot-like arthropathy in rheumatoid arthritis. Consequence of overuse of a joint repeatedly injected with hydrocortisone. JAMA *193*:1052, 1965.
32. Beetham WP Jr, Kaye RL, Polley HF: Charcot joints. A case of extensive polyarticular involvement, and discussion of certain clinical and pathologic features. Ann Intern Med *58*:1002, 1963.
33. Key JA: Clinical observations on tabetic arthropathies (Charcot joints). Am J Syph *16*:429, 1932.
34. Pomeranz MM, Rothberg AS: A review of 58 cases of tabetic arthropathy. Am J Syph *25*:103, 1941.
35. Frewin DB, Downey JA, Feldman F, Myers SJ: Neuropathic arthropathy: A report of two cases. Aust NZ J Med *3*:587, 1973.
36. Brain R, Wilkinson M: Cervical arthropathy in syringomyelia, tabes dorsalis, and diabetes. Brain *81*:275, 1958.
37. Campbell DJ, Doyle JO: Tabetic Charcot's spine: Report of 8 cases. Br Med J *1*:1018, 1954.
38. Herndon RF: Three cases of tabetic Charcot's spine. J Bone Joint Surg *9*:605, 1927.
39. Holland HW: Tabetic spinal arthropathy. Proc R Soc Med *46*:747, 1953.
40. Thomas DF: Vertebral osteoarthropathy or Charcot's disease of the spine. Review of the literature and a report of two cases. J Bone Joint Surg *34B*:248, 1952.
41. Cutting PEJ: A case of Charcot's disease of the cervical spine. Br Med J *1*:311, 1949.
42. McNeel DP, Ehni G: Charcot joint of the lumbar spine. J Neurosurg *30*:55, 1969.
43. Ramani PS, Sengupta RP: Cauda equina compression due to tabetic arthropathy of the spine. J Neurol Neurosurg Psychiatry *36*:260, 1973.
44. Meyer GA, Stein J, Poppel MH: Rapid osseous changes in syringomyelia. Radiology *69*:415, 1957.
45. Skall-Jansen J: Osteoarthropathy in syringomyelia. Analysis of seven cases. Acta Radiol *38*:382, 1952.
46. Tully JC Jr, Latteri A: Paraplegia, syringomyelia tarda and neuropathic arthrosis of the shoulder: A triad. Clin Orthop Rel Res *134*: 244, 1978.
47. Villiaumey J, Caron JP, Larget-Piet B, Haddad A: Arthropathie destructive de l'épaule révélatrice d'un syndrome syringomyélique chez un malade atteint d'une paraplégie post-traumatique. Rev Rhum Mal Osteoartic *40*:279, 1973.
48. Von Cube N, Lincke HO: Akuter Verlauf bei Arthropathia Syringomyelica. Ein kasuistischer Beitrag zur Differentialdiagnose der akuten Schultergelenksaffektion. Z Orthop *116*:745, 1978.
49. Heyser K, Günther E, Rumpf P: Progrediente Nekrose am Humeruskopf bei Syringomyelie. Fortschr Geb Roentgenstr Nuklearmed *123*:280, 1975.
50. Sackellares JC, Swift TR: Shoulder enlargement as the presenting sign in syringomyelia. JAMA *236*:2878, 1976.
51. Sheppe WM: Neuropathic (Charcot) joints occurring in diabetes mellitus. Ann Intern Med *39*:625, 1953.
52. Clouse ME, Gramm HF, Legg M, Flood T: Diabetic osteoarthropathy: Clinical and roentgenographic observations in 90 cases. Am J Roentgenol *121*:22, 1974.
53. Pogonowska MJ, Collins LC, Dobson HL: Diabetic osteopathy. Radiology *89*:265, 1971.
54. Kraft E, Spyropoulos E, Finby N: Neurogenic disorders of the foot in diabetes mellitus. Am J Roentgenol *124*:17, 1975.
55. Shagan BP, Friedman SA, Allesandri R: Diabetic osteopathy: Report of a relentlessly progressive case with clinico-pathologic correlations. J Am Geriatr Soc *21*:561, 1973.
56. Forgacs S: Stages and roentgenological picture of diabetic osteoarthropathy. Fortschr Geb Roentgenstr Nuklearmed *126*:36, 1977.
57. Gray RG, Gottlieb NL: Rheumatic disorders associated with diabetes mellitus: Literature review. Semin Arthritis Rheum *6*:19, 1976.
58. Meltzer AD, Skversky N, Ostrum BJ: Radiographic evaluation of soft-tissue necrosis in diabetics. Radiology *90*:300, 1968.
59. Campbell WL, Feldman F: Bone and soft tissue abnormalities of the upper extremity in diabetes mellitus. Am J Roentgenol *124*:7, 1975.
60. Lippmann HI, Perotto A, Farrar R: The neuropathic foot of the diabetic. Bull NY Acad Med *52*:1159, 1976.
61. Clouse ME, Gramm HF, Legg M, Flood T: Diabetic osteoarthropathy. Clinical and roentgenographic observations in 90 cases. Am J Roentgenol *121*:22, 1974.
62. Gondos B: Roentgen observations in diabetic osteopathy. Radiology *91*:6, 1968.
63. Gondos B: The pointed tubular bone. Its significance and pathogenesis. Radiology *105*:541, 1972.
64. Schwarz GS, Berenyi MR, Siegel MW: Atrophic arthropathy and diabetic neuritis. Am J Roentgenol *106*:523, 1969.
65. Giesecke SB, Dalinka MK, Kyle GC: Lisfranc's fracture-dislocation: A manifestation of peripheral neuropathy. Am J Roentgenol *131*:139, 1978.
66. Jordan WR: Neuritic manifestations in diabetes mellitus. Arch Intern Med *57*:307, 1936.
67. Bailey CC, Root HF: Neuropathic foot lesions in diabetes mellitus. N Engl J Med *236*:397, 1947.
68. Eichenholtz SN: Charcot Joints. Springfield, Ill, Charles C Thomas, 1966.
69. Parsons H, Norton WS: Management of diabetic neuropathic joints. N Engl J Med *244*:935, 1951.
70. Boehm HJ Jr: Diabetic Charcot joints. N Engl J Med *267*:185, 1962.
71. Lippman EM, Grow JL: Neurogenic arthropathy associated with diabetes mellitus. J Bone Joint Surg *37A*:971, 1955.
72. Robillard R, Gagnon PA, Alarie P: Diabetic neuroarthropathy. Report of 4 cases. Can Med Assoc J *91*:795, 1974.
73. Ellenberg M: Diabetic neuropathy of upper extremities. J Mt Sinai Hosp *35*:134, 1968.
74. Chochinov RH, Ullyot GLE, Moorhouse JA: Sensory perception thresholds in patients with juvenile diabetes and their close relatives. N Engl J Med *286*:1233, 1972.
75. Zucker G, Marder MJ: Charcot spine due to diabetic neuropathy. Am J Med *12*:118, 1952.
76. King ESJ: On some aspects of the pathology of hypertrophic Charcot's joints. Br J Surg *18*:113, 1930.
77. Lister J, Maudsley RH: Charcot joints in diabetic neuropathy. Lancet *2*:1110, 1951.
78. Fagerberg SE: Diabetic neuropathy: Clinical and histological study on the significance of vascular affections. Acta Med Scand Suppl *345*:1, 1959.
79. Woltman HW, Wilder RM: Diabetes mellitus: Pathologic changes in spinal cord and peripheral nerves. Arch Intern Med *44*:576, 1929.
80. Thornhill HL, Richter RW, Shelton ML, Johnson CA: Neuropathic arthropathy (Charcot forefeet) in alcoholics. Orthop Clin North Am *4*:7, 1973.
81. Chappet V, Mouriquand G: Arthropathies nerveuses et maux perforants

de causes diverses (tabes, diabete, alcoolisme). Bull Soc Med Hôp Lyon *2*:523, 1903.
82. Classon JN: Neuropathic arthropathy with ulceration. Ann Surg *159*:891, 1964.
83. Schlesinger AS, Duggins VA, Masucci EF: Peripheral neuropathy in familial primary amyloidosis. Brain *85*:357, 1962.
84. Andrade C: A peculiar form of peripheral neuropathy. Brain *75*:408, 1952.
85. Scott RB, Elmore SM, Brackett NC, Harris WU Jr, Still WJS: Neuropathic joint disease (Charcot joints) in Waldenström's macroglobulinemia with amyloidosis. Am J Med *54*:535, 1973.
86. Peitzman SJ, Miller JL, Ortega L, Schumacher HR, Fernandez PC: Charcot arthropathy secondary to amyloid neuropathy. JAMA *235*:1345, 1976.
87. Dearborn GV: A case of congenital general pure analgesia. J Nerv Ment Dis *75*:612, 1932.
88. Feindel W: Note on the nerve endings in a subject with arthropathy and congenital absence of pain. J Bone Joint Surg *35B*:402, 1953.
89. Murray RO: Congenital indifference to pain with special reference to skeletal changes. Br J Radiol *30*:2, 1957.
90. Silverman FN, Gilden JJ: Congenital insensitivity to pain; a neurologic syndrome with bizarre skeletal lesions. Radiology *72*:176, 1959.
91. Sandell LJ: Congenital indifference to pain. J Fac Radiol 9:50, 1958.
92. Franklyn PP: Congenital indifference to pain. Ann Radiol *15*:343, 1972.
93. Siegelman S, Heimann WG, Manin MC: Congenital indifference to pain. Am J Roentgenol *97*:242, 1966.
94. Drummond RP, Rose GK: A twenty-one year review of a case of congenital indifference to pain. J Bone Joint Surg *57B*:241, 1975.
95. Schneider R, Goldman AB, Bohne WH: Neuropathic injuries to the lower extremities in children. Radiology *128*:713, 1978.
96. Van der Houwen H: A case of neuropathic arthritis caused by indifference to pain. J Bone Joint Surg *43B*:314, 1961.
97. Riley CR: Familial autonomic dysfunction. JAMA *149*:1532, 1952.
98. Kirkpatrick RH, Riley CR: Roentgenographic findings in familial dysautonomia. Radiology *68*:654, 1957.
99. Levine DB, Axelrod F: The occurrence of spinal deformities in familial dysautonomia (Abstr). Clin Orthop Rel Res *105*:298, 1974.
100. Pinsky L, DiGeorge AM: Congenital familial sensory neuropathy with anhidrosis. J Pediatr *68*:1, 1966.
101. Gold RH, Mirra JM: Case report 45. Skel Radiol *2*:127, 1977.
102. Heller IH, Robb P: Hereditary sensory neuropathy. Neurology *5*:15, 1955.
103. Pallis C, Schneeweiss J: Hereditary sensory radicular neuropathy. Am J Med *32*:110, 1962.
104. Banna M, Foster JB: Roentgenologic features of acrodystrophic neuropathy. Am J Roentgenol *115*:186, 1972.
105. Gyepes MT, Newbern DH, Neuhauser EBD: Metaphyseal and physeal injuries in children with spina bifida and meningomyeloceles. Am J Roentgenol *95*:168, 1965.
106. Korhonen BJ: Fractures in myelodysplasia. Clin Orthop Rel Res *79*:145, 1971.
107. Brunt PW: Unusual cause of Charcot's joints in early adolescence (Riley-Day syndrome). Br Med J *4*:277, 1967.
108. Nellhaus G: Neurogenic arthropathies (Charcot's joints) in children. Description of a case traced to occult spinal dysraphism. Clin Pediatr *14*:647, 1975.
109. Edvardsen P: Physeo-epiphyseal injuries of lower extremities in myelomeningocele. Acta Orthop Scand *43*:550, 1972.
110. Slabaugh PB, Smith TK: Neuropathic spine after spinal cord injury. J Bone Joint Surg *60A*:1005, 1978.
111. Halonen PI, Jarvinen KAJ: On the occurrence of neuropathic arthropathies in pernicious anaemia. Ann Rheum Dis *7*:152, 1948.
112. Bruckner FE, Kendall BE: Neuroarthropathy in Charcot-Marie-Tooth disease. Ann Rheum Dis *28*:577, 1969.
113. Wolfgang GL: Neurotrophic arthropathy of the shoulder — a complication of progressive adhesive arachnoiditis. A case report. Clin Orthop Rel Res *87*:217, 1972.
114. Nissenbaum M: Neurotrophic arthropathy of the shoulder secondary to tuberculous arachnoiditis. A case report. Clin Orthop Rel Res *118*:169, 1976.
115. Meyn M Jr, Yablon IG: Idiopathic arthropathy of the elbow. Clin Orthop Rel Res *97*:90, 1973.
116. Blanford AT, Keane SP, McCarty DJ, Albers JW: Idiopathic Charcot joint of the elbow. Arthritis Rheum *21*:723, 1978.
117. Shahriaree H, Kotcamp WW, Sheikh S, Sajdi K: Hereditary perforating ulcers of the foot. "Hereditary sensory radicular neuropathy." Clin Orthop Rel Res *140*:189, 1979.
118. William B: Orthopaedic features in the presentation of syringomyelia. J Bone Joint Surg *61B*:314, 1979.
119. El-Khoury GY, Kathol MH: Neuropathic fractures in patients with diabetes mellitus. Radiology *134*:313, 1980.
120. Newman JH: Spontaneous dislocation in diabetic neuropathy. A report of six cases. J Bone Joint Surg *61B*:484, 1979.
121. Vardy PA, Greenberg LW, Kachel C, deLeon GF: Congenital insensitivity to pain with anhydrosis. Am J Dis Child *133*:1153, 1979.
122. Roberts JM, Taylor J, Burke S: Recurrent dislocation of the hip in congenital indifference to pain. J Bone Joint Surg *62A*:829, 1980.
123. Townsend PF, Cowell HR, Steg NL: Lower extremity fractures simulating infection in myelomeningocele. Clin Orthop Rel Res *144*:255, 1979.
124. Wenger DR, Jeffcoat BT, Herring JA: The guarded prognosis of physeal injury in paraplegic children. J Bone Joint Surg *62A*:241, 1980.
125. Brower AC, Allman RM: The pathogenesis of the neurotrophic joint. Neurotraumatic versus neurovascular. Radiology (in press).
126. Klawans HL: Neurological manifestations of systemic diseases. *In* PJ Vinken, GW Bruyn (Eds): Handbook of Clinical Neurology. New York, North Holland Publishing Co, 1979, Chapter 18, p 431.
127. Rubinow A, Spark EC, Canoso JJ: Septic arthritis in a Charcot Joint. Clin Orthop Rel Res *147*:203, 1980.

SECTION XV

CONGENITAL DISEASES

71

CONGENITAL DYSPLASIA OF THE HIP

by John A. Ogden, M.D.

Congenital dysplasia of the hip (CDH) is an extremely variable morphologic disease that often appears quite confusing to orthopaedists and radiologists alike. Although the ideal would be detection and immediate inception of treatment of this entity at birth by appropriate neonatal clinical and roentgenographic examinations, the diagnosis still is missed in many children, who subsequently present for evaluation and treatment at several months to years of age. At any stage of initial diagnosis, no matter how old the child, the primary goal must be to adequately delineate the specific morphologic pathology in a manner that will more effectively define treatment. In order to accomplish such a goal, an understanding of the three-dimensional pathobiologic (morphologic) changes that occur with time — the fourth dimension — is absolutely necessary. Such transformational changes may have profound effect upon the outcome of any treatment modality.

Subluxation and dislocation of the developing hip represent arbitrary definitions of relatively static stages within a spectrum of dynamic morphologic changes that are often insidious in onset, subtle in the initial clinical and roentgenographic changes, and potentially devastating in short- and long-term results if the entity is not adequately diagnosed and treated in the earliest stages of structural deformation. Early diagnosis should be accomplished during the neonatal period. Unfortunately, during this time routine radiography of the chondro-osseous hip does not always afford a great deal of diagnostic assistance.[4, 30, 39]

Treatment modalities differ significantly for incompletely (subluxated) and completely dislocated hips. One of the major problems confronting the diagnostician is that routine roentgenograms may not show the profound differences in soft tissue morphology that affect the acetabular cartilage, capsule, and iliopsoas tendon. Figure 71–1 shows radiographs from children initially examined at about 6 months of age. These roentgenograms illustrate the basic problem: Are these hips truly dislocated or only partially displaced (subluxated)? Are the deformities fixed, or can the hips be anatomically reduced? There are obvious changes of lateralization and superior displacement of the proximal femoral metaphysis. There is delay in development of the capital femoral ossification center and deformation of the osseous roof of the acetabulum (ilium). Yet, without an appreciation of the degree of change in the soft tissue components that are not visible radiologically, one cannot make an accurate statement regarding the exact pathologic condition present in these cases. Arthrography provides a means of obtaining such information, and it certainly is a very effective means of evaluating the type of deformation of the acetabular margin, the reducibility of the displaced proximal femur and, to some extent, the need for nonoperative or operative intervention.[1, 21, 29, 35] Later in this chapter arthrography will be discussed in more detail, and the specific arthrograms from the patients in Figure 71–1 will be presented.

The interpretation of roentgenograms from patients with the various diseases affecting the developing hip has a major drawback — namely, a pau-

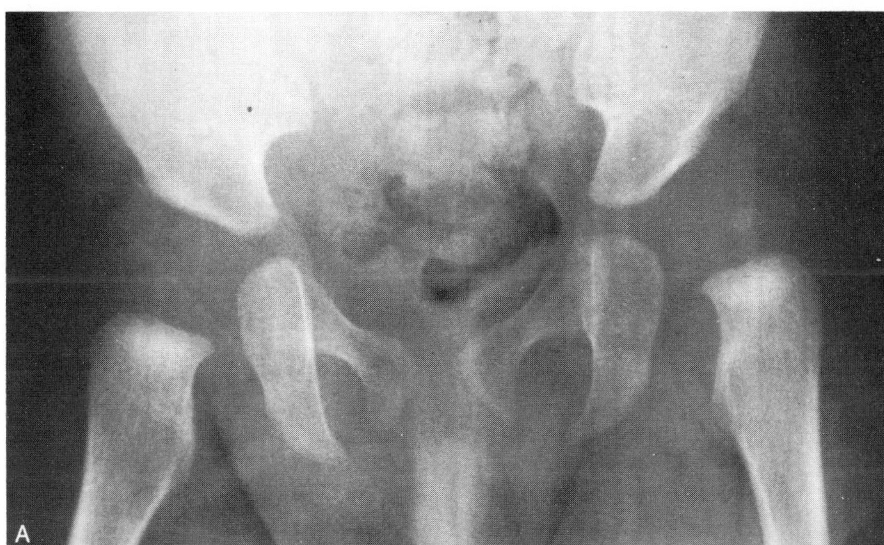

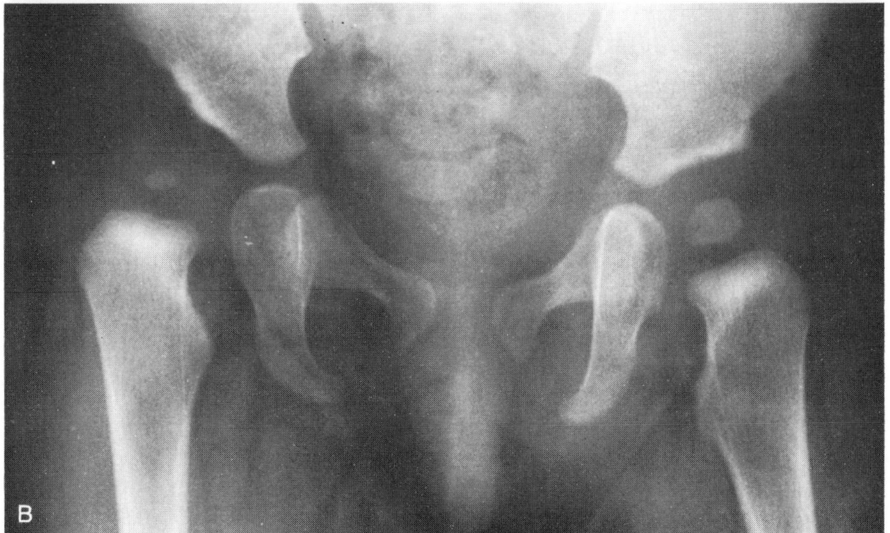

Figure 71–1. *Four examples of dysplastic hips.* **A**, *A 4 month old female;* **B**, *a 7 month old female.*

Illustration continued on the following page

city of adequately documented specimen material that the radiologist and pediatric orthopaedist may use as a reference base.[2, 5, 9, 10, 14, 20, 25, 26, 32, 37, 38, 42] Certainly our understanding of diseases affecting the mature hip has been immensely improved by correlative pathoanatomic/roentgenographic studies. Unfortunately, similar material is not readily available for developmental hip disorders.

This chapter will concentrate on the continually changing pathobiology and the accompanying variable roentgenologic manifestations of congenital dysplasia of the hip. I have deliberately chosen the term "dysplasia" as the best description of the highly variable plastic deformation that affects both the proximal femur and the acetabulum. The term should not be construed to mean a primary pathologic change in the acetabulum. The structural changes affect *both* sides of the hip joint, but to varying degrees. The initial changes are often quite subtle, and hardly seem to presage the changes that will result if treatment is not introduced. The deformations affecting the two primary elements of the hip joint — femoral head and acetabulum — may begin in utero or may not take place until some time in the postnatal period. External factors, whether ante natal or post natal, may have a significant role in the progressive deformation that inexorably occurs if the condition is not recognized clinically and radio-

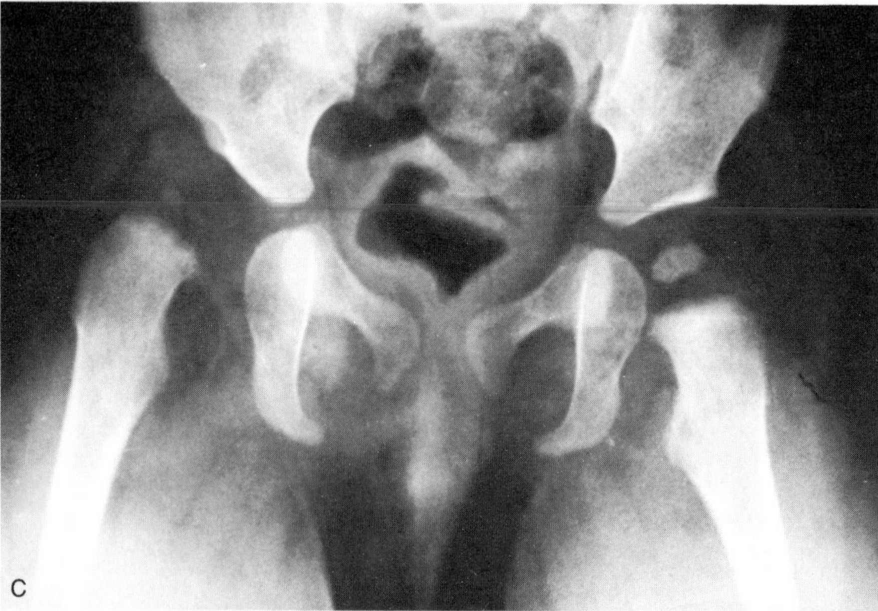

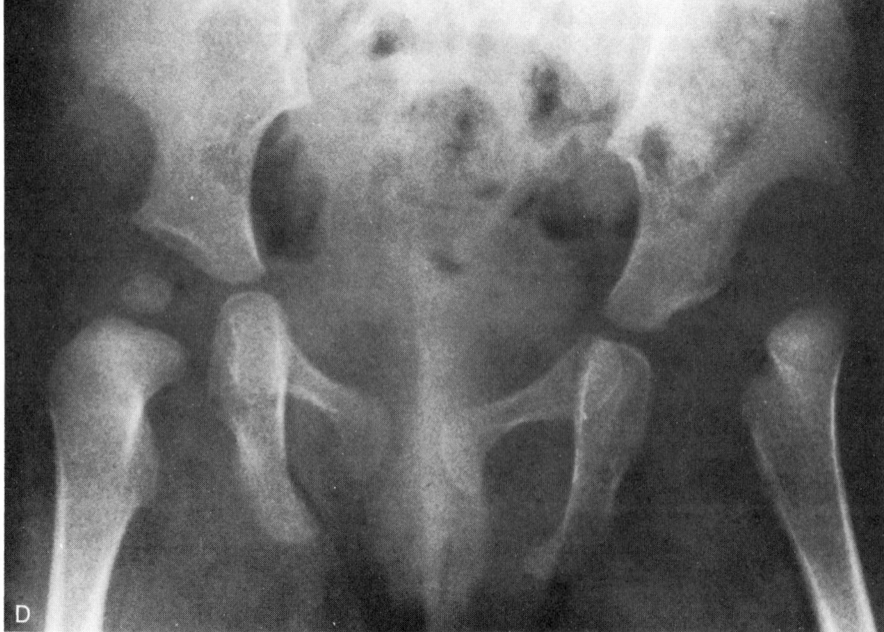

Figure 71–1. Continued
C, *A 6 month old female;* **D**, *an 11 month old female with bilateral foot polydactyly and a brother with congenital dysplasia of the hip. Throughout the anatomic presentations in this chapter these varying roentgenographic presentations should be kept in mind. In the clinical section of this chapter the arthrograms of these patients will be shown to define the specific deformities in each case.*

graphically. Such factors may be breech presentation, anteversion of the femur, and hip joint contractures (specifically adduction and flexion).[37]

When certain factors external to the hip joint per se are present, particularly neuromuscular diseases such as myelomeningocele and arthrogryposis multiplex congenita, the term "teratologic hip" often is applied. Although such an arbitrary differentiation has significance from a treatment standpoint, the morphologic changes are comparable in all types of CDH and depend upon both the severity of the external deformation forces and the time in prenatal and postnatal development when such forces began to adversely affect hitherto normal hip joint development. This concept may be further emphasized and exemplified by a disease such as cerebral palsy. In patients with this disorder the hips presumably develop in a normal fashion, and at birth show the usual degree of anteversion. Once the disease process begins it affects particular muscles with varying degrees of spasticity or flaccidity; the hip components subsequently may readily and progressively become deformed, subluxated and, if left untreated, eventually dislocated. Spasticity in the adductors and iliopsoas exposes the developing hip to intrinsic muscular forces that predispose to subluxation. These same muscles are involved in nonteratogenic CDH. The roentgenographic manifestations in CDH complicating cerebral palsy may be indistinguishable from those of any other type of CDH.

Congenital hip disease is a highly variable entity, frequently referred to as a "dysplasia," a term that connotes anatomic malformation. However, a true congenital malformation is a structural change arising during the embryonic period of organogenesis, prior to eight weeks of gestation, and represents a major alteration of the involved organ system (in this case the musculoskeletal system). With the exception of rare entities such as femoral duplication, proximal femoral focal deficiency, and phocomelia, true biologic malformations affecting the hip joint are extremely rare. To better understand changes affecting the developing hip, Dunn introduced the concept of "congenital deformation" or "fetopathy," which may be defined as the progressive deformation of an initially normally formed structure during the subsequent fetal period, rather than during the embryonic period.[7-9] Factors that place normal mechanical stress on components of the developing musculoskeletal system may readily and variably alter their shape. This same phenomenon of gradual deformation also may occur postnatally, especially during the neonatal period, when extrinsic as well as intrinsic mechanical factors may act adversely on a hip that either is normal or has been rendered susceptible to instability by the prevailing intrauterine conditions. Dunn stipulated that gentle mechanical forces, if persistently applied, may lead to gradual but progressive deformation, and that such deformation occurred much more readily in periods of excessively rapid growth.[7-9] This certainly occurs during the first year of life, a time when unstable (subluxating) hips may become true dislocated hips. The fetus is particularly susceptible to deformation because of the rapid rate of growth and the relative plasticity of the chondro-osseous skeleton.[27]

Prenatal deforming forces may be intrinsic, such as the position of the skeletal components and muscle imbalance, or extrinsic, such as intrauterine muscle tone, amount of amniotic fluid, and presence of more than one fetus.[8, 14, 18, 33] The extrinsic forces may become more prevalent during the last trimester, owing to increasing fetal size and a relative decrease in the amniotic fluid volume. As the fetus grows, it becomes increasingly exposed to pressure from the uterine musculature, the maternal spinal column, and the maternal abdominal wall. During this period of development the skeletal system is gradually becoming less plastic as a result of progressive primary ossification and is more able to resist some types of deformation, although the hip capsule is an exception, as it may be altered physiochemically by maternal hormonal changes during the last trimester of pregnancy.

Figure 71–2 shows hips from a fetus of approximately 24 weeks' gestation with polycystic kidneys and other urinary tract abnormalities. One hip was displaced and one was normal. As can be seen from the radiography of the pelvis, the osseous contributions of the ilium to the acetabular roof were normal, with a normal, symmetric acetabular index on each side. However, the cartilage-air interface technique of this film shows that despite normal osseous morphology, there was significant deformation of the acetabulum in both the soft tissue and the cartilaginous portions. It is important to realize that the acetabular index, which has wide variation, from 20 to 40 degrees,[4, 39] may be perfectly normal and yet there may be a significant dysplasia of the hip. Apparently many of the changes associated with an increased acetabular index do not occur until the postnatal phase, when the hip gradually loses its intrauterine flexion contracture, and continued pressure from the femoral head causes increased pressure on this lateral area and both a gradual osteoclastic resorption of the bone and a delay of normal endochondral bone formation at the lateral margin of the ossified portion of the acetabular roof (Fig. 71–3). Furthermore, the finding of early hypertrophy of the hyaline-fibrocartilage margin of the labrum, despite obvious marginal eversion of the bulk of this structure, suggests that the hypertrophied limbus may develop by continued tissue remodeling, rather than by abrupt inversion.

Before embarking upon a detailed description of the various pathologic changes encountered in the neonatal and postnatal periods, several important facets and definitions of normal hip development need to be presented. This material should serve as a

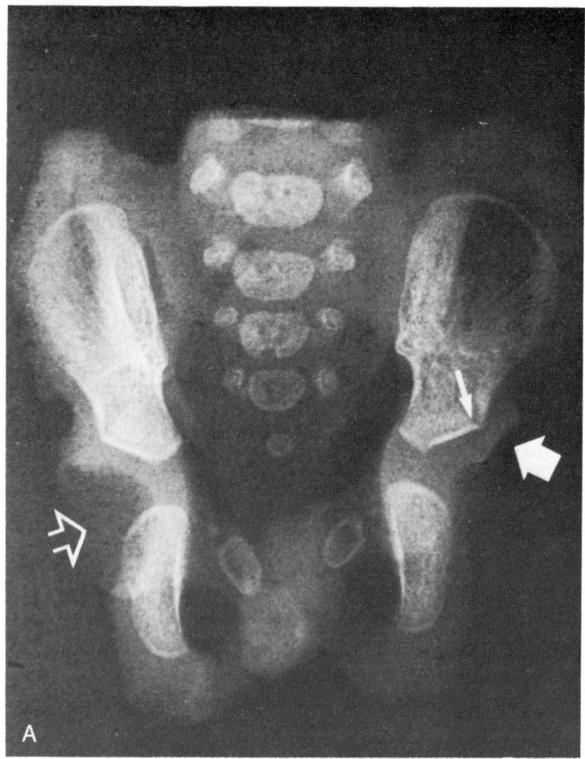

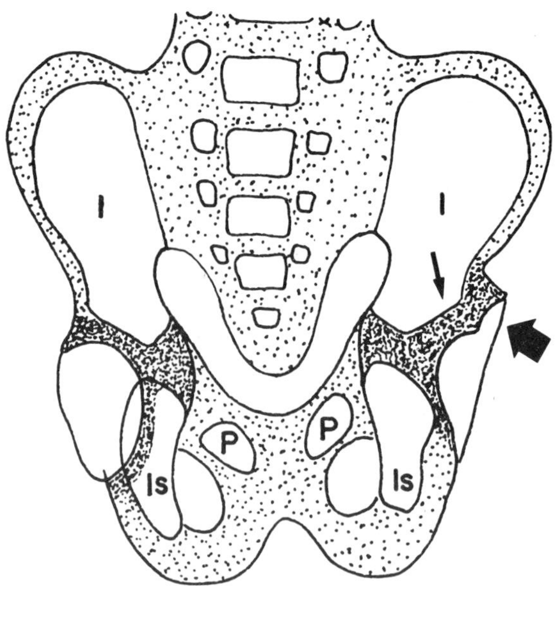

Figure 71–2. Roentgenogram **(A)** and schematic diagram **(B)** of pelvis of a stillborn male with polycystic kidneys. The right hip was normal; the left had a pathologically hypertrophied, inverted fibrocartilaginous labrum. The acetabular indices are normal, yet major cartilaginous changes are evident. The normal acetabular cavity is well outlined on the roentgenogram (open arrow). The small solid arrow depicts the normal lateral acetabular roof, while the larger solid arrow shows the labrum deformity. The iliac (I), ischial (Is) and pubic (P) ossification centers are identified. The light stippling indicates hyaline cartilage and emphasizes the early continuity of the cartilage throughout the pelvis. The darker stippling indicates the acetabular and triradiate cartilage.

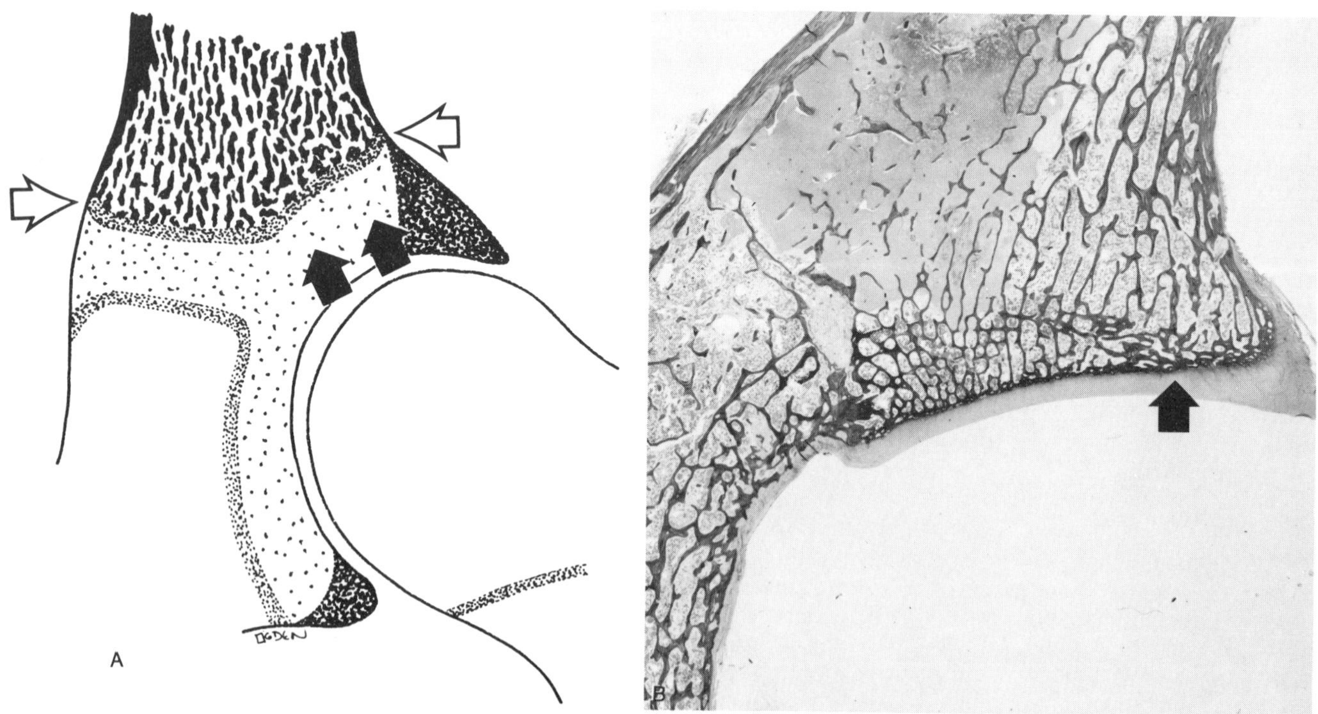

Figure 71–3. **A,** Schematic diagram of acetabular–capital femoral relationships. The solid arrows show the direction of the normal joint reaction force toward the portion of the iliac ossification center that forms the osseous acetabular roof. The open arrows depict the medial and lateral extent of the iliac physis. If the joint reaction force is shifted laterally, excess pressure concentration on the lateral physis may impede endochondral ossification and increase the acclivity of the osseous portion as the more medial aspect continues to grow. **B,** Mature acetabular roof in a 14 year old girl, showing the combined longitudinal and transverse trabecular pattern that must develop. Notice the density of the trabeculae laterally (arrow).

basic framework to better understand the morphologic changes that will be described subsequently.

DEVELOPMENTAL ANATOMY

The neonatal proximal femur is a large, radiolucent chondroepiphyseal unit that is a composite of femoral head, greater trochanter, and lesser trochanter. The common physis (growth plate) initially is relatively transversely oriented and primarily extracapsular (Fig. 71–4). With subsequent postnatal growth, the various characteristic regions and contours will become defined more clearly. However, for much of postnatal development the cartilaginous interrelationships of the three proximal femoral components will be maintained, an important factor allowing integrated patterns of growth (Fig. 71–5).

The proximal femur develops two major regions of morphologic differentiation. These are the greater trochanter and femoral head. Initially these two

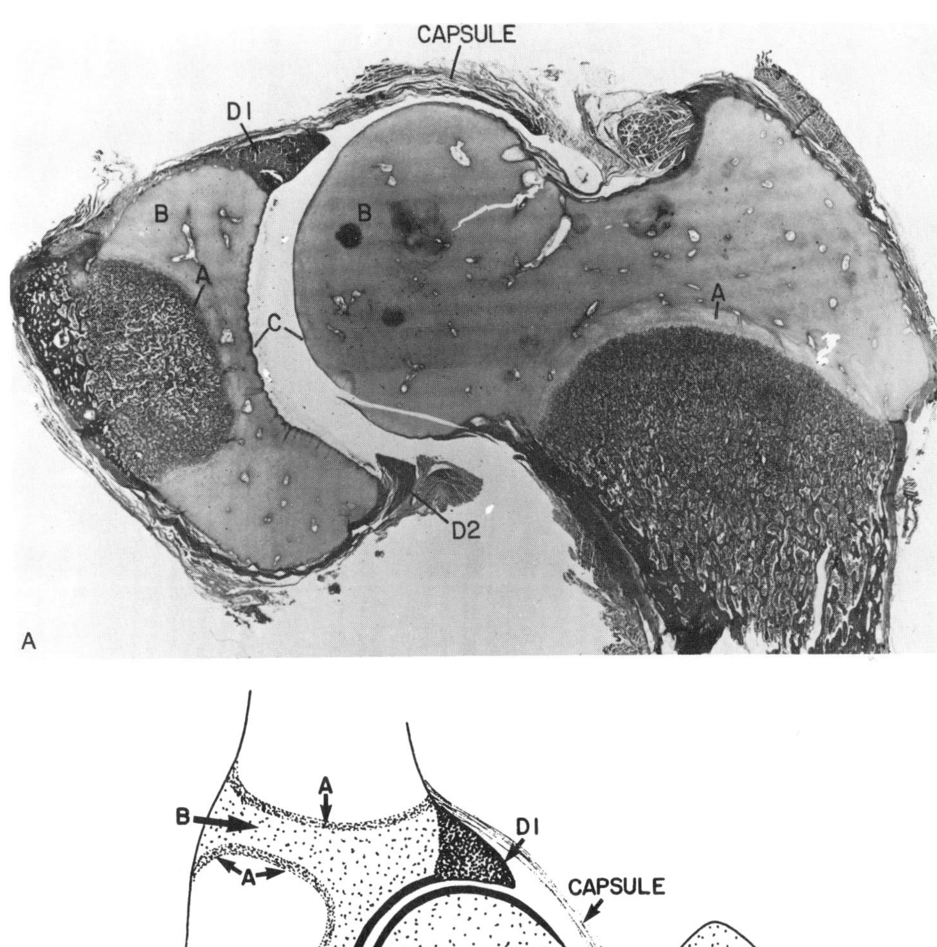

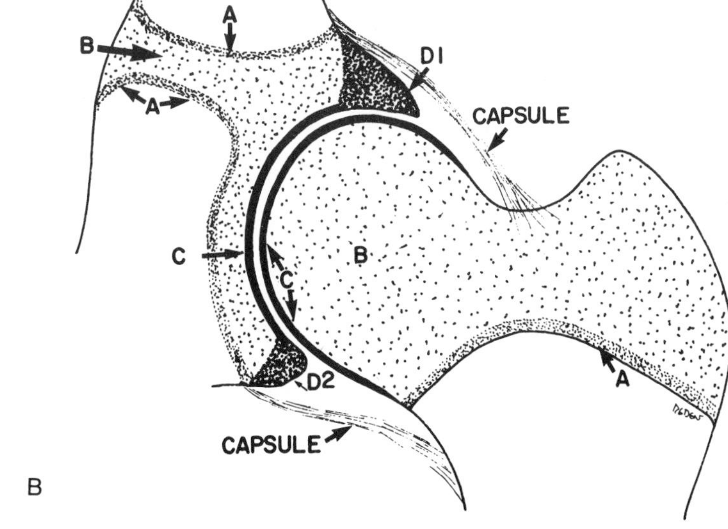

Figure 71–4. *Histologic* **(A)** *and schematic* **(B)** *sections of neonatal hip showing relatively transverse, single physis under the common chondroepiphysis of the femoral head and greater trochanter. The cartilage canals are readily evident throughout the femoral and acetabular cartilage. Several different types of cartilage are present:* A, *physeal cartilage;* B, *hyaline cartilage;* C, *articular cartilage;* D, *fibrocartilage of the acetabular labrum* (D1) *and transverse acetabular ligament* (D2).

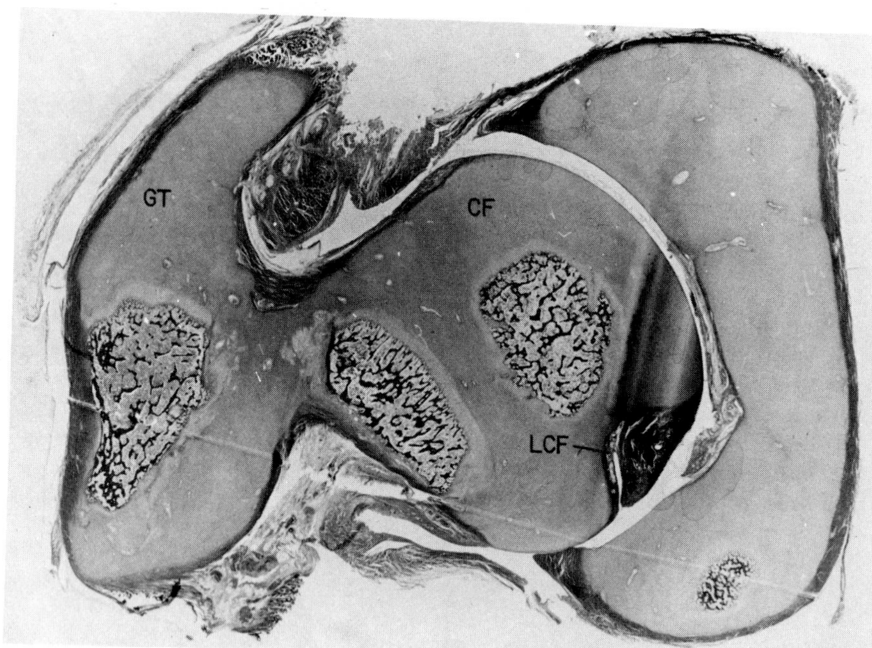

Figure 71–5. **A,** *Posterior section from 8 month old infant showing continuity of the epiphyseal cartilage of the head of the femur* (CF), *greater trochanter* (GT), *and lesser trochanter. The indentation for the ligamentum capitis femoris* (LCF) *is evident.*

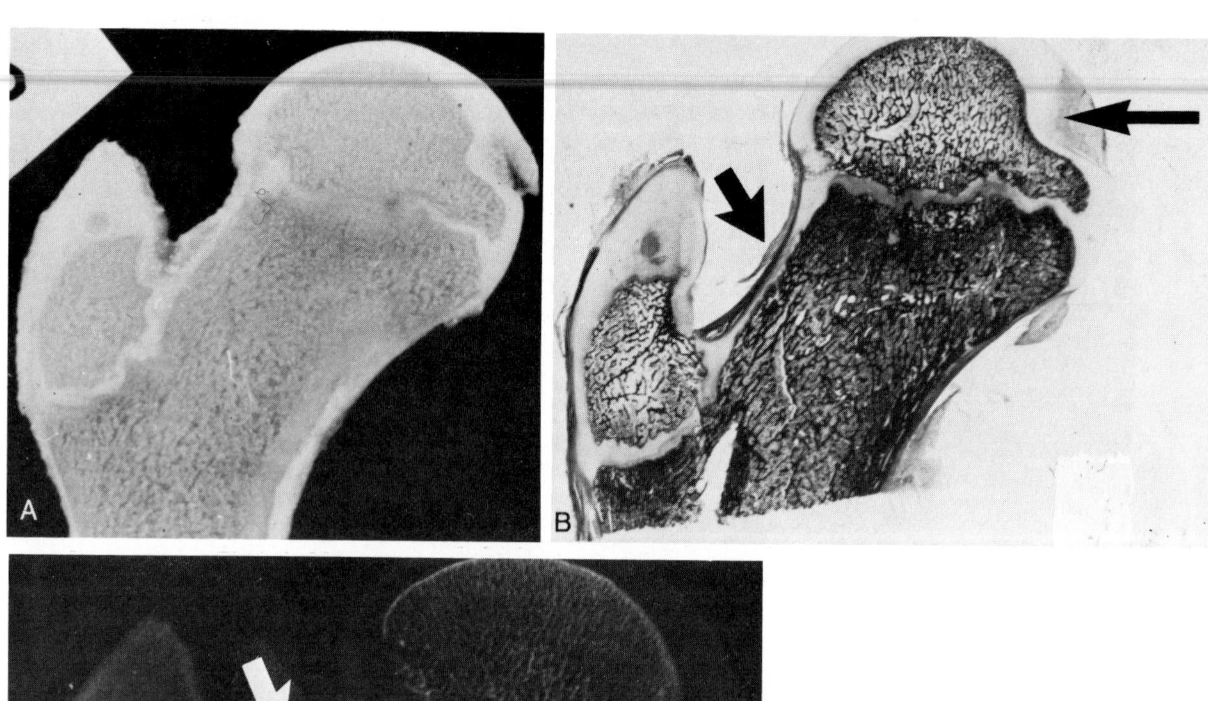

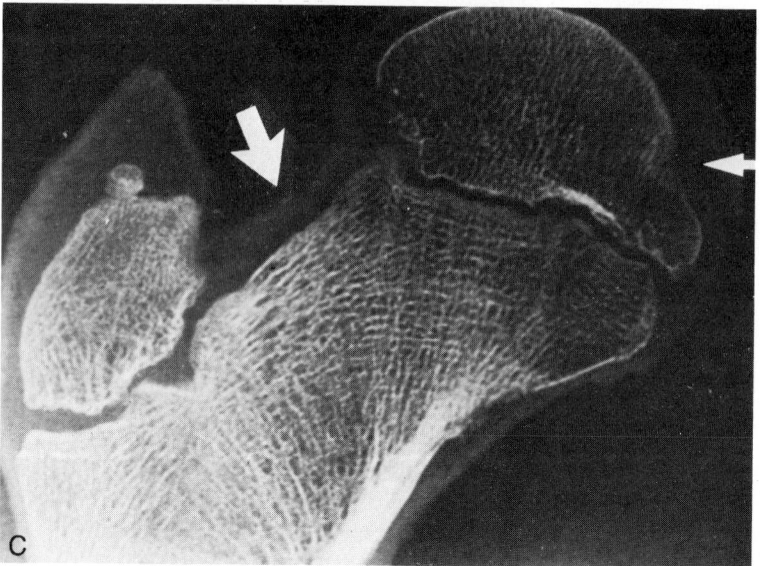

Figure 71–6. *Gross pathologic* **(A)**, *histologic* **(B)**, *and roentgenographic* **(C)** *sections from an 8 year old child showing that cartilage still exists along the posterosuperior femoral neck (heavy arrow). Note the indentation of the ossification center caused by the insertion of the ligamentum capitis femoris (thin arrow). An accessory ossification center is evident in the greater trochanter.*

regions are part of a unitary chondroepiphysis, but with continued postnatal development the femoral head will progressively "grow away" from the trochanter, effectively establishing the femoral neck characteristic of the adult. Since the chondroepiphysis is a composite unit there is an extensive connection of epiphyseal cartilage between the trochanter and head of the femur. As the femoral neck develops, this region becomes less prominent morphologically (Fig. 71–6). However, throughout most of the skeletal developmental period there is some epiphyseal cartilage along the posterior and superior regions of the femoral neck, an area that is generally radiolucent, but which must be considered in evaluating hip dysplasia. This intertrochanteric portion of the original chondroepiphysis is necessary for continued formation of an adequate femoral neck. If growth is disturbed in this region, major deformation of the femoral neck may accompany problems in the development of the femoral head. The pattern of growth in a posterosuperior direction from this particular segment of growth cells also is integral to the gradual decrease in the degree of anteversion.

Anteversion is a term frequently applied to the hips of young and older children. By definition it represents the relationship of the knee (bicondylar) axis to a similar axis drawn through the neck of the femur.[36] Since an elongated, anatomically defined, and radiographically measurable femoral neck is not present in the neonatal period, anteversion is difficult to quantitate radiologically. By 4 to 6 months of age, commensurate with development of the capital femoral ossification center, selective endochondral ossification in the medial and intertrochanteric portions (especially the latter) leads to a more readily defined femoral neck (Fig. 71–7). Measurement of the neck axis is easy in anatomic specimens, but it is not at all easy in roentgenograms, since these show only the ossified regions, which certainly are not indicative of the entire chondro-osseous neck width or length. As the child grows older and the intraepiphyseal cartilage becomes thinner along the superoposterior neck, defining the femoral neck axis becomes easier, although the large number of articles and mathematical conversion tables available suggest that measurement of the axis of the femoral neck is not completely foolproof. Documentation of the absolute degrees of anteversion is not necessary before approximately 18 months of age, when surgical approaches such as femoral osteotomies become more useful corrective procedures. However, despite the earlier statements, anteversion of the capital femoral chondroepiphysis relative to the trochanters and bicondylar distal femoral axis exists in the newborn and even occurs prenatally (Fig. 71–8), and this probably is a major factor in the development of anterior acetabular deficiency and external rotation-adduction contracture deformities of the femur, alterations that will be shown to be of major significance in the development of the secondary acetabular cartilaginous and osseous changes that precede and predispose to subluxation and dislocation of the head of the femur.

The greater trochanter initially forms a large

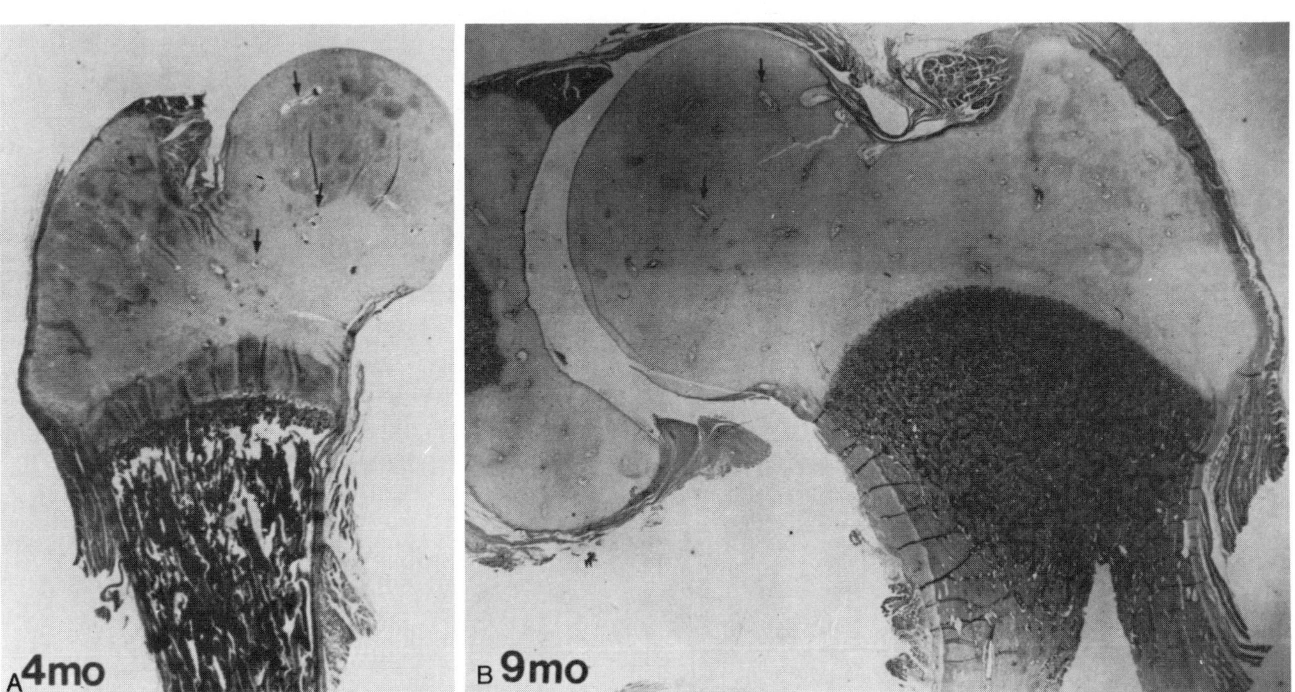

Figure 71–7. Histologic sections at 4 months' gestation **(A)** and at full term **(B)** showing early changes in physeal contour, but without the establishment of a roentgenographically measurable neck.

Illustration continued on the following page

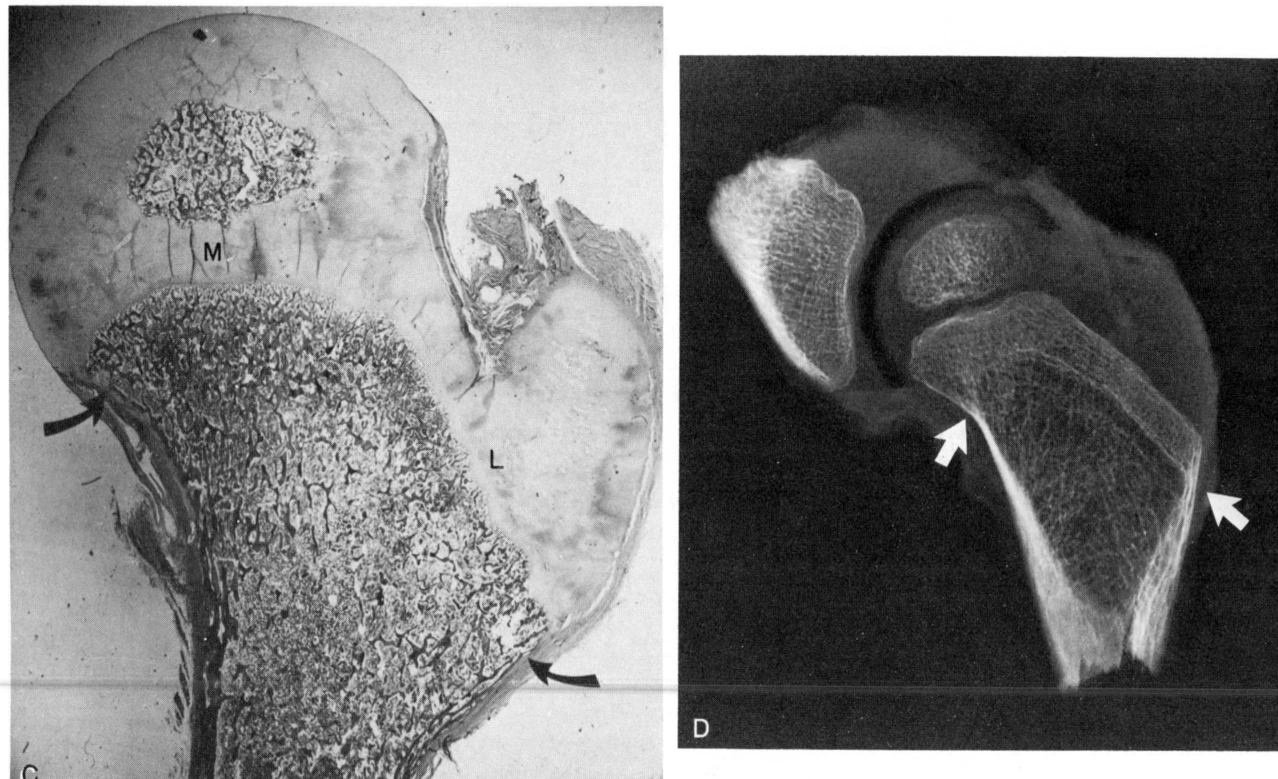

Figure 71–7. Continued

C, *By 7 months after birth, differential growth of the medial physis (M) at a faster rate than the lateral physis (L) has created a femoral neck. Arrows point to the fenestrated metaphyseal cortex that allows intertrabecular infection to penetrate easily into the subperiosteal space.* **D,** *Roentgenogram of 16 month old child showing Harris growth line (arrows).*

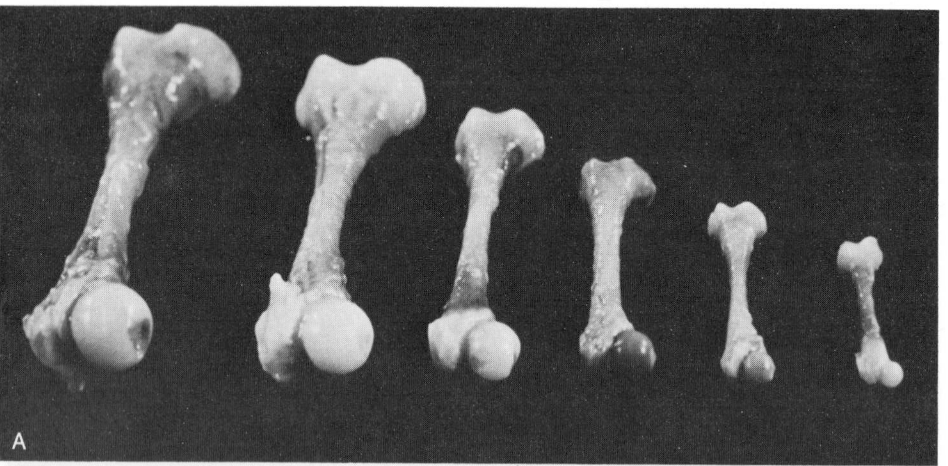

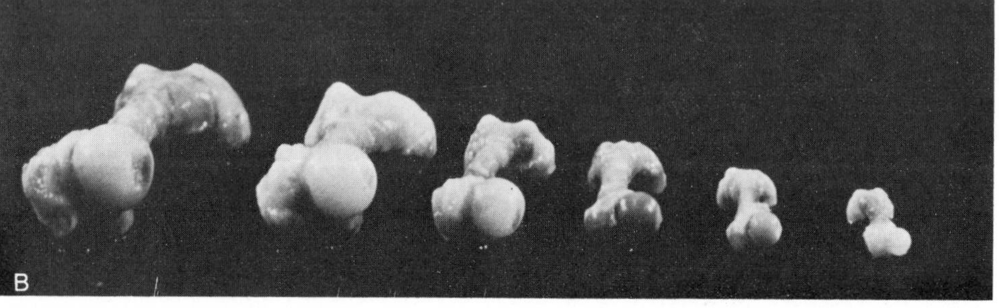

Figure 71–8. *Series of fetal femora ranging from 3 months (right) to full term (left), showing the variable degrees of anteversion. (Femoral heads located at bottom of each specimen as if viewed from the pelvis.)*

cartilaginous element and continues to enlarge in this tissue mode until the child is 5 to 6 years of age, when secondary ossification eventually begins. The initial ossification occurs in a region near the physis and then progressively extends proximally into the preexistent epiphyseal cartilage (Fig. 71–9). This pattern of development gives rise to certain misconceptions regarding radiographic measurements, particularly that of the articulotrochanteric distance, which often is used to define whether a relative coxa vara exists, especially in dealing with growth deformity secondary to complicating ischemic necrosis. It should be remembered that a large cartilaginous component always exists, and that ossification progressively extends into this region. There is some longitudinal growth from the proximal portion of the greater trochanter.

The composite physis (growth plate) extends from the lateral margin under the greater trochanter, along the developing femoral neck under the intraepiphyseal region, and finally under the head of the femur. Initially this growth plate is relatively transverse (Figs. 71–10 and 71–11). However, as the femoral neck develops, the growth plate assumes greater degrees of angulation relative to the longitudinal axis of the femur, and the region under the femoral head begins to turn until it is approximately perpendicular to the developing neck axis. At the medial region, the growth plate curves retrogradely toward the calcar. These contour changes are a reflection and response of the physeal growth cells to the genetic message determining the development of the human femur as well as a response to biomechanical stress. If the normal biologic stresses are altered, as in a hip that is being subjected to pathologic muscular contractures or which is being progressively subluxated or dislocated, abnormal stress is being applied, and the appropriate stimulus to growth in certain directions is lessened, if not negated. This may result in failure of the growth plate to begin development of the posterosuperior region of the femoral neck, leaving residual anteversion. Also, there is a decreased stimulus for the region under the head of the femur to begin its more medial angulation. This will accordingly affect development of the femoral neck and accentuate valgus direction.

The femoral head is the largest portion that develops from the initially composite proximal femoral chondroepiphysis. This region requires contiguity and a certain degree of congruency with the

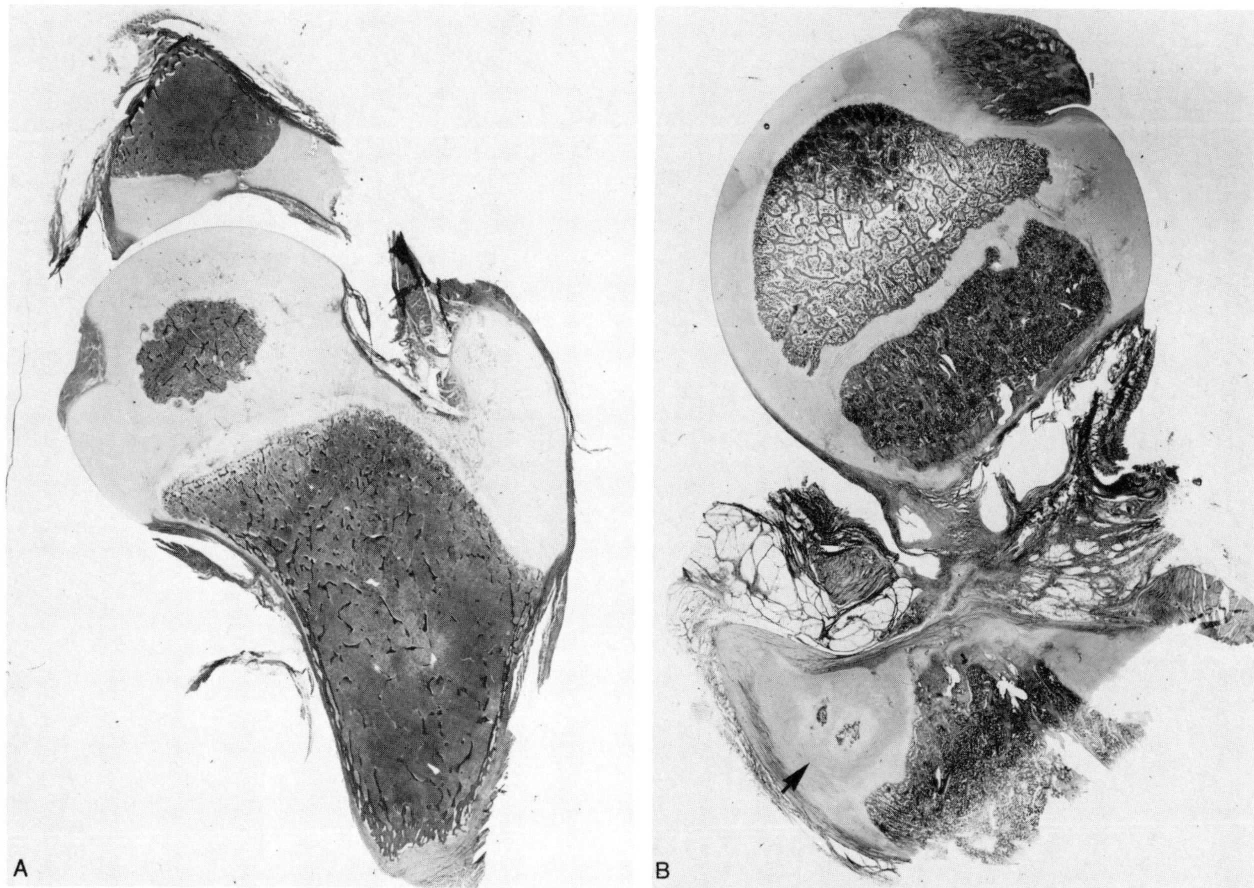

Figure 71–9. *Development of the trochanter.* **A,** *Ten month old infant with well-established chondroepiphysis.* **B,** *Early ossification in a 7 year old child (arrow).*

Illustration continued on the following page

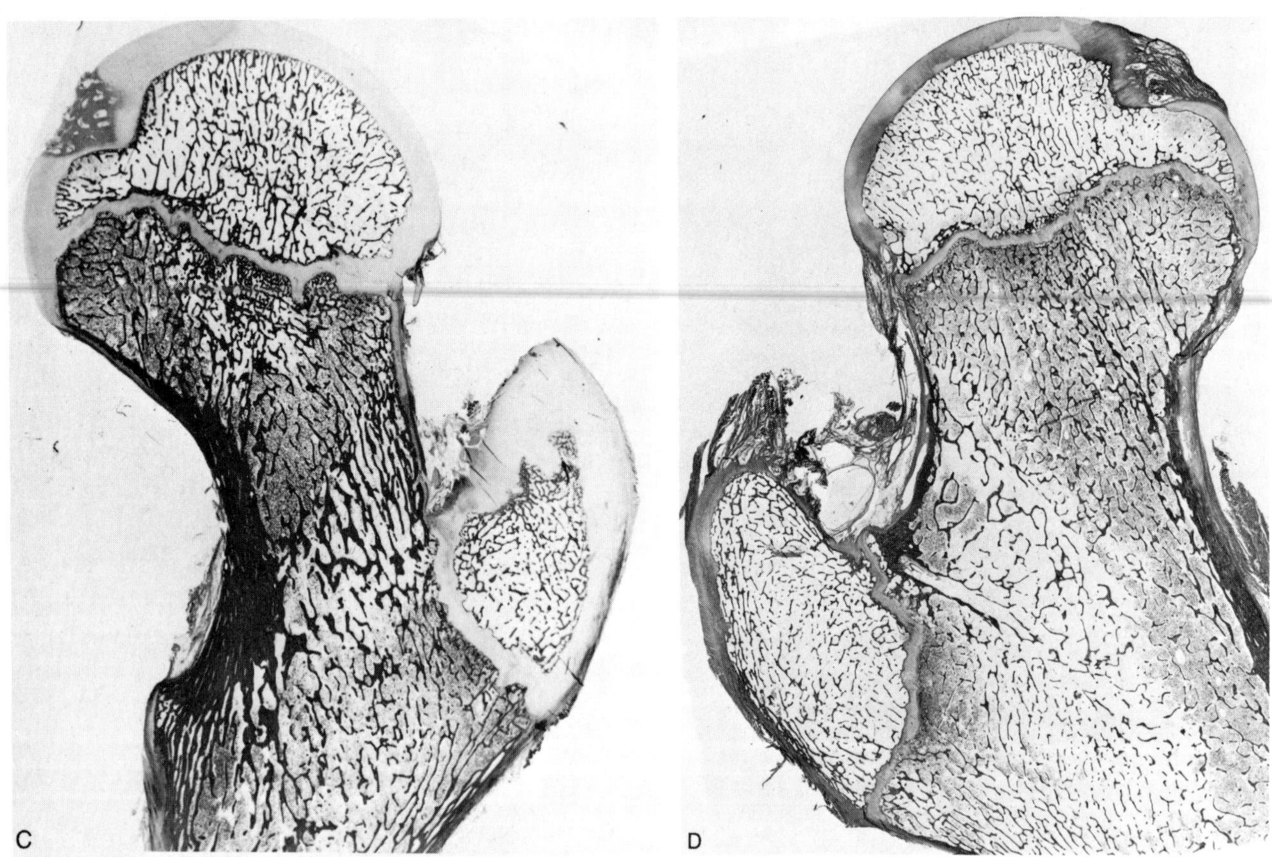

Figure 71–9. Continued
C, *Established ossification in a 10 year old child.* **D,** *Relatively complete ossification in a 14 year old adolescent.*

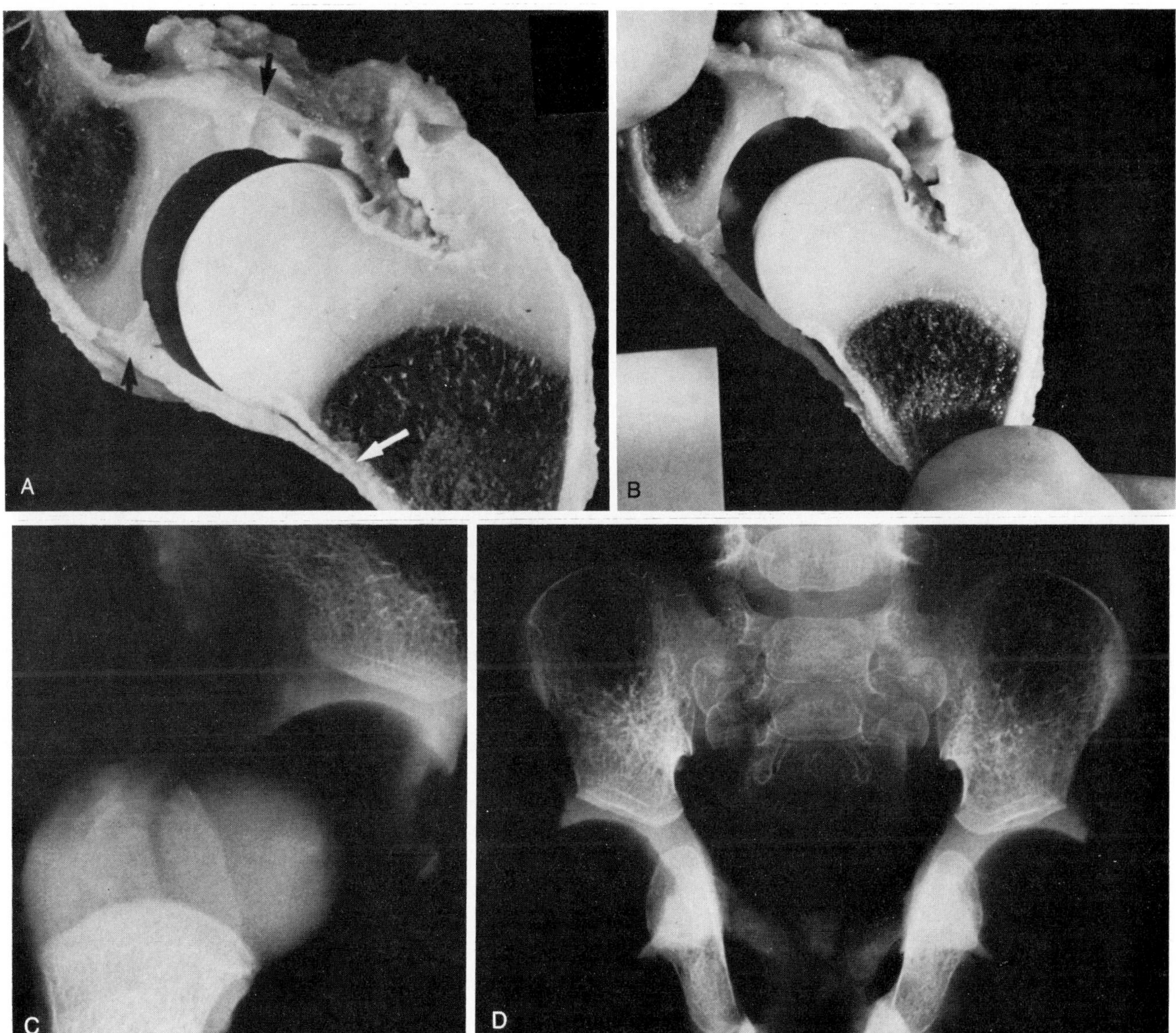

Figure 71–10. *Hip from a 2 month old infant.* **A,** *Slab section showing attachment of capsule to metaphysis (white arrow), making part of neck intracapsular, and to the acetabulum beyond the labrum (black arrows), making this structure also intracapsular, a fact readily evident on arthrography ("rose thorn" sign).* **B,** *The hip components have been separated (capsule intact) to duplicate displacement that may occur in an unstable hip or in a septic hip of infancy.* **C,** *Roentgenogram of proximal femur illustrating normally radiolucent chondroepiphysis.* **D,** *Roentgenogram of pelvis showing normally radiolucent acetabular cartilage.*

acetabular articular surface in order to develop its normal hemispheric shape. Again, if the proximal femur is being progressively subluxated or is even completely dislocated from the acetabulum, the appropriate and necessary integral joint surface will not be present, and pathologic pressure will be applied to the posterior and superior regions of the femoral head, leading to structural deformation of the posterior region. In these early stages of development, and certainly within the first 12 to 18 months after birth, the femoral head is primarily a cartilaginous structure, and as such is capable of a considerable degree of plastic deformation, which is, to a certain extent, reversible.

A secondary center of ossification develops within the head of the femur. Initially this forms as a solitary focus of ossification, although multiple foci occasionally may be present. The development of this ossification center requires a preexistent and adequately functioning blood supply (Fig. 71–12).

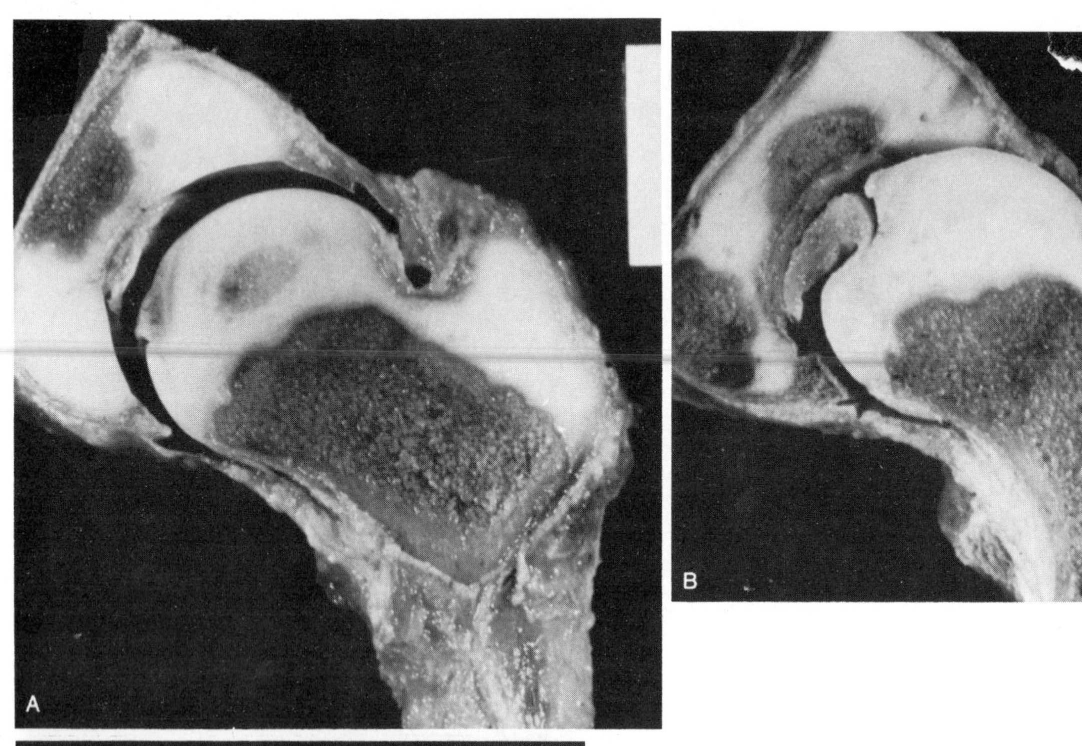

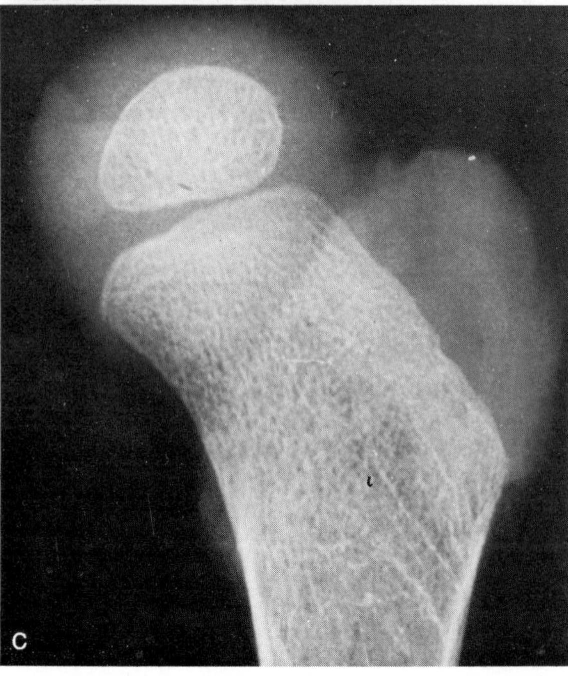

Figure 71–11. *Hip from 16 month old child. Compare development of the femoral neck with that in the neonate in Figure 71–10.* **A,** *Midsagittal section showing initial undulations of physis.* **B,** *Posterosagittal section showing attachment of ligamentum capitis femoris.* **C,** *Roentgenogram of proximal femur demonstrating cartilage.*

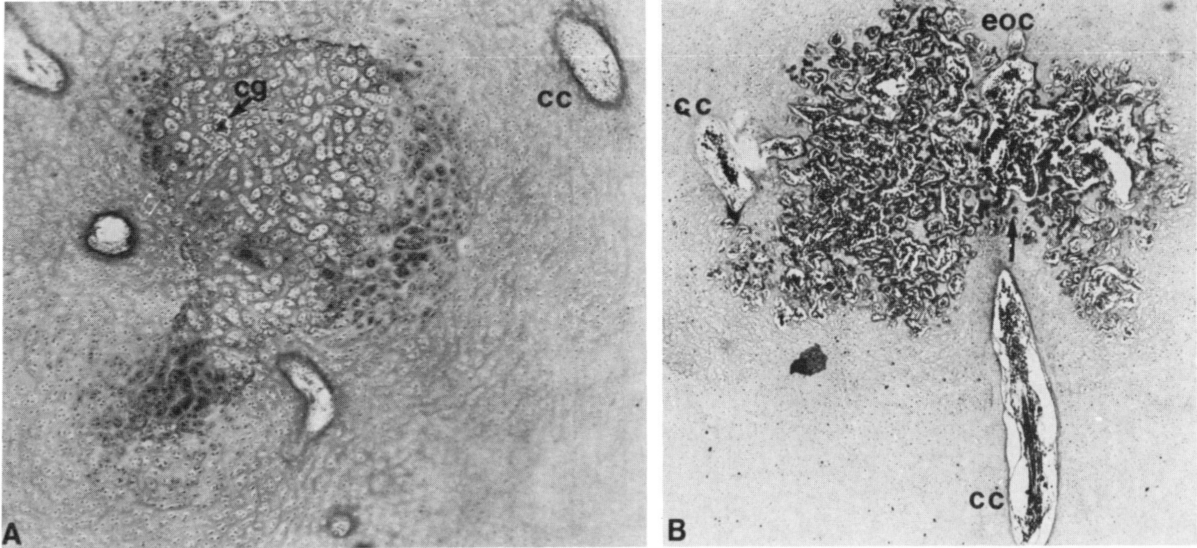

Figure 71–12. *Early development of ossification center.* **A**, *Preossification center with cartilage hypertrophy within several cartilage canals* (cc). *A small capillary glomerulus* (cg) *is present within the cartilage, a necessary prerequisite to ossification.* **B**, *Radiation of ossification center* (eoc) *away from the site of initial vascular invasion* (cc, *arrow*).

The formation of the secondary center is a modified endochondral ossification process. One small blood vessel from one of the cartilage canal systems enters the hypertrophic cartilage region, comparable to the irruption artery of primary ossification, and begins the transformation of epiphyseal cartilage to bone. The continued enlargement of the ossification center (Fig. 71–13) also is dependent on a continued vascular supply. Interference with this blood supply at either microvascular or macrovascular (extracapsular) levels may lead to ischemic (avascular) damage to the proximal femur.

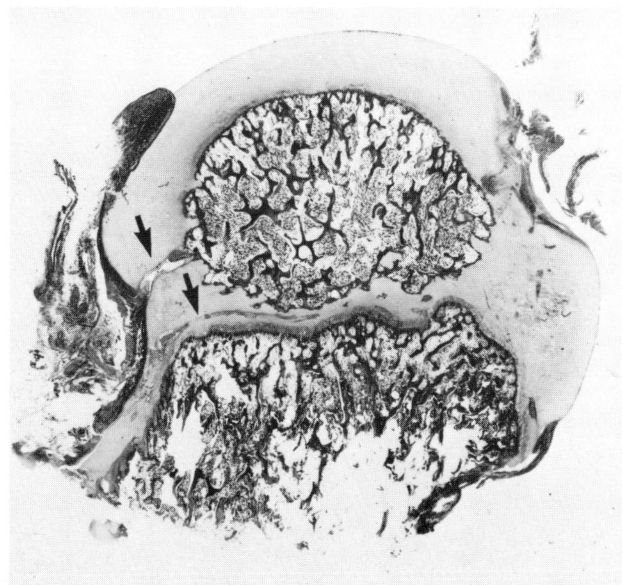

Figure 71–13. *Vessels entering femoral head in a 4 year old child (arrows). This posterosuperior vessel is the primary supply to the capital femoral ossification center, and its compromise may lead to ischemic necrosis.*

As in the development of the physis, the appearance of the secondary ossification center of the femoral head, although to some extent genetically predetermined, also is highly contingent upon the appropriate biomechanical stimuli. If the hip is unstable, there is delayed development of this ossification center. It is not uncommon to see asymmetric ossification (right versus left; Fig. 71–14) as one of the primary diagnostic determinants of an unstable hip, although a certain degree of asymmetry is normal. If there is asymmetric ossification coupled with significant clinical findings and some subtle changes in the development of the acetabular rim, it is reasonable to make a diagnosis of congenital hip dysplasia.

The acetabulum is equally complex in its development and involves several major areas that are of importance to the understanding of congenital hip dysplasia. The acetabulum is a composite of chondro-osseous elements of the iliac, ischial, and pubic bones. The cartilaginous "ends" of each of these three bones, analogous to the epiphyses of a long bone, meet as the triradiate cartilage (Fig. 71–15). This cartilage allows integrated development of the three pelvic bones and increasing enlargement of the hemispheric shape of the acetabulum. Eventually secondary centers of ossification will form within the triradiate cartilage and contribute to closure (fusion) of all three bones (Fig. 71–16).

The bulk of the triradiate cartilage and acetabular surface is composed of hyaline cartilage. However, at the margin of the joint there is a his-

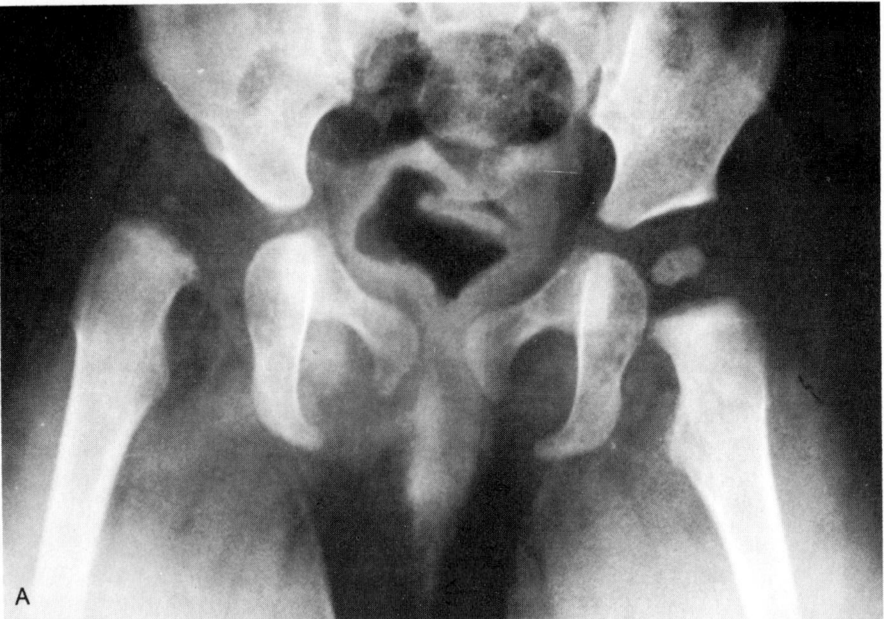

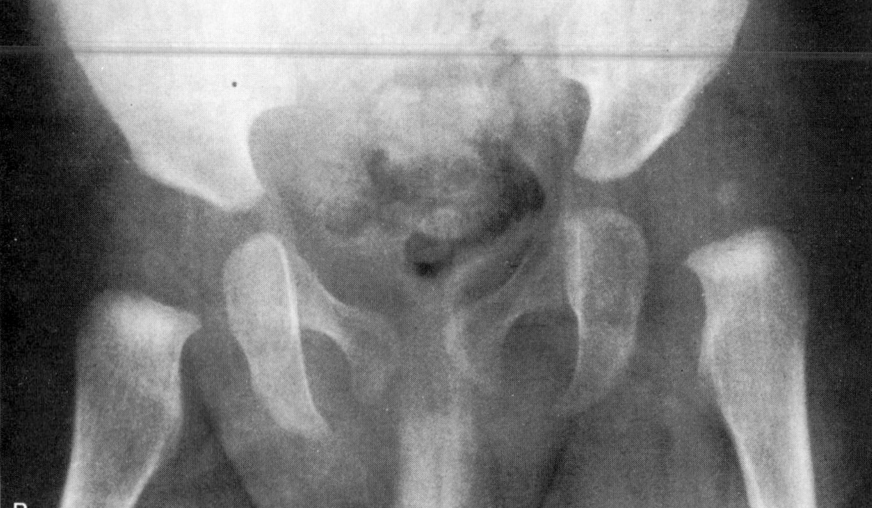

Figure 71–14. *Asymmetric ossification of the femoral head.* **A,** *Usually the dysplastic side (right side) is developmentally delayed.* **B,** *However, the more mature side also may be the dysplastic side (left side). Asymmetric ossification also may be normal, but its presence should alert the physician to possible problems.*

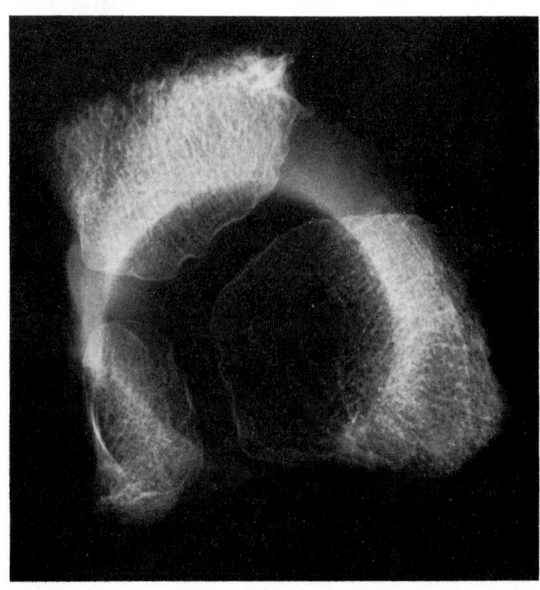

Figure 71–15. *Acetabulum from a 3 year old child showing the triradiate cartilage.*

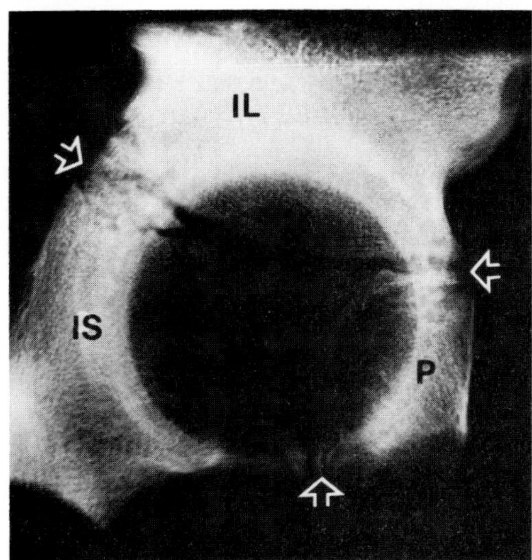

Figure 71–16. *Triradiate cartilage from 14 year old patient showing development of secondary ossification centers (arrows) within the cartilage. These are analogous to epiphyseal secondary ossification centers. IL, Ilium; IS, ischium; P, pubis.*

tologically different cartilage, fibrocartilage, which makes up the acetabular labrum and its continuity, the transverse acetabular ligament (Figs. 71–17 and 71–18). The latter structure is simply the same fibrocartilaginous tissue traversing an area devoid of underlying hyaline cartilage. The traversed area is filled with a fibrofatty tissue in which can be found the attachments of the ligamentum capitis femoris and its blood supply. The acetabular labrum is extremely pliable and may be structurally deformed by excessive pressure from the femoral head, leading to eversion or inversion of the fibrocartilage. If it inverts and undergoes subsequent pathologic cellular hypertrophy, it becomes an impediment to reduction of the proximal femur into the acetabulum and may be defined as a *limbus* (Fig. 71–30).

The joint capsule attaches at the junction of the fibrocartilaginous labrum with the adjacent hyaline cartilage, making the labrum completely intracapsular. If the capsule is attenuated and elongated, allowing the hip to subluxate or dislocate, the proximal femur may progress beyond the limits of the labrum (but yet still be intracapsular). The capsule attaches to the proximal femur along the margins of the intertrochanteric groove. Development of the femoral neck thus makes it an increasingly intracapsular structure (Fig. 71–17).

One of the areas of major significance in diagnosis of CDH is the concept of acetabular acclivity,

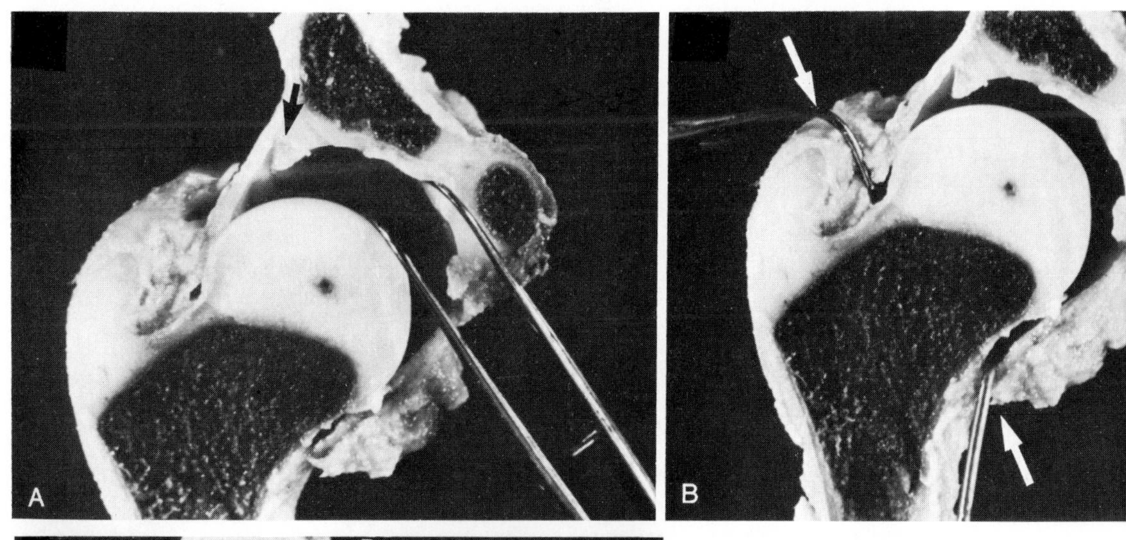

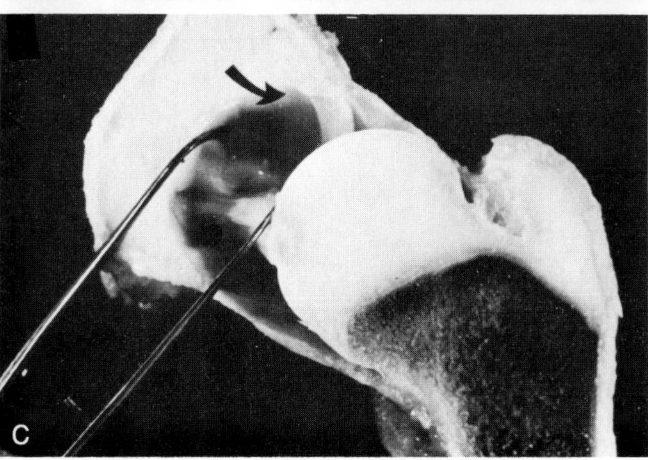

Figure 71–17. *Hip from a 4 month old infant. Note early development of the secondary ossification center.* **A,** *Extent of lateral displacement easily allowed by capsular laxity is demonstrated. The acetabular labrum is intracapsular (arrow).* **B,** *The capsule attaches to the base of the neck (arrows), making much of the medial metaphysis intracapsular.* **C,** *The fibrocartilage of the labrum (arrow) is grossly distinguishable from the articular surface of the acetabulum.*

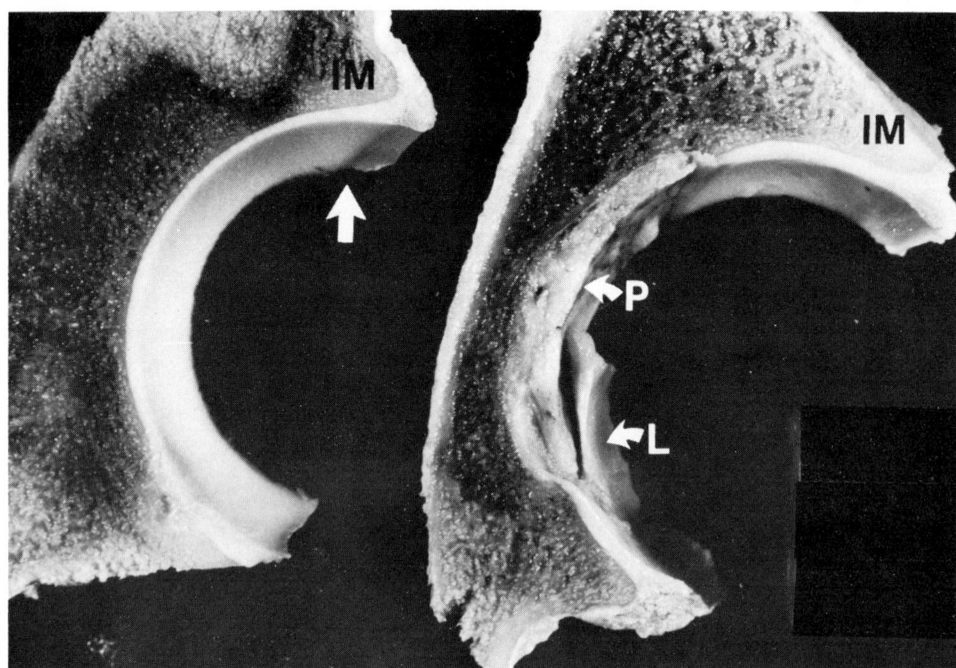

Figure 71–18. *Sagittal sections of acetabulum from a 14 year old patient showing junction of fibrocartilage and articular cartilage (arrow).* IM, *Iliac metaphysis;* P, *pulvinar;* L, *ligamentum capitis femoris.*

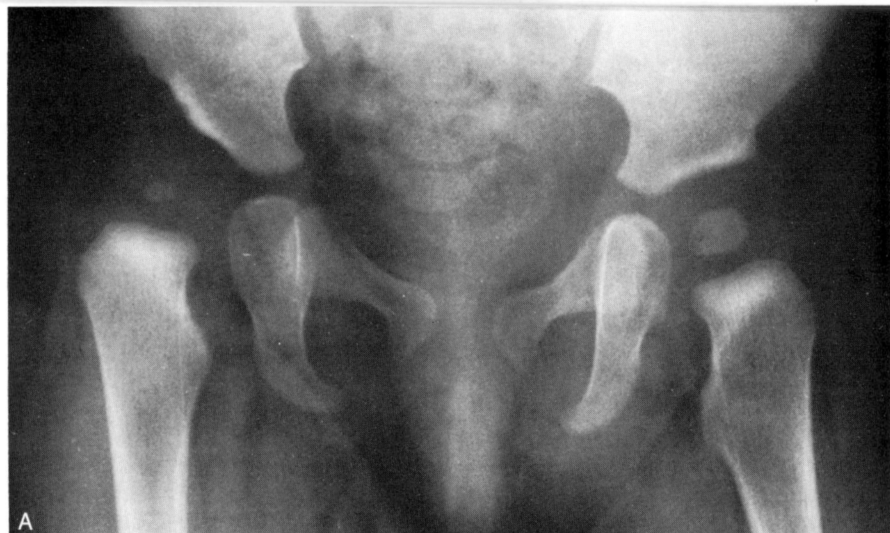

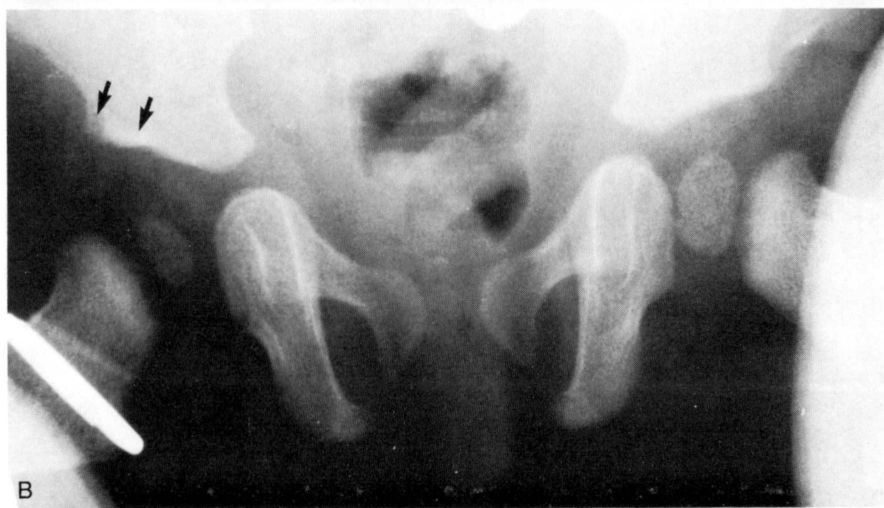

Figure 71–19. **A,** *Seven month old female infant with dysplastic right hip and increased acetabular acclivity.* **B,** *Six months after active treatment in a Pavlik harness, the lateral acetabular roof has filled in (arrows) to create a more normal acetabulum.*

involving the lateral osseous roof. This region is analogous to a metaphysis and as such is capable of extensive remodeling in response to biologic stress. The area is composed of trabecular bone and does not normally have a dense subchondral plate in the neonatal period. If abnormal pressure is applied to this region, soft tissue development (that is, cartilaginous) may continue, but the appropriate stimulus for normal endochondral transformation will be delayed or impeded. This is most evident on an arthrogram in which there is an obviously large segment of radiolucent cartilage between the joint surface and the radiopaque osseous elements (Fig. 71–19*A*). When treatment of CDH is progressing satisfactorily, this lateral margin will fill in very rapidly and have a more acceptable radiographic appearance (Fig. 71–19*B*).

To a certain degree, the femoral head is maintained in its relationship with the acetabulum by a suction effect, but the ligamentum capitis femoris also plays a role in keeping the hip stable in certain positions. This is normally a flat, ribbon-like structure, rather than the rounded structure often shown in anatomy textbooks. It will generally follow the contour of the head, but in CDH may become pathologically elongated and hypertrophied and serve as an additional impediment to normal reduction.

The blood supply to the proximal femur is constantly changing[6, 22] at both micro- and macrovascular levels. The primary blood supply is derived from the medial circumflex artery, which sends off two major branches in its course along the posterior femoral neck. These are the posteroinferior and posterosuperior branches, which become intracapsular structures. Both are susceptible to compromise, as is the main medial circumflex artery, and any impingement on the normal flow of blood through these particular vessels may result in ischemic changes.[3, 11, 13, 23, 24, 34] These vascular patterns in the normal and abnormal states are described in more detail elsewhere.[3, 23]

PATHOBIOLOGY

Before embarking on a description of the pathologic changes in the various types of hip dysplasia, it is necessary to introduce some basic definitions. Classification may be based upon two criteria: primary causes and secondary changes. From an etiologic standpoint, congenital hip disease may be classified as teratologic or typical. The use of these terms implies known etiology, usually of a neuromuscular nature, in contradistinction to an idiopathic problem that probably arises due to intrauterine positioning and physiologic changes of the last trimester (e.g., capsular response to hormonal changes). The teratologic hip frequently is severely subluxated or completely dislocated at birth, and the degree of malposition may worsen during the postnatal period owing to continued abnormal biomechanics, particularly if the deformity is the result of a significant neurologic disorder. A child with a high level myelomeningocele may have considerable deformation of the hip at birth, whereas a child with a lower level myelomeningocele may not begin to manifest hip deformity until the postnatal period. Similarly, teratologic hip displacement in a child with cerebral palsy will occur in a hip that has developed normally throughout gestation, which only begins to deform postnatally in accordance with the type of palsy (e.g., flaccid versus spastic) and the degree of muscular involvement. In contrast, only rarely is the typical "dislocated hip" truly dislocated at birth. In reality this type of hip is unstable in some positions and stable in others. It should be "reducible" in appropriate positions of flexion and abduction. It should be realized that the arbitrary terms of "typical" and "teratologic" refer only to etiology.

Leveuf and co-workers emphasized that CDH should be divided into two distinct categories — subluxation and luxation.[16, 17] According to their criteria, the acetabular rim is forced superiorly (everted) against the ilium in subluxation, whereas the rim is inverted into the true acetabulum in a luxation or true dislocation. These investigators referred to this acetabular rim as the limbus in both the normal hip and the two types of CDH. However, prevailing use of the term "limbus" should perhaps be confined to the pathologically hypertrophied, inverted acetabular margin of the complete dislocation. As demonstrated by several authors, this fibrocartilaginous acetabular rim is grossly and histologically distinct from the hyaline cartilage of the acetabulum, and is easily deformed by applied pressure, whether acute or chronic.[12, 15, 23, 26, 28, 31] Unfortunately, this classification is simplistic, especially with regard to the labrum, which probably does not invert acutely. Instead, it appears more likely that eccentric pressure from the lateralized, but still located, femoral head induces "flow" in the fibrocartilage, causing redirection of a portion of the tissue into the acetabulum, and an appearance of inversion during arthrography or during open reduction. This phenomenon will be discussed in more detail in ensuing sections.

Dunn performed a detailed study of neonatal hips and devised a classification scheme based primarily upon the shape of the acetabular margin, eversion or inversion of the limbus, and gross contour of the femoral head.[8, 9] These three types, as well as the normal, are illustrated schematically in Figure 71–20, and respectively represent positional instability or subluxatability (type 1), subluxation (type 2), and dislocation (type 3). The following description of the types of CDH is based upon a study of pathologic material derived from available fetal and child cadavers. This description serves to emphasize the variability of the radiographic and

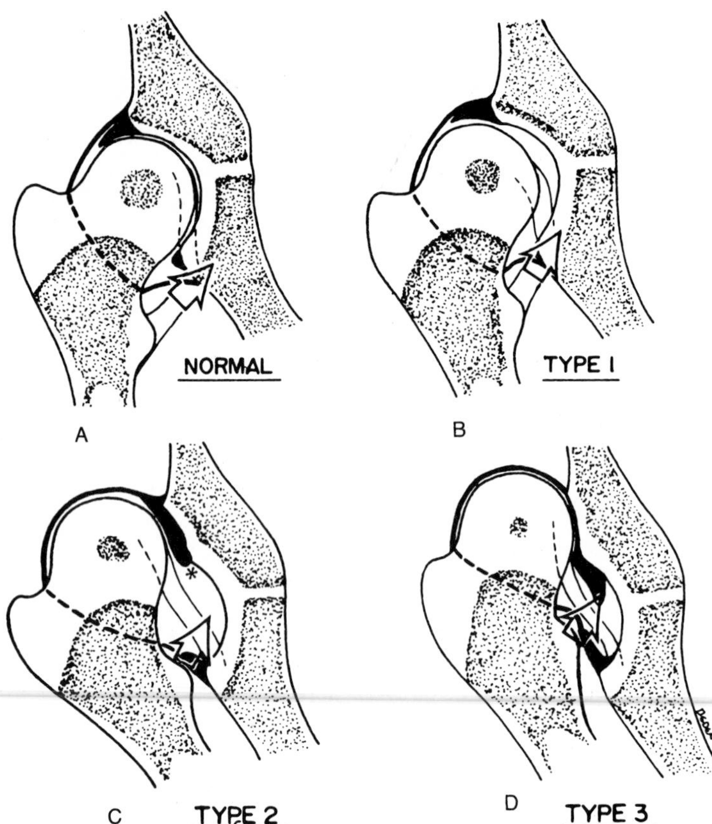

Figure 71–20. *Schematic diagram of hip dysplasia patterns.* **A**, *Normal.* **B**, *Type 1 —positionally unstable or subluxatable hip. The pliable labrum may be slightly deformed.* **C**, *Type 2 —subluxated hip, with eversion of the fibrocartilaginous labrum, which may exhibit some inversion (asterisk). This hip may be reduced relatively easily in flexion.* **D**, *Type 3 —dislocated hip, with inversion and hypertrophy of the limbus, which present an impediment to reduction.*

pathologic features of CDH. It will be followed by a discussion of pertinent clinical correlates.

Type 1

Probably 80 to 90 per cent of patients in the CDH classification have this pattern, especially during the neonatal period, which may be defined as a *subluxatable or positionally unstable hip.* Usually there are mild marginal changes in the acetabulum, while the femoral head is anteverted but spherically normal. There are mild adduction and flexion contractures attributed to the muscles (adductors), although much of the soft tissue change may be in the anterior and inferior joint capsule. If left untreated, this is probably the type of hip that may either progress to more severe deformity or, more likely, become the subluxated/anteverted hip of the older child. This type of hip probably would not manifest a true Ortolani sign (i.e., an emphatic "clunk"), but it certainly would exhibit lack of abduction.

Several positionally unstable hips were found among stillborn fetuses. All had unilateral involvement. All had flexion and adduction contractures that were not easily corrected to anatomic position even after all muscles were removed. The capsule, rather than the musculature, very obviously appeared to be the major limiting factor to complete abduction and extension. The femoral heads did not exhibit any gross contour deformities other than anteversion, which ranged from 60 to 90 degrees. In each case the obvious structural deformities involved the acetabulum (Fig. 71–21). All had mild, variable changes in the acetabular rim, involving both the hyaline and fibrocartilage components. Each involved acetabulum was shallow relative to the contralateral one. Figure 71–21*A* demonstrates limited involvement of the anterior and superior walls and virtually no involvement of the posterior wall. Figure 71–21*B* shows anterior and posterior wall deficiency, with eversion and enlargement of the superior rim; this patient also demonstrated minimal "inversion" of the fibrocartilage-hyaline cartilage junction posteriorly, despite eversion of the bulk of the fibrocartilaginous labrum. The last example (Fig. 71–21C) shows anterior deficiency with posterior eversion (again with a suggestion of minimal marginal "inversion" at the junction of articular surface and labrum). When the femora were placed in the acetabula, it was evident that the anteverted femoral heads were placing pressure on the deformed superior and posterior rims, whereas the anterior deformity appeared to result from pressure from the lesser trochanter and medial femoral metaphysis as well as the femoral head (Fig. 71–22). If the femur was placed in a position of flexion and moderate abduction of less than 60 degrees (a standard treatment position attainable by multiple diapers, Frejka pillow, Pavlik harness, and similar equipment), the

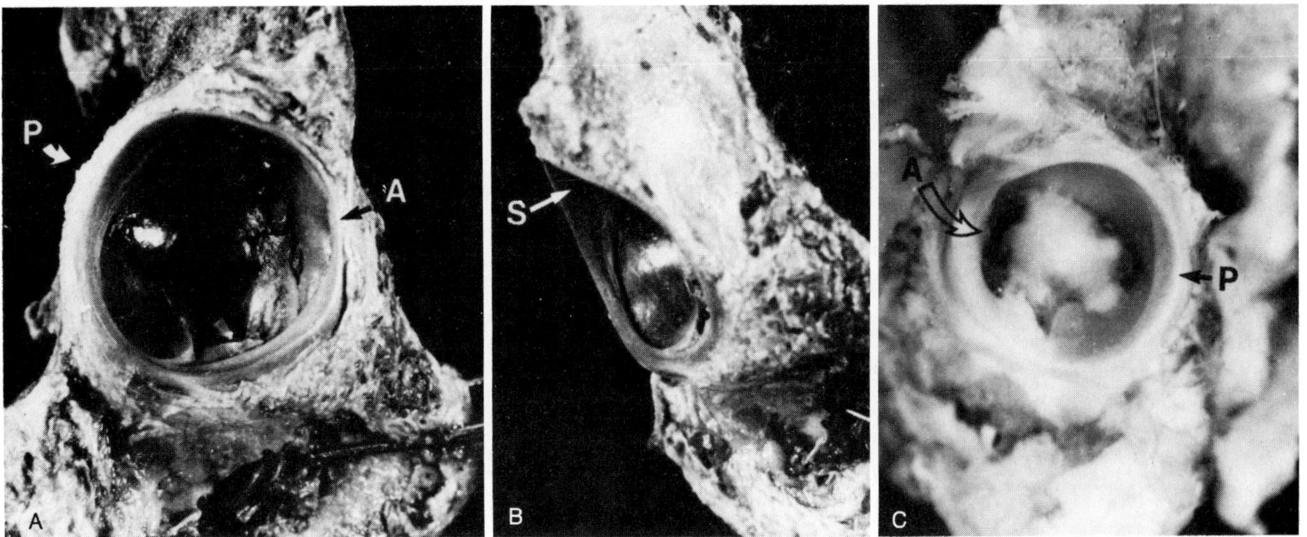

Figure 71–21. Type 1 variations. **A**, Narrowing of anterior labrum (A) and minimal eversion of posterosuperior labrum (P). **B**, Mild eversion of superior (S) labrum associated with anterior wall deficiency. **C**, Shallow anterior labrum (A) associated with posterior eversion (P) and normal superior rim.

femoral head could be directed more centrally and appeared to place less eccentric pressure on the superior and posterior rims. Further, in this position the femoral metaphysis and lesser trochanter were no longer resting against the deficient anterior rim (Fig. 71–23). Similar mild soft tissue changes may exist in the slightly older child, and appear to be the cause of marginal osseous changes seen during roentgenography (Fig. 71–23).

These fetuses demonstrate that mild changes along the acetabular margins lessen femoral head coverage and allow variable instability in certain positions, especially extension and adduction. All had significant femoral anteversion. The apparent intrauterine positions were such that excessive pressure was directed at the anterior wall by the lesser trochanter, iliopsoas tendon, and femoral head and metaphysis, causing anterior marginal deficiency. Because of soft tissue contractures (primarily capsular), the anteverted femoral head also placed excessive pressure on the superior and posterior margins, causing the fibrocartilaginous labrum to evert.

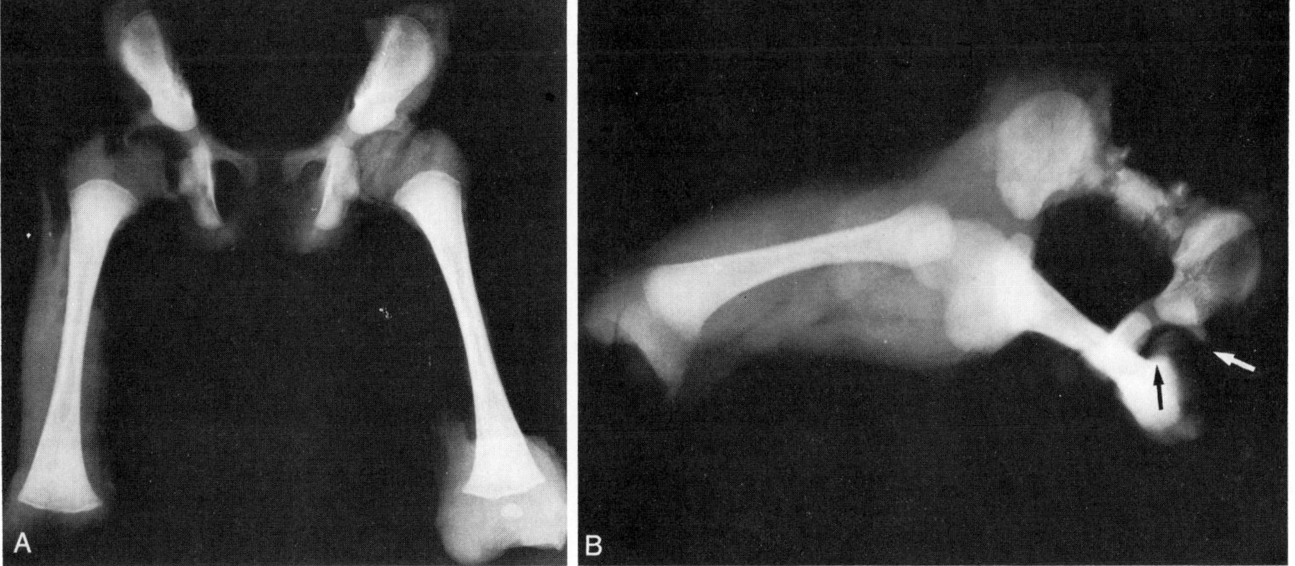

Figure 71–22. Pelvis of stillborn fetus with type 1 dysplasia (bilateral). **A**, Air has been introduced to outline the joint space on the left. On the right the hip has been displaced laterally. **B**, The left hip has been flexed and abducted to show how metaphysis lies against anterior rim (black arrow) and the head of the femur tends to be displaced posterosuperiorly (white arrow).

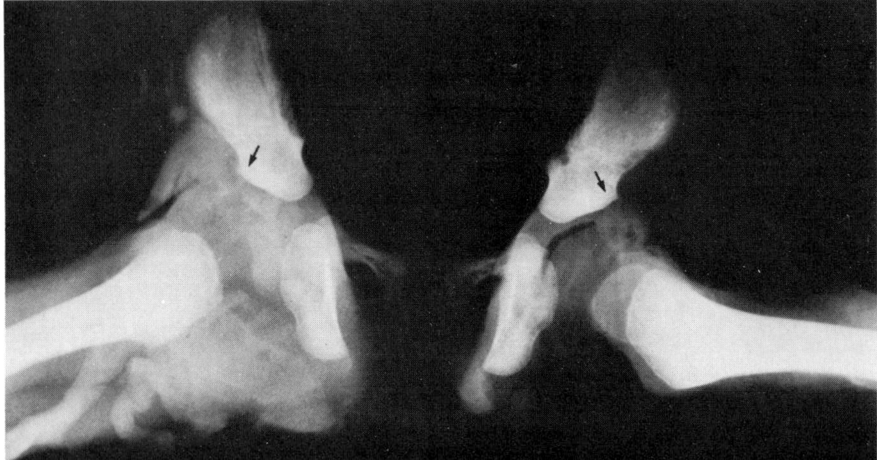

Figure 71–23. *Pelvis from a 2 month old infant with myelomeningocele. Minimal type 1 changes were evident grossly. The roentgenogram shows increased acclivity only of the lateral acetabular roof (arrows). Such subtle changes may be detected in clinical radiographs, and should make one suspect an unstable hip.*

However, while the majority of the posterior/superior labrum was everting, small portions of the fibrocartilage were noted to be hypertrophic and suggested that early, concomitant inversion may not be an acute phenomenon but rather a gradual, tectonic change.[19, 26] Placement of the hips in a flexion-abduction position created better coverage of the femoral head and directed pressure centrally rather than eccentrically. These positions decreased potentially deforming contact along the anterior margin and lessened lateralized contact superiorly. Both the anterior deficiency and the increased pressure from the anteverted, subluxatable femoral head undoubtedly contribute to the decreased ossification of the acetabular roof that manifests itself as an increased acetabular index (steepness or acclivity).

Type 2

This type of hip, which can be considered *subluxated,* will begin to show loss of sphericity of the femoral head as well as anteversion. Owing to pressure from different portions of the femoral head, the acetabulum is more shallow, has a significant narrowing of the anterior margin, and is beginning to show superior and posterior marginal deformities, primarily eversion of the labrum. The eversional soft tissue changes are accompanied by osseous chang-

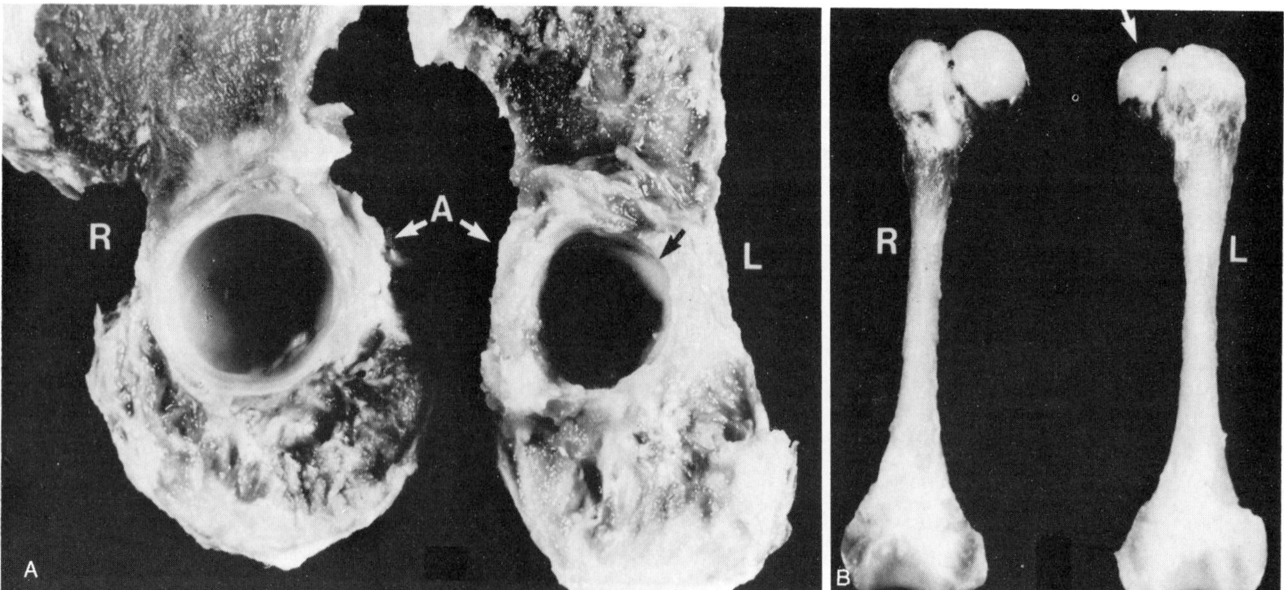

Figure 71–24. *Type 2 deformity in a stillborn infant.* **A,** *Acetabula;* **B,** *proximal femurs (R, right; L, left). The proximal femur had a mild varus deformity. The left acetabulum had a deficient anterior wall (A) and eversion of the posterior wall (black arrow). There is obvious loss of normal sphericity of the femoral head (white arrow).*

es — the acetabular roof fails to ossify laterally, leading to increased acetabular acclivity, which is an early roentgenographic sign. If untreated, this hip pattern probably progresses to a more severe subluxation or even complete dislocation. The hip usually has more severe flexion and adduction contractures. As the extensor-abductor groups (especially the gluteus medius and gluteus minimus muscles) become more active postnatally, they may pull the positionally susceptible proximal femur superiorly or posteriorly, or both, accentuating the marginal eversion. During this stage the first traces of inversion of the limbus may be discerned. As previously noted, it appears that inversion may not be an abrupt phenomenon, but rather a gradual process of hypertrophy and ingrowth of that portion of the fibrocartilaginous labrum adjacent to the hyaline cartilage. At this stage the inversional hypertrophy, which is associated with eversion of most of the labrum, is undoubtedly reversible. This type of hip probably exhibits a "clicking" sensation during an Ortolani maneuver, as well as loss of full abduction.

The acetabula were more deformed, particularly showing increased eversion of the posterosuperior margin, which contributed, along with the anterior labral deficiency, to shallow acetabula (Fig. 71–24*A*). The femoral heads again demonstrated significant anteversion and were beginning to show loss of sphericity (Fig. 71–24*B*). Attempts to place the hips in various treatment positions were not so successful as for type 1, owing to slightly increased incongruency between femoral head and acetabulum. The hips removed from an older child (3 months post partum) showed marked eversion of the posterosuperior rim on gross examination and increased acclivity on roentgenography (Fig. 71–25*A*). When air was introduced into the hip joint for roentgenographic contrast, the superior displacement and distended capsule became quite evident (Fig. 71–25*B*, *C*). Attempted reduction was not successful, owing to the presence of fibrofatty tissue in the acetabulum and flattening of the acetabulum, which caused incongruency of the components.

The hips in this category demonstrated a change

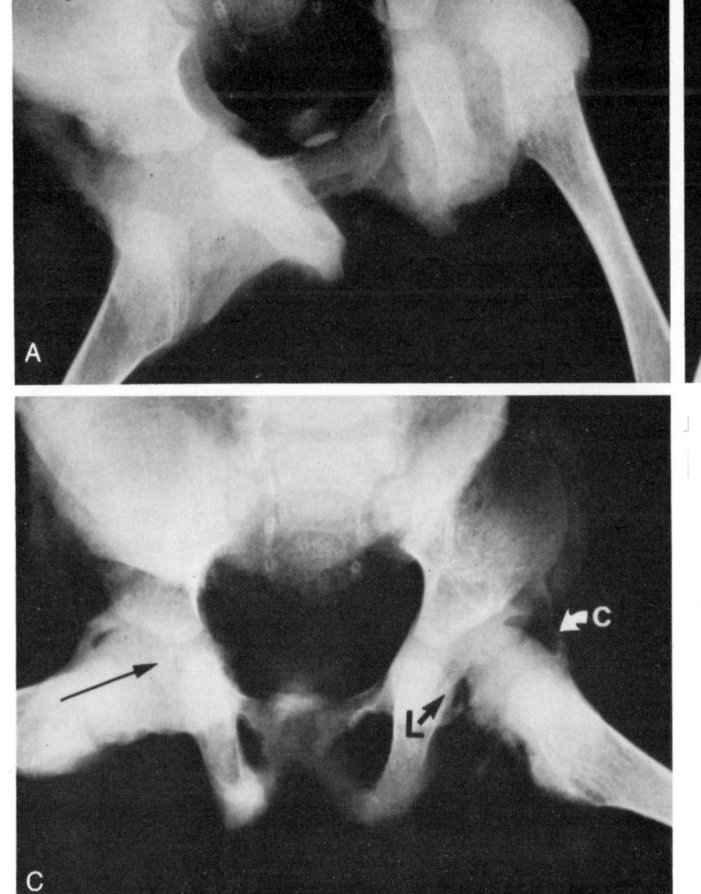

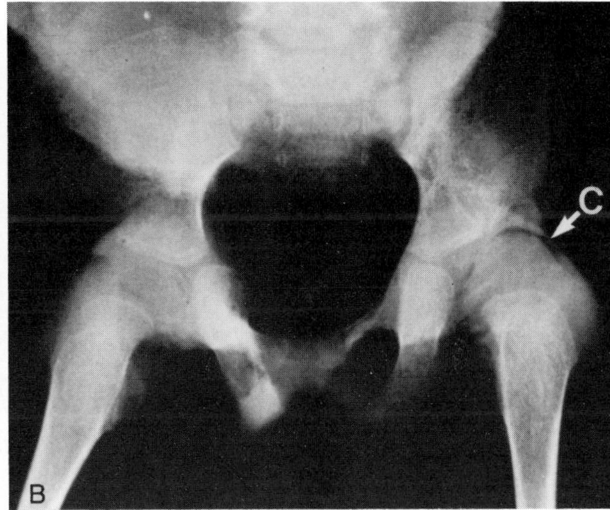

Figure 71–25. *Specimen roentgenogram of pelvis from a 3 month old infant with bilateral type 2 lesions.* **A,** *Increased acclivity of the acetabular roof, with some accompanying sclerosis (black arrow). The displacing femoral head is indicated by the open arrow.* **B,** *Air has been introduced to delineate the joint space and elongated, attenuated capsule (C).* **C,** *The proximal femur has been flexed and abducted, partially reducing the head into the acetabulum. Capsular (c) redundancy is evident. L, Ligamentum capitis femoris.*

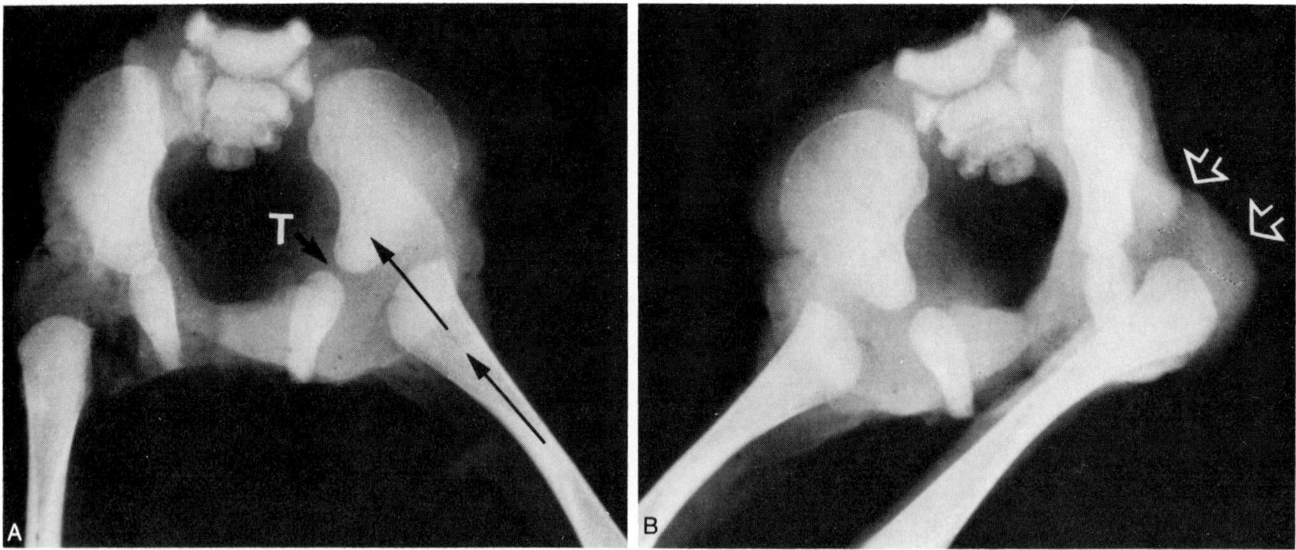

Figure 71–26. Specimen exhibiting type 3 deformity. **A,** Abduction fails to reduce the hip (T, triradiate cartilage). **B,** Adduction illustrates the posterosuperior displacement of the hip (arrows). Open reduction and removal of soft tissue would have been necessary to correct the deformity.

in gradation manifested by femoral head deformity and eversion of the posterosuperior labrum. In type 1, the mildly deformed acetabulum was elliptical in shape. In type 2, eccentric eversion and hypertrophy made the marginal contours much more irregular. Reduction was less satisfactory in type 2, but placement in usual treatment positions did lessen eccentric contact between femoral head and acetabulum.

Type 3

This type of hip is the most severely involved, with significant deformation of the acetabular margin and femoral head and a posterosuperior displacement of the head to form a false acetabulum by eversion of the labrum. Inversional hypertrophy of the fibrocartilage to form the limbus posterosuperiorly causes the acetabulum to be more incongruent in relation to the femoral head. Furthermore, the more hypertrophied the limbus, the more pressure it will apply to the femoral head, causing secondary indentations and continued loss of sphericity. The ligamentum capitis femoris is elongated, and it also is pulled up from its normal origin, bringing along with it the transverse acetabular ligament, which compromises acetabular volume and further precludes complete reduction. During the first 24 to 48 hours there is frequently sufficient laxity to manifest a "clunking" sensation during an Ortolani maneuver, with a concomitant dislocation during the Barlow maneuver.

The most severe deformations of the acetabular margins were encountered in this group. Figure 71–26 shows roentgenographic findings in a child

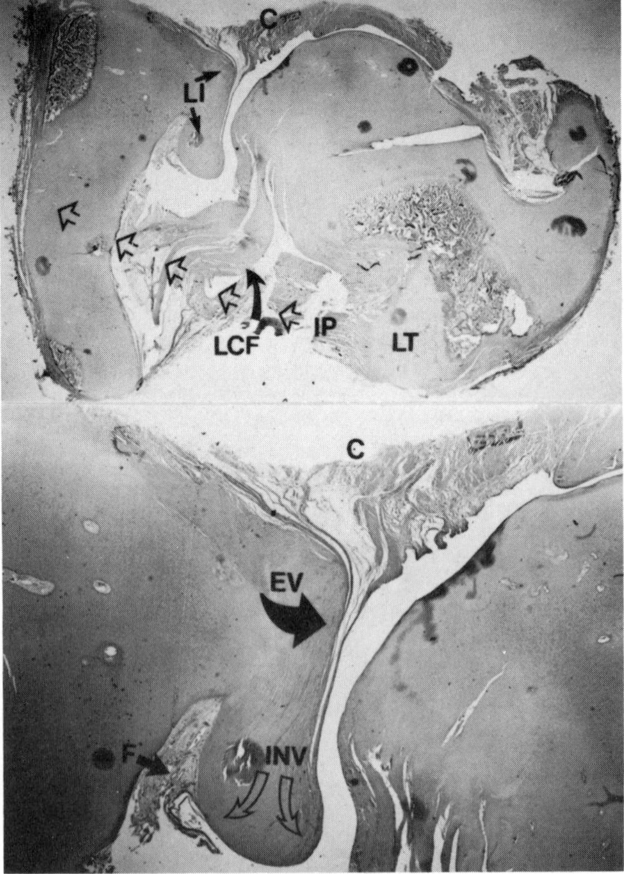

Figure 71–27. Histologic sections of type 3 dislocation with inversional hypertrophy and mild eversion of limbus. C, *Capsule;* LI, *limbus;* LT, *lesser trochanter;* LCF, *ligamentum capitis femoris;* IP, *iliopsoas tendon (open arrows indicate its course across the acetabulum);* EV, *everted labrum;* INV, *inverted labrum (limbus);* F, *fibrovascular pulvinar.*

who died several days after birth. It was impossible to acutely reduce this hip owing to contractures of the capsule (all muscles had been removed). Following capsulotomy, reduction was still unsatisfactory owing to loss of femoral head sphericity and extreme acetabular deformity. Other completely dislocated neonatal hips demonstrated that marginal changes of inversion really were a combination of (presumed) initial eversion followed by inversional hypertrophy, filling the vacated acetabulum (Fig. 71–27). The ligamentum capitis femoris was elongated in these cases and was pulled up from its normal origin, along with the transverse acetabular ligament.

These type 3 cases showed the most dramatic changes, with incongruency incompatible with acute, stable reduction. However, placement in treatment positions suggested that rearrangement of joint reaction forces might possibly reverse the inversional hypertrophy. This raises the possibility that excision of the limbus may not always be necessary. However, reversion of the changes may take an exceedingly long time. As in the other types, a major impediment to reduction was the presence of capsular rather than muscular contractures.

Although the less severe anatomic types appeared to be associated with typical CDH and the more severe anatomic changes were associated with teratologic CDH, the findings in this pathoanatomic study strongly suggest that there is an overlap of pathologic changes in this concatenate disease. Furthermore, many teratologic dislocations occur postnatally in previously normal hips, a situation not unlike the untreated typical CDH found only after the child begins to walk. The major differences between typical and teratologic types are the chronicity and degree of muscular deforming forces and the time of initial displacement. Because each etiologic type in the neonatal period has at least three recognizable anatomic types, it is imperative that the treating physician define the pathologic changes as accurately as possible and direct treatment appropriately.

The times of maximum susceptibility to hip subluxation and dislocation appear to be the last trimester and the neonatal period. Ráliš and McKibbin have shown that the depth of the acetabulum and the overall coverage of the femoral head gradually decrease to a minimum around full term.[33] The femoral head has a significant effect on the contour of the acetabulum and may profoundly change the acetabular shape owing to intrauterine position, thereby accentuating the normal process of decreasing acetabular depth.

Postnatal Pathobiology

The changes that take place in the perinatal period form a spectrum of deformities involving both sides of the hip joint. These changes have been classified arbitrarily into three types. The subluxatable hip (type 1), by far the most commonly encountered during neonatal examination, shows minimal acetabular and no femoral head changes (other than anteversion) and adequate correction of presumed deforming forces by flexion-mild abduction treatment. The subluxated hip (type 2) also shows improvement potential by these treatment positions, but concomitant femoral head changes also are becoming evident. The most deformed hips are the true dislocations (type 3). One of the most important structural changes is the development of the limbus. However, this appears consequent to "flow" of the biologically plastic fibrocartilage, rather than to abrupt inversion, raising the possibility that even these changes might be gradually reversible. As the child becomes older, the pull of the gluteus muscles against the adducted proximal femur appears to be a major factor accentuating the posterior (and to some degree, superior) deformity. In fact, if the hip, with its attendant capsular contractures, is brought toward extension, the proximal femur tends to piston posterosuperiorly out of the acetabulum, regardless of whether it is of type 1, 2, or 3 deformity. Finally, there is *no* correlation between typical or teratologic hip and severity of anatomic changes.

From a clinical standpoint the subluxating or dislocated hip becomes increasingly difficult to diagnose and manage after the first 3 to 4 months of life, as cartilaginous deformation and soft tissue contractures worsen. Of those hips available for detailed pathologic study, only a few from the perinatal period demonstrated major structural deformities. The majority of the perinatal cases exhibited mild to moderate anteversion, some posteromedial flattening of the femoral head, and marginal changes along the anterior and superior acetabular rims, but these did not always appear to be irreversible deformities, even in the teratologic hips.

The first year of life is characterized by a growth rate that gradually decreases until it becomes static. This equilibrium rate will be maintained for several years, until the child enters the first growth spurt between the ages of 4 and 7 years.[28] Although the prenatal and perinatal periods are associated with rapid rates of growth that lead to the femoral and acetabular deformities, the slower postnatal growth rates imply that structural changes will occur more gradually. This applies to both the progression of deformity in the unrecognized or untreated CDH and the gradual correction in the child treated by nonoperative or operative measures. Surgical methods are directed at acute correction of the deformity, and it should be realized that nonoperative methods (cast, splint, brace) may take many months to years to manifest acceptable and significant changes.

Available pathologic material from the infancy and childhood periods is extremely rare. Milgram and Tachdjian described the hip removed at autopsy

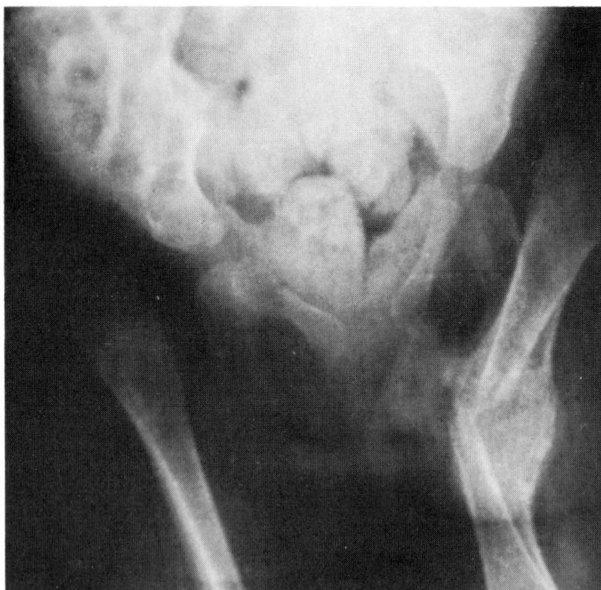

Figure 71–28. Roentgenogram of 5 month old infant with arthrogryposis, bilateral congenital dysplasia of the hip, and a healing femoral fracture. Ten months later the child died from multiple episodes of pneumonia. Pathologic specimens from this infant are shown in Figures 71–29 to 71–32.

from a 10 month old child.[20] The femur was displaced anterosuperiorly into a false acetabulum. Anteversion was only 20 degrees. Despite the chronicity of dislocation, the proximal femur was only mildly deformed, whereas the acetabulum was much more adversely affected. The appearance of the limbus suggested gradual ingrowth rather than abrupt inversion. A comparable case from a 15 month old girl showed similar mild to moderate deformities: Because of multiple recurrent medical problems (pneumonitis) this child had never been treated for a bilateral dislocation that had been present from birth (Fig. 71–28). The correlative gross and roentgenographic findings of the right hip have been described elsewhere.[25] The right and left hips were almost comparable in degree of dislocation and structural changes. Gross examination (Fig. 71–29) of the left hip revealed an anterosuperior displacement and marked anteversion (of 70 degrees; however, the femur had been fractured 10 months prior to death). The capsule was contracted anteriorly and inferiorly and was attenuated posterosuperiorly. The iliopsoas tendon crossed the true acetabulum to reach the lesser trochanter, causing a significant indentation of the attenuated, contracted inferior capsule. Specimen roentgenography showed an obvious dislocation (Fig. 71–30); the soft tissue technique revealed the outline of the laterally displaced femoral head. Air was introduced into the capsule to outline the joint (Fig. 71–30*B*). This very readily demonstrated apparent inversion of the acetabular margin. The hips were then disarticulated (Fig. 71–31). The proximal femora were mildly deformed but still retained most of their sphericity. Flattening was evident along the posterior portion of the femoral head. Both femora had significant valgus deformity and anteversion. The true acetabulum initially appeared inadequate to accommodate the femoral head in any position of reduction, but once the reactive soft tissue (pulvinar) was removed from the femoral head, there was

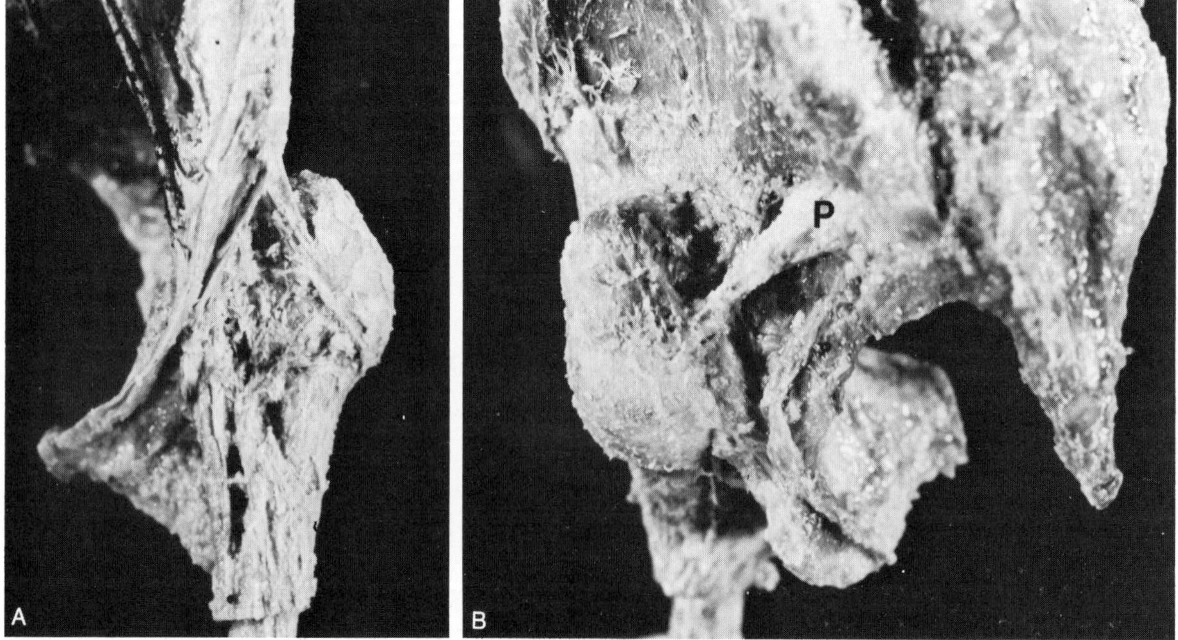

Figure 71–29. **A**, Anterior view of gross specimen showing posterosuperior displacement. **B**, Posterior view showing contracted piriformis (P).

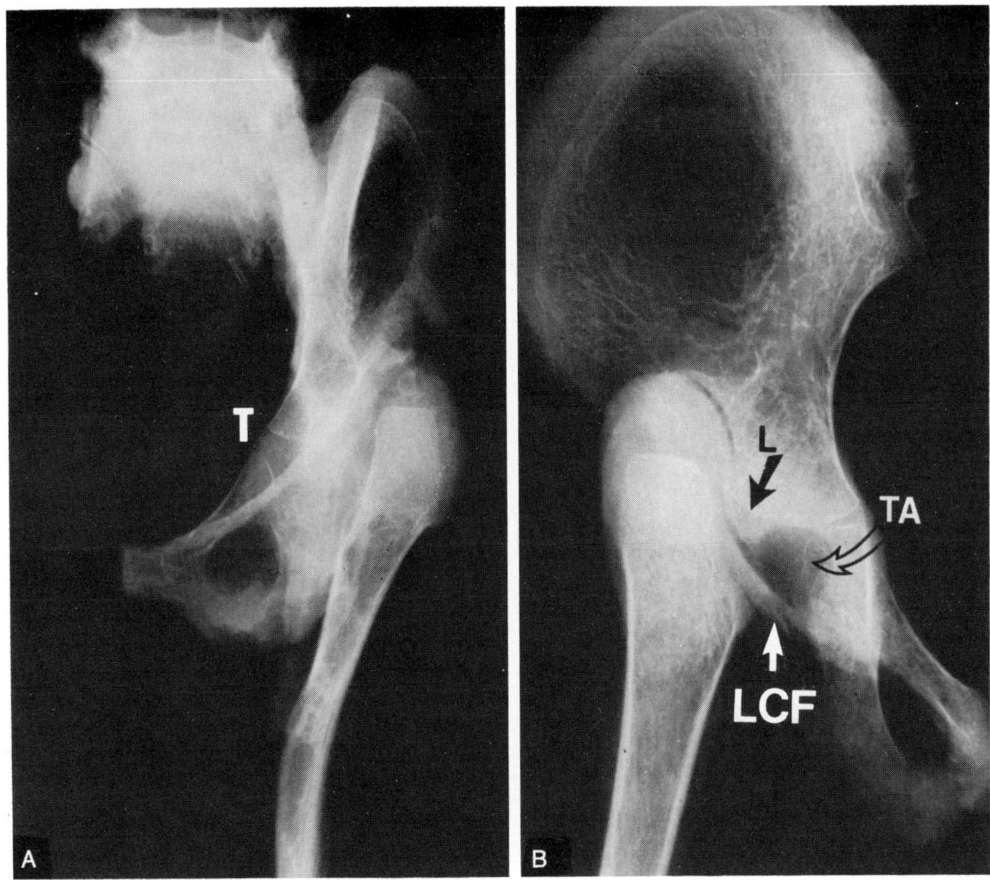

Figure 71–30. *Specimen roentgenography of left* **(A)** *and right* **(B)** *hips.* T, *Triradiate cartilage;* L, *limbus;* TA, *true acetabulum,* LCF, *ligamentum capitis femoris.*

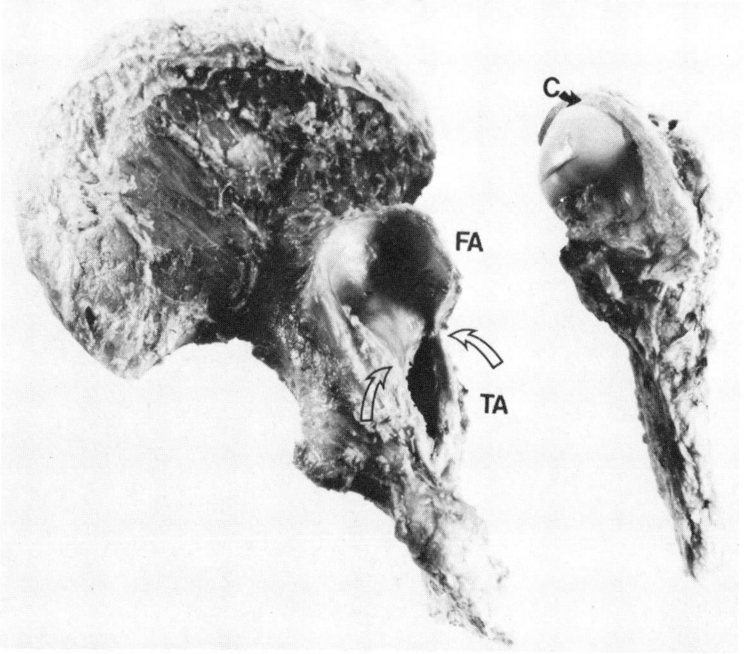

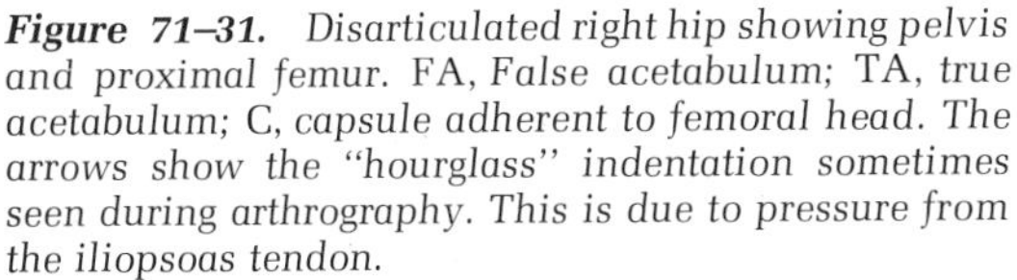

Figure 71–31. *Disarticulated right hip showing pelvis and proximal femur.* FA, *False acetabulum;* TA, *true acetabulum;* C, *capsule adherent to femoral head. The arrows show the "hourglass" indentation sometimes seen during arthrography. This is due to pressure from the iliopsoas tendon.*

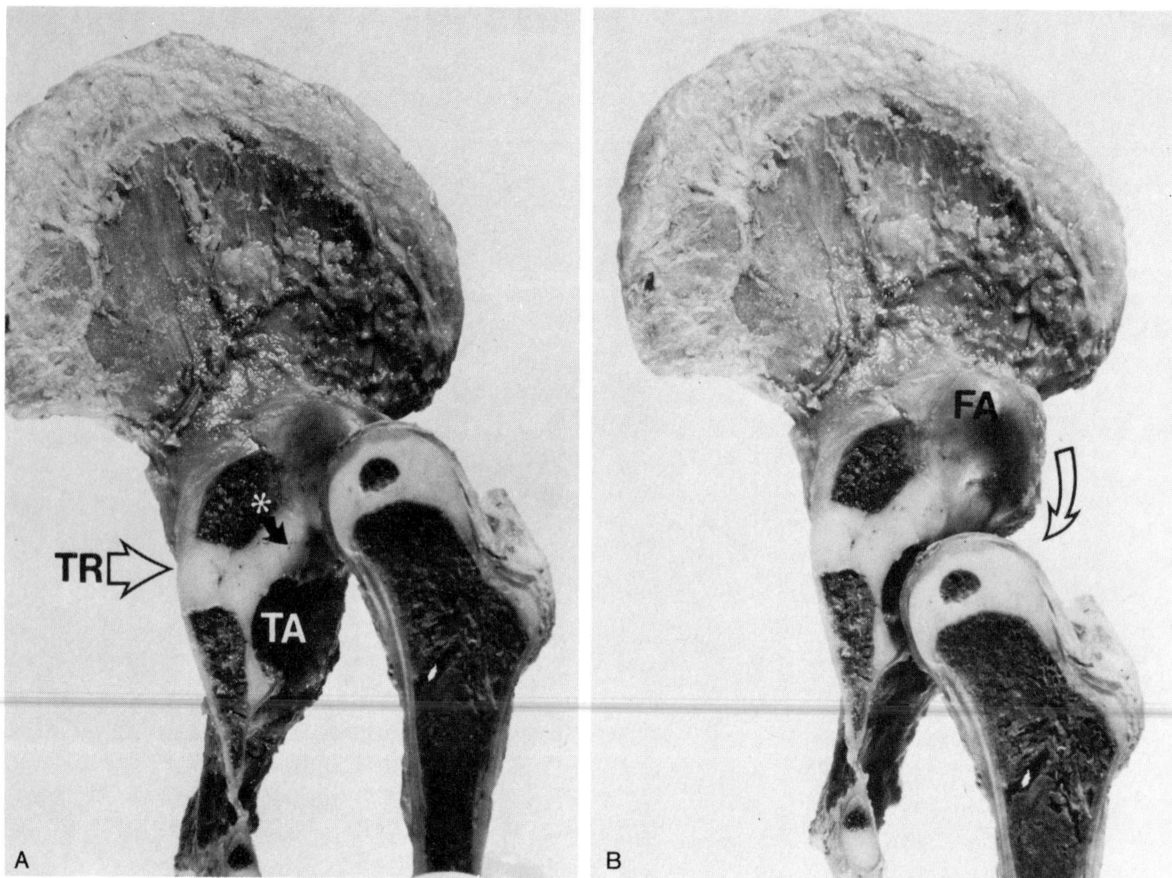

Figure 71–32. *Sagittal sections of right hip in dislocated* **(A)** *and correct* **(B)** *positions.* TR, *Triradiate cartilage;* TA, *true acetabulum;* FA, *false acetabulum; asterisk, limbus.*

increased acetabular depth and a reasonable, although imperfect, reduction was possible. An obvious false acetabulum was in continuity with the true acetabulum. This resulted from a gradual, progressive, upward displacement of the femur, with the capsule and labrum being pushed against the ilium and causing secondary osseous remodeling (increased acetabular index). Some of the most informative views were obtained by removing parts of the femur and pelvis to show chondro-osseous relationships (Fig. 71–32). The acetabular margin (labrum) was primarily everted, but there were regions where hypertrophic ingrowth was occurring. These areas of ingrowth could easily be discerned as an inverted labrum, or limbus, especially on roentgenography (Fig. 71–30).

Thus, despite 15 months of dislocation postnatally, and an unknown time period of changes in utero, both hips showed moderate changes that probably could have been reversed with appropriate treatment. In the flexed, abducted position, the femoral head was reasonably covered. These hips were unusual in the degree of symmetric deformity. In general, in bilateral cases one side is more involved than the other.

The hips from two older children, in the 7 to 11 year age range, also were studied. Both children had gone through the first major growth spurt and showed very significant deformations of both the acetabulum and proximal femur that would have an adverse effect on any treatment modality.

The first specimen was removed from a 7 year old child with a myelomeningocele. The gross specimen showed a posterosuperior dislocation (Fig. 71–33). The adductors did not have a significant contracture (in fact, the hip was in mild abduction). The hip capsule was attenuated in the direction of dislocation (superiorly and posteriorly) and contracted anteriorly and inferiorly. The lesser trochanter abutted the superior portion of the pubic ramus and caused marked indentation of the bone anterior to the true acetabulum, accentuating the anterior deficiency of this structure (Fig. 71–33*B*). The proximal femur had over 110 degrees of anteversion, as well as marked valgus deformity (over 180 degrees in the true anteroposterior plane). The lesser trochanter, in response to the iliopsoas tone, was overgrown and much more prominent than in a normal femur (Fig. 71–33*C*). The femoral head was deformed in all areas and had lost all sphericity (Fig. 71–34*A*). The chronic pressure from the ligamentum capitis femoris had eroded away all articular cartilage in the medial region of the femoral head. The acetabular labrum was variably deformed (Fig. 71–34*B*). There were obvious areas of eversion, and other areas, especially posterior structures, suggestive of inversion. The irregularity of the margin between true and false acetabula had obviously contributed to deformity in the femoral head. Roentgenography showed a shallow true acetabulum and a well-formed false acetabulum (Fig. 71–35). The medial circumflex artery had shifted concomitantly with the iliopsoas and coursed between the iliopsoas tendon and the pubic ramus. The capsule was indented into the true acetabulum by the translocated tendon. This area had a moderate amount of reactive tissue and contracture that made isolation of the artery difficult.

This specimen demonstrated several significant features that may be seen in the older child, whether the hip is considered to have typical or teratologic dislocation. First, there were positional shifts of the vessels that would render the medial circumflex artery more susceptible to occlusion or transection. Particularly, the cephalad shift of the proximal femur brought the lesser trochanter closer to the pubic ramus, and the iliopsoas tendon had a longer course over bone, with both factors increasing risk of vascular compromise. Second, the femur was twist-

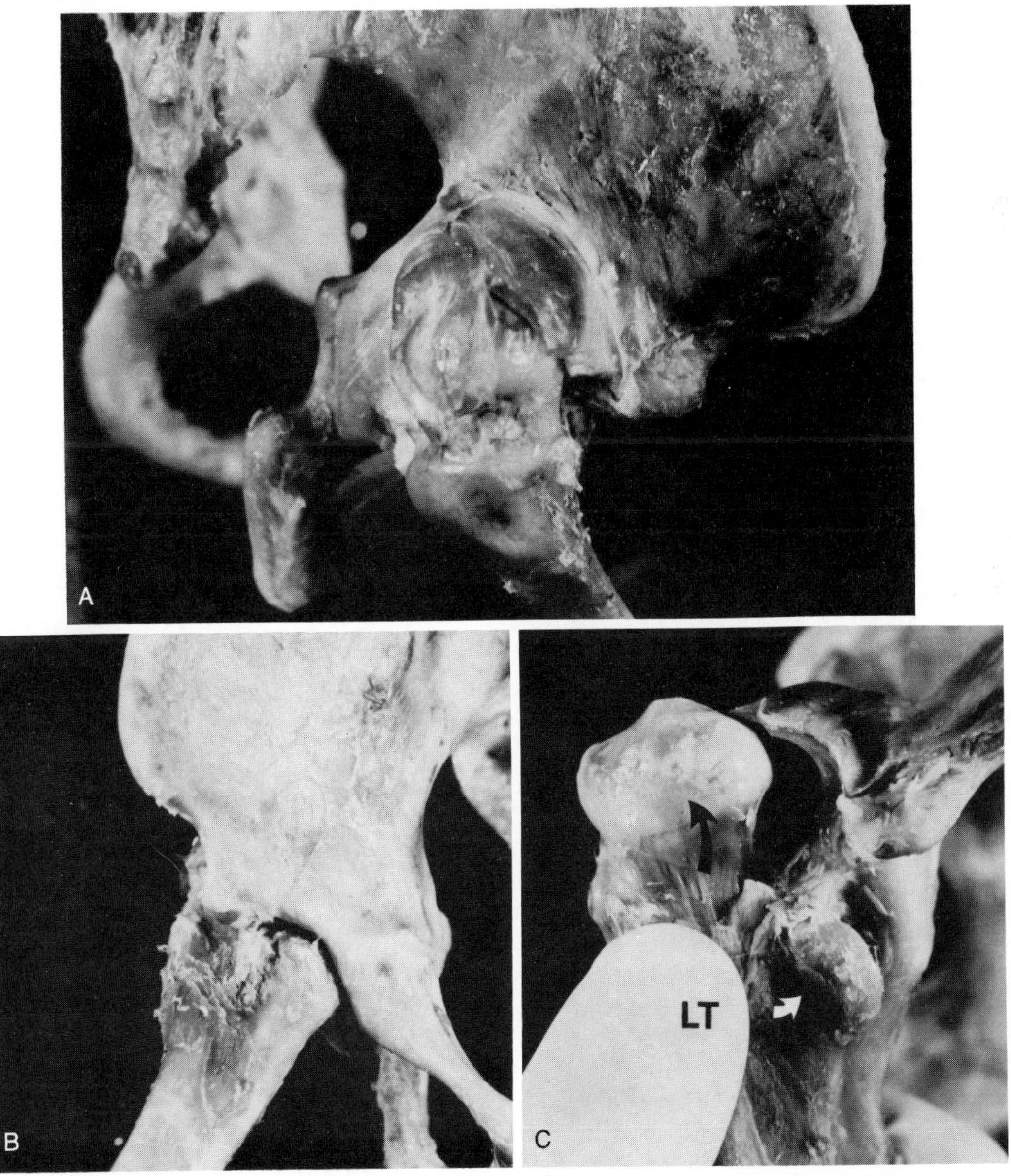

Figure 71–33. *Severe type 3 dislocation.* **A,** *Posterosuperior dislocation.* **B,** *Overgrowth of lesser trochanter to articulate with the pubic ramus.* **C,** *Hypertrophied lesser trochanter (LT) and severe valgus deformity of the femoral head. (See also Figures 71–34 and 71–35.)*

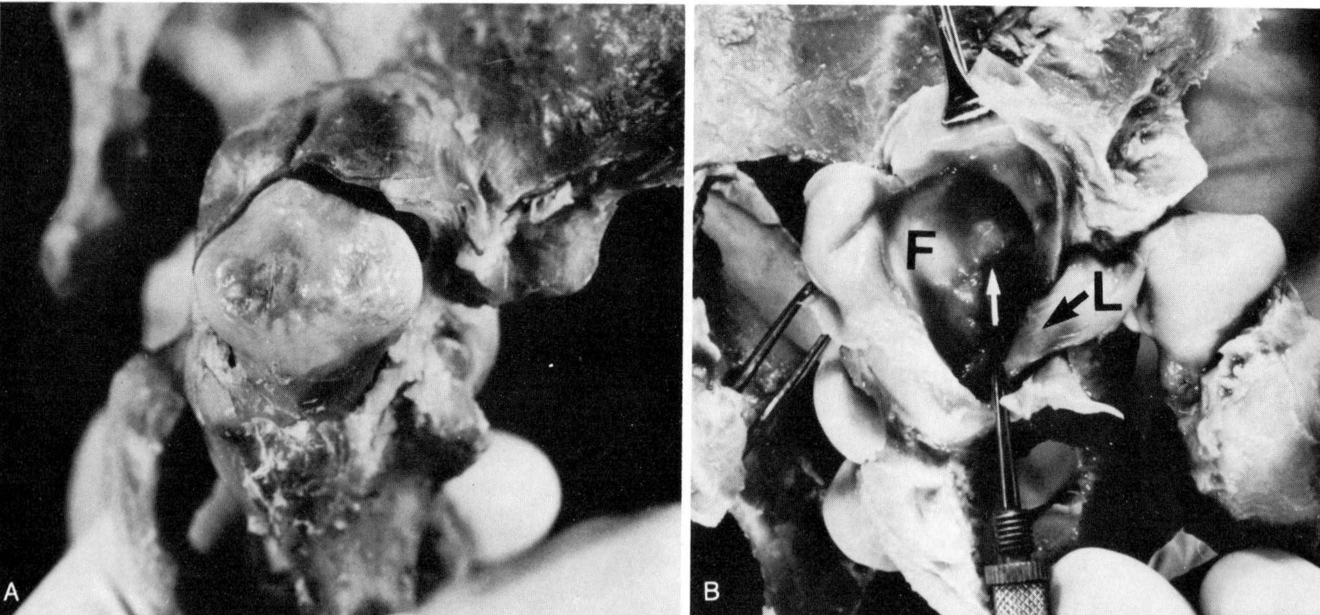

Figure 71–34. **A,** *Irregular contour of femoral head.* **B,** *Irregular margin of acetabular rim (white arrow). F, False acetabulum; L, ligamentum capitis femoris, with black arrow indicating course of ligament down into true acetabulum.*

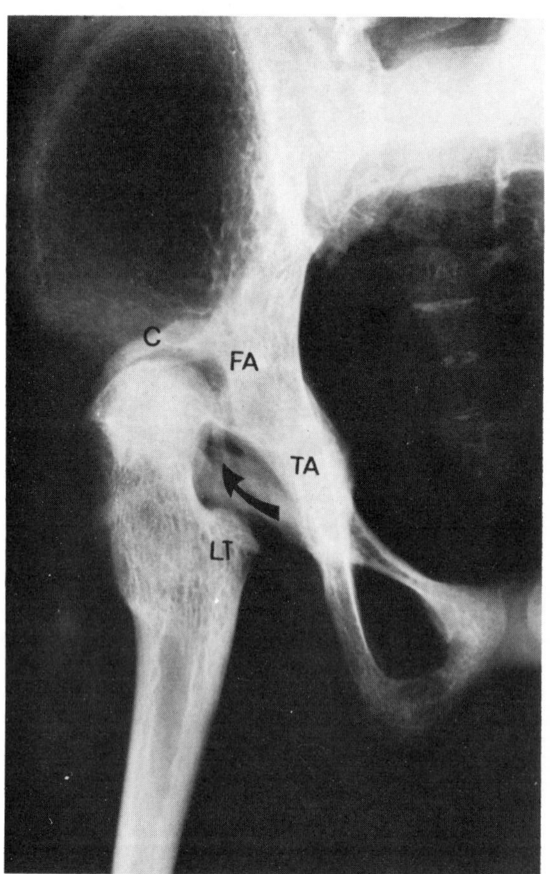

Figure 71–35. *Roentgenogram of specimen in Figure 71–34. C, Capsule; FA, false acetabulum; TA, true acetabulum; LT, lesser trochanter; arrow, ligamentum capitis femoris.*

ed into extreme anteversion (beyond 90 degrees) and showed valgus deformity (beyond 180 degrees). These deformities obviously occurred over an extended period of time in response to biologic plasticity. Also, the lesser trochanter showed deformed overgrowth that only compounded the deformity. Third, the femoral head was grossly deformed, whereas the acetabulum was less involved, except for the irregular marginal deformity. The primary acetabular deformity appeared to be lack of normal depth.

The second specimen was removed from an 11 year old child without known musculoskeletal pathology. The proximal femur was dislocated superiorly and slightly anteriorly and had an approximately 30 degree flexion and 10 degree adduction contracture. The iliopsoas tendon crossed the true acetabulum and depressed the inferior capsule into the acetabulum (Fig. 71–36). The transverse acetabular ligament was hypertrophied and displaced into the acetabulum. The ligamentum capitis femoris was elongated and could be followed from the false acetabulum into the true acetabulum (Fig. 71–37). The medial circumflex artery was displaced superiorly along with the iliopsoas tendon and was in close proximity to the pubic ramus. The femoral head was not as severely deformed as in the previous child, but there certainly was moderate posterior flattening and 80 degrees of anteversion. In contrast, the opposite hip was located, but showed increased anteversion to 90 degrees, valgus deformity, and a shallow acetabulum with anterior marginal deficiency. Roentgenography demonstrated the true acetabulum

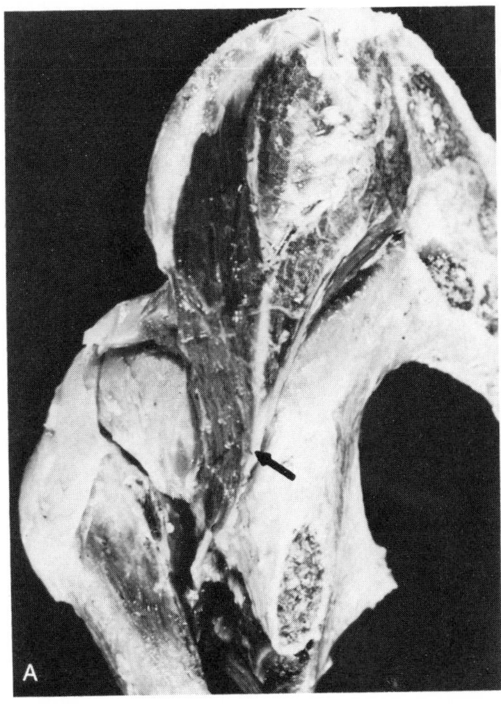

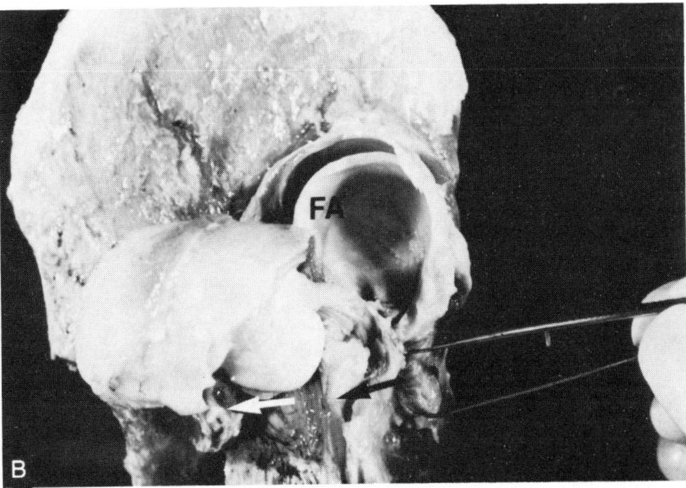

Figure 71–36. **A,** *Specimen showing posterosuperior dislocation in an 11 year old child. The course of the iliopsoas tendon is shifted laterally (arrow).* **B,** *Forceps surround proximal half of iliopsoas tendon, the course of which is depicted by the arrows, indenting the capsule into the true acetabulum. FA, False acetabulum. (See also Figures 71–37 and 71–38.)*

with irregular ossification of the roof, false acetabulum with increased soft tissue between the capsule and ilium, and femoral valgus deformity and moderate deformation of the femoral ossification center (Fig. 71–38).

This specimen, especially the proximal femur, proved to be less deformed than in the previously described child, corroborating the observation that pathologic structural changes are unpredictably variable. However, the basic patterns of change in these two specimens from older children were comparable and certainly would have made reduction and construction of an acetabular roof difficult.

The foregoing case presentations and discussions have focused on the concept that intrauterine and postnatal factors may predispose the hip to progressive subluxation and eventual dislocation. However, it is conceivable that many hips so affected during early development will not actually become dislocated, but rather may retain some mild deformity and be classified as chronic subluxation.

A set of hips was obtained from a 2 year old

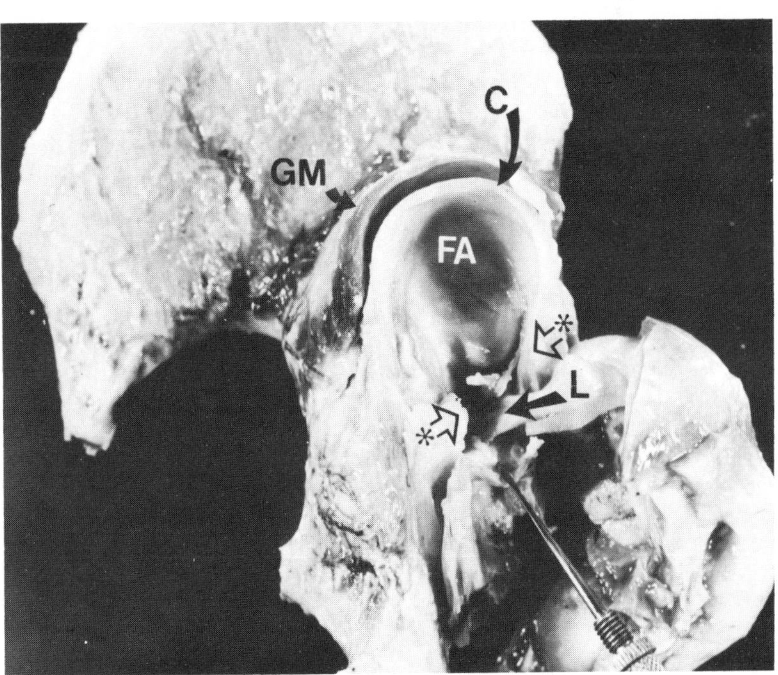

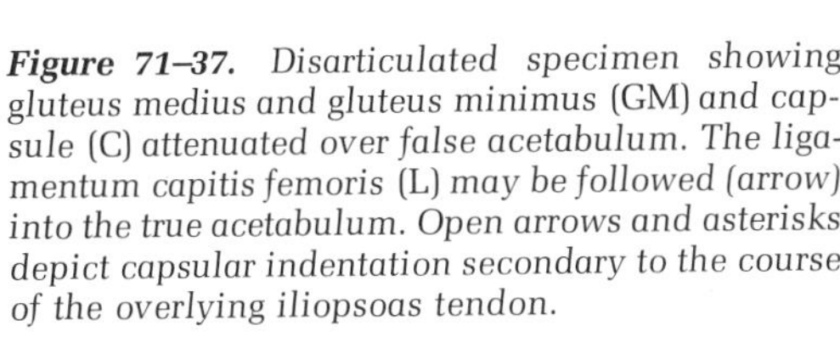
Figure 71–37. *Disarticulated specimen showing gluteus medius and gluteus minimus (GM) and capsule (C) attenuated over false acetabulum. The ligamentum capitis femoris (L) may be followed (arrow) into the true acetabulum. Open arrows and asterisks depict capsular indentation secondary to the course of the overlying iliopsoas tendon.*

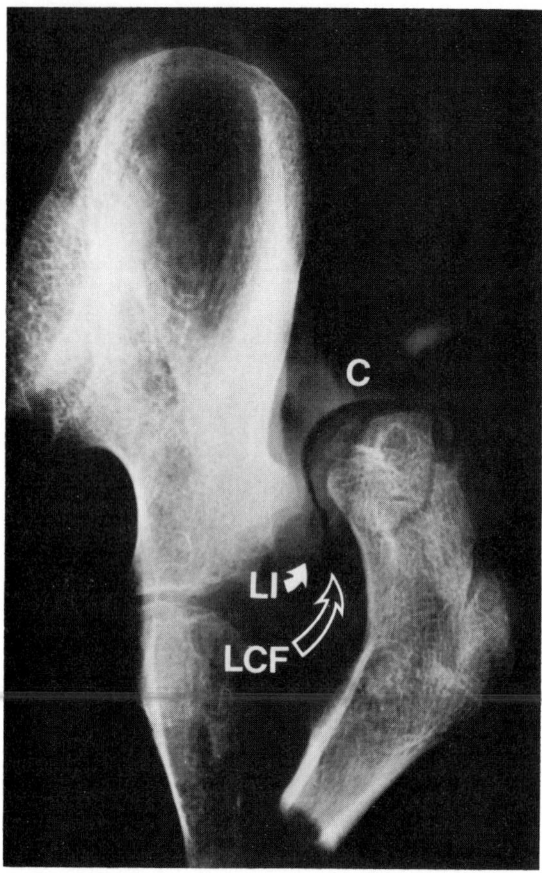

Figure 71–38. Roentgenogram of specimen in Figure 71–37. C, Capsule; LI, limbus; LCF, ligamentum capitis femoris.

girl. The right hip was normal, although the proximal femur was slightly anteverted (50 degrees). The left hip had several structural differences. The acetabulum was more shallow than that on the right side and had a very narrow anterior wall, as well as thinning of the superior labrum. The acetabulum was slightly ovoid in a superior-inferior direction. The proximal femur showed approximately 70 to 80 degrees of anteversion. There was a significant posteromedial flattening and indentation of the femoral head (Fig. 71–39). When the femur was placed in the acetabulum there was an obvious lack of coverage anteriorly compared with the other side (Fig. 71–40). Roentgenograms (Fig. 71–41) showed that there were structural deformities in both the osseous and cartilaginous elements of the left hip, but not on the right. However, despite the obvious gross changes, the acetabular indices appeared relatively normal, with just a slight marginal eversion of the osseous roof on the left.

This case very succinctly demonstrated a mild, unilateral deformity with many CDH characteristics, and it may be the type of mild hip deformation that predisposes to adult-onset arthritic changes, even though a significant superior displacement did not occur.

This child also illustrated mild acetabular dysplasia that included superior-inferior elongation, anterior wall deficiency, and mild eversion of the superior hyaline component, in conjunction with an anteverted, deformed femoral head. In the apparent functional, resting position the femoral head was uncovered anteriorly and the areas of deformity of the acetabulum and femoral head were the sites of chronic contact that had deformed as a result of biologic plasticity. Why this hip, which had some of the findings presumed to predispose to eventual dislocation, did not dislocate is not certain. Such chronically subluxated hips may represent the long-term consequences of a type 1 or type 2 dysplasia, which usually stabilizes rapidly simply with abduction treatment (although anteversion generally persists).

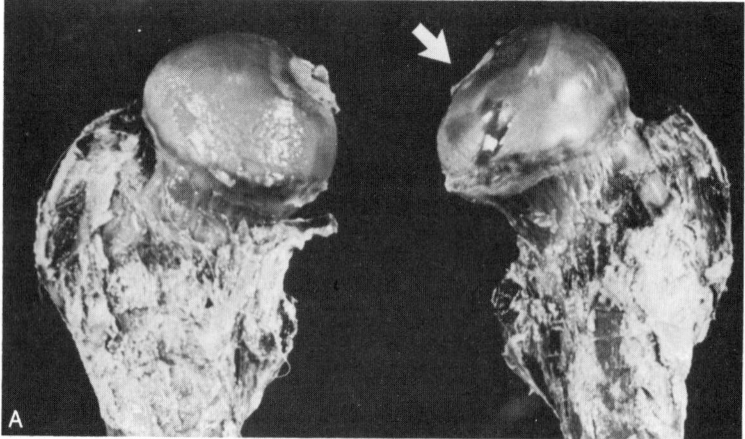

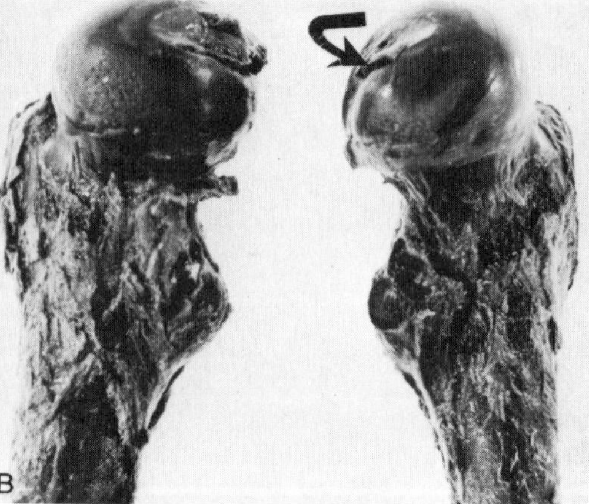

Figure 71–39. Chronic subluxation. Femoral heads depict a normal right side and posteromedial flattening of the left side (arrow) consequent to persistent anteversion and pressure against a mildly deformed acetabulum. **A,** Neutral rotation. **B,** External rotation. (See also Figures 71–40 and 71–41.)

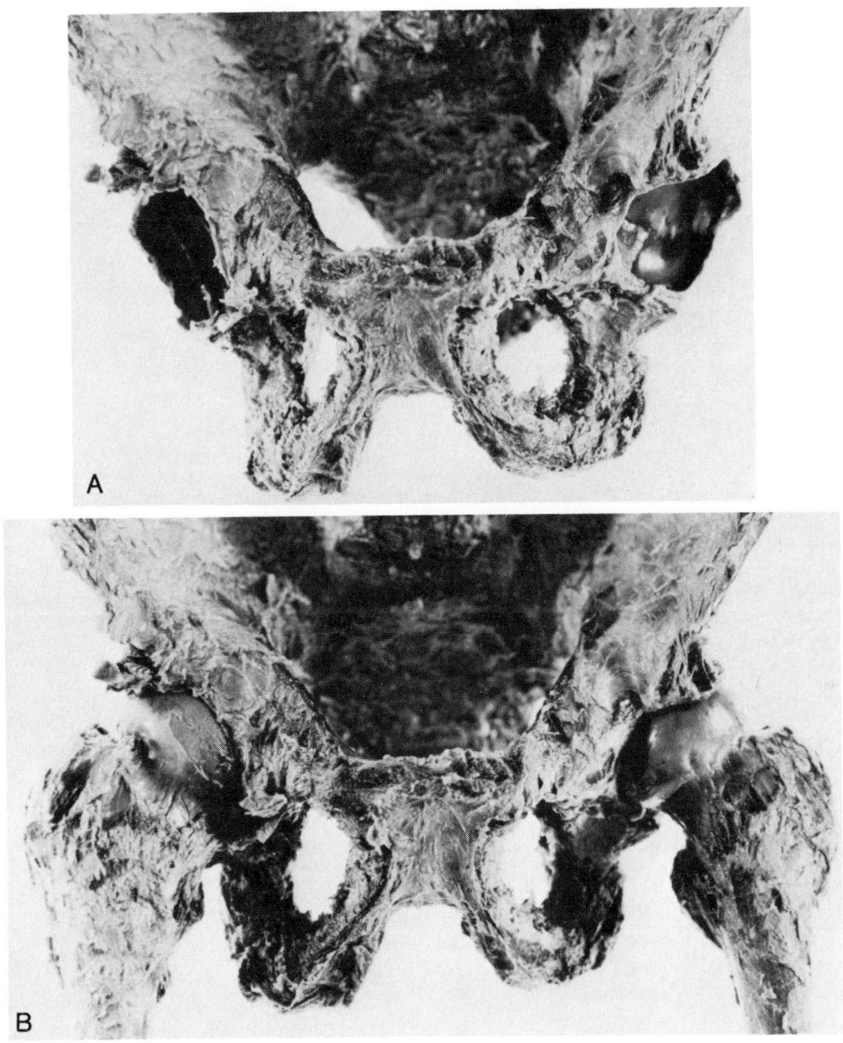

Figure 71–40. *Chronic subluxation.* **A,** *The involved left acetabulum has a deficient anterior wall.* **B,** *The left femoral head exhibits a greater degree of uncovering.*

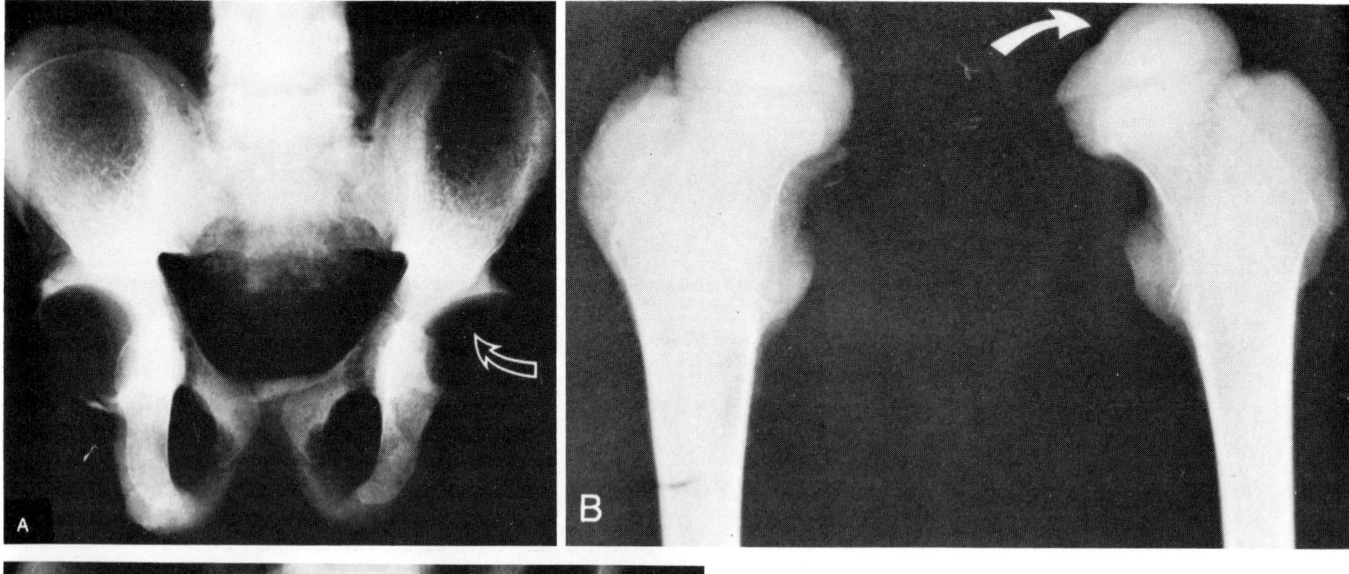

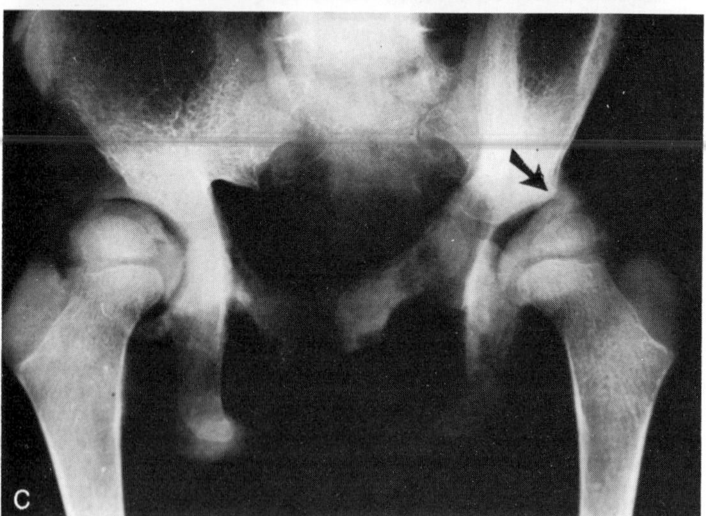

Figure 71–41. *Roentgenogram illustrating loss of sphericity of the acetabulum* **(A)** *and femoral head* **(B)** *on the left (arrows).* **C,** *Composite roentgenogram showing mild incongruency of femoral head and acetabulum in slight internal rotation (arrow).*

CLINICAL CORRELATIONS

The most reliable methods for diagnosing CDH in the neonatal period are clinical ones: the Ortolani and Barlow maneuvers. Basically the Ortolani test assesses proximal femoral reduction into the acetabulum by progressive abduction. The Barlow test is the reverse — the proximal femur is displaced by progressive adduction. These maneuvers are usually done together. These tests are positive for only a few days after birth. In most neonates, whether the hip is normal, subluxated, or dislocated, there is sufficient joint laxity to permit full abduction even if the femoral head cannot be reduced into the acetabulum. However, within a few weeks, if the hip remains subluxated or dislocated, limitation of abduction becomes a much more consistent finding.

Since the child with undiagnosed CDH grows relatively rapidly during the first year, certain clinical findings become more obvious. Anatomically the surrounding soft tissues and chondro-osseous components gradually adapt to the abnormal relationship between femoral head and acetabulum. Reduction of the femoral head becomes progressively more difficult, and the Ortolani and Barlow tests become negative. Major muscle groups become shortened and contracted; adductor tightness becomes increasingly apparent.

Routine radiologic evaluation of the neonate is not dependable. Even if clinical examination reveals an obviously dislocated hip, the radiolucent areas (reflecting the sites of unossified cartilage) are difficult to assess, and roentgenograms may not appear to reveal CDH. *However, negative findings on roentgenographic examination do not indicate the presence or absence of subluxation or dislocation.* If a teratologic hip dislocation is present, neonatal films may be more reliably diagnostic.

By 4 to 6 weeks of age more reliable radiologic changes are developing. Characteristic findings include (1) proximal or lateral migration of the femoral neck relative to the ilium, (2) a shallow, incompletely developed acetabulum, especially superiorly, (3) development of a false acetabulum, and (4) delayed ossification of the femoral head ossification center. However, even the latter is not an unequivocal finding, since the unstable side may have a greater degree of femoral head ossification (Fig. 71–14).

Several roentgenographic patterns have been described in an attempt to distinguish the normal from the dysplastic hip.[4, 30, 39, 40] Various lines and angles may be superimposed on the anteroposterior roentgenogram (Fig. 71–42). Accurate positioning is imperative, with the lower extremities aligned longitudinally in neutral rotation and as extended as possible. The most helpful parameters are the following:

1. *Acetabular index.* This is a measurement of the slope of the ossified portion of the acetabular roof, which averages 27.5 degrees in the neonate, although an upper limit of 30 degrees generally is acceptable as normal. Higher values should make one suspicious, as should significant asymmetry (difference of greater than 5 degrees).

2. *Lateral migration.* Displacement of the femoral metaphysis (and secondary ossification center, if present) may be measured by using the horizontal *line of Hilgenreiner* through the triradiate cartilage, and its intersection with *Perkin's line,* a vertical line drawn downward from the lateral margin of the ossified rim of the acetabular roof. The intersection of these lines divides the hip joint into quadrants. If the capital femoral ossification center or medial metaphysis is in the outer lower quadrant, subluxation is likely; if it is in the outer upper quadrant, dislocation is likely. The identification of any portion of the ossification center within the inner two quadrants probably indicates that a stable hip is present.

3. *Superior migration.* Proximal (upward) migration of the femoral metaphysis or ossification center may be measured by shortening of the vertical distance from Hilgenreiner's line.

4. *Shenton's line.* A curved line is drawn along the medial border of the femoral metaphysis and the superior border of the obturator foramen. In the normal hip this line is a smooth curve. In a subluxated or dislocated hip, it is broken and interrupted.

Because many of the changes that can be detected radiographically are subtle and slow to develop, there are misconceptions regarding the relevance of neonatal films. First, screening films are beneficial, if only to rule out unusual causes of shortness of the leg, limitation of movement, and instability, such as femoral hypoplasia or proximal femoral focal deficiency. If the dysplasia has been present for a significant period (probably greater than 1 month) in utero, the acetabulum probably will not be as well developed as in the normal full term child. In particular, the lateral margin may be deficient, leading either to an angular change at the lateral margin or to increased overall acclivity (Fig. 71–23). *Marginal lateral acclivity* is important to recognize, especially in the hip considered to be at risk, for it implies that the femoral head has not been seated sufficiently in the acetabulum in utero to stimulate normal patterns of chondro-osseous transformation in the ilium above the acetabulum.

Dislocation (type 3) is infrequent in the neonatal period; subluxatable (type 1) and subluxated (type 2)

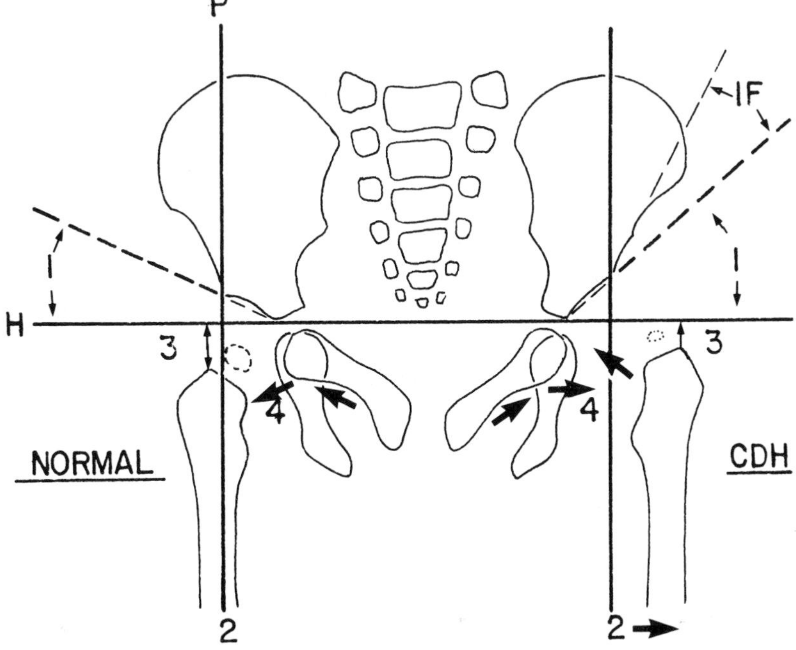

Figure 71–42. *Roentgenographic indications of congenital dysplasia of the hip (left side — abnormal).* 1, *Acetabular index;* IF, *additional index of false acetabulum;* 2, *lateral migration;* H, *Hilgenreiner's line;* P, *Perkin's line;* 3, *superior migration;* 4, *Shenton's line. See text for details.*

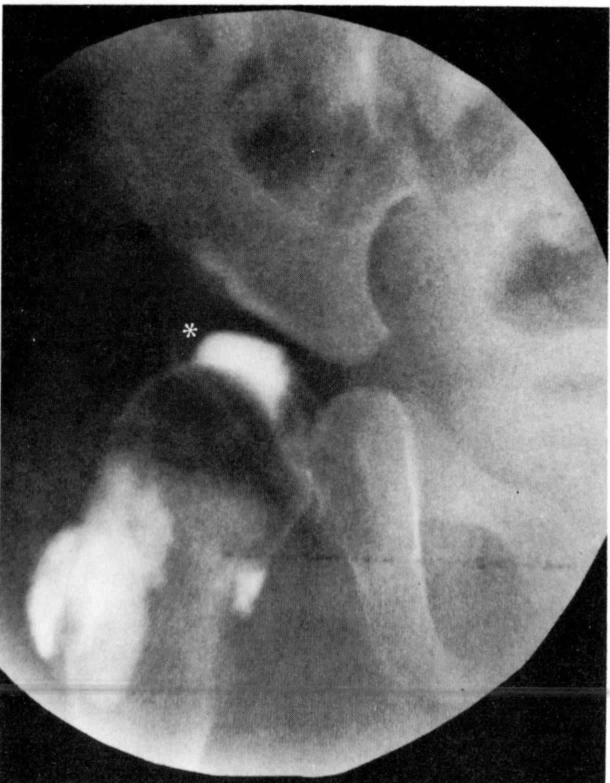

Figure 71–43. Arthrogram of patient in Figure 71–1**B.** This pull film shows the degree of capsular laxity, leading to superior pooling of dye. The acetabular rim folds down (asterisk) in this view, but does not invert into the joint. This hip therefore represents a type 2 congenital dysplasia of the hip and responded very effectively to nonoperative treatment with a Pavlik harness.

hips constitute the majority (probably 95 per cent) of unstable hips detected in the neonate. The best screening film is an anteroposterior film with the legs together in neutral rotation and the normal degree of hip flexion (do not push legs down or the pelvis will tilt, affecting measurements). This will show acetabular acclivity and lateralization. A frog-leg lateral view is of *no* benefit in the initial evaluation of hip dysplasia in the neonate. In such a position of abduction, the proximal femur in CDH usually readily seats in the acetabulum. Only if the hip is totally dislocated will there be any displacement detected in the lateral films.

ARTHROGRAPHY

As emphasized throughout this chapter, definition of specific pathology is essential in choosing the most appropriate methods of treatment. Arthrography is extremely helpful in visualizing major as well as subtle joint changes in CDH, such as an inverted limbus or hourglass capsular configuration.[1, 21, 24, 29, 35] *Routine arthrography in every case seldom is indicated.* However, arthrography is particularly useful in the child (1) who has not had an obviously satisfactory reduction, (2) who has unclear reducibility even under routine fluoroscopy, (3) who needs definition of possible efficacy of dynamic treatment methods (e.g., Pavlik harness), and (4)

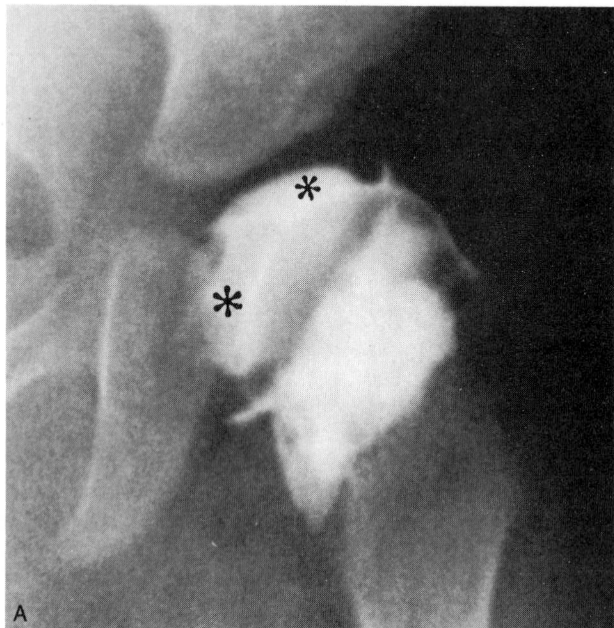

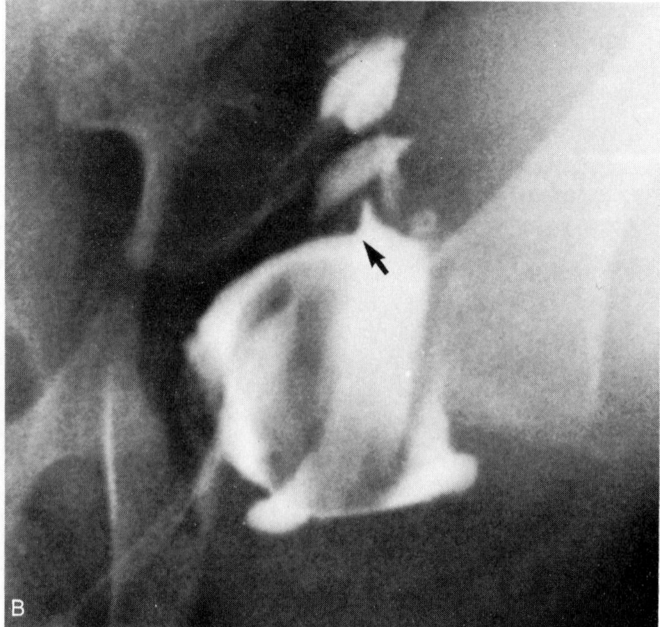

Figure 71–44. Arthrogram of patient in Figure 71–1**A.** The pull film **(A)** shows superior pooling, as in Figure 71–43, but also a greater tendency to lateral displacement and pooling of dye (asterisk). The acetabular labrum also exhibits a tendency to turn down, but not to invert. **B,** With flexion and mild abduction the femoral head reduced adequately and restored acetabular contour at the labrum (arrow). This child is being treated with a Pavlik harness.

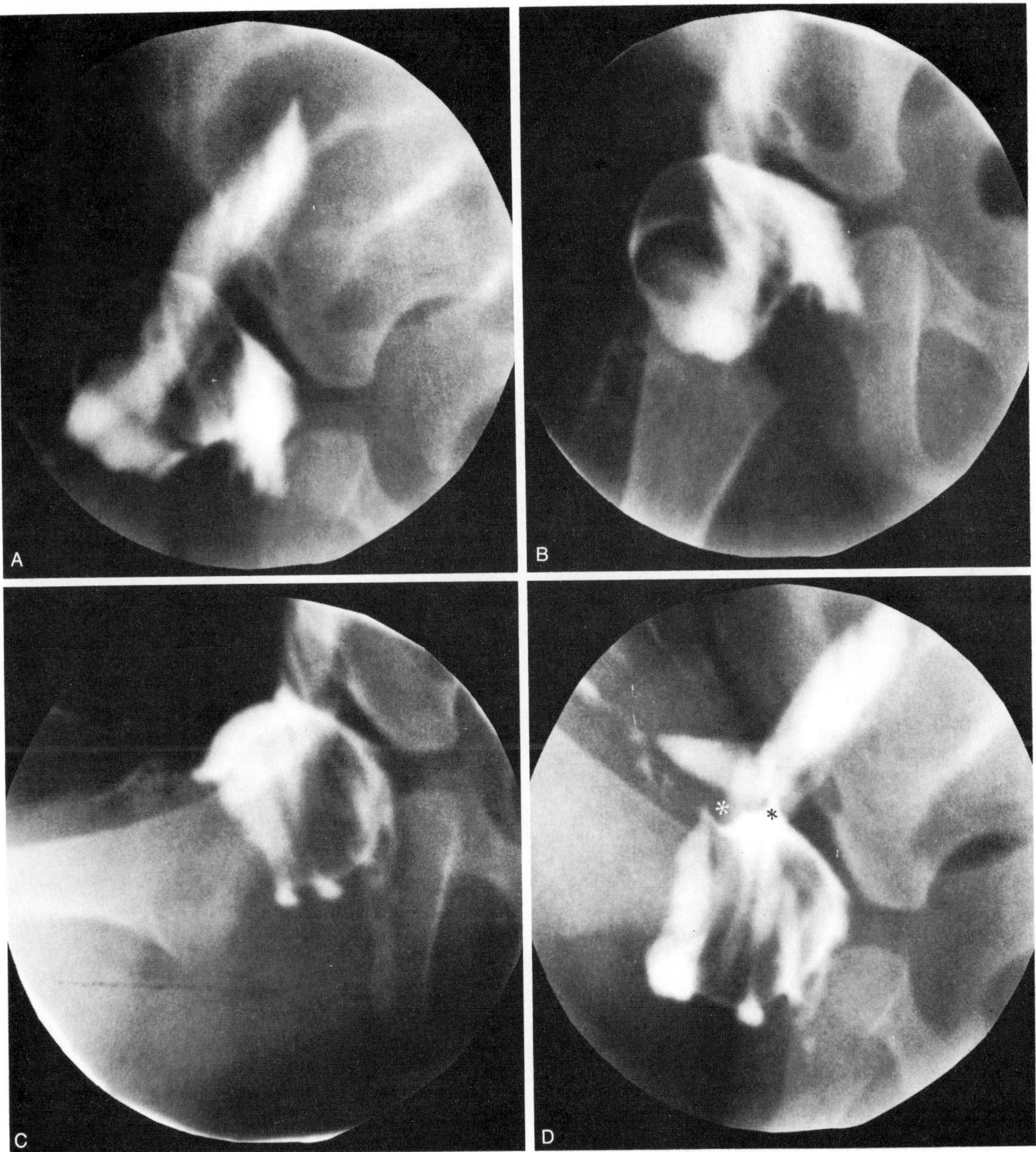

Figure 71–45. *Arthrogram of patient in Figure 71–1C.* **A,** *Proximal femur in the displaced position showing absence of a well-defined acetabular rim, suggesting gradual eversion and displacement over several months.* **B,** *The femur is pulled down as far as capsular contractures will permit. Thus, even near an extended position, soft tissue changes suggest the hip is not reducible.* **C,** *The hip is placed in a frog-leg position and there still is medial pooling of dye and incomplete reduction.* **D,** *The optimum treatment position was flexion and mild abduction, which allowed relaxation of the capsule (white asterisk) and redirection of the femoral head into the acetabulum. The acetabular cartilage contour is steep, but not inverted, and the normal recess between labrum and capsule is evident (black asterisk). This evaluation allowed nonoperative, active treatment with a Pavlik harness of a patient who might have been treated by rigid cast immobilization or even surgical reduction.*

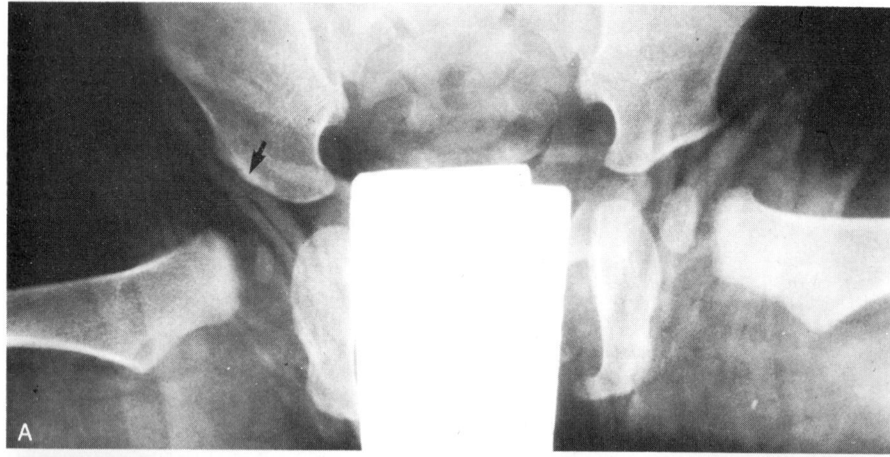

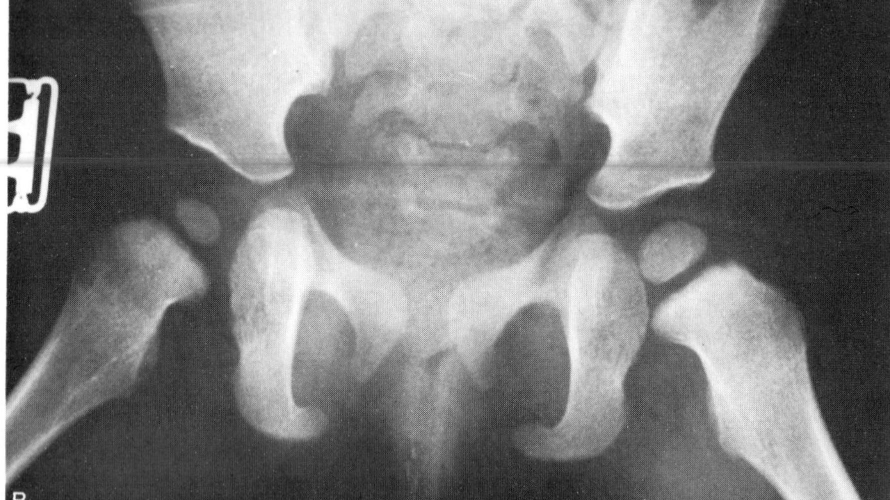

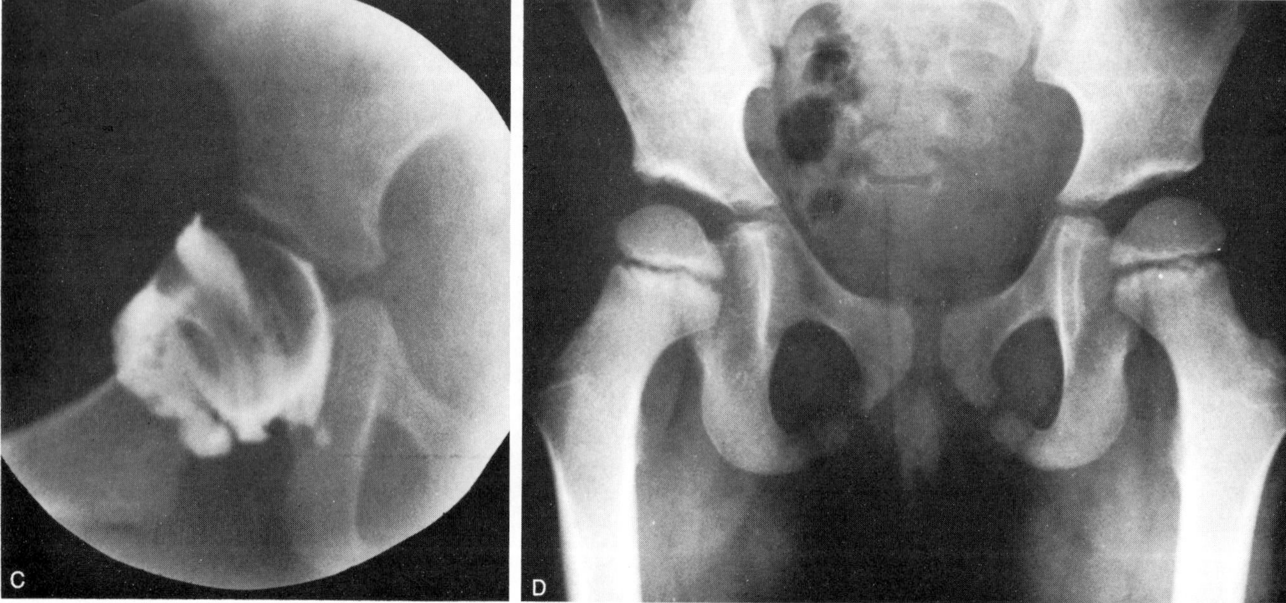

Figure 71–46. *Follow-up of patient in Figure 71–45.* **A,** *Within 6 weeks of inception of dynamic splinting, the hip is clinically stable and extensive ossification has occurred at the lateral acetabular rim (arrow).* **B,** *Four months after inception of treatment, the hip is developing well, although capital femoral ossification is still asymmetric.* **C,** *At this time a repeat arthrogram shows a stable hip with a good "rose-thorn" appearance to the acetabular labrum. The patient was now switched to an Ilfeld bar, which allowed increasing hip motion and ambulation, but still kept the hip in a protected position.* **D,** *At 4 years of age, the hip is essentially normal.*

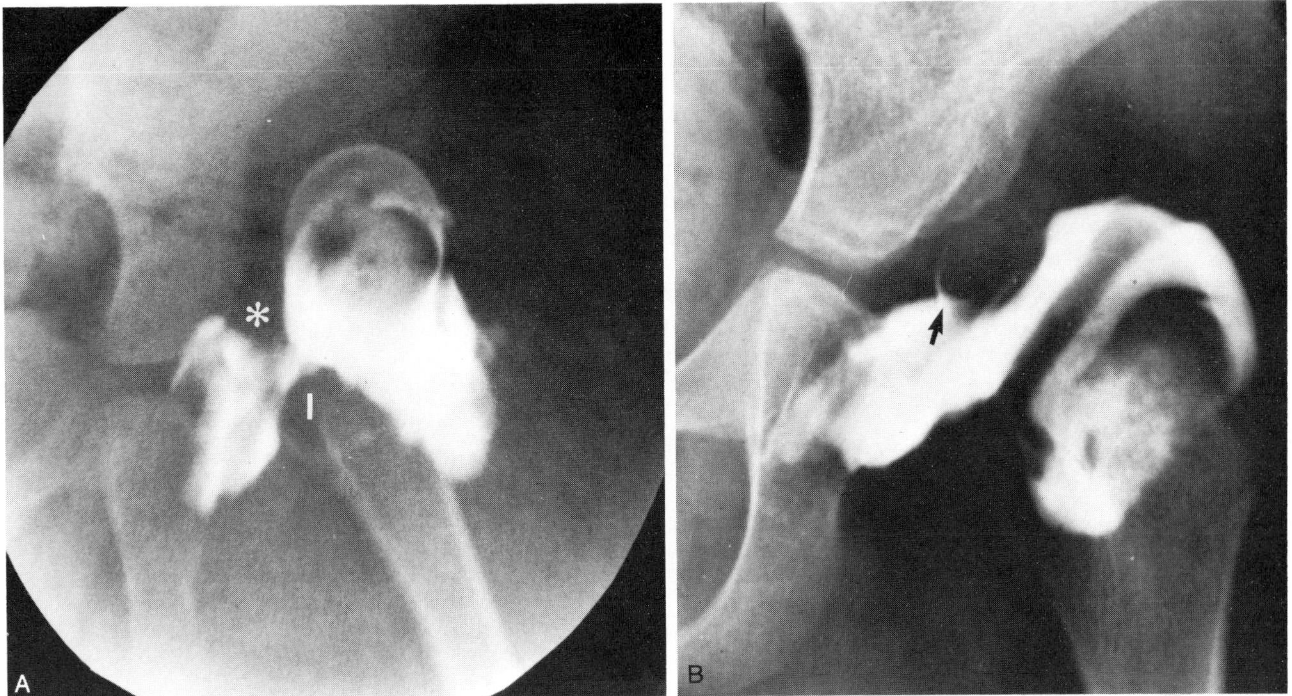

Figure 71–47. **A,** *Arthrogram of patient in Figure 71–1***D.** *A hypertrophic limbus (asterisk) and iliopsoas tendon (I) have created the "hourglass" constriction impeding reduction. Open reduction was necessary.* **B,** *Older patient (2 years at initial diagnosis) with large limbus and recess (arrow) between limbus and the rest of the acetabulum.*

whose hips have redislocated following what appeared to be an adequate closed reduction.

Arthrography, which is undertaken *only* after 2 to 3 weeks of traction to loosen soft tissue contractures, is done under a general anesthetic that will allow muscle relaxation and a proper assessment of reducibility. After sterile preparation of the skin, a narrow (20 gauge) spinal needle is introduced into the hip joint under fluoroscopic control. A small trial injection ascertains whether the hip capsule is satisfactorily penetrated. A small amount of contrast material (1 to 2 milliliters) is then injected, again using fluoroscopy to determine satisfactory filling. The needle is then removed and the hip is manipu-

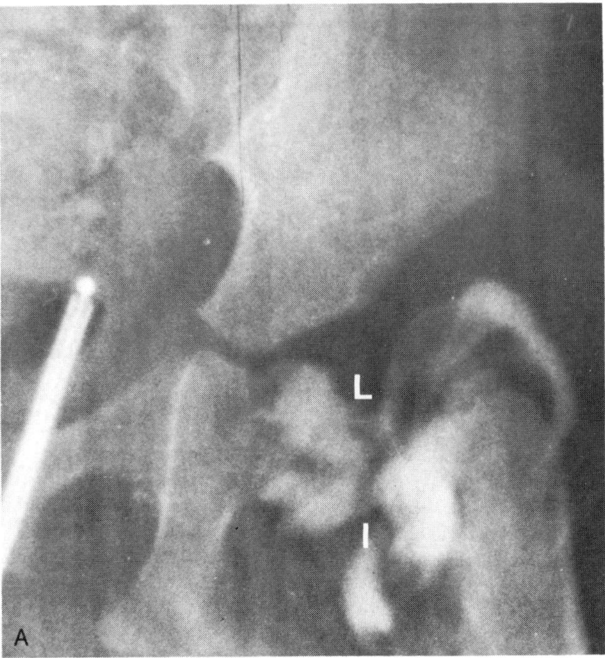

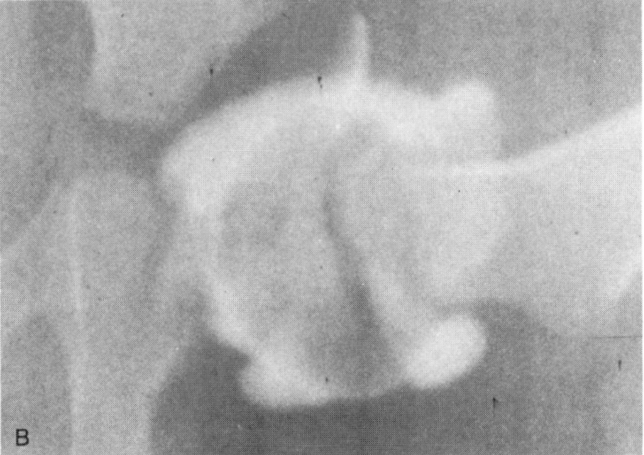

Figure 71–48. **A,** *Operative arthrogram showing an apparent limbus (L) and iliopsoas tendon indentation (I).* **B,** *The iliopsoas tendon was released from the lesser trochanter and the hip could be reduced, with the acetabular labrum assuming an everted appearance. Capsulotomy and open reduction, with the exception of the iliopsoas tenotomy, were not necessary. Again, arthrography and definition of pathology permitted intraoperative decisions minimizing surgical insult to the hip joint.*

lated under fluoroscopy to determine reducibility and appropriate positions that maintain reduction. Spot films (anteroposterior views) are then taken in the following positions: (1) extension-external rotation, (2) extension-neutral rotation, (3) extension-internal rotation, (4) abduction-neutral rotation, (5) abduction-internal rotation, (6) abduction-flexion, (7) adduction, (8) adduction-push, and (9) adduction-pull (Figs. 71–43 to 71–46).

Two major impediments to closed reduction may be encountered. The "inverted" limbus is maintained between the femoral head and the articular surface. The characteristic "rose thorn" appearance of the normal labrum is lost (Fig. 71–47). Translocation of the iliopsoas tendon may narrow the joint capsule and create an *hourglass configuration* (Figs. 71–47 and 71–48).

COMPLICATIONS

Early (preferably neonatal) diagnosis and reduction of CDH is directed at reestablishing normal chondro-osseous development of the hip. If the hip remains significantly subluxated or dislocated, progressive changes will create a false acetabulum incapable of withstanding prolonged use. Eventually secondary osteoarthritis will supervene and probably necessitate reconstructive surgery at some time during adult life, although the hip may not "wear out" until the patient is in the 5th or 6th decade of life. This is important to consider before embarking on any treatment when a child, particularly one who is over 1 year of age, presents with a unilateral or bilateral dislocation.

Perhaps the major complication of closed or open reduction is ischemic necrosis of the femoral head, which may lead to severe roentgenographic changes and a painful, dysfunctional hip in early adult life. This complication appears avoidable by appropriate definition of the specific pathology in each case, adequate pretreatment traction, and the selection of the most appropriate treatment modality, which, in large part, will be based on delineation of soft tissue changes.[3, 23, 41]

SUMMARY

Increased familiarity with the normal and abnormal gross morphology and roentgenographic appearance, as depicted in this chapter, can only increase the confidence and facility with which the radiologist and orthopaedist may effectively diagnose and treat the child with congenital hip disease.

Supported in part by the Easter Seal Research Foundation and the National Institutes of Health (RO1-HD-10854 and KO4-AM-00300).

REFERENCES

1. Astley R: Arthrography in congenital dislocation of the hip. Clin Radiol *18*:253, 1967.
2. Bernbeck R.: Zur Pathologie der Luxatio coxae congenita. Virchows Arch (Pathol Anat) *320*:238, 1951.
3. Bucholz RW, Ogden JA: Patterns of ischemic necrosis of the proximal femur in non-operatively treated congenital hip disease. *In* The Hip: Proceedings of the 6th Open Scientific Meeting of the Hip Society. St Louis, CV Mosby, 1978, p 43.
4. Caffey J: Pediatric X-Ray Diagnosis. 6th Ed. Chicago, Year Book Medical Publishers, 1972.
5. Campos DaPaz A Jr, Kalil RK: Congenital dislocation of the hip in the newborn. A correlation of clinical, roentgenographic and anatomical findings. Ital J Orthop Traumatol *2*:261, 1976.
6. Chung, SMK: The arterial supply of the developing proximal end of the human femur. J Bone Joint Surg *58A*:961, 1976.
7. Dunn PM: Congenital dislocation of the hip (CDH): Necropsy studies at birth. Proc R Soc Med *62*:1035, 1969.
8. Dunn PM: Perinatal observations on the etiology of congenital dislocation of the hip. Clin Orthop Rel Res *119*:11, 1976.
9. Dunn PM: The anatomy and pathology of congenital dislocation of the hip. Clin Orthop Rel Res *119*:23, 1976.
10. Fairbank HAT: Congenital dislocation of the hip: With special reference to the anatomy. Br J Surg *17*:380, 1930.
11. Gage J, Winter R: Avascular necrosis of the capital femoral epiphysis as a complication of closed reduction of congenital dislocation of the hip. J Bone Joint Surg *54A*:373, 1972.
12. Gardner E, Gray DJ: Prenatal development of the human hip joint. Am J Anat *87*:163, 1950.
13. Gore DR: Iatrogenic avascular necrosis of the hip in young children. J Bone Joint Surg *56A*:493, 1974.
14. Laurenson RD: Bilateral anomalous development of the hip joint. Post mortem study of a human fetus twenty-six weeks old. J Bone Joint Surg *46A*:283, 1964.
15. Laurenson RD: Development of the acetabular roof in the fetal hip. An arthrographic and histological study. J Bone Joint Surg *47A*:975, 1965.
16. Leveuf J, Bertrand P: Luxations et subluxations congénitales de la hanche. Leur traitment basé sur l'arthrographie. Paris, Doin, 1946.
17. Leveuf J: Primary congenital subluxation of the hip. J Bone Joint Surg *29*:149, 1947.
18. McKibbin B: Anatomical factors in the stability of the hip joint in the newborn. J Bone Joint Surg *52B*:148, 1970.
19. Michelsson JE, Langenskiöld A: Dislocation or subluxation of the hip. Regular sequels of immobilization of the knee in extension in young rabbits. J Bone Joint Surg *54A*:1177, 1972.
20. Milgram JW, Tachdjian MO: Pathology of the limbus in untreated teratologic congenital dislocation of the hip. A case report of a ten-month-old infant. Clin Orthop Rel Res *119*:107, 1976.
21. Mitchell GP: Arthrography in congenital displacement of the hip. J Bone Joint Surg *45B*:88, 1963.
22. Ogden, JA: Changing patterns of proximal femoral vascularity. J Bone Joint Surg *56A*:941, 1974.
23. Ogden JA: Anatomic and histologic study of factors affecting development and evolution of avascular necrosis in congenital hip dislocation. *In* The Hip: Proceedings of the Second Open Scientific Meeting of the Hip Society. St Louis, CV Mosby, 1974, p 125.
24. Ogden JA: Treatment positions for congenital dysplasia of the hip. J Pediatr *86*:732, 1975.
25. Ogden JA, Jensen PS: Roentgenography of congenital dislocation of the hip. Radiology *119*:189, 1976.
26. Ogden JA, Moss HL: Pathologic anatomy of congenital hip disease. *In* Progress in Orthopaedic Surgery. Vol 2. Berlin, Springer-Verlag, 1978.
27. Ogden JA: The development and growth of the musculoskeletal system. *In* JA Albright, RA Brand: Scientific Basis of Orthopaedics. New York, Appleton-Century-Crofts, 1979.
28. Ogden JA: Prenatal and postnatal development of the hip. *In* R Siffert, J Katz: Hip Disorders in Children. Philadelphia, JB Lippincott (in press).

29. Ozonoff MB: Controlled arthrography of the hip: A technic of fluoroscopic monitoring and recording. Clin Orthop Rel Res *93*:260, 1973.
30. Ozonoff, MB: Pediatric Orthopaedic Radiology. Philadelphia, WB Saunders Co, 1979.
31. Ponseti IV: Growth and development of the acetabulum in the normal child. Anatomical, histological and roentgenographic studies. J Bone Joint Surg *60A*:575, 1978.
32. Ponseti IV: Morphology of the acetabulum in congenital dislocation of the hip. J Bone Joint Surg *60A*:586, 1978.
33. Ráliš Z, McKibbin B: Changes in shape of the human hip joint during its development and their relation to its stability. J Bone Joint Surg *55B*:780, 1973.
34. Salter RB, Kostuik J, Dallas S: Avascular necrosis of the femoral head as a complication of treatment for congenital dislocation of the hip in young children. Can J Surg *12*:44, 1969.
35. Severin E: Arthrography in congenital dislocation of the hip. J Bone Joint Surg *21*:304, 1939.
36. Somerville EW: Development of congenital dislocation of the hip. J Bone Joint Surg *35B*:568, 1953.
37. Stanisavljevic S, Mitchell CL: Congenital dysplasia, subluxation, and dislocation of the hip in stillborn and newborn infants. J Bone Joint Surg *45A*:1147, 1963.
38. Stanisavljevic S: Diagnosis and Treatment of Congenital Hip Pathology in the Newborn. Baltimore, Williams & Wilkins, 1964.
39. Tonnis D: Normal values of the hip joint for the evaluation of x-rays in children and adults. Clin Orthop Rel Res *119*:39, 1976.
40. Zsernaviczky J, Turk G: Two new radiological signs in the early diagnosis of congenital dysplasia of the hip joint. Int Orthop *2*:223, 1978.
41. Kalamchi A, MacEwen GD: Avascular necrosis following treatment of congenital dislocation of the hip. J Bone Joint Surg *62A*:876, 1980.
42. Walker JM: Morphological variants in the human fetal hip joint. Their significance in congenital hip disease. J Bone Joint Surg *62A*:1073, 1980.

72

COLLAGEN DISEASES, EPIPHYSEAL DYSPLASIAS, AND RELATED CONDITIONS

by Amy Beth Goldman, M.D.

This chapter covers a group of disorders, many of which are associated with precocious osteoarthritis.

The Marfan syndrome, homocystinuria, the Ehlers-Danlos syndrome, and osteogenesis imperfecta are all disorders of connective tissue synthesis. In varying degrees they involve the skin, ligaments, tendons, eyes, cardiovascular system, and skeleton. The joints of the extremities are not primarily affected by the connective tissue abnormalities. However, incongruity resulting from the skeletal abnormalities and repetitive subclinical trauma resulting from ligamentous laxity combine to produce precocious osteoarthritis. Myositis ossificans progressiva is also a primary disorder of connective tissues. However, it affects the joints of the extremities by causing peripheral ossification, the reverse of the other disorders in this category. Fibrogenesis imperfecta and pseudoxanthoma elasticum do not result in joint changes, but are included in this category because of possible similarities in pathogenesis.

The epiphyseal dysplasias are a heterogeneous group of inherited diseases, all of which result in abnormalities of the epiphyseal ends of the bones. Alterations in the contours of the articular surfaces result in incongruity and eventually in premature degeneration of the hyaline cartilage. Degenerative joint disease is frequently the clinical complaint that brings these patients to medical attention.

Macrodystrophia lipomatosa and the Klippel-Trenaunay-Weber syndrome are two of the causes of congenital macrodactyly. The digital enlargement may be accompanied by articular changes. In macrodystrophia lipomatosa, secondary degenerative changes are dramatic and render the involved digit useless. In the Klippel-Trenaunay-Weber syndrome, the articular changes result from an associated bleeding diathesis.

THE MARFAN SYNDROME

The Marfan syndrome is a familial disorder of connective tissue that primarily involves the eye, the skeleton, and the cardiovascular system. It is usually an inherited autosomal dominant disorder with a high degree of penetrance. Sporadic cases do occur, but rarely, and have been related to advanced paternal age.

The Marfan syndrome is classifed by McKusick[21] as a disorder that primarily affects the fibrous component of connective tissue. Other diseases in this category include the Ehlers-Danlos syndrome, osteogenesis imperfecta, and cutis laxa.

This syndrome was first described by Marfan in 1896.[19] However, his original patient no longer fits the definition of the disease owing to the associated joint contractures he had; in retrospect, the patient probably suffered from another familiar disorder, which today is referred to as congenital contractural arachnodactyly.

The Marfan syndrome has also been referred to as arachnodactyly and dolichostenomelia.

Pathology and Pathophysiology

The nature of the defect in the connective tissues of patients with the Marfan syndrome remains unknown, and it is uncertain whether the abnormality involves collagen, elastic fibers, or both. Chromosome studies and hormonal assays have all been negative. Various investigators have described a decrease in circulating mucopolysaccharides,[1] an increase in urinary hydroxyproline,[14] and an increase in the urinary contents of chondroitin sulfate.[14] However, the latter findings remain unsubstantiated by other studies.[20, 21] Recent investigations concerning the aldehyde cross-linkages of collagen in patients with various connective tissue defects[7] have demonstrated an increase in the soluble fraction of skin collagen in patients with the Marfan syndrome. Research on normal and abnormal cross-linkages of collagen may provide information concerning the pathophysiology of this disease.

Pathologic changes in the tunica media of the aorta are part of the characteristic findings of the Marfan syndrome. Accumulation of collagenous and mucoid material and fragmentation of elastic fibers predispose these patients to dissection and rupture. The changes are most prominent in the ascending aorta, and early dilatation of the proximal portion frequently results in incompetence of the aortic valve and dilatation of the coronary sinuses. Medial necrosis of the main pulmonary artery segment has also been described.

In addition to the abnormalities of the great vessels, fibromyxomatous changes may occur in the anulus, leaflets, and chordae tendineae of the aortic and mitral valves. They result in left-sided insufficiency related to the "floppy valve" syndrome.

The bilateral ectopia lentis that occurs in a majority of patients with the Marfan syndrome has been related to changes in the suspensory ligaments of the lens. As with changes elsewhere in the body, the primary connective tissue defect is unknown.

Many patients with the Marfan syndrome have severe muscle hypotonia. The changes do not appear to be related to a primary defect in the muscle fibers themselves, since the serum creatinine level is normal. However, atrophy of type I muscle fibers may result from lack of tension.[10]

The etiology and pathology of the skeletal changes are the most puzzling of all. None of the current theories concerning a defect in collagen synthesis can adequately explain the skeletal overgrowth that characterizes this disorder.

Clinical Findings

There is no sexual or racial predisposition for the Marfan syndrome. Patients are characteristically tall and thin. The limbs are disproportionately elongated in relation to the trunk (Fig. 72–1*A*) and arm span can exceed height. The lower extremities are more severely affected than the trunk or upper extremities. The increased length of the extremities is most exaggerated distally, particularly in the hands and feet. This gives the patient the typical appearance of "arachnodactyly" (Fig. 72–1*B*). Chest deformities (pectus carinatum or excavatum) and scoliosis (Fig. 72–1*A*) accentuate the limb-trunk discrepancy. Absence of normal subcutaneous fat and muscle atrophy also contribute to the appearance of abnormally long extremities. The skull is typically

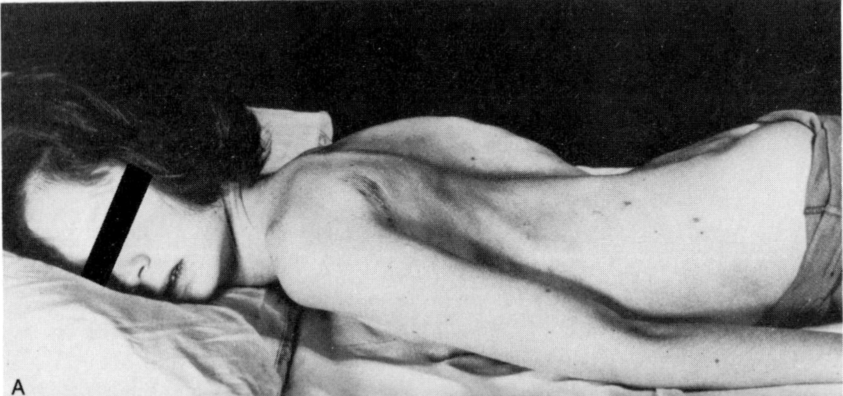

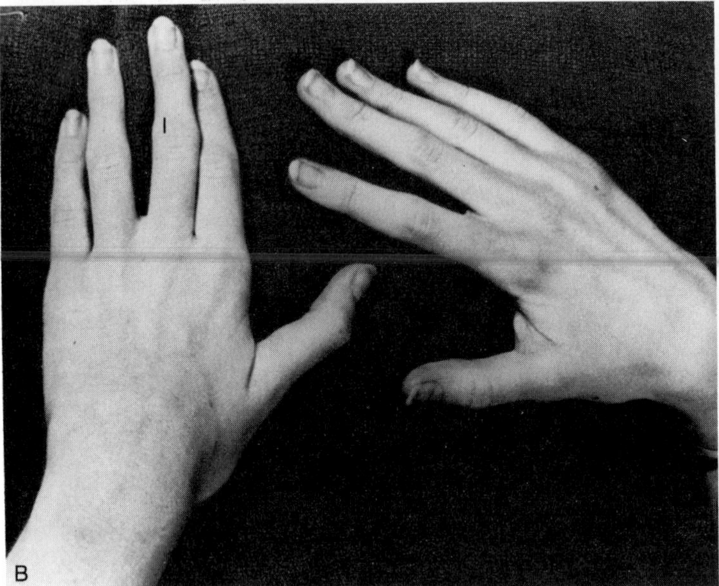

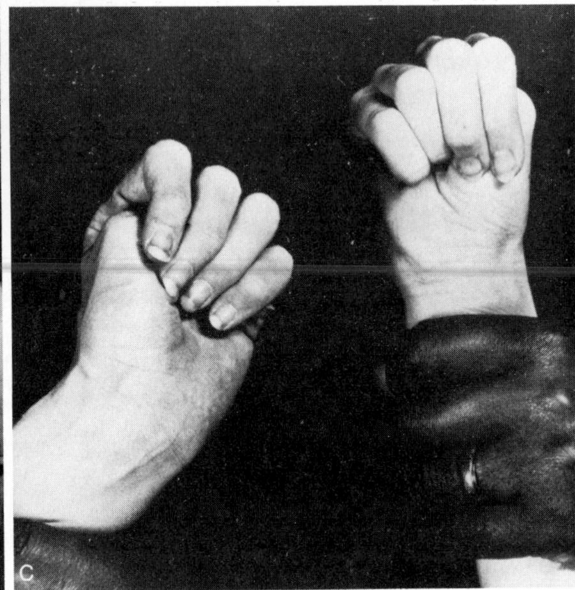

Figure 72–1. *Marfan syndrome: Adolescent girl.* **A,** *A prone view demonstrates disproportionately long arms and a thoracic kyphoscoliosis.* **B,** *The digits of the hands are elongated, and the thumb protrudes beyond the clenched fist* **(C)**.

dolichocephalic, the face elongated, the jaw prominent, and the palate high and arched. Blue sclerae and poor dentition are sometimes present. Intelligence is normal.

The most common ocular abnormalities are bilateral ectopia lentis and myopia, but there may also be strabismus and retinal detachments. Cataracts occur late in the course of the disease and are secondary to the lens detachments.

The cardiac abnormalities are responsible for the shortened life expectancy of patients with the Marfan syndrome. Cystic medial necrosis of the aorta or pulmonary artery occurs in a majority of patients and predisposes to dissection and rupture. Aortic and mitral insufficiency may result from the aortic dilatation, from a "floppy valve" syndrome, or from both. Septal defects and sinus of Valsava aneurysms are also associated with the Marfan syndrome.

Some of the confusion associated with the Marfan syndrome is due to the difficulty in establishing the diagnosis. There is marked variation in expressivity of this congenital disorder, and no single clinical or pathologic finding is invariably present. In one orthopedic series, reported by Robins and co-workers, bilateral dislocation of the lens occurred in 57 per cent of cases, arachnodactyly in 89 per cent of cases, and aortic murmurs in 62 per cent of cases.[29] Two clinical tests and one roentgenologic test have been advocated as a means of establishing the diagnosis by quantitating the osseous changes. The first is the "thumb sign" described by Steinberg,[30] in which the protrusion of the thumb beyond the confines of a clenched fist is used to reflect the narrow palm and long thumb that characterize arachnodactyly (Fig. 72–1C). The second test is the segmental measurement reported by Keech and associates.[16] The distance from the pubic symphysis to the floor and the distance from the top of the head to the floor are measured and a ratio is calculated. In normal adults, this ratio is less than 0.85. In patients with the Marfan syndrome and dolichostenomelia, the ratio is increased (Figs. 72–2, and 72–3). Skeletal proportions vary with age, and a table is necessary[15] to calculate the segmental index in children. The third test is the metacarpal index described by Par-

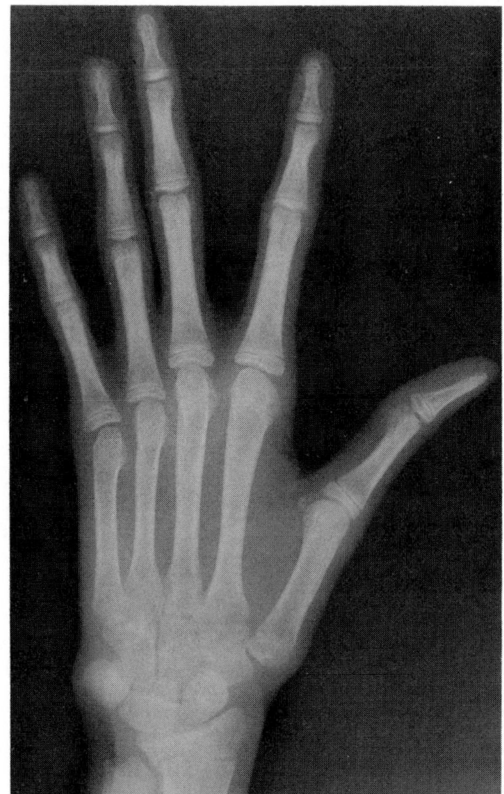

Figure 72–2. *Marfan syndrome. Posteroanterior view of the hand demonstrates absence of subcutaneous fat, elongation of phalanges and metacarpals, and normal bone density.*

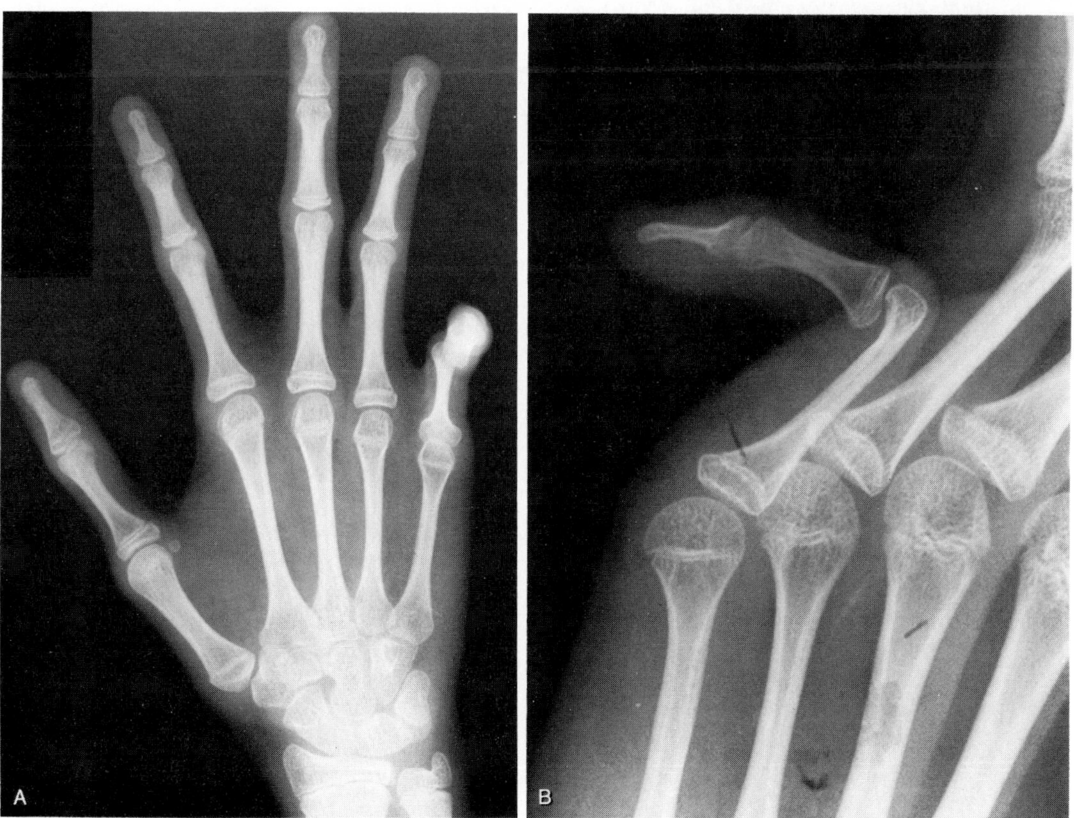

Figure 72–3. *Marfan syndrome. Frontal* **(A)** *and oblique* **(B)** *views of hand revealing 90 degree flexion contracture of fifth digit and arachnodactyly.*

rish,[26] which is based on the lengths of the second through fifth metacarpals and is measured on roentgenograms of the hand. The lengths of the metacarpals are then divided by the respective width of each diaphysis, and ratios are obtained. The four ratios are then averaged. In normal men, the metacarpal index is less than 8.8; in normal women, it is less than 9.4. McKusick[20] does not rely on the osseous findings to establish the diagnosis, but instead defines the Marfan syndrome on the basis of the ocular findings and on the family history. He has also subdivided the syndrome into asthenic, nonasthenic, and hypermobility syndromes.

Definition of the Marfan syndrome is further complicated by the occurrence of formes frustes and by reports of syndromes with features of osteogenesis imperfecta and Ehlers-Danlos syndrome coexisting with arachnodactyly.

Roentgenographic Findings

The diagnosis of the Marfan syndrome is usually made after the child has begun to walk. Roentgenograms of the hands and feet of patients with the Marfan syndrome demonstrate arachnodactyly with elongation of both the metacarpals and the phalanges (Figs. 72–2 and 72–3). In adults, the metacarpal index exceeds 8.8 in men and 9.4 in women. There is frequently a 90 degree flexion deformity of one or both fifth digits of the hands (Fig. 72–3), and there may be a disproportionate elongation of the first digit of the foot. Bone age is normal or advanced. Other deformities in the hands and feet include hallux valgus, hammer toes, club feet, and calcaneal spurs. Pes planus deformities result from ligamentous laxity.

The extremities of patients with the Marfan syndrome demonstrate a marked diminution of soft tissue owing to both muscular atrophy and sparse subcutaneous fat (Figs. 72–2 and 72–3). The long bones are slender and gracile. Osteoporosis is not present. Limb length discrepancies can occur. There is an increased incidence of slipped capital femoral epiphyses. Joints are hypermobile, predisposing to deformities (genu recurvatum, patella alta), dislocations (patellae, hips, clavicles, mandible) and joint instability. The hyperlaxity is also responsible for abnormal joint mechanics, repetitive subclinical trauma, and premature degenerative joint disease.

Scoliosis occurs in a high proportion of patients with the Marfan syndrome. The curve pattern is similar to that of idiopathic scoliosis (Fig. 72–4). However, the scoliosis of the Marfan syndrome begins earlier than the idiopathic form and does not have the female predominance of the idiopathic type. The spinal deformity is progressive and may be painful. Posterior scalloping of the vertebral bodies has been reported and is attributed to dural ectasia.

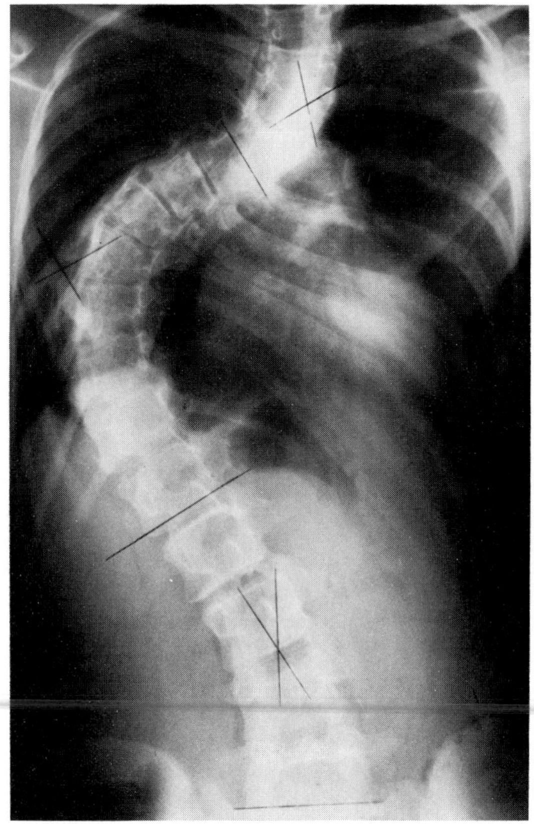

Figure 72–4. *Marfan syndrome: Scoliosis. The roentgenographic appearance is indistinguishable from that of idiopathic scoliosis.*

There is also an increased incidence of Scheuermann's disease and spondylolysis.

Chest deformities associated with the Marfan syndrome include pectus excavatum resulting from elongation of the ribs.

Cystic disease of the lung has also been reported in association with this syndrome.

The roentgenographic differential diagnosis relies on clinical correlation because "marfanoid" skeletal changes occur in several other syndromes. Homocystinuria, a congenital disorder of methionine metabolism, is characterized by arachnodactyly, scoliosis, sternal deformities, and ligamentous laxity. However, patients are mentally retarded, and the skeleton is osteoporotic. Congenital contractural arachnodactyly, another inherited disorder of connective tissue, is also characterized by long, thin limbs. However, the absence of eye and cardiac changes and the presence of joint contractures and deformed ears distinguish the two entities. Slowly progressive myopathies, particularly nemaline myopathy, is another differential possibility. However, muscle biopsies and electromyographic studies will be positive for primary abnormalities of the muscle fibers. Type IIb multiple endocrine neoplasia syndrome (mucosal neuromas, pheochromocytoma, medullary carcinoma of the thyroid) is also associated with marfanoid features, as is the Ehlers-Danlos syndrome. With both diseases, clinical history is necessary to establish the correct diagnosis.

HOMOCYSTINURIA

The term homocystinuria encompasses a group of disorders characterized by inborn defects in methionine metabolism. The best known of these entities is the syndrome associated with a deficiency in the enzyme cystathionine synthetase. It is inherited on an autosomal recessive basis and affects the eye, skeleton, central nervous system, and vascular structures. It is classified by McKusick[48] as a secondary disorder of the fibrous component of connective tissue and is grouped with alkaptonuria, Menkes' syndrome, and pseudoxanthoma elasticum. Cystathionine synthetase deficiency is not a homogeneous disorder but is related to multiple alleles at a single locus. Clinical manifestations are extremely variable, and the disease has been further subdivided into the vitamin B_6 (pyridoxine)–responsive and vitamin B_6–unresponsive forms.

The syndrome of homocystinuria was first described in 1962 by two separate groups of investigators.[36, 42] It is also referred to as cystathionine synthetase deficiency.

Pathology and Pathophysiology

The enzyme cystathionine synthetase catalyzes the conversion of serine and homocysteine to cystathionine. One of the results of this defect is a deficiency in the substance that follows the metabolic block, and cystathionine is decreased in the brain, skin, and liver. The second result is an abnormal accumulation of the substance that precedes the defective enzyme — i.e., homocysteine. The latter product of methionine metabolism accumulates in the tissues and may undergo methylation back to methionine or oxidation to disulfite homocystine. Homocysteine, homocystine, and methionine accumulate in the plasma, and excessive homocysteine is excreted in the urine.

Vitamin B_6 (pyridoxine) is a coenzyme in two steps of the methionine metabolic pathway. In some cases of homocystinuria, the clinical and chemical abnormalities can be altered by massive doses of this vitamin. The patients who respond to vitamin B_6 tend to have some cystathionine synthetase activity detectable in the skin or liver prior to treatment, whereas those who do not respond tend to have a more severe enzymatic deficit.

The three other enzyme deficiencies associated with homocystinuria do not have as marked elevations in homocysteine concentration and are not characterized by ocular abnormalities.

Experimental evidence, reported by Francis and co-workers,[38] Hurwitz and associates,[44] and Kang and Trelstad,[45] indicates that homocystinuria is associated with a defect in collagen synthesis. Studies of skin collagen have demonstrated an abnormal increase in the soluble component and an abnormal decrease in polymeric collagen. It is currently postulated that high levels of homocysteine bind with and interfere with the formation of the aldehyde cross-linkages that stabilize the collagen macromolecule. A similar defect is thought to occur in the Marfan syndrome, a disorder that shares many of the clinical findings of homocystinuria.

Arterial and venous thromboses complicate the course of homocystinuria and are the result of an increase in platelet "stickiness." The abnormal aggregation of platelets results from changes in the vessel walls and from the presence of unstable collagen. Elevated levels of plasma homocysteine and homocystine have no direct effect. As in the Marfan syndrome, cystic medial necrosis and fragmentation of elastic fibers are found in the aortas of patients with homocystinuria. However, unlike the Marfan syndrome, similar changes occur in the media of all elastic arteries and are uniquely accompanied by the presence of patchy intimal pads or ridges. In addition, despite thinning of the media, aortic dissections are not a characteristic feature of homocystinuria.

Both mental retardation and seizures occur as a result of cystathionine synthetase deficiency. Cystathionine, a major free amino acid in the brain, is decreased in amount. However, the exact etiology of the central nervous system abnormalities is not yet known. Investigations are complicated by the coexisting changes of venous and arterial thromboses.

The most characteristic ocular abnormality of homocystinuria is bilateral dislocation of the lens. Described pathologic findings include thickening of the basement membrane of the ciliary body and atrophy of nonpigmented epithelium.

Other pathologic abnormalities reported in patients with homocystinuria include fatty changes in the liver and electromicroscopic abnormalities in the hepatocytes. Muscle disturbances with changes in the electromyogram have also been described.

Clinical Findings

Homocystinuria occurs most commonly in northern Europeans from Sweden, Germany, Holland, England, Ireland, and Scotland.

Patients seem normal at birth and during infancy, the sole clinical finding being irritability. However, in early childhood, motor development slows or even regresses. Patients with homocystinuria tend to have thin skin with prominent venous markings. Striae occur over the buttocks and shoulders. A malar flush is frequently present and "cigarette paper" scars occur with minor trauma. Hair is thin and sparse. A high, arched palate and poor dentition are both characteristic of this disorder.

The most frequent physical finding is bilateral lens dislocations, which may be present at birth, but which are not obvious until later. Other, less frequent eye abnormalities include cataracts, optic atrophy, microphthalmus, and congenital glaucoma.

The degree of mental retardation varies and may be modified by therapy. Epileptic seizures and vascular accidents also produce symptoms referable to the central nervous system.

Spontaneous venous and arterial thromboses complicate the clinical course of homocystinuria and are frequently life-threatening. Common sites of arterial clotting are the intermediate-sized vessels, including the coronary, renal, and carotid arteries and the other major branches of the aorta. Venous thromboses frequently involve the mesenteric vessels, the vena cava, the iliac vessels, and the pulmonary veins. Surgery may precipitate a major vascular accident.

Twenty-five[35] to 60[34] per cent of patients with homocystinuria have skeletal abnormalities that resemble those of the Marfan syndrome. Patients are tall, with disproportionately long extremities, a "duck-like" gait, scoliosis, pectus excavatum, and joint laxity. However, several clinical findings differentiate these two entities. First, mental retardation, the malar flush, and vascular thromboses are not found in the Marfan syndrome. Second, although both entities are characterized by bilateral lens dislocations, this sign can be detected in infancy in patients with homocystinuria. Third, in the Marfan syndrome, contractures occur only in the fifth digits of the hands, whereas in homocystinuria, contractures occur in multiple digits as well as in the elbows and knees. Lastly, unlike the Marfan syndrome, there are positive and specific laboratory findings in homocystinuria. The plasma levels of homocysteine, homocystine, and methionine are all elevated, and the urine contains abnormal amounts of homocysteine, which, like cystine, gives a positive result on the nitroprusside test. Cystine and homocysteine can be differentiated by paper electrophoresis. Liver and skin biopsies are necessary for a specific enzymatic diagnosis.

Roentgenographic Findings

There are no roentgenographic abnormalities present at birth in this disorder. Skeletal changes occur gradually during childhood and do not appear to correlate with the severity of the enzymatic defect or with its response to vitamin B_6.

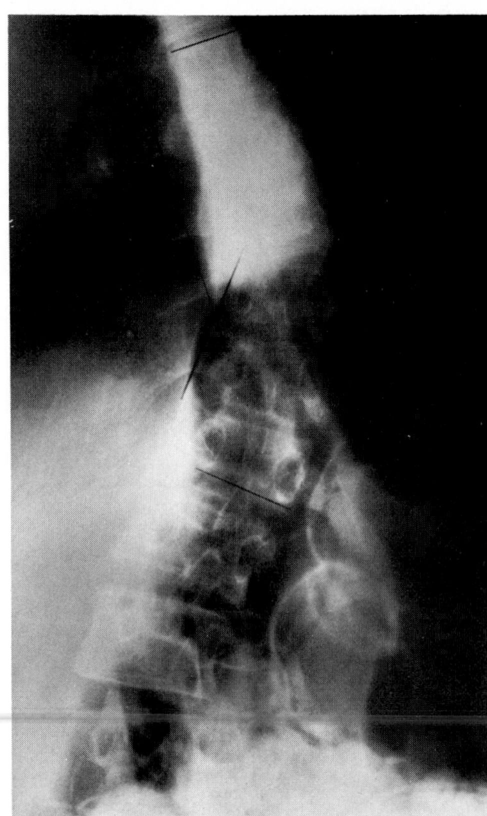

Figure 72–5. *Homocystinuria. Scoliosis and osteoporosis in the spine of a patient with homocystinuria.*

Examination of the axial skeleton can reveal generalized osteoporosis, enlarged sinuses, and scoliosis (Fig. 72–5). The vertebral bodies have an increased anteroposterior diameter and may be biconcave in shape. Compression fractures are frequent. Posterior scalloping of the vertebral bodies and premature degenerative disc disease have also been described.

Changes in the extremities include dolichostenomelia, osteoporosis, and multiple growth arrest lines (Fig. 72–6). Frequent deformities include flattening of the femoral heads and varus deformities of the humeri. There can be a characteristic stippled appearance in the growth plates of the distal radii and ulnae, which contain punctate areas of ossification. Joint findings are variable. Abnormal laxity may be present and result in genu valgum deformities and patella alta (Fig. 72–6). However, coexisting with laxity of some joints are flexion contractures of others, particularly in the digits, the elbows, and the knees.

Characteristic roentgenographic changes in the hands include arachnodactyly (Fig. 72–7) and carpal deformities. Bone age may be normal, accelerated, or retarded.

The nonosseous roentgenographic abnormalities of homocystinuria include venous calcifications and an increased incidence of medullary sponge kidney.

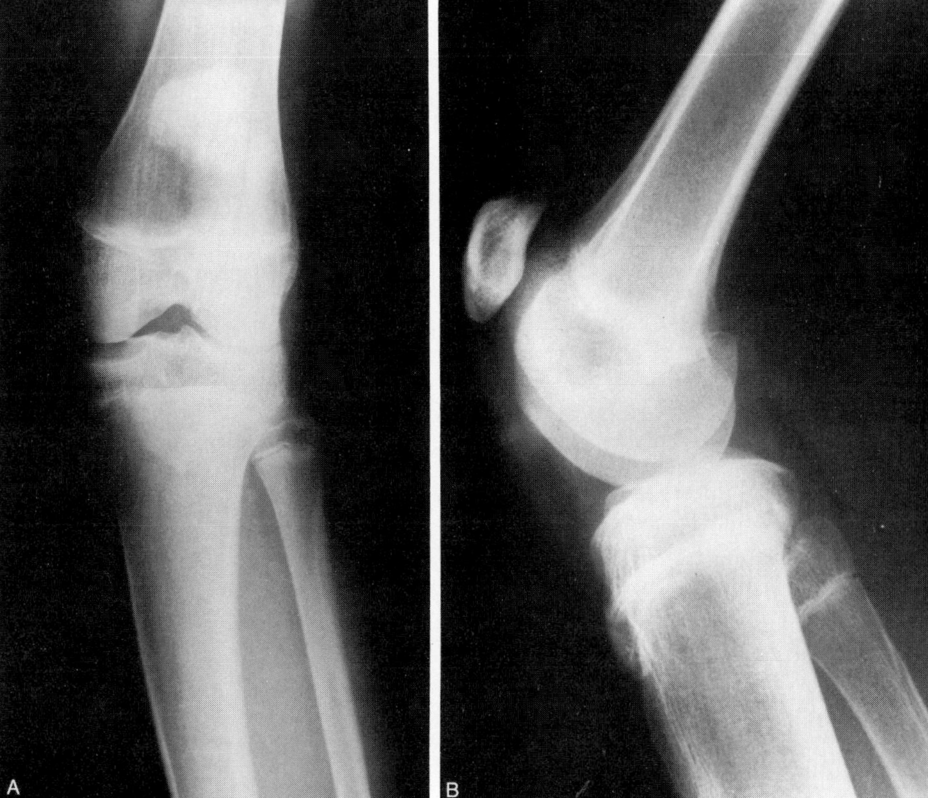

Figure 72–6. *Homocystinuria. Anteroposterior* **(A)** *and lateral* **(B)** *views of knee demonstrate an elongated limb, a genu valgum deformity, and patella alta. The bones are osteoporotic and the metaphyses are flared. Multiple growth arrest lines are present, although not well shown here.*

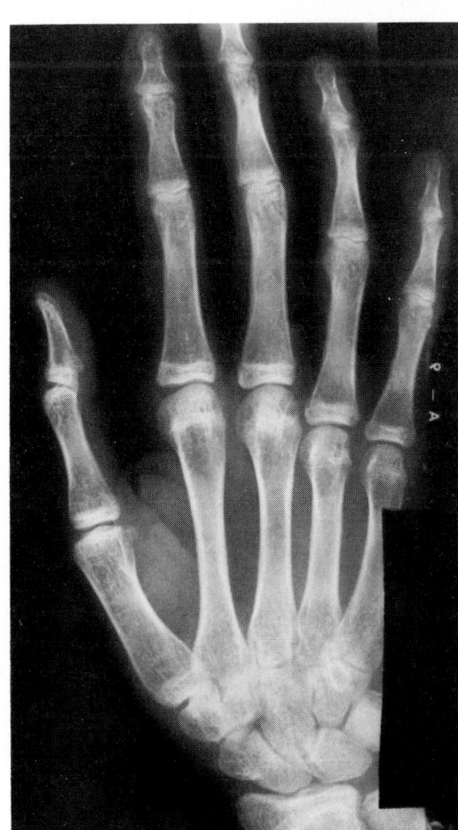

Figure 72–7. *Homocystinuria. Frontal view of the hand reveals arachnodactyly and osteoporosis.*

The major roentgenographic differential diagnosis of homocystinuria involves the Marfan syndrome. The presence of osteoporosis, metaphyseal flaring, and multiple contractures should distinguish the radiographic appearance of dolichostenomelia in a patient with homocystinuria from that in a patient with the Marfan syndrome.

THE EHLERS–DANLOS SYNDROME

The Ehlers–Danlos syndrome is a familial disorder of connective tissue that is characterized by hyperelasticity and fragility of the skin, hyperlaxity of the joints, and a bleeding diathesis. The eye, the gastrointestinal tract, the bronchopulmonary tree, and the cardiovascular system may also be affected by this primary defect in mesenchyme.

This syndrome is not a single homogeneous disorder but a group of related entities, which share, in varying degrees, the same complex of clinical abnormalities. The majority of cases are associated with an autosomal dominant pattern of inheritance, with extremely variable penetrance. However, cases are also reported with an autosomal recessive or an X-linked recessive pattern of inheritance.

Beighton and co-workers[54] and McKusick[68] have recognized seven distinct clinical forms of the Ehlers-Danlos syndrome. Type I is the full-blown clinical syndrome. It is characterized by dramatic joint hypermobility, hyperextensible skin, and easy bruisability. Type II is a milder syndrome, with minimal cutaneous and joint manifestations. Skin friability is absent. Type III is characterized by the predominance of joint findings, Type IV by the predominance of vascular fragility (autosomal recessive), and Type V (the X-linked recessive form) is dominated by skin stretching. Type VI (autosomal recessive) has a known defect in collagen synthesis and the clinical picture is dominated by ocular abnormalities. Type VII (autosomal recessive) is characterized by short stature and congenital dislocations.

This syndrome has also been referred to as cutis hyperelastica and dermatorrhexis. The first documented case is attributed to van Meeker in 1682.[68]

Pathology and Pathophysiology

The skin of patients with the Ehlers-Danlos syndrome is abnormally thin and demonstrates a marked decrease in tensile strength. The hair follicles and sebaceous glands are normal. The primary histologic defect in the structure of the skin is a matter of dispute, as various histologic studies have described the elastic fiber content of the dermis to be increased, decreased, and normal.[74] Still others[54, 64, 68, 74] have theorized that the Ehlers-Danlos syndrome is a defect in collagen synthesis and that the observed changes in elastic fibers are only a secondary, variable phenomenon. Reported changes in the collagen include abnormal organization of the collagen bundles with defective cross-linkages and abnormal shortening of the collagen chains. Collagen turnover is normal, but in Types VI and VII Ehlers-Danlos syndrome, enzymatic defects in collagen synthesis have been isolated (lysyl hydroxylase and procollagen protease). Other defects, as yet unrecognized, may exist in the other clinical types of the disease.

The mesenchymal defect involves the joint capsules, the ligaments, and the paravertebral supporting tissues. No primary osseous abnormality has been reported in clinical studies of the Ehlers-Danlos syndrome. However, immunofluoroscent studies have shown a defect in tetracycline uptake, substantiating the theory of a primary abnormality in collagen production.

The molluscoid fibrous tumors, found on the pressure points of the body, are composed of proliferating connective tissue and degenerated fat. The vasculature is increased. Subcutaneous spherules of necrotic fat are also found in the skin and are thought to be related to subclinical trauma.

The bleeding diathesis associated with the Ehlers-Danlos syndrome is ascribed to abnormalities in the vessel walls as well as to defects in the supporting perivascular tissues. Abnormal platelets and coagulation defects have also been reported in patients with the Ehlers-Danlos syndrome. However, it is uncertain whether the latter cases represent another manifestation of the connective tissue disorder or whether they are coincidental findings.

Clinical Findings

The Ehlers-Danlos syndrome occurs most frequently in Caucasians of European origin. There is a male predominance, and many of the patients are of tall stature. Typical facial characteristics include lop ears, redundant skin folds around the eyes, poor dentition, and a high, arched palate. As in osteogenesis imperfecta, blue sclerae may be seen. Mental retardation is not present. Patients affected with the Ehlers-Danlos syndrome walk with a characteristic gait that results from hyperextension of the hips in order to compensate for genu recurvatum deformities. The gait disturbance is exacerbated by the presence of pes planus deformities and may be mistaken for tabes dorsalis.

The skin is velvety, thin, and hyperelastic. It can be raised in high folds and, unlike cases of cutis laxa, it retracts spontaneously. However, with advancing age and a concomitant decrease in the hyperelasticity of the skin, the folds become permanent, and the skin lax. The skin is also easily bruised and tends to split with minor trauma. Scars are large and are covered by thin skin. The appearance of these scars has been compared to "cigarette paper." Repeated hemorrhage results in a purple discoloration to the pretibial areas. Stitches hold very poorly, and surgery should be avoided. Three types of skin nodules complicate the changes of the Ehlers-Danlos syndrome: Molluscoid tumors occur at presssure points, spherules of fat necrosis occur in the subcutaneous tissues, and hematomas produce calcified masses.

The passive and active hypermobility of joints in the Ehlers-Danlos syndrome has provided many a circus with an "India rubber man." The elbows and knees hyperextend. Patients are able to touch their thumbs to their forearms (Fig. 72–8). Spontaneous dislocations are frequent and correlate with the degree of laxity. Patients are frequently able to reduce these dislocations themselves. Ligamentous as well as capsular laxity is present and results in kyphoscoliosis, pes planus, and inguinal and hiatal hernias. The ligamentous and capsular laxity is exacerbated by pregnancy and decreases with advancing age. Ligamentous laxity and recurrent dislocations lead to premature degenerative joint disease. Older patients complain of stiffness of hands, knees, and shoulders.

The fragility of the vessel walls and lack of tamponade can result in bleeding from the gastrointestinal tract, the bronchopulmonary tree, or the gums. Dissecting aneurysms of the aorta and sponta-

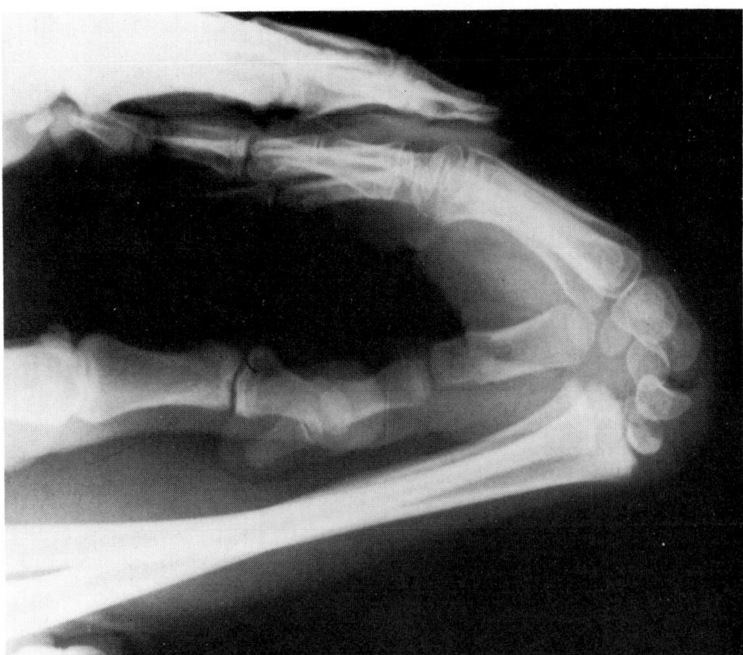

Figure 72–8. *Ehlers-Danlos syndrome. Lateral view of the wrist shows a vacuum phenomenon in lunate-capitate articulation secondary to joint laxity. Patient is able to touch the forearm with the thumb.*

neous ruptures of the large vessels may occur and frequently result in death.

Ocular abnormalities involve the cornea, sclera, fundus, and suspensory mechanism of the lens. Reported changes include strabismus, ectopia lentis, and retinal detachments.

Muscular weakness and easy fatigability are also features of the Ehlers-Danlos syndrome. Infants may be hypotonic and older children frequently complain of muscle cramps.

Visceral manifestations include segmental ectasia of the alimentary canal and respiratory tract. Spontaneous ruptures of bowel and bronchi have been reported. Raynaud's phenomenon also occurs. Cardiac abnormalities include "floppy" mitral and tricuspid valves.

Roentgenographic Findings

Calcification of fatty spherules produces multiple subcutaneous dense lesions that are visible on roentgenograms. They occur primarily in the forearms and shins and measure 2 to 8 mm in diameter. These calcifications usually have a dense rim and resemble phleboliths. Other soft tissue calcifications result from scarring, hematomas, and myositis ossificans.

Joint findings include persistent effusions or hemarthroses (Fig. 72–9). The fluid is thought to result from ligamentous and capsular laxity, which, in turn, produces repetitive subclinical trauma. Olecranon and prepatellar bursitis results from a similar process. The joint spaces may widen with minor stress (Fig. 72–8), and dislocations frequently complicate the clinical course (Fig. 72–10). The most frequent sites of dislocation are the shoulder joints, the patellofemoral joints, the temporomandibular joints, the radial heads, and the sternoclavicular and acromioclavicular joints. There is an increase in the incidence of congenital hip dislocations (Fig. 72–11). Precocious osteoarthritis is the sequela of the repetitive minor trauma associated with capsular laxity and of the repetitive major trauma associated with dislocations. The incidence of degenerative changes correlates with the severity of the laxity.

Ligamentous laxity also results in pes planus deformities (Fig. 72–12) and abnormalities of the axial skeleton. The thorax can be asymmetric, with pectus carinatum (Fig. 72–13) and prominence of the costochondral junctions. The upper ribs may slant sharply downward (Fig.72–13), giving the cervical spine an elongated appearance. A kyphoscoliosis is frequently present at the thoracolumbar junction (Fig. 72–13) and in older patients is associated with anterior wedging of the vertebrae. As in neurofibromatosis, posterior scalloping of the vertebral bodies (secondary to dural ectasia) has been reported. If there is an associated Raynaud's disease, acro-osteolysis may be present.

The roentgenograms can also demonstrate congenital anomalies associated with the Ehlers-Danlos syndrome, including arachnodactyly, triphalangeal thumbs, radioulnar synostoses, club feet, supernumerary teeth, delayed cranial ossification, spondylolysis (Fig. 72–14), elongation of the ulnar styloid, and a short fifth proximal phalanx.

The roentgenographic differential diagnosis of joint laxity includes the Marfan syndrome, Larsen's syndrome, cachexia, Down's syndrome, and neuro-

Text continued on page 2505

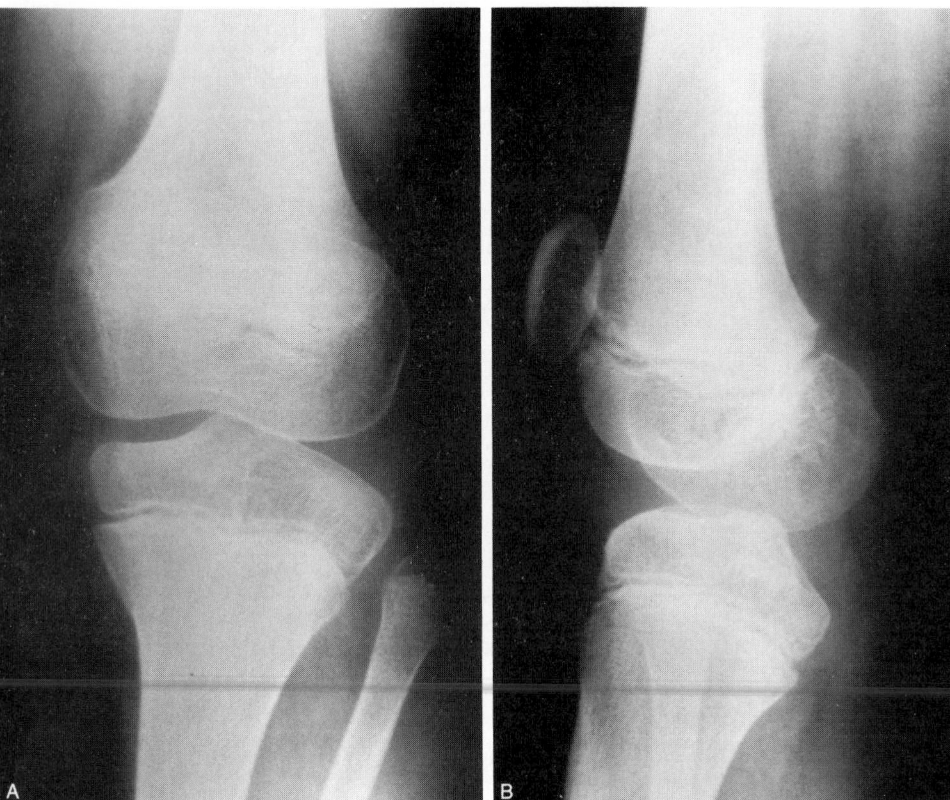

Figure 72–9. Ehlers-Danlos syndrome. Anteroposterior **(A)** and lateral **(B)** views of the knee reveal effusion and genu recurvatum deformity. Also noted is soft tissue prominence in the region of the prepatellar bursa.

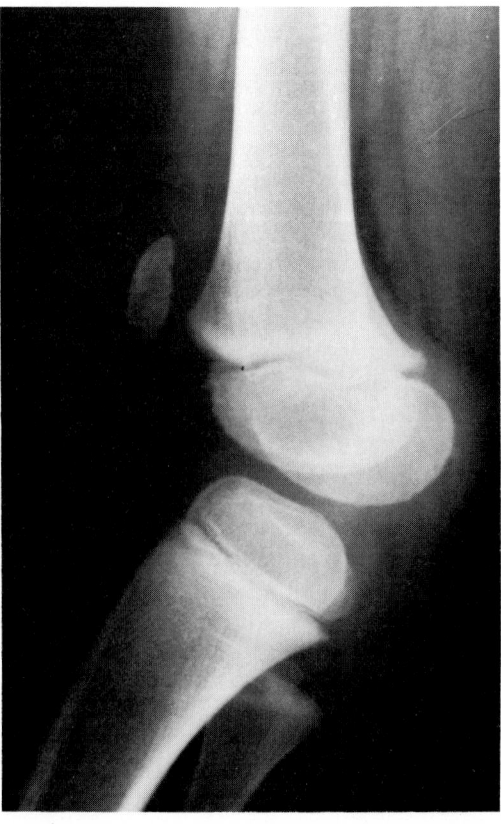

Figure 72–10. Ehlers-Danlos syndrome. Lateral view of the knee shows fibular head dislocation and genu recurvatum deformity.

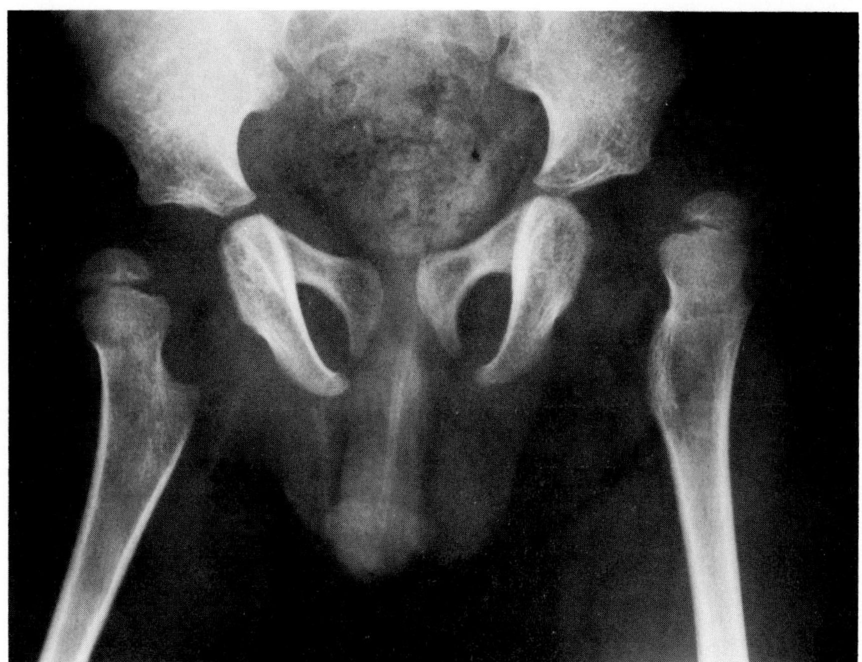

Figure 72–11. *Ehlers-Danlos syndrome: Bilateral congenital hip dislocations.*

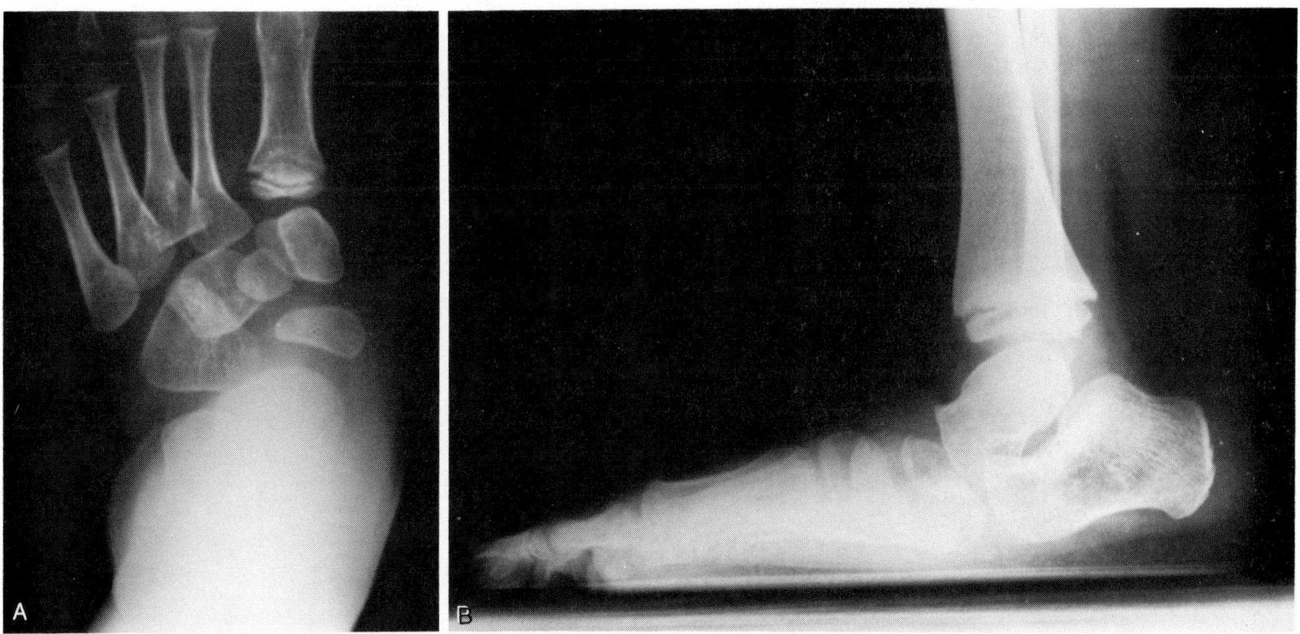

Figure 72–12. *Ehlers-Danlos syndrome. Anterposterior* **(A)** *and lateral* **(B)** *views of the foot reveal severe hindfoot valgus with pes planus deformity.*

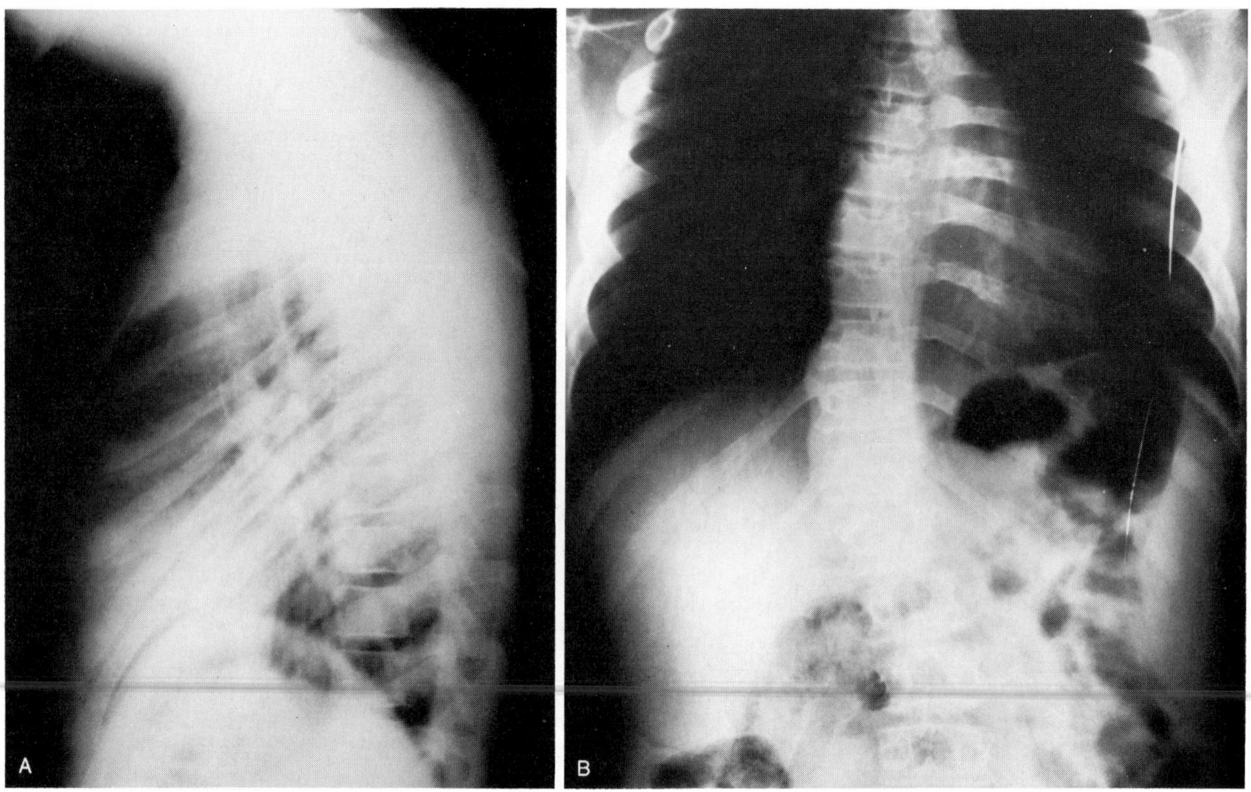

Figure 72–13. *Ehlers-Danlos syndrome: Axial deformities include pectus carinatum* **(A)**, *thoracolumbar scoliosis* **(A, B)**, *and an exaggerated downward slant to ribs* **(B)**.

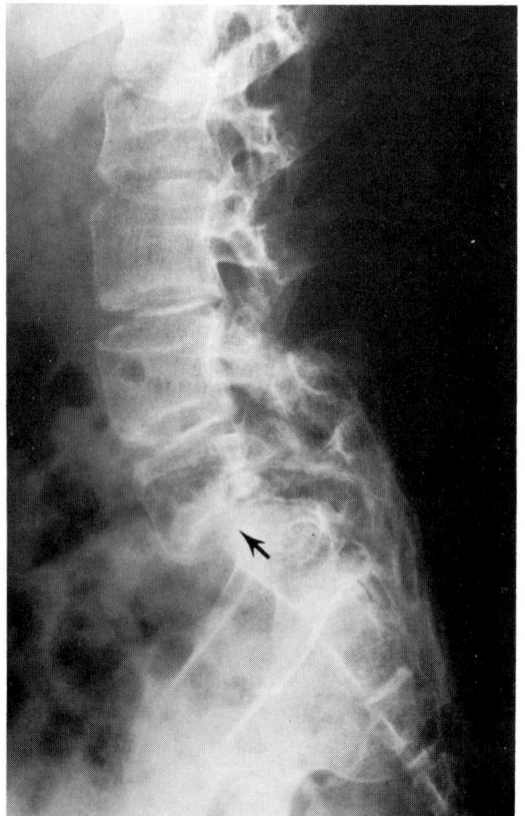

Figure 72–14. *Ehlers-Danlos syndrome: Lateral view of the lumbar spine shows a spondylolysis and spondylolisthesis (arrow).*

muscular disorders. A syndrome of hereditary ligamentous laxity also occurs. In the absence of the characteristic subcutaneous calcifications, the clinical history of skin changes may be necessary to establish the diagnosis.

The soft tissue calcifications of the Ehlers-Danlos syndrome may be confused with cysticercosis, vascular tumors, phleboliths, or collagen diseases. Their predilection for the lower extremities and their location in the subcutaneous tissues in the Ehlers-Danlos syndrome should help in establishing the correct diagnosis.

OSTEOGENESIS IMPERFECTA

Osteogenesis imperfecta is an inherited disorder of connective tissue that affects the skeleton, ligaments, skin, sclerae, and dentin. It is thought to be characterized by the abnormal maturation of collagen in both mineralized and nonmineralized tissues.[88, 89, 102] Some authors have postulated abnormalities in the adenosine triphosphate energy mechanism,[99] but this theory remains unsubtantiated.

The three major clinical criteria are (1) osteoporosis with abnormal fragility of the skeleton, (2) blue sclerae, and (3) dentinogenesis imperfecta. The presence of two of these abnormalities confirms the diagnosis. Other features are premature otosclerosis, ligamentous laxity, episodic diaphoresis with abnormal temperature regulation, easy bruisability, constipation, hyperplastic scars, premature vascular calcifications, and inappropriate euphoria.

Osteogenesis imperfecta has been subclassified into two syndromes: the congenita form, which has a high infant mortality rate, and the tarda form, which has a normal life expectancy. The distinction between these two forms of the disease was initially based on the age at the time of the first fracture.[86] However, clinical investigators have altered the definitions, and the terms congenita and tarda now refer to the presence or absence of osseous deformities.[76, 86] Bowing of the long bones is a useful guide to the severity of the disorder because it correlates with both the number of fractures and the probability of ambulation. The classification employed at the Hospital for Special Surgery in New York City defines the congenita type by the presence of upper and lower extremity bowing at the time of birth (Fig. 72–15). The tarda group is subclassified into type I, with acquired bowing, and type II, with no bowing deformities. The terms tarda and congenita remain descriptive because it is as yet uncertain whether osteogenesis imperfecta is a single disorder or a group of related entities. Spranger[100] and Sillence and co-workers[206] have offered new classifications, which correlate the clinical findings with genetic patterns of inheritance. In the future these newer classifications may replace the ones that are currently in use. Most patients with the tarda form have a family history consistent with an autosomal dominant mode of transmission. Penetrance of the abnormal gene is extremely variable. Patients with the less common congenita form may have had spontaneous mutations or have an autosomal recessive pattern of inheritance.

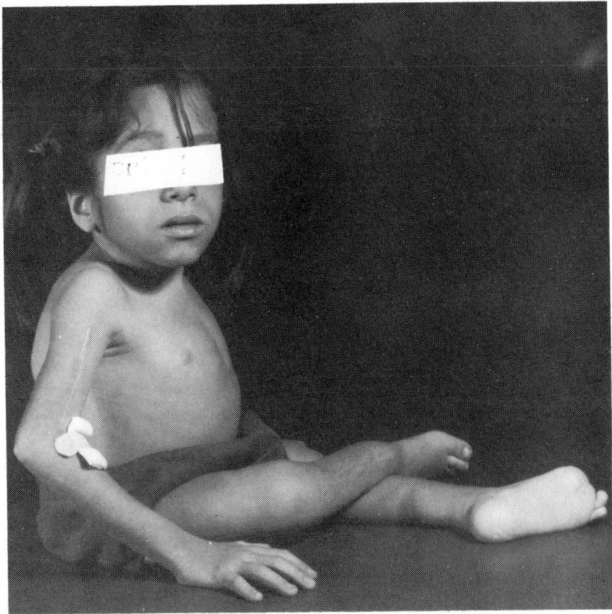

Figure 72–15. *Osteogenesis imperfecta: Congenita form. The limbs are disproportionately short and there is bowing of all four extremities. Thoracic deformities are also present.*

Other names used in reference to osteogenesis imperfecta include fragilitas ossium, la maladie de Lobstein, and van der Hoeve's syndrome.

Pathology and Pathophysiology

Osteogenesis imperfecta is a generalized connective tissue disorder characterized by abnormal maturation of collagen. Reported defects include a decrease in the rate of collagen synthesis,[89, 94, 97] alterations in the aldehyde cross-linkages of the collagen macromolecule, and changes in the normal proportions of the type I and type II collagen molecules.[89, 94, 102] The abnormalities in synthesis and aggregation result in the formation of an unstable fetal collagen.[89, 91, 94, 97] Spranger[100] has identified four different patterns of abnormalities in collagen synthesis. Recent studies[86, 99] have also suggested the presence of abnormalities in the adenosine triphosphate energy mechanism.

The skeletal changes of osteogenesis imperfecta are characterized by a primary defect in the bone matrix. Periosteal bone formation is decreased, which disturbs the normal circumferential growth of the bones.[94, 97] Osteoblastic activity is slowed,[86, 96] and there is a failure to replace fetal bone with normal lamellar bone,[80, 85, 88, 94, 99] which leaves the cortex thinned and mechanically weakened. Immature collagen in the bone matrix results in irregular granular calcification.[76, 88, 99] The number of osteoblasts and osteocytes, per unit matrix, is actually increased, as is the rate of bone turnover.

The sclerae are thin and also contain abnormal collagen. The blue color results from the brown choroid shining through the abnormal outer layer.[96]

Immature collagen has also been observed in the pulp of the teeth and is associated with the clinically observed abnormality in calcification.[22]

The disturbance of the cellular ATPase mechanism is thought to be related to abnormal temperature regulation[96, 99] and to defective platelet aggregation.[99] The exact reason for conduction or nerve deafness remains unknown.

Clinical Findings

Osteogenesis imperfecta occurs in all races. Some series report an equal sex incidence,[96] whereas others have observed a slight female predominance.[76, 84, 92] The congenita cases have high intrauterine and infant mortality rates owing to the complications of intracerebral hemorrhage or a flail chest.

Facial characteristics include temporal bulging, flattening of the features, micrognathia and hypertelorism. Blue sclerae occur in over 90 per cent of cases,[78, 86] and intensity of the hue can vary with the patient's emotional status. A small ring of sclera surrounding the cornea can retain a normal white color and is called a "Saturn's ring." Abnormal dentition with opalescent gray teeth is termed dentinogenesis imperfecta. The primary abnormality originates in the pulp canal.[96] It is not so frequent a clinical finding as blue sclerae, but it is specific for osteogenesis imperfecta.

Growth retardation occurs in most cases,[94] and severely affected individuals are dwarfed (Fig. 72–15). The short stature is due to both microscopic defects in collagen synthesis and the gross fracture deformities. Growth disturbances have been detected in utero. The limbs are more involved than the trunk and the lower extremities are more shortened than the upper extremities (Fig. 72–15). Skeletal deformities include kyphoscoliosis and bowing of the long bones, which exacerbates the limb-trunk discrepancy.

Multiple fractures, resulting from normal daily activities or minor trauma, are the predominant clinical finding in osteogenesis imperfecta. In congenita cases, the fractures occur even in the protected environment of the uterus. The frequency of the pathologic fractures appears to decrease after puberty owing to either hormonal factors or the patient's increased awareness of the condition.

Otosclerosis can occur prior to the age of 40 years, and aside from the early age of onset, it is indistinguishable from the idiopathic form of conduction deafness.

As in other hereditary disorders of collagen synthesis (the Marfan syndrome, Ehlers-Danlos syndrome, homocystinuria), the clinical abnormalities of osteogenesis imperfecta include thin skin, a tendency to form hyperplastic scars, premature vascular calcifications, joint laxity, a high incidence of hernias, and platelet abnormalities.

The central nervous system can also be affected. Basilar impression effectively decreases the volume of the posterior fossa and can result in hydrocephalus. Intracranial hemorrhage results from osseous injury and platelet abnormalities, which are associated with the increased incidence of pituitary deficiency.[96] The causes of hyperthermia and inappropriate euphoria are as yet unknown.

Roentgenographic Findings

The most characteristic roentgenographic finding of osteogenesis imperfecta is a diffuse decrease in osseous density (Figs. 72–16 to 72–18), which

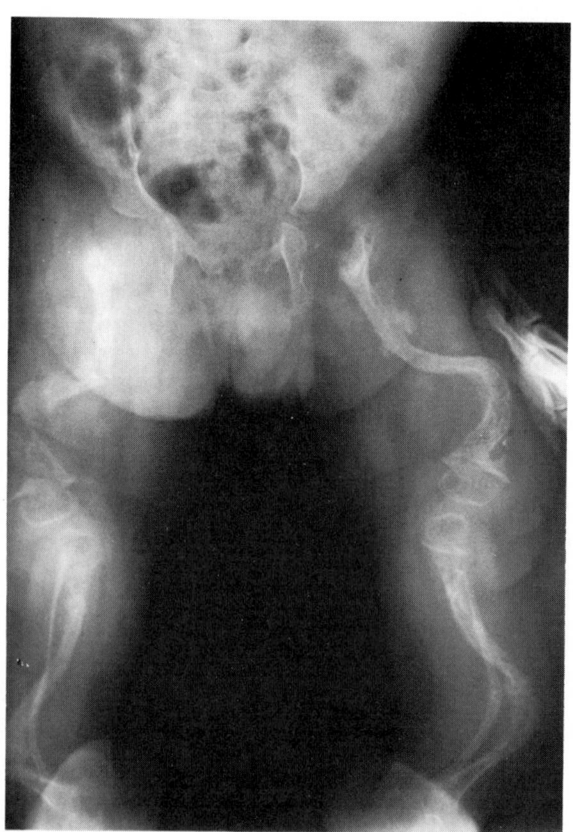

Figure 72–16. *Osteogenesis imperfecta. Anteroposterior view of pelvis and lower extremities reveals a decrease in osseous density associated with thin, gracile long bones. Multiple fractures in various stages of healing are present. The long bones are bowed.*

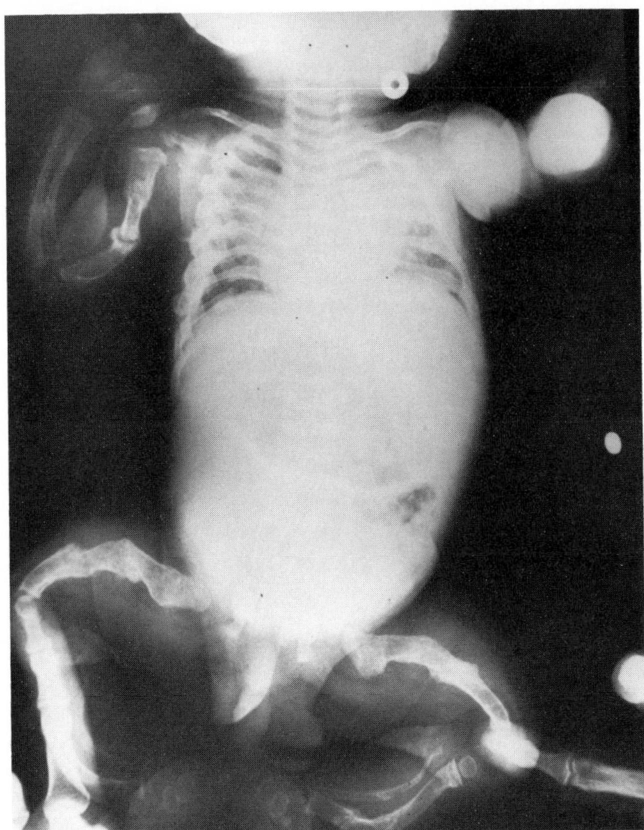

Figure 72–17. *Osteogenesis imperfecta. Anteroposterior view of the skeleton shows a decrease in osseous density associated with short thick bones and telescoping fractures. Bowing of the extremities is present. Fractures are seen in all long bones and ribs.*

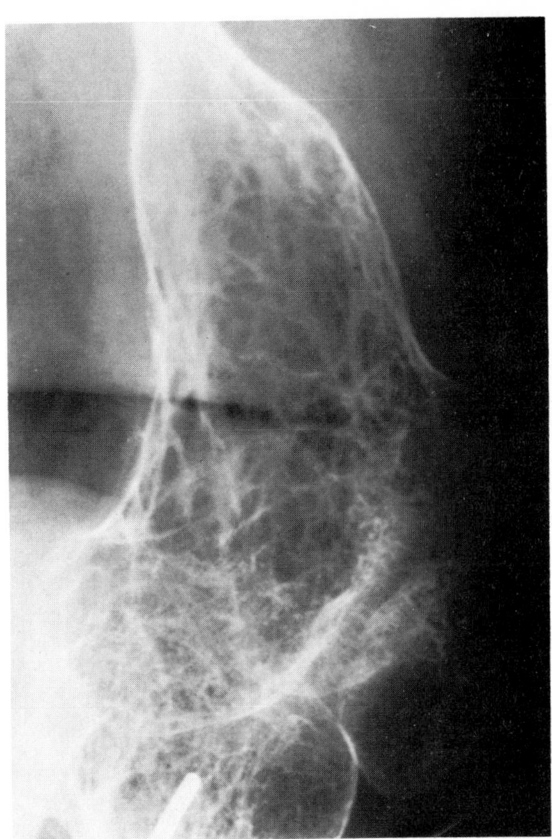

Figure 72–18. *Osteogenesis imperfecta. Lateral view of knee demonstrating the rare cystic type of disease. The metaphyses are flared and honeycombed by thick, coarse trabeculae.*

involves equally the axial and appendicular portions of the skeleton. By definition, the decrease in osseous density is classified as a form of hereditary osteoporosis, since the primary abnormality involves synthesis of collagen matrix. However, in osteogenesis imperfecta, the primary defect in matrix is accompanied by a secondary alteration in mineralization. Therefore, the roentgenographic changes are not exclusively those of osteoporosis.

Based on the roentgenographic appearance of the extremities, Fairbank[84] has subclassified patients with osteogenesis imperfecta into three groups. The first category encompasses those cases with thin, gracile bones (Fig. 72–16). This is the most common expression of the disease and includes most of the patients in the tarda type I and tarda type II clinical categories. The second group includes the patients with short, thick limbs (Fig. 72–17). This type of roentgenographic appearance occurs almost exclusively in patients with a congenita form of the disease and, as with congenital bowing of the extremities, it is usually associated with severe micromelia (Fig. 72–17) and a poor prognosis. Third, and least frequent, is a group of cases with cystic changes in the extremities (Fig. 72–18). The roentgenographic findings in this category are characterized by flared metaphyses, which are hyperlucent and transversed by a honeycomb of coarse trabeculae (Fig. 72–18). As with the clinical categories, the roentgenographic classification is purely descriptive. Frequently during periods of active growth, a patient may show change from one appearance to another. Congenita patients who survive infancy often undergo change from the thick limb type to the cystic or gracile type. Considerable variation also exists within each category, since the roentgenographic appearance reflects a dynamic balance between the microscopic abnormalities and the gross fracture deformities. The cortices of the long bones may be either abnormally thin (Figs. 72–16 to 72–18) or abnormally thick (Fig. 72–19). The metaphyses may be flared (Fig. 72–18) or undermodeled (Fig. 72–16), and the shafts can be straight (Fig. 72–19) or bowed (Figs. 72–16 and 72–17).

The fractures that complicate the course of osteogenesis imperfecta occur most frequently in the lower extremities and are usually transverse in direction (Fig. 72–19). Avulsion injuries are common and result from normal muscle pull. Micromelia and bowing deformities are the sequelae of multiple telescoping fractures, which begin to occur during gestation (Fig. 72–17). Fracture healing is usually

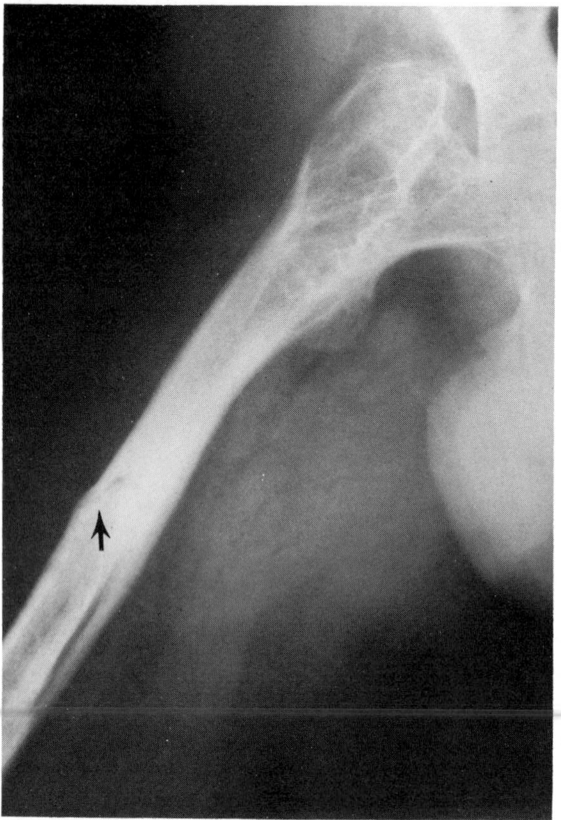

Figure 72–19. Osteogenesis imperfecta. Oblique view of the femur showing characteristic transverse fracture (arrow). Although the general density of the bone is decreased, the cortices are thickened as a result of previous trauma and bowing deformities.

normal, but tumoral callus (Fig. 72–20) and pseudarthroses (Fig. 72–21) may occur. In children with severe osteogenesis imperfecta, the metaphyses or epiphyses of the long bones may contain multiple scalloped radiolucent areas with sclerotic margins (Fig. 72–22). The latter appearance is referred to as "popcorn calcifications" and it is thought to result from the traumatic fragmentation of the cartilage growth plate.[205]

The joints of the extremities are affected by two separate processes, both of which lead to premature degenerative joint disease. First, fracture deformities distort the articular surfaces and result in incongruity (Fig. 72–23). The incongruity eventually leads to premature degeneration of the articular surfaces. Second, ligamentous and capsular laxity produces repetitive minor trauma, which also results in damage to the hyaline cartilage (Figs. 72–24 and 72–25). In recent years, use of the Sofield procedure,[98] multiple osteotomies, and intramedullary rodding has changed the course of this disease. Correction of bowing deformities has increased the probability of ambulation, particularly in congenita patients. There is greater weight-bearing stress on the joints, as well as possible intra-articular protrusion of the rods, which may increase the incidence of joint changes.

Roentgenograms of the skull demonstrate persistent wormian bones (Fig. 72–26) and, as in homocystinuria, enlargement of the sinuses. Platybasia, with or without basilar impression, is a frequent deformity. The spine studies reveal flattening of the vertebral bodies, which are either biconcave in shape or wedge-shaped anteriorly (Fig. 72–27). Severe kyphoscoliosis results from the combination of ligamentous laxity, osteoporosis, and posttraumatic deformities (Fig. 72–28). The pelvis is narrowed and frequently triradiate in shape (Fig. 72–29). Protrusion deformities of the acetabuli (Figs. 72–29 and 72–30) and shepherd's crook deformities of the femora may be present. Premature vascular calcifications can be seen in the soft tissues.

The differential diagnosis of osteogenesis imperfecta includes other entities with multiple fractures, such as the battered child syndrome and congenital indifference to pain. The relatively normal bone density at uninvolved sites and the absence of eye or dental abnormalities should differentiate these latter disorders from fragilitas ossium. Other differential diagnostic possibilities are diseases that produce a generalized decrease in osseous density. Hypophosphatasia is associated with lucent bones and bowing deformities of the extremities, but the metaphyseal changes of rickets are also present, distinguishing it from osteogenesis imperfecta. The roentgenographic findings of juvenile osteoporosis

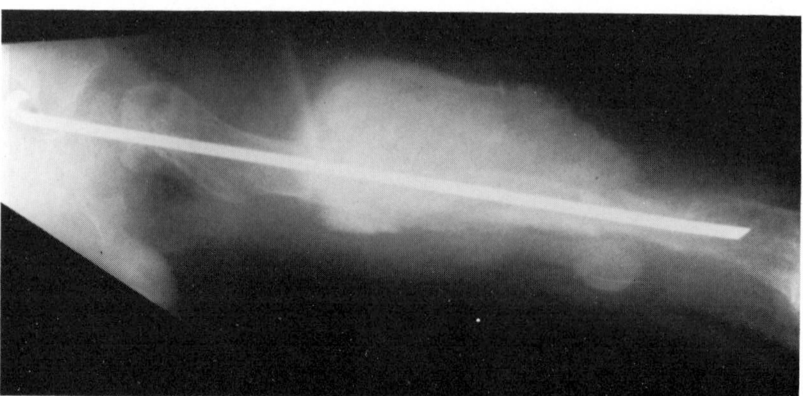

Figure 72–20. Osteogenesis imperfecta. Tumoral callus formation around Sofield osteotomies.

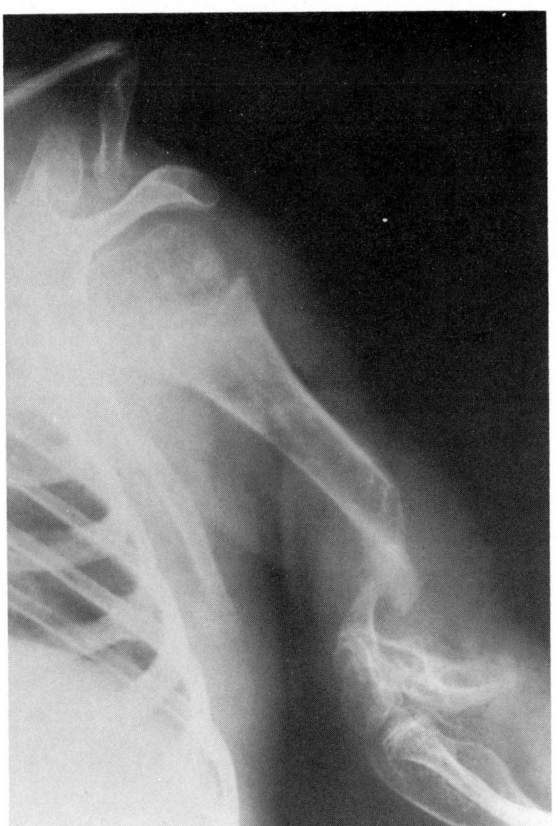

Figure 72–21. *Osteogenesis imperfecta. Pseudarthroses of the humerus and clavicle complicating fractures.*

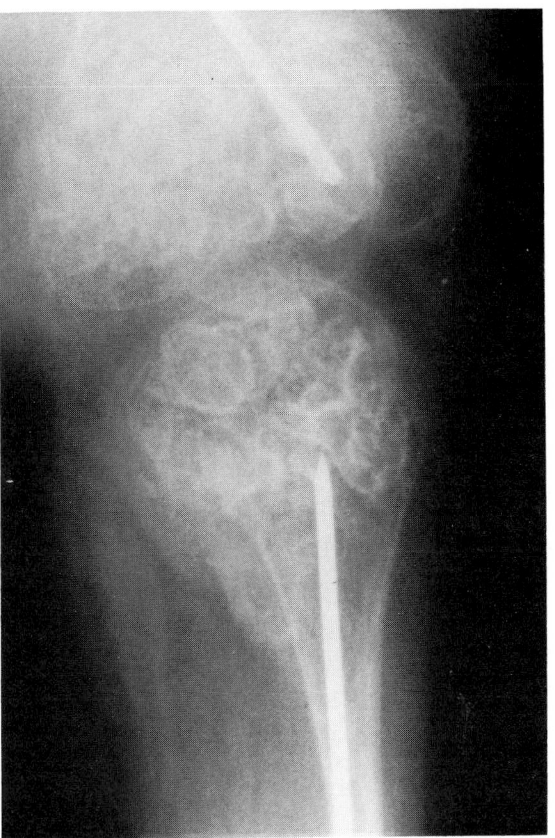

Figure 72–22. *Osteogenesis imperfecta. Oblique view of the knee showing "popcorn calcifications." These lucencies with sclerotic margins are associated with absence of a normal horizontal growth plate. Sofield procedures have been performed.*

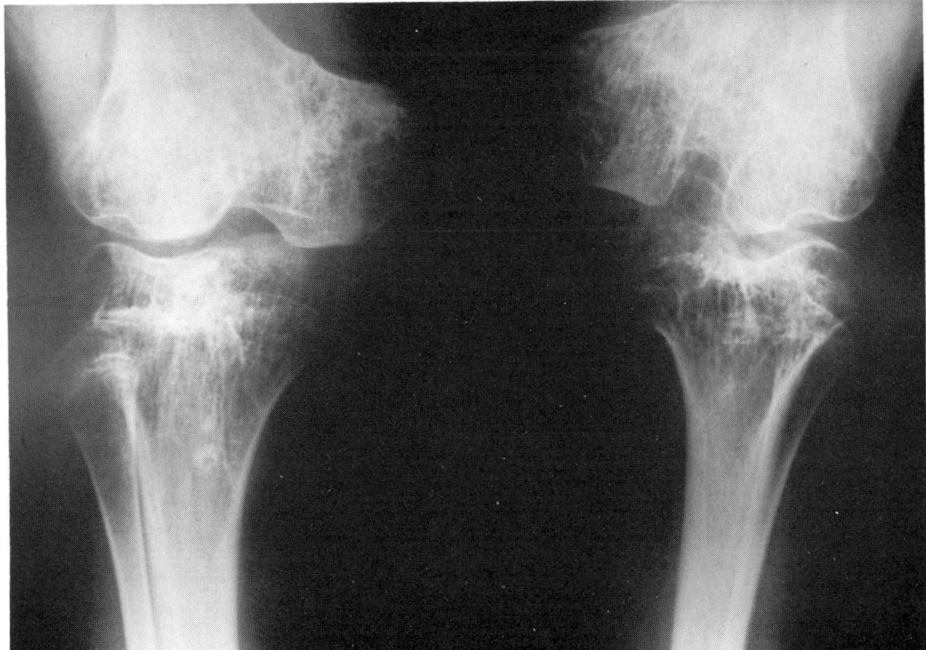

Figure 72–23. *Osteogenesis imperfecta. Posttraumatic deformities result in irregularity of the articular surfaces of the knees.*

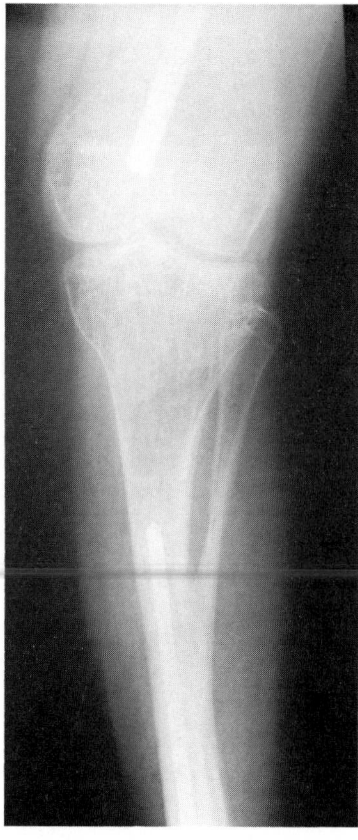

Figure 72–24. Osteogenesis *imperfecta. Anteroposterior view of the knee revealing genu valgum.*

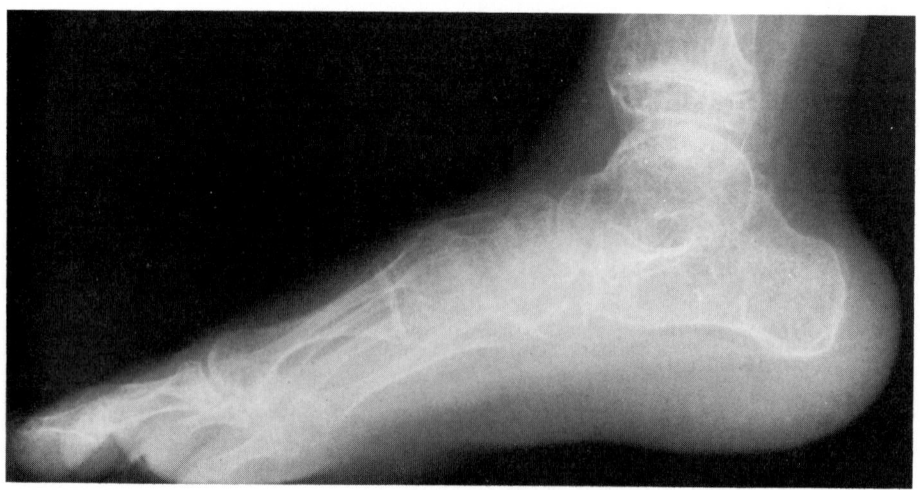

Figure 72–25. Osteogenesis *imperfecta. Lateral view of foot demonstrates pes planus deformity.*

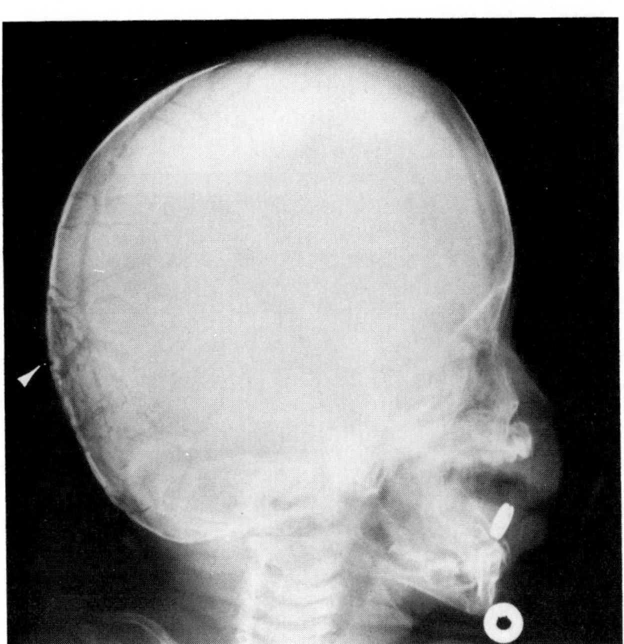

Figure 72–26. *Osteogenesis imperfecta. Lateral view of the skull shows decreased osseous density, thinning of both tables, and multiple wormian bones (arrowhead).*

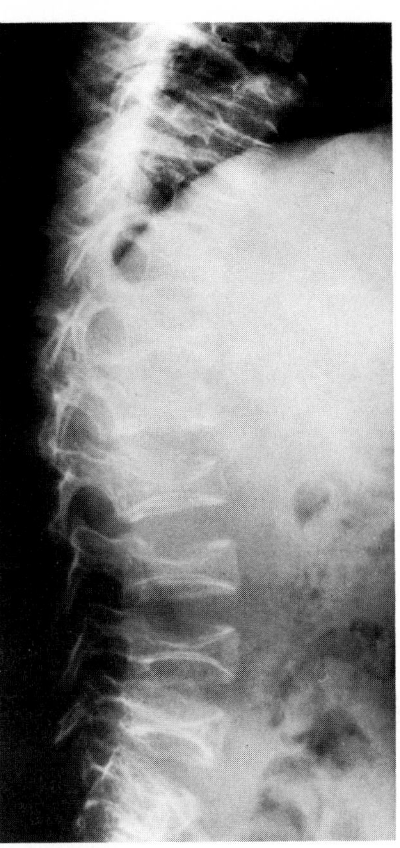

Figure 72–27. *Osteogenesis imperfecta. Lateral view of the spine shows both biconcave vertebrae and vertebrae with anterior wedge deformities.*

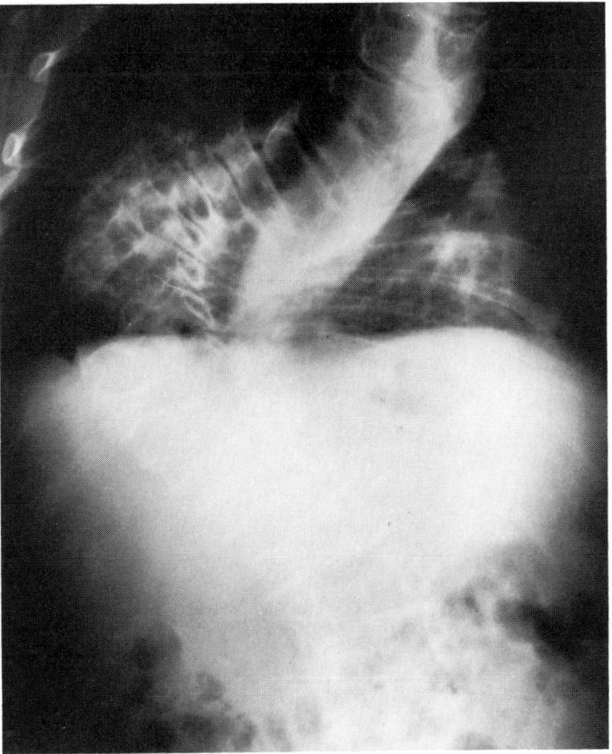

Figure 72–28. *Osteogenesis imperfecta. Anteroposterior view of the spine reveals a severe kyphoscoliosis, decreased osseous density, and flattening of the vertebral bodies.*

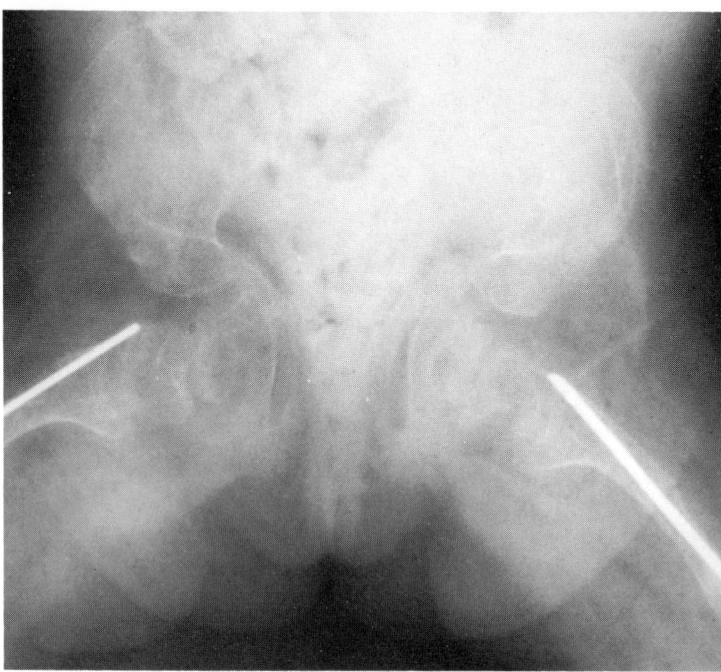

Figure 72–29. Osteogenesis imperfecta. Anteroposterior view of the pelvis showing a triradiate shape and protrusio acetabuli deformities. Sofield procedures have been performed in the femora.

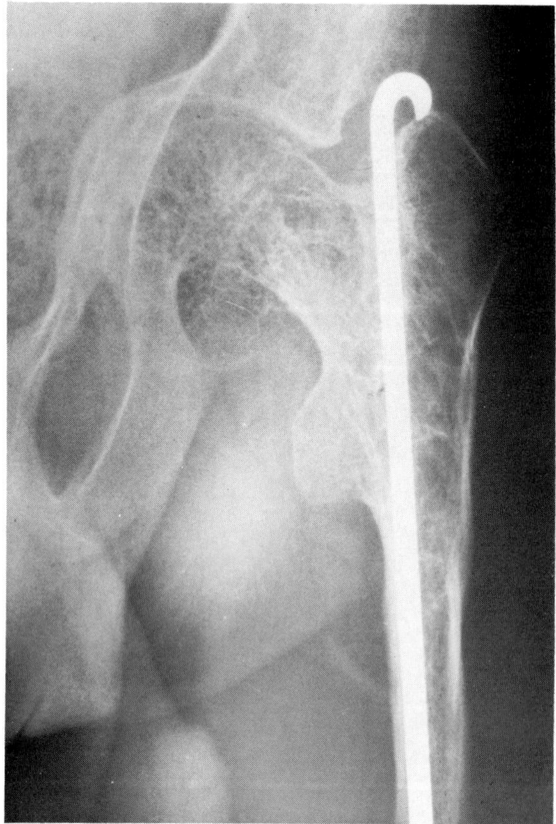

Figure 72–30. Osteogenesis imperfecta. Anteroposterior view of the hip demonstrating a protrusio acetabuli deformity and a coxa vara deformity. A Sofield procedure has been performed.

and Cushing's disease may be indistinguishable from those of osteogenesis imperfecta, and in these instances clinical correlation is necessary.

MYOSITIS OSSIFICANS PROGRESSIVA

Myositis ossificans progressiva is a hereditary mesodermal disorder characterized by progressive ossification of striated muscles, tendons, ligaments, and fasciae. The pattern of inheritance remains unknown. McKusick[113] has theorized that it is an autosomal dominant trait with a wide range of expressivity. However, most reported cases are spontaneous mutations.

This syndrome was first described in 1692 by Patin, who reported the case of a young woman who in his words "turned to wood." It was Münchmeyer who reported the first series of cases, and this disorder is often referred to as Münchmeyer's disease. It is also called fibrogenesis ossificans progressiva.

Pathology and Pathophysiology

The etiology of myositis ossificans progressiva is unknown. It is classified as a hereditary disorder on the basis of two pieces of evidence. First, there have been two sets of homozygous twins with the

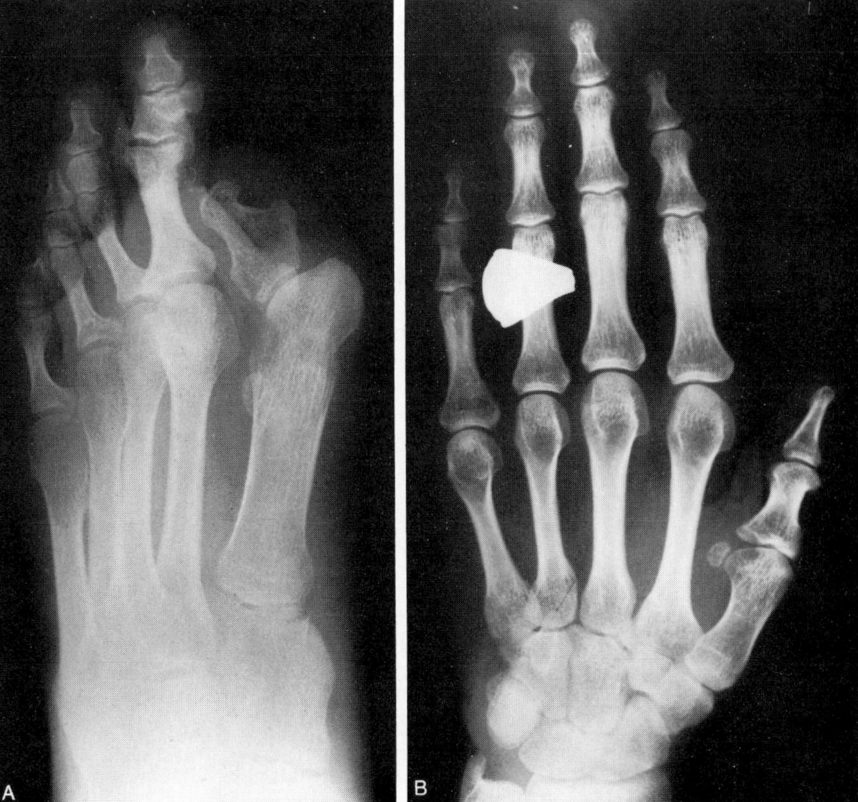

Figure 72–31. *Myositis ossificans progressiva. Frontal views of the foot* **(A)** *and hand* **(B)** *demonstrating microdactyly of the first digits with hypoplasia and fusion of the phalanges.*

disease.[109] Second, there is a high association of congenital digital anomalies. Seventy-five per cent of patients with myositis ossificans progressiva and 5 per cent of their families have bilateral microdactyly of the first toes with synostosis of the phalanges (Figs. 72–31 and 72–32).

Blood chemistry values, serum alkaline phosphatase concentrations, renal function, and parathormone levels are all within normal limits.[112] Calcium kinetic studies, using radioactive tracers, have indicated only the expected increase in the rates of bone deposition and bone resorption, with a disproportionate increase in deposition.[112] Even the target tissue is uncertain. The prevailing theory, supported by McKusick,[113] postulates that the disease affects primarily the interstitial tissues and that muscle damage is secondary to pressure atrophy. Involvement of skin, tendons, and ligaments, which contain no muscle fibers, as well as the detectable localized increase in alkaline phosphatase supports the concept of a fibrous tissue defect. The abnormal deposition of calcium salts has been attributed either to absence of a circulating inhibitor[112] or to a primary defect in the collagen itself.[113] However, other investigators remain convinced that the mesenchymal defect is primarily in the muscles themselves. Electromyographic studies, performed on unossified areas, have revealed abnormalities consistent with a myopathy.[106, 115] Histochemical studies have demonstrated variability in muscle fiber size and a decrease

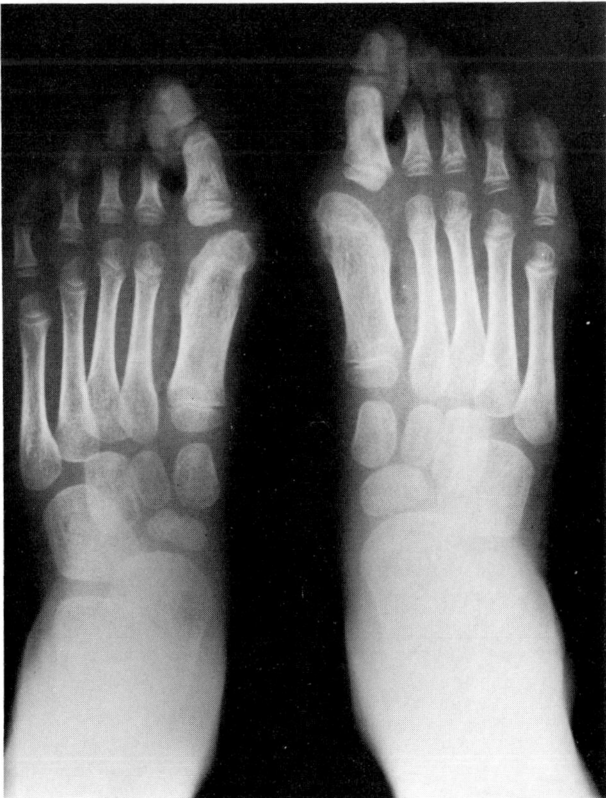

Figure 72–32. *Myositis ossificans progressiva. Anteroposterior view of both feet showing the characteristic congenital anomalies of the first digits.*

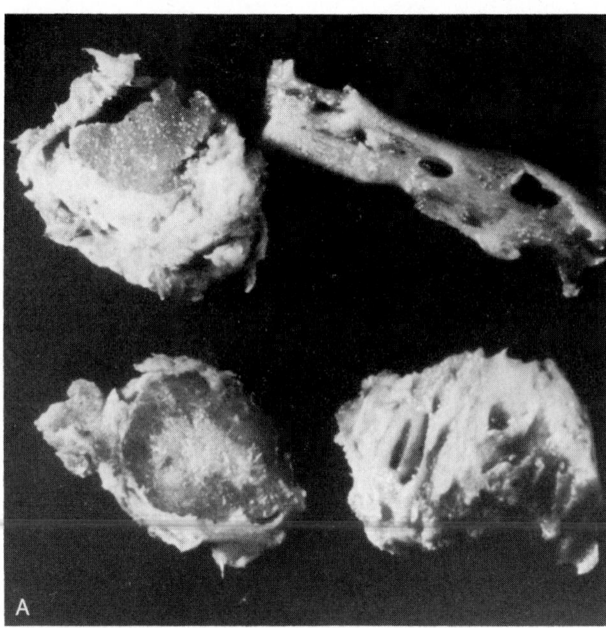

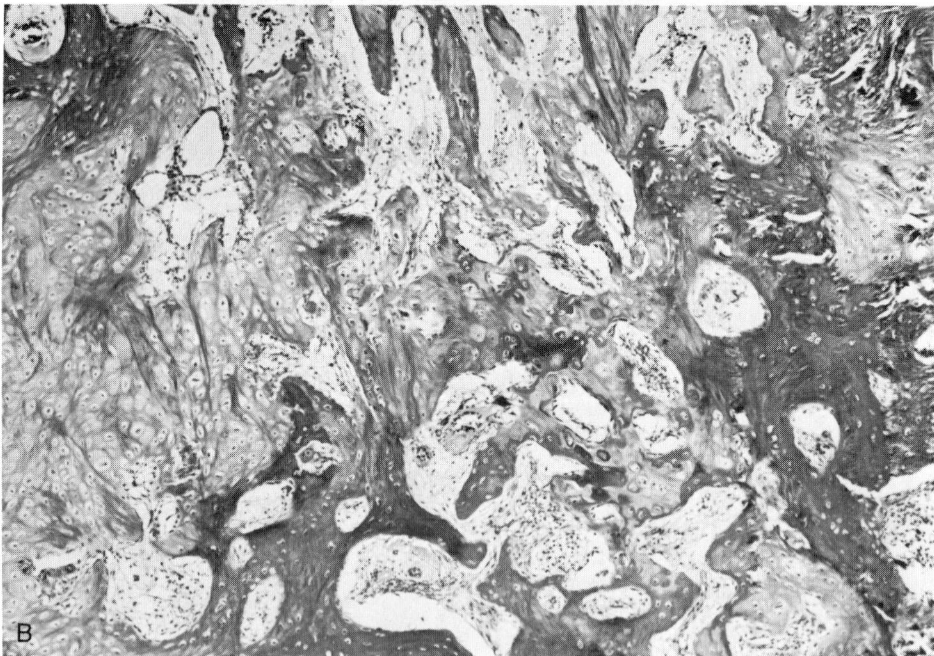

Figure 72–33. *Myositis ossificans progressiva.* **A,** *Irregular pieces of new bone removed from the soft tissues surrounding the hip of a patient with myositis ossificans progressiva. Microscopic sections with unpolarized* **(B)** *and polarized* **(C)** *light show irregular collagen fibers and sheets of lamellar bone. Islands of woven bone are also present.*

Illustration continued on the opposite page

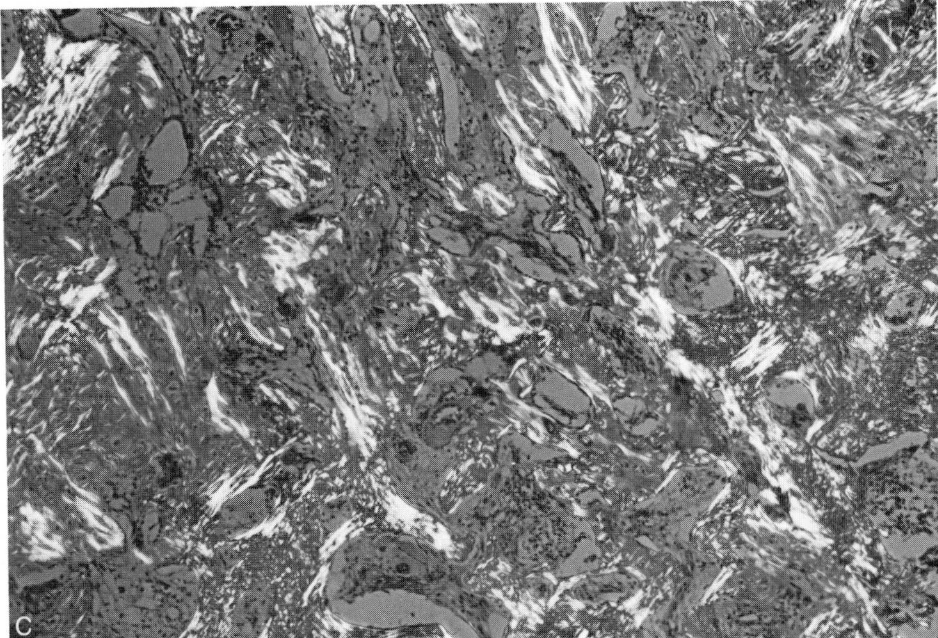

Figure 72–33. Continued

in ATPase activity, which predates ossification.[106, 115] Thus, the location of the metabolic error is still to be decided upon.

The pathologic abnormalities that characterize the individual lesions are similar to those of myositis ossificans circumscripta. The earliest histologic changes are edema and an inflammatory exudate. Mesenchymal proliferation then results in the formation of a large mass of collagen, which, unlike normal collagen, is capable of accepting the deposition of calcium salts. Eventually, the lesion is transformed into irregular masses of lamellar and woven bone (Fig. 72–33).

Clinical Findings

Myositis ossificans progressiva has no known sexual predilection. Although the onset of symptoms is usually in the first decade of life, ossification is not present at the time of birth. The most frequent presenting symptom is torticollis resulting from a painful mass within the sternocleidomastoid muscle. The disease usually progresses from the shoulder girdle to the upper arms, spine, and pelvis (Fig. 72–34). The distal extremities are involved late in the course of the disease. The heart, diaphragm, larynx, tongue, and sphincters are spared, as are all smooth muscle structures. The natural history of myositis ossificans progressiva is one of remissions and exacerbations. A new episode of ossification is frequently precipitated by minor trauma. As an area becomes involved, the first symptoms are heat, edema, and a painful mass. The local changes may be accompanied by fever. The pain gradually decreases and the mass gradually hardens as new bone formation occurs. Joint ankylosis and conductive hearing loss are common complications. Death is inevitable and may be secondary to respiratory failure with constriction of the chest wall, or it may

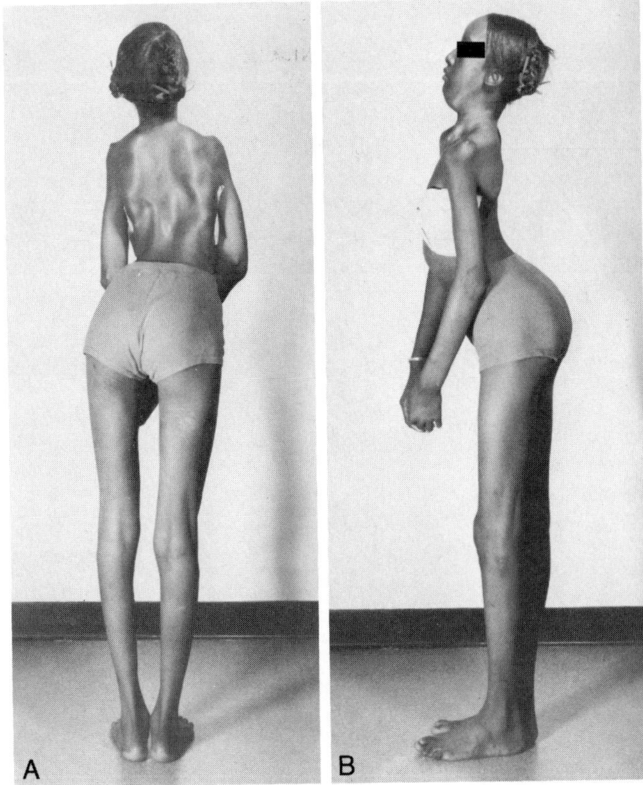

Figure 72–34. *Myositis ossificans progressiva. Posterior* **(A)** *and lateral* **(B)** *views of an adolescent girl with myositis ossificans progressiva show the shoulder girdle and spine to be most affected.*

result from starvation with ossification of the masseter muscles.

Roentgenographic Findings

Digital anomalies are present at birth and precede the soft tissue ossification. The most common abnormality is microdactyly of the first toes, with hypoplasia and synostosis of the phalanges (Figs. 72–31 and 72–32). Total absence of the first toes has also been reported. Similar abnormalities less frequently involve the thumbs (Fig. 72–31*B*). Other congenital anomalies associated with myositis ossificans progressiva are hallux valgus deformities (Fig. 72–31*A*), broad femoral necks, shortening of all the digits and clinodactyly. In children with this disease, the epiphyses may be larger than normal.

After the onset of symptoms, the roentgenographic findings in the individual locations are similar to those of the traumatic form of myositis ossificans. The first radiographic finding is a soft tissue mass. The lesion gradually shrinks in size and ossifies. The final appearance of the myositis ossificans may be that of a column of solid new bone replacing the entire muscle (Figs. 72–35 and 72–36) or a plate of new bone with a "dotted veil" pattern outlining the fascial planes. The zonal phenomenon, a characteristic feature of myositis ossificans circumscripta,

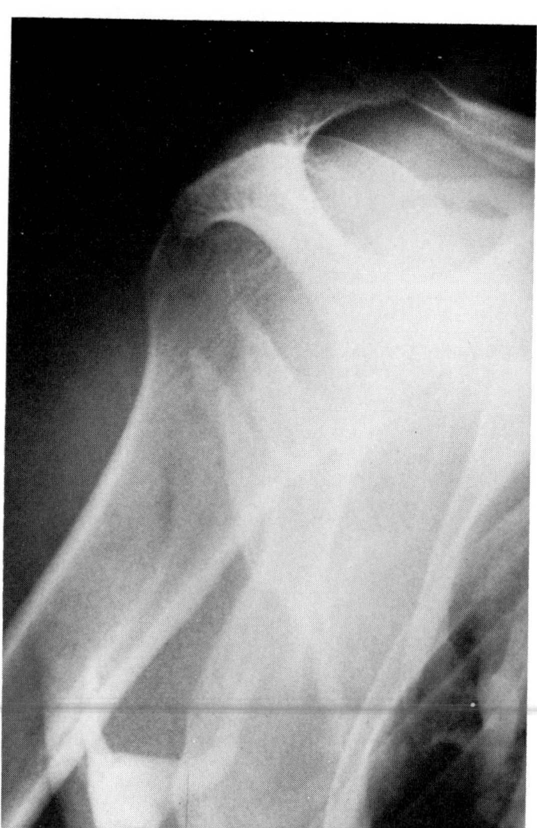

Figure 72–36. *Myositis ossificans progressiva. Anteroposterior view of the shoulder demonstrating columns of mature bone replacing the normal soft tissue structures.*

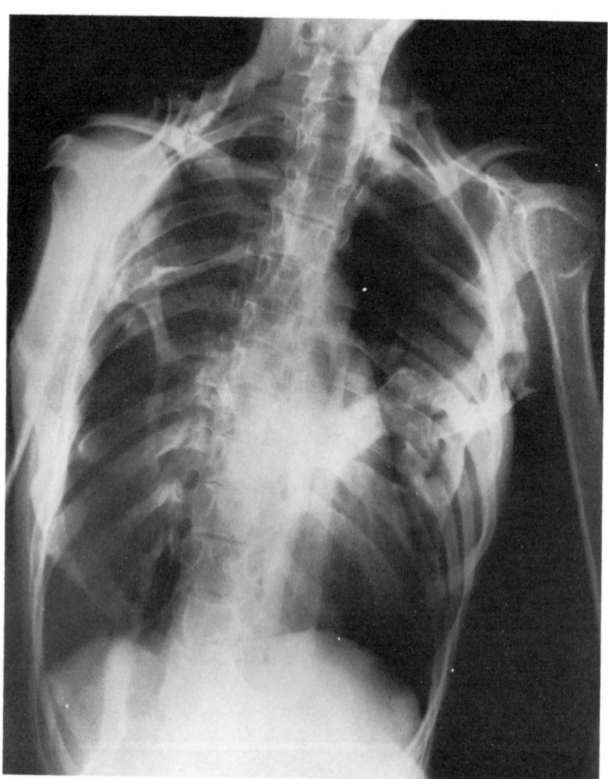

Figure 72–35. *Myositis ossificans progressiva. An anteroposterior view of the thorax showing the early distribution of soft tissue ossification: shoulders, neck, and cervical spine.*

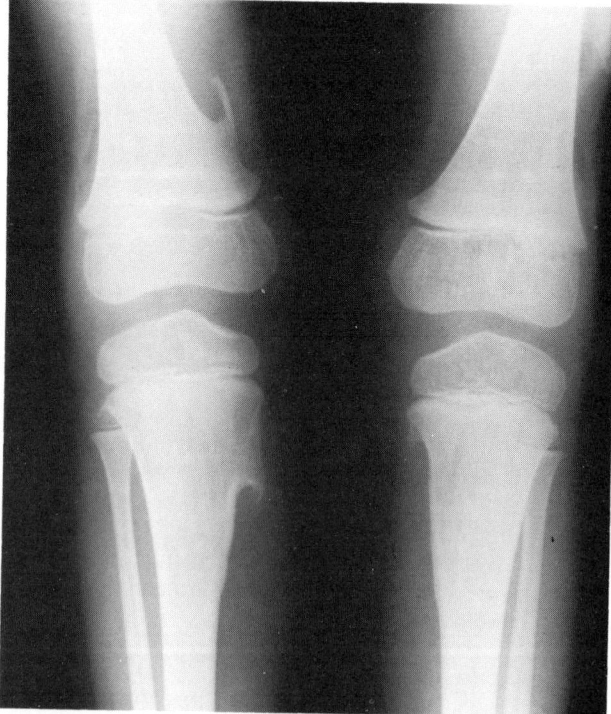

Figure 72–37. *Myositis ossificans progressiva. Ossification of ligamentous insertions results in metaphyseal "exostoses."*

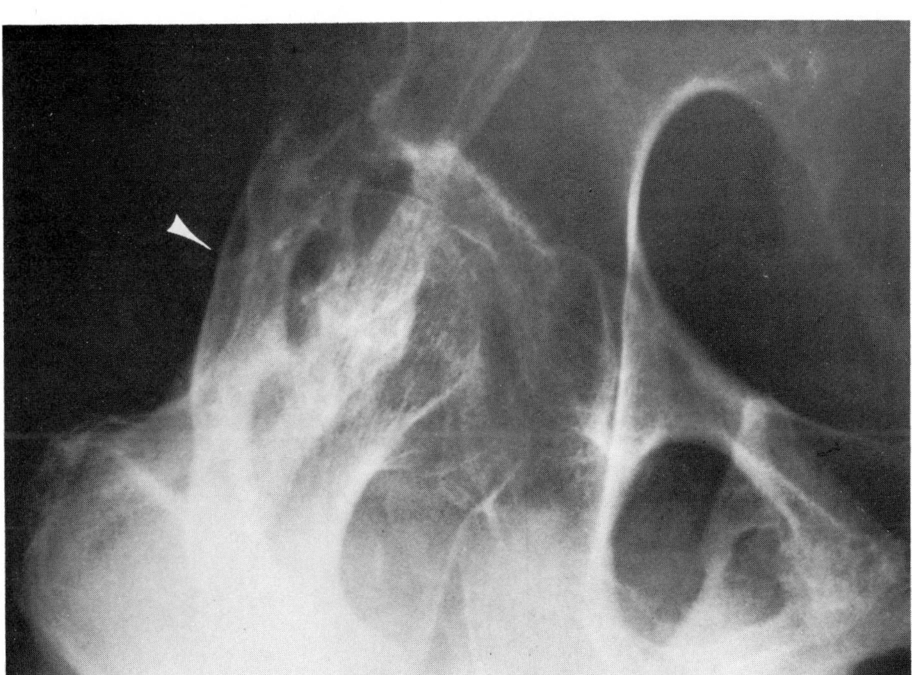

Figure 72–38. *Myositis ossificans progressiva. Anteroposterior view of the hip shows joint ankylosis resulting from ossification of periarticular soft tissues (arrowhead).*

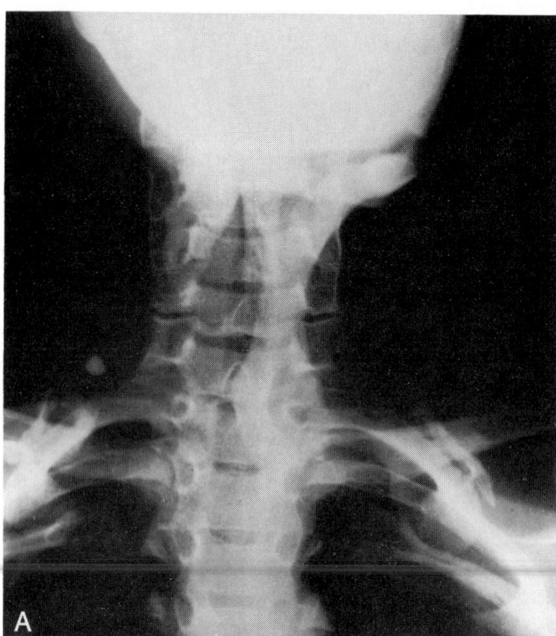

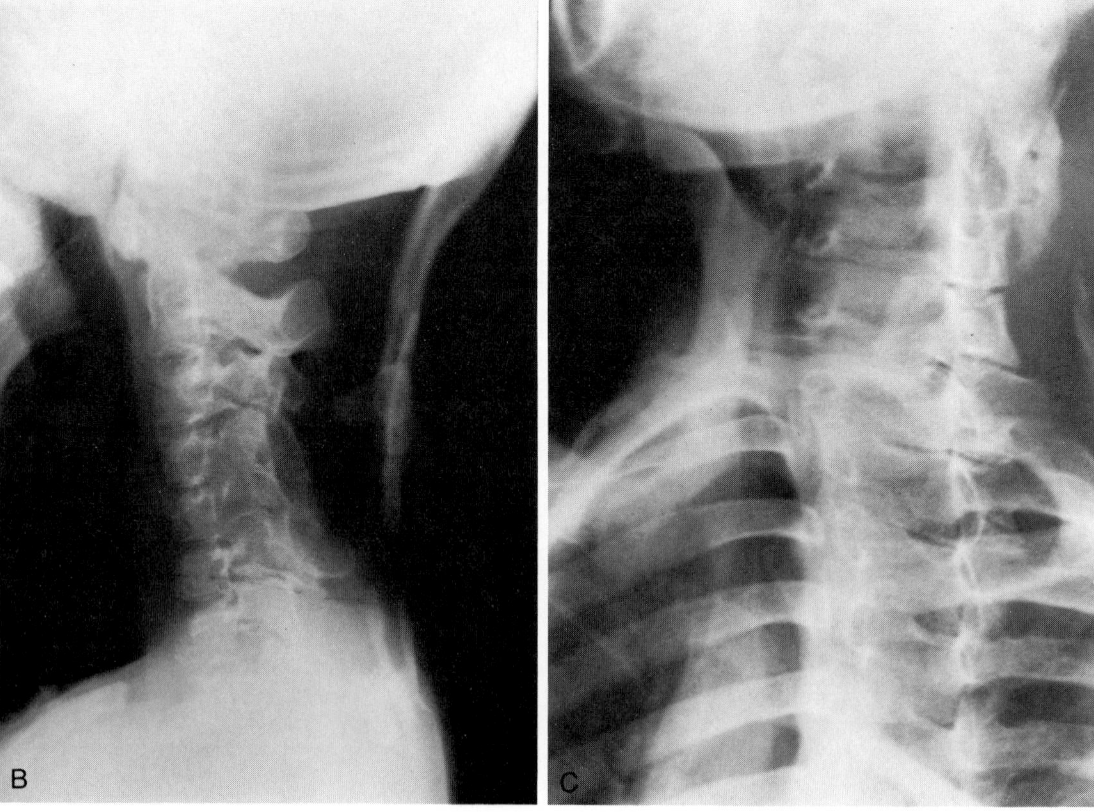

Figure 72–39. *Myositis ossificans progressiva. Anteroposterior* **(A)**, *lateral* **(B)**, *and oblique* **(C)** *views of the cervical spine reveal ossification of the soft tissues and fusion of the apophyseal joints.*

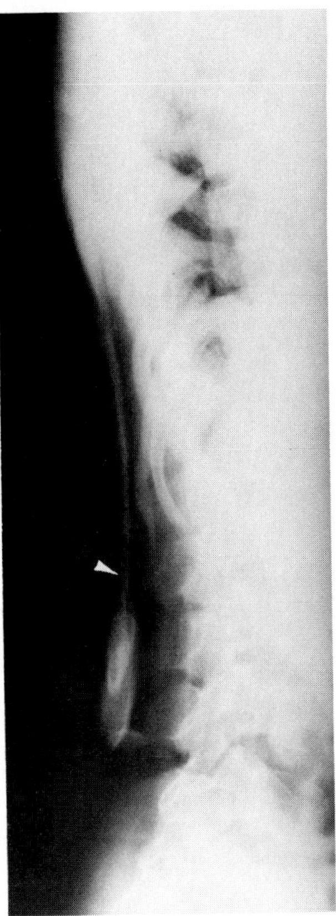

Figure 72–40. *Myositis ossificans progressiva. Lateral view of the thoracic and lumbar spine shows ridge of bone resulting from involvement of the paraspinal ligaments (arrowhead).*

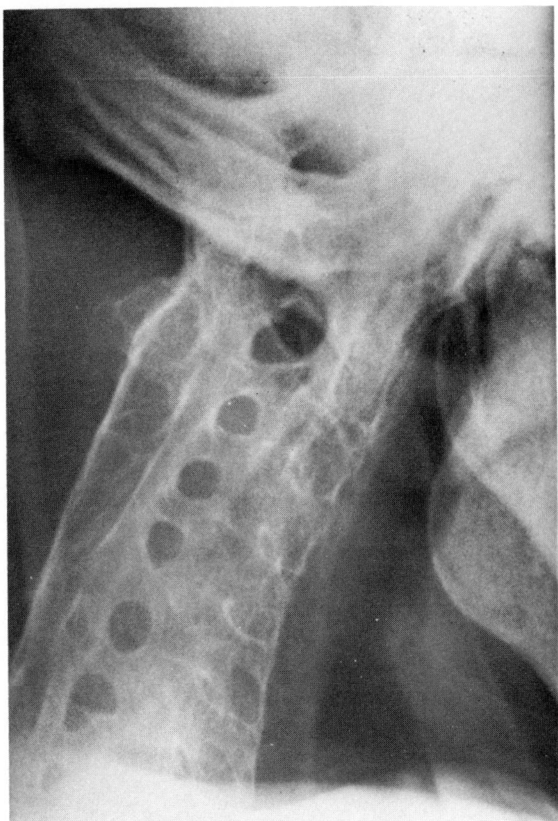

Figure 72–41. *Myositis ossificans progressiva. Lateral view of the cervical spine showing the late changes of the disease with fusion of both apophyseal joints and vertebral bodies.*

is not present in progressiva cases. Involvement of the insertions of fasciae, ligaments, and tendons produces "exostoses" (Fig. 72–37), which arise from the metaphyses of the long bones, the occiput, and the calcaneus. Sesamoids that may fuse to the digits are another cause of "exostoses." Joint ankylosis (Fig. 72–38) results from ossification of the surrounding soft tissue structures.

Abnormalities in the spine occur as a result of loss of motion. Ossification of the soft tissues is followed by fusion of the apophyseal joints (Figs. 72–39 and 72–40) and finally the vertebral bodies (Fig. 72–41).

The roentgenographic differential diagnosis includes the causes of metastatic calcifications — e.g., calcinosis universalis, dermatomyositis, tumoral calcinosis, and disorders of calcium metabolism. However, in all these conditions, the dense lesions remain calcific and do not mature into trabecular bone.

PSEUDOXANTHOMA ELASTICUM

Pseudoxanthoma elasticum is an inherited disorder characterized by a defect in elastic fibers that involves the skin, eyes, and cardiovascular system. The exact nature of the abnormality is unknown, but the elastic fibers have a tendency to calcify. Most patients have a family history consistent with an autosomal recessive mode of inheritance, but there are also documented cases with autosomal dominant inheritance.

McKusick[123] attributes the first pathologic description to Darier, who reported a case in 1896 and who coined the term pseudoxanthoma elasticum. Other names used in reference to this entity are elastorrhexis and the Grönblad-Strandberg syndrome, named for the authors who first recognized the association between the ocular and dermatologic findings.

Pathology and Pathophysiology

Skin biopsies of patients with pseudoxanthoma elasticum demonstrate granular or rod-like material occupying the deep and middle layers of the corium. The material shows staining properties similar to those of elastic fibers[116, 121, 123] and is calcified or ossified. Collections of giant cells surround areas of degeneration. The epidermis is normal. The earliest changes are thought to include calcification and fragmentation of elastic fibers, but the nature of the primary defect remains unknown.

The ocular changes are characterized by angioid streaks, which represent the fissuring and scarring of the membrane beneath the retina. They are thought to be related either to sclerosis of the choroidal arteries or to tears of the lamina elastica of Bruch's membrane.

Narrowing and occlusion of the large muscular arteries of the extremities, viscera, and central nervous system are also findings of pseudoxanthoma elasticum. The pathologic changes include fragmentation of the external elastic membrane, thinning of the intima, and fibrous proliferation in the media. The vascular stage of clotting is also abnormal.

Clinical Findings

Pseudoxanthoma elasticum occurs in all races, and there is a slight female predominance.[123, 128] It is not a homogeneous disorder and four separate clinical-genetic variants have been identified,[120, 126] with a predominance of the skin, ocular, or cardiovascular abnormalities, or a combination of all three findings.

Skin abnormalities usually become apparent in the second decade of life, although there is a wide range in the age of onset. Changes involve primarily those areas that are subjected to mechanical wear and tear, including the face, the axillary and inguinal folds, the cubital areas, and the periumbilical region. Also affected are the heart and soft palate and the mucosae of the mouth, gastrointestinal tract, and vagina. The earliest clinical finding is accentuation of the normal skin lines. Later, the skin becomes thickened, redundant, deeply grooved, and hyperextensible. The most characteristic clinical feature is the yellow papules that occur between the thickened folds. These raised, abnormally colored areas give the skin a "pebbly" texture or a "peau d'orange" appearance.[120]

The angioid streaks, which characterize the ocular findings of pseudoxanthoma elasticum, also begin in the second decade of life. They appear as gray, red, or brown streaks, which eventually involve the maculae and decrease central visual acuity. Angioid streaks also occur in Paget's disease, sickle cell anemia, and the Ehlers-Danlos syndrome. Chorioretinitis, a more severe threat to vision, is a second ocular abnormality that may occur in pseudoxanthoma elasticum.

Involvement of the muscular arteries usually occurs in the third decade of life and may result in life-threatening complications. Resultant symptoms include intermittent claudication in both the upper and lower extremities, coronary insufficiency, abdominal angina, hypertension, and bleeding from almost every organ. The gastrointestinal tract is the most frequent location of hemorrhage, but the subarachnoid space, the retinal arteries, the genitourinary tract, and the nasal passages are also subject to bleeding. Petechiae occur, but bleeding from superficial lacerations is not a problem in this disorder. Peripheral pulses are weak or absent, and cardiac changes result from both hypertension and coronary artery disease. The early age of the onset of symptoms, plus the upper extremity involvement, differentiates these patients from those with atherosclerosis. High serum cholesterol and serum triglyceride levels have been reported in patients with pseudoxanthoma elasticum.[117]

Psychiatric disturbances are another complication of this disease.

Roentgenographic Findings

Roentgenograms of the skull frequently demonstrate premature calcification of the falx, the tentorium, the choroid plexus, and the petroclinoid ligaments. Thickening of the calvarium and the base of the skull has also been reported.[127] Films of the extremities may demonstrate a variety of calcifications. Most typically, abnormal dense lesions are observed in the middle and deep layers of the dermis, the site of the pathologic abnormalities. Calcifications also occur (1) within tendons and ligaments, (2) around the metacarpophalangeal joints, the hip joints, or the elbow joints, and (3) within both large peripheral veins and arteries. Angiography of the extremities demonstrates occlusion and narrowing of large arteries as well as the formation of localized aneurysms and arteriovenous malformations. Resorption of the tufts of the distal phalanges may result from the latter vascular changes. Osseous abnormalities, including osteoporosis, bowing, metaphyseal ectasia, and abnormal lucent areas, have also been reported in association with four cases of pseudoxanthoma elasticum.[127] However, it is difficult to understand why other such cases have not been recognized in large clinical series. It is possible that these osseous changes may represent only a coincidental dysplasia.

Unlike the hereditary diseases of collagen synthesis, this primary disorder of elastic fibers does not affect the joints of the extremities.

The roentgenographic differential diagnosis includes other entities with both soft tissue and vascular calcification. Both renal disease and collagen vascular disease can produce calcifications in soft tissues as well as erosion of the distal tufts of the phalanges. However, in the latter two disorders, there are coexisting articular and osseous abnormalities, which should differentiate them from pseudoxanthoma elasticum. The Ehlers-Danlos syndrome and parasitic disorders can also produce soft tissue calcifications, but their distribution differs from that of pseudoxanthoma elasticum.

FIBROGENESIS IMPERFECTA OSSIUM

Fibrogenesis imperfecta ossium is a rare disorder of collagen synthesis. The etiology is unknown and changes are limited to the skeleton. The entity was first described by Baker and Turnbull in 1950.[130]

Pathology and Pathophysiology

The characteristic pathologic abnormality of this disorder is the presence of abnormal collagen in the lamellar bones. Unlike normal collagen, the fibrils are not birefringent when viewed with the polarizing microscope. The collagen defect, in turn, results in incomplete mineralization of the bone and in wide osteoid seams. Superficially, the changes may resemble those of osteomalacia.

Clinical Findings

This disorder presents late in adult life. The onset of symptoms is heralded by spontaneous fractures. Changes are rapidly progressive, with eventual debilitation of the patient. Serum calcium and phosphorus levels are normal. There may, however, be elevation of the serum alkaline phosphatase level. The most characteristic laboratory abnormality is the excessive fecal excretion of calcium, with levels approaching those of hyperparathyroidism. Changes in the bone marrow distribution have also been reported.[134] The diagnosis is established on the basis of the roentgen changes.

Roentgenographic Findings

The roentgenographic changes in fibrogenesis imperfecta ossium are found in the entire skeleton except the skull. There is a generalized decrease in osseous density, and changes are most marked in the axial skeleton or around the joints. There is a decrease in the number of trabeculae, but those that remain are coarse and dense. The cortices are replaced by a network of abnormal trabeculae, and there are multiple fracture deformities. The contours of the bones are normal. The vertebral end-plates are dense, mimicking a rugger jersey spine.

The roentgenographic differential diagnosis includes advanced osteitis fibrosa cystica (hyperparathyroidism), Paget's disease, and atypical axial osteomalacia. The latter disorder is rare and produces radiographic changes almost identical to those of fibrogenesis imperfecta ossium. The principal differences are the abnormal collagen, which is found in fibrogenesis imperfecta ossium but not in the atypical form of osteomalacia, and the distribution of the roentgenographic changes. In fibrogenesis imperfecta ossium, the skeletal changes are generalized. In atypical axial osteomalacia, the changes occur only in the central skeleton.

THE MULTIPLE EPIPHYSEAL DYSPLASIAS

Spranger[164] has defined the term multiple epiphyseal dysplasia as "a group of heterogeneous disorders characterized by defective or excessive bone formation in the secondary ossification centers of the tubular bones and sometimes vertebrae." Unlike the mucopolysaccharidoses and hypothyroidism, which are both characterized by irregular ossification of articular surfaces, the epiphyseal dysplasias have no known etiology. Therefore, these disorders are grouped together and are subclassified on the basis of morphologic changes. Rubin[161] has divided the epiphyseal dysplasias into two large categories: the spondyloepiphyseal dysplasias (with universal platyspondyly or beaking) and multiple epiphyseal dysplasias (with minimal or no spinal changes). The category of multiple epiphyseal dysplasias is far from homogeneous and contains isolated epiphyseal dysplasias, epiphyseal dysplasias associated with ocular, auditory, or endocrine abnormalities, and those which combine the findings of epiphyseal and metaphyseal dysostoses. The problem of understanding epiphyseal dysplasias is further exacerbated by the multiple classifications and definitions used in various publications. For this textbook, the entity referred to as dysplasia epiphysealis multiplex (multiple epiphyseal dysplasia tarda) is considered as the prototype of the epiphyseal dysplasias. At the end of this section, chondrodystrophia calcificans (multiple epiphyseal dysplasia congenita) and Meyer's dysplasia are discussed in brief.

In 1937, Ribbing[160] published a description of a multiple epiphyseal dysplasia with mild osseous abnormalities and with an autosomal dominant mode of inheritance. Ten years later, Fairbank[139] reported similar, but more severe, osseous changes in 20 additional cases and coined the term dysplasia epiphysealis multiplex. Since these original reports, this disease has been shown to be a classic example of genetic heterogeneity. Most affected families have an inheritance pattern consistent with an autosomal dominant gene with high penetrance. However, cases of spontaneous mutation and cases with autosomal recessive inheritance have also been reported.

Other terms used in reference to this entity are Fairbank-Ribbing disease, multiple epiphyseal dysplasia tarda and dysplasia polyepiphysaire.

Pathology and Pathophysiology

The primary defect in dysplasia epiphysealis multiplex appears to involve the epiphyseal chondrocyte.[138, 144, 146, 153] On gross specimens, the growth plate is found to be widened and has an irregular metaphyseal margin. Tongues of cartilage extend into the osseous metaphysis and there is irregularity of the peripheral trabeculae. Histologic specimens of the growth plate demonstrate a decrease in the number of chondrocytes in all zones, invasion of vessels into the cartilage, and loss of the normal columnar arrangement of the chondrocytes. There is excessive matrix as well as areas of degeneration and cleft formation. Bars of calcified fibrous tissue extend from the epiphysis to the metaphysis. The collagen within the growth plate is normal but there is a decrease in mucopolysaccharide content, specifically in galactosamine.[146] The result of these abnormalities is delayed and disorderly ossification of the epiphyseal ends of the bones. The midportion of the secondary ossification centers contains woven bone and the peripheries are irregular in contour. Joint incongruity inevitably leads to secondary degenerative joint disease (Fig. 72–42).

Clinical Findings

Dysplasia epiphysealis multiplex affects both sexes equally and intelligence is normal. There is

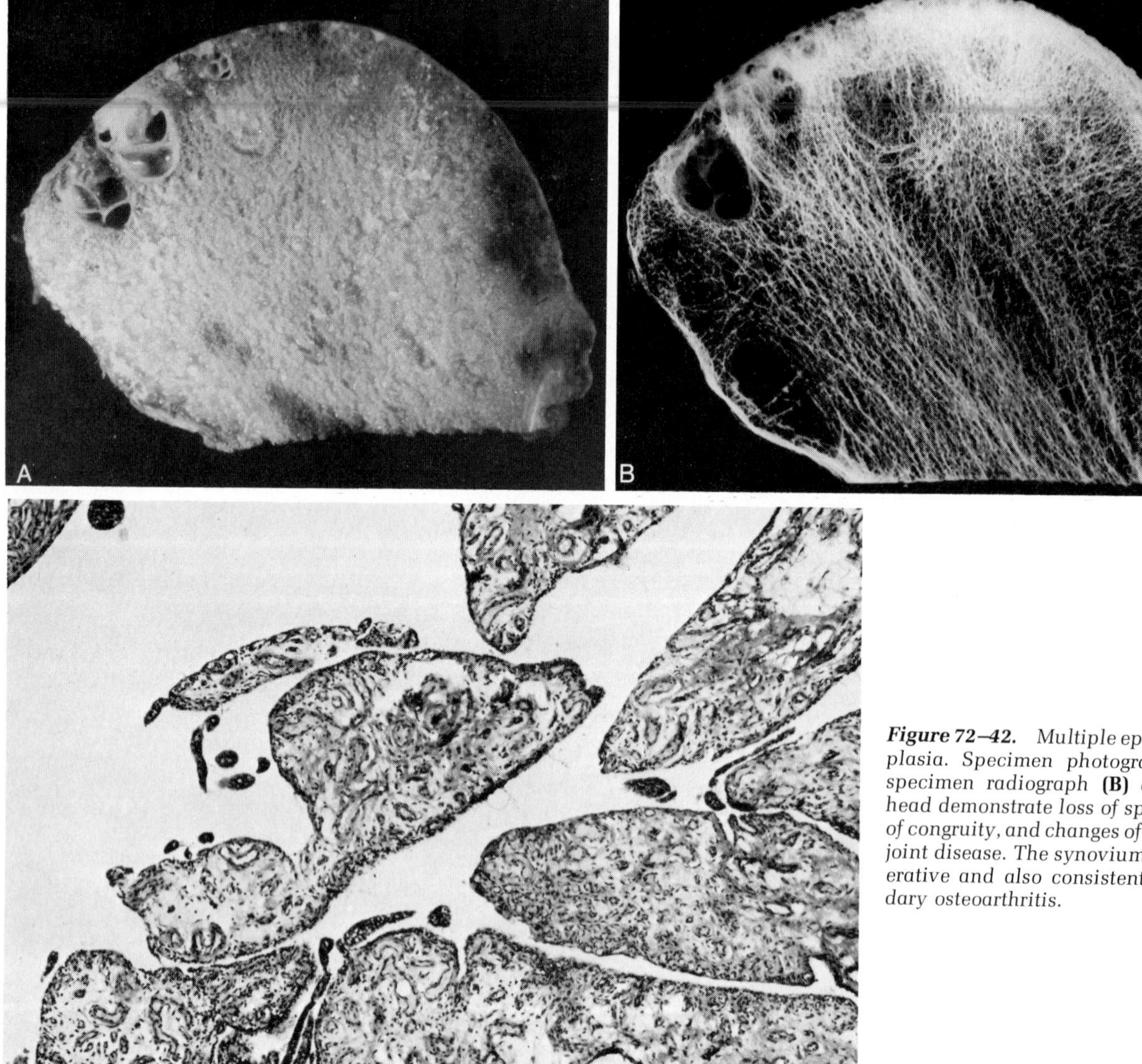

Figure 72–42. Multiple epiphyseal dysplasia. Specimen photograph **(A)** and specimen radiograph **(B)** of a femoral head demonstrate loss of sphericity, loss of congruity, and changes of degenerative joint disease. The synovium **(C)** is proliferative and also consistent with secondary osteoarthritis.

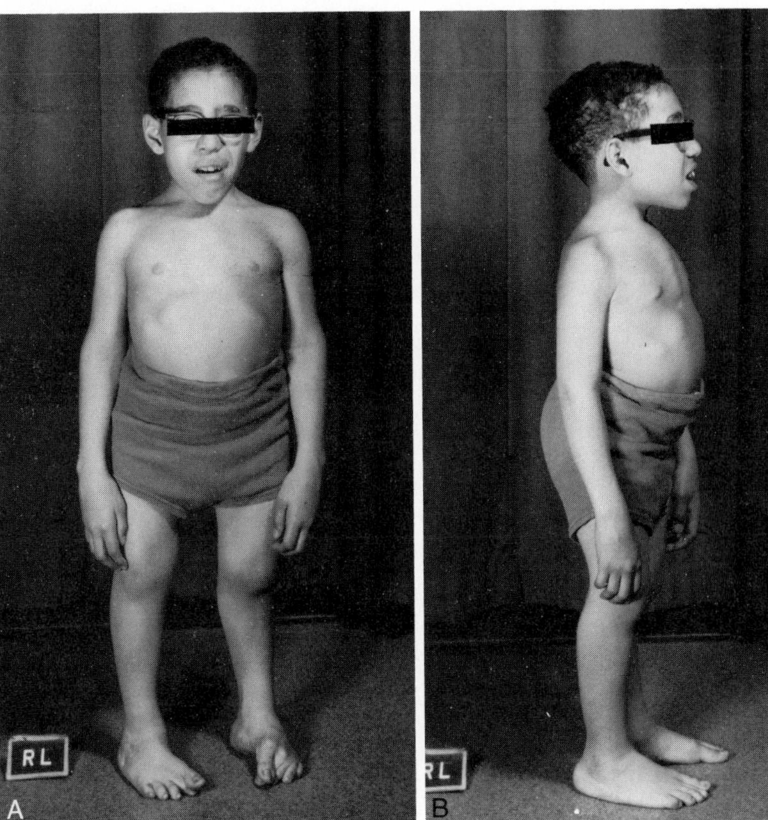

Figure 72–43. *Multiple epiphyseal dysplasia. Frontal* **(A)** *and lateral* **(B)** *views of patient with this disease revealing short stature, protuberant joints, and scoliosis.*

considerable variation in the severity of the disease even among members of the same family. The most frequent sites of involvement are the hips, knees, shoulders, ankles, and wrists. The onset of symptoms is usually early in childhood, and common presenting complaints include gait disturbances and difficulty in running and climbing stairs. In milder cases, symptoms may not occur until adulthood, when secondary degenerative joint disease supervenes.

Physical examination reveals short stature, but only in severe cases is dwarfing present (Fig. 72–43). The growth disturbance may lead to symmetric shortening of the skeleton, if the spine is involved, or to micromelia if only the limbs are affected (Fig. 72–43). The hands and feet have a characteristic stubby appearance. A waddling gait is common and associated deformities include genu valgum, genu varum, or tibiotalar slants. In older patients, precocious degenerative joint disease leads to stiffness and decreased range of motion. Hematologic and urinary studies are normal. The diagnosis is established on the basis of the roentgenographic findings.

Roentgenographic Findings

Roentgenographic abnormalities appear in the second or third year of life and are most marked in the hips, knees, wrists, and ankles. The number of joints affected and the degree of severity vary even among members of the same family. Osseous involvement is always bilaterally symmetric.

In young children, the epiphyseal centers of the long bones are late in appearing, and when they begin to ossify they are irregularly fragmented (Figs. 72–44 to 72–46). The epiphyses frequently ossify from multiple centers and have a mulberry-like appearance (Fig. 72–44). The secondary centers are small in size (Figs. 72–44 to 72–46) or flattened (Fig. 72–47). Rarely, the ends of the bones may be enlarged and mushroom-shaped (Fig. 72–48). In older children, slipped epiphyses complicate the coxa vara deformities (Fig. 72–49). Fusion of epiphyseal centers is also delayed.

In the adolescent and adult, the articular surfaces of the long bones are irregular and abnormal in shape (Figs. 72–45 to 72–50). The femoral heads and femoral condyles are flattened (Figs. 72–50 and 72–51). The talar articular surface is also flat. Differential growth rates within the same epiphyseal plate result in wedge-shaped epiphyses and eventually in angular deformities of the articular surfaces. Common abnormalities include coxa vara (Figs. 72–44 and 72–49), genu valgum (Fig. 72–52), genu varum (Fig. 72–53), tibio-talar slant (Fig. 72–54), and V-shaped deformities of the wrists (Fig. 72–55). In the third and fourth decades of life, changes of secondary degenerative joint disease complicate the

Text continued on page 2530

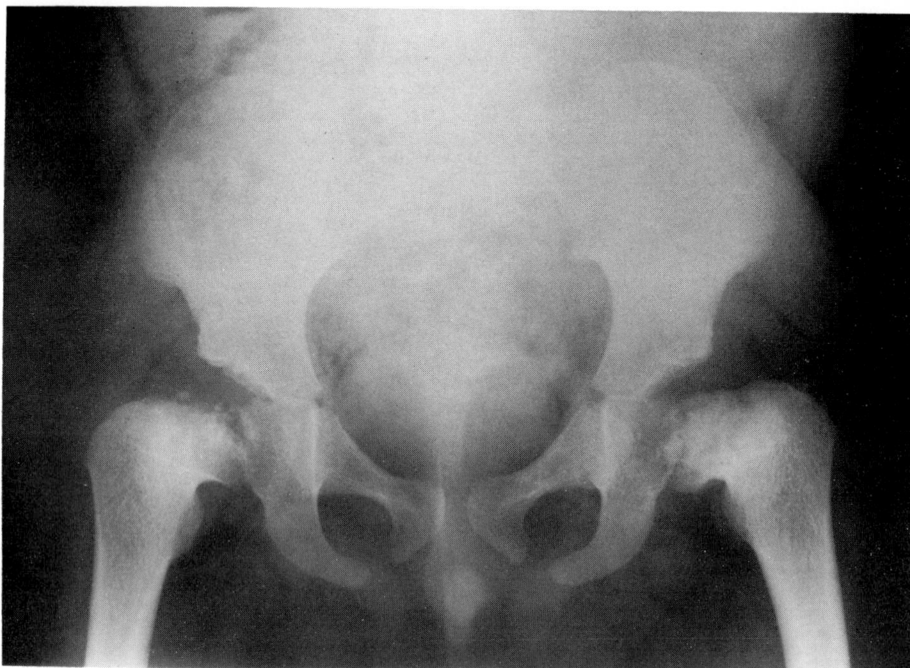

Figure 72–44. *Multiple epiphyseal dysplasia. Anteroposterior view of the pelvis showing irregular femoral epiphyses and multiple epiphyseal ossification centers. There are bilateral coxa vara deformities. Mild irregularity of the metaphyses is also noted, and the acetabula show minimal irregularities.*

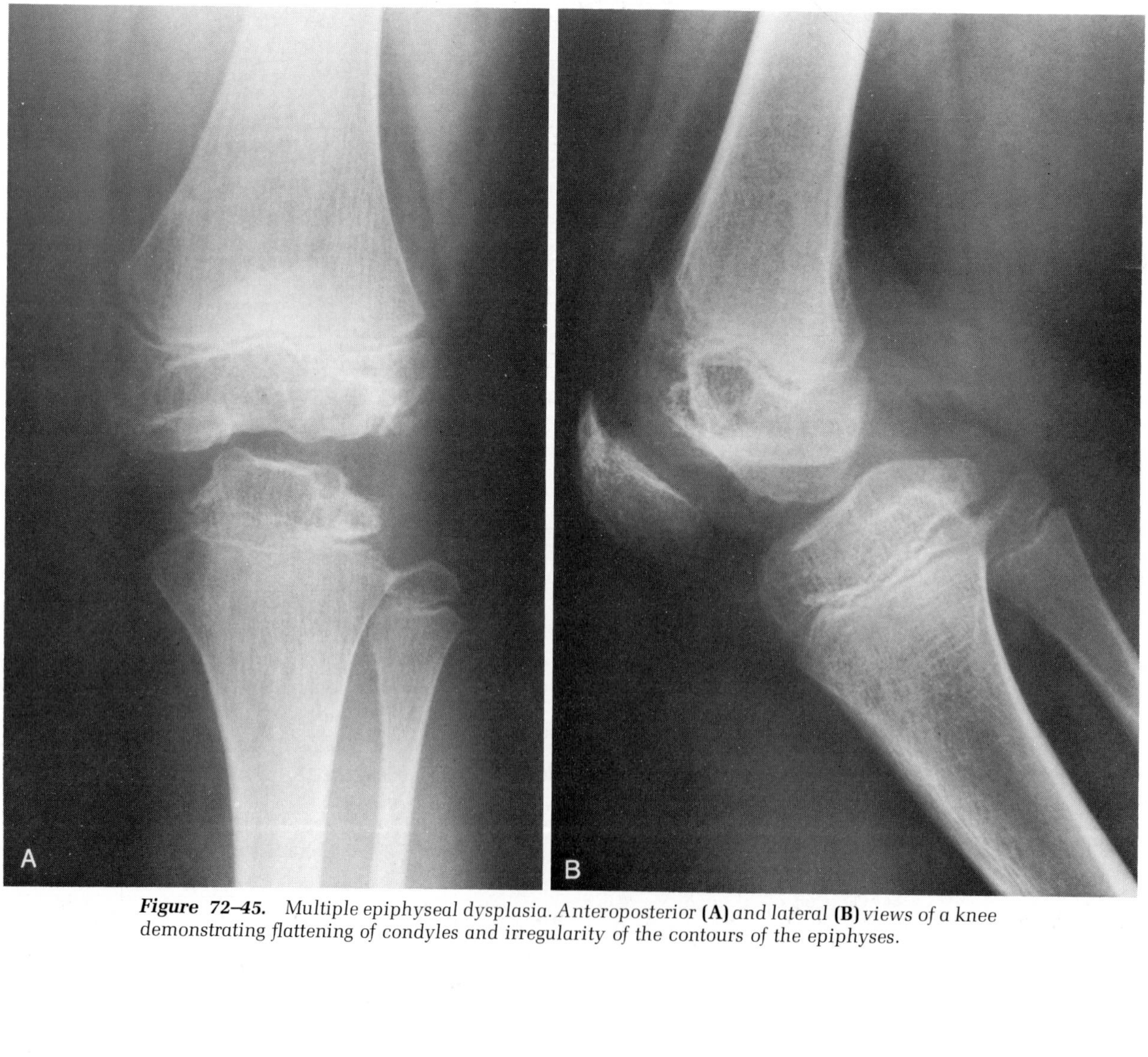

Figure 72–45. *Multiple epiphyseal dysplasia. Anteroposterior* **(A)** *and lateral* **(B)** *views of a knee demonstrating flattening of condyles and irregularity of the contours of the epiphyses.*

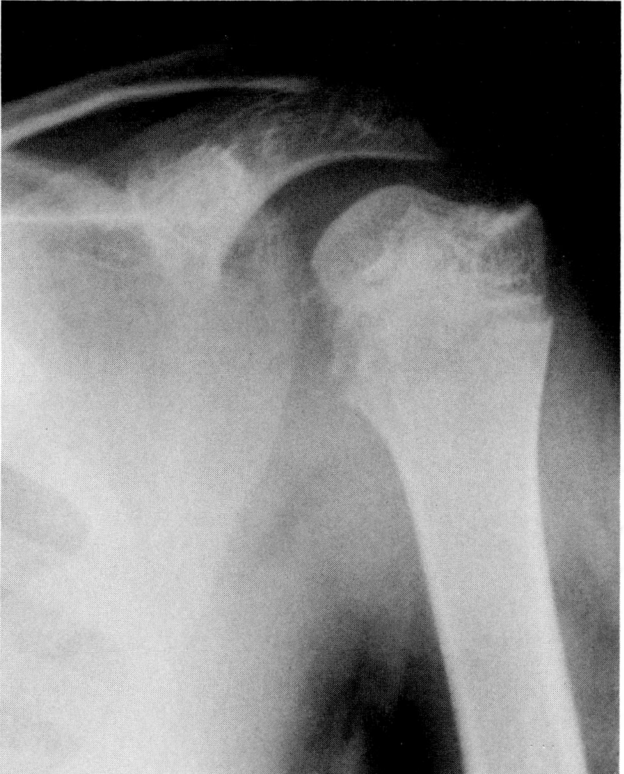

Figure 72–46. *Multiple epiphyseal dysplasia. Anteroposterior view of a shoulder revealing an irregular contour and abnormal shape to the humeral head.*

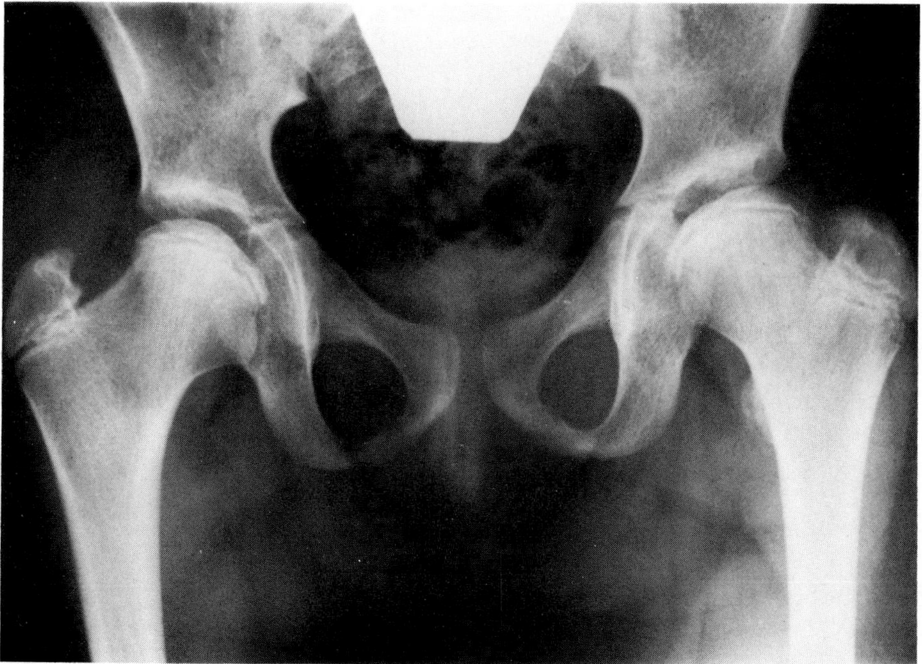

Figure 72–47. *Multiple epiphyseal dysplasia. Anteroposterior view of both hips shows flattening of the femoral heads and irregularity of the acetabular margins.*

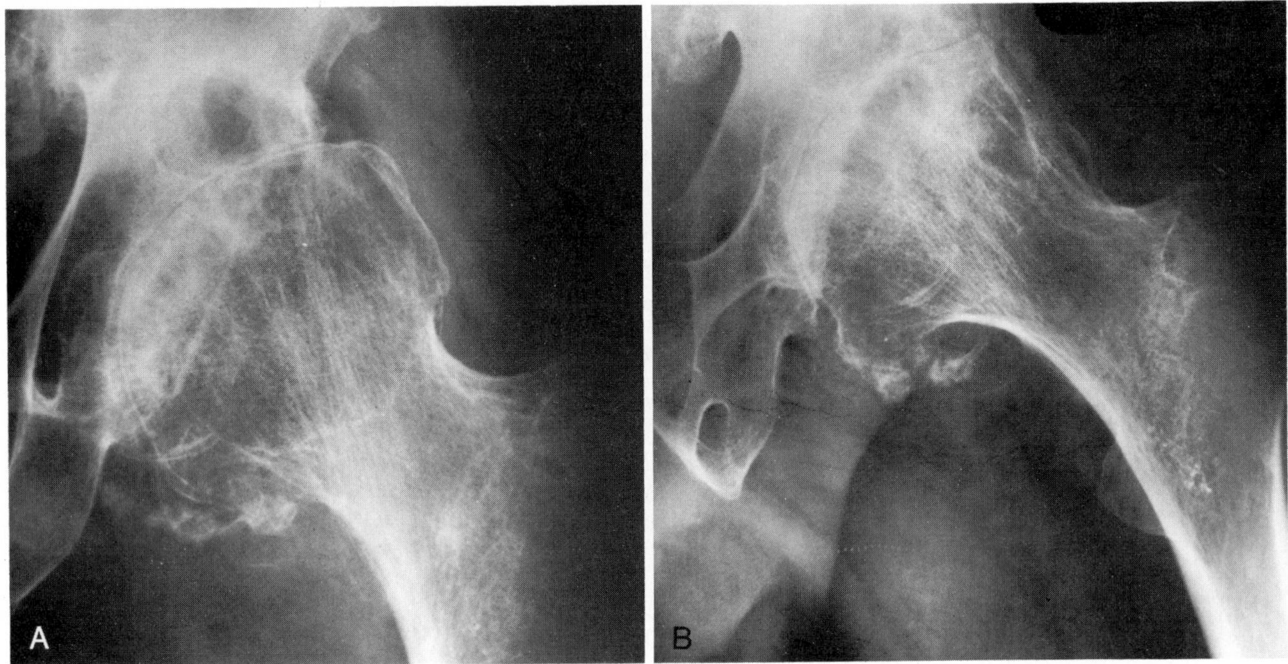

Figure 72–48. *Multiple epiphyseal dysplasia. Anteroposterior* **(A)** *and "frog-leg" lateral* **(B)** *views of the hip showing enlargement of the epiphyses. Premature degenerative joint disease is present.*

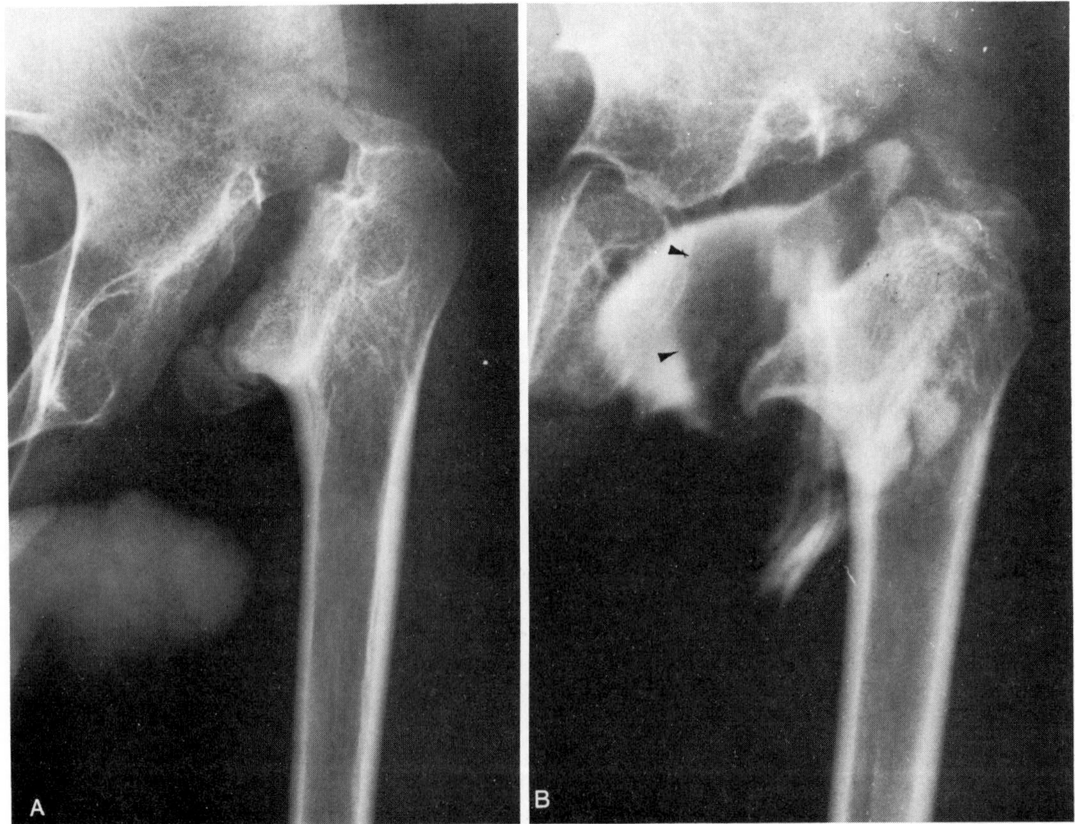

Figure 72–49. *Multiple epiphyseal dysplasia.* **A,** *Anteroposterior view of hip shows small irregular femoral head and marked coxa vara deformity.* **B,** *The arthrogram reveals displacement of the cartilaginous femoral head (arrowheads) associated with a slipped epiphysis.*

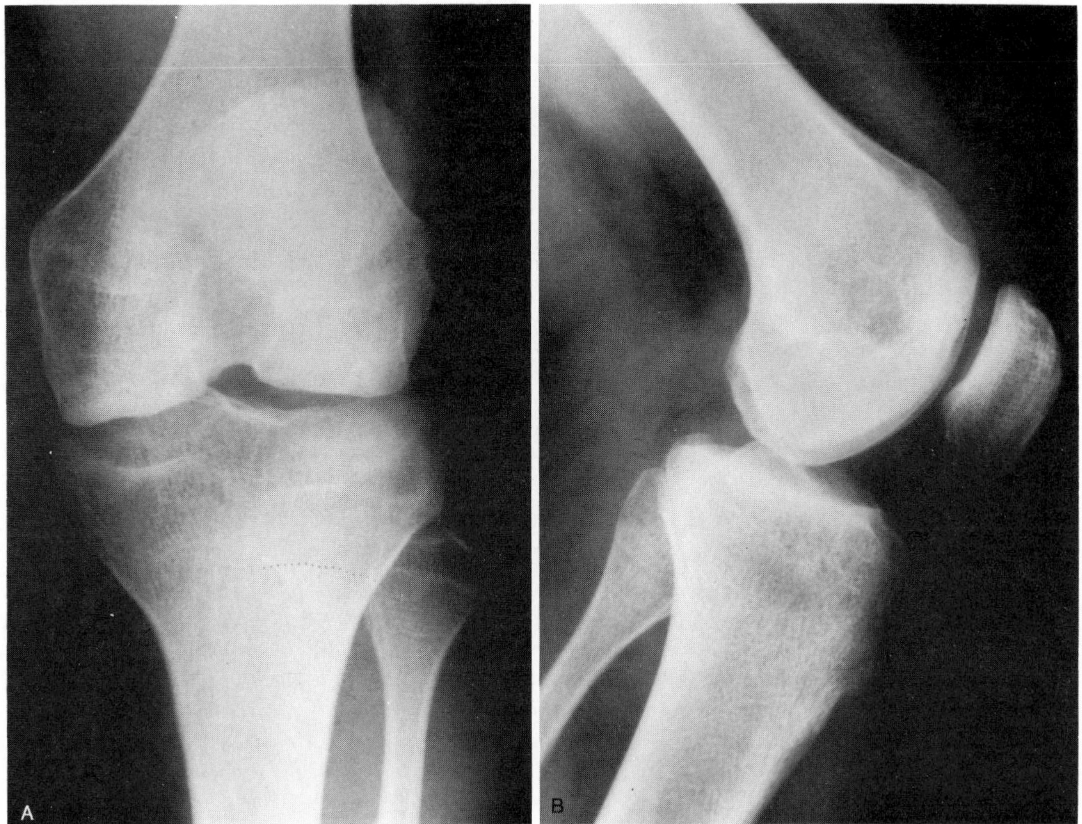

Figure 72–50. *Multiple epiphyseal dysplasia. Anteroposterior* **(A)** *and lateral* **(B)** *views of the knee reveal flattening of the femoral condyles and irregularities of the articular surfaces.*

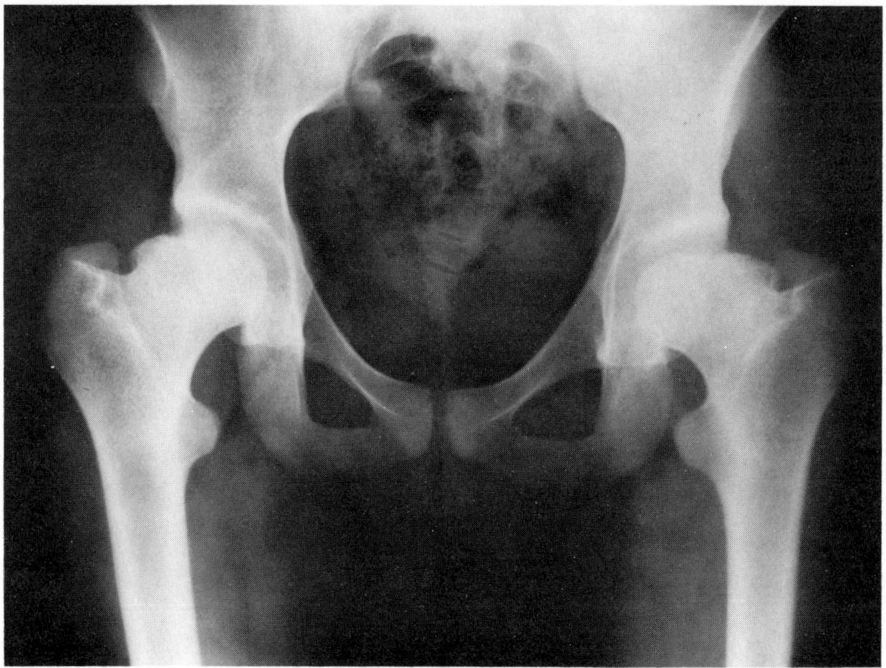

Figure 72–51. *Multiple epiphyseal dysplasia. Anteroposterior view of the pelvis demonstrates flattening and irregularity of the articular surfaces of the femoral heads.*

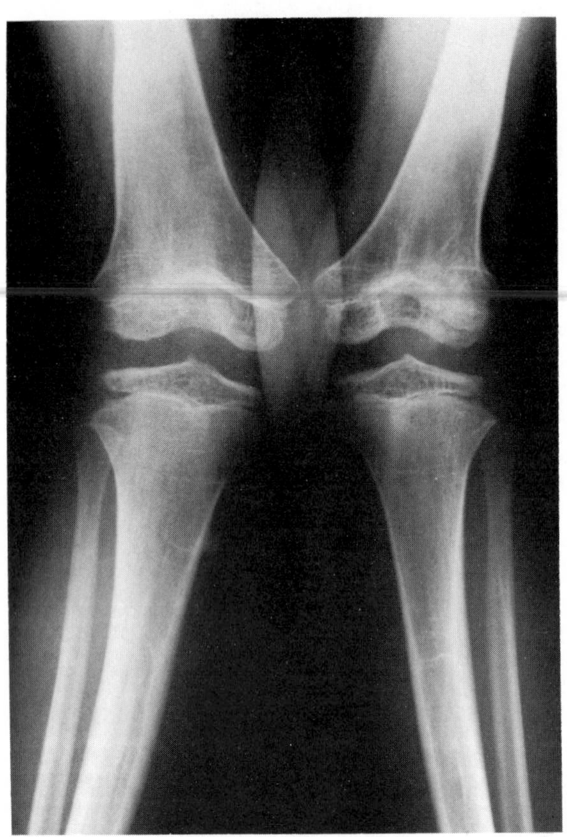

Figure 72–52. *Multiple epiphyseal dysplasia. Anteroposterior standing view of knees with irregularity of epiphyses and genu valgum deformities.*

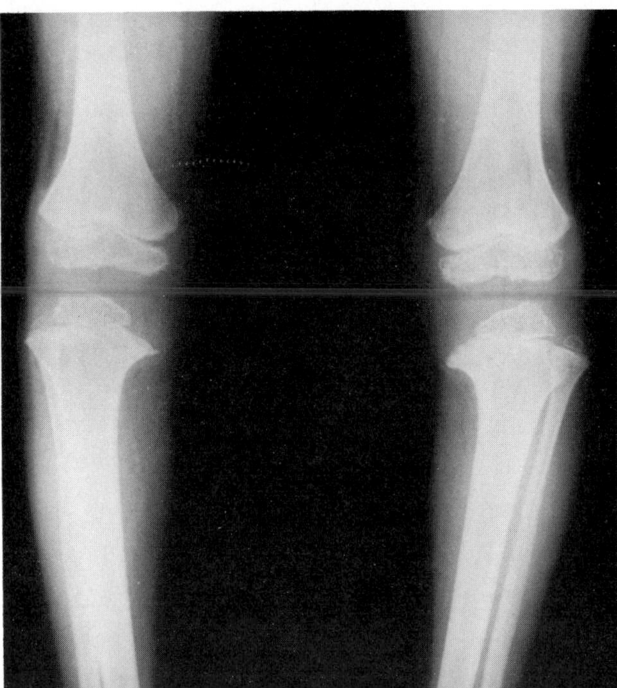

Figure 72–53. *Multiple epiphyseal dysplasia. Anteroposterior standing view of knees with genu varum deformity and early beaking of proximal tibial metaphyses. Epiphyses show characteristic irregularities of ossification.*

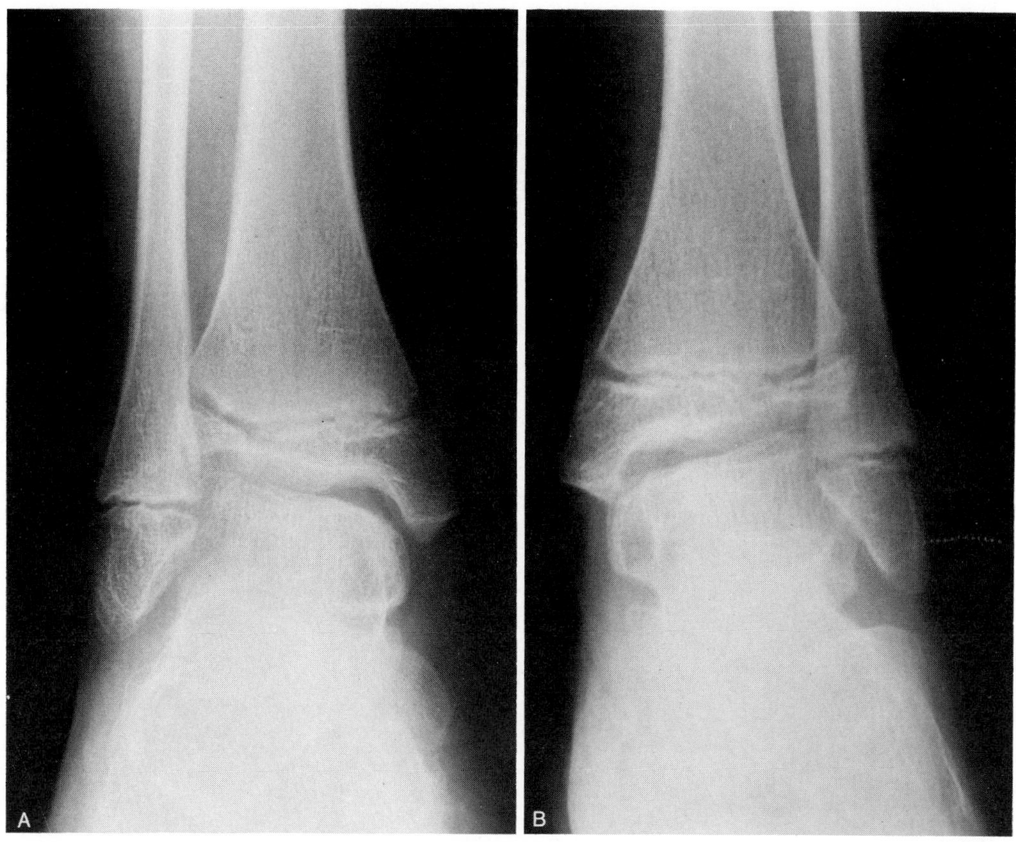

Figure 72–54. *Multiple epiphyseal dysplasia. Anteroposterior views of both ankles demonstrate tibiotalar slants with wedge-shaped distal tibial epiphyses.*

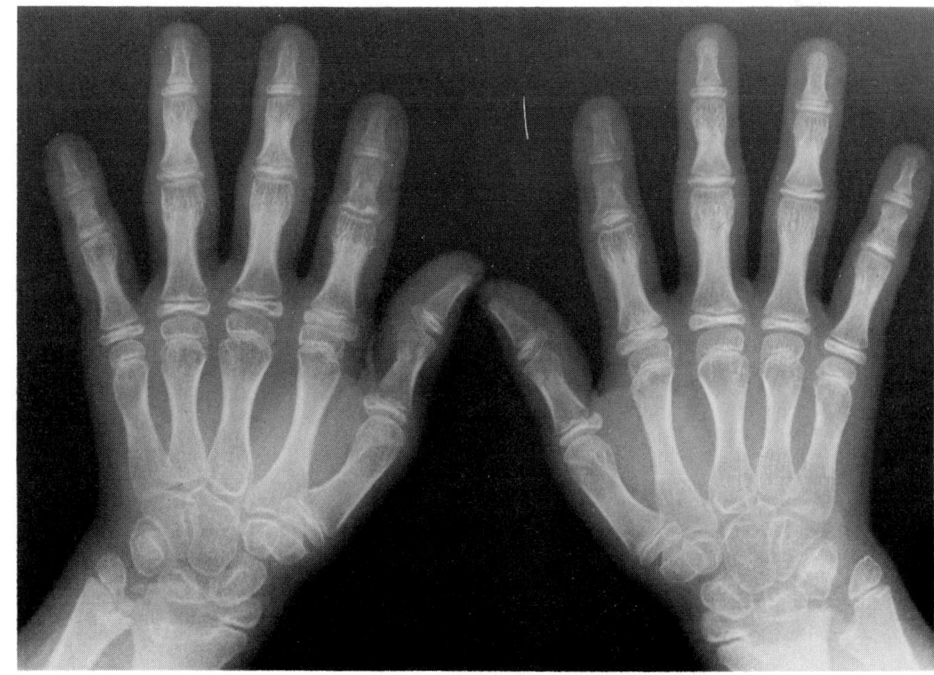

Figure 72–55. *Multiple epiphyseal dysplasia. Frontal view of both hands showing the characteristic stubby phalanges and a V-shaped deformity of the wrists. The epiphyses of the radii and ulnae have an abnormal wedge shape.*

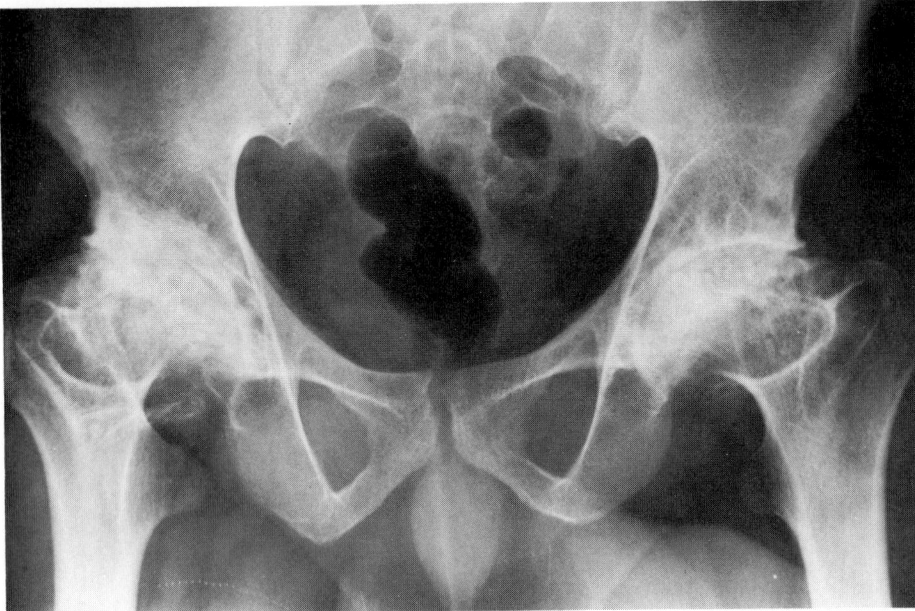

Figure 72–56. Multiple epiphyseal dysplasia. Anteroposterior view of hips showing secondary degenerative changes complicating the epiphyseal dysplasia.

osseous abnormalities (Fig. 72–56). Cartilage changes result from a combination of joint incongruity owing to the abnormal shape of the articular surfaces and abnormal weight-bearing forces owing to the malalignment of the joint surfaces. In some cases, there may be mild flaring and irregularity of the metaphyses (Fig. 72–44). However, if there are gross metaphyseal changes, the diagnosis should be changed to metaepiphyseal or epimetaphyseal dysplasia.

The hands and feet of patients with dysplasia epiphysealis multiplex demonstrate small, broad phalanges, sometimes with irregularity of both epiphyseal and nonepiphyseal ends of the bones (Figs. 72–55 and 72–57).

The spine is affected in two thirds of patients,[145, 146] and the roentgenographic changes are similar to those of Scheuermann's disease (Fig. 72–58). The incidence of spinal involvement does not correlate with the severity of the peripheral changes. The vertebral abnormalities associated with this entity include irregularity of the anterior aspects of the vertebral end-plates, anterior wedging of the vertebral bodies, mild platyspondyly, and scoliosis. In rare cases, the odontoid process is missing.[151]

The roentgenographic differential diagnosis in-

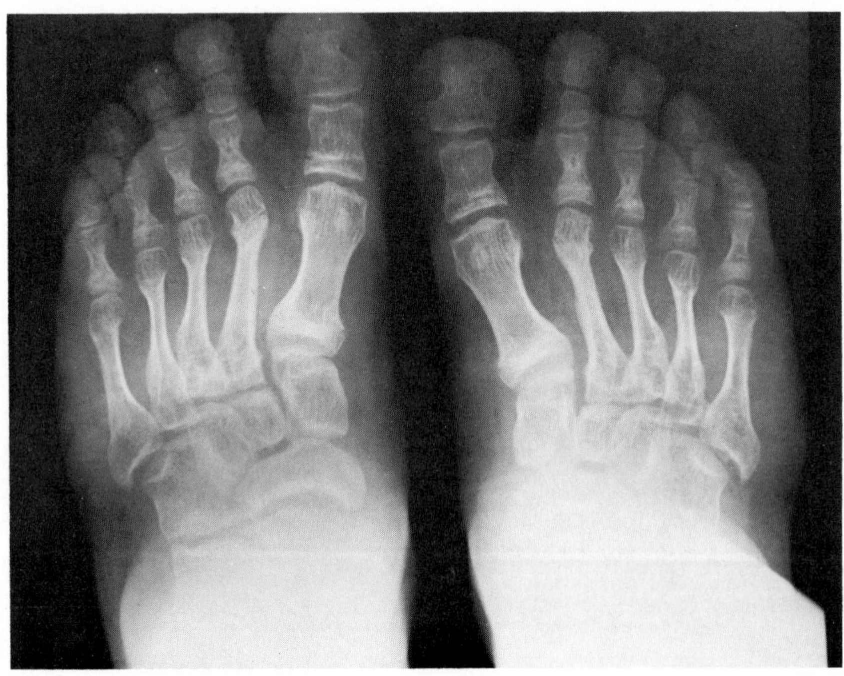

Figure 72–57. Multiple epiphyseal dysplasia. Anteroposterior view of feet with epiphyseal irregularity, forefoot adductus deformities, and stubby phalanges.

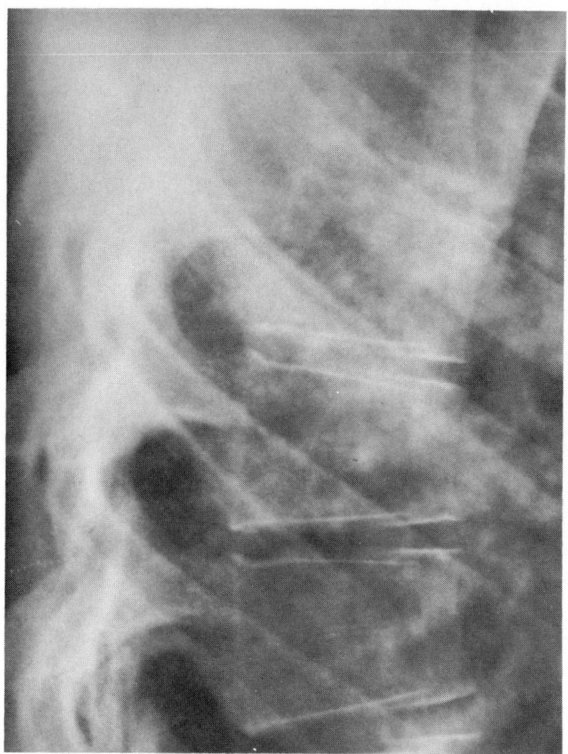

Figure 72–58. *Multiple epiphyseal dysplasia. Lateral view of spine shows the mild changes that are associated with epiphyseal dysplasias. The vertebral bodies and intervertebral discs are wedge-shaped and there are minor irregularities of the vertebral end-plates.*

cludes other causes of irregular articular surfaces, such as inflammatory arthritides, osteonecrosis, cretinism, the mucopolysaccharidoses, the Stickler syndrome, and other dysplasias. Still's disease may produce abnormalities of the epiphyses; however, the osseous changes are not always symmetric and are accompanied by effusions and juxta-articular osteoporosis. In 10 per cent of cases, Legg-Calvé-Perthes' disease is bilateral. However, the roentgenographic changes are not symmetric and are limited to the hips. In addition, early changes of osteonecrosis are isolated to the superolateral aspect of the epiphysis, whereas epiphyseal dysplasias involve the entire articular surface. Cretinism is also associated with epiphyseal irregularities, but there is retardation of bone age, generalized osteoporosis, wormian bones, and broad femoral necks. The Stickler syndrome has many features of an epiphyseal dysplasia, but they are combined with marfanoid osseous abnormalities and dislocation of the lens. The roentgenographic findings of spondyloepiphyseal dysplasias and the mucopolysaccharidoses are characterized by more severe spinal changes than those noted in epiphysealis dysplasia multiplex. Beaking of the vertebral bodies and universal platyspondyly differentiate the former entities from the latter, but roentgenographic differentiation is not always clear-cut. There are dysplasias that combine epiphyseal and metaphyseal abnormalities. In general, these problem syndromes are grouped together under the name metaepiphyseal dysplasia or epimetaphyseal dysplasia.[154]

Chondrodysplasia Punctata

Chondrodysplasia punctata is a form of multiple epiphyseal dysplasia that is characterized by the calcification of the cartilaginous epiphyseal centers during the first year of life (Fig. 72–59). Also referred to as multiple epiphyseal dysplasia congenita, this entity presents at birth and has a broad spectrum of clinical signs and symptoms. Spranger[164] has subclassified this disorder into two syndromes. First is the Conradi-Hünermann syndrome, which is associated with an autosomal dominant mode of transmission and has a normal life expectancy. Second is the rhizomelic form, which follows an autosomal recessive pattern of inheritance and is lethal in early childhood. Both forms may result from spontaneous mutations. The Conradi-Hünermann syndrome is also associated with maternal use of warfarin sodium. Cases which combine features of both syndromes have been reported.[154]

Described pathologic findings in the epiphyseal centers include mucoid degeneration, cyst formation, and calcification. Calcifications, although present at birth, are resorbed during the first year of life, but during growth the epiphyses ossify in an irregular fashion. The abnormalities preceding cartilage degeneration are unknown. However, studies performed on Beagle puppies, who have a form of chondrodysplasia punctata, suggest a three-stage process. In the animals, the first pathologic findings are areas of abnormal matrix with large amounts of free chondroitin sulfate. During the second stage, there is coalescence of the abnormal matrix with liquefaction and cyst formation. In the third stage, calcification occurs both in the contents of the cyst and in the surrounding abnormal cartilage.

The clinical findings include shortening of the extremities, scoliosis, a flattened face due to malar hypoplasia, wide-set eyes, and a saddle nose deformity. In the Conradi-Hünermann syndrome, the involvement of the limbs is asymmetric, spine changes are prominent (Fig. 72–60) and there is a low incidence of cataracts, joint contractures, and skin changes (Fig. 72–59). The intelligence of these patients is normal. In the rhizomelic form of the disease, limb changes are symmetric and the spine is not involved. There is a high incidence of cataracts forming in the first months of life, and optic atrophy is common. Other findings include mental retardation, fibrous joint contractures, alopecia, and ichthyosiform rashes.

The roentgenographic changes differ in the two syndromes. In the milder form, roentgenograms

Text continued on page 2535

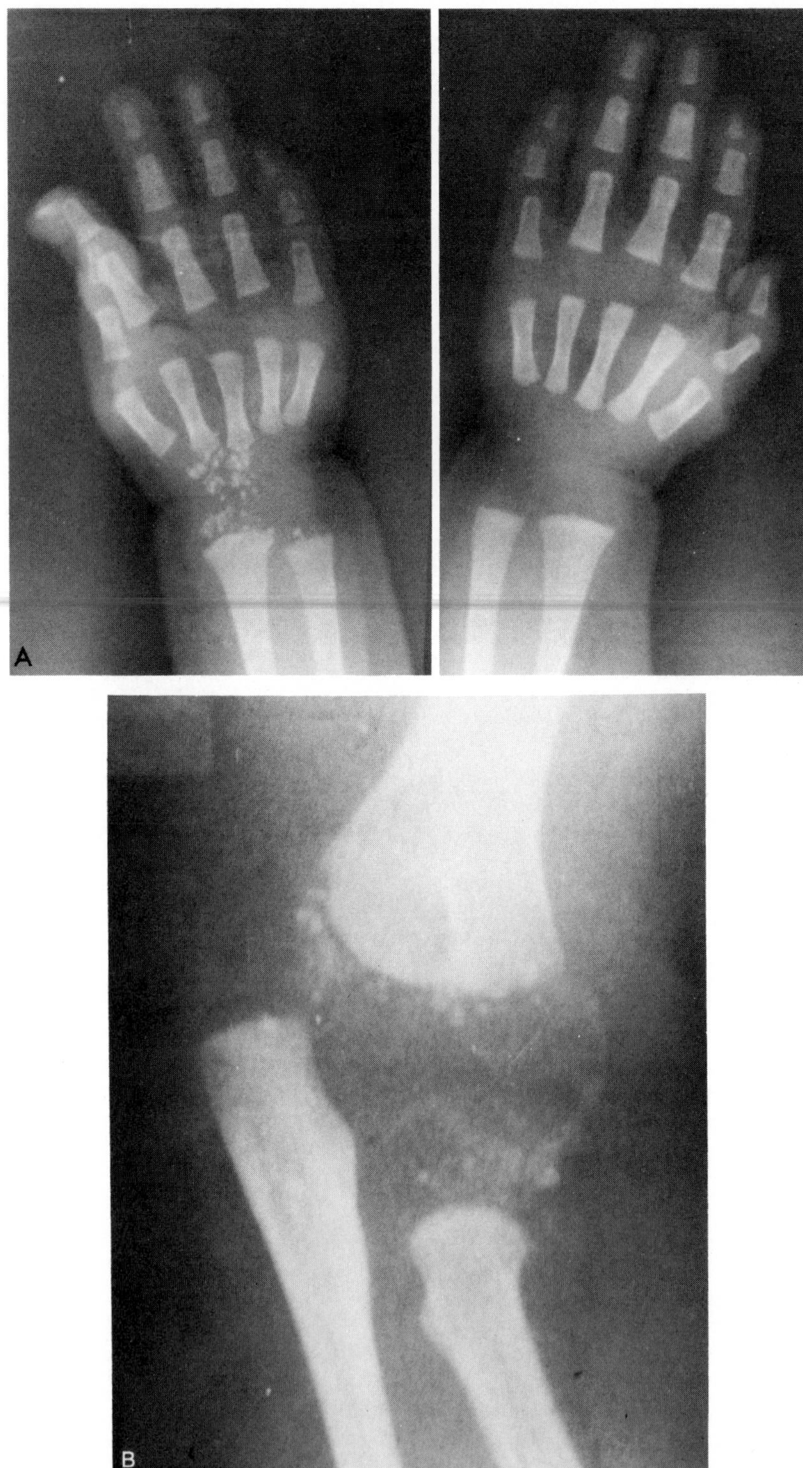

Figure 72–59. *Chondrodysplasia punctata.* **A,** *Posteroanterior views of hands obtained at birth demonstrate asymmetric stippling of cartilage epiphyses.* **B,** *Anteroposterior view of elbow shows similar changes.*

Illustration continued on the opposite page

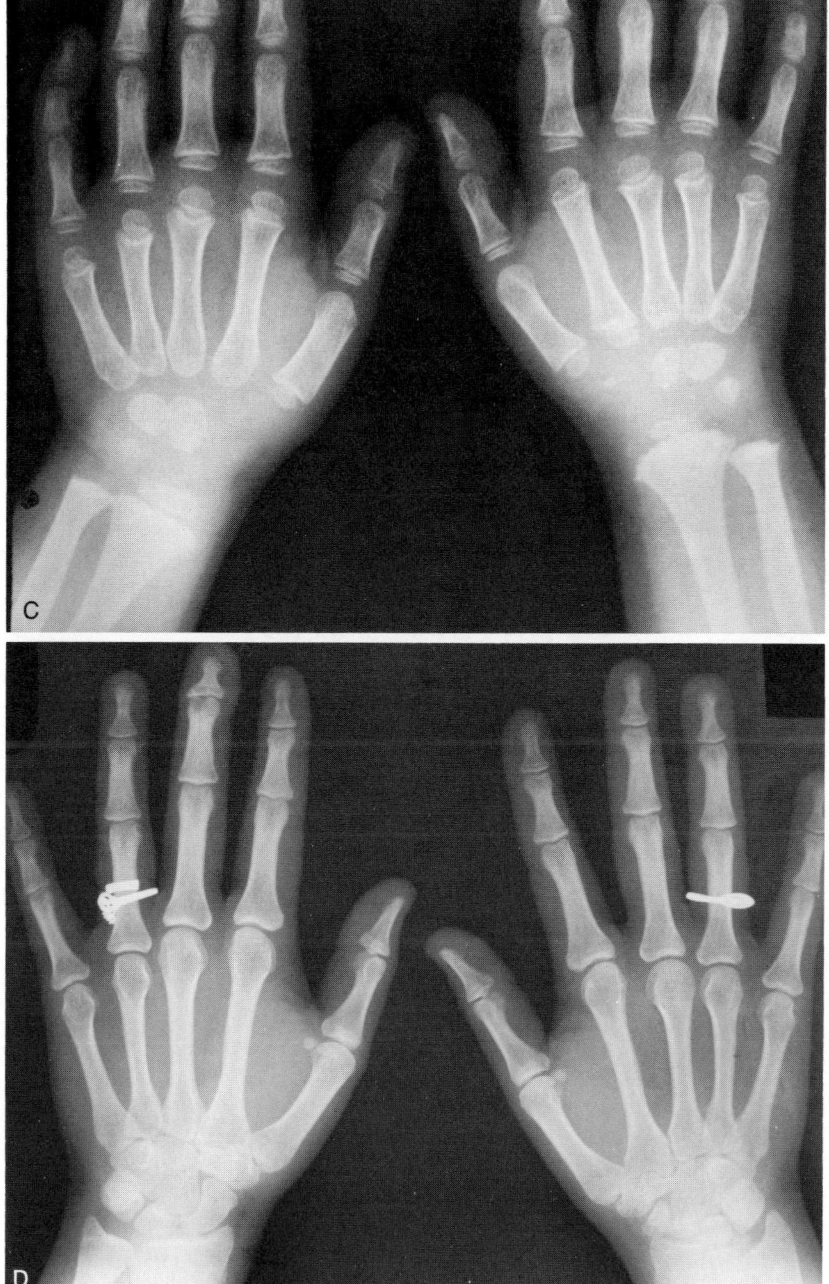

Figure 72–59. Continued

C, *Posteroanterior views of hands obtained at 3 years of age show minimal calcifications remaining.* **D**, *Posteroanterior views of hands at 13 years of age demonstrate almost normal ossification. Only the carpal scaphoid remains abnormal.*

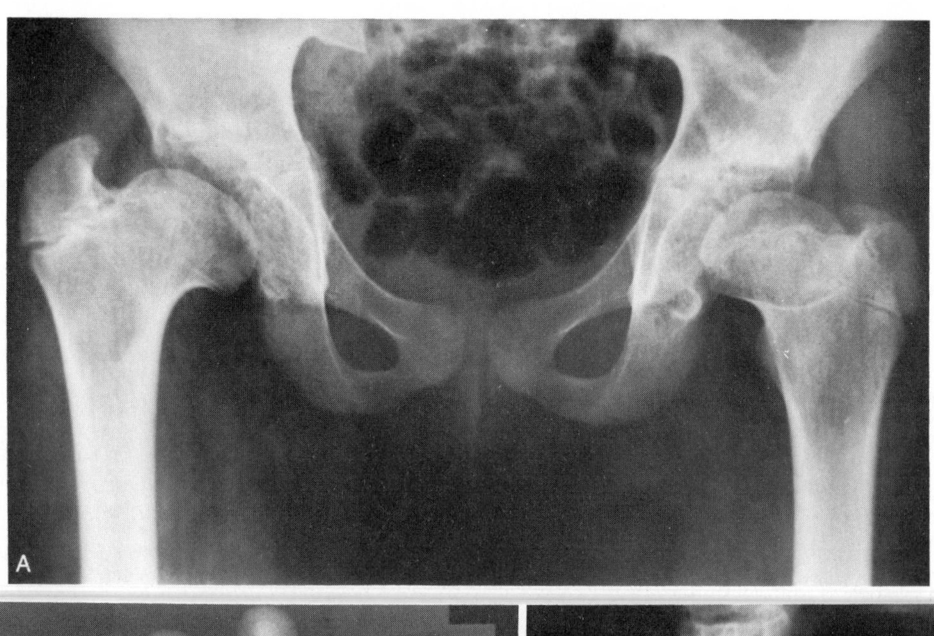

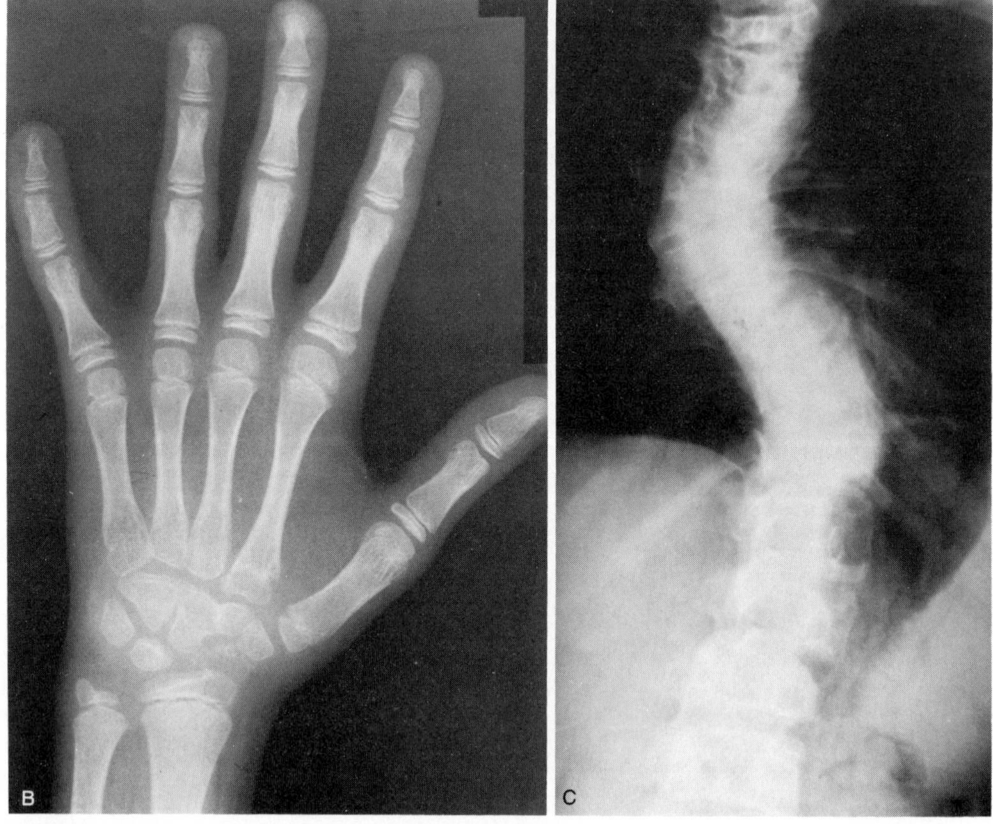

Figure 72–60. *Chondrodysplasia punctata.* **A**, *Anteroposterior view of hips shows epiphyseal dysplasia resulting from the Conradi-Hünermann syndrome.* **B**, *Patient's wrist has suffered delayed ossification and residual stippling of the scaphoid.* **C**, *Anteroposterior view of spine revealing severe scoliotic deformity.*

obtained in the first year of life demonstrate punctate or stippled calcifications at the ends of the long bones (Fig. 72–59), at the ends of the short tubular bones, in the vertebral end-plates, in the cartilage rings of the trachea, and in the cartilage structures of the pharynx. Later in life, roentgenograms demonstrate a diffuse asymmetric epiphyseal dysplasia (Fig. 72–60). The metaphyses and shafts of the long bones are normal. A kyphoscoliosis frequently results from the irregular shape of the vertebral bodies. In the severe recessive form of chondrodysplasia punctata, the stippled calcifications occur primarily in the hips and shoulders. Shortening of the extremities is symmetric and more severe proximally than distally. The metaphyses are flared, and the shafts of the long bones are bowed. The vertebral bodies show a characteristic coronal cleft, which results from failure of the normal ossification centers to fuse. Spinal deformities are not so severe as they are in the dominant Conradi-Hünermann syndrome. If the patient survives infancy, roentgenograms show irregularity of the cartilaginous growth plate and abnormal contours of the secondary ossification centers.

The roentgenographic differential diagnosis of

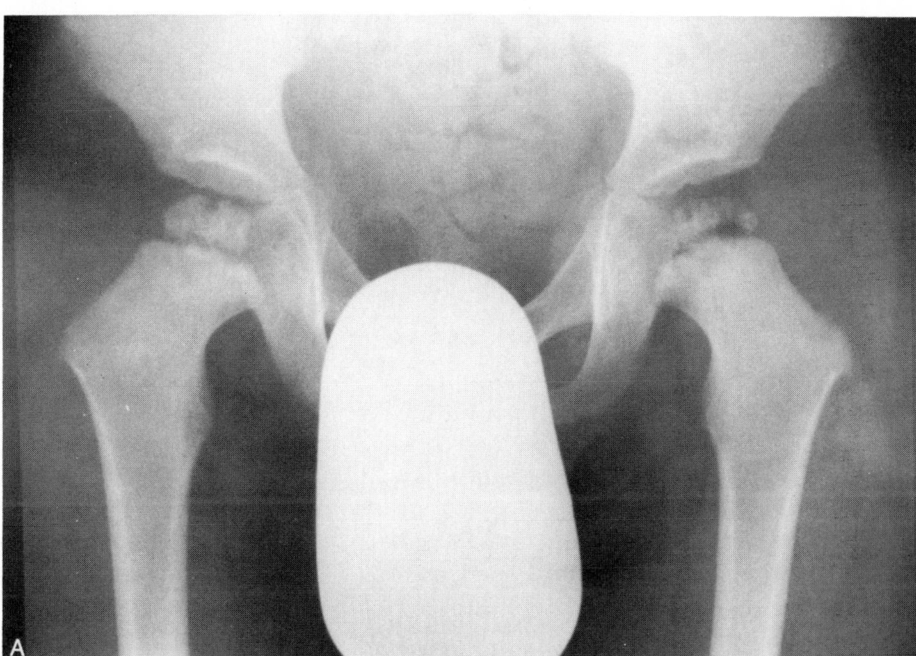

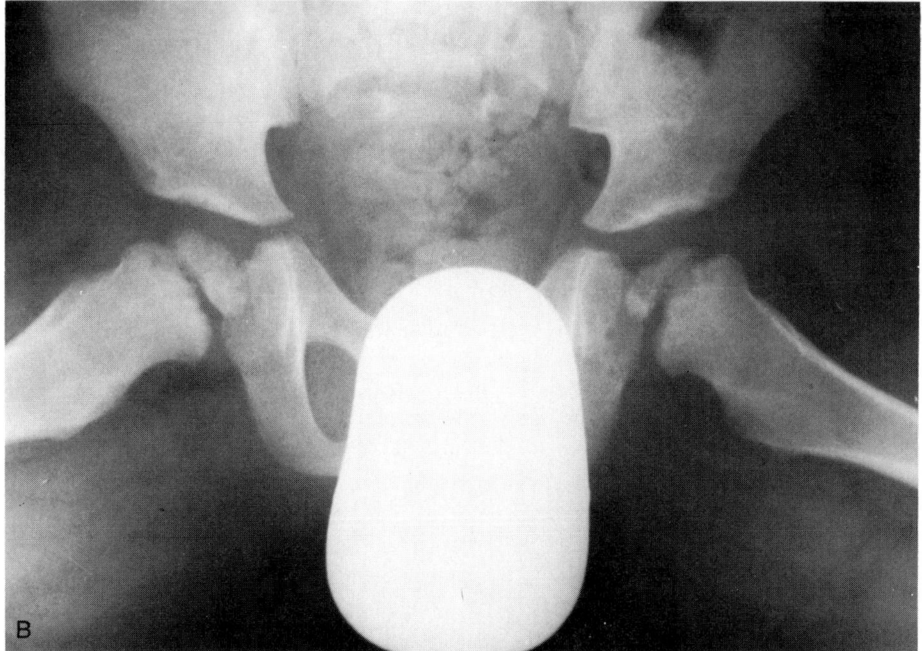

Figure 72–61. *Meyer's dysplasia. Anteroposterior* **(A)** *and "frog-leg" lateral* **(B)** *views of pelvis demonstrate irregular ossification of both femoral heads. The irregularity involves the entire epiphysis, and the changes are symmetric. The femoral heads are of normal density.*

chondrodystrophia punctata includes other causes of "stippled epiphyses," such as the gangliosidoses, infections, and the Fanconi-Albertini-Zellweger syndrome.

Meyer's Dysplasia

Meyer's dysplasia is a localized epiphyseal dysplasia that affects only the femoral heads. Family members are not at risk for developing a diffuse epiphyseal dysplasia. The nature of the pathologic changes is unknown. The symptoms associated with this disorder are mild and the most serious problem encountered is the risk of misdiagnosing the condition as Legg-Calvé-Perthes' disease. Roentgenographic studies obtained during childhood demonstrate irregular ossifications and flattening of the femoral capital epiphyses (Fig. 72–61). Unlike osteonecrosis, the changes are bilaterally symmetric, there is no predilection for the superior aspect of the femoral heads, and the children are usually younger in age (Fig. 72–61).

MACRODYSTROPHIA LIPOMATOSA PROGRESSIVA

Macrodystrophia lipomatosa progressiva is a rare form of localized gigantism characterized by a congenital and progressive overgrowth of all the mesenchymal elements of a digit, with a disproportionate increase in the fibroadipose tissue. It is classified as a developmental anomaly and is not hereditary.

In 1967, Barsky defined true macrodactyly as "a rare congenital malformation characterized by an increase in the size of all elements or structures of a digit or digits."[167] By this definition, only 56 reported cases and seven of his own patients could be said to have true macrodactyly. According to Kelikian,[173] it was Feriz, in 1925, who coined the term macrodystrophia lipomatosa progressiva, referring to only localized gigantism in the lower extremity. In 1966, Ranawat and co-workers[181] accepted macrodystrophia lipomatosa as a term applicable to gigantism in the upper extremity.

Dramatic proliferation of fatty tissue associated with localized gigantism has been described in the literature under many titles, including partial acromegaly, macrosomia, elephantiasis, megalodactyly, dactylomegaly, macrodactyly macroceir, and club finger.

Pathology and Pathophysiology

The etiology of macrodystrophia lipomatosa remains obscure, and theories include lipomatous degeneration,[173] disturbed fetal circulation,[174] an error in segmentation,[174] the trophic influence of a tumefied nerve[7] and the in utero disturbance of a growth-limiting factor.[167] Several authors postulate that macrodystrophia lipomatosa is an expression of neurofibromatosis.[178, 184] The evidence supporting this theory includes (1) the distribution in the hand corresponding to the territory of the median nerve, (2) the pathologic similarities, including neural enlargement, (3) the predominant involvement of those mesenchymal elements that are under neural control, and (4) the observation that macrodactyly is known to occur in patients with documented neurofibromatosis.

The evidence against the association of macrodystrophia lipomatosa and neurofibromatosis is based on (1) the lack of neurocutaneous or other systemic abnormalities in patients with macrodystrophia lipomatosa, (2) the absence of an increased incidence of localized gigantism or other anomalies in family members, in contrast to neurofibromatosis, which is clearly hereditary, (3) the neural enlargement, which is not present in all cases and which is the result of fibrosis of the sheath, not neural tumefaction, (4) the disproportionate increase in adipose tissue, and (5) the difference in the roentgenographic appearance. On the basis of the latter evidence, most investigators[167, 170, 173, 177] postulate that in the absence of the cutaneous findings of neurofibromatosis, isolated congenital macrodactyly is an independent pathologic process.

The most dramatic pathologic finding is the increase in adipose tissue, interspersed in a fine mesh of fibrous tissue, which involves the bone marrow, periosteum, muscles, nerve sheaths, and the subcutaneous tissues (Fig. 72–62). Neural enlargement and irregularity may be prominent, most frequently involving the median nerve in the hand and the plantar nerve in the foot. On microscopic sections, the increase in size of the nerve is noted to be due to infiltration of the sheath by fibroadipose tissue, not by an increase in the number of axons. The phalanges are enlarged by both endosteal and periosteal deposition of bone. The periosteum is studded with nodules approximately 1 mm in diameter that consist of chondroblasts and osteoblasts and that become larger and more numerous toward the distal ends of the phalanges. This probably accounts for the predominantly distal enlargement of the osseous structures.

Clinical Findings

The localized gigantism associated with macrodystrophia lipomatosa is recognizable at birth. There is no known sexual predilection. The rate of accelerated growth varies from patient to patient and even digit to digit. Involvement is almost always unilateral, although there may be enlargement of one

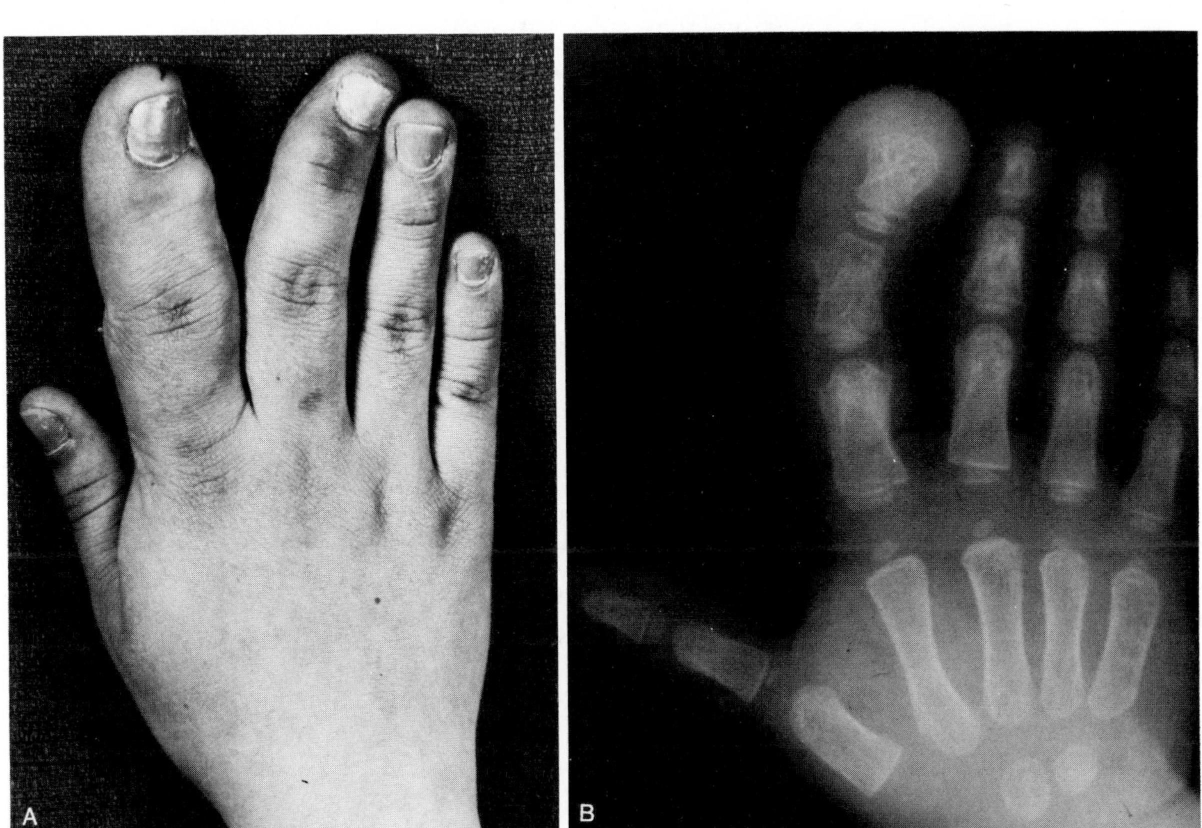

Figure 72–62. *Macrodystrophia lipomatosa.* **A,** *Clinical appearance of involvement of the second and third digits of hand.* **B,** *Posteroanterior roentgenogram shows osseous and soft tissue enlargement, predominantly affecting the distal end of the second digit, and splaying of the ends of the phalanges.*

Illustration continued on the following page

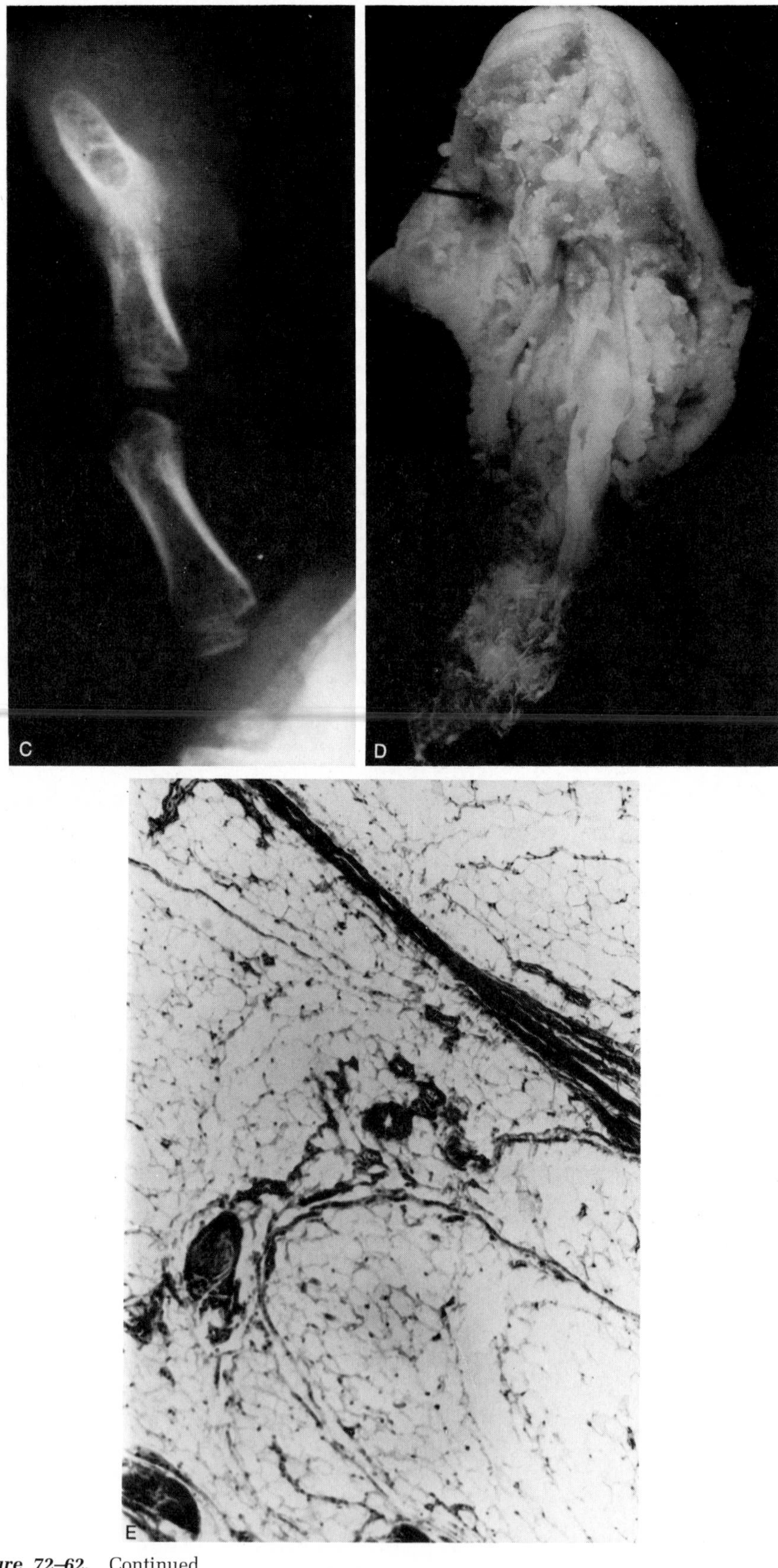

Figure 72–62. Continued

C, *Lateral roentgenogram demonstrates dorsal angulation produced by volar enlargement of soft tissues, and soft tissue lucent areas.* **D,** *Gross specimen and section of specimen* **(E)** *showing bulk of digit to be composed of fat. Enlarged nerve is seen in gross specimen. (From Goldman AB, Kaye JJ: Am J Roentgenol 128:101, 1977. Copyright 1977, American Roentgen Ray Society.)*

or more adjacent digits in the same extremity (Figs. 72–62 and 72–63). The lower extremity is more commonly involved than the upper extremity, and the second and third digits are the favored sites in both upper and lower extremities (Figs. 72–62 and 72–63). The usual reason for seeking surgical correction is cosmetic. Mechanical problems are not encountered until adolescence, when secondary degenerative joint disease reduces function and large osteophytes result in compression of the neurovascular structures. Rarely, the patient presents with a carpal tunnel syndrome.

The affected part is increased in both length and girth. The skin is thickened, pale, and glossy. Growth of the digit ceases at puberty.

Roentgenographic Findings

Roentgenograms of patients with macrodystrophia lipomatosa demonstrate abnormalities in both the soft tissues and osseous structures (Figs. 72–62 and 72–63). The soft tissue overgrowth is most

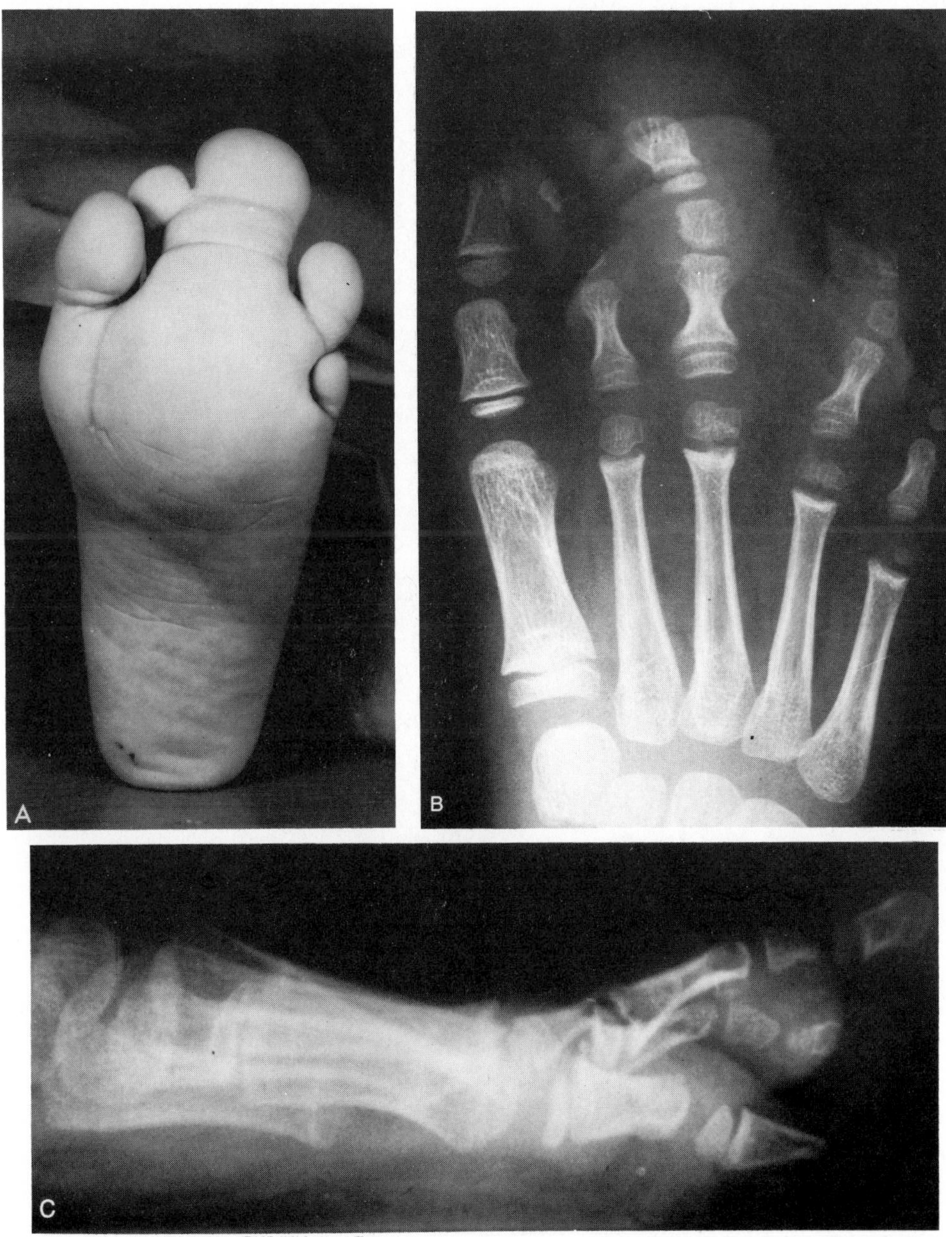

Figure 72–63. *Macrodystrophia lipomatosa.* **A,** *Clinical appearance of involvement of the second and third digits of foot with soft tissue syndactyly. Anteroposterior* **(B)** *and lateral* **(C)** *roentgenograms demonstrate soft tissue and osseous overgrowth with predominant involvement of the distal ends of the digits and the volar surface of the foot. Soft tissue lucent areas are apparent.*

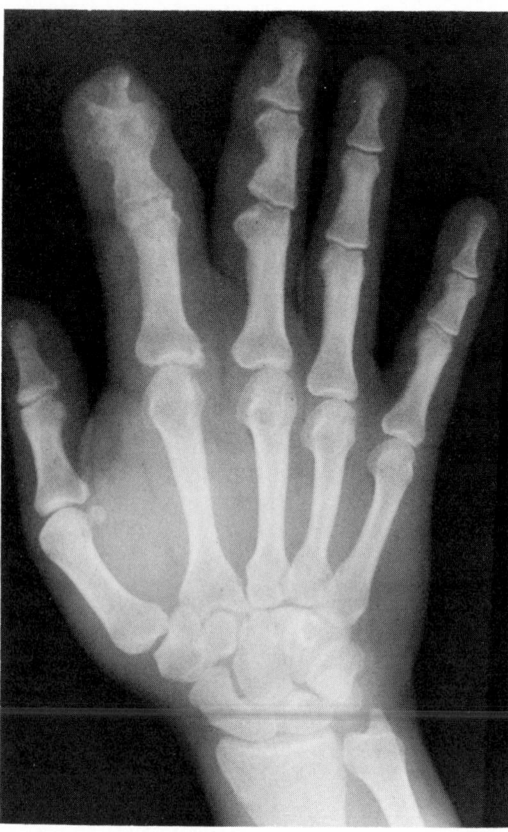

Figure 72–64. Macrodystrophia lipomatosa. Adult patient with involvement of second and third digits of hand. Roentgenogram demonstrates osseous overgrowth and exuberant secondary degenerative joint disease.

marked at the distal end of the digit and along its volar aspect. Volar overgrowth produces dorsal deviation of the affected parts (Figs. 72–62 and 72–63). Small lucent areas reflecting overgrowth of fat are usually detectable within the soft tissues (Figs. 72–62 and 72–63). The phalanges are long, broad, and often splayed at their distal ends (Figs. 72–62 and 72–63). The articular surfaces may slant, and, late in childhood, severe secondary degenerative joint disease supervenes (Fig. 72–64). The osteophytes and reactive new bone are disproportionately large in relation to the joint space narrowing, which may be the result of the periosteal nodules associated with overgrowth (Fig. 72–64). There is a high incidence of associated local anomalies, including syndactyly (Fig. 72–63) and polydactyly. Clinodactyly is almost invariably present, as a result of the side-to-side variations in the accelerated rate of growth.

The roentgenographic differential diagnosis of localized gigantism includes both acquired and congenital disorders. On the basis of the history, the acquired causes (dactylitis secondary to infection, infarction, or Still's disease, osteoid osteoma, melorheostosis) can be eliminated from the differential diagnosis of macrodystrophia lipomatosa. The majority of congenital causes can also be excluded. Hyperemia, secondary to tumorous overgrowth of hemangiomatous and lymphangiomatous elements, produces soft tissue hypertrophy and symmetric overgrowth of the bones. The Klippel-Trenaunay-Weber syndrome has obvious cutaneous abnormali-

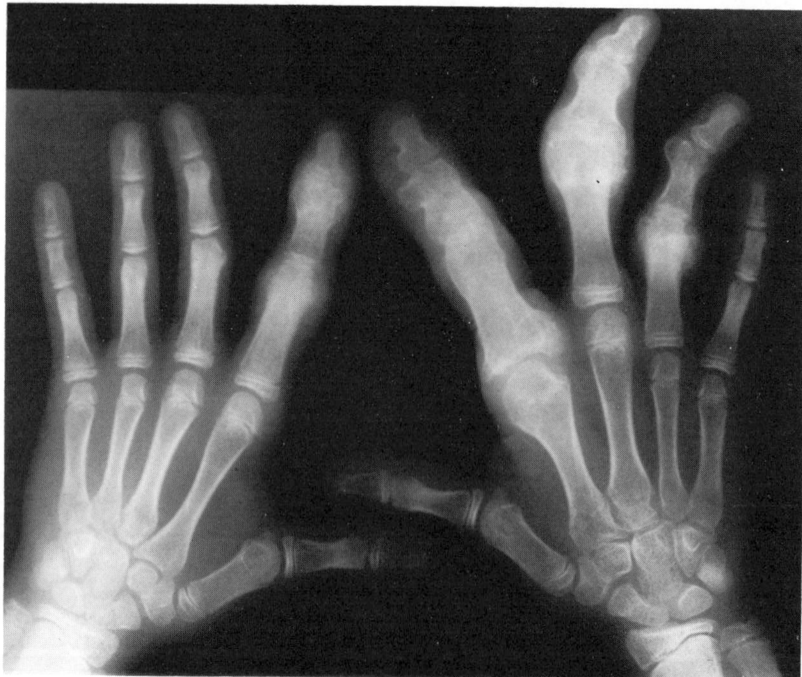

Figure 72–65. Neurofibromatosis. Bilateral macrodactyly can be evident in this disease. (From Goldman AB, Kaye JJ: Am J Roentgenol 128:101, 1977. Copyright 1977, American Roentgen Ray Society.)

ties. The absence of enchondromas eliminates the possibility of Ollier's disease.

The most difficult differential diagnosis on roentgenograms, as on pathologic examination, involves neurofibromatosis (Fig. 72–65). Macrodactyly in patients with von Recklinghausen's disease is the result of plexiform neurofibromas (with hemangiomatous and lymphangiomatous elements), combined with a mesodermal dysplasia. Several roentgenographic findings can help to differentiate macrodystrophia lipomatosa from neurofibromatosis. First, the distribution of localized gigantism in neurofibromatosis is not identical to that of macrodystrophia lipomatosa. In neurofibromatosis, the enlarged digits may be bilateral, involvement of one extremity does not necessarily involve contiguous digits, and the distal phalanges are not the most severely affected (Fig. 72–65). Second, the hemangiomatous elements of the plexiform neurofibroma can produce premature fusion of the growth plates. Growth in a digit involved by macrodystrophia lipomatosa ceases with puberty. Third, the enlarged osseous structures in neurofibromatosis may have a wavy cortex and an elongated, sinuous appearance (Fig. 72–65). The latter deformity is related to the periosteal abnormalities in neurofibromatosis. Last, the observation of soft tissue lucent areas has not been reported in patients with macrodactyly who have the neurocutaneous manifestations of neurofibromatosis.

THE KLIPPEL-TRENAUNAY-WEBER SYNDROME

The Klippel-Trenaunay-Weber syndrome is characterized by a clinical triad that includes unilateral cutaneous capillary hemangiomas, varicose veins, and local gigantism with both soft tissue and osseous overgrowth (Fig. 72–66).

It is not a familial disorder, although involvement of twins has been observed.

The association of limb hypertrophy and port wine hemangiomas was reported independently by Klippel and Trenaunay in 1900[196] and by Parke-Weber in 1907.[203] The latter author, in a later publication, described additional cases with associated arteriovenous malformations. Some investigators[198, 199] prefer to split the syndrome into two forms: those without arteriovenous malformations (Klippel-Trenaunay syndrome) and those with arteriovenous malformations (Parke-Weber syndrome), but most consider them as a single entity under the umbrella term Klippel-Trenaunay-Weber syndrome. Other

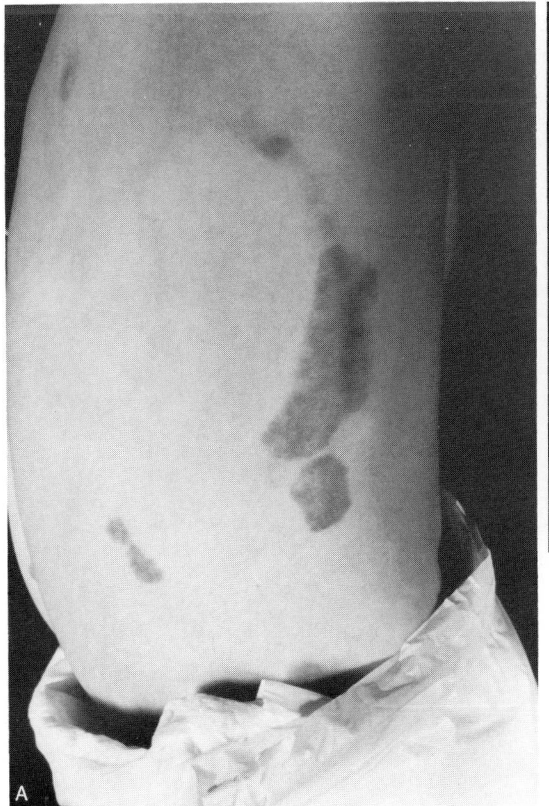

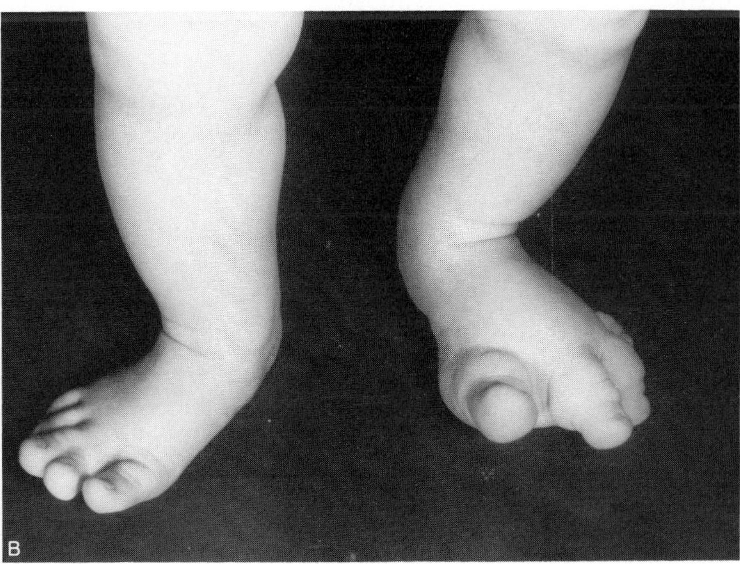

Figure 72–66. Klippel-Trenaunay-Weber syndrome. **A**, Photograph of abdomen shows unilateral cutaneous hemangiomas and prominent venous markings. **B**, View of legs demonstrates overgrowth of extremity.

Illustration continued on the following page

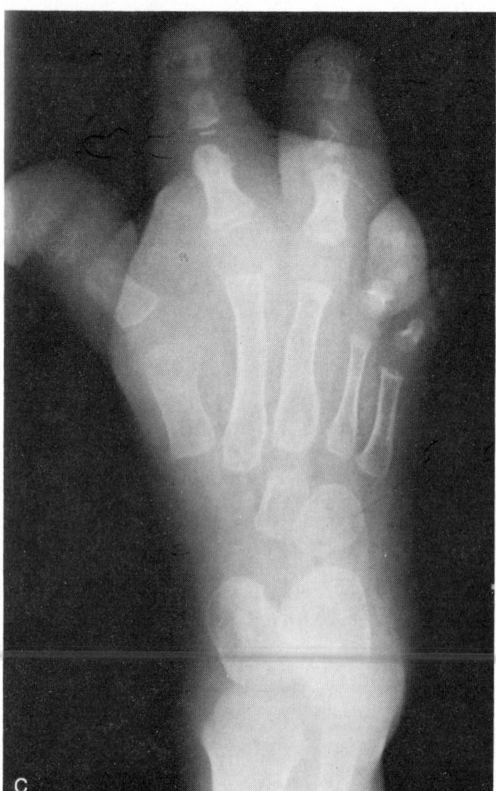

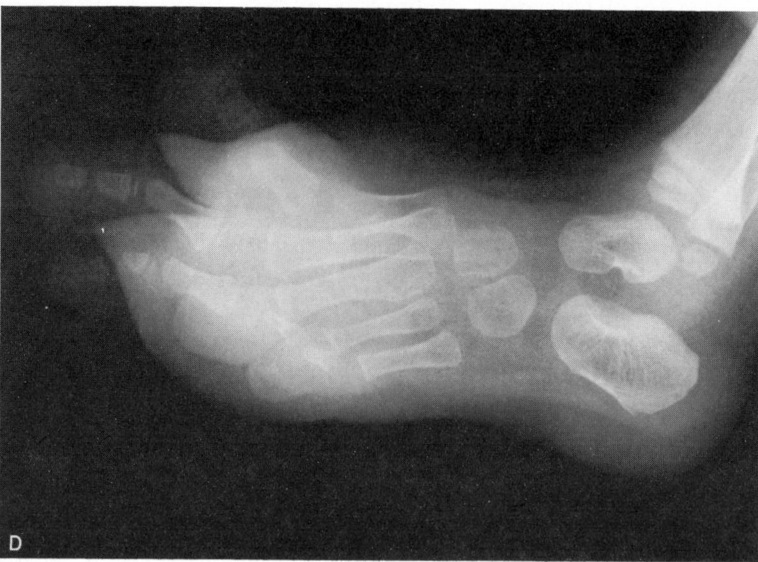

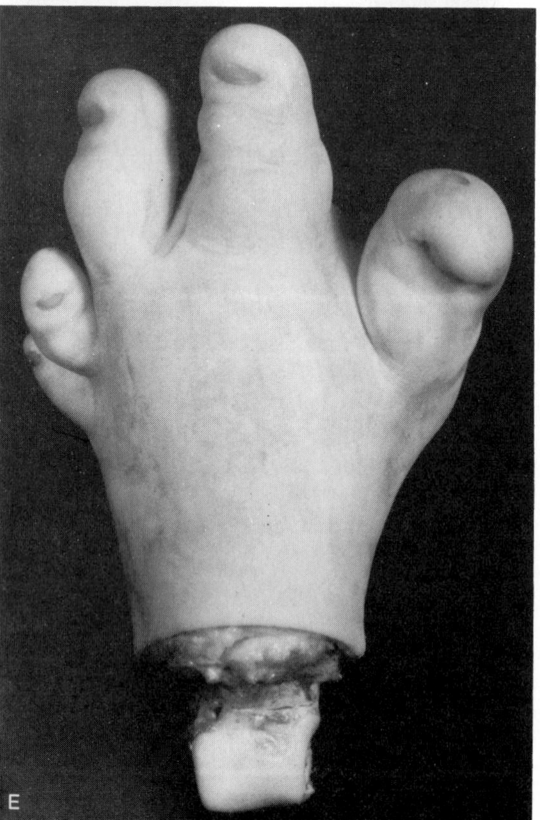

Figure 72–66. Continued
Anteroposterior **(C)** *and lateral* **(D)** *views of foot reveal both osseous and soft tissue overgrowth.* **E,** *Amputation specimen.*

names used in reference to this disease are angio-osteohypertrophy, acro-osteochondral hypertrophy, partial hypertrophy with angioectasia, and nevus varicosis osteohypertrophicus.

Pathology and Pathophysiology

The Klippel-Trenaunay-Weber syndrome is thought to result from a disturbance in embryogenesis. It is associated with a variety of vascular abnormalities, including superficial blue and pigmented hemangiomas, varicose veins, arteriovenous fistulas, lymphangiomas, and absence of the deep venous system. Skin biopsies of affected limbs have revealed scattered groups of thin-walled vessels and increased collagen proliferation.[195] The arteriovenous malformations, if present, provide a low resistance pathway for the cardiac output. They dilate progressively with age and can result in both local and systemic complications (bleeding, high output failure). A high incidence of spinal arteriovenous fistulas has been observed, and Djindjian and coworkers[188] have suggested that these are traceable to the embryogenesis of the vascular supplies of the spine and skin, which originate from the paired dorsolateral arteries.

The osseous and soft tissue overgrowth that characterizes the Klippel-Trenaunay-Weber syndrome occurs in the same area as the vascular malformations (Fig. 72–66). There seem to be no specific primary osseous abnormalities, and local gigantism is attributed to the abnormal vascular supply.[191, 197, 203] Brooksaler,[187] on the basis of studies of animal models, has suggested that the osseous overgrowth is related to paralysis of the normal vasoconstrictor mechanism. Lindenauer[198, 199] observed that in patients with arteriovenous malformations, the augmented rate of blood flow may be a primary factor contributing to excessive growth.

Clinical Findings

The Klippel-Trenaunay-Weber syndrome has no sex predilection. It is usually unilateral and most frequently affects the lower extremities (Fig. 72–66). However, the vascular anomalies may occur in the upper extremity, in two ipsilateral extremities, in the face, or in the trunk. Hemihypertrophy, bilateral involvement, and crossed forms are rare. No abnormalities are present at birth, and in one series,[198] the average age of the patients when seeking medical attention was 13.2 years. The most frequent presenting complaint is related to the varicosities.

The port-wine cutaneous hemangiomas (nevus flammeus) represent the earliest clinical finding (Fig. 72–66). They may be present at birth or appear in the first months of life. The color of the skin lesions varies from bright orange to faintly pink. Associated with the cutaneous angiomas are increased skin temperature, altered sweating, hair loss, and dyskeratosis. Involvement of the face may result in alterations of lacrimation and salivation.

Varicose veins become obvious when the child begins to walk (Fig. 72–66). They vary in size from slightly dilated to finger thickness. Ulcerations and lymphedema further complicate the venous changes. Pulmonary varices can also occur in association with this syndrome.

Localized gigantism develops early in childhood and may involve all or only a part of an extremity (Fig. 72–66). Periods of rapid growth alternate with periods of no change. If the upper extremity is involved, a carpal tunnel syndrome may result from the combination of tissue hypertrophy and augmented blood supply. Facial involvement usually affects the mandible and maxilla, with unilateral exophthalmus and premature eruption of permanent teeth.

Arteriovenous malformations create both local and systemic complications. In the extremities, vascular fistulas may produce intermittent claudication or high output congestive heart failure. Physical examination may reveal thrills, bruits, or pulsatile masses. Visceral vascular malformations have been reported in the colon, producing hematochezia and ulcerations. In the bladder, they result in hematuria and in the spinal canal they create subarachnoid hemorrhages.

Formes frustes of the Klippel-Trenaunay-Weber syndrome have also been described, and are subclassified into neviforme, osteohypertrophic, and avaricose types. Angio-osteohypertrophy may also occur in combination with the bleeding diathesis of the Kasabach-Merritt syndrome.

Roentgenographic Findings

The gigantism associated with the Klippel-Trenaunay-Weber syndrome may involve an entire extremity or only the distal digits. Increases occur in the soft tissues as well as in the length and girth of the affected part (Fig. 72–66). Radionuclide bone scans have demonstrated an increase in the rate of bone turnover at the growth plates. The phalanges, metatarsals, and metacarpals are all increased in size (Fig. 72–66) and may demonstrate cortical thickening. The limb with the angiomatous anomalies is rarely shorter than the normal limb. Congenital osseous abnormalities are frequent and include syndactyly, polydactyly, and congenital hip dislocations. A scoliotic deformity may be present owing to leg length discrepancies.

Venograms performed on patients with the Klippel-Trenaunay-Weber syndrome have demonstrated a variety of abnormalities, including ectasia, deformity secondary to compression by fibrous cords, and total absence of the deep system, frequently involving the femoral and popliteal veins, but rarely the deep calf veins. Phleboliths within the varicosities produce multiple soft tissue calcifications.

Arteriovenous malformations also produce skeletal changes, including multiple lytic lesions. Those involving the viscera may be detected on plain films by the presence of a fixed collection of phleboliths. Unlike phleboliths that occur in normal adults, these dense structures are found in children and are located in atypical sites. Barium studies performed on patients with colonic hemangiomas have revealed thickened folds secondary to varices, extrinsic compression by a soft tissue mass, infiltration of the bowel wall, and secondary mucosal ulcerations.

Lung nodules can be hamartomas or pulmonary varices.

If there are coexisting changes of the Kasabach-Merritt syndrome, joint findings occur and resemble those of hemophilia.

The major roentgenographic differential diagnoses involve Maffucci's syndrome and macrodystrophia lipomatosa. The former entity does exhibit vascular soft tissue calcifications and brachydactyly with multiple enchondromas. The latter entity is distinguished from the Klippel-Trenaunay-Weber syndrome because overgrowth is limited to the digits. Enlargement is worse around the distal phalanges, and soft tissue overgrowth is accompanied by lucent areas representing fat deposits.

SUMMARY

Certain disorders of connective tissue that can lead to significant radiologic alterations have been discussed. Included in this discussion are diseases of connective tissue synthesis and disorders of epiphyses. The roentgenographic changes are diverse, ranging from joint incongruity with secondary degeneration to soft tissue calcification or ossification with or without osseous overgrowth. Although clinical and laboratory features exist for some of these diseases that provide important clues to the correct diagnosis, an awareness of the radiographic alterations will allow early and appropriate assessment in cases in which the diagnosis may be more obscure.

REFERENCES

The Marfan Syndrome

1. Bacchus H: A quantitative abnormality in serum mucoproteins in the Marfan syndrome. Am J Med *25*:744, 1958.
2. Baer RW, Taussig HB, Oppenheimer, FH: Congenital aneurysmal dilatation of aorta associated with arachnodactyly. Bull Johns Hopkins Hosp *72*:309, 1943.
3. Bjerkreim I, Skogland LB, Trygstad O: Congenital contractural arachnodactyly. Acta Orthop Scand *47*:250, 1976.
4. Brenton DP, Dow CJ: Homocystinuria and Marfan syndrome. A comparison. J Bone Joint Surg *54B*:277, 1972.
5. Case records of the Massachusetts General Hospital. N Engl J Med *277*:92, 1967.
6. Epstein CJ, Graham CB, Hodgkin WE, Hecht F, Motulsky AG: Hereditary dysplasia of bone with kyphoscoliosis, contractures and abnormally shaped ears. J Pediatr *73*:379, 1968.
7. Francis MJO, Smith DP, Smith R: Polymeric collagen of skin in osteogenesis imperfecta, homocystinuria, and Ehlers-Danlos and Marfan syndromes. Birth Defects *11*:15, 1975.
8. Forsman PJ, Jenkins ME: Medullary carcinoma of the thyroid with Marfan-like habitus. Pediatrics *52*:188, 1973.
9. Ghosh S: Marfan syndrome or variant. J Pediatr *74*:840, 1969.
10. Goebel HH, Muller J, DeMyer W: Myopathy associated with Marfan syndrome. Fine structural and histochemical observations. Neurology *23*:1257, 1973.
11. Goodman RM, Wooley CF, Frazier RL, Covault L: Ehlers-Danlos syndrome occurring together with the Marfan syndrome. N Engl J Med *273*:514, 1965.
12. Gutjahr P, Spranger J: Thyroidectomy in type IIb multiple-endocrine-neoplasia syndrome. Lancet *1*:1149, 1977.
13. Heldrich FJ Jr, Wright CE: Marfan syndrome. Diagnosis in the neonate. Am J Dis Child *114*:419, 1967.
14. Hirst AE, Gore I: Marfan syndrome: A review. Progr Cardiovasc Dis *16*: 187, 1973.
15. Joseph MC, Meadow SR: The metacarpal index of infants. Arch Dis Child *44*:515, 1969.
16. Keech MR, Wendt VE, Reed RC, Bistue AR, Bianchi FA: Family studies of the Marfan syndrome. J Chronic Dis *19*:57, 1966.
17. Lee JD: Marfan syndrome. JAMA *218*:597, 1961.
18. MacLeod PM, Fraser C: Congenital contractural arachnodactyly. A heritable disorder of connective tissue distinct from Marfan syndrome. Am J Dis Child *126*:810, 1973.
19. Marfan AB: Un cas de déformation congénitale des quatre membres, tres prononcée aux extrémitiés caracterisée par d'allongement des os avec un certain degré d'amincissement. Bull Mém Soc Méd Hôp Paris, 3rd Series, *13*:220, 1896.
20. McKusick VA: Heritable Disorders of Connective Tissue. 4th Ed. St Louis, CV Mosby Co, 1972, p 61.
21. McKusick VA: The classification of heritable disorders of connective tissue. Birth Defects *11*:1, 1975.
22. McKusick VA: More speculation on Marfan syndrome. J Pediatr *80*:530, 1972.
23. Murdoch JL, Walker BA, Halpern BL, Kuzma LW, McKusick VA: Life expectancy and causes of death in Marfan syndrome. N Engl J Med *286*:804, 1972.
24. Ogden JA, Southwick WO: Contraposed curve patterns in monozygotic twins. Clin Orthop Rel Res *116*:35, 1976.
25. Papioannou AC, Matsaniotis N, Cantez T, Durst MD: Marfan syndrome. Onset and development of cardiovascular lesions in Marfan syndrome. Angiology *21*:580, 1970.
26. Parrish JG: Heritable disorders of connective tissue. Proc R Soc Med *53*:515, 1960.
27. Payvandi MN, Kerber RE, Phelps CD, Tudisch GF, El-Khoury G, Schrott HG: Cardiac, skeletal and ophthalmologic abnormalities in relatives of patients with Marfan syndrome. Circulation *55*:797, 1977.
28. Phornphutkeil C, Rosenthal A, Nadas AS: Cardiac manifestations of Marfan syndrome in infancy and childhood. Circulation *47*:587, 1973.
29. Robins PR, Moe JH, Winter RB: Scoliosis in Marfan syndrome. Its characteristics and results of treatment in thirty-five patients. J Bone Joint Surg *57A*:358, 1975.
30. Steinberg I: A simple screening test for the Marfan syndrome. Am J Roentgenol *97*:118, 1966.
31. Stinson HK, Cruess RL: Marfan syndrome with marked limb-length discrepancy. J Bone Joint Surg *49A*:735, 1967.
32. Walker BA, Beighton PH, Murdock JL: The marfanoid hypermobility syndrome. Ann Intern Med *71*:349, 1969.

Homocystinuria

33. Beals RK: Homocystinuria. A report of two cases and review of the literature. J Bone Joint Surg *51A*:1561, 1969.
34. Brenton DP, Dow CJ, James JIP, Hay RL, Wynne Davis R: Homo-

cystinuria and Marfan's syndrome. A comparison. J Bone Joint Surg *54B*:277, 1972.
35. Brill PW, Mitty JA, Gaull GE: Homocystinuria due to cystathionine synthetase deficiency: Clinical roentgenologic correlations. Am J roentgenol *121*:45, 1974.
36. Carson NAJ, Dent CE, Field CMB, Gaull GE: Homocystinuria clinical and pathological review of ten cases. J Pediatr *66*:565, 1965.
37. Davis JW, Flournoy LD, Phillips PE: Amino acids and collagen-induced platelet aggregation. Lack of effect of three amino acids that are elevated in homocystinuria. Am J Dis Child *129*:1020, 1975.
38. Francis MJO, Smith DP, Smith R: Polymeric collagen of skin in osteogenesis imperfecta, homocystinuria, and Ehlers-Danlos and Marfan syndromes. Birth Defects *11*:15, 1975.
39. Gaull GE: Homocystinuria, vitamin B_6 and folate: Metabolic interrelationships and clinical significance. J Pediatr *81*:1014, 1972.
40. Gaull G, Sturman JA, Schaffner F: Homocystinuria due to cystathionine synthase deficiency: Enzymatic and ultrastructural studies. J Pediatr *84*:381, 1974.
41. Gibson JB, Carson MDJ, Neill DW: Pathological findings in homocystinuria. J Clin Pathol *17*:427, 1964.
42. Gerittsen T, Waisman HA: Homocystinuria, an error in metabolism of methionine. Pediatrics *33*:413, 1964.
43. Hunter KR: Homocystinuria or Marfan's syndrome. Lancet *1*:842, 1969.
44. Hurwitz LJ, Chopra JS, Carson NAJ: Electromyographic evidence of a muscle lesion in homocystinuria. Acta Paediatr Scand *57*:401, 1968.
45. Kang AH, Trelstad RL: A collagen defect in homocystinuria. J Clin Invest *52*:2571, 1973.
46. Leonard MS: Homocystinuria: A differential diagnosis of Marfan syndrome. Oral Surg *36*:214, 1973.
47. London Letter: Can Med Assoc J *99*:1013, 1968.
48. McKusick VA: The classification of heritable disorders of connective tissue. Birth Defects *11*:1, 1975.
49. McKusick VA: Heritable Disorders of Connective Tissue. 4th Ed. St Louis, CV Mosby Co, 1972, p 224.
50. Schimke RN, McKusick VA, Pollack AD: Homocystinuria simulating the Marfan syndrome. Trans Assoc Am Physicians *78*:60, 1965.
51. Shulman JD, Agarwal B, Mudd HS, Shulman NR: Pulmonary embolism in homocystinuria patient during treatment with Dipyridamole and acetylsalicylic acid 661. N Engl J Med *299*:661, 1978.
52. Smith SW: Roentgen findings in homocystinuria. Am J Roentgenol *100*:147, 1967.

The Ehlers-Danlos Syndrome

53. Beighton P, Horan F: Orthopaedic aspects of the Ehlers-Danlos syndrome. J Bone Joint Surg *51B*:444, 1969.
54. Beighton P, Trice A, Lord T, Dickson E: Variants of Ehlers-Danlos syndrome. Clinical, biochemical, haematological and chromosomal features of 100 patients. Ann Rheum Dis *28*:251, 1969.
55. Beighton P, Thomas ML: The radiology of Ehlers-Danlos syndrome. Clin Radiol *20*:354, 1969.
56. Brown A, Stock VF: Dermatorrhexis: Report of a case. Am J Dis Child *54*:956, 1967.
57. Carter C, Sweetran R: Familial joint laxity and recurrent dislocation of the patella. J Bone Joint Surg *40B*:664, 1958.
58. Carter C, Sweetran R: Recurrent dislocation of the patella and of the shoulder. Their association with familial joint laxity. J Bone Joint Surg *42B*:721, 1960.
59. Carter C, Wilkinson T: Persistent joint laxity and congenital dislocation of the hip. J Bone Joint Surg *46B*:40, 1964.
60. Coventry MB: Some skeletal changes in the Ehlers-Danlos syndrome. A report of two cases. J Bone Joint Surg *43A*:855, 1961.
61. Francis MJO, Smith DP, Smith R: Polymeric collagen of skin in osteogenesis imperfecta, homocystinuria, Ehlers-Danlos and Marfan syndromes. Birth Defects *11*:15, 1975.
62. Freeman JT: Ehlers-Danlos syndrome. Am J Dis Child *79*:1049, 1950.
63. Holt JF: The Ehlers-Danlos syndrome. Am J Roentgenol *55*:420, 1946.
64. Jansen LH: The structure of the connective tissue, an explanation of the symptoms of the Ehlers-Danlos syndrome. Dermatologica *110*:108, 1955.
65. Katz I, Stuner K: Ehlers-Danlos syndrome with ectopic bone formation. Radiology *65*:352, 1955.
66. Kirk JA, Ansell BM, Bywaters EGL: The hypermobility syndrome — musculoskeletal complaints associated with generalized joint hypermobility. Ann Rheum Dis *26*:419, 1967.
67. McKusick VA: The classification of heritable disorders of connective tissue. Birth Defects *11*:1, 1975.
68. McKusick VA: Heritable Disorders of Connective Tissue. St Louis, CV Mosby Co, 1972, p 292.
69. Mitchell GE, Lourie H, Berne AS: The various causes of scalloped vertebrae with notes on their pathogenesis. Radiology *89*:67, 1967.
70. Newton TH, Carpenter ME: The Ehlers-Danlos syndrome with acro-osteolysis. Br J Radiol *32*:739, 1959.
71. Olsen GA, Allan LH: The lateral stability of the spine. Clin Orthop Rel Res *65*:143, 1969.
72. Rybka FJ, O'Hara ET: The surgical significance of Ehlers-Danlos syndrome. Am J Surg *113*:431, 1967.
73. Sutro CJ: Hypermobility of bones due to "overlengthened" capsular and ligamentous tissue. A case for recurrent intra-articular effusions. Surgery *21*:67, 1947.
74. Svane S: Ehlers-Danlos syndrome. A case with some skeletal changes. Acta Orthop Scand *37*:49, 1966.

Osteogenesis Imperfecta

75. Bailey JA: Forms of dwarfism recognized at birth. Clin Orthop Rel Res *76*:150, 1971.
76. Bauze RJ, Smith R, Francis MJO: A new look at osteogenesis imperfecta. J Bone Joint Surg *57B*:2, 1975.
77. Brailsford JF: The Radiology of Bones and Joints. Baltimore, Williams & Wilkins Co, 1948, p 547.
78. Caffee J: Pediatric X-Ray Diagnosis. 6th Ed. Chicago, Year Book Medical Publishers, 1973, pp. 54, 1037.
79. Castells S: New approaches to treatment of osteogenesis imperfecta. Clin Orthop Rel Res *93*:239, 1973.
80. Doty SB, Mathews RS: Electron microscope and histochemical investigation of osteogenesis imperfecta tarda. Clin Orthop Rel Res *80*:191, 1971.
81. Ederken J, Hodes PJ: Roentgen Diagnosis of Diseases of Bone. 2nd Ed. Baltimore, Williams & Wilkins Co, 1973, p 145.
82. Elias S, Simpson JL, Griffin LP: Intrauterine growth retardation in osteogenesis imperfecta. JAMA *239*:23, 1978.
83. Engfeldt B, Engstrom A, Zetterstorm R: Bio-physical studies of bone tissue in osteogenesis imperfecta. J Bone Joint Surg *36B*:654, 1954.
84. Fairbank T: Atlas of General Affectations of the Skeleton. Edinburgh, E & S Livingstone, 1951.
85. Falvo KA, Bullough PG: Osteogenesis imperfecta: A histometric analysis. J Bone Joint Surg *55A*:275, 1973.
86. Falvo KA, Root L, Bullough PG: Osteogenesis imperfecta: Clinical evaluation and management. J Bone Joint Surg *56A*:783, 1974.
87. Falvo KA, Root L: Osteogenesis imperfecta tarda. J Hosp Special Surg *1*:44, 1975.
88. Francis MJO: Polymeric collagen of skin in osteogenesis imperfecta, homocystinuria, and Ehlers-Danlos and Marfan syndromes. Birth Defects *11*:15, 1975.
89. Fugi K, Tanzer ML: Osteogenesis imperfecta: Biochemical studies of bone collagen. Clin Orthop Rel Res *124*:271, 1977.
90. Greenfield GB: Radiology of Bone Disease. Philadelphia, JB Lippincott Co, 1979, p 209.
91. Halbara H, Yamasaki Y, Kyogoku M: An autopsy case of osteogenesis imperfecta congenita — histochemical and electron microscopical studies. Acta Pathol Jap *19*:377, 1967.
92. Ibsen KH: Distinct varieties of osteogenesis imperfecta. Clin Orthop Rel Res *50*:279, 1967.
93. Currano G, Brooksaler F: Osteogenesis imperfecta. *In* HJ Kaufman (Ed): Intrinsic Disease of Bones. Progress in Pediatric Radiology, Vol 4. Basel, S Karger, 1973, p 346.
94. King JD, Bobechko WP: Osteogenesis imperfecta. An orthopedic description and surgical review. J Bone Joint Surg *53B*:72, 1971.
95. Laurent LE, Salenius P: Hyperplastic callus formation in osteogenesis imperfecta. Report of a case simulating sarcoma. Acta Orthop Scand *38*:280, 1967.
96. McKusick VA: Heritable Disorders of Connective Tissue. 4th Ed. St Louis, CV Mosby Co, 1972, p 390.
97. Ramser JR, Villanueva AR, Pirok D, Frost HM: Tetracycline-based measurement of bone dynamics in 3 women with osteogenesis imperfecta. Clin Orthop Rel Res *49*:151, 1966.
98. Sofield HA, Millar EA: Fragmentation realignment and intramedullary rod fixation of deformities of the long bones in children. A ten year appraisal. J Bone Joint Surg *41A*:1371, 1959.
99. Solomons CC, Millar EA: Osteogenesis imperfecta — new perspectives. Clin Orthop Rel Res *96*:299, 1973.
100. Spranger J: Osteogenesis imperfecta and related disorders. International Skeletal Society, 6th Annual Refresher Course, August 31–September 2, 1979 (in press).
101. Spencer AT: A histochemical study of long bones in osteogenesis imperfecta. J Pathol Bacteriol *83*:423, 1962.
102. Sykes B, Francis MJO, Smith R: Altered relation of two collagen types in osteogenesis imperfecta. N Engl J Med *296*:1200, 1977.
103. Wright PG, Gernsetter SL, Greenblatt RB: Therapeutic acceleration of bone age in osteogenesis imperfecta. A case report. J Bone Joint Surg *36B*:654, 1954.

Myositis Ossificans Progressiva

104. Ackerman LV: Extraosseous localized non-neoplastic bone and cartilage formation (so-called myositis ossificans). Clinical and pathological confusion with malignant neoplasms. J Bone Joint Surg *40A*:279, 1958.
105. Adams RC, Denny-Brown D, Pearson CM: Diseases of Muscle: A Study of Pathology. 2nd Ed. New York, Harper & Row, 1962.
106. Fletcher E, Moss MS: Myositis ossificans progressiva. Ann Rheum Dis *24*:267, 1965.
107. Gwinn JL: Radiological case of the month. Progressive myostitis ossificans. Am J Dis Child *116*:655, 1968.
108. Illingworth RS: Myositis ossificans progressiva (Münchmeyer's disease). Brief review with report of 2 cases treated with corticosteroids and observed for 16 years. Arch Dis Child *46*:264, 1971.
109. Letts RM: Myositis ossificans progressiva. A report of two cases with chromosome studies. Can Med Assoc J *99*:856, 1976.
110. Letts RM: Myositis ossificans progressiva. Can Med Assoc J *100*:133, 1969.
111. Ludman H, Hamilton EBD, Eade AWT: Deafness in myositis ossificans progressiva. J Laryngol *82*:57, 1968.
112. Ludwak L: Myositis ossificans progressiva. Mineral, metabolic, and radioactive calcium studies of the effects of hormones. Am J Med *37*:269, 1964.
113. McKusick VA: Fibrodysplasia ossificans progressiva. *In* Heritable Disorders of Connective Tissue. 4th Ed. St Louis, CV Mosby Co, 1972, p 687.
114. Simpson AJ, Friedman S: Myositis ossificans progressiva. Mt Sinai J Med *38*:416, 1971.
115. Smith DM, Zerman W, Johnston CC, Deiss WP: Myositis ossificans progressiva. Case report with metabolic and histochemical studies. Metabolism *15*:521, 1966.

Pseudoxanthoma Elasticum

116. Akhtar M, Brody H: Elastic tissue in pseudoxanthoma elasticum. Ultrastructural study of endocardial lesions. Arch Pathol *99*:667, 1975.
117. Alinder I, Boström H: Clinical studies on a Swedish material of pseudoxanthoma elasticum. Acta Med Scand *191*:273, 1972.
118. Cocco AE, Grayer DI, Walker BA, Martyn LJ: The stomach in pseudoxanthoma elasticum. JAMA *210*:2381, 1972.
119. Eng AM: Pseudoxanthoma elasticum in hyperphosphatasia. Arch Dermatol *111*:271, 1975.
120. Engelman MW, Fliegelman MT: Pseudoxanthoma elasticum. Cutis *21*:837, 1978.
121. Fellner MJ, Chen AS, McCabe JB: Pseudoxanthoma elasticum. Arch Dermatol *114*:288, 1978.
122. Hogan JF, Heaton CL: Angioid streaks and systemic disease. Br J Dermatol *89*:411, 1973.
123. McKusick VA: Heritable Disorders of Connective Tissue. 4th Ed. St Louis, CV Mosby Co, 1972, p 475.
124. Mehta HK: Grönblad-Strandberg syndrome. Proc R Soc Med *61*:548, 1968.
125. Najjar SS, Farah FS, Kurban AK, Melhem RE, Khatchadouria AK: Tumoral calcinosis and pseudoxanthoma elasticum. J Pediatr *72*:243, 1968.
126. Pope FM: Two types of autosomal recessive pseudoxanthoma elasticum. Arch Dermatol *110*:209, 1974.
127. Prick JJG, Thijssen HDM: Radiodiagnostic signs in pseudoxanthoma elasticum generalisatum (dysgenesis elastofibrillaris mineralisans). Clin Radiol *28*:549, 1977.
128. Schachner L, Young D: Pseudoxanthoma elasticum with severe cardiovascular disease in a child. Am J Dis Child *127*:571, 1974.
129. Shevick M: Pseudoxanthoma elasticum. Angiology *122*:629, 1971.

Fibrogenesis Imperfecta

130. Baker SL, Turnbull HM: Two cases of a hitherto undescribed disease characterized by a gross defect in collagen matrix. J Pathol Bacteriol *62*:132, 1950.
131. Baker SL: Fibrogenesis imperfecta ossium. J Bone Joint Surg *34B*:378, 1956.
132. Baker SL, Dent CE, Freidman M, Watson L: Fibrogenesis imperfecta ossium. J Bone Joint Surg *48B*:804, 1966.
133. Frost HM, Frame B, Ormond RS, Hunter RB: Atypical axial osteomalacia. A report of three cases. Clin Orthop *23*:283, 1962.
134. Golde D, Greipp P, Sanzenbacher L, Gralnick HR: Hematologic abnormalities in fibrogenesis imperfecta ossium. J Bone Joint Surg *53A*:365, 1971.
135. Golding FC: Fibrogenesis imperfecta. J Bone Joint Surg *50B*:619, 1968.
136. Murray RO, Jacobson JG: The Radiology of Skeletal Disorders. 2nd Ed. Edinburgh, Churchill Livingstone, 1977, p 1170.

Multiple Epiphyseal Dysplasias

137. Bailey JA II: Forms of dwarfism recognizable at birth. Clin Orthop *76*:150, 1971.
138. Berg PK: Dysplasia epiphysialis multiplex. Am J Roentgenol *97*:31, 1966.
139. Fairbank T: Dysplasia epiphysialis multiplex. Br J Surg *34*:225, 1947.
140. Felman AH: Multiple epiphyseal dysplasia. Three cases with unusual vertebral anomalies. Radiology *93*:119, 1969.
141. Gamboa I, Lisker R: Multiple epiphyseal dysplasia tarda. A family with autosomal recessive inheritance. Clin Genet *6*:15, 1974.
142. Gwinn JL, Lee FA: Radiological case of the month. Am J Dis Child *129*:287, 1975.
143. Herring JA: Rapidly progressive scoliosis in multiple epiphyseal dysplasia. J Bone Joint Surg *50A*:703, 1976.
144. Hoefnagel D, Sycamore LK, Russel SW, Bucknall WE: Hereditary multiple epiphyseal dysplasia. Ann Hum Genet *30*:201, 1967.
145. Hulvey JT, Keats T: Multiple epiphyseal dysplasia. A contribution to the problem of spinal involvement. Am J Roentgenol *106*:170, 1969.
146. Hunt DD, Ponseti IV, Pedrine-Mille A, Pedrini V: Multiple epiphyseal dysplasia in two siblings. J Bone Joint Surg *49A*:1611, 1967.
147. Juberg RC, Holt JF: Inheritance of multiple epiphyseal dysplasia tarda. Am J Hum Genet *20*:549, 1968.
148. Juberg RC: Hereditary and multiple epiphyseal dysplasia. JAMA *237*:2600, 1977.
149. Koslowski K, Lipska E: Hereditary dysplasia epiphysealis multiplex. Clin Radiol *18*:330, 1967.
150. Koslowski K, Budzinska A: Combined metaphyseal and epiphyseal dystosis. Report of two cases — one in which metaphyseal changes predominate, and a second one in which epiphyseal changes are more marked. Am J Roentgenol *97*:21, 1966.
151. Lie SO, Siggers DC, Dorst JP, Kopits SE: Unusual multiple epiphyseal dysplasia. Birth Defects *10*:165, 1974.
152. Mansoor IA: Dysplasia epiphysealis multiplex. Clin Orthop Rel Res *72*:287, 1970.
153. Maroteaux P: Epiphyseal dysplasia, multiple. *In* D Bergsma (Ed): Birth Defects Compendium. New York, National Foundation, March of Dimes, Alan R Liss Inc, 1979, p 409.
154. Mason RC, Kozlowski K: Chondrodysplasia punctata. A report of 10 cases. Radiology *109*:145, 1973.
155. Mena HR, Pearson EO: Multiple epiphyseal dysplasia. JAMA *236*:2629, 1976.
156. Meyer J: Dysplasia epiphysealis capitis femoris. A clinico-radiological syndrome and its relationship to Legg-Calvé-Perthes' disease. Acta Orthop Scand *34*:183, 1964.
157. Pfeiffer RA, Jünemann G, Polster J, Bauer H: Epiphyseal dysplasia of the femoral head, severe myopia and perceptive hearing loss in three brothers. Clin Genet *4*:141, 1973.
158. Rasmussen PG, Reimann I: Multiple epiphyseal dysplasia with special reference to histologic findings. Acta Pathol Microbiol Scand *81*:381, 1973.
159. Rasmussen PG: Multiple epiphyseal dysplasia. Two morphological and histochemical investigation of cartilage matrix, particularly in the precalcification stage. Acta Pathol Microbiol Scand *83*:493, 1975.
160. Ribbings S: Studien über hereditäre, multiple Epiphysenstörungen. Acta Radiol Suppl *34*:1, 1937.
161. Rubin P: Dynamic Classification of Bone Dysplasias. Chicago, Year Book Medical Publishers, 1964, p 120.
162. Sensenbrenner JA: Probable multiple epiphyseal dysplasia. Birth Defects *10*:419, 1974.
163. Shaul WL, Emery J, Hall JG: Chondrodysplasia punctata and maternal warfarin use during pregnancy. Am J Dis Child *129*:360, 1975.
164. Spranger J: The epiphyseal dysplasias. Clin Orthop Rel Res *114*:46, 1976.
165. Sugarman GI: Chondrodysplasia punctata (rhizomelic type): Case report and pathologic findings. Birth Defects *10*:399, 1974.
166. Wolcott ED, Rallison ML: Infancy-onset diabetes mellitus and multiple epiphyseal dysplasia. J Pediatr *80*:292, 1972.

Macrodystrophia Lipomatosa Progressiva

167. Barsky AJ: Macrodactyly. J Bone Joint Surg *49A*:1255, 1967.
168. Ben-Bassat M, Casper J, Kaplan I, Laron Z: Congenital macrodactyly. A case report with three-year follow-up. J Bone Joint Surg *48B*:359, 1966.
169. Cockshott WP: Dactylitis and growth disorders. Br J Radiol *36*:19, 1963.
170. Goldman AB, Kaye JJ: Macrodystrophia lipomatosa: Radiographic diagnosis. Am J Roentgenol *128*:101, 1977.
171. Inglis K: Local gigantism (a manifestation of neurofibromatosis): Its relation to general gigantism and to acromegaly. Illustrating the influence of intrinsic factors in disease when development of the body is abnormal. Am J Pathol *26*:1059, 1950.
172. Johnson EW, Ghormley RK, Dockerty MB: Hemangiomas of the extremities. Surg Gynecol Obstet *102*:531, 1956.

173. Kelikian H: Macrodactyly. *In* Congenital Deformities of the Hand and Forearm. Philadelphia, WB Saunders Co, 1974, p 610.
174. Littler JW, Cramer LM, Smith JW: Symposium on Reconstructive Hand Surgery. St Louis, CV Mosby Co, 1974, p 218.
175. McCarthy DM, Dorr CA, Mackintosh CE: Unilateral localized gigantism of the extremities with lipomatosis, arthropathy, and psoriasis. J Bone Joint Surg *51B*:348, 1969.
176. Meszaros WT, Guzzo F, Schorsch H: Neurofibromatosis. Am J Roentgenol *98*:557, 1966.
177. Minkowitz S, Minkowitz F: A morphological study of macrodactylism. A case report. J Pathol Bacteriol *90*:323, 1965.
178. Moore BH: Macrodactylism and associated peripheral nerve changes associated with congenital deformities. J Bone Joint Surg *26*:282, 1944.
179. Pitt MJ, Mosher JF, Edeiken J: Abnormal periosteum and bone in neurofibromatosis. Radiology *103*:143, 1972.
180. Posnanski AK: The Hand in Radiologic Diagnosis. Philadelphia, WB Saunders Co, 1974, pp 193, 328, 416.
181. Ranawat CS, Arora MM, Singh RG: Macrodystrophia lipomatosa with carpal tunnel syndrome. A case report. J Bone Joint Surg *50A*:1242, 1968.
182. Rosborough D: Osteoid osteoma. Report of a lesion in the terminal phalanx of a finger. J Bone Joint Surg *48B*:485, 1966.
183. Thorne FL, Posch JL, Mladick RA: Megalodactyly. Plast Reconstr Surg *41*:232, 1968.
184. Tuli SM, Khanna NN, Sinha GP: Congenital macrodactyly. Br J Plast Surg *22*:237, 1969.

Klippel-Trenaunay-Weber Syndrome

185. Baar AJ: Klippel-Trenaunay's syndrome in connection with a possible teratogenic effect of butobarbital. Dermatologica *154*:314, 1977.
186. Belovic B, Nethercott J, Donsky HJ: An unusual variant of Klippel-Trenaunay-Weber syndrome. Can Med Assoc J *111*:439, 1974.
187. Brooksaler F: The angioosteohypertrophy syndrome, Klippel-Trenaunay-Weber syndrome. Am J Dis Child *112*:161, 1966.
188. Djindjian M, Djindjian R, Hurth M, Rey A, Houdart R: Spinal cord arteriovenous malformations and Klippel-Trenaunay-Weber syndrome. Surg Neurol *8*:229, 1977.
189. Gamsu G: The Klippel-Trenaunay syndrome. A case report. J Can Assoc Radiol *21*:287, 1970.
190. Ghahremani GG, Kangarloo H, Volberg F, Meyers MA: Diffuse cavernous hemangioma of the colon in the Klippel-Trenaunay syndrome. Radiology *118*:673, 1976.
191. Gellis SS, Feingold M: Picture of the month. Klippel-Trenaunay-Weber syndrome (angioosteohypertrophy). Am J Dis Child *128*:213, 1974.
192. Gwinn DL, Lee FA: Radiologic case of the month. Am J Dis Child *131*:89, 1977.
193. Hall BD: Bladder hemangiomas in Klippel-Trenaunay-Weber syndrome. N Engl J Med *285*:1032, 1971.
194. Harper PS, Horton WA: Klippel-Trenaunay-Weber syndrome. Birth Defects *78*:315, 1971.
195. Inui M, Chiba R, Shike S: An autopsy case of Klippel-Trenaunay-Weber disease. Acta Pathol Jap *19*:251, 1969.
196. Klippel M, Trenaunay P: Du naevus variqueux ostéohypertrophique. Arch Gen Med *3*:641, 1900.
197. Letts RM: Orthopaedic treatment of hemangiomatous hypertrophy of the lower extremity. J Bone Joint Surg *59A*:777, 1977.
198. Lindenauer SM: Congenital arteriovenous fistula and the Klippel-Trenaunay syndrome. Ann Surg *174*:248, 1971.
199. Lindenauer SM: The Klippel-Trenaunay syndrome: Varicosity, hypertrophy and hemangioma with no arteriovenous fistula. Ann Surg *162*:303, 1965.
200. MacPherson RI, Letts RM: Skeletal disease associated with angiomatosis. J Can Assoc Radiol *29*:90, 1978.
201. Moynahan JA: Nevoid hypertrophy of the lower limbs, with gigantism of digits (Klippel-Weber-Trenaunay syndrome). Proc R Soc Med *54*:695, 1961.
202. Owens DW, Garcia E, Pierce RR, Castrow FF II: Klippel-Trenaunay-Weber syndrome with pulmonary vein varicosity. Arch Dermatol *108*:111, 1973.
203. Parke-Weber F: Angioma formation in connection with hypertrophy of the limbs and hemihypertrophy. Br J Dermatol *19*:231, 1907.
204. Sehgal VN, Aggarwal SP, Gupta RC: Klippel-Trenaunay-Parke-Weber syndrome. Derm Int *7*:212, 1968.

Others

205. Goldman AB, Davidson D, Pavlov H, Bullough PG: "Popcorn" calcifications: a prognostic sign in osteogenesis imperfecta. Radiology *136*:351, 1980.
206. Sillence DO, Senn A, Danks DM: Genetic heterogeneity in osteogenesis imperfecta. J Med Genet *16*:101, 1979.

ADDITIONAL CONGENITAL OR HERITABLE ANOMALIES AND SYNDROMES

by Donald Resnick, M.D.

73

In Chapter 72, important congenital and inherited disorders, including diseases of collagen and developing epiphyses, are discussed. In the following pages, additional anomalies and syndromes are outlined that may lead to significant abnormalities in the growing skeleton and that, in some cases, may produce clinical and radiologic alterations that simulate those of certain acquired conditions. The discussion of each entity is brief, and the interested reader should consult standard textbooks that are currently available for more detailed analysis.[1-5]

SKELETAL APLASIA AND HYPOPLASIA

The entire bone or a portion thereof may not form in the normal fashion, producing a variety of congenital deficiencies.[462] These have been extensively studied and classified by Frantz and O'Rahilly[6] and later by other investigators.[7, 8] Initially, in 1961,[6] deficiencies were subdivided into two basic types: terminal deficiencies, in which there was absence of all skeletal elements distally along a designated axis; and intercalary deficiencies, in which there was an absence of parts ordinarily interposed between the proximal and distal aspects of the remaining limb. Each of these two types was further divided into transverse and longitudinal varieties based upon whether the absent bone(s) extended across the width of a limb or ran parallel to the long axis of the limb.[8] This schema was subsequently changed in 1966,[7] at which time the general term meromelia was utilized to describe all partial absences. The four major categories that had been previously described — terminal, intercalary, transverse, and longitudinal — were again utilized, and a new category, central defects, was added. In 1974, an international classification system was formulated.[9, 10] In it, all limb deficiencies were classified as transverse or longitudinal. The transverse category encompassed those congenital anomalies that had previously been described as terminal transverse deficiencies, and the longitudinal category consisted of all the remaining deficiencies.

Of the major tubular bones, aplasia or hypoplasia affects the fibula, radius, femur, ulna, and humerus in order of descending frequency.

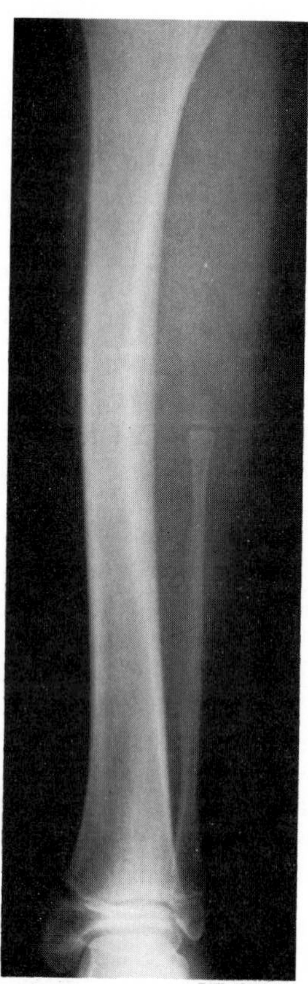

Figure 73–1. *Hypoplasia: Fibula. Note severe hypoplasia of the fibula with medial bowing of the midshaft of the tibia.*

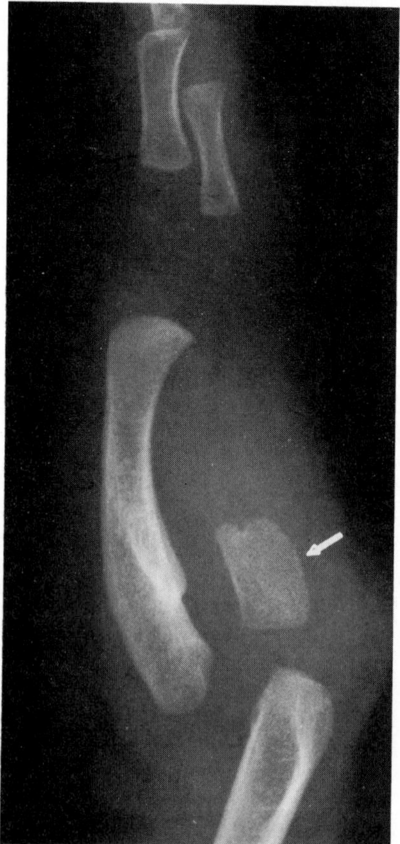

Figure 73–2. *Hypoplasia: Radius. Severe hypoplasia of the radius (arrow) is associated with a deformed ulna and absence of some bones in the hand and the wrist.*

Fibular Aplasia and Hypoplasia

The severity of this most common osseous deficiency is variable.[11-15, 452] Congenital absence or severe hypoplasia of the fibula can be combined with ventral and medial bowing of the companion tibia, a skin dimple at the apex of the bow, an equinovalgus foot, absence of one or two of the lateral rays of the foot, tarsal aplasia or fusion, and retarded development or shortening of the ipsilateral femur (Fig. 73–1). Milder varieties of fibular hypoplasia may also be more difficult to recognize. Distal or proximal deficiencies can be seen; distal fibular hypoplasia may be associated with a valgus deformity of the ankle, whereas proximal fibular hypoplasia can be accompanied by valgus knee deformity and instability at the proximal tibiofibular articulation.[16]

Radial and Ulnar Aplasia and Hypoplasia

Radial anomalies may include total or partial aplasia or hypoplasia (Fig. 73–2). Bilateral abnormalities are common and may be combined with hypoplasia or absence of the thumb or radial carpal bones. Such radial lesions can be associated with systemic disorders in some cases. These include the vertebral-anal-tracheo-esophageal-radial-renal syndrome (VATER syndrome) (Fig. 73–3); cardiac abnormalities, including ventricular septal defect, atrial septal defect, pulmonary artery atresia, and patent ductus arteriosus; and thrombocytopenia.[17-20]

Ulnar deficiency is less frequent and severe than that of the radius. Three types of deformity are recognized: hypoplasia, partial aplasia, and total aplasia.[21] There is ulnar deviation of the hand, suggesting that a tethering effect exists in which a radiographically invisible fibrocartilaginous band attaches distally to the distal radial epiphysis, the ulnar side of the carpus, or both, extending from the proximal ulnar primary ossification center. Resection of this band may reduce the angular growth deformities.

Proximal Femoral Focal Deficiency (PFFD)

This term is applied to a spectrum of conditions characterized by partial absence and shortening of the proximal femur.[22-26] Additional designations for this congenital but not inherited disorder are dysgenesis of the proximal femur, congenital short femur, congenital hypoplasia of the upper femur, and femoral hypoplasia with coxa vara. PFFD is distinguished from total femoral agenesis and coxa vara without shortening of the femoral shaft.[463] Although some cases of PFFD are associated with other skeletal defects, it is usually an isolated occurrence, apearing in a unilateral fashion in 90 per cent of patients. A variety of classification systems have been suggested, based on the presence and location of the femoral head and neck[23] (Table 73–1) (Figs. 73–4 and 73–5). The designation of a specific type of PFFD in an individual patient may require both radiography and arthrography. Roentgenograms of a newborn infant demonstrate a short femur that is displaced superiorly, posteriorly, and laterally to the iliac crest. The distal end of the femur is usually normal. Ossification of the femoral capital epiphysis is invariably delayed. After the second year of life, affected children reveal either dysgenesis or absence of subtrochanteric ossification, the severity of the abnormalities varying with the type of PFFD that is present. At skeletal maturity, changes include subtrochanteric varus deformity or pseudarthrosis, a large unossified gap between the femoral capital epiphysis and dysplastic shaft, or ossification of only the distal femoral epiphysis.[22] Secondary abnormalities of the pelvis and acetabulum are common, correlating with the degree of femoral head deformity or hypoplasia. The major differential diagnosis of the radiographic findings is developmental coxa vara, in which familial and bilateral characteristics may be seen and in which abnormalities are less severe, delayed in appearance, progressive, and related to a true decrease in the neck-shaft angle as opposed to the subtrochanteric varus that appears in PFFD.

The etiology of this disorder is obscure. It has been suggested that the condition arises from a cellular nutritional disturbance at the time of cell division (4 to 6 weeks after ovulation).[27] The occurrence of some cases of PFFD in children of diabetic mothers and the production of similar osseous defects in chick embryos by the injection of insulin suggest that an abnormality of carbohydrate metabolism may be important in this malformation.[22, 23, 28] Additional possible pathogeneses include vascular damage to mesenchymal tissue in the upper femur or mechanical injury.[23, 29]

Sacrococcygeal Agenesis (Caudal Regression Syndrome)

This well-known anomaly leads to absence of one or more segments of the sacrum, which may be combined with aplasia of the lower thoracic and upper lumbar spine[30-33, 450, 451] (Fig. 73–6). Approximately 20 per cent of individuals with this syndrome are the children of diabetic mothers. Associated abnormalities include hip dislocations, flexion contractures of the knees and hips, and foot deformities. Radiographic findings vary with the severity of

Text continued on page 2555

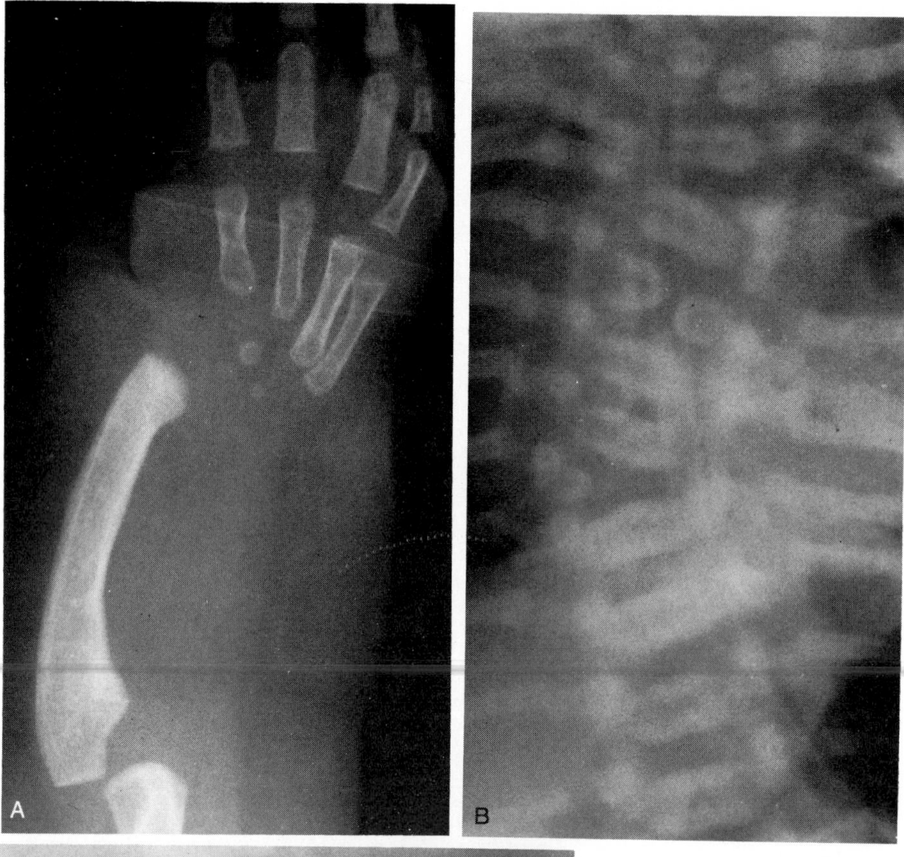

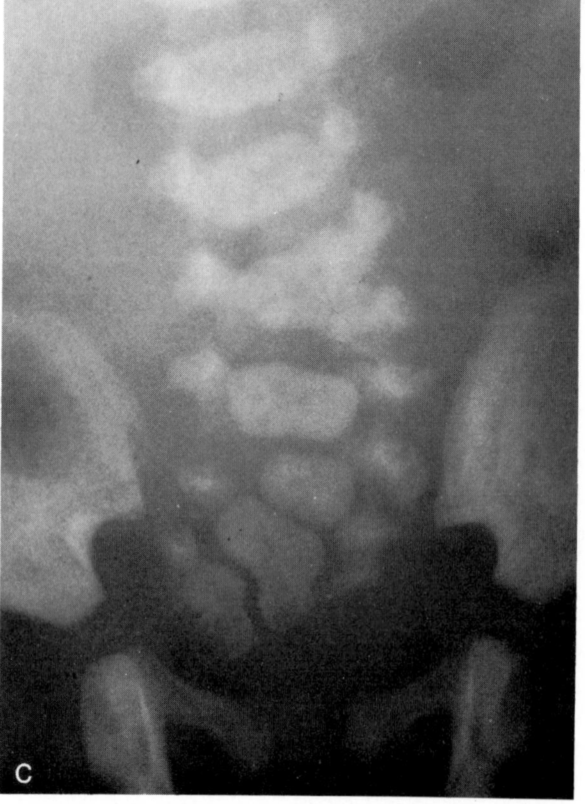

Figure 73–3. *Vertebral-anal-tracheo-esophageal-radial-renal (VATER) syndrome. This 2½ year old child demonstrates radial aplasia, absence of the thumb, and severe spinal anomalies. Additional abnormalities included a tracheoesophageal fistula and renal and anal anomalies.*

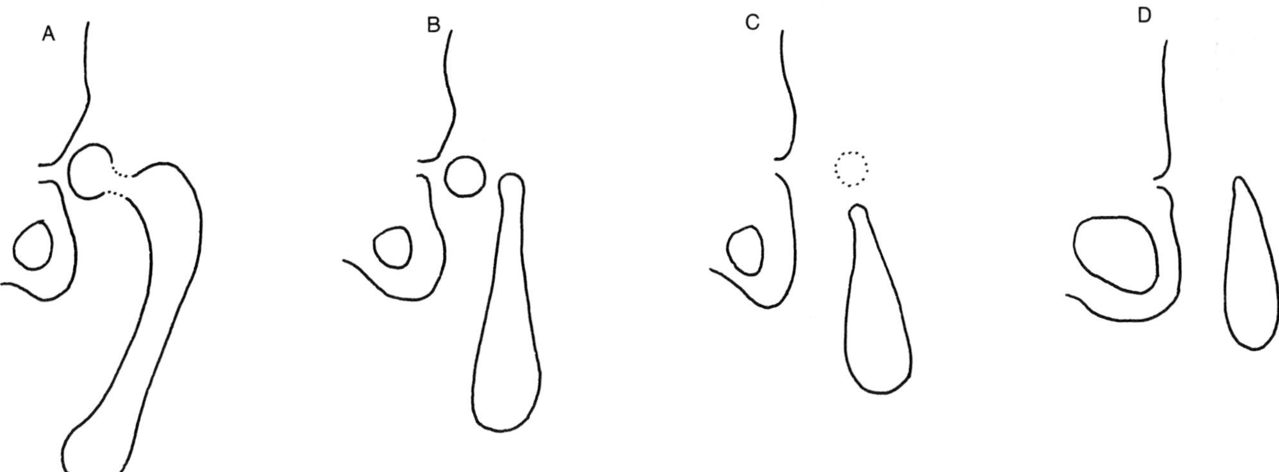

Figure 73–4. *Proximal femoral focal deficiency (PFFD): Classification system. Classes A to D are described. In all classes, there is a very short femoral shaft. Dashed lines indicate structures that will (Class A) or may (Class C) ossify at a later date. (After Levinson ED, et al: Radiology 125:197, 1977.)*

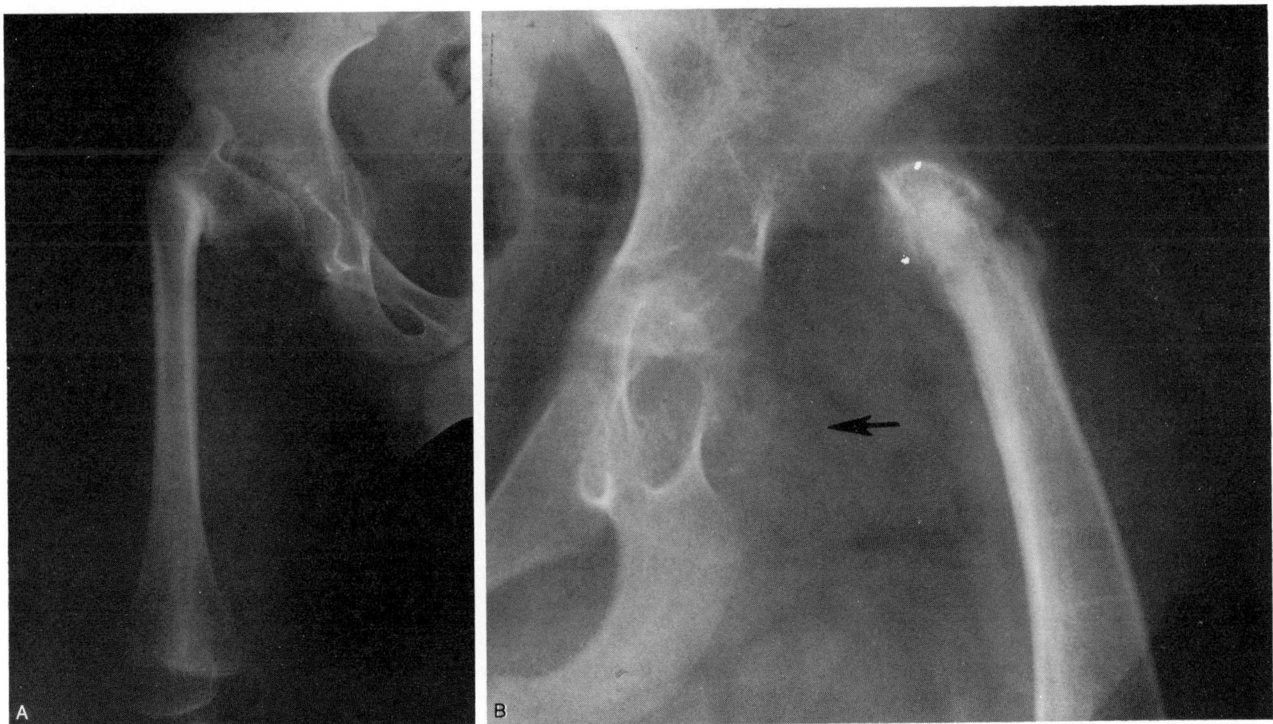

Figure 73–5. *Proximal femoral focal deficiency (PFFD): Types of involvement.*

A *Class A. The short right femoral shaft, continuity of head and shaft, femoroacetabular articulation, and subtrochanteric varus are characteristic.*

B *Class B. The left femoral shaft is short. The femoral head (arrow) is seated in the acetabulum, but there is no bony communication between head and shaft.*

Illustration continued on the following page

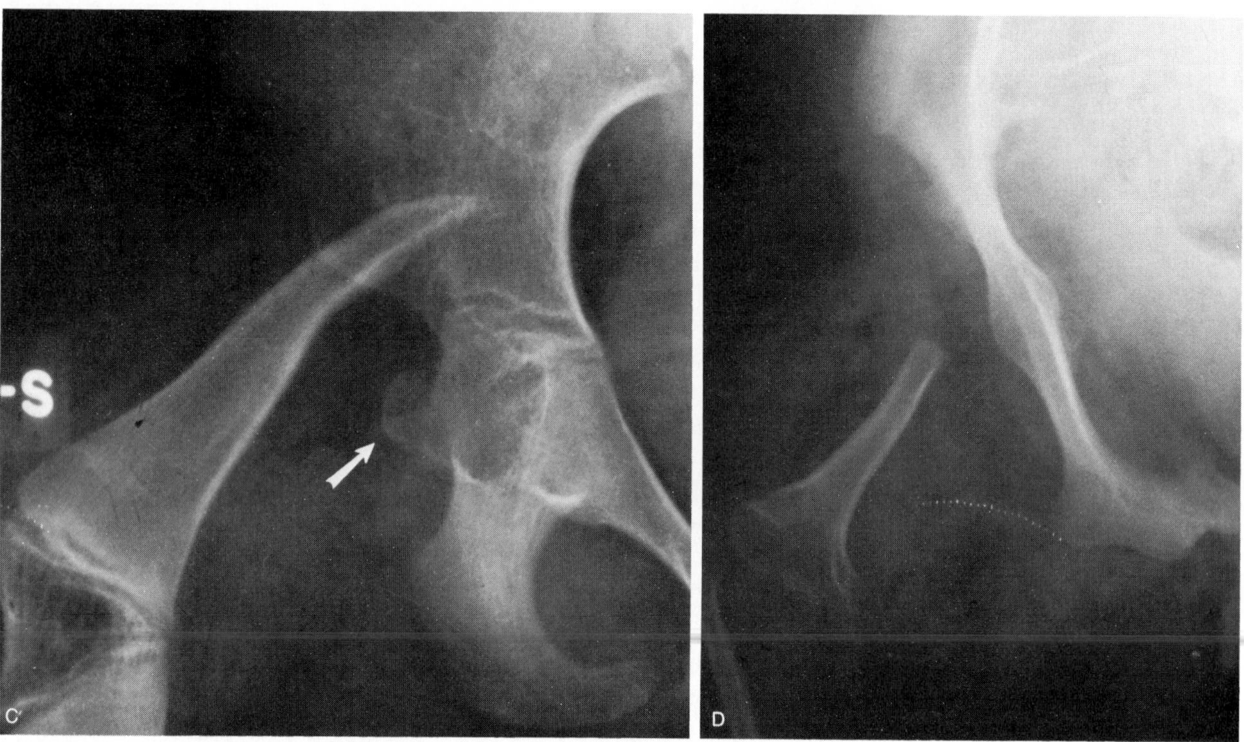

Figure 73–5. Continued

C *Class C. The right femoral shaft is short, tapered, and elevated. No femoral head is evident. The dysplastic acetabulum contains a bony protuberance, which, on other views, represented a part of the acetabulum. A right knee fusion had previously been performed.*

D *Class D. Complete absence of the acetabulum and femoral head is apparent. Note the changes in the knee.*

(**A–C,** *From Levinson ED, et al: Radiology 125:197, 1977.*)

Table 73–1

CLASSIFICATION OF PROXIMAL FEMORAL FOCAL DEFICIENCY

Class	Head of Femur	Acetabulum	Femoral Segment	Relationship Among Components of Femur and Acetabulum at Skeletal Maturity
A	Present	Adequate	Short	Bony connection between components of femur; head in acetabulum; subtrochanteric varus, often with pseudarthrosis
B	Present	Adequate or moderately dysplastic	Short; usually proximal bony tuft	No osseous connection between head and shaft; head in acetabulum
C	Absent or represented by ossicle	Severely dysplastic	Short; usually proximally tapered	May be osseous connection between shaft and proximal ossicle; no osseous connection between femur and acetabulum
D	Absent	Absent; obturator foramen enlarged; pelvis squared in bilateral cases	Short, deformed	

(Courtesy of Levinson ED, Ozonoff MB, Royen PM: Proximal femoral focal deficiency (PFFD). Radiology *125*:197–203, 1977.)

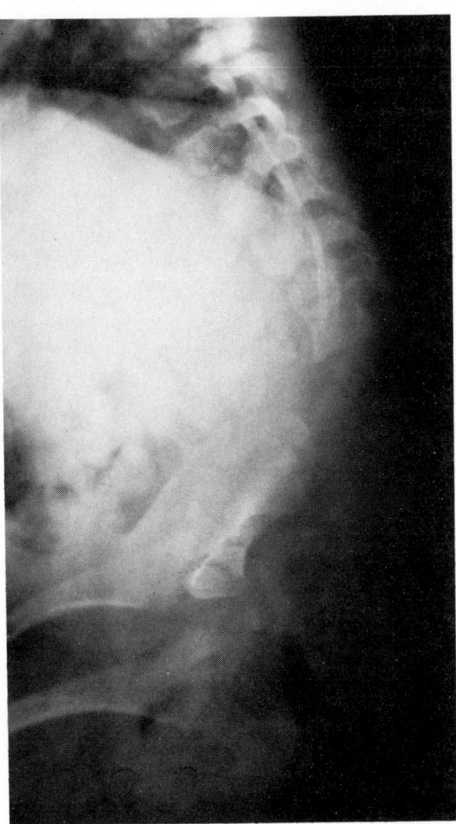

Figure 73–6. *Sacrococcygeal agenesis (caudal regression syndrome). In this child of a diabetic mother, observe absence of much of the lumbar spine and all of the sacrum. Deformity of the ilia is evident.*

the anomaly. Complete sacral agenesis is combined with deformed ilia that may articulate with each other or with the lowest vertebral body or that fuse in the midline. Partial agenesis may lead to a deformed and sickle-shaped sacrum through which an anterior meningocele may protrude. Central sacral defects may be combined with hereditary presacral teratoma.[34]

The detection of associated skeletal and visceral abnormalities requires myelography, urography, cystography, and contrast studies of the gastrointestinal tract in addition to plain film radiography.[35, 36]

SKELETAL HYPERPLASIA

Congenital enlargement may involve a single bone, a portion of a limb, or the entire limb. In some instances, one half of the body can be affected. Soft tissue hypertrophy generally accompanies the osseous abnormality. Although idiopathic in a large number of cases, similar changes can be evident in a wide variety of disorders, including neurofibromatosis, lipomatosis, hemangiomatosis, lymphangiomatosis, arteriovenous malformations, endocrine disorders, cerebral gigantism, Wilm's tumor, and neoplasms of the adrenal glands.[37-39] Localized osseous overgrowth can be noted in response to hyperemia in articular and inflammatory disorders, such as hemophilia, juvenile chronic arthritis, and osteomyelitis.

MALSEGMENTATIONS AND FUSIONS

Errors in segmentation are frequently inherited and result in osseous fusion of neighboring bones, such as the radius and ulna. Bony ankylosis can also occur between longitudinally arranged bones, as in the digits of the hand and the foot. On the opposite side of the spectrum, hypersegmentation and duplication anomalies exist. In both of these situations, radiographs are particularly helpful, outlining the presence and characteristics of the malformation.

Hyperphalangism and Polydactyly

Extra phalanges in humans are virtually confined to the thumb (Fig. 73–7). The triphalangeal thumb is a rare familial disorder[40, 41] that leads to a small or large ossicle in the abnormal digit. Al-

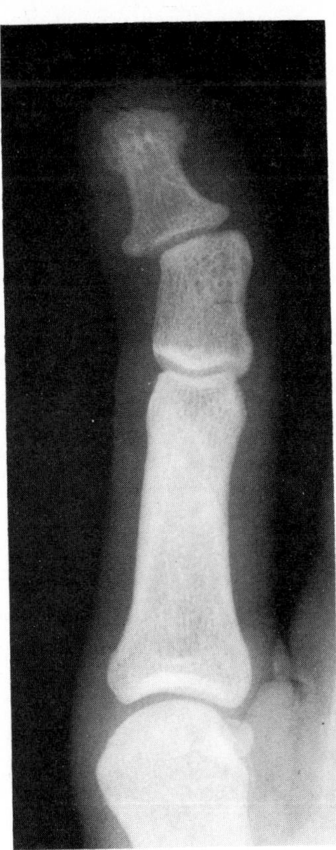

Figure 73–7. *Hyperphalangism: Thumb. In this patient with the Holt-Oram syndrome, observe three separate phalanges in the thumb.*

though the anomaly can occur as an isolated finding, it may also be associated with other anomalies, including polydactyly, duplications, and absent bones, and with certain syndromes, including Holt-Oram syndrome, trisomy 13-15, and Blackfan-Diamond anemia.[42] Accessory phalanges should be differentiated from pseudoepiphyses of the digits that may accompany certain syndromes, such as cleidocranial dysostosis and hypothyroidism.

Polydactyly, representing an increased number of digits, can appear in the hand or the foot (Fig. 73–8). Polydactyly is more common in blacks than in whites, and the presence and pattern of its inheritance are dependent upon the type of anomaly that is evident. Its appearance on the radial side of the hand is termed preaxial polydactyly, and its existence on the ulnar side of the hand is known as postaxial polydactyly. Preaxial polydactyly may be associated with acrocephalosyndactyly, brachydactyly B, acropectorovertebral dysplasia, Fanconi's syndrome, Holt-Oram syndrome, and other conditions; postaxial polydactyly can appear in chondroectodermal dysplasia (Ellis-van Creveld syndrome), Laurence-Moon-Biedl syndrome, trisomy 13, asphyxiating thoracic dystrophy, Goltz's focal dermal hypoplasia, and other diseases.[42]

Syndactyly

This common anomaly relates to a lack of differentiation between two or more digits.[43] It may be subdivided into cases with soft tissue or osseous involvement and classified into partial (involving the proximal segments of a digit) or complete (involving the entire digit) types. Other classification systems are also utilized.[42] Most cases are inherited, although some appear in a sporadic fashion. Men are more commonly affected than women. A large number of syndromes have been associated with syndactyly.[42] Included in this list is Poland's syndrome, in which there is syndactyly and absence of the pectoral muscles[44] (Fig. 73–9). Additional anomalies in this nonhereditary syndrome are hypoplasia of the hand, the nipple, or the ribs, pectus excavatum, pectus carinatum, elevated scapulae, and scoliosis. A possible association of Poland's syndrome with leukemia has been noted.[45, 46]

Symphalangism

This anomaly represents a fusion of one phalanx to another within the same digit, presumably due to a failure of differentiation of the intervening articulation.[47, 48] It is usually inherited as a dominant trait. On radiographs in the infant, the anomaly may be difficult to recognize owing to the "invisible" nature of the cartilaginous tissue. However, hypoplasia of the joint and an adjacent abnormal epiphysis represent roentgenographic clues even at this early age. Typical sites of involvement include the proximal interphalangeal joints of the fingers and the distal interphalangeal joints of the toes, with predilection for the ulnar side of the hand.[42] The thumb is rarely affected. Additional abnormalities may include shortening and flattening of the metacarpals and carpal and tarsal fusions.[49] Associated syndromes include diastrophic dwarfism, Bell's brachydactyly types A and C, popliteal pterygium syndrome, and certain acrocephalosyndactyly syndromes.[42]

It is important to differentiate this anomaly from acquired intra-articular fusions accompanying various arthritides, including juvenile chronic arthritis and psoriatic arthritis. With congenital symphalangism, the proximal and middle phalanges may be joined by a smooth osseous contour, although a slight expansion of the bony margin may be encountered at the level of the affected joint. Furthermore, a small lucent cleft at the site of fusion and hypoplasia of distal phalanges and metacarpal heads are helpful signs.

Carpal Fusion (Coalition)

Carpal fusion or coalition is a relatively common abnormality that may occur as an isolated phenomenon or as part of a generalized congenital malformation syndrome. As a rule, isolated fusions involve bones in the same carpal row (proximal or distal), whereas syndrome-related fusions may affect bones in different rows (proximal and distal).[42, 50]

The most common site of the isolated fusion is between the triquetrum and the lunate bones, occurring in 0.1 to 1.6 per cent of the general population, more frequently in men and in blacks,[51] and having little or no clinical significance[52] (Fig. 73–10). Less common isolated coalitions that may be encountered include capitate-hamate fusion,[53] trapezium-trapezoid fusion, and pisiform-hamate fusion,[54] and, in fact, isolated fusions have been described in almost all possible combinations.[55] The presence and exact location of coalition are not always easy to identify on radiographic examination. This difficulty relates to the partial or incomplete nature of the ankylosis in some cases, the necessity for multiple projections owing to the obliquity of the osseous surfaces of the normal carpal bones, and the requirement that differentiation of congenital and acquired coalition must be accomplished. In most cases, symptoms and signs are entirely lacking, although a definite risk of fracture exists in the presence of a fused carpus.[56, 57]

Massive carpal fusion usually indicates the presence of other anomalies. Similarly, fusion between bones of the proximal and distal carpal rows or between the carpal bones and radius or ulna is

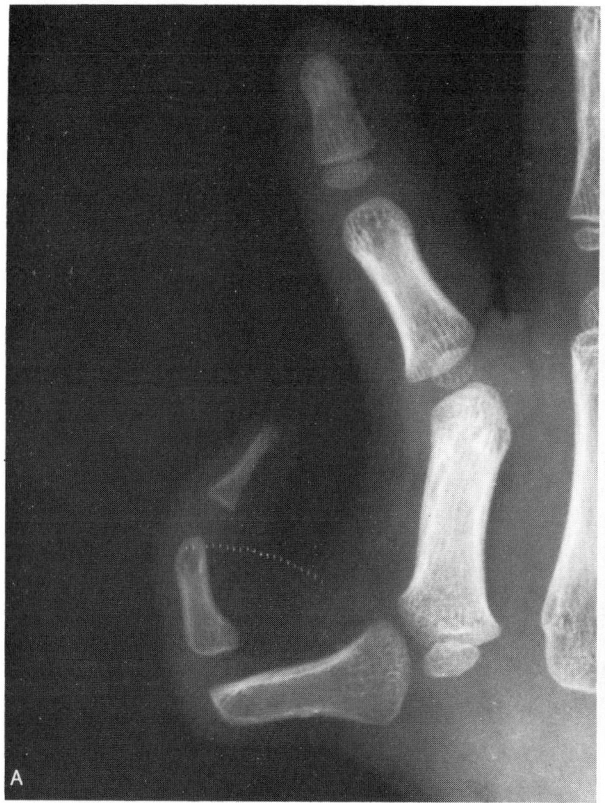

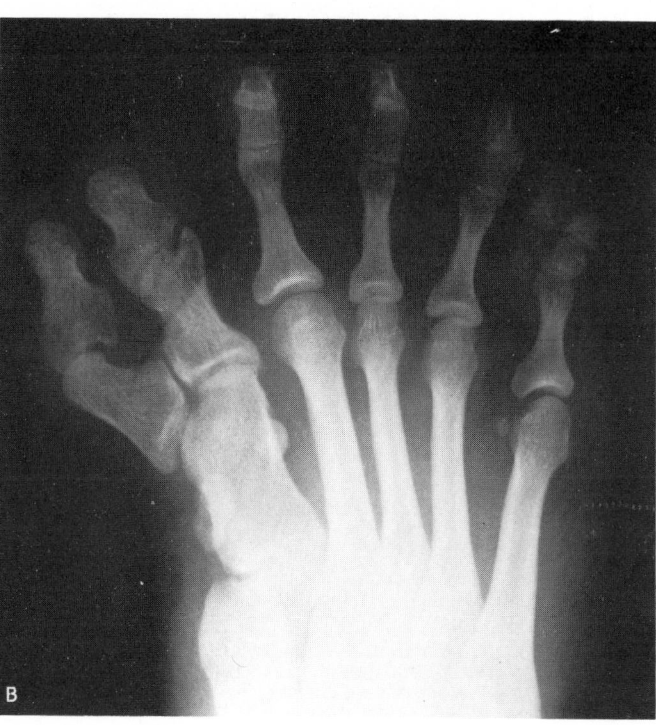

Figure 73–8. Polydactyly.

A *Hand: Preaxial polydactyly has resulted in an extra digit adjacent to the thumb.*

B *Foot: Observe the extra digit medial to the great toe, which is associated with deformity of the adjacent phalanges, metatarsals, and tarsal bones. Also note extra phalanges in the fifth toe.*

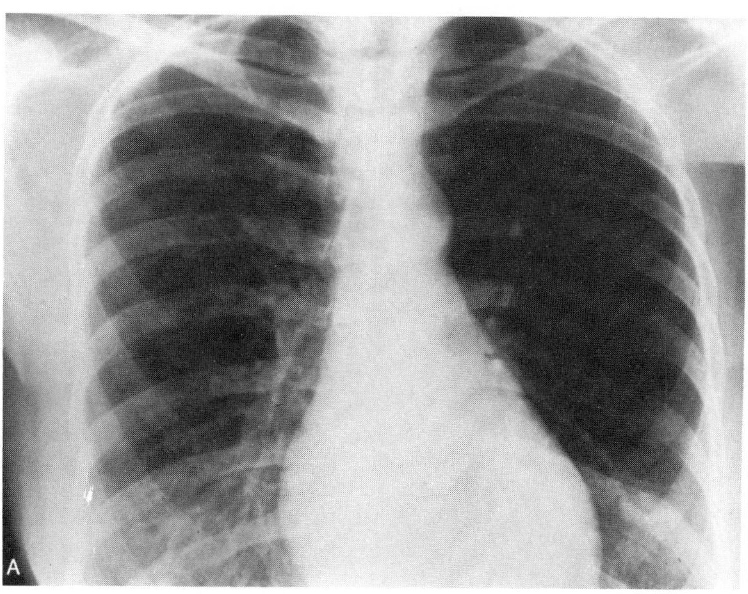

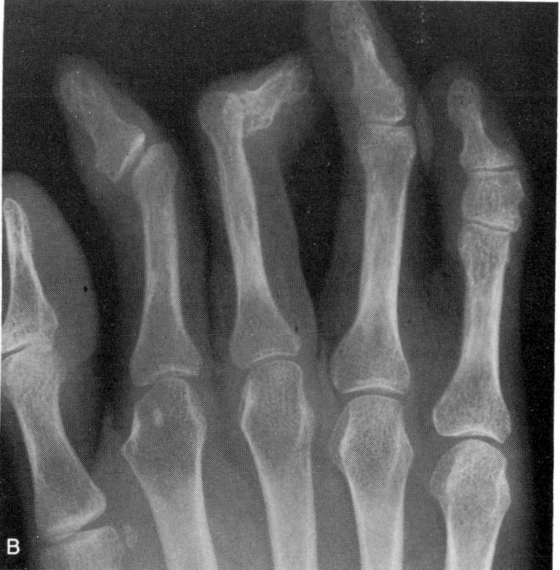

Figure 73–9. Poland's syndrome.

A *Note the absence of the left pectoral muscles, creating increased lucency of the left hemithorax. Elevation of the scapula and deformity of the ribs are also seen.*

B *The involved hand reveals aplasia (second, third, and fourth digits) and hypoplasia (fifth digit) of the middle phalanges, partial soft tissue syndactyly between the fourth and fifth and between the second and third fingers, and osseous deformities.*

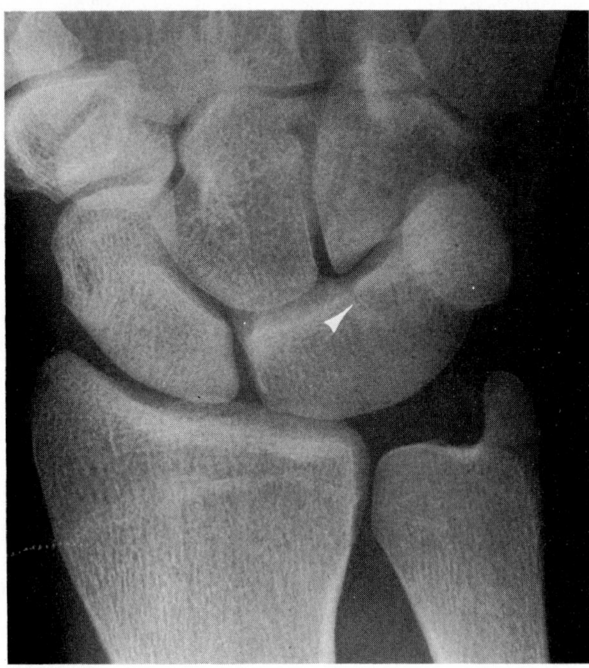

Figure 73–10. Carpal fusion (coalition). Note the bony fusion between the lunate and the triquetrum with a small cleft (arrowhead) at the site of ankylosis.

generally associated with additional malformations. The associated alterations may include tarsal coalition or one of a variety of congenital syndromes, such as acrocephalosyndactyly syndrome, arthrogryposis, diastrophic dwarfism, Ellis-van Creveld syndrome, hand-foot-uterus syndrome, Holt-Oram syndrome, oto-palato-digital syndrome, Turner's syndrome, or symphalangism.[42] Many such carpal fusions are familial.

The anomaly develops from a failure of segmentation of the primitive cartilaginous canals with absence of joint formation.[53, 58] The osseous centers of the involved carpus coalesce at variable ages, usually between 6 and 15 years of age. On radiographs, continuous trabeculae can be traced from one bone to the next, although a small notch or cleft may remain at the site of coalition. The changes can usually be differentiated from acquired ankylosis that may accompany infection, certain arthritides, such as juvenile chronic arthritis and rheumatoid arthritis, trauma, and surgery.

Accessory Carpal Bones

A number of extra ossification centers may appear in the wrist adjacent to the eight normal carpal bones. These have been well described by Poznanski.[42] Although they produce no symptoms or signs, they must be differentiated from chip fractures. In addition, certain ossicles are associated with specific malformation syndromes. Accessory bones in the distal carpal row can accompany diastrophic dwarfism, Ellis-van Creveld syndrome, Larson's syndrome, oto-palato-digital syndrome, and brachydactyly A-1. The os centrale or remnant of a central row of carpal bones can be noted in the hand-foot-uterus syndrome, Holt-Oram syndrome, oto-palato-digital syndrome, and Larsen's syndrome.

Radioulnar Synostosis

A common site of osseous fusion in the tubular bones of the extremities is between the proximal radius and ulna[59] (Fig. 73–11). Two distinct types are recognized: proximal or true radioulnar synostosis, in which the radius and ulna are smoothly fused at their proximal borders for a distance of about 2 to 6 cm; and a second variety, in which fusion just distal to the proximal radial epiphysis is associated with congenital dislocation of the radial head.[60] In both types, there is interference with normal forearm supination. The condition is bilateral in distribution in approximately 60 per cent of patients, affecting men and women equally. Sporadically occurring examples appear more often than familial cases. Radioulnar synostosis is regarded as an anomaly of longitudinal segmentation in which, instead of the formation of the superior radioulnar joint space, the interzonal mesenchyme persists, undergoing chondrification and ossification.

Additional anomalies that may accompany radioulnar synostosis are clubbed feet, congenital dislocation of the hip, knee anomalies, hypoplasia of the thumb, carpal fusion, symphalangism, and Madelung's deformity. Radioulnar synostosis may also appear as part of arthrogryposis, multiple hereditary exostosis, acrocephalopolysyndactyly, acrocephalosyndactyly, Holt-Oram syndrome, mandibulofacial dysostosis, Nievergelt-Pearlman syndrome, Klinefelter's syndrome, and other chromosomal aberrations, including those with excessive X chromosomes (XXXXY, XXXY, or XXYY).[60, 61] Furthermore, such synostosis can be acquired when osseous proliferation of one or both bones appears in the course of infection or infantile cortical hyperostosis.

The diagnosis of congenital radioulnar synostosis is not difficult when the ossified bridge has formed, appearing as a bar that may eventually engulf the radial head. Prior to such ossification, the continuous cartilaginous tissue extending between the proximal radius and ulna is radiographically invisible, although abnormal traction or tethering can produce secondary changes in the adjacent osseous tissue. Lateral bowing of the distal radius may accompany this synostosis.

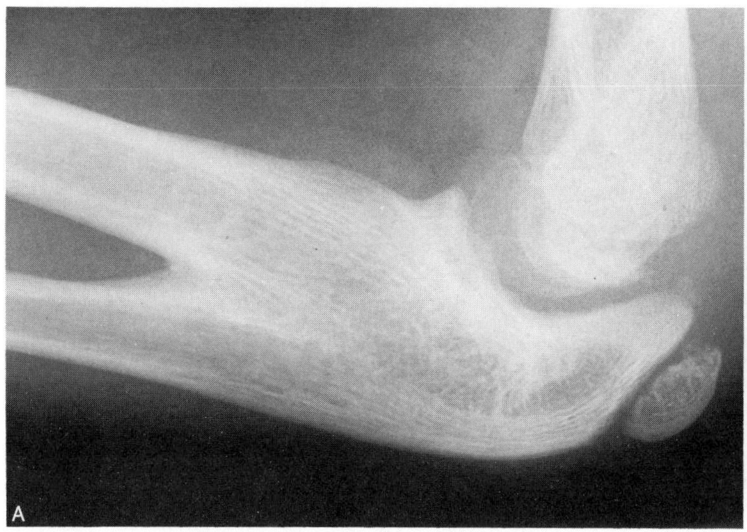

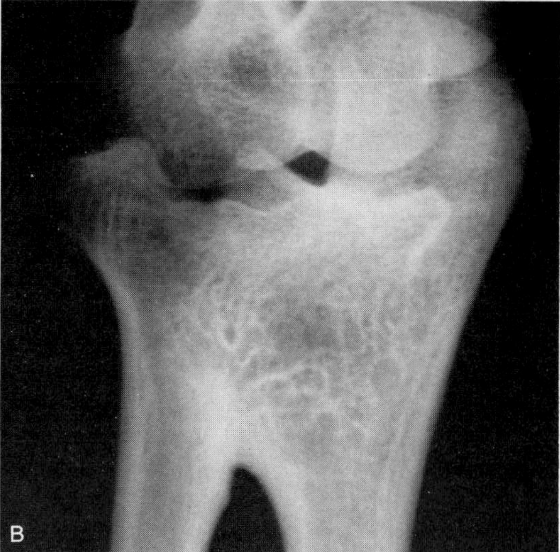

Figure 73–11. *Radioulnar synostosis.*

A *In this patient, note smooth osseous fusion of the proximal segments of the radius and the ulna.*

B *In a different patient; fusion has occurred just distal to the proximal border of the radius, and there is a congenital dislocation of the radial head.*

Tarsal Fusion (Coalition)

Tarsal coalition represents an abnormal fusion of one or more of the tarsalia. The union may be fibrous, cartilaginous, or osseous and can be congenital or acquired in response to infection, trauma, articular disorders, or surgery.

Congenital tarsal coalition is of unknown etiology. It appears to arise on the basis of a failure of differentiation and segmentation of the primitive mesenchyme that results in lack of formation of intervening articulations, a theory that gains support from the identification of such anomalies in the fetus,[62] although in 1896, Pfitzner[63] proposed that tarsal coalitions were caused by the incorporation of accessory ossicles into adjacent tarsal bones, a suggestion that was supported at least in part by later investigators.[64-67] The observation of similar changes in fetuses discounts such a proposal. In some cases, a familial history of identical abnormalities is obtained.[68-70] In fact, Leonard[71] reported that 39 per cent of 98 first-degree relatives of 31 patients with peroneal spastic flatfoot and partial coalition had some type of fusion, although the presence and degree of symptoms and signs and the pattern of ankylosis varied among some patients and relatives. He suggested that the disorder was of autosomal dominant inheritance with genetic variability of expression. It appears that familial factors are indeed important in some cases, particularly those with massive tarsal fusions.

The condition dates from antiquity, cases having been found in pre-Columbian Indian skeletons.[72] Despite an early description of peroneal spastic flatfoot by Sir Robert Jones in 1897,[73] it was not until 1921 that a relationship of this clinical entity and tarsal coalition was documented.[64] This association is now well recognized,[65, 74] although it is not uniform in all cases of peroneal spastic flatfoot; other conditions, such as juvenile chronic arthritis, tuberculosis, osteoarthritis, and fracture can cause a similar clinical problem. Typically, symptoms and signs of tarsal coalition appear in the second or third decades of life; an earlier age of onset is rare, perhaps owing to the fact that the fusion is fibrous or cartilaginous in the young child or adolescent, and only with the appearance of ossification do pain and restricted motion become evident. Following minor trauma or unusual activity, the affected individual complains of vague pain in the foot, aggravated by prolonged standing or athletic endeavor.[75] Limited subtalar motion, pes planus, and shortening with persistent or intermittent spasm of the peroneal muscles are seen on physical examination. The rigid foot may be held in a valgus attitude, although anterior tibial spasm can lead to varus deformity.[76, 77] Coalition can also present with a cavus foot[78, 79] or as an incidental finding in an asymptomatic individual.

Isolated partial coalitions can be classified according to the bones that are affected; calcaneonavicular, talocalcaneal, talonavicular, and calcaneocuboid fusions, in order of decreasing frequency, can be detected. Tarsal fusions accompanying multiple malformation syndromes may have "atypical" patterns or may involve the entire tarsus.[80] In the oto-palato-digital syndrome and the hand-foot-uterus syndrome, coalition among the cuneiforms and metatarsal bases may be encountered.[81, 82] Tarsal fusions may also accompany hereditary symphalangism,[48, 83] arthrogryposis,[84] acrocephalosyndactyly (Apert's syndrome),[85] and many other disorders.[1, 2] Identification of the nature and extent of a coalition frequently requires routine radiography supplemented with special views, tomography, and even arthrography.[75, 86-88]

Calcaneonavicular Coalition. This type of coalition is one of the most frequent and can be asymptomatic or associated with rigid flatfoot. In general, symptoms and signs are less severe than those accompanying talocalcaneal coalitions, and "secondary" radiographic abnormalities may be less marked. Coalition is optimally identified on a 45 degree medial-oblique view of the foot and may, in fact, be completely overlooked on anteroposterior and lateral projections[89] (Fig. 73–12). The diagnosis is simplified by the presence of a solid bony bar extending between the calcaneus and the navicular bone but is more difficult in cases of cartilaginous or fibrous coalition. Normally, an articulation does not exist between the two bones; a close approximation of their bony contours, especially if adjacent eburnation or sclerosis is evident, should raise the possibility of a nonosseous coalition. Bony fusion may be identified between the ages of 8 and 12 years. A secondary roentgenographic sign of calcaneonavicular coalition is hypoplasia of the head of the talus.[90] Talar "beaking" is uncommon and, when present, may be the result of an associated talocalcaneal fusion.

Talocalcaneal Coalition. This represents the other common type of tarsal coalition. Almost all such fusion occurs at the middle facet, between the talus and sustentaculum tali (Fig. 73–13); ankylosis of the posterior subtalar joint or of the anterior facets is far less frequent (Fig. 73–14). The condition is more common in boys than in girls and is bilateral in 20 to 25 per cent of patients. Cartilaginous, fibrous, or bony bridges may be identified, although radiographic evaluation often requires special views in addition to standard anteroposterior and lateral projections. A penetrated axial radiograph (Harris-Beath view) obtained with varying degrees of beam angulation, oblique roentgenograms, and anterior and lateral tomograms may be necessary. These techniques may identify the actual site of osseous fusion, although closely apposed and irregular bony articular surfaces can indicate the presence of bridging fibrous or cartilaginous tissue. In the latter instances, arthrography of the talocalcaneonavicular articulation may be helpful; contrast medium introduced into the talonavicular space of this joint will fail to flow beneath the anterior aspect of the talus and over the sustentaculum tali owing to the abnormal tissue elements[91] (see Chapter 15).

Fortunately, a number of secondary radiograph-

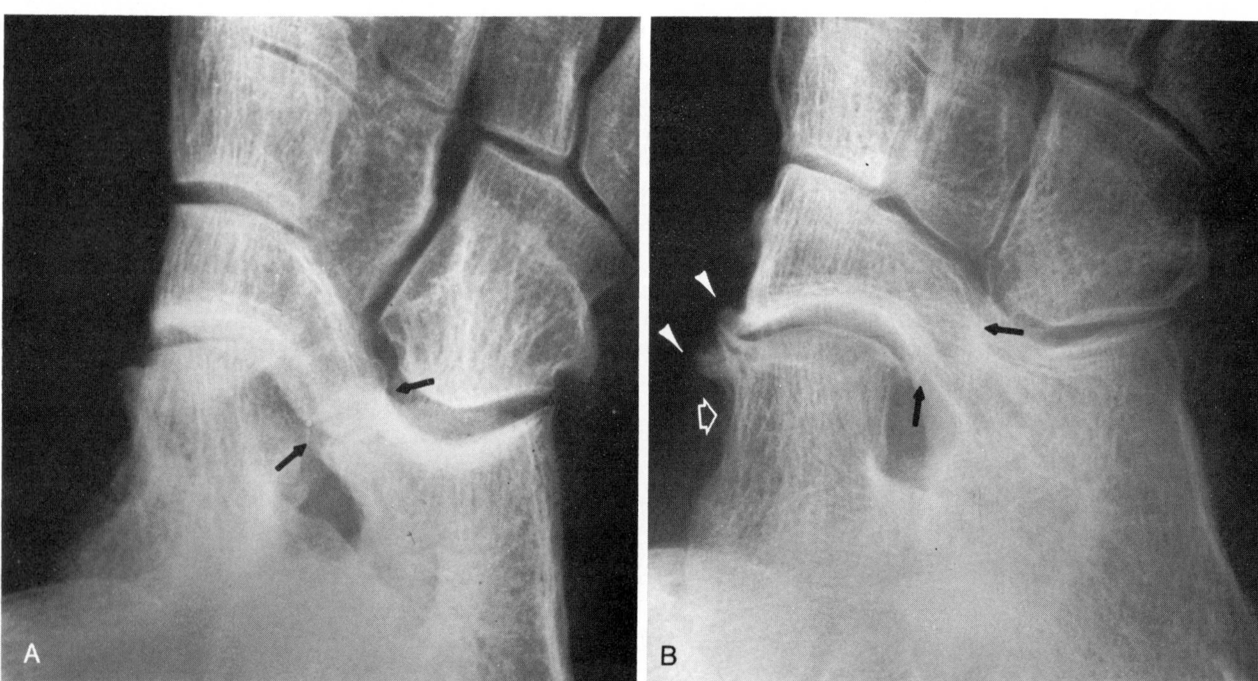

Figure 73–12. *Calcaneonavicular tarsal coalition.*

A *Observe the approximation of the osseous surfaces of the calcaneus and navicular bone (arrows) on the medial oblique view. Mild abnormalities are apparent at the calcaneocuboid articulation.*

B *In this patient, a complete osseous coalition (solid arrows) is evident on the medial oblique view. Observe the bony excrescences at the talonavicular joint space (arrowheads) and hypoplasia of the distal aspect of the talus (open arrow).*

Illustration continued on the opposite page

ic signs have been described in association with talocalcaneal coalition[75, 86] (Fig. 73–13). These include the following:

1. Talar beaking: Dorsal subluxation of the navicular bone produced by subtalar rigidity leads to elevation of the periosteum below the talonavicular ligament with subperiosteal proliferation and the production of a beak or excrescence at the dorsal surface of the talar head adjacent to the talonavicular space, best identified on lateral projections. A similar but less constant outgrowth occurs on the adjacent navicular bone. This "beak" is not pathognomonic of talocalcaneal coalition; it may be identified in other conditions associated with abnormal motion at the talonavicular space, such as rheumatoid arthritis. A similar beak may be identified in diffuse idiopathic skeletal hyperostosis and acromegaly. Osseous excrescences at the talonavicular space or on the dorsal aspect of the proximal navicular bone related to osteoarthritis of the midfoot or ankle (respectively) are easily differentiated from the talar beak of talocalcaneal coalition.

2. Broadening of the lateral process of the talus: Broadening or rounding of this process is easily identified when comparison views of the opposite

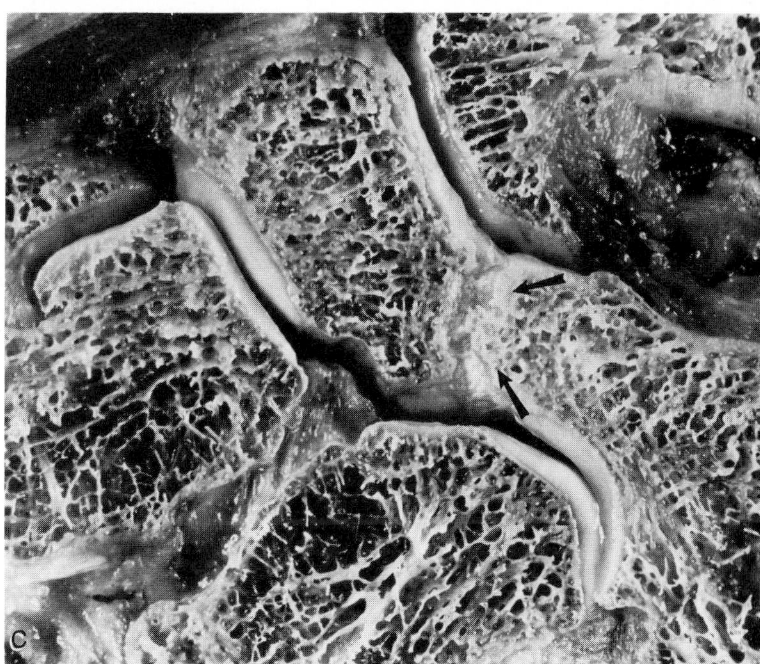

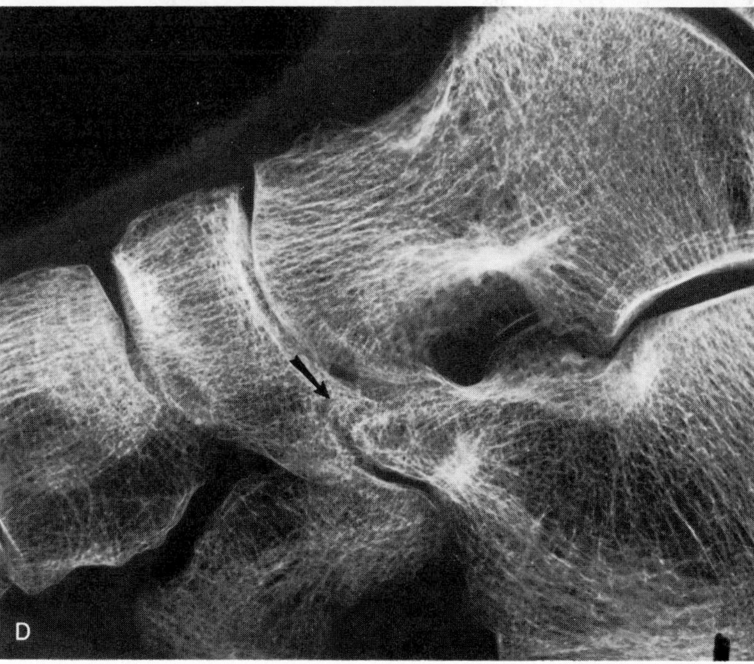

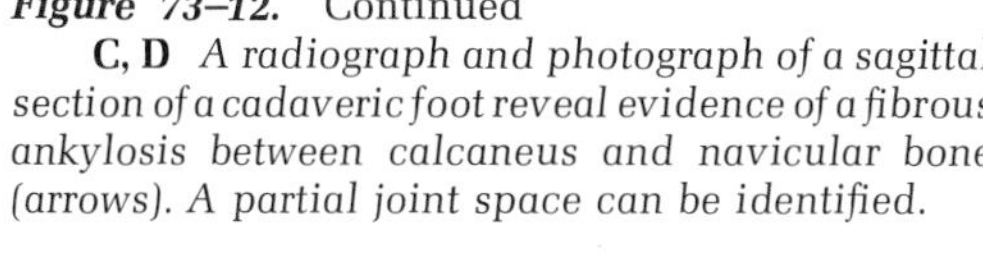

Figure 73–12. Continued

C, D *A radiograph and photograph of a sagittal section of a cadaveric foot reveal evidence of a fibrous ankylosis between calcaneus and navicular bone (arrows). A partial joint space can be identified.*

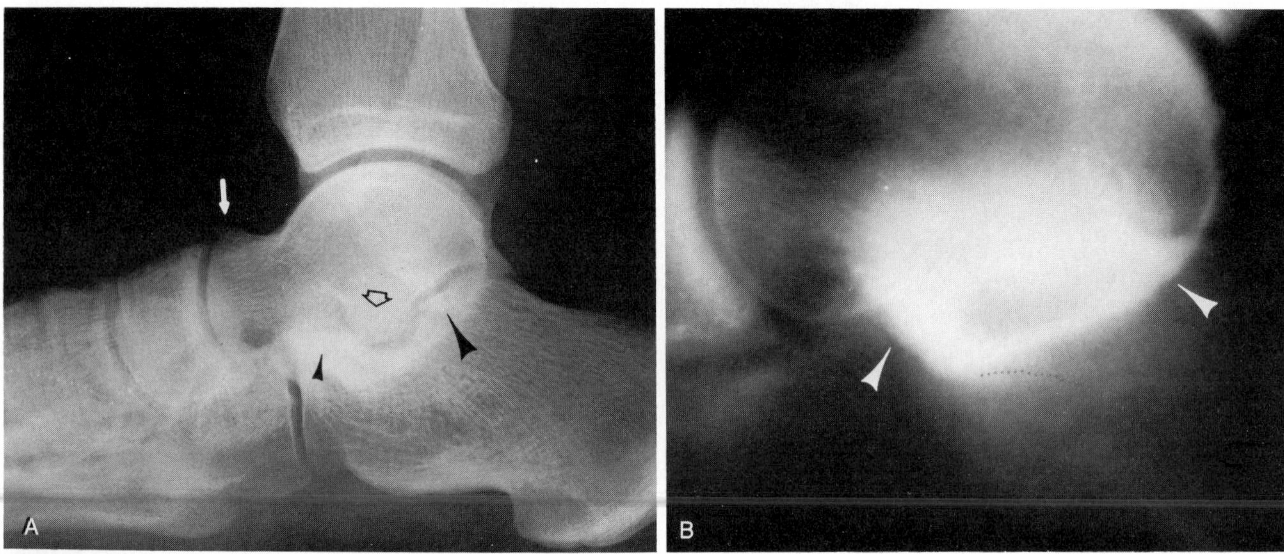

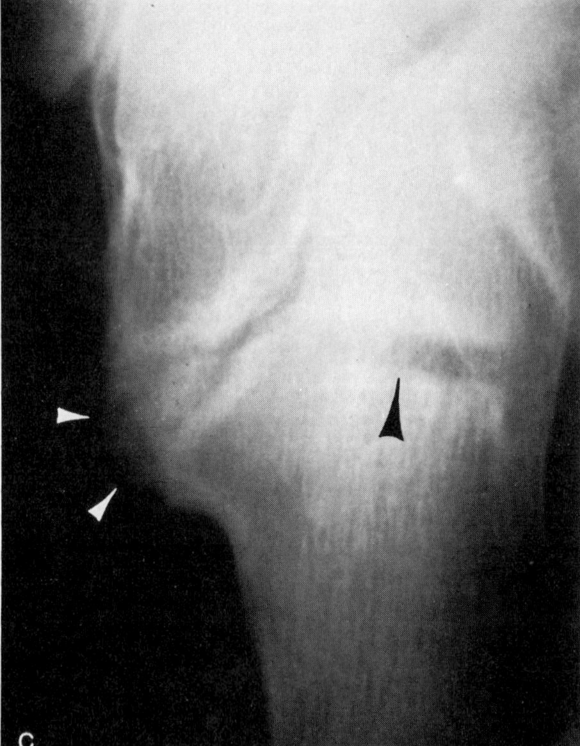

Figure 73–13. *Talocalcaneal tarsal coalition: Middle facet.*

A *A lateral radiograph reveals talar beaking (solid arrow), broadening of the lateral process of the talus (open arrow), narrowing of the posterior subtalar joint (large arrowhead), and absence of visualization of the space between the sustentaculum tali and talus ("middle" subtalar joint) (small arrowhead).*

B *A lateral tomogram identifies the bony bridge between talus and calcaneus (arrowheads).*

C *In a different patient, a Harris-Beath view outlines partial bony ankylosis (small arrowheads) between the sustentaculum tali and talus. Note the intact posterior subtalar joint (large arrowhead).*

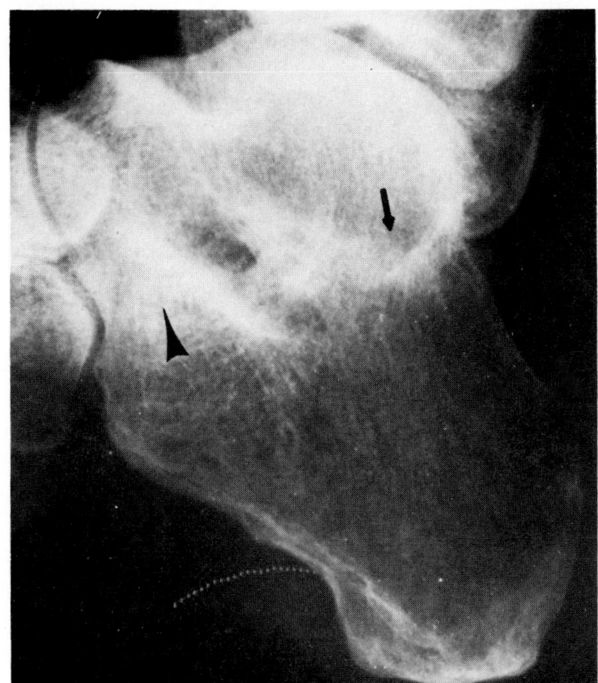

Figure 73–14. *Talocalcaneal tarsal coalition: Anterior, middle, and posterior facets. Observe bony ankylosis of the anterior and middle facets (arrowhead) and the posterior facet (arrow). A calcaneus deformity of the hindfoot is evident.*

(uninvolved) foot are part of the roentgenographic examination. It is present in 40 to 60 per cent of patients, may occur in the absence of a talar beak, and is apparently related to a valgus angulation of the calcaneus.

3. Narrowing of the posterior subtalar joint: This finding can be evident in as many as 50 to 60 per cent of patients with or without additional secondary signs of coalition and represents degenerative arthritis or a nontangential position of the articular surface due to calcaneal eversion.

4. Concave undersurface of the talar neck and asymmetry of the talocalcaneonavicular joint: Comparison views are helpful in the detection of this sign, although care must be taken to insure that similar projections are available on both sides.

5. Failure of visualization of the "middle" subtalar joint: The inability to identify this articulation on lateral views is a useful finding but is one that is difficult to apply in some cases owing to a faulty position of the foot.

6. Ball and socket ankle joint: A rounded, convex appearance of the proximal talar articular surface and a concomitant concave appearance of the distal tibia may accompany talocalcaneal coalition, presumably owing to an adaptation of the ankle joint to provide the inversion and eversion function that is restricted at the talocalcaneal articulations[92-95] (Fig. 73–15). This change may also accompany other congenital anomalies, including short extremities and hypoplasia or aplasia of the fibula. Ball and socket ankle joints may also result from acquired disorders of the midfoot, although the degree and smoothness of the deformity are less in the acquired conditions (Fig. 73–16).

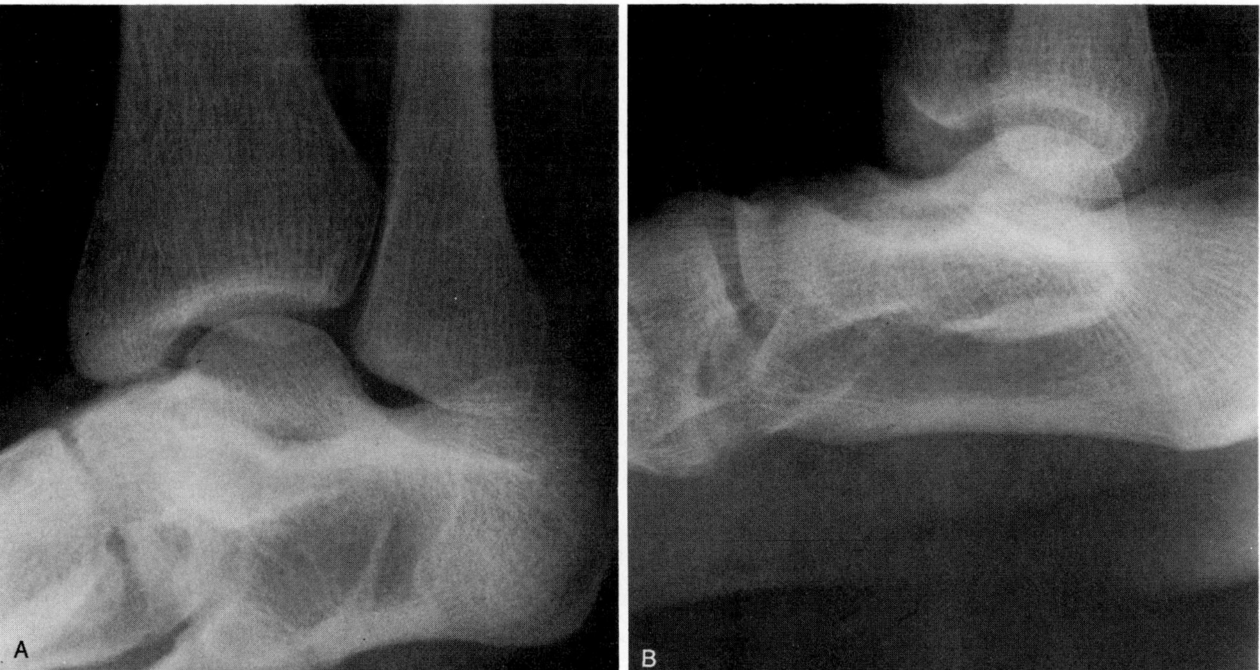

Figure 73–15. *Tarsal coalition with ball-and-socket ankle joint (congenital coalition).*

A, B *Oblique and lateral radiographs outline bony coalition among most of the tarsal bones, including the talocalcaneal articulations. Note the ball-and-socket appearance of the ankle with associated deformity of the distal fibula.*

Illustration continued on the following page

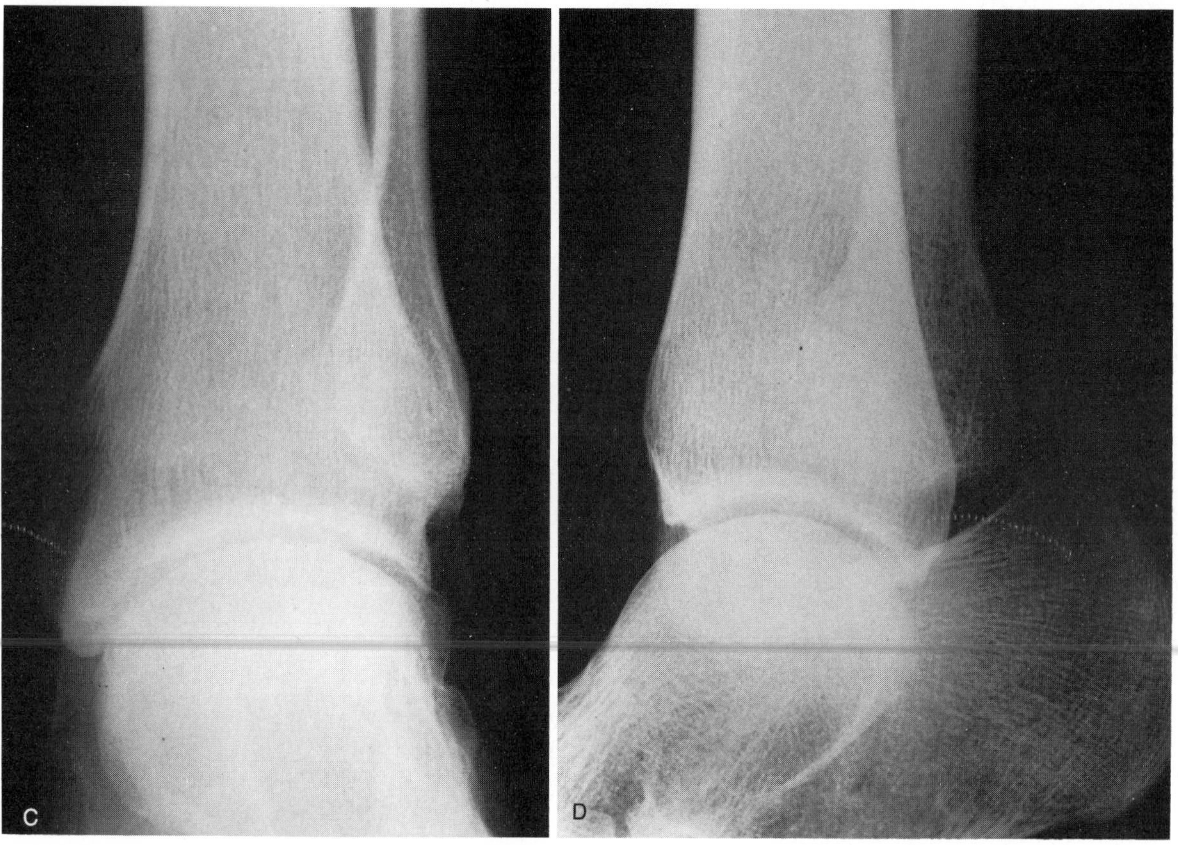

Figure 73–15. Continued

C, D *In a different patient, talocalcaneal coalition is again associated with a ball-and-socket ankle joint and with a shortened fibula.* (**C, D,** Courtesy of *Dr. F. Brahme, University Hospital, University of California, San Diego, California.*)

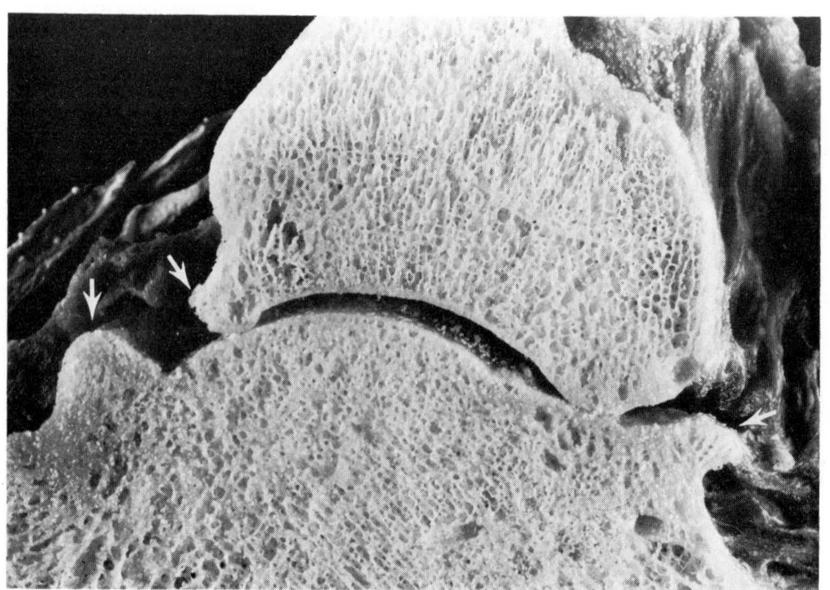

Figure 73–16. *Tarsal coalition with ball-and-socket ankle joint (acquired coalition). A surgical fusion of the talocalcaneal articulations can be associated with deformity of the ankle. The degree of deformity is greater in those cases in which ankylosis occurs at a young age. In this case, a photograph of a sagittal section of the ankle of the cadaver indicates rounding of the talar surface and spur formation (arrows).*

Talonavicular Coalition. This is an uncommon type of coalition that may reveal an autosomal dominant[96, 97] or recessive[98] hereditary transmission and an association with anomalies of the little finger.[97] Patients may be asymptomatic or may have peroneal spasm. Radiography usually outlines the osseous bridge, and little difficulty in diagnosis is encountered (Fig. 73–17).

Other Coalitions. Calcaneocuboid coalitions are very rare, are readily identified on radiographs, and may be asymptomatic or associated with peroneal spasm.[99-101] A bilateral or unilateral distribution can be seen, and other anomalies may coexist. Isolated examples of cubonavicular and naviculocuneiform coalitions have been reported.[102-105]

Klippel-Feil Syndrome

The term Klippel-Feil deformity is loosely applied to many types of congenital fusions of the cervical vertebrae, yet the original syndrome, as described by Klippel and Feil in 1912,[106, 107] consisted of a triad of signs: a short neck, a low posterior hairline, and a limitation of movement of the neck. These easily recognized clinical manifestations are present at birth, yet the relatively minor nature of the affliction may delay the patient's presentation to a physician until the second or third decade of life. At this time, in addition to the physical signs noted previously, neurologic abnormalities may be present. As currently applied, the designation of the Klippel-Feil syndrome indicates a congenital fusion of two or more cervical vertebrae, yet the classic triad is not apparent in more than 50 per cent of such patients.

The reported incidence of congenital cervical vertebral fusion has varied considerably. Some investigators regard the finding as exceedingly rare,[108] whereas others report its occurence in almost 0.5 per cent of spinal roentgenograms.[109] Men and women are affected with approximately equal frequency. The level and extent of cervical involvement are not constant. In most cases, fusion begins at the occiput and the first cervical vertebra, at the first and second cervical vertebrae, or at the second and third cervical vertebrae[110] (Fig. 73–18). With involvement of the upper cervical region, the segment of the second and third vertebrae represents a typical distal location of the fusion; with involvement of the lower cervical region, it is the segment between the sixth and seventh vertebrae that generally denotes the distal extent of disease. The joints of the second and third and fifth and sixth cervical vertebrae are most frequently altered. Occasionally, cases involve upper thoracic vertebrae as well, usually ending at the fourth and fifth thoracic levels. These findings are not constant, nor is the fusion solid throughout its extent. In some instances, one or more intervening levels may not be affected. This allows for some degree of motion in involved spinal segments.

Patients with a Klippel-Feil or related deformity usually do not reveal evidence of a familial history of disease; exceptions to this rule occur, as evidenced by several reports.[111, 112] On clinical examination, the patient has a short neck, which, when the syndrome is severe, may create the illusion that the head is resting directly on the thorax. Restriction of motion may be marked, particularly that of lateral motion rather than flexion and extension. Torticollis can be present in some cases. Neurologic abnormalities are variable and may include spasticity, hyperreflexia, pain, muscle atrophy, oculomotor disturbances,

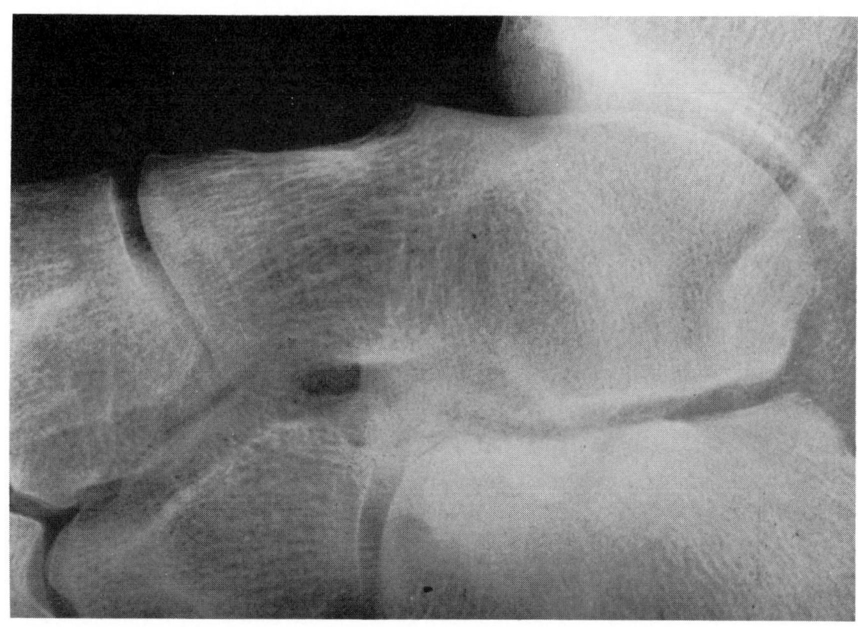

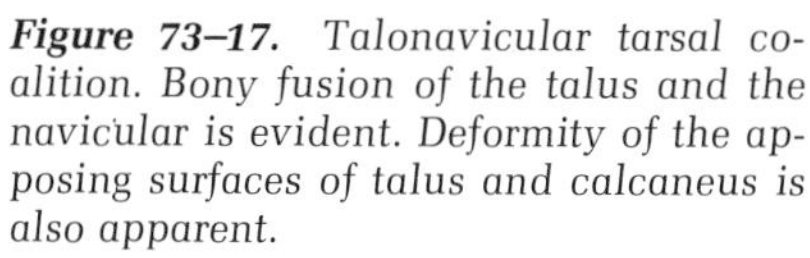

Figure 73–17. *Talonavicular tarsal coalition. Bony fusion of the talus and the navicular is evident. Deformity of the apposing surfaces of talus and calcaneus is also apparent.*

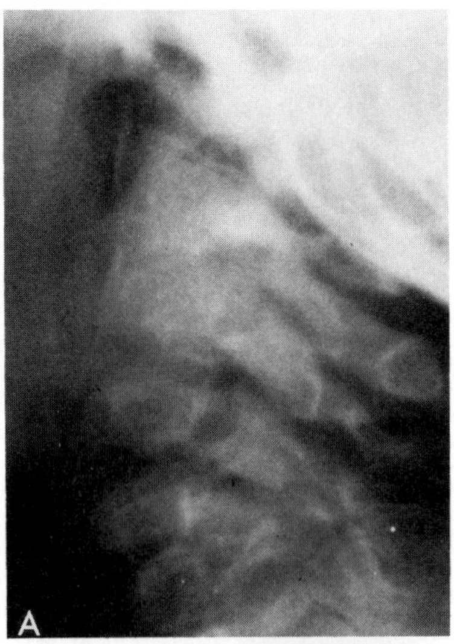

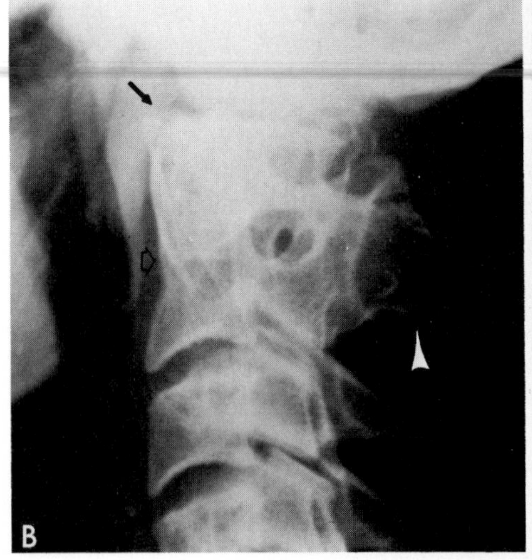

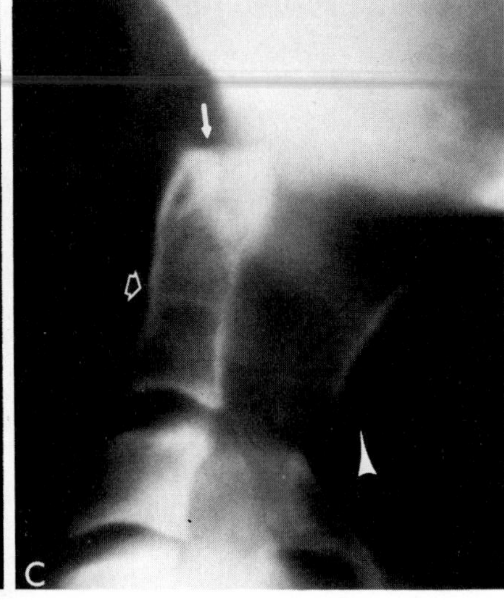

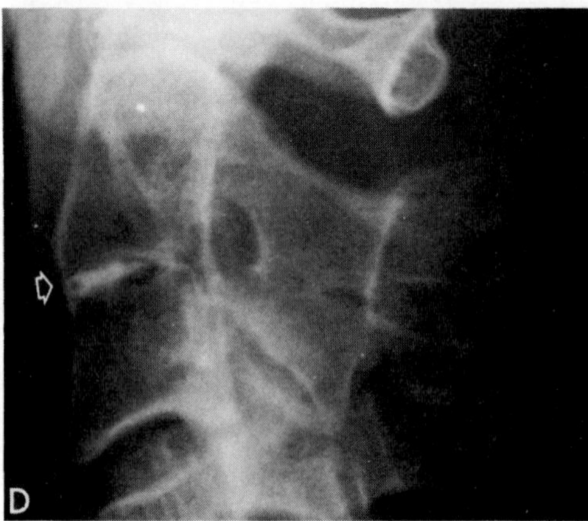

Figure 73–18. Klippel-Feil syndrome.

A *Observe bony fusion of the atlas and the axis with deformity of the base of the skull. Both the vertebral bodies and the posterior elements are involved.*

B, C *In a different patient, lateral radiography and tomography indicate osseous fusion of cervical vertebrae. Note the incorporation of the odontoid process into the anterior arch of the atlas (solid arrow), the narrowed "waist" of the fused vertebral bodies (open arrow), and ankylosis of the posterior elements including the spinous processes (arrowhead).*

D *In a third patient, fusion of the second and third cervical vertebrae is seen. Note the ankylosis of the posterior elements and the atrophic intervertebral disc containing calcification (open arrow).*

pyramidal tract findings, paralysis, anesthesia, and paresthesia. In the presence of high cervical fusions, neurologic findings tend to be more prominent and appear earlier in the course of the disease.

Many associated malformations have been described.[110]

1. Sprengel's deformity: Unilateral or bilateral elevation of the scapula is present in approximately 20 to 25 per cent of cases, especially in those with high and extensive cervical fusions (Fig. 73–19). It may be associated with an omovertebral bone connecting the scapula and vertebrae. This bone, which is present in approximately 30 to 40 per cent of cases of fixed elevated scapula, is not always ossified.[453] It may consist of osseous, cartilaginous, or fibrous tissue, and the connection between scapula and omovertebral element may be cartilaginous, bony, or fibrous[472] in nature, or possess a true joint. The connection is usually at the middle to lower portion of the vertebral border of the scapula. Alterations of the adjacent clavicle may be evident.

2. Cervical ribs: Anomalous ribs are evident in approximately 10 to 15 per cent of cases, most frequently in women.

3. Webbed neck (pterygium colli): Webbing of the soft tissues on each side may accentuate the shortness of the neck and may involve the skin, muscles, and fascia. Reports of cervical spinal fusions and webbed necks in patients with Turner's syndrome have also appeared.[113]

4. Hemivertebrae: This manifestation is present in approximately 15 to 20 per cent of cases and can lead to scoliosis.

5. Spina bifida: Anterior or posterior spina bifida is frequent in patients with cervical fusions. The abnormalities may be apparent in one or more levels in the cervical or thoracic regions.

6. Other anomalies: Kyphosis, scoliosis, fused, absent, or deformed ribs, basilar impression, cranial asymmetry, deformed dens, cleft palate, supernumerary lobes of the lung, patent foramen ovale, interventricular septal defect, renal anomalies, and enteric cysts or duplications represent some of the additional malformations that may be apparent.[114-116]

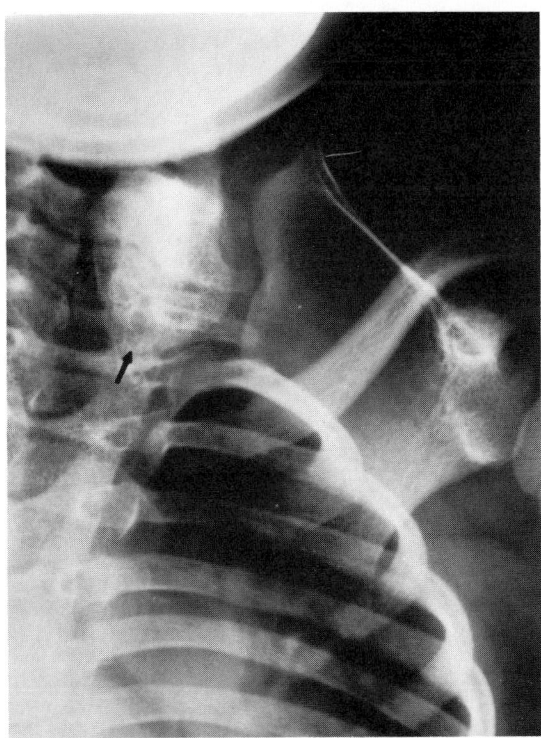

Figure 73–19. *Klippel-Feil syndrome with Sprengel's deformity. Note the elevated position of the scapula, an omovertebral bone (arrow), and cervical spinal abnormalities.*

On roentgenograms, the fusion may be partial or complete and may affect the vertebral bodies, the pedicles, the laminae, or the spinous processes (Fig. 73–18). Initially detected changes may progress in severity and extent on serial roentgenograms.[118, 467] With fusion of the vertebral bodies, small atrophic intervertebral discs may be apparent, which can contain calcification. The anteroposterior diameter of the vertebral bodies at the level of an affected discovertebral junction may be smaller than that at the superior and inferior limits of the vertebrae adjacent to uninvolved discs. The resulting trapezoidal shape of the vertebral body is very suggestive of a congenital fusion or at least one that has occurred at an early age, as it is related to the interference with normal growth at the site of fusion; continued growth at the unaffected aspects of the vertebrae then produces the altered vertebral shape that is characteristic of the condition.

The Klippel-Feil deformity apparently results from an insult to the developing fetus, preventing normal embryogenesis. Oxygen deprivation in rabbits during the 9th to 11th days of gestation can lead to vertebral anomalies in the offspring, a period corresponding to the 25th day of gestation in humans.[116] Gardner and Collis[117] have postulated that overdistention of the neural tube in embryonal life is a common factor in the pathogenesis of the Klippel-Feil syndrome, syringomyelia, diastematomyelia, meningomyelocele, and the Arnold-Chiari syndrome, although this theory may be an oversimplification of the processes leading to varied spinal malformations.[110] Additional factors, such as hereditary effects and chromosomal abnormalities, have yet to be fully explored.

The radiographic features of a congenital fusion of cervical vertebral bodies must be distinguished from those in acquired cases of ankylosis (Fig. 73–20). Although this is not always possible, the following signs are helpful in the diagnosis of Klippel-Feil syndrome and related anomalies: trapezoidal shape of vertebral bodies with intervening atrophic intervertebral discs, irregularity of the intervertebral foramina, and fusion of both the anterior (vertebral bodies and intervertebral discs) and posterior (pedicles, laminae, spinous processes) columns of the spine. Application of these criteria in the evaluation of spinal radiographs may allow differentiation of congenital fusion from other processes, particularly juvenile chronic arthritis, yet a review of some of the earlier reports of Klippel-Feil syndrome indicates that cases of juvenile chronic arthritis were included in the analyses. Although it is the clinical history that is most helpful in differentiation between these two conditions, the radiographic findings of juvenile chronic arthritis do not include ankylosis of adjacent spinous processes. Furthermore, in this articular disease, abnormalities of other skeletal sites are apparent, and an elevated position of the scapula is not seen. In ankylosing spondylitis, ankylosis of vertebral bodies and apophyseal joints is noted, but the size of the vertebrae and intervertebral discs is not diminutive. Differentiation of congenital cervical fusion from tuberculosis and traumatic and surgical changes is usually not difficult.

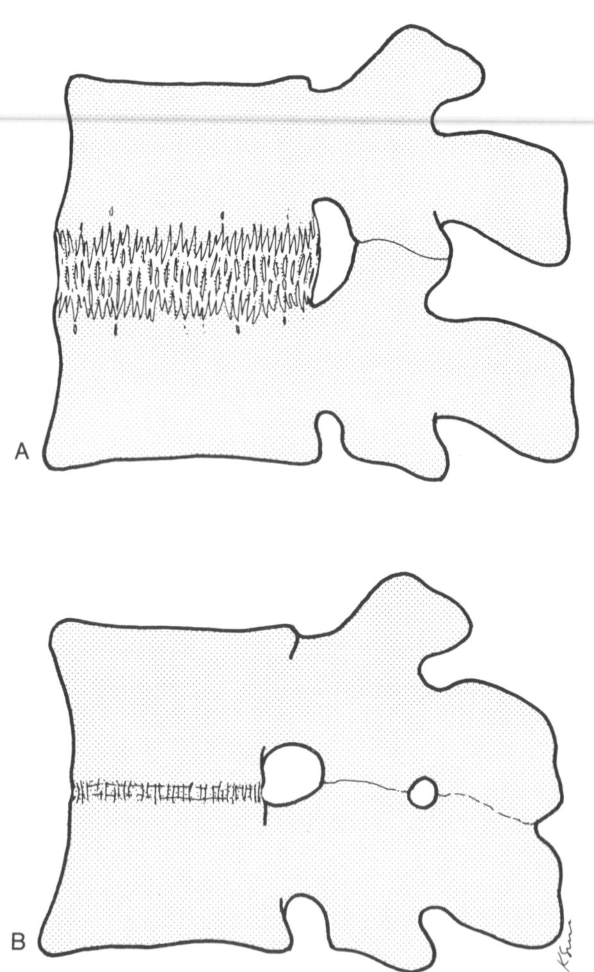

Figure 73–20. Acquired versus congenital vertebral fusion.

A Acquired ankylosis. Note the absence of constriction at the level of the intervertebral disc and the absence of posterior element fusion.

B Congenital ankylosis. A constricted appearance at the level of the intervertebral disc has produced a trapezoidal shape of the bony mass. The posterior elements are also ankylosed, and the intervertebral disc is atrophic.

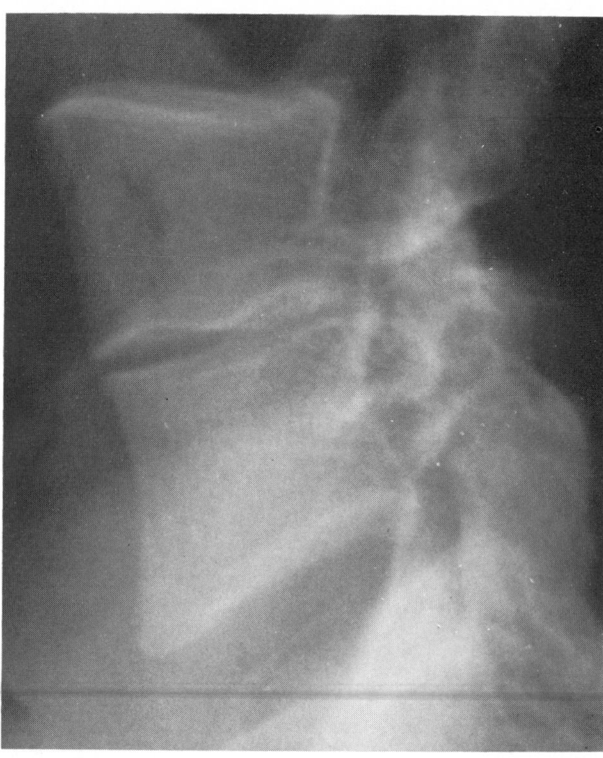

Figure 73–21. Congenital block vertebrae: Lumbar spine. Note incomplete fusion between the fourth and fifth lumbar vertebral bodies. The intervertebral disc is atrophic and the anteroposterior width of the vertebral bodies at the site of fusion is less than at the uninvolved portions of the bodies, creating a trapezoidal vertebral shape.

Congenital Block Vertebrae

Congenital synostosis of vertebrae in the thoracic and lumbar spine may also be encountered, again related to a derangement of embryologic development (Fig. 73–21). The anomaly is usually limited in extent, affecting two adjacent vertebrae, and is commonly asymptomatic, being discovered on roentgenograms obtained for other reasons. The fusion typically affects the vertebral bodies, although the posterior elements can also be incorporated into an ossified mass. The intervening intervertebral disc is atrophic and calcified or completely obliterated. Partial fusion of one side of the vertebrae can lead to scoliosis or other abnormalities of spinal curvature. The same radiographic guidelines noted in the discussion of the Klippel-Feil syndrome apply to the recognition of congenital fusion of thoracic and lumbar vertebrae.

ARTICULAR ABNORMALITIES

Madelung's Deformity

In 1878, Madelung[119] described a painful wrist deformity in a young woman that he considered the result of an overloading of an articulation that was already predisposed to malformation. Subsequently, Madelung's deformity has attracted the attention of numerous investigators.[120-125] The primary deformity is a bowing of the distal end of the radius. Typically, the radial bowing occurs in a volar direction while the ulna continues to grow in a straight fashion. The curvature and growth disturbance of the radius result in its being shorter than the ulna. Thus, the ulna is relatively long in comparison to its osseous neighbor, and the carpal angle, formed by the intersection of two lines (the first tangent to the proximal surfaces of the scaphoid and the lunate bones, the second tangent to the proximal margins of the triquetrum and the lunate bones), which normally is 130 to 137°, is decreased[126, 127] (Table 73–2). In recent years, numerous roentgenographic alterations have been reported in Madelung's deformity[124] (Fig. 73–22).

1. Radial abnormalities: Dorsal and ulnar curvature, decreased length, triangularization of the distal radial epiphysis with unequal growth of the eipiphysis, premature fusion of the medial half of the radial epiphysis, a localized area of lucency along the ulnar border of the radius, osteophytosis along the inferior ulnar portion of the radius, and ulnar and volar angulation of the distal radial articular surface have been reported.
2. Ulnar abnormalities: Dorsal subluxation, enlargement and distortion of the ulnar head, and changes in length have been observed.
3. Carpal abnormalities: Wedging of the carpus between the deformed radius and protruding ulna, triangular configuration with the lunate at the apex, and arched curvature in the lateral projection as a direct continuation of the arch of posterior bowing of the radial epiphysis have occurred.

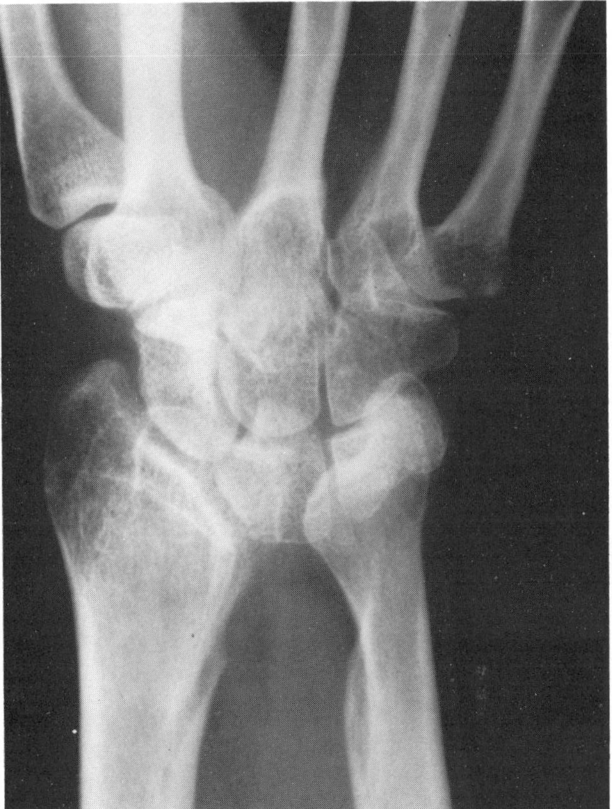

Figure 73–22. *Madelung's deformity. Abnormalities include increased width between the distal radius and distal ulna, a relatively long ulna compared to the length of the radius, a decreased carpal angle, triangularization of the distal radial epiphysis, osseous excrescences on apposing metaphyseal regions of radius and ulna, distortion of the ulnar head, and wedging of the carpus between the deformed radius and protruding ulna, with the lunate at the apex of the wedge.*

Table 73–2

SYNDROMES ASSOCIATED WITH ABNORMALITY OF THE CARPAL ANGLE

Decreased	Increased
Madelung's deformity	Arthrogryposis
Dyschondrosteosis	Diastrophic dwarfism
Turner's syndrome	Epiphyseal dysplasias
Morquio's syndrome	Frontometaphyseal dysplasia
Hurler's syndrome	Oto-palatal-digital syndrome
	Pfeiffer's syndrome
	Spondyloepiphyseal dysplasia
	Trisomy 21

(Courtesy of Poznanski AK: The Hand in Radiologic Diagnosis. Philadelphia, W. B. Saunders Co., 1974, p. 140.)

There has been much confusion regarding the etiology of this deformity. Some of this confusion was stimulated by the report in 1929 by Léri and Weill,[128] in which a case of hereditary dwarfism was characterized by a wrist alteration that appeared identical to Madelung's deformity. In addition, the forearms and the lower legs were shorter than the proximal and distal parts of the extremities. This mesomelic variety of dwarfism has become known as dyschondrosteosis, and additional reports of this disease have confirmed the constant and prominent role that Madelung's deformity assumes in its radiographic features. Considerable debate has existed regarding the relationship of dyschondrosteosis and Madelung's deformity. At the extremes are the opinions that the two are not related[129] and that they are identical syndromes.[130] It appears that this wrist deformity is frequent in patients with dyschondrosteosis but that it is also evident as an isolated phenomenon without associated dwarfism. Whether

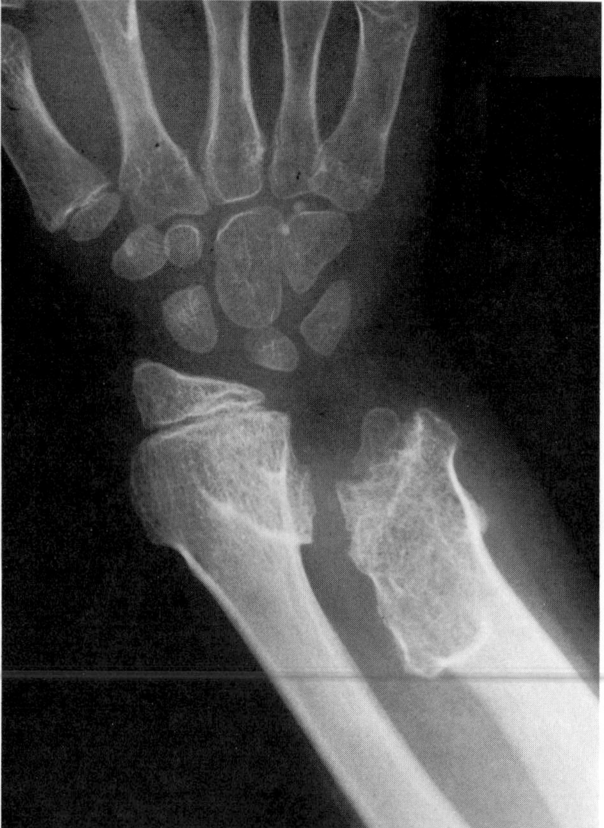

Figure 73–23. Wrist deformity in multiple hereditary exostosis. Observe broad-based exostoses of the radius and ulna with metaphyseal widening. The ulna is relatively short compared to the radius. The distal radial epiphysis is triangular in shape.

this latter pattern represents a forme fruste of dyschondrosteosis cannot be ascertained with certainty. Golding and Blackburne[129] believe that isolated Madelung's deformity is not hereditable and is restricted to women, whereas dyschondrosteosis is confined to men. Recently, Madelung's deformity has been classified into several types, including post-traumatic (due to extension injuries to the radial epiphysis), dysplastic (due to dyschondrosteosis and multiple hereditary exostoses) (Fig. 73–23), genetic (in association with Turner's syndrome), and idiopathic.[125] This classification system is complicated by the fact that the wrist abnormality in some of these conditions is not a typical Madelung's deformity but rather a "reverse" deformity in which the distal end of the radius is tilted dorsally, the carpus is shifted dorsally, and the distal end of the ulna appears to be dislocated anteriorly.

The isolated variety of Madelung's deformity is more commonly bilateral than unilateral, is asymmetrical in severity, and, if not isolated to women, is at least three to five times more common in female patients. Clinical manifestations usually become evident in the adolescent or young adult, in whom visible deformity, pain, fatigue, and limited range of motion, especially dorsal extension, ulnar deviation, and supination, are noted. After several years of progressive symptoms and signs, the findings may become stationary, and the pain may actually decrease, although in some cases, surgical intervention is required. Rarely, spontaneous rupture of extensor tendons may be evident.[131]

Congenital Subluxation and Hyperextension of the Knee

This is a rare congenital deformity in which the tibia and femur are abnormally related.[132-135] There is a definite female preponderance in a reported ratio of approximately 3:1. Hereditary factors appear to be important in some cases based upon a familial history of the deformity;[136, 137] associated congenital

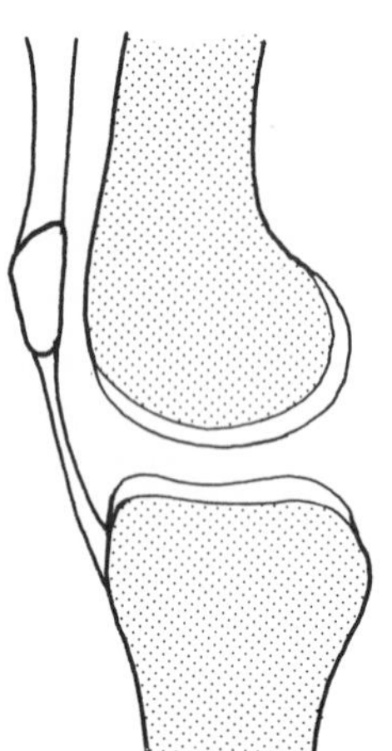

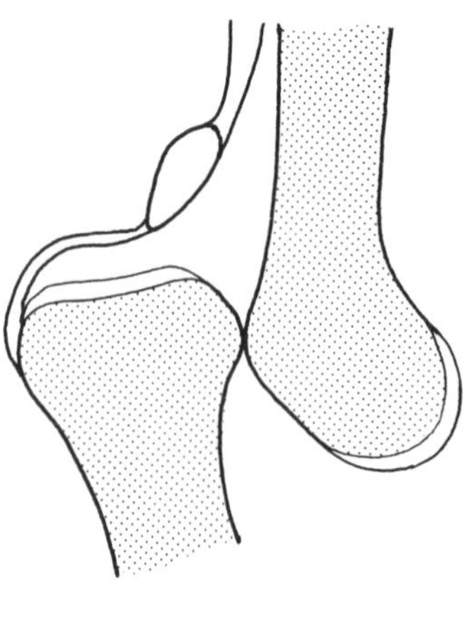

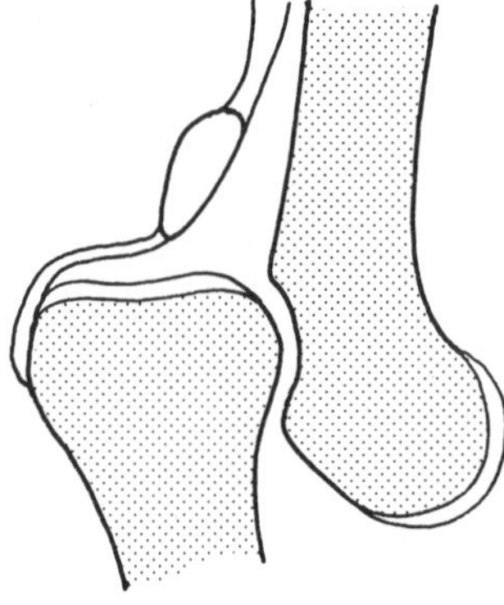

Figure 73–24. Congenital subluxation and hyperextension of the knee. Variable patterns can be encountered. Mild subluxation or frank dislocation with anterior femoral erosion may be seen.

deformities include dislocation of the hip, foot abnormalities, and dislocation of the elbow, in order of decreasing frequency.[138] Other factors that may be important in the etiology of this condition include abnormal fetal position during pregnancy,[139] perinatal injury, quadriceps contracture,[140] and absence or hypoplasia of the cruciate ligaments.[138] The last two findings may be the result of, rather than the cause of, the knee malposition.

The severity of the deformity is variable[141] (Fig. 73–24). Hyperextension can occur without tibial malposition; tibial subluxation or dislocation can appear without hyperextension; or both hyperextension and subluxation or dislocation may occur together. At birth, an affected infant frequently reveals a hyperextended knee or knees with limited flexion capabilities and anterior transverse skin folds or creases at the point of hyperextension. Radiographs confirm the anterior position of the proximal tibia with respect to the distal femur and, possibly, lateral subluxation and valgus deformity of the knee. Anterior tibial bowing and patellar hypoplasia may also be seen. Arthrography can delineate flattening of the chondral surface in the posterior tibial epiphysis and obliteration of the suprapatellar pouch secondary to local fibrous adherence to the quadriceps muscle.

This condition should be distinguished from genu recurvatum due to ligament laxity, acquired quadriceps contracture, and traumatic changes.

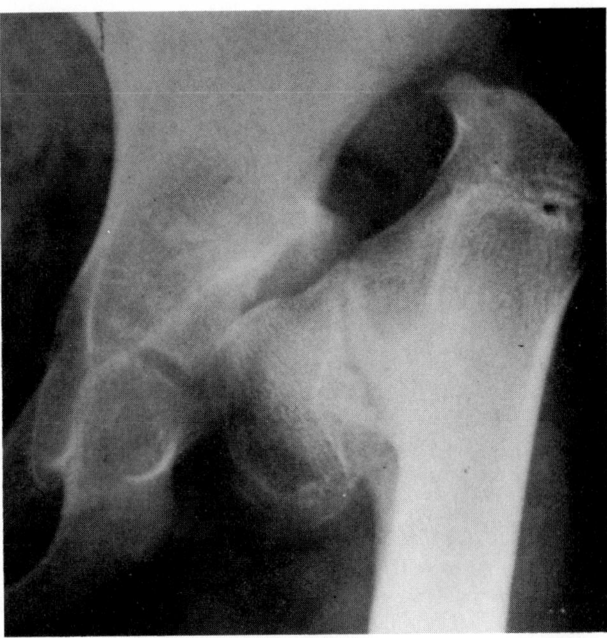

Figure 73–25. *Infantile coxa vara. Note the severe varus deformity of the proximal femur, the vertically located and irregular growth plate, thickening of the medial cortex of the femoral neck, a prominent greater trochanter, and acetabular flattening.*

Infantile Coxa Vara

Normally, the angle of intersection of the axis of the femoral neck and that of the femoral shaft varies with age but is approximately 150° at birth and 120 to 130° in the adult. The relative valgus position in the infant's femur is due to an increased growth of the medial portion of the cartilage plate in the prenatal period. With an acceleration of growth in the lateral portion of the plate in the child, a more varus position becomes apparent.

The term coxa vara indicates a neck-shaft angle that is less than 120° despite the variation of normal values that occurs in different age groups. Coxa vara may accompany various processes, including proximal femoral focal deficiency, osteogenesis imperfecta, renal osteodystrophy, rickets, and fibrous dysplasia.[142] Infantile or developmental coxa vara is a designation of a proximal femoral deformity that usually becomes apparent in the first few years of life, especially the age at which the child first walks. Boys and girls are affected with approximately equal frequency, and the condition is unilateral in 60 to 75 per cent of cases. Clinically, the affected child presents with a painless lurching gait or, in the case of bilateral involvement, a "duck-waddle" gait.[143-148] Limited joint motion is also seen. Additional features include a short stature and excessive lumbar lordosis.

Roentgenograms reveal a decrease in the femoral shaft-neck angle and a medially located triangular piece of bone in the neck adjacent to the head that is bounded by two radiolucent bands traversing the neck and forming an inverted V. The growth plate itself is widened, and its alignment is more vertical than normal. With further growth, the varus deformity frequently progresses, probably related to the forces of weight-bearing (Fig. 73–25). The triangular piece of bone may merge with the shaft, remodeling thickens the medial cortex of the femoral neck, the greater trochanter enlarges, and secondary degenerative joint disease can appear.

The precise etiology of this condition has not been delineated. A familial incidence of the deformity is noted in some cases, suggesting a genetic etiology or predisposition.[148-152] Additional mechanisms that have been proposed in infantile coxa vara are a juvenile osteochondrosis similar to Legg-Calvé-Perthes disease,[143] a pathologic ossification of the femoral neck, an embryonic interference with blood supply to the proximal femur,[153] and a traumatic insult.[154] Experimentally, coxa vara can be produced by inducing growth arrest in the capital femoral epiphysis.[155]

The differential diagnosis of infantile coxa vara includes proximal femoral focal deficiency, slipped capital femoral epiphysis, septic arthritis and osteomyelitis, rickets, and fibrous dysplasia.[454]

Primary Protrusion of the Acetabulum

Acetabulum protrusion refers to intrapelvic displacement of the medial wall of the acetabulum. It may be evident in many articular and nonarticular disorders, including rheumatoid arthritis, ankylosing spondylitis, septic arthritis, degenerative joint disease, osteomalacia, Paget's disease, neoplasm, trauma, and as an effect of irradiation. Protrusion of the acetabulum can also appear in the absence of any recognizable cause, and, in such a case, it is termed primary acetabular protrusion. The primary variety was first recognized by Otto in 1824[156] and is sometimes referred to as Otto pelvis.

The etiology of primary acetabular protrusion is unknown. A failure of ossification[157, 158] or premature fusion[159] of the Y cartilage has been offered as a possible etiologic agent. Alexander[160] suggested that the deep acetabulum was unrelated to any pathologic process in the joint, the adjacent bone, or the Y cartilage, but was a direct consequence of normal stress on the Y cartilage; under normal circumstances, the protrusion was reversible owing to the diminishing stresses after the age of 8 years, but under abnormal circumstances, a failure of correction of the protrusion resulted in its persistence into adult life. This investigator postulated that factors that might lead to acetabular protrusion were the female sex, premature fusion, and coxa vara. He also noted persistent beaking of the Y cartilage as a feature in young children that was associated with acetabular protrusion in the adult. Thus, according to Alexander, the deformity was the direct result of a failure of normal acetabular remodeling. A familial nature of the disorder was first emphasized by Rechtman in 1936[161] and subsequently was confirmed in numerous reports.[162-164]

Primary acetabular protrusion usually affects both hips and is much more frequent in women than in men. Hooper and Jones[165] divided the patients with the disorder into three subgroups: a juvenile group, in which boys and girls were affected in equal numbers, a family history was frequent, and symptoms and signs occurred in adolescence, progressed rapidly, and became incapacitating; a middle-aged group, in which symptoms and signs appeared later in life and in which osteoarthritis was not uncommon; and an elderly group, in which osteoarthritis was invariable. These investigators noted that the deformity was aggravated during periods of rapid hormone flux, namely at puberty and following menopause.

The predictive value of beaking of the Y cartilage of the acetabular region may be somewhat limited. Such a change is not infrequent in the developing skeleton, probably resulting from medial displacement of the Y synchondrosis due to normal weightbearing, and is reversible in most individuals. Marked beaking combined with abnormal varus angulation of the femoral neck or premature fusion of the Y cartilage is a more alarming finding that may later be accompanied by protrusion of the acetabulum. Such protrusion is readily confirmed on radiographic examination, although appropriate criteria that differ in the male and female patient must be applied (see Chapter 3).

With progressive protrusion deformity, the femoral head assumes an intrapelvic location, and the joint space may be normal, narrowed, or obliterated. Pathologic examination confirms fibrocartilaginous replacement and osteophytosis of the femoral head.[164]

Acetabular deformity in mild cases of primary protrusion must be distinguished from normal variations in acetabular depth. The radiographic diagnosis of abnormal protrusion based upon the mere "crossing" of the acetabular line and ilioischial line is inadequate; rather, an abnormal situation exists in the adult pelvis when the distance between the

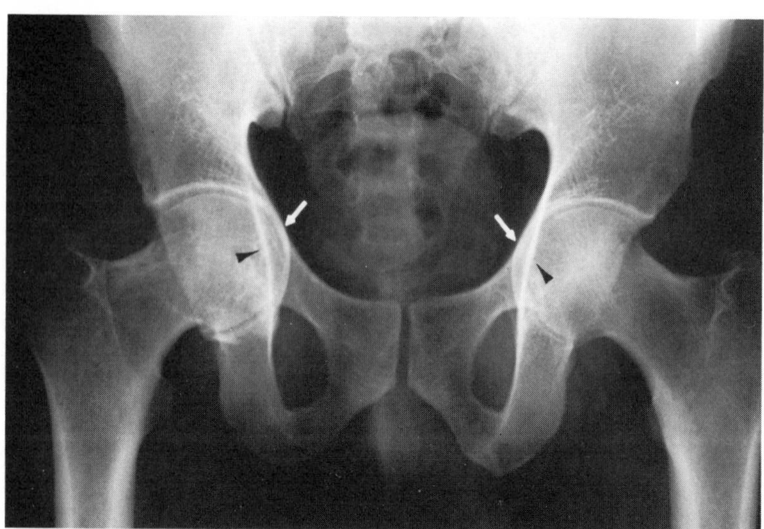

Figure 73–26. *Primary protrusion of the acetabulum. This 30 year old man reveals bilateral acetabular protrusion with concentric loss of joint space. Note that the acetabular line (arrows) is located medial to the ilioischial line (arrowheads) by a considerable distance.*

medially located acetabular line and the laterally located ilioischial line is 6 mm or more in women and 3 mm or more in men (Fig. 73–26). With the onset of joint degeneration and narrowing in primary acetabular protrusion, the findings must be distinguished from other articular disorders of the hip. The joint space loss in idiopathic acetabular protrusion usually results in axial or medial migration of the femoral head with respect to the acetabulum. In osteoarthritis alone, superior or, less commonly, medial migration of the femoral head is typical. Axial migration of the femoral head is seen in rheumatoid arthritis, ankylosing spondylitis, chondrolysis, chondral atrophy due to immobilization, and calcium pyrophosphate dihydrate crystal deposition disease, but other radiographic features insure accurate diagnosis of these conditions.

Foot Deformities

Although a detailed discussion of the complexities of the deformed foot is well beyond the scope of this textbook, a brief summary of the major foot deformities is included. The interested reader should consult the excellent radiographic reviews provided by Ozonoff,[166] Freiberger and colleagues,[167] and Ritchie and Keim,[168] from which many of the following observations are derived. Proper roentgenographic analysis requires both anteroposterior and lateral projections exposed during weight-bearing. The anteroposterior projection is obtained with the sagittal plane of the leg perpendicular to the film and with the knees together; the lateral view is exposed with the foot in maximal dorsiflexion, a technique that usually requires the utilization of a support beneath the plantar surface of the foot. The following terms are applied to the deformities.

Talipes: a long-established name for congenital deformities of the foot (for example, talipes equinovarus).

Pes: a name that should be restricted to acquired deformities of the foot (such as pes equinovarus).

Valgus: the bones distal to a specified joint are oriented in a plane away from the midline of the body.

Varus: the opposite of valgus, in which the bones distal to a specified joint are oriented in a plane toward the midline of the body.

Equinus: fixed plantar flexion of the hindfoot.

Calcaneus: fixed dorsiflexion of the hindfoot.

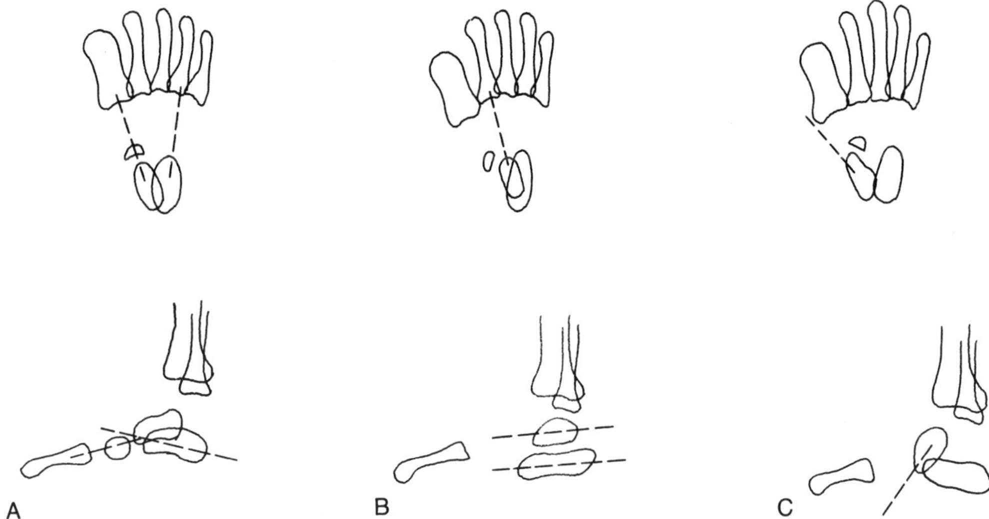

Figure 73–27. *Foot: Normal and abnormal hindfoot and forefoot relationship.*

A *Normal. On an anteroposterior radiograph, the talar axis intersects or points slightly medial to the first metatarsal, and the navicular bone is situated directly opposite the head of the talus. The calcaneus points toward the fourth metatarsal, creating a talocalcaneal angle of approximately 35 degrees in the adult and somewhat greater in the infant. On a lateral radiograph, the anterior portion of the talus is mildly flexed in a plantar direction, and the calcaneus is slightly dorsiflexed. An extended line through the longitudinal axis of the talus is directed along the axis of the first metatarsal. The talocalcaneal angle is approximately 35 degrees.*

B *Hindfoot varus deformity. The anteroposterior radiograph reveals a decrease in the talocalcaneal angle as the two bones lie closely together and more parallel to each other. The navicular bone is displaced medially, and the talar axis points laterad to the first metatarsal base. In the lateral projection, the talus and the calcaneus are both more horizontal and parallel with each other.*

C *Hindfoot valgus deformity. On the anteroposterior radiograph, the talocalcaneal angle is increased, with the navicular bone and remaining tarsal bones being located lateral to the talus. The talar axial line passes medial to the first metatarsal. On the lateral radiograph, the talus is oriented more vertically, and the long axis of the talus and that of the first metatarsal angulate in a plantar direction.*

(After Ozonoff MB: Pediatric Orthopedic Radiology. Philadelphia, WB Saunders Co, 1979.)

Cavus: a raised longitudinal arch of the foot.

Planus: a flattened longitudinal arch of the foot.

Adduction: displacement in a transverse plane toward the axis of the body.

Abduction: displacement in a transverse plane away from the axis of the body.

The normal alignment of the foot is inferred from the information obtained on anteroposterior and lateral radiographs utilizing, in large part, the relationship of the talus and the calcaneus (Figs. 73–27 and 73–28). In the anteroposterior projection, a line through the long axis of the talus extended distally will fall on, or close to, the medial border of the first metatarsal, and one through the long axis of the calcaneus falls at the base of the fourth metatarsal. The angle between the two lines, the talocalcaneal angle, averages approximately 35° in the adult and is somewhat greater in the infant. The axes of the metatarsals are roughly parallel and fan out slightly in a distal direction. In the lateral projection, the foot can be dorsiflexed to such an extent that an angle between it and the lower leg is considerably less than 90°. In neutral position, the long axis of the calcaneus extends dorsally from posterior to anterior, and the long axis of the talus is flexed in a plantar direction and is mildly angulated with the long axis of the first metatarsal. The talocalcaneal angle averages approximately 35° and is about equal to that noted on the anteroposterior view. The longitudinal axes of the metatarsals are approximately parallel, with the fifth metatarsal being most plantar, the others superimposed, and the first metatarsal being most dorsal in location.

The talus is utilized as the point of reference in the description of foot deformities. It is generally assumed that the talus is relatively fixed with relationship to the lower leg, so that a change in the relationship of the talus and the calcaneus reflects a movement of the latter bone. The calcaneus can abduct, increasing the talocalcaneal angle, or adduct, decreasing the talocalcaneal angle.

In *hindfoot (heel) valgus* (Fig. 73–27), an anteroposterior projection reveals an increase in the talocalcaneal angle. An extended line through the longitudinal axis of the talus will fall medial to the first metatarsal, and the navicular and other tarsal bones will be displaced laterally to the talus. On the lateral projection, the talus will be tilted more vertically than normal owing to the abduction of the calcaneus, which decreases the plantar support on the anterior portion of the talus. The long axis of the talus and that of the first metatarsal will angulate plantarward.

In *hindfoot (heel) varus* (Fig. 73–27), on anteroposterior views, the long axis of the talus falls lateral to the base of the first metatarsal owing to the adduction of the anterior end of the calcaneus. The

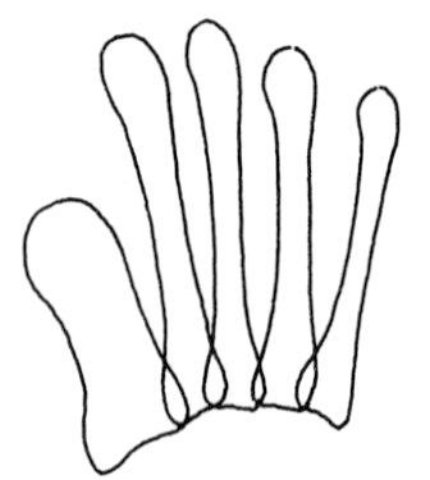

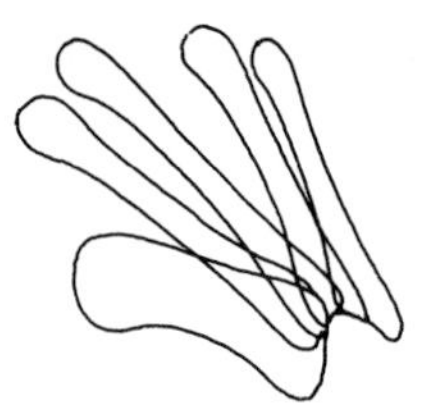

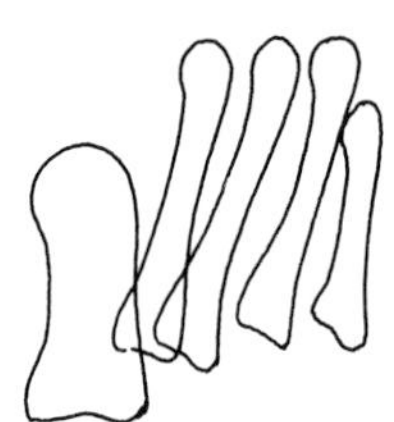

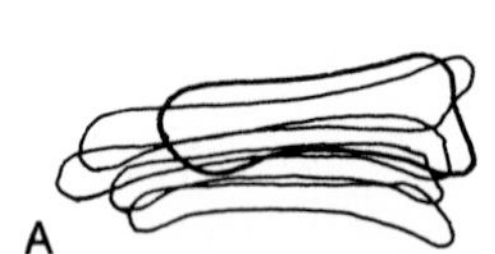

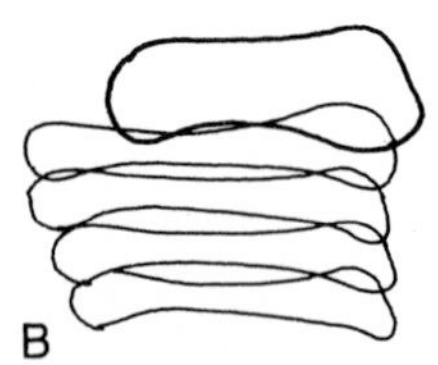

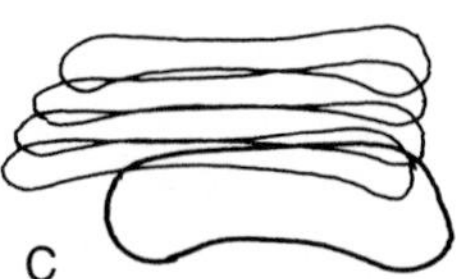

Figure 73–28. *Foot: Normal and abnormal forefoot alignment.*

A *Normal. On the anteroposterior roentgenogram, the metatarsals converge proximally with overlapping at their bases. On the lateral projection, the fifth metatarsal is in the most plantar position, with the other metatarsals being superimposed.*

B *Forefoot varus deformity. On the frontal radiograph, the forefoot is narrowed, with increased convergence at the bases, resulting in more overlap than normal. On the lateral radiograph, a ladder-like arrangement is seen, with the first metatarsal being most dorsal.*

C *Forefoot valgus deformity. The forefoot is broadened, with the metatarsals being more prominent than normal and with decreased overlap at the metatarsal bases. In the lateral projection, a ladder-like arrangement can be noted in some cases, with the first metatarsal being in the most plantar position.*

(After Ozonoff MB: Pediatric Orthopedic Radiology. Philadelphia, WB Saunders Co, 1979.)

talocalcaneal angle is decreased, and the talus and calcaneus are more parallel to each other than in the normal foot. The navicular bone is displaced medially. On the lateral view, the calcaneus and talus are both more horizontal and parallel with each other.

Hindfoot or heel valgus is present in flatfoot, metatarsus varus, congenital vertical talus, and certain congenital and neurologic deformities of the foot. Hindfoot or heel varus is commonly visible in talipes equinovarus and some paralytic deformities.

In *hindfoot equinus*, in the lateral projection, the calcaneus is flexed in a plantar direction so that the angle between the axes of the calcaneus and the tibia is greater than 90°. This deformity accompanies talipes equinovarus and congenital vertical talus.

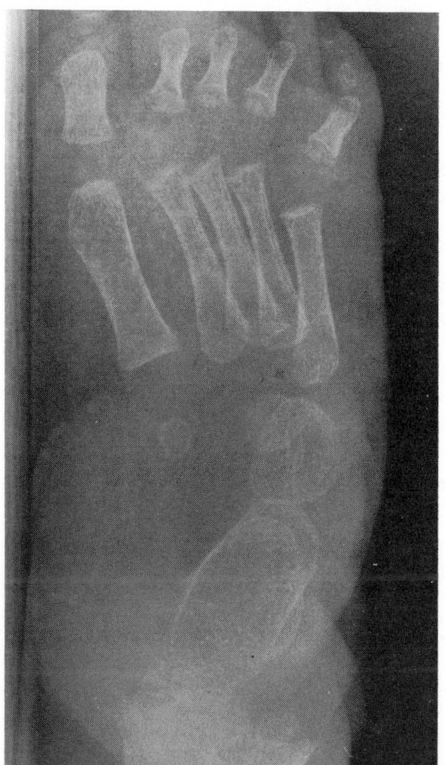

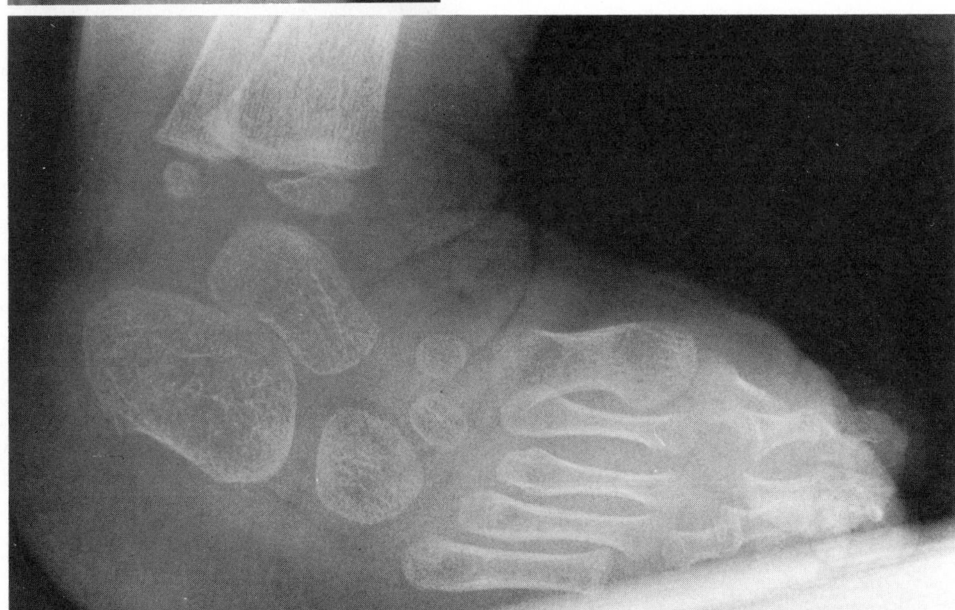

Figure 73–29. *Clubfoot (equinovarus) deformity.*

A *Anteroposterior projection. The hindfoot is in marked varus position, with superimposition of the talar and calcaneal centers. A line drawn through the talus will pass far laterally to the first metatarsal. The navicular is not ossified, but its abnormal position can be inferred from the location of the first metatarsal base and the first cuneiform center. The forefoot is narrowed, with increased overlap of the metatarsal bases.*

B *Lateral projection. The talus and the calcaneus are more parallel than normal. The calcaneus is in equinus position, abnormally flexed in a plantar direction. Forefoot inversion with a ladder-like arrangement of the metatarsals is apparent.*

(From Ozonoff MB: Pediatric Orthopedic Radiology. Philadelphia, WB Saunders Co, 1979.)

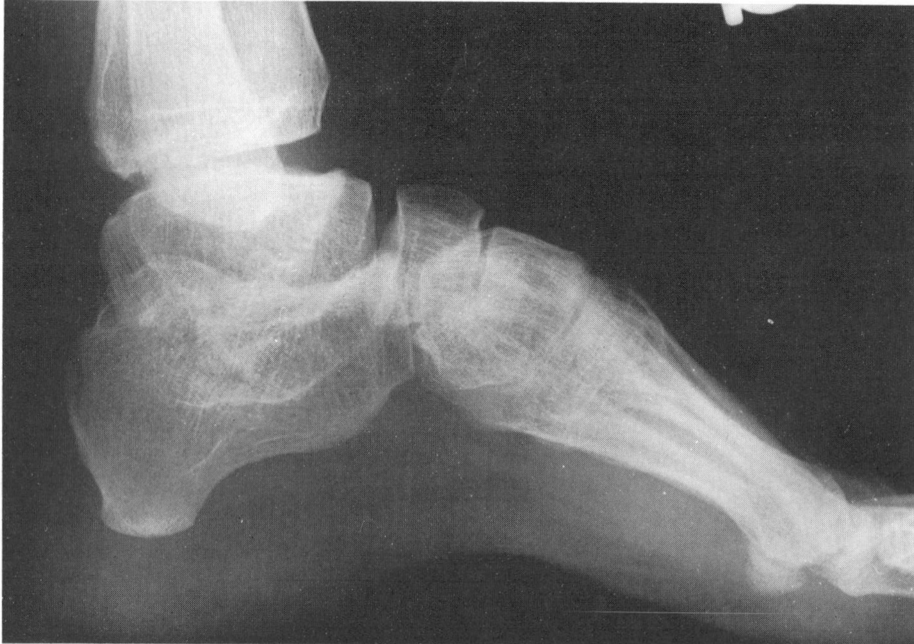

Figure 73–30. Corrected clubfoot (equinovarus) deformity with flat-topped talus. Note also the flattening of the articular surface of the tibia. A cavus arch is apparent. (From Ozonoff MB: Pediatric Orthopedic Radiology. Philadelphia, WB Saunders Co, 1979.)

Equinus of the entire foot is evident in various neuromuscular disorders. In *calcaneal hindfoot deformity,* in the lateral projection, the calcaneus is abnormally dorsiflexed so that its anterior end has a more superior position, and the bone possesses a "box-like" appearance. Calcaneal positions of the calcaneus appear in association with cavus deformities of the foot.

The term *clubfoot* represents a condition associated with equinovarus foot deformity and hindfoot varus (Fig. 73–29). Thus, the anteroposterior radiograph reveals a decreased talocalcaneal angle, and the talus and calcaneus are roughly parallel. The forefoot is adducted and in varus. On the lateral radiograph, an equinus heel and a plantar flexed forefoot are evident. Again, the axes of the talus and calcaneus are roughly parallel. The clubfoot deformity is relatively common, occurs more frequently in male children, and can be unilateral or bilateral in distribution. Its exact etiology is not clear, although a considerable number of theories have been proposed: defective connective tissue with ligamentous laxity, muscular imbalance, intrauterine position deformity, central nervous system or vascular abnormality, and persistence of early normal fetal relationships.[166, 455, 464] Anatomic studies in some cases have revealed a small talus containing a talar dome that is less convex than normal and a neck that is dislocated in a medial and plantar direction.[169] These changes result in an articular surface between the talus and the navicular bone that faces medially with the subtalar surface tilted in varus, equinus, and medial rotation.[166] The calcaneus may be diminished in size and displaced into varus, equinus, and internal rotation. This produces talonavicular and calcaneocuboid spaces that are located in a vertical line.[166]

Following inadequate or improper treatment of the clubfoot, certain deformities may remain. These include the rocker-bottom deformity, which is due to correction of the foot dorsiflexion before the equinus, and the flattop talus, which is due to

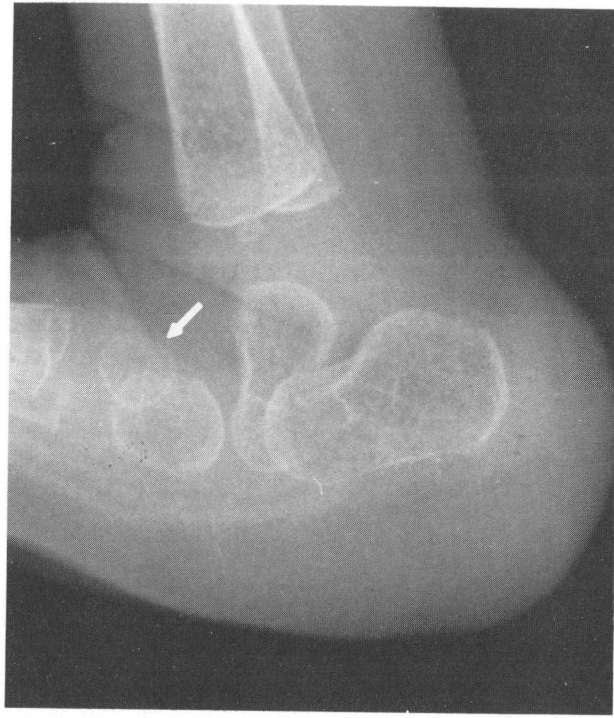

Figure 73–31. Congenital vertical talus. The talar axis is markedly vertical in orientation, and the calcaneus is in equinus position, producing an inferior convexity to the plantar surface of the foot. The navicular is unossified, but, because of the position of the ossified third cuneiform (arrow), it should be displaced dorsally, occupying the space between the cuneiform and the talus.

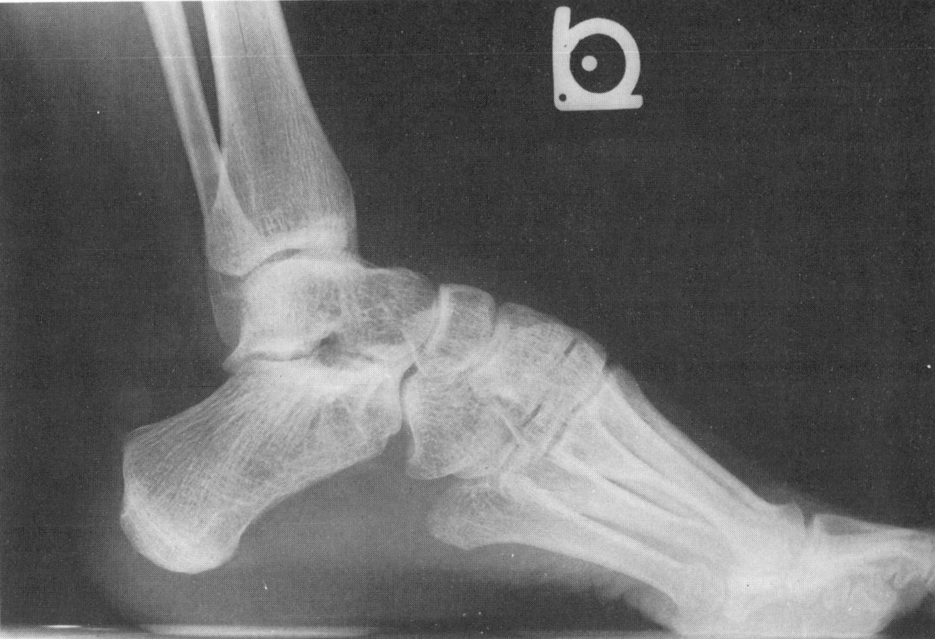

Figure 73–32. Cavus foot. Following polio, this 18 year old girl reveals an increased plantar arch with a calcaneus position of the os calcis and increased plantar flexion of the forefoot. (From Ozonoff MB: Pediatric Orthopedic Radiology. Philadelphia, WB Saunders Co, 1979.)

flattening of the superior surface of the plantar flexed talus that is articulating with the tibia (Fig. 73–30).

A *congenital vertical talus* (congenital flatfoot with talonavicular dislocation) can occur as an isolated condition or as part of a generalized malformation syndrome or disorder. It is frequently associated with myelomeningocele. On the anteroposterior radiograph, severe heel valgus and forefoot abduction result in an increased talocalcaneal angle with the talar axis lying medial to the first metatarsal. On the lateral radiograph, an equinus heel with plantar flexion of both the calcaneus and the talus is evident (Fig. 73–31). In fact, the talar axis is almost vertical in orientation, producing an increase in the talocalcaneal angle. The forefoot is dorsiflexed at the midtarsal level, resulting in a convex plantar surface of the foot, the rocker-bottom deformity. The navicular bone is dorsally dislocated, locking the talus into its plantar flexed position. With ossification of the navicular bone, the talonavicular dislocation becomes visible.

The *cavus foot deformity* is a frequent accompaniment of neurologic or muscular disorders, such as peroneal muscular atrophy, poliomyelitis, and meningomyelocele.[170] There is an abnormally high longitudinal arch of the foot, as the calcaneus is dorsiflexed (calcaneus position) and the metatarsals are plantar flexed (Fig. 73–32).

The *flexible flatfoot deformity* is associated, on the anteroposterior view, with an increase in the talocalcaneal angle, heel valgus, and forefoot abduction. The midtarsal transverse arch is flattened, and the metatarsals are approximately parallel in their orientation. On the lateral projection, hindfoot valgus is again noted with the talus in a more vertical attitude than normal (Fig. 73–33). The calcaneus and the metatarsals are horizontally aligned, and the plantar arch is flattened. Although the resulting radiographic picture may superficially resemble that seen in congenital vertical talus, the flexible flatfoot deformity is not associated with equinus, and the navicular bone retains its normal

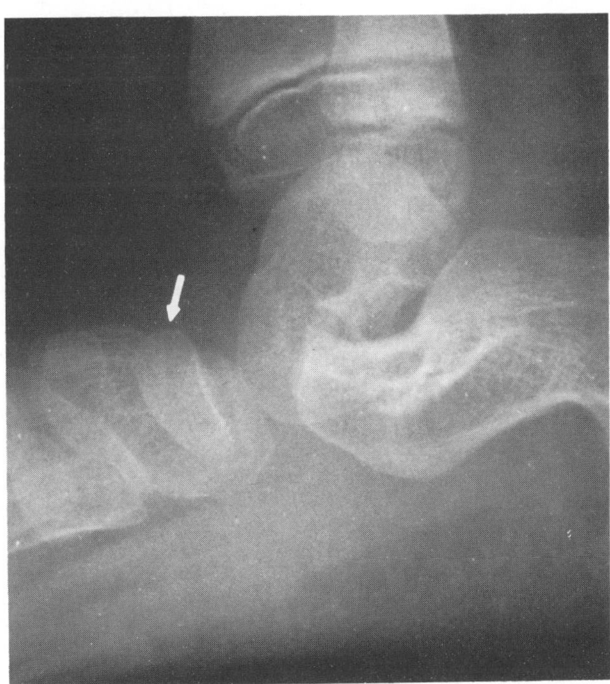

Figure 73–33. Flexible flatfoot (pronated foot). A lateral radiograph demonstrates an increased vertical position of the talus. The calcaneus and metatarsals are more horizontal than normal, flattening the plantar arch. Note the relatively normal position of the tarsal navicular (arrow). An anteroposterior view revealed hindfoot valgus deformity, with an increased talocalcaneal angle.

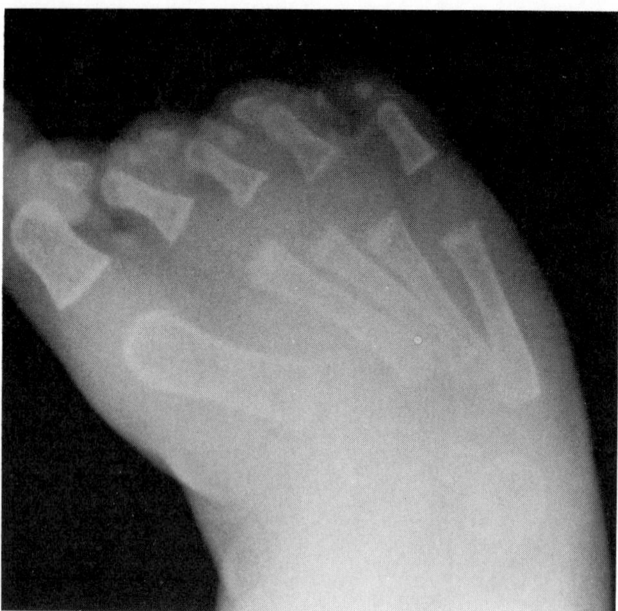

Figure 73–34. *Metatarsus adductus and metatarsus varus. Note the adducted varus position of the forefoot, with a concave medial border and convex lateral border.*

position with regard to the distal surface of the talus.

Metatarsus adductus and varus is a common deformity of unknown etiology (Fig. 73–34). The forefoot is adducted and in varus with a concave medial border, convex lateral border, and high arch. The hindfoot is normal in mild cases and is in valgus in severe cases. Dorsiflexion of the foot is normal or exaggerated.

Peroneal spastic flatfoot is a deformity that is frequently associated with a tarsal coalition (previously discussed).

SPECIFIC MALFORMATION SYNDROMES

Some specific malformation syndromes, predominantly those that involve the epiphysis, are discussed in the previous chapter. An outline of additional important syndromes is included in the following pages. Their manner of organization is

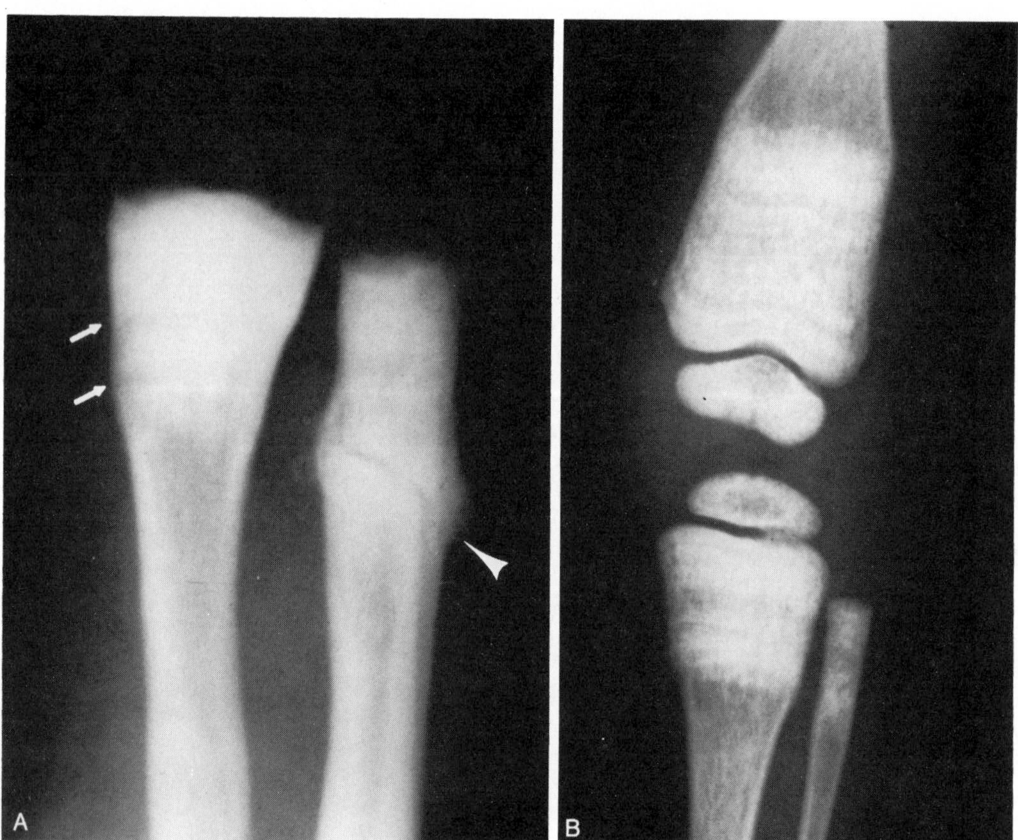

Figure 73–35. *Osteopetrosis with precocious manifestations.*

A *This infant reveals increased radiodensity of the distal radius and distal ulna, with metaphyseal flaring or widening. Radiolucent bands can also be identified (arrows), and a pathologic fracture is seen (arrowhead).*

B *In this child, note bands of increased density in the metaphyses, sclerosis of the epiphyses, and metaphyseal widening.*

similar to that utilized by Spranger and colleagues.[2]

Skeletal Dysplasias with Increased Bone Density

OSTEOPETROSIS. *Osteopetrosis with precocious manifestations* is an autosomal recessive disorder that becomes evident during infancy.[171-174] Clinical findings include small stature, spontaneous bruising, abnormal bleeding, hepatosplenomegaly, anemia, bone fragility, and diminished resistance to infection. Delayed dentition, palsies of the facial, optic, and oculomotor nerves, and macrocephaly are additional findings.[473] Death in the first decades of life is common, although occasionally individuals survive into adulthood. The etiology and pathogenesis of the condition are not clear. Experimental and histologic studies are consistent with the conclusion that the skeletal lesions result from a decrease in the rate of bone and cartilage resorption with little or no change in the rate of bone and cartilage formation.[456] A cellular defect in the osteoclast may be important, and this cell may subsequently be unable to resorb bone or cartilage or respond normally to parathyroid hormone.[456]

The radiographic picture is dominated by increased bone density (Fig. 73–35). Transverse radiodense metaphyseal bands and longitudinal radiodense diaphyseal striations or widespread osteosclerosis are evident, frequently combined with metaphyseal flaring and club-shaped or flask-shaped tubular bones. Sclerotic foci can lead to a "bone within bone" appearance as well as "sandwich" vertebrae. Thickening and sclerosis of the cranial base and vault and poor pneumatization of the mastoid and paranasal sinuses can be apparent. Complications include fractures, osteomyelitis, and coxa vara deformity.[175]

Osteopetrosis with delayed manifestations (Albers-Schönberg disease) appears to be transmitted as an autosomal dominant trait in the majority of cases, although there is considerable interfamilial variation.[176-178] Affected individuals may remain totally asymptomatic, the diagnosis being established by chance on roentgenograms obtained for other reasons. Other patients reveal anemia, facial palsy or deafness, hepatosplenomegaly, and fractures. Tooth extraction may be followed by osteomyelitis.

At birth, radiographs may be entirely normal, but sclerosis becomes increasingly apparent during childhood and adolescence. Widespread and symmetrical osseous alterations are the rule, as trabecular architecture is obliterated. Calvarial thickening and eburnation and sinus obliteration can be seen, and a "bone-within-bone" appearance may be encountered in the axial and appendicular skeleton (Fig. 73–36). The degree of metaphyseal flaring is variable and predilects the distal ends of the femora. Tuftal erosion[179] and premature degenerative joint disease[180] can be noted in some cases.

PYKNODYSOSTOSIS. Pyknodysostosis, defined by Maroteaux and Lamy in 1962,[181] is predominantly characterized by osteosclerosis and dwarfism. It is inherited as an autosomal recessive trait.[182] Disproportionate short stature usually becomes evident in early childhood. Affected individuals have a small face, hooked nose, receding chin, carious teeth, large calvarium, fronto-occipital bulging, and open anterior fontanelle. Terminal phalanges appear short, and the fingernails are dysplastic. Increased bone fragility, kyphosis, scoliosis, thoracic narrowing, and genu valgum deformity can be noted. An example of a patient with the clinical manifestations of pyknodysostosis is provided by the painter Toulouse-Lautrec.[183]

The roentgenographic features include persistence of the anterior fontanelle, multiple wormian bones, hypoplastic facial bones and sinuses, and an obtuse mandibular angle[184] (Fig. 73–37). Osseous eburnation appears during childhood and increases in severity and extent thereafter. Skeletal modeling is only mildly abnormal, and radiodense striations and a "bone-within-bone" appearance are usually not evident. Hypoplasia of the terminal phalanges of the fingers and toes and lateral end of the clavicle, coxa valga, shallow acetabulae, fractures, spinal anomalies, and disappearance of the hyoid bone have all been noted in this syndrome.[185]

SCLEROSTEOSIS. This disorder was first delineated by Truswell in 1958,[186] and the designation "sclerosteosis" was introduced by Hansen in 1967.[187] It is an autosomal recessive disorder that usually becomes evident in infancy or early childhood.[188-190, 422] Clinical findings are excessive height and weight, peculiar facies with a broad, flat nasal bridge, ocular hypertelorism, mandibular prominence, deafness, facial palsy, cutaneous or bony syndactyly of the second and third fingers, absent or dysplastic nails, and radial deviation of the terminal phalanges. In adults, headaches due to elevation of intracranial pressure have been described.

Radiographs outline hyperostosis of the skull and mandible and sclerosis of the cortices of the tubular bones and, perhaps, the pelvis and pedicles. There is a lack of normal diaphyseal constriction of the tubular bones. Pathologic fractures do not generally occur.[457]

ENDOSTEAL HYPEROSTOSIS. Endosteal hyperostosis of recessive type, van Buchem's disease, and hyperostosis corticalis generalisata are designations applied to a sclerotic disease first described by van Buchem and co-workers in 1955.[191] It is an autosomal recessive disorder that generally becomes evident at the end of the first decade of life[192-197] (Fig. 73–38*A*). Clinical manifestations include overgrowth and distortion of the mandible and brow,

Text continued on page 2583

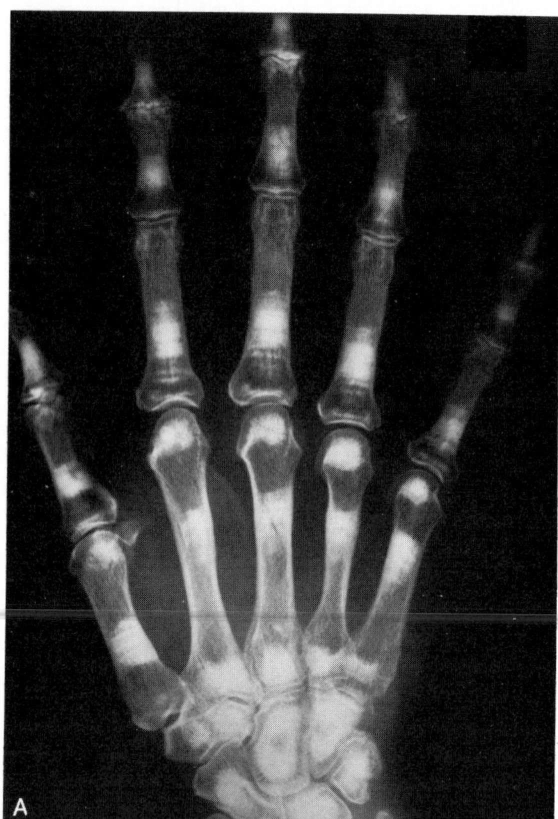

Figure 73–36. Osteopetrosis with delayed manifestations (Albers-Schönberg disease). This 78 year old woman had had multiple previous pathologic fractures of tubular bones. She presented with an acute fracture of the left femur.

A Osteosclerotic foci are evident in the metaphyses and epiphyses of metacarpals and phalanges, as well as in the carpus, radius, and ulna.

B, C Similar abnormalities are evident in the foot. Note the "bone-within-bone" appearance in the tarsus, especially the calcaneus.

Illustration continued on the opposite page

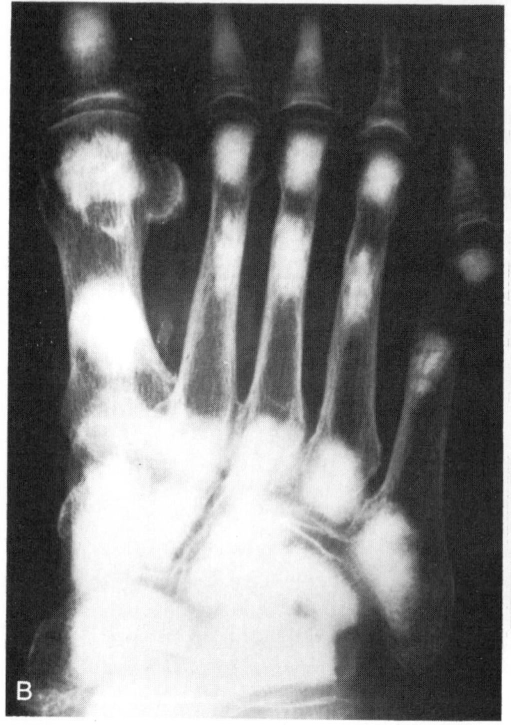

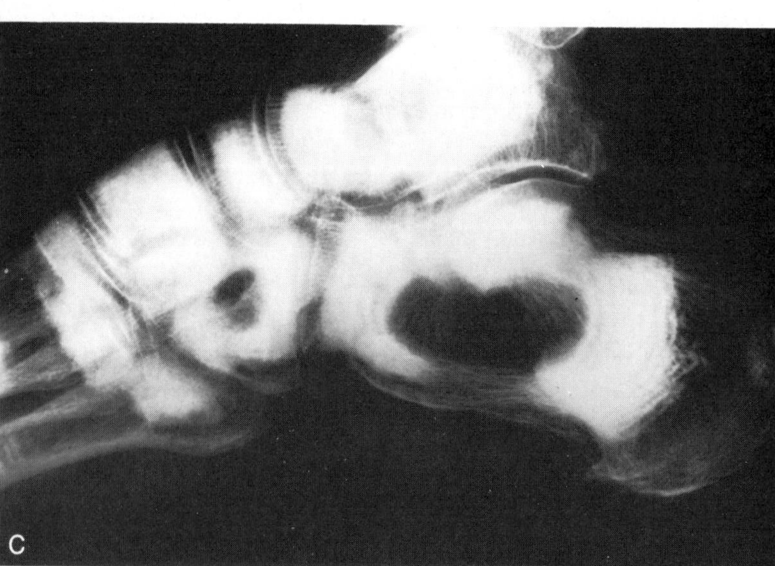

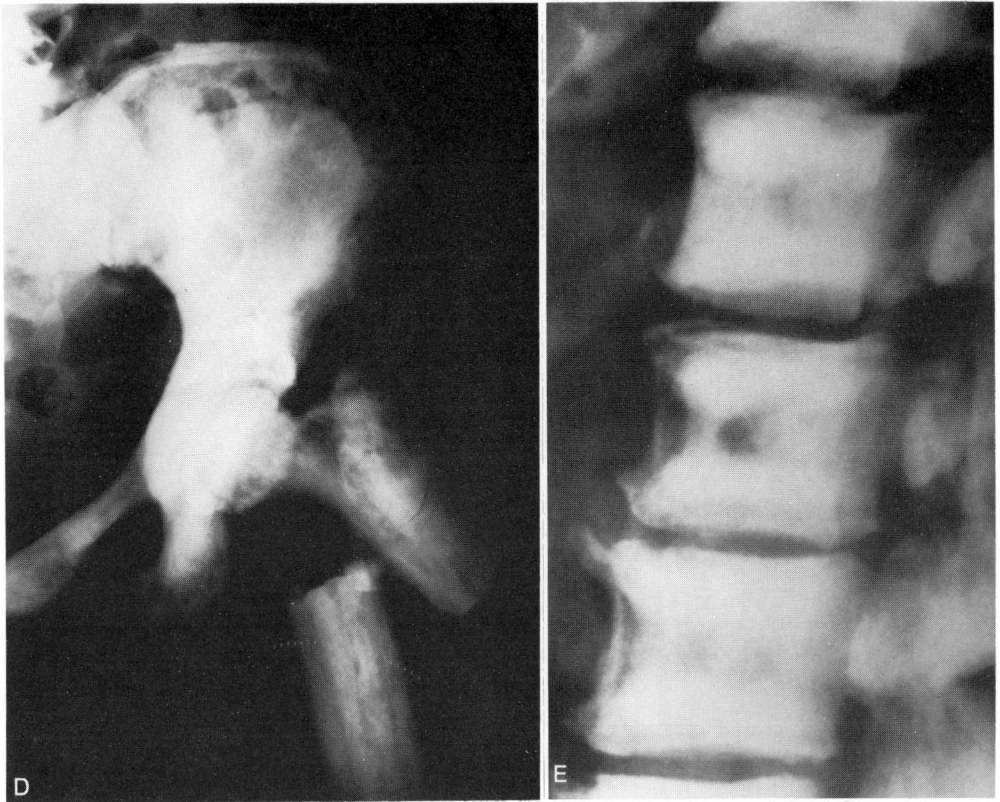

Figure 73–36. Continued
D *A pathologic displaced fracture of the left femur is evident.*
E *Note the sclerosis of multiple vertebrae and "sandwich" vertebral bodies.*
(Courtesy of Dr. D. Sauser, Loma Linda University, Loma Linda, California.)

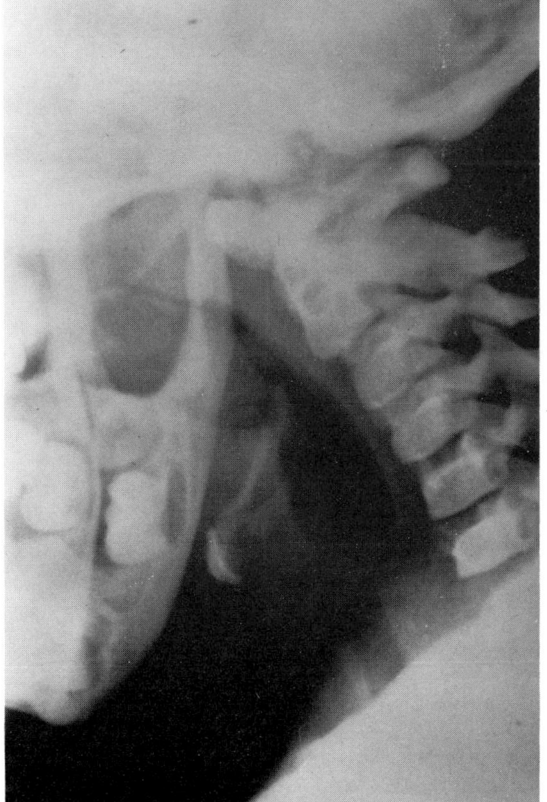

Figure 73–37. Pyknodysostosis. *Note the increased radiodensity of the facial bones and cervical spine and the flattened mandibular angle.*

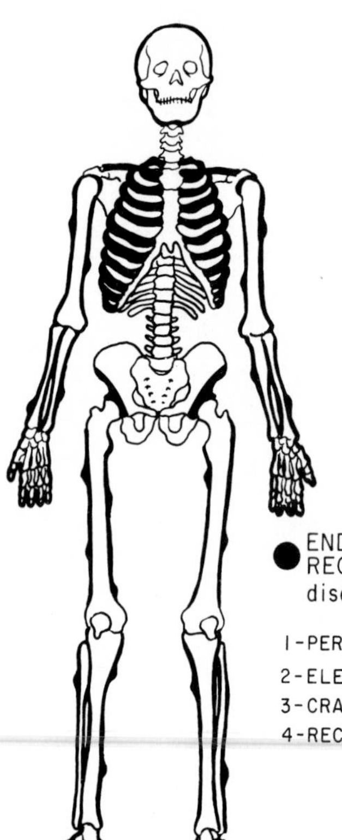

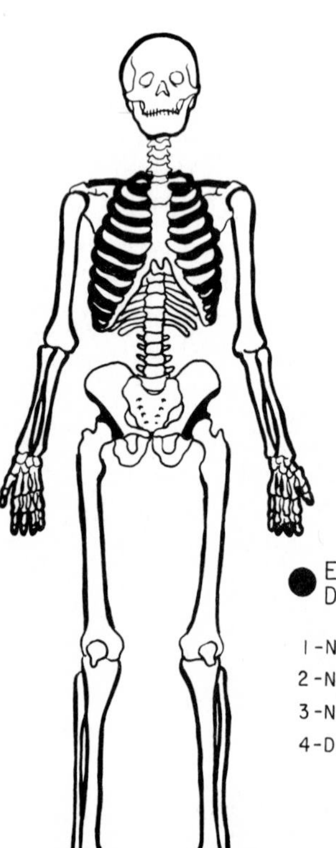

Figure 73–38. *Endosteal hyperostosis: Recessive versus dominant type.*

A, B *Major alterations allowing differentiation of recessive (van Buchem's disease) and dominant type of endosteal hyperostosis are outlined.*

Illustration continued on the opposite page

clavicular thickening, and facial palsy and deafness. The serum alkaline phosphatase level may be elevated. Radiographic abnormalities include widening and sclerosis of the calvarium, cranial base, and mandible and underpneumatization of the sinuses. Endosteal thickening of the diaphyseal regions of the tubular bones, widening of the medial portions of the clavicles, and increased density of the spinous processes of the vertebrae can be seen.

An autosomal dominant variety of endosteal hyperostosis was noted by Worth and Wollin in 1966[198] and subsequently by other investigators.[199-201] Although radiographic features are somewhat similar to those of van Buchem's disease, the clinical course is milder, and cranial nerve involvement is rarely seen (Fig. 73–38). A widened and deepened mandible with an increased gonial angle is evident. Roentgenograms reveal bilateral symmetrical cortical thickening of the diaphyses of the tubular bones and thickening and sclerosis of the calvarium, mandible, shoulder and pelvic girdles, and thoracic cage. Unlike van Buchem's disease, periosteal excrescences are not observed, the basal foramina are not encroached upon, and serum alkaline phosphatase levels are normal.

Metaphyseal Dysplasia (Pyle's Disease). This rare autosomal recessive disorder becomes manifest at a variable age with mild clinical

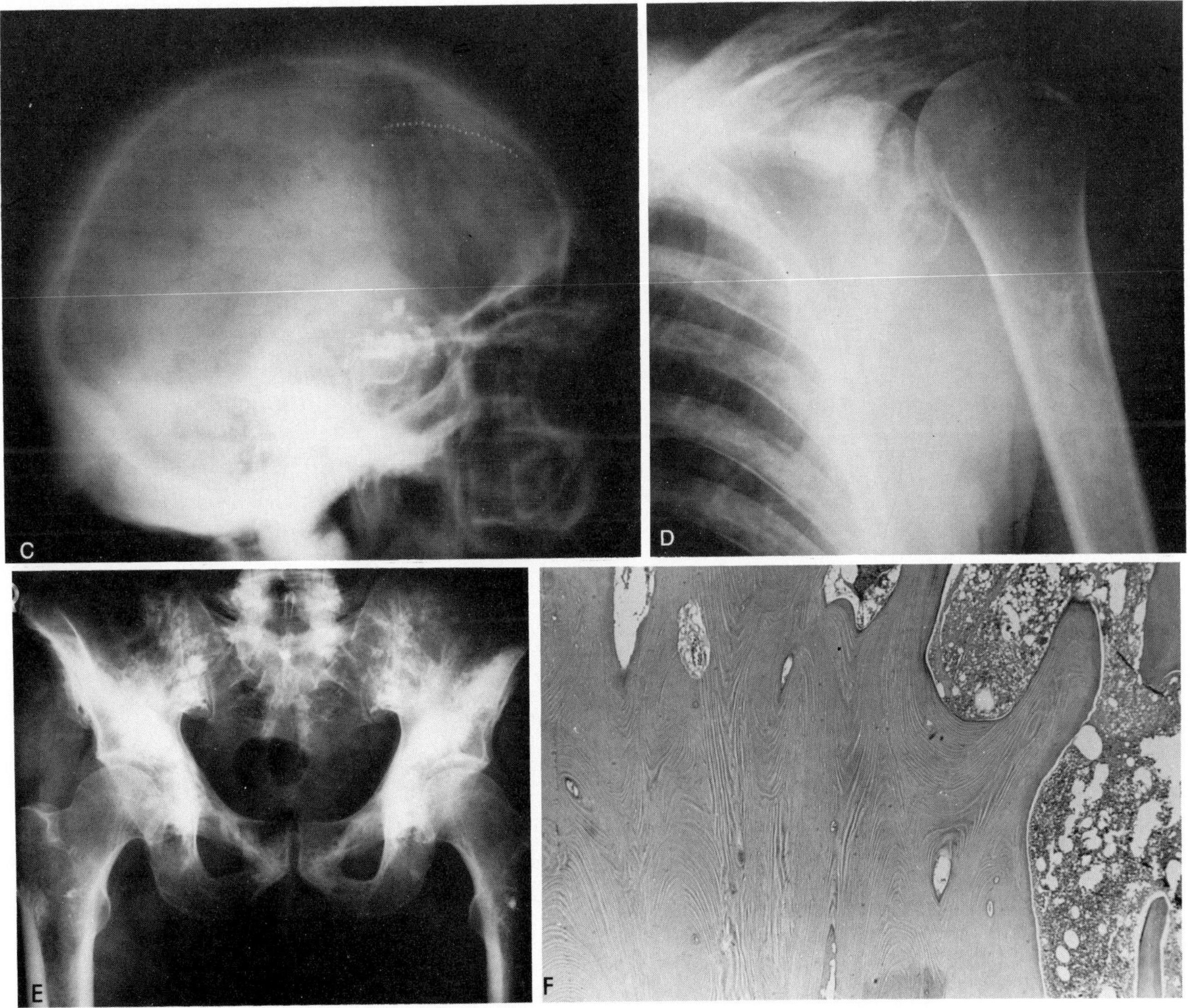

Figure 73–38. Continued

C–F *Endosteal hyperostosis: Dominant type. This 57 year old man had had a prior diagnosis of Paget's disease. Serum calcium, phosphorus, and alkaline phosphatase determinations yielded normal results. Radiographs reveal thickening of the calvarium, especially at the base and petrous portions of the skull, with residual iophendylate material from a previous myelogram* **(C)***; coarsening and thickening of the trabecular pattern of the clavicle, acromion, and glenoid* **(D)***; and prominence of the trabecular pattern throughout the pelvis, and cortical thickening of the proximal femora* **(E)***. An acromial biopsy* **(F)** *demonstrates thickened but normal mature lamellar bone.*

Illustration continued on the following page

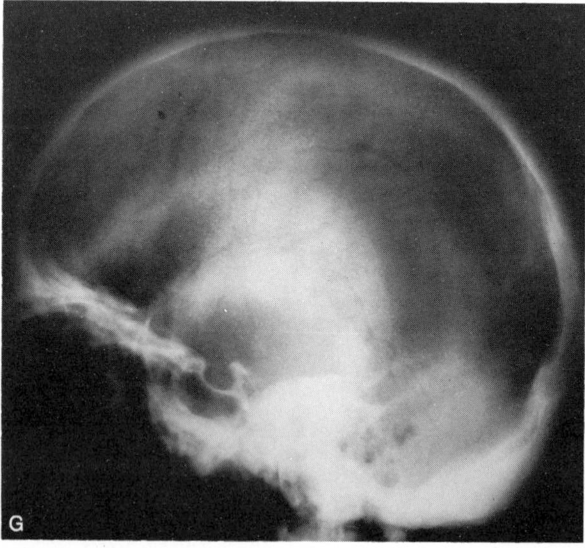

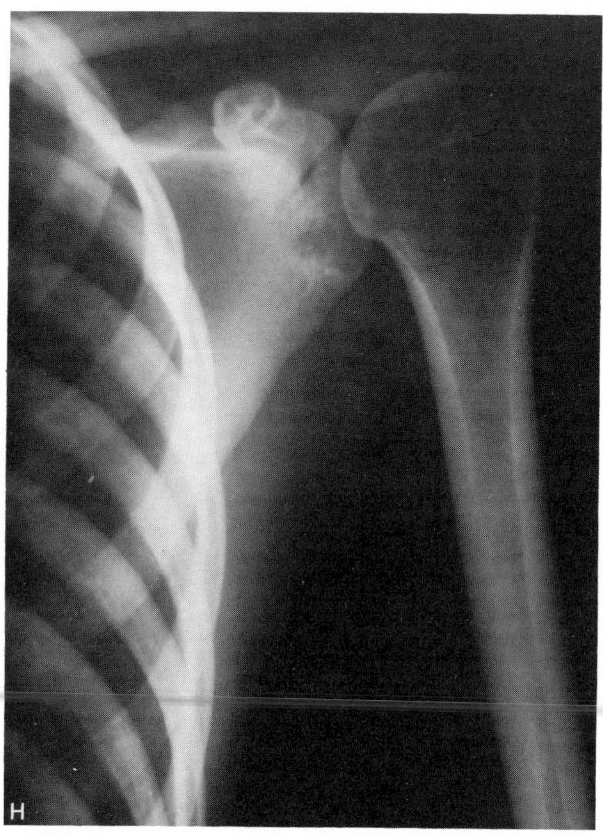

Figure 73–38. Continued

G, H *The 37 year old daughter of the patient described in* **C** *through* **F** *reveals similar abnormalities of the skull, shoulder girdle, ribs, and humerus.*

(From Gelman MI: Radiology 125:289, 1977.)

symptoms and signs, including joint pain, muscular weakness, scoliosis, genu valgum deformity, dental malocclusion, and bone fragility.[202-205] The radiographic abnormalities are striking (Fig. 73–39). Marked expansion of the metaphyseal segments of tubular bones leads to an "Erlenmeyer flask" appearance, especially in the distal femur and proximal tibia and fibula. Changes in the upper extremity are similar but less extensive. In both locations, a rather abrupt transition exists between the cylindrical and flared portions of the bone. Minor alterations in the skull include supraorbital prominence, an

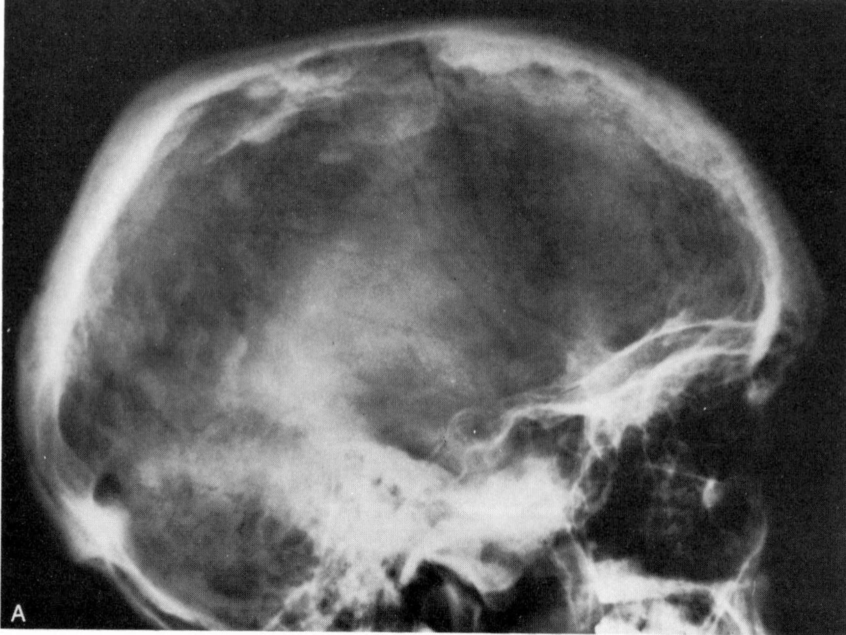

Figure 73–39. *Metaphyseal dysplasia (Pyle's disease).*

A *Note hyperostosis of the cranial vault.*

Illustration continued on the opposite page

obtuse angle of the jaw, and mild sclerosis of the cranial vault. The bones of the pelvis and thoracic cage are expanded.

Frontometaphyseal Dysplasia. This dysplasia was initially described by Gorlin and Cohen in 1969[206] and encompasses cranial hyperostosis, abnormal tubulation of cylindrical bone, and additional skeletal and extraskeletal abnormalities.[207-211] Clinical manifestations include childhood onset, prominent horn-like supraorbital ridges, micrognathia, defective dentition, a wide nasal bridge, a high arched palate, hearing loss, visual disturbances, a

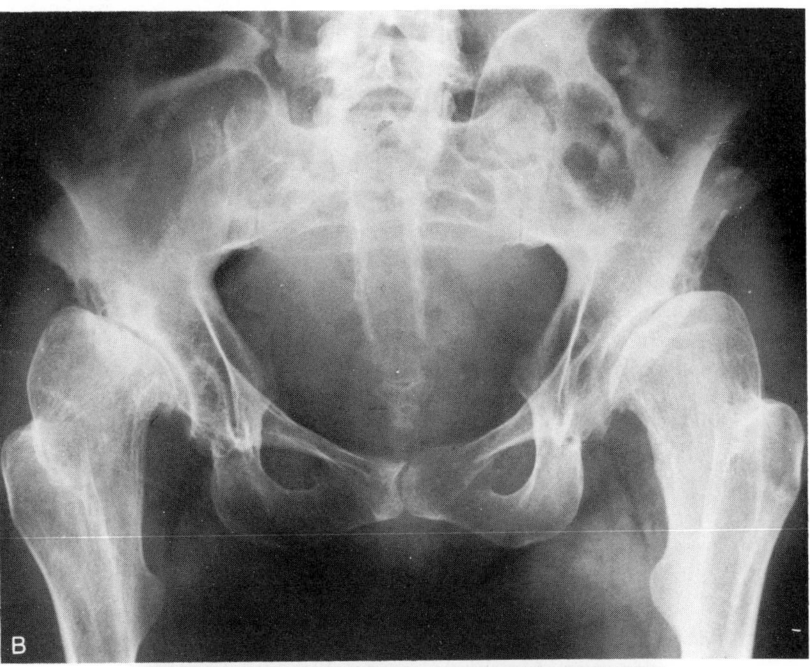

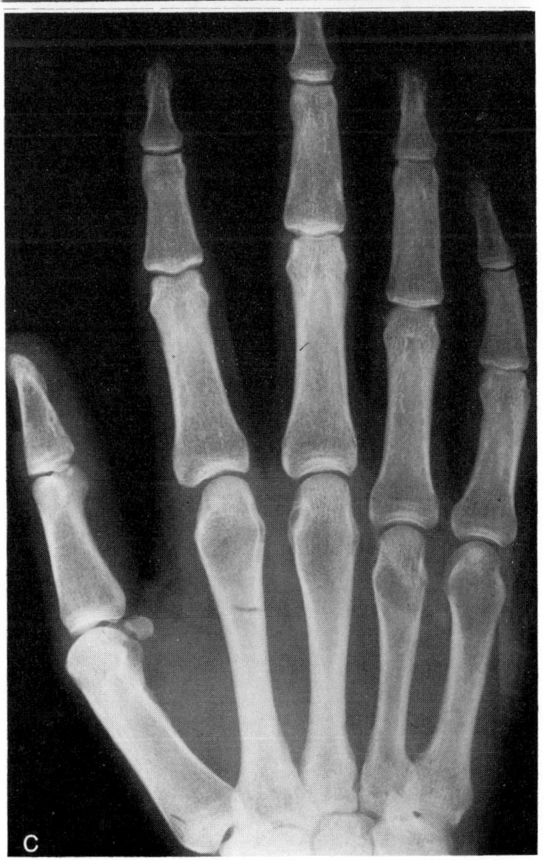

Figure 73–39. Continued

B *The proximal ends of the femora are expanded. The femoral necks are in valgus position, and secondary degenerative joint disease of both hips is seen. Expansion of both ischia is also evident.*

C *Minor abnormalities of the hand include slight expansion of the metacarpals and phalanges with small cystic changes.*

(Courtesy of Dr. A. Goldman, Hospital for Special Surgery, New York, New York.)

short trunk with long extremities, elongated fingers with ulnar deviation of the hands, genu valgum, decreased joint mobility, and contractures. The initial manifestations are usually related to the craniofacial abnormalities. A dominant mode of inheritance is likely but is not definite.

Radiographic features are a prominent supraorbital ridge, calvarial hyperostosis, absent frontal sinuses, micrognathia, dental malformations, accentuated flare of the iliac bones, undertubulation of the metaphyses of the tubular bones, waviness and bowing of the tibias and fibulas with genu valgum, tibia recurvatum, and elongation or widening of metacarpals and phalanges. In older patients, progressive erosion and fusion of the carpus and tarsus have been noted, which may simulate the findings in juvenile chronic arthritis or various osteolytic syndromes.[211]

Although the exact relationship of this entity to other craniotubular disorders is not clear, the presence of prominent cranial abnormalities allows its differentiation from Pyle's disease. Its features resemble those in *craniometaphyseal dysplasia*,[212, 213] although it has been suggested that facial and occipital bone involvement and a normal pelvic contour in the latter condition allow separation of the two disorders.[2]

Diaphyseal Dysplasia (Camurati-Engelmann Disease). This is a rare generalized bilaterally symmetrical dysplasia of bone that is characterized by cortical thickening, increased diameter, and a narrowed medullary cavity in the diaphyses of the tubular bones with epiphyseal sparing.[214-219] Diaphyseal dysplasia is an autosomal dominant disorder with considerable variability of expression and occasionally complete lack of penetrance. The clinical manifestations are variable. Some patients initially present in the first decade of life, whereas others are discovered in the second to fourth decades.[458] A reduction of muscle mass and subcutaneous fat, muscular weakness, abnormal gait, bony enlargement, and leg pain may be evident. Occasionally, the erythrocyte sedimentation rate is elevated. Characteristic roentgenographic features include cortical thickening and sclerosis of the diaphyses of the tubular bones (Fig. 73–40). In order of decreasing frequency, the tibia, the femur, the humerus, the ulna, the radius, and the bones of the hands and feet are affected. In addition, the fibula, the clavicle, the ribs, the pelvis, and the spine can be altered. A symmetrical distribution is typical but not uniform. Both the endosteum and the periosteum are active in this disease. Calvarial hyperostosis and sclerosis of the base of the skull are also encountered.

The course is variable. Progressive findings are common, but spontaneous improvement in adolescence has also been recognized. Increased intracranial pressure and encroachment on cranial nerves can lead to significant complications in some individuals.

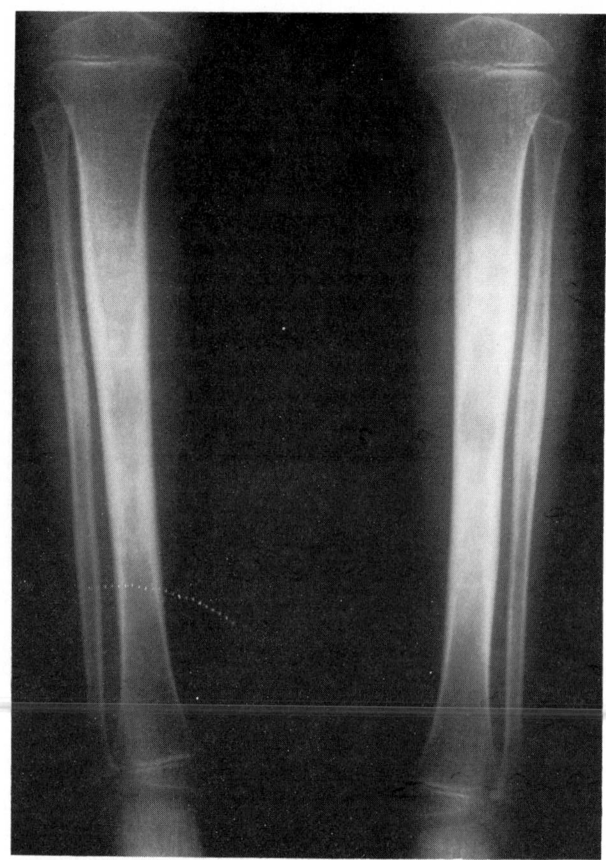

Figure 73–40. *Diaphyseal dysplasia (Camurati-Engelmann disease). Radiographic findings include symmetrically distributed increased sclerosis of the diaphyses of both tibiae and fibulae, with endosteal and periosteal bone formation. Fusiform widening and a wavy bony contour are apparent.*

Ribbing in 1949[220] and Paul in 1953[221] described a familial disorder that was similar to Engelmann's disease. This disorder, which is known as *Ribbing's disease*, appears to have an autosomal recessive inheritance and is associated with radiographic changes that, as in diaphyseal dysplasia, are characterized by sclerosis and cortical thickening of tubular bones. The distribution is asymmetrical, however, and pain is not uncommon.

Craniodiaphyseal dysplasia is a term introduced by Joseph and colleagues in 1958,[222] who described a rare dysplasia characterized by severe sclerosis and hyperostosis of the skull and facial bones, diaphyseal expansion of the tubular bones, and widening of the ribs and clavicles.[223, 224] Infants and children reveal progressive thickening and distortion of the facies, small stature, mental retardation, deafness, and visual disturbances, and death ensues in the first two decades of life.

Hereditary Hyperphosphatasia. This disorder, which is also known as juvenile Paget's

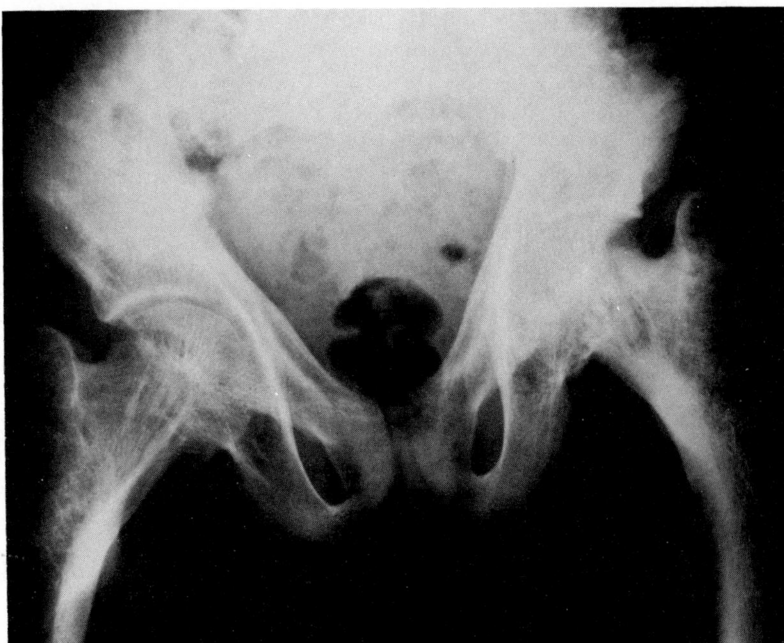

Figure 73–41. *Hereditary hyperphosphatasia. Pagetoid alterations are evident in the pelvis and proximal femora, consisting of trabecular thickening and osseous widening.*

disease, chronic osteopathy with hyperphosphatasia, and osteoectasia with hyperphosphatasia, is a rare disorder of infancy and childhood characterized by generalized cortical thickening of bones and chronic sustained elevation of the level of serum alkaline phosphatase.[225-232] It was first described by Bakwin and Elger in 1956[233] and is detected in early life because of an abnormal modeling of bones that leads to marked skeletal deformity. An autosomal recessive inheritance seems to exist with considerable variability of expression. Involvement may be severe or mild, and clinical variation is evident even in a single family. Overproduction of bone and bone collagen by osteocytes and failure of primitive fibrous tissue to mature into compact lamellar bone can be noted. Affected children have a small stature, large skull, fusiform swelling and bowing of the tubular bones, and a tendency toward fractures. They may reveal severely limited motion and may be unable to walk, crawl, or sit up. Laboratory abnormalities, in addition to elevation of the serum alkaline phosphatase level, include raised serum levels of acid phosphatase, uric acid, and leucine aminopeptidase, and elevation of urinary peptide–bound hydroxyproline and uric acid levels. On radiographic analysis, virtually every bone is affected (Fig. 73–41). Calvarial thickening and mottling, osteopenia, and osseous bowing and widening are discovered. A lack of a discrete cortical shadow is noteworthy. By the second and third decades of life, most patients are severely deformed and incapacitated. Much recent attention has been directed toward the utilization of thyrocalcitonin in the treatment of this disease.

Other Syndromes. *Dysosteosclerosis* is an autosomal recessive disorder manifest in early childhood as small stature, dental anomalies, increased bone fragility, and, occasionally, neurologic abnormalities.[234] Although thickening and sclerosis of the cranial vault, base of the skull, ribs, clavicles, and tubular bones may resemble the findings in osteopetrosis, the presence of platyspondyly and lucency about expanded diametaphyseal segments of long bones allows differentiation of this syndrome.

Tubular stenosis with periodic hypocalcemia (congenital medullary stenosis of the tubular bones) is a disorder of infancy, perhaps of autosomal dominant inheritance, that leads to dwarfism, episodic hypocalcemic tetany and convulsions, transient hypocalcemia and hyperphosphatemia, and radiographically apparent narrowing of the medullary cavities of the tubular bones with normal or increased cortical thickness, reduced diameter of the diaphyses of the bones, and calvarial abnormalities.[2, 235]

Skeletal Dysplasias with Major Involvement of One or More Specific Regions or Segments

Cleidocranial Dysostosis. This is a rare autosomal dominant disorder that leads to abnormality in the development of membranous and cartilaginous bones.[236-241] The disorder becomes manifest at birth; major clinical findings include a large head with delayed closure of sutures, a small face, dental dysplasia with late eruption and impaction of permanent teeth, mobile shoulder girdles, a narrow pelvis, joint hypermobility, short fingers, and hypo-

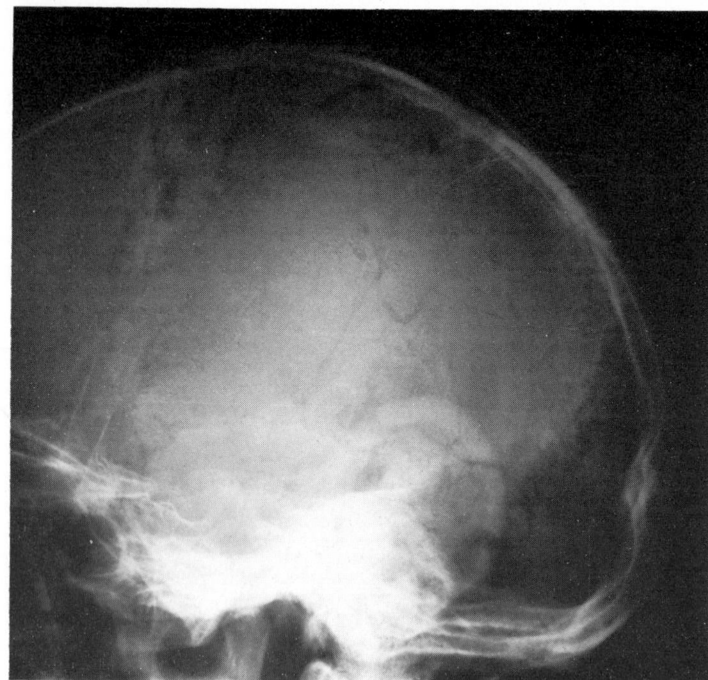

Figure 73–42. *Cleidocranial dysostosis: Cranial abnormalities. Observe multiple wormian bones creating osseous islands within the sutures. Platybasia is also present.*

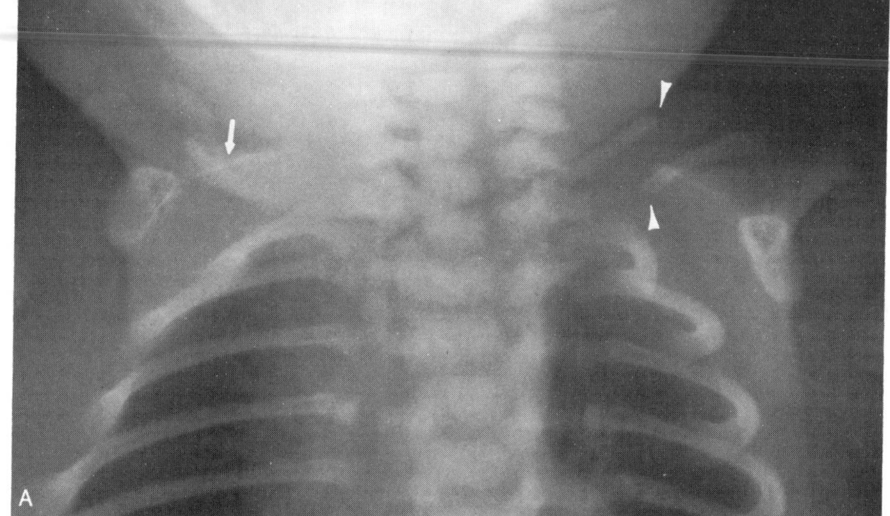

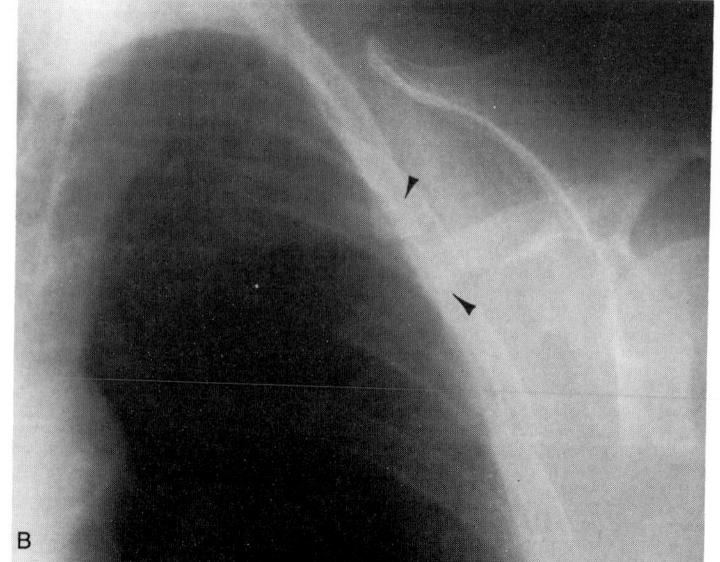

Figure 73–43. *Cleidocranial dysostosis: Clavicular abnormalities.*

A *In this infant, marked hypoplasia of the right clavicle (arrow) and lack of osseous fusion of the lateral and medial portions of the left clavicle (arrowheads) are apparent. Spinal and scapular alterations are also present.*

B *In this adult, lack of osseous fusion and hypoplasia of the lateral and medial ends of the clavicle (arrowheads) and an abnormal scapular position are noted.*

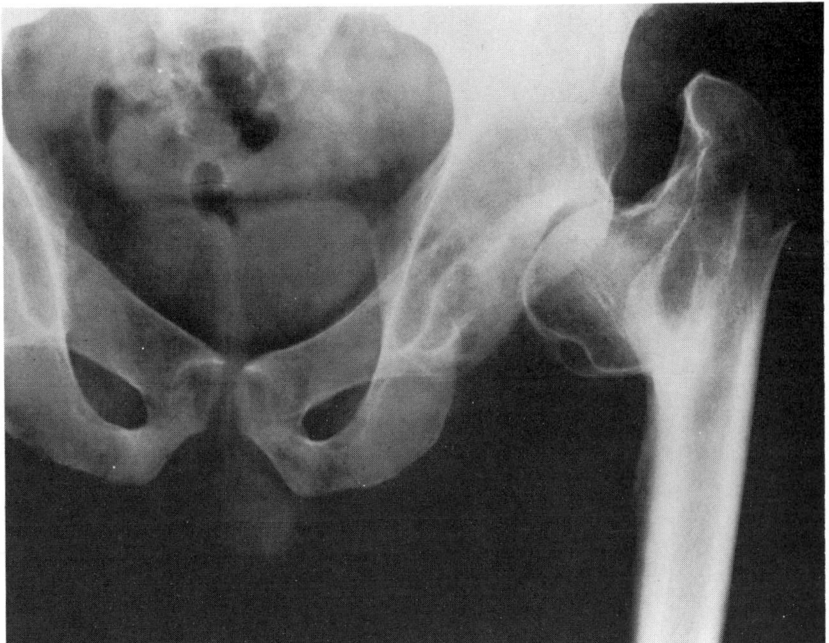

Figure 73–44. Cleidocranial dysostosis: Pelvic and femoral abnormalities. Findings include acetabular malformation and hypoplasia of the pubic bones with widening of the symphysis pubis as well as coxa vara with broadening of the femoral head and enlargement of the greater trochanter. (Courtesy of Dr. R. Freiberger, Hospital for Special Surgery, New York, New York.)

plastic nails. Hearing loss represents one significant complication of the disease, apparently related to structural abnormalities of the ossicles.[239]

Roentgenographic abnormalities are characteristic. Brachycephaly, hypertelorism, open sutures with numerous wormian bones, thickening of the supraorbital portion of the frontal bone, the squama of the temporal bones, and the occipital bone, and deformity of the foramen magnum with platybasia are recognized cranial changes (Fig. 73–42). Clavicular alterations vary in severity but are a constant part of the syndrome (Fig. 73–43). Flaring or absence of the medial third of the bone may represent a subtle abnormality in some patients, but in others, there is partial or total unilateral or bilateral clavicular aplasia, especially in the middle and lateral segments. Marked pseudarthroses can be seen with the formation of a joint just lateral to the midpoint of the clavicle. The scapulae may be small or deformed.

Spinal alterations include neural arch defects, hemivertebrae, and spondylolysis and spondylolisthesis. The thorax may be cone-shaped. In the pelvis, ossification of the pubic bones is absent or delayed until the age of approximately 25 years, and these bones may be distorted or sclerotic in the adult patient (Fig. 73–44). Hypoplasia of the iliac wings,

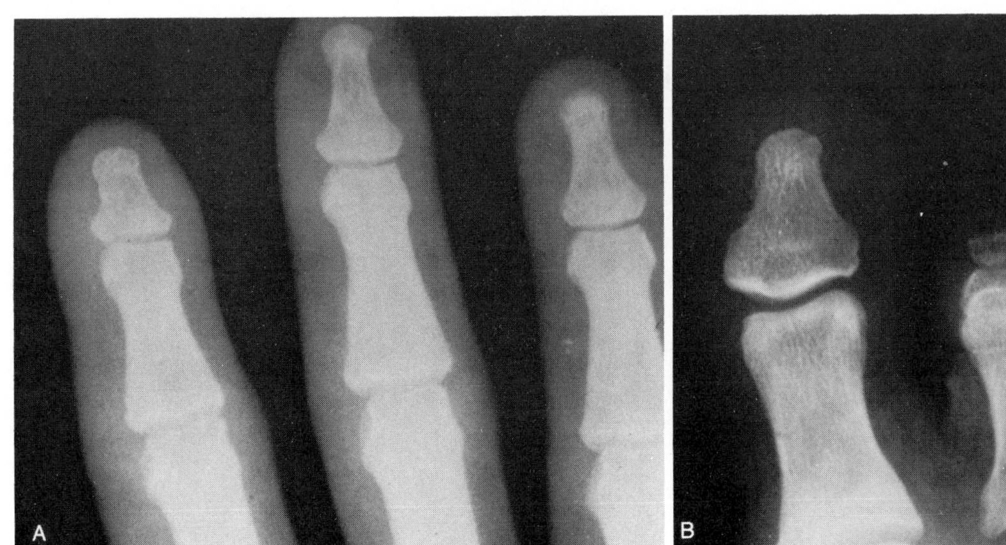

Figure 73–45. Cleidocranial dyostosis: Phalangeal abnormalities. Findings in the hand and feet include shortening of the phalanges, especially the terminal phalanges, with tuftal deformity. (Courtesy of Dr. R. Freiberger, Hospital for Special Surgery, New York, New York.)

widening of the sacroiliac joint, and prominence of the Y cartilage of the acetabulum can be encountered. Valgus or varus deformities of the femoral neck and broadening of the femoral head may also be seen (Fig. 73–44).

In the hands and feet, the distal phalanges may be shortened with pointed tufts, especially in the thumbs, and clinodactyly, brachymesophalangia, accessory metacarpal and metatarsal epiphyses, dysplasia of the middle phalanx of the fifth finger, and retarded ossification of carpal and tarsal bones can be evident (Fig. 73–45). Narrowed epiphyses and expanded metaphyses of tubular bones have also been noted.

Although life expectancy is normal, dental anomalies, hearing loss, dislocation of the shoulder, radial head, and hip, and scoliosis represent important complications of this syndrome.

OSTEO-ONYCHODYSOSTOSIS. This autosomal dominant disorder is also referred to as the nail-patella syndrome, hereditary osteo-onychodysplasia (HOOD), and Fong's syndrome.[242-249] It is characterized by dysplastic fingernails, hypoplastic or absent patellae, additional bony deformities, particularly about the pelvis and elbows, iliac horns, widespread soft tissue changes, and renal dysplasia.[250] Proteinuria and, occasionally, hematuria may be present in infancy, although significant renal impairment is usually not evident until adulthood. Renal osteodystrophy[243] and death can result from the kidney disease. The exact nature of the renal changes is not clear; a characteristic abnormality of the glomerular basement membrane can be evident with electron microscopy, and an enzymatic defect in collagen metabolism may be the common link to the skeletal and renal lesions.[251-253]

Clinical manifestations can become evident in the child, adolescent, or adult but are most frequently seen in the second and third decades of life. Hypoplasia or splitting of fingernails, palpable absence of the patellae and presence of iliac protuberances, increased carrying angle of the elbow, abnormal pigmentation of the iris, and proteinuria may be recognized on initial clinical examination. Laboratory analysis can confirm more severe renal dysfunction.

The roentgenographic changes are highly characteristic and may allow accurate diagnosis

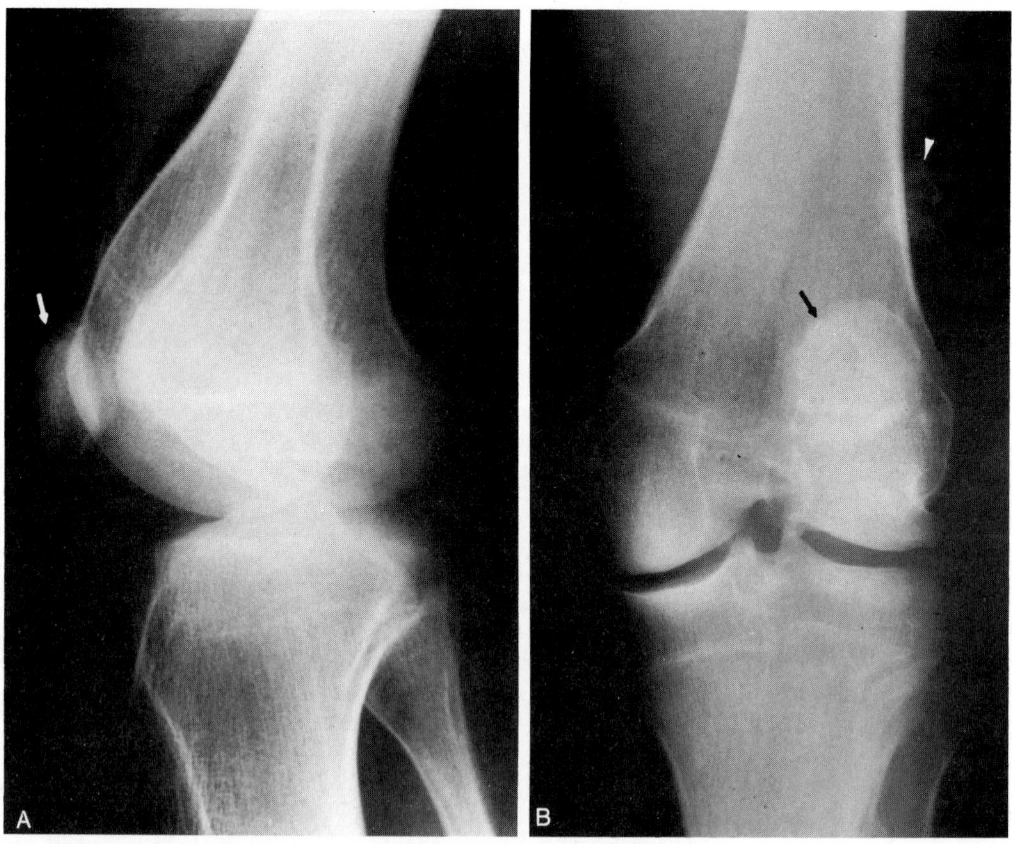

Figure 73–46. *Osteo-onychodysostosis: Knee abnormalities.*

A *Observe the hypoplastic patella (arrow). (Courtesy of Dr. A. Goldman, Hospital for Special Surgery, New York, New York.)*

B *In a different patient, the patella is hypoplastic (arrow), the lateral condyle of the femur is relatively small in comparison to the medial condyle, and an intra-articular osseous body within the suprapatellar pouch (arrowhead) can be seen. (Courtesy of Dr. V. Vint, Scripp's Clinic, La Jolla, California.)*

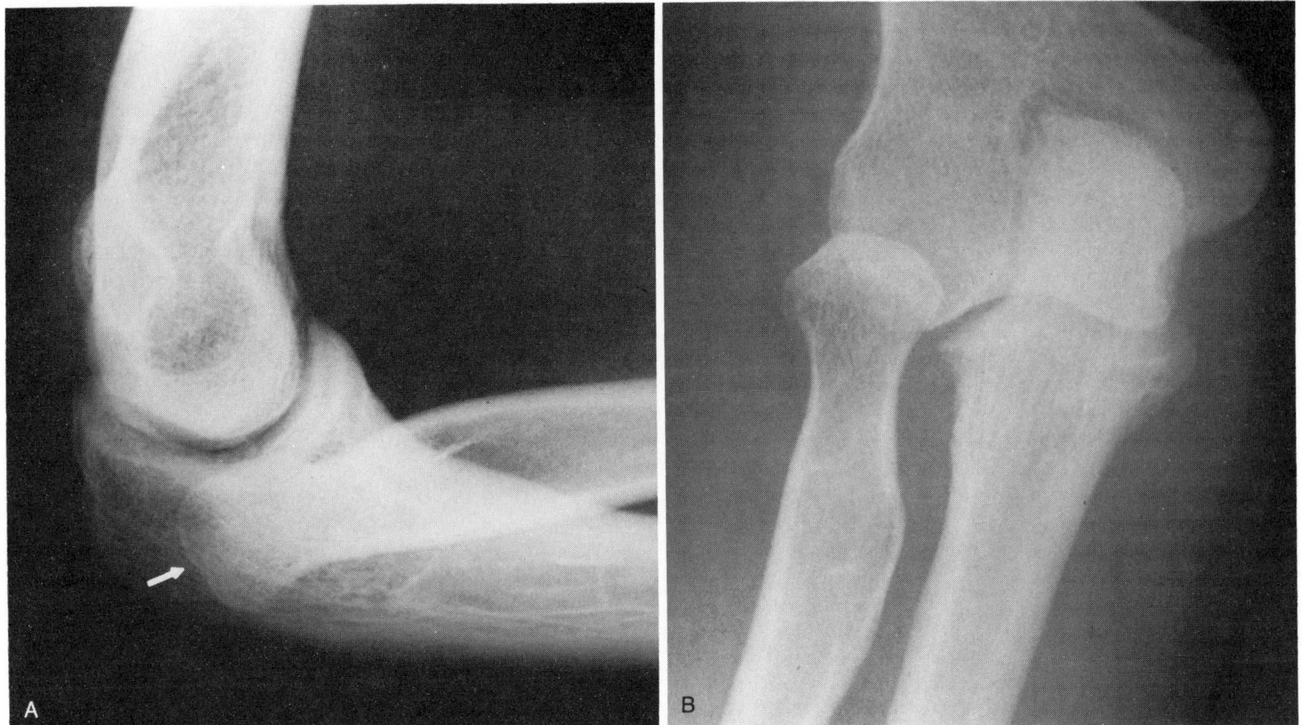

Figure 73–47. *Osteo-onychodysostosis: Elbow abnormalities.*

A *The dislocation and deformity of the proximal radius (arrow) and irregularity of the humeral condyles can be seen. (Courtesy of Dr. A. Goldman, Hospital for Special Surgery, New York, New York.)*

B *In another individual, observe subluxation and deformity of the proximal radius and hypoplasia of the distal lateral portion of the humerus.*

even in the absence of clinical suspicion of the disease. Thus, in infancy, the demonstration of posterior iliac horns allows identification of this dysplasia.[249] Skeletal changes are also apparent in other regions of the body. In the knee, absence or hypoplasia of the patella, asymmetrical development of the femoral condyles with hypoplasia of the lateral condyle and an apparent or true enlargement of the medial condyle and a sloping tibial plateau with a prominent tibial tubercle are identified (Fig. 73–46). These changes can lead to deformity, abnormal gait, patellar instability, and genu valgum. In the elbow, asymmetrical development of the humeral condyles, hypoplasia of the capitulum, and subluxation or dislocation of the radial head are the major changes (Fig. 73–47).

Abnormalities of the pelvis consist of dysplasia of the iliac wings and the presence of iliac horns

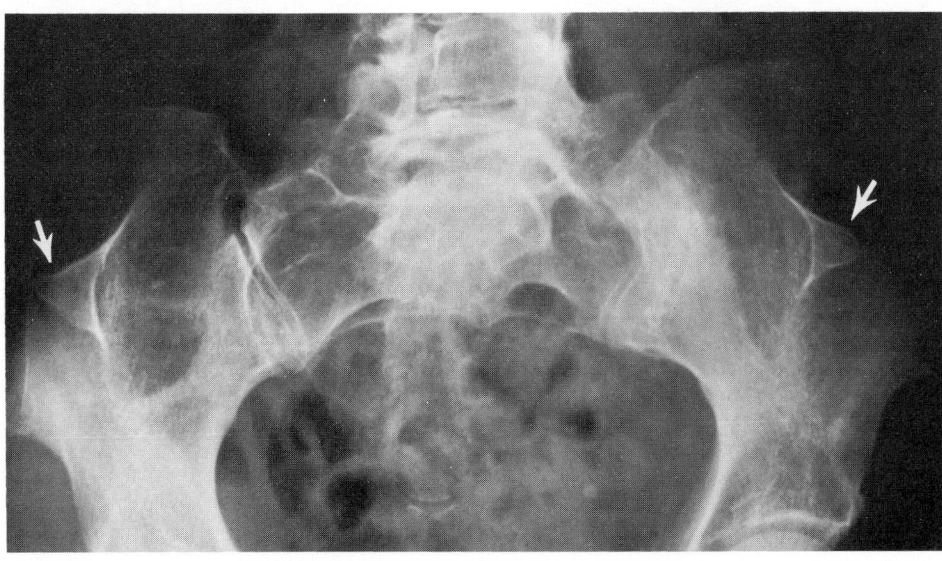

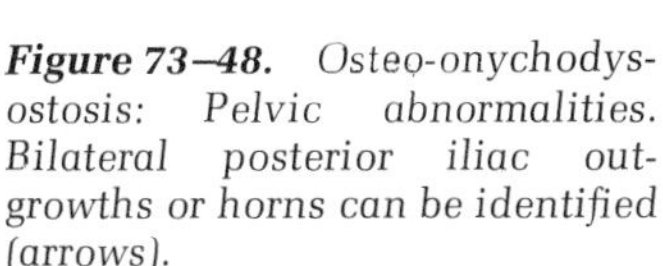

Figure 73–48. *Osteo-onychodysostosis: Pelvic abnormalities. Bilateral posterior iliac outgrowths or horns can be identified (arrows).*

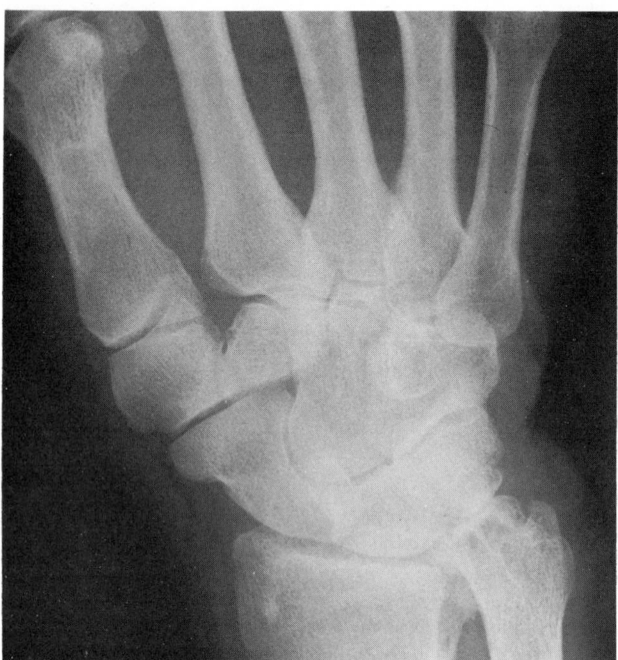

Figure 73–49. Osteo-onychodysostosis: Wrist abnormalities. Relative overgrowth of the distal ulna with secondary degenerative joint disease can be seen.

(Fig. 73–48). Iliac horns were first described by Kieser in 1939[254] and Fong in 1946.[255] Their association with nail, elbow, and knee dysplasia was recognized by Mino and co-workers in 1948.[256] Bilateral outgrowths from the posterior ilium, which are occasionally capped by an epiphysis, are virtually pathognomonic of osteo-onychodysostosis, although they are absent in a small percentage of cases. Unilateral iliac horns apparently can be unassociated with additional skeletal abnormalities.[257]

Additional bony changes can be evident in the shoulder, wrist, ankle, and subtalar joints, emphasizing the generalized nature of this dysplasia (Fig. 73–49). Soft tissue alterations include flexion contractures of the hip, knee, elbow, fingers, and foot, web formation, and deltoid, triceps, and quadriceps hypoplasia.[244]

The basic defect is not known. An abnormality in the connective tissue due to an alteration of the enzymatic system of the ground substance has been suggested.[258] Other mechanisms have also been proposed and are summarized by Valdueza.[244]

Larsen's Syndrome. In 1950, Larsen and co-workers[259] described the association of multiple congenital dislocations and a characteristic facial abnormality. Subsequently, numerous reports have documented the existence of this syndrome.[260-271] The disorder is inherited, although the pattern of inheritance is heterogenetic; in some instances, the trait appears to be dominant, whereas in others, an autosomal recessive transmission is more probable.[2] Larsen's syndrome is evident at birth. Prominent clinical findings include a peculiar flattened facies with prominent forehead, low nasal bridge, widely spaced eyes, and cleft palate or uvula. Joint dislocations are typical, frequently multiple, and affect predominantly the knees, the hips, and the elbows (Fig. 73–50). Laxity of costochondral cartilage, abnormal hands with cylindrical fingers, and foot deformities may be seen. Radiographs confirm the dislocation and deformity of various joints and reveal an extracalcaneal ossification center (which may later fuse with the parent bone), supernumerary carpal bones, and distortion of metacarpals and phalanges. Abnormal spinal curvature, segmentation, and instability, which can lead to cord compression and even death, have been noted. Craniofacial disproportionism has, in some instances, been associated with hydrocephalus. Premature degenerative disease may complicate the articular abnormalities. Laryngeal malformations can lead to respiratory distress.

Multiple joint dislocations can also occur in arthrogryposis, Ehlers-Danlos syndrome, congenital laxity,[272-274] Down's syndrome (mongolism), other chromosomal aberrations, diastrophic dwarfism, and the oto-palato-digital syndrome, but clinical and radiographic characteristics usually allow an accurate differential diagnosis.

Dyschondrosteosis (Léri-Weill Disease). In 1929, Léri and Weill[128] described a young woman with drawfism and Madelung-like wrist deformities, and they designated the disorder as dyschondrosteosis. Despite the rarity of the condition, numerous descriptions exist of its clinical and radiologic features.[275-280] It is an autosomal dominant disorder and expresses itself more severely in female patients. The clinical findings of short stature, especially of the lower legs and forearms, and wrist deformity usually become apparent in late childhood or adolescence. Endocrine disturbances, such as goiter, diabetes mellitus, and hyperthyroidism, have been noted in some individuals.[281]

Radiographic findings include a bayonet-wrist deformity with a shortened radius in relationship to the ulna, an ulnar and palmar slant of the radial articular surface, triangular distal radial epiphysis and carpal bones, and dorsal subluxation of the distal ulna. In the leg, the tibia is shortened, and its medial portion is prominent.

The exact relationship of Madelung's deformity and dyschondrosteosis is a matter of much debate (p. 2569). Other differential diagnostic conditions include Turner's syndrome, mesomelic dwarfism of the Nievergelt or Langer types,[282, 283] and ulnofibular dysplasia.[2]

Other Syndromes. *Tricho-rhino-phalangeal dysplasia,* which has been divided into two distinct types,[2] presents in infancy or early childhood with characteristic hair, nose, and hand changes.[284-285] Although the radiographic features vary between the two subgroups, findings include shortening of phalanges and metacarpals, epiphyseal deformities and fragmentation that may resemble Legg-Calvé-Perthes or Thiemann's disease, and exostoses similar to those of hereditary multiple exostoses (Fig. 73–51).[449]

The oto-palato-digital syndrome may lead to mental retardation, cleft palate, distinctive facies, short stature, joint subluxation, and changes in the hands and feet in male infants, and less severe clinical findings in females.[286, 287] Its radiologic features include, among others, a prominent supraorbital ridge, small facial structures and mandible, short and broad distal phalanges, accessory carpal bones, foot anomalies, joint dislocations, and deformities of the pelvis and spine. Some of the clinical and radiologic features resemble those found in Larsen's syndrome.

The Weismann-Netter-Stuhl syndrome (toxopachyostéose diaphysaire tibio-péronière) is a rare inherited disorder leading to anterior bowing of the tibia and fibula with posterior cortical thickening, usually in a bilateral and symmetrical fashion, associated with short stature, pelvic deformity, and, possibly, mental retardation, dural calcification, and radial abnormalities.[288, 289] The alterations of the lower leg may resemble the "saber shin" of syphilis or the bowing changes of rickets. The posterior cortical

Text continued on page 2597

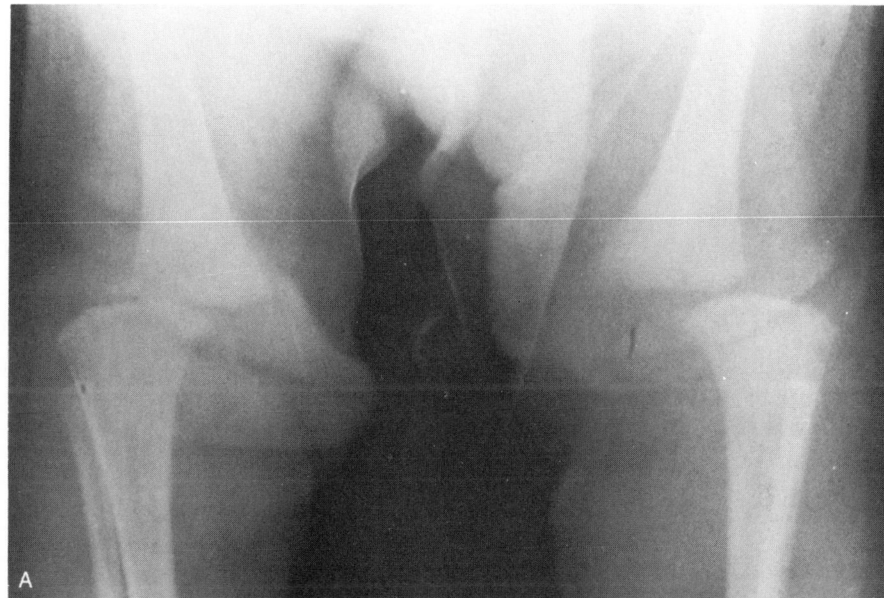

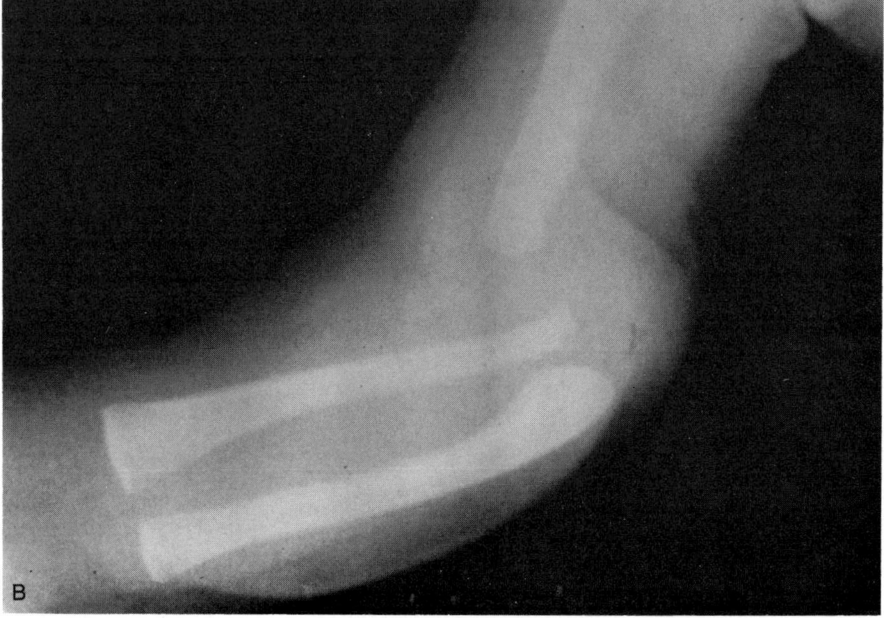

Figure 73–50. *Larsen's syndrome. In this disorder, dislocation of multiple joints is characteristic. Note the lateral displacement of tibiae and fibulae and the posterior dislocation of the elbow. (Courtesy of Dr. R. Freiberger, Hospital for Special Surgery, New York, New York.)*

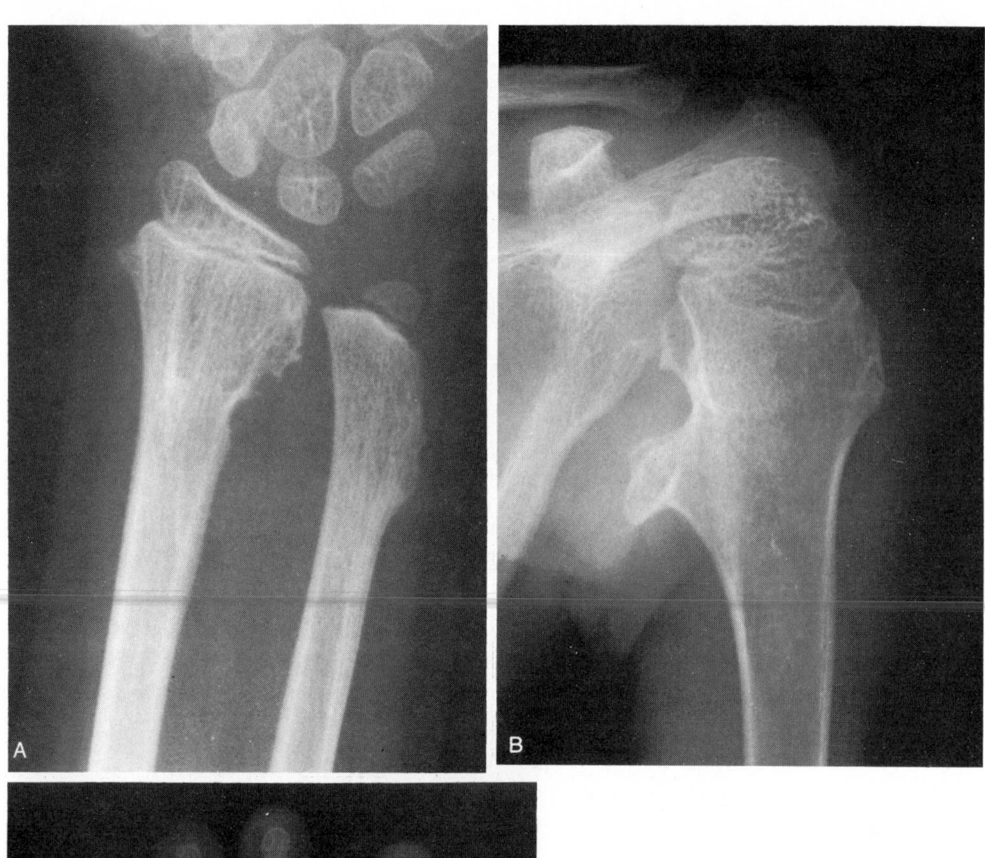

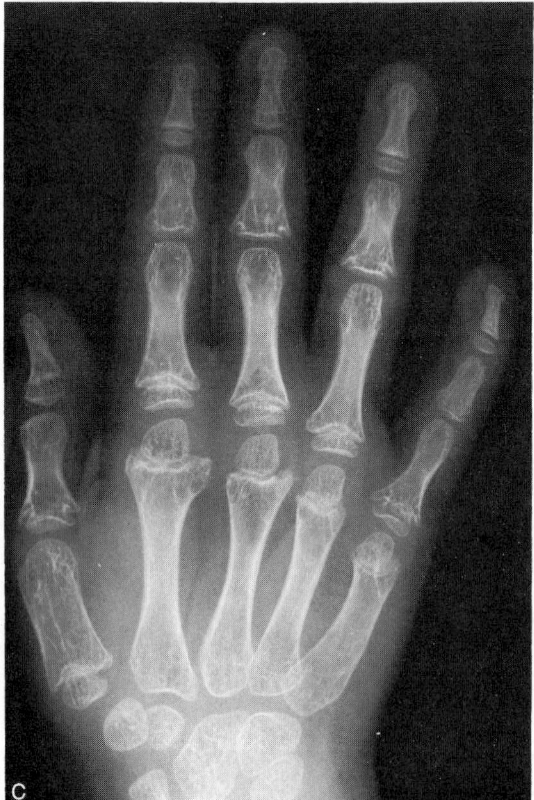

Figure 73–51. *Tricho-rhino-phalangeal dysplasia (Type II). In this 12 year old boy with small stature, sparse hair, protruding ears, and peculiarly shaped nose and upper lip, observe exostoses of the distal radius, distal ulna, and proximal humerus and cone-shaped epiphyses of the metacarpals and phalanges.*

Table 73–3
CLASSIFICATION OF THE CRANIOSTENOSIS-SYNDACTYLISM SYNDROMES

	SKULL				HANDS			FEET					
No. Eponym	Acrocephaly	Hypo-plastic Maxilla	Hypo-plastic Mandible	Asym-metry	Osseous Fusion	First Phalangeal Deformity	Hypoplasia (Aplasia) of Middle Phalanx	Osseous Fusion	First Phalangeal Deformity	Hypoplasia (Aplasia) of Middle Phalanx	Numerical Abnormalities	Associated Features	Genetic Trans-mission
I Apert	severe	+	–	–	+	+	+	+	+	+	occasionally duplication first toe	—	autosomal dominant
II Chotzen	mild	+	–	+	–	–	–	–	–	–	—	short stature cryptorchism seizures	autosomal dominant
III Waardenburg	mild, distinct, delayed ossification	–	+	–	–	+	+	–	–	+	oligodactyly feet	short stature, pericardial cyst, contractures, rectal prolapse, deformed ears	?
IV Pfeiffer	mild	+	–	–	–	+	+	–	+	+	occasionally duplication first toe	—	autosomal dominant
V Summit	mild, distinct	+	–	–	±	–	+	±	±	±	—	obesity	autosomal recessive
Acrocephalopolysyndactyly													
I Carpenter	severe, distinct	–	+	–	–	–	+	–	+	+	polydactyly feet	obesity, hypogenitalism, absent coccyx	autosomal recessive

(Courtesy of Spranger JW, Langer LO, Wiedemann HR: Bone Dysplasias: An Atlas of Constitutional Disorders of Skeletal Development. Philadelphia, WB Saunders Co, 1974, pp 262–263.)

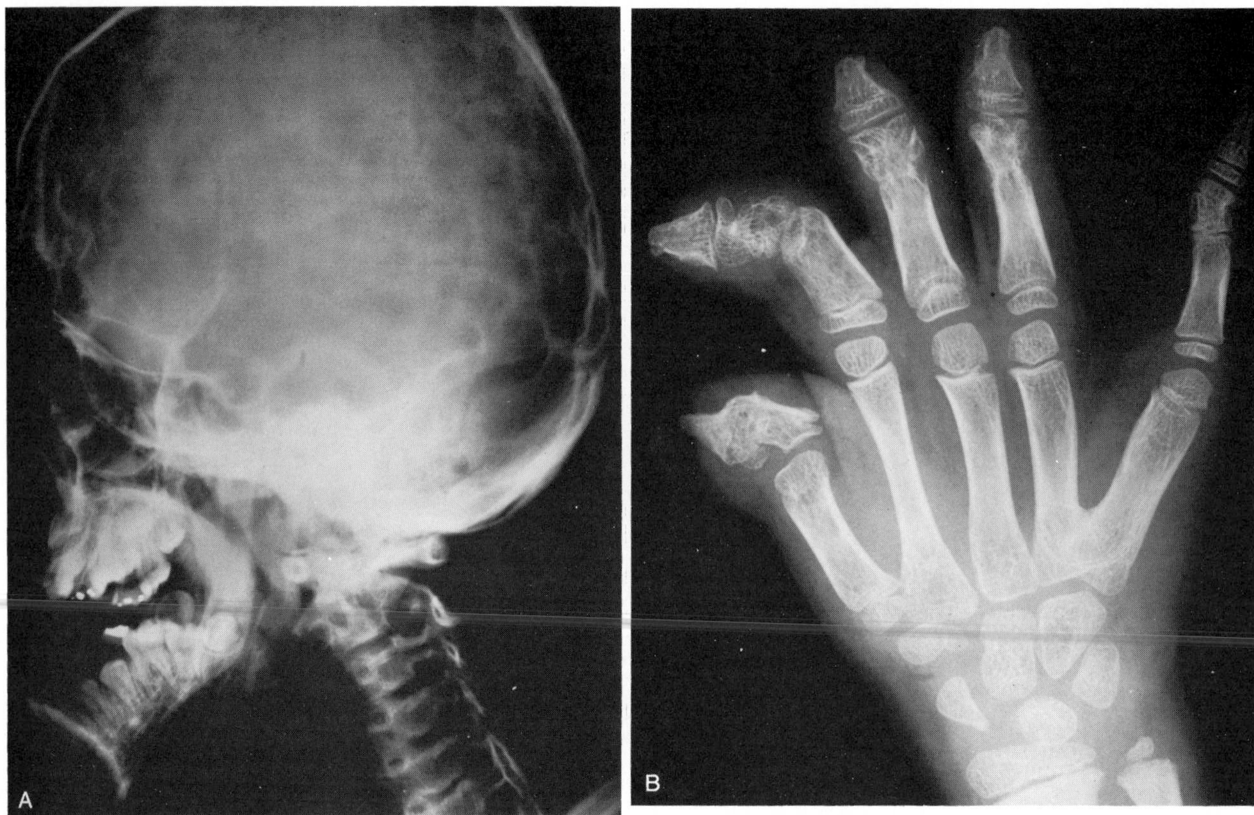

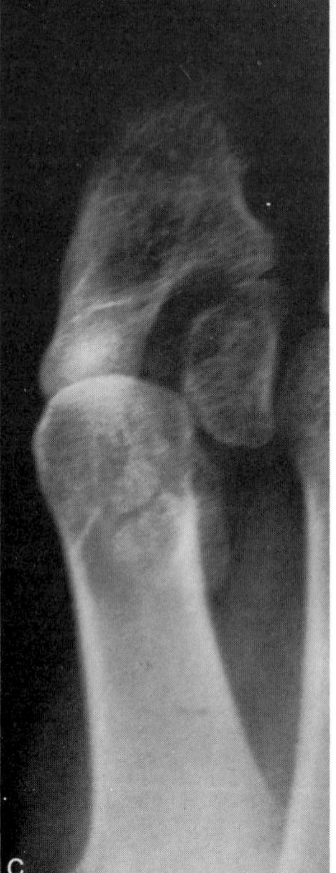

Figure 73–52. *Acrocephalosyndactyly syndrome: Type I — Apert syndrome.*

A *There is an increased vertical diameter and a decreased anteroposterior diameter of the skull. The occiput is flat and the maxilla is hypoplastic.*

B *The changes in the hand include soft tissue syndactyly, symphalangism, and bizarre deformity of the phalanges of the thumb.*

C *In the great toe, note the delta-shaped proximal phalanx and the deformed distal phalanx.*

(Courtesy of Dr. R. Freiberger, Hospital for Special Surgery, New York, New York.)

thickening of the tibia and fibula in this syndrome differs from the anterior osseous changes in syphilis.

There exists a group of *acrocephalosyndactyly syndromes* that are characterized by the combination of craniosynostosis and malformations of the hands and feet.[290-294] These can be classified into six major types: Apert syndrome, Chotzen syndrome, Waardenburg syndrome, Pfeiffer syndrome, Summit syndrome, and Carpenter syndrome.[2] They can be differentiated by the severity of the findings, the presence and type of hand and foot deformity, and the pattern of genetic transmission (Table 73–3) (Fig. 73–52). It is suspected that additional distinct varieties of acrocephalo(poly)syndactyly will be recognized.

Mucopolysaccharidoses and Mucolipidoses

The term mucopolysaccharidosis (MPS) was first utilized in 1952 by Brante[295] in a description of the histologic findings in patients with gargoylism, which included swollen collagen tissues filled with water-soluble material. The same material was discovered in other sites and organs. Later studies

Table 73–4
THE GENETIC MUCOPOLYSACCHARIDOSES (AS CLASSIFIED IN 1972)

	Designation	Clinical Features	Genetics	Excessive Urinary MPS	Substance Deficient
MPS I-H	Hurler syndrome	Early clouding of cornea, grave manifestations, death usually before age 10	Homozygous for MPS I gene	Dermatan sulfate Heparan sulfate	α-L-iduronidase (formerly called Hurler corrective factor)
MPS I-S	Scheie syndrome	Stiff joints, cloudy cornea, aortic regurgitation, normal intelligence, ?normal life-span	Homozygous for MPS IS gene	Dermatan sulfate Heparan sulfate	α-L-iduronidase
MPS I-H/S	Hurler-Scheie compound	Phenotype intermediate between Hurler and Scheie	Genetic compound of MPS IH and IS genes	Dermatan sulfate Heparan sulfate	α-L-iduronidase
MPS II-A	Hunter syndrome, severe	No clouding of cornea, milder course than in MPS IH but death usually before age 15 years	Hemizygous for X-linked gene	Dermatan sulfate Heparan sulfate	Hunter corrective factor
MPS II-B	Hunter syndrome, mild	Survival to 30's to 50's, fair intelligence	Hemizygous for X-linked allele for mild form	Dermatan sulfate Heparan sulfate	Hunter corrective factor
MPS III-A	Sanfilippo syndrome A	Identical phenotype Mild somatic, severe central nervous system effects	Homozygous for Sanfilippo A gene	Heparan sulfate	Heparan sulfate sulfatase
MPS III-B	Sanfilippo syndrome B		Homozygous for Sanfilippo B (at different locus)	Heparan sulfate	N-acetyl-α-D-glucosaminidase
MPS IV	Morquio syndrome (probably more than one allelic form)	Severe bone changes of distinctive type, cloudy cornea, aortic regurgitation	Homozygous for Morquio gene	Keratan sulfate	Unknown
MPS V	(Scheie syndrome may be classified as MPS V or MPS I-S, as above.)				
MPS VI-A	Maroteaux-Lamy syndrome, classic form	Severe osseous and corneal change, normal intellect	Homozygous for M-L gene	Dermatan sulfate	Maroteaux-Lamy corrective factor
MPS VI-B	Maroteaux-Lamy syndrome, mild form	Milder osseous and corneal change, normal intellect	Homozygous for allele at M-L locus	Dermatan sulfate	Maroteaux-Lamy corrective factor
MPS VII	β-glucuronidase deficiency (more than one allelic form?)	Hepatosplenomegaly, dysostosis multiplex, white cell inclusions, mental retardation	Homozygous for mutant gene at beta-glucuronidase locus	Dermatan sulfate Chondroitin sulfate A Chondroitin sulfate C	β-glucuronidase

(Courtesy of McKusick VA: Heritable Disorders of Connective Tissue. 4th Ed. St Louis, The CV Mosby Co, 1972, p 525.)

indicated extensive amounts of certain mucopolysaccharides in the urine of affected patients.[296] In the ensuing years, the detection of different chemical substances in the urine of patients with similar varieties of dwarfism led to the delineation of closely related but distinct disorders. Currently, the MPS are classified into six or seven types,[3] and there are recognized additional diseases, some of which are mucolipidoses, that demonstrate similar clinical and radiologic findings (Table 73–4). Common to the MPS and mucolipidoses are the following general roentgenographic characteristics.[2]

General osseous structure: osteoporosis with coarsened trabeculation.

Skull: macrocephaly, dyscephaly, J-shaped sella, thick calvaria.

Chest: oar-shaped ribs, widened clavicles, plump scapulae.

Spine: oval-shaped and hook-shaped vertebral bodies.

Pelvis: overconstriction of iliac bodies, wide iliac flare, dysplasia of capital femoral epiphysis, coxa valga.

Long tubular bones: shortening, epiphyseal dysplasia, metaphyseal widening, proximal tapering of second to fifth metacarpals.

A more precise diagnosis requires clinical information, including the pattern of genetic transmission, and biochemical data, including the pattern of increased urinary excretion of acid mucopolysaccharides.

MPS-I (Hurler Syndrome). This autosomal recessive disorder presents in the first few years of life.[297] Patients reveal distinctive facies, mental retardation, deafness, dwarfism, corneal opacities, hepatosplenomegaly, cardiomegaly, and cardiac murmurs. Laboratory analysis reveals increased urinary excretion of dermatan sulfate and heparan sulfate, abnormal mucopolysaccharide accumulation in the bone marrow and peripheral leukocytes, and low or absent activity of α-L-iduronidase in various tissues.[2] Radiographs reveal macrocephaly, craniostenosis, J-shaped sella, widening of the anterior portion of the ribs, ovoid vertebral bodies with hypoplasia of vertebrae about the thoracolumbar junction resulting in kyphosis, hypoplasia and stenosis of the bases of the ilia with pseudoenlargement of the acetabulum and coxa valga, shortening and widening of the shafts of the long tubular bones, pointing of the proximal portions of the metacarpals, and osteoporosis (Fig. 73–53). Mental retardation and skeletal deformities may be progressive, leading to considerable disability.

Rarely, patients are discovered with Hurler disease phenotypes who do not excrete excessive amounts of mucopolysaccharides in the urine.[298]

MPS-II (Hunter Syndrome). This X-linked recessive disorder is differentiated from MPS-I by its occurrence only in males, mild mental retardation, absence of corneal clouding, less significant hearing impairment, and a relatively benign clinical course.[299, 300] Two forms of the disease exist. In the milder variety, survival into middle age and beyond is not infrequent. Chemical values reveal abnormalities identical to those in MPS-I, and roentgenographic changes are similar but not so extensive.

MPS-III (Sanfilippo Syndrome). This autosomal recessive disorder becomes evident in early childhood with mild somatic and moderate to severe neurologic abnormalities.[301-302] These include pro-

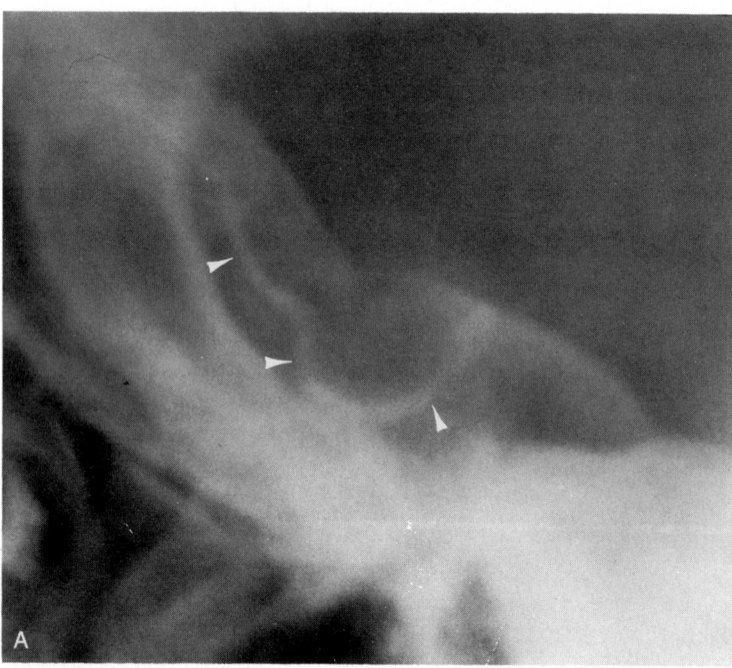

Figure 73–53. *Mucopolysaccharidosis I: Hurler syndrome (3 year old child).*

A *A coned-down lateral radiograph of the skull reveals a J-shaped sella turcica (arrowheads).*

Illustration continued on the opposite page

gressive mental retardation, motor overactivity, coarse facial features, hirsutism, and, rarely, clouding of the cornea. Two clinically indistinguishable but biochemically different forms are recognized. Radiographic findings are similar to but milder than MPS-I with the most diagnostic signs being present in the hands, the pelvis, and the spine. Increased urinary excretion of heparan sulfate is seen.

MPS-IV (Morquio Syndrome). This is a rare autosomal recessive disorder that becomes manifest in early childhood.[303, 304] Clinical manifestations include dwarfism, facial deformity, fine corneal opacities, impaired hearing, dental hypoplasia, sternal protrusion, ligamentous laxity, and hepatomegaly. Urinary excretion of excess amounts of keratan sulfate is observed. Radiographic analysis reveals platyspon-

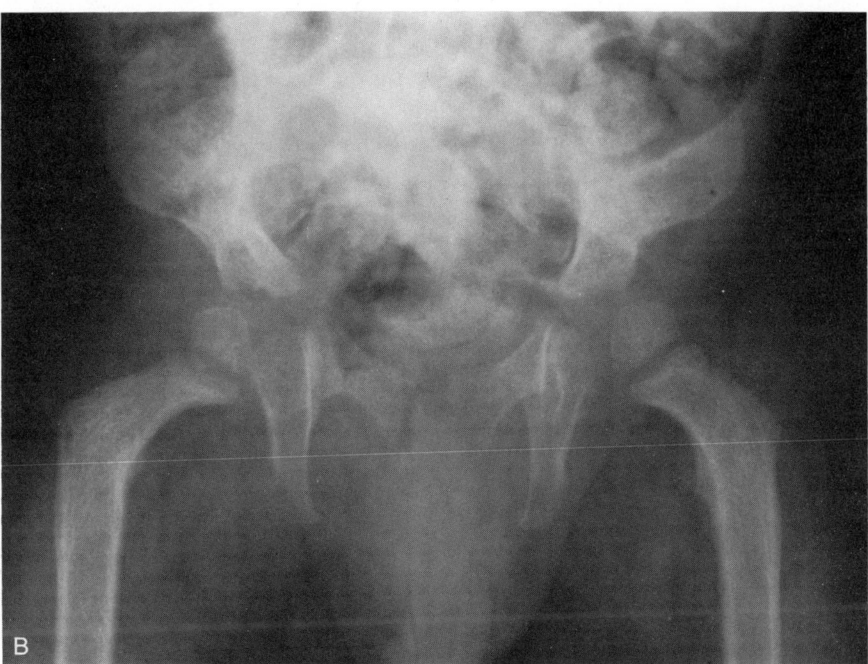

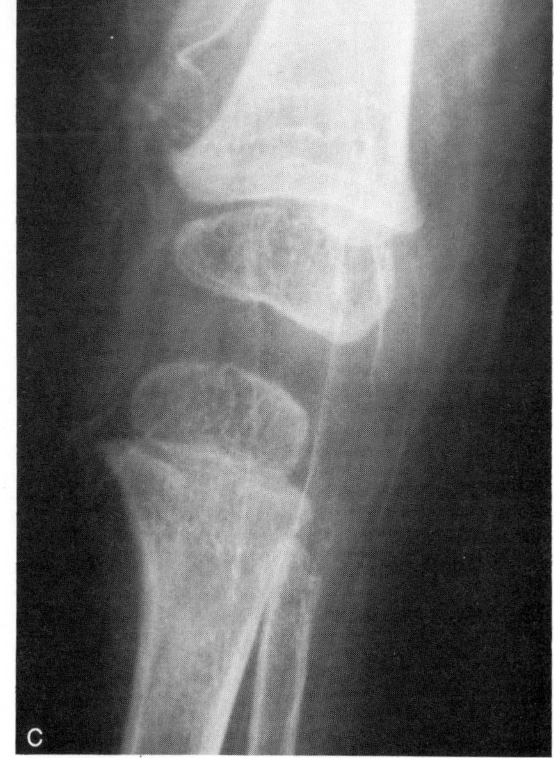

Figure 73–53. Continued
B *In the pelvis, hypoplasia of the basilar portions of the iliac bones, flared iliac wings, and dysplastic proximal capital femoral epiphyses can be noted.*
C *In the knee, osteoporosis, lack of normal modeling of the shaft, and slanting of the proximal tibial growth plate are seen.*

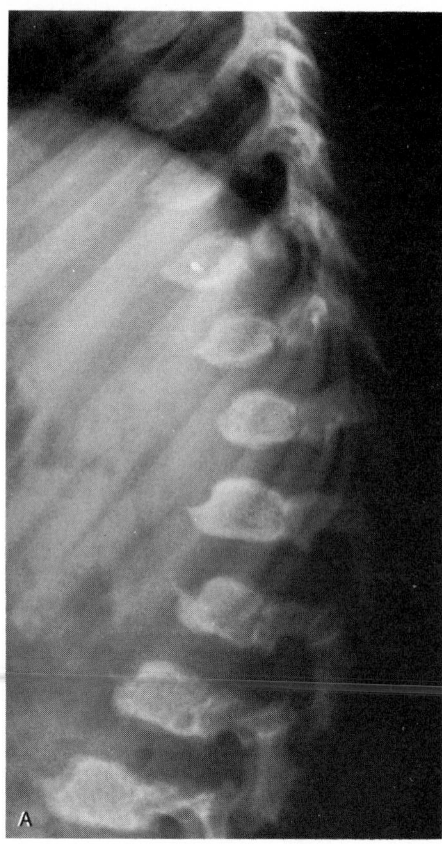

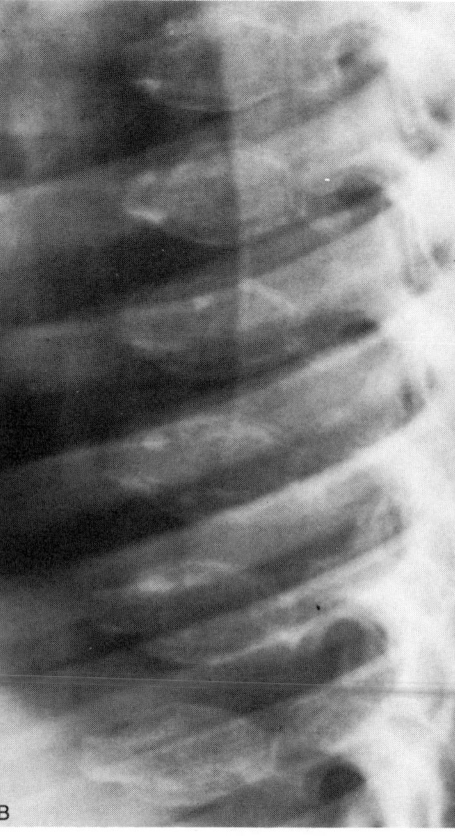

Figure 73–54. *Mucopolysaccharidosis IV: Morquio disease —spinal abnormalities. Two examples showing the platyspondyly that characterizes this condition. Note the flattened vertebral bodies, the anterior central beaks and, in one case, an exaggerated kyphosis.*

dyly with central beaking of vertebral bodies, odontoid hypoplasia with atlanto-axial subluxation, cone-shaped bases of the second to fifth metacarpals, hypoplasia of the lateral aspects of the acetabular roof, and coxa valga[2, 305] (Figs. 73–54 to 73–56). Additional findings may include errors of modeling of the large tubular bones and widened ribs. Rarely, cases of apparent Morquio syndrome do not reveal typical urinary findings.[306]

MPS-V (Scheie Syndrome—MPS I-S). An autosomal recessive disorder, MPS-V, or I-S, is characterized by peripheral clouding of the cornea, normal mentality, normal or slightly reduced stature, stiff joints, hirsutism, flexion of the hands, and aortic regurgitation.[3] Increased excretion of dermatan sulfate and heparan sulfate is evident. Radiographs outline proximal tapering of the metacarpals, widening of the ribs, and mild alterations of the spine and skull. This disorder is closely related to MPS-I, explaining its frequent classification as MPS I-S, although it is less common than Hurler syndrome and its clinical and radiologic features are less striking.

MPS-VI (Maroteaux-Lamy Syndrome). This syndrome, which is an autosomal recessive disorder, is characterized by short stature that usually becomes evident at about two years of age in association with lumbar kyphosis, sternal protrusion, knock knees, abnormal facies, hepatosplenomegaly, and joint contractures.[307, 308] Corneal opacification and normal intelligence are additional clinical findings. Dermatan sulfate excretion is increased. Radiographs reveal macrocephaly, an enlarged sella turcica, ilial hypoplasia, flared iliac crests, dysplasia of capital femoral epiphyses, coxa valga, biconvexity of vertebral end-plates, deformities of long tubular bones, and shortening, widening, and proximal tapering of metacarpal bones.[2]

MPS-VII (Beta-glucuronidase Deficiency). This is a recently reported new variety of MPS in which growth retardation, hepatosplenomegaly, mental retardation, and pulmonary infections are observed.[421]

MPS-like Disorders. The *Winchester syndrome*[309] reveals an autosomal recessive pattern of inheritance that can lead to rheumatoid-like radiographic changes. Some investigators believe it is incorrectly classified as a MPS (see Chapter 28).

Dyggve-Melchior-Clausen disease is an autosomal recessive disorder presenting in infancy or early childhood with short trunk dwarfism, small hands and feet, hepatosplenomegaly, and mental retardation.[310, 311] Vertebral body flattening and notching, ilial hypoplasia, abnormalities of the growth plate of the proximal femora, delayed ossification of the femoral epiphyses, and shortening of the tubular bones with irregular epiphyseal or metaphyseal ossification are the recognized radiographic findings.[2] Although some studies indicate abnormal mu-

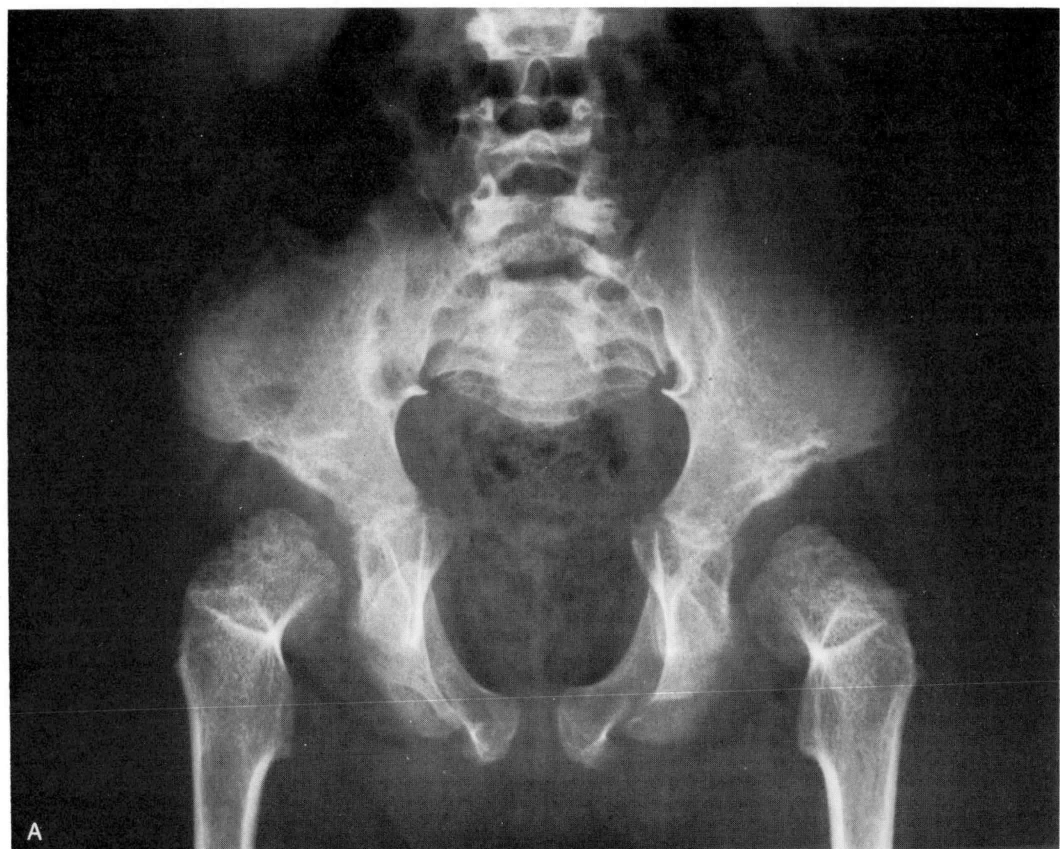

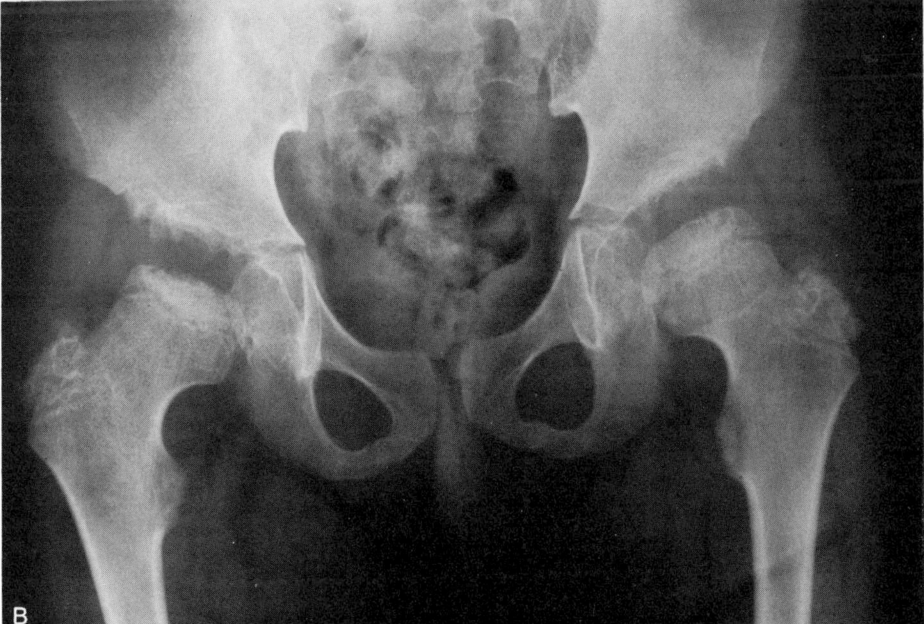

Figure 73–55. *Mucopolysaccharidosis IV: Morquio disease — pelvic abnormalities.*

A *In this child, there is flaring of the iliac wings, poor ossification of the superior aspect of the acetabula, prominent sacroiliac articular spaces, coxa valga, and irregularity of the proximal capital femoral epiphyses.*

B *In an older child, a similar pelvic configuration is noted. Observe the irregularity of the ossified proximal capital femoral epiphyses.*

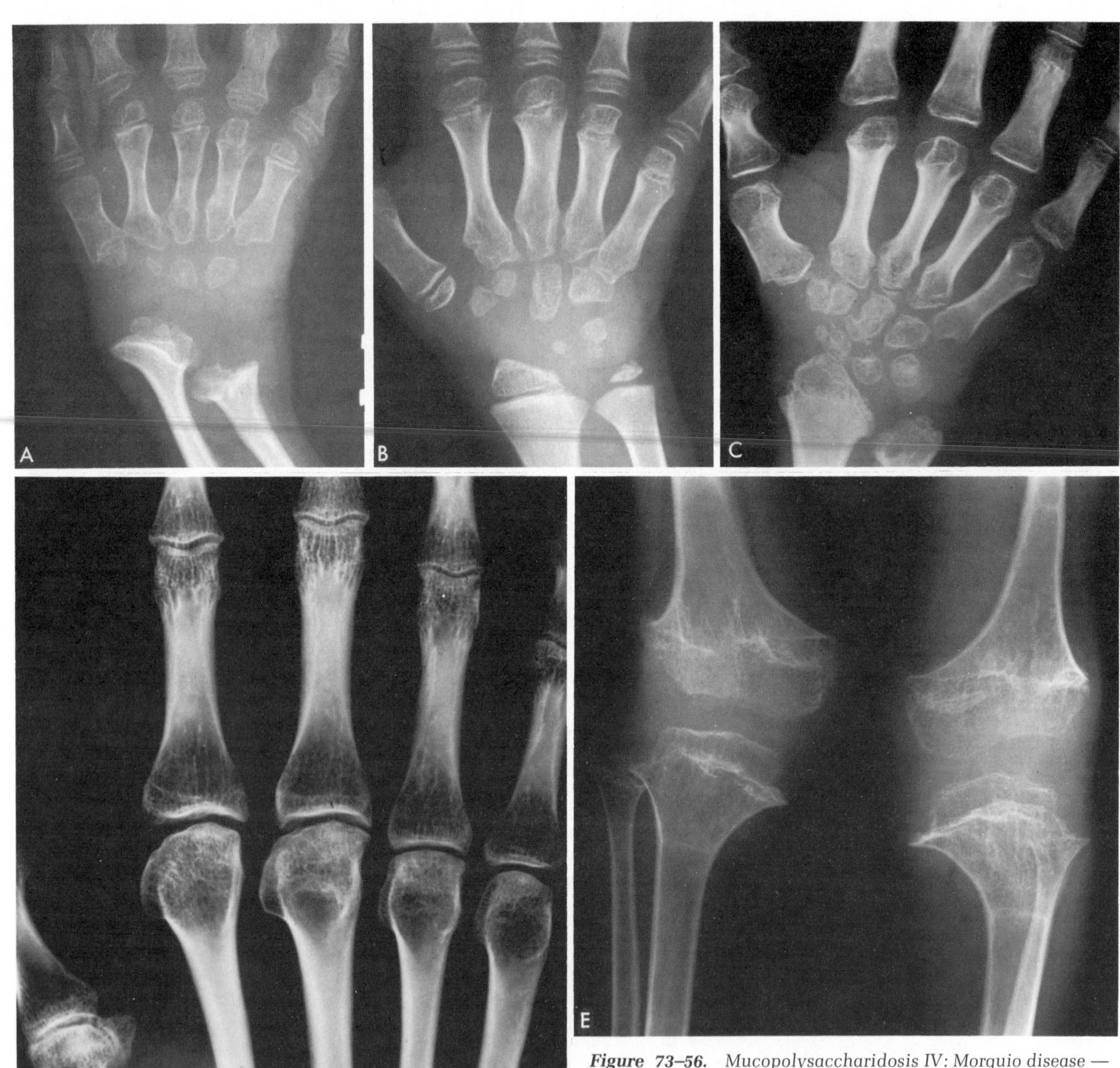

Figure 73–56. Mucopolysaccharidosis IV: Morquio disease — appendicular skeletal abnormalities.

A–C In these three examples of Morquio disease in children and adolescents, note the conical bases of the metacarpals, irregularity of the epiphyses and growth plates of the distal radius and distal ulna, and deformities of the carpus and phalanges.

D In an adult, flattening of the metacarpal heads, joint space narrowing at the metacarpophalangeal articulations, and osteoporosis are evident.

E In the knee, osteoporosis, relative enlargement of the medial femoral condyle, and genu valgum can be seen.

copolysaccharide excretion, this is not a constant feature.

Mucolipidosis I. This autosomal recessive disorder reveals clinical findings of varied severity.[2] A mild type causes no neurologic or fundoscopic changes, whereas a severe variety can be associated with mental retardation, neurologic degeneration, cherry-red macular spots, and hepatosplenomegaly. Urinary excretion of acid mucopolysaccharides is normal, and lysosomal enzymatic activity in the liver is increased. Calvarial thickening, ilial hypoplasia, rib expansion, and abnormalities of the vertebrae and tubular bones can be seen.

Mucolipidosis II (I-Cell Disease). Clinical and radiologic features of this autosomal recessive disorder simulate those of Hurler's syndrome.[312-315, 459] However, normal urinary excretion of acid mucopolysaccharides is evident. A peculiar feature is a high incidence of congenital dislocation of the hip. Additional roentgenographic abnormalities in early infancy are osteoporosis, periosteal bony deposition of long tubular bones, metaphyseal irregularity, and vertebral anomalies; in later infancy and childhood, pelvic bone hypoplasia, shortening and deformity of long tubular bones, and retardation of ossification in the carpus and tarsus are seen.

Mucolipidosis III (Pseudo-Hurler Polydystrophy). This autosomal recessive disorder is characterized by mucopolysaccharides in the fibroblasts, viscera, and mesenchymal tissue, normal urinary excretion of mucopolysaccharides, dwarfism, restricted joint mobility, peculiar facies, corneal opacities, and mild or moderate mental retardation.[316-318] Radiographic abnormalities simulate those in MPS-I and MPS-II and are of variable severity. Claw hands, flattening of the femoral epiphyses, platyspondyly, and iliac wing flaring are described.

Mucolipidosis-like Disorders. *Mannosidosis* is a storage disorder associated with a deficiency of the enzyme α-mannosidase in the liver.[319] This deficiency results in the intracellular accumulation and excessive urinary excretion of mannose-containing oligosaccharides. Radiographs reveal calvarial thickening, flattening and deformity of vertebral bodies, ilial hypoplasia, and mild expansion of the tubular bones of the hand.

Fucosidosis is a lysosomal storage disorder that leads to psychomotor deterioration and even death. A deficiency of alpha-L-fucosidase enzyme allows abnormal accumulation of fucosyl components in the lysosomes.[320, 321] Radiographic features, which include calvarial thickening, premature sutural closure, poorly developed sinuses, rib expansion, hypoplastic odontoid process, and kyphosis, are not specific. Of interest, intervertebral disc space "vacuum" phenomena and calcification have been described in some cases.

Gangliosidosis (neurovisceral lipidosis) is an autosomal recessive disorder presenting in infancy and childhood with Hurler-like facies, hepatosplenomegaly, joint rigidity, and cherry-red macular spots.[322-324] Accumulation of ganglioside in the brain, liver, and spleen is seen. Radiographic features are virtually identical to those found in I-cell disease.[469]

Skeletal Dysplasias with Predominant Metaphyseal Involvement

Achondrogenesis. This rare type of congenital micromelic dwarfism was first recognized in 1936 by Parenti[325] and was designated as achondrogenesis by Fraccaro in 1952.[326] An autosomal recessive pattern of inheritance has been documented. The disorder becomes manifest in early infancy (Table 73–5). A premature or stillborn product of a pregnancy frequency complicated by polyhydramnios reveals short limbs and trunk, abdominal swelling, and a relatively large head.[327] Radiographs outline extremely shortened limbs, gross retardation of development and ossification of vertebral bodies, hypoplasia of the pelvic bones, absence of ossification of the talus, the calcaneus, the sacrum, and the sternum, and flared metaphyses of the tubular bones (Fig. 73–57). Affected infants who are not stillborn die shortly after birth. Postmortem histologic studies reveal findings that are quite variable and that are dependent upon the specific type of achondrogenesis that is evident.[460] In this regard, there appear to be two different forms of the disease, with varying clinical, radiologic, and pathologic findings.

Thanatophoric Dwarfism. This disorder was first recognized in 1967,[328] and its method of inheritance has not been clearly defined. It is associated with characteristic clinical features and death in early infancy, frequently from cardiopulmonary complications. Shortened limbs, a trunk of normal length, a constricted thorax, a protuberant abdomen, and a disproportionately large head are seen.[329, 330] Hypo-

Table 73–5

LETHAL AND NONLETHAL TYPES OF NEONATAL SHORT-LIMBED DWARFISM

Lethal	Nonlethal
Achondrogenesis	Achondroplasia
Campomelic dwarfism	Asphyxiating thoracic dystrophy (ATD — Jeune Syndrome)
Chondrodysplasia punctata, Rhizomelic type	Chondrodysplasia punctata, Conradi-Hunermann type
Homozygous achondroplasia	Chondroectodermal dysplasia (Ellis-van Creveld syndrome — EVC)
Hypophosphatasia (severe)	Diastrophic dwarfism
Osteogenesis imperfecta (severe)	Hypochondroplasia
Thanatophoric dwarfism	Metatropic dwarfism
	Spondyloepiphyseal dysplasia congenita (SED congenita)

(Courtesy of Saldino RM: Med Radiogr Photogr *49*:61, 1973.)

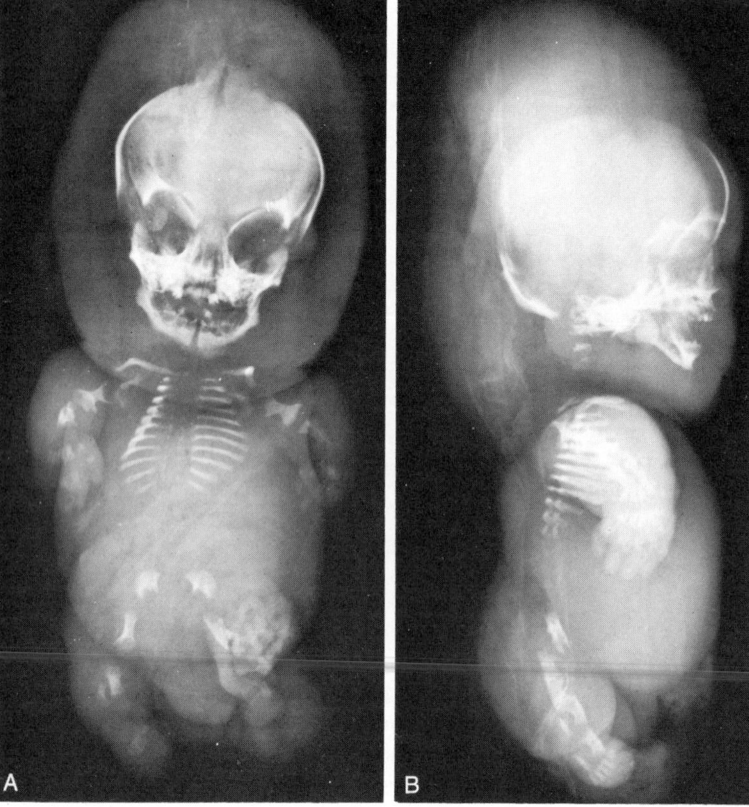

Figure 73–57. *Achondrogenesis. Findings in this stillborn infant include edematous soft tissue, especially about the head, extreme lack of ossification of the vertebral column, shortened limbs, and flared metaphyses. Note femoral bowing. (From Saldino RM: Med Radiogr Photogr 49:61, 1973.)*

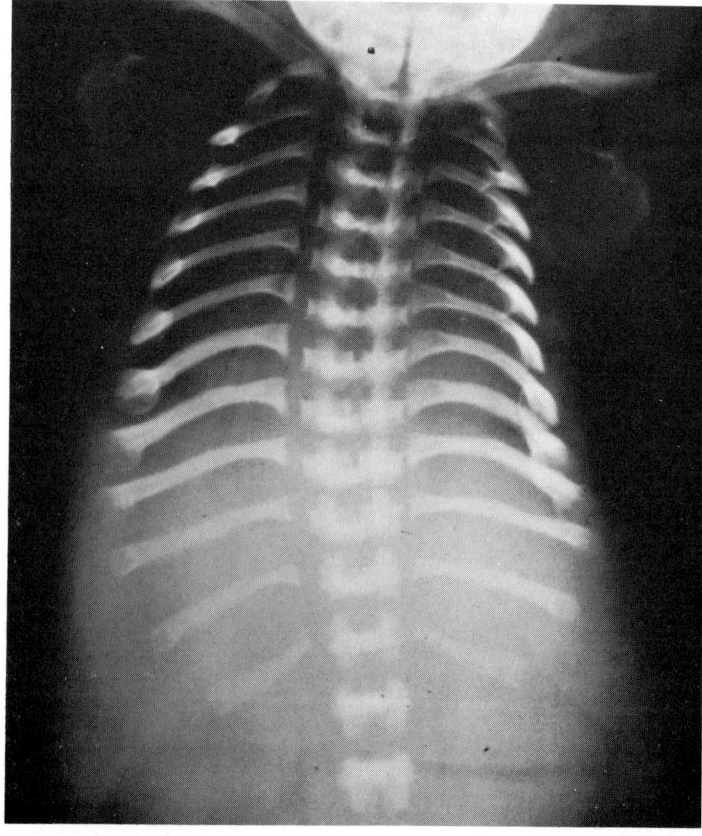

Figure 73–58. *Thanatophoric dwarfism. Extreme platyspondyly and short ribs with widened anterior ends are characteristic findings.*

tonia, thickened skin, depression of the nasal bridge, and visceral anomalies are also encountered. A cloverleaf skull (kleeblattschadel), extreme platyspondyly, ilial hypoplasia, hypoplastic femora with incurvation, and shortening of all tubular bones can be detected on radiographs (Fig. 73–58).

ASPHYXIATING THORACIC DYSTROPHY (JEUNE SYNDROME). This autosomal recessive disorder was first noted in 1954 by Jeune and colleagues.[331] It becomes manifest at birth owing to respiratory distress promoted by a small thoracic cage and underdevelopment of the lungs, a complication that can lead to the infant's death. In some instances, less severe involvement is compatible with survival into and beyond adolescence.[330] Clinical findings include a long and narrow thoracic cage, protuberant abdomen, reduction in limb length, polydactyly, and renal anomalies.[332] Radiographic changes predominate in the ribs and pelvis; shortened ribs with bulbous anterior ends, short iliac wings, and horizontal acetabular margins with bony spikes are seen (Fig. 73–59). Short extremities with metaphyseal irregularities and polydactyly and cone-shaped epiphyses are also apparent. Hypoplasia of the lungs and pneumonia can be evident on chest roentgenograms. The radiographic features in this syndrome closely resemble those found in the Ellis-van Creveld syndrome.

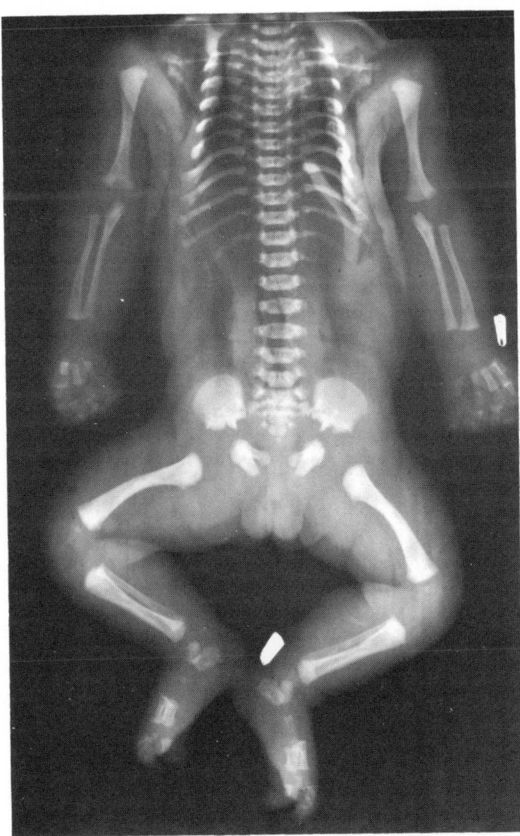

Figure 73–59. *Asphyxiating thoracic dystrophy (Jeune syndrome). This postmortem radiograph of a newborn with asphyxiating thoracic dystrophy reveals a normal vertebral column, mild shortening of the limbs and ribs, and short iliac wings with horizontal acetabular margins containing bony spikes. The pelvic abnormalities are identical to those of the Ellis–van Creveld syndrome. (From Saldino RM: Med Radiogr Photogr 49:61, 1973.)*

CHONDROECTODERMAL DYSPLASIA (ELLIS-VAN CREVELD SYNDROME). This variety of short-limbed dwarfism is characterized by ectodermal dysplasia, polydactyly, and congenital heart disease.[333, 334] It is autosomal recessive and is manifest at birth. Short stature, distal shortening of limbs, polydactyly, absent or hypoplastic fingernails or toenails, dysplastic teeth, upper lip anomalies, and, less commonly, cardiac defects (atrial septal defect or a single atrium) are clinical features of the disease. In addition, renal abnormalities and hydrocephalus have been noted in some individuals. The radiographic features resemble those of familial asphyxiating thoracic dystrophy and include an elongated chest, shortened ribs with anterior osseous expansion, hypoplastic ilia, a trident pelvis, shortening of the tubular bones, especially the phalanges, polydactyly, carpal fusion, cone-shaped epiphyses, swelling of the proximal end of the ulna and distal end of the radius ("drumstick" appearance), anterior dislocation of the radial head, slanting proximal tibial metaphyses, medial tibial diaphyseal exostoses, and genu valgum[330] (Fig. 73–60). The skull and spine are usually normal.

Death in childhood is common owing to cardiac and pulmonary complications, although survival into adulthood may be seen.

HOMOZYGOUS ACHONDROPLASIA. This is an extremely rare type of congenital short-limbed dwarfism that is lethal; an affected infant dies within the first days or weeks of life.[335] The condition results from a mating of two achondroplastic dwarfs. A large cranium, depressed nasal bridge, and limb shortening in an infant with respiratory distress represent characteristic clinical features of the disease. The radiographs outline changes that are more severe than classic (heterozygous) achondroplasia, simulating the findings in thanatophoric dwarfism[330] (Fig. 73–61).

CLASSIC (HETEROZYGOUS) ACHONDROPLASIA. This is a common and well-recognized autosomal dominant disorder that is compatible with a long life span.[336-340] Manifest at birth, achondroplasia is associated with shortening of the limbs that is most exaggerated in proximal segments (rhizomelic micromelia), a prominent forehead and large cranium with a depressed nasal bridge, thoracolumbar kyphosis, prominent buttocks, and flexion contractures of the hips. Additional clinical manifestations are genu varum, restricted elbow motion, and trident hands with short fingers. Neurologic problems can be prominent at all ages owing to hydrocephalus in the infant and to compression of the spinal cord and nerve roots from a narrow spinal canal, herniated intervertebral

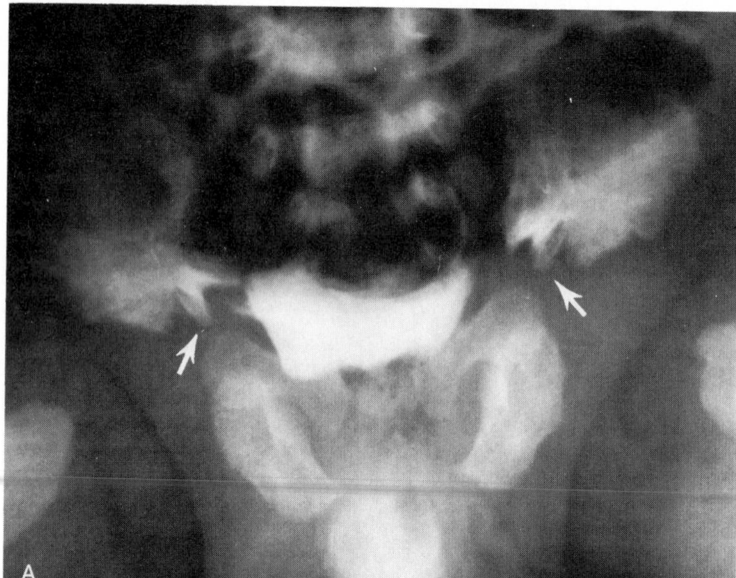

Figure 73–60. Chondroectodermal dysplasia (Ellis-van Creveld syndrome).

A *Observe the flattened acetabular roofs and the elongated bony protuberances at the inferior margin of the sacrosciatic notches (arrows). Contrast opacification of the bladder following an intravenous pyelogram is evident.*

B, C *In the hands and feet, typical findings include polydactyly, progressive hypoplasia of the phalanges as one proceeds in a distal direction, and cone-shaped epiphyses.*

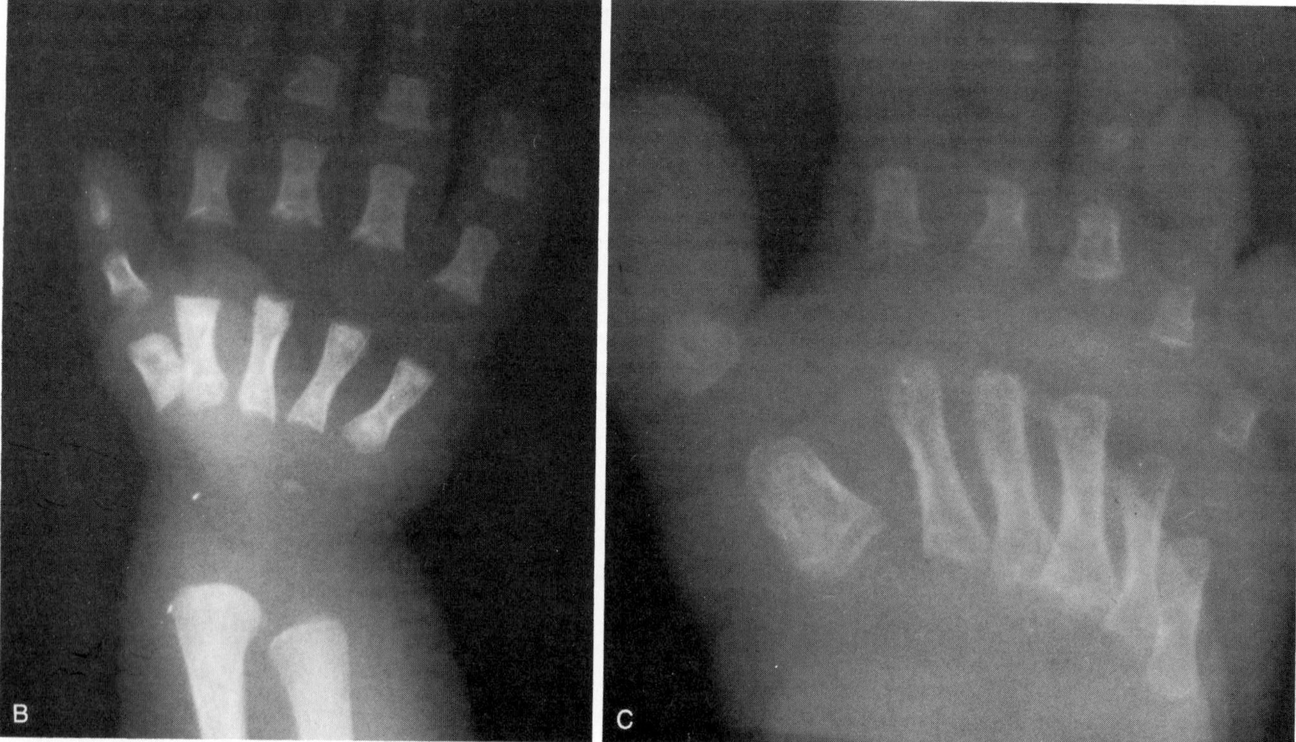

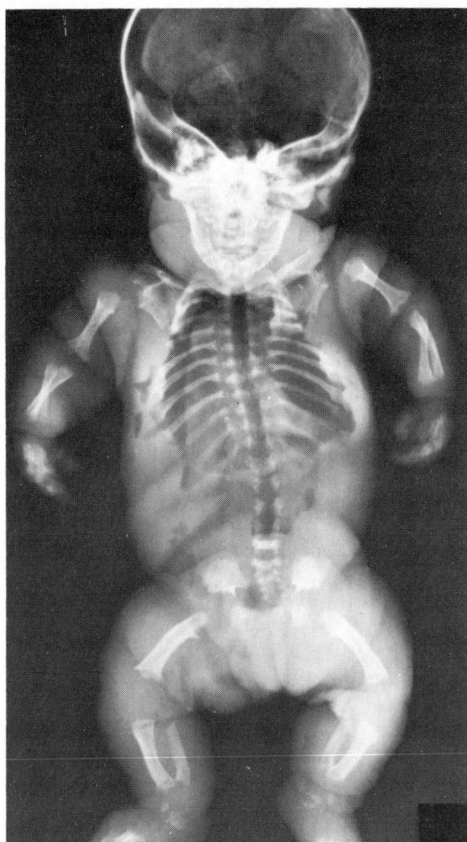

Figure 73–61. *Homozygous achondroplasia. An anteroposterior postmortem radiograph of a 2 day old infant following removal of most of the vertebrae reveals short ribs, limb shortening, and pelvic alterations, as well as other findings. (From Saldino RM: Med Radiogr Photogr 49:61, 1973.)*

disc, or angular deformity[341, 342] (see Chapter 14). The cause of hydrocephalus in achondroplasia may be obstructive or nonobstructive.[343]

The most diagnostic radiographic features occur in the skull, vertebrae, pelvis, and limbs [330] (Fig. 73–62). Lumbar vertebrae reveal short pedicles, posterior scalloping of vertebral bodies, increase in the size of the intervertebral disc spaces, and, in older patients, exaggerated lumbar lordosis. The distance between the lumbar pedicles, as noted on anteroposterior roentgenograms, narrows as one proceeds distally. The iliac bones are flat and round with lack of normal flaring. The superior acetabular margins are broad and horizontally oriented, and the sacrosciatic notches are small. The tubular bones may be significantly shortened. This is especially prominent in the humerus and, less constantly, in the femur. An oval area of radiolucency may be seen in the proximal femoral metaphysis, and the growth plate in the distal femoral metaphysis is not horizontal. A lateral radiograph of the skull reveals an enlarged cranium, a prominent frontal bone, and a small base with a constricted foramen magnum. Basilar impression is also frequent. Additionally, the phalanges and ribs may be shortened.

The skeletal abnormalities of achondroplasia are the result of a generalized defect in the process of endochondral bone formation. Although the histologic features of endochondral bone formation may be only slightly altered, the rate of such formation appears to be depressed.[344]

Hypochondroplasia. This autosomal dominant disorder presents in childhood with clinical and radiologic findings that are similar to but less severe than achondroplasia.[345, 346, 470] Thus, small stature, increased lumbar lordosis, bowlegs, and limited elbow extension may be noted on clinical evaluation; narrowing of the interpedicular distances and exaggerated posterior concavity of vertebral bodies in the lumbar region, shortening of the tubular bones, and a short, broad femoral neck can be seen on radiologic examination. The skull is not significantly affected, although macrocephaly has been noted in some cases.[461]

Hypophosphatasia. Both lethal and tarda autosomal recessive varieties of this disorder have been described.[2, 347] It has been suggested that both forms of the disease are due to the same genetic mutation.[348] In the lethal form, clinical manifestations become evident at birth, and respiratory distress or intracranial hemorrhage leads to death of the infant within a few days.[347, 348] Serum alkaline phosphatase levels are low, and there is increased urinary excretion of phosphoethanolamine. The absence of ossification of the bones of the calvarium and face is striking. The tubular bones are shortened, irregularly ossified, and contain ill-defined metaphyseal segments that resemble the changes of rickets. Poor ossification of the ribs, flat bones, and vertebrae is also apparent.

In the tarda form, death may occur in the first year of life owing to cardiorespiratory failure and increased intracranial pressure, or infants may survive into childhood or adulthood with rickets-like skeletal deformities, defective gait, mental retardation, dental anomalies, joint pain, and increased bone fragility[2, 347, 349] (Fig. 73–63). Laboratory findings include low or absent serum alkaline phosphatase activity, hypercalcemia, and high urinary excretion of phosphoethanolamine. In infancy, radiographs delineate late ossification of the cranial vault and base and metaphyseal ossification defects in the tubular bones. Craniostenosis, bowing, and ectopic calcification may be seen in childhood and adulthood.

Metaphyseal Chondrodysplasia (Metaphyseal Dysostosis). Several types of metaphyseal chondrodysplasia have been recognized. The *Jansen type* is an autosomal dominant disorder, presenting in infancy or childhood, characterized by short-limbed dwarfism, enlarged and relatively immobile joints, and a prominent skull and face.[350] Hypercalcemia is present on laboratory analysis. In addition to osteopenia, metaphyseal cupping and irregularity in infants are reminiscent of findings in rickets or hyperparathyroidism. Cranial ossification may be defective, leading to a reticular or striated

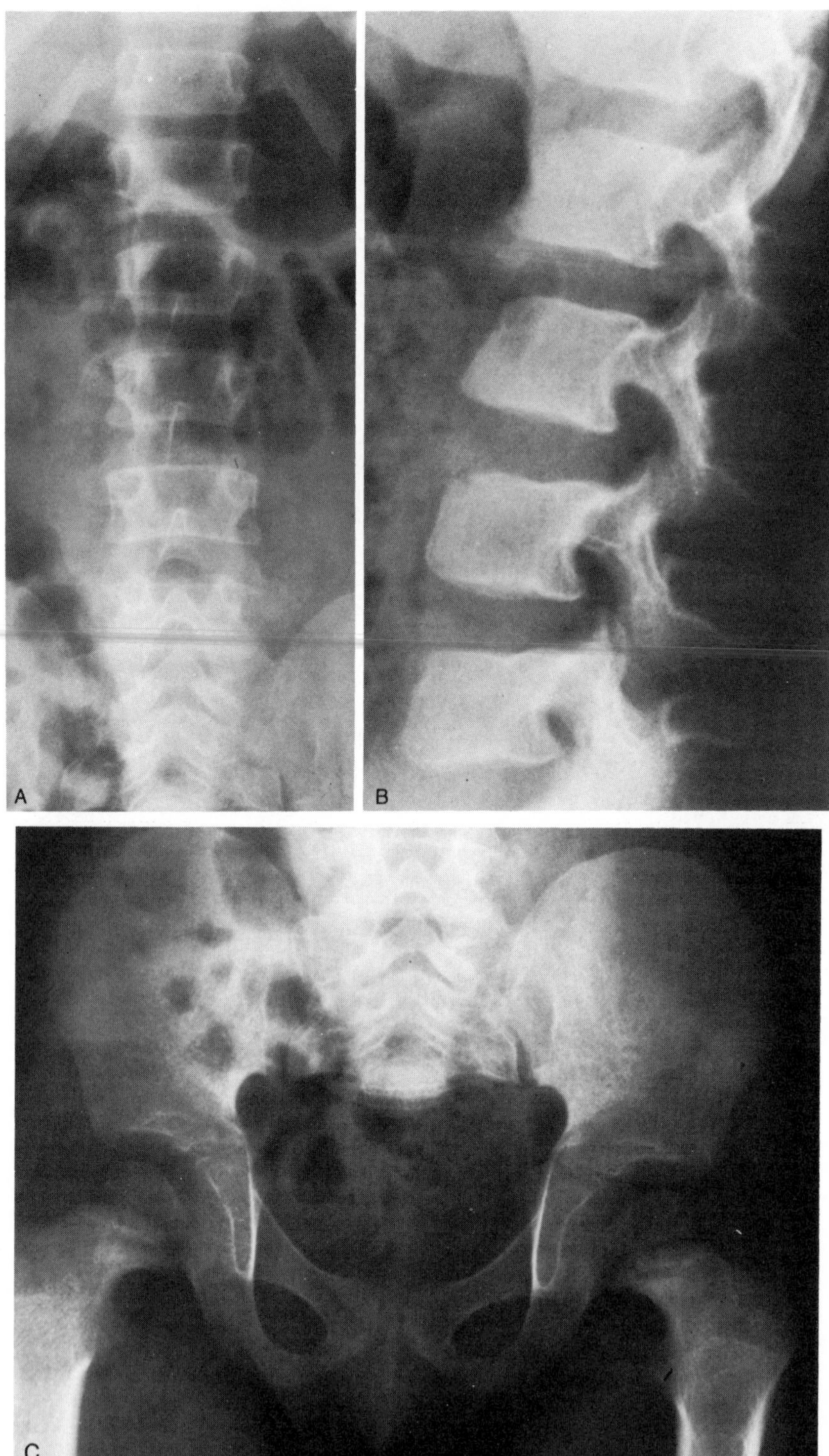

Figure 73–62. Classic achondroplasia. Radiographs of a 5 year old girl with classic achondroplasia are shown.

A, B Spinal abnormalities. Note the decreasing interpedicular distance on the anteroposterior roentgenogram as one proceeds caudad. The intervertebral disc spaces are prominent and there is exaggerated posterior concavity of the vertebral bodies.

C Pelvic abnormalities. Observe a low, broad pelvic contour, horizontally oriented acetabular margins, and a "champagne glass" inner pelvic margin.

Illustration continued on the opposite page

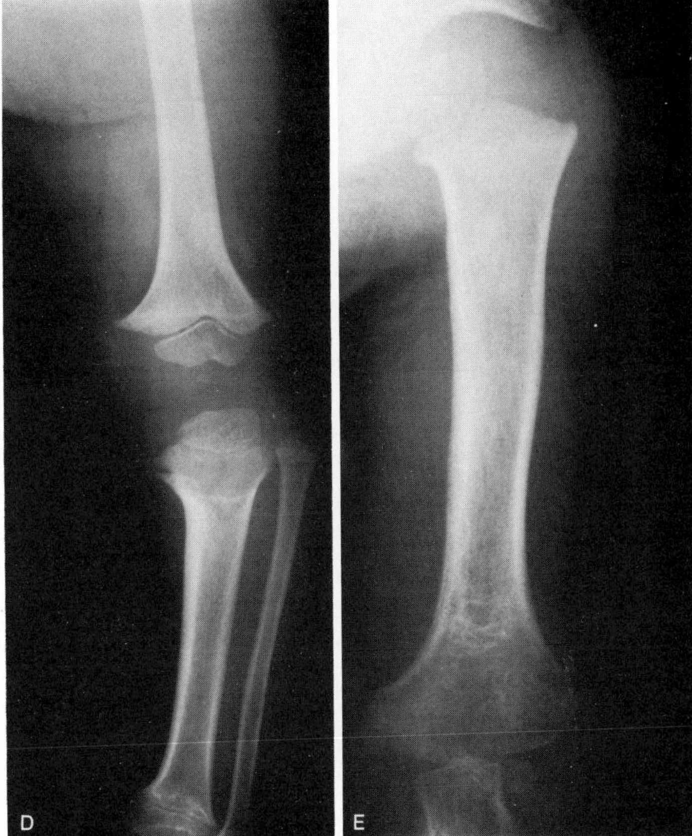

Figure 73–62. Continued
D, E *Tubular bone abnormalities. The bones are significantly shortened, especially the humerus and the femur. A "ball-and-cup" or V-shaped distal femoral growth plate is seen.*

appearance. In older individuals, shortening and bowing of tubular bones, metaphyseal flaring, and calvarial hyperostosis are seen. In the *Schmid type,* abnormalities are usually evident by the second year of life.[351] Clinical and radiologic findings are less striking. A small stature and shortened, bowed limbs may be seen in both children and adults with this autosomal dominant disorder. The metaphyseal alterations consist of rickets-like irregularity, cupping, and widening, and, in the proximal femur, coxa vara and a short femoral neck can be evident (Fig. 73–64).

Cartilage-hair hypoplasia is an additional variant of metaphyseal dysostosis.[352-354] Short-limbed dwarf-

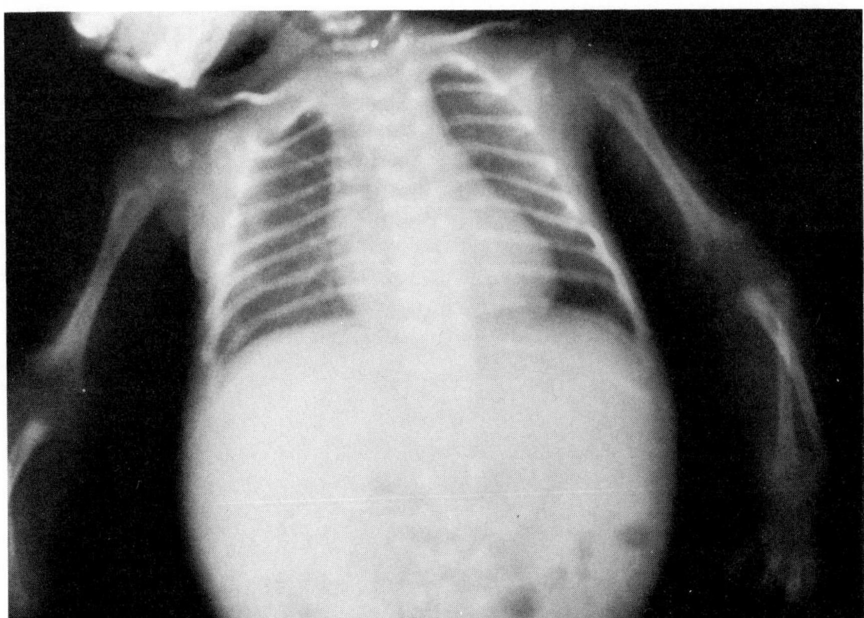

Figure 73–63. *Hypophosphatasia tarda. Defective ossification is most striking in the metaphyseal areas where rickets-like skeletal changes are apparent.*

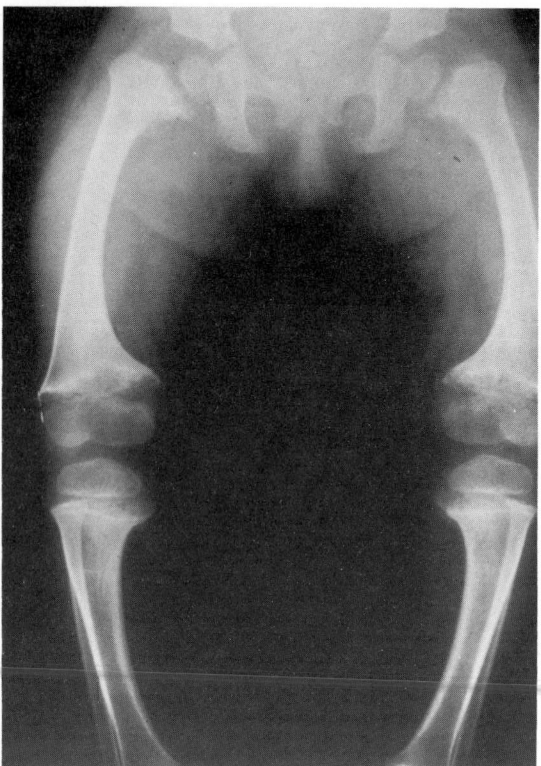

Figure 73–64. Metaphyseal chondrodysplasia (metaphyseal dysostosis): Schmid type. The lower limbs are bowed, and rickets-like abnormalities are evident in all of the metaphyses.

ism, metaphyseal irregularities in the tubular bones, sparse, fine, blond hair, normal intelligence, and transmission by an autosomal recessive inheritance are features of this syndrome. A peculiar predilection for the Amish has been noted. Ligamentous laxity, malabsorption syndrome, and an aganglionic colon have also been noted. Radiographs outline irregularity and widening of the growth plate in the long bones, especially about the knee, elongation of the distal portion of the fibula, normal or increased vertebral height, an increase in the lumbosacral angle, and a normal skull. Biopsy of the growth plate reveals a paucity of maturing cartilage cells and their failure to form orderly columns. Although life span may be normal in some patients, gastrointestinal problems, impaired cellular immunity, and severe reaction to varicella and smallpox vaccination have been recorded.

A *Spahr type* of metaphyseal dysostosis occurring as an autosomal recessive disorder has also been described.[3]

The metaphyseal dysostoses are an interesting group of disorders. The resemblance of the skeletal alterations in infants with the Jansen variety of the disease to hyperparathyroidism may indicate that parathyroid dysfunction is important in the pathogenesis of the disease. The association of metaphyseal irregularities, immunologic defects, intestinal disorders, and ectodermal dysplasia in some affected individuals may indicate the presence of widespread

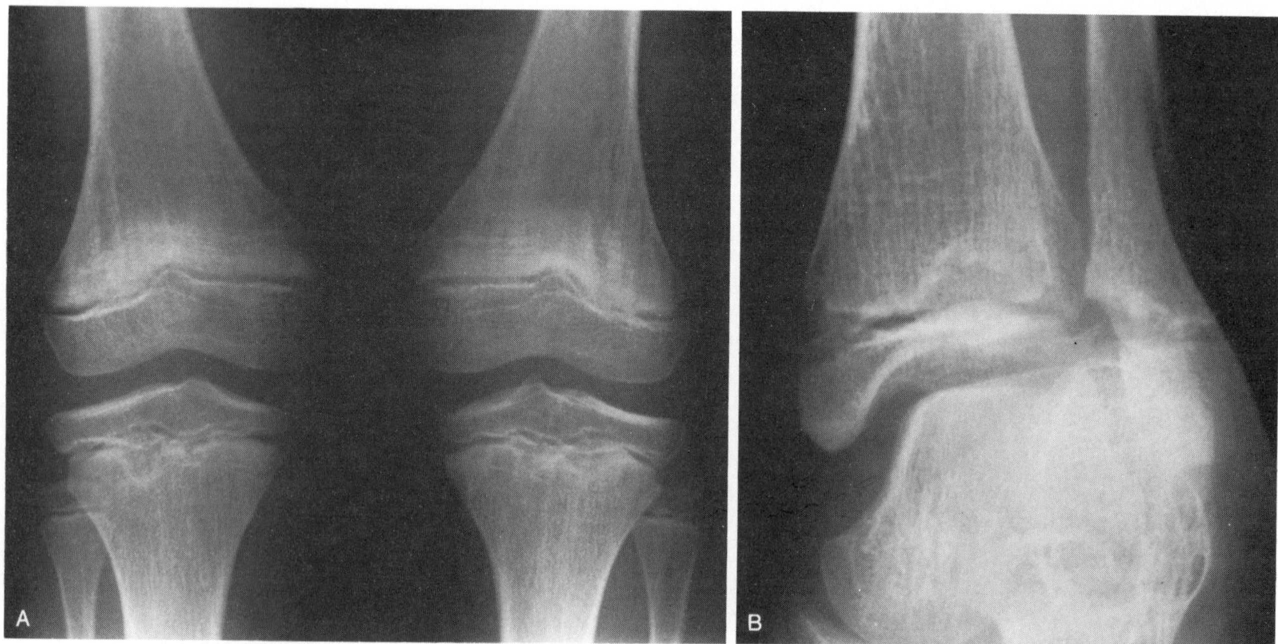

Figure 73–65. Shwachman-Diamond syndrome. This is a 10 year old boy with metaphyseal dysostosis, anemia, thrombocytopenia, and decreased physical development. Pancreatic exocrine function was slightly abnormal.

A, B Minor irregularity of the metaphyses about the knees and the ankle is observed.

Illustration continued on the opposite page

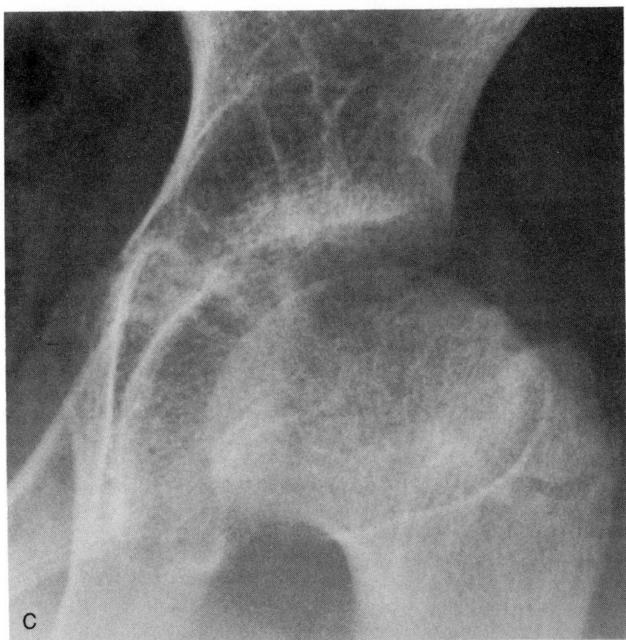

Figure 73–65. Continued
C *Coxa vara is apparent.*

mesenchymal defects controlled by the same genetic anomalies. A combination of metaphyseal irregularity, pancreatic insufficiency, and hematologic abnormalities has also been recorded[355] (Fig. 73–65).

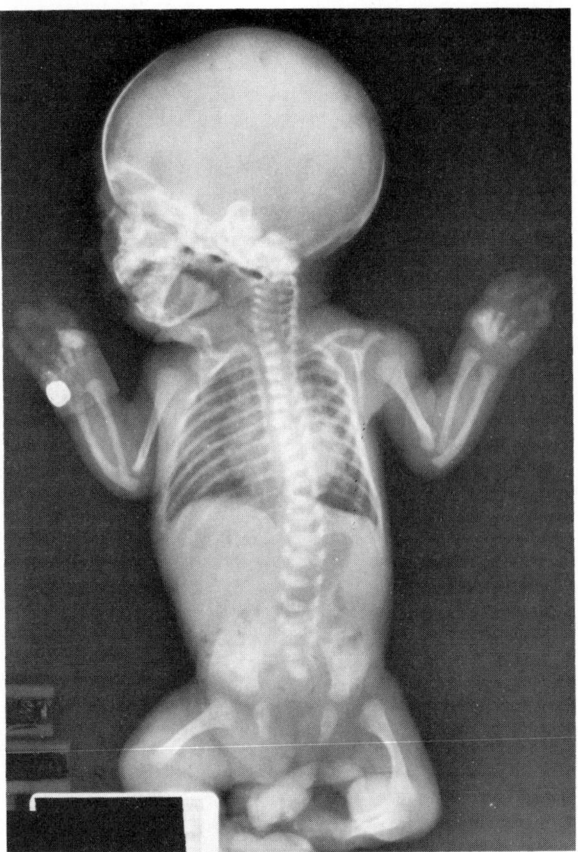

Figure 73–66. Diastrophic dwarfism. In a newborn infant, all the limbs are short, the radial heads are dislocated, and the midcervical vertebral bodies are hypoplastic. (From Saldino RM: Med Radiogr Photogr 49:61, 1973.)

Skeletal Dysplasias With Major Involvement of the Spine

DIASTROPHIC DWARFISM. Diastrophic means twisted and is descriptive of the severe deformities of the spine and peripheral skeleton that accompany this autosomal recessive dysplasia. It was identified as a disorder distinct from achondroplasia by Lamy and Maroteaux in 1960.[356] At birth, certain clinical manifestations usually allow identification of infants with diastrophic dwarfism.[357] Small stature, short limbs, clubbed feet, cleft palate, inflammation of the pinna, hypermobile abducted thumbs (hitch-hiker's thumb), stiff interphalangeal joints, and deafness are commonly seen. Progressive kyphoscoliosis is evident in some cases. Although death in infancy can occur owing to respiratory problems, survival into adulthood is not uncommon and is frequently associated with severe deformities and disability. Mental retardation is not present.

Radiographic features include short phalanges, metacarpals, and metatarsals, oval-shaped first metacarpals, clubfoot deformity, shortened tubular bones with flaring of the metaphyses, short, broad femoral necks with wide trochanteric regions, and spinal abnormalities, such as thoracolumbar kyphoscoliosis, irregular deformities of the vertebral bodies, and cervical kyphosis[358, 359] (Fig. 73–66). In the knee, a flat and irregular ossified distal femoral epiphysis and medial placement of the proximal tibial epiphysis are useful radiographic signs.[330]

METATROPIC DWARFISM. This type of dwarfism was described by Maroteaux and co-workers in 1966.[360] It is very rare, and its mode of inheritance has not been defined.[330] At birth, affected individuals reveal a trunk of normal length and shortened extremities. The chest is narrow, and articulations are prominent with restricted motion. Subsequently, progressive kyphoscoliosis and spinal shortening appear, and a peculiar tail-like appendage in the region of the coccyx can be detected. Metaphyseal regions of tubular bones are palpably enlarged. On radiographs, metaphyseal enlargement is especially characteristic[361, 362] (Fig. 73–67). It is evident at multiple sites but may be most prominent in the femurs. A "trumpet-like" appearance of the expanded metaphyses is typical. Shortening of the tubular bones, flexion contractures, hypoplasia of the ilia, and small and deformed femoral epiphyses can also be noted. In the spine, platyspondyly, anterior wedging of vertebral bodies, narrowing of the intervertebral spaces in the lower lumbar region, and kyphoscoliosis are the

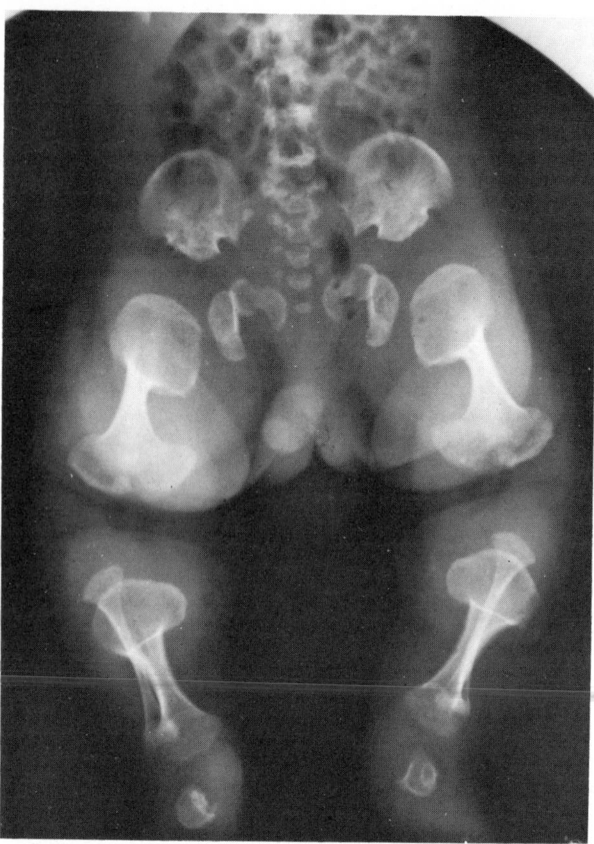

Figure 73–67. Metatropic dwarfism. In this infant, note the bizarre expansion of all the metaphyses, especially in the femora and tibiae. The supra-acetabular notches are prominent, and platyspondyly is seen. (From Saldino RM: Med Radiogr Photogr 49:61, 1973.)

observed roentgenographic features. Additional manifestations include a long narrow cylindrical thorax, long and slender fingers, and a relatively normal cranium.

PARASTREMMATIC DWARFISM. The designation parastremmatic dwarfism was applied by Langer and co-workers[363] to a condition that was characterized by severe dwarfism, marked kyphoscoliosis, and asymmetrical deformities of the lower extremities with joint contractures. It appears to represent an autosomal dominant or X-chromosomal dominant disorder. Joint stiffening and spinal deformity are evident at birth, leading to a delay in walking and an abnormal gait.[363, 364] Dwarfism results from kyphoscoliosis, platyspondyly, and shortness of tubular bones. The neck is diminutive, and the thorax reveals an increase in anteroposterior diameter. Bowing deformities, including genu varum or valgum, are seen.

Radiographs reveal platyspondyly, irregular ossification of the vertebral end-plates, hypoplastic iliac wings, grossly expanded metaphyseal and epiphyseal segments of tubular bones, and, in general, a "flocky" skeletal appearance due to alternating areas of radiolucency and sclerosis. Affected patients may survive into adulthood with decrease or disappearance of the irregular ossification pattern.[2]

KNIEST DISEASE (SWISS CHEESE CARTILAGE SYNDROME). In 1952, Kniest[365] described a young girl who revealed disproportionate dwarfism, kyphoscoliosis, peculiar facies, deformed extremities, and enlarged joints with restricted motion. Based upon this and additional reports,[366-368] a well-defined syndrome has emerged. Clinical features, which may be evident in infancy, include a flattened midface with a depressed nasal bridge, a high arched palate, hearing loss, a short trunk with dorsal kyphosis, an accentuated lumbar lordosis, and short extremities with enlarged joints. Myopia, retinal detachment, clubfeet, and a broad thorax may also be apparent. Abnormal mucopolysacchariduria has been identified in some patients.[369] Radiography outlines platyspondyly, kyphoscoliosis, vertebral irregularity, pelvic deformity, broad ilia, flat femoral heads with broad and short femoral necks, and short tubular bones with enlarged metaphyses and deformed epiphyses. In the hands, periarticular osseous enlargement may produce findings similar to Heberden's and Bouchard's nodes that appear in degenerative joint disease.[468] In some patients, progressive joint problems may require orthopedic attention.[2]

Histologic evaluation reveals friable cartilage with irregularity in both cellular size and matrix staining.[366, 370] The combination of hypertrophic cartilage cells and surrounding loose matrix containing large holes resembles Swiss cheese. A basic defect in collagen metabolism has been proposed as the abnormality in this syndrome.

SPONDYLOEPIPHYSEAL DYSPLASIA (SED) CONGENITA. SED congenita is recognized at birth by short limbs, delayed ossification, and distinctive alterations in the pelvis, the vertebrae, and the proximal ends of the femur.[330] It is an autosomal dominant disorder with considerable variability of expression.[371] Clinical findings include a flat facies, severe myopia, retinal detachment, prominent eyes, cleft palate, loss of hearing, disproportionate dwarfism with a short spine and neck, barrel chest with pectus carinatum, diminished muscle tone with delayed motor development and a waddling gait, flexion contractures of the hip, knock-knee deformity, and normal sized hands and feet.[2, 330, 372, 373] The major roentgenographic changes are identified in the pelvis and vertebral column (Figs. 73–68 and 73–69). Retarded ossification of the pelvis with horizontal acetabular roofs, short iliac wings, flattening of all the vertebral bodies, and hypoplasia of the odontoid process are seen. The ossification of the femoral head and neck is retarded or absent, and severe coxa vara and bowing of the femoral shafts can be encountered. The epiphyses and metaphyses of the long tubular bones are commonly abnormal. Rhizomelic shortening of the limbs is occasionally seen.

Although SED congenita has been confused with

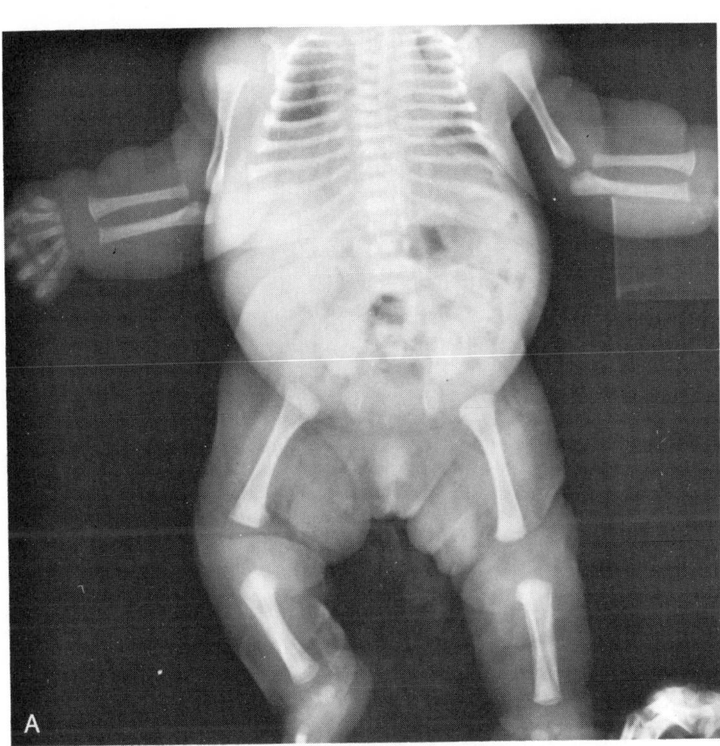

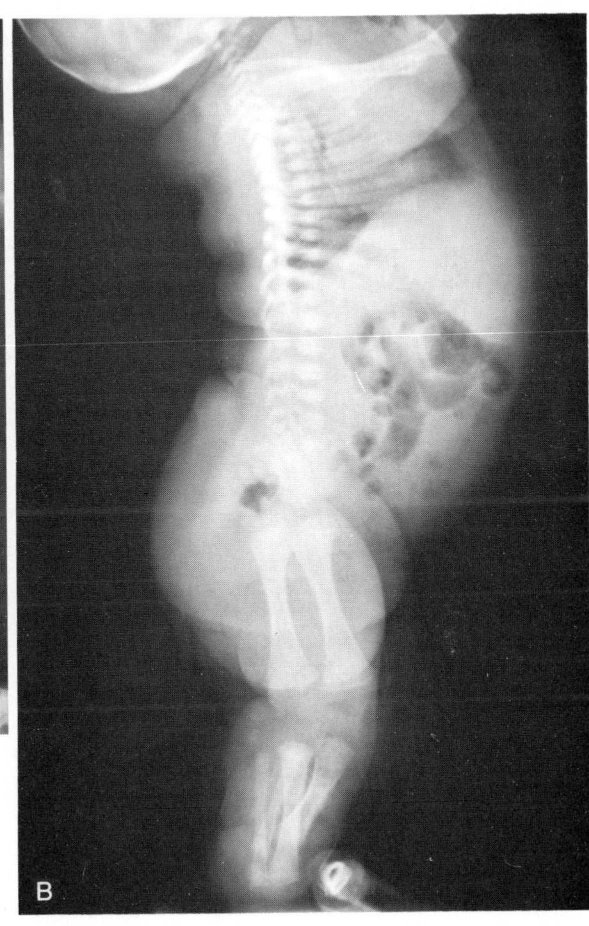

Figure 73–68. *Spondyloepiphyseal dysplasia (SED) congenita. In this 15 day old infant, note the absence of ossification of the pubic bones and the delayed ossification of the epiphyses of the knees. The bodies of the thoracic vertebrae are flattened posteriorly, and the ribs and the long bones are moderately shortened. (From Saldino RM: Med Radiogr Photogr 49:61, 1973.)*

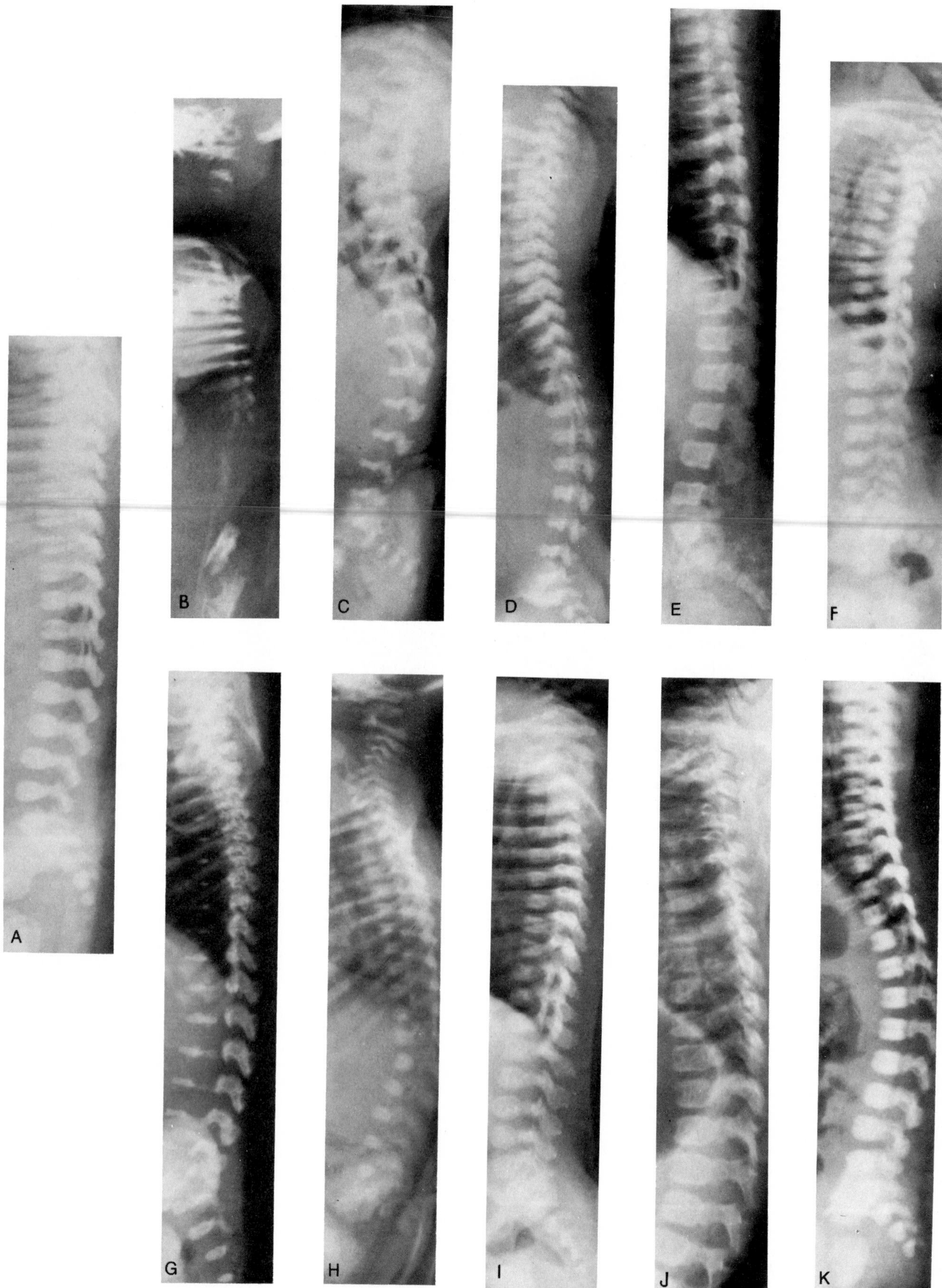

Figure 73–69. See legend on opposite page

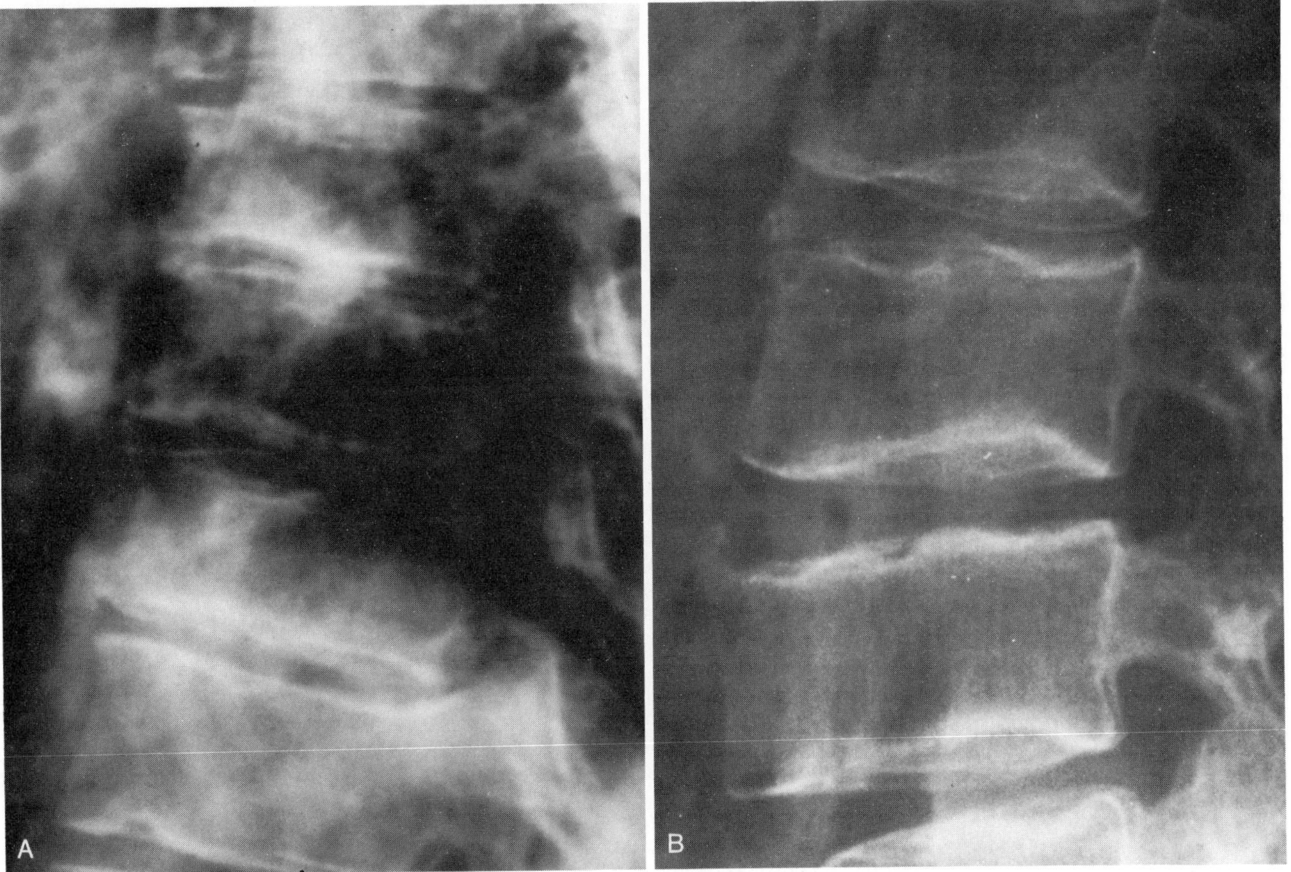

Figure 73–70. *Spondyloepiphyseal dysplasia (SED) tarda. This is a 37 year old woman who developed premature degenerative joint disease, especially of the hips and the knees.*

A, B *Lateral radiographs of the thoracic and lumbar spine reveal generalized flattening of the vertebrae with irregularity of vertebral contour.*

Illustration continued on the following page

Figure 73–69. *Spinal abnormalities in neonatal short-limbed dwarfism. Lateral radiographs of the thoracolumbar area of the vertebral column of a normal infant and infants with different types of short-limbed dwarfism are submitted.*

A *Normal.*
B *Achondrogenesis.*
C *Thanatophoric dwarfism.*
D *Homozygous achondroplasia.*
E *Achondroplasia.*
F *Spondyloepiphyseal dysplasia (SED) congenita.*
G *Metatropic dwarfism.*
H *Diastrophic dwarfism.*
I *Congenital epiphyseal dysplasia punctata (Conradi-Hünermann type).*
J *Asphyxiating thoracic dystrophy (Jeune syndrome).*
K *Chondroectodermal dysplasia (Ellis–van Creveld syndrome).*
(From Saldino RM: Med Radiogr Photogr 49:61, 1973.)

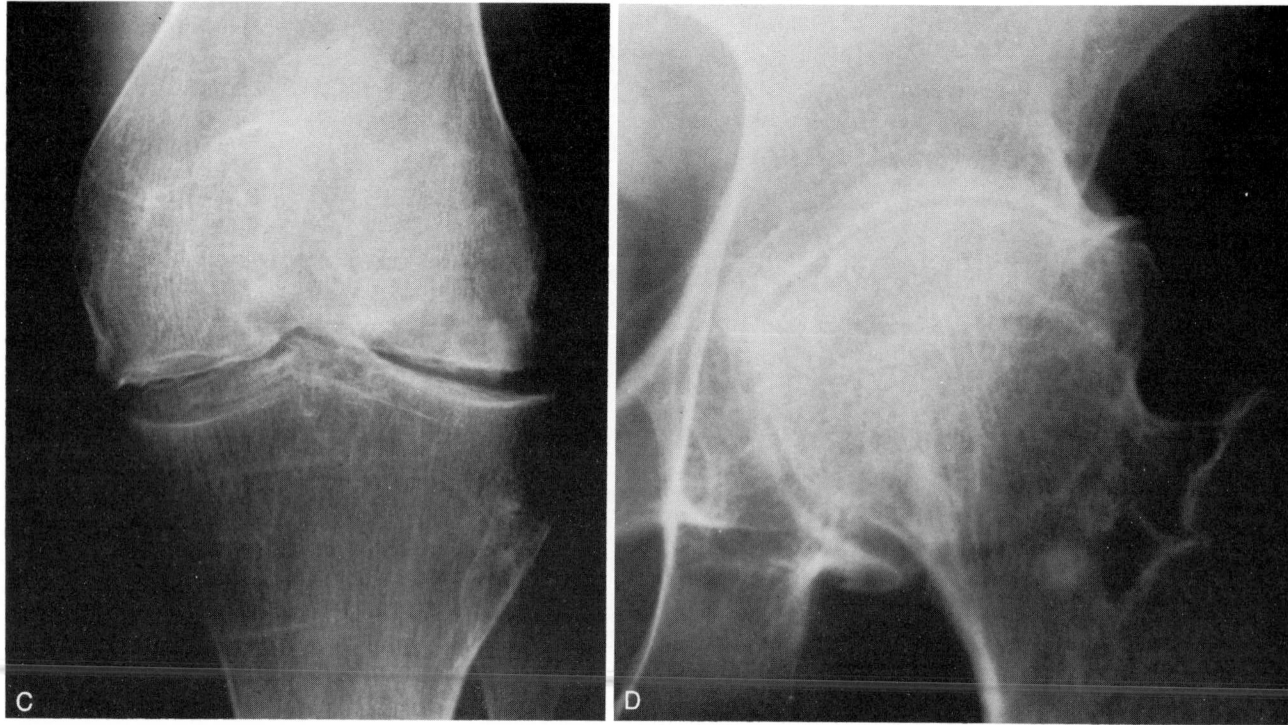

Figure 73–70. Continued
C, D *Premature degenerative joint disease is evident in the knee and the hip, characterized by articular space narrowing, osteophytosis, and sclerosis.*
(Courtesy of Dr. J. Wild, San Antonio, Texas.)

Morquio's syndrome, it is a separate disorder.[330] Morquio's syndrome is not manifest at birth, and in Morquio's syndrome, the hands and feet are affected and corneal clouding, mucopolysacchariduria, and an autosomal recessive pattern of inheritance are typical.

Spondyloepiphyseal Dysplasia (SED) Tarda. This X-chromosomal recessive disorder becomes manifest in late childhood as short stature with spinal abnormalities, sternal protrusion, and a broad thorax.[374, 375] In later life, premature osteoarthritis, especially of the hips and the shoulders, is common. Radiographs reveal generalized flattening of the vertebral bodies with irregularity of vertebral contour, intervertebral disc space narrowing, cartilaginous nodes, small iliac bones, and mild dysplastic changes of the articular surfaces of the large joints that may lead to secondary degenerative joint disease (Fig. 73–70). Although the appendicular skeletal changes resemble those in multiple epiphyseal dysplasia, the involvement of the spine and the lack of significant changes in the epiphyses of bones in the distal extremities allow differentiation of these disorders. The dwarfism in SED tarda is less severe than in SED congenita, and the findings are usually not manifest until late childhood. The vertebral alterations in SED tarda simulate those in Scheuermann's disease.

Spondylometaphyseal Dysplasia. In 1967, Kozlowski and colleagues[376] described a short trunk type of dwarfism with prominent spinal and metaphyseal alterations. It is an autosomal dominant disorder that usually presents in early childhood with dwarfism, waddling gait, kyphoscoliosis, and restricted joint mobility.[377-379, 423] Platyspondyly, kyphosis, scoliosis, shortening of the femoral neck, coxa vara, and metaphyseal abnormalities predominate. The epiphyses are normal or mildly affected.

Chromosomal Disorders

Down's Syndrome — Trisomy 21 (Mongolism). In 1959, Lejeune and co-workers[380] observed that patients with certain phenotypic characteristics of the Down's syndrome had 47 chromosomes. Ninety to 95 per cent of individuals with this syndrome possess the extra chromosome, which is designated as number 21. Patients with this syndrome are identified at birth owing to ocular abnormalities (which include oblique palpebral fissures, epicanthal folds, cataracts, Brushfield spots, nystagmus, and strabismus), hypotonia, brachycephaly, mental retardation, and a large tongue. Congenital hip dysplasia is evident in approximately 40 per cent of individuals, and gastrointestinal abnormalities, including duodenal atresia, are well recognized. Dermatoglyphic alterations are also characteristic.

Radiographs of the pelvis reveal flared iliac wings and flattened acetabular roots[381, 382] (Fig. 73–

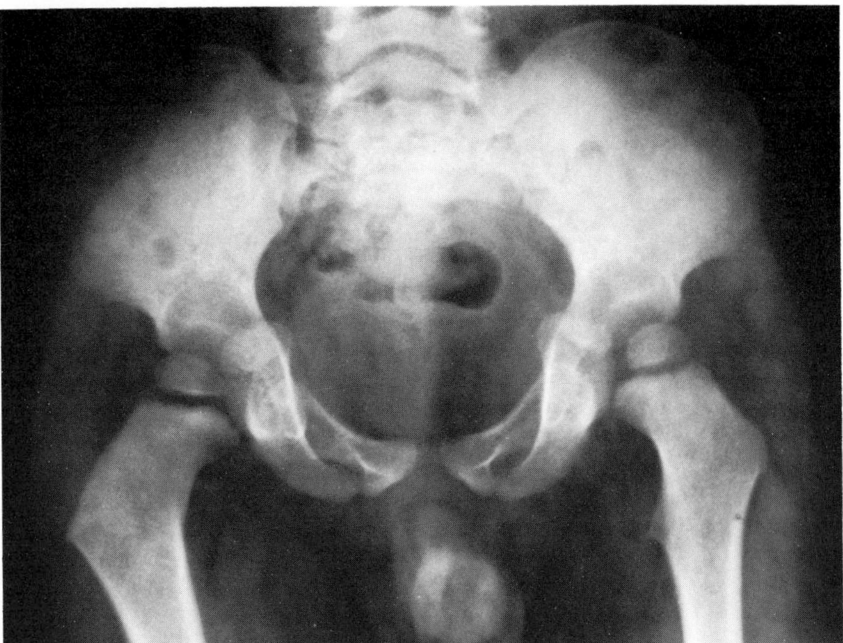

Figure 73–71. Down's syndrome — trisomy 21. Findings include flared iliac wings and flattened acetabular roofs. Mild lateral subluxation of the hips can be noted.

71). Hypoplasia of the middle phalanx of the fifth finger with clinodactyly, short and irregular metacarpals, accessory epiphyses, an extramanubrial ossification center, cuboid vertebral bodies, 11 pairs of ribs, microcephaly, high arched palate, delayed sutural closure, and sinus hypoplasia may be identified. These abnormalities vary in severity, related in part to whether patients have trisomy 21 or translocation and mosaicism.[383]

Atlanto-axial instability and myelopathy can lead to significant neurologic deficits.[384, 385, 466] The exact mechanism for neurologic symptoms and signs is not certain, although a high degree of ligamentous laxity, especially of the transverse atlantal ligament, is suspect.[386, 387] Additional factors that are responsible for atlanto-axial instability may include trauma, pharyngeal infection, and osseous abnormalities of the odontoid process. This instability may decrease with increasing age of the patient.

Trisomy 18 Syndrome. In 1960, Edwards and associates[388] published the first case report of trisomy 18. The increased age of mothers of infants with trisomy 18 is similar to that which is noted in Down's syndrome. Affected infants are of low birth weight and possess a narrow head, prominent occiput, malformed ears, micrognathia, high arched palate, finger deformities, hypertonicity, and hernias.[381, 389] Cardiac and renal anomalies, mental retardation, and early death are other features of this syndrome. Radiographs of the hand reveal adduction of the thumb, superimposition of the second and third fingers, and hypoplasia of the first metacarpal. "Rocker-bottom" feet, metatarsus varus, shortened first toe, hypoplastic terminal phalanges of the toes, hypoplasia of ribs, clavicles, and sternum, and pelvic deformities complete the radiographic picture (Fig. 73–72).

Trisomy 13 Syndrome. This is a clearly defined chromosomal disorder first described in 1960 by Patau and associates.[390] Affected infants have severe anomalies with mental retardation, seizures, and apnea. A small skull, arrhinencephaly, holopros-

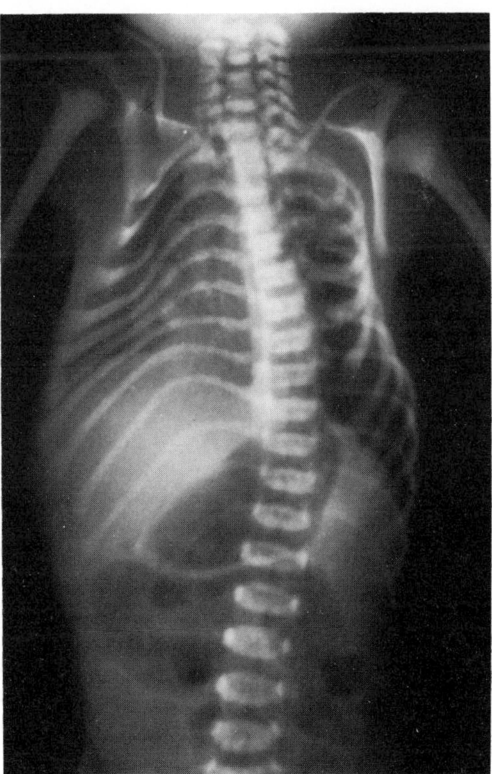

Figure 73–72. Trisomy 18 syndrome. This 5 day old infant demonstrated malformed ears and palate, a small tongue, and bilateral inguinal hernias. Observe defective ossification of ribs and clavicles with wavy, hypoplastic osseous contours.

encephaly, abnormal eyes and ears, cleft lip and palate, cutaneous hemangiomas, flexion deformities of fingers, and congenital heart disease are evident. The most common skeletal alterations are polydactyly, syndactyly, asymmetry of the thorax, prominence of the calcaneus, midline craniofacial anomalies, and widened sutures.[391]

Other Trisomy Syndromes. *Trisomy 8* can result in malformed pinnae, mental retardation, restricted joint motion, micrognathia or retrognathia, high arched palate, a long and slender trunk, and an abnormal nose and ears.[392] Osteoporosis, joint subluxations, hypoplastic pelvic and shoulder girdles, and coxa valga are among the radiographic findings.

Trisomy 9-p is associated with growth and mental retardation, hypertelorism, a large nose, cup-shaped ears, kyphoscoliosis, small hands and feet with short digits, clinodactyly, syndactyly, hypoplastic terminal phalanges and nails, and characteristic dermatoglyphic patterns.[393] Radiographic findings are evident in the feet, hands, and pelvis during the period of epiphyseal growth and consist of retardation of osseous maturation, pseudoepiphyses, and hypoplasia of the pubic bones.[394] By contrast, trisomy for the entire chromosome 9 reveals a different pattern of facial and limb alterations.

The Cat Cry Syndrome. Deletion of the short arm of chromosome 5 results in this well-known syndrome named after the characteristics of the cry made by affected patients. Mental retardation is severe, growth is slow, and microcephaly, a round face, hypertelorism, epicanthal folds, and an antimongoloid slant of the palpebral fissures are seen.[381, 395] Nonspecific roentgenographic features include microcephaly, hypertelorism, abnormal development of long bones, perhaps owing to muscular hypotonia, scoliosis, shortening of carpal and tarsal bones, and small iliac wings.

Wolf's Syndrome. Patients with deletion of the short arm of chromosome 4 reveal mental and growth retardation, seizures, eye deformities, cleft lip and palate, hypoplastic dermal ridges, and nonspecific skeletal alterations, including microcephaly, hypertelorism, foot deformities, and delayed pelvic ossification.[381, 396] A widened interpubic distance and deficiencies of ossification in the cervical spine may be prominent radiographic findings.[448]

Turner's Syndrome. This syndrome is produced when there exists a normal complement of autosomes but only one sex chromosome, X (45, X). Most fetuses with this combination of chromosomes are aborted in the first trimester of pregnancy; rarely, a live infant is produced, which has a female phenotype. During subsequent development of the child and adolescent, secondary sex characteristics do not appear, primary amenorrhea is frequent, and the ovaries consist of fibrous tissue. Clinical manifestations include lymphedema of the lower extremities, loose skin about the neck, congenital anomalies of the heart, great vessels, and kidney, short stature, and laterally displaced nipples on a shield-like chest.[381, 397,398]

There are many radiographic abnormalities that may be evident in this syndrome.[397-401] Osteoporosis characterized by an increased percentage of bone surface undergoing resorption is similar to that observed in postmenopausal osteoporosis and may be related to an estrogen deficiency early in life.[399] The decreased bone density is most pronounced in the spine, carpus, and tarsus. Although skeletal maturation may appear to proceed normally, epiphyseal

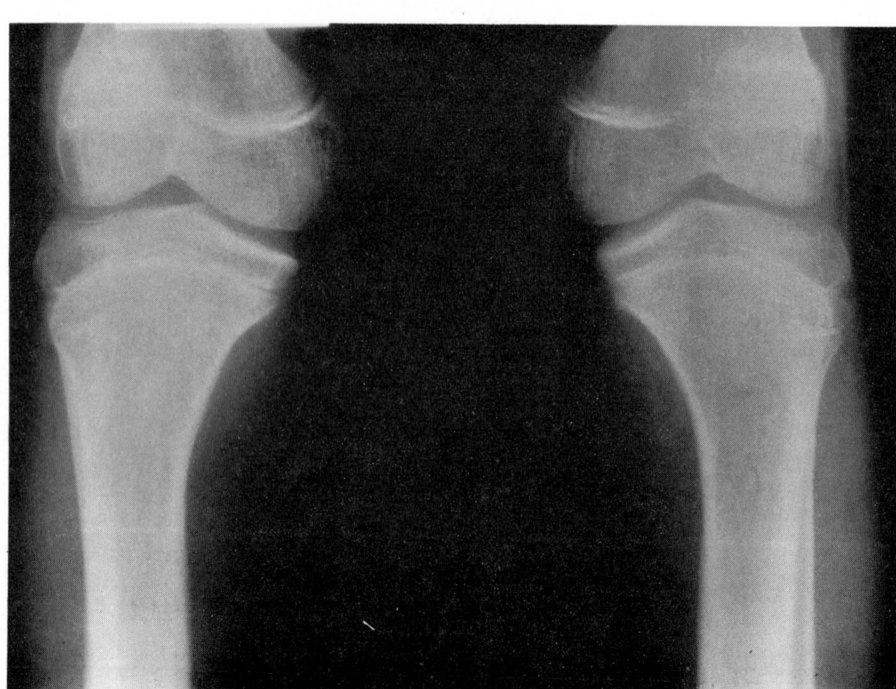

Figure 73–73. *Turner's syndrome. Findings include overgrowth of the medial femoral condyle and flattening of the medial tibial plateau.*

fusion is delayed and may not occur until the third decade of life. Shortening of the metacarpals, especially the fourth, and the metatarsals can be evident. Although a decrease in the carpal angle has been noted in this syndrome, it does not appear to be a useful radiographic sign.[402] Deformities of the knees with flattening of the medial tibial plateau, beaking of the proximal tibia, and enlargement of the medial femoral condyle are observed (Fig. 73–73). Cubitus valgus, Madelung-like deformities, thin clavicles and ribs, vertebral body irregularities, and odontoid and atlas abnormalities have also been described.

KLINEFELTER'S SYNDROME. This syndrome is usually due to the presence of two or more X chromosomes and a Y chromosome, although a number of variant chromosomal patterns are also recognized, such as XXYY.[403] Muscular weakness, mental retardation, delayed puberty, azospermia, and infertility are frequent. A variety of nonspecific radiographic changes has been outlined, including metacarpal shortening, clinodactyly, accessory epiphyses, a flattened ulnar styloid process, pointed phalangeal tufts, radioulnar synostosis, and retarded bone age.

Miscellaneous Syndromes and Conditions

PROGERIA. This rare syndrome was described by Hutchinson in 1886.[404] Infants appear normal at birth, and typical clinical manifestations become evident within the first few years of life. Dwarfism, alopecia, brown pigmentation of the trunk, atrophic skin, loss of subcutaneous fat, impaired extension at the hips and knees, a receding chin, a beaked nose, and exophthalmos are seen.[405] Radiographic findings include hypoplastic facial bones and mandible, delay of cranial sutural closure, and coxa valga. Acro-osteolysis of the terminal phalanges of the hands and feet and of the clavicles is a distinctive finding.[406, 407] Progressive dissolution of these bones and others, including the ribs and humerus, can lead to pathologic fractures. The pattern and degree of osteolysis may be reminiscent of that in hyperparathyroidism or massive osteolysis of Gorham in some cases.

HEREDITARY MULTIPLE EXOSTOSES. This autosomal dominant disorder leads to clinical abnormalities in the first or second decades of life and characteristic roentgenographic changes.[408] Palpable osseous protuberances or masses and secondary deformities due to shortening and bowing of bones and joint restriction are common. Osteochondromas arise from the expanded metaphyses of the tubular bones as well as from the flat bones (Fig. 73–74). Changes in the vertebrae are less frequent but can lead to spinal cord compression.[409, 410] The excrescences usually increase in size during childhood and adolescence, but new exostoses do not appear and existing exostoses do not enlarge following closure of the neighboring growth plate. A variety of complications may be encountered (Figs. 73–75 to 73–77). These include growth disturbances, compression and irritation of adjacent nerves, vessels, and tendons, urinary or intestinal obstruction, and sarcomatous degeneration (1 to 20 per cent of cases).[411-413, 424] Malignant degeneration is usually evident in the hip or shoulder region and is associated with clinically evident pain and an enlarging mass, and radiographically evident growth and irregularity of the excrescence (Fig. 73–78). Bone scintigraphy and computed tomography may be useful in evaluating patients with hereditary exostoses for possible malignancy.[414, 415]

OLLIER'S DISEASE. This syndrome, consisting of multiple enchondromas, is *not hereditary* in nature. Clinical manifestations usually appear in the first decade of life and consist of palpable bony masses, asymmetrical shortening of the extremities, and pathologic fractures.[416] On radiographs, linear or columnar translucencies in the metaphyses, which may reveal calcification, represent persistent cartilaginous tissue (Fig. 73–79). Any bone can be affected, although changes predominate in the tubular structures of the arm and the leg. Asymmetry is common. Dwarfism due to impaired epiphyseal function and expansile lesions, especially in the hands, are noted. Some of the lesions may regress during the years of growth, being replaced by normal bone, and may even disappear completely, although persistent growth disturbances are common. Following cessation of normal growth, lesions do not increase in size unless malignant degeneration has occurred. This complication has been noted in 5 to 20 per cent of cases, an incidence that is increased when enchondromas are combined with hemangiomas of the soft tissue (Maffucci's syndrome).[425] The only condition that enters into the differential diagnosis of radiographic features in this syndrome is fibrous dysplasia.

ARTHROGRYPOSIS MULTIPLEX CONGENITA. The term arthrogryposis is derived from two Greek words meaning curved joints[417] and is an appropriate name for this disorder. The role of hereditary factors in arthrogryposis has long been disputed, and a precise mode of inheritance has not been documented.[418] Numerous causes of the condition have been proposed, including mechanical, neurologic,[471] and infectious abnormalities, but none has been substantiated. At birth, affected individuals display multiple and frequently symmetrical joint contractures involving many of the peripheral articulations, with limitation of both active and passive motion. A "diamond deformity" of the lower extremities is typical, with the hips abducted, flexed, and externally rotated and with the knees flexed. Sensation is intact.

Roentgenographic features include decreased muscle mass and contractures. Equinovarus deformity of the foot, clubhand in ulnar deviation, carpal fusion, and dislocation of the hips are frequent[419, 420] (Fig. 73–80). Fractures are not unusual, and scoliosis

Text continued on page 2627

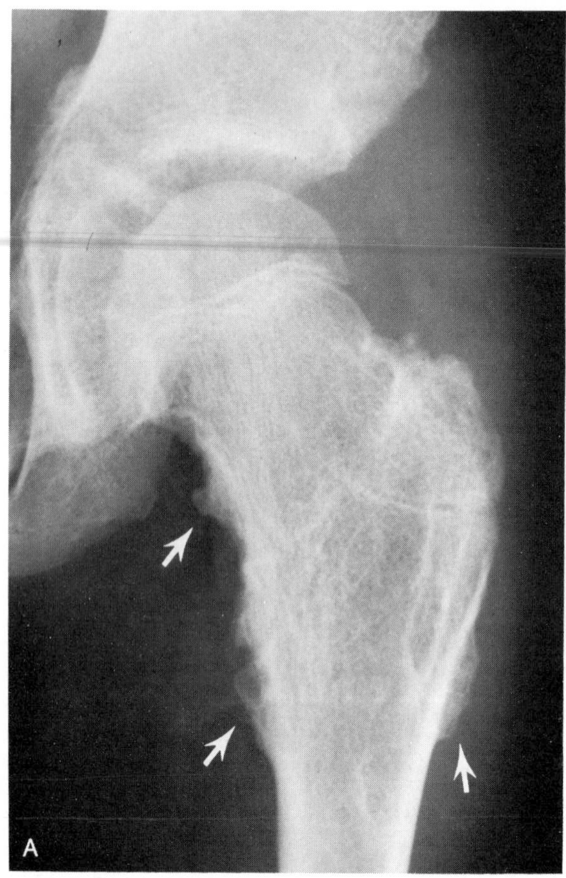

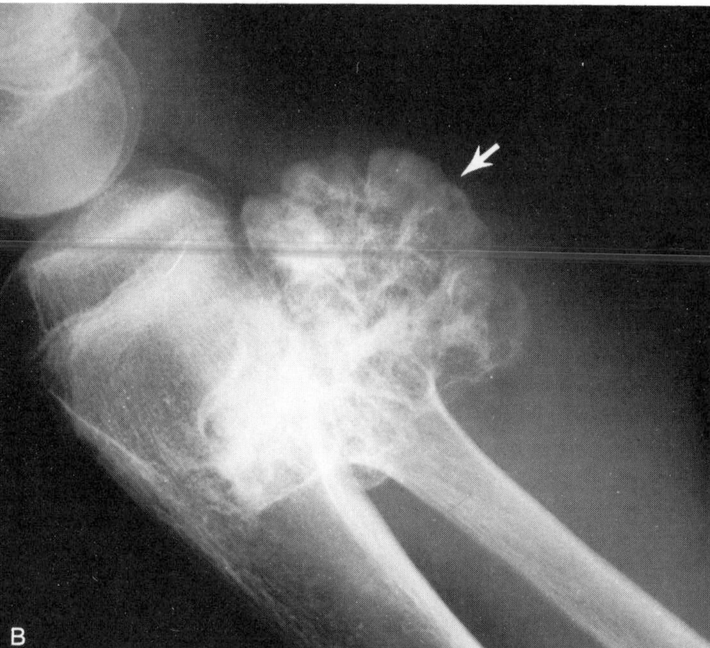

Figure 73–74. *Hereditary multiple exostoses. Examples of osteochondromas of the metaphyses of the proximal femur and proximal fibula (arrows) are given. The wide metaphyseal contour of the femoral neck is particularly characteristic.*

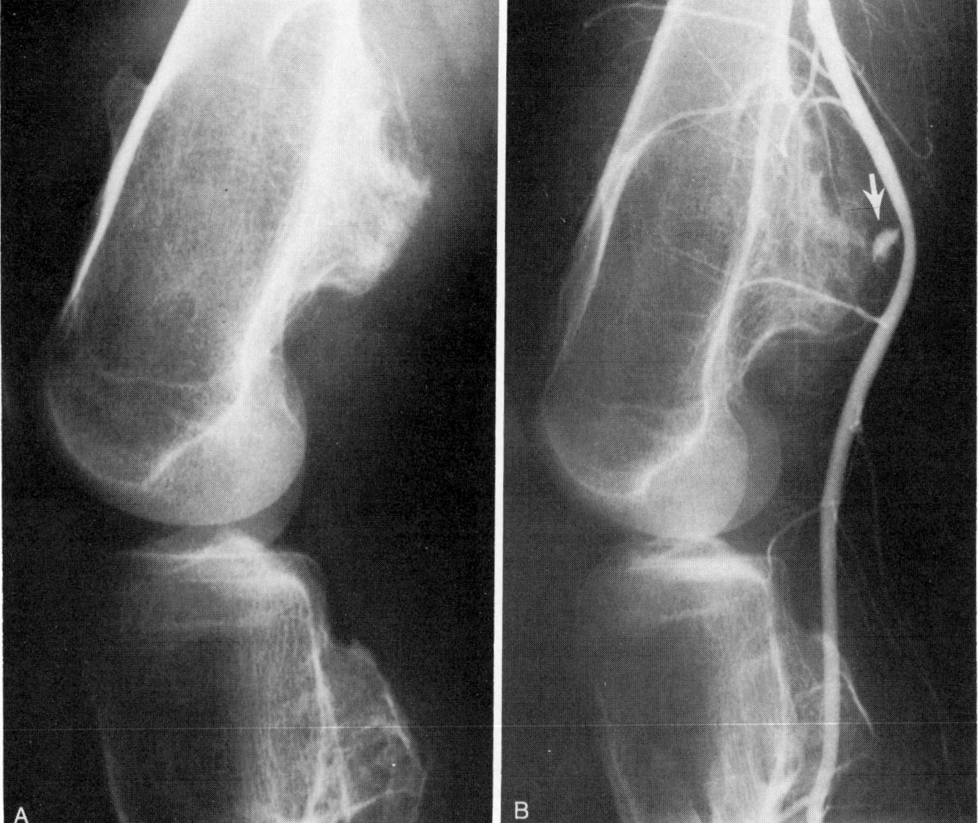

Figure 73–75. *Hereditary multiple exostoses: Complications — vascular injury. In this 16 year old girl, a posterior osteochondroma of the distal femur has produced compression of the popliteal artery with extravasation of contrast medium into a pseudoaneurysm (arrow). (From Greenway G, et al: Am J Roentgenol 132:294, 1979. Copyright 1979, American Roentgen Ray Society.)*

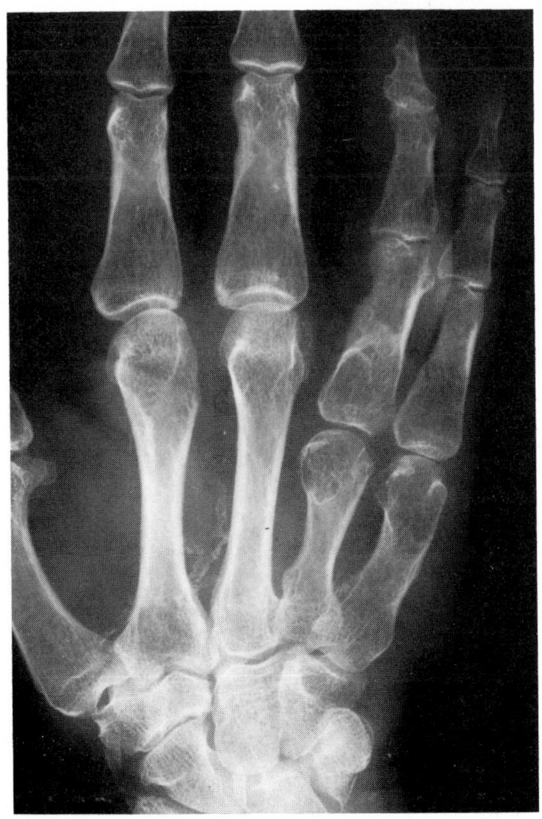

Figure 73–76. *Hereditary multiple exostoses: Complications — growth disturbance. In addition to osteochondromas, observe the shortening of the fourth and fifth metacarpals. Vascular calcification is present.*

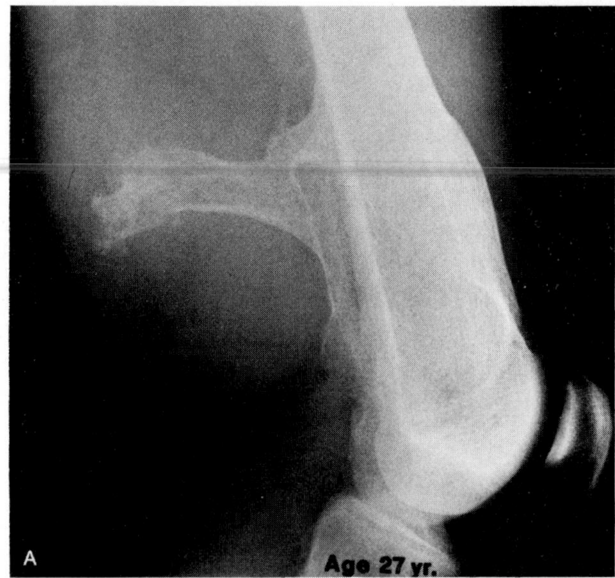

Figure 73–77. Hereditary multiple exostoses: *Complications* — bursitis. *A 27 year old man developed increasing swelling and pain in the popliteal bursa.*

A *A lateral radiograph outlines a large osteochondroma of the distal posterior femur with irregularity of the tip and a soft tissue mass. The appearance of the outgrowth had changed when compared to an earlier film, and the possibility of malignant degeneration was raised.*

Illustration continued on the opposite page

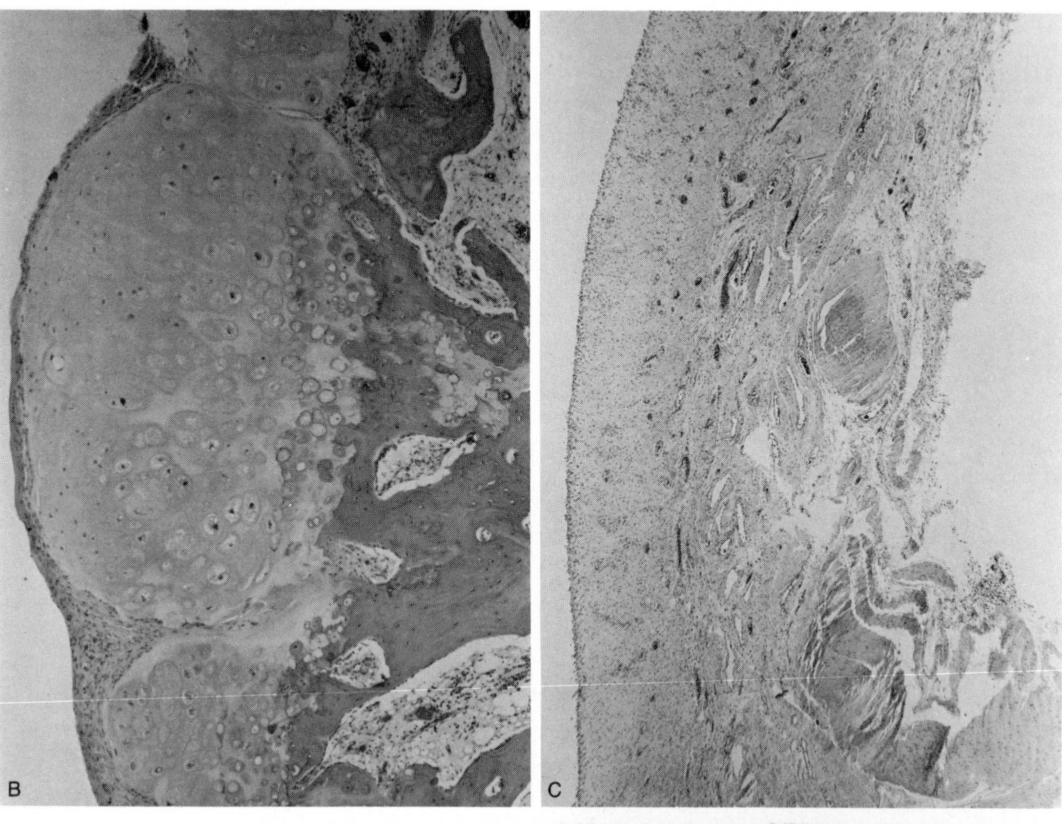

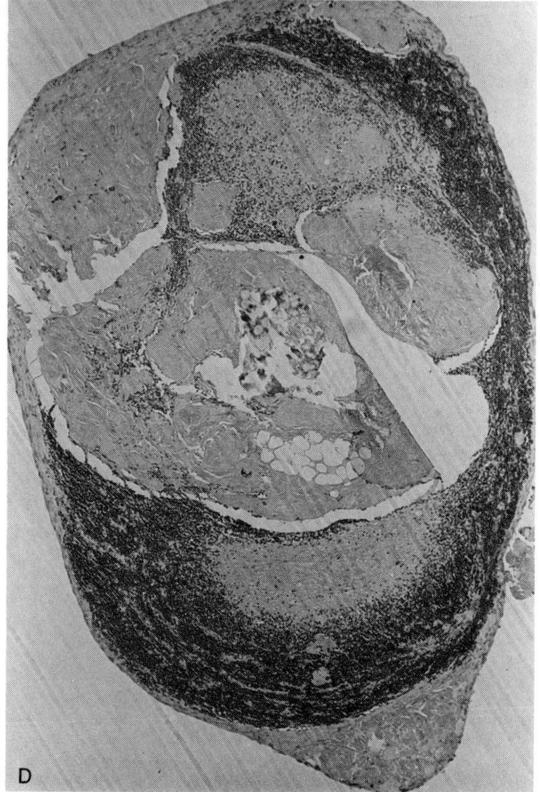

***Figure** 73–77.* Continued

B *A section of the osteochondroma reveals a moderately cellular cartilage cap overlying viable bony trabeculae.*

C *The wall of a large bursa surrounding the osteochondroma is composed of dense fibrous tissue lined by mesothelial cells. Foci of lymphocytes and hemosiderin deposits are present.*

D *The bursa contains "loose" bodies consisting of encapsulated fibrous tissue with centers of calcified cartilage.*

(From El-Khoury GY, Bassett GS: Am J Roentgenol 133:895, 1979. Copyright 1979, American Roentgen Ray Society.)

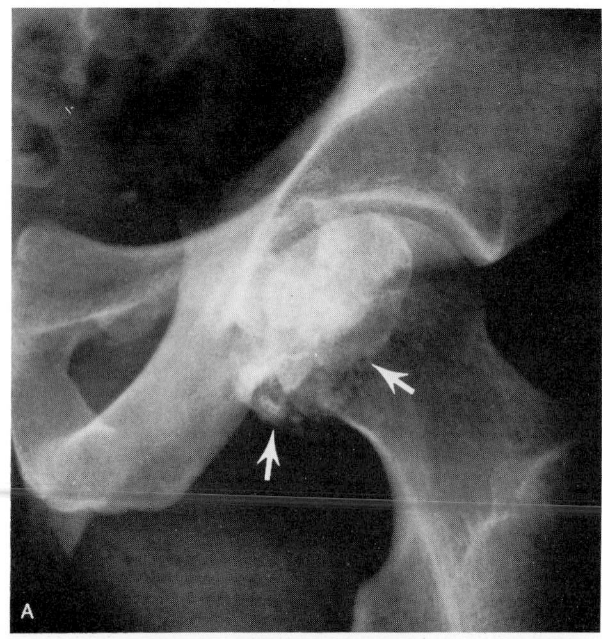

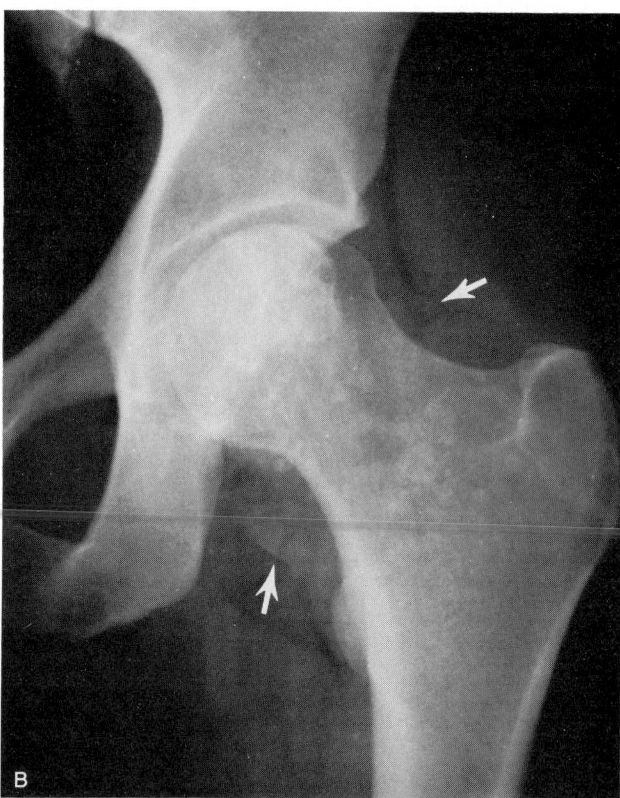

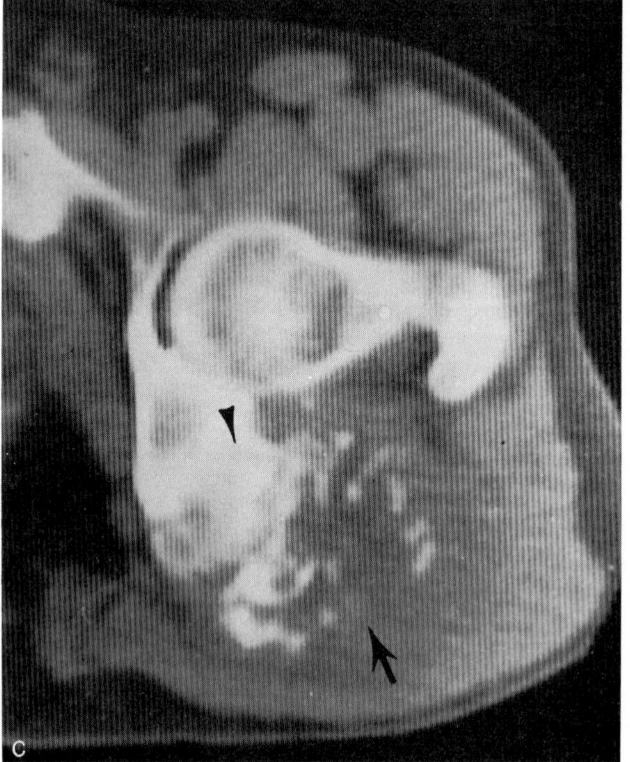

Figure 73–78. *Solitary exostosis. Complications — malignant degeneration (chondrosarcoma). A 35 year old man developed an enlarging mass on the posterior aspect of the thigh.*

A *A radiograph obtained two years prior to admission reveals a partially calcified or ossified dense lesion overlying the left hip (arrows).*

B *On admission, the changing nature of the radiodense area is evident (arrows).*

C *On computed tomography, an osteochondroma is found to be arising from the ischium (arrowhead). It is associated with a soft tissue mass containing irregular calcification (arrow).*

Illustration continued on the opposite page

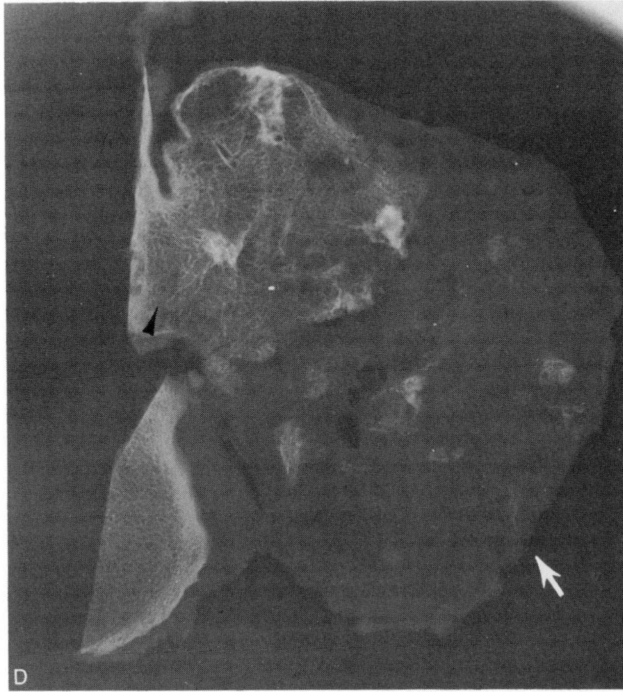

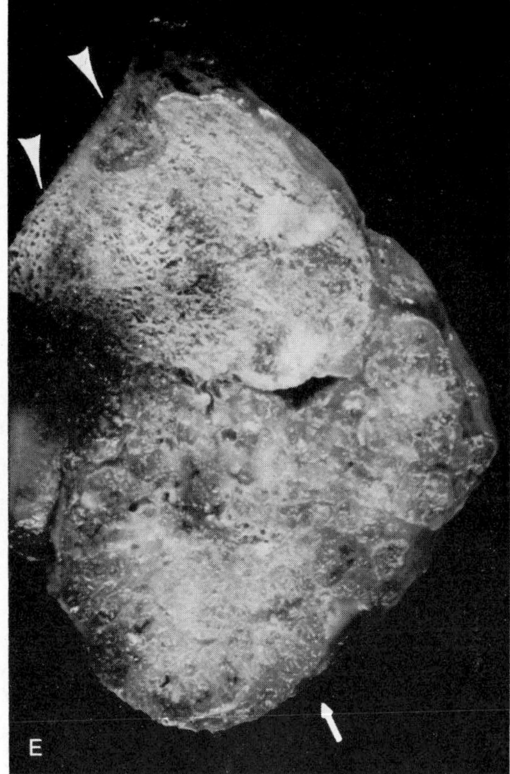

Figure 73–78. Continued

D *A radiograph of a section of the specimen delineates the site of attachment of the osteochondroma (arrowhead) and the calcified tumor mass (arrow).*

E *A photograph of the section outlines the site of osseous attachment (arrowheads) and the tumor (arrow). A typical chondrosarcoma was revealed on histologic examination.*

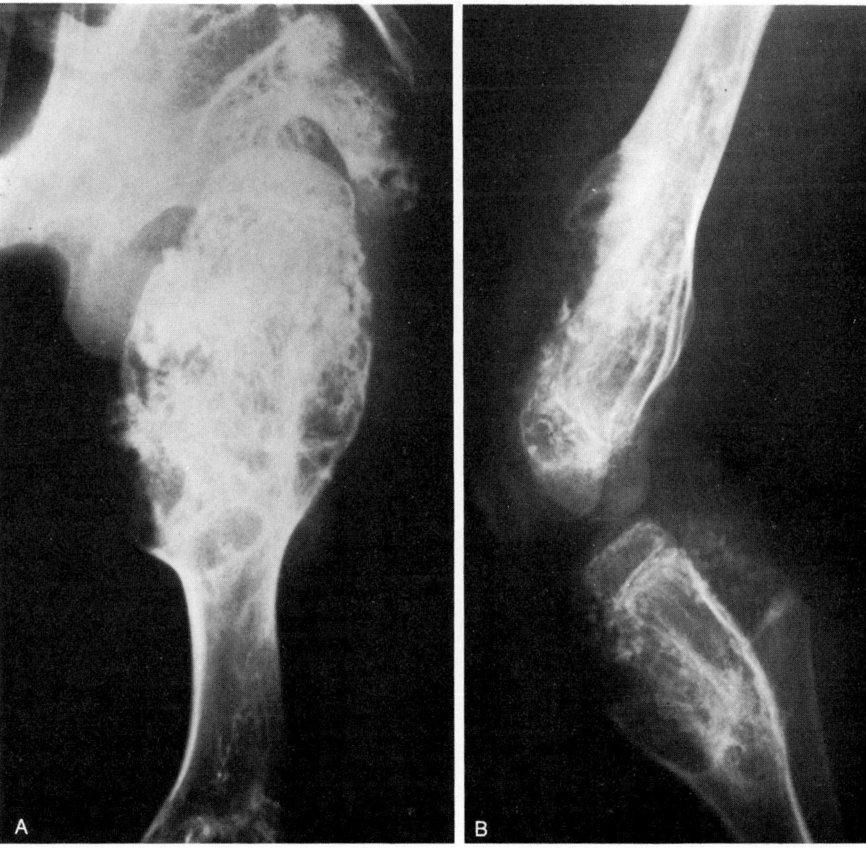

Figure 73–79. *Ollier's disease.*

A, B *In this young girl, bizarre calcified lesions are present in the metaphyses of multiple bones, where they have produced osseous expansion.*

Illustration continued on the following page

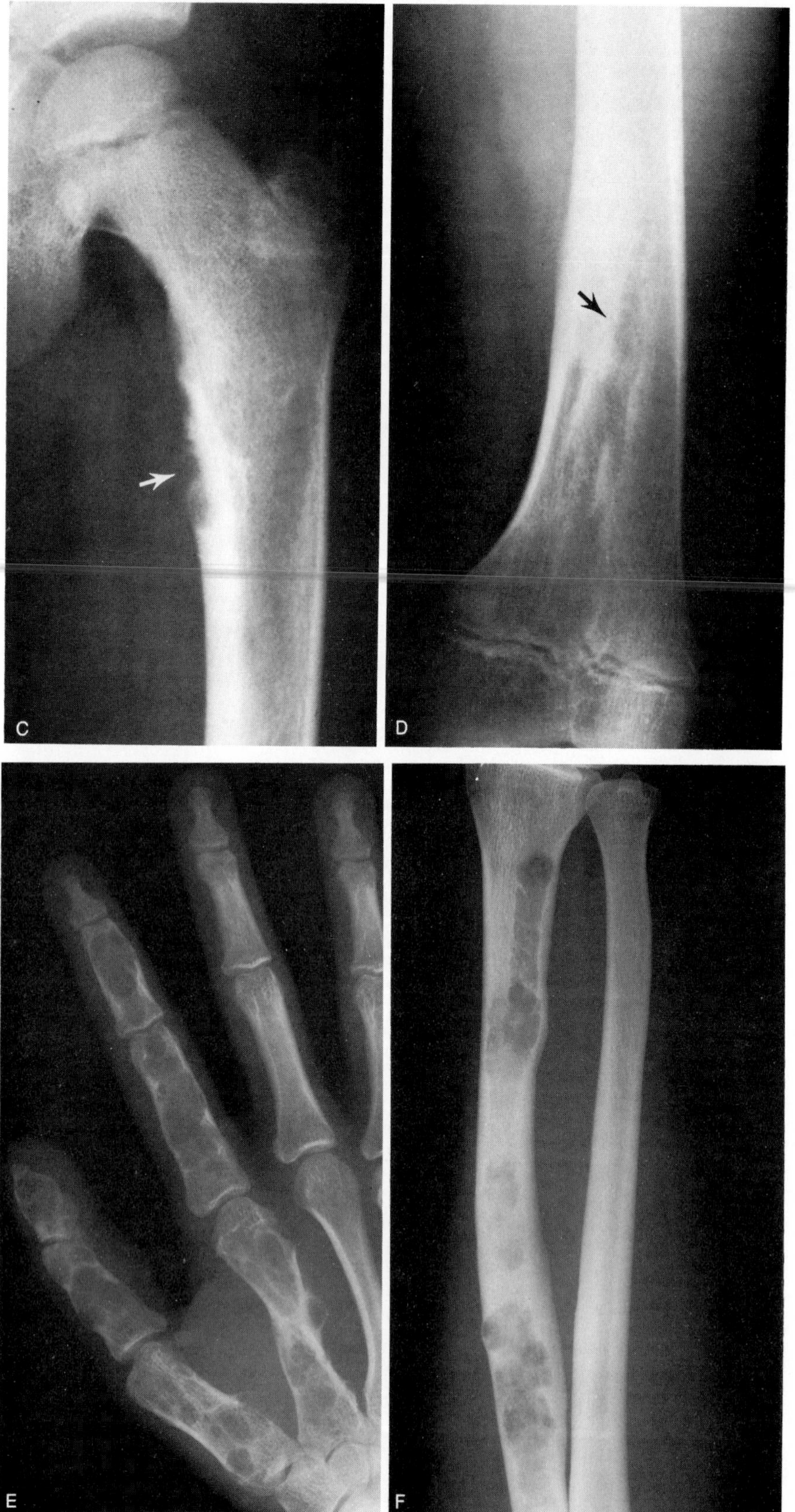

Figure 73–79. Continued

C, D *In another child, linear radiolucent areas (arrow) are evident, predominantly in the metaphyses or adjacent diaphysis of the femur. Leg length discrepancy had resulted.*

E, F *In two adult patients, multiple circular radiolucent lesions have produced endosteal erosion, osseous expansion, and deformity.*

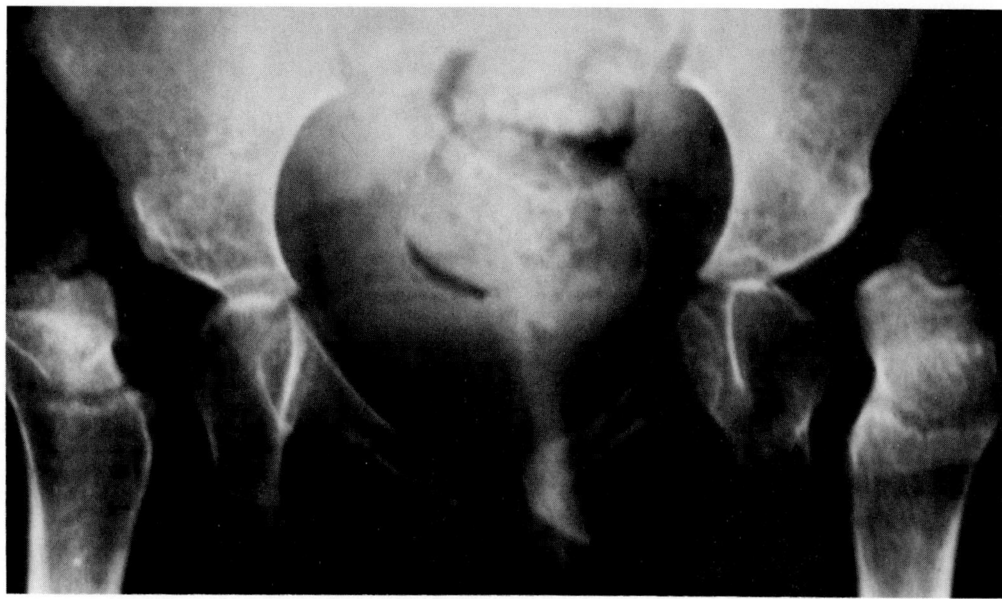

Figure 73–80. Arthrogryposis multiplex congenita. Note bilateral dislocations of the hip.

can be detected in many individuals. Multiple surgical procedures may be required, although a high incidence of recurrence of deformities is apparent.

WERNER'S SYNDROME. Werner's syndrome is named after the investigator who, in 1904, described four siblings with similar clinical findings: shortness of stature, premature aging, scleroderma-like skin changes, and cataracts.[443] Werner attributed the peculiar clinical abnormalities to a failure of ectoderm-derived cells. Since this original description, more than 100 cases have been documented, which are well summarized in the classic review by Epstein and collaborators.[444] Werner's syndrome is similar to but distinct from progeria. Its principal clinical manifestations include a symmetric retardation of growth with absence of the adolescent growth spurt, graying and loss of the hair, voice alterations, cataracts, skin ulcerations, and, in some cases, mild diabetes mellitus.[444] Additional changes are vascular and soft tissue calcifications, generalized osteoporosis, atrophy of muscle and fat, and hypogonadism with small genitalia and decreased libido and potency in men, and small breasts and menstrual abnormalities in women. Neoplasms, especially sarcomas and meningiomas, may complicate the clinical picture. The prognosis is guarded, as many patients succumb by the fourth or fifth decade of life to complications of cardiovascular involvement, including myocardial infarction and stroke. Genetic studies in Werner's syndrome reveal findings compatible with an autosomal recessive mode of inheritance. Although it has been suggested that a defect in a single protein or enzyme could account for the findings, the exact nature of the disorder remains elusive.[444]

Radiographic evaluation reveals patchy or generalized osteoporosis.[445-447] Extensive arterial calcifications may be evident, particularly in the vessels of the extremities, coronary arteries, and aorta. Aortic and mitral valvular calcification may also be apparent in association with cardiac enlargement and congestive heart failure. Soft tissue calcification is observed in approximately one third of cases and predominates about bony protuberances, including the distal ends of the tibia and fibula, and areas about the knees, feet, and hands (Fig. 73–81). Soft tissue atrophy may also be apparent. Destructive osseous lesions related to osteomyelitis and septic arthritis and neurotrophic changes in the feet resembling the findings of diabetes mellitus can be evident.[445] Degenerative changes in the spine have also been described.

Clinically, Werner's syndrome resembles progeria, although cataracts, hyperkeratosis, skin ulcerations, and diabetes mellitus are not characteristics of this latter syndrome.[444] Werner's syndrome also bears some resemblance to Rothmund's syndrome, myotonic dystrophy, scleroderma, and the Cockayne syndrome. Radiographically, the findings are most reminiscent of those in collagen vascular disorders and hyperparathyroidism.

CONGENITAL PSEUDARTHROSIS. This is an unusual condition associated with fracture followed by a nonunion. It is most typically identified in the tibia,[426-428] although pseudarthroses may also be seen in the fibula, femur, clavicle, humerus, ulna, rib,

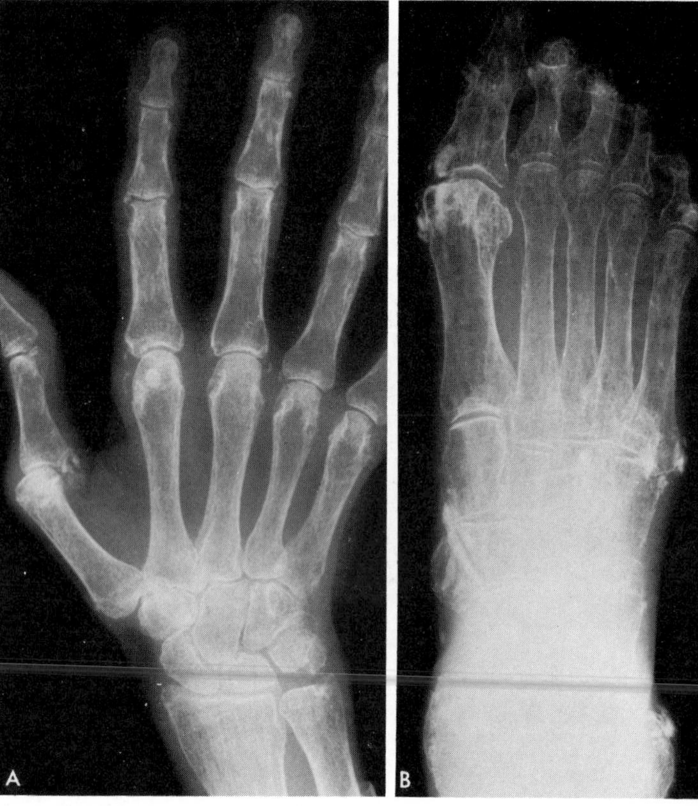

Figure 73–81. Werner's syndrome. Observe osteoporosis and soft tissue calcifications, most prominent in periarticular locations. (Courtesy of Dr. Paul Major, Winnipeg, Manitoba.)

and, rarely, other bones.[429-432] Its classification and pathogenesis have been the source of a great deal of confusion and debate. In some patients, pseudarthroses are present at birth (true congenital pseudarthrosis), whereas in other patients, they develop in the first few years of life (infantile pseudarthrosis).[1,433] Some affected individuals may have stigmata of neurofibromatosis or fibrous dysplasia,[429] although others do not; the reported incidence of neurofibromatosis in cases of pseudarthrosis has varied considerably (0 to 70 per cent), in part related to the criteria utilized to substantiate the diagnosis of neurofibromatosis. Histologic evaluation of the affected site may reveal interosseous tissue that appears to be representative of a neurofibroma or schwannoma, although ultrastructural characteristics may demonstrate subtle differences between the dense cellular tissue of a pseudarthrosis and the tissue of a neural tumor.[434] Thus, the precise relationships among congenital pseudarthrosis, neurofibromatosis, and fibrous dysplasia remain a mystery, although in some cases, pseudarthrosis can apparently represent a localized and isolated phenomenon.

It is the more common infantile variety of the disease as it appears in the tibia that has attracted the most attention in the literature. This lesion usually develops in the first or second year of life, although, occasionally, it may appear after this time and, rarely, may be delayed until the eighth to eleventh years of life. Unilateral changes predominate. Initially, anterior bowing of the lower half of the tibia is recognized with or without abnormality of the adjacent fibula. At the apex of the curve, sclerosis, narrowing of the medullary canal, and cystic abnormality may indicate impending fracture and pseudarthrosis. These early pre-fracture findings have been emphasized by Lloyd-Roberts and others,[435] and have been attributed to an abnormality of the primary cartilaginous anlage by some investigators. Badgley and collaborators[436] noted that the site of tibial angulation coincided with the location of the primary ossification center, suggesting that cartilaginous changes in this center could produce the typical osseous defect, a theory that was supported by histologic data derived from later clinical and laboratory investigations.[437-439] Although additional theories abound, including those that suggest that the tibial pseudarthrosis is related to trauma, amnionic bands, genetic aberration, vascular anomalies, and nutritional or metabolic disturbance, the possibility of a primary alteration in the cartilaginous anlage producing this lesion is attractive and could possibly explain the development of similar defects at other sites, such as the clavicle and proximal femur.[439] Once the fracture appears, the margins of the adjacent bone ends taper further (Fig. 73–82). The prognosis for ultimate union at the fracture site varies with the age of the patient (fractures developing before 2 years of age carry a poor prognosis) and the type of therapy that is employed[429]; if a graft is applied, healing may be expected in approximately 25 to 35 per cent of patients.

Congenital pseudarthrosis of the clavicle occurs almost exclusively on the right side of the body, although it may be bilateral in distribution in 10 per cent of cases.[432, 465] Its occurrence on the left side may be associated with dextrocardia, suggesting that the position of adjacent vascular structures such as the subclavian artery may be important in the pathogenesis of this osseous defect; the pulsation of a nearby artery located between the clavicle and first rib or cervical rib could conceivably produce bony resorption.[440] Other theories emphasize the role of trauma, a defect in the primary ossification center of the clavicle, or a failure of coalescence of two centers of clavicular ossification.[441, 442] A familial incidence of the disorder is occasionally noted. The lesion is usually discovered within the first few months of life owing to the presence of a painless lump over the middle one third of the clavicle. On radiographs, the medial end of the clavicle is superior to the lateral end, osseous discontinuity is evident, and callus formation is absent. It is the absence of pain and visible callus that usually allows differentiation from a posttraumatic pseudarthrosis. A third disorder leading to similar clavicular changes is cleidocranial dysostosis. On pathologic examination of the clavicle in cases of congenital pseudarthrosis, fibrous tissue separates the two cartilage-covered bone ends, and there is no evidence of neurofibromatosis or fibrous dysplasia.[442]

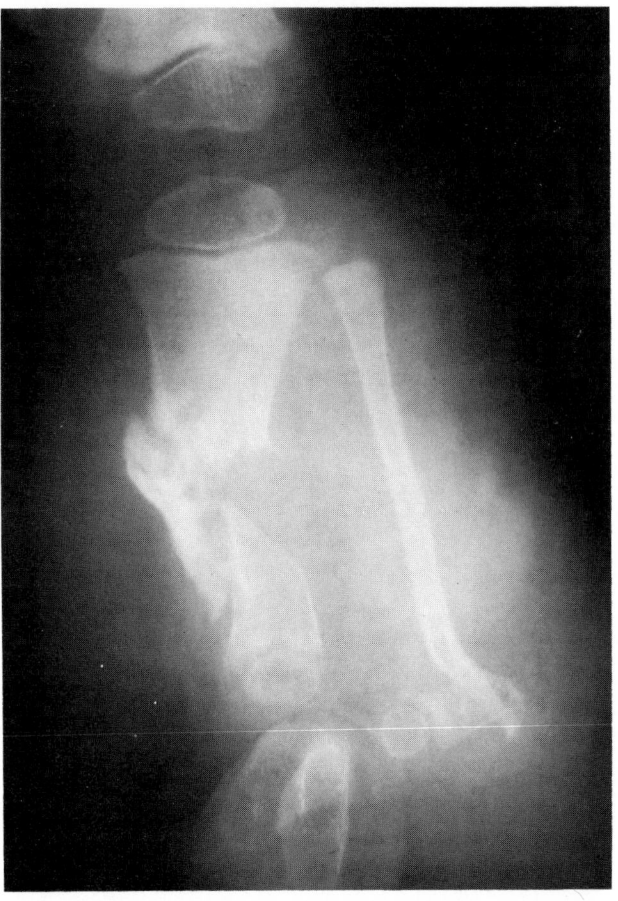

Figure 73–82. *Congenital pseudarthrosis. Fractures with pseudarthroses are observed in the middle third of the tibia and the lower third of the fibula. Some of the ends of the fractured bones are tapered. Considerable soft tissue swelling and hypertrophy are evident, although this child had no clinical evidence of neurofibromatosis.*

SUMMARY

A summary of the many congenital and inherited disorders of the skeleton has been undertaken. It is evident that these present with varied clinical and radiologic manifestations. In some instances, radiographic features are entirely specific, whereas in others, they must be interpreted with knowledge of clinical abnormalities in order to arrive at a correct diagnosis.

REFERENCES

1. Caffey JP: Pediatric X-ray Diagnosis. 7th ed. Chicago, Year Book Medical Publishers, 1978.
2. Spranger JW, Langer LO Jr, Wiedemann HR: Bone Dysplasias. An Atlas of Constitutional Disorders of Skeletal Development. Philadelphia, WB Saunders Co, 1974.
3. McKusick VA: Heritable Disorders of Connective Tissue. St. Louis, The CV Mosby Co, 1972.
4. Rubin P: Dynamic Classification of Bone Dysplasias. Chicago, Year Book Medical Publishers, 1964.

5. Bailey JA: Disproportionate Short Stature. Diagnosis and Management. Philadelphia, WB Saunders Co, 1973.
6. Frantz CH, O'Rahilly R: Congenital skeletal limb deficiencies. J Bone Joint Surg *43A*:1202, 1961.
7. Burtch RL, Fishman S, Kay HW: Nomenclature for congenital skeletal limb deficiencies, a revision of the Frantz and O'Rahilly classification. Artif Limbs *10*:24, 1966.
8. Mital MA: Limb deficiencies: Classification and treatment. Orthop Clin North Am *7*:457, 1976.
9. Kay HW: A proposed international terminology for the classification of congenital limb deficiencies. Interclinic Information Bull *13*:1, 1974.
10. Kay HW: A proposed international terminology for the classification of congenital limb deficiencies. Orthot Prosth *28*:33, 1974.
11. Coventry MB, Johnson EW Jr: Congenital absence of the fibula. J Bone Joint Surg *34A*:941, 1952.
12. Kruger LM, Talbott RD: Amputation and prosthesis as definitive treatment in congenital absence of the fibula. J Bone Joint Surg *43A*:625, 1961.
13. Achterman C, Kalamchi A: Congenital deficiency of the fibula. J Bone Joint Surg *61B*:133, 1979.
14. Jansen K, Andersen KS: Congenital absence of the fibula. Acta Orthop Scand *45*:446, 1974.
15. Westin GW, Sakai DN, Wood WL: Congenital longitudinal deficiency of the fibula. Follow-up of treatment by Syme amputation. J Bone Joint Surg *58A*:492, 1976.
16. Ogden JA: Proximal fibular growth deformities. Skel Radiol *3*:223, 1979.
17. Barnes JC, Smith WL: The VATER association. Radiology *126*:445, 1978.
18. Simcha A: Congenital heart disease in radial clubbed hand syndrome. Arch Dis Child *46*:345, 1971.
19. Hall JG, Levin J, Kuhn JP, Ottenheimer EJ, Van Berkum KAP, McKusick VA: Thrombocytopenia with absent radius (TAR). Medicine *48*:411, 1969.
20. Omenn GS, Figley MM, Graham CB, Heinrichs WL: Prospects for radiographic intrauterine diagnosis — the syndrome of thrombocytopenia with absent radii. N Engl J Med *288*:777, 1973.
21. Ogden JA, Watson HK, Bohne W: Ulnar dysmelia. J Bone Joint Surg *58A*:467, 1976.
22. Goldman AB, Schneider R, Wilson PD Jr: Proximal focal femoral deficiency. J Can Assoc Radiol *29*:101, 1978.
23. Levinson ED, Ozonoff MB, Royen PM: Proximal femoral focal deficiency (PFFD). Radiology *125*:197, 1977.
24. Lange DR, Schoenecker PL, Baker CL: Proximal femoral focal deficiency: Treatment and classification in forty-two cases. Clin Orthop Rel Res *135*:15, 1978.
25. Panting AL, Williams PF: Proximal femoral focal deficiency. J Bone Joint Surg *60B*:46, 1978.
26. Fixsen JA, Lloyd-Roberts GC: The natural history and early treatment of proximal femoral dysplasia. J Bone Joint Surg *56B*:86, 1974.
27. Shands AR Jr, MacEwen GD: Congenital abnormalities of the femur. Acta Orthop Scand *32*:307, 1962.
28. Pedersen LM, Tygstrup I, Pedersen J: Congenital malformations in newborn infants of diabetic women. Correlation with maternal diabetic vascular complications. Lancet *1*:1124, 1964.
29. Holden CEA: Congenital shortening of one femur in one identical twin. Postgrad Med J *44*:813, 1968.
30. Blumel J, Evans EB, Eggers GWN: Partial and complete agenesis or malformation of the sacrum and associated anomalies. J Bone Joint Surg *41A*:497, 1958.
31. Banta JV, Nichols O: Sacral agenesis. J Bone Joint Surg *51A*:693, 1969.
32. Passarge E, Lenz W: Syndrome of caudal regression in infants of diabetic mothers: Observations of further cases. Pediatrics *37*:672, 1966.
33. Renshaw TS: Sacral agenesis: A classification and review of twenty-three cases. J Bone Joint Surg *60A*:373, 1978.
34. Hunt PT, Davidson KC, Ashcraft KW, Holder TM: Radiography of hereditary presacral teratoma. Radiology *122*:187, 1977.
35. Wilkinson RH, Strand RD: Congenital anomalies and normal variants. Semin Roentgenol *13*:7, 1979.
36. Dounis E: Sacrococcygeal agenesis. A report of four new cases. Acta Orthop Scand *49*:475, 1978.
37. Poznanski AK, Stephenson JM: Radiographic findings in hypothalamic acceleration of growth associated with cerebral atrophy and mental retardation (cerebral gigantism). Radiology *88*:446, 1967.
38. Inglis K: Local gigantism (a manifestation of neurofibromatosis): Its relation to general gigantism and to acromegaly. Illustrating the incidence of intrinsic factors in disease when development of the body is abnormal. Am J Pathol *26*:1059. 1950.
39. Barsky AJ: Macrodactyly. J Bone Joint Surg *49A*:1255, 1967.
40. Poznanski AK, Garn SM, Holt JF: The thumb in the congenital malformation syndromes. Radiology *100*:115, 1971.
41. Swanson AB, Brown KS: Hereditary triphalangeal thumb. J Hered *53*:259, 1962.
42. Poznanski AK: The Hand in Radiologic Diagnosis. Philadelphia, WB Saunders Co, 1974.
43. Warkany J: Congenital Malformations: Notes and Comments. Chicago, Year Book Medical Publishers, 1971.
44. Ireland DCR, Takayama N, Flatt AE: Poland's syndrome. A review of forty-three cases. J Bone Joint Surg *58A*:52, 1976.
45. Hoefnagel D, Rozycki A, Worster-Hill D, Stern P, Gregory D: Leukaemia and Poland's syndrome. Lancet *2*:1038, 1972.
46. Mace JW, Kaplan JM, Schanberger JE, Gotlin RW: Poland's syndrome: Report of seven cases and review of the literature. Clin Pediatr *11*:98, 1972.
47. Elkington SG, Huntsman RG: The Talbot fingers: A study in symphalangism. Br Med J *1*:407, 1967.
48. Strasberger AK, Hawkins MR, Eldridge R, Hargrave RL, McKusick VA: Symphalangism: Genetic and clinical aspects. Johns Hopkins Med J *117*:108, 1965.
49. Harle TS, Stevenson JR: Hereditary symphalangism associated with carpal and tarsal fusions. Radiology *89*:91, 1967.
50. Cope JR: Carpal coalition. Clin Radiol *25*:261, 1974.
51. Garn SM, Frisancho AR, Poznanski AK, Schweitzer J, McCann MB: Analysis of triquetral-lunate fusion. Am J Phys Anthropol *34*:431, 1971.
52. Dean RFA, Jones PRM: Fusion of triquetral and lunate bones shown in several radiographs. Am J Phys Anthropal *17*:279, 1959.
53. Cockshott WP: Carpal fusions. Am J Roentgenol *89*:1260, 1963.
54. Cockshott WP: Pisiform hamate fusion. J Bone Joint Surg *51A*:778, 1969.
55. O'Rahilly R: A survey of carpal and tarsal anomalies. J Bone Joint Surg *35A*:626, 1953.
56. McGoey PF: Fracture-dislocation of fused triangular and lunate (congenital). Report of a case. J Bone Joint Surg *25*:928, 1943.
57. Smitham JH: Some observations on certain congenital abnormalities of the hand in African natives. Br J Radiol *21*:513, 1948.
58. McCredie J: Congenital fusion of bones: Radiology, embryology, and pathogenesis. Clin Radiol *26*:47, 1975.
59. Green WT, Mital MA: Congenital radio-ulnar synostosis: Surgical treatment. J Bone Joint Surg *61A*:738, 1979.
60. Mital MA: Congenital radioulnar synostosis and congenital dislocation of the radial head. Orthop Clin North Am *7*:375, 1976.
61. Davenport CB, Taylor HL, Nelson LA: Radio-ulnar synostosis. Arch Surg *8*:705, 1924.
62. Harris BJ: Anomalous structures in the developing human foot. Anat Rec *121*:399, 1955.
63. Pfitzner W: Die Variationen im Aufbau des Fussskelets. Morphol Arb *6*:245, 1896.
64. Slomann HC: On coalitio calcaneo-navicularis. J Orthop Surg *3*:586, 1921.
65. Harris RI, Beath T: Etiology of peroneal spastic flat foot. J Bone Joint Surg *30B*:624, 1948.
66. Chambers CH: Congenital anomalies of the tarsal navicular with particular reference to calcaneo-navicular coalition. Br J Radiol *23*:580, 1950.
67. Hark FW: Congenital anomalies of the tarsal bones. Clin Orthop *16*:21, 1960.
68. Rothberg AS, Feldman JW, Schuster OF: Congenital fusion of astragalus and scaphoid: Bilateral, inherited. NY State Med J *35*:29, 1935.
69. Webster FS, Roberts WM: Tarsal anomalies and peroneal spastic flatfoot. JAMA *146*:1099, 1951.
70. Bersani FA, Samilson RL: Massive familial tarsal synostosis. J Bone Joint Surg *39A*:1187, 1957.
71. Leonard MA: The inheritance of tarsal coalition and its relationship to spastic flat foot. J Bone Joint Surg *56B*:520, 1974.
72. Heiple KG, Lovejoy CO: The antiquity of tarsal coalition. J Bone Joint Surg *51A*:979, 1969.
73. Jones Sir R: Peroneal spasm and its treatment. Report of a meeting of the Liverpool Medical Institution. Liverpool Med Chir J *17*:442, 1897.
74. Badgley CE: Coalition of the calcaneus and the navicular. Arch Surg *15*:75, 1927.
75. Conway JJ, Cowell HR: Tarsal coalition: Clinical significance and roentgenographic demonstration. Radiology *92*:799, 1969.
76. Kendrick JI: Treatment of calcaneonavicular bar. JAMA *172*:1242, 1960.
77. Simmons EH: Tibialis spastic varus foot with tarsal coalition. J Bone Joint Surg *47B*:533, 1965.

78. Schmidt F: Über eine symmetrische Synostosis calcaneo-navicularis bei gleichzeitigem Klumphohlfub. Arch Orthop Unfallchir *30*:289, 1931.
79. Lapidus PW: Spastic flat foot. J Bone Joint Surg *28*:126, 1946.
80. Poznanski AK: Foot manifestations of the congenital malformation syndromes. Semin Roentgenol *5*:354, 1970.
81. Poznanski AK, Stern AM, Gall JC Jr: Radiographic findings in the hand-foot-uterus syndrome (HFUS). Radiology *95*:129, 1970.
82. Langer LO Jr: The roentgenographic features of the oto-palato-digital (OPD) syndrome. Am J Roentgenol *100*:63, 1967.
83. Geelhoed GW, Neel JV, Davidson RT: Symphalangism and tarsal coalitions: A hereditary syndrome. A report on two families. J Bone Joint Surg *51B*:278, 1969.
84. Poznanski AK, LaRowe PC: Radiographic manifestations of the arthrogryposis syndrome. Radiology *95*:353, 1970.
85. Schauerte EW, St. Aubin PM: Progressive synostosis in Apert's syndrome (acrocephalosyndactyly), with a description of roentgenographic changes in the feet. Am J Roentgenol *97*:67, 1966.
86. Beckly DE, Anderson PW, Pedegana LR: The radiology of the subtalar joint with special reference to talo-calcaneal coalition. Clin Radiol *26*:333, 1975.
87. Jack EA: Bone anomalies of the tarsus in relation to "peroneal spastic flat foot." J Bone Joint Surg *36B*:530, 1954.
88. Feist JH, Mankin JH: The tarsus. I. Basic relationships and motions in the adult and definition of optimal recumbent oblique projection. Radiology *79*:250, 1962.
89. Herschel H, von Ronnen JR: The occurrence of calcaneonavicular synosteosis in pes valgus contractus. J Bone Joint Surg *32A*:280, 1950.
90. Braddock GTF: A prolonged follow-up of peroneal spastic flat foot. J Bone Joint Surg *43B*:734, 1961.
91. Kaye JJ, Ghelman B, Schneider R: Talocalcaneonavicular joint arthrography for sustentacular-talar tarsal coalitions. Radiology *115*:730, 1975.
92. Brahme F: Upper talar enarthrosis. Acta Radiol *55*:221, 1961.
93. Schrieber RR: Congenital and acquired ball-and-socket ankle joint. Radiology *84*:940, 1965.
94. Lamb D: The ball and socket ankle joint — a congenital abnormality. J Bone Joint Surg *40B*:240, 1958.
95. Channon GM, Brotherton BJ: The ball and socket ankle joint. J Bone Joint Surg *61B*:85, 1979.
96. Boyd HB: Congenital talonavicular synostosis. J Bone Joint Surg *26*:682, 1944.
97. Challis J: Hereditary transmission of talonavicular coalition in association with anomaly of the little finger. J Bone Joint Surg *56A*:1273, 1974.
98. Zeide MS, Wiesel SW, Terry RL: Talonavicular coalition. Clin Orthop Rel Res *126*:225, 1977.
99. Mahaffey HW: Bilateral congenital calcaneocuboid synostosis, a case report. J Bone Joint Surg *27*:164, 1945.
100. Veneruso LC: Unilateral congenital calcaneocuboid synostosis with complete absence of a metatarsal and toe, a case report. J Bone Joint Surg *27*:718, 1945.
101. Outland T, Murphy ID: Relation of tarsal anomalies to spastic and rigid flatfeet. Clin Orthop Rel Res *1*:217, 1953.
102. Waugh W: Partial cubo-navicular coalition as a cause of peroneal spastic flat foot. J Bone Joint Surg *39B*:520, 1957.
103. Lusby HLJ: Naviculo-cuneiform synostosis. J Bone Joint Surg *41B*:150, 1959.
104. Gregersen HN: Naviculocuneiform coalition. J Bone Joint Surg *59A*:128, 1977.
105. Del Sel JM, Grand NE: Cubo-navicular synostosis. A rare tarsal anomaly. J Bone Joint Surg *41B*:149, 1959.
106. Klippel MM, Feil A: Absence de colonne cervicale. Cage thoracique remontant jusqu' à la base du crâne. Presse Med *20*:411, 1912.
107. Klippel M, Feil A: Anomalie de la colonne vertébrale par absence des vertèbres cervicales; cage thoracique remontant jusqu' à la base du crâne. Bull Mem Soc Anat Paris *87*:185, 1912.
108. Luftman II, Weintraub S: Klippel-Feil syndrome in a full term stillborn infant. NY State J Med *51*:2035, 1951.
109. Shands AR Jr, Bundens WD: Congenital deformities of the spine. An analysis of the roentgenograms of 700 children. Bull Hosp Joint Dis *17*:110, 1956.
110. Gray SW, Romaine CB, Skandalakis JE: Congenital fusion of the cervical vertebrae. Surg Gynecol Obstet *118*:373, 1964.
111. Sicard JA, Lermoyez J: II. Formes fruste, évolutive, familiale du syndrome de Klippel-Feil. Rev Neurol Paris *39*:71, 1923.
112. Masi A, Vichi GF: La sindrome di Klippel-Feil j contributo statistics e clinico radiologico. Riv Clin Pediatr *65*:22, 1960.
113. Haddad HM, Wilkins L: Congenital anomalies associated with gonadal aplasia, review of 55 cases. Pediatrics *23*:885, 1959.
114. Hensinger RN, Lang JE, MacEwen GD: Klippel-Feil syndrome. A constellation of associated anomalies. J Bone Joint Surg *56A*:1246, 1974.
115. Ramsay J, Bliznak J: Klippel-Feil syndrome with renal agenesis and other anomalies. Am J Roentgenol *113*:460, 1971.
116. Degenhardt KH, Kladetsky J: Malformaciones de la columna vertebrale y del esbozo de la corda dorsalis. Arch Pediatr *7*:1, 1956.
117. Gardner WJ, Collins JS: Klippel-Feil syndrome. Syringomyelia, diastematomyelia and myelomeningolocele — one disease? Arch Surg *83*:638, 1961.
118. Fietti VG Jr, Fielding JW: The Klippel-Feil syndrome: Early roentgenographic appearance and progression of the deformity. J Bone Joint Surg *58A*:891, 1976.
119. Madelung OW: Die spontane Subluxation der Hand nach vorne. Verh Dtsch Ges Chir *7*:259, 1878.
120. Anton JI, Reitz GB, Spiegel MB: Madelung's deformity. Ann Surg *108*:411, 1938.
121. Felman AH, Kirkpatrick JA Jr: Madelung's deformity: Observations in 17 patients. Radiology *93*:1037, 1969.
122. Nielsen JB: Madelung's deformity: A follow-up study of 26 cases and a review of the literature. Acta Orthop Scand *48*:379, 1977.
123. Dannenburg M, Anton JI, Spiegel MB: Madelung's deformity. Consideration of its roentgenological diagnostic criteria. Am J Roentgenol *42*:671, 1939.
124. Ranawat CS, DeFiore J, Straub LR: Madelung's deformity. An end-result study of surgical treatment. J Bone Joint Surg *57A*:772, 1975.
125. Henry A, Thorburn MJ: Madelung's deformity. A clinical and cytogenetic study. J Bone Joint Surg *49B*:66, 1967.
126. Kosowicz J: The Carpal sign in gonadal dysgenesis. J Clin Endocrinol Metab *22*:949, 1962.
127. Kosowicz J: The roentgen appearance of hand and wrist in gonadal dysgenesis. Am J Roentgenol *93*:354, 1965.
128. Léri A, Weill J: Une affection congénitale et symétrique du développement osseux: La dyschondrostéose. Bull Mem Soc Hop Paris *53*:1491, 1929.
129. Golding JSR, Blackburne JS: Madelung's disease of the wrist and dyschondrosteosis. J Bone Joint Surg *58B*:350, 1976.
130. Herdman RC, Langer LO, Good R: Dyschondrosteosis, the most common cause of Madelung's deformity. J Pediatr *68*:432, 1966.
131. Goodwin DRA, Michels CH, Weissman SL: Spontaneous rupture of extensor tendons in Madelung's deformity. Hand *11*:72, 1979.
132. Niebauer JJ, King DE: Congenital dislocation of the knee. J Bone Joint Surg *42A*:207, 1960.
133. Carlson DH, O'Connor J: Congenital dislocation of the knee. Am J Roentgenol *127*:465, 1976.
134. Laurence M: Genu recurvatum congenitum. J Bone Joint Surg *49B*:121, 1967.
135. Curtis BH, Fisher RL: Congenital hyperextension with anterior subluxation of the knee. J Bone Joint Surg *51A*:255, 1969.
136. McFarlane AL: A report on four cases of congenital genu recurvation occurring in one family. Br J Surg *34*:388, 1947.
137. Provenzano RW: Congenital dislocation of the knee. Report of a case. N Engl J Med *236*:360, 1947.
138. Katz MP, Grogono BJS, Soper KC: The etiology and treatment of congenital dislocation of the knee. J Bone Joint Surg *49B*:112, 1967.
139. Shattock SG: Genu recurvatum in a foetus at term. Trans Pathol Soc Lond *42*:280, 1891.
140. Middleton DS: The pathology of congenital genu recurvatum. Br J Surg *22*:696, 1935.
141. Ahmadi B, Shahriaree H, Silver CM: Severe congenital genu recurvatum. Case report. J Bone Joint Surg *61A*:622, 1979.
142. Calhoun JD, Pierret G: Infantile coxa vara. Am J Roentgenol *115*:561, 1972.
143. Babb FS, Ghormley RK, Chatterton CC: Congenital coxa vara. J Bone Joint Surg *31A*:115, 1949.
144. Hark FW: Congenital coxa vara. Am J Surg *80*:305, 1950.
145. Johanning K: Coxa vara infantum. I. Clinical appearance and aetiological problems. Acta Orthop Scand *21*:273, 1951.
146. Zadek I: Congenital coxa vara. Arch Surg *30*:62, 1935.
147. Golding FC: Congenital coxa vara. J Bone Joint Surg *30B*:161, 1948.
148. Fisher FL, Waskowitz WJ: Familial developmental coxa vara. Clin Orthop Rel Res *86*:2, 1972.
149. Letts RM, Shokeir MHK: Mirror-image coxa vara in identical twins. J Bone Joint Surg *57A*:117, 1975.
150. Almond HG: Familial infantile coxa vara. J Bone Joint Surg *38B*:539, 1956.
151. Barrington-Ward LE: Double coxa vara with other deformities occurring in brother and sister. Lancet *1*:157, 1912.
152. Say B, Taysi K, Pirnar T, Tokgözoğlu N, Inan E: Dominant congenital coxa vara. J Bone Joint Surg *56B*:78, 1974.
153. Morgan JD, Somerville EW: Normal and abnormal growth at the upper end of the femur. J Bone Joint Surg *42B*:264, 1960.
154. Magnusson R: Coxa vara infantum. Acta Orthop Scand *23*:284, 1953.

155. Compere EL, Garrison M, Fahey JJ: Deformities of the femur resulting from arrestment of growth of capital and greater trochanteric epiphysis. J Bone Joint Surg *22*:909, 1940.
156. Otto AW, EinBecken: Mit hagelformig aus gedehnten pfannen. *In* Neue seltene Beobachtungen zur Anatomie, Physiologie, und Pathologie gehörig. Berlin, August Rücker, 1824.
157. Eppinger H: Pelvis-Chrobak: Coxathrolisthesis-Becken (Festschir R Chrobak). Beitr Geb Gynakol *2*:176, 1903.
158. Golding FC: Protrusio acetabuli (central luxation). Br J Surg *22*:56, 1934.
159. Gilmour J: Adolescent deformities of the acetabulum and investigation into the nature of protrusio acetabuli. Br J Surg *26*:670, 1939.
160. Alexander C: The aetiology of primary protrusio acetabuli. Br J Radiol *38*:567, 1965.
161. Rechtman AM: Etiology of deep acetabulum and intrapelvic protrusion. Arch Surg *33*:122, 1936.
162. Macdonald D: Primary protrusio acetabuli. Report of an affected family. J Bone Joint Surg *53B*:30, 1971.
163. Bilfield BS, Janecki CJ, Evarts CM: Primary protrusion of the acetabulum. Report of affected identical twins. Clin Orthop Rel Res *94*:257, 1973.
164. D'Arcy K, Ansell BM, Bywaters EGL: A family with primary protrusio acetabuli. Ann Rheum Dis *37*:53, 1978.
165. Hooper JC, Jones EW: Primary protrusion of the acetabulum. J Bone Joint Surg *53B*:23, 1971.
166. Ozonoff MB: Pediatric Orthopedic Radiology. Philadelphia, WB Saunders Co, 1979.
167. Freiberger RH, Hersh A, Harrison MO: Roentgen examination of the deformed foot. Semin Roentgenol *5*:341, 1970.
168. Ritchie GW, Keim HA: A radiographic analysis of major foot deformities. Can Med Assoc J *91*:840, 1964.
169. Settle GW: The anatomy of congenital talipes equinovarus: Sixteen dissected specimens. J Bone Joint Surg *45A*:1341, 1963.
170. Brewerton DA, Sandifer PH, Sweetnam DR: "Idiopathic" pes cavus. An investigation into its etiology. Br Med J *2*:659, 1963.
171. Beighton PH, Horan FT, Hamersma H: A review of the osteopetroses. Postgrad Med J *53*:507, 1977.
172. Loría-Cortés R, Quesada-Calvo E, Cordero-Chaverri C: Osteopetrosis in children. A report of 26 cases. J Pediatr *91*:43, 1977.
173. Horan FT, Beighton PH: "Osteopetrosis" in the Fairbank collection. J Bone Joint Surg *60B*:53, 1978.
174. Dent EC, Smellie JM, Watson L: Studies in osteopetrosis. Arch Dis Child *40*:7, 1965.
175. King RE, Lovejoy JF Jr: Familial osteopetrosis with coxa vara. A case report. J Bone Joint Surg *55A*:381, 1973.
176. Johnston CC Jr, Lavy N, Lord T, Vellios F, Merritt AD, Deiss WP Jr: Osteopetrosis. A clinical, genetic, metabolic and morphologic study of the dominant inherited benign form. Medicine *47*:149, 1968.
177. Piatt AD, Erhard GA, Araj JS: Benign osteopetrosis. Report of 9 cases. Am J Roentgenol *76*:1119, 1956.
178. Hinkel CL, Beiler DD: Osteopetrosis in adults. Am J Roentgenol *74*:46, 1955.
179. Moss AA, Mainzer F: Osteopetrosis: An unusual cause of terminal-tuft erosion. Radiology *97*:631, 1970.
180. Cameron HU, Dewar FP: Degenerative osteoarthritis associated with osteopetrosis. Clin Orthop Rel Res *127*:148, 1977.
181. Maroteaux P, Lamy M: La pycnodysostose. Presse Med *70*:999, 1962.
182. Sedano HD, Gorlin RJ, Anderson VE: Pycnodysostosis. Clinical and genetic considerations. Am J Dis Child *116*:70, 1968.
183. Maroteaux P, Lamy M: The malady of Toulouse-Lautrec. JAMA *191*:715, 1965.
184. Dusenberry JF Jr, Kane JJ: Pycnodysostosis. Report of three new cases. Am J Roentgenol *99*:717, 1967.
185. Theander G: Partial disappearance of the hyoid bone in pyknodysostosis. Report of a case. Acta Radiol (Diagn) *19*:237, 1978.
186. Truswell AS: Osteoporosis with syndactyly. A morphological variant of Albers-Schönberg's disease. J Bone Joint Surg *40*:208, 1958.
187. Hansen HG: Sklerosteose. *In* H Opitz, F Schmid (Eds): Handbuch der Kinderheilkunde. Vol. 6. Berlin, Springer-Verlag, 1967, p 351.
188. Beighton PH, Cremin BJ, Hamersma H: The radiology of sclerosteosis. Br J Radiol *49*:934, 1976.
189. Beighton PH, Davidson J, Durr L, Hamersma H: Sclerosteosis — an autosomal recessive disorder. Clin Genet *11*:1, 1977.
190. Sugiura Y, Yasuhara T: Sclerosteosis. A case report. J Bone Joint Surg *57A*:273, 1975.
191. van Buchem FSP, Hadders HN, Ubbens R: An uncommon familial systemic disease of the skeleton: Hyperostosis corticalis generalisata familiaris. Acta Radiol *44*:109, 1955.
192. van Buchem FSP, Hadders HN, Hansen JF, Woldring MG: Hyperostosis corticalis generalisata. Report of seven cases. Am J Med *33*:387, 1962.
193. Owen RH: van Buchem's disease (hyperostosis corticalis generalisata). Br J Radiol *49*:126, 1976.
194. Jacobs P: van Buchem disease. Postgrad Med J *53*:497, 1977.
195. Beals RK: Endosteal hyperostosis. J Bone Joint Surg *58A*:1172, 1976.
196. Eastman JR, Bixler D: Generalized cortical hyperostosis (van Buchem disease): Nosologic considerations. Radiology *125*:297, 1977.
197. Fosmoe RJ, Holm RS, Hildreth RC: van Buchem's disease (hyperostosis corticalis generalisata familiaris). A case report. Radiology *90*:771, 1968.
198. Worth HM, Wollin DG: Hyperostosis corticalis generalisata congenita. J Can Assoc Radiol *17*:67, 1966.
199. Maroteaux P, Fontaine G, Scharfman W, Farriaux JP: L'hyperostose corticale généralisée; à transmission dominante. Arch Fr Pediatr *28*:685, 1971.
200. Gelman MI: Autosomal dominant osteosclerosis. Radiology *125*:289, 1977.
201. Gorlin RJ, Glass L: Autosomal dominant osteosclerosis. Radiology *125*:547, 1977.
202. Pyle E: A case of unusual bone development. J Bone Joint Surg *13*:874, 1931.
203. Gorlin RJ, Koszalka MF, Spranger J: Pyle's disease (familial metaphyseal dysplasia). A presentation of two cases and argument for its separation from craniometaphyseal dysplasia. J Bone Joint Surg *52A*:347, 1970.
204. Mabille J-P, Benoit J-P, Castera D: Dysplasie métaphysaire de Pyle. Ann Radiol *16*:723, 1973.
205. Heselson NG, Raad MS, Hamersma H, Cremin BJ, Beighton P: The radiological manifestations of metaphyseal dysplasia (Pyle disease). Br J Radiol *52*:431, 1979.
206. Gorlin RJ, Cohen MM Jr: Frontometaphyseal dysplasia: A new syndrome. Am J Dis Child *118*:487, 1969.
207. Sauvegrain J, Lombard M, Garel L, Truscelli D: Dysplasie frontométaphysaire. Ann Radiol *18*:155, 1975.
208. Kassner EG, Haller JO, Reddy H, Mitarotundo A, Katz I: Frontometaphyseal dysplasia; evidence for autosomal dominant inheritance. Am J Roentgenol *127*:927, 1976.
209. Medlar RC, Crawford AH: Frontometaphyseal dysplasia presenting as scoliosis. A report of a family with four cases. J Bone Joint Surg *60A*:392, 1978.
210. Holt JF, Thompson GR, Arenberg IK: Frontometaphyseal dysplasia. Radiol Clin North Am *10*:225, 1972.
211. Danks DM, Mayne V, Hall RK, McKinnon MC: Fronto-metaphyseal dysplasia. A progressive disease of bone and connective tissue. Am J Dis Child *123*:254, 1972.
212. Holt JF: The evolution of cranio-metaphyseal dysplasia. Ann Radiol *9*:209, 1966.
213. Saper JR, Holt JF: Cranial metaphyseal dysplasia. A cause of recurrent bilateral facial palsy. Arch Neurol *31*:204, 1974.
214. Engelmann G: Ein Fall von Osteopathia hyperostotica (sclerotisans) multiplex infantilis. Fortschr Geb Roentgenstr Nuklearmed *39*:1101, 1929.
215. Camurati M: Di un rara caso di osteite simmetrica ereditaria delgi arti inferiori. Chir Organi Mov *6*:662, 1922.
216. Hundley JC, Wilson FC: Progressive diaphyseal dysplasia. Review of the literature and report of seven cases in one family. J Bone Joint Surg *55A*:461, 1973.
217. Neuhauser EBD, Schwachman H, Wittenborg M, Cohen J: Progressive diaphyseal dysplasia. Radiology *51*:11, 1948.
218. Sparkes RS, Graham CB: Camurati-Engelmann disease: Genetics and clinical manifestations with a review of the literature. J Med Genet *9*:73, 1972.
219. Lennon EA, Schechter MM, Hornabrook RW: Engelmann's disease. Report of a case with a review of the literature. J Bone Joint Surg *43B*:273, 1961.
220. Ribbing S: Hereditary, multiple, diaphyseal sclerosis. Acta Radiol *31*:522, 1949.
221. Paul LW: Hereditary multiple diaphyseal sclerosis (Ribbing). Radiology *60*:412, 1953.
222. Joseph R, Lefebrvre J, Guy E, Job JC: Dysplasie craniodiaphysaire progressive. Ann Radiol *1*:477, 1958.
223. Gorlin RJ, Spranger J, Koszalka MF: Genetic craniotubular bone dysplasias and hyperostoses: A critical analysis. Birth Defects 5(4):79, 1969.
224. Tucker AS, Klein L, Antony GJ: Craniodiaphyseal dysplasia: Evolution over a five-year period. Skel Radiol *1*:47, 1976.
225. McNulty JF, Pim P: Hyperphosphatasia. Report of a case with 30 year follow-up. Am J Roentgenol *115*:614, 1972.

226. Mitsudo SM: Chronic idiopathic hyperphosphatasia associated with pseudoxanthoma elasticum. J Bone Joint Surg *53A*:303, 1971.
227. Eroglu M, Taneli NN: Congenital hyperphosphatasia (juvenile Paget's disease). Eleven years follow-up of 3 sisters. Ann Radiol *20*:145, 1977.
228. Blanco O, Stivel M, Mautalen C, Schajowicz F: Familial idiopathic hyperphosphatasia. A study of two young siblings treated with porcine calcitonin. J Bone Joint Surg *59B*:421, 1977.
229. Dunn V, Condon VR, Rallison ML: Familial hyperphosphatasemia: Diagnosis in early infancy and response to human thyrocalcitonin therapy. Am J Roentgenol *132*:541, 1979.
230. Doyle FH, Woodhouse NJY, Glen ACA, Joplin GF, MacIntyre I: Healing of bones in juvenile Paget's disease treated by human calcitonin. Br J Radiol *47*:9, 1974.
231. Whalen JP, Horwith M, Krook L, MacIntyre I, Mena E, Viteri F, Torun B, Nunez EA: Calcitonin treatment in hereditary bone dysplasia with hyperphosphatasemia: A radiographic and histologic study of bone. Am J Roentgenol *129*:29, 1977.
232. Eyring EJ, Eisenberg E: Congenital hyperphosphatasia. A clinical, pathological, and biochemical study of two cases. J Bone Joint Surg *50A*:1099, 1968.
233. Bakwin H, Elger MS: Fragile bones with macrocranium. J Pediatr *49*:558, 1956.
234. Roy C, Maroteaux P, Kremp L, Courtecuisse V, Alagille D: Un nouveau syndrome osseux avec anomalies cutanée et troubles neurologiques. Arch Fr Pediatr *25*:983, 1968.
235. Kenny FM, Linarelli L: Dwarfism and cortical thickening of tubular bones. Transient hypocalcemia in a mother and son. Am J Dis Child *111*:201, 1966.
236. Forland M: Cleidocranial dysostosis. A review of the syndrome and report of a sporadic case with hereditary transmission. Am J Med *33*:792, 1962.
237. Jarvis JL, Keats TE: Cleidocranial dysostosis. A review of 40 new cases. Am J Roentgenol *121*:5, 1974.
238. Lasker GW: Inheritance of cleidocranial dysostosis. Hum Biol *18*:103, 1946.
239. Hawkins HB, Shapiro R, Petrillo CJ: The association of cleidocranial dysostosis with hearing loss. Am J Roentgenol *125*:944, 1975.
240. Eventov I, Reider-Grosswasser I, Weiss S, Legum C, Schorr S: Cleidocranial dysplasia. A family study. Clin Radiol *30*:323, 1979.
241. Keats TE: Cleidocranial dysostosis. Some atypical roentgen manifestations. Am J Roentgenol *100*:71, 1967.
242. Turner JW: A hereditary arthrodysplasia associated with hereditary dystrophy of the nails. JAMA *100*:882, 1933.
243. Eisenberg KS, Potter DE, Bovill EG Jr: Osteo-onychodystrophy with nephropathy and renal osteodystrophy. A case report. J Bone Joint Surg *54A*:1301, 1972.
244. Valdueza AF: The nail-patella syndrome. A report of 3 families. J Bone Joint Surg *55B*:145, 1973.
245. Gilula LA, Kantor OS: Familial colon carcinoma in nail-patella syndrome. Am J Roentgenol *123*:783, 1975.
246. Preger L, Miller EH, Winfield JS, Choy SH: Hereditary onycho-osteoarthrodysplasia. Am J Roentgenol *100*:546, 1967.
247. Darlington D, Hawkins CF: Nail-patella syndrome with iliac horns and hereditary nephropathy. Necropsy report and anatomical dissection. J Bone Joint Surg *49B*:164, 1967.
248. Palacios E: Hereditary osteo-onycho-dysplasia. The nail-patella syndrome. Am J Roentgenol *101*:842, 1967.
249. Williams HJ, Hoyer JR: Radiographic diagnosis of osteo-onychodysostosis in infancy. Radiology *109*:151, 1973.
250. Hawkins CF, Smith OE: Renal dysplasia in a family with multiple hereditary abnormalities including iliac horns. Lancet *1*:803, 1950.
251. Hoyer JR, Michael AF, Vernier RL: Renal disease in nail-patella syndrome: Clinical and morphologic studies. Kidney Int *2*:231, 1972.
252. Ben-Bassat M, Cohen L, Rosenfeld J: The glomerular basement membrane in the nail-patella syndrome. Arch Pathol *92*:350, 1971.
253. Uranga VM, Simmons RL, Høyer SR, Kjellstrand CM, Buselmeier TJ, Najarian JS: Renal transplantation for the nail patella syndrome. Am J Surg *125*:777, 1973.
254. Keiser W: Die sog. Flughaut beim Menschen. Ihre Beziehung zum Status dysraphicus und ihre Erblichkeit (Dargestellt an der sippe fr). Z Menschl Vererb Konstitutionslehre *23*:594, 1939.
255. Fong EE: "Iliac horns" (symmetrical bilateral central posterior iliac processes). A case report. Radiology *47*:517, 1946.
256. Mino RA, Mino VH, Livingstone RG: Osseous dysplasia and dystrophy of the nails. Review of the literature and report of a case. Am J Roentgenol *60*:633, 1948.
257. Wasserman D: Unilateral iliac horn (central posterior iliac process). Case report. Radiology *120*:562, 1976.
258. Cosack G: Hereditäre Arthro-Osteo-Onycho-Dysplasie mit Beckenhörnern ("Turner-Kieser-Syndrom") in Verbindung mit Hyposiderämie. Z Kinderheilk *75*:449, 1954.
259. Larsen LJ, Schottstaedt ER, Bost FC: Multiple congenital dislocations associated with characteristic facial abnormality. J Pediatr *37*:574, 1950.
260. Silverman FN: Larsen's syndrome: Congenital dislocation of the knees and other joints, distinctive facies, and, frequently, cleft palate. Ann Radiol *15*:297, 1972.
261. Habermann ET, Sterling A, Dennis RI: Larsen's syndrome: A heritable disorder. J Bone Joint Surg *58A*:558, 1976.
262. Steel HH, Kohl EJ: Multiple congenital dislocations associated with other skeletal anomalies (Larsen's syndrome) in three siblings. J Bone Joint Surg *54A*:75, 1972.
263. Bartsocas CS, Dimitriou JK: Multiple joint dislocations in mother and child. J Pediatr *80*:299, 1972.
264. Lee PA: Multiple joint dislocations and peculiar facies. Am J Dis Child *126*:828, 1973.
265. Robertson FW, Kozlowski K, Middleton RW: Larsen's syndrome. Three cases with multiple congenital joint dislocations and distinctive facies. Clin Pediatr *14*:53, 1975.
266. Oki T, Terashima Y, Murachi S, Nogami H: Clinical features and treatment of joint dislocations in Larsen's syndrome. Report of three cases in one family. Clin Orthop *119*:206, 1976.
267. Trigueros AP, Vazquez JLV, DeMiguel GFD: Larsen's syndrome. Report of three cases in the one family, mother and two offspring. Acta Orthop Scand *49*:582, 1978.
268. Ronningen H, Bjerkreim I: Larsen's syndrome. Acta Orthop Scand *49*:138, 1978.
269. Haarmeyer A: Larsen-Syndrom — Symptomatik und Therapie. Fallberichte von drei Kindern. Z Orthop *116*:802, 1978.
270. Latta RJ, Graham CB, Aase J, Scham SM, Smith DW: Larsen's syndrome: A skeletal dysplasia with multiple joint dislocations and unusual facies. J Pediatr *78*:291, 1971.
271. Micheli LJ, Hall JE, Watts HG: Spinal instability in Larsen's syndrome. Report of three cases. J Bone Joint Surg *58A*:562, 1976.
272. Carter C, Wilkinson J: Persistent joint laxity and congenital dislocation of the hip. J Bone Joint Surg *46B*:40, 1964.
273. Owen JR, Elson RA, Grech P: Generalized hypermobility of joints. Arthrochalasis multiplex congenita. Arch Dis Child *48*:487, 1973.
274. Kirk JA, Ansell BM, Bywaters EGL: The hypermobility syndrome. Musculoskeletal complaints associated with generalized joint hypermobility. Ann Rheum Dis *26*:419, 1967.
275. Lamy M, Maroteaux P: Les Chondrodystrophies Génotypiques. Paris, L'expansion Scientifique Française, 1960, p. 33.
276. Berdon WE, Grossman H, Baker DH: Dyschondrostéose (Léri-Weill syndrome): Congenital short forearms, Madelung-type wrist deformities, and moderate dwarfism. Radiology *85*:677, 1965.
277. Langer LO Jr: Dyschondrosteosis, a heritable bone dysplasia with characteristic roentgenographic features. Am J Roentgenol *95*:178, 1965.
278. Hoeffel JC, Brauer B, Jimenez J, Hoeffel F: Radiographic patterns of dyschondrosteosis (Léri-Weill disease). Radiol Clin Biol *42*:366, 1973.
279. Hoeffel JC, Brauer B, Jimenez J, Hoeffel F: The radiographic patterns in dyschondrosteosis. Aust Paediatr J *8*:191, 1972.
280. Beals RK, Lovrien EW: Dyschondrosteosis and Madelung's deformity. Report of three kindreds and review of the literature. Clin Orthop Rel Res *116*:24, 1976.
281. Oikawa K, Yamaguchi T, Kato K, Takenouchi T, Yasuda K, Yamamoto M, Sato T, Okuyama M, Sakurada T, Saito S, Onodera S, Yoshinaga K, Ito H: Dyschondrosteosis associated with endocrine dysfunctions and mental deficiency. Tohoku J Exp Med *114*:287, 1974.
282. Solonen KA, Sulamaa N: Nievergelt syndrome and its treatment. Ann Chir Gynaecol Fenn *47*:142, 1958.
283. Langer LO Jr: Mesomelic dwafism of the hypoplastic ulna, fibula, mandible type. Radiology *89*:654, 1967.
284. Giedion A, Burdea M, Fruchter Z, Meloni T, Trosc V: Autosomal-dominant transmission of the tricho-rhino-phalangeal syndrome. Report of 4 unrelated families, review of 60 cases. Helv Paediatr Acta *28*:249, 1973.
285. Gorlin RJ, Cohen MM Jr, Wolfson J: Tricho-rhino-phalangeal syndrome. Am J Dis Child *118*:595, 1969.
286. Langer LO Jr: The roentgenographic features of the oto-palato-digital (OPD) syndrome. Am J Roentgenol *100*:63, 1967.
287. Dudding BA, Gorlin RJ, Langer LO: The oto-palato-digital syndrome. A new symptom-complex consisting of deafness, dwarfism, cleft palate, characteristic facies, and a generalized bone dysplasia. Am J Dis Child *113*:214, 1967.

288. Alavi SM, Keats TE: Toxopachyostéose diaphysaire tibiopéronière — Weismann-Netter syndrome. Am J Roentgenol *188*:314, 1973.
289. Azimi F, Bryan PJ: Weissman-Netter-Stuhl syndrome (toxopachyostéose diaphysaire tibio-péronière). Br J Radiol *47*:618, 1974.
290. Palacios E, Schimke RN: Craniosynostosis-syndactylism. Am J Roentgenol *106*:144, 1969.
291. Saldino R, Steinbach HL, Epstein CJ: Familial acrocephalosyndactyly (Pfeiffer syndrome). Am J Roentgenol *116*:609, 1972.
292. Duggan CA, Keener EB, Gay BB Jr: Secondary craniosynostosis. Am J Roentgenol *109*:277, 1970.
293. Blank CE: Apert's syndrome (a type of acrocephalosyndactyly). Observations on a British series of thirty-nine cases. Ann Hum Genet *24*:151, 1960.
294. Hoover GH, Flatt AE, Weiss MW: The hand and Apert's syndrome. J Bone Joint Surg *52A*:878, 1970.
295. Brante G: Gargoylism: A mucopolysaccharidosis. Scand J Clin Lab Invest *4*:43, 1952.
296. Dorfman A, Lorincz AE: Occurrence of urinary acid mucopolysaccharides in the Hurler syndrome. Proc Natl Acad Sci *43*:443, 1957.
297. Hurler G: Über einen Typ multipler Abartungen, vorwiegend am Skelettsystem. Z Kinderheilkd *24*:220, 1919.
298. Steinbach HL, Preger L, Williams HE, Cohen P: The Hurler syndrome without abnormal mucopolysacchariduria. Radiology *90*:472, 1968.
299. Hunter C: A rare disease in two brothers. Proc R Soc Med *10*:104, 1971.
300. Njae A: A sex-linked type of gargoylism. Acta Paediatr *33*:267, 1946.
301. Sanfilippo SJ, Podosin R, Langer LO, Good R: Mental retardation associated with acid mucopolysacchariduria heparitin sulfate type. J Pediatr *63*:837, 1963.
302. Langer LO: The radiographic manifestations of the HS-mucopolysaccharidosis of Sanfilippo. Ann Radiol *7*:315, 1964.
303. Morquio L: Sur une forme de dystrophie osseuse familiale. Bull Soc Pediatr *27*:145, 1929.
304. Maroteaux P, Lamy M, Foucher M: La maladie de Morquio; Étude clinique, radiologique et biologique. Presse Med *71*:2091, 1963.
305. Kozlowski K, Bartkowiak K, Chmielowa M: Mucopolysaccharidosis IV (Morquio's disease) in a twenty-months old child. Australas Radiol *15*:362, 1971.
306. Jenkins P, Davies GR, Harper PS: Morquio-Brailsford disease. A report of four affected sisters with absence of excessive keratin sulphate in the urine. Br J Radiol *46*:668, 1973.
307. Maroteaux P, Levêque B, Marie J, Lamy M: Une nouvelle dysostose avec élimination urinaire de chondroitine-sulfate B. Presse Med *71*:1849, 1963.
308. Spranger JW, Koch F, McKusick VA, Natzschka J, Wiedemann HR, Zellweger H; Mucopolysaccharidosis VI (Maroteaux-Lamy's disease). Helv Paediatr Acta *25*:337, 1970.
309. Winchester P, Grossman H, Lim WN, Danes BS: A new acid mucopolysaccharidosis with skeletal deformities simulating rheumatoid arthritis. Am J Roentgenol *106*:121, 1969.
310. Dyggve HV, Melchior JC, Clausen J: Morquio-Ullrich's disease. An inborn error of metabolism? Arch Dis Child *37*:525, 1962.
311. Clausen J, Dyggve HV, Melchior JC: Chemical and enzymatic studies of a family with skeletal abnormalities associated with mental retardation. Clin Chim Acta *29*:197, 1970.
312. Leroy JG, Ho MW, MacBrinn MC, Zielke K, Jacob J, O'Brien JS: I-cell disease: Biochemical studies. Pediatr Res *6*:752, 1972.
313. Spritz RA, Doughty RA, Spackman TJ, Murnane MJ, Coates PM, Koldovsky O, Zackai EH: Neonatal presentation of I-cell disease. J Pediatr *93*:954, 1978.
314. Taber P, Gyepes MT, Philippart M, Ling S: Roentgenographic manifestations of Leroy's I-cell disease. Am J Roentgenol *118*:213, 1973.
315. Patriquin HB, Kaplan P, Kind HP, Giedion A: Neonatal mucolipidosis II (I-cell disease): Clinical and radiologic features in three cases. Am J Roentgenol *129*:37, 1977.
316. Maroteaux P, Lamy M: La pseudo-polydystrophie de Hurler. Presse Med *74*:2889, 1966.
317. Melhem R, Dorst JP, Scott CI Jr, McKusick VA: Roentgen findings in mucolipidosis III (pseudo-Hurler polydystrophy). Radiology *106*:153, 1973.
318. Nolte K, Spranger J: Early skeletal changes in mucolipidosis III. Ann Radiol *19*:151, 1976.
319. Spranger J, Gehler J, Cantz M: The radiographic features of mannosidosis. Radiology *119*:401, 1976.
320. Lee FA, Donnell GN, Gwinn JL: Radiographic features of fucosidosis. Pediatr Radiol *5*:204, 1977.
321. Brill PW, Beratis NG, Kousseff BG, Hirschhorn K: Roentgenographic findings in fucosidosis type 2. Am J Roentgenol *124*:75, 1975.
322. Grossman H, Danes BS: Neurovisceral storage disease: Roentgenographic features and mode of inheritance. Am J Roentgenol *103*:149, 1968.
323. O'Brien J: Generalized gangliosidosis. J Pediatr *75*:167, 1969.
324. Rabinowitz JG, Sacher M: Gangliosidosis (GM). A re-evaluation of the vertebral deformity. Am J Roentgenol *121*:155, 1974.
325. Parenti GC: La anosteogenesi (una varietà della osteogenesi imperfetta). Pathologica *28*:447, 1936.
326. Fraccaro M: Contributo allo studio delle malattie del mesenchima osteopoietico. L'acondrogenesi. Folia Hered Pathol *1*:190, 1952.
327. Saldino RM: Lethal short-limbed dwarfism: Achondrogenesis and thanatophoric dwarfism. Am J Roentgenol *112*:185, 1971.
328. Maroteaux P, Lamy M, Robert J-M: Le nanisme thanatophore. Presse Med *75*:2519, 1967.
329. Callaghan KA: Thanatophoric dwarfism. A case report. Australas Radiol *14*:435, 1970.
330. Saldino RM: Radiographic diagnosis of neonatal short-limbed dwarfism. Med Radiogr Photogr *49*:61, 1973.
331. Jeune M, Carron R, Beraud C, Loaec Y: Polychondrodystrophie avec blocage thoracique d'évolution fatale. Pediatrie *9*:390, 1954.
332. Keats TE, Riddervold HO, Michaelis LL: Thanatophoric dwarfism. Am J Roentgenol *108*:473, 1970.
333. Ellis RWB, van Creveld S: A syndrome characterized by ectodermal dysplasia, polydactyly, chondro-dysplasia and congenital morbus cordis. Report of three cases. Arch Dis Child *15*:65, 1940.
334. Jéquier S, Dunbar JS: The Ellis-van Creveld syndrome. *In* Progress in Pediatric Radiology. Vol 4. Intrinsic Diseases of Bones. Basel, S Karger, 1973, p 167.
335. Hall JG, Dorst JP, Taybi H, Scott CI, Langer LO Jr, McKusick VA: Two probable cases of homozygosity for the achondroplasia gene. Birth Defects *5*(4):24, 1969.
336. Bailey JA II: Orthopedic aspects of achondroplasia. J Bone Joint Surg *52A*:1285, 1970.
337. Caffey J: Achondroplasia of the pelvis and lumbosacral spine. Some roentgenographic features. Am J Roentgenol *80*:449, 1958.
338. Langer LO Jr, Baumann PA, Gorlin RJ: Achondroplasia. Am J Roentgenol *100*:12, 1967.
339. Silverman FN: A differential diagnosis of achondroplasia. Radiol Clin North Am *6*:223, 1968.
340. Ponseti IV: Skeletal growth in achondroplasia. J Bone Joint Surg *52A*:701, 1970.
341. Cohen ME, Rosenthal AD, Matson DD: Neurological abnormalities in achondroplastic children. J Pediatr *71*:367, 1967.
342. Alexander E Jr: Significance of the small lumbar spinal canal: Cauda equina compression syndromes due to spondylosis. Part 5: Achondroplasia. J Neurosurg *31*:513, 1969.
343. Wise BL, Sondheimer F, Kaufman S: Achondroplasia and hydrocephalus. Neuropaediatrie *3*:106, 1971.
344. Rimoin DL, Hughes GN, Kaufman RL, Rosenthal RE, McAlister WH, Silberberg R: Endochondral ossification in achondroplastic dwarfism. N Engl J Med *283*:728, 1970.
345. Beals RK: Hypochondroplasia. A report of five kindreds. J Bone Joint Surg *51A*:728, 1969.
346. Walker BA, Murdoch JL, McKusick VA, Langer LO, Beals RK: Hypochondroplasia. Am J Dis Child *122*:95, 1971.
347. Currarino G, Neuhauser EBD, Reyersbach GC, Sobel EH: Hypophosphatasia. Am J Roentgenol *78*:392, 1957.
348. MacPherson RI, Kroeker M, Houston CS: Hypophosphatasia. J Assoc Can Radiol *23*:16, 1972.
349. Fraser D: Hypophosphatasia. Am J Med *22*:730, 1957.
350. Jansen M: Über atypische Chondrodystrophie (Achondroplasie) und über eine noch nicht beschriebene angeborene Wachstumsstörung des Knochensystems: Metaphysäre Dysostosis. Z Orthop Chir *61*:253, 1934.
351. Schmid F: Beitrag zur Dysostosis enchondralis metaphysaria. Monatsschr Kinderheilkd *97*:393, 1949.
352. Irwin GAL: Cartilage-hair hypoplasia (CHH) variant of familial metaphyseal dysostosis. Radiology *86*:926, 1966.
353. Beals RK: Cartilage-hair hypoplasia. A case report. J Bone Joint Surg *50A*:1245, 1968.
354. McKusick VA: Metaphyseal dysostosis and thin hair. A "new" recessively inherited syndrome? Letter to Editor. Lancet *1*:832, 1964.
355. Taybi H, Mitchell AD, Friedman GD: Metaphyseal dysostosis and the associated syndrome of pancreatic insufficiency and blood disorders. Radiology *93*:563, 1969.
356. Lamy M, Maroteaux P: Le nanisme diastrophique. Presse Med *68*:1977, 1960.
357. Walker BA, Scott CI, Hall JG, Murdoch JL, McKusick VA: Diastrophic dwarfism. Medicine *51*:41, 1972.

358. Stover CN, Hayes JT, Holt JF: Diastrophic dwarfism. Am J Roentgenol *89*:914, 1963.
359. Cremin BJ, Jarrett J: Diastrophic dwarfism. Australas Radiol *14*:84, 1970.
360. Maroteaux P, Spranger J, Wiedemann H-R: Der metatropische Zwergwuchs. Arch Kinderheilkd *173*:211, 1966.
361. Larose JH, Bay BB Jr: Metatropic dwarfism. Am J Roentgenol *106*:156, 1969.
362. Jenkins P, Smith MB, McKinnell JS: Metatropic dwarfism. Br J Radiol *43*:561, 1970.
363. Langer LO, Petersen D, Spranger J: An unusual bone dysplasia: Parastremmatic dwarfism. Am J Roentgenol *110*:550, 1970.
364. Horan F, Beighton P: Parastremmatic dwarfism. J Bone Joint Surg *58B*:343, 1976.
365. Kniest W: Zur Abgrenzung der Dysostosis enchondralis von der Chondrodystrophie. Z Kinderheilkd *70*:633, 1952.
366. Rimoin DL, Hollister DW, Silberberg R, Lachman RS, McAlister W, Kaufman R: Kniest (Swiss cheese cartilage) syndrome: Clinical, radiographic, histologic and ultrastructural studies (Abstr). Clin Res *21*:296, 1973.
367. Lachman RS, Rimoin DL, Hollister DW, Dorst J, Siggers D, McAlister W, Kaufman RL, Langer LO: The Kniest syndrome. Am J Roentgenol *123*:805, 1975.
368. Frayha R, Melhem R, Idriss H: The Kniest (Swiss cheese cartilage) syndrome. Description of a distinct arthropathy. Arthritis Rheum *22*:286, 1979.
369. Brill PW, Kim HJ, Beratis NG, Hirschhorn K: Skeletal abnormalities in the Kniest syndrome with mucopolysacchariduria. Am J Roentgenol *125*:731, 1975.
370. Rimoin DL, Hollister DW, Siggers D, Silberberg R, Lachman RS, McAlister W, Kaufman R, McKusick VA, Dorst J: Clinical, radiologic, histologic and ultrastructural definition of Kniest syndrome (Abstr). Pediatr Res *7*:348, 1973.
371. Fraser GR, Friedmann AI, Maroteaux P, Glen-Bott AM, Mittwoch U: Dysplasia spondyloepiphysaria congenita and related generalized skeletal dysplasias among children with severe visual handicaps. Arch Dis Child *44*:490, 1969.
372. Spranger JW, Langer LO Jr: Spondyloepiphyseal dysplasia congenita. Radiology *94*:313, 1970.
373. Spranger J, Wiedemann HR: Dysplasia spondyloepiphysaria congenita. Helv Paediatr Acta *21*:598, 1966.
374. Maroteaux P, Lamy M, Bernard J: La dysplasie spondylo-epiphysaire tardive. Presse Med *65*:1205, 1957.
375. Langer LO Jr: Spondyloepiphyseal dysplasia tarda. Hereditary chondrodysplasia with characteristic vertebral configuration in the adult. Radiology *82*:833, 1964.
376. Kozlowski K, Maroteaux P, Spranger J: La dysostose spondylométaphysaire. Presse Med *75*:2769, 1967.
377. Riggs W Jr, Summit RL: Spondylometaphyseal dysplasia (Kozlowski). Report of affected mother and son. Radiology *101*:375, 1971.
378. Thomas PS, Nevin NC: Spondylometaphyseal dysplasia. Am J Roentgenol *128*:89, 1977.
379. Lachman R, Zonana J, Khajavi A, Rimoin D: The spondylometaphyseal dysplasias. Clinical, radiologic and pathologic correlation. Ann Radiol *22*:125, 1979.
380. Lejeune J, Gautier M, Turpin R: Étude des chromosomes somatiques de neuf enfants mongoliens. C R Acad Sci *248*:1721, 1959.
381. Weiss L, Reynolds WA: Osseous malformations associated with chromosome abnormalities. Orthop Clin North Am *3*:713, 1972.
382. Mortensson W, Hall B: Abnormal pelvis in newborn infants with Down's syndrome. Acta Radiol (Diagn) *12*:847, 1972.
383. Willich E, Fuhr U, Kroll W: Skeletal manifestations in Down's syndrome. Correlation between roentgenologic and cytogenetic findings. Ann Radiol *18*:355, 1975.
384. Semine AA, Ertel An, Goldberg MJ, Bull MJ: Cervical-spine instability in children with Down syndrome (trisomy 21). J Bone Joint Surg *60A*:649, 1978.
385. Giblin PE, Micheli LJ: The management of atlanto-axial subluxation with neurologic involvement in Down's syndrome: A report of two cases and review of the literature. Clin Orthop Rel Res *140*:66, 1979.
386. Tishler JM, Martel W: Dislocation of the atlas in mongolism. A preliminary report. Radiology *84*:904, 1965.
387. Martel W, Tishler JM: Observations on the spine in mongoloidism. Am J Roentgenol 97:630, 1966.
388. Edwards JH, Harnden DG, Cameron AH, Crosse VM, Wolff OH: A new trisomic syndrome. Lancet *1*:787, 1960.
389. James AE Jr, Belcourt CL, Atkins L, Janower ML: Trisomy 18. Radiology *92*:37, 1969.
390. Patau K, Smith DW, Therman E, Inhorn SL, Wagner HP: Multiple congenital anomaly caused by an extra autosome. Lancet *1*:790, 1960.
391. James AE Jr, Belcourt CL, Atkins L, Janower ML: Trisomy 13–15. Radiology *92*:44, 1969.
392. Lai CC, Gorlin RJ: Trisomy 8 syndrome. Clin Orthop Rel Res *110*:239, 1975.
393. Schinzel A: Autosomal chromosome aberrations. A review of the clinical syndromes caused by structural chromosome aberrations, mosaic-trisomies 8 and 9, and triploidy. Ergeb Inn Med Kinderheilkd *38*:37, 1976.
394. Schinzel A: Trisomy 9p, a chromosome aberration with distinct cadiologic findings. Radiology *130*:125, 1979.
395. James AE Jr, Atkins L, Feingold M, Janower ML: The cri du chat syndrome. Radiology *92*:50, 1969.
396. Wolf U, Reinwein H, Porsch R, Schröter R, Baitsch H: Defizienz an den kurzen Armen eines Chromosoms nummern 4. Humangenetik *1*:397, 1965.
397. Finby N, Archibald RM: Skeletal abnormalities associated with gonadal dysgenesis. Am J Roentgenol *89*:1222, 1963.
398. Baker DH, Berdon WE, Morishima A, Conte F: Turner's syndrome and pseudo-Turner's syndrome. Am J Roentgenol *100*:40, 1967.
399. Brown DM, Jowsey J, Bradford DS: Osteoporosis in ovarian dysgenesis. J Pediatr *84*:816, 1974.
400. Beals RK: Orthopedic aspects of the XO (Turner's) syndrome. Clin Orthop Rel Res *97*:19, 1973.
401. Preger L, Steinbach HL, Moskowitz P, Scully AL, Goldberg MB: Roentgenographic abnormalities in phenotypic females with gonadal dysgenesis. A comparison of chromatin positive patients and chromatin negative patients. Am J Roentgenol *104*:899, 1968.
402. Poznanski AK, Garn SM, Shaw HA: The carpal angle in the congenital malformation syndromes. Ann Radiol *19*:141, 1976.
403. Ohsawa T, Furuse M, Kikuchi Y, Suda Y, Tamiya T, Hikita M: Roentgenographic manifestations of Klinefelter's syndrome. Am J Roentgenol *112*:178, 1971.
404. Hutchinson J: Congenital absence of hair and mammary glands: With atrophic condition of skin and its appendages in a boy whose mother had been almost wholly bald from alopecia areata from the age of six. Med Chir Trans *69*:473, 1886.
405. Margolin FR, Steinbach HL: Progeria. Hutchinson-Gilford syndrome. Am J Roentgenol *103*:173, 1968.
406. Franklyn PP: Progeria in siblings. Clin Radiol *27*:327, 1976.
407. Ozonoff MB, Clemett AR: Progressive osteolysis in progeria. Am J Roentgenol *100*:75, 1967.
408. Solomon L: Hereditary multiple exostosis. J Bone Joint Surg *45B*:292, 1963.
409. Vinstein AL, Franken EA Jr: Hereditary multiple exostoses. Report of a case with spinal cord compression. Am J Roentgenol *112*:405, 1971.
410. Madigan R, Worrall T, McClain EJ: Cervical cord compression in hereditary multiple exostosis. Review of the literature and report of a case. J Bone Joint Surg *56A*:401, 1974.
411. Solomon L: Chondrosarcoma in hereditary multiple exostosis. S Afr Med J *48*:671, 1974.
412. Greenway G, Resnick D, Bookstein JJ: Popliteal pseudoaneurysm as a complication of an adjacent osteochondroma: Angiographic diagnosis. Am J Roentgenol *132*:294, 1979.
413. Signargout J, Guégan Y, LeMarec B, Simon J: Les paraplégies de la maladie des exostoses multiples. A propos de deux observations. J Radiol Electrol Med Nucl *54*:403, 1973.
414. Epstein DA, Levin EJ: Bone scintigraphy in hereditary multiple exostoses. Am J Roentgenol *130*:331, 1978.
415. El-Khoury GAY, Bonfiglio M: Case report 60. Skel Radiol *3*:49, 1978.
416. Fairbank HAT: Dyschondroplasia. Synonyms: Ollier's disease, multiple enchondromata. J Bone Joint Surg *30B*:689, 1948.
417. Lewin P: Arthrogryposis multiplex congenita. J Bone Joint Surg *7*:630, 1925.
418. Friedlander HL, Westin GW, Wood WL Jr: Arthrogryposis multiplex congenita. A review of forty-five cases. J Bone Joint Surg *50A*:89, 1968.
419. Poznanski AK, LaRowe PC: Radiographic manifestations of arthrogryposis syndrome. Radiology *95*:353, 1970.
420. Bléry M, Pannier S, Barre JL: Étude radiologique de l'arthrogrypose. A propos de 28 cas. J Radiol Electrol Med Nucl *58*:597, 1977.
421. Sly WS, Quinton BA, McAlister WH, Rimoin DL: Beta glucuronidase deficiency: Report of clinical, radiologic, and biochemical features of a new mucopolysaccharidosis. J Pediatr *82*:249, 1973.
422. Beighton P, Hamersma H: Sclerosteosis in South Africa. S Afr Med J *55*:783, 1979.
423. Kozlowski K, Prokop BE, Scougall JS, Silink M, Vines RH: Spondylo-

metaphyseal dysplasia (report of a case of common type and three cases of "new varieties"). Fortschr Geb Roentgenstr Nuklearmed *130*:222, 1979.

424. Shapiro F, Simon S, Glimcher MJ: Hereditary multiple exostoses. Anthropometric, roentgenographic, and clinical aspects. J Bone Joint Surg *61A*:815, 1979.
425. Bender BL, Yunis E: Fibrocartilaginous lesions of bone and hemangiomas and lipomas of soft tissue resembling Maffucci's syndrome. A case report. J Bone Joint Surg *61A*:1104, 1979.
426. Andersen KS: Congenital angulation of the lower leg and congenital pseudarthrosis of the tibia in Denmark. Acta Orthop Scand *43*:539, 1972.
427. Andersen KS: Radiological classification of congenital pseudarthrosis of the tibia. Acta Orthop Scand *44*:719, 1973.
428. Boyd HB, Sage FB: Congenital pseudarthrosis of the tibia. J Bone Joint Surg *40A*:1245, 1958.
429. Brown GA, Osebold WR, Ponseti IV: Congenital pseudarthrosis of long bones. A clinical, radiographic, histologic, and ultrastructural study. Clin Orth Rel Res *128*:228, 1977.
430. Gibson DA, Carroll N: Congenital pseudarthrosis of the clavicle. J Bone Joint Surg *52B*:629, 1970.
431. Owen R: Congenital pseudarthrosis of the clavicle. J Bone Joint Surg *52B*:644, 1970.
432. Ahmadi B, Steel HH: Congenital pseudarthrosis of the clavicle. Clin Orth Rel Res *126*:130, 1977.
433. VanNes CP: Congenital pseudarthrosis of the leg. J Bone Joint Surg *48A*:1467, 1966.
434. Briner J, Yunis E: Ultrastructure of congenital pseudarthrosis of the tibia. Arch Pathol *95*:97, 1973.
435. Lloyd-Roberts GC, Shaw NE: The prevention of pseudarthrosis in congenital kyphosis of the tibia. J Bone Joint Surg *51B*:100, 1969.
436. Badgley CE, O'Connor SJ, Kudner DF: Congenital kyphoscoliotic tibia. J Bone Joint Surg *34A*:349, 1952.
437. Duraiswami PK: Comparison of congenital defects induced in developing chickens by certain teratogenic agents with those caused by insulin. J Bone Joint Surg *37A*:277, 1955.
438. Dunn AW, Aponte GE: Congenital bowing of the tibia and femur. J Bone Joint Surg *44A*:737, 1962.
439. Newell RLM, Durbin FC: The aetiology of congenital angulation of tubular bones with constriction of the medullary canal and its relationship to congenital pseudarthrosis. J Bone Joint Surg *58B*:444, 1976.
440. Lloyd-Roberts GC, Apley AG, Owen R: Reflection upon the etiology of congenital pseudarthrosis of the clavicle. J Bone Joint Surg *57B*:24, 1975.
441. Wall JJ: Congenital pseudarthrosis of the clavicle. J Bone Joint Surg *52B*:1003, 1970.
442. Manashil G, Laufer S: Congenital pseudarthrosis of the clavicle: Report of three cases. Am J Roentgenol *132*:678, 1979.
443. Werner O: Uber katarakt in verbindung mit sklerodermie. (Doctoral dissertation, Kiel University). Kiel, Schmidt & Klaunig, 1904.
444. Epstein CJ, Martin GM, Schultze AL, Motulsky AG: Werner's syndrome. A review of its symptomatology, natural history, pathologic features, genetics and relationship to the natural aging process. Medicine *45*:177, 1966.
445. Jacobson HG, Rifkin H, Zucker-Franklin D: Werner's syndrome: A clinical-roentgen entity. Radiology *74*:373, 1960.
446. Rosen RS, Cuwini R, Cablentz D: Werner's syndrome. Br J Radiol *43*:193, 1970.
447. Herstone ST, Bower J: Werner's syndrome. Am J Roentgenol *51*:639, 1944.
448. Magill HL, Shackelford GD, McAlister WH, Graviss ER: 4p- (Wolf-Hirschhorn) syndrome. Am J Roentgenol *135*:283, 1980.
449. Miki T, Kohno H, Miyata H, Oka M, Shima M, Tanaka S: Multiple exostoses–mental retardation (MEMR) syndrome: Report of a case. Clin Orthop Rel Res *150*:207, 1980.
450. Abraham E: Sacral agenesis with associated anomalies (caudal regression syndrome): Autopsy case report. Clin Orthop Rel Res *145*:168, 1979.
451. Stanley JK, Owen R, Koff S: Congenital sacral anomalies. J Bone Joint Surg *61B*:401, 1979.
452. Hootnick DR, Levinsohn EM, Packard DS Jr: Midline metatarsal dysplasia associated with absent fibula. Clin Orthop Rel Res *150*:203, 1980.
453. Ogden JA, Conlogue GJ, Phillips SB, Bronson ML: Sprengel's deformity. Radiology of the pathologic deformation. Skel Radiol *4*:204, 1979.
454. Pavlov H, Goldman AB, Freiberger RH: Infantile coxa vara. Radiology *135*:631, 1980.
455. Ippolito E, Ponseti IV: Congenital club foot in the human fetus. A histological study. J Bone Joint Surg *62A*:8, 1980.
456. Shapiro F, Glimcher MJ, Holtrop ME, Tashjian AH, Brickley-Parsons D, Kenzora JE: Human osteopetrosis. J Bone Joint Surg *62A*:384, 1980.
457. Cremin BJ: Sclerosteosis in children. Pediatr Radiol *8*:173, 1979.
458. Fallon MD, Whyte MP, Murphy WA: Progressive diaphyseal dysplasia (Engelmann's disease). Report of a sporadic case of the mild form. J Bone Joint Surg *62A*:465, 1980.
459. Cipolloni C, Boldrini A, Donti E, Maiorana A, Coppa GV: Neonatal mucolipidosis II (I-cell disease): Clinical, radiological, and biochemical studies in a case. Helv Paediatr Acta *35*:85, 1980.
460. Dorfman HD, Lorenzo J: Case report 122. Skel Radiol *5*:189, 1980.
461. Hall BD, Spranger J: Hypochondroplasia: Clinical and radiological aspects in 39 cases. Radiology *133*:95, 1979.
462. Lenz W: Genetics and limb deficiencies. Clin Orthop Rel Res *148*:9, 1980.
463. Hamanishi: C: Congenital short femur. J Bone Joint Surg *62B*:307, 1980.
464. Atlas S, Menacho LCS, Ures S: Some new aspects in the pathology of clubfoot. Clin Orthop Rel Res *149*:224, 1980.
465. Quinlan WR, Brady PG, Regan BF: Congenital pseudarthrosis of the clavicle. Acta Orthop Scand *51*:489, 1980.
466. Whaley WJ: Atlanto-axial dislocation and Down's syndrome. Can Med Assoc J *123*:35, 1980.
467. Southwell RB, Reynolds AF, Badger VM, Sherman FC: Klippel-Feil syndrome with cervical cord compression resulting from cervical subluxation in association with an omo-vertebral bone. Spine *5*:480, 1980.
468. Frayha RA, Frayha H, Melhem R: Hand arthropathy: A clue to the diagnosis of the Kniest (Swiss cheese cartilage) dysplasia. Rheumatol Rehab *19*:167, 1980.
469. Owman T, Sjöblad St, Göthlin J: Radiological skeletal changes in juvenile GM_1-gangliosidosis. Fortschr Geb Roentgenstr Nuklearmed *132*:682, 1980.
470. Gemme G, Pinelli G, Bonioli E, Sbolgi P, Bonzano MA: Aspetti clinici e radiologici dell'iponcondroplasia. Minerva Pediatr *32*:237, 1980.
471. Brown LM, Robson MJ, Sharrard WJW: The pathophysiology of arthrogryposis multiplex congenita neurologica. J Bone Joint Surg *62B*:291, 1980.
472. Wilkinson JA, Campbell D: Scapular osteotoma for Sprengel's deformity. J Bone Joint Surg *62B*:486, 1980.
473. Miyamoto RT, House WF, Brackmann DE: Neurotologic manifestations of the osteopetroses. Arch Otolaryngol *106*:210, 1980.

SECTION XVI

TUMORS AND TUMOR-LIKE CONDITIONS

TUMORS AND TUMOR-LIKE LESIONS OF BONE

by Donald Resnick, M.D.

74A

An accurate diagnosis of the nature of a solitary bone lesion on the basis of its radiographic characteristics often is not possible. However, the precise morphology of a lesion does provide reliable information regarding its "aggressiveness" or rate of growth,[1] and this information coupled with data reflecting the site of the lesion and the age of the patient allows the formulation of a reasonable diagnosis in most cases. The solitary bone lesion is often a tumor or is tumor-like in nature, although congenital, inflammatory, ischemic, and traumatic disorders of bone can also present in this fashion. In this text, which is devoted primarily to a discussion of articular disorders, a detailed analysis of neoplastic and neoplastic-like skeletal diseases is not indicated. This information is readily available to the interested reader.[2-4] The role of other diagnostic modalities such as xeroradiography,[5] scintigraphy,[6-8] and computed tomography[9-11] in the evaluation of musculoskeletal neoplasms has been commented upon in earlier chapters and will not be repeated here.[225-258, 264, 265] Rather, a summary of morphologic characteristics and location of some of the more important tumors and tumor-like lesions will be given.

MORPHOLOGY

Morphologic features that aid in the differential diagnosis of tumors and tumor-like osseous lesions

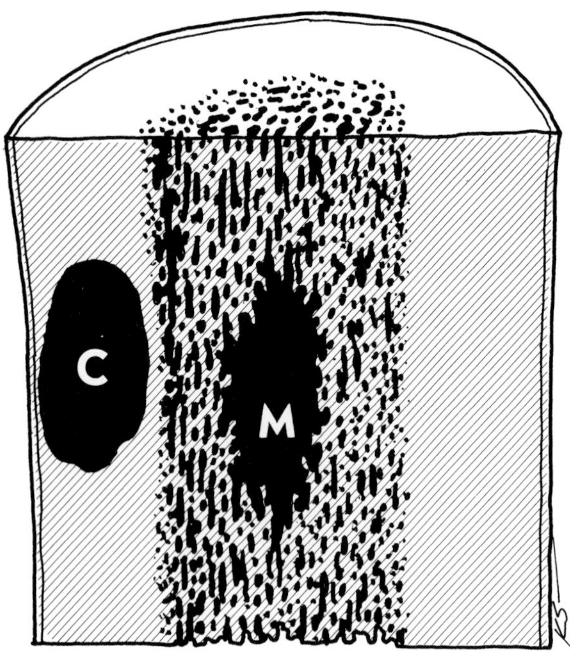

Figure 74–1. Cortical versus medullary involvement. A lesion in the medullary bone (M) may be more difficult to recognize than one in the cortical bone (C). In addition, a nonaggressive cortical lesion will produce a sharp interface with the surrounding bone, whereas such a lesion in the medullary bone may not.

include, among others, the pattern of bone destruction, the presence and nature of visible tumor matrix or periosteal response, the pattern of cortical erosion, expansion, or penetration, and the presence and characteristics of an adjacent soft tissue mass. These features have been extremely well summarized by Lodwick,[12] who applied them to the computer analysis of bone and joint neoplasms. Many of Lodwick's concepts are included in this discussion.

Pattern of Bone Destruction

The radiograph is not extremely sensitive in the detection of small amounts of bone destruction, especially if the destructive focus is located in cancellous bone. Cortical lesions are more readily detected (Fig. 74–1). In certain sites, such as the ribs and spine, technical factors, including the size or thickness of the body part, and the presence of considerable overlying shadows accentuate the radiograph's insensitivity in delineating small lesions.

Three radiographic patterns of bone destruction have been identified: geographic, motheaten, and permeative.[12]

GEOGRAPHIC BONE DESTRUCTION (Fig. 74–2). This is the least aggressive pattern of bone destruction, as it is generally indicative of a slow-growing lesion. The margin of the lesion is well defined and easily separated from the surrounding normal bone. This margin may be smooth or irregular, but in either instance, it is usually clearly demarcated with a short zone of transition from normal to abnormal bone. Benign bone tumors usually demonstrate geographic bone destruction.

"MOTHEATEN" BONE DESTRUCTION (Fig. 74–3). This is a more aggressive pattern of bone destruction, characteristic of a lesion that is more rapidly growing than one that demonstrates geographic bone destruction. The motheaten pattern

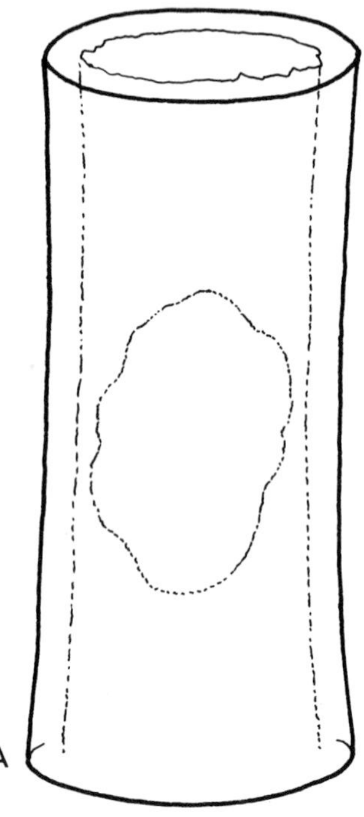

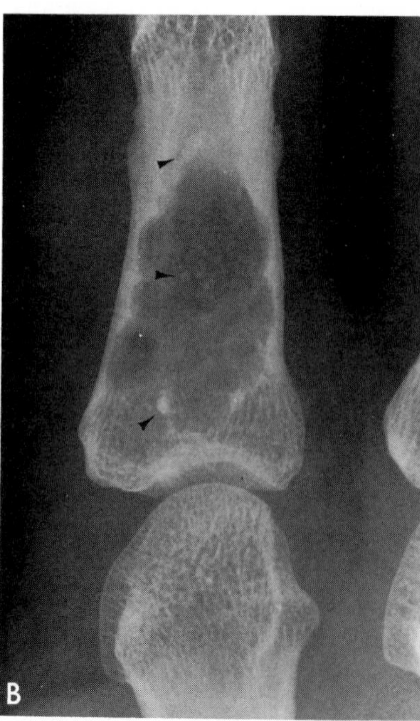

Figure 74–2. Geographic bone destruction.

A *This pattern of bone destruction is characterized by well-defined lesional margins and a short zone of transition from normal to abnormal bone.*

B *The lesion in the proximal phalanx demonstrates geographic bone destruction, a central location, lobulated margins, and small foci of calcification (arrowheads). (Final diagnosis —enchondroma.)*

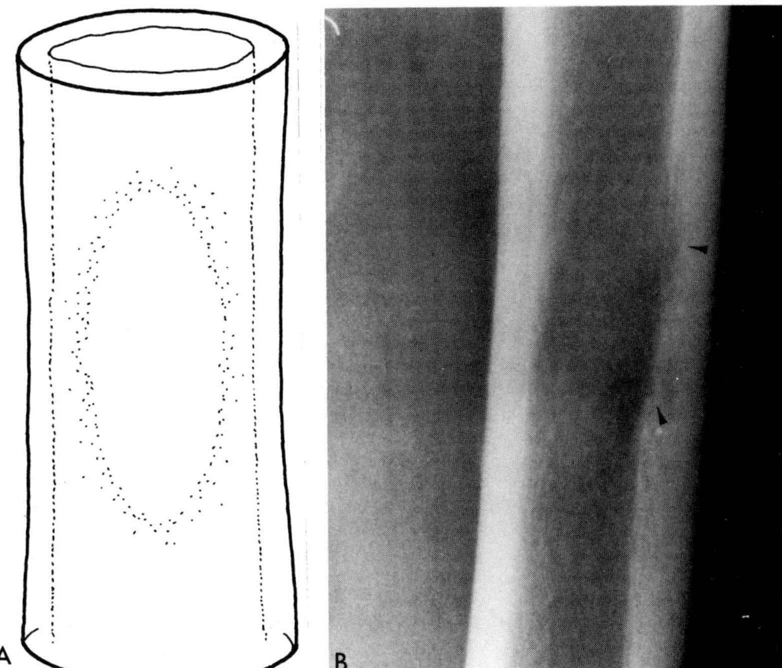

Figure 74–3. "Motheaten" bone destruction.

A *This pattern of bone destruction is associated with lesional margins that are less well defined and a longer zone of transition from normal to abnormal bone.*

B *A lesion with "motheaten" bone destruction is identified in this femur. Note its ill-defined margins and its erosion of the endosteal margin of the cortex (arrowheads). (Final diagnosis —reticulum cell sarcoma.)*

of bone destruction is associated with a less well defined or demarcated lesional margin and with a longer zone of transition from normal to abnormal bone. Malignant bone tumors and osteomyelitis may demonstrate the motheaten pattern of bone destruction.

Permeative Bone Destruction (Fig. 74–4). This pattern indicates an aggressive bone lesion

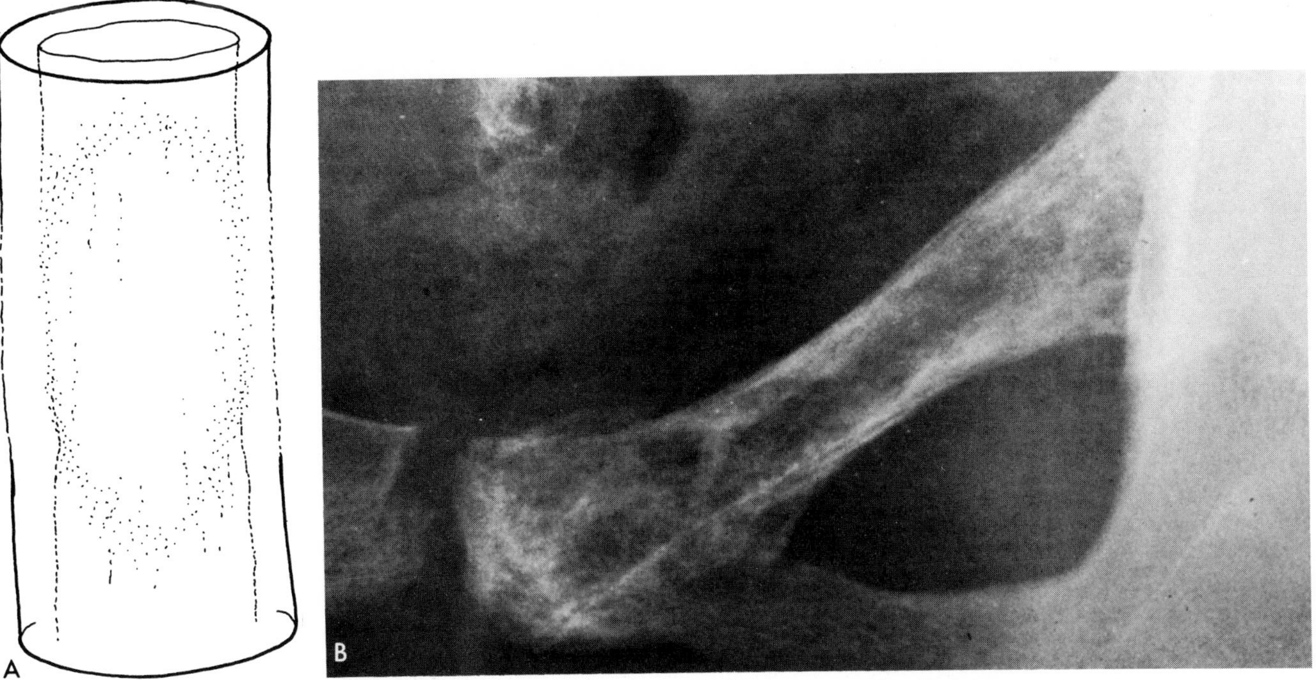

Figure 74–4. Permeative bone destruction.

A *This pattern of bone destruction is associated with very poorly defined lesional margins and a very long zone of transition from normal to abnormal bone.*

B *The lesion in the superior pubic ramus reveals permeative bone destruction with cortical erosion, periostitis, and a soft tissue mass. (Final diagnosis —reticulum cell sarcoma.)*

with rapid growth potential. The lesion is poorly demarcated and not easily separated from the surrounding normal bone. In fact, it may imperceptibly merge with uninvolved osseous segments, creating a zone of transition that is very long. Certain malignant bone tumors, such as Ewing's sarcoma, may demonstrate permeative bone destruction.

Size, Shape, and Margin of Lesion

Lodwick[12] has indicated that certain features regarding the size and shape of the lesion can be useful in differential diagnosis. In general, primary malignant tumors of bone are larger than benign tumors and may be greater than 6 cm in size when first discovered. Although the shape of a lesion is a relatively poor guide to its nature, elongated lesions, in which the greatest lesional diameter is at least 1.5 times the least diameter, may be indicative of Ewing's sarcoma, reticulum cell sarcoma, chondrosarcoma, and angiosarcoma.

Slowly growing lesions can be associated with reactive sclerosis of the surrounding normal bone. The sclerotic margin can be of variable thickness and may partially or completely surround the bone lesion. A vigorous bony reaction is especially characteristic of cortical osteoid osteomas, and this reaction may obscure the radiolucent nidus of the tumor.

Presence and Nature of Visible Tumor Matrix

Certain tumors produce matrix that calcifies or ossifies.[12] The resulting radiodense areas must be distinguished from calcification that may develop in regions of necrotic or degenerative tissue, from callus formation that may indicate the presence of a pathologic fracture, and from a sclerotic response of non-neoplastic bone to the adjacent tumorous deposit.

Certain cartilage tumors are associated with matrix calcification. These include chondromas, chondroblastomas, chondrosarcomas, and, less frequently, chondromyxoid fibromas. In most instances, the incidence and extent of pathologically evident calcification are greater than the incidence and extent of radiographically evident calcification. Cartilage matrix calcification is frequently centrally located and may appear as ring-like, flocculent, or fleck-like radiodense areas.[12] Similar findings can be apparent within the cartilaginous cap of an osteochondroma.

Visible tumor matrix is also associated with neoplastic bone.[12] Examples of neoplasms producing such tumor matrix are osteogenic sarcomas, parosteal osteogenic sarcomas, ossifying fibromas, osteomas, and osteoblastomas. The resulting radiodense collections are of variable size; they may occupy an entire lesion or a part of a lesion and can be inhomogeneous or homogeneous in nature.

Certain lesions, such as fibrous dysplasia, can be accompanied by a uniform increase in radiodensity, an appearance that is called the ground-glass pattern. This pattern is associated with obscuration or obliteration of neighboring trabeculae.

Internal or External Trabeculation

Within or around the lesion, trabeculated shadows may be identified on the radiograph. In some instances, these reflect the location of residual trabeculae that have been modified or displaced by the neighboring tumor. In other instances, the trabeculation represents new bone formation evoked as a response to the presence of a nearby neoplasm. Such bony proliferation is frequently located at the interface between the endosteal and periosteal envelopes.[12] The location and appearance of the trabeculation provide information regarding the nature of the neoplasm (Table 74–1). For example, giant cell tumors are commonly associated with delicate or thin trabeculae (Fig. 74–5*A*), chondromyxoid fibromas can be accompanied by coarse or thick trabeculae, and aneursymal bone cysts can be characterized by horizontally oriented, delicate trabeculation extending into the surrounding soft tissues. Hemangiomas can stimulate a coarse periosteal response leading to a honeycombed, striated, or radiating appearance (Fig. 74–5*B*), and nonossifying fibromas may reveal lobulated trabeculation (Fig. 74–5*C*).

Cortical Erosion, Penetration, and Expansion

The bony cortex can serve as an effective barrier to the further lateral growth of certain tumors, whereas in other instances, the neoplasm may par-

Table 74–1
TRABECULATED LESIONS

Lesion	Pattern
Giant cell tumor	Delicate, thin
Chondromyxoid fibroma	Coarse, thick
Nonossifying fibroma	Loculated
Aneurysmal bone cyst	Delicate, horizontally oriented
Hemangioma	Striated, radiating

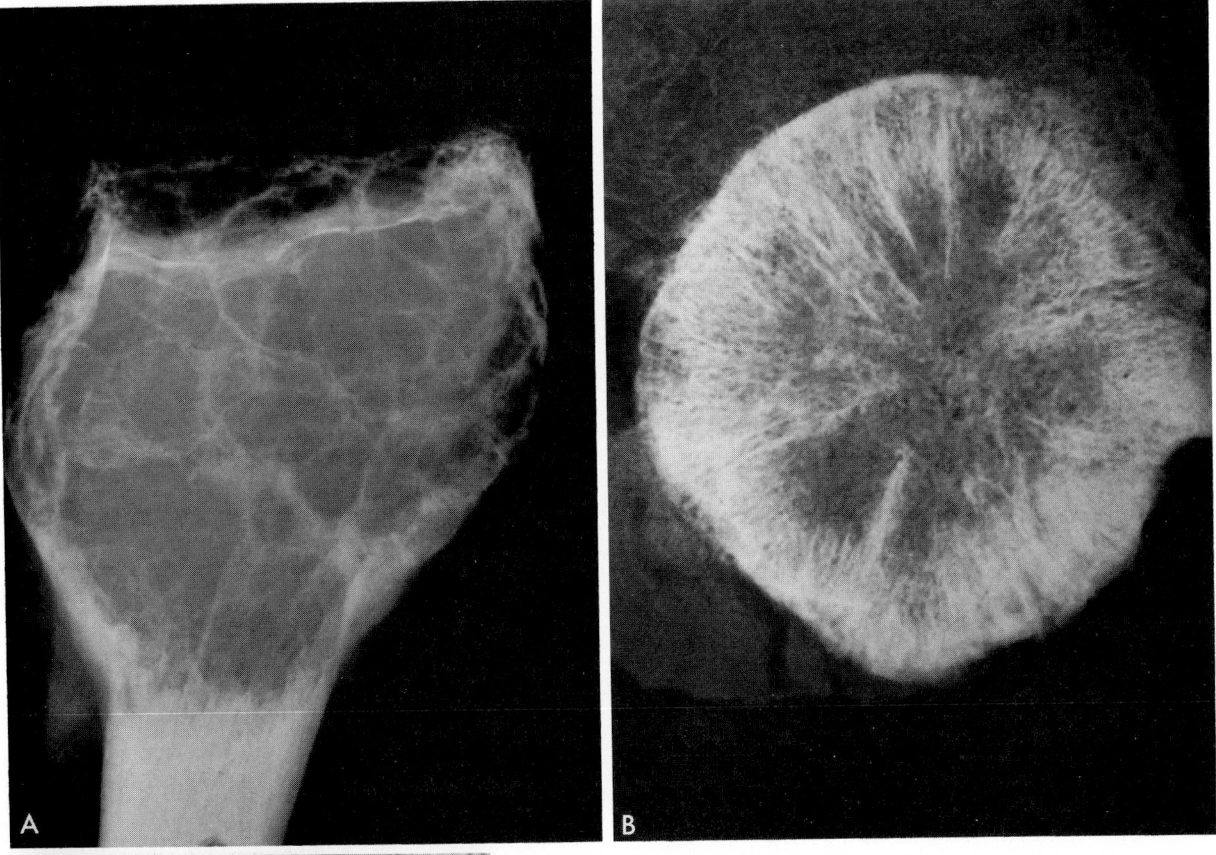

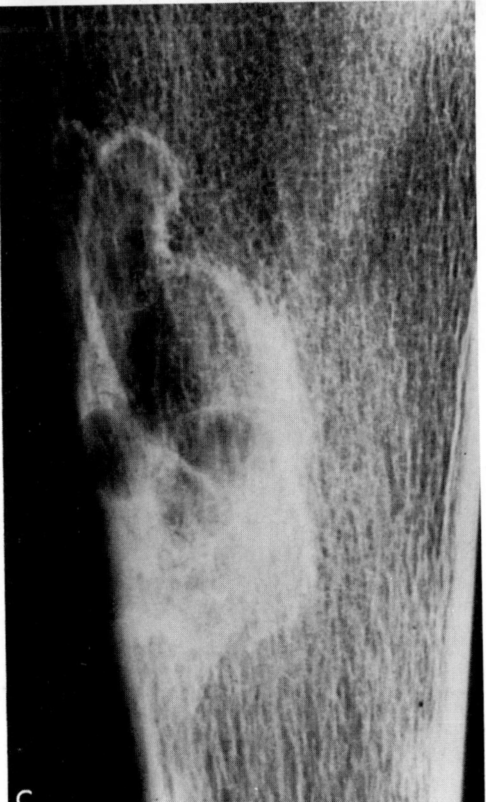

Figure 74–5. *Trabeculation.*

A *Giant cell tumor. Note delicate trabeculae that extend through and around this lesion of the distal radius (specimen radiograph).*

B *Hemangioma. Observe the radiating pattern of trabeculation associated with this lesion of the cranial vault (specimen radiograph).*

C *Nonossifying fibroma. A lobulated pattern of trabeculation characterizes this lesion of the proximal tibia (specimen radiograph).*

tially or completely penetrate the cortex. Nonaggressive medullary lesions may provoke little change in the endosteal surface of the cortex and, in fact, may extend in a path of least resistance within the medullary canal. Other slow-growing lesions, such as enchondromas, can lead to lobulated erosion of the inner margin of the cortex, producing a scalloped endosteal margin, which may be associated with uniform periosteal proliferation or buttressing of the outer cortical surface. If progressive endosteal erosion is associated with periosteal bone deposition, an expanded osseous contour can be created. The rate of bone expansion is variable. Certain tumors expand bone very slowly, and the accompanying periosteal response may eventually produce a surrounding cortical shell of such thickness that further expansion of the cortex is resisted. Other lesions such as the aneurysmal bone cyst expand bone very rapidly.

Aggressive bone lesions can penetrate the entire thickness of the cortex in one or more places. As the tumor reaches the outer aspect of the cortex, the periosteal membrane may be elevated, leading to a variety of patterns of periosteal new bone formation.

Periosteal Response (Fig. 74–6)

Lodwick[12] has characterized the various patterns of periosteal response to adjacent tumor. A slowly growing tumor that is eroding or penetrating the cortex can evoke a periosteal response in which additional layers of new bone are added to the exterior, creating an expanded osseous contour. In these instances, the ultimate thickness of the surrounding cortical bone is dependent upon the extent of endosteal erosion and periosteal proliferation. It can be of diminished or of "normal" thickness when compared to the original thickness of the cortex, or the new cortex can be thickened in a uniform or nonuniform fashion. If the interface between the normal and expanded cortex is "filled in" with bone, a buttressed pattern has evolved. With more rapid tumor growth, the periosteal response may be characterized by delicate layers of new bone. Single or multiple laminated bone formation may be identified. Multiple concentric layers of periosteal new bone produce the "onion-peel" pattern,[12] which has been interpreted by some investigators to indicate alternating periods of rapid and slow growth,[13] although others regard it as indicating only an acceleration of the normal periosteal bone response.[14] The "onion-peel" pattern can be identified in some cases of Ewing's sarcoma and osteogenic sarcoma.

At the edges or periphery of a neoplasm or an infective focus, a triangular elevation of the periosteum may be identified, termed Codman's triangle. In these cases, histologic evaluation will frequently confirm that the periosteum has been elevated by adjacent neoplasm, although the subperiosteal area in the region of the Codman's triangle is itself free of tumor.

In some patients with aggressive bone tumors, delicate rays of periosteal bone formation can form, separated by spaces containing blood vessels.[12] In certain neoplasms, such as osteogenic sarcoma, the rays extend away from the bone in a radiating or "sunburst" pattern, emanating from a single focus in the bone; in other neoplasms, such as Ewing's sarcoma, the rays extend in a direction perpendicular to the underlying bone, creating a "hair-on-end" periosteal pattern.

Soft Tissue Mass

Soft tissue masses are not infrequently associated with malignant bone neoplasms. In some tumors, such as reticulum cell sarcoma, the masses may be quite large at the time of clinical presentation, as other physical signs and symptoms are not marked. In other tumors, considerable pain and tenderness may quickly lead a patient to the hospital, so that a small mass or even no mass cannot be regarded as a uniformly good prognostic sign. Osteomyelitis is also associated with a soft tissue mass or swelling. Although radiographic characteristics have been formulated that may separate an inflammatory mass from a neoplastic mass, these are not extremely reliable and often depend upon the modification of radiographic technique to optimize soft tissue detail or the use of other diagnostic modalities, such as low KV radiography or xeroradiography.[15] A soft tissue mass related to tumor may reveal displacement of adjacent soft tissue planes, whereas one related to infection may be associated with distortion or obliteration of these planes.

DISTRIBUTION

The distribution of a solitary lesion within a bone provides an important clue to the correct diagnosis. Lodwick's analysis,[12] which is summarized here, is based predominantly on lesions in tubular bones, although the analysis can be extended to involvement of flat bones in some instances.

Position of Lesion in Transverse Plane (Fig. 74–7)

The identification of a lesion's center is of fundamental importance in establishing a correct diagnosis. The position of the center of a lesion can frequently be identified as of central, eccentric, corti-

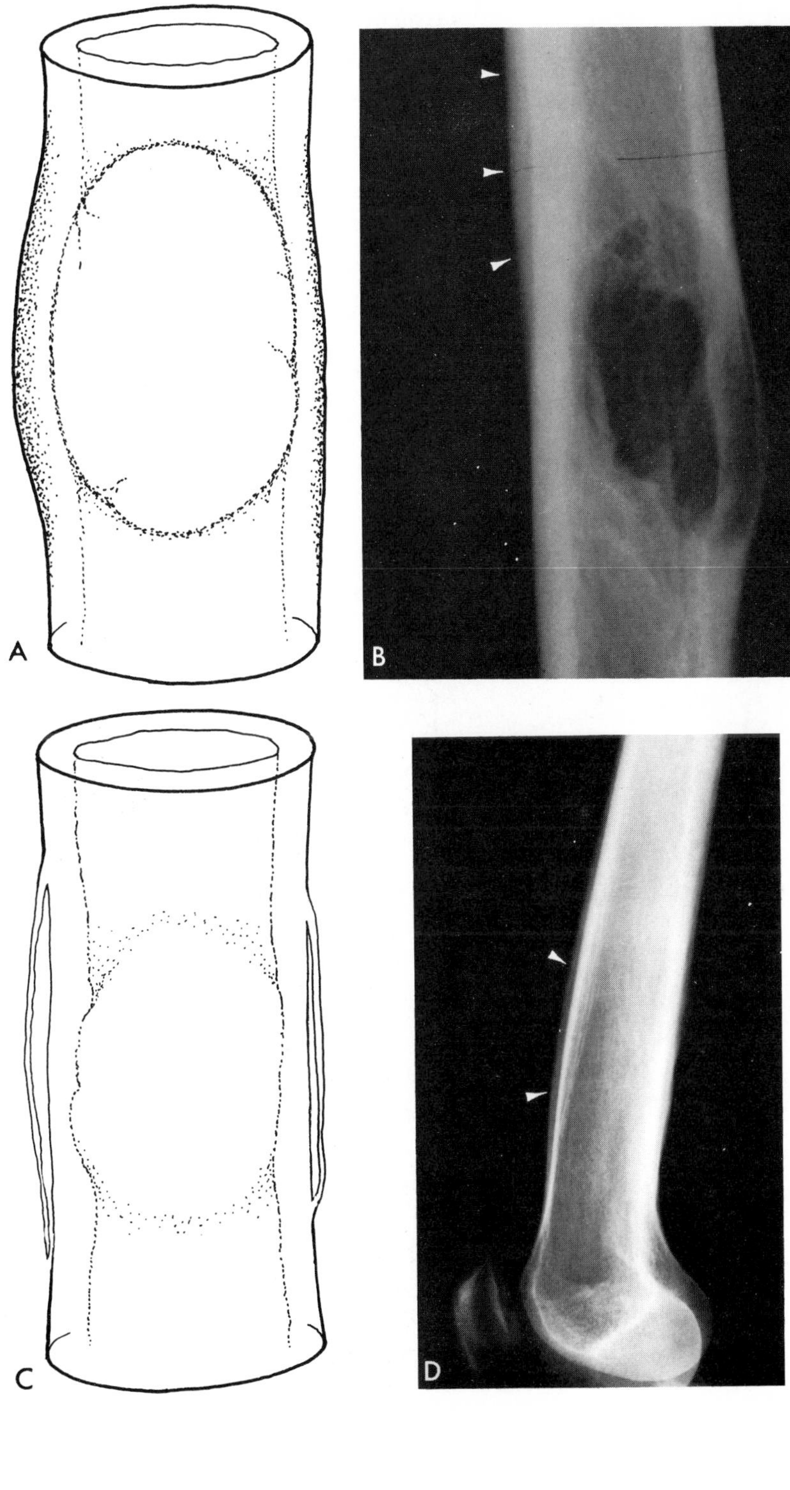

A

B

C

D

Figure 74–6. *Periosteal response.*

A, B *Periosteal buttressing. The diagram* **(A)** *indicates that periosteal bone formation in response to a lesion may merge with the underlying cortex, producing a buttressed appearance. On the radiograph* **(B)**, *a thick single layer of periosteal bone (arrowheads) about this femoral lesion is still separated from the underlying cortex. The thickness of the periosteal response would indicate a relatively slow-growing lesion. (Final diagnosis — solitary bone cyst.)*

C, D *Single layer of periosteal bone. The diagram* **(C)** *demonstrates the appearance of a single thin layer of periosteal bone about a lesion, separated from the underlying bone. The radiograph* **(D)** *indicates a single layer of periosteal bone on both the anterior and posterior surfaces of the femur. Anteriorly, the periosteal layer is quite thick and still separated from the underlying bone (arrowheads). Posteriorly, the periosteal bone has merged with the femur.*

Illustration continued on the following page

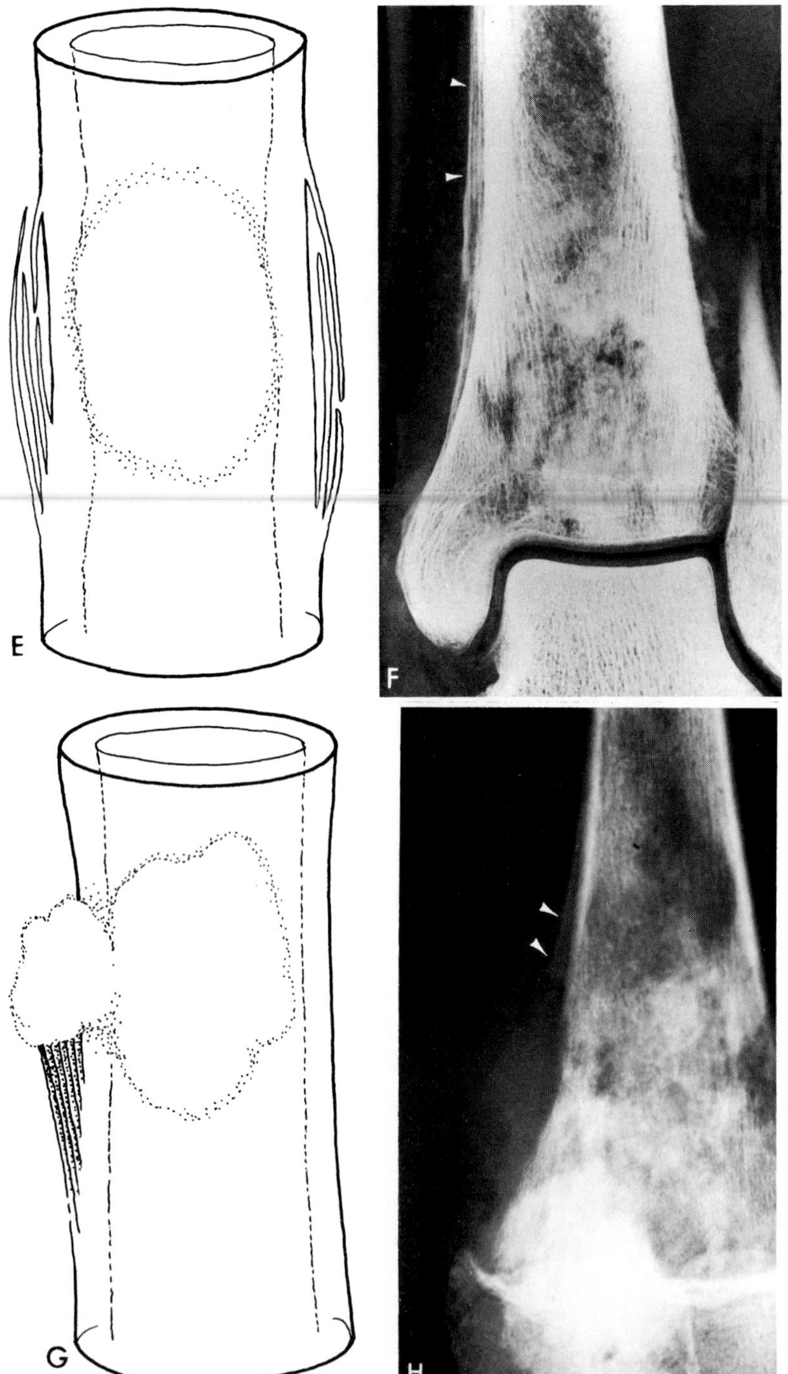

Figure 74–6. Continued

E, F *Multiple layers of periosteal bone: Onion-peel pattern. The diagram* **(E)** *indicates multiple concentric layers of periosteal bone about the lesion. The specimen radiograph* **(F)** *shows such a pattern along one side of the distal tibia (arrowheads). On the other side of the bone, a more complex pattern of periostitis is seen. The medullary lesion contains radiopaque foci. (Final diagnosis — osteogenic sarcoma.)*

G, H *Codman's triangle. The diagram* **(G)** *reveals triangular elevation of the periosteum beneath an aggressive lesion that is penetrating the cortex. The specimen radiograph* **(H)** *shows such a Codman's triangle (arrowheads). Note the medullary and cortical bone destruction, soft tissue mass, and radiodense foci within the lesion. (Final diagnosis — osteogenic sarcoma.)*

Illustration continued on the opposite page

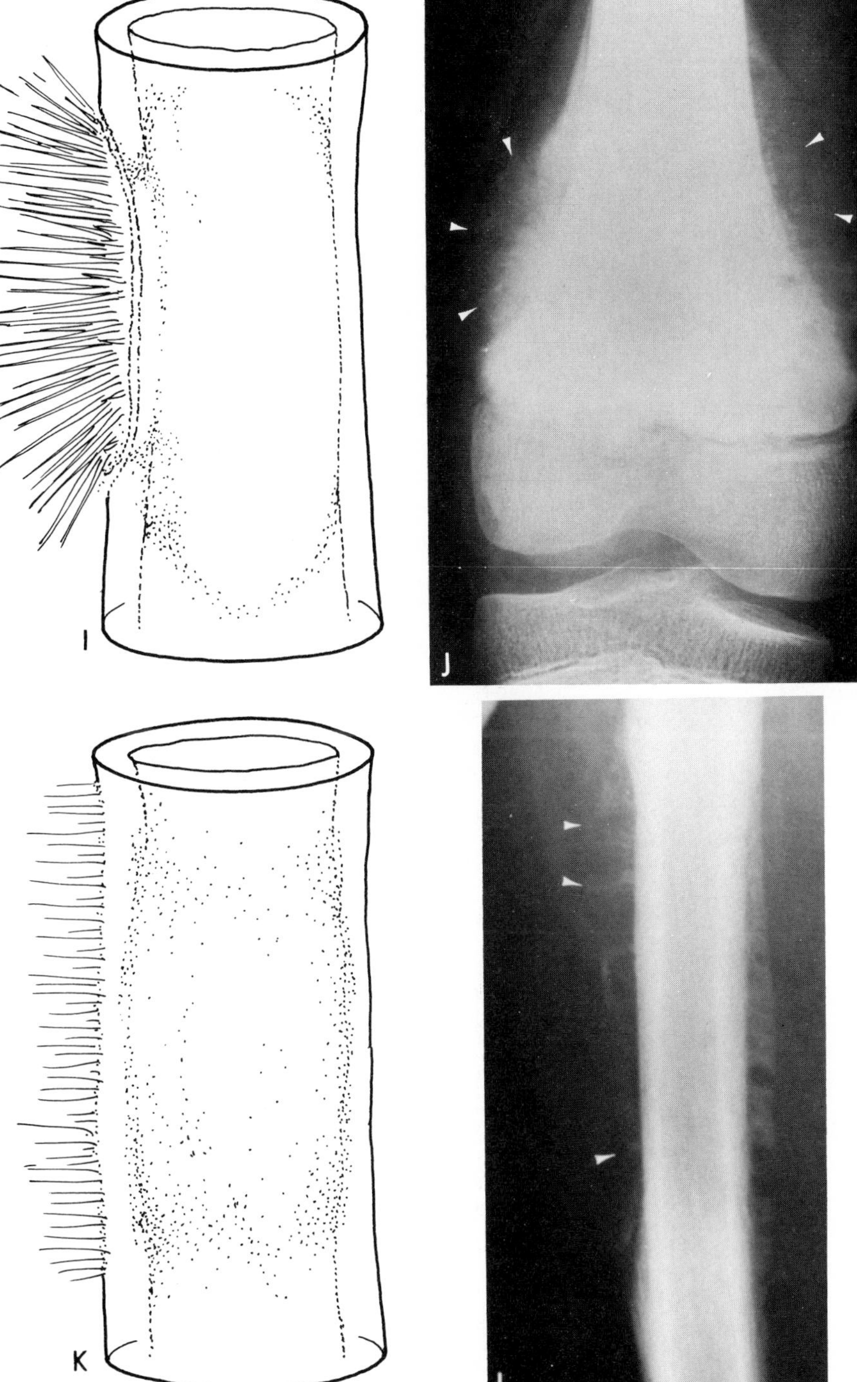

Figure 74–6. Continued

I, J *Radiating spicules of periosteal bone: Sunburst pattern. The diagram* **(I)** *shows radiating spicules that emanate from a single focus within the bone. The radiograph* **(J)** *indicates such a sunburst pattern of periosteal bone (arrowheads), which is intermixed with tumor bone formation. Note the radiodense lesion in the medullary bone and the Codman's triangle. (Final diagnosis — osteogenic sarcoma.)*

K, L *Radiating spicules of periosteal bone: Hair-on-end pattern. The diagram* **(K)** *demonstrates the parallel horizontal spicules that emanate from the underlying bone. The radiograph* **(L)** *indicates a femoral lesion characterized by a hair-on-end pattern (arrowheads). The individual striations of periosteal bone have created an inhomogeneous band of radiodensity on the opposite side of the bone. (Final diagnosis — Ewing's sarcoma.)*

cal, juxtacortical (parosteal), or soft tissue location. This analysis is facilitated when the lesion is not of great size, as the center may be more difficult to define when a large lesion is encountered. Furthermore, establishing the position of the center of a lesion is less reliable when a small tubular bone, such as the fibula, is the site of involvement, as eccentric lesions in small tubular bones soon appear central in location.

Some lesions characteristically lie on or close to the central axis of the bone (i.e., central lesions) within the medullary canal. These include, among others, enchondromas and solitary bone cysts. Other lesions arise to one side of the central axis of the bone, still within the medullary canal (i.e., eccentric lesions) or within the cortex (i.e., cortical lesions). It may be difficult to differentiate a lesion arising in a subcortical location from one originating in the

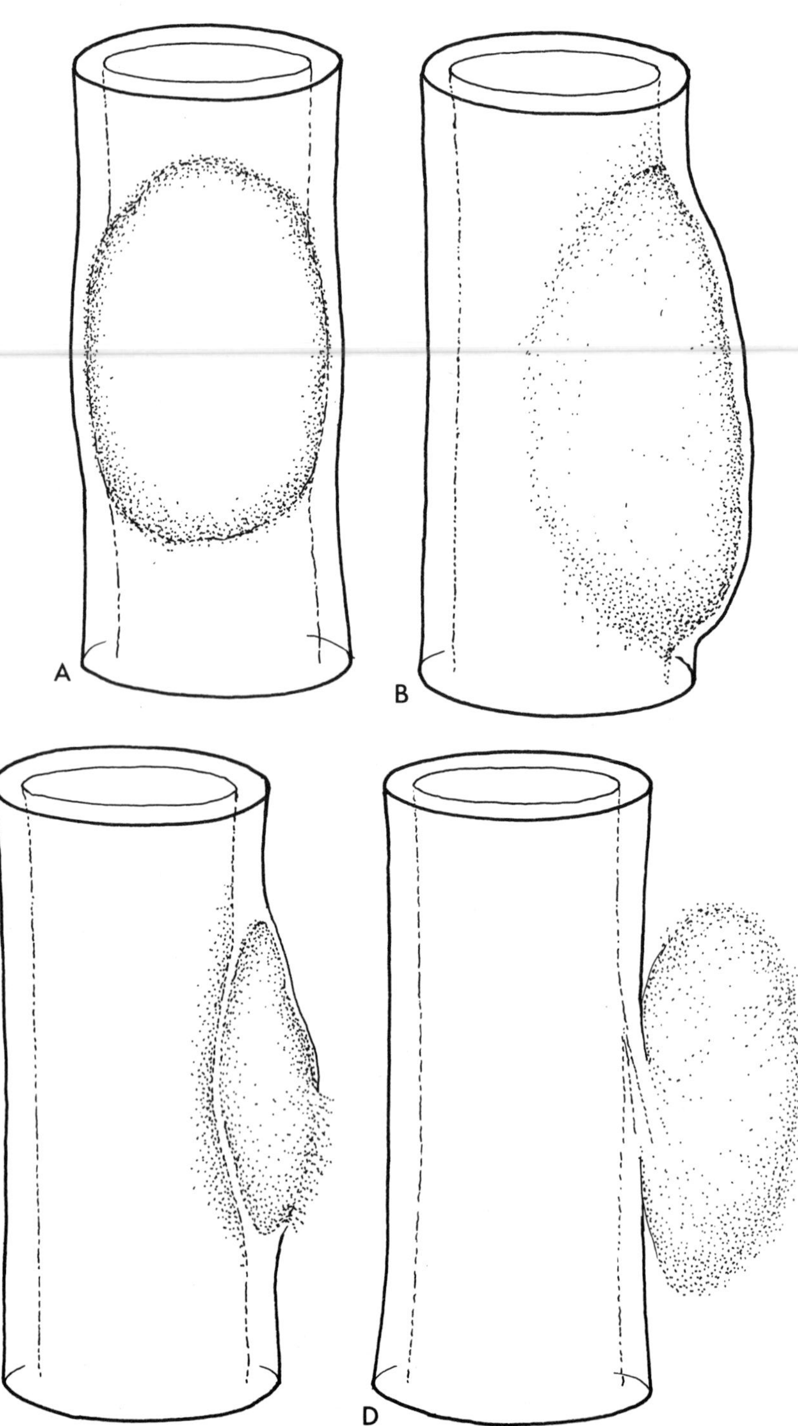

Figure 74–7. *Position of lesion in transverse plane. Lesions may be central* **(A)**, *eccentric* **(B)**, *cortical* **(C)**, *or parosteal* **(D)**. *Identification of the precise position of the lesion requires that radiographs be obtained in more than one projection.*

cortex. Eccentric lesions include giant cell tumors, mesenchymal sarcomas, such as osteogenic sarcoma, chondrosarcoma, and fibrosarcoma, and chondromyxoid fibromas. Cortical lesions include nonossifying fibromas and osteoid osteomas. Lesions arising adjacent to the outer surface of the cortex are parosteal or juxtacortical in location. Typical examples are juxtacortical chondromas, osteochondromas, and parosteal osteogenic sarcomas. Soft tissue lesions are of many types and are discussed in Chapter 85. Some kinds of lesions, such as osteogenic sarcomas, chondrosarcomas, fibrosarcomas, and osteoblastomas, may arise from any one of these locations.[12]

Position of Lesion in Longitudinal Plane

Certain solitary lesions in the tubular bones show a remarkable propensity to develop in specific anatomic locations, such as the epiphysis, metaphysis, and diaphysis. Examples of epiphyseal lesions include chondroblastoma, which typically develops within an epiphysis prior to closure of the growth plate, and intra-osseous ganglion. Although originating in the metaphysis, giant cell tumors quickly penetrate the closed growth plate, involving the epiphysis with extension to the subchondral bone adjacent to the joint. Metaphyseal lesions include nonossifying fibroma, which characteristically develops at a short distance from the growth plate, chondromyxoid fibroma, which abuts the growth plate, solitary bone cyst, osteochondroma, Brodie's abscess, and mesenchymal sarcomas, such as osteogenic sarcoma and chondrosarcoma (Table 74–2). Lesions that may develop in a diaphysis include round cell tumors, such as Ewing's sarcoma. Nonaggressive lesions that may appear in the diaphysis of a tubular bone include nonossifying fibromas, solitary bone cysts, aneurysmal bone cysts, enchondromas, osteoblastomas, and fibrous dysplasia. Although these anatomic divisions are not so accurately applied to lesions in flat bones,[12] epiphyseal equivalent areas exist beneath the articular cartilage in the bones of the pelvic and shoulder girdles, such that lesions within these areas are commonly those that show predilection for the epiphyses in the tubular bones. Similar "epiphyseal" lesions may develop in the small bones of the wrist and midfoot and in the patella.

Specific Bones

Certain neoplasms show predilection for specific skeletal sites. Examples include adamantinomas and ossifying fibromas, which may appear in the tibia; hemangiomas, plasma cell myelomas, and skeletal metastases, which are frequent in the spine; chordomas, which predominate in the clivus and sacral region; and enchondromas, which are quite common in the small bones of the hand.

SPECIFIC TUMORS AND TUMOR-LIKE LESIONS

Cartilage-Forming Tumors

Benign Tumors

Enchondroma (Fig. 74–8). The solitary enchondroma is a tumor that develops in the medullary cavity and is composed of lobules of hyaline cartilage.[16-20] The neoplasm is usually discovered in the third or fourth decade of life and is equally frequent in men and women. The most common site of involvement is a bone in the hand, especially the metacarpals or the proximal or middle phalanges. Other sites include the bones of the foot, the long tubular bones, such as the humerus, femur, and tibia, and the ribs. Lesions, particularly those in the hand, are usually asymptomatic or associated with painless swelling. The appearance of pain should arouse suspicion of malignant transformation, a complication that, although infrequent, is more commonly noted in the long tubular bones, especially those about the pelvic and shoulder girdles. Radiographs generally reveal a well-defined medullary lesion with some degree of calcification. A lobulated con-

Table 74–2

MESENCHYMAL SARCOMA VERSUS ROUND CELL SARCOMA*

	Mesenchymal	Round Cell
Examples	Osteogenic sarcoma, chondrosarcoma, fibrosarcoma	Ewing's sarcoma, leukemias
Location in tubular bones	Metaphyseal	Metadiaphyseal
Types of bone destruction	Motheaten pattern	Permeative pattern
Visible tumor matrix	Common (osteogenic sarcoma, chondrosarcoma)	Rare
Periostitis	Sunburst, Codman's triangle	Onion-peel, hair-on-end, Codman's triangle

*Classic features are indicated for each type of sarcoma, although considerable variability can be evident.

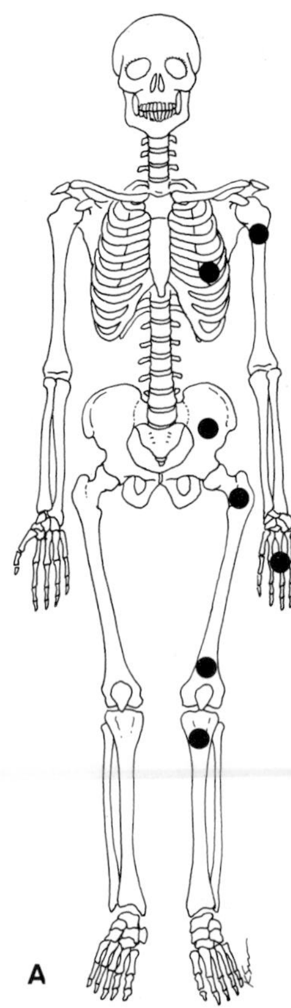

Figure 74–8. Enchondroma.

A *Characteristic distribution. (In this diagram and others that appear later in this chapter, the markers indicate the most common skeletal sites of the tumor. They do not necessarily indicate the specific location in the bone that is involved.)*

B *An enchondroma of a proximal phalanx is associated with geographic bone destruction, a central location, a lobulated contour, and central calcifications.*

C *An enchondroma of the distal femur reveals punctate calcifications.*

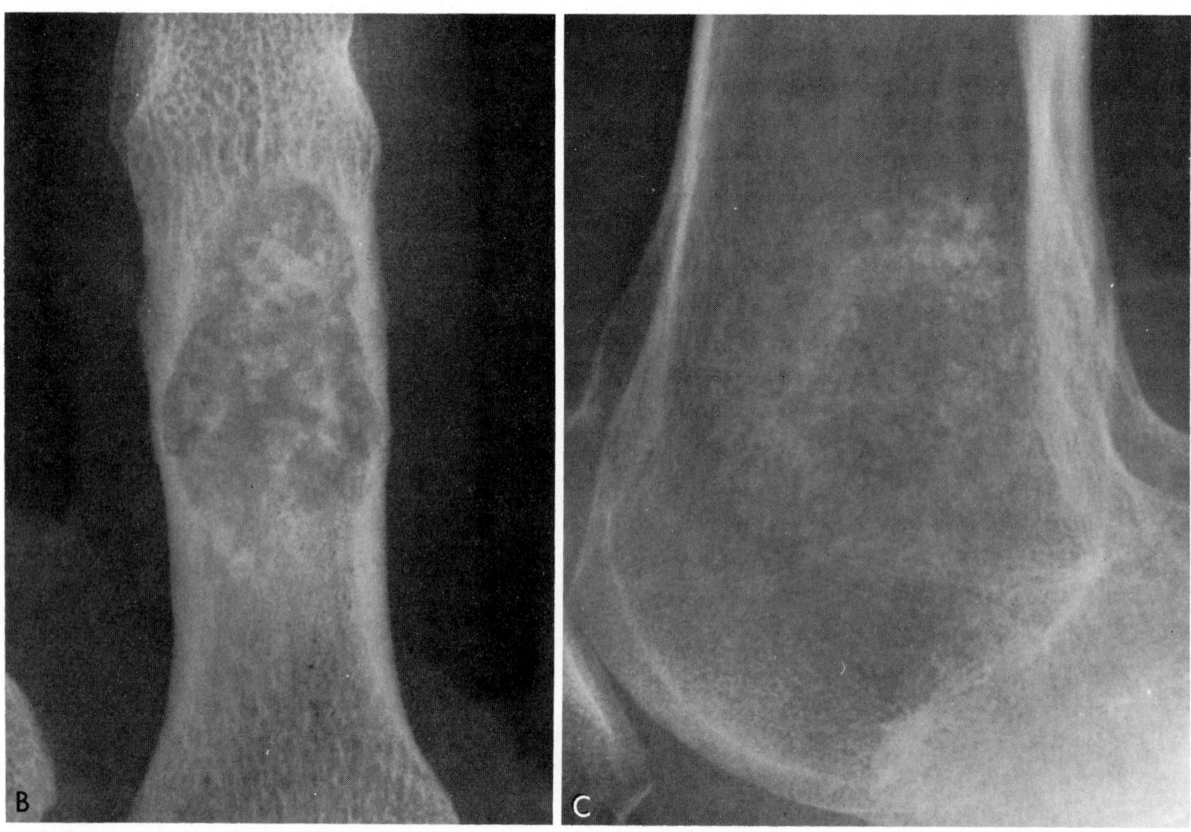

tour, endosteal erosion, cortical expansion or thickening, and a pathologic fracture are other potential radiographic characteristics. In a tubular bone, a metaphyseal or diametaphyseal location is typical.

Multiple enchondromatosis is called Ollier's disease. The combination of enchondromatosis and hemangiomatosis is termed Maffucci's syndrome. These conditions are discussed elsewhere in this text.

Parosteal (Juxtacortical) Chondroma (Fig. 74–9). This tumor, composed of hyaline cartilage, develops adjacent to the cortical surface, beneath the periosteal membrane.[21-24] It may be discovered in children as well as in adults, men and women being affected with equal frequency. The most common sites of involvement are the small tubular bones of the hands and the feet, although long tubular bones, flat bones, clavicles, and ribs can be affected. Pain and swelling may be evident, as opposed to the infrequency of these clinical findings in cases of enchondroma. Radiographically, a soft tissue mass with erosion or "saucerization" of the adjacent cortex is evident. Medullary sclerosis and periostitis may be seen. Calcification within the lesion is evident in approximately 50 per cent of cases.

Chondroblastoma (Fig. 74–10). This relatively rare cartilage tumor consists of polyhedral cells, giant cells, and fine calcifications; small foci of osteoid and bone and hemorrhagic areas may be identified.[25-27] The microscopic features may resemble those of a chondromyxoid fibroma. Chondroblastomas are most frequent in the second and third decades of life.[28, 29] Men are affected more commonly than women in an approximate ratio of 2:1. The tumors characteristically arise within an epiphysis of a long tubular bone, particularly that in the proximal end of the femur, humerus, or tibia. Less common sites of involvement are apophyses (such as that in the greater trochanter), the innominate bones, particularly near the triradiate cartilage, and tarsus.[30] Extension of a neoplasm from the epiphyseal region to the metaphysis is observed and, in rare instances, a tumor isolated in the metaphysis may be discovered.[31, 32] Clinical findings may include mild pain and tenderness, swelling, and limitation of motion. Pathologic fracture and joint effusion are less typical features of this neoplasm. Radiographs reveal a lytic lesion of an epiphysis, usually less than 5 or 6 cm in size, which is well defined and spheroid or oval in shape. Calcification within the lesion (approximately 50 per cent of cases) and periostitis of the adjacent metaphysis or diaphysis (approximately 30 per cent of cases) can be seen. In some cases, extreme calcification or ossification may produce a radiopaque lesion that may be mistaken for an osteoblastoma.[33] Cortical expansion, metaphyseal or intra-articular extension, and accentuated maturation and premature fusion of the growth plate are additional poten-

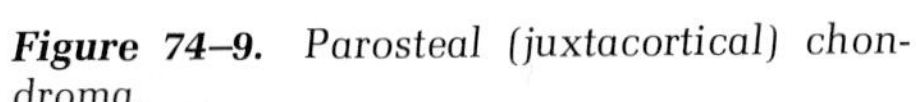

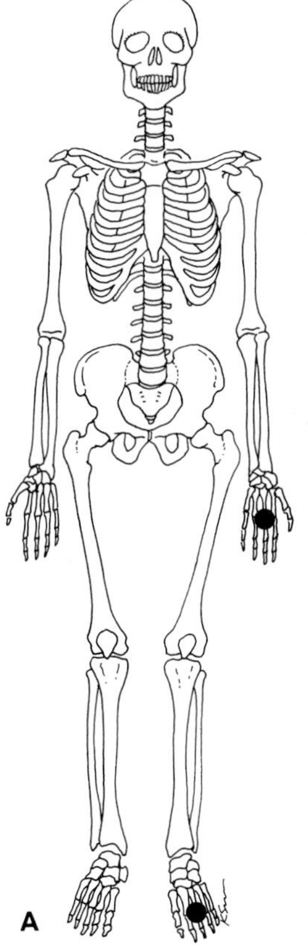

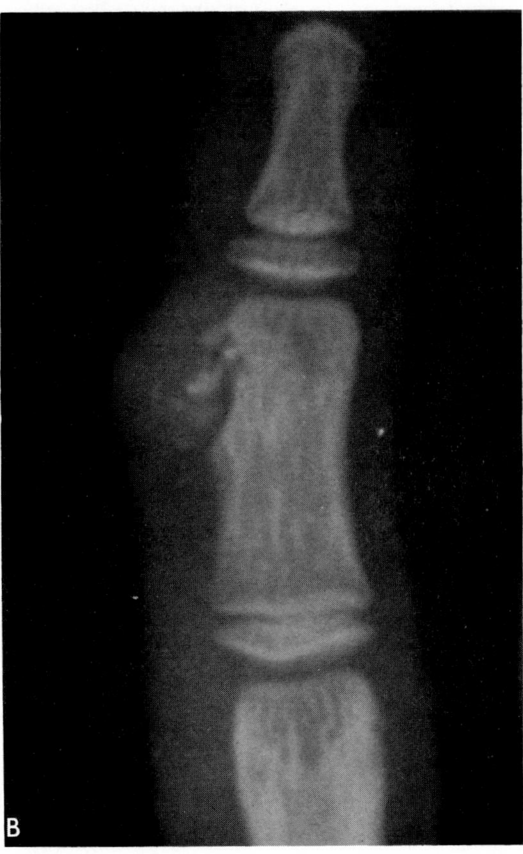

Figure 74–9. *Parosteal (juxtacortical) chondroma.*

A *Characteristic distribution.*

B *A parosteal chondroma of a finger has created a soft tissue mass containing calcification. Cortical excavation can be seen in association with neighboring periosteal response.*

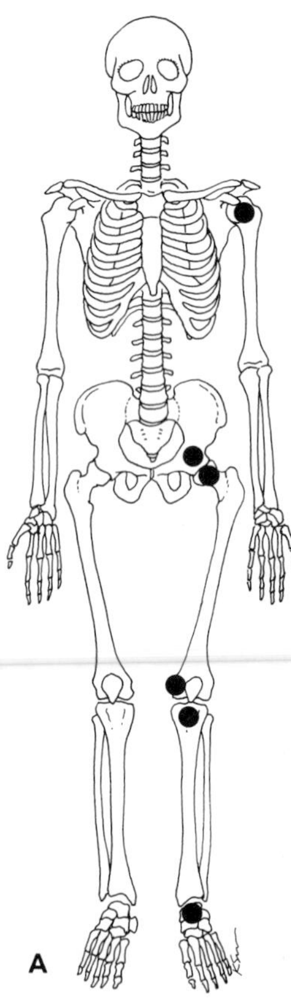

Figure 74–10. Chondroblastoma.

A Characteristic distribution.

B *A lytic lesion of the distal femur (arrowheads) demonstrates geographic bone destruction and small calcific foci.*

C *An osteolytic lesion of the talus (arrowheads) reveals geographic bone destruction. Calcific foci cannot be definitely delineated. (**C,** Courtesy of Dr. Thomas Goergen, San Diego, California.)*

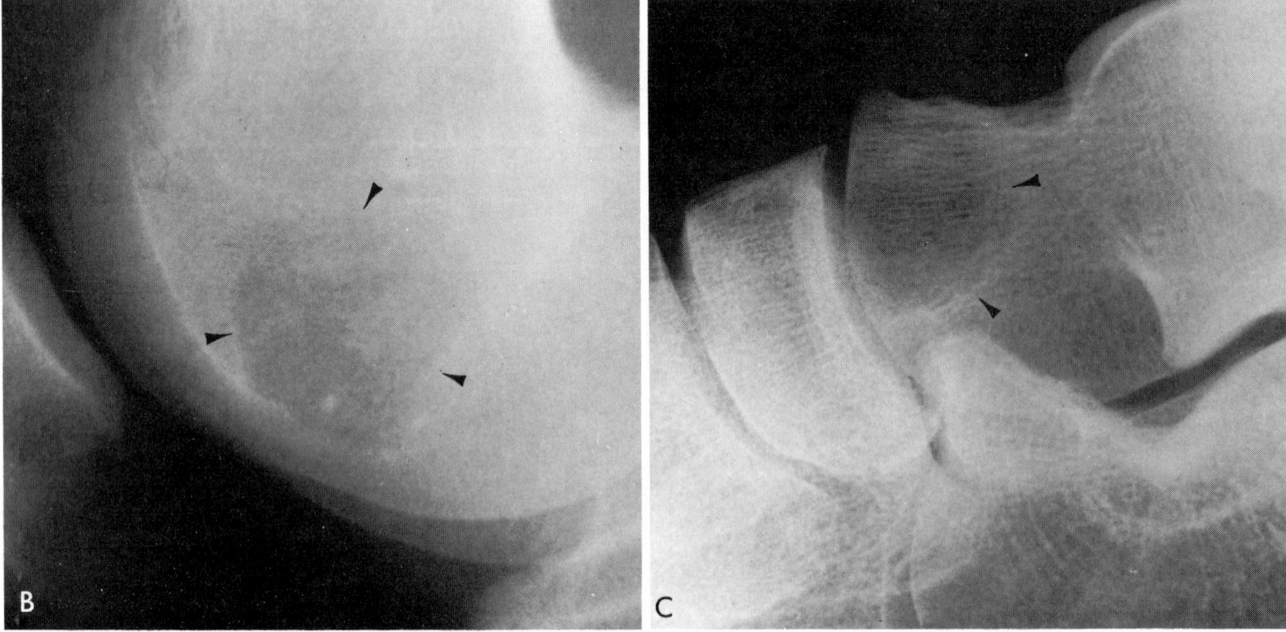

tial findings. Very rarely, "benign" lesions may metastasize to the lungs, or malignant transformation may be evident.[34-38]

Chondromyxoid Fibroma (Fig. 74–11). Chondromyxoid fibroma is a benign bone tumor composed of cartilaginous, fibrous, and myxoid tissue in varying amounts.[39, 40] The tumor is most common in the second and third decades of life, affecting men slightly more commonly than women. Slowly progressive pain, tenderness, swelling, and restriction of motion may be evident on clinical evaluation. The most frequent sites of involvement are the proximal end of the tibia, proximal and distal ends of the femur and fibula, and small bones of the foot.[41] In a tubular bone, a metaphyseal focus is favored, with extension into the neighboring epiphysis and diaphysis. Chondromyxoid fibromas are frequently eccentrically located and elongated in shape, ranging in size from 2 to 9 cm. Cortical expansion, exuberant endosteal sclerosis, and coarse trabeculation may characterize its radiographic appearance. Calcification and pathologic fractures are rare. Malignant degeneration of a chondromyxoid fibroma is distinctly unusual, and such cases may indeed represent primary myxoid chondrosarcomas.

Osteochondroma (Fig. 74–12). The solitary osteochondroma or exostosis is a cartilage-capped bony excrescence that arises from the surface of a bone. Osteochondromas are most frequently discovered in the first, second, or third decade of life. There may be a slight predilection for men to develop this neoplasm. The tumor is extremely common, and it is typically encountered in the metaphysis of a long tubular bone, especially in the proximal portion of the humerus, proximal and distal portions of the femur and tibia, and distal portion of the radius. Flat and irregular bones may also be affected, especially the scapula, ribs, and innominate bones. In a tubular bone, the osteochondroma arises adjacent to the growth plate and eventually is directed toward the metaphysis and diaphysis. The lesions are of variable shape and size, although their growth usually ceases at puberty with fusion of the adjacent growth plate. Radiographic features are diagnostic. The cortex and spongiosa of the lesion are continuous with those of the underlying bone. Calcification or ossification or both may appear at the periphery of the outgrowth and may become so prominent as to obliterate much of the lesion. Metaphyseal widening is also prominent, a sign that is much more frequent in the hereditary form of the disease. Pathologically, a cartilage cap is identified containing a basal surface that exhibits endochondral ossification. This cellular activity usually ceases with the completion of bone growth. Malignant transformation in cases of solitary osteochondromas is rare. The incidence of

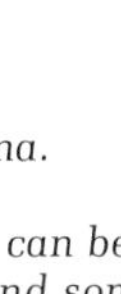

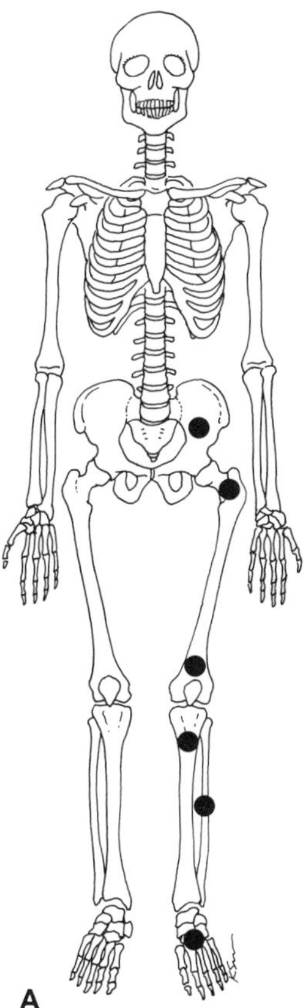

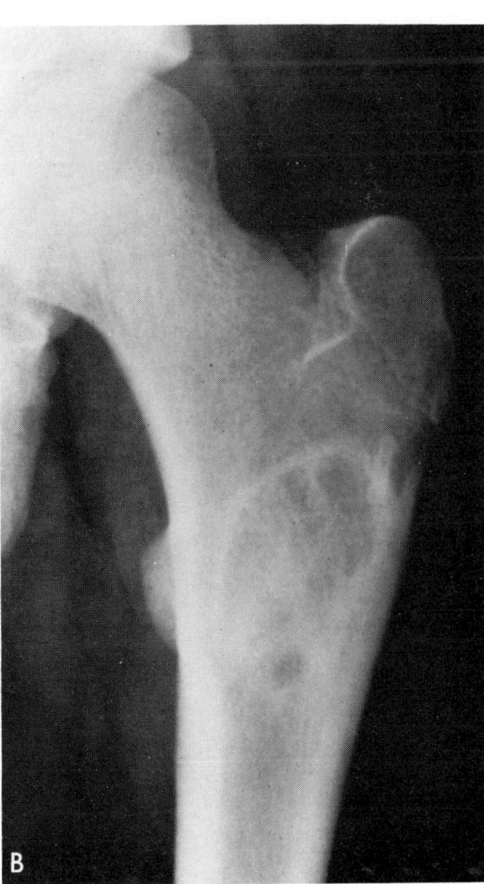

Figure 74–11. *Chondromyxoid fibroma.*
A *Characteristic distribution.*
B *A lesion of the proximal femur can be identified. It possesses a sclerotic margin and some trabeculation.*

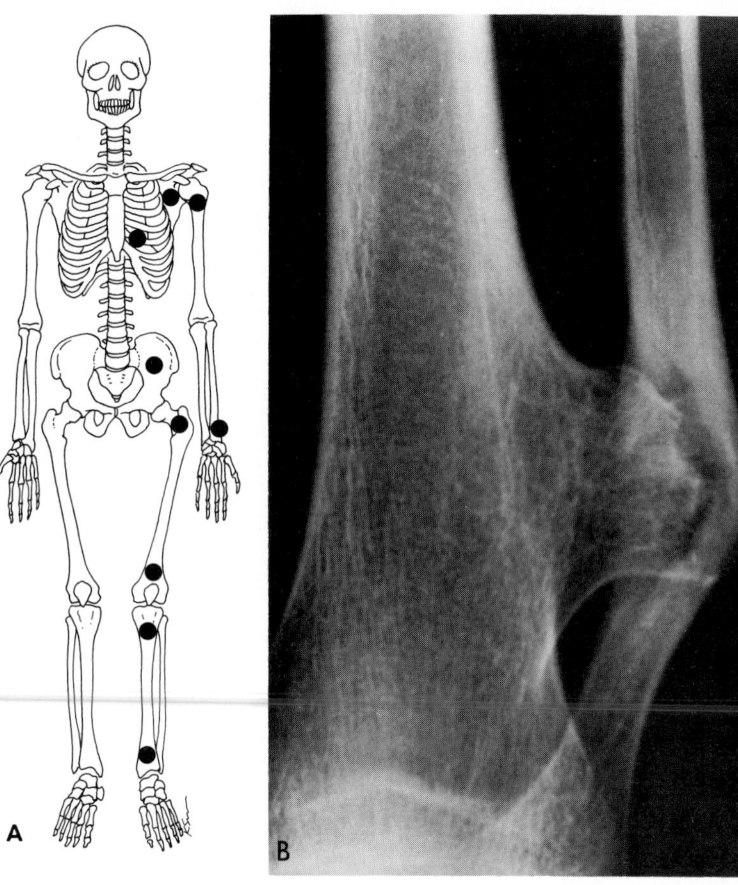

Figure 74–12. Osteochondroma.
A *Characteristic distribution.*
B *An ostechondroma is arising from the distal tibia, producing deformity of the adjacent fibula. Note that the cortex and spongiosa of the lesion are continuous with those of the underlying bone.* (**B**, *Courtesy of Dr. Jack Slivka, San Diego, California.*)

chondrosarcomatous degeneration is probably less than 1 per cent and, when present, is usually discovered in adult life. As symptoms and signs related to a benign osteochondroma are infrequent and mild, the presence of an enlarging soft tissue mass and pain should arouse suspicion of the possibility of malignant degeneration, although similar symptoms and signs can indicate a fracture, overlying bursitis, or injury to neighboring vessels or nerves.[249] Spinal cord compression can result from osteochondromas developing in the vertebral column or ribs.[42-44, 253]

Special varieties of osteochondromas include hereditary multiple exostoses (diaphyseal aclasis), Trevor's disease (epiphyseal aclasis), postirradiation osteochondroma, and subungual exostosis developing in the region of a phalangeal tuft. These lesions are discussed elsewhere in this book.[45]

Malignant Tumors

Chondrosarcoma (Fig. 74–13). This frequent malignant tumor is composed of sarcomatous stroma that is producing cartilage.[46, 47] Chondrosarcomas may arise de novo (primary chondrosarcoma) or as a complication of a preexisting skeletal abnormality such as an osteochondroma, enchondroma, or parosteal chondroma (secondary chondrosarcoma). The usual age of onset is during the fifth and sixth decades of life, although the age range is quite variable and is influenced by the type of chondrosarcoma that is being considered. Men are more commonly affected than women (1.5:1). The most common sites of involvement are the pelvis, femur, tibia, humerus, ribs, skull, and facial bones. Clinical findings include pain, swelling, and a mass, although many tumors are entirely asymptomatic.

Chondrosarcomas can be further classified according to their point of origin. They may be central, arising in the medullary bone, peripheral, originating within an osteochondroma, or juxtacortical (parosteal), or they may arise within soft tissue. Central chondrosarcomas[48] are grossly destructive lesions commonly containing one or more foci of calcification that may be better demonstrated on conventional tomography than on plain film radiography. Erosion of the endosteal margin of the cortex, with endosteal scalloping and cortical thickening, and a large soft tissue mass may be observed. Cortical disruption, periostitis, and a pathologic fracture are additional radiographic features. Peripheral chondrosarcomas produce destruction and enlargement of an osteochondroma with extension into the adjacent soft tissues. Periostitis and soft tissue calcification and ossification are seen. Juxtacortical chondrosarcomas[49] arise from the external surface of the bone and appear to represent the malignant counterpart of the parosteal chondroma. These le-

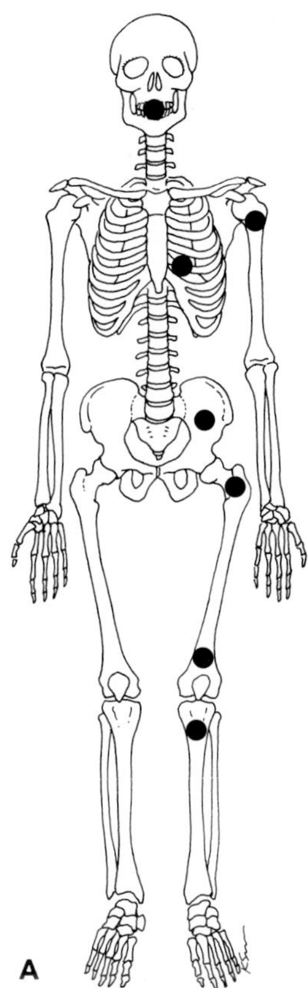

Figure 74–13. Chondrosarcoma.

A Characteristic distribution.

B, C Preoperative and specimen radiographs demonstrate the features of a chondrosarcoma of the proximal tibia. The tumor reveals a metaphyseal localization, motheaten pattern of bone destruction, matrix calcification, a soft tissue calcified mass, and mild periosteal response.

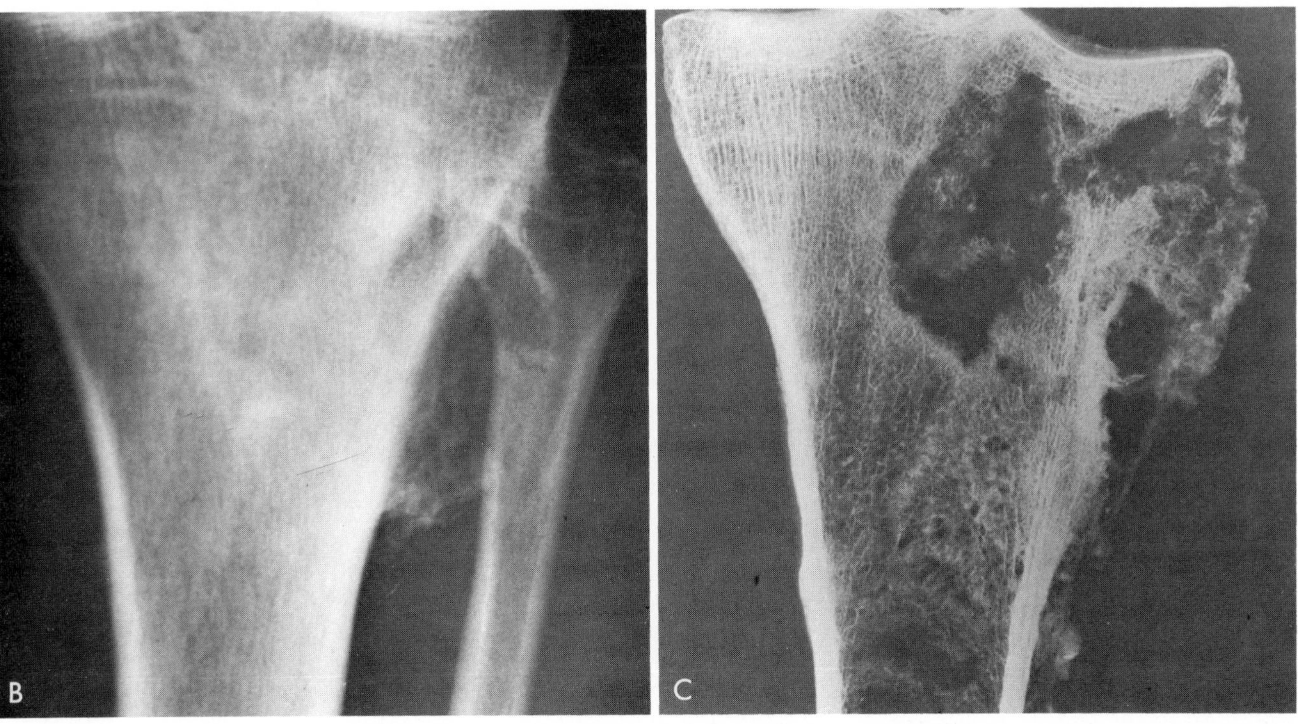

sions may be identical to the periosteal type of osteogenic sarcoma, appearing as destructive foci within the outer portions of the cortex, with calcification, periostitis, and a soft tissue mass. Extraosseous or soft tissue chondrosarcomas[54] are discussed elsewhere in this book.

Elaborate histologic grading systems utilized in describing chondrosarcoma of bone underscore difficulty in accurate assessment of the lesion and variability in its cell type.[50] Special varieties of chondrosarcomas include the clear cell type (which affects secondary centers of ossification in the epiphyses and which may be related to chondroblastoma)[51] and the mesenchymal type (which commonly arises in the soft tissues and which contains various types of connective tissue).[52, 53]

Bone-Forming Tumors

Benign Tumors

Osteoma. These benign lesions, usually arising from membranous bones and composed of dense compact osseous tissue, are discussed elsewhere in this book. They may be associated with intestinal polyposis, producing Gardner's syndrome.

Osteoid Osteoma (Fig. 74–14). These distinctive osteoblastic lesions contain a central nidus, which is characterized by osteoid and highly vascular fibrous tissue.[55] The nidus is usually less than 1 cm in size and is surrounded by a zone of reactive sclerosis. The etiology of osteoid osteoma is debated. The lesion may be a tumor or an inflammatory process. Osteoid osteomas are most frequently observed in the second and third decades of life, more commonly in men than women, in a ratio of approximately 2:1. The most frequent sites of involvement are the femur, tibia, humerus, and spine, although virtually any bone may be affected. Pain, worse at night and relieved by aspirin, can occur, and spinal osteoid osteomas may be associated with scoliosis.[56, 57] Muscle wasting and growth disturbance may also be evident.[58, 59] Osteoid osteomas may be classified according to their location within a bone: cortical, medullary, or parosteal. On radiographs, cortical osteoid osteomas produce a round or oval area of lucency surrounded by significant sclerosis and periostitis. The nidus may be entirely lucent or may be partially or totally calcified. Such cortical lesions may occasionally possess more than a single nidus, may recur, or may evoke periosteal reaction in a closely situated neighboring bone.[60-62] Rarely, a second nidus can be located in an adjacent bone.[63] The identification of the lesion may be difficult because of the degree of surrounding bony proliferation. Computed tomography, arteriography, and scintigraphy can be useful additional diagnostic modalities.[64-69, 263] During surgery, radiography of the bone specimen can document that the nidus has been removed.

Medullary osteoid osteomas may be associated with a lucent defect in bone or one that is partially or completely calcified. The degree of bony reaction is less striking and, when present, the reactive bone may be located at a considerable distance from the nidus. Parosteal osteoid osteomas produce cortical erosion and reactive sclerosis. Osteoid osteomas arising in the spine are commonly located in the posterior elements, including the pedicles, laminae, and spinous and transverse processes. An increase in density of the corresponding neural arch may be identified, which may be located along the concave aspect at the apex of an accompanying scoliotic curve. Osteoid osteomas arising in a vertebral body can extend across the adjacent intervertebral disc space.[70] In an intra-articular location, an osteoid osteoma can produce significant joint symptoms and signs, including a lymphofollicular synovitis with accumulation of articular fluid.[71] The clinical and radiographic appearance can simulate that of an infection or rheumatoid arthritis.[72]

Osteoblastoma (Fig. 74–15). An osteoblastoma is a lesion that is closely related to an osteoid osteoma.[73] It is usually larger in size than an osteoid osteoma and is associated with a lesser degree of bone reaction. Subtle histologic characteristics may also be differentiated from those of an osteoid osteoma: osteoid trabeculae are more discontinuous and bone formation is more irregular, fibrous stromal reaction is more abundant, and multinucleated giant

Figure 74–14. *Osteoid osteoma.*

A *Characteristic distribution.*

B *An osteoid osteoma of the distal tibia (arrowhead) can be recognized. Note the lucent nidus, which is surrounded by periostitis and cortical thickening. A periosteal response of the adjacent fibula can be seen.*

C *An osteoid osteoma within the olecranon fossa of the distal humerus (arrowhead) is associated with a calcified nidus, soft tissue swelling, and osteoporosis of neighboring bones.*

D *This osteoid osteoma (arrowhead) involves the posterior elements of a lower cervical vertebra.*

(**C, D,** Courtesy of *Dr. Robert Freiberger, New York, New York.*)

E *An osteoid osteoma of the medial portion of the femoral neck is obscured by adjacent reactive bone formation (arrows). Note the osteophytosis of the femur at the femoral head–femoral neck junction (arrowheads).* (**E,** Courtesy of *Dr. J. E. L. Desautels, Calgary, Alberta.*)

See illustration on the opposite page

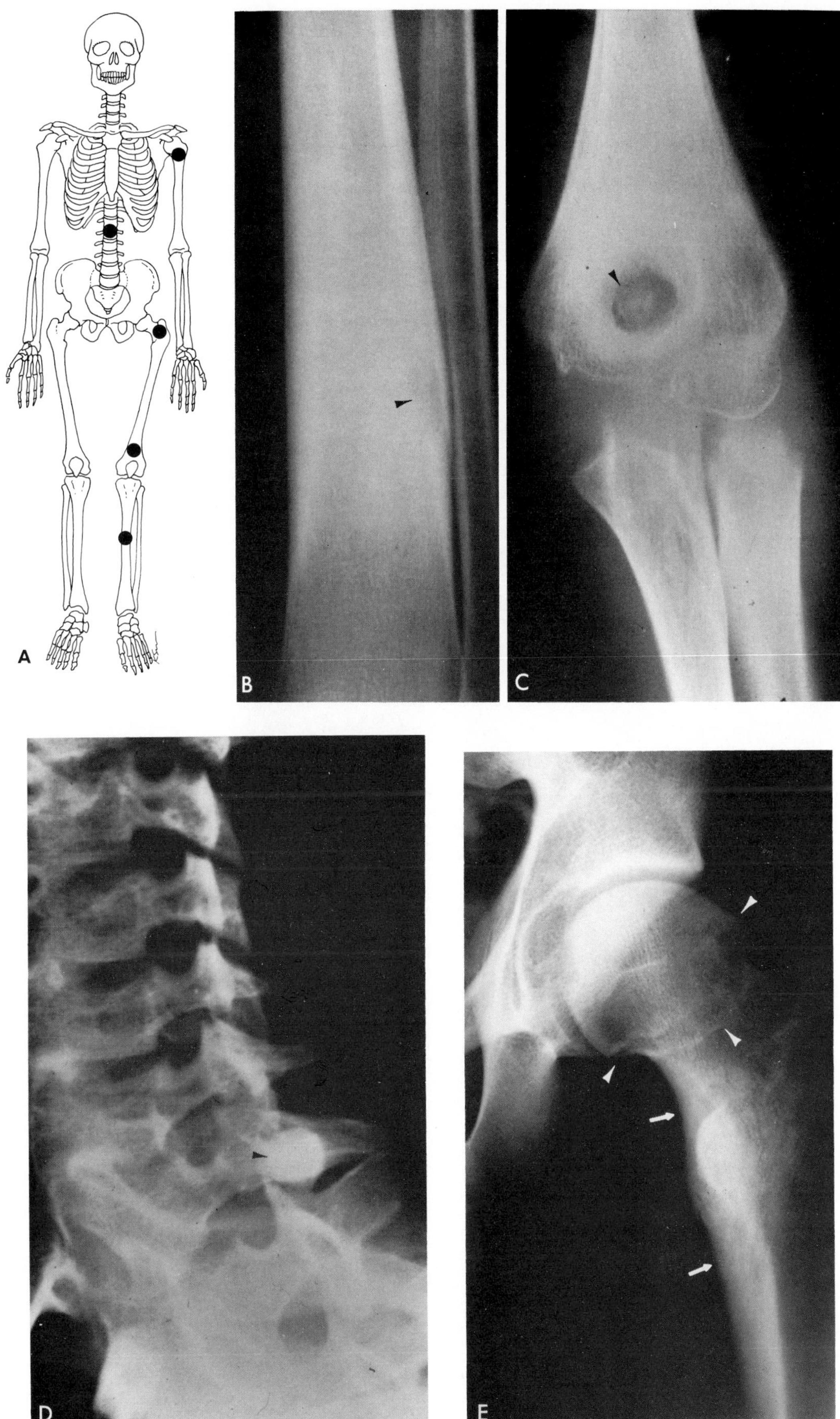

Figure 74–14. See legend on opposite page

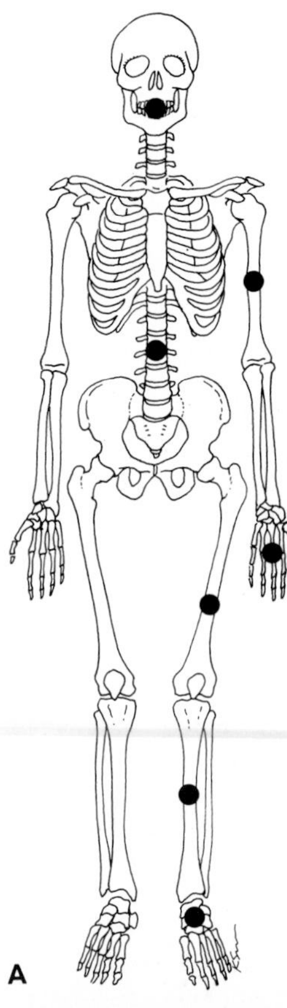

Figure 74–15. Osteoblastoma.

A *Characteristic distribution.*

B *An osteoblastoma has produced an expansile radiodense lesion (arrowheads) of the transverse process of the fourth lumbar vertebra.*

(Courtesy of Dr. Robert Freiberger, New York, New York.)

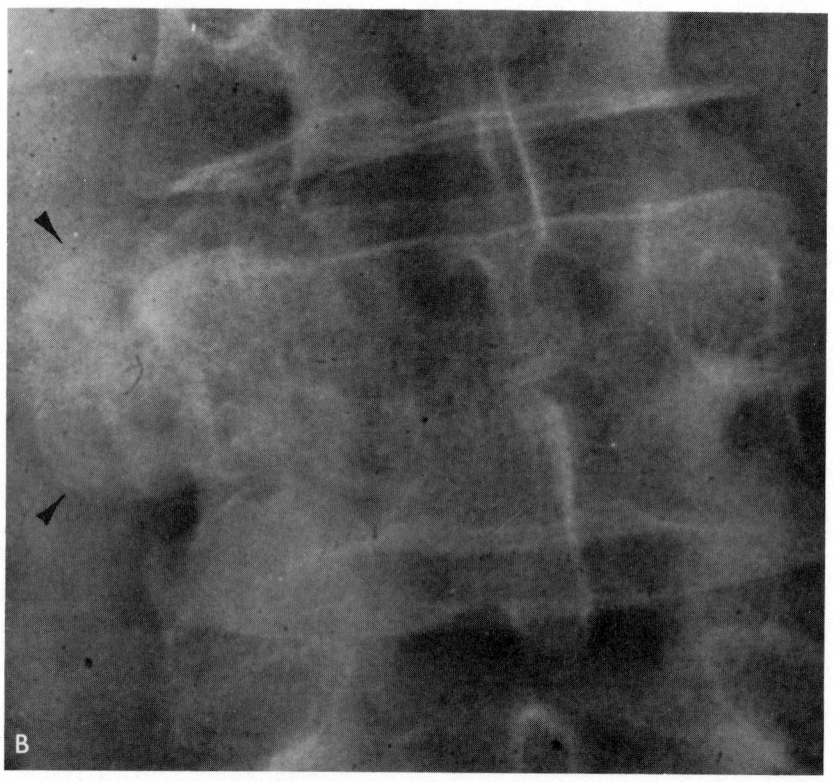

cells are more numerous.[3] Clinical manifestations may be less prominent in patients with osteoblastomas than in those with osteoid osteomas, consisting of mild to moderate localized pain and tenderness. This rare lesion is usually identified in patients in the second and third decades of life, with approximate equal frequency in men and women. Osteoblastomas are usually encountered in the spine (30 to 40 per cent), the long tubular bones of the extremities including the femur, tibia, and humerus (30 per cent), facial bones, including the mandible, and the small bones of the hands and feet (15 per cent).[74, 75] In the spine, the lesion shows predilection for the posterior elements, whereas in the tubular bones, diaphyseal or metaphyseal localization is typical. In the tubular bones, cortical, medullary, or parosteal lesions may be identified.[76] Rare reports have indicated multicentric or multifocal lesions.

Radiologic characteristics of osteoblastoma are quite variable and generally nonspecific. In the vertebral column, radiolucent or radiopaque lesions may be encountered, most typically in the posterior elements but occasionally in the vertebral bodies.[77] They are usually well circumscribed and commonly expansile in nature. Intralesional calcification can be seen, and a scoliotic curve, although not so common as in cases of osteoid osteoma, may be evident. In the appendicular skeleton, osteoblastomas are usually osteolytic, although some evoke a considerable amount of adjacent bone sclerosis. Occasionally, the lesion is radiopaque, appearing as a focal inhomogeneous or homogeneous dense area. Locally aggressive behavior and recurrence can characterize osteoblastoma and, rarely, malignant transformation has been described.[78, 79, 250]

Ossifying Fibroma (Fig. 74–16). This fibro-osseous lesion is closely related radiographically and pathologically to fibrous dysplasia and, possibly, adamantinoma. It is usually encountered in the second, third, and fourth decades of life, predominantly in women. Most ossifying fibromas arise in

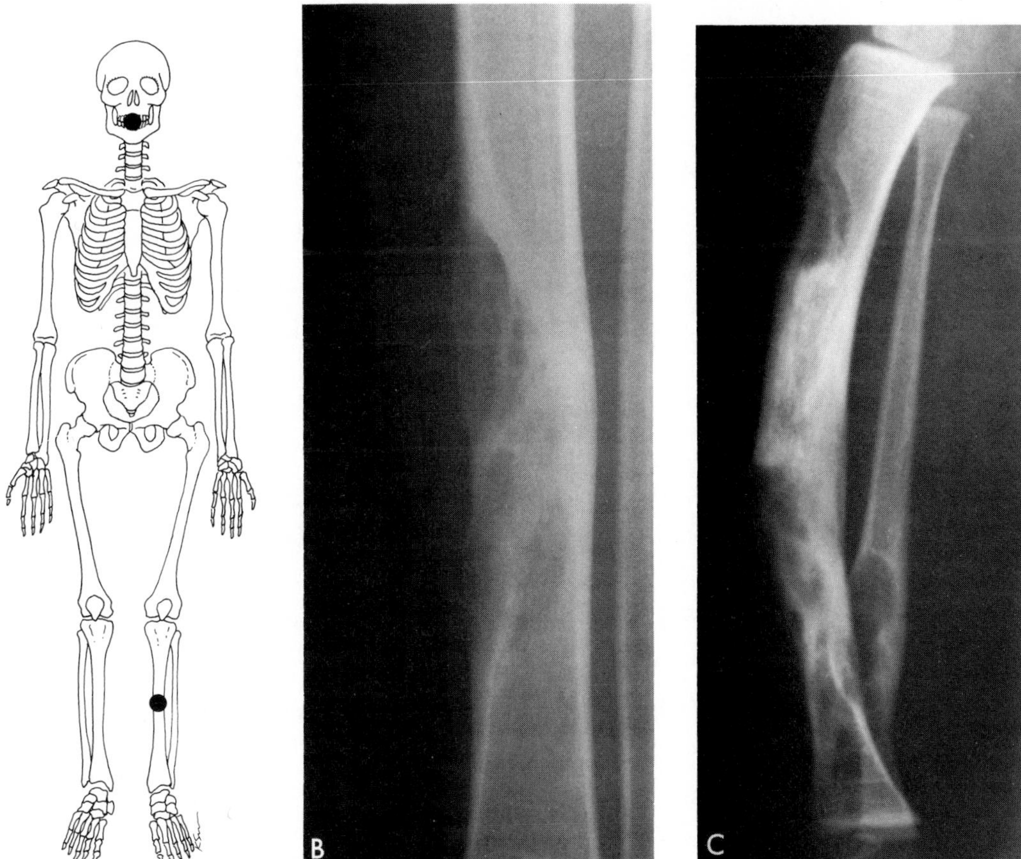

Figure 74–16. *Ossifying fibroma.*

A *Characteristic distribution.*

B *An eccentric and elongated radiolucent lesion with a ground-glass appearance is seen in the distal tibia. Osseous expansion and mild periosteal response are evident.*

C *In this 2 year old child, note the multiloculated, eccentric cortical lesion of the tibia with an additional lesion of the fibula. Other bones were not affected. Although the biopsy indicated only "fibrous" tissue, the appearance is compatible with osteofibrous dysplasia (see text). (**C**, Courtesy of Dr. J. E. L. Desautels, Calgary, Alberta.)*

the facial bones, particularly in the mandible and the maxilla, although the tumor can appear in a tubular bone, almost exclusively the tibia. Tibial involvement can be associated with adjacent abnormality of the fibula. On pathologic examination, the lesion is often well marginated and expansive, possessing cellular fibrous spindle cells. Osteoblastic activity may be pronounced, and a capsule is often evident. These latter histologic features may be helpful in distinguishing ossifying fibromas from fibrous dysplasia. On radiographs, lesions in the facial bones present as well-circumscribed, round or oval tumors with moderate expansion of the cortex.[80] The tumor matrix is usually of homogeneous density, without bony reaction, and the overlying cortex is intact. Occasionally, the lesion is sclerotic or possesses a mixed pattern of lysis and sclerosis. In the tubular bones, an eccentric, ground-glass lesion simulates the appearance of fibrous dysplasia.[81] Recurrences are frequent and may be associated with more extensive involvement of the bone, osseous expansion, and periosteal reaction. Lobulated lesions with cortical components may be identified.

Recently, an additional slowly progressive lesion of the tibia has been identified.[246, 247] This lesion, which is termed osteofibrous dysplasia, involves infants and children, and leads to anterior bowing of the lower leg, with a painless mass. Radiographs reveal a lucent, expansile cortical lesion of the lower diaphysis of the tibia with or without similar abnormality of the adjacent fibula (Fig. 74–16C). Bowing may be prominent. Histologically or radiographically osteofibrous dysplasia resembles other lesions, including ossifying fibroma, fibrous dysplasia, non-ossifying fibroma, and generalized fibromatosis.

Malignant Tumors

Classic Osteogenic Sarcoma (Fig. 74–17). Osteogenic sarcoma is a frequently occurring malignant tumor that is characterized histologically by a proliferating spindle cell stroma that produces osteoid or immature bone.[3, 82] Most patients with osteogenic sarcoma are in the second and third decades of life,[83-85] although cases in patients after the age of 50 years have also been identified.[86] Men are affected slightly more frequently than women, in a ratio of approximately 1.5:1. Pain and swelling, restriction of motion, and pyrexia can be evident as clinical manifestations of this neoplasm. The most typical sites of involvement are the tubular bones in the appendicular skeleton, particularly the femur (40 per cent), the tibia (16 per cent), and the humerus (15 per cent).[3] Nearly one half of all cases develop in osseous structures about the knee. However, any bone of the skeleton can be affected.[262] Examples of osteogenic sarcoma appearing at multiple sites are recorded. In some instances, this phenomenon represents the simultaneous occurrence of multiple foci of neoplasm, whereas in other instances, multiple foci originate as metastatic lesions from a single osteogenic sarcoma[87] or develop in a patient with Paget's disease. Multiple, simultaneously developing osteogenic sarcomas are often referred to as sclerosing osteogenic sarcoma and usually appear in the first decade of life.[88, 89] They may have a symmetric distribution, affecting the metaphyseal regions of tubular bones, where they appear as radiodense lesions. Flat bones such as those in the pelvis, thorax, and skull can be involved. Sclerosing osteogenic sarcoma has a uniformly poor prognosis, with rapid development of the lesion and early death of the patient. Occasionally, multiple osteogenic sarcomas can become evident in several bones at different times, each lesion behaving clinically and radiographically like a primary tumor.[90] These metachronous osteogenic sarcomas may represent sites of skeletal metastasis despite the absence of visceral evidence of metastases, or they may represent a multicentric origin of the sarcomatous tumor.

Radiographically, an osteogenic sarcoma usually arises eccentrically in the metaphysis of a tubular bone. It is associated with a motheaten pattern of bone destruction, cortical disruption, periostitis, and a soft tissue mass. Lytic areas represent sites of neoplastic osteoid tissue and are combined with sclerotic areas resulting from tumor bone formation. The classic radiographic picture may be modified in the presence of specific types of osteogenic sarcoma. For example, a telangiectatic osteogenic sarcoma,[91] characterized on gross pathologic examination by a cystic tumor and on histologic examination by aneurysmally dilated, blood-filled spaces, may be associated with a predominantly lytic lesion on the radiograph with little or no evidence of tumor bone formation. In other instances, an osteogenic sarcoma within the medullary canal may possess a relatively benign radiographic appearance characterized by a fairly well circumscribed radiodense focus[92] or a cyst-like expanded lesion.

Of interest, secondary lymph node or visceral deposits from osteogenic sarcoma may appear as ossified lesions on the radiograph,[93, 94] and pulmonary metastatic foci can be associated with a spontaneous pneumothorax.

Periosteal Osteogenic Sarcoma (Fig. 74–18). This rare variety of osteogenic sarcoma is most commonly observed in the second decade of life.[95-97] The tibia is the most frequently affected bone, followed in order of frequency by the femur. Metaphyseal or diaphyseal localization is seen. Although it resembles the more common parosteal (juxtacortical) osteogenic sarcoma, this tumor is limited to the periphery of the cortex. The medullary canal and endosteal margin of the cortex are normal. Periosteal osteogenic sarcomas are usually small, are associated with varying degrees of calcification and ossification, and produce cortical

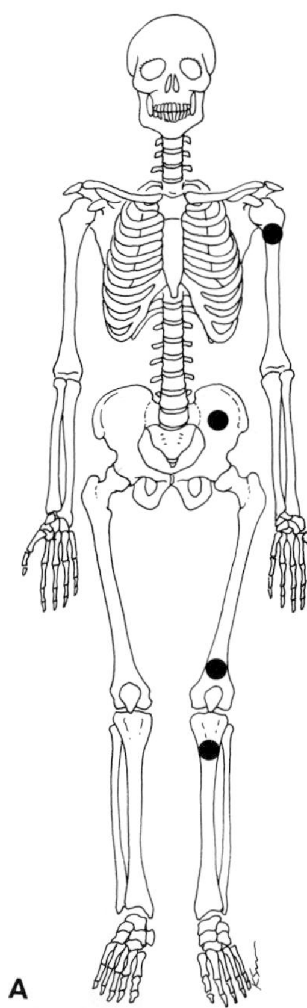

Figure 74–17. *Classic osteogenic sarcoma.*

A *Characteristic distribution.*

B *An elongated medullary lesion with a motheaten pattern of bone destruction is associated with erosion and penetration of the cortex and a soft tissue mass. Exuberant periosteal response is identified in the form of radiating osseous spicules and Codman's triangles. Ossifying tumor matrix can be seen.*

C *This osteogenic sarcoma of the proximal humerus has produced motheaten or permeative bone destruction and a large ossifying soft tissue mass.*

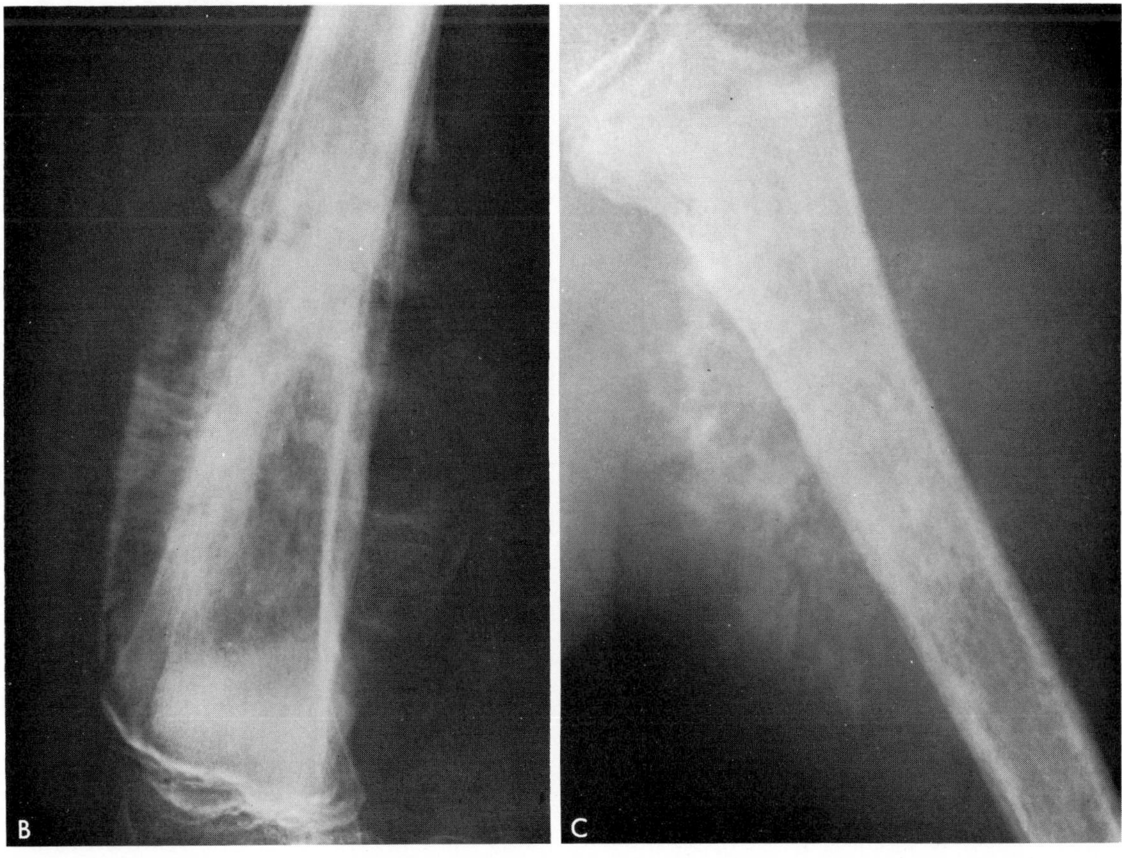

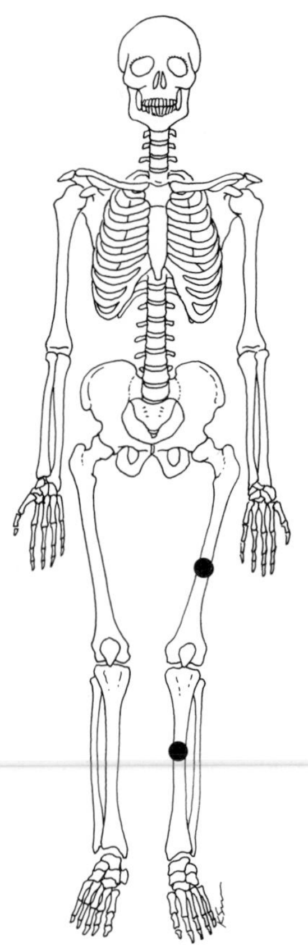

Figure 74–18. *Periosteal osteogenic sarcoma. Characteristic distribution.*

tubular bones, especially those around the knee. Diaphyseal extension of metaphyseal tumors may be identified, although a diaphyseal site of origin is unusual. The posterior aspect of the distal end of the femur is the most characteristic site of involvement, accounting for approximately 50 per cent of the lesions.[3] Other common sites of involvement are the tibia, humerus, radius, and ulna. These slowly growing lesions may produce few symptoms and signs for a long period of time. Gradually increasing pain and tenderness associated with swelling or a palpable mass can eventually be noted.

Radiographic features are quite characteristic.[101-103] Initially a lobulated soft tissue mass containing small foci of ossification is seen. The radiodense areas progress in number and size, particularly centrally within the lesion, and may eventually produce a homogeneously radiodense lesion. In 30 to 40 per cent of cases, this lesion is initially separated from the underlying bone by a thin radiolucent zone or cleavage plane. The cleavage plane may later be obliterated as the neoplasm attaches to and wraps around the

thickening and adjacent periosteal reaction. Radiating spicules of bone or a Codman's triangle can be seen. The tumor may spread into the soft tissues. Pathologically, periosteal osteogenic sarcoma is characterized by masses of abnormal-appearing cartilage and osteoid, which extend from the cortical surface into the adjacent soft tissue.

Parosteal (Juxtacortical) Osteogenic Sarcoma (Fig. 74–19). This neoplasm arises adjacent to the bone, in close relationship to the periosteum or parosteal connective tissue.[3] Its pathologic features vary considerably, depending upon the extent and appearance of fibrous, osseous, and cartilaginous elements; some neoplasms possess benign-appearing fibrous stroma, whereas others reveal frankly sarcomatous stroma that is actively forming new bone.[98-100] Similarly, the osseous and cartilaginous stromata within the lesion vary greatly in their appearance. As opposed to the situation in myositis ossificans, in which the periphery of the lesion may appear quite mature, it is the peripheral areas of the parosteal osteogenic sarcoma that frequently demonstrate the greatest cellular activity.

Parosteal osteogenic sarcomas are most common in the third and fourth decades of life and are of equal frequency in men and women. The most typical skeletal location is about the metaphyses of the long

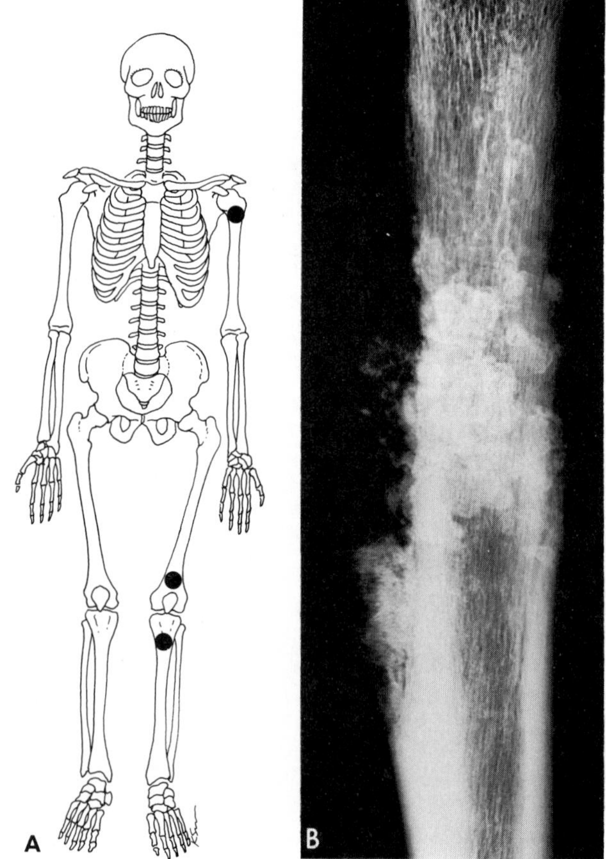

Figure 74–19. *Parosteal (juxtacortical) osteogenic sarcoma.*

A *Characteristic distribution.*

B *A specimen radiograph reveals a parosteal osteogenic sarcoma of the proximal tibia. Note the ossific foci within the soft tissues adjacent to the cortex. Cortical excavation and periosteal response can be identified.*

parent bone. Adjacent periostitis is unusual. Although the prognosis of this lesion is better than that in classic osteogenic sarcoma, cortical infiltration and medullary involvement, which are evident pathologically in some cases, indicate a poor prognosis.[251]

Tumors Arising from or Forming Fibrous Connective Tissue

BENIGN TUMORS

Nonossifying Fibroma (Fig. 74–20). Nonossifying fibroma and the related fibrocortical defect are common lesions composed histologically of whorled bundles of connective tissue cells. The cellularity of the stroma and the prominence of multinucleated giant cells and foamy xanthomatous cells vary among the lesions.[2, 3] The giant cells and the spindly stromal cells can contain hemosiderin. Nonossifying fibromas appear regularly in children in the first and second decades of life, and it has been suggested that 30 to 40 per cent of normal children older than 2 years of age have one or more lesions.[104] Their infrequency in adults supports the concept that most lesions heal by being replaced by normal bone, although some become quite large and may lead to pathologic fracture.[107] It is these latter lesions that may produce local symptoms and signs and that may require orthopedic intervention. An association of nonossifying fibromas and neurofibromatosis has been suggested.[254]

Nonossifying fibromas are most frequently discovered in the metaphyseal regions of one (75 per cent) or more (25 per cent) long tubular bones, especially the femur, tibia, and fibula.[105, 106] Many of the lesions are located about the knees; fewer than 10 per cent are found in the bones of the upper extremity. They possess diagnostic radiographic characteristics, including an eccentric location in the metaphysis frequently separated slightly from the growth plate, an elongated radiolucent lesion with trabeculation and a sclerotic rim, and cortical thinning or expansion. Although they are usually less than 2 cm in size, they occasionally become larger and may become located in the diaphysis. Sclerotic foci may appear which eventually obliterate portions of the lesion.

Periosteal (Juxtacortical) Desmoid (Fig. 74–21). A periosteal desmoid represents a tumor-like alteration of the periosteum characterized by fibroblastic proliferation analogous to that which occurs in a desmoplastic fibroma.[108] It is usually apparent in patients between the ages of 15 and 20 years and may show a slight male predilection. Almost all cases are localized to the posteromedial cortex of the distal end of the femur, adjacent to the femoral condyle.[109-111] Most patients are asymptomatic, although occasionally mild pain is present. A history of localized trauma is frequent. The radiographic characteristics of a periosteal desmoid include soft tissue swelling, a saucer-like radiolucent defect of the cortex with adjacent sclerosis, and periostitis. The periosteal response can be exuberant and irregular in outline, leading to an appearance which, for the radiologist unfamiliar with the lesion, might be mistaken for a malignant tumor.

The periosteal desmoid is probably not a neoplasm but a reaction to trauma occurring at the musculotendinous insertion site of the adductor magnus muscle.[110, 252]

Desmoplastic Fibroma (Fig. 74–22). This is a rare benign neoplasm characterized by abundant collagen formation and the absence of significant cellularity and pleomorphism.[3] The histologic characteristics of this lesion resemble those in periosteal and soft tissue desmoids, central fibromas and nonodontogenic fibromas of the jaws, and juvenile aponeurotic fibromas. Desmoplastic fibromas are most frequent in the second and third decades of life and occur in men and women with similar frequency. Although virtually any bone may be affected, the most common sites of involvement are the innominate bones, mandible, tubular bones, particularly the humerus and tibia, and scapula. In tubular bones, metaphyseal localization is more typical than diaphyseal or epiphyseal localization. Clinical manifestations include slowly progressive pain and local tenderness or acute pain related to a pathologic fracture (approximately 10 per cent of lesions).

The radiographic features indicate the presence of an aggressive lesion of variable size.[112-114] Desmoplastic fibromas are osteolytic in nature, producing destruction of medullary bone with cortical erosion and expansion, trabeculation, and pathologic fracture. Bone reaction is unusual, although mild adjacent sclerosis can be seen. Periostitis is rare. The radiographic alterations can simulate those of a malignant process, especially a fibrosarcoma or an osteolytic type of an osteogenic sarcoma. Local recurrence of the tumor is not uncommon.

MALIGNANT TUMORS

Fibrosarcoma (Fig. 74–23). This malignant tumor of bone is characterized histologically by poorly differentiated to well-differentiated fibrous tissue proliferation that is not associated with the production of cartilage, osteoid, or bone. The appearance of the tumor varies from a well-organized herringbone pattern of proliferation to one that exhibits less organization and more anaplasia of fibroblasts, with pleomorphism, abnormal mitoses, and giant cells. Hemorrhagic, necrotic, and calcific foci can be apparent as well.

Fibrosarcomas of bone are most frequent in the third, fourth, fifth, and sixth decades of life, affecting men and women with equal frequency. The most frequent sites of involvement are the pelvis, facial bones, and long tubular bones, particularly those about the knee, although the selection of a specific site is influenced by the type of tumor that is being

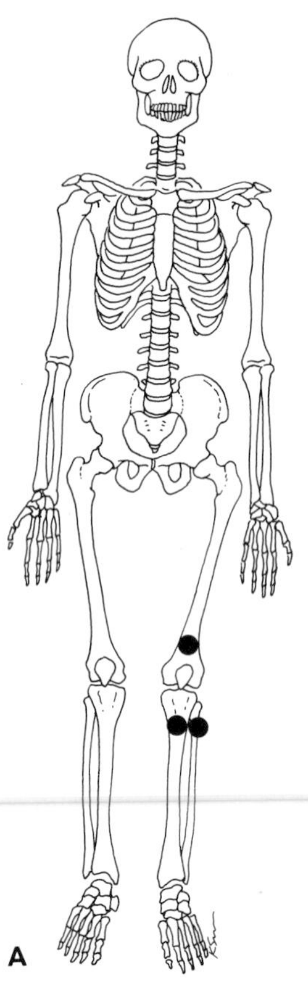

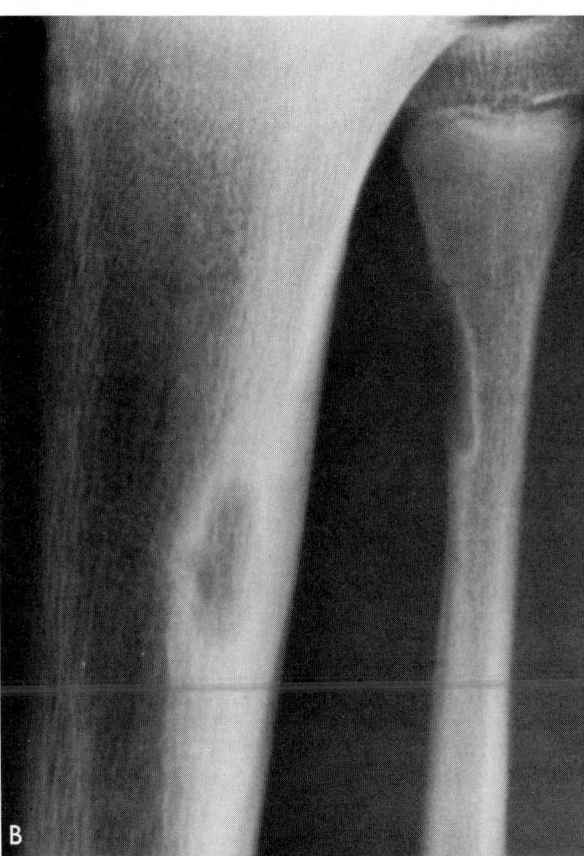

Figure 74–20. *Nonossifying fibroma.*

A *Characteristic distribution.*

B *Nonossifying fibromas or cortical defects are identified in the proximal tibia and fibula. Note their eccentric location and the geographic bone destruction. The nonossifying fibroma of the fibula is located at a short distance from the neighboring growth plate.*

C *A large, nonossifying fibroma of the distal tibia has produced deformity of the adjacent fibula. Note the eccentric location, geographic bone destruction, radiolucent lesion with lobulated trabeculation, internal sclerotic border, and cortical expansion. This lesion is located at a short distance from the neighboring growth plate.*

D *This large, nonossifying fibroma of the distal femur has led to a spontaneous fracture. Its upper border indicates its eccentric location.*

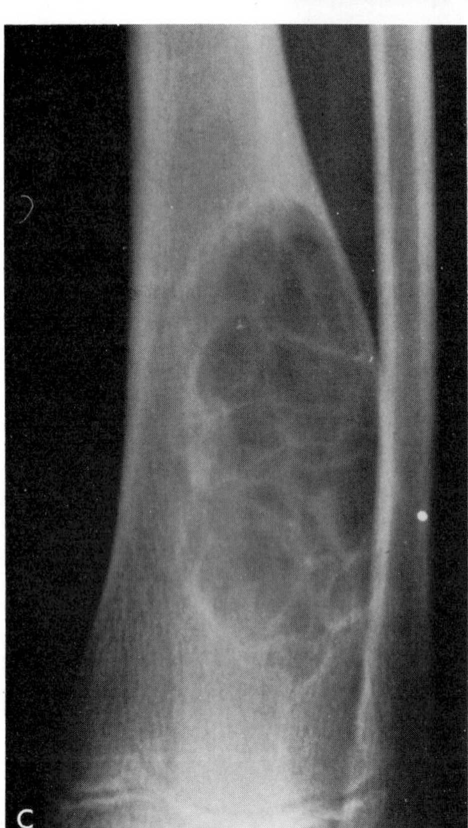

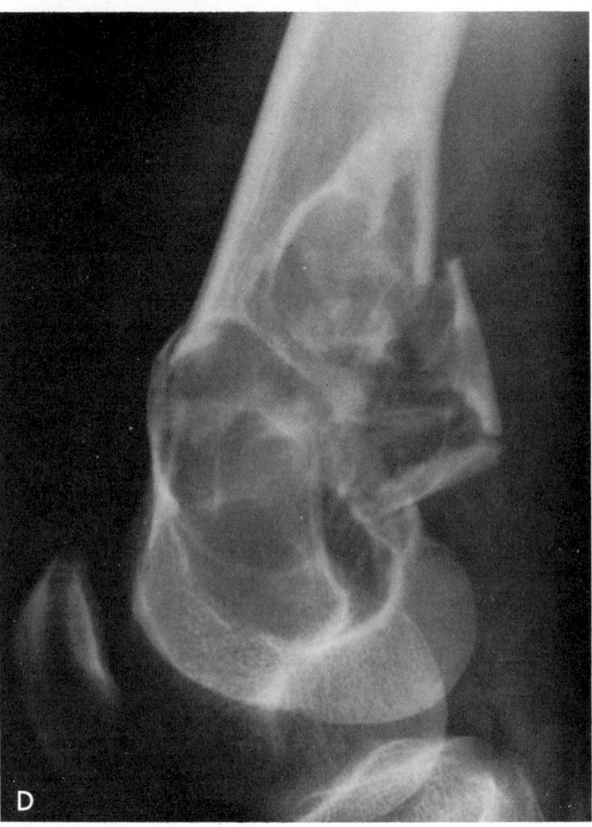

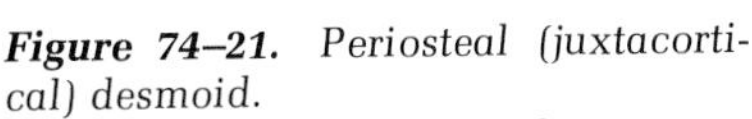

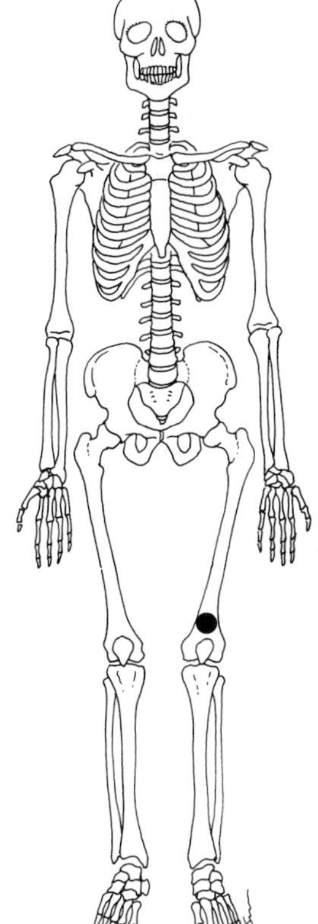

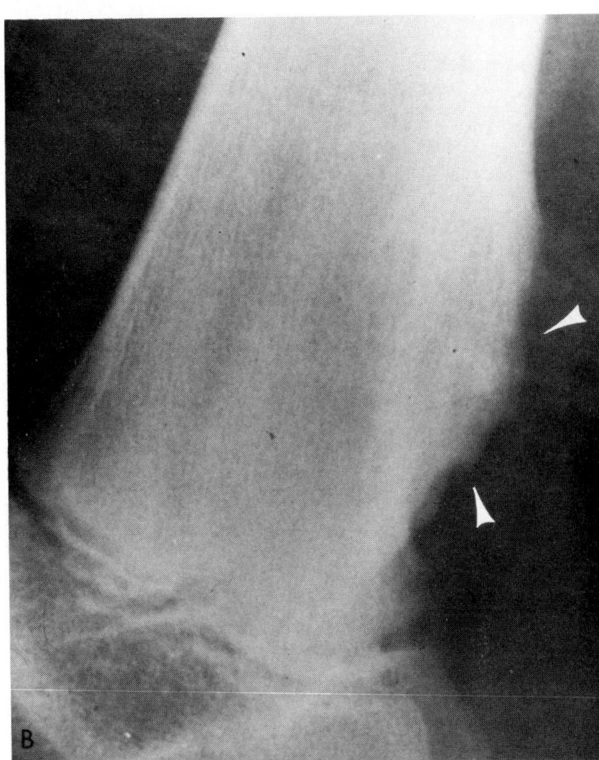

Figure 74–21. Periosteal (juxtacortical) desmoid.

A *Characteristic distribution.*

B *A lateral radiograph of the distal femur demonstrates the typical location and appearance of a periosteal desmoid (arrowheads). It involves the posteromedial cortex of the distal end of the femur and is associated with a periosteal response creating an expanded and irregular osseous contour. This response is probably related to traction at the site of osseous insertion of the adductor magnus muscle.*

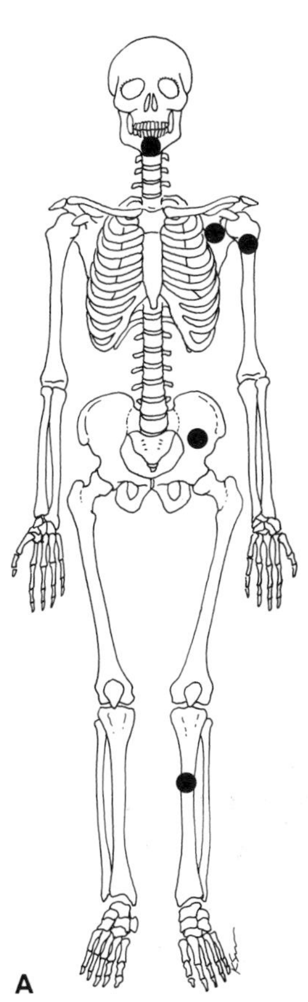

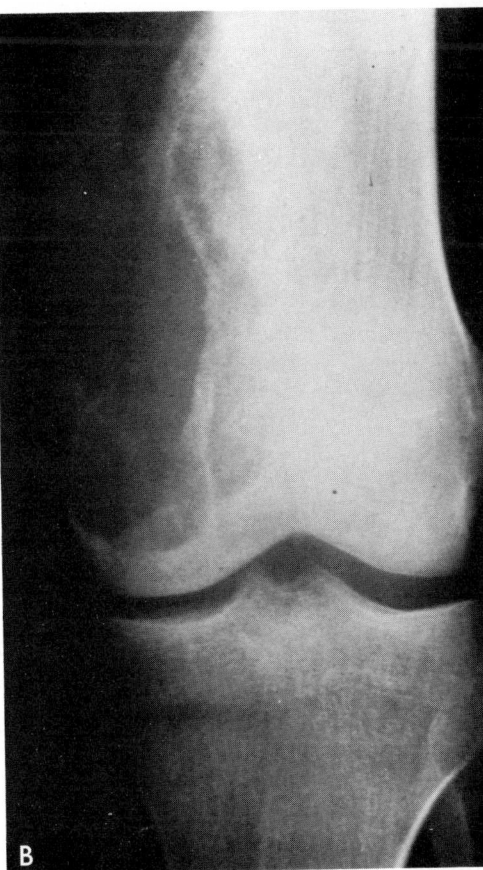

Figure 74–22. Desmoplastic fibroma.

A *Characteristic distribution.*

B *An aggressive lesion of the metaphyseal region of the distal femur can be identified. It is associated with an eccentric location, motheaten pattern of bone destruction, cortical erosion, and a soft tissue mass. No significant sclerosis is apparent.*

(Courtesy of Dr. Robert Freiberger, New York, New York.)

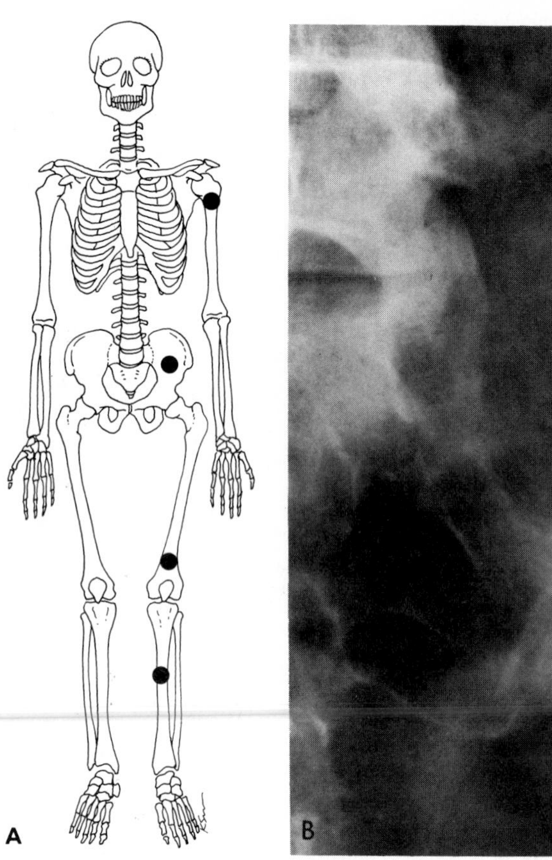

Figure 74–23. *Fibrosarcoma.*
A *Characteristic distribution.*
B *An osteolytic lesion of the ilium and adjacent sacrum is seen. No bony reaction can be identified.*

encountered; for example, fibrosarcomas of medullary bone (approximately 67 per cent) commonly localize in the tubular bones, whereas those in periosteal locations (approximately 33 per cent) have a more widespread distribution.[3] Of the tubular bones, the femur, tibia, and humerus are most commonly involved, and diametaphyseal localization is typical. Pain and swelling of several months' duration are usually present.

Fibrosarcomas are characterized radiographically by lytic foci of a motheaten pattern or, less frequently, permeative bone destruction and by little sclerosis or periostitis.[115] In fact, the degree of bone destruction and the absence of osseous reaction can be striking. Cortical destruction and soft tissue masses are seen. Visible tumor matrix is not evident, although dystrophic calcification may be encountered. Solitary bone lesions are the rule, although multiple or diffuse tumors are occasionally reported,[116] an appearance that may also indicate skeletal metastases from a single neoplastic focus.[117]

Tumors of Histiocytic or Fibrohistiocytic Origin

Locally Aggressive Tumors

Giant Cell Tumor (Fig. 74–24). This relatively common and locally aggressive lesion is composed of connective tissue, stromal cells, and giant cells, which vary in amount and appearance (Table 74–3). The stromal cells are mononuclear, spindle-shaped or ovoid cells with indistinct margins. The multinucleated giant cells are interspersed among the mononuclear cells. The proportions of mononuclear and giant cells are variable and may be utilized to classify the lesion, although such tissue typing is unreliable as a guide to prognosis. In fact, no consistently predictable microscopic features are available to forecast the "aggressiveness" of the lesion, its propensity to recur, or its malignant behavior.[3] Malignant transformation of a "benign" giant cell tumor generally occurs within the first five years, and the resulting neoplasm may be classified as a fibrosarcoma or osteogenic sarcoma. To further complicate accurate clinical appraisal and treatment of giant cell tumors, primary malignant giant cell tumors and "benign" metastasizing giant cell tumors are also recognized.[3, 118]

Giant cell tumors are usually discovered in the third and fourth decades of life, although they may appear in older patients as well as younger individuals who have not yet ceased growing.[119-122] The incidence of all types of giant cell tumors is approximately the same in men and women; there is a female preponderance (3:2) with regard to benign giant cell tumors and a male preponderance (3:1) with regard to malignant giant cell tumors.[3] Giant cell tumors are usually observed at an end of a long tubular bone, especially the distal aspect of the femur and radius

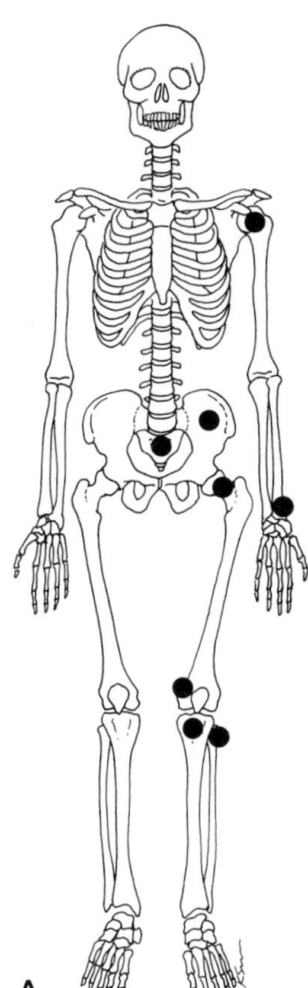

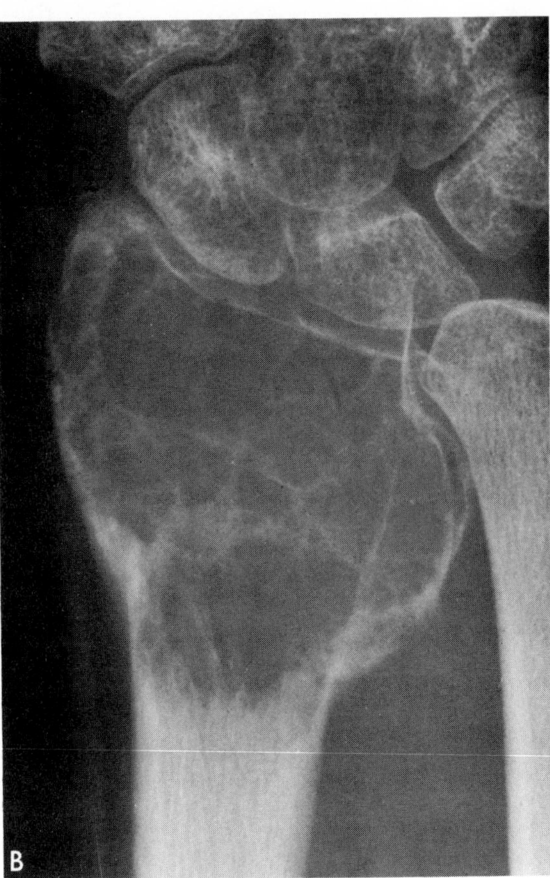

Figure 74–24. Giant cell tumor.

A Characteristic distribution.

B A typical giant cell tumor of the distal radius is evident. It is radiolucent, possesses a trabeculated architecture, and extends to the subchondral bone. The cortex is expanded.

C In this example, a giant cell tumor has produced destruction of a large segment of the patella.

D An aggressive giant cell tumor of the distal femur has penetrated the posterior cortex and produced a large soft tissue mass. Note that the lesion extends to the subchondral bone of the femur.

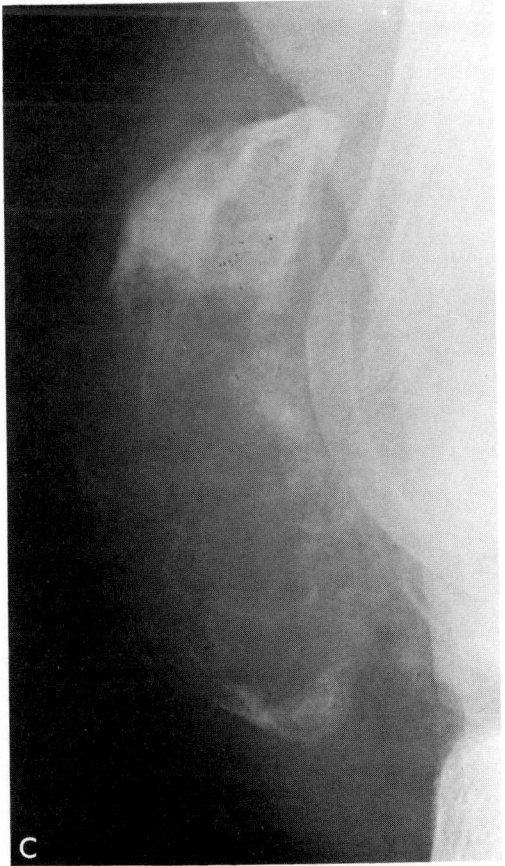

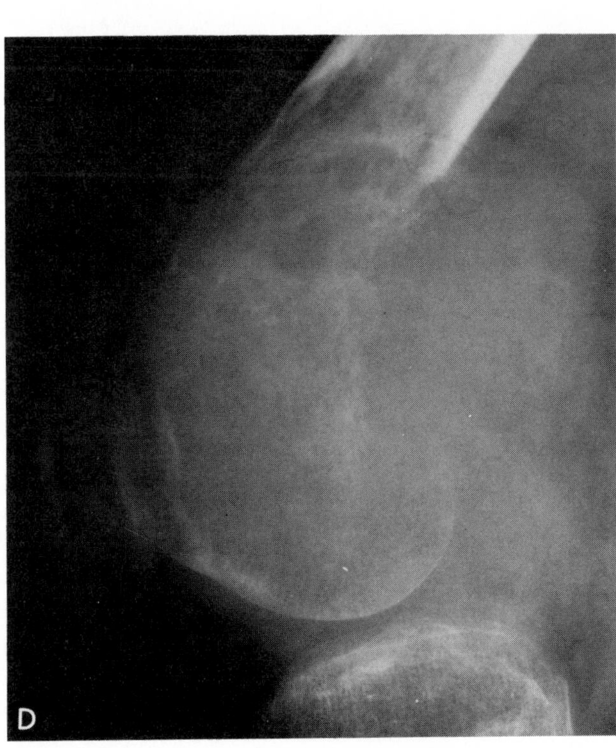

and the proximal aspect of the tibia, humerus, fibula, and femur. Approximately 50 to 60 per cent of tumors are found in the bones about the knee. Flat bone involvement is also seen, particularly of the pelvis and sacrum.[129] Giant cell tumors of the vertebral column above the sacrum are unusual; in the spine, either the vertebral bodies or posterior elements can be affected. In the hand, giant cell tumors may be observed in the metacarpal head or adjacent portion of the proximal phalanx.[128] A single bone is generally involved; however, occasional examples of giant cell tumors affecting multiple sites have been documented,[123-126, 130] although in such a situation, the possibility of hyperparathyroidism with brown tumors must be considered. In any site, pain, swelling, and limitation of motion may be identified, frequently associated with a history of trauma.

The radiographic appearance of a giant cell tumor is highly characteristic. In a long tubular bone, an eccentric osteolytic lesion extending to subchondral bone is seen, producing cortical thinning and expansion, and possessing a delicate trabecular pattern. The margins of the lesion may be well or poorly defined, although an extensive sclerotic rim and periostitis are generally not evident. Occasionally, a giant cell tumor may extend from one bone across an articulation to involve a neighboring bone. The epiphyseal involvement and extension to subarticular bone are the findings that represent the most typical features of a giant cell tumor. These findings suggest to most observers that the tumor should be considered epiphyseal in origin, although others regard them as metaphyseal in origin, citing the occurrence of metaphyseal giant cell tumors in the immature skeleton prior to closure of the growth plate.[127] In any age group, giant cell tumors may involve a large part of the metaphysis and even a portion of the diaphysis. The aggressive nature of giant cell tumors must also be recognized. Frequently, they extend into the adjacent soft tissues, creating apparent disruption of the cortex. The radiographic characteristics are a poor guide to the histologic composition and clinical behavior of the lesion.

In flat bones, such as those of the pelvis, an "epiphyseal" focus is again favored. Thus, giant cell tumors may originate adjacent to the sacroiliac or hip

Table 74–3
DIFFERENTIAL DIAGNOSIS OF GIANT CELL LESIONS OF BONE*

	Most Common Age Group	Location in Bone	Radiologic Appearance	Gross Features	Microscopic Features	
					GIANT CELLS	STROMAL CELLS
Giant cell tumor	Third and fourth decades	Epiphysis	Eccentric expanded radiolucency	Fleshy soft tissue	Abundant number uniformly distributed	Plump and polyhedral with abundant cytoplasm
Nonossifying fibroma	First decade	Metaphysis	Eccentric oval defects	Fleshy soft tissue	Focal distribution, small with few nuclei	Slender and spindly with little cytoplasm
Aneurysmal bone cyst	First and second decades	Vertebral column or metaphysis of long bone	Eccentric blow-out "soap bubble" appearance	Cavity filled with blood	Focally around vascular channels	Large vascular channels; slender to plump cells with hemosiderin granules
Brown tumor of hyperparathyroidism	Any age	Anywhere in bone	Absent lamina dura of teeth	Fleshy tissue or cystic spaces	Focal around hemosiderin pigment	Fibrous stroma with slender cells
Unicameral bone cyst	First and second decades	Metaphysis (proximal humerus)	Trabeculations in radiolucency	Cyst filled with clear fluid	Focal around cholesterol clefts	Cyst wall is fibrous tissue
Chondroblastoma	Second decade	Epiphysis	Radiolucency with spotty opacities	Firm to fleshy tissue	Few and focal	Large, plump, and round cells with pericellular calcifications
Fibrous dysplasia	First and second decades	Metaphysis (proximal femur)	Ground-glass appearance	Firm and gritty	Few and focal	Woven bone and fibrous tissue
Giant cell reparative granuloma	Second and third decades	Maxilla and mandible	Radiolucent focus	Soft fleshy tissue	Abundant around hemosiderin pigment	Slender or plump cells
Ossifying fibroma	Second and third decades	Maxilla and mandible	Radiopaque	Bony hard tissue	Few and focal	Lamellar bony trabeculae in fibrous tissue
Osteogenic sarcoma	Second and third decades	Metaphysis	Radiolucent	Soft or firm	Focal distribution	Malignant spindle cells with direct osteoid formation
Chondromyxoid fibroma	Second and third decades	Metaphysis	Eccentric with expanded cortex	Soft to firm	Focal distribution	Chondroid and myxoid components
Osteoblastoma	Second and third decades	Vertebral column	Radiolucent or dense	Soft to firm	Focal distribution	Abundant osteoblasts between osteoid trabeculae

*Modified from Ghandur-Mnaymneh L, Mnaymneh WA: J Med Liban *25*:91, 1972.

articulation. Sacral and spinal giant cell tumors are relatively nonspecific on radiographic examination.[129]

MALIGNANT TUMORS

Malignant Fibrous Histiocytoma (Malignant Fibrous Xanthoma) (Fig. 74–25). This rare malignant bone tumor of probable histiocytic origin consists of densely collagenized fibrous areas adjacent to foci of poorly differentiated, spindle-shaped fibrogenic cells, with additional cellular elements, including xanthomatous histiocytic cells.[3] Inflammatory cells, including lymphocytes, plasma cells, and eosinophils, can also be evident.[131-136]

The ages of patients with malignant fibrous histiocytomas vary; subjects may be in the first through eighth decades of life, although the average age is approximately 50 years. Men are affected more frequently than women. Clinical findings consist of local pain and a soft tissue mass; the duration of these findings is varied, although rapid soft tissue enlargement, perhaps related to a pathologic fracture, can be evident. Indeed, pathologic fractures are quite common, occurring in as many as 50 per cent of lesions.[132] The most common sites of involvement, in descending order of frequency, are the femur, tibia, humerus, ribs, and craniofacial bones.[3]

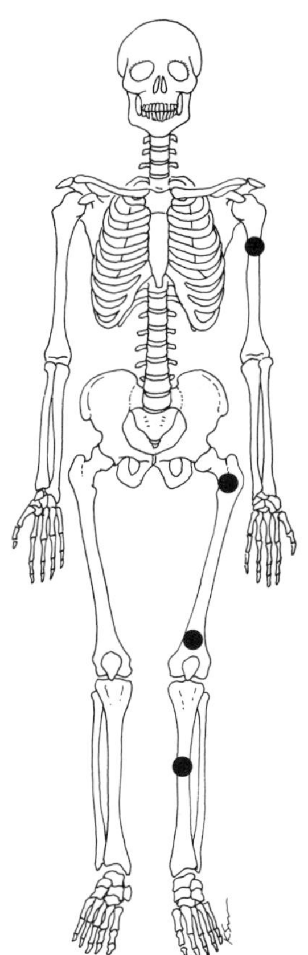

Figure 74–25. *Malignant fibrous histiocytoma. Characteristic distribution.*

The roentgenographic appearance is generally not specific. Osteolytic lesions predominate; they can be from 2.5 to 10.0 cm in diameter and frequently appear smaller on radiographic examination than on pathologic examination. In the long tubular bones, these lesions are most frequent in the metaphyseal region, with secondary extension into the diaphyseal and epiphyseal areas. Ill-defined margins and cortical destruction or permeation are typical. Periosteal and endosteal bone production is infrequent in the absence of a pathologic fracture. Rarely, more extensive sclerosis or irregular calcification may be seen. A soft tissue mass of variable size is commonly detected.

Tumors of Fatty Tissue Origin

BENIGN TUMORS

Intraosseous Lipoma (Fig. 74–26). Intraosseous lipomas are rare benign lesions arising within the bone marrow and containing mature fat cells without evidence of cellular atypism. Bony trabeculae may be interspersed within the fat, and surrounding areas of bone infarction may be identified. The pathogenesis of this lesion is debated. Some investigators believe intraosseous lipomas represent tumors, whereas others regard them as a degenerative phenomenon related to trauma or infection. The ages of individuals with intraosseous lipomas show wide variations, and both men and women are affected with approximately equal frequency. The tumor may localize at almost any skeletal site, including the tubular bones (especially the tibia, fibula, humerus, and femur), skull, mandible, sacrum, ribs, and calcaneus.[137-142] In tubular bones, a metaphyseal localization is favored. Spinal involvement is unusual. Radiologically, a well-defined radiolucent lesion is observed. Trabeculae within the lesion may produce a loculated or septated appearance. Cortical expansion is not infrequent, but cortical disruption, periostitis, and a soft tissue mass are unusual. Calcific or ossific foci within the lesion have been identified, particularly in those lipomas that arise within the calcaneus.[261]

Parosteal Lipoma (Fig. 74–27). This rare lesion arises adjacent to a bone, in intimate relationship with the periosteum.[143] It is firmly attached to the subjacent cortex, and consists of lobulated fatty tissue with intervening fibrous tissue on histologic examination. Its precise nature and manner of development are unknown. These lesions show no specific age or sex predilection. Uusually a long tubular bone is affected, most commonly the femur, humerus, or tibia. On radiographic examination, a radiolucent soft tissue mass containing linear and curvilinear osseous spicules is seen. Adjacent periostitis may be evident (see Fig. 74–45).

MALIGNANT TUMORS

Intraosseous Liposarcoma. Liposarcoma originating in bone is distinctly unusual despite the fact

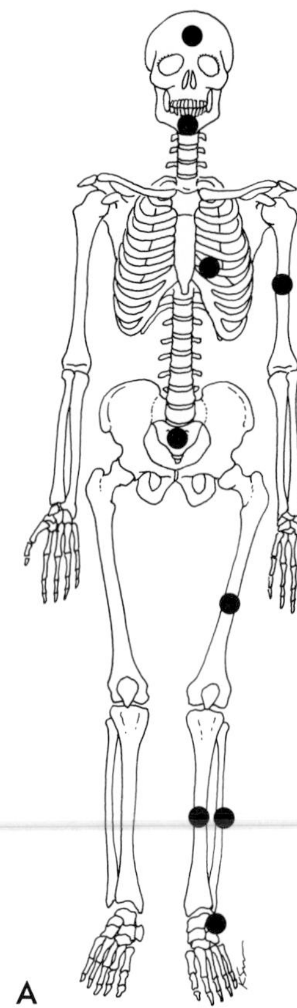

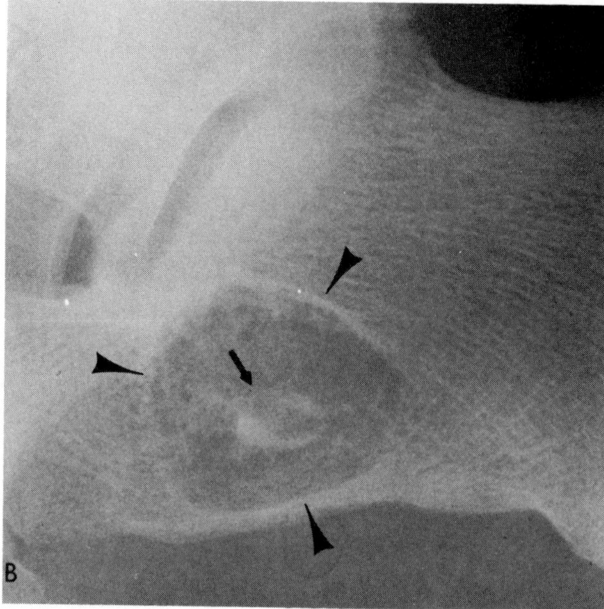

Figure 74–26. Intraosseous lipoma.
A *Characteristic distribution.*
B *A radiolucent lesion (arrowheads) of the calcaneus is associated with a central radiodense focal area (arrow). Although these lesions are commonly interpreted as lipomas, their relationship to solitary bone cysts, which occur in the same area of the calcaneus, is questioned.*

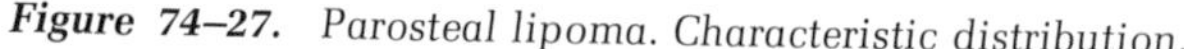

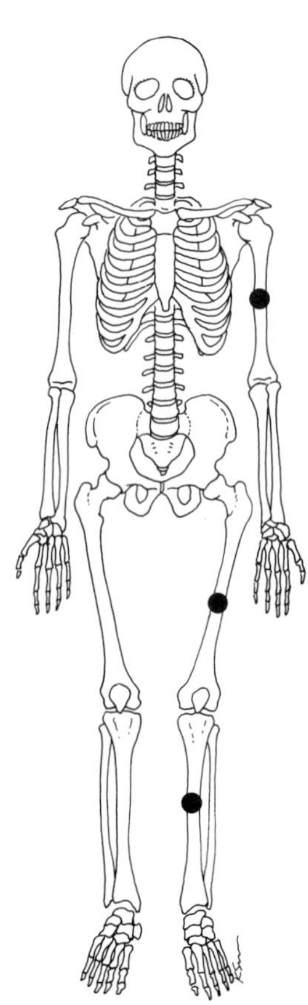

Figure 74–27. Parosteal lipoma. Characteristic distribution.

that bone marrow is rich in adipose tissue.[144, 248] Histologically, these lesions are composed of large fat-containing cells with vacuolated cytoplasm and hyperchromatic nucleii. Tubular or flat bones may be involved. The radiographic appearance is not diagnostic, consisting of an osteolytic lesion that may be well or poorly defined.[145, 146]

Tumors of Vascular Origin

Benign Tumors

Hemangioma (Fig. 74–28). Hemangiomas of bone are lesions composed of vascular channels that are cavernous, capillary, or venous in type. Cavernous hemangiomas consist of large vessels and sinuses interspersed among trabeculae or embedded in a connective tissue matrix; capillary hemangiomas are composed of fine capillary loops[147]; and venous hemangiomas contain thick-walled venous vessels intermixed with arterioles, capillaries, or large-caliber feeding vessels that are lined by endothelial cells.[3] The origin of hemangiomas is contested; they are variously regarded as benign neoplasms or congenital vascular malformations. The lesion is brown or red in color on gross pathologic examination and consists of a cystic space containing or surrounded by thickened osseous trabeculae. It is these trabeculae that produce a "honeycomb" or "spoke-wheel" appearance on the radiograph that is virtually diagnostic.

Hemangiomas are usually identified in middle-aged patients, particularly those in the fourth and fifth decades of life. Women are affected almost twice as frequently as men. Although they are asymptomatic in most cases, hemangiomas may be associated with soft tissue swelling or pain, particularly in the presence of a pathologic fracture. Vertebral hemangiomas may extend into the spinal canal, leading to neurologic symptoms and signs.

Single lesions predominate, although examples of multiple primary hemangiomas of bone are recorded.[148] The two most common sites of involvement are the vertebrae and the skull or facial bones. In the spine, changes predominate in the thoracic segment and in the vertebral bodies in comparison to the posterior elements. In this location, a coarse vertical trabecular pattern is identified in the vertebral body that may extend into the pedicles and laminae. Soft tissue and intraspinal extension of tumor or secondary hemorrhage can produce paraspinal masses.[149] Vertebral fracture is unusual. Hemangioma of the craniofacial bones predominates in the cranial vault or mandible. A radiolucent, slightly expansile, and well-defined lesion is typically accompanied by a radiating trabecular pattern.

Hemangiomas in other locations are rare. The innominate bones, ribs, and clavicle can be affected. In tubular bones, a metaphyseal or diaphyseal focus is preferred, although epiphyseal lesions also occur. Intracortical and periosteal hemangiomas have been described.[150, 151, 259] In any extravertebral location, occasional examples with a motheaten pattern of bone destruction, sclerosis, significant osseous expansion, soft tissue extension, or radiating periostitis can resemble changes in a malignant process.

Glomus Tumor (Fig. 74–29). A glomus tumor (angioglomoid tumor) is a rare benign lesion of bone composed of cells intimately associated with vascular structures and derived from the neuromyoarterial glomus.[3] Although patients of any age can be affected, many are in the fourth and fifth decades of life. Pain may be a prominent symptom. Intraosseous glomus tumors appear as lytic lesions and are almost invariably located in the terminal phalanx.[159, 160]

Lymphangioma (Fig. 74–30). Lymphangiomas are composed of dilated lymphatic vessels and rarely may produce single or multiple intraosseous lesions.[152-154] The osseous defect is generally medullary in location, is lytic in nature, can affect flat[260] or tubular bones, and may lead to pathologic fracture. Children or adolescents are usually affected, although older patients with lymphangiomas of bone have also been described. A diffuse form of the disease, lymphangiomatosis, is recognized, in which multiple cystic skeletal lesions can be combined with widespread soft tissue abnormalities and involvement of other organ systems.[155-157] Associated abnormalities include lymphedema and chylous pleural effusions. Lymphangiography may document the lymphatic nature of the skeletal changes, with intraosseous accumulation of contrast material.[158]

Cystic Angiomatosis (Fig. 74–31). This rare skeletal disorder, which may be related to lymphangiomatosis of bone, is characterized by diffuse cystic skeletal lesions that are frequently combined with visceral involvement.[161-165] It is the latter involvement that is usually responsible for the patient's symptoms and signs, although the skeletal lesions themselves can produce pain and swelling, especially if a pathologic fracture has developed or if the neighboring soft tissues are also altered. Patients are usually in the first, second, or third decade of life. Men are affected about twice as often as women. The femur, pelvis, ribs, humerus, skull, vertebrae, scapula, tibia, and clavicle, in descending order of frequency, are most typically involved.[165] Other sites of disease are also noted, with predilection for the axial skeleton, although changes in the tubular bones of the hands and feet are probably rare. On radiographic examination, well-defined lytic lesions are usually seen, surrounded by a rim of sclerotic bone. Medullary involvement predominates, and cortical invasion and periostitis are unusual. In some cases, the lesions appear sclerotic, simulating skeletal metastases from prostatic carcinoma. Histologically, a cystic lesion is identified, frequently lined by endothelial cells and containing either erythrocytes or a homogeneous, pink-staining coagulum.[161] The cysts are dilated vascular channels of blood vessel or lymphatic origin.

Text continued on page 2676

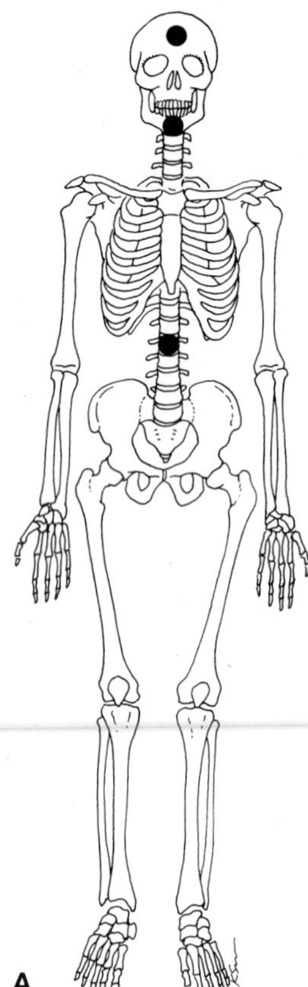

Figure 74–28. Hemangioma.

A *Characteristic distribution.*

B *A typical hemangioma of a vertebral body is demonstrated. Note the radiolucency of the vertebra and the accentuation of vertical trabeculation. The neighboring vertebral body possessed a similar hemangioma.*

C *A large expansile lesion of the mandible represents a hemangioma. Note the radiating trabeculation within the lesion, typical of a hemangioma.*

Illustration continued on the opposite page

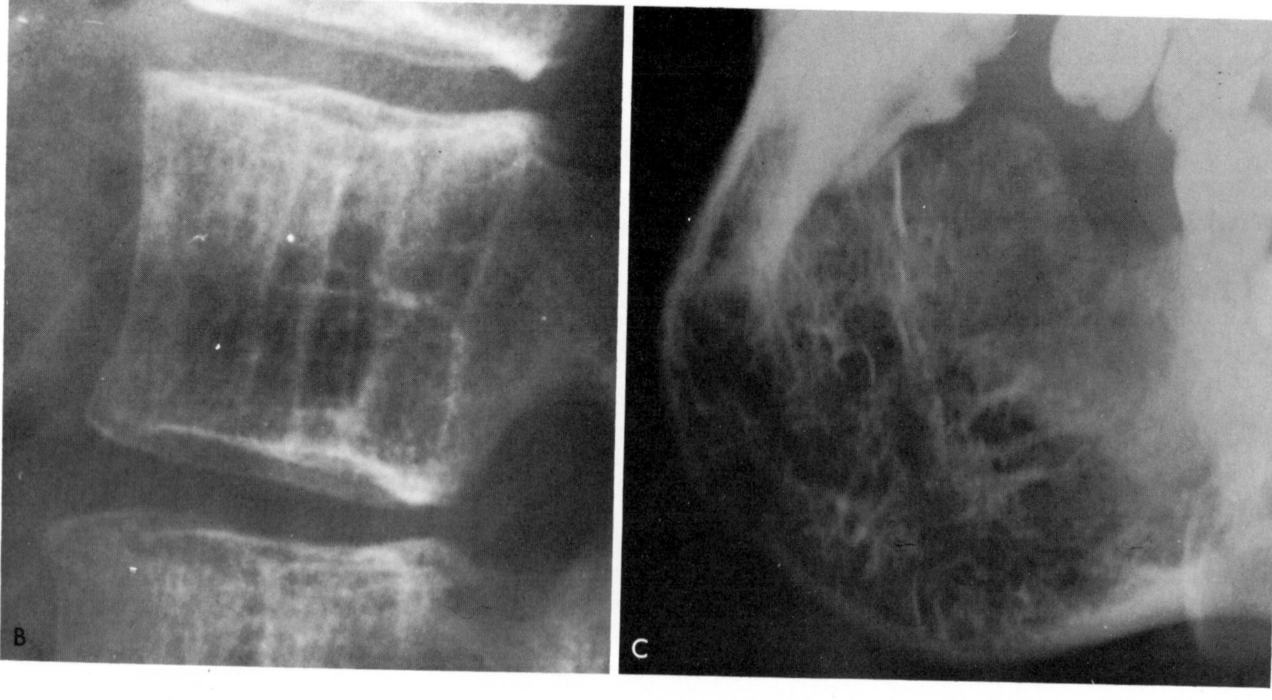

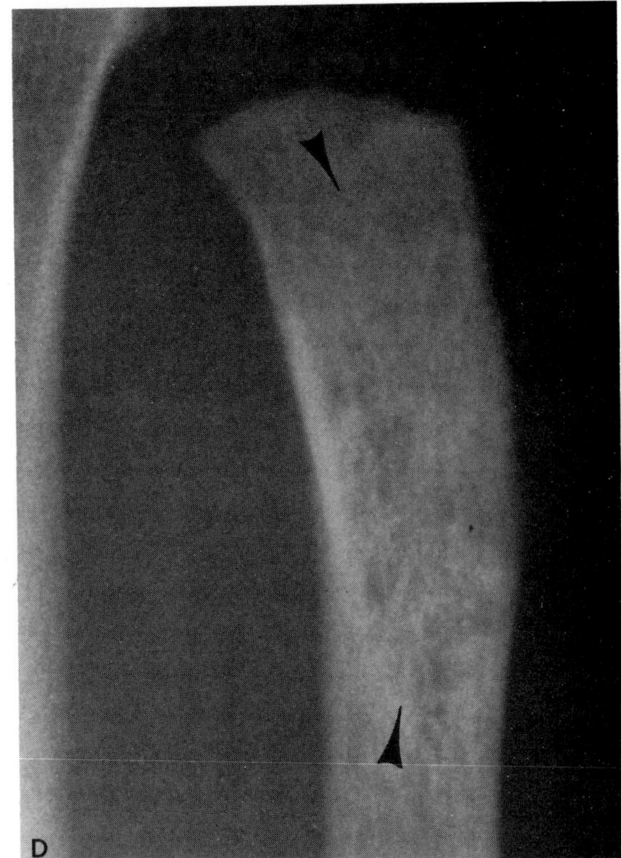

Figure 74–28. Continued
D *This hemangioma of the ulna has produced a coarsened trabecular pattern (arrowheads). Mild osseous expansion is evident.*

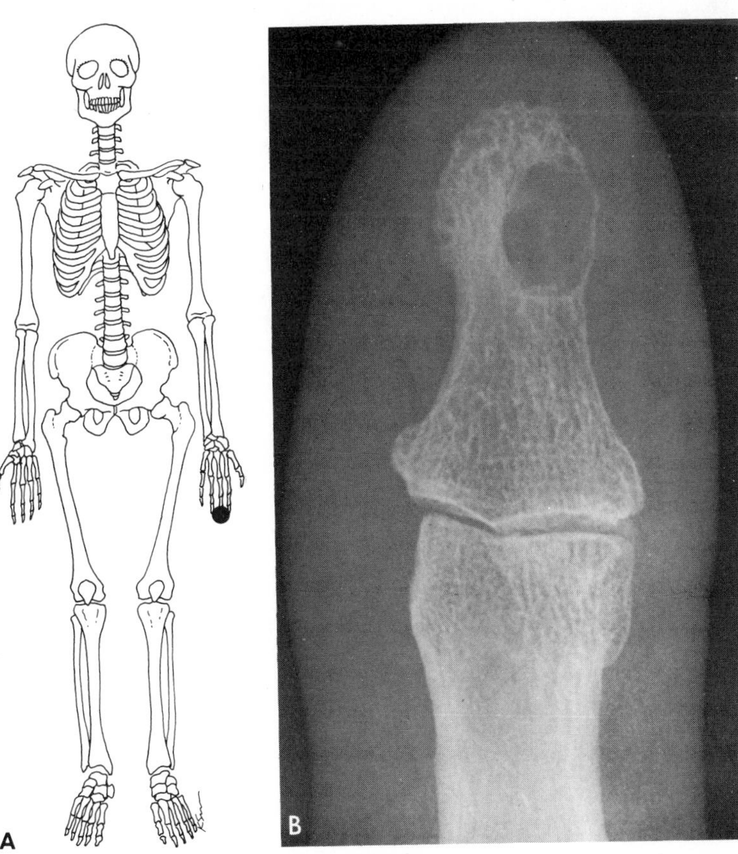

Figure 74–29. Glomus tumor.
A *Characteristic distribution.*
B *An eccentric lytic lesion of the terminal phalanx is associated with geographic bone destruction. This is a typical appearance of a glomus tumor.*

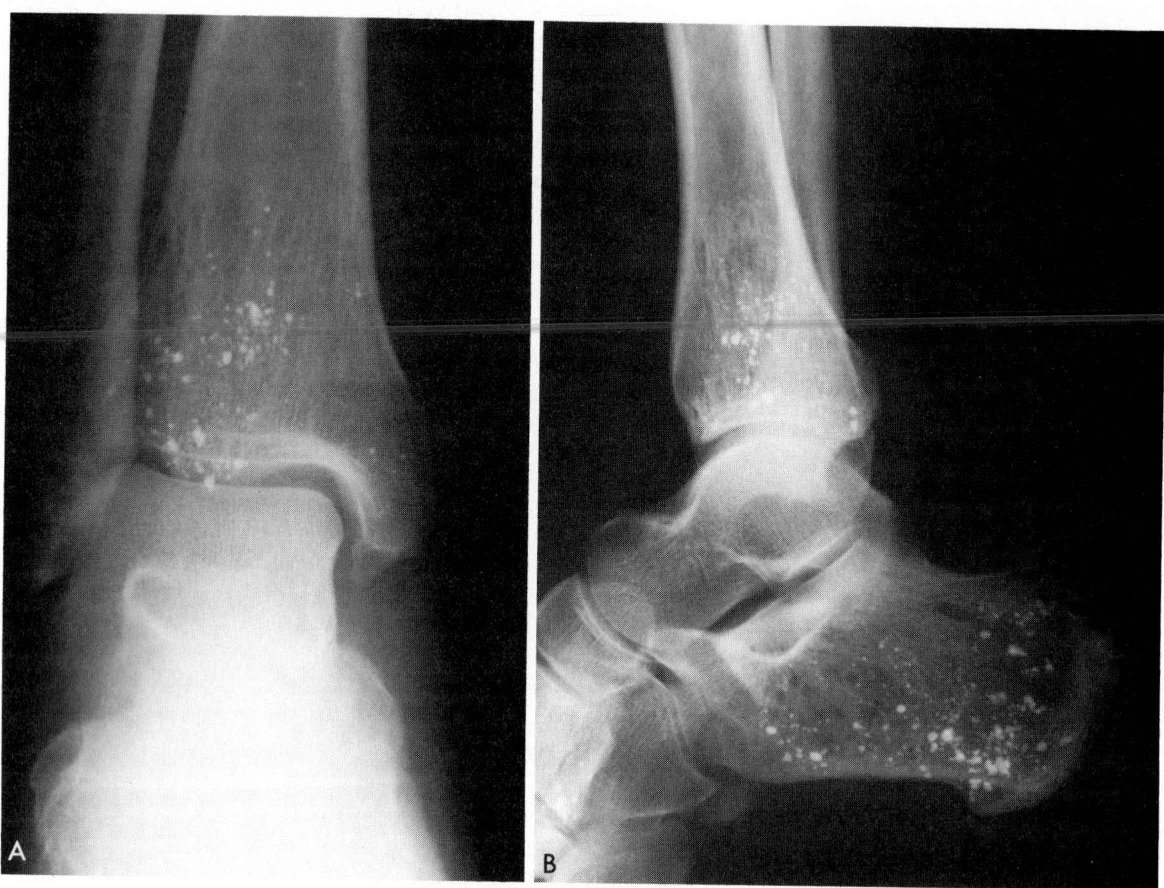

Figure 74–30. Lymphangioma. *Frontal and lateral radiographs of the ankle indicate the presence of lymphangiomas, especially in the distal tibia and calcaneus. They have produced small cystic lesions within the bone. The radiodense areas represent contrast material that had collected within the lymphangiomas during a previous lymphangiogram.*

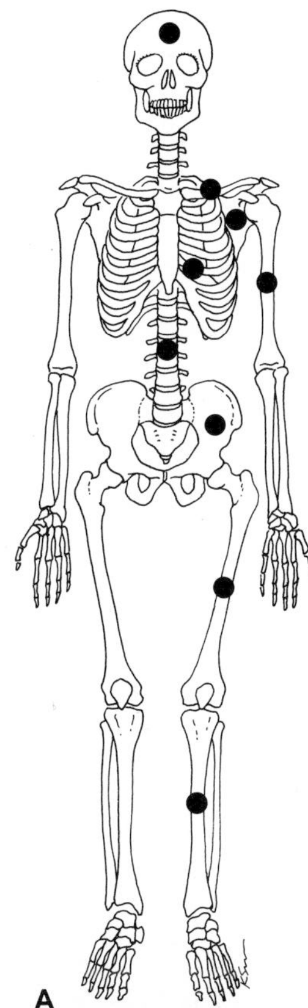

Figure 74–31. Cystic angiomatosis.

A *Characteristic distribution.*

B, C *In this patient, widespread skeletal lesions can be identified. Within the ribs, the lesions are well defined and lytic in nature, surrounded by a rim of sclerotic bone. In the pelvis, the circular lesions appear more radiodense but possess a central radiolucent zone.*

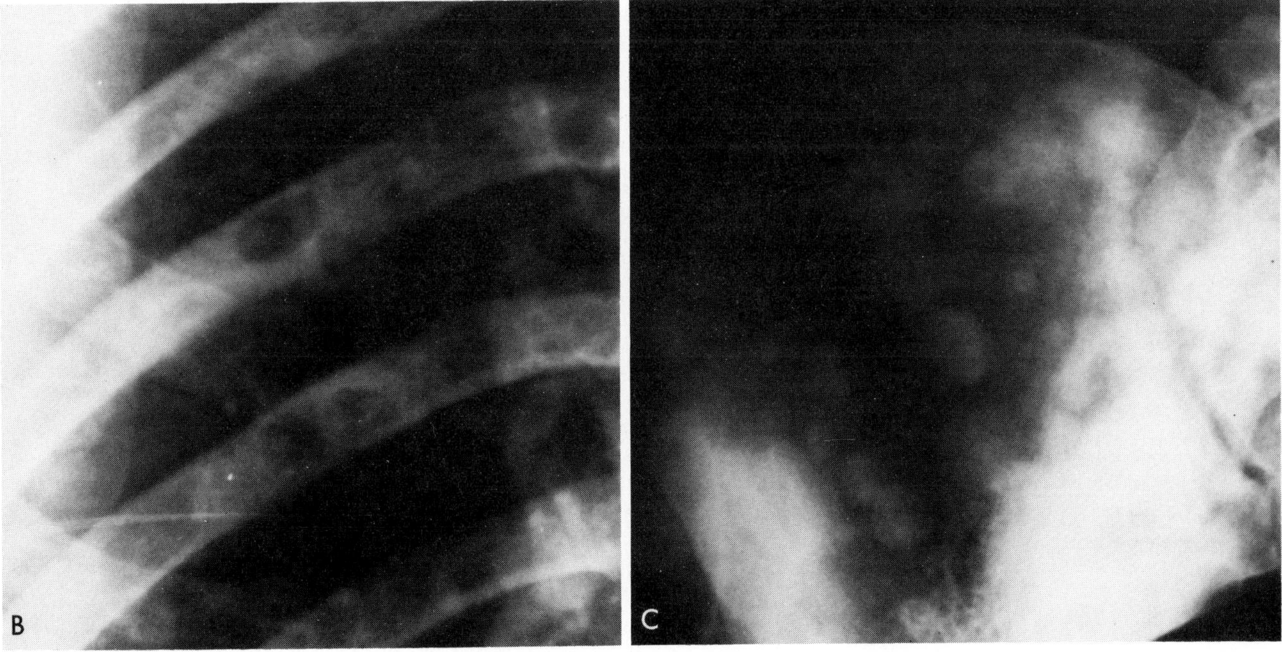

Benign or Malignant Tumors

Hemangiopericytoma. Hemangiopericytomas of bone are extremely rare.[166-168] They may behave as benign lesions, be locally aggressive, or possess malignant characteristics. Most patients are middle-aged, in the fourth or fifth decade of life. Involvement of the axial skeleton and proximal long bones is usually evident. The radiographic appearance is not specific.

Malignant Tumors

Angiosarcoma (Hemangioendothelioma) (Fig. 74–32). This rare lesion of bone is composed of irregular anastomosing vascular channels lined by one or several layers of atypical endothelial cells with an anaplastic, immature appearance.[3] Either solitary or multifocal lesions may be discovered. Angiosarcomas can occur in any age group, but are most frequent in the fourth and fifth decades of life; patients affected by multifocal disease are usually about 10 years younger than those possessing single lesions.[3] Men are involved more frequently than women, particularly with regard to multifocal disease. Of the tubular bones, the femur, tibia, and humerus are affected most constantly. Of the flat bones, those in the pelvis and skull are most typically altered. Spinal involvement is also recorded, with destruction of one or more vertebral bodies. With multifocal disease, a regional distribution may be encountered, with involvement of the tubular bones of a single extremity. The lesions are usually osteolytic in appearance, producing thinning, expansion, or disruption of the cortex. In the tubular bones, metaphyseal localization is preferred.[169-175]

Tumors of Neural Origin

Benign Tumors

Solitary Neurofibroma. Although multiple neurogenic tumors are well recognized as part of neurofibromatosis, solitary neurofibromas of the skeleton are quite rare.[2] Spinal and mandibular involvement is most typical; however, tubular bones can also be affected. Intraosseous or subperiosteal localization may be seen. The intraosseous neurofibroma produces a nonspecific osteolytic lesion. In periosteal locations, neurofibromas produce cortical erosion and periosteal reaction.

Neurilemoma. Neurilemomas, arising from a nerve sheath, rarely originate in bone.[176-179] Solitary lesions predominate. The most frequently reported sites of involvement are the mandible, sacrum, and humerus, in descending order of frequency. Three modes of presentation are encountered: central involvement characterized as a cystic osteolytic focus with a sclerotic margin; localization to the nutrient

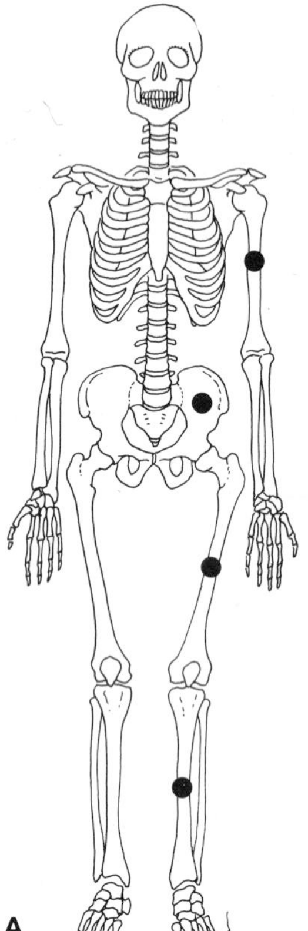

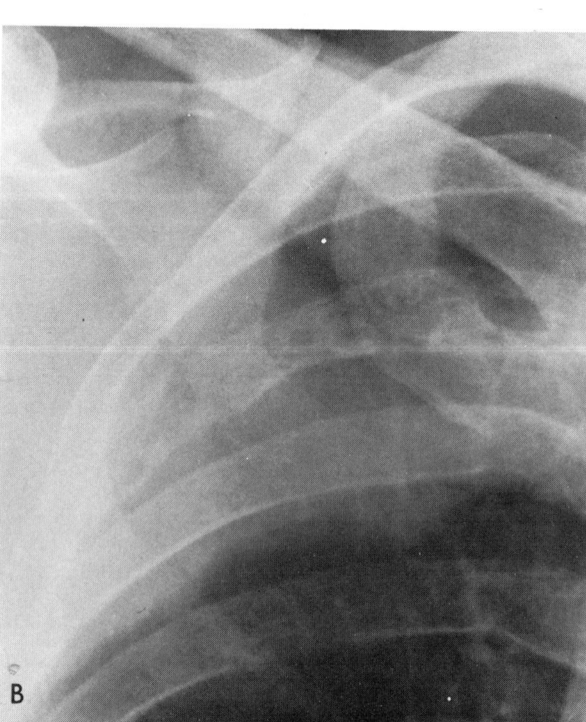

Figure 74–32. *Angiosarcoma (hemangioendothelioma).*

A *Characteristic distribution.*

B *An ill-defined lesion of the posterior aspect of the fourth rib is associated with a coarsened trabecular pattern and a large soft tissue mass. The osseous changes are consistent with a vascular lesion. The extent of the soft tissue enlargement would suggest an aggressive process.*

canal with production of a dumbbell lesion; and periosteal involvement producing cortical erosion or excavation.[176]

MALIGNANT TUMORS

Neurogenic Sarcoma (Malignant Schwannoma). Malignant bone lesions of Schwann cell origin are unusual,[2] and some investigators maintain that such lesions are not truly related to nerve tissue but arise from fibrous elements (fibrosarcoma) or fascial and other tissues adjacent to the nerve. The lesions have a variable histologic appearance, perhaps related to the versatility of Schwann cells, which, through metaplasia, can produce cartilage, bone, fat, and muscle.[2] The malignant schwannoma of bone usually appears in a patient in the third, fourth, or fifth decade of life as an ill-defined osteolytic process with soft tissue extension.[180] It may be seen in patients with generalized neurofibromatosis.

Tumors of Notochord Origin

LOCALLY AGGRESSIVE TUMORS

Chordoma (Fig. 74–33). Chordoma is a rare "malignant" lesion of notochord origin characterized by a lobular arrangement and a composition of highly vacuolated (physaliferous) cells and mucoid intercellular material.[3] Areas of hemorrhage or calcification may also be identified. It is a locally aggressive tumor that grows slowly, invades surrounding soft tissue structures, and infrequently metastasizes (approximately 10 to 20 per cent of tumors). Chordomas can become evident at any age, although most patients are in the fifth and sixth decades of life; chordomas are rare prior to the third decade of life. Men and women are affected with equal frequency.

Chordomas, arising from notochordal remnants, are encountered anywhere in the vertebral column.[181-188] Favored locations are the sacrococcygeal region (50 to 70 per cent), spheno-occipital region (15 to 25 per cent), and other spinal regions (15 to 20 per cent). In the spine, some predilection may exist for involvement of the second cervical vertebra, with cervical, lumbar, and thoracic localization, in descending order of frequency. Symptoms and signs can be prominent although initial nonspecific and mild manifestations may lead to delay in diagnosis. Intracranial chordomas can produce headache, visual disturbance, and neurologic findings. With tumors of the nasopharynx, nasal obstruction or discharge can be evident.[3] In sacrococcygeal and vertebral sites, chordomas can compress the adjacent spinal cord and nerves and produce pressure on neighboring organs, such as the rectum and bladder.

On radiographic examination, sacrococcygeal and vertebral chordomas produce lytic bone destruction with calcific foci and a soft tissue mass. Initially, destruction of the vertebral body is unaccompanied by loss of height of the adjacent intervertebral disc. Subsequently, osteosclerosis may become prominent, and contiguous vertebral bodies may be affected, with involvement of intervertebral discs.[181, 185] Vertebral collapse and radiodense vertebral bodies ("ivory" vertebrae) are additional manifestations of this tumor. Intraspinal extension is readily apparent during myelography. Intracranial chordomas are associated with destruction of the clivus and sella turcica, with a soft tissue mass that is readily apparent during pneumoencephalography. Extension of tumor to petrous and sphenoid bones is seen, and a nasopharyngeal mass can become evident. Calcification within the lesion may be detected in 20 to 70 per cent of cases. At the base of the skull, chordomas exhibiting cartilaginous features have been identified, termed "chondroid" chordomas.[189, 190] These lesions may have a better prognosis than the classic chordomas seen elsewhere in the skeleton.

Tumors of Hematopoietic Origin

MALIGNANT TUMORS

Non-Hodgkin's Lymphomas (Lymphosarcoma, Reticulum Cell Sarcoma), Hodgkin's Disease, Leukemias. The skeletal manifestations of these tumors are discussed in Chapter 58.

Plasma Cell Dyscrasias

LOCALLY AGGRESSIVE OR MALIGNANT TUMORS

Plasmacytoma, Multiple Myeloma. These and other plasma cell dyscrasias are discussed in Chapter 56.

Tumors and Tumor-Like Lesions of Miscellaneous or Unknown Origin

BENIGN TUMORS

Solitary (Simple or Unicameral) Bone Cyst (Fig. 74–34). The solitary bone cyst is a common lesion that generally becomes evident in the first and second decades of life, affecting boys with greater frequency than girls (2:1), and showing remarkable predilection for the proximal end of both the humerus and the femur (60 to 70 per cent of cases). Histologically, a fluid-filled cavity within bone is surrounded by a lining containing a layer of flattened to plump cells, with giant cells and loose fibrous tissue.[191] The pathogenesis of this lesion is unknown. Proposed theories implicate trauma with hematoma formation, infection, abnormal hyperplasia of osteoclasts, or faulty calcium metabolism. More recently, it has been suggested that solitary bone cysts develop as a result of blockage of interstitial fluid drainage in a rapidly growing and remodeling area of cancellous bone.[192, 193] The lining cells of the cyst resemble

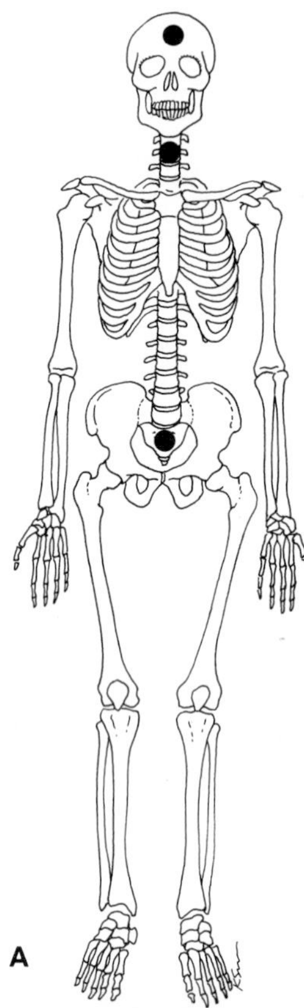

Figure 74–33. Chordoma.

A Characteristic distribution.

B Within the sacrum, this large chordoma has produced lytic destruction of bone and contains calcific foci.

C This chordoma of a cervical vertebral body is associated with nonspecific destruction of the vertebra (arrows). The adjacent intervertebral discs appear slightly narrowed and there is some irregularity of the vertebral bodies on either side of that containing the lesion.

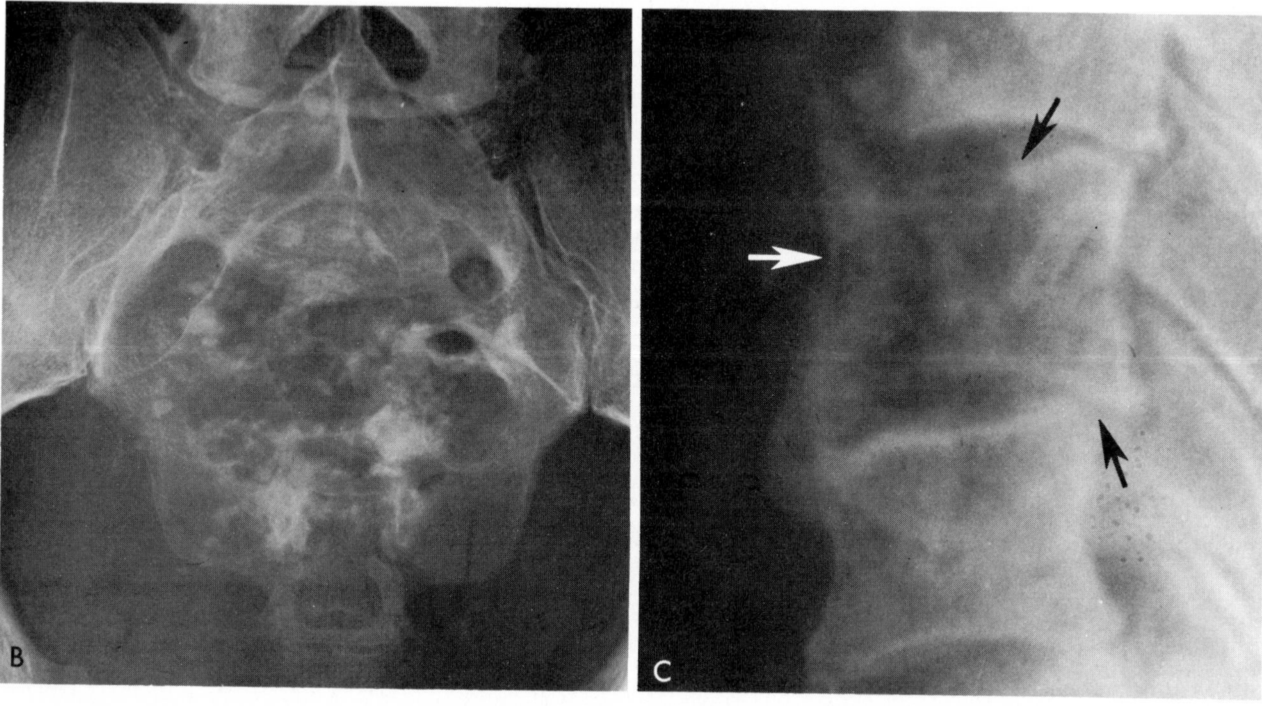

the cells lining the villi of normal synovium in morphology, suggesting that the lesion may be an intraosseous synovial cyst, arising when a small nest of synovium becomes trapped within a bone as a result of traumatic or developmental factors.[191] Synovial cell entrapment might be expected to occur in the metaphyseal region of bone at the synovium-capsular bone reflection.

Solitary bone cysts are rarely symptomatic unless a pathologic fracture has occurred. Such fractures are not infrequent and may be associated with intracystic dislocation of a piece of the surrounding bony cortex. The displaced bony spicule may migrate to the inferior aspect of the lesion, creating the "fallen fragment" sign.[194] In young patients, a metaphyseal localization in tubular bones is characteristic, especially in the proximal humerus and proximal femur. In older patients, flat bones, such as those in the pelvis, and small bones, such as the calcaneus, are not uncommonly involved. Solitary bone cysts located adjacent to the growth plate have been considered "active" because of their capacity for growth, whereas those that have "migrated" away from the plate have been considered "latent."[195] This division

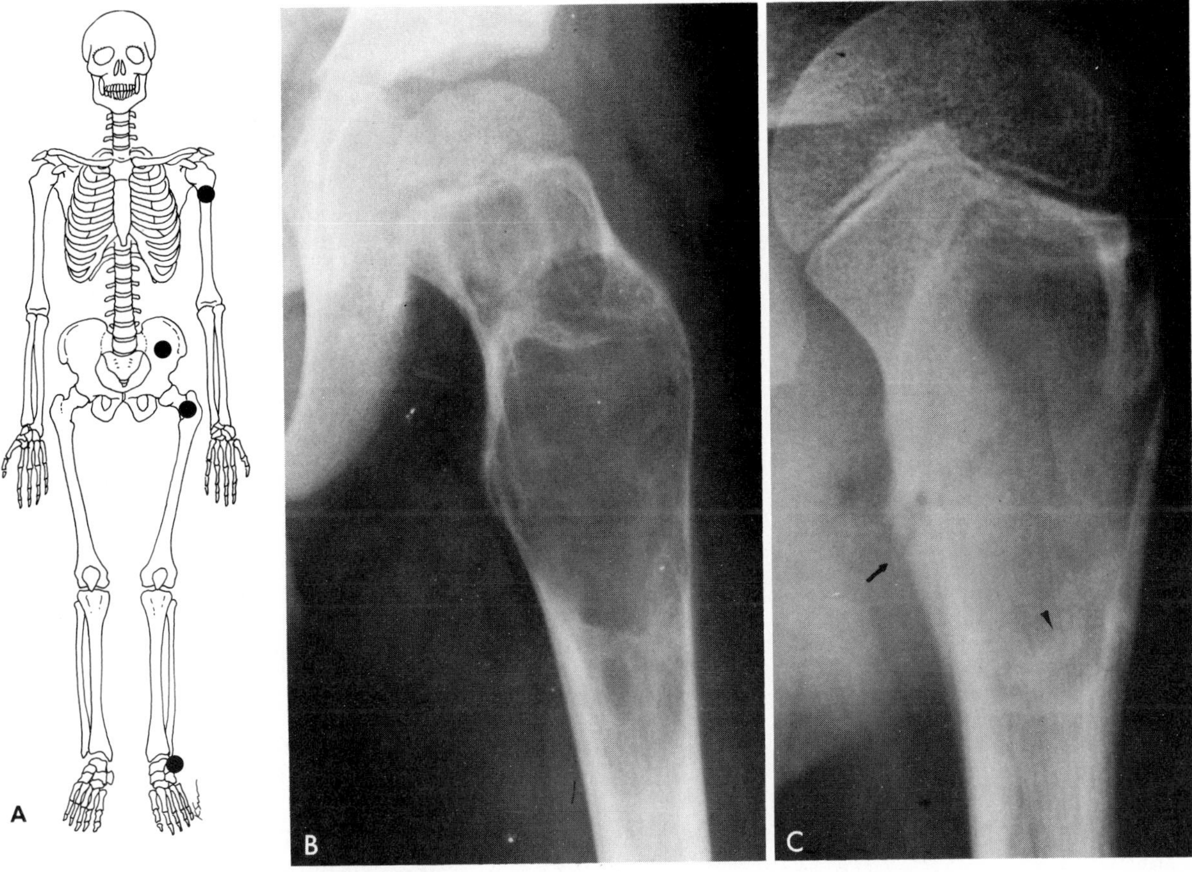

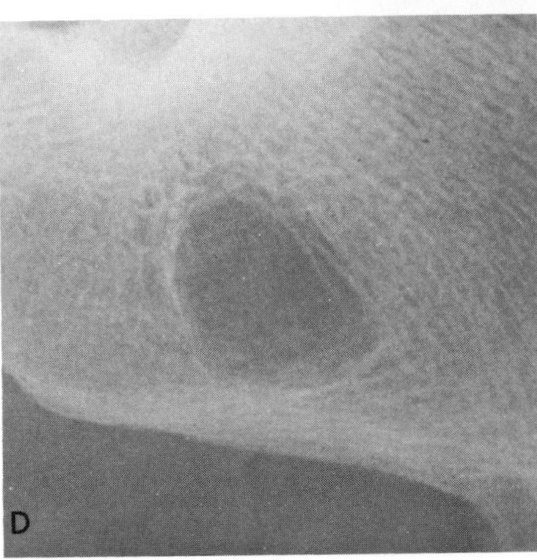

Figure 74–34. Solitary bone cyst.

A *Characteristic distribution.*

B *A typical solitary bone cyst of the proximal femur in a child is illustrated. Note its central location and geographic pattern of bone destruction. The lesion is lucent and is associated with endosteal erosion and mild cortical expansion. It has a multiloculated appearance.*

C *This solitary bone cyst of the proximal humerus involves the metaphysis. It shows geographic bone destruction and is centrally located. A pathologic fracture (arrow) through the lesion can be identified. A radiodense collection (arrowhead) at the inferior aspect of the lesion may represent a "fallen fragment" sign, in which a piece of the fractured cortex has migrated to the inferior aspect of this cystic lesion.*

D *A typical solitary bone cyst of the calcaneus is shown. (Compare with Figure 74–26B.)*

of solitary bone cysts into active and latent forms based upon location in the bone is not entirely accurate; examples of active cysts in the diaphysis are recorded.[196] Such activity appears to correlate better with the age of the patients; the recurrence rate of these lesions is much greater in patients below the age of 10 years.[196, 199, 200]

On radiographs, solitary bone cysts produce centrally located radiolucent lesions with cortical thinning and mild osseous expansion. Some may possess a multilocular appearance. Patchy marginal sclerosis may be evident, related to ossification of fibrin clot lining the cystic cavity.[197] Curvilinear calcification and ossification of calcaneal cysts have been reported,[198] creating an appearance identical to that of a lipoma. Indeed, the two lesions may be closely related. In the calcaneus, solitary bone cysts are constantly located at the base of the calcaneal neck just inferior to the anterior portion of the posterior facet.[201]

Rarely, sarcomas may develop in the wall of a solitary bone cyst.[202-204]

Epidermoid Cyst (Fig. 74–35). Epidermoid cysts of bone are uncommon. In most reported cases, the calvarium or the terminal phalanges of the fingers or, much less frequently, the toes have been involved.[205-207] Long tubular bones are rarely affected.[208] Patients are usually in the second, third, or fourth decade of life. Histologic evaluation reveals squamous epithelium, keratin, and cholesterol crystals. A well-defined osteolytic lesion is observed, which may be calcified or ossified. Soft tissue swelling can also be evident. Although their pathogenesis is debated, epidermoid cysts of the fingers are usually associated with a history of trauma.

Aneurysmal Bone Cyst (Fig. 74–36). An aneurysmal bone cyst is an expansile lesion containing thin-walled, blood-filled cystic cavities. Large vascular channels are associated with slender to plump cells with hemosiderin granules and surrounding giant cells.[3] Aneurysmal bone cysts are generally regarded as non-neoplastic in nature; trauma appears to be important in their pathogenesis. They may exist as a primary abnormality of bone or as a secondary phenomenon superimposed on a preexisting osseous lesion. The nature of the underlying bone disorder is quite variable; examples of aneurysmal bone cysts superimposed on chondroblastomas, giant cell tumors, and osteoblastomas have been recorded.

Aneurysmal bone cysts are usually seen in the first, second, or third decade of life, affecting men and women with equal frequency. They may arise in almost any bone, although most reports indicate their predilection for the spine, innominate bones, and metaphyses of long tubular bones (femur, humerus, tibia, fibula). Small tubular bones in the hands and

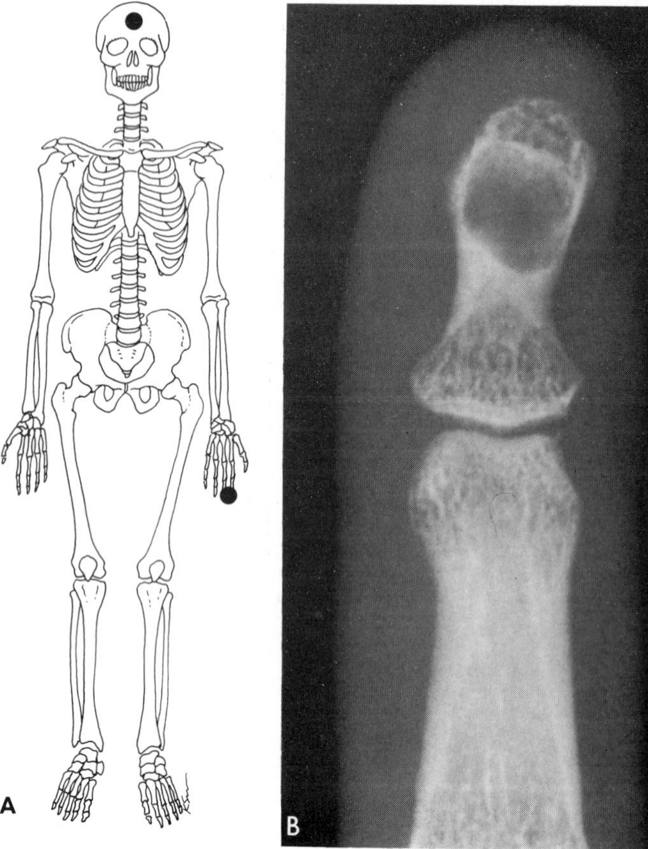

Figure 74–35. *Epidermoid cyst.*
A *Characteristic distribution.*
B *A well-defined osteolytic lesion of the terminal phalanx is typical of this lesion.*

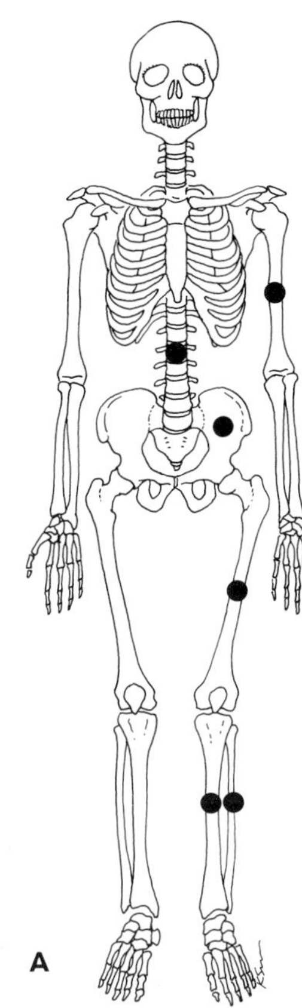

Figure 74–36. *Aneurysmal bone cyst.*

A *Characteristic distribution.*

B *Observe the expansile osteolytic lesion of the metaphyseal and diaphyseal portions of the proximal humerus in this child. The lesion possesses a trabecular structure producing curvilinear and circular radiodense shadows. Note the shell of bone that encloses this expansile lesion.*

C *This aggressive lesion of the metacarpal represents an aneurysmal bone cyst. Osteolytic destruction of a large portion of the bone is associated with a soft tissue mass. A calcific shell (arrowheads) can be identified around the mass, and faint horizontal trabeculae (open arrow) can also be seen. These latter features suggest the diagnosis of an aneurysmal bone cyst.*

(Courtesy of Balboa Naval Hospital, San Diego, California.)

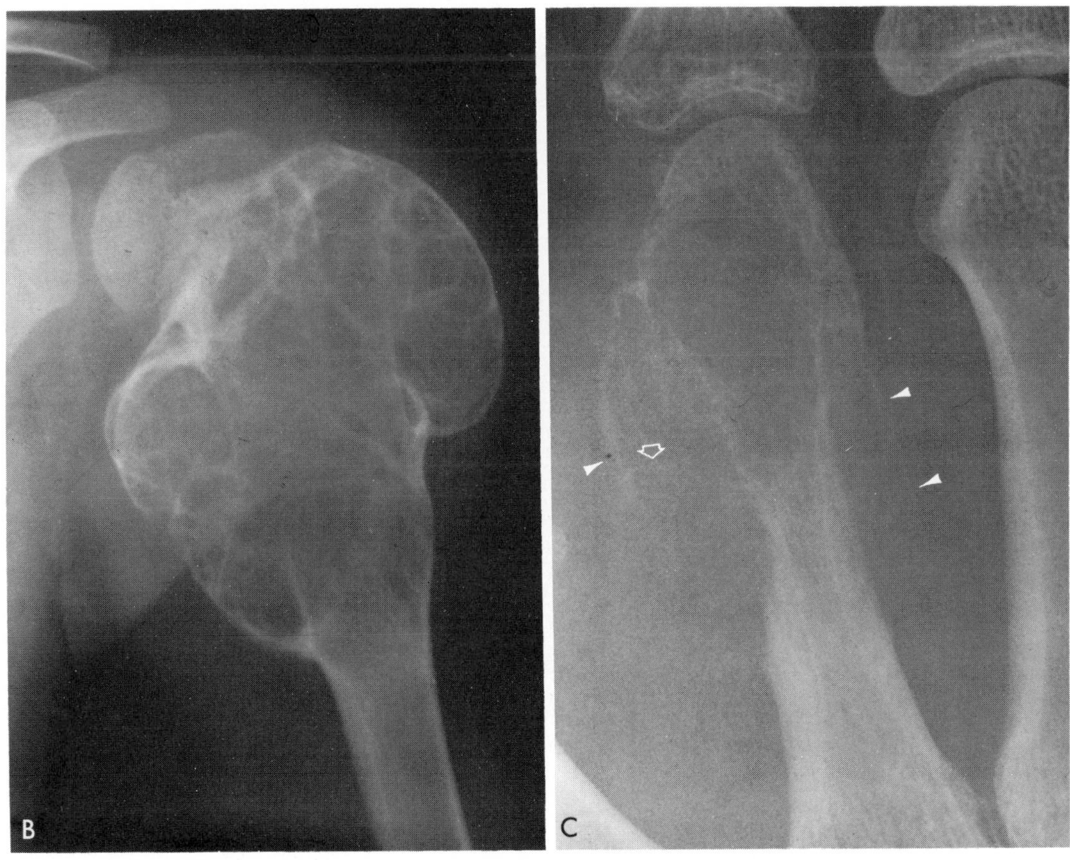

feet, and additional flat or irregular bones, such as the scapula, clavicle, ribs, calcaneus, mandible, maxilla, and calvarium, can be affected.[209-215] Radiographically, in the appendicular skeleton, an eccentric osteolytic and expansile lesion is evident, which displaces and obscures the cortex. Horizontally oriented trabeculae may extend into the adjacent soft tissue. Eventually a shell of bone may surround the lesion, although at early stages, the shell can be absent, and the aggressive appearance may simulate that of a malignant process. In the spine, the posterior elements are generally affected,[209, 214] and an expansile lucent lesion is seen. Extension into or primary involvement of a vertebral body can also be evident in some cases.

Locally Aggressive Tumors

Ameloblastoma (Fig. 74–37). An ameloblastoma is an invasive tumor of unknown origin that affects the maxilla and mandible. Its histologic characteristics are variable; some lesions are follicular in type, possessing columnar cells, whereas others are plexiform in type, with irregular masses of epithelial tissue surrounded by cuboidal or columnar cells. The source of the cells within this tumor is unknown; they may originate from the epithelial lining of an odontogenic cyst, the dental lamina or enamel, the stratified squamous epithelium of the oral cavity, or the dental epithelial remnants.[216, 217] Most patients with ameloblastomas are in the fourth and fifth decades of life. Men and women are affected with approximately equal frequency. A gradually enlarging mass with or without pain is common.

Mandibular involvement is approximately three or four times more frequent than maxillary involvement.[218] The angle of the mandible is commonly affected. A radiolucent unilocular or multilocular cystic lesion with cortical expansion is typical.[219, 220] The margin of the lesion may be scalloped, and resorption of the root or roots of neighboring teeth may be identified. Recurrent lesions may appear even more aggressive, with perforation of the cortical plate.

Locally Aggressive or Malignant Tumors

Aaamantinoma (Angioblastoma) (Fig. 74–38). This locally aggressive or malignant lesion of unknown pathogenesis is composed of rows of stellate cells arranged in anastomosing elongated masses supported by a dense, fibrous stroma.[221] Areas may show squamous transformation, or tubular, alveolar, or vessel transformation. Vascularity is prominent, with hyperplastic endothelial lining cells. An angioblastic origin of this lesion has been suggested.[3] A relationship with fibrous dysplasia has also been

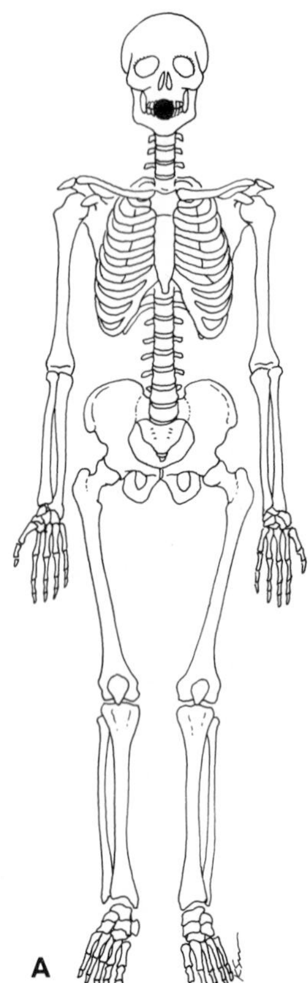

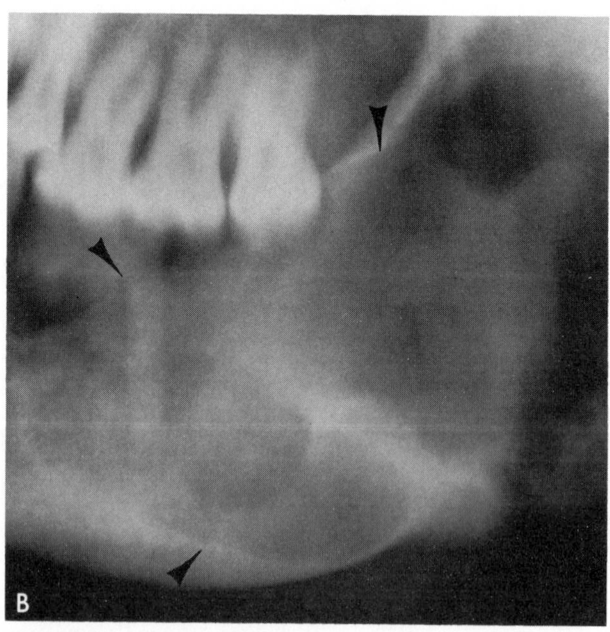

Figure 74–37. *Ameloblastoma.*
A *Characteristic distribution.*
B *A tomogram defines a large expansile osteolytic lesion involving the mandible (arrowheads). It has a multilocular appearance.*

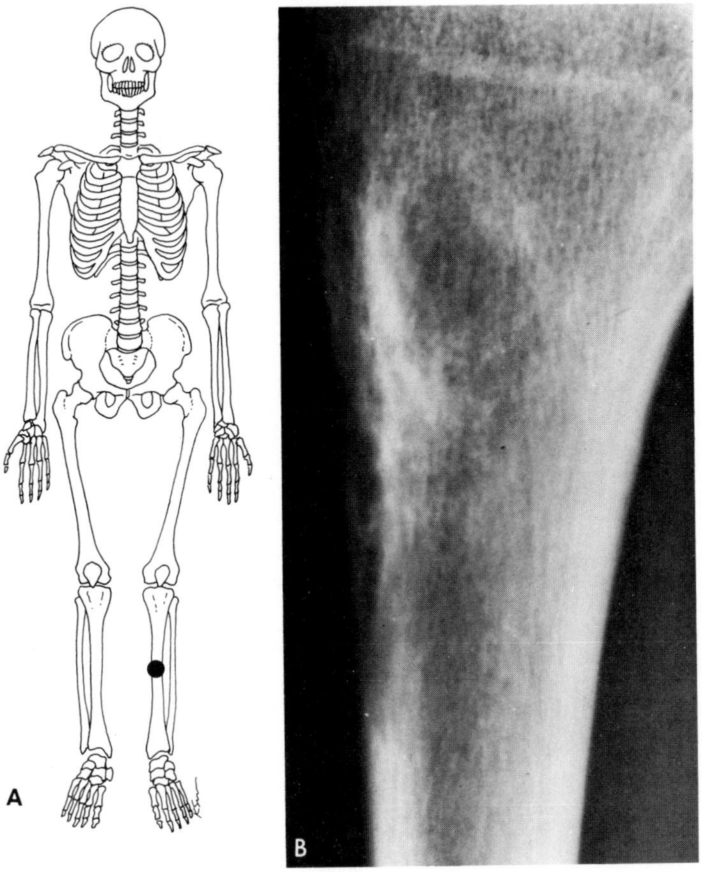

Figure 74–38. *Adamantinoma (angioblastoma).*
A *Characteristic distribution.*
B *This lesion of the proximal tibia has an eccentric location and is associated with cortical involvement and reactive sclerosis. Periostitis is absent.*
(Courtesy of Dr. Robert Freiberger, New York, New York.)

noted, as the two lesions may coexist in the same bone,[222] although this occurrence may actually indicate the misinterpretation of the prominent fibrous tissue element that characterizes the adamantinoma.[223, 224]

Although the age range of patients with this lesion is variable, most individuals are in the fourth and fifth decades of life. A history of trauma is frequent, and many patients describe local swelling with or witout pain as the major clinical finding. The tibia is, by far, the most common site of tumor involvement, although other long tubular bones, such as the femur, ulna, humerus, and fibula, can be affected.[225-230] The small bones of the hands and feet and flat bones are rarely involved.[231] In the tibia, the lesion is usually localized in the middle third of the bone. An eccentric location and a sharply delineated osteolytic lesion are characteristic of adamantinoma. Reactive sclerosis and small satellite radiolucent foci in direct continuity with the major lesion may be identified. In fact, changes in the adjacent fibula can be seen. Periostitis is usually not apparent in the absence of a pathologic fracture. Occasionally, cortical disruption, exuberant periostitis, and a soft tissue mass are noted. In other tubular bones, the roentgenographic characteristics of the lesion are generally the same as in the tibia. Diametaphyseal localization is most common. Following resection, recurrence is frequent, and distant metastases may be evident.

Malignant Tumors

Ewing's Sarcoma (Fig. 74–39). This relatively common malignant tumor of bone has a varied histologic pattern. The tumor cells are arranged in broad sheets. Some cells have a larger, lightly stained, finely granular nucleus with pale, ill-defined cytoplasm, whereas others possess small, darker staining nuclear chromatin feltwork with a rim of moderately well delineated cytoplasm; cells may be located about vessels in a perithelial arrangement.[3] A large-cell variety has also been described.[242] The origin of Ewing's sarcoma is unknown; it may be derived[3] from mesenchymal cells of the bone marrow,[232] from immature reticulum cells,[233] or from vascular[234] or myelogenic[235] elements.

Ewing's sarcoma is identified in patients in the first, second, or third decade of life; the ratio of affected men to affected women is approximately 3:2 (Table 74–4). Localized pain and swelling may be combined with fever, weight loss, anemia, and leukocytosis, simulating the clinical findings of an infection. Any skeletal site can be involved, although the

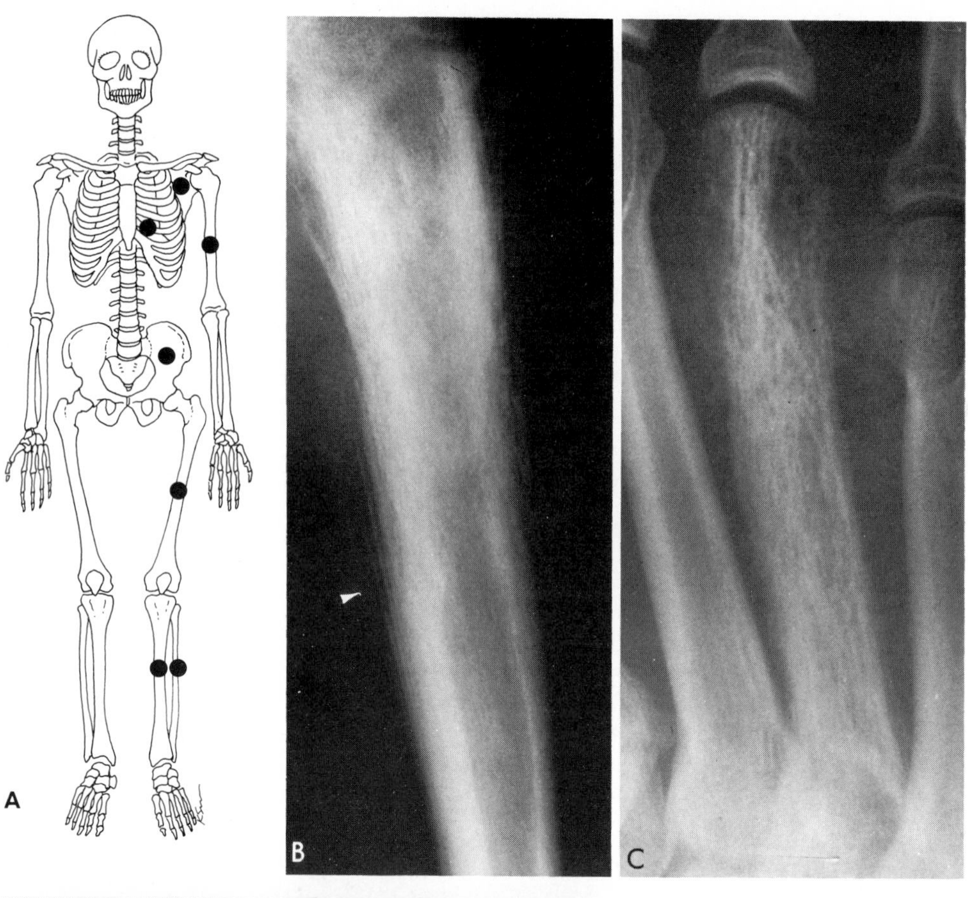

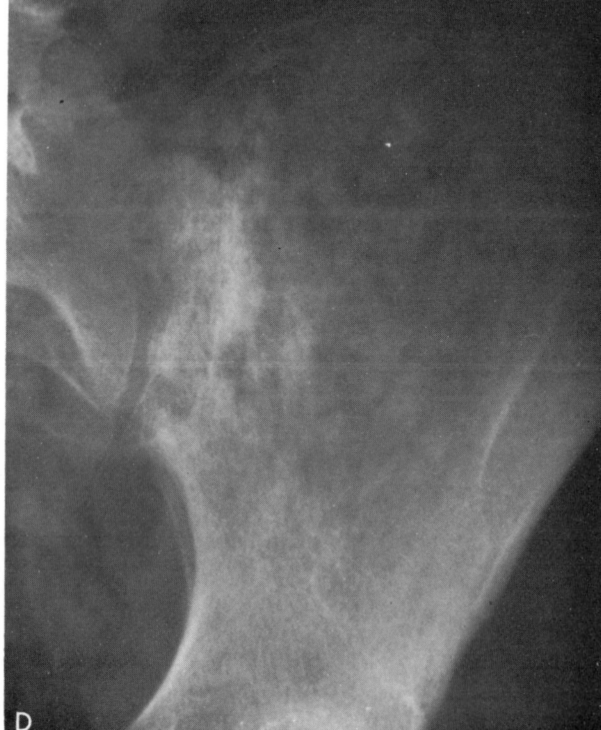

Figure 74–39. *Ewing's sarcoma.*

A *Characteristic distribution.*

B *An aggressive lesion of the proximal humerus is associated with permeative bone destruction, mild sclerosis, and an onion-peel pattern of periostitis (arrowhead).*

C *A Ewing's sarcoma of the metatarsal is characterized by permeative bone destruction, cortical invasion and erosion, soft tissue swelling, and periostitis. The entire bone is affected.*

D *This Ewing's sarcoma of the ilium has produced a motheaten pattern of bone destruction with both osteolysis and osteosclerosis.*

Table 74–4

DIFFERENTIAL DIAGNOSIS OF SMALL CELL SARCOMA OF BONE IN CHILDREN*

Ewing's Sarcoma	Non-Hodgkin's Lymphoma
Most common in second decade (but frequently occurs below 10 years of age) Rare in blacks Pain is most common presenting symptom Flat bones (ribs, scapula, pelvis) are common sites Femur is most common site Diaphyseal lesion in long bones Diffuse osteolytic lesion of entire shaft Large soft tissue mass (originating in bone) May give positive stain for glycogen granules (PAS)	No age or race predilection in children Long bones most common (femur and tibia) Diffuse metaphyseal lesion, usually mixed osteolytic and osteosclerotic areas Lymphadenopathy and splenomegaly may be present Early diffuse bone marrow involvement in children Reticulum fibers demonstrable with special stain Cell nuclei somewhat larger and rounder than in Ewing's sarcoma Cytoplasmic border more distinct than in Ewing's sarcoma
Metastatic Neuroblastoma	**Embryonal Rhabdomyosarcoma**
Usually in children less than 5 years of age Long bones are frequently symmetrically involved Lytic lesions can be very extensive with a paucity of soft tissue mass Bone marrow aspiration can show clumps of extrinsic cells ("rosettes") Presence of primary tumor; abnormal intravenous pyelogram or paraspinal mass Urine may be positive for vanillylmandelic acid or catecholamines	Lesions of the trunk and extremity can frequently involve bone Usually presents with soft tissue swelling rather than pain as the predominant symptom The soft tissue mass usually invades bone secondarily Systemic symptoms are rare Lesions in the head and neck area are usually primary, not metastatic Cells have a predominance of pink cytoplasm occasionally exhibiting striations on higher magnification (rhabdomyoblast)

*From Rosen G: Pediatr Clin North Am *23*:183, 1976.

frequent sites of involvement are the long tubular bones (femur, tibia, humerus, fibula), the pelvic girdle, the vertebrae, the ribs, and the scapula.[236-238] Flat bone involvement is more frequent in patients over the age of 18 years.[237] Ewing's tumor in the craniofacial region[239] and small bones of the hand and foot[240, 241] is less typical.

In the tubular bones, Ewing's sarcoma shows predilection for the diaphyseal or diametaphyseal region. It is characterized by a long permeative osteolytic lesion with poorly defined margins, cortical disruption, and periosteal reaction. The periostitis is frequently described as "onion-peel" or "hair-on-end" in type. Pathologic fractures are identified in 5 to 10 per cent of cases. Saucerization and excavation of the cortex are also noted in some tumors, and this feature may be the most prominent radiographic finding. In some of these cases, an eccentric or cortical location of the tumor may be apparent on pathologic examination. In the flat bones, permeative destruction is also typical. In this location, the amount of new bone formation may be striking. In the vertebral column, the sacrum, lumbar spine, thoracic spine, and cervical spine are involved, in descending order of frequency. Osteolysis and vertebral collapse predominate. Occasionally uniform sclerosis of a vertebral body may be seen.[238] Tumor extension into the posterior elements can be evident. Paravertebral masses, loss of height of intervertebral disc spaces, and spread to contiguous vertebral bodies are additional radiographic features of spinal involvement.

Skeletal and extraskeletal metastasis due to Ewing's sarcoma is frequent. Osseous changes in these cases may simulate those in leukemias, lymphomas, or metastatic neuroblastomas.

Other Malignant Tumors. Rare examples of osseous leiomyosarcoma,[243, 244] rhabdomyosarcoma,[245] and malignant granular cell myoblastoma (alveolar soft-part sarcoma)[2] are described.

SUMMARY

Many different types of tumors and tumor-like lesions involve the skeleton. Morphologic characteristics provide important radiographic clues to a precise diagnosis in some cases, although, more importantly, they indicate the "aggressiveness" of the lesion. In this regard, the pattern of bone destruction (geographic, motheaten, permeative) is of primary importance. This feature when combined with others (size and shape of lesion; presence and nature of visible tumor matrix, trabeculation, and periosteal response; and specific location) forms the foundation for proper radiographic interpretation.

REFERENCES

1. Lodwick GS, Wilson AJ, Farrell C, Virtama, P, Smeltzer FM, Dittrich F: Estimating rate of growth in bone lesions: Observer performace and error. Radiology *134*:585, 1980.
2. Lichtenstein L: Bone Tumors. 4th Ed. St Louis, CV Mosby Co, 1972.
3. Huvos AG: Bone Tumors: Diagnosis, Treatment, Prognosis. Philadelphia, WB Saunders Co, 1979.
4. Dahlin DC: Bone Tumors: General Aspects and Data on 6,221 Cases. 3rd Ed. Springfield, Ill, Charles C Thomas, 1978.
5. Nessi R, de Yoldi GC: Xeroradiography of bone tumors. Skel Radiol *2*:143, 1978.
6. Gilday DL, Ash JM, Reilly BJ: Radionuclide skeletal survey for pediatric neoplasms. Radiology *123*:399, 1977.
7. Telfer N: Nuclear medicine in the management of musculoskeletal tumors. Orthop Clin North Am *8*:1011, 1977.
8. Siddiqui AR, Oseas R, Wellman HN, Doerr DR, Baehner RL: Evaluation of bone-marrow scanning with technetium-99m sulfur colloid in pediatric oncology. J Nucl Med *20*:379, 1979.
9. Levine E, Lee KR, Neff JR, Maklad NF, Robinson RG, Preston DF: Comparison of computed tomography and other imaging modalities in the evaluation of musculoskeletal tumors. Radiology *131*:431, 1979.
10. de Santos LA, Goldstein HM, Murray JA, Wallace S: Computed tomography in the evaluation of musculoskeletal neoplasms. Radiology *128*:89, 1978.
11. Berger PE, Kuhn JP: Computed tomography of tumors of the musculoskeletal system in children. Clinical applications. Radiology *127*:171, 1978.
12. Lodwick GS: The Bones and Joints. *In* PJ Hodes (Ed): Atlas of Tumor Radiology. Chicago, Year Book Medical Publishers, 1971.
13. Braunschwig A, Harman PH: Studies in bone sarcoma, III. An experimental and pathological study of role of the periosteum in formation of bone in various primary bone tumors. Surg Gynecol Obstet *60*:30, 1935.
14. Volberg FM Jr, Whalen JP, Krook L, Winchester P: Lamellated periosteal reactions: A radiologic and histologic investigation. Am J Roentgenol *128*:85, 1977.
15. Nessi R, de Yoldi GC: Xeroradiography of bone tumors. Skel Radiol *2*:143, 1978.
16. Takigawa K: Chondroma of the bones of the hand. A review of 110 cases. J Bone Joint Surg *53A*:1591, 1971.
17. McFarland GB Jr, Morden ML: Benign cartilaginous lesions. Orthop Clin North Am *8*:737, 1977.
18. Pandey S: Giant chondromas arising from the ribs. A report of four cases. J Bone Joint Surg *57B*:519, 1975.
19. Takigawa K: Carpal chondroma. Report of a case. J Bone Joint Surg *53A*:1601, 1971.
20. Jaffe HL, Lichtenstein L: Solitary benign enchondroma of bone. Arch Surg *46*:480, 1943.
21. Lichtenstein L, Hall JE: Periosteal chondroma, a distinctive benign cartilage tumor. J Bone Joint Surg *34A*:691, 1952.
22. Jaffe HL: Juxtacortical chondroma. Bull Hosp Joint Dis *17*:20, 1956.
23. Kirchner SG, Pavlov H, Heller RM, Kaye JJ: Periosteal chondromas of the anterior tibial tubercle: Two cases. Am J Roentgenol *131*:1088, 1978.
24. Cooke GM, Pearce JG: Periosteal chondroma. Report of two cases with atypical radiologic features. J Can Assoc Radiol *27*:301, 1976.
25. Huvos AG, Marcove RC: Chondroblastoma of bone. A critical review. Clin Orthop Rel Res *95*:300, 1973.
26. Dahlin DC, Ivins JC: Benign chondroblastoma. A study of 125 cases. Cancer *30*:401, 1972.
27. Schajowicz F, Gallardo H: Epiphysial chondroblastoma of bone. A clinicopathological study of sixty-nine cases. J Bone Joint Surg *52B*:205, 1970.
28. Nolan DJ, Middlemiss H: Chondroblastoma of bone. Clin Radiol *26*:343, 1975.
29. McLeod RA, Beabout JW: The roentgenographic features of chondroblastoma. Am J Roentgenol *118*:464, 1973.
30. Kricun ME, Kricun R, Haskin ME: Chondroblastoma of the calcaneus: Radiographic features with emphasis on location. Am J Roentgenol *128*:613, 1977.
31. Aronsohn RS, Hart WR, Martel W: Metaphyseal chondroblastoma of bone. Am J Roentgenol *127*:686, 1976.
32. Fechner RE, Wilde HD: Chondroblastoma in the metaphysis of the femoral neck. A case report and review of the literature. J Bone Joint Surg *56A*:413, 1974.
33. Gravanis MB, Giansanti JS: Benign chondroblastoma. Report of four cases with a discussion of the presence of ossification. Am J Clin Pathol *55*:624, 1971.
34. Riddell RJ, Bromberger NA: Pulmonary metastasis from chondroblastoma of the tibia. Report of a case. J Bone Joint Surg *55B*:848, 1973.
35. Sirsat MV, Doctor VM: Benign chondroblastoma of bone. Report of a case of malignant transformation. J Bone Joint Surg *52B*:741, 1970.
36. Green P, Whittaker RP: Benign chondroblastoma. Case report with pulmonary metastasis. J Bone Joint Surg *57A*:416, 1975.
37. Hall MT, Gonzalez-Crussi F, DeRosa GP, Graul RS: Aggressive chondroblastoma. Report of a case with multiple bone and soft tissue involvement. Clin Orthop Rel Res *126*:261, 1977.
38. Huvos AG, Higinbotham NL, Marcove RC, O'Leary P: Aggressive chondroblastoma. Review of the literature on aggressive behavior and metastases with report of one new case. Clin Orthop Rel Res *126*:266, 1977.
39. Jaffe HL, Lichtenstein L: Chondromyxoid fibroma of bone: A distinctive benign tumor likely to be mistaken especially for chondrosarcoma. Arch Pathol *45*:541, 1948.
40. Schajowicz, F, Gallardo H: Chondromyxoid fibroma (fibromyxoid chondroma) of bone. A clinico-pathological study of thirty-two cases. J Bone Joint Surg *53B*:198, 1971.
41. Feldman F, Hecht HL, Johnston AD: Chondromyxoid fibroma of bone. Radiology *94*:249, 1970.
42. Twersky J, Kassner EG, Tenner MS, Camera A: Vertebral and costal osteochondromas causing spinal cord compression. Am J Roentgenol *124*:124, 1975.
43. Julien J, Riemens V, Vital CI, Lagueny A, Miet G: Cervical cord compression by solitary osteochondroma of the atlas. J Neurol Neurosurg Psychiatry *41*:479, 1978.
44. Becker MH, Epstein F: Case report 77. Skel Radiol *3*:197, 1978.
45. Landon GC, Johnson KA, Dahlin DC: Subungual exostoses. J Bone Joint Surg *61A*:256, 1979.
46. Erlandson RA, Huvos AG: Chondrosarcoma: A light and electron microscopic study. Cancer *34*:1642, 1974.
47. Dahlin DC, Salvador AH: Chondrosarcomas of bones of the hands and feet — a study of 30 cases. Cancer *34*:755, 1974.
48. Reiter FB, Ackerman LV, Staple TW: Central chondrosarcoma of the appendicular skeleton. Radiology *105*:525, 1972.
49. Schajowicz F: Juxtacortical chondrosarcoma. J Bone Joint Surg *59B*:473, 1977.
50. Mankin HJ, Cantley KP, Lippiello L, Schiller AL, Campbell CJ: The biology of human chondrosarcoma. Parts I and II. J Bone Joint Surg *62A*:160, 176, 1980.
51. Unni KK, Dahlin DC, Beabout JW, Sim FH: Chondrosarcoma: Clear-cell variant. J Bone Joint Surg *58A*:676, 1976.
52. Dahlin DC, Henderson ED: Mesenchymal chondrosarcoma. Further observations on a new entity. Cancer *15*:410, 1962.
53. Salvador AH, Beabout JW, Dahlin DC: Mesenchymal chondrosarcoma — observations on 30 new cases. Cancer *28*:605, 1971.
54. Wu KK, Collon DJ, Guise ER: Extra-osseous chondrosarcoma. Report of five cases and review of the literature. J Bone Joint Surg *62A*:189, 1980.
55. Jaffe HL: Osteoid-osteoma of bone. Radiology *45*:319, 1945.
56. Caldicott WJH: Diagnosis of spinal osteoid osteoma. Radiology *92*:1192, 1969.
57. Keim HA, Reina EG: Osteoid-osteoma as a cause of scoliosis. J Bone Joint Surg *57A*:159, 1975.
58. Norman A, Dorfman HD: Osteoid-osteoma inducing pronounced overgrowth and deformity of bone. Clin Orthop Rel Res *110*:233, 1975.
59. Giustra PE, Freiberger RH: Severe growth disturbance with osteoid osteoma. A report of two cases involving the femoral neck. Radiology *96*:285, 1970.
60. Glynn JJ, Lichtenstein L: Osteoid osteoma with multicentric nidus. A report of two cases. J Bone Joint Surg *55A*:855, 1973.
61. Greenspan A, Elguezabel A, Bryk D: Multifocal osteoid osteoma. A case report and review of the literature. Am J Roentgenol *121*:103, 1974.
62. Worland RL, Ryder CT, Johnston AD: Recurrent osteoid-osteoma. Report of a case. J Bone Joint Surg *57A*:277, 1975.
63. O'Dell CW Jr, Resnick D, Niwayama G, Goergen TG, Linovitz RJ: Osteoid osteomas arising in adjacent bones: Report of a case. J Can Assoc Radiol *27*:298, 1976.
64. Mitnick JS, Braunstein P, Genieser NB: Osteoid osteoma of the hip: Unusual isotopic appearance. Am J Roentgenol *133*:322, 1979.
65. Lisbona R, Rosenthall L: Role of radionuclide imaging in osteoid osteoma. Am J Roentgenol *132*:77, 1979.
66. Winter PF, Johnson PM, Hilal SK, Felman F: Scintigraphic detection of osteoid osteoma. Radiology *122*:177, 1977.
67. Goldstein HA, Treves S: Bone scintigraphy of osteoid osteoma: A clinical review. Clin Nucl Med *3*:359, 1978.
68. Lateur L, Baert AL: Localization and diagnosis of osteoid osteoma of the carpal area by angiography. Skel Radiol *2*:75, 1977.
69. O'Hara JP III, Tegtmeyer C, Sweet DE, McCue FC: Angiography in the

diagnosis of osteoid-osteoma of the hand. J Bone Joint Surg *57A*:163, 1975.

70. Heiman ML, Cooley CJ, Bradford DS: Osteoid osteoma of a vertebral body. Report of a case with extension across the intervertebral disk. Clin Orthop Rel Res *118*:159, 1976.
71. Snarr JW, Abell MR, Martel W: Lymphofollicular synovitis with osteoid osteoma. Radiology *106*:557, 1973.
72. Corbett JM, Wilde AH, McCormack LJ, Evarts CM: Intra-articular osteoid osteoma. A diagnostic problem. Clin Orthop Rel Res *98*:225, 1974.
73. Jackson RP, Reckling FW, Mantz FA: Osteoid osteoma and osteoblastoma. Similar histologic lesions with different natural histories. Clin Orthop Rel Res *128*:303, 1977.
74. McLeod RA, Dahlin DC, Beabout JW: The spectrum of osteoblastoma. Am J Roentgenol *126*:321, 1976.
75. Marsh BW, Bonfiglio M, Brady LP, Enneking WF: Benign osteoblastoma: Range of manifestations. J Bone Joint Surg *57A*:1, 1975.
76. Goldman RL: The periosteal counterpart of benign osteoblastoma. Am J Clin Pathol *56*:73, 1971.
77. De Souza Dias L, Frost HM: Osteoblastoma of the spine. A review and report of eight new cases. Clin Orthop Rel Res *91*:141, 1973.
78. Jackson RP: Recurrent osteoblastoma. A review. Clin Orthop Rel Res *131*:229, 1978.
79. Schajowicz F, Lemos C: Malignant osteoblastoma. J Bone Joint Surg *58B*:202, 1976.
80. Schwartz E: Ossifying fibroma of the face and skull. Am J Roentgenol *91*:1012, 1964.
81. Goergen TG, Dickman PS, Resnick D, Saltzstein SL, O'Dell CW, Akeson WH: Long bone ossifying fibroma. Cancer *39*:2067, 1977.
82. Dahlin DC: Pathology of osteosarcoma. Clin Orthop Rel Res *111*:23, 1975.
83. Marcove RC, Mike V, Hajek JV, Levin AG, Hutter RVP: Osteogenic sarcoma under the age of twenty-one. J Bone Joint Surg *52A*:411, 1970.
84. Wu KK, Guise ER, Frost HM, Mitchell CL: Osteogenic sarcoma. Report of one hundred and fifty-seven cases. Henry Ford Hosp Med J *24*:213, 1976.
85. Enneking WF, Springfield DS: Osteosarcoma. Orthop Clin North Am *8*:785, 1977.
86. de Santos LA, Rosengren JE, Wooten WB, Murray JA: Osteogenic sarcoma after the age of 50: A radiographic evaluation. Am J Roentgenol *131*:481, 1978.
87. Thayer C, Rogers LF: Unicentric osteosarcoma of bone with subsequent skeletal metastases. Skel Radiol *4*:148, 1979.
88. Reider-Grosswasser I, Grunebaum M: Metaphyseal multifocal osteosarcoma. Br J Radiol *51*:671, 1978.
89. Mahoney JP, Spanier SS, Morris JL: Multifocal osteosarcoma. A case report with review of the literature. Cancer *44*:1897, 1979.
90. Fitzgerald RH Jr, Dahlin DC, Sim FH: Multiple metachronous osteogenic sarcoma. J Bone Joint Surg *55A*:595, 1973.
91. Larsson SE, Lorentzon R, Boquist L: Telangiectatic osteosarcoma. Acta Orthop Scand *49*:589, 1978.
92. Ellman H, Gold RH, Mirra JM: Roentgenographically "benign" but rapidly lethal diaphyseal osteosarcoma. A case report. J Bone Joint Surg *56A*:1267, 1974.
93. Goldstein C, Ambos MA, Bosniak MA: Multiple ossified metastases to the kidney from osteogenic sarcoma. Am J Roentgenol *128*:148, 1977.
94. Madsen EH: Lymph node metastases from osteoblastic osteogenic sarcoma visible on plain films. Skel Radiol *4*:216, 1979.
95. de Santos LA, Murray JA, Finklestein JB, Spjut HJ, Ayala AG: The radiographic spectrum of periosteal osteosarcoma. Radiology *127*:123, 1978.
96. Dahlin DC: Case report 27. Skel Radiol *1*:249, 1977.
97. Unni KK, Dahlin DC, Beabout JW: Periosteal osteogenic sarcoma. Cancer *37*:2476, 1976.
98. Farr GH, Huvos AG: Juxtacortical osteogenic sarcoma. An analysis of fourteen cases. J Bone Joint Surg *54A*:1205, 1972.
99. Ahuja SC, Villacin AB, Smith JS, Bullough PG, Huvos AG, Marcove RC: Juxtacortical (parosteal) osteogenic sarcoma. Histologic grading and prognosis. J Bone Joint Surg *59A*:632, 1977.
100. Unni KK, Dahlin DC, Beabout JW, Ivins JC: Parosteal osteogenic sarcoma. Cancer *37*:2466, 1976.
101. Edeiken J, Farrel C, Ackerman LV, Spjut HJ: Parosteal sarcoma. Am J Roentgenol *111*:579, 1971.
102. Ranniger K, Altner PC: Parosteal osteoid sarcoma. Radiology *86*:648, 1966.
103. Smith J, Ahuja SC, Huvos AG, Bullough PG: Parosteal (juxtacortical) osteogenic sarcoma. A roentgenological study of 30 patients. J Can Assoc Radiol *29*:167, 1978.
104. Caffey J: On fibrous defects in cortical walls of growing tubular bones: Their radiologic appearance, structure, prevalence, natural course, and diagnostic significance. Adv Pediatr *7*:13, 1955.
105. Mubarak S, Saltzstein SL, Daniel DM: Non-ossifying fibroma. Report of an intact lesion. J Clin Pathol *61*:697, 1974.
106. Allman RM: RPC of the month from the AFIP. Radiology *93*:167, 1969.
107. Drennan DB, Maylahn DJ, Fahey JJ: Fractures through large non-ossifying fibromas. Clin Orthop Rel Res *103*:82, 1974.
108. Kirkpatrick JA, Wilkinson RH: Case report 52. Skel Radiol *2*:189, 1978.
109. Young DW, Nogrady MB, Dunbar JS, Wiglesworth FW: Benign cortical irregularities in the distal femur of children. J Can Assoc Radiol *23*:107, 1972.
110. Barnes GR Jr, Gwinn JL: Distal irregularities of the femur simulating malignancy. Am J Roentgenol *122*:180, 1974.
111. Brower AC, Culver JE Jr, Keats TE: Histological nature of the cortical irregularity of the medial posterior distal femoral metaphysis in children. Radiology *99*:389, 1971.
112. Rabhan WN, Rosai J: Desmoplastic fibroma. Report of ten cases and review of the literature. J Bone Joint Surg *50A*:487, 1968.
113. Sugiura I: Desmoplastic fibroma. Case report and review of the literature. J. Bone Joint Surg *58A*:126, 1976.
114. Hardy R, Lehrer H: Desmoplastic fibroma vs desmoid tumor of bone. Two cases illustrating a problem in differential diagnosis and classification. Radiology *88*:899, 1967.
115. Larsson SE, Lorentzon R, Boquist L: Fibrosarcoma of bone. J Bone Joint Surg *58B*:412, 1976.
116. Hernandez FJ, Fernandez BB: Multiple diffuse fibrosarcoma of bone. Cancer *37*:939, 1976.
117. Jeffree GM, Price CHG: Metastatic spread of fibrosarcoma of bone. J Bone Joint Surg *58B*:418, 1976.
118. Nascimento AG, Huvos AH, Marcove RC: Primary malignant giant cell tumor of bone. A study of eight cases and review of the literature. Cancer *44*:1393, 1979.
119. McGrath PJ: Giant cell tumor of bone. An analysis of fifty-two cases. J Bone Joint Surg *54B*:216, 1972.
120. Goldenberg RR, Campbell CJ, Bonfiglio M: Giant cell tumor of bone. An analysis of two hundred and eighteen cases. J Bone Joint Surg *52A*:619, 1970.
121. Larsson SE, Lorentzon R, Boquist L: Giant-cell tumor of bone. J Bone Joint Surg *57A*:167, 1975.
122. McInerney DP, Middlemiss JH: Giant-cell tumor of bone. Skel Radiol *2*:195, 1978.
123. Sim FH, Dahlin DC, Beabout JW: Multicentric giant-cell tumor of bone. J Bone Joint Surg *59A*:1052, 1977.
124. Sybrandy S, De la Fuente AA: Multiple giant-cell tumour of bone. Report of a case. J Bone Joint Surg *55B*:350, 1973.
125. Kaufman SM, Isaac PC: Multiple giant cell tumors. South Med J *70*:105, 1977.
126. Tornberg DN, Dick HM, Johnston AD: Multicentric giant-cell tumors in the long bones. A case report. J Bone Joint Surg *57A*:420, 1975.
127. Peison B, Feigenbaum J: Metaphyseal giant-cell tumor in a girl of 14. Radiology *118*:145, 1976.
128. Averill RM, Smith RJ, Campbell CJ: Giant-cell tumors of the bones of the hand. J Hand Surg *5*:39, 1980.
129. Smith J, Wixon D, Watson RC: Giant-cell tumor of the sacrum. Clinical and radiological features in 13 patients. J Can Assoc Radiol *30*:34, 1979.
130. Peimer CA, Schiller AL, Mankin HJ, Smith RJ: Multicentric giant-cell tumor of bone. J Bone Joint Surg *62A*:652, 1980.
131. Spanier SS, Enneking WF, Enriquez P: Primary malignant fibrous histiocytoma of bone. Cancer *36*:2084, 1975.
132. Feldman F, Lattes R: Primary malignant fibrous histiocytoma (fibrous xanthoma) of bone. Skel Radiol *1*:145, 1977.
133. Huvos AG: Primary malignant fibrous histiocytoma of bone. Clinicopathologic study of 18 patients. NY State J Med *76*:552, 1976.
134. Feldman F, Norman D: Intra- and extraosseous malignant histiocytoma (malignant fibrous xanthoma). Radiology *104*:497, 1972.
135. Spanier SS: Malignant fibrous histiocytoma of bone. Orthop Clin North Am *8*:947, 1977.
136. Hudson TM, Hawkins IF Jr, Spanier SS, Enneking WF: Angiography of malignant fibrous histiocytoma of bone. Radiology *131*:9, 1979.
137. Hart JAL: Intraosseous lipoma. J Bone Joint Surg *55B*:624, 1973.
138. Appenzeller J, Weitzner S: Intraosseous lipoma of the os calcis. Clin Orthop Rel Res *101*:171, 1974.
139. Poussa M, Holmström T: Intraosseous lipoma of the calcaneus. Acta Orthop Scand *47*:570, 1976.
140. DeLee JC: Intra-osseous lipoma of the proximal part of the femur. Case report. J Bone Joint Surg *61A*:601, 1979.
141. Hanelin LG, Sclamberg EL, Bardsley JL: Intraosseous lipoma of the coccyx. Report of a case. Radiology *114*:343, 1975.
142. Matsubayashi T, Nakajima M, Tsukada M: Case report 118. Skel Radiol *5*:131, 1980.

143. Jacobs P: Parosteal lipoma with hyperostosis. Clin Radiol *23*:196, 1972.
144. Larsson SE, Lorentzon R, Boquist L: Primary liposarcoma of bone. Acta Orthop Scand *46*:869, 1975.
145. Schwartz A, Shuster M, Becker SM: Liposarcoma of bone. Report of a case and review of the literature. J Bone Joint Surg *52A*:171, 1970.
146. Catto M, Stevens J: Liposarcoma of bone. J Pathol Bacteriol *86*:248, 1963.
147. Feldman F: Case report 104. Skeletal Radiol *4*:245, 1979.
148. Karlin CA, Brower AC: Multiple primary hemangiomas of bone. Am J Roentgenol *129*:162, 1977.
149. Krieger AJ: Hemangioma of fifth cervical vertebra with intermittent spinal cord dysfunction. South Med J *70*:1008, 1977.
150. Schajowicz F, Rebecchini AC, Bosch-Mayol G: Intracortical haemangioma simulating osteoid osteoma. J Bone Joint Surg *61B*:94, 1979.
151. Sugiura I: Tibial periosteal hemangioma. Clin Orthop Rel Res *106*:242, 1975.
152. Rosenquist CJ, Wolfe DC: Lymphangioma of bone. J Bone Joint Surg *50A*:158, 1968.
153. Bullough PG: Solitary lymphangioma of bone. A case report. J Bone Joint Surg *58A*:418, 1976.
154. Rogers HM, Chou SN: Lymphangioma of the craniocervical junction. Case report. J Neurosurg *38*:510, 1973.
155. Kittredge RD, Finby N: The many facets of lymphangioma. Am J Roentgenol *95*:56, 1965.
156. Steiner GM, Farman J, Lawson JP: Lymphangiomatosis of bone. Radiology *93*:1093, 1969.
157. Gilsanz V, Yeh HC, Baron MG: Multiple lymphangiomas of the neck, axilla, mediastinum and bones in an adult. Radiology *120*:161, 1976.
158. Nixon GW: Lymphangiomatosis of bone demonstrated by lymphangiography. Am J Roentgenol *110*:582, 1970.
159. Carroll RE, Berman AT: Glomus tumors of the hand. Review of the literature and report of twenty-eight cases. J Bone Joint Surg *54A*:691, 1972.
160. Sugiura I: Intra-osseous glomus tumour. A case report. J Bone Joint Surg *58B*:245, 1976.
161. Boyle WJ: Cystic angiomatosis of bone. A report of three cases and review of the literature. J Bone Joint Surg *54B*:626, 1972.
162. Schajowicz F, Aiello CL, Francone MV, Giannini RE: Cystic angiomatosis (hamartous haemolymphangiomatosis) of bone. A clinicopathological study of three cases. J Bone Joint Surg *60B*:100, 1978.
163. Brower AC, Cluver JE Jr, Keats TE: Diffuse cystic angiomatosis of bone. Report of two cases. Am J Roentgenol *118*:456, 1973.
164. Singh R, Grewal DS, Bannerjee AK, Bansal VP: Haemangiomatosis of the skeleton. Report of a case. J Bone Joint Surg *56B*:136, 1974.
165. Graham DY, Gonzales J, Kothari SM: Diffuse skeletal angiomatosis. Skel Radiol *2*:131, 1978.
166. Stout AP: Hemangiopericytoma. A study of twenty-five cases. Cancer *2*:1027, 1949.
167. Marcial-Rojas RA: Primary hemangiopericytoma of bone. Cancer *13*:308, 1960.
168. Anderson C, Rorabeck CH: Skeletal metastases of an intracranial malignant hemangiopericytoma. J Bone Joint Surg *62A*:145, 1980.
169. Stout AP: Hemangioendothelioma. A tumor of blood vessels featuring vascular endothelial cells. Ann Surg *118*:445, 1943.
170. Dunlop J: Malignant hemangioendothelioma of bone. Case report of en bloc resection and prosthetic hip replacement. J Bone Joint Surg *59A*:832, 1977.
171. Srinivasan CK, Patel MR, Pearlman HS, Silver JW: Malignant hemangioendothelioma of bone. Review of the literature and report of two cases. J Bone Joint Surg *60A*:696, 1978.
172. Beabout JW: Case report 11. Skel Radiol *1*:121, 1976.
173. Dalinka MK, Brennan RE, Patchefsky AS: Case report 3. Skel Radiol *1*:59, 1976.
174. Milgram JW, Riley LH Jr: Hemangioendothelioma of the proximal part of the humerus. A case report. J Bone Joint Surg *54A*:1543, 1972.
175. Larsson SE, Lorentzon R, Boquist L: Malignant hemangioendothelioma of bone. J Bone Joint Surg *57A*:84, 1975.
176. Morrison MJ, Ivins JC: Case report 47. Skel Radiol *2*:177, 1978.
177. Dalinka MK, Cannino C, Patchefsky AS, Romisher GP: Case report 12. Skel Radiol *1*:123, 1976.
178. Dickson JH, Waltz TA, Fechner RE: Intraosseous neurilemoma of the third lumbar vertebra. J Bone Joint Surg *53A*:349, 1971.
179. Fawcett KJ, Dahlin DC: Neurilemmoma of bone. Am J Clin Pathol *47*:959, 1967.
180. Peers JH: Primary intramedullary neurogenic sarcoma of the ulna. Am J Pathol *10*:811, 1934.
181. Firooznia H, Pinto RS, Lin JP, Baruch HH, Zusner J: Chordoma: Radiologic evaluation of 20 cases. Am J Roentgenol *127*:797, 1976.
182. Pinto RS, Lin JP, Firooznia H, Lefleur RS: The osseous and angiographic features of vertebral chordomas. Neuroradiology 9:231, 1975.
183. Schechter MM, Liebeskind AL, Azar-kia B: Intracranial chordomas. Neuroradiology *8*:67, 1974.
184. Sundaresan N, Galicich JH, Chu FCH, Huvos AG: Spinal chordomas. J Neurosurg *50*:312, 1979.
185. Heaston DK, Gelman MI: Case report 74. Skel Radiol *3*:186, 1978.
186. Paavolainer P, Teppo L: Chordoma in Finland. Acta Orthop Scand *47*:46, 1976.
187. Wu KK, Mitchell DC, Guise ER: Chordoma of the atlas. J Bone Joint Surg *61A*:140, 1979.
188. Fox JE, Batsakis JG, Owano LR: Unusual manifestations of chordoma. A report of two cases. J Bone Joint Surg *50A*:1618, 1968.
189. Falconer MA, Bailey IC, Duchen LW: Surgical treatment of chordoma and chondroma of the skull base. J Neurosurg *29*:261, 1968.
190. Heffelfinger MJ, Dahlin DC, MacCarty CS, Beabout JW: Chordomas and cartilaginous tumors at the skull base. Cancer *32*:410, 1973.
191. Mirra JM, Bernard GW, Bullough PG, Johnston W, Mink G: Cementum-like bone production in solitary bone cysts (so-called "cementoma" of long bones). Clin Orthop Rel Res *135*:295, 1978.
192. Cohen J: Simple bone cysts fluid in 6 cases with a theory of pathogenesis. J Bone Joint Surg *42A*:609, 1960.
193. Cohen J: Etiology of simple bone cyst. J Bone Joint Surg *52A*:1493, 1970.
194. Reynolds J: The "fallen fragment sign" in the diagnosis of unicameral bone cysts. Radiology *92*:949, 1969.
195. Jaffe HL: Tumors and Tumorous Conditions of the Bones and Joints. Philadelphia, Lea & Febiger, 1958, p 70.
196. Norman A, Schiffman M: Simple bone cysts: factors of age dependency. Radiology *124*:779, 1977.
197. Sanerkin NG: Old fibrin coagula and their ossification in simple bone cysts. J Bone Joint Surg *61B*:195, 1979.
198. Linthoudt DV, Lagier R: Calcaneal cysts. A radiological and anatomico-pathological study. Acta Orthop Scand *49*:310, 1978.
199. Spence KF Jr, Bright RW, Fitzgerald SP, Sell KW: Solitary unicameral bone cyst: Treatment with freeze-dried crushed cortical bone allograft. J Bone Joint Surg *58A*:636, 1976.
200. Fahey JJ, O'Brien ET: Subtotal resection and grafting in selected cases of solitary unicameral bone cyst. J Bone Joint Surg *55A*:59, 1973.
201. Smith RW, Smith CF: Solitary unicameral bone cyst of the calcaneus. A review of twenty cases. J Bone Joint Surg *56A*:49, 1974.
202. Johnson LC, Vetter H, Putschar WGJ: Sarcomas arising in bone cysts. Virchows Arch (Pathol Anat) *335*:428, 1962.
203. Grabias S, Mankin HJ: Chondrosarcoma arising in histologically proved unicameral bone cyst. A case report. J Bone Joint Surg *56A*:1501, 1974.
204. Cohen J: Unicameral bone cysts. A current synthesis of reported cases. Orthop Clin North Am *8*:715, 1977.
205. Trias A, Beauregard G: Epidermoid cyst of bone. Can J Surg *17*:1, 1974.
206. Lerner MR, Southwick WO: Keratin cysts in phalangeal bone. Report of an unusual case. J Bone Joint Surg *50A*:365, 1968.
207. Svenes KJ, Halleraker B: Epidermal bone cyst of the finger. A case report. Acta Orthop Scand *48*:29, 1977.
208. Exner G, Hort W, Boger A: Epidermoidzyste der Tibia. Z Orthop *116*:362, 1978.
209. Carlson DH, Wilkinson RH, Bhakkaviziam A: Aneurysmal bone cysts in children. Am J Roentgenol *116*:644, 1972.
210. Robinson AE, Thomas RL, Manson DM: Aneurysmal bone cyst of the rib. A report of two unusual cases. Am J Roentgenol *100*:526, 1967.
211. Cacdac MA, Malis LI, Anderson PJ: Aneurysmal parietal bone cyst. Case report. J Neurosurgery *37*:237, 1972.
212. Clough JR, Price CHG: Aneurysmal bone cyst: Pathogenesis and long term results of treatment. Clin Orthop Rel Res *97*:52, 1973.
213. Oliver LP: Aneurysmal bone cyst. Report of a case. Oral Surg *35*:67, 1973.
214. Koskinen EVS, Visuri TI, Holmstrom T, Roukkula MA: Aneurysmal bone cyst. Clin Orthop Rel Res *118*:136, 1976.
215. Sherman RS, Soong KY: Aneurysmal bone cyst: Its roentgen diagnosis. Radiology *68*:54, 1957.
216. Hinds EC, Pleasants JE, Snyder PL: Management of ameloblastoma. Oral Surg *7*:1169, 1954.
217. Gorlin RJ, Chaudhry AP, Pindborg JJ: Odontogenic tumors. Cancer *14*:73, 1961.
218. Sehdev MK, Huvos AG, Strong EW, Gerold FP, Willis GW: Ameloblastoma of maxilla and mandible. Cancer *33*:324, 1974.
219. McIvor J: The radiological features of ameloblastoma. Clin Radiol *25*:237, 1974.
220. Eversole LR, Rovin S: Differential radiographic diagnosis of lesions of the jawbones. Radiology *105*:277, 1972.
221. Huvos AG, Marcove RC: Adamantinoma of long bones. A clinicopathological study of fourteen cases with vascular origin suggested. J Bone Joint Surg *57A*:148, 1975.

222. Cohen DM, Dahlin DC, Pugh DG: Fibrous dysplasia associated with adamantinoma of the long bones. Cancer *15*:515, 1962.
223. Unni KK, Dahlin DC, Beabout JW, Ivins JC: Adamantinomas of long bones. Cancer *34*:1796, 1974.
224. Weiss SW, Dorfman HD: Adamantinoma of long bone. Hum Pathol *8*:141, 1977.
225. Braidwood AS, McDougall A: Adamantinoma of the tibia. Report of two cases. J Bone Joint Surg *56B*:735, 1974.
226. Besemann EF, Perez MA: Malignant angioblastoma, so-called adamantinoma involving the humerus. A case report. Am J Roentgenol *100*:538, 1967.
227. Dameron TB Jr: Adamantinoma of the appendicular skeleton. Johns Hopkins Med J *145*:107, 1979.
228. Stoker DJ: Case report 22. Skel Radiol *1*:187, 1977.
229. Beabout JW: Case report 29. Skel Radiol *1*:257, 1977.
230. Freiberger RH, Bullough PG: Case report 8. Skel Radiol *1*:112, 1976.
231. Lasda NA, Hughes EC Jr: Adamantinoma of the ischium. J Bone Joint Surg *61A*:599, 1979.
232. Llombart-Bosch A, Blache R, Peydro-Olaya A: Ultrastructural study of 28 cases of Ewing's sarcoma: Typical and atypical forms. Cancer *41*:1362, 1978.
233. Friedman B, Gold H: Ultrastructure of Ewing's sarcoma of bone. Cancer *22*:307, 1968.
234. Povysil C, Matejovsky Z: Ultrastructure of Ewing's tumour. Virchows Arch (Pathol Anat) *374*:303, 1977.
235. Kadin ME, Bensch KG: On the origin of Ewing's tumor. Cancer *27*:257, 1971.
236. Larsson SE, Boquist L, Bergdahl L: Ewing's sarcoma. Clin Orthop Rel Res *95*:263, 1973.
237. Lavallee G, Lemarbre L, Bouchard R, Beauregard CG, Dussault R: Ewing's sarcoma in adults. J Can Assoc Radiol *30*:223, 1979.
238. Whitehouse GH, Griffiths GJ: Roentgenologic aspects of spinal involvement by primary and metastatic Ewing's tumor. J Can Assoc Radiol *27*:290, 1976.
239. de Santos LA, Jing BS: Radiographic findings of Ewing's sarcoma of the jaws. Br J Radiol *51*:682, 1978.
240. Dick HM, Francis KC, Johnston AD: Ewing's sarcoma of the hand. J Bone Joint Surg *53A*:345, 1971.
241. Dunn EJ, Yaska KH, Judge DM, Garner FL, Varano LA: Ewing's sarcoma of the great toe. A case report. Clin Orthop Rel Res *116*:203, 1976.
242. Nascimento AG, Cooper KL, Unni KK, Dahlin DC, Pritchard DJ: A clinicopathologic study of 20 cases of large cell (atypical) Ewing's sarcoma of bone. Am J Surg Pathol *4*:29, 1980.
243. Evans DMD, Sanerkin NG: Primary leiomyosarcoma of bone. J Pathol *90*:348, 1965.
244. Meister P, Konrad E, Gokel JM, Remberger K: Case report 59. Skel Radiol *2*:265, 1978.
245. Pasquel PM, Levet SN, DeLeon B: Primary rhabdomyosarcoma of bone. A case report. J Bone Joint Surg *58A*:1176, 1976.
246. Capusten BM, Rochon L, Rosman MA, Marton D: Osteofibrous dysplasia. J Can Assoc Radiol *31*:50, 1980.
247. Campanacci M: Osteofibrous dysplasia of long bones: A new clinical entity. Ital J Orthop Traumatol *2*:221, 1976.
248. Schneider HM, Wunderlich TH, Puls P: The primary liposarcoma of the bone. Arch Orthop Traumat Surg *96*:235, 1980.
249. Israels SJ, Downs AR: Traumatic aneurysm of the popliteal artery due to an osteochondroma of the femur. Can J Surg *23*:270, 1980.
250. Merryweather R, Middlemiss JH, Sanerkin NG: Malignant transformation of osteoblastoma. J Bone Joint Surg *62B*:381, 1980.
251. Dunham WK, Wilborn WH, Zarzour RJ: A large parosteal osteosarcoma with transformation to high-grade osteosarcoma. A case report. Cancer *44*:1495, 1979.
252. Dunham WK, Marcus NW, Enneking WF, Haun C: Developmental defects of the distal femoral metaphysis. J Bone Joint Surg *62A*:801, 1980.
253. Palmer FJ, Blum PW: Osteochondroma with spinal cord compression. Report of three cases. J Neurosurg *52*:842, 1980.
254. Schwartz AM, Ramos RM: Neurofibromatosis and multiple nonossifying fibromas. Am J Roentgenol *135*:617, 1980.
255. Hughes S: Radionuclides in orthopaedic surgery. J Bone Joint Surg *62B*:141, 1980.
256. Cheng TH, Holman BL: Increased skeletal:renal uptake ratio. Etiology and characteristics. Radiology *136*:455, 1980.
257. Schutte HE: The influence of bone pain on the results of bone scans. Cancer *44*:2039, 1979.
258. Kirks DR, McCook TA, Merten DF, Sullivan DC: The value of radionuclide bone imaging in selected patients with osteogenic sarcoma metastatic to lung. Pediatr Radiol *9*:139, 1980.
259. Hall FM, Goldberg RP, Kasdon EJ, White AA III: Case report 131. Skel Radiol *5*:275, 1980.
260. Ellis GL, Brannon RB: Intraosseous lymphangiomas of the mandible. Skel Radiol *5*:253, 1980.
261. Lagier R: Case report 128. Skel Radiol *5*:267, 1980.
262. Barwick KW, Huvos AG, Smith J: Primary osteogenic sarcoma of the vertebral column. Cancer *46*:595, 1980.
263. Smith FW, Gilday DL: Scintigraphic appearances of osteoid osteoma. Radiology *137*:191, 1980.
264. Humphry A, Gilday DL, Brown RG: Bone scintigraphy in chondroblastoma. Radiology *137*:497, 1980.
265. Simon MA, Kirchner PT: Scintigraphic evaluation of primary bone tumors. J Bone Joint Surg *62A*:758, 1980.

TUMORS AND TUMOR-LIKE LESIONS IN OR ABOUT JOINTS

by John E. Madewell, M.D., and Donald E. Sweet, M.D.

74B

Numerous tumors and tumor-like lesions of the soft tissues have been described with a variety of clinical and radiographic patterns.[1-15] They range from the common (lipoma and liposarcoma) to the rare (glomus tumor). A number of these lesions are of interest because of their dominant clinical features, such as the production of pain (glomus tumors, leiomyomas, and multiple, painful lipomatosis). The soft tissue tumors may be benign or malignant and vary greatly in size, especially the fatty tumors. Each lesion usually has a characteristic clinical, pathologic, and radiographic pattern. In this chapter those soft tissue tumors and tumor-like lesions that present as masses in or about the joint will be discussed. Some of these lesions are also discussed elsewhere in the book (see Chapter 85), but they are emphasized here since a consideration of periarticular masses is fundamental in the analysis of joint disease.

The opinions or assertions contained herein are the private views of the authors, and are not to be construed as official or as reflecting the views of the United States Departments of the Army, Air Force, Navy, or Defense.

DIAGNOSTIC MODALITIES

Soft tissue tumors and tumor-like lesions usually present with a soft tissue mass or swelling. A variety of imaging techniques are useful in evaluation of the mass.[16-19] All techniques assist in determination of the anatomic extent and effect on structures adjacent to the lesion. Such findings, which are accurately predicted by radiographic technique, are extremely helpful in planning management, which is usually surgical.[20-28] A definite diagnosis using radiographic features alone is usually not possible. However, specific radiographic findings, such as phleboliths, fat and cartilage mineralization, are very important clues to the lesion's identity.

Plain Film Radiography. The plain film radiographs, when obtained with technical excellence and special attention to soft tissue detail, are most helpful in showing these soft tissue masses and their effect on bone.[19, 29-31] Overpenetrated views may be helpful in demonstrating less obvious abnormalities of the adjacent bone. Tomography is also of assistance by delineating soft tissue abnormalities adjacent to complex bony structures (pelvis and shoulder) and augments but does not replace the plain film examination.[19, 32] The plain film is still superior to other techniques in predicting the presence and nature of bone involvement.[32] When bone is involved by a slow-growing soft tissue mass, local pressure by the mass results in a scalloped appearance with a well-defined sclerotic margin. This is most frequently seen in benign processes. Irregular cortical destruction is usually associated with fast-growing and frequently malignant lesions. Obliteration or displacement, or both, of the normal fascial planes due to soft tissue infiltration is common in both benign and malignant tumors. Occasionally, this interface may be lobulated and smooth, suggesting an encapsulated tumor. This is usually pseudoencapsulation, since most of the lesions will invade locally. Thus, the margin about soft tissue tumors, either benign or malignant, can be deceptive, and inaccurate information may be disseminated if the presence of a smooth margin is always equated with benign, noninfiltrating tumors. In the evaluation of patients with soft tissue masses, an integration of radiographic procedures plus clinical correlation is necessary for adequate diagnosis and management.

Xeroradiography and Arthrography. These techniques may characterize the soft tissue mass by the process of edge enhancement. Xeroradiographs demonstrate fine structures adjacent to the soft tissue lesion, especially fascial planes and musculotendinous structures.[33, 34] This definition enables the xeroradiogram to show soft tissue displacement by the tumor. However, it is still questionable whether the information is greater than that obtained with conventional radiography under optimal techniques.[19] Arthrography is also a useful radiographic technique for demonstrating synovial lesions and secondary involvement of the synovium by adjacent soft tissue or bony tumors (see Chapter 15).

Radionuclide Scanning. Radionuclide scanning with phosphate agents may demonstrate uptake in soft tissue tumors. However, results are inconsistent and if isotopic uptake occurs, the margins and local extent of the lesion are poorly defined.[32, 35-43] Invasion of the adjacent bone may also be detected but this is best shown on plain film radiographs. Scanning is most helpful in demonstrating additional skeletal or soft tissue lesions that may not be detected on conventional radiographs.[32] Such findings are significant for patient management, since they may alter the therapeutic procedure.

Sonography. Sonography provides an accurate method of determining the size of soft tissue masses in the extremities.[32] It is less reliable when the mass occurs in complex locations, such as the pelvis, or is located deep in the soft tissue adjacent to bone. With the sonographic image, the precise anatomic relationships and tumor margins have less detail than with other modalities, such as angiography or computed tomography. However, ultrasound can be very useful in following soft tissue mass size on serial studies or the response of the mass to treatment by nonsurgical means, such as chemotherapy or radiation therapy.[32]

Angiography. This modality is most helpful in evaluating soft tissue masses, especially those in the peripheral extremities, where fatty tissue is sparse.[19, 22, 32, 44-56] It provides information about the anatomic extent of the tumor, its effect on adjacent structures, the vascular anatomy, and the venous drainage. These features influence the choice of operative procedure and thus angiography is a valuable adjunct in patient management.[22] Malignant soft tissue tumors are frequently heterogeneous, with areas appearing histologically benign, hemorrhagic, and necrotic. If these sites are biopsied, confusing and erroneous data may be obtained. These sites tend to be less vascular on angiography, whereas the most malignant sites tend to have the greatest vascularity.[51, 55, 432] Thus, angiography can be helpful in localizing an area within the soft tissue tumor that will be likely to yield the most accurate biopsy data. Unsuspected satellite tumors may be uncovered by this method.[53] Although certain angiographic patterns are suggestive of specific histologic diagnoses (hemangiomas), an absolute pathologic diagnosis cannot be made. It is also difficult to definitely differentiate benign from malignant soft tissue tumors.[19, 22, 56] Thus, biopsy and histologic confirmation of the suspected diagnosis remain essential.

Computed Tomography. Computed tomography has proved to be extremely helpful in planning the management of soft tissue tumors.[32, 57-67] Computed tomography is most useful in defining the extent of the soft tissue mass and its relationship to adjacent structures, even in complex bony areas like the pelvis. Occasionally it may help establish a diagnosis, especially with regard to fatty tumors. Contrast enhancement is of value in determining the vascularity of the soft tissue mass.

In the surgical management of soft tissue tumors of an extremity, several factors are important and influence the choice of operative procedure and its results. These factors include histologic diagnosis, determination of anatomic extent of the tumor, and prevention of tumor spread during the operative procedure.[22] Data pertaining to the latter two factors are best obtained through utilization of the multiple diagnostic imaging systems outlined previously. The integration of these procedures will be of great importance in future soft tissue tumor studies.[18]

It is important to understand that even though all these modalities assist in obtaining significant morphologic information about the soft tissue mass, the preoperative diagnosis remains speculative and, almost invariably, a biopsy is required to establish a histologic diagnosis.

BENIGN SOFT TISSUE TUMORS

Lipomatous Tumors

Lipomas. Lipomas arise from fatty tissue and are among the most common and widely distributed soft tissue tumors of mesenchymal origin.[14, 68-70] They are usually solitary but occasionally cases of multiple lipomas have been encountered. Lipomas may occur in any soft tissue that contains fat such as subcutaneous fat,[70] muscle,[71, 72] nerves,[73, 74] synovium,[75] or adjacent to bone in the periosteum.[76-79] Lipomas located deep within the limb grow within muscles (intramuscular type) or between muscles (intermuscular type).[71] Lipomas most commonly occur in the extremities of adult women as a movable, soft, compressible, asymptomatic, slow-growing, subcutaneous soft tissue mass[1] (Fig. 74–40). They are infrequent in the hands or feet,[80-82] and if present are rarely identified prior to surgery.[83] Lipomas are uncommon in children[14, 81] and are rarely congenital or familial.[84, 85]

Rarely, lipomas may be painful (lipoma dolorosa).[86] This type is usually associated with multiple nonsymmetric lipomatosis, in which one tumor after another becomes symptomatic. Lipomas occurring in dependent areas tend to become large and pedunculated.[87] Lipomas may occasionally be associated with nerve paralysis,[76, 88] macrodactyly,[89, 90] and carpal tunnel syndrome.[91] Deep lipomas in the extremities, which commonly occur in the shoulder or thigh, are less readily recognized by clinical examination[71] (Fig. 74–41). These tumors usually change shape with muscular contraction and rarely cause dysfunction of the involved muscle.[71] However, if they develop in a closed fascial space, a firm mass may be palpable even when the muscle is relaxed. This contrasts with the typical pliable consistency of most lipomas.

Lipomas represent a local collection of adipose tissue and some appear related to disturbances in fat metabolism.[14] The adipose tissue in lipomas is histologically and chemically similar to normal fat, but it is not available for normal metabolism, as evidenced by the fact that it maintains its size or

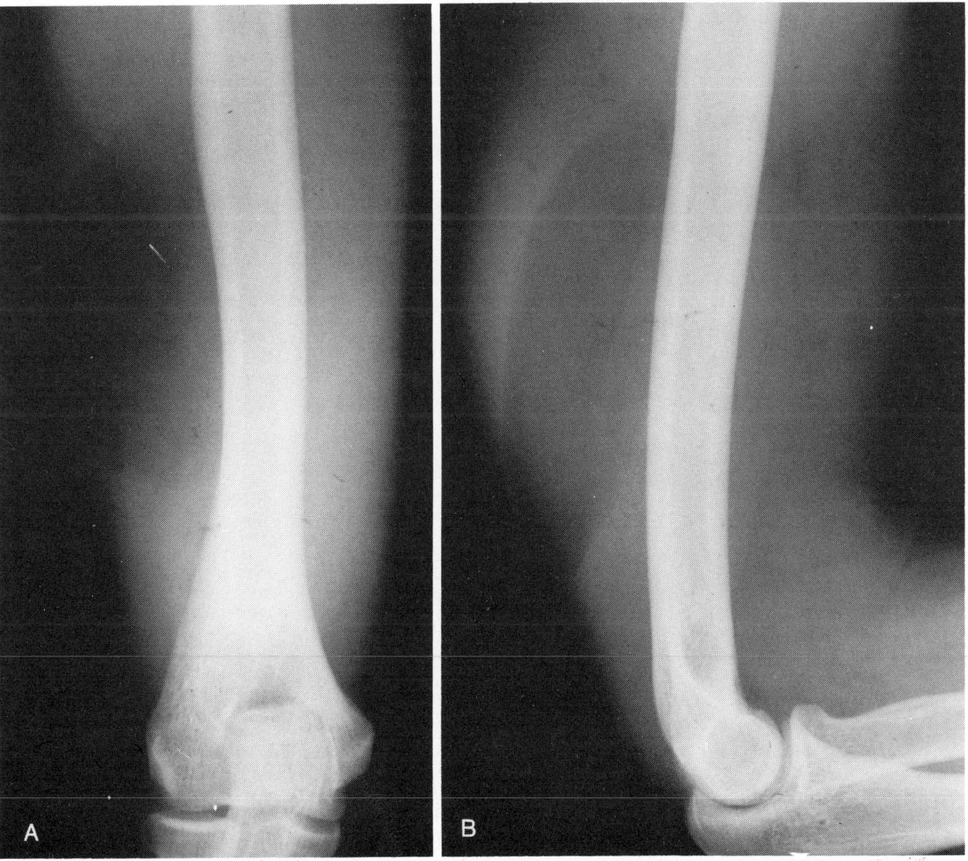

Figure 74–40. *Intermuscular lipoma. Arm with typical radiographic appearance and changing shape. This patient presented with a palpable soft tissue mass.*

A *Anteroposterior radiograph shows a sharply circumscribed, homogeneous, radiolucent fatty mass.*

B *On the lateral radiograph the shape of the lipoma changes with muscular contraction.* (Armed Forces Institute of Pathology Neg. Nos. 72-6580-1,2.)

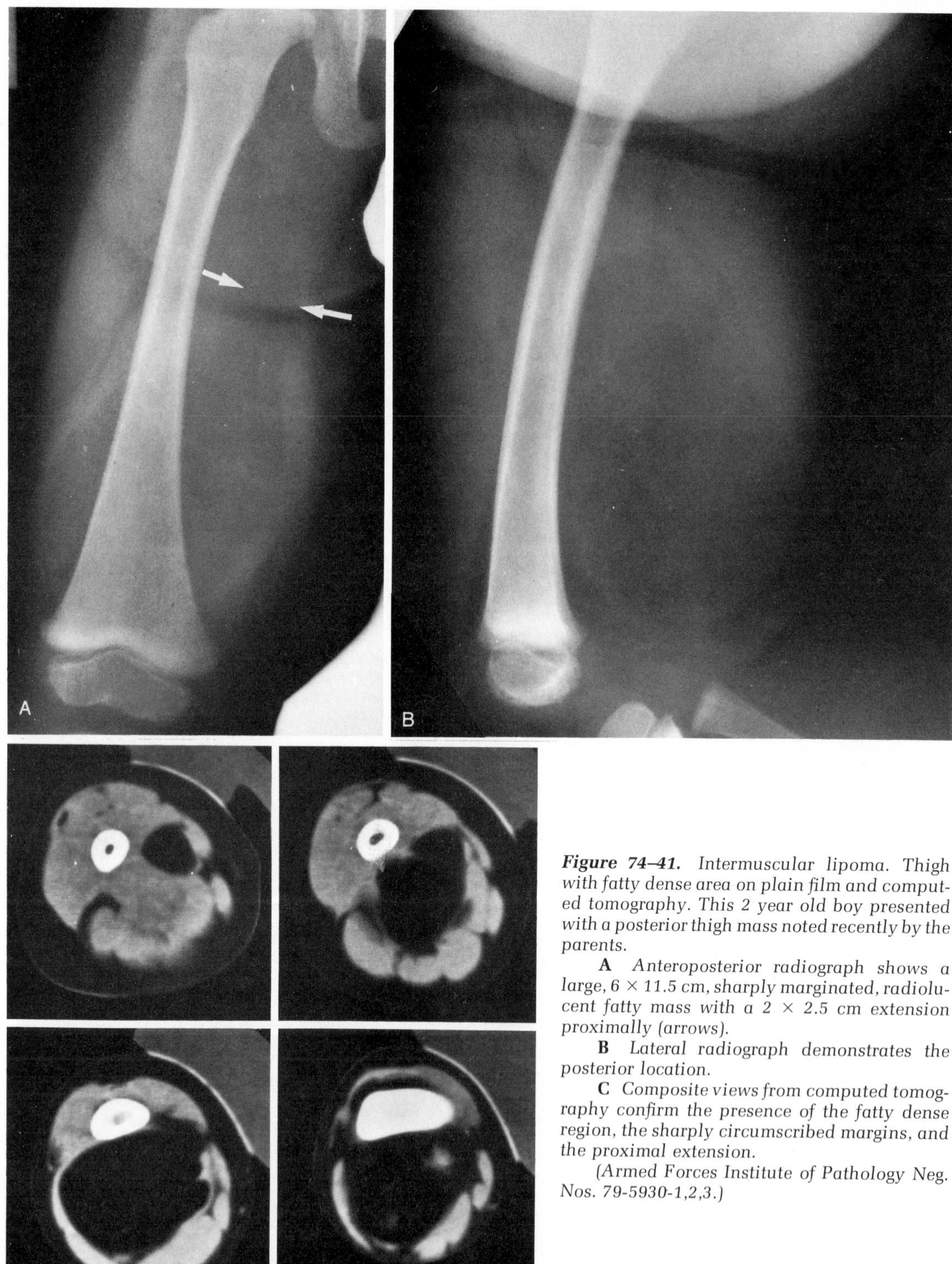

Figure 74–41. *Intermuscular lipoma. Thigh with fatty dense area on plain film and computed tomography. This 2 year old boy presented with a posterior thigh mass noted recently by the parents.*

A *Anteroposterior radiograph shows a large, 6 × 11.5 cm, sharply marginated, radiolucent fatty mass with a 2 × 2.5 cm extension proximally (arrows).*

B *Lateral radiograph demonstrates the posterior location.*

C *Composite views from computed tomography confirm the presence of the fatty dense region, the sharply circumscribed margins, and the proximal extension.*

(Armed Forces Institute of Pathology Neg. Nos. 79-5930-1,2,3.)

amount during starvation.[1, 92] Grossly, intermuscular and subcutaneous lipomas are usually well-defined masses with smooth rounded or lobular surfaces, which may grow to considerable size[71, 87, 93, 94] (Fig. 74–42). In contrast, intramuscular lipomas grossly are ill-defined lesions with extensive infiltration both locally and into adjacent muscles[71] (Fig. 74–43). Huge lipomas, which may weigh more than the patient, seldom occur in the extremities. The lipoma is arranged in lobules with many fibrous septa and is surrounded by a delicate capsule. The latter, which is the boundary between the lipoma and surrounding tissue, may be indistinct and difficult to identify in surgery, especially when it is located within normal adipose tissue.

Microscopically, lipomas consist of aggregates of mature fat cells with trabeculated fibrous septa. They may occasionally contain bone (ossifying lipoma),[95-98] cartilage,[99] or bone marrow (myelolipoma.)[100] An admixture of other mesenchymal structures can occur, such as embryonic fat, blood vessels, and fibrous tissue. Whether they are deep or subcutaneous, lipomas rarely undergo malignant change.[14, 101-103]

An interesting form of lipoma is the spindle cell lipoma.[104] In contrast to most lipomas, it occurs chiefly in men over the age of 45 years. The spindle cell lipoma has a predilection for the shoulder and posterior neck, although it is occasionally seen in the extremities. These tumors usually present in the dermis or subcutaneous tissue as a slow-growing, well-circumscribed, painless mass. Histologically, they contain an intricate mixture of lipocytes with uniform spindle cells and a matrix of mucinous material traversed by birefringent collagen fibers.[104] This pattern can easily be mistaken for a liposarcoma. However, the spindle cell lipomas have a uniformly favorable clinical course.

The lipomas, either subcutaneous or deep, are of special radiographic interest because of their fat density. When these fatty tumors are surrounded by tissues of water density, as in deep locations, the radiograph shows a pathognomonic homogeneous radiolucent mass with sharp margins (Fig. 74–40).

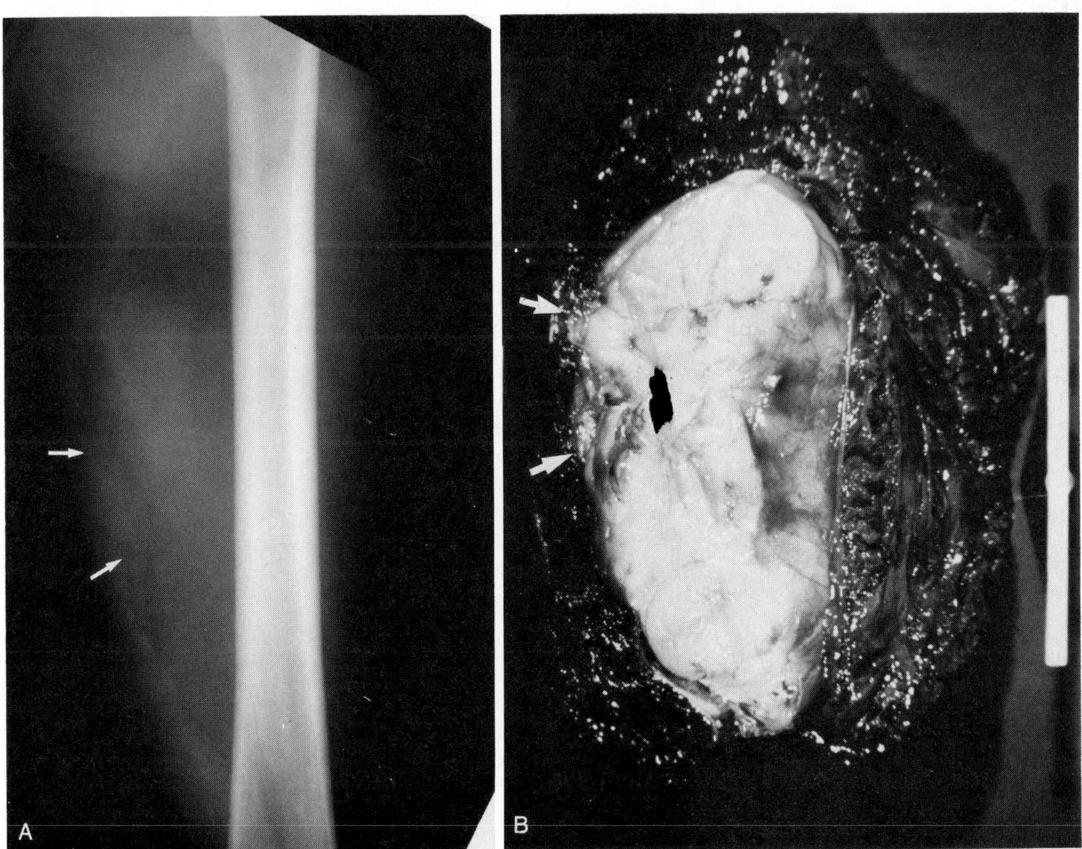

Figure 74–42. *Intermuscular lipoma. Thigh with focal ill-defined margin. This 38 year old man presented with progressive swelling of the thigh of 15 months' duration.*

A *Oblique radiograph shows a fatty mass which is sharply circumscribed except for an ill-defined medial border (arrows). Note the area of water density adjacent to the ill-defined margin.*

B *Gross specimen confirms these findings, with focal infiltration into adjacent muscle (arrows). The well-defined margin and pseudocapsule are also appreciated about most of the lesion.*

(Armed Forces Institute of Pathology Neg. Nos. 74-5340-2, 74-5656-1.)

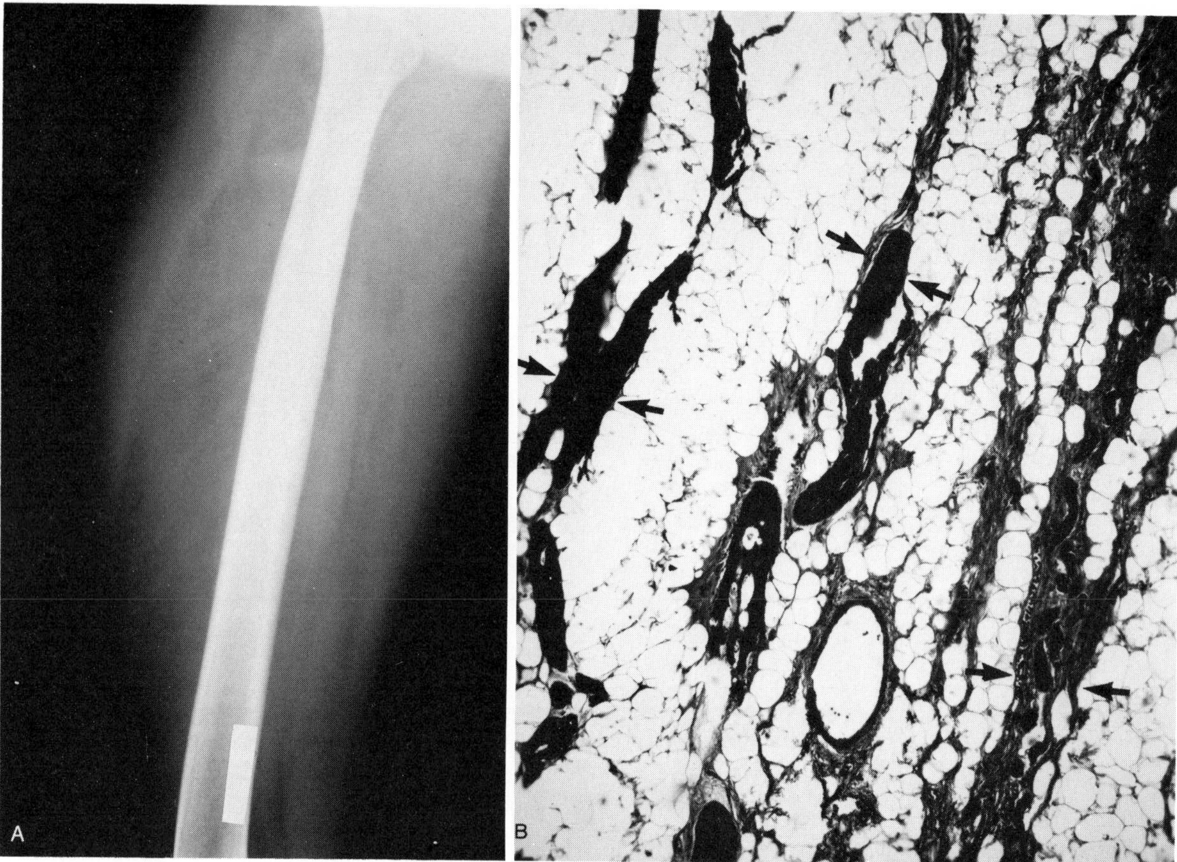

Figure 74–43. *Intramuscular lipoma. Thigh with nonhomogeneous radiolucent mass. This 37 year old woman presented with a painless mass in the thigh.*

A *Oblique radiograph demonstrates a well-circumscribed, nonhomogeneous fatty mass with oblique streaks of water density.*

B *Photomicrograph (63×) reveals the fatty tumor to have infiltrated and entrapped muscle bundles (arrows). This pattern is reflected in the radiograph by the water-dense streaks.*

(Armed Forces Institute of Pathology Neg. Nos. 69-5538, 79-16648.)

Lipomas in the usual subcutaneous location presenting with characteristic clinical findings are not a diagnostic problem and may not be studied radiographically. However, the radiograph can easily confirm the fatty nature of the mass. The deep lipomas of the intermuscular or intramuscular types are not as readily identified by clinical examination but are easily diagnosed radiologically.[16, 71] They are more radiolucent than the surrounding tissue and have two patterns. The intermuscular lipoma is a well-circumscribed, homogeneous, radiolucent mass with only occasional focal irregularity of the margin[71, 105] (Fig. 74–42). Intramuscular lipomas frequently have an inhomogeneous radiolucent appearance because they may contain streaks of muscle bundles of higher density that traverse the mass (Fig. 74–43). Since the lipomas, either in the subcutaneous or deeper soft tissue, are soft, muscular contraction or local compression may change the lipoma's shape and be documented on soft tissue radiographs (Fig. 74–40).

The homogeneous radiolucency of lipomas may be disturbed by metaplastic bone or cartilage formation.[96-99] The mineralized matrix can appear plaque-like or as a homogeneous dense area. The latter is seen in the ossifying lipoma and is due to extensive bone formation. The demonstration of bone and cartilage within the lipoma is not an indication of malignancy[97]; however, bone and cartilage are probably more frequent in liposarcomas.[16]

The nonhomogeneous fatty tumor, whether resulting from water-density collagen or muscle or from calcified cartilage or bone, always presents a bothersome pattern on radiography. An identical inhomogeneous pattern is frequently seen in liposarcomas and, therefore, when it is encountered, histologic confirmation of the nature of the mass is essential. Arteriograms of the lipoma, whether superficial or deep in location, reveal displacement of normal vessels and absent neovascularity, early venous filling, or hypervascularity.[71, 106] Lipomas usually appear on computed tomography as homogeneous, sharply marginated, low-density masses with EMI numbers usually in the −50 to −60 range (Fig. 74–41). Occasionally, the fibrous capsule separating the fatty mass from the adjacent soft tissue may be seen on computed tomography. These lesions are not enhanced on post–contrast computed tomographic scans.[61]

Synovial lipomas are rare and occur almost exclusively in the knee joint, producing nonspecific symptoms.[75, 107, 108] They are solitary round to oval masses of mature fat located intra-articularly, with a covering synovium. The gross specimen reveals the fatty nature of the mass and osseous metaplasia can be encountered.[75] On plain films, synovial lipomas present as a swelling about the knee, and fat may be seen. Arthrography demonstrates a smooth, lobular synovial mass. Computed tomography should confirm the fatty nature of the tumor. This lesion is different from the more common lipoma arborescens, which is also monoarticular and most commonly found in the knee[109] (Fig. 74–44). Lipoma arborescens is characterized by numerous, swollen synovial villous projections of fatty tissue. It may begin de novo but is frequently associated with degenerative joint disease, chronic rheumatoid arthritis, or posttraumatic conditions.[75, 109-112] The plain film radiograph shows soft tissue swelling that may or may not be radiolucent, and the lesion may be seen only on arthrography as multiple, sharply marginated filling defects.[110]

Lipomas originating in the periosteum are also rare (Fig. 74–45). They present as large soft tissue masses and occasionally are accompanied by nerve paralysis.[76, 78, 88, 113] The plain film radiograph has a characteristic appearance, with a deep, radiolucent soft tissue mass adjacent to bone, which is frequently associated with cortical hyperostosis.[113] Calcifications may be present as broad spicules extending out into the fatty mass or patchy homogeneous bony dense areas with a trabecular appearance. The dense shadows are due to osteoid formation with mineralization.

ANGIOLIPOMAS. The angiolipomas are rare benign fatty tumors with a distinct cellular composition.[114-120] They are composed of mature lipocytes with many areas of angiomatous elements, interposed within normal tissue. Most commonly, the lesions are found in young adults. Firmness is more apparent in these lesions than in the ordinary lipoma. These tumors have been divided into (1) noninfiltrating and (2) infiltrating types.[118] The noninfiltrating type is more common and usually is located in subcutaneous tissue. These tumors present as firm, painful, and sometimes multiple masses in the upper extremity. A thin capsule is frequently found. Enucleation of the mass is appropriate, and recurrence is rare. The infiltrating type of angiolipoma usually is found within the deep soft tissue and is less common than the noninfiltrating type. These tumors are ill-defined masses with infiltration of adjacent structures. Although the lesions are histologically benign, local invasion and recurrence are a problem[116, 118] and wide excision is usually necessary.

Radiographically, the angiolipoma, especially the infiltrating type, presents as a soft tissue mass with an inhomogeneous appearance owing to intermixed water- and fatty-density tissues, and it has ill-defined margins. Ossification[61] and phleboliths have been noted. Unlike typical lipomas, angiolipomas have coarse, irregular hypervascularity, show mottled staining during the capillary phase of arteriography, and lack precapillary arteriovenous shunts.[121] Although they are benign, angiolipomas may be misdiagnosed as malignant on arteriography. Computed tomography demonstrates a poorly defined, heterogeneous mass with elements of both fat- and water-density and infiltration of the mass into adjacent tissue.[61] Contrast-enhanced studies may confirm the hypervascularity of the mass.

HIBERNOMAS. Hibernomas are an interesting variant of benign lipoma (Fig. 74–46). They are thought to be a manifestation of a vestigial fat storage organ analogous to the dorsal fat pad of hibernating animals.[122-126] They usually present in the 30 to 50 year age group as a firm, movable, asymptomatic mass that occurs more frequently in women. Occasionally, the prominent vascularity of the tumor will be detected in the overlying skin as an area of warmth compared with the adjacent normal skin.[127] They grow slowly, but rapid enlargement can occur.[128] Microscopically, they are composed of large, polyhedral cells with vacuolated, coarsely granular cytoplasm and central nuclei. On plain films, the hibernoma resembles an inhomogeneous lipoma. On angiography, however, the hibernoma is very vascular, with irregular vessels, an intense homogeneous vascular blush during the capillary phase,[71, 127] and early venous filling. With these findings the hibernoma may be misdiagnosed as malignant preoperatively. Computed tomography also demonstrates the inhomogeneity and fairly well defined margins of the lesion. Malignant degeneration has not been described in this entity.

Lipomatosis

Multiple lipomas (lipomatosis) can occur and are usually randomly distributed throughout the soft tissue. Rarely, however, they are symmetrically deposited and in this case are referred to as multiple symmetric lipomatosis.[14, 129] Affected patients have a striking, bizarre appearance, with masses resembling overdeveloped and unusually located muscles.[14] Lipomas may also be multiple and nonsymmetric in distribution, and these are called nonsymmetric lipomatosis. Some patients may have lipoma dolorosa, characterized by pain which develops in one lipoma after another.[14] The cause of this pain is unknown.

DIFFUSE LIPOMATOSIS. Diffuse lipomatosis is a disorder of fat tissue in which part or all of a limb

Text continued on page 2702

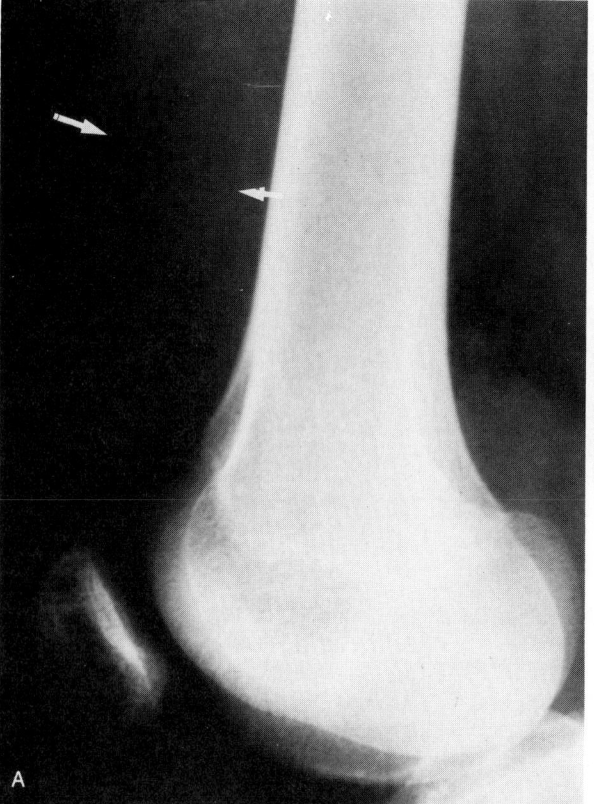

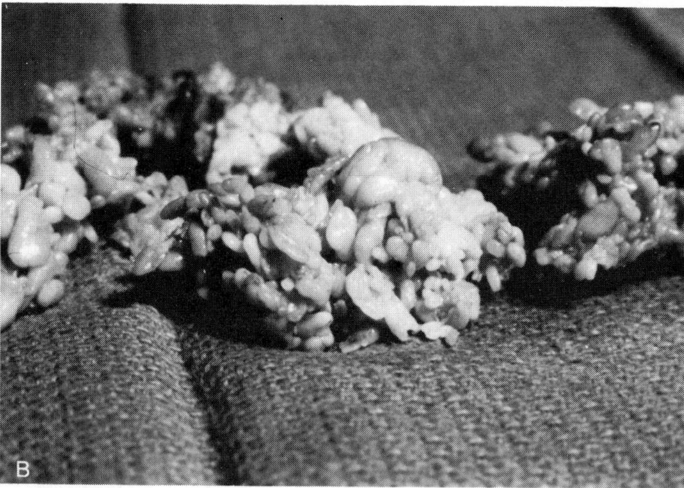

Figure 74–44. *Lipomatosis of synovium (lipoma arborescens). This 18 year old man presented with right knee pain and effusion. There was no evidence of rheumatoid arthritis, osteoarthritis, or trauma.*

A *Lateral radiograph shows a fatty, radiolucent suprapatellar swelling (arrows).*

B *Gross specimen demonstrates prominent villous projections of variable size.*

C *Low power photomicrograph (3×) reveals fatty infiltration throughout the synovium and adjacent capsule.*

D *High power photomicrograph (15×) confirms the fatty engorgement of villi.*

(Armed Forces Institute of Pathology Neg. Nos. 79-2792-5, 80-231, 80-225, 80-226.)

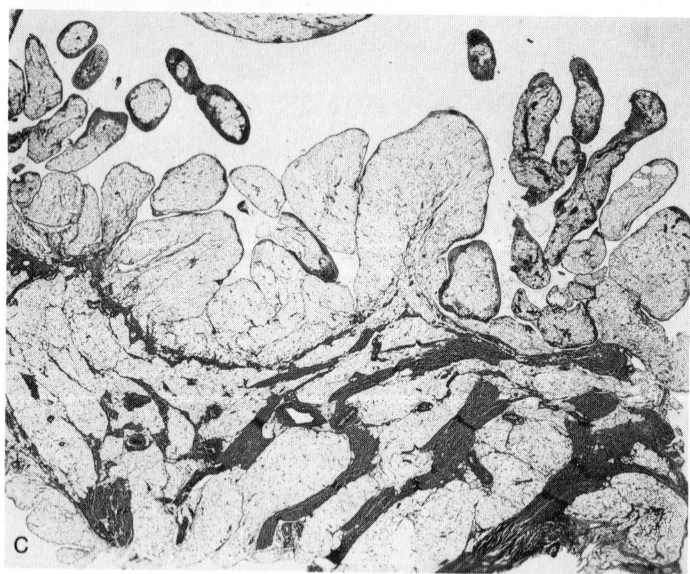

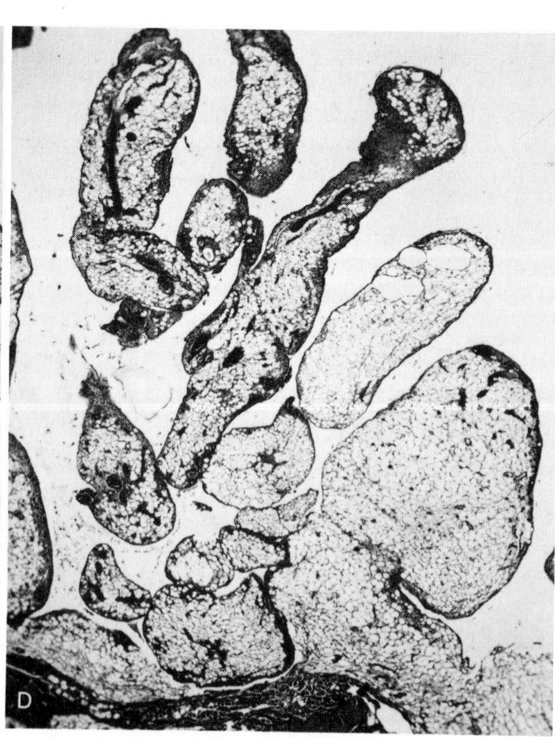

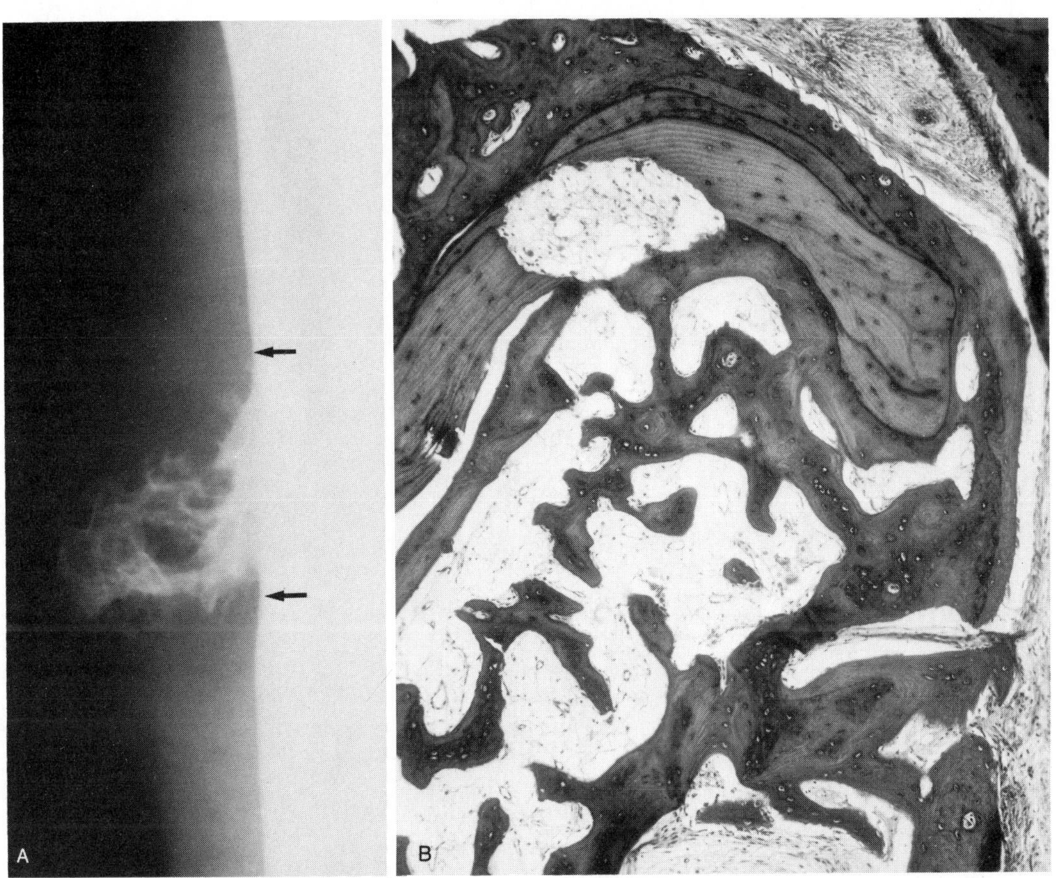

Figure 74–45. *Lipoma of the periosteum of the femur. This 51 year old man presented with symptoms of local pressure due to a thigh mass since childhood.*

A *Anteroposterior coned radiograph of the proximal thigh shows a 9 × 4 cm, sharply marginated, radiolucent fatty mass with a central area of structured density. This dense area has both cortical margins and trabeculae, representing mature bone formation. Note its origin from the bony surface and secondary cortical scalloping (arrows).*

B *Photomicrograph (15×) is characterized by a centrally located trabeculum of mature lamellar bone encased by successive layers of less mature bone. Note the focus of active bone resorption within the mature trabeculum.*

(Armed Forces Institute of Pathology Neg. Nos. 68-7665, 80-219.)

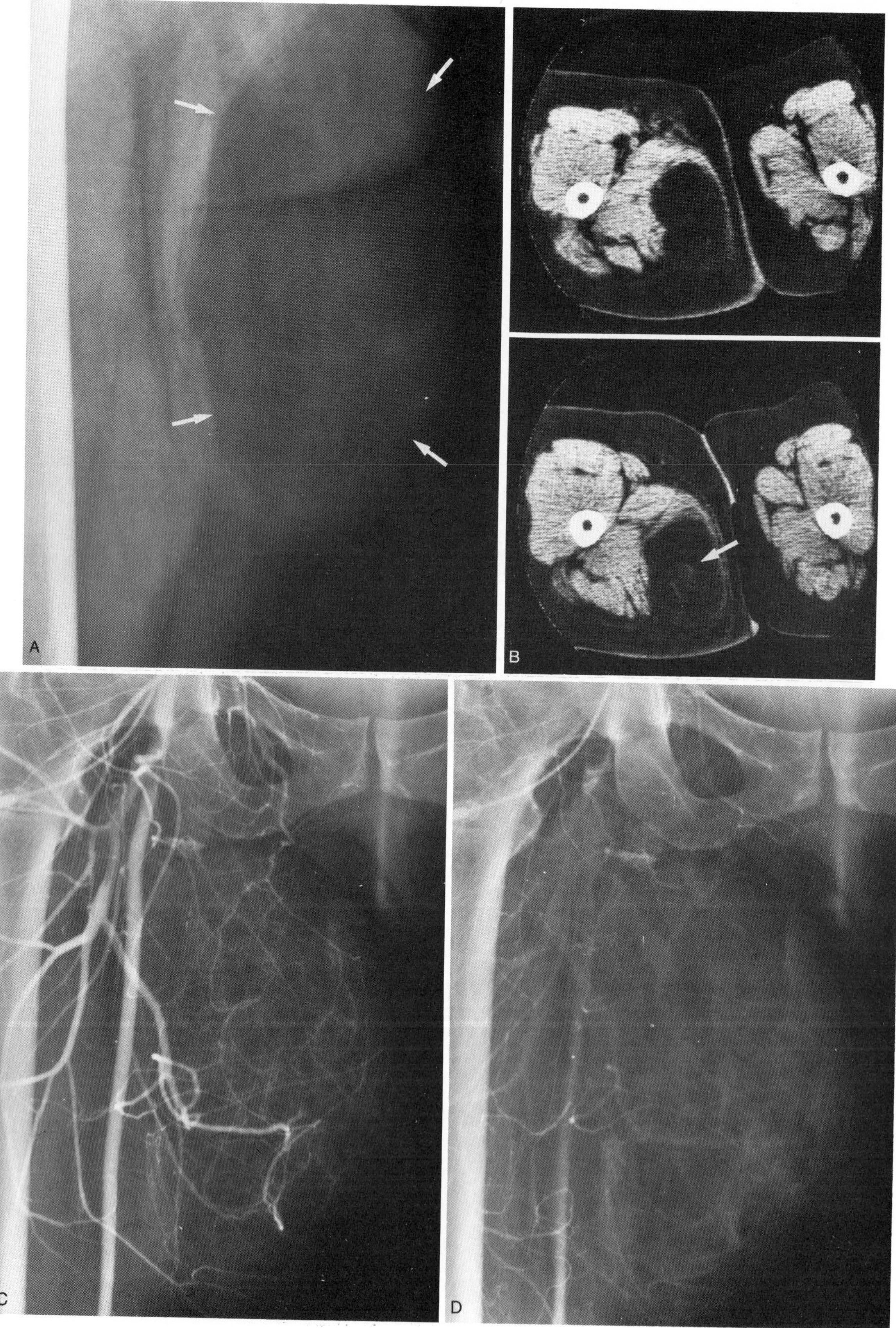

Figure 74–46. See legend on opposite page

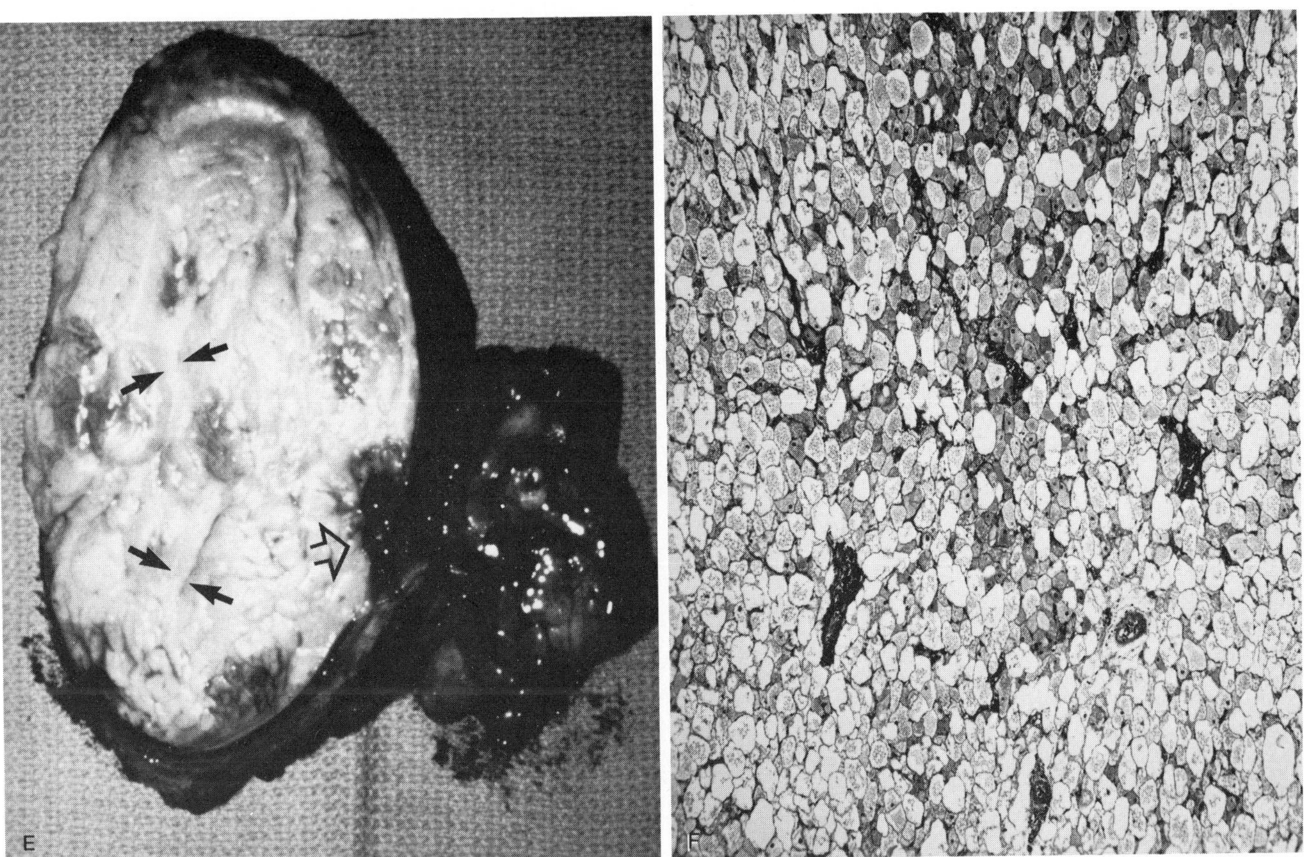

Figure 74–46. *Hibernoma of the thigh. This 30 year old woman presented with recent dull, aching pain in a thigh mass that had been present for several years.*

A *Anteroposterior radiograph shows an ill-defined, nonhomogeneous mass of less than water density (arrows) in the medial thigh.*

B *Composite computed tomography demonstrates a low attenuation coefficient (fatty) mass with well-delineated but not sharply circumscribed margins. The nonhomogeneous dense area is characterized by water-dense streaks throughout the lesion (arrow).*

C *A hypervascular lesion with neovascularity is noted on the arteriogram (arterial phase).*

D *Arteriogram (late arterial phase) reveals a nonhomogeneous parenchymal blush within the mass.*

E *The fatty nature of the lesion is confirmed on the gross specimen. Note the well-delineated margin and streaks (arrows) of fibrovascular tissue seen on the radiographic studies. An old biopsy site is also seen (open arrow).*

F *Photomicrograph (63 ×) shows the typical large, polyhedral cells with vacuolated, coarsely granular cytoplasm.*

(Armed Forces Institute of Pathology Neg. Nos. 79-2565-1,2,3,4; 79-14847-2; 80-230.)

may be extensively infiltrated by adipose tissue.[130-132] This fatty infiltration may extend into subcutaneous tissue, muscle, fascia, or even bone.[133] Diffuse lipomatosis is found most frequently in children and rarely occurs in adults. It is considered a congenital disorder and frequently presents clinically with overgrowth of the soft tissues and bone of the affected limb[89, 90, 130, 132, 134-143] (Fig. 74–47). The overgrowth is referred to as macrodystrophia lipomatosa. It is progressive, and it involves all mesenchymal elements, with a disproportionate increase in fibroadipose tissue. Macrodystrophia lipomatosa is usually found at birth, and growth is variable. Cessation of growth occurs at puberty. Usually one or more adjacent digits are involved in the affected extremity.

Radiographically, diffuse lipomatosis is neither circumscribed nor homogeneous. Diffuse swelling of the soft tissue and overgrowth of the bone with severe deformity are frequent. Mottled lucent areas are usually apparent in the soft tissue. An unusual form of diffuse lipomatosis may affect the leg following poliomyelitis,[133] with diffuse infiltration of fat into subcutaneous tissue, muscle, fascia, and bone, and associated enlargement of the osseous elements.

Lipoblastomatosis. This is a rare type of embryonal fatty tumor.[84, 144-148] These tumors are mostly limited to the pediatric age group, especially during the first year of life, and are rare in adults.[14, 145] In most instances the tumor is located superficially in the extremities[144] and presents as a soft tissue swelling (Fig. 74–48). It may be confused with liposarcoma on histology, but the latter is extremely rare in children. These lesions may present as

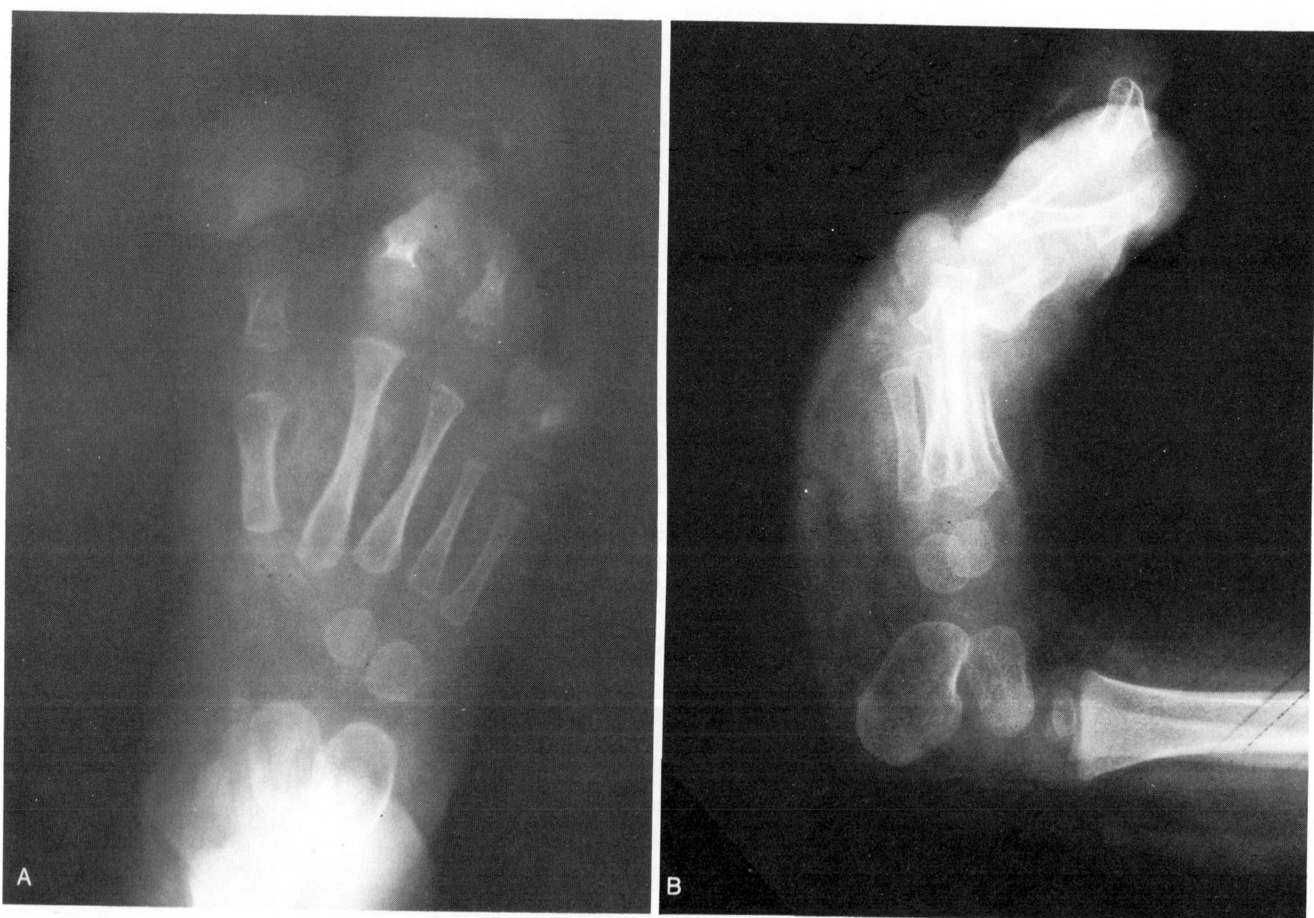

Figure 74–47. *Diffuse lipomatosis in foot with macrodystrophia lipomatosa. Eleven month old girl with deformity of the right foot since birth.*

A *Anteroposterior radiograph shows a disproportionately enlarged foot consisting of both soft tissue and bony overgrowth.*

B *Lateral radiograph (oriented to facilitate comparison with* **A***) more clearly demonstrates the nonhomogeneous (fatty and water density) consistency of the soft tissue.*

(Armed Forces Institute of Pathology Neg. Nos. 73-3477-1,2.)

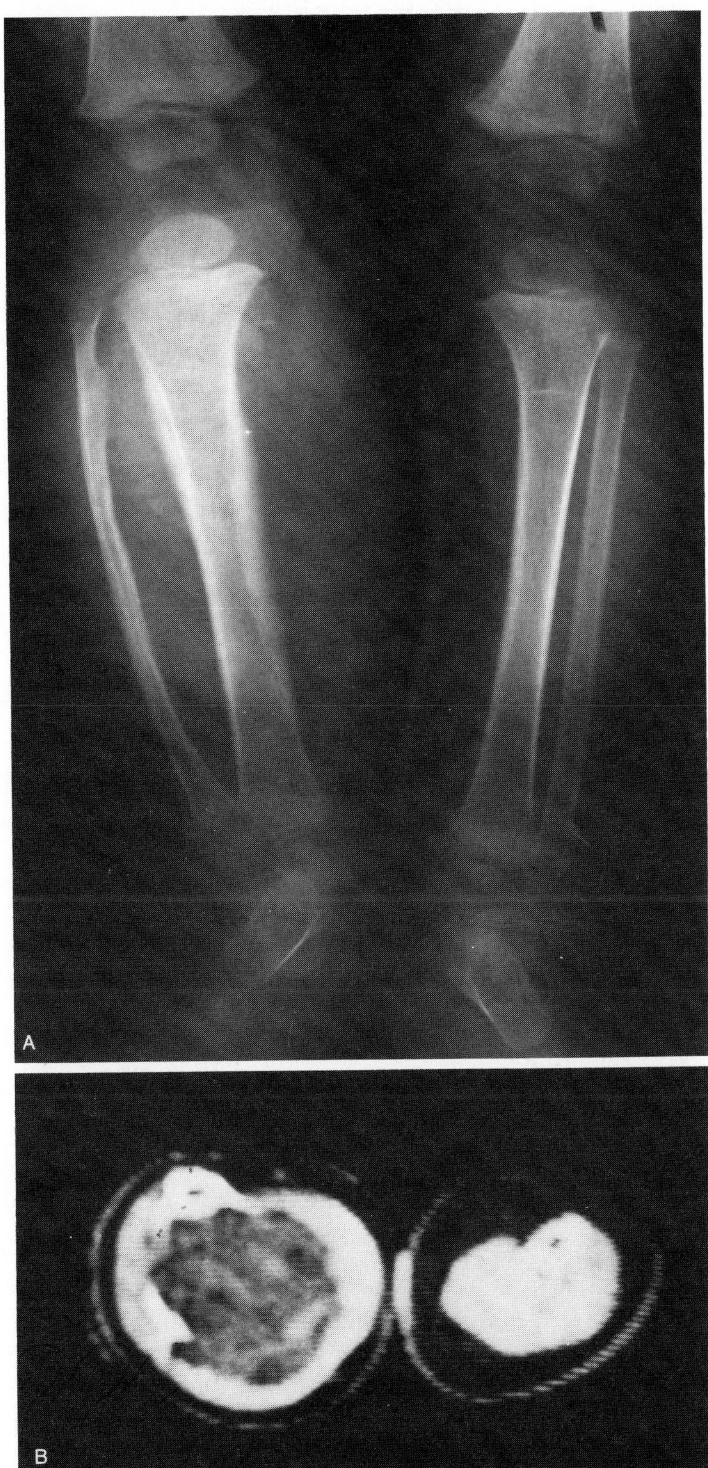

Figure 74–48. *Lipoblastomatosis of the right calf. This 9 month old boy presented with an increasing right calf size.*

A *Anteroposterior radiograph shows large ill-defined nonhomogeneous mass with deformity, erosion, and periosteal new bone formation in the adjacent tibia and fibula.*

B *The ill-defined nonhomogeneous low attenuation coefficient character of the mass is verified on an early generation computed tomographic study.*

(Armed Forces Institute of Pathology Neg. Nos. 76-11506-2, 76-11324.)

circumscribed or diffuse swellings. Recurrence and continued growth of the tumor following surgery are a particular problem, especially in the diffuse form of the tumor.

Vascular Tumors

The etiology and classification of vascular lesions are complicated problems, and agreement on them is not universal.[14, 18, 149-159] The most common vascular tumor is the hemangioma, which occurs in all tissues but is especially common in the skin, where it is usually seen at birth or within the first several years of life.[14] The majority of these cutaneous hemangiomas are asymptomatic and regress spontaneously before the seventh year of life. These lesions are infrequently studied radiographically because of their obvious clinical manifestations. However, the less common, deeper soft tissue hemangiomas can be recognized and easily studied radiographically.

Hemangiomas. The majority of deeper soft tissue hemangiomas are asymptomatic and usually remain so until late childhood or early adult life. Less commonly, they may present prior to the age of 30 years with nonspecific symptoms, such as a mass, pain, or swelling, perhaps requiring cosmetic correction.[149, 155] On rare occasions, in the adult woman, they will become clinically apparent during pregnancy.[154] The lesions are frequently associated with overlying skin abnormalities, such as reddish-blue discoloration, enlarged veins, or even cutaneous hemangiomas.[156, 160] The mass may vary its size spontaneously, independently of position. Occasionally enlargement with a color change will occur in the dependent position, and rarely pulsations and bruits may be found.[161] The deeper soft tissue hemangiomas may involve any soft tissue, such as muscle, tendon, connective tissue, fatty tissue, synovium, or bone, and involvement of a combination of these sites is not uncommon[162-176] (Fig. 74–49). They are relatively common in skeletal muscle, with the highest incidence in young adult women, particularly in the third decade of life[149, 154, 155, 177-180] (Fig. 74–50). A predilection for the limbs, especially distal to the elbows and knees, is noted.[149, 155] These lesions are usually cured by local excision; however, recurrence can take place.[181]

Hemangiomas are associated with a variety of clinical problems, such as consumption coagulopathy, cardiac decompensation, gangrene, discrepancies in extremity growth, osteomalacia, varicose veins, massive osteolysis, Maffucci's syndrome, and Klippel-Trenaunay-Weber syndrome. In 1940, Kasabach and Merritt described a syndrome bearing their names, marked by the association of capillary hemangiomas with extensive purpura.[182] This syndrome usually affects infants up to 1 year of age. It is characterized by an asymptomatic hemangioma, commonly located in the extremities, which suddenly increases in size and is accompanied by a generalized bleeding tendency, usually manifested by bruising, petechiae, and purpura. Thrombocytopenia and hypofibrinogenemia are noted.[183] The vascular lesion may be either a cavernous or a capillary hemangioma or even a hemangioendothelioma.[183-191] The clinical and laboratory findings result from trapping of platelets and deposition of fibrin clot in the vascular spaces of the tumor, which provoke intravascular hemolysis and red cell fragmentation.[192-195] Massive precapillary arteriovenous shunting of blood may result in cardiac decompensation[153, 196, 197] as well as cyanosis and, on rare occasions, even gangrene of the soft tissue distal to the lesion.[153] Growth discrepancies associated with vascular lesions are not uncommon, frequently reflected by overgrowth and less commonly atrophy or shortening of the involved extremity.[153, 197-199] This feature may be seen as a part of the Klippel-Trenaunay-Weber syndrome (varicose veins, soft tissue and bony hypertrophy, and cutaneous hemangiomas).[200] On physical examination, these extremities are typically found to be warm, with dilated superficial veins and cutaneous hemangiomas. The bony hypertrophy is manifested clinically by discrepancy in leg length.[197, 201, 202] Other bony changes can be noted with hemangiomas, such as osteomalacia,[203-207] massive osteolysis,[208, 209] and Maffucci's syndrome.[210]

The hemangioma presenting as a soft tissue mass may be characterized as a poorly circumscribed, localized or diffuse swelling on gross inspection. These tumors vary in size from less than 4 cm to over 20 cm, but most are less than 9 cm in diameter.[149] Hemangiomas may recur locally but do not metastasize.

Hemangiomas are benign lesions classically divided into capillary and cavernous types,[14] dependent upon their composition. Capillary hemangiomas are composed of capillaries with a sparse fibrous stroma and are arranged haphazardly, whereas cavernous hemangiomas are composed of large, dilated, blood-filled spaces lined by flat endothelium. In fact, a large number of hemangiomas exhibit a continuous spectrum ranging from pure capillary hemangiomas through mixed cavernous and capillary types to the pure cavernous type of hemangioma.[149]

Hemangioendotheliomas are rare tumors that occur most frequently in infants and young children but may present in the adult.[1, 14] A thick endothelial layer is found within the capillaries. This layer is formed by proliferation of endothelial cells, which assume a rounded to cuboidal shape instead of the typical flattened shape. This results in a relatively solid mass of large cells about narrow blood channels, which needs to be distinguished from a malignant tumor.

Radiographically, hemangiomas present as a nonhomogeneous, water-density mass or swelling that may be localized or diffuse. Single or multiple focal discrete nodules may be seen. These usually

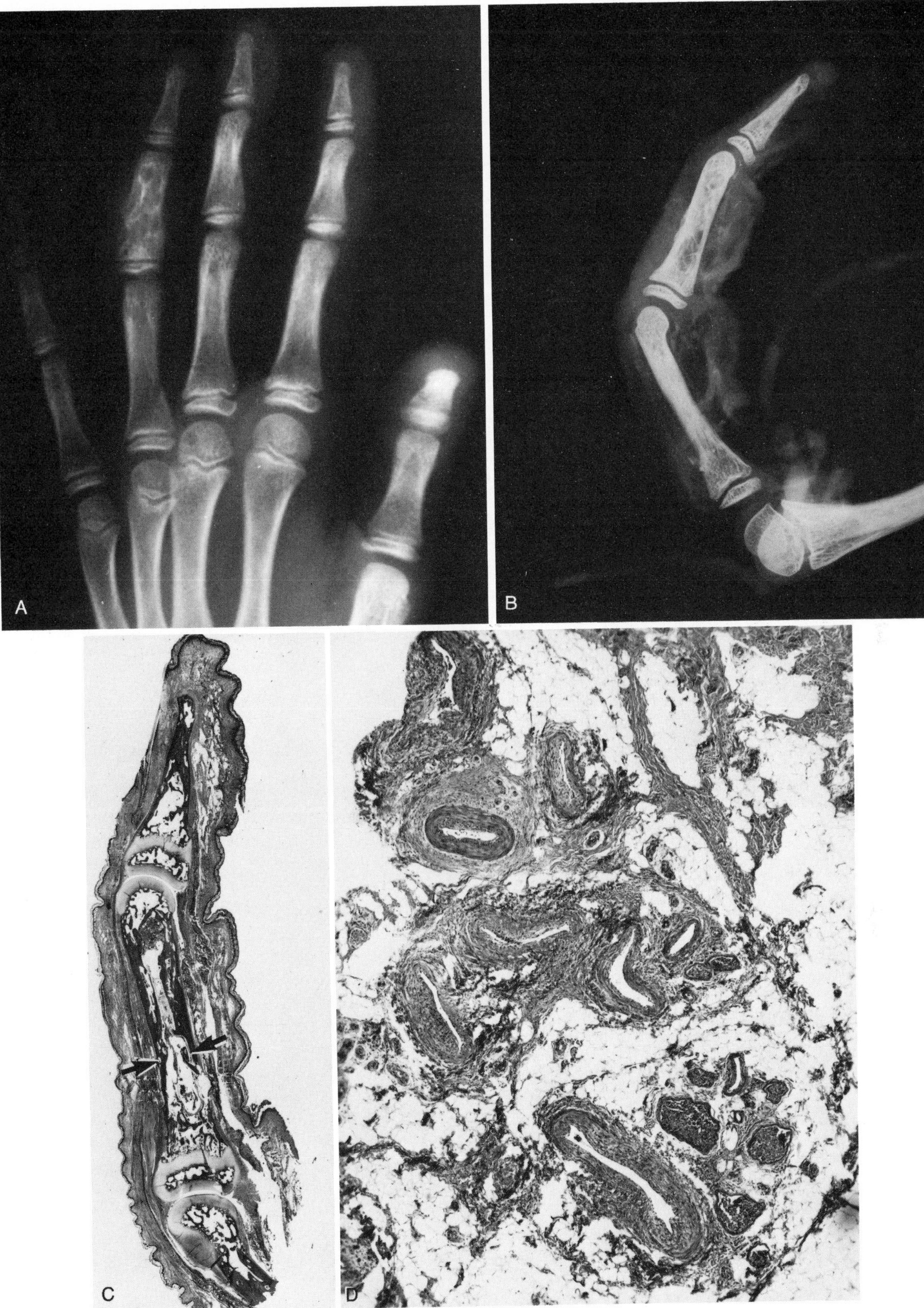

Figure 74–49. *Hemangioma of soft tissue and bone of the ring finger. This 8 year old girl presented with a swollen ring finger.*

A *Oblique radiograph shows multiple, sharply circumscribed lytic lesions involving the middle phalanx, with sclerotic margins and extension into the adjacent soft tissue.*

B *Specimen radiograph confirms the intraosseous lysis.*

C *Macrophotomicrograph (1.5×) shows the intraosseous hemangioma (arrows). Note the areas of cortical thickening (distally) and thinning (proximally).*

D *Photomicrograph (25×) demonstrates a cluster of varying sized thickened vessels in the adjacent soft tissue.*

(Armed Forces Institute of Pathology Neg. Nos. 78-6162-1, 78-6162-2, 80-221, 80-220.)

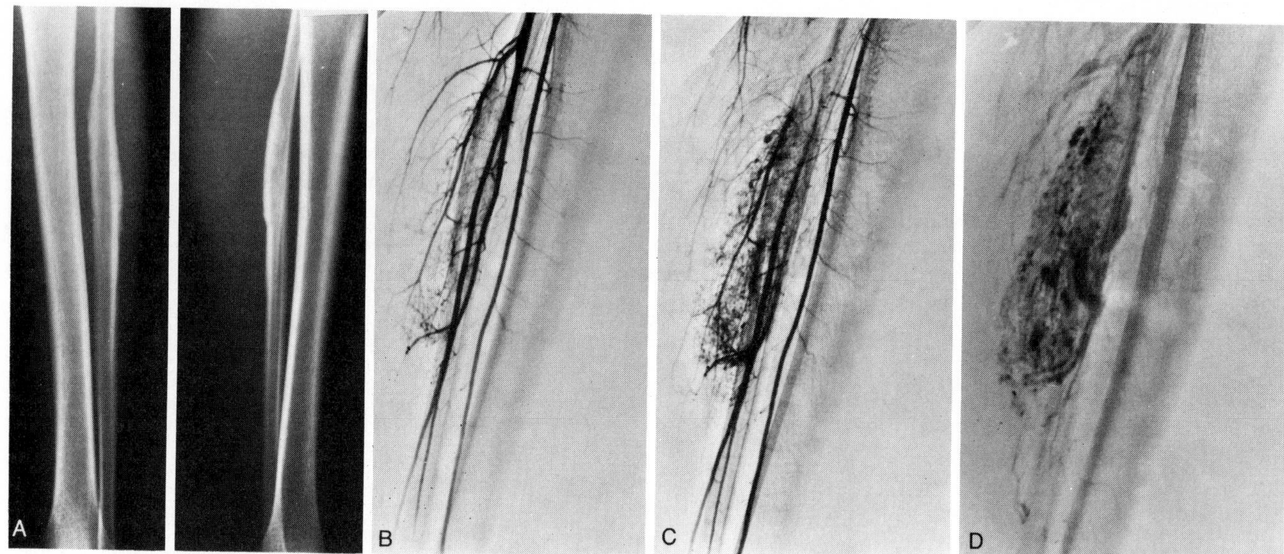

Figure 74–50. *Intramuscular hemangioma of the calf. This 19 year old man presented with calf pain on ambulation.*

A *Composite anteroposterior and lateral radiographs show cortical hyperostosis of the fibula.*

B *Arteriogram (arterial phase) shows vessel displacement with hypervascularity.*

C *Arteriogram (late arterial phase) demonstrates tumor blush and involvement of adjacent fibular cortex.*

D *Arteriogram (venous phase) reveals arteriovenous shunting and contrast puddling in small venous channels.*

(Armed Forces Institute of Pathology Neg. Nos. 79-1343-1,2,3,4.)

vary in size and are due to focal proliferation of hemangiomatous tissue. The margin is typically poorly defined, especially in the diffuse type, but occasionally a sharp interface between the tumor and adjacent soft tissue is seen. Tortuous channels of water density representing the arterial supply and venous drainage of the tumor may occasionally be demonstrated radiographically within the adjacent subcutaneous fat. Calcification within the hemangioma is common and may be of three types. The nonspecific type is either amorphous or, at times, curvilinear. The second type, which is more specific and the most frequent (49 per cent) type of calcification, is the phlebolith[161, 211-213] (Fig. 74–51). Phleboliths are rounded calcific masses frequently demonstrating a laminated structure. Occasionally, metaplastic ossification may be found in hemangiomas, and this is the third type of calcification.[155] Adjacent smooth bone erosions can occur, especially with the deep hemangiomas. This may be due to the localized pressure effect of the adjacent consolidated mass or the hypertrophied vessels of the soft tissue, periosteum, cortex, or marrow cavity (Fig. 74–49). Overgrowth of the bone and soft tissue of the extremity is seen with hemangiomas, especially if they are diffuse or extensive. In these patients, bone scans usually show increased activity in the growth plates on the involved side.[197] Rarely, periosteal new bone, cortical hyperostosis, or regional osteoporosis may be found.

Arteriography in vascular tumors is extremely helpful in patient management by defining the lesion's extent, degree of vascularity, and vascular supply.[22, 153, 156, 214-217] It also helps in differentiating among the several types of vascular masses: hemangiomas, arteriovenous malformations, and venous malformations.[156] These types have been referred to under the broad descriptive term "angiodysplasia."[153, 218] Regardless of the terms applied, arteriography is a helpful tool in the evaluation of vascular tumors. Hemangiomas are hypervascular, usually with fine-caliber vessels, and reveal homogeneous contrast opacification or staining (Fig. 74–50). Occasionally coarse, irregular vessels are seen and the vascular pattern may be indistinguishable from that of malignant soft tissue tumors.[156] Large hemangiomas may be painful, and partial embolization has been successful in controlling pain in unresectable lesions.[219] Arteriovenous malformations are composed of large tortuous and coarse arterial and venous vessels and thick-walled capillaries. Arteriographically, large vessels with densely opacified vascular spaces and early filling of draining veins are seen[153, 156] (Fig. 74–52). The vessels of the arteriovenous malformations may be regularly arranged and parallel to each other along the fiber bundle axis of an involved muscle. This striation suggests benignancy, since malignant tumors rarely leave muscle bundles intact.[151] Venous malformations consist of large dilated venous spaces, which have very slow blood flow within the enlarged vascular spaces, and the feeding vessels may be thrombosed. These two features may explain why

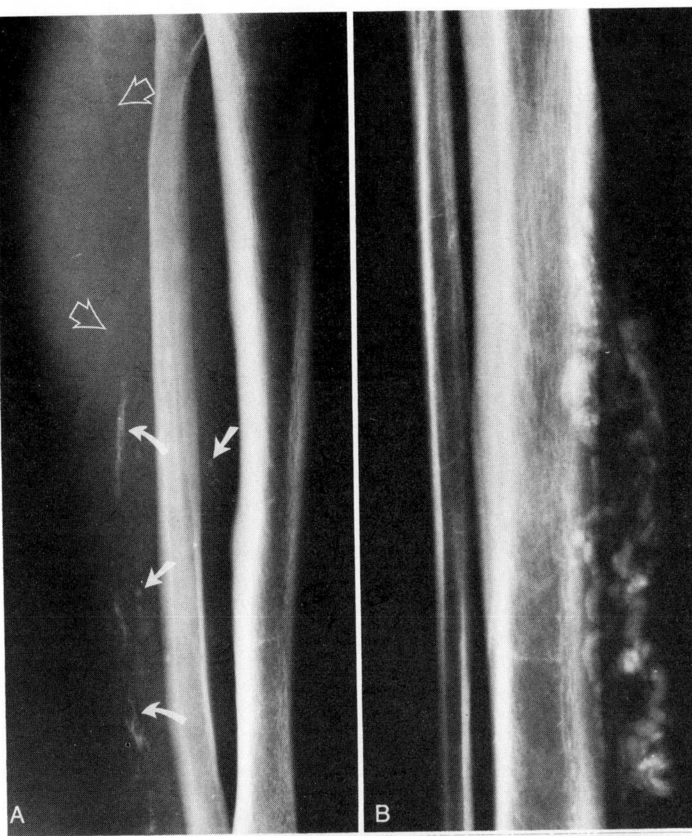

Figure 74–51. Intramuscular hemangioma of the calf with phleboliths. This 25 year old man presented with recurrent swelling and calf pain.

A *Lateral radiograph shows two patterns of calcification: small circular dense lesions (straight arrows) and linear dense areas with a central lucent core (curved arrows). Both are due to dystrophic calcification* **(D)** *of organized thrombi (phlebolith). The channels of water density (open arrows) result from dilated subcutaneous veins. Note the smooth pressure erosion of the tibia posteriorly.*

B *Arteriogram (late arterial phase) demonstrates arteriovenous shunting into tortuous dilated venous channels, which are patent and do not contain phleboliths. Their close proximity to bone may occasionally cause pressure erosion* **(A)**.

C *Specimen radiograph confirms the phleboliths as small calcifications — one lamellated and two with central lucent cores.*

D *Photomicrograph displays large dilated venous channels with thrombi in different stages of organization. The largest thrombus is attached in part to the vessel wall. Spotty dystrophic calcification (straight arrows) is present in the old organized portion of the thrombus. Note the propagating clot (curved arrow) emanating from a more recently organized portion of the thrombus. The eventual dystrophic calcification within the propagating thrombus produces the linear density pattern* **(A)**.

(Armed Forces Institute of Pathology Neg. Nos. 75-2058-3, 75-2058-2, 75-2059, 79-16646.)

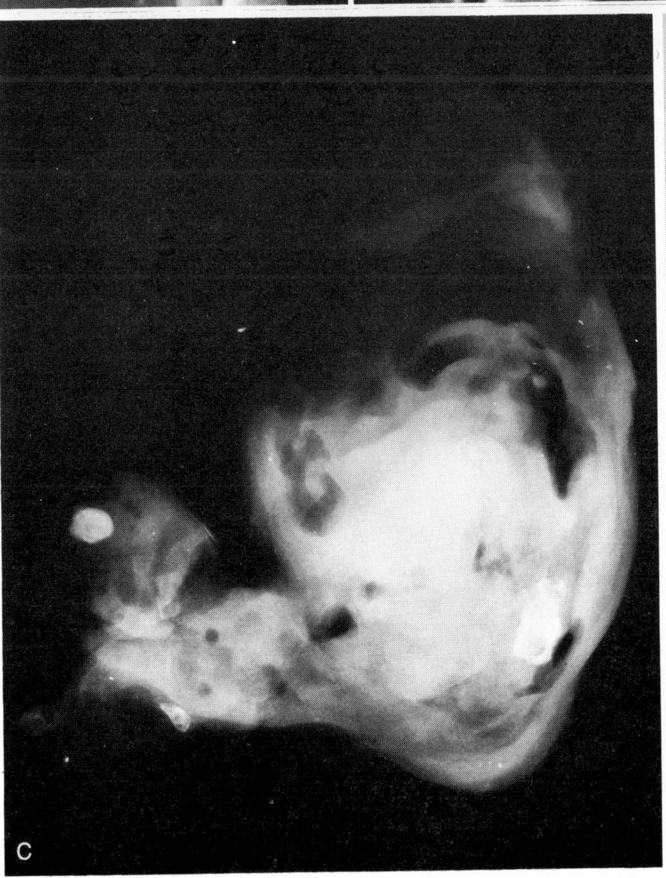

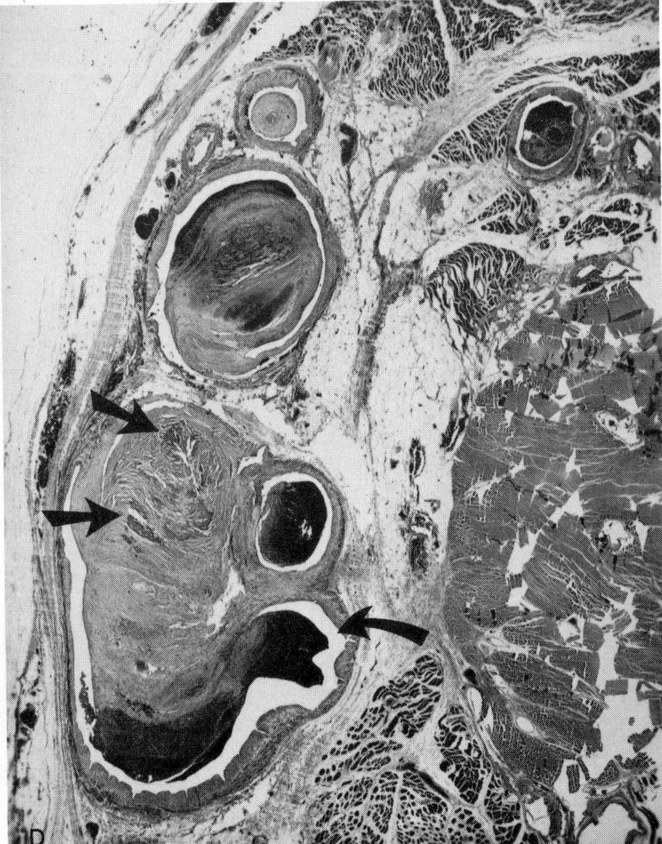

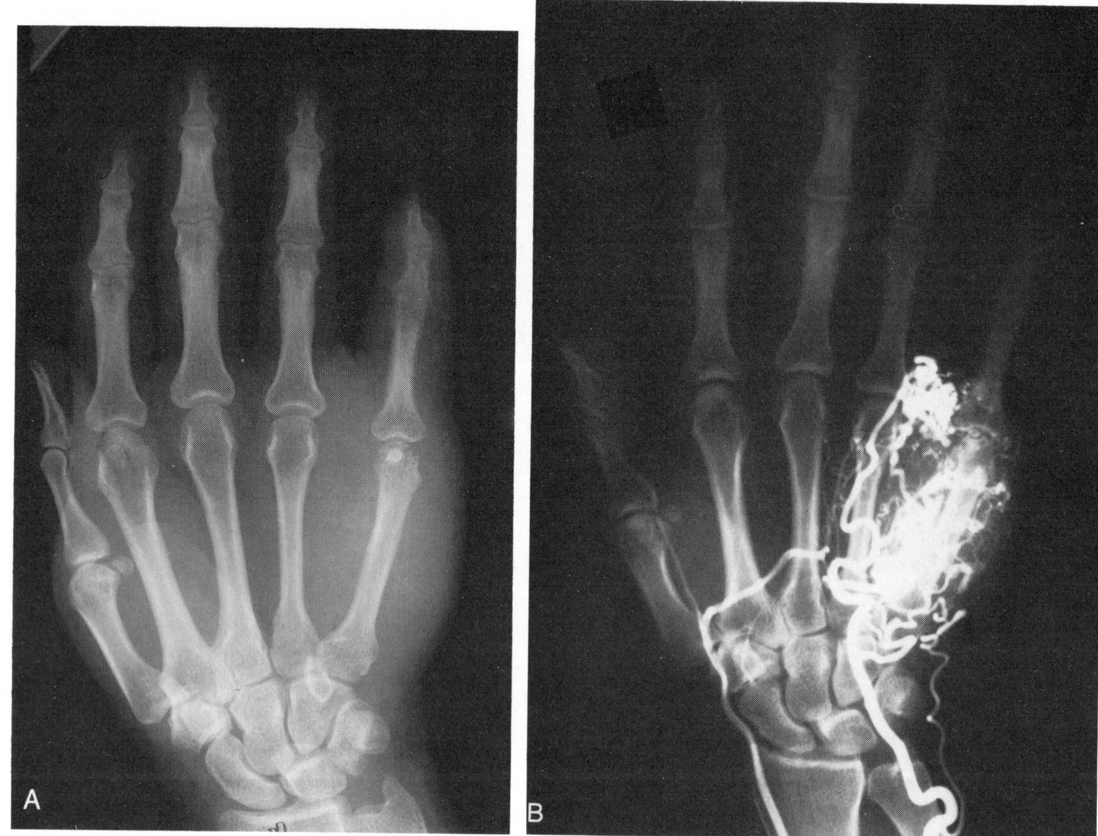

Figure 74–52. *Arteriovenous malformation of the hand. This 36 year old woman presented with spontaneous swelling of the hypothenar eminence and little finger.*

A *Frontal film shows diffuse soft tissue swelling about the fifth metacarpal and phalanges in association with erosions and osteoporosis of the underlying bone.*

B *Arteriogram (arterial phase) demonstrates an enlarged ulnar artery and mass of tortuous vessels predominantly about the fifth metacarpal.*

Illustration continued on the opposite page

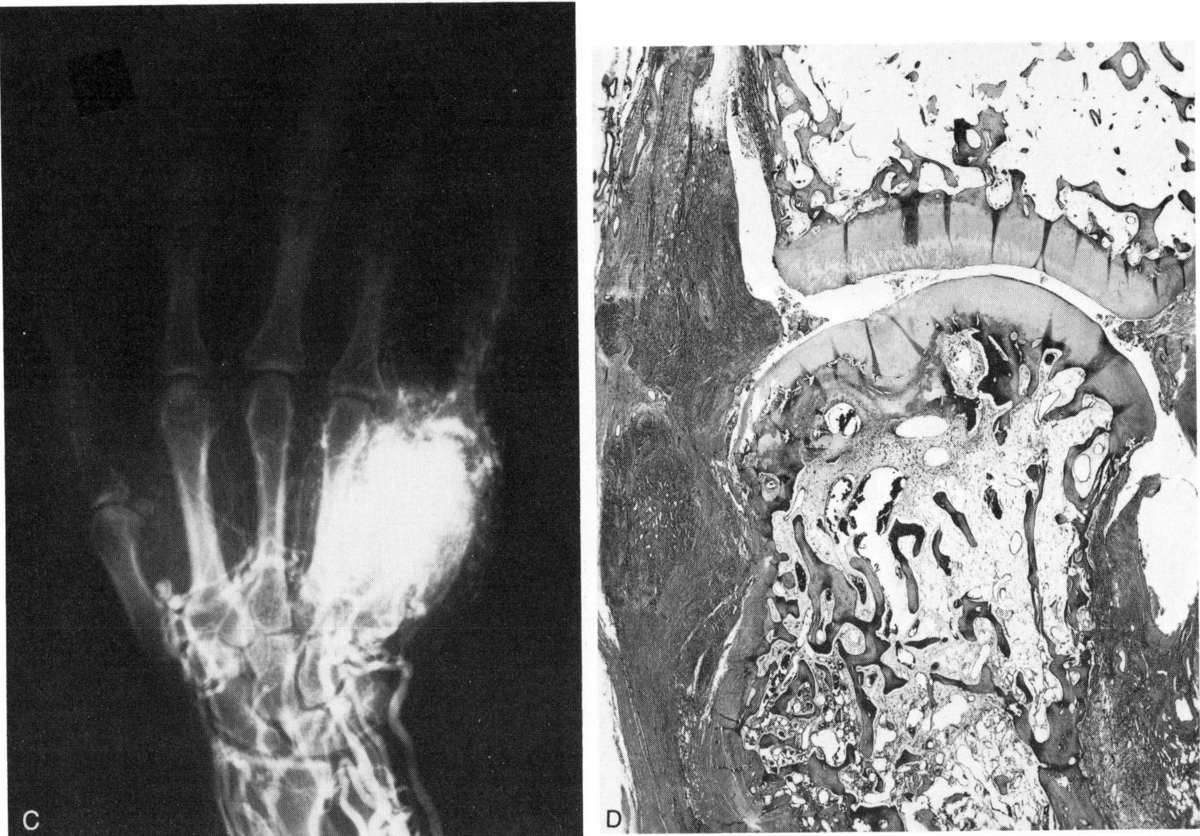

Figure 74–52. Continued

C *Arteriogram (late arterial phase) reveals an intense blush, with arteriovenous shunting. Note the extensive hypervascularity extending beyond the blush into adjacent soft tissue and to the tip of the little finger.*

D *Photomicrograph (7×) of the metacarpophalangeal joint shows densely packed small vessels with extensive involvement of the periarticular soft tissue and synovium. These findings are responsible for the intense arteriographic blush and cortical erosions. The dilated intraosseous vascular channels account for the localized areas of trabecular loss.*

(Armed Forces Institute of Pathology Neg. Nos. 78-8767-3, 78-8767-2, 78-8767-7, 80-227.)

venous malformations are uncommonly seen on arteriography. Venography, including direct injection, may be necessary to demonstrate the lesion and determine its extent.[153] These vascular deformities are commonly associated with lymphatic abnormalities, which may be related to secondary hypertrophy or which may be part of the original vessel anomaly or neoplasm.[220] Thus, lymphangiography may be helpful and frequently demonstrates hypoplasia or aplasia of lymph vessels, vesicles, lymph fistulae, and cysts. These findings are usually seen when the venous elements are dominant and in conjunction with the Klippel-Trenaunay-Weber syndrome. Hyperplastic lymph pathways on lymphangiography are typically seen in the arteriovenous shunts and malformations. Computed tomography, especially with contrast enhancement, augments the arteriographic findings by displaying tumor extent and relationship to adjacent structures as well as prominent areas of vascularity. It also shows the infiltrative margins of the tumor. Sometimes enhanced computed tomography of hemangiomas may show no recognizable change when compared with nonenhanced studies.[66]

SYNOVIAL HEMANGIOMAS. Hemangiomas of the synovium are uncommon tumors, occurring most frequently in the knee. They are invariably unilateral (Fig. 74–53) and are rarely found in other joints or in synovial tendon sheaths.[202, 221-223] Synovial hemangiomas usually occur in adolescent or young adult women and are frequently symptomatic, with pain, swelling, and decreased range of motion. They are commonly associated with adjacent cutaneous and deeper soft tissue hemangiomas.[224]

Pathologically, there are two morphologic patterns. One is the localized, pedunculated synovial mass, which may cause mechanical problems with locking of the joint[225] and which is easily excised. The other pattern is diffuse, with intermittent pain, hemarthrosis, and occasionally increase in limb length. These lesions are difficult to excise, may recur, and may also be associated with visceral and cutaneous vascular lesions. The synovial proliferation accompanying the diffuse synovial hemangio-

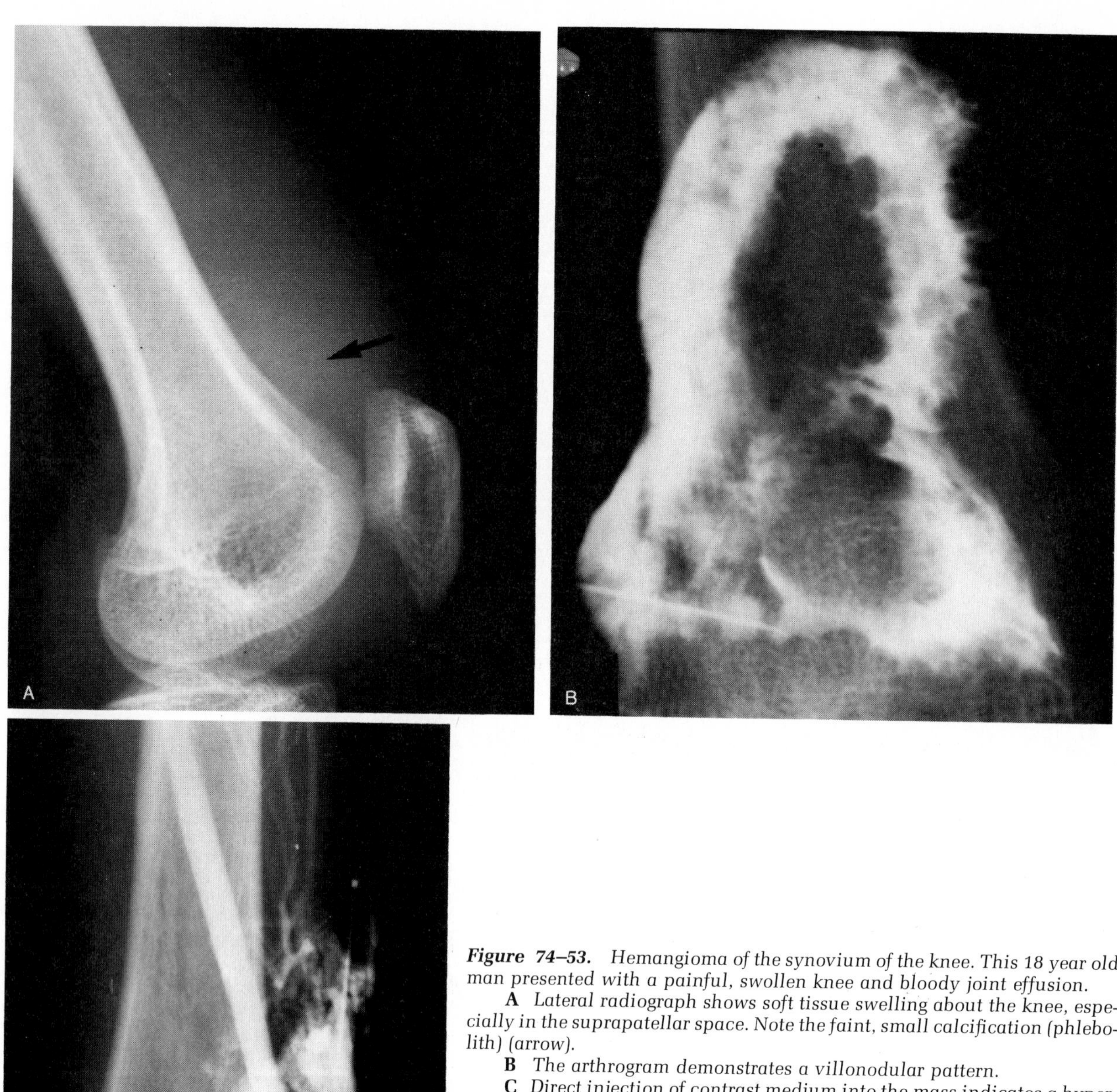

Figure 74–53. *Hemangioma of the synovium of the knee. This 18 year old man presented with a painful, swollen knee and bloody joint effusion.*

A *Lateral radiograph shows soft tissue swelling about the knee, especially in the suprapatellar space. Note the faint, small calcification (phlebolith) (arrow).*

B *The arthrogram demonstrates a villonodular pattern.*

C *Direct injection of contrast medium into the mass indicates a hypervascular lesion and venous shunting.*

Illustration continued on the opposite page

ma can be quite similar to that seen in hemophilia.[202, 226]

The plain film radiographs usually show soft tissue swelling or a mass about the involved joint,[222, 227-229] occasionally with phleboliths[227-229] (Fig. 74–53). Advanced maturity of the epiphysis, discrepancy in limb length, periosteal new bone, and articular destruction may be seen[229] (see Chapter

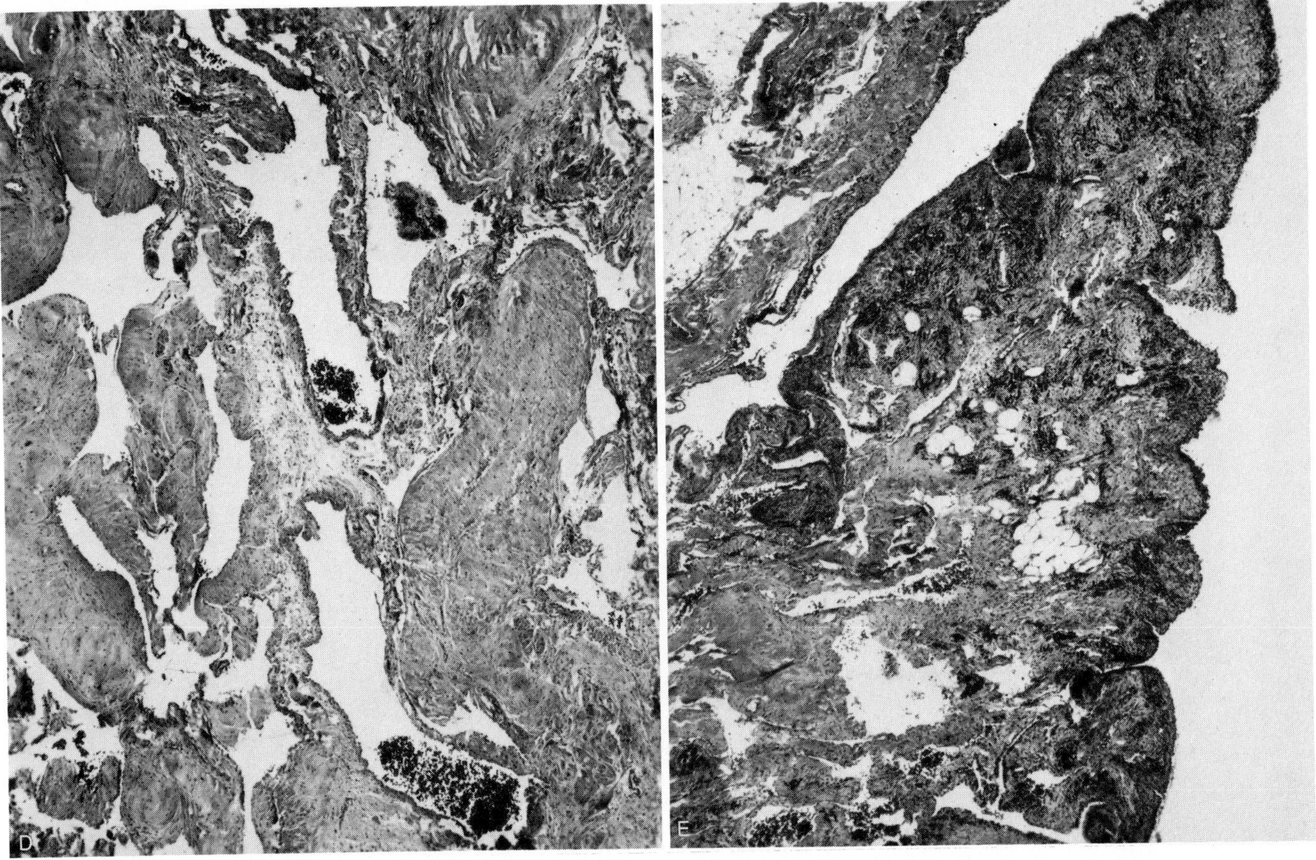

Figure 74–53. Continued
D *Photomicrograph (40×) reveals dilated vascular channels in the joint capsule.*
E *Photomicrograph (40×) of the synovium shows a villus with proliferation of the synovial membrane, increased vascularity, and extensive hemosiderin deposition.*
(Armed Forces Institute of Pathology Neg. Nos. 77-4645-7, 77-4645-6, 77-4645-2, 80-223, 80-222.)

59). Arthrography usually shows the intra-articular mass as multiple filling defects with a villous configuration. The lesions are hypervascular on arteriography, with a fine vascular pattern and staining.[230] Thermography may also help in assessing the hemangioma's extrasynovial extent when it is unsuspected clinically.[231]

Hemangiopericytomas. These are vascular tumors of the soft tissue that are believed to originate from the pericytes of Zimmerman, which surround the capillary wall[14, 232-237] (Fig. 74–54). These tumors most frequently present in adults and are located in the deep soft tissue of the thigh.[237-241] A slowly growing, painless mass (with a median size of 6.5 cm) is the most frequent clinical symptom. Because of the tumor's striking hypervascularity, its surgical removal is frequently complicated by hemorrhage. The majority of hemangiopericytomas act in a benign fashion, although occasionally malignant lesions have been encountered. Grossly, the hemangiopericytoma is a well-circumscribed mass with a frequent covering of large plexiform vessels about its periphery. Microscopically, there is proliferation of rounded or elongated cells just outside of the capillary reticular sheath. This relation is best seen on silver reticulin stain.

The plain film radiograph is nonspecific, revealing a focal homogeneous soft tissue mass with a variable margin. The tumors may occasionally demonstrate calcification and bone erosion. Arteriography demonstrates an extremely hypervascular tumor with lobular growth, tumor vessels, and striking heterogeneous blush[242-248] (Fig. 74–54). Occasionally, the tumor can function as an arteriovenous shunt.[249]

A closer look at the pattern of hypervascularity demonstrates that the main arteries, early in the arterial phase, are displaced by the tumor. Later, the feeding arteries spread around the tumor before entering it. Occasionally, the vessels will coalesce into a vascular pedicle and enter the outer margin of the mass, whereupon the vessels branch and encircle the tumor. This peripheral distribution of arteries correlates well with the gross findings of a plexiform meshwork of vessels covering the tumor.[238] This angiographic pattern is highly suggestive of hemangiopericytoma.[248]

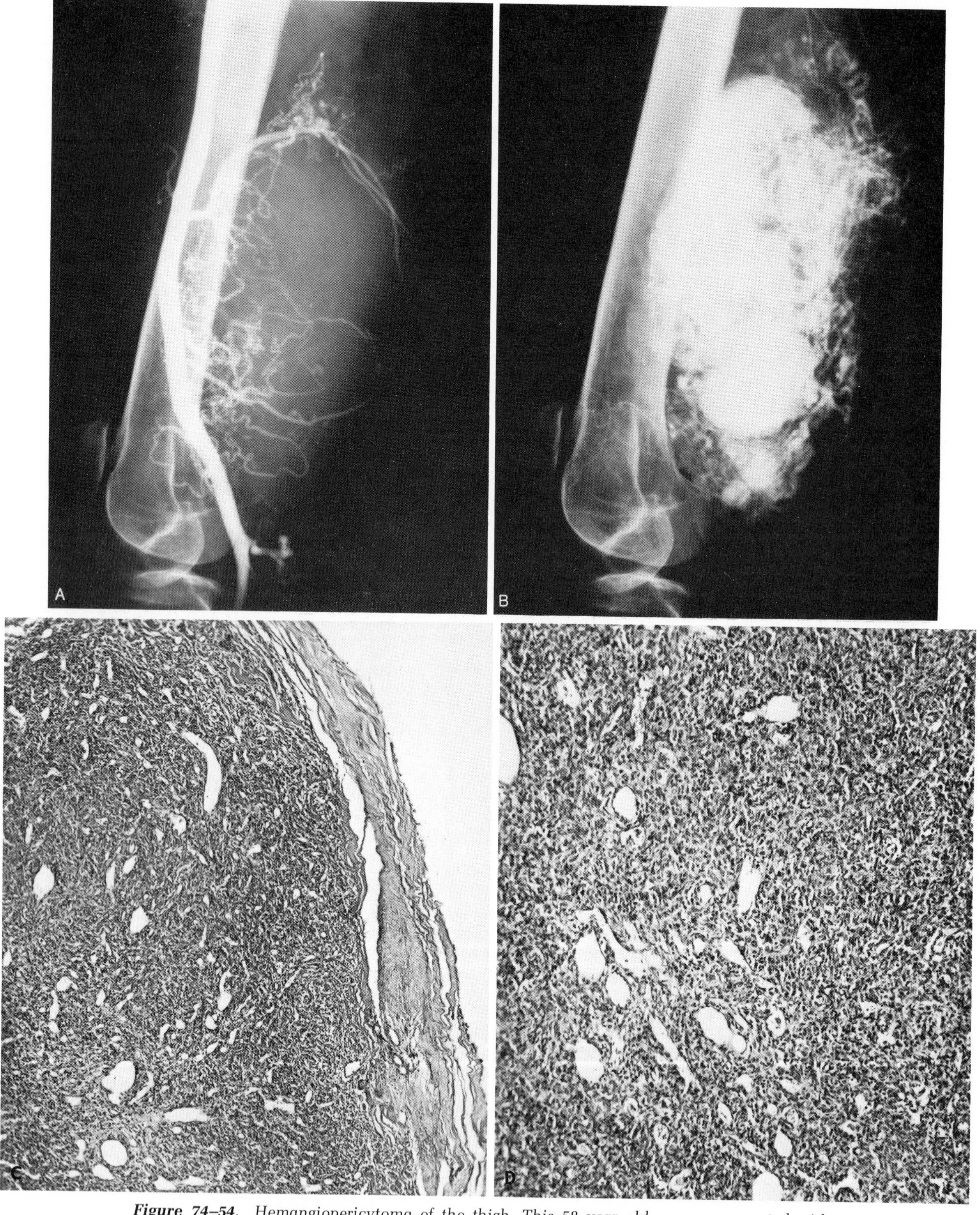

Figure 74–54. *Hemangiopericytoma of the thigh. This 58 year old woman presented with a painful mass in the leg of 1 year's duration.*

A *Arteriogram (arterial phase) shows a large hypervascular mass displacing the femoropopliteal artery anteriorly. The vascularity is concentrated around the periphery in a plexiform arrangement.*

B *Arteriogram (late arterial phase) demonstrates a dense heterogeneous blush, neovascularity, and a lobular configuration, which was also seen in the gross specimen.*

C *Photomicrograph (low power view) reveals cellular proliferation about vascular spaces of varying sizes.*

D *Photomicrograph (63×) shows an intricate network of small, thin-walled branching vascular channels separated by rounded and sometimes elongated cells.*

(Armed Forces Institute of Pathology Neg. Nos. 69-11422-1,2; 71-2102-1; 80-232.)

Lymphangiomas. Lymphangiomas are rare tumors, which are composed of multiple lymph-filled vessels and cystic spaces, with occasional foci of lymphoid tissue.[250-252] They usually occur in the skin and subcutaneous tissue and are frequently noted at birth or by 1 year of age. Local invasion into adjacent tissues is common, and there is a high recurrence rate after local excision. Wide excision is recommended, leaving a margin of normal tissue.[250] The lesions are poorly defined, with infiltrative margins, and are only rarely localized. Inspection of the gross tissue shows a diffuse, spongy, compressible mass. Microscopically, there is proliferation of lymph vessels with dilated lymph channels, which may form cysts.[14] The plain film radiograph is nonspecific but may demonstrate a diffuse, ill-defined, poorly marginated mass.

Cartilage Tumors

Chondromas are cartilage proliferations of the soft tissue, usually composed of well-differentiated hyaline cartilage and frequently demonstrating endochondral bone formation. They most commonly arise from synovium of joints and occasionally from a tendon sheath or bursa. In these sites they are referred to as (idiopathic) synovial (osteo)chondromatosis.[8, 253-262] Less commonly, benign cartilage proliferations (chondromas) of other soft parts are encountered. The exact origin of these latter tumors is unknown, but they are commonly attached to a tendon and could also represent a tenosynovial process.[263-266]

Synovial (Osteo)Chondromatosis. Synovial chondromatosis represents cartilage formation by the synovial membrane.[8, 258] The etiology is unknown, but it most likely represents a metaplasia or neoplasia.[254, 267] This disorder is almost invariably a monoarticular disease with a chronic progressive course.[258] Rarely, spontaneous regression has been reported.[253, 268, 269] The most common joints affected are the knee, hip, and elbow.[259] However, any joint can be involved.[270-294] It is twice as common in men as in women and is usually found in the third to fifth decades of life.[267] Clinically, patients present with a several-year history of joint pain with limitation of motion.[259] Joint effusion is rare but when present may be bloody. Intra-articular loose body formation is common and may lead to mechanical destruction of the articular cartilage, with resultant osteoarthritis.[254, 267, 295-297] Joint instability can also occur and be responsible for pain.[294] Focal recurrence after surgery is not uncommon and usually necessitates many surgical procedures. Synovial chondromatosis may rarely become malignant.[260, 267, 297-302, 587]

The synovium in synovial chondromatosis is hyperplastic, with foci of cartilage metaplasia. Grossly, the synovium has many villous or nodular projections. These cartilage nodules usually have an upper limit of 2 to 3 cm in size. Rarely, a large dominant nodule will be found.[303] As these cartilage nodules continue to grow they may project into the joint space by means of a delicate pedicle. Endochondral bone formation within these cartilage nodules occurs frequently and requires an intact blood supply through the pedicle. With slight trauma, the pedicle breaks and the nodule becomes a loose body.[259, 297] The loose bodies are white to gray in color and oval to round or faceted in shape.[304-306] While the body is free within the joint space with its vascular supply disrupted, the cartilage component may increase in size by continuous cartilage proliferation on the surface, which is nourished by synovial fluid. The loose body may become reattached to the thickened synovium.[259] With reestablishment of a vascular supply at this new site, the nodule may again grow and form bone or be resorbed. The cartilage nodules may extend through the joint capsule and continue to proliferate within the adjacent soft tissue.[267, 298] Microscopically, numerous circumscribed nodules of cartilage may be myxoid in type but more commonly are composed of hyaline cartilage. Mineralization of chondroid matrix is common and bone, when present, frequently develops fatty marrow. Considerable cellular proliferation with atypical nuclei is common in the subcapsular cartilage areas, and while this is often misinterpreted as a sign of aggressiveness, this pattern is still compatible with a benign process.[267, 307-309]

Radiographically, synovial chondromatosis commonly presents with multiple juxta-articular radiodense shadows (Fig. 74–55). They range in size from a few millimeters to several centimeters and show varying degrees of mineralization (chondrification or ossification) within each lesion.[275, 296, 310-316] The typical pattern of mineralization ranges from small specks of calcification to large calcified bodies with peripheral linear dense areas and radiolucent centers. Bony trabeculation can be seen in the mature osteoid areas of the nodules. Some nodules may be of water density and seen only as soft tissue masses in or about the joint. The nodules may cause erosions of the adjacent bone and widening of the joint space (Fig. 74–56). Noncalcified lesions are best seen on arthrography as they displace the contrast medium and produce multiple filling defects (Fig. 74–57). In the late stages, many loose bodies will be found, and secondary osteoarthritis is common. The joint space at this time will be narrow, with eburnation and osteophyte formation consistent with secondary osteoarthritis.

Soft Tissue Chondromas. Chondromas of the soft parts are less common than synovial chondromatosis.[263-266, 317, 318] They occur more frequently in men and are seen predominantly in the third and fourth decades of life. These tumors present as slow-growing masses that are lobular and well demarcated and almost invariably occur in the extremities, especially in the hands and feet.[263] These masses shell out easily at surgery and thus

Text continued on page 2719

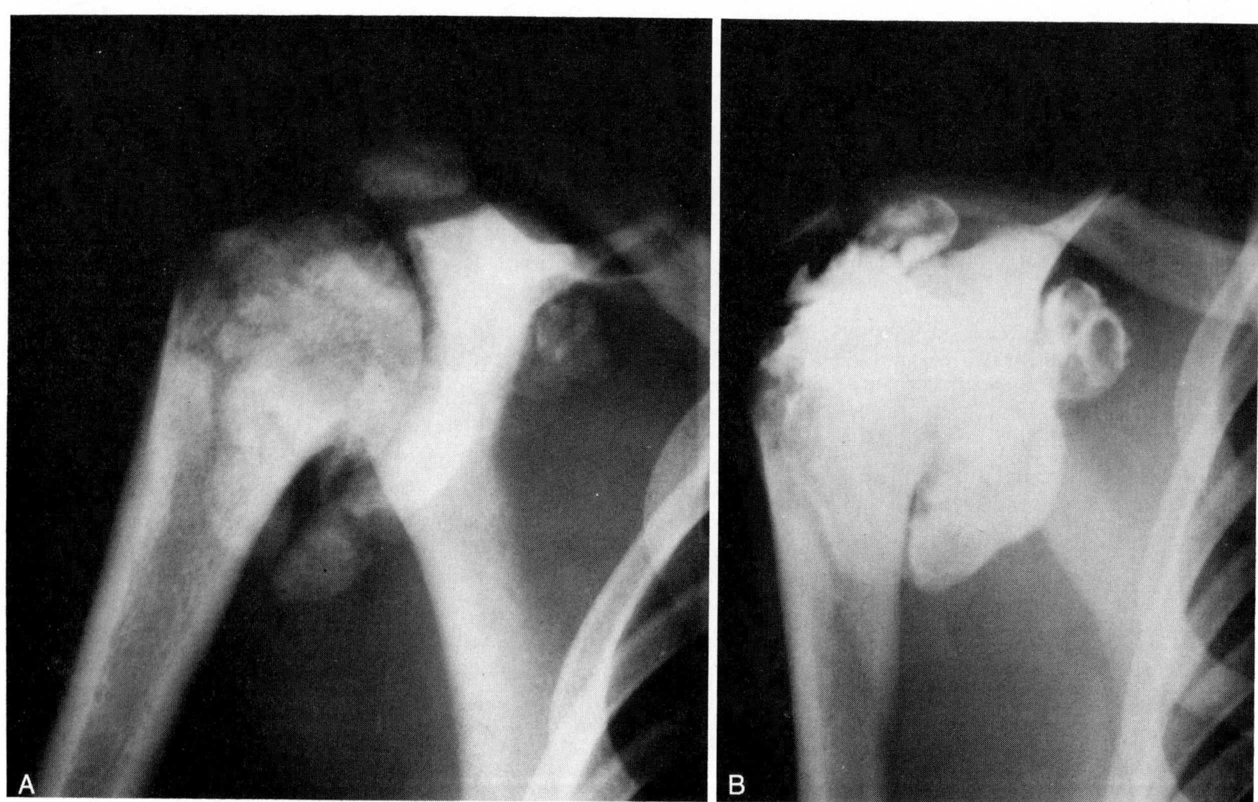

Figure 74–55. Synovial chondromatosis of the shoulder. This 20 year old man presented with shoulder pain and limitation of motion.

A Frontal radiograph shows multiple calcific nodules distributed throughout the joint. These nodules have smooth margins with a nonhomogeneous trabeculated pattern. Note the extensive secondary osteoarthritis with joint space narrowing, eburnation, and osteophytes.

B Arthrography reveals a multinodular pattern, confirming the intra-articular location of the nodules.

Illustration continued on the opposite page

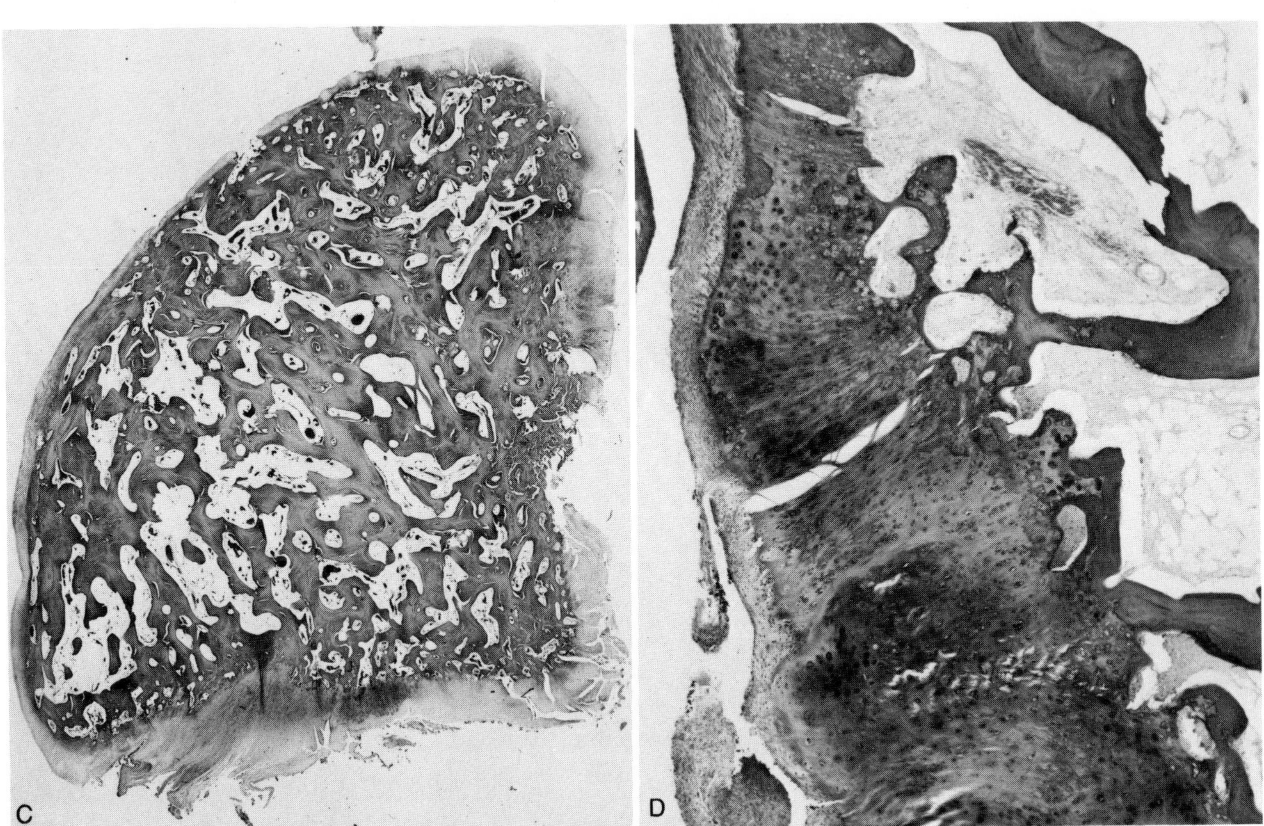

Figure 74–55. Continued

C *Macroslide of an intra-articular nodule shows a coarse trabecular pattern encased by a predominantly smooth fibrocartilaginous capsule.*

D *Photomicrograph (×43) of the capsule documents its cartilaginous nature. Areas of hyaline cartilage with endochondral bone formation and fibrocartilage are noted.*

(Armed Forces Institute of Pathology Neg. Nos. 76-268-2,5; 79-16663; 80-224.)

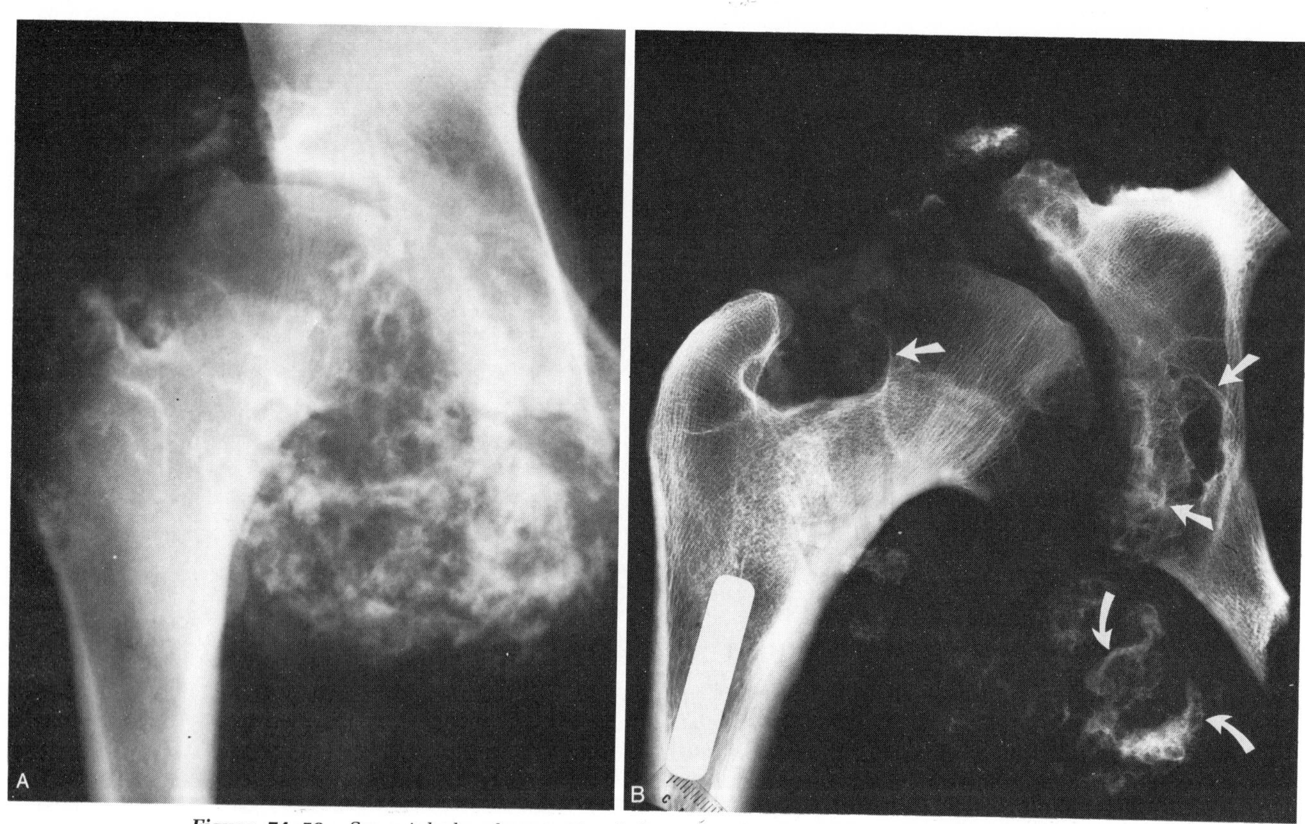

Figure 74–56. *Synovial chondromatosis of the hip. This 29 year old man presented with a slow-growing hip mass of 15 years' duration.*

A *Anteroposterior radiograph shows a large joint mass with stipples, rings, and arcs of calcification. The femoral head is displaced laterally and osteoarthritic changes are present. Bony erosions are also noted.*

B *Specimen radiograph demonstrates bony erosions (arrows) and bone formation (curved arrows) within the mass.*

Illustration continued on the opposite page

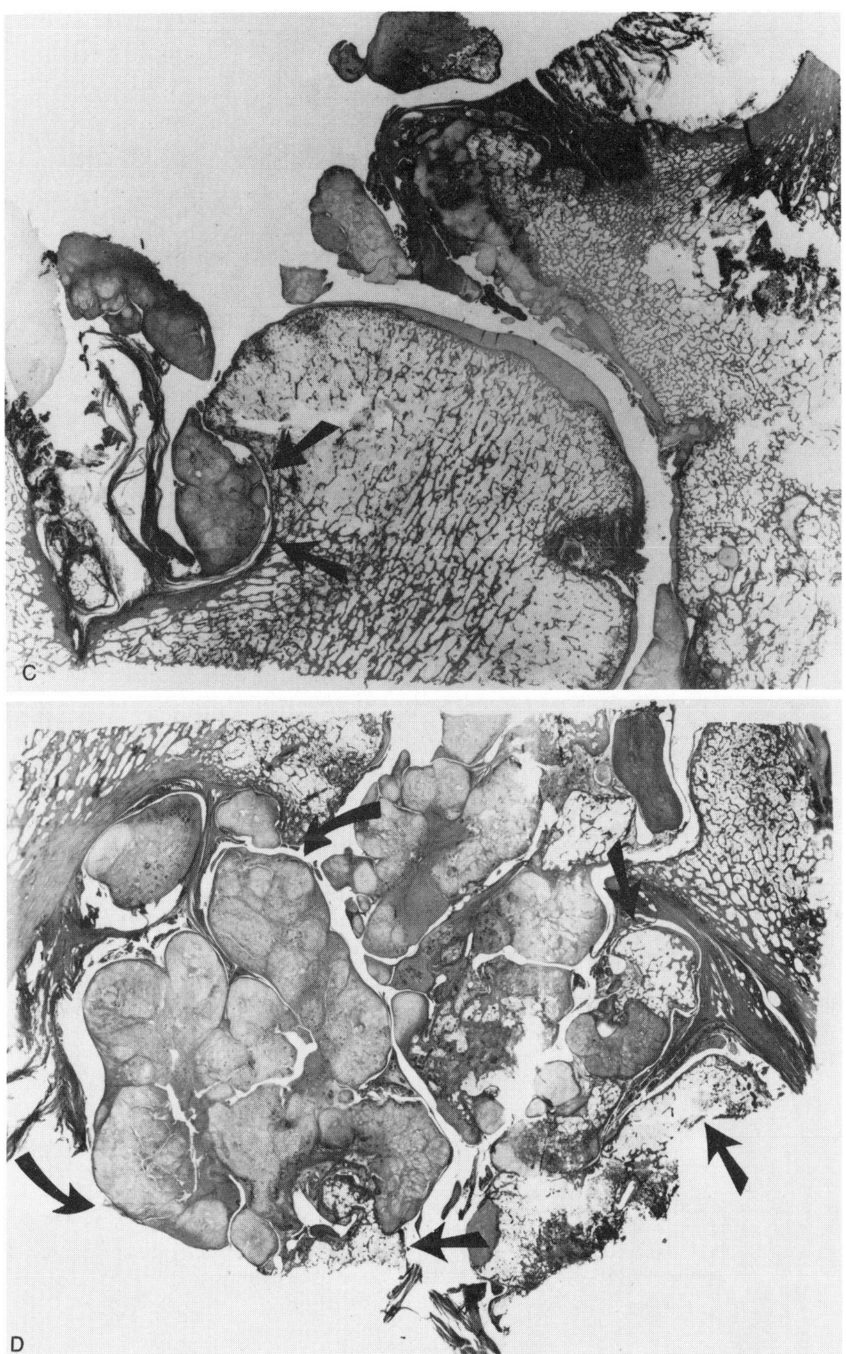

Figure 74–56. Continued

C *Macroslide of the upper femur and acetabulum shows evidence of joint remodeling and cartilage nodules in the adjacent soft tissue, one of which is causing a smooth bony erosion (arrows).*

D *Macroslide of the lower femur and inferior portion of the mass reveals the characteristic multilobular pattern of cartilage proliferation with (straight arrows) and without (curved arrows) bone formation.*

(Armed Forces Institute of Pathology Neg. Nos. 74-12924-2,1; 76-5768-1; 76-5769.)

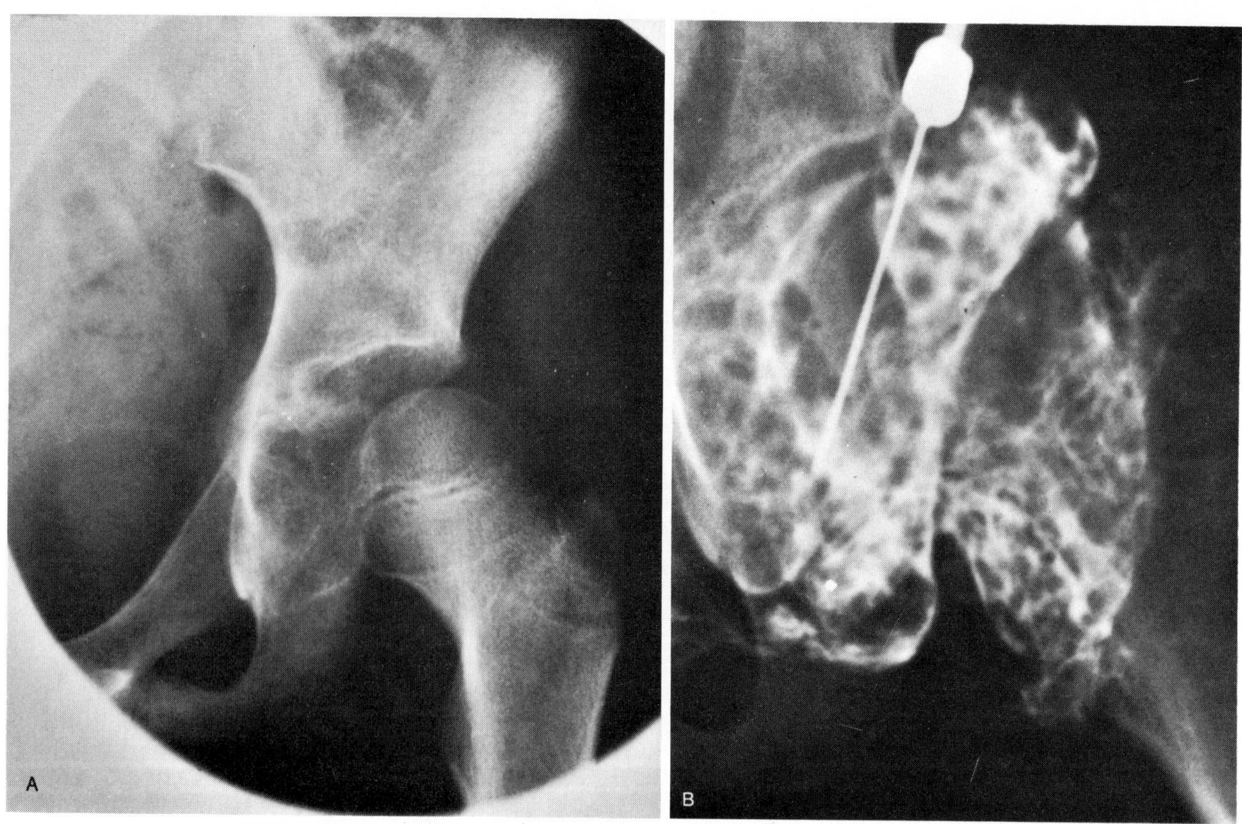

Figure 74–57. *Synovial chondromatosis of the hip. This 7 year old girl presented with a painless limp.*

A *Anteroposterior radiograph of the hip shows a widened joint space with lateral displacement of the femoral head. There is no evidence of soft tissue calcification.*

B *Arthrogram demonstrates multiple noncalcified nodules filling the joint.*

Illustration continued on the opposite page

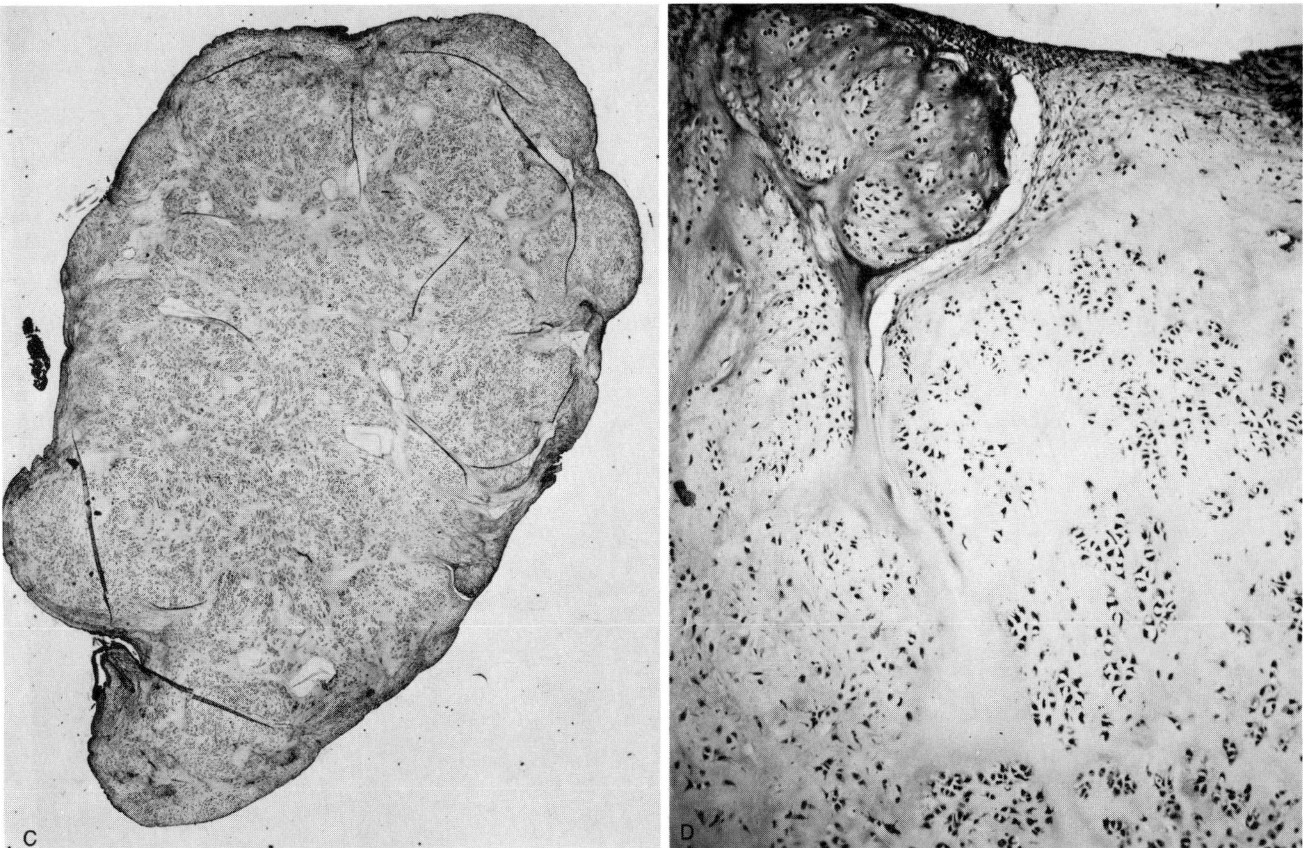

Figure 74–57. Continued
C *Photomicrograph (7×) of a single nodule shows the lobulated appearance of proliferating cartilage.*
D *Photomicrograph (63×) of the nodule's surface reveals the increased cellularity and variability of the cartilage.*
(Armed Forces Institute of Pathology Neg. Nos. 79-2001-1,2; 80-229; 80-228.)

attest to their having circumscribed margins. They are rubbery to firm in consistency and rarely exceed 2 cm in size. Microscopically, they are composed of adult type hyaline cartilage with some areas of ossification and calcification. They may have spindle-shaped nuclei that vary in size and shape, as well as mitotic figures. This pattern may be confused with chondrosarcoma if the pathologist is not aware of the range of histologic findings in this lesion.[263]

Radiographs show a nonspecific soft tissue mass, often with coarse specks of calcification. Occasionally, a lacy or trabecular pattern, which corresponds to areas of ossification, will be demonstrated. The mass can also cause extrinsic pressure erosion of the adjacent bone, with scalloping and a sclerotic margin.

Fibrous Tumors

Fibrous tumors of soft tissue represent a numerous and heterogeneous group of lesions, which have been supplied with a variety of terms and classifications.[14, 319-325] Benign forms of fibrous proliferative "tumors" are encountered with some frequency in the deeper soft and subcutaneous tissues. They have been termed "fibromatosis" to distinguish them from persistent hyperplasia or reparative scar tissue. The latter is usually self-limiting. Two principal groups of fibromatosis are recognized.[322, 323] In one group the disorder occurs as a congenital lesion or is diagnosed during childhood. From this group, some lesions can be differentiated by anatomic location and microscopic appearance into specific diagnoses, such as juvenile aponeurotic fibroma, infantile dermal fibromatosis, aggressive infantile fibromatosis, and congenital generalized fibromatosis.[320-323] These lesions will be discussed in more detail because of their frequency of presentation in the extremities. The other group of lesions may present at any time during life but is usually found in the adult. In this group of cellular fibroblastic lesions, it is difficult to separate specific diagnostic types and, in some cases, to differentiate them on a morphologic basis from adult fibrosarcoma.

Juvenile Aponeurotic Fibroma. This is a specialized form of fibromatosis that occurs in children or adolescents, with a male predominance.[14, 326-336] It usually arises in the aponeurotic tissue of the hands and feet, especially in the palms and soles,[326, 329] and presents as a painless, poorly circumscribed soft tissue mass, which is frequently firm and fixed. The tumor grows slowly with infiltration, and tends to calcify. The mass is usually less than 4 cm in diameter, and local recurrence is common as a result of its infiltrative nature.[326, 331]

Infantile Dermal Fibromatosis. This tumor is a benign fibrous proliferative lesion that almost exclusively involves the extensor surfaces of fingers and toes.[321, 337-343] It appears within the first 2 years of life and is frequently discovered at birth. Boys are predominantly affected. Classically, several digits are involved by multiple nodules, which are well circumscribed and firmly attached to skin. If they are large enough, they may also attach to the adjacent fascia or periosteum. Clinically, there may be a reddish appearance to the nodules. Grossly, they are whitish and usually less than 1 cm in diameter. The histologic appearance typically is of uniformly arranged interlacing bundles of fibroblasts, compressed by abundant birefringent collagen with incorporated adnexal structures.[321] Recurrence is frequent following surgery.

Radiologically, multiple soft tissue masses or swellings are noted on the extensor surface of the digits. The fingers may be deformed with flexion contractures, and rarely bone erosions are found.[344]

Aggressive Infantile Fibromatosis. This lesion presents as painless soft tissue swellings or masses in the extremities, usually during the first 2 years of life (Fig. 74–58). They are slightly more prominent in boys. Clinically, the tumor remains stationary for long periods of time and rarely, if ever, metastasizes.[321, 345] Grossly, these tumors are aggressive, infiltrating into local muscles, vessels, nerves, fasciae, tendons, and subcutaneous fat. Microscopically, the level of mitotic activity varies greatly among the interlacing bundles of fusiform and spindle-shaped cells and reticulin and collagen fibers. The histologic features make differentiation from fibrosarcoma difficult.[321] The lesions tend to recur following surgery. The radiographs demonstrate a soft tissue mass or swelling with an occasional bone deformity and scalloped defect.

Congenital Generalized Fibromatosis. This disorder is a disseminated disease that develops in utero and is usually fatal shortly after birth, if the infant is not stillborn.[321, 346-356] It consists of multiple nodular lesions of fibroblastic proliferation, in superficial soft tissue, muscle, viscera, and bone. It has been recently reported in a solitary

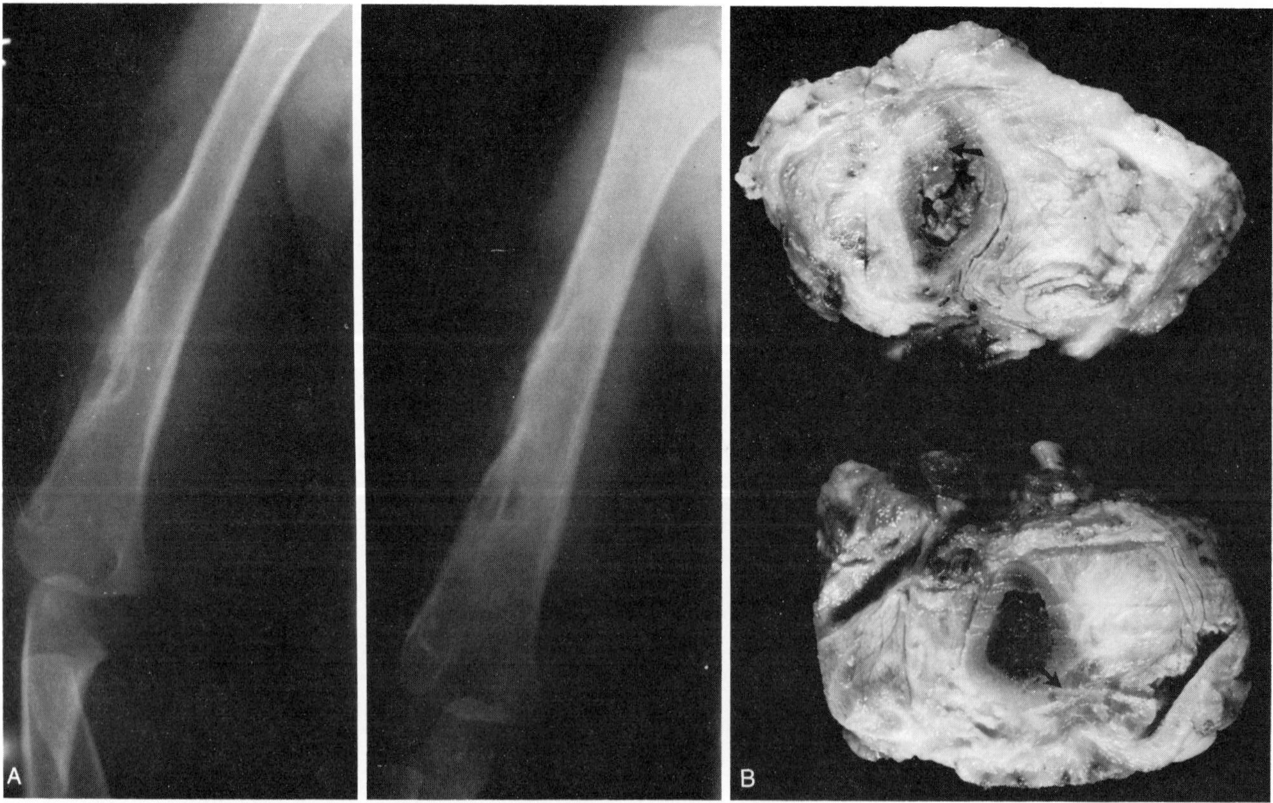

Figure 74–58. *Aggressive infantile fibromatosis of the upper arm. This 5 month old female infant presented with a rapidly growing mass attached to the periosteum.*

A *Anteroposterior and oblique radiographs show bony erosions with areas of cortical hyperostosis.*

B *Gross specimen demonstrates the large soft tissue mass and its extension into bone (arrows).*

(Armed Forces Institute of Pathology Neg. Nos. 67-6597-1, 67-6444.)

form.[350-352] Familial occurrences have been noted.[14, 357] The nodules are subcutaneous, firm, unencapsulated, and yellowish to white in color when removed from the body. Microscopically, there are curving fascicles of comparatively large elongated fibroblasts with a somewhat immature appearance.[321] The radiograph shows soft tissue swelling or masses and frequently multiple lytic lesions in bone.[358-360] Another form with no visceral involvement is now known (congenital multiple fibromatosis); it has a much better prognosis.[354-356] Regression with resolution of the lytic bone lesions in this type can occur[354, 356] (see Chapter 85).

Other Benign Soft Tissue Tumors

Although many additional soft tissue tumors exist (see Chapter 85), a few deserve special emphasis.

GANGLIONS. Ganglions are cystic masses, usually attached to tendon sheaths of the hands and feet.[14] Occasionally, they may be found within tendons, muscles, subcutaneous tissue at the fingertips, and semilunar cartilages. These lesions are characterized by unilocular or multilocular cystic spaces with a myxoid matrix. The lesion rarely communicates with the synovium of a tendon sheath or a joint in the unoperated patient, and it is not lined by synovium. Radiographically, it appears as a soft tissue mass, and if large enough, the fluid-filled space may be demonstrated by sonography or computed tomography. Angiography shows the mass to be avascular.[51]

MYXOMAS. Myxomas are soft, gelatinous growths; most frequently they are encountered in the heart, but not uncommonly they occur in subcutaneous soft tissues or within muscular structures.[14, 361-364] They are usually painless masses, presenting in the 50 to 60 year old age range. These lesions are uncommon in young adults and rare in children. The mass is poorly defined and unencapsulated, and it infiltrates adjacent structures, for which reason it may be difficult to eradicate. Microscopically, there is a fairly uniform consistency of poorly vascular, richly mucoid tumor, containing scattered stellate cells and minimal fibrosis. In contrast to ganglions, myxomas are rarely cystic. The radiograph usually demonstrates a nonspecific, ill-defined soft tissue mass. However, with computed tomography, the mucoid material should have an attenuation coefficient less than that of water.

LEIOMYOMAS. Leiomyomas are uncommon outside of the uterus and gastrointestinal tract but may be found in the skin and subcutaneous soft tissue.[14, 365-367] One type, the vascular leiomyoma, arises from small blood vessels of smooth muscle. These tumors may be solitary or multiple and are usually seen in the skin or deep soft tissues. The superficial lesions may present with paroxysmal pain. Because of the tumor's prominent vascularity, radiographic techniques, such as arteriography or contrast-enhanced computed tomography, may demonstrate the lesion.

Other lesions occurring in soft tissue include histiocytoma,[368] xanthomatosis,[369, 370] rhabdomyoma,[371-373] and myoblastoma.[14, 371] These lesions have no specific radiographic findings (see Chapter 85).

MALIGNANT SOFT TISSUE TUMORS

Liposarcoma

Liposarcoma is a common soft tissue malignancy.[1, 14, 374-387] It is seen most frequently in adults (fifth decade) but may occur at any age. Young children have a more favorable prognosis.[377, 388] The tumors are usually located in the fat-containing or deep soft tissues of the buttock, thigh, lower leg, and retroperitoneum, and there is a slight male predominance.[1, 14] Clinically, these lesions present as either poorly defined or well-circumscribed swellings or masses. Recurrence after surgery is common. While the duration of symptoms may be long, thus suggesting origin from an antecedent benign lesion as a possibility, it is generally agreed that liposarcomas arise de novo rather than from benign lipomas.[1, 14] The usual treatment is surgery, but local recurrence is common. The most common sites for metastasis are the lungs, pleurae, and liver.[14]

Liposarcomas are often large, bulky tumors. They not infrequently appear grossly as a circumscribed or encapsulated lesion, but they usually infiltrate into adjacent soft tissue[14, 92] (Fig. 74–59). Several different histologic types occur. The most common type found in the extremities, especially the thigh and popliteal area, is the well-differentiated myxoid form of liposarcoma.[1, 376-378, 388]

Radiographically, the liposarcoma usually presents as a nonhomogeneous, ill-defined mass that may calcify.[19, 61] However, the mass may be well circumscribed with obvious fatty content on plain films. The latter finding is most frequently seen in the well-differentiated liposarcoma[61, 389] (Fig. 74–60). Computed tomography may demonstrate their fatty character as a nonhomogeneous, fat-containing mass, with water density structures and poor margins (Fig. 74–61). The portions of water density will usually show enhancement on computed tomography after intravenous injection of contrast medium and correspond to the hypervascular areas. Occasionally, nonlipogenic tumors may infiltrate normal fat tissue, trapping the fat and producing a mottled appearance. This pattern can be confused with liposarcoma; however, it usually does not have the bulky

Text continued on page 2727

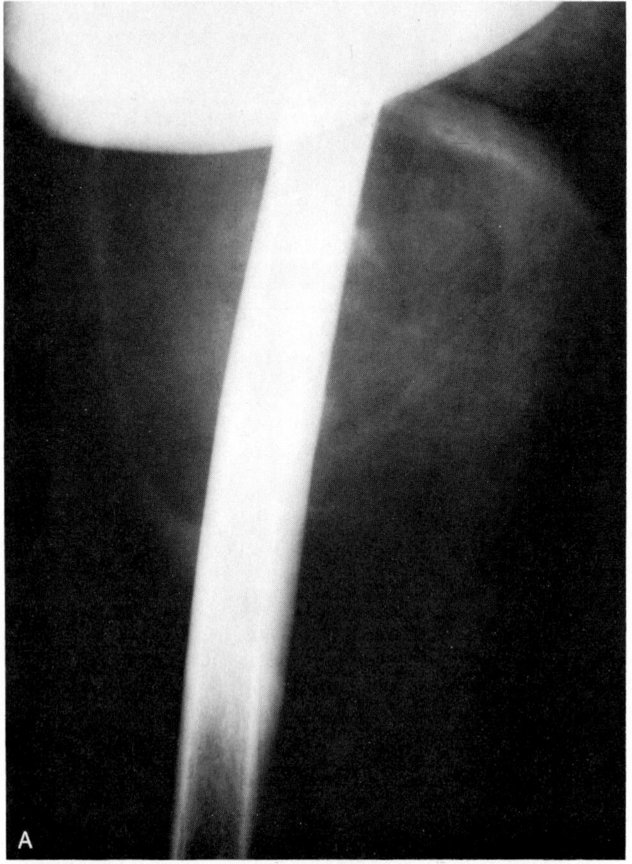

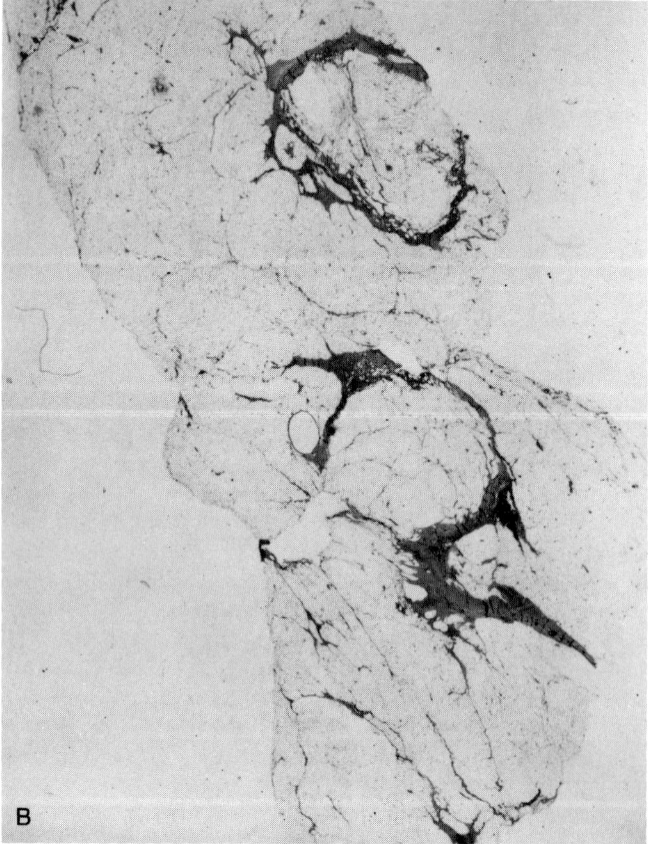

Figure 74–59. *Liposarcoma of the thigh, well-differentiated type. This 44 year old woman presented with a progressively enlarging thigh mass of 2 years' duration.*

A *Oblique radiograph shows a large, sharply circumscribed, nonhomogeneous fatty mass with a water-dense linear component.*

B *Photomicrograph (low power view) confirms the fatty nature and fibrous septa of the tumor. The latter causes the nonhomogeneous radiographic feature.*

Illustration continued on the opposite page

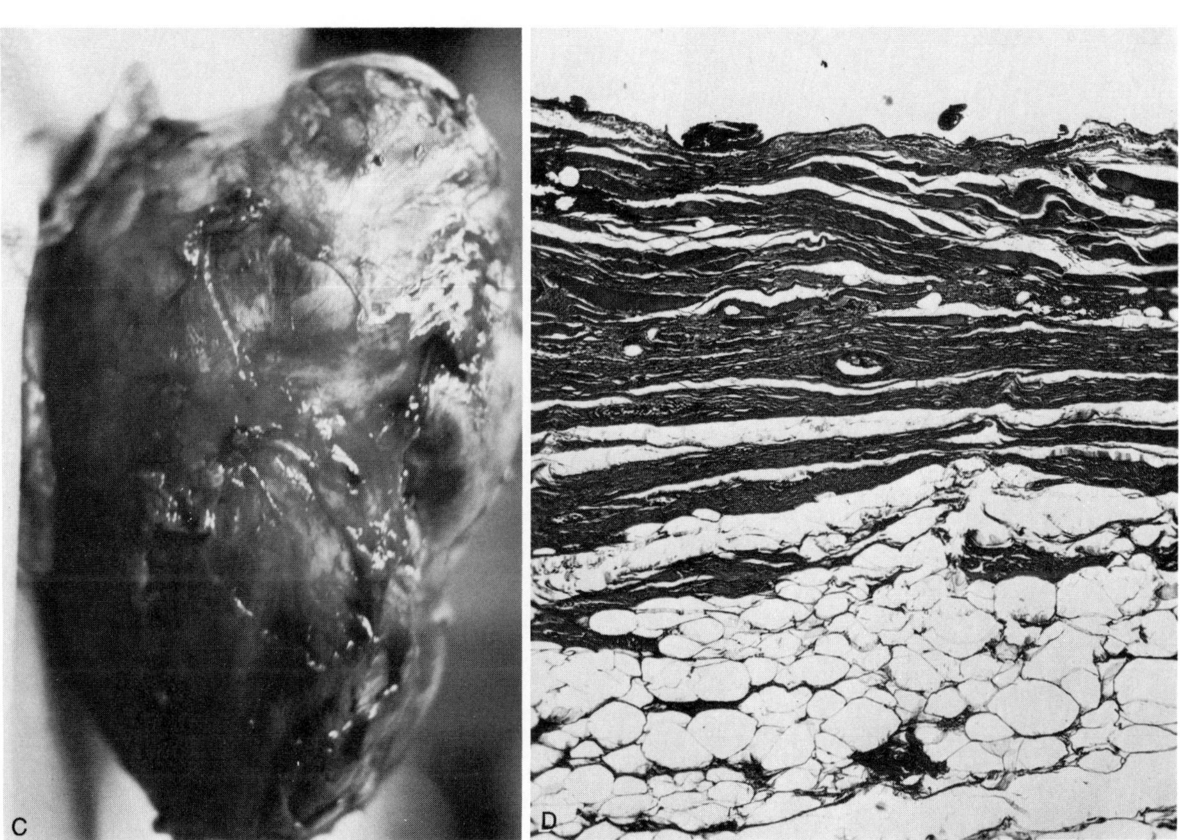

Figure 74–59. Continued

C *Gross specimen demonstrates the sharp, well-delineated peripheral margin.*

D *Photomicrograph (high power view) reveals a fibrous pseudocapsule about the periphery of the tumor.*

(Armed Forces Institute of Pathology Neg. Nos. 73-11119-1, 76-5775-1, 73-11241-1, 76-5785-1.)

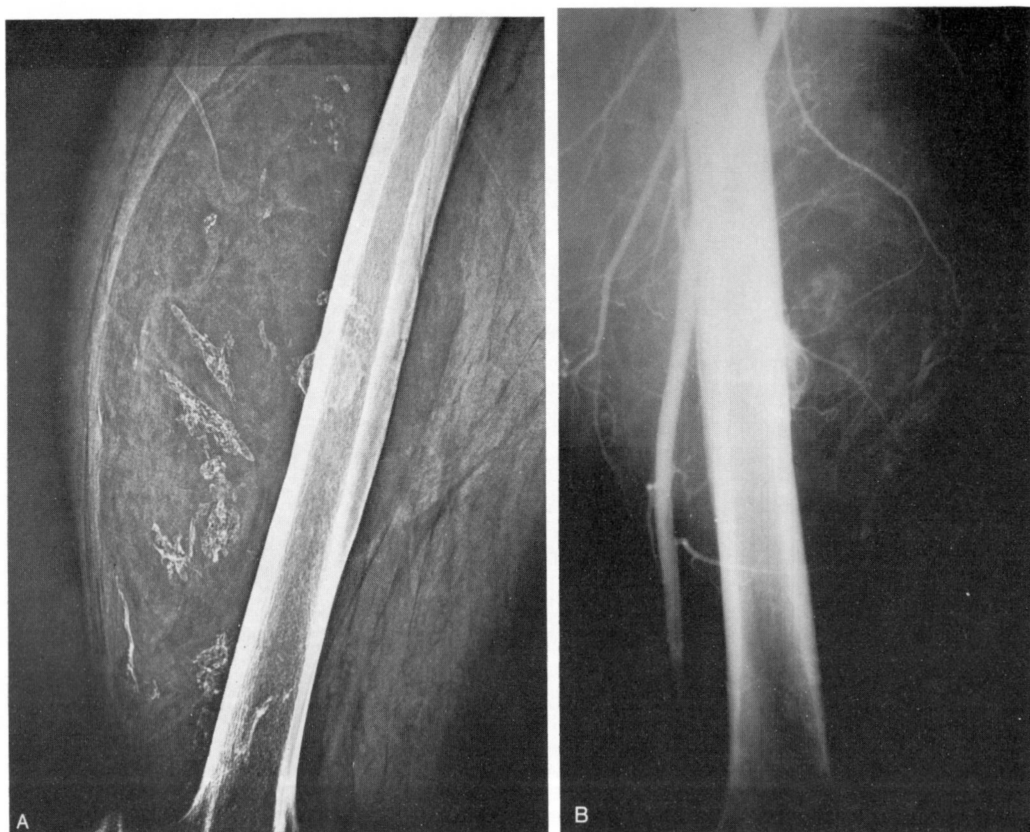

Figure 74–60. *Liposarcoma of the thigh, well-differentiated type. This 45 year old man presented with a rapidly growing soft tissue mass in the thigh.*

A *Lateral xeroradiograph shows the sharply circumscribed, fatty mass with multiple calcifications. Some dense areas have a trabecular pattern and represent ossification.*

B *Arteriogram (arterial phase) demonstrates a relatively hypervascular lesion with vessel displacement and neovascularity.*

Illustration continued on the opposite page

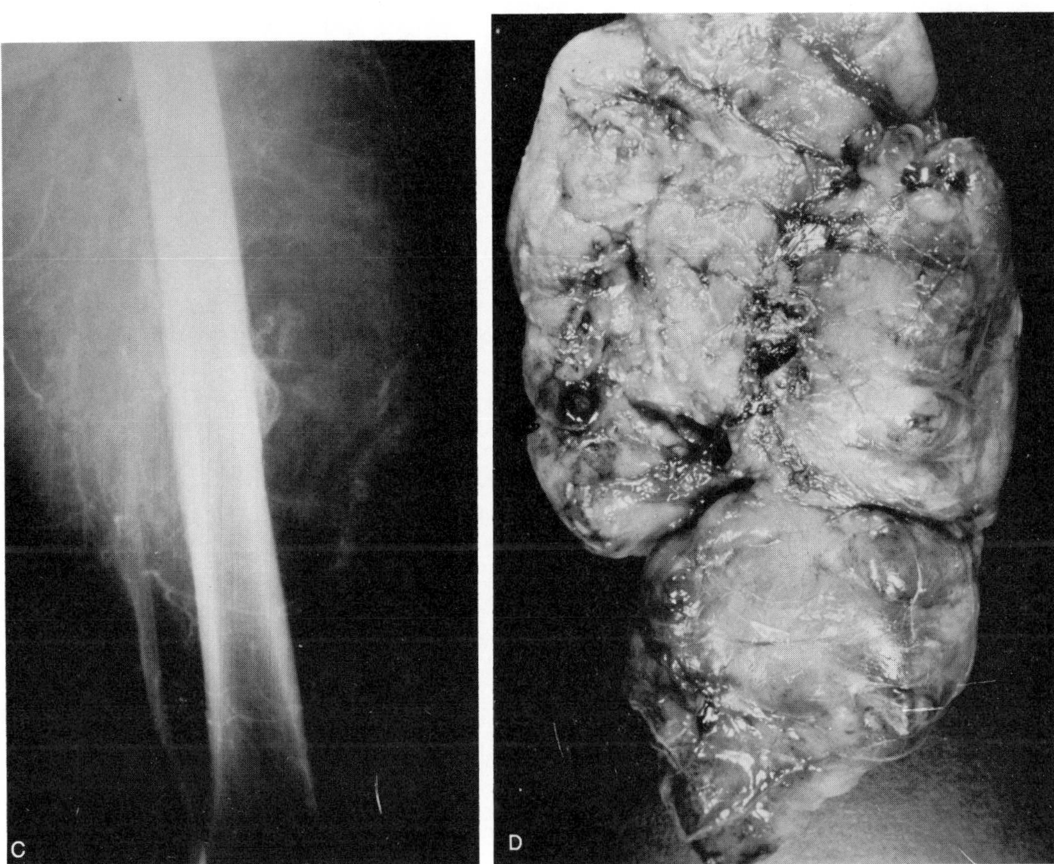

Figure 74–60. Continued
C *Arteriogram (late arterial phase) reveals a nonhomogeneous blush.*
D *Gross specimen demonstrates the well-delineated tumor margin.*
(Armed Forces Institute of Pathology Neg. Nos. 77-7859-4,2,3; 77-7820.)

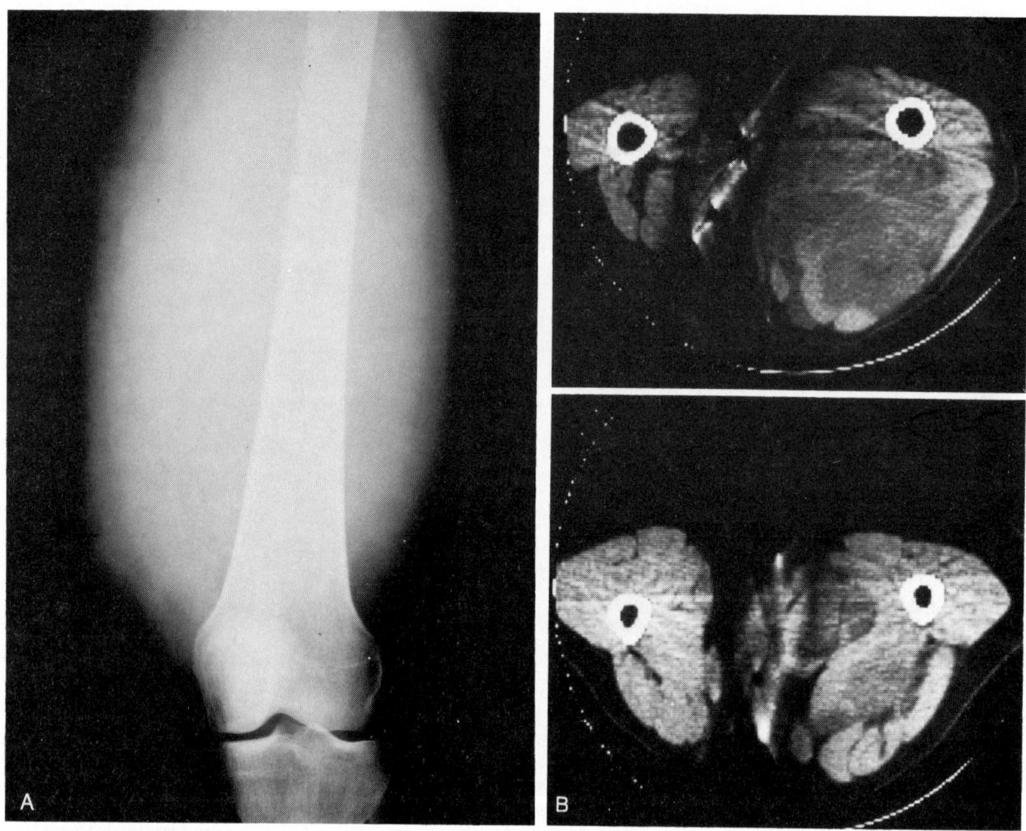

Figure 74–61. *Liposarcoma of the thigh, myxoid type. This 30 year old woman presented with a large, hard mass in the thigh.*

A *Anteroposterior radiograph shows a large water-dense mass with an ill-defined margin medially.*

B *A nonhomogeneous, low attenuation coefficient mass is noted on computed tomography. This finding suggests a fatty component not appreciated on plain film* **(A)**. *The margin is irregular, with infiltration into adjacent soft tissue.*

Illustration continued on the opposite page

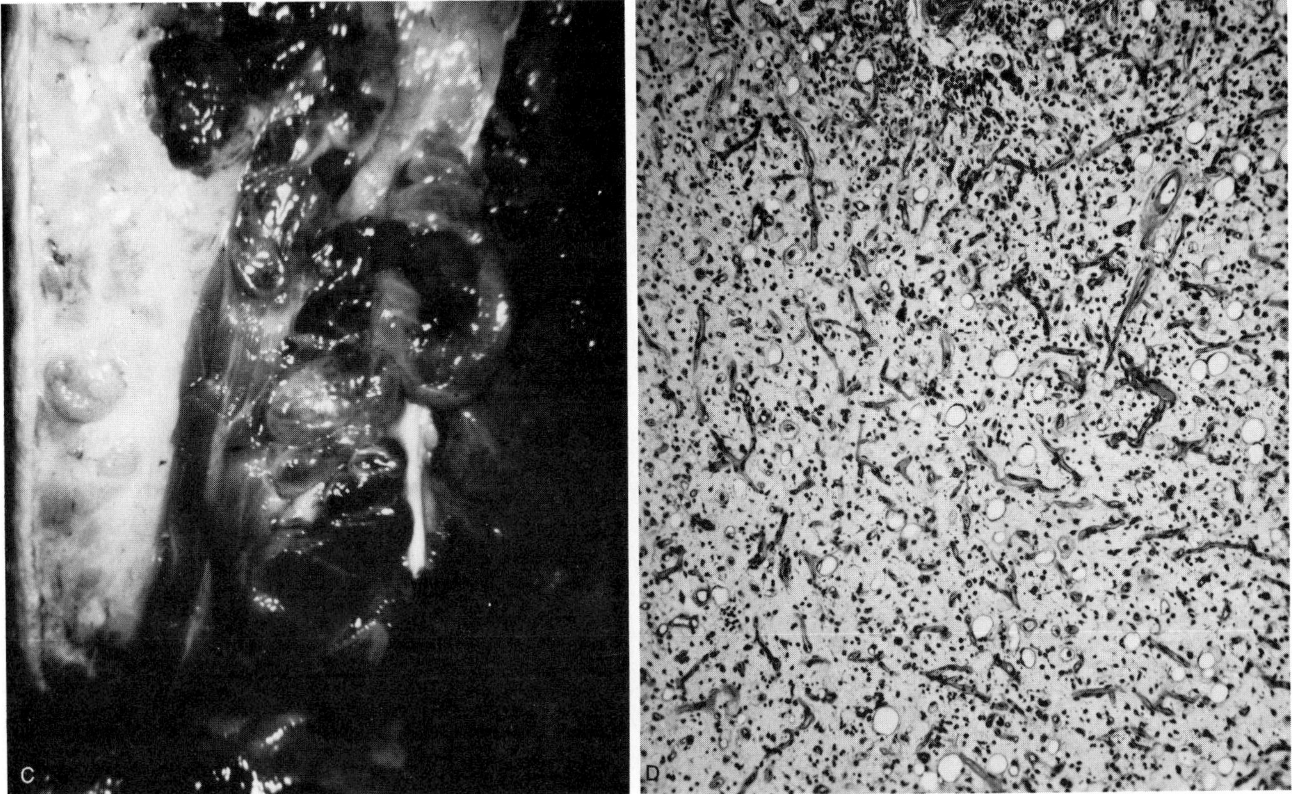

Figure 74–61. Continued
C *Gross specimen confirms the fatty nature and infiltrative features of the tumor.*
D *Photomicrograph (63 ×) demonstrates delicate vascular channels, loose myxoid stroma, and lipoblasts.*
(Armed Forces Institute of Pathology Neg. Nos. 77-9059-4,7; 77-7931-5; 79-16670.)

fatty component seen in well-differentiated liposarcoma.

Synovial Sarcoma

Synovial sarcoma is an uncommon malignant tumor, which is most frequently located in the soft tissue of the extremities[390-399] (Fig. 74–62). The lower extremities are more commonly affected than the upper extremities, with the knee, ankle, and foot most frequently involved. The neoplasms generally arise adjacent to a joint, bursa, or tendon sheath. However, fewer than 10 per cent are primarily located within the joint cavity.[377] Occasionally, the synovial membrane is involved by direct extension. Synovial sarcomas occur at all ages but are most frequent in the young adult and rare in infants.[14, 400, 401]

Clinically, patients present with a painful swelling or mass. Rarely, cutaneous pain will be present without a palpable tumor mass.[402, 403] The tumor usually grows slowly, with the duration of symptoms from onset to death varying from 5 months to 16 years.[14, 404, 405] Metastasis, when present, usually occurs to the lungs. Local recurrence following surgery is common and is associated with a poor prognosis.[1]

The tumors are grossly solid, with sharply circumscribed margins, appearing encapsulated. Adjacent soft tissue structures are usually displaced, and local extension occurs. Microscopically, the tumors usually have a biphasic histologic appearance.[14, 406-408] One phase demonstrates slightly enlarged polygonal cells and occasional cylindrical cells growing in cords arranged around clefts or slits, resulting in an adenomatous or pseudoglandular appearance. The other phase shows spindle-shaped cells (fibrous-appearing), filling in the areas between the slits.[14] Occasionally, one cell type will predominate, giving the tumor a monophasic appearance. These histologic patterns have been subclassified into (1) pseudoglandular, (2) fibrosarcoma, and (3) endothelioid types. The first two patterns may have a more favorable prognosis.[377]

Radiographically, a soft tissue mass possessing a variable peripheral margin, ranging from smooth to indistinct, is usually present.[409, 410] Spotty calcification is common, occurring in about one third of lesions.[390, 411] The tumor can also cause adjacent bony osteoporosis or destruction. In slow-growing lesions, bone destruction appears as an extrinsic

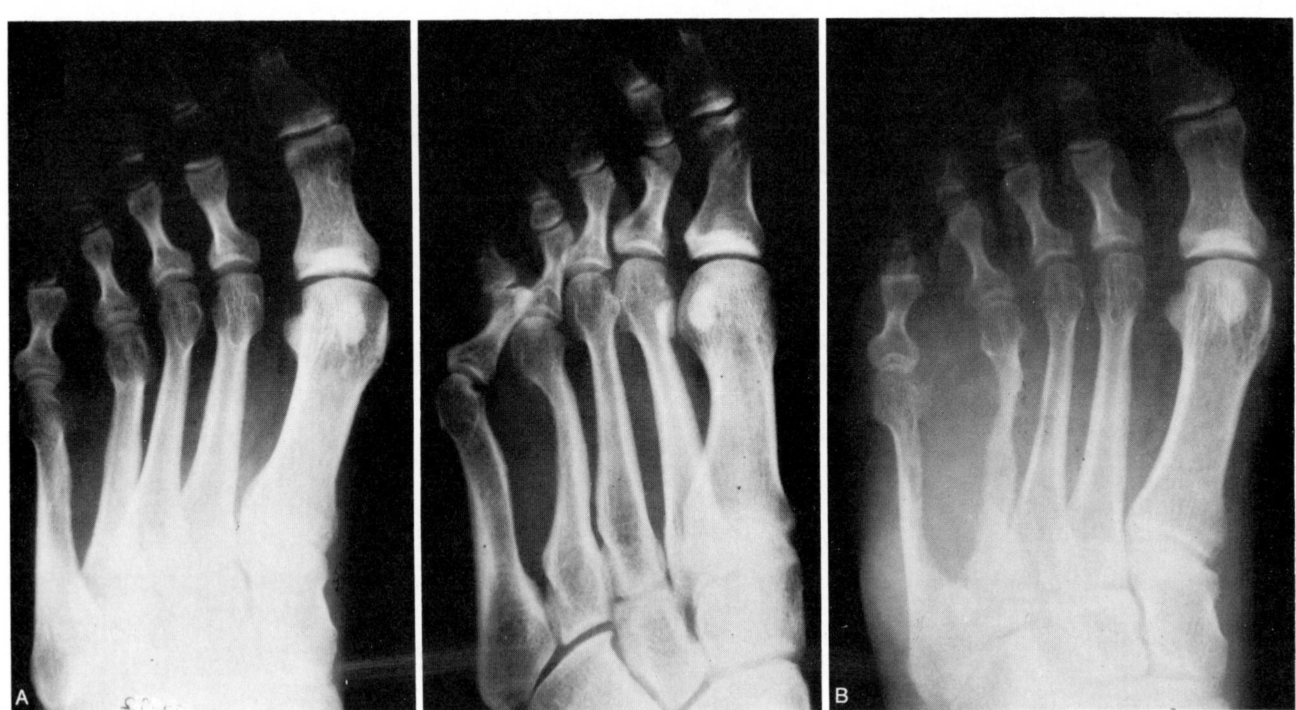

Figure 74–62. *Synovial sarcoma of the foot. This 40 year old man presented with a mass of the foot that grew slowly over the last 9 months.*

A *Initial anteroposterior and oblique radiographs show the mass with secondary pressure erosion of the fourth metatarsal.*

B *Anteroposterior radiograph 9 months later demonstrates aggressive destruction and infiltration of the fourth and fifth metatarsals.*

Illustration continued on the opposite page

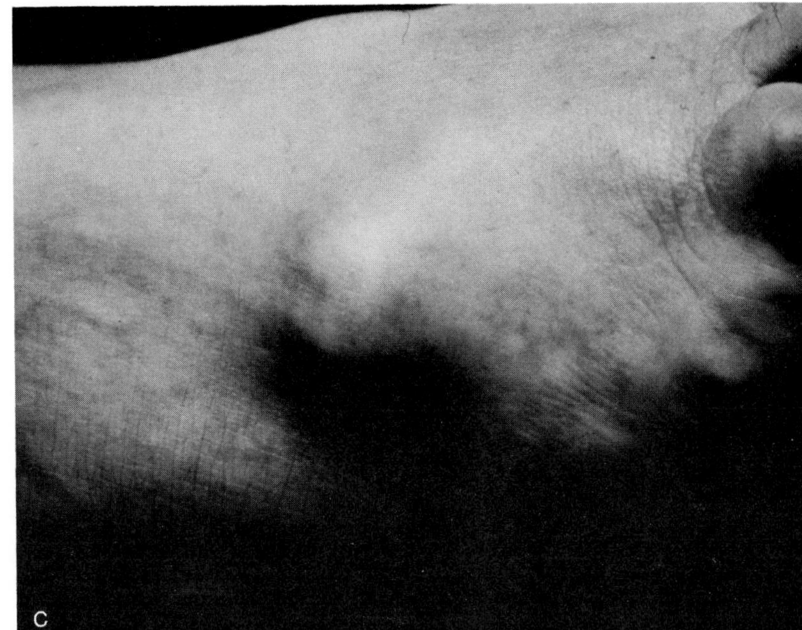

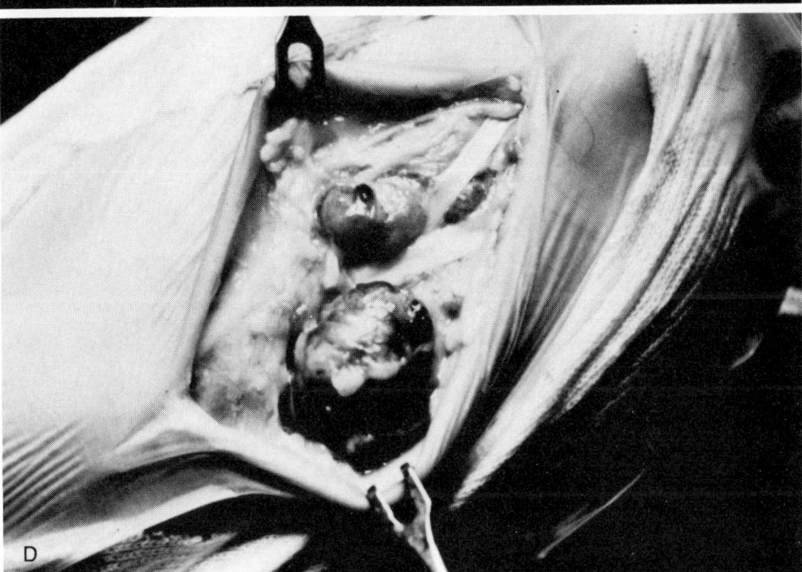

Figure 74–62. Continued

C *Clinical photograph outlines the soft tissue mass.*

D *At surgery, the tumor was infiltrating the adjacent soft tissues and extending around the dorsal ligaments and tendons of the foot.*

(Armed Forces Institute of Pathology Neg. Nos. 74-19670-1,2; 74-12420-3,6.)

pressure erosion (Fig. 74–62). However, if the bone has been invaded, an aggressive pattern of irregular destruction is seen. Arteriography in synovial sarcoma usually demonstrates a hypervascular lesion with neovascularity and nonhomogeneous staining. Occasionally the lesion is hypovascular. Computed tomography shows a soft tissue mass, which may infiltrate adjacent structures. Because of its extensive vascular supply, the synovial sarcoma should be enhanced after contrast injection.

Rhabdomyosarcoma

Rhabdomyosarcoma is a common malignant soft tissue tumor of muscle origin, which has an exceedingly poor prognosis.[412-422] There are two distinct groups, one found in children and the other in adults. In children, the mass is frequently found in the head and neck or genitourinary tract. Tumors in adult patients most commonly occur in the deep soft tissues of the extremities. Grossly, the lesions have a soft consistency. Infiltration of local tissues is common and is probably responsible for the frequent recurrence after initial surgery. Distant spread to the lungs and occasionally lymph nodes is also common. There are three histologic types: embryonal, alveolar, and pleomorphic. The embryonic type is the most common type and typically occurs in children. This histologic pattern is uncommon in the extremities. The alveolar type tends to affect older children and young adults, and is frequently found in the extremities. The pleomorphic type is the least common and predominates in the skeletal muscles of adults. Radiographically, these tumors present as an ill-defined soft tissue mass. They tend to involve adjacent bone by local extension, resulting in either destruction, saucerization, or, occasionally, sclerosis of the cortex. Calcification within the tumor may also occur and is more common than generally appreciated.[16, 417] The rhabdomyosarcoma is usually hypervascular on arteriography.

Fibrosarcoma

Fibrosarcoma presents as a swelling or mass among the fibrous supportive structures of muscles, tendons, ligaments, and fasciae.[423-427] These tumors are most frequent in the external soft tissues of the extremities, such as the thigh,[428] and occasionally develop in cicatrices following trauma or irradiation.[14] Fibrosarcoma is found both in adults and in children and has a male predominance. It is less often fatal when present in children.[429, 430] The tumor infiltrates the adjacent soft tissue, and therefore recurrence following surgery is frequent.

Grossly, fibrosarcomas are firm, with ill-defined margins, and vary widely in size. The histologic differentiation between fibromatosis and well-differentiated fibrosarcoma can be difficult.[14] In the latter tumor, there are fewer fibers; disproportionate cell size and mitoses are found without difficulty.

The fibrosarcoma appears as a nonspecific soft tissue mass on the plain film radiograph. Infiltration into adjacent bone with destruction and calcification, although not common, can be seen. Arteriography demonstrates hypervascularity with neovascularity. The angioarchitecture is usually uneven due to the heterogeneous arrangement of the fibrosarcoma.[428] The more vascular tumors generally reflect a higher grade sarcoma and a poorer prognosis.[428, 431, 432]

The fibrosarcomas in infants are unique and differ from the fibrosarcomas of adults.[429, 430, 433-437] They usually present as a mass within the first 2 years of life, frequently at birth, and have a better prognosis (Fig. 74–63). These tumors are more common in boys and chiefly affect the distal areas of the lower and upper extremities. Like the adult type, they are poorly marginated and infiltrate adjacent tissues. After treatment, which is usually wide local excision or amputation, late recurrence and meta-

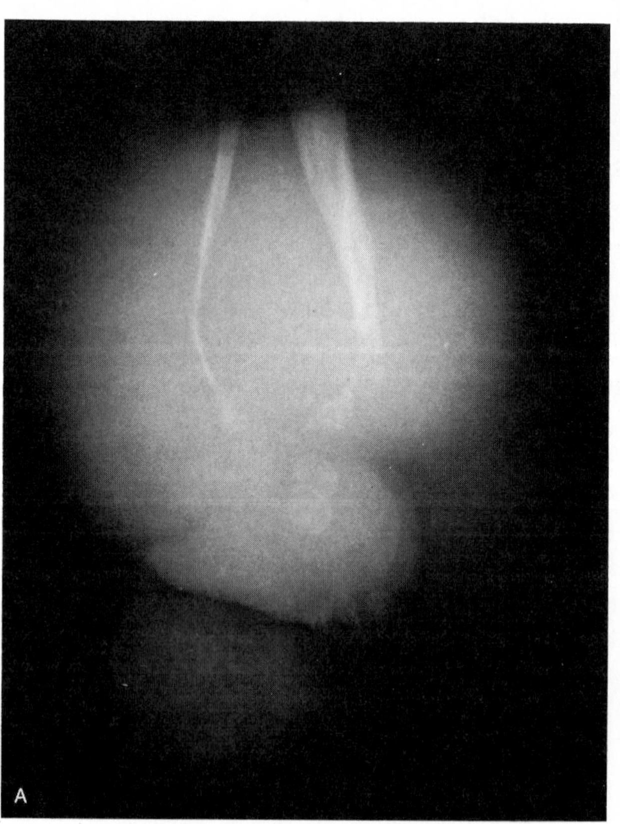

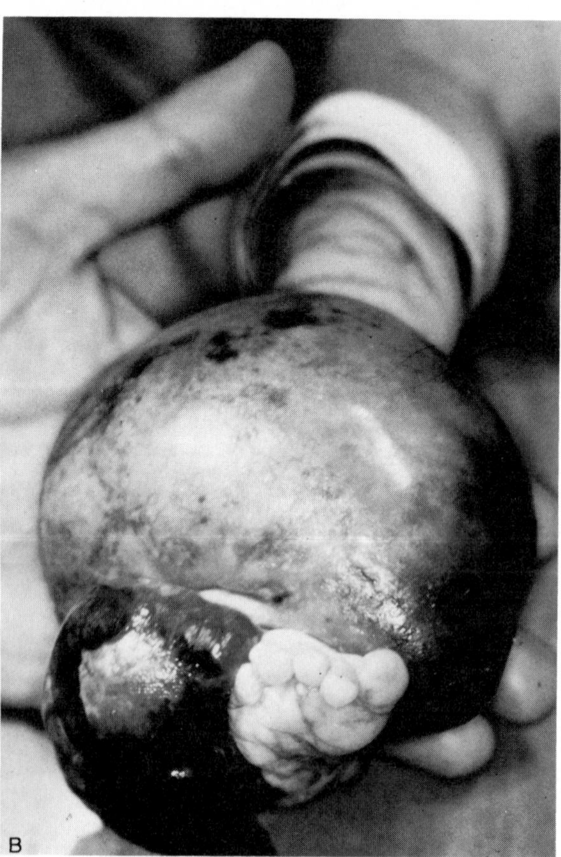

Figure 74–63. *Infantile fibrosarcoma of the leg. This 3 day old female infant presented with a large, friable, bleeding mass at birth.*

A *Tomography of the leg shows a large water-dense mass with displacement, deformity, and erosion of the tibia and fibula.*

B *The mass with its bleeding surface is seen on the clinical photograph.*

Illustration continued on the opposite page

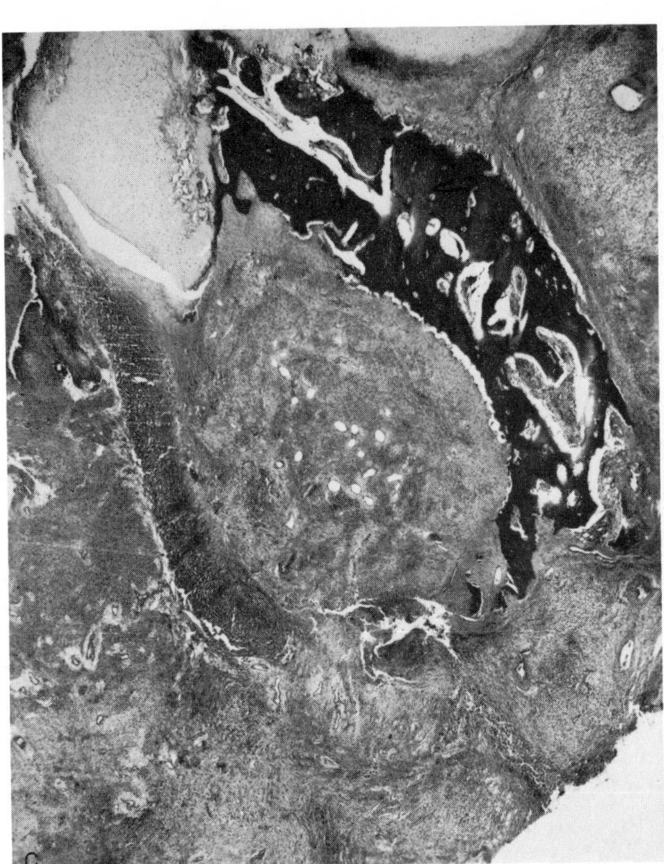

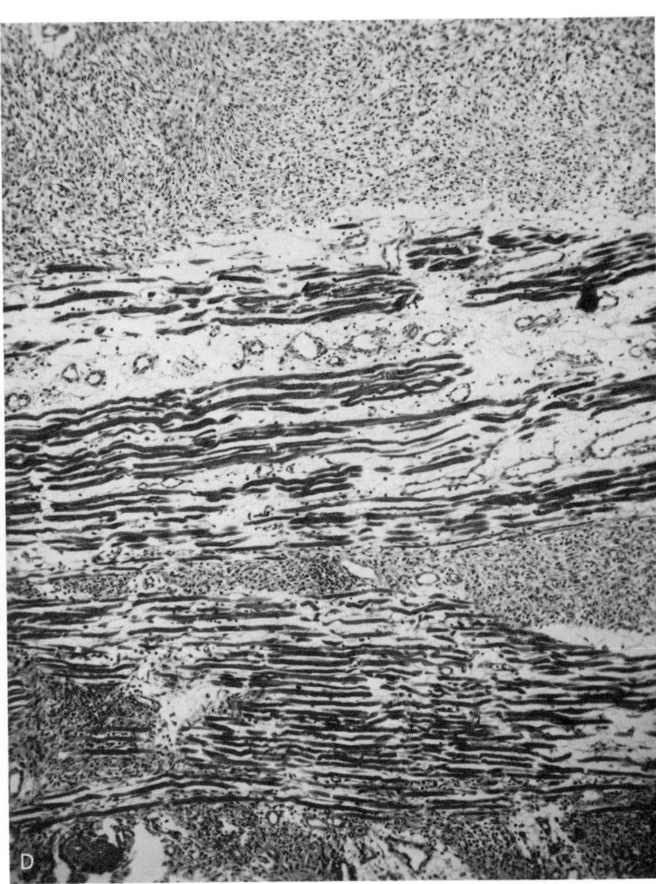

Figure 74–63. Continued
C *Photomicrograph (15×) demonstrates the tumor infiltrating bone, as seen in the radiograph* **(A)**.
D *Photomicrograph (63×) taken from the soft tissue component of the mass shows tumor infiltrating muscle.*
(Armed Forces Institute of Pathology Neg. No. 77-477-9, 77-432-2, 79-16668, 79-16665.)

static disease can occur. Thus, long-term follow-up is necessary. Radiographically, a soft tissue mass is seen, and frequently severe deformity and marked erosions of adjacent bone are noted (Fig. 74–63).

Other Malignant Soft Tissue Tumors

Other malignant soft tissue tumors may be considered in the differential diagnosis of soft tissue masses in and about the joint; among these are malignant schwannoma,[1] leiomyosarcoma,[1, 438-441] extraskeletal osteogenic sarcoma,[14, 442-444] extraskeletal chondrosarcoma,[14, 443-451] mesenchymoma,[1, 14] epithelioid sarcoma,[1] and malignant fibrous histiocytoma[14, 452-455] (see Chapter 85).

The malignant schwannoma and leiomyosarcoma are found uncommonly in the extremities, with the exception of malignant schwannoma associated with neurofibromatosis.[1] Extraskeletal osteogenic sarcoma and extraskeletal chondrosarcoma occur in the deeper soft tissues of the extremities. Mineralized osteoid with a homogeneous pattern may be seen in the former and a stippled calcification pattern, suggesting chondroid matrix, in the latter. The malignant fibrous histiocytoma, mesenchymoma, and epithelioid sarcoma will also be found in the extremities. However, these lesions are associated with no specific radiographic findings.

SOFT TISSUE TUMOR–LIKE LESIONS

Myositis Ossificans

Localized myositis ossificans is a tumor-like heterotopic formation of bone and cartilage in soft tissue, usually muscles, but also tendons, ligaments, fasciae, aponeuroses, and joint capsules.[1, 14, 456-467] Patients of any age or either sex may be affected. They usually present with a mass following trauma, although ossification is also encountered with some frequency, especially about the knee, thigh, and hips, in paraplegic patients.[1, 462] The mass may be doughy, painful, and warm during its early development. With time, the lesion shrinks to a firm and definable mass attached to the adjacent soft tissues or bone.[1, 459] Growth of the mass occurs during this

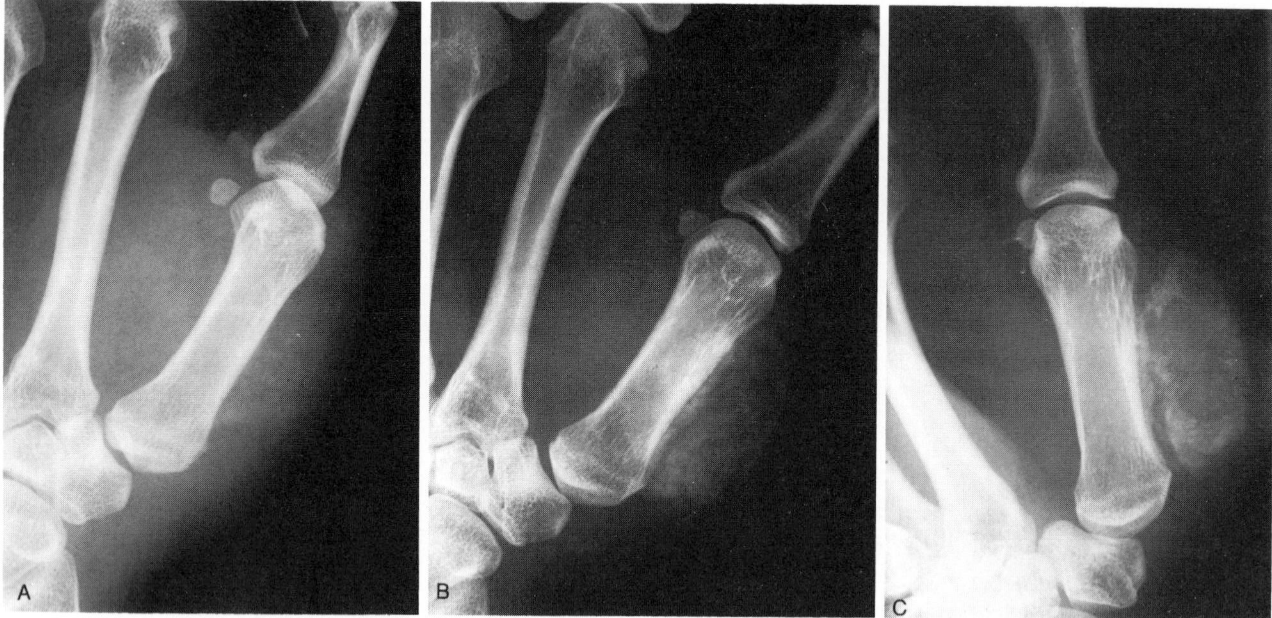

Figure 74–64. Myositis ossificans of the hand with serial radiographic changes. This 24 year old woman presented with swelling adjacent to the first metacarpal of 2 months' duration.

A Initial film shows soft tissue swelling with ill-defined calcification.

B Follow-up film 3 weeks later demonstrates an organized calcification pattern. The lesion has a peripheral shell of increased density with a less dense center. Also noted is periosteal reaction and attachment of the process to the adjacent bone.

C The attachment and peripheral shell of bone are best seen on this oblique radiograph. (Armed Forces Institute of Pathology Neg. Nos. 73-3602-2,5,1.)

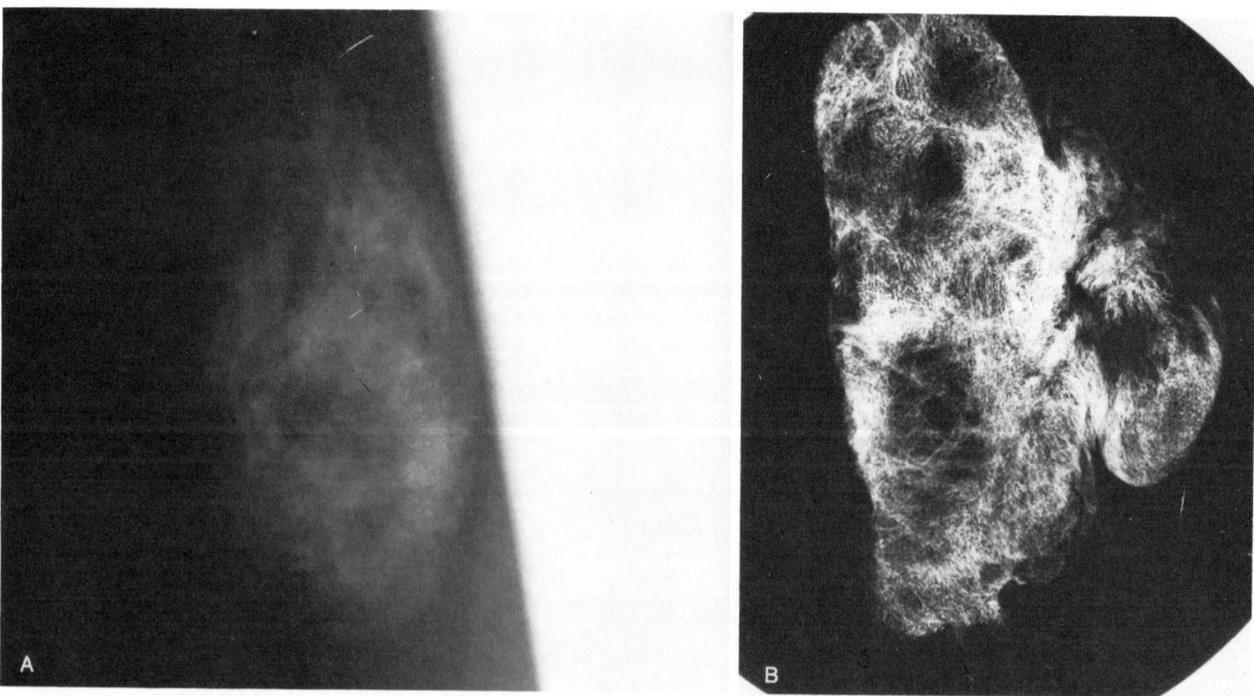

Figure 74–65. Myositis ossificans of the thigh. This 25 year old man initially presented with a swollen thigh following trauma. A small nodule was palpated several months later.

A Anteroposterior radiograph taken several months after the injury shows an oval calcified soft tissue mass with a peripheral shell.

B The peripheral shell, bony trabecular pattern, and less dense (lucent) areas are noted on the specimen radiograph.

Illustration continued on the opposite page

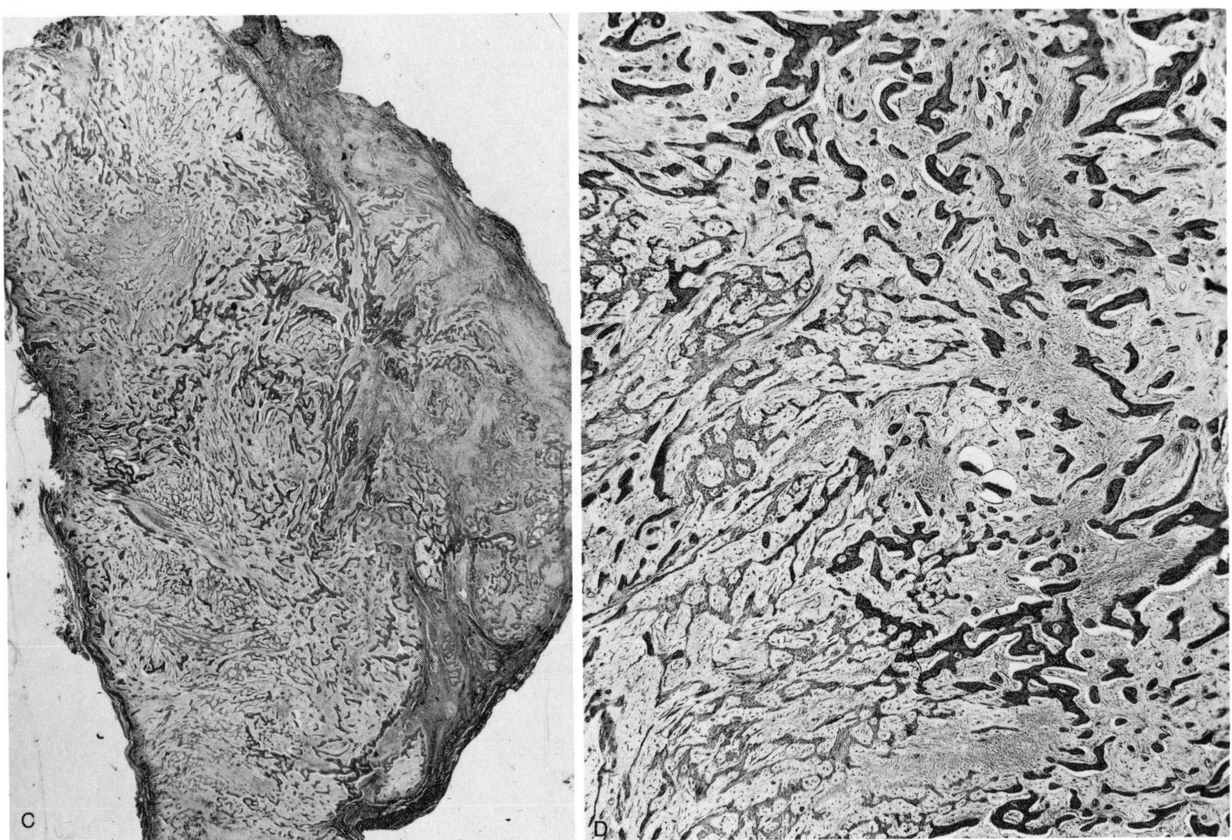

Figure 74–65. Continued

C *Macroslide shows an admixture of fibrous tissue and varying degrees of maturing bone trabeculae surrounded by a bony shell.*

D *Photomicrograph (11×) more clearly demonstrates varying degrees of bone maturation.*

(Armed Forces Institute of Pathology Neg. Nos. 74-8835-1,3; 75-3853; 75-3852.)

active proliferative phase and is self-limited.[14] Although lesions are usually small, occasionally they may be quite large — up to 10 cm in diameter.[14] The proliferating tissue, including osteoid, interdigitates with the muscle bundles. During this active phase, the florid osteoblastic repair tissue may be mistaken for an osteosarcoma on biopsy.[14, 456, 468] Rarely an osteosarcoma may arise from this otherwise benign process.[469, 470] Eventually, the lesion develops into a mass of mature bone with a cortical shell surrounding central cancellous, less mature tissue.[471]

Serial radiographs are required to appreciate a dynamic changing pattern[49, 468, 472-475] (Fig. 74–64). Initially, a nonspecific, ill-defined soft tissue mass without calcification is seen. As cell proliferation and maturation occur, the peripheral zone produces osteoid, which in turn will mineralize. This change appears from 4 to 6 weeks following injury and results in a well-developed ossified shell at 8 to 10 weeks post injury, surrounding a central radiolucent, usually cystic area (Fig. 74–65). Sonography data are similar to those obtained with plain film radiography.[472] Myositis ossificans, if associated with a deep injury, may involve the periosteum and attach to bone with superficial erosion or thickening of the cortex (Fig. 74–65). If adjacent bones are closely apposed, myositis ossificans in the intervening soft tissue may produce bony struts with synostosis. Joint ligaments and capsules may also be involved, producing external ankylosis. Arteriographic findings in myositis ossificans vary during the different phases of the disease.[474] In the acute phase, the lesion is hypervascular with fine vessels and staining on late films. In the healing phase, the lesion is usually avascular.

Villonodular Synovitis

Villonodular synovitis is a proliferative disorder of the synovium, which frequently is localized or nodular.[476-498] The mass is thought to arise in the synovial lining of joints, tendon sheaths, fascial planes, or ligamentous tissue. It usually involves young adults and is slightly more common in men. The lesions present as nonpainful soft tissue masses, frequently located in the digits of the hands and feet (Fig. 74–66). Other joints and tendon sheath areas can be involved, especially the knee.[586] A monoarticular distribution is the rule, but rare polyarticular involve-

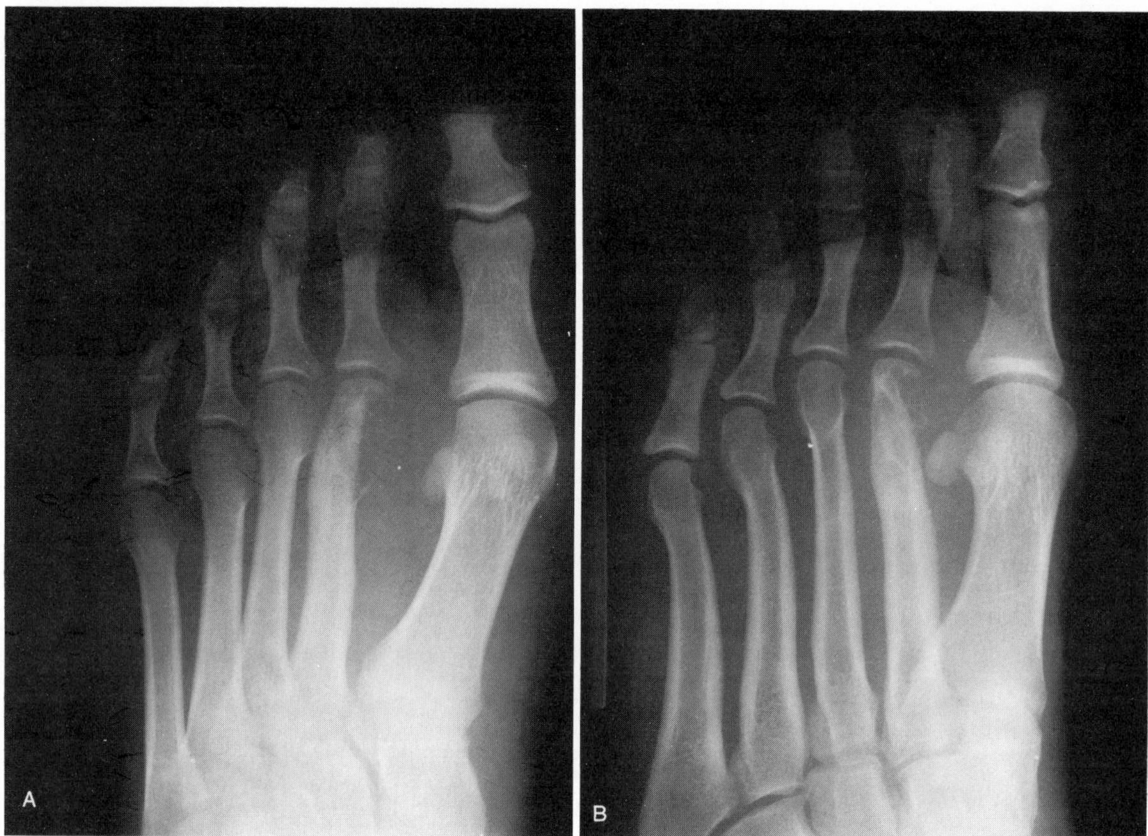

Figure 74–66. Villonodular synovitis of the foot. This 17 year old man presented with a mass on the volar aspect of the foot.

A Anteroposterior radiograph shows a soft tissue mass widening the space between the first and second metatarsals and bony erosions.

B Oblique radiograph reveals multiple, well-circumscribed bony erosions with sclerotic margins involving the second metatarsal head.

Illustration continued on the opposite page

ment occurs. The etiology is unknown;[499-502] some investigators consider it an inflammatory response,[503] whereas others consider it a neoplasm.[14]

Grossly localized villonodular synovitis is a firm, nodular mass, with a gray or yellowish appearance. Microscopically, there is a considerable variability in the histologic pattern. Low power views reflect an accentuated villous and nodular morphologic appearance. Higher magnification reveals extensive cellular (stromal cell) proliferation in association with fibroblastic tissue, multinucleated giant cells, xanthoma cells, lymphocytes, and variable amounts of hemosiderin deposition. The varying histology has resulted in a number of synonyms, such as giant cell tumor, fibroma, fibroxanthoma, or xanthoma of the tendon sheath.

The localized nodular lesion described previously probably should be differentiated from a more diffuse pigmented villonodular synovitis.[504, 505] The latter is less common and usually involves the larger joints, especially the knee. Grossly, the specimen is brown owing to extensive hemosiderin deposition. It is often associated with hemorrhagic effusions and is thought by some observers to represent a vascular anomaly,[505] distinguishing it from villonodular synovitis, which may be either a reactive or a true neoplastic process. Such differentiation between villonodular synovitis and pigmented villonodular synovitis is not always possible on histologic grounds.[504] Thus, some authorities use the term pigmented villonodular synovitis to encompass all of these various synovial processes.[506]

On radiographs, localized villonodular synovitis presents as a soft tissue mass, frequently associated with bony erosions[507-514] (Fig. 74–66). These erosions have a well-defined sclerotic margin and are a sign not of malignancy but of direct extension and pressure effect.[515] Diffuse intra-articular pigmented villonodular synovitis produces a joint effusion. Usually, the joint space is normal in width and osteoporosis is absent or mild. Bony erosions can occur in juxta-articular locations and are variable in size. Such osseous defects are more frequent in "tight" articulations, such as the hip, the elbow, and the wrist. Calcification is not typical, although cartilaginous and osseous metaplasia of the synovial lining has been encountered on rare occasions. If hemosiderin deposition is extensive, it can be de-

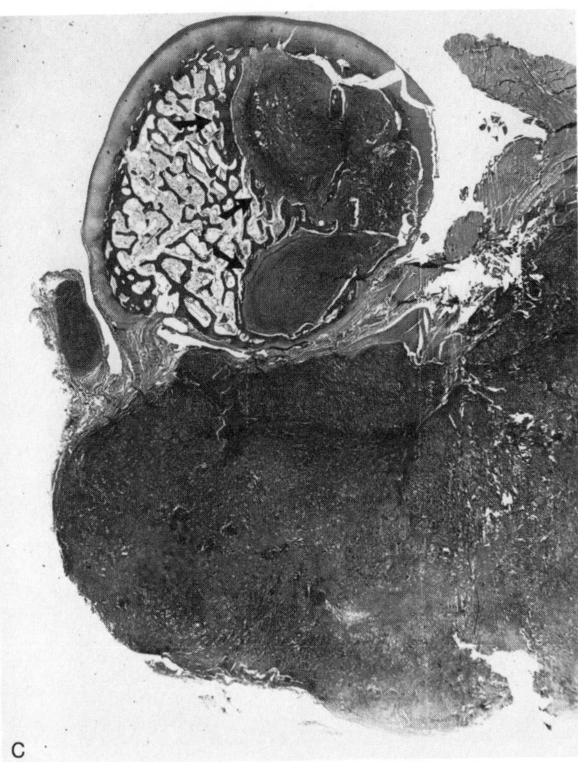

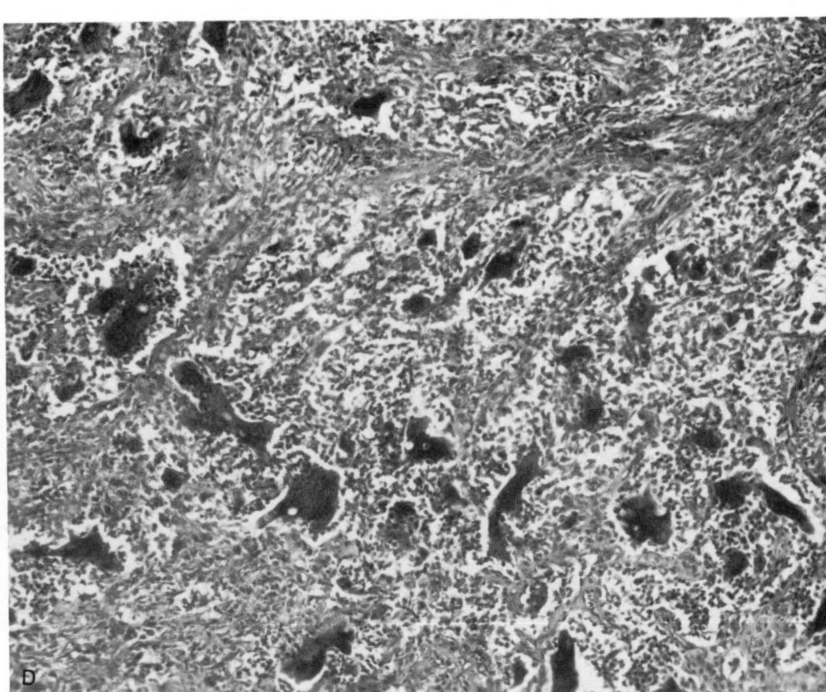

Figure 74–66. Continued

C *Macroscopic coronal cut through the distal second metatarsal head demonstrates the large volar mass with erosion into bone. Note the sclerotic bony margins (arrows) about the intraosseous extension.*

D *Photomicrograph (63×) documents the proliferative stromal cells, giant cells, and fibrous components that characterize this lesion.*

(Armed Forces Institute of Pathology Neg. Nos. 66-2598-1,2; 71-3116-1; 71-3118.)

monstrable on computed tomography as increased attenuation values.[516] Arteriography usually shows a hypervascular lesion. However, in the late stages, or if fibrosis dominates, the lesion may appear avascular. Arthrography will also show the lesion and its extent as a localized nodule or a diffuse villonodular mass.[517-520]

The differential diagnosis of the radiographic features of localized nodular synovitis includes other soft tissue tumors and tumor-like lesions. Diffuse pigmented villonodular synovitis must be differentiated from idiopathic synovial osteochondromatosis (in which calcification and ossification may appear), infection (in which osteoporosis, joint space loss, and ill-defined bony erosions may be seen), and other articular disorders.

Tumoral Calcinosis

Tumoral calcinosis is a rare condition, consisting of calcium salt deposition in extracapsular soft tissues about joints[521-527] (Fig. 74–67). The masses are painless and occur most frequently in children and adolescents. An increased incidence in blacks and a familial tendency are recognized.[529] These lesions are most commonly found about the shoulders, hips, and elbows. They are usually idiopathic, but metabolic defects, collagen vascular disorders, and trauma have been suggested in their pathogenesis.[528] Since the masses are extracapsular, there is little limitation of motion at the joint unless the tumors are exceedingly large. The cutaneous surface over the masses occasionally breaks down, and a draining sinus with chalky material will be found. This draining sinus may become secondarily infected if it is not treated adequately. The deposits tend to grow and recur after incomplete excision. Rarely, the serum alkaline phosphatase and phosphate levels will be elevated.[530-532]

At surgery, the masses are found to be encapsulated, multilocular spaces with dense, fibrous walls. The spaces are filled with very viscous semifluid calcium salts and white particles. Microscopically, these cysts are lined by giant cells with adjacent lymphocytic infiltration.[10, 533-535]

The masses of tumoral calcinosis usually appear extremely dense, homogeneous, and loculated on the radiograph[536-541] (Fig. 74–67). However, initially, there may be only faint calcification within the multiloculated lesions, with radiolucent septa of water density separating the lobules of calcification. The peripheral margin is smooth and bosselated. Fluid calcium layers on an upright film may rarely be seen.[542, 543] Adjacent bone erosion from pressure by the mass occurs but is rare.

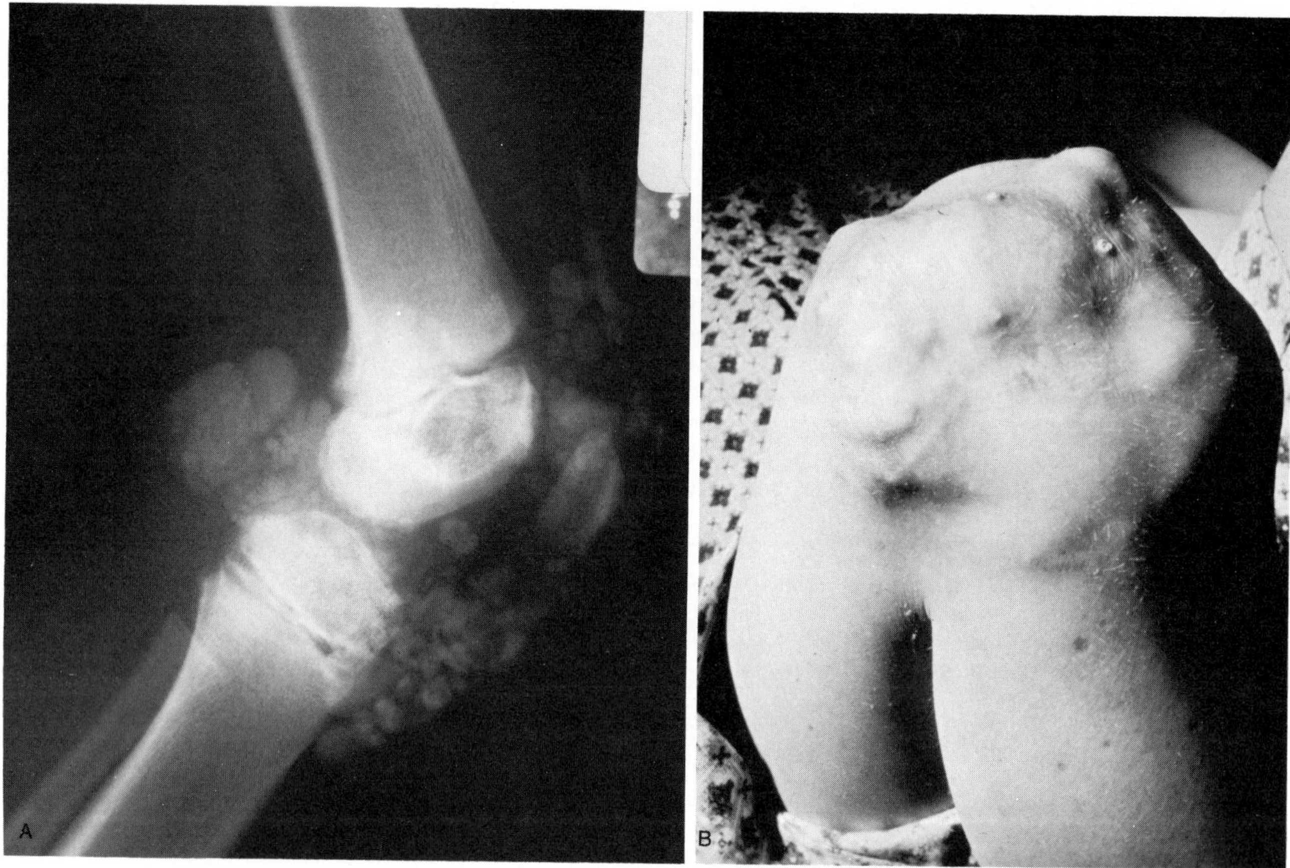

Figure 74–67. Tumoral calcinosis.

A, B Knee. This 7 year old boy presented with a swollen knee of 2 years' duration. There was no evidence of pain, trauma or infection. **A,** Lateral radiograph shows homogeneous calcific dense nodules about the knee joint. **B,** The clinical photograph demonstrates the knee in a flexed position, indicating little limitation of motion. Note the nodular surface of the skin, with areas of draining sinus tracts, old cutaneous scars, and pointing of a few nodules. These represent cutaneous complications from the subcutaneous nodules.

Illustration continued on the opposite page

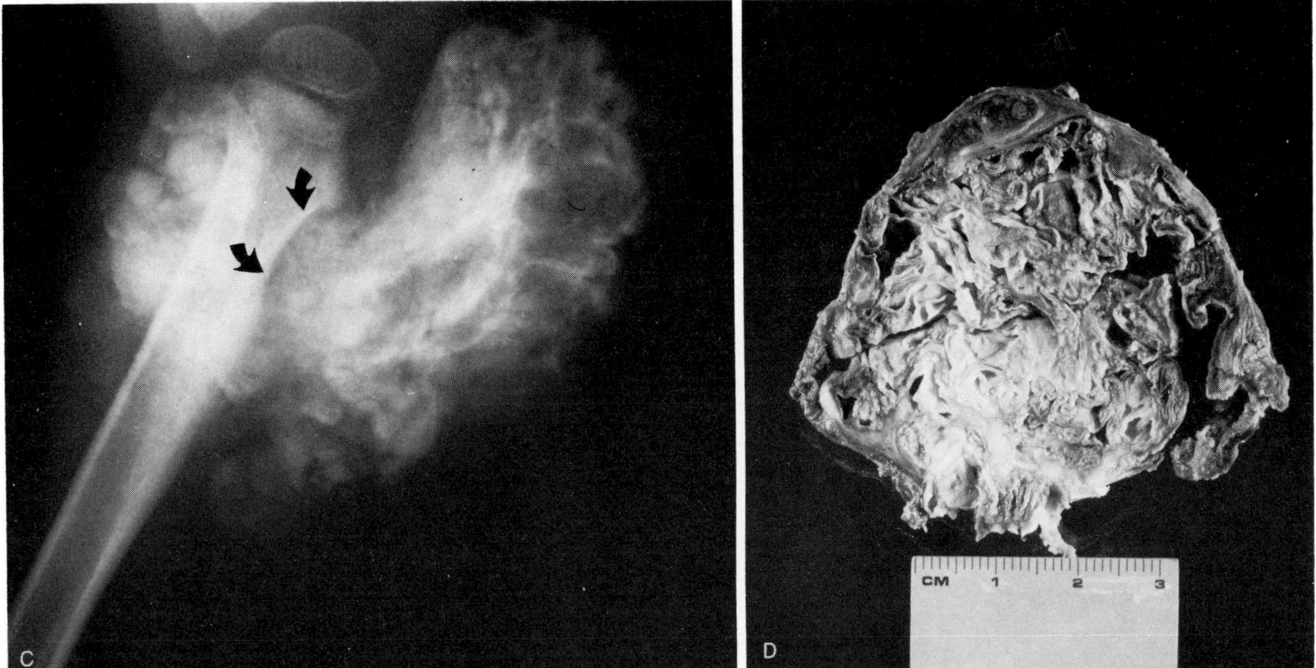

Figure 74–67. Continued

C, D *Shoulder. This patient is a 2 year old child with a shoulder mass of 6 months' duration.* **C,** *Axillary radiograph demonstrates a nonhomogeneous, dense, multilocular appearing mass about the shoulder with humeral erosions (arrows).* **D,** *Gross specimen confirms the multilocular configuration, fibrous septa, and grumous material within these locules.*

(Armed Forces Institute of Pathology Neg. Nos. 74-8966-2, 74-11906-1, 78-1059-2, 77-8127-2.)

Aneurysms

Popliteal artery aneurysm is the most common aneurysm found in the extremities.[544-547] Patients usually present in the fifth or sixth decade of life with pain and claudication; however, ischemia and swelling in the lower leg and neurologic symptoms resulting from pressure on the sciatic nerve can also be noted. Rarely a patient is asymptomatic. The aneurysm is usually palpated on physical examination. It is commonly associated with additional aneurysms, especially of the contralateral popliteal artery or of the abdominal aorta. Complications are usually arterial in origin, such as thrombosis, rupture of the aneurysm, or embolic occlusion of the artery distal to the aneurysm.

Radiographically, the aneurysm presents as a pulsatile soft tissue mass in the popliteal space. Curvilinear calcification may be noted in the aneurysm wall. The aneurysm may also erode adjacent bone, causing scalloping of the cortex. Arteriography is extremely helpful in evaluating the arterial and venous vascular beds and in demonstrating the vascular origin of the soft tissue mass. Occasionally partial occlusion by venous thrombosis of the popliteal vein may be demonstrated. Sonography, Doppler studies, radionuclide venography, and computed tomography may also establish the diagnosis.

Granulomatous Synovitis

Advanced granulomatous synovitis, especially tuberculous synovitis, which results from chronic infection, produces such a proliferative granulomatous pannus that it may cause a soft tissue mass in or about the joint (Fig. 74–68). The process is insidious and progressive, with ultimate destruction of the joint. The organisms usually reach the joint by hematogenous spread, but occasionally extend directly from an adjacent bony focus. The primary site is usually the lung. However, the chest radiograph frequently fails to show extensive disease.[548, 549]

The patients present with a painful, swollen, tender, doughy joint and occasionally will have a draining sinus tract. This clinical setting can easily be misinterpreted as evidence of a tumor, because these patients usually do not have toxic symptoms. Granulomatous synovitis is a monoarticular disease most commonly involving the hip, knee, elbow, and ankle.

The gross appearance may resemble an infiltrating tumor, with a mass that involves a joint and extends into the adjacent soft tissue, causing extensive tissue destruction and fibrotic reaction. Microscopic evaluation, however, will document the granulomatous nature of the process and therefore correctly characterize the lesion.

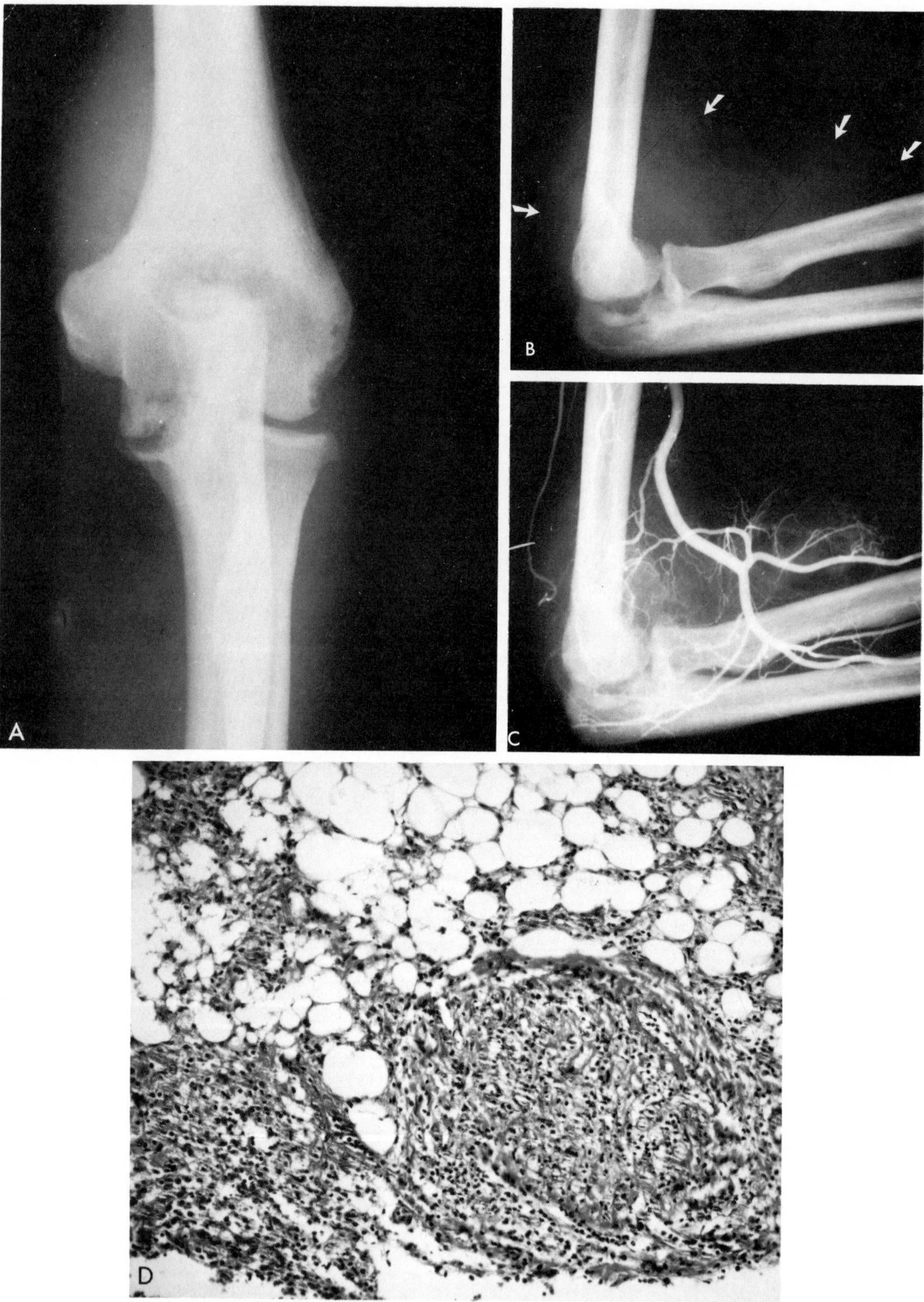

Figure 74–68. *Tuberculous synovitis of the elbow. This 61 year old man presented with pain and a doughy mass about the elbow of 6 months' duration.*

A *Anteroposterior radiograph shows para-articular bony erosions with relative sparing of the joint space.*

B *Lateral radiograph demonstrates a large mass (arrows) and bony erosions.*

C *The mass is hypervascular, with neovascularity and vessel displacement demonstrated on arteriography.*

D *Photomicrograph (157×) confirms the presence of a granulomatous synovitis.*

(Armed Forces Institute of Pathology Neg. Nos. 73-7980-3,4,2; 80-233.)

The radiographic findings depend on the stage of development.[550-554] Early disease is manifested as nonspecific soft tissue swelling. Arteriography at this time may show a hypervascular inflammatory synovitis (Fig. 74–68). With progression, however, the findings become more specific, with a soft tissue mass, juxta-articular osteoporosis, and marginal bony erosions in the non–weight-bearing surfaces. Eventually, the articular cartilage and subarticular bony plate will be destroyed. With repair, the extensive soft tissue, articular, and bony destruction may heal, with subsequent soft tissue calcification and bony ankylosis.

BONE TUMORS

Benign Bone Tumors

Bone tumors may involve the adjacent soft tissue and should be a consideration in the differential diagnosis of soft tissue tumors in and about the joint. Usually there is obvious bony change on the radiograph to indicate the origin of the lesion. These bony changes may be seen in both benign and malignant bone tumors. Benign bone tumors involving soft tissue usually arise from the bone surface and include osteochondroma, periosteal (juxtacortical) chondroma, articular chondroma (Trevor's disease), and osteoid osteoma. Occasionally, benign intraosseous lesions such as giant cell tumor (Fig. 74–69) and chondroblastoma will extend beyond the confines of the bony cortex into the adjacent soft tissue. Postoperative recurrences of benign bone tumors frequently will involve the soft tissue and are most commonly seen with giant cell tumor.

Benign cartilage tumors of bone arising as proliferative lesions from the bony cortex, periosteum, or articular cartilage are labeled osteochondroma, periosteal chondroma, and articular chondroma (Trevor's disease), respectively.

Osteochondromas. Osteochondromas consist of hyperplastic displaced or aberrant growth plate cartilage and are characterized by a cartilage cap, perichondrium, and bony stalk. The lesions may be solitary or multiple and are usually located in the metaphyseal end of the long bone. The patients are usually asymptomatic, unless the adjacent soft tissue structures are disturbed or traumatized. The lesions are found most commonly about the knee and usually point away from the joint. Pain and rapid growth suggest malignancy, especially after the third decade of life. However, these symptoms may also be associated with symptomatic bursitis[555, 556] or pseudoaneurysm, especially of the popliteal artery.[557, 558] Grossly, osteochondromas can be of two types, sessile or pedunculated. The cortex and spongiosa of the lesion are derived from the growing cartilage cap and are in direct continuity with the parent bone. The cartilage cap may be considerably thickened or may demonstrate endochondral bone fomation with mineralization. The radiograph usually shows a bony projection from the normal bone with a varying-sized cartilage cap (Fig. 74–70). The latter may have areas of stippled calcification.

Periosteal (Juxtacortical) Chondromas. Periosteal chondromas result from the growth of displaced or metaplastic cartilage within the periosteum.[559-566] They are most frequently found about the hand and foot, proximal humerus, ankle, proximal tibia, and proximal femur and are usually discovered in the third to fifth decades of life. Pathologically, these lesions are located on the cortical surface of bone and are covered by a fibrous capsule (perichondrium). Microscopically, myxoid degeneration, pleomorphism, and double nuclei are found and underscore the importance of the pathologist's being aware of the presence of the tumor, as it frequently resembles more ominous cartilaginous neoplasms.

Radiographs show a soft tissue mass, with scalloping of the adjacent bony cortex. The intact cortical margin is sclerotic and separates the lesion from the adjacent marrow cavity. A small periosteal buttress on either side of the lesion is frequent. Stippled calcification within the mass is also common.

Articular Chondromas. Articular chondromas, often referred to as dysplasia epiphysealis hemimelica or Trevor's disease,[567-572] also represent a form of cartilage proliferation. The lesion is an osteocartilaginous growth involving single or multiple epiphyses on one side of the body. It is more frequent in boys and is usually discovered during the first decade of life. Deformity, limitation of motion, and joint pain are common symptoms. The lesions commonly occur on the talus and distal femoral or distal tibial epiphysis. Severe deformity and even joint fusion may occur postoperatively.[568] The condition may be hereditary and associated with chondromas elsewhere in the skeleton.[570] Grossly, the focal overgrowth or pedunculated mass of hyaline cartilage involving the epiphysis results in a misshapen articular surface. Microscopically, the findings are identical to those of other osteocartilaginous masses. Radiographically, there is a lobular mass arising from the epiphysis, usually with calcification (Fig. 74–71). Initially mineralized portions of the lesion may be separated from the underlying bone by nonmineralized cartilage. As the lesion matures, the calcification becomes confluent with the adjacent epiphyseal bone, as is seen in osteochondromas. The ossification centers may appear prematurely in affected bones.

Osteoid Osteomas. Osteoid osteoma is a common benign bone lesion of unknown etiology that usually arises in the midshaft of long bones and presents with intermittent local pain, particularly at night.[573-580] It may produce joint swelling if it involves a segment of bone confined by a joint capsule.

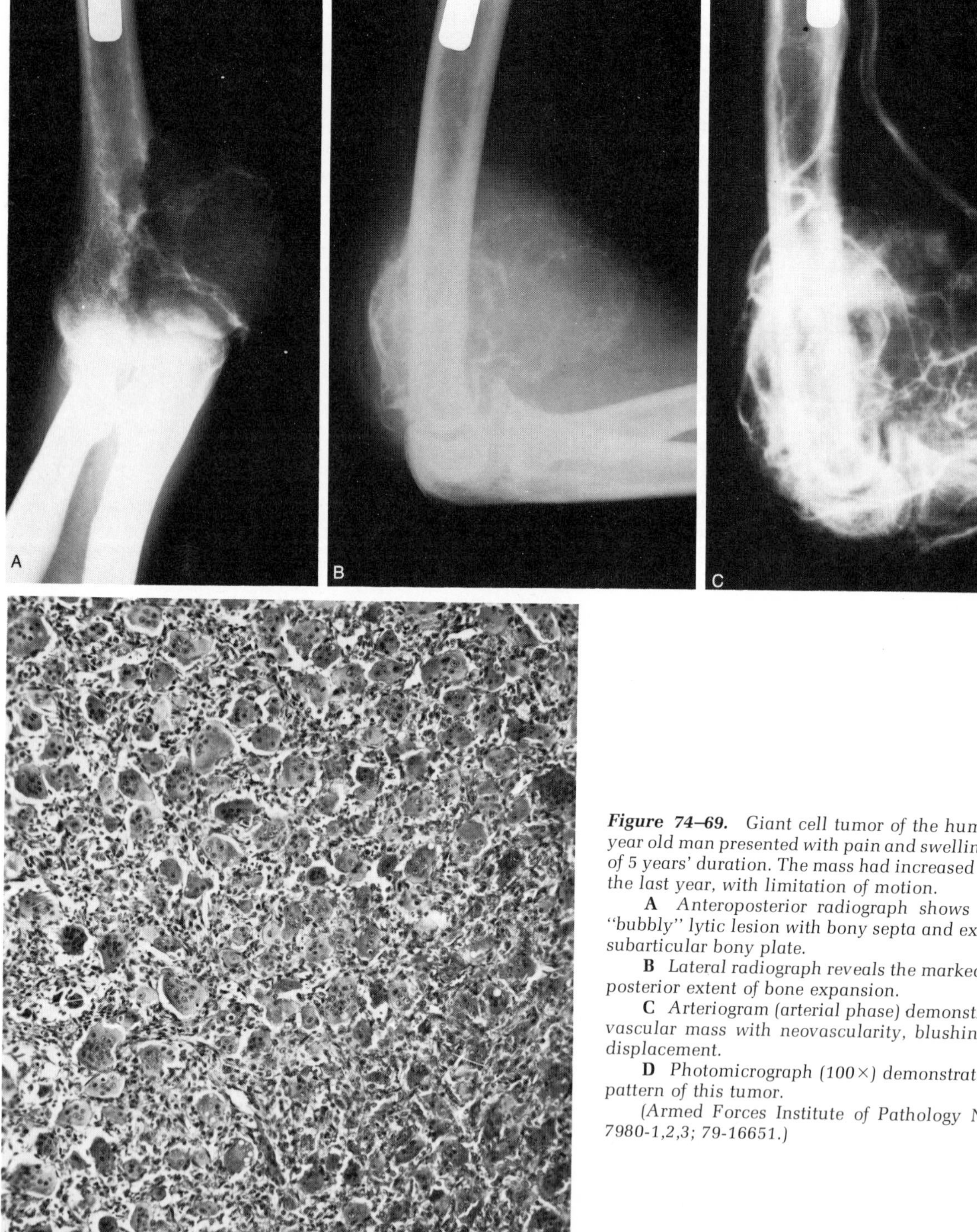

Figure 74–69. *Giant cell tumor of the humerus. This 37 year old man presented with pain and swelling in the elbow of 5 years' duration. The mass had increased in size during the last year, with limitation of motion.*

A *Anteroposterior radiograph shows an expansile "bubbly" lytic lesion with bony septa and extension to the subarticular bony plate.*

B *Lateral radiograph reveals the marked anterior and posterior extent of bone expansion.*

C *Arteriogram (arterial phase) demonstrates a hypervascular mass with neovascularity, blushing, and vessel displacement.*

D *Photomicrograph (100×) demonstrates the typical pattern of this tumor.*

(Armed Forces Institute of Pathology Neg. Nos. 73-7980-1,2,3; 79-16651.)

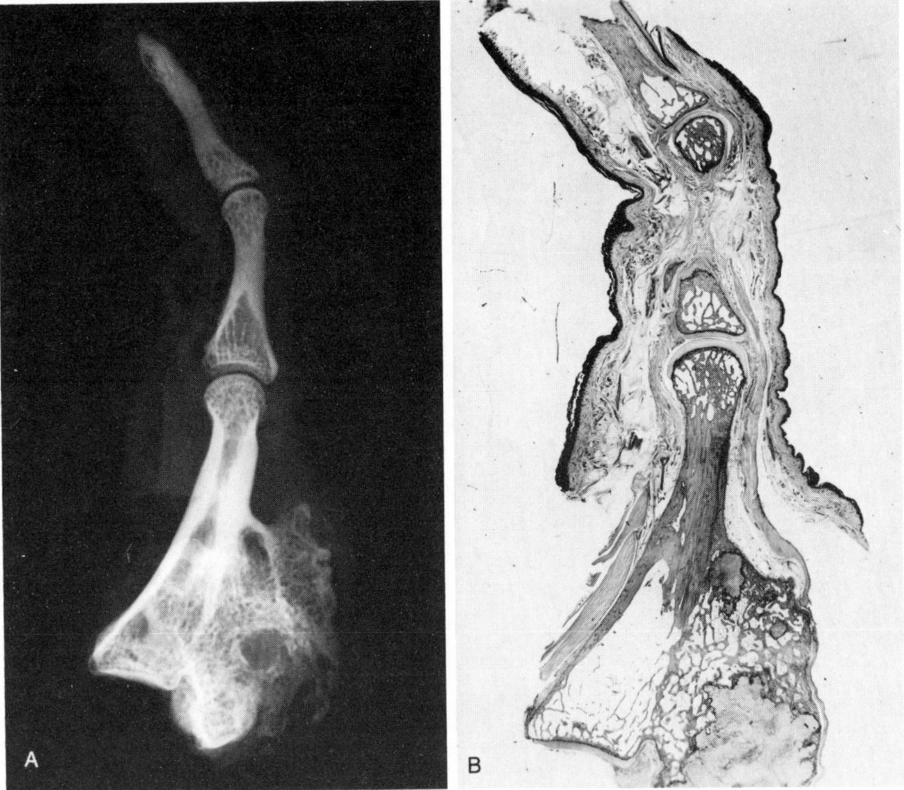

Figure 74–70. Osteochondroma of the proximal phalanx. The patient presented with recent growth of a mass of long duration on the finger.

A *Lateral specimen radiograph shows a bony growth with an irregular surface and lucent areas. Note the trabecular pattern of the lesion and its continuity with the adjacent normal marrow space of the involved phalanx.*

B *Macroslide demonstrates an exophytic growth consisting of a bony stalk (trabecular pattern) and foci of cartilage of varying sizes (lucent areas).*

(Armed Forces Institute of Pathology Neg. Nos. 59-6685, 72-3066.)

Under this circumstance, the lesion will present as a monoarticular arthritis with an inflammatory synovitis and loss of range of motion. It is more frequent in men, usually occurring during the second or third decade of life. Pathologically, osteoid osteoma is characterized by a central nidus of atypical-appearing osteoid and adjacent sclerotic bone formation.

On radiographs, extra-articular cortical lesions evoke a significant degree of reactive sclerosis, although intra-articular osteoid osteomas may present as very subtle lucent areas with little or no adjacent

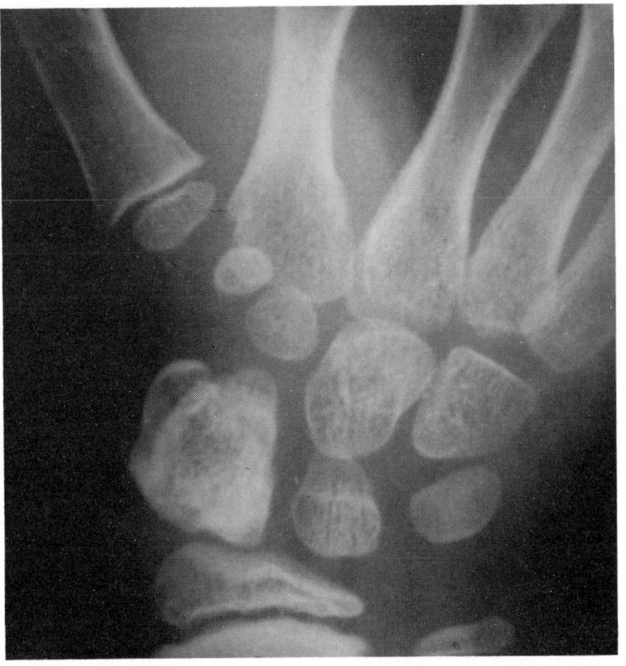

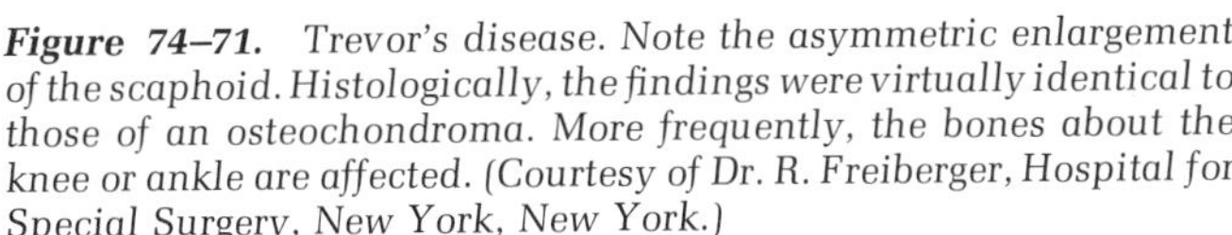

Figure 74–71. Trevor's disease. Note the asymmetric enlargement of the scaphoid. Histologically, the findings were virtually identical to those of an osteochondroma. More frequently, the bones about the knee or ankle are affected. (Courtesy of Dr. R. Freiberger, Hospital for Special Surgery, New York, New York.)

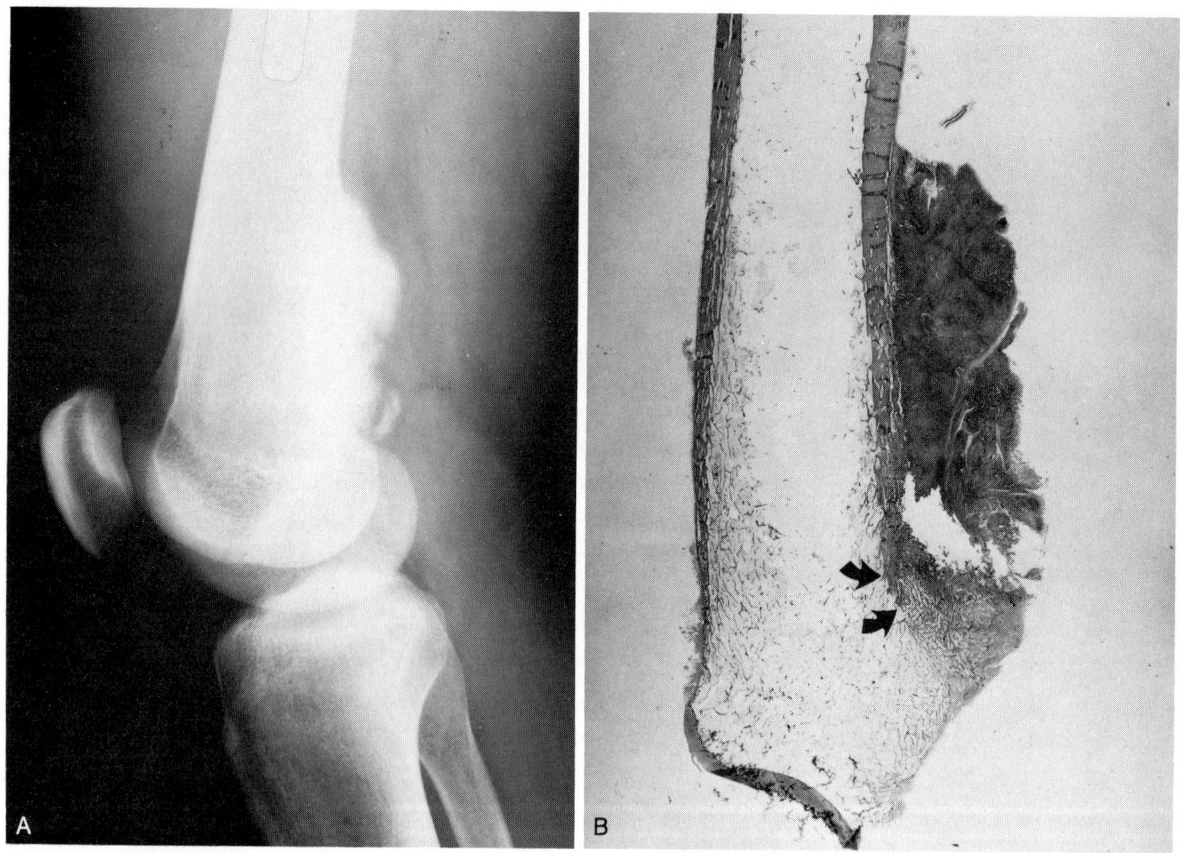

Figure 74–72. *Parosteal sarcoma of the femur. This 24 year old man presented with pain and tenderness on the posterior aspect of the knee of 1 year's duration.*

A *Lateral radiograph shows a dense homogeneous mass with an irregular margin arising from the posterior surface of the distal femur.*

B *Sagittal cut macroslide corresponding to the radiograph in* **A** *demonstrates a tumor mass arising from the posterior femoral cortical surface with minimal growth (arrows) into the bone distally. This location is typical of parosteal sarcomas.*

Illustration continued on the opposite page

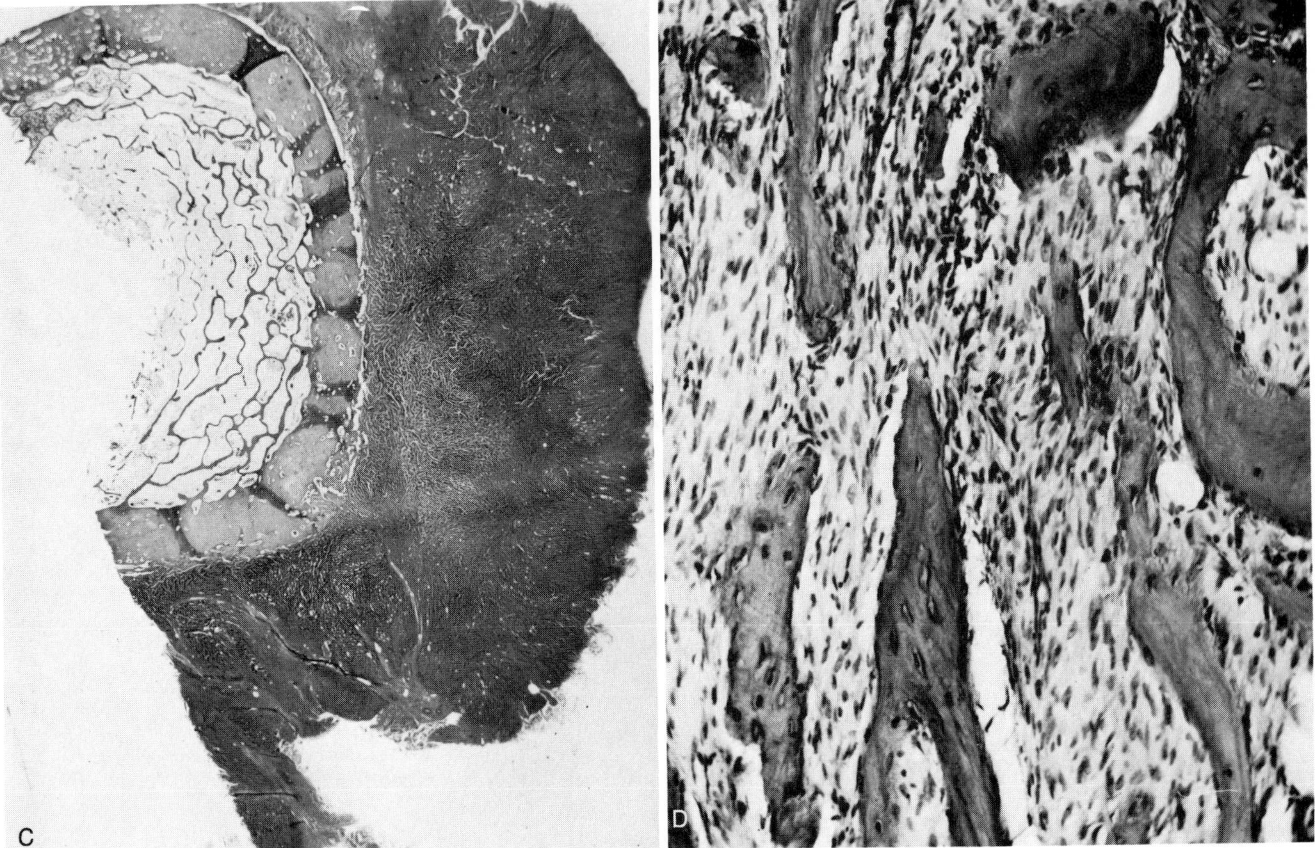

Figure 74–72. Continued

C *A cross sectional macroslide confirms the bone nature of the lesion that accounts for the homogeneous dense area on the radiograph.*

D *Photomicrograph (165×) reveals irregular and slightly atypical bone trabeculae separated by an excessively cellular spindle cell pattern. This is also typical of parosteal sarcomas.*

(Armed Forces Institute of Pathology Neg. Nos. 52-7554, 72-4251, 72-4253, 72-4254.)

sclerosis. The joint is swollen, and periarticular osteoporosis is common if symptoms have been present for some time. The nidus may be difficult to see on plain films but is readily apparent on bone scan as a photodense area[581-583] or on the arteriogram as a small hypervascular focus.[584, 585]

Malignant Bone Tumors

Malignant bone tumors frequently extend into the adjacent soft tissue. This extension is commonly seen with primary skeletal malignancies, such as osteosarcoma, chondrosarcoma, and Ewing's tumor, and it reflects the aggressive growth characteristics. The extraosseous extension can be evaluated by plain films, arteriography, and computed tomography and is easily differentiated from primary soft tissue lesions. However, parosteal sarcoma, a malignant tumor developing from the periosteum, may be confused with soft tissue tumor. Typically it is a slow-growing, low-grade malignancy; however, rapid aggressive growth with early death can occur. These lesions have few symptoms and usually present as gradually enlarging masses. They most commonly involve the posterior aspect of the distal femur. Grossly, these tumors are attached to cortical bone and grow into the adjacent soft tissue. Most parosteal sarcomas demonstrate some degree of osseous, cartilaginous or collagenous matrix production. This provides the basis for labeling them as parosteal osteosarcoma, parosteal chondrosarcoma, or parosteal fibrosarcoma. The matrix patterns may appear very mature in some areas and frankly malignant in others.

Radiographically, parosteal osteosarcoma is the most common tumor and usually shows a dense, homogenous calcific mass on the cortical surface of the distal femur (Fig. 74–72). Calcification extends into the adjacent soft tissue, with an irregular margin. The tumor may occasionally grow into the adjacent medullary space.

SUMMARY

A discussion of tumors and tumor-like lesions that appear about joints emphasizes the diverse nature of the processes that can lead to periarticular masses. In most cases, careful evaluation of the clinical history and routine radiographs provides a single, most likely diagnosis, although, at times, additional modalities, such as scintigraphy, sonography, arteriography, and computed tomography, must be utilized.

REFERENCES

1. Aegerter E, Kirkpatrick JA Jr: Orthopedic Diseases: Physiology, Pathology, Radiology. 4th Ed. Philadelphia, WB Saunders, 1975, p. 721.
2. Brindley HH: Malignant tumors of the soft tissues of the extremity. South Med J *56*:868, 1963.
3. Collins DH: The Pathology of Articular and Spinal Diseases. Baltimore, Williams & Wilkins Co, 1950.
4. Enzinger FM, Lattes R, Torloni H: Histological Typing of Soft Tissue Tumors. International Classification of Tumors, No. 3. Geneva, World Health Organization, 1969.
5. Gerner RE, Moore GE, Pickren JW: Soft tissue sarcomas. Ann Surg *181*:803, 1975.
6. Hare HF, Cerny MD Jr: Soft tissue sarcoma. A review of 200 cases. Cancer *16*:1332, 1963.
7. Horn RC Jr: Sarcomas of soft tissues. JAMA *183*:511, 1963.
8. Jaffe HL: Tumors and Tumorous Conditions of the Bones and Joints. Philadelphia, Lea & Febiger, 1958, p. 502.
9. Pack GT, Anglem TJ: Tumors of the soft somatic tissues in infancy and childhood. J Pediatr *15*:372, 1939.
10. Spjut HJ, Dorfman HD, Fechner RE, Ackerman LV: Tumors of Bone and Cartilage. Atlas of Tumor Pathology. Second Series, Fascicle 5. Washington, D.C., Armed Forces Institute of Pathology, 1971, p. 391.
11. Suit HD, Russell WO, Martin RG: Sarcoma of soft tissue — clinical and histopathologic parameters and response to treatment. Cancer *35*:1478, 1975.
12. Stout AP: Pathology and classification of tumors of the soft tissues. Am J Roentgenol *66*:903, 1951.
13. Stout AP: Sarcomas of the soft parts. J Mo Med Assoc *44*:329, 1947.
14. Stout AP, Lattes R: Tumors of the Soft Tissues. Atlas of Tumor Pathology. Second Series, Fascicle 1. Washington DC, Armed Forces Institute of Pathology, 1967, p. 11.
15. Thompson DE, Frost HM, Hendrick JW, Horn RC Jr: Soft tissue sarcomas involving the extremities and limb girdles: A review. South Med J *64*:33, 1971.
16. Cavanagh RC: Tumors of the soft tissues of the extremities. Semin Roentgenol *8*:73, 1973.
17. Forrester DM, Becker TS: The radiology of bone and soft tissue sarcomas. Orthop Clin North Am *8*:973, 1977.
18. Levine E, Lee KR, Neff JR, Maklad NF, Robinson RG, Preston DF: Comparison of computed tomography and other imaging modalities in the evaluation of musculoskeletal tumors. Radiology *131*:431, 1979.
19. Martel W, Abell MR: Radiologic evaluation of soft tissue tumors. Cancer *32*:352, 1973.
20. Das Gupta TK, Ghosh BC: Principles of diagnosis and management of soft tissue sarcomas. Surg Annu *7*:115, 1975.
21. Fortner JG, Kim DK, Shiu MH: Limb-preserving vascular surgery for malignant tumors of the lower extremity. Arch Surg *112*:391, 1977.
22. Hudson TM, Hass G, Enneking WF, Hawkins IF Jr: Angiography in the management of musculoskeletal tumors. Surg Gynecol Obstet *141*:11, 1975.
23. Krementz ET, Shaver, JO: Behavior and treatment of soft tissue sarcomas. Ann Surg *157*:770, 1963.
24. Morton DL, Eilber FR, Townsend CM Jr, Grant TT, Mirra J, Weisenburger TH: Limb salvage from a multidisciplinary treatment approach for skeletal and soft tissue sarcomas of the extremity. Ann Surg *184*:268, 1976.
25. Rosenberg JC: The value of arteriography in the treatment of soft tissue tumors of the extremities. J Int Coll Surg *41*:405, 1964.
26. Shiu MH, Castro ER, Hajdu SI, Fortner JG: Surgical treatment of 297 soft tissue sarcomas of the lower extremity. Ann Surg *182*:597, 1975.
27. Simon MA, Enneking WF: The management of soft tissue sarcomas of the extremities. J Bone Joint Surg *58A*:317, 1976.
28. Suit HD, Russell WO, Martin RG: Management of patients with sarcomas of soft tissue in an extremity. Cancer *31*:1247, 1973.
29. Frantzell A: Soft tissue radiography. Acta Radiol Suppl *85*:1, 1951.
30. Melson GL, Staple TW, Evens, RG: Soft tissue radiographic technique. Semin Roentgenol *8*:19, 1973.
31. Pirkey EL, Hurt J: Roentgen evaluation of the soft tissues in orthopedics. Am J Roentgenol *82*:271, 1959.
32. Levine E, Lee KR, Neff JR, Maklad NF, Robinson RG, Preston DF: Comparison of computed tomography and other imaging modalities in the evaluation of musculoskeletal tumors. Radiology *131*:431, 1979.
33. Nessi R: La xeroradiografia nello studio delle parti molli. Radiol Med (Torino) *63*:1083, 1977.
34. Wolfe JN: Xeroradiography of the bones, joints, and soft tissues. Radiology *93*:583, 1969.
35. Blatt CJ, Hayt DB, Desai M, Freeman LM: Soft tissue sarcomas imaged with technetium-99m pyrophosphate. NY State J Med *77*:2118, 1977.
36. Chaudhuri IK, Chaudhuri TK, Go RT, Taube RR, Christie JH: Uptake of ^{87m}Sr by liver metastasis from carcinoma of colon. J Nucl Med *14*:293, 1973.
37. Matsui K, Yamada H, Chiba K, Iio M: Visualization of soft tissue malignancies by using ^{99m}Tc polyphosphate, pyrophosphate and diphosphonate (^{99m}TcP). J Nucl Med *14*:632, 1973.
38. Nolan NG: Intense uptake of ^{99m}Tc-diphosphonate by an extra-osseous neurofibroma. J Nucl Med *15*:1207, 1974.
39. Papavasilious C, Kostamis P, Angelakis P, Constantinides C: Localization of ^{87m}Sr in extra-osseous tumors. J Nucl Med *12*:265, 1971.
40. Rosenthall L, Hawkins D: Radionuclide joint imaging in the diagnosis of synovial disease. Semin Arthritis Rheum *7*:49, 1977.
41. Samuels LD: Detection and localization of extraskeletal malignant neoplasms of children with strontium-87m. Am J Roentgenol *115*:777, 1972.
42. Telfer N: Nuclear medicine in the management of musculoskeletal tumors. Orthop Clin North Am *8*:1011, 1977.
43. Wenzel WW, Heasty RG: Uptake of ^{99m}Tc-stannous polyphosphate in an area of cerebral infarction. J Nucl Med *15*:207, 1974.
44. Cockshott WP, Evans KT: The place of soft tissue arteriography. Br J Radiol *37*:367, 1964.
45. Finck EJ, Moore TM: Angiography for mass lesions of bone, joint, and soft tissue. Orthop Clin North Am *8*:999, 1977.
46. Gronner AT: Muscle necrosis simulating a malignant tumor angiographically. Case report. Radiology *103*:309, 1972.
47. Hawkins IF Jr, Hudson T: Priscoline in bone and soft-tissue angiography. Radiology *110*:541, 1974.
48. Herzberg DL, Schreiber MH: Angiography in mass lesions of the extremities. Am J Roentgenol *111*:541, 1971.
49. Hutcheson J, Klatte EC, Kremp R: The angiographic appearance of myositis ossificans circumscripta. A case report. Radiology *102*:57, 1972.
50. Lagergren C, Lindbom A: Angiography of peripheral tumors. Radiology *79*:371, 1962.
51. Levin DC, Watson RC, Baltaxe HA: Arteriography in the diagnosis and management of acquired peripheral soft-tissue masses. Radiology *104*:53, 1972.
52. Margulis AR, Murphy TO: Arteriography in neoplasms of extremities. Am J Roentgenol *80*:330, 1958.
53. Stanley P, Miller JA: Angiography of extremity masses in children. Am J Roentgenol *130*:1119, 1978.
54. Steckel RJ: Usefulness of extremity arteriography in special situations. Radiology *86*:293, 1966.
55. Templeton AW, Stevens E, Jansen C: Arteriographic evaluation of soft tissue masses. South Med J *59*:1255, 1966.
56. Viamonte M Jr, Roen S, Le Page J: Nonspecificity of abnormal vascularity in the angiographic diagnosis of malignant neoplasms. Radiology *106*:59, 1973.
57. Berger PE, Kuhn JP: Computed tomography of tumors of the musculoskeletal system in children. Radiology *127*:171, 1978.
58. deSantos LA, Goldstein HM, Murray JA, Wallace S: Computed tomography in the evaluation of musculoskeletal neoplasms. Radiology *128*:89, 1978.
59. Heelan RT, Watson RC, Smith J: Computed tomography of lower extremity tumors. Am J Roentgenol *132*:933, 1979.
60. Hermann G, Rose JS: Computed tomography in bone and soft tissue pathology of the extremities. J Comput Assist Tomogr *3*:58, 1979.
61. Hunter JC, Johnston WH, Genant HK: Computed tomography evaluation of fatty tumors of the somatic soft tissues: Clinical utility and radiologic-pathologic correlation. Skel Radiol *4*:79, 1979.
62. Levinsohn EM, Bryan PJ: Computed tomography in unilateral extremity swelling of unusual cause. J Comput Assist Tomogr *3*:67, 1979.
63. Levitt RG, Sagel SS, Stanley RJ, Evens RG: Computed tomography of the pelvis. Semin Roentgenol *13*:193, 1978.
64. McLeod RA, Gisvold JJ, Stephens DH, Beabout JW, Sheedy PF II: Computed tomography of soft tissues and breast. Semin Roentgenol *13*:267, 1978.
65. Schumacher IM, Genant HK, Korobkin M, Bovill EG Jr: Computed

tomography: Its use in space-occupying lesions of the musculoskeletal system. J Bone Joint Surg *60A*:600, 1978.
66. Wilson JS, Korobkin M, Genant HK, Bovill EG Jr: Computed tomography of musculoskeletal disorders. Am J Roentgenol *131*:55, 1978.
67. Weinberger G, Levinsohn EM: Computed tomography in evaluation of sarcomatous tumors of the thigh. Am J Roentgenol *130*:115, 1978.
68. Regan JM, Bickel WH, Broders AC: Infiltrating benign lipomas of the extremities. West J Surg Obstet Gynecol *54*:87, 1946.
69. Geschickter CF: Lipoid tumors. Am J Cancer *21*:617, 1934.
70. Robbins SL, Cotran RS: Pathologic Basis of Disease. 2nd Ed. Philadelphia, WB Saunders Co, 1979.
71. Kindblom LG, Angervall L, Stener B, Wickbom I: Intermuscular and intramuscular lipomas and hibernomas, a clinical, roentgenologic, histologic, and prognostic study of 46 cases. Cancer *33*:754, 1974.
72. Dempster WH: Intermuscular lipomata. Br J Radiol *25*:553, 1952.
73. Rowland SA: Case report: Ten year follow-up of lipofibroma of the median nerve in the palm. J Hand Surg *2*:316, 1977.
74. Terzis JK, Daniel RK, Williams HB, Spencer PS: Benign fatty tumors of the peripheral nerves. Ann Plast Surg *1*:193, 1978.
75. Pudlowski RM, Gilula LA, Kyriakos M: Intra-articular lipoma with osseous metaplasia: Radiographic pathologic correlation. Am J Roentgenol *132*:471, 1979.
76. Berry JB, Moiel RH: Parosteal lipoma producing paralysis of the deep radial nerve. Southern Med J *66*:1298, 1973.
77. Kenin A, Levine J, Spinner M: Parosteal lipoma, a report of two cases with associated bone changes. J Bone Joint Surg *41A*:1122, 1959.
78. Khan AA: Parosteal lipoma. J Indian Med Assoc *63*:285, 1974.
79. Rosen H: Parosteal lipoma. Bull Hosp Joint Dis *20*:96, 1959.
80. Booher RJ: Lipoblastic tumors of the hands and feet. Review of the literature and report of thirty-three cases. J Bone Joint Surg *47A*:727, 1965.
81. Kalisman M, Beck AR: Lipoma of the thumb in a child. Ann Plast Surg *2*:165, 1979.
82. Leffert RD: Lipomas of the upper extremity. J Bone Joint Surg *54A*:1262, 1972.
83. Straus FH: Deep lipomas of the hand. Ann Surg *94*:269, 1931.
84. Kauffman SL, Stout AP: Lipoblastic tumors of children. Cancer *12*:912, 1959.
85. Elsahy NI, Lorimer A: Congenital fibrolipomata in both heels. Case report. Plast Reconstr Surg *59*:434, 1977.
86. Wohl MG, Pastor N: Adiposis dolorosa (Dercum's disease); treatment of asthenic phase with prostigmine and aminoacetic acid. JAMA *110*:1261, 1938.
87. Bellemore C: Massive pedunculated lipoma. Aust N Z J Surg *32*:83, 1962.
88. Wu KT, Jordan FR, Eckert C: Lipoma, a cause of paralysis of deep radial (posterior interosseous) nerve: Report of a case and review of the literature. Surgery *75*:790, 1974.
89. Goldman AB, Kaye JJ: Macrodystrophia lipomatosa: Radiographic diagnosis. Am J Roentgenol *128*:101, 1977.
90. Yaghmai I, McKowne F, Alizadeh, A: Macrodactylia fibrolipomatosis. Southern Med J *69*:1565, 1976.
91. Engeron O, Stallings JO: An unusual cause of carpal tunnel syndrome. J Iowa Med Soc *65*:25, 1975.
92. Wells HG: Adipose tissue, a neglected subject. JAMA *114*:2177, 1940.
93. Bartis JR: Massive lipoma of the foot — a case report. J Am Podiatry Assoc *64*:874, 1974.
94. Delamater J: Mammoth tumor. Cleveland Med Gaz *1*:31, 1859.
95. Louis DS, Dick HM: Ossifying lipofibroma of the median nerve. J Bone Joint Surg *55A*:1082, 1973.
96. Murphy NB: Ossifying lipoma. Br J Radiol *47*:97, 1974.
97. Plaut GS, Salm R, Truscott DE: Three cases of ossifying lipoma. J Pathol Bacteriol *78*:292, 1959.
98. Robson PN: A large calcified lipoma of the thigh. Report of a case. J Bone Joint Surg *32B*:384, 1950.
99. McAndrews PG, Greenspan JS: Lipoma of the lip with cartilage formation. Br Dent J *140*:239, 1976.
100. Dodge OG, Evans DM: Haemopoiesis in a presacral fatty tumour (myelolipoma). J Pathol Bacteriol *72*:313, 1956.
101. Sampson CC, Saunders EH, Green WE, Laurey JR: Liposarcoma developing in a lipoma. Arch Pathol *69*:506, 1960.
102. Sternberg SS: Liposarcoma arising within a subcutaneous lipoma. Cancer *5*:975, 1952.
103. Wright CJE: Liposarcoma arising in a simple lipoma. J Pathol Bacteriol *60*:483, 1948.
104. Enzinger FM, Harvey DA: Spindle cell lipoma. Cancer *36*:1852, 1975.
105. Greenberg SD, Isensee C, Gonzalez-Angulo A, Wallace SA: Infiltrating lipomas of the thigh. Am J Clin Pathol *39*:66, 1963.
106. Schobinger RA, Ruzicka FF Jr: Vascular Roentgenology. New York, Macmillan Co, 1964.
107. Jaffe H: Tumors and Tumorous Conditions of the Bones and Joints. Philadelphia, Lea & Febiger, 1974, p 574.
108. Smillie IS: Diseases of the Knee Joint. Edinburgh, Churchill Livingstone, 1974.
109. Arzimanoglu A: Bilateral arborescent lipoma of the knee — a case report. J Bone Joint Surg *39A*:976, 1957.
110. Burgan DW: Lipoma arborescens of the knee: Another cause of filling defects on knee arthrogram. Radiology *101*:583, 1971.
111. Weitzman G: Lipoma arborescens of the knee. Report of a case. J Bone Joint Surg *47A*:1030, 1965.
112. Weston WJ: The intra-synovial fatty masses in chronic rheumatoid arthritis. Br J Radiol *46*:213, 1973.
113. Jacobs P: Parosteal lipoma with hyperostosis. Clin Radiol *23*:196, 1972.
114. Bradley RL, Klein MM: Angiolipoma. Am J Surg *108*:887, 1964.
115. Dionne GP, Seemayer TA: Infiltrating lipomas and angiolipomas revisited. Cancer *33*:732, 1974.
116. Gonzalez-Crussi F, Enneking WF, Arean VM: Infiltrating angiolipoma. J Bone Joint Surg *48A*:1111, 1966.
117. Howard WR, Helwig EB: Angiolipoma. Arch Dermatol *82*:924, 1960.
118. Lin JJ, Lin F: Two entities in angiolipoma. A study of 459 cases of lipoma with review of literature on infiltrating angiolipoma. Cancer *34*:720, 1974.
119. Räsänen O, Nohteri H, Dammert K: Angiolipoma and lipoma. Acta Chir Scand *133*:461, 1967.
120. Stimpson N: Infiltrating angiolipomata of skeletal muscle. Br J Surg *58*:464, 1971.
121. Finberg HJ, Levin DC: Angiolipoma: A rare benign soft tissue tumor with a malignant arteriographic appearance. Am J Roentgenol *128*:697, 1977.
122. Angervall L, Björntorp P, Stener B: The lipid composition of hibernoma as compared with that of lipoma and of mouse brown fat. Cancer Res *25*:408, 1965.
123. Brines OA, Johnson MH: Hibernoma, a special fatty tumor: Report of a case. Am J Pathol *25*:467, 1949.
124. Fentiman IS, Davies EE, Ramsay GS: Hibernoma of the thigh. Clin Oncol *1*:71, 1975.
125. Hull D, Segall MM: Distinction of brown from white adipose tissue. Nature *212*:469, 1966.
126. Rasmussen AT: The so-called hibernating gland. J Morphol *38*:147, 1923.
127. McLane RC, Meyer LC: Axillary hibernoma: Review of the literature with report of a case examined angiographically. Radiology *127*:673, 1978.
128. Lawson W, Biller HF: Cervical hibernoma. Laryngoscope *86*:1258, 1976.
129. Kodish ME: Alsever RN, Block MB: Benign symmetric lipomatosis: Functional sympathetic denervation of adipose tissue and possible hypertrophy of brown fat. Metabolism *23*:937, 1974.
130. Lewis D, Geschickter CF: Diffuse lipoma of the right upper extremity. Prolan A and B yielded by bio-assay of fat. Ann Surg *102*:154, 1935.
131. Lippitt DA, Johnston JR: Diffuse lipomatosis of lower extremities. Report of a case. Bull Ayer Clin Lab Penn Hosp *4*:55, 1954.
132. Oosthuizen SF, Barnetson J: Two cases of lipomatosis involving bone. Br J Radiol *20*:426, 1947.
133. Kindblom L-G, Möller-Nielsen J: Diffuse lipomatosis in the leg after poliomyelitis. Acta Pathol Microbiol Scand (A) *83*:339, 1975.
134. Barsky AJ: Macrodactyly. J Bone Joint Surg *49A*:1255, 1967.
135. Ben-Bassat M, Kaplan I, Laron Z, Tikva P: Congenital macrodactyly: A case report with a three-year follow-up. J Bone Joint Surg *48B*:359, 1966.
136. Inglis K: Local gigantism (a manifestation of neurofibromatosis): Its relation to general gigantism and to acromegaly illustrating the influence of intrinsic factors in disease when development of the body is abnormal. Am J Pathol *26*:1059, 1950.
137. Minkowitz S, Minkowitz F: A morphological study of macrodactylism: A case report. J Pathol *90*:323, 1965.
138. Moore BH: Macrodactyly and associated peripheral nerve changes. J Bone Joint Surg *24*:617, 1942.
139. Moore BH: Peripheral-nerve changes, associated with congenital deformities. J Bone Joint Surg *26*:282, 1944.
140. Ranawat CS, Arora MM, Singh RG: Macrodystrophia lipomatosa with carpal-tunnel syndrome. A case report. J Bone Joint Surg *50A*:1242, 1968.
141. Thorne FL, Posch JL, Miladick RA: Megalodactyly. Plast Reconstr Surg *41*:232, 1968.
142. Tuli SM, Khanna NN, Sinha GP: Congenital macrodactyly. Br J Plast Surg *22*:237, 1969.
143. Adair FE, Pack GT, Farrior JH: Lipomas. Am J Cancer *16*:1104, 1932.
144. Chung EB, Enzinger FM: Benign lipoblastomatosis. An analysis of 35 cases. Cancer *32*:482, 1973.
145. Gibbs MK, Soule EH, Hayles AB, Telander RL: Lipoblastomatosis: A tumor of children. Pediatrics *60*:235, 1977.

146. Langloh JT, Reing CM, Chun BK, Grant E: Lipoblastomatosis: A case report. J Bone Joint Surg *60A*:130, 1978.
147. Paarlberg D, Linscheid RL, Soule EH: Lipomas of the hand: Including a case of lipoblastomatosis in a child. Mayo Clin Proc *47*:121, 1972.
148. Vellios F, Baez J, Schumacker HB: Lipoblastomatosis: A tumor of fetal fat different from hibernoma. Am J Pathol *34*:1149, 1958.
149. Allen PW, Enzinger FM: Hemangioma of skeletal muscle, an analysis of 89 cases. Cancer *29*:8, 1972.
150. Andervont HB, Grady HG, Edwards JE: Induction of hepatic lesions, hepatomas, pulmonary tumors and hemangio-endotheliomas in mice with O-Amino-azotoluene. J Natl Cancer Inst *3*:131, 1942.
151. Angervall L, Nielsen JM, Stener B, Svendsen P: Concomitant arteriovenous vascular malformation in skeletal muscle: A clinical angiographic and histologic study. Cancer *44*:232, 1979.
152. Ben-Menachem Y, Epstein MJ: Post-traumatic capillary hemangioma of the hand. A case report. J Bone Joint Surg *56A*:1741, 1974.
153. Bliznak J, Staple TW: Radiology of angiodysplasias of the limb. Radiology *110*:35, 1974.
154. Goidanich IF, Campanacci M: Vascular hamartomata and infantile angioectatic osteohyperplasia of the extremities. J Bone Joint Surg *44A*:815, 1962.
155. Heitzman ER, Jones JB: Roentgen characteristics of cavernous hemangioma of striated muscle. Radiology *74*:420, 1960.
156. Levin DC, Gordon DH, McSweeney J: Arteriography of peripheral hemangiomas. Radiology *121*:625, 1976.
157. Thomas ML, Andress MR: Angiography in venous dysplasias of the limbs. Am J Roentgenol *113*:722, 1971.
158. Malan E, Puglionisi A: Congenital angiodysplasias of the extremities. Note 2. Arterial, arterial and venous, and haemolymphatic dysplasias. J Cardiovasc Surg *6*:255, 1975.
159. Malan E, Puglionisi A: Congenital angiodysplasias of the extremities. Note 1. Generalities and classification; venous dysplasias. J Cardiovasc Surg *5*:87, 1964.
160. Fergusson ILC: Haemangiomata of skeletal muscle. Br J Surg *59*:634, 1972.
161. Fulton MN, Sosman MC: Venous angiomas of skeletal muscle; report of 4 cases. JAMA *119*:319, 1942.
162. Bendeck TE, Lichtenberg F: Cavernous hemangioma of striated muscle. Review of the literature and report of 2 cases. Ann Surg *146*:1011, 1957.
163. Borden JI, Shea TP: Cavernous hemangioma of the foot. A case report and review. J Am Podiatry Assoc *66*:484, 1976.
164. Brodsky AE: Synovial hemangioma of the knee joint. Bull Hosp Joint Dis *17*:58, 1956.
165. Cobey MC: Hemangioma of joints. Arch Surg *46*:465, 1943.
166. Harkins HN: Hemangioma of tendon or tendon sheath. Report of a case with a study of twenty-four cases from the literature. Arch Surg *34*:12, 1937.
167. Jacobs JE, Lee FW: Hemangioma of the knee joint. J Bone Joint Surg *31A*:831, 1949.
168. Karlholm S, Stjernswärd J: Hemangioma of the knee joint. Acta Orthop Scand *33*:306, 1963.
169. Perras P, Boulianne P: Multiple congenital hemangiomatosis. J Can Assoc Radiol *24*:231, 1973.
170. Politz MJ: Hemangioma of the digits. Two cases. J Am Podiatry Assoc *66*:515, 1976.
171. Sugiura I: Tibial periosteal hemangioma. Clin Orthop Rel Res *106*:242, 1975.
172. Sutherland AD: Equinus deformity due to haemangioma of calf muscle. J Bone Joint Surg *57B*:104, 1975.
173. Stevens J, Katz PL, Archer FL, McCarty DJ: Synovial hemangioma of the knee. Arthritis Rheum *12*:647, 1969.
174. Szilagyi DE, Smith RF, Elliott JP, Hageman JH: Congenital arteriovenus anomalies of the limbs. Arch Surg *111*:423, 1976.
175. Weaver JB: Hemangiomata of the lower extremities. With special reference to those of the knee-joint capsule and the phenomenon of spontaneous obliteration. J Bone Joint Surg *20*:731, 1938.
176. Wind ES, Pillari G: Deep soft tissue hemangioma of infancy: Kasabach-Merritt syndrome. NY State J Med *79*:373, 1979.
177. Jenkins HP, Delaney PA: Benign angiomatous tumors of skeletal muscles. Surg Gynecol Obstet *55*:464, 1932.
178. Jones KG: Cavernous hemangioma of striated muscle — a review of the literature and a report of four cases. J Bone Joint Surg *35A*:717, 1953.
179. Scott JES: Hemangiomata in skeletal muscle. Br J Surg *44*:496, 1957.
180. Shallow TA, Eger SA, Wagner FB Jr: Primary hemangiomatous tumors of skeletal muscle. Ann Surg *119*:700, 1944.
181. Oldmixon WJ: Hemangioma. Case for diagnosis. Milit Med *142*:434, 1977.
182. Kasabach HH, Merritt KK: Capillary hemangioma with extensive purpura. Report of a case. Am J Dis Child *59*:1063, 1940.
183. Sutherland DA, Clark H: Hemangioma associated with thrombocytopenia. Report of a case and review of the literature. Am J Med *33*:150, 1962.
184. Carnelli U, Bellini F, Ferrari M, Rossi E, Masera G: Giant hemangioma with consumption coagulopathy: Sustained response to heparin and radiotherapy. J Pediatr *91*:504, 1977.
185. Dadash-Zadeh M, Czapek EE, Schwartz AD: Skeletal and splenic hemangiomatosis with consumption coagulopathy: Response to splenectomy. Pediatrics *57*:803, 1976.
186. Evan J, Batchelor ADR, Stark G, Uttley WS: Haemangioma with coagulopathy: Sustained response to prednisone. Arch Dis Child *50*:809, 1975.
187. Hagerman LJ, Czapek EE, Donnellan WL, Schwartz AD: Giant hemangioma with consumption coagulopathy. J Pediatr *87*:766, 1975.
188. Inceman S, Tangün Y: Chronic defibrination syndrome due to a giant hemangioma associated with microangiopathic hemolytic anemia. Am J Med *46*:997, 1969.
189. Lee JH Jr, Kirk RF: Pregnancy associated with giant hemangiomata, thrombocytopenia, and fibrinogenopenia (Kasabach-Merritt syndrome). Report of a case. Obstet Gynecol *29*:24, 1967.
190. Rodriguez-Erdmann F, Button L, Murray JE, Moloney WC: Kasabach-Merrit syndrome: Coagulo-analytical observations. Am J Med Sci *261*:9, 1971.
191. Thompson LR, Umlauf HJ Jr: Hemangioma associated with thrombocytopenia: Report of two cases and review of the literature with emphasis on methods of therapy. Milit Med *129*:652, 1964.
192. Blix S, Aas K: Giant hemangioma, thrombocytopenia, fibrinogenopenia, and fibrinolytic activity. Acta Med Scand *169*:63, 1961.
193. Hillman RS, Phillips LL: Clotting — fibrinolysis in a cavernous hemangioma. Am J Dis Child *113*:649, 1967.
194. Lozman J, Holmblad J: Cavernous hemangiomas associated with scoliosis and a localized consumption coagulopathy. A case report. J Bone Joint Surg *58A*:1021, 1976.
195. Propp RP, Scharfman WB: Hemangioma-thrombocytopenia syndrome associated with microangiopathic hemolytic anemia. Blood *28*:623, 1966.
196. Keller L, Bluhm JF III: Diffuse neonatal hemangiomatosis. A case with heart failure and thrombocytopenia. Cutis *23*:295, 1979.
197. Letts RM: Orthopaedic treatment of hemangiomatous hypertrophy of the lower extremity. J Bone Joint Surg *59A*:777, 1977.
198. Cohen J, Cashman WF: Hemihypertrophy of lower extremity associated with multifocal intraosseous hemangioma. Clin Orthop Rel Res *109*:155, 1975.
199. Milikow E, Asch T: Hemangiomatosis, localized growth disturbance and intravascular coagulation disorder presenting with an unusual arthritis resembling hemophilia. Radiology *97*:387, 1970.
200. Klippel M, Trenaunay P: Du naevus variqueux ostéo-hypertrophique. Arch Gen Med *185*:641, 1900.
201. Lindenauer SM: The Klippel-Trenaunay syndrome: Varicosity, hypertrophy and hemangioma with no arteriovenous fistula. Ann Surg *162*:303, 1965.
202. Resnick D, Oliphant M: Hemophilia-like arthropathy of the knee associated with cutaneous and synovial hemangiomas. Report of 3 cases and review of the literature. Radiology *114*:323, 1975.
203. Evans DJ, Azzopardi JG: Distinctive tumours of bone and soft tissue causing acquired Vitamin D resistant osteomalacia. Lancet *1*:353, 1972.
204. Linovitz RJ, Resnick D, Keissling P, Kondon JJ, Sehler B, Nejdi RJ, Rowe JH, Deftos LJ: Tumor-induced osteomalacia and rickets: A surgically curable syndrome, a report of two cases. J Bone Joint Surg *58A*:419, 1976.
205. Renton P, Shaw DG: Hypophosphatemic osteomalacia secondary to vascular tumors of bone and soft tissue. Skel Radiol *1*:21, 1976.
206. Salassa RM, Jowsey J, Arnaud CD: Hypophosphatemic osteomalacia associated with "nonendocrine tumors." N Engl J Med *283*:65, 1970.
207. Turner ML, Dalinka MK: Osteomalacia: Uncommon causes. Am J Roentgenol *133*:539, 1979.
208. Gorham LW, Stout AP: Hemangiomatosis and its relation to massive osteolysis. Trans Assoc Am Phys *67*:302, 1954.
209. Yamamoto K, Ueki J: Proceedings: Massive osteolysis with periosteal hemangiomatosis, report of a case. Calcif Tissue Res *15*:160, 1974.
210. Lewis RJ, Ketcham AS: Maffucci's syndrome: Functional and neoplastic significance. Case report and review of the literature. J Bone Joint Surg *55A*:1456, 1973.
211. Schwartz A, Salz N: Cavernous hemangioma associated with phleboliths in the masseter muscle. Acta Radiol *43*:233, 1955.
212. Shallow TA, Eger SA, Wagner FB Jr: Primary hemangiomatous tumours of skeletal muscle. Ann Surg *119*:700, 1944.
213. Teller WH, Soliscohen T, Levine S: Cavernous hemangioma of the leg. Radiology *22*:369, 1934.
214. McNeill TW, Chan GE, Capek V, Ray RD: The value of angiography in the surgical management of deep hemangiomas. Clin Orthop Rel Res *101*:176, 1974.
215. Bartley O, Wickbom I: Angiography in soft tissue hemangiomas. Acta Radiol *51*:81, 1959.
216. Olcott C IV, Newton TH, Stoney RJ, Ehrenfeld WK: Intra-arterial

embolization in the management of arteriovenous malformations. Surgery *79*:3, 1976.
217. Piyachon C: Radiology of peripheral arteriovenous malformations. Australas Radiol *21*:246, 1977.
218. Thomas ML, Andress MR: Angiography in venous dysplasias of the limbs. Am J Roentgenol *113*:722, 1971.
219. Mitty HA, Kleiger B: Partial embolization of large peripheral hemangioma for pain control. Radiology *127*:671, 1978.
220. Kinmonth JB, Young AE, Edwards JM, O'Donnell TF, Thomas ML: Mixed vascular deformities of the lower limbs, with particular reference to lymphography and surgical treatment. Br J Surg *63*:899, 1976.
221. Larsen IJ, Landry RM: Hemangioma of the synovial membrane. J Bone Joint Surg *51A*:1210, 1969.
222. Lewis RC Jr, Coventry MB, Sowle EH: Hemangioma of the synovial membrane. J Bone Joint Surg *41A*:264, 1959.
223. Waddell GF: A haemangioma involving tendons. J Bone Joint Surg *49B*:138, 1967.
224. Moon NF: Synovial hemangioma of the knee joint. A review of previously reported cases and inclusion of two new cases. Clin Orthop Rel Res *90*:183, 1973.
225. Bennett GE, Cobey MC: Hemangioma of joints. Report of five cases. Arch Surg *38*:487, 1939.
226. Wynne-Roberts C, Anderson C: Synovial haemangioma of the knee: Light and electron microscopic findings. J Pathol *123*:247, 1977.
227. DePalma AF, Mauler GG: Hemangioma of synovial membrane. Clin Orthop Rel Res *32*:93, 1964.
228. Forrest J, Staple TW: Synovial hemangioma of the knee. Demonstration by arthrography and arteriography. Am J Roentgenol *112*:512, 1971.
229. Halborg A, Hansen H, Sneppen HO: Haemangioma of the knee joint. Acta Orthop Scand *39*:209, 1968.
230. Mahadevan H, Ozonoff MB, Joki P: Arteriographic findings in synovial hemangioma of the knee. Radiology *106*:627, 1973.
231. McInerney D, Park WM: Thermographic assessment of synovial hemangioma. Clin Radiol *29*:469, 1978.
232. Kauffman SL, Stout AP: Hemangiopericytoma in children. Cancer *13*:695, 1960.
233. McCormack LJ, Gallivan WF: Hemangiopericytoma. Cancer *7*:595, 1954.
234. McMaster MJ, Soule EH, Ivins JC: Hemangiopericytoma. A clinicopathologic study and long term follow-up of 60 patients. Cancer *36*:2232, 1975.
235. Stout AP: Hemangiopericytoma. A study of twenty-five new cases. Cancer *2*:1027, 1949.
236. Stout AP: Tumors featuring pericytes; glomus tumor and hemangiopericytoma. Lab Invest *5*:217, 1956.
237. Stout AP, Murray MR: Hemangiopericytoma. A vascular tumor featuring Zimmermann's pericytes. Ann Surg *116*:26, 1942.
238. Enzinger FM, Smith BH: Hemangiopericytoma. An analysis of 106 cases. Hum Pathol *7*:61, 1976.
239. Kennedy JC, Fisher JH: Haemangiopericytoma: its orthopaedic manifestations. J Bone Joint Surg *42B*:80, 1960.
240. Reynolds FC, Lansche WE: Hemangiopericytoma of the lower extremity, a case report. J Bone Joint Surg *40A*:921, 1958.
241. Daeke DA, Lindorfer DB: Malignant retroperitoneal hemangiopericytoma with associated hypoglycemia. Treatment via radiotherapy. Wis Med J *73*:S92, 1974.
242. Angervall L, Kindblom LG, Nielsen JM, Stener B, Svendsen P: Hemangiopericytoma: A clinicopathologic, angiographic and microangiographic study. Cancer *42*:2412, 1978.
243. Ayella RJ: Hemangiopericytoma: A case report with arteriographic findings. Radiology *97*:611, 1970.
244. Gerstmann KE, Nimberg GA: Hemangiopericytoma with angiographic studies. A case report. Clin Orthop Rel Res *68*:108, 1970.
245. Hoeffel IL, Chardot C, Parache R, Brauer B, Delagoutte J, Henry M: Radiologic patterns of hemangiopericytoma of the leg. Am J Surg *123*:591, 1972.
246. Joffe N: Haemangiopericytoma: Angiographic findings. Br J Radiol *33*:614, 1960.
247. Mujahed Z, Vasilas A, Evans JA: Hemangiopericytoma; report of four cases with a review of the literature. Am J Roentgenol *82*:658, 1959.
248. Yaghmai I: Angiographic manifestations of soft-tissue and osseous hemangiopericytomas. Radiology *126*:653, 1978.
249. Gensler S, Caplan LH, Laufman H: Giant benign hemangiopericytoma functioning as an arteriovenous shunt. JAMA *198*:85, 1966.
250. Harkins GA, Sabiston DC Jr: Lymphangioma in infancy and childhood. Surgery *47*:811, 1960.
251. Hill JT, Briggs JD: Lymphangioma. West J Surg Obstet Gynecol *69*:78, 1961.
252. Nix JT: Lymphangioma. Essential data in forty-two cases from Charity Hospital of Louisiana at New Orleans. Am Surg *20*:556, 1954.
253. Freund E: Chondromatosis of the joints. Arch Surg *34*:670, 1937.
254. Jeffreys TE: Synovial chondromatosis. J Bone Joint Surg *49B*:530, 1967.
255. Lichtenstein L, Goldman RL: Cartilage tumors in soft tissue, particularly in the hand and foot. Cancer *17*:1203, 1964.
256. Mallory TB: A group of metaplastic and neoplastic bone- and cartilage-containing tumors of soft parts. Am J Pathol *9*:765, 1933.
257. Murphy AF, Wilson JN: Tenosynovial osteochondroma in the hand. J Bone Joint Surg *40A*:1236, 1958.
258. Murphy FP, Dahlin DC, Sullivan CR: Articular synovial chondromatosis. J Bone Joint Surg *44A*:77, 1962.
259. Mussey RD Jr, Henderson MS: Osteochondromatosis. J Bone Joint Surg *31A*:619, 1949.
260. Nixon JE, Frank GR, Chambers G: Synovial osteochondromatosis with report of four cases, one showing malignant change. US Armed Forces Med J *11*:1434, 1960.
261. Symeonides P: Bursal chondromatosis. J Bone Joint Surg *48B*:371, 1966.
262. Wilmoth CL: Osteochondromatosis. J Bone Joint Surg *23*:367, 1941.
263. Chung EB, Enzinger FM: Chondroma of soft parts. Cancer *41*:1414, 1978.
264. Dellon AL, Weiss SW, Mitch WE: Bilateral extraosseous chondromas of the hand in a patient with chronic renal failure. J Hand Surg *3*:139, 1978.
265. Sim FH, Dahlin DC, Ivins JC: Extra-articular synovial chondromatosis. J Bone Joint Surg *59A*:492, 1977.
266. Wells TJ, Hooker SP, Roche WC: Osteochondroma cutis: Report of a case. J Oral Surg *35*:144, 1977.
267. Spjut HJ, Dorfman HD, Fechner RE, Ackerman LV: Tumors of Bone and Cartilage. *In* Atlas of Tumor Pathology. Second Series, Fascicle 5. Washington DC, Armed Forces Institute of Pathology, 1971, p 391.
268. Someren A, Merritt WH: Tenosynovial chondroma of the hand: A case report with a brief review of the literature. Hum Pathol *9*:476, 1978.
269. Swan EF, Owens WF Jr: Synovial chondrometaplasia, a case report with spontaneous regression and a review of the literature. South Med J *65*:1496, 1972.
270. Akhtar M, Mahajan S, Kott E: Synovial chondromatosis of the temporomandibular joint. Report of a case. J Bone Joint Surg *59A*:266, 1977.
271. Bloom R, Pattinson JN: Osteochondromatosis of hip joint. J Bone Joint Surg *33B*:80, 1954.
272. Brahms MA, Fumich RM: Chondroma within the flexor hallucis longus tendon sheath. A case report and literature review. Am J Sport Med *6*:143, 1978.
273. Christensen JH, Poulsen JO: Synovial chondromatosis. Acta Orthop Scand *46*:919, 1975.
274. Constant E, Harebottle NH, Davis DG: Synovial chondromatosis of the hand. Case report. Plast Reconstr Surg *54*:353, 1974.
275. Giustra PE, Furman RS, Roberts L, Killoran PJ: Synovial chondromatosis involving the elbow. Am J Roentgenol *127*:347, 1976.
276. Ishizuki M, Isobe Y, Arai T, Nagatsuka Y, Tanabe K, Okumura S: Osteochondromatosis of the finger joints. Hand *9*:198, 1977.
277. Kettlekamp DB, Dolan J: Synovial chondromatosis of an interphalangeal joint of a finger. Report of a case. J Bone Joint Surg *48A*:329, 1966.
278. Lewis MM, Marshall JL, Mirra JM: Synovial chondromatosis of the thumb. A case report and review of the literature. J Bone Joint Surg *56A*:180, 1974.
279. Lynn MD, Lee J: Periarticular tenosynovial chondrometaplasia. Report of a case at the wrist. J Bone Joint Surg *54A*:650, 1972.
280. Lyritis G: Synovial chondromatosis of the inferior radial ulnar joint. Acta Orthop Scand *47*:373, 1976.
281. McBryde AM Jr: Benign (intracapsular) tumors of the hip. *In* JP Ahstrom Jr (Ed): Current Practice in Orthopaedic Surgery, Vol 7. St Louis, CV Mosby Co, 1977, p 154.
282. Miller AS, Harwick RD, Daley DJ: Temporomandibular joint synovial chondromatosis: Report of a case. J Oral Surg *36*:467, 1978.
283. Mishra KP: Synovial chondromatosis of shoulder joint. A case report and review of literature. East Afr Med J *55*:130, 1978.
284. Moazzez K: Osteochondromatosis of the hip joint. Report of a case. Acta Med Iran *18*:35, 1975.
285. Mosher JF, Kettelkamp DB, Campbell CJ: Intracapsular or para-articular chondroma. A report of three cases. J Bone Joint Surg *48A*:1561, 1966.
286. Paul RG, Leach RE: Synovial chondromatosis of the shoulder. Clin Orthop Rel Res *68*:130, 1970.
287. Ronald JB, Keller EE, Weiland LH: Synovial chondromatosis of the temporomandibular joint. J Oral Surg *36*:13, 1978.
288. Rosen PS, Pritzker KPH, Greenbaum J, Holgate RC, Noyek AM: Synovial chondromatosis affecting the temporomandibular joint. Case report and literature review. Arthritis Rheum *20*:736, 1977.
289. Szepesi J: Synovial chondromatosis of the metacarpophalangeal joint. Acta Orthop Scand *46*:926, 1975.
290. Thomas S.: Synovial chondromatosis of the hip: Case with long-term follow up. SD J Med *30*:7, 1977.
291. Tormes FR, Hardin NJ, Pledger SR: Synovial chondromatosis of the shoulder: Case report. Milit Med *143*:872, 1978.

292. Trias A, Quintana O: Synovial chondrometaplasia: Review of world literature and a study of 18 Canadian cases. Can J Surg *19*:151, 1976.
293. Varma BP, Ramakrishna YJ: Synovial chondromatosis of the shoulder. Aust NZ J Surg *46*:44, 1976.
294. Weiss C, Averbuch PF, Steiner GC, Rusoff JH: Synovial chondromatosis and instability of the proximal tibiofibular joint. Clin Orthop Rel Res *108*:187, 1975.
295. Collins DH: The Pathology of Articular and Spinal Diseases. Baltimore, Williams & Wilkins Co, 1950.
296. Jacob RA, Campbell WP, Niemann KMW: Synovial chondrometaplasia. A case report. Clin Orthop Rel Res *109*:152, 1975.
297. Jones HT: Loose body formation in synovial osteochondromatosis with specific reference to the etiology and pathology. J Bone Joint Surg *6*:407, 1924.
298. Dunn AW, Whisler JH: Synovial chondromatosis of the knee with associated extracapsular chondromas. J Bone Joint Surg *55A*:1747, 1973.
299. Goldman RL, Lichtenstein L: Synovial chondrosarcoma. Cancer *17*: 1233, 1964.
300. King JW, Spjut HJ, Fechner RE, Vanderpool DW: Synovial chondrosarcoma of the knee joint. J Bone Joint Surg *49A*:1389, 1967.
301. Milgram JW, Addison RG: Synovial osteochondromatosis of the knee. Chondromatosis recurrence with possible chondrosarcomatous degeneration. J Bone Joint Surg *58A*:264, 1976.
302. Mullins F, Berard CW, Eisenberg SH: Chondrosarcoma following synovial chondromatosis. A case study. Cancer *18*:1180, 1965.
303. Sarmiento A, Elkins RW: Giant intra-articular osteochondroma of the knee, a case report. J Bone Joint Surg *57A*:560, 1975.
304. Fisher AGT: A study of loose bodies composed of cartilage or of cartilage and bone occurring in joints. With special reference to their pathology and etiology. Br J Surg *8*:493, 1921.
305. Halstead AE: Floating bodies in joints. Ann Surg *22*:327, 1895.
306. Milgram JW: The classification of loose bodies in human joints. Clin Orthop Rel Res *124*:282, 1977.
307. Holm CL: Primary synovial chondromatosis of the ankle. A case report. J Bone Joint Surg *58A*:878, 1976.
308. Milgram JW: Synovial osteochondromatosis. A histopathological study of thirty cases. J Bone Joint Surg *59A*:792, 1977.
309. Strong ML Jr: Chondromas of the tendon sheath of the hand. Report of a case and review of the literature. J Bone Joint Surg *57A*:1164, 1975.
310. Crittenden JJ, Jones DM, Santarelli AG: Knee arthrogram in synovial chondromatosis. Radiology *94*:133, 1970.
311. Goldberg RP, Genant HK: Calcified bodies in popliteal cysts: A characteristic radiographic appearance. Am J Roentgenol *131*:857, 1978.
312. Henderson MS, Jones HT: Loose bodies in joints and bursae due to synovial osteochondromatosis. J Bone Joint Surg *5*:400, 1923.
313. Leydig SM, Odell RT: Synovial osteochondromatosis. Surg Gynecol Obstet *89*:457, 1949.
314. Noyek AM, Holgate RC, Fireman SM, Rosen P, Pritzker KPH: The radiologic findings in synovial chondromatosis (chondrometaplasia) of the temporomandibular joint. J Otolaryngol *6*:45, 1977.
315. Prager RJ, Mall JC: Arthrographic diagnosis of synovial chondromatosis. Am J Roentgenol *127*:344, 1976.
316. Zimmerman C, Sayegh V: Roentgen manifestations of synovial osteochondromatosis. Am J Roentgenol *83*:680, 1960.
317. Dahlin DC, Salvador AH: Cartilaginous tumor of the soft tissues of the hands and feet. Mayo Clin Proc *49*:721, 1974.
318. Shellito JG, Dockerty MB: Cartilaginous tumors of the hand. Surg Gynecol Obstet *86*:465, 1948.
319. Allen PW: The fibromatoses: A clinicopathologic classification based on 140 cases. Am J Surg Pathol *1*:255, 1977.
320. Dehner LP, Askin FB: Tumors of fibrous tissue origin in childhood. A clinicopathologic study of cutaneous and soft tissue neoplasms in 66 children. Cancer *38*:888, 1976.
321. Enzinger FM: Fibrous tumors of infancy. *In* Tumors of Bone and Soft Tissue. 8th Annual Clinical Conference on Cancer, MD Anderson Hospital and Tumor Institute, 1963. Chicago, Year Book Medical Publishers, 1965, p 375.
322. MacKenzie DH: The fibromatoses — a clinicopathological concept. Br Med J *4*:277, 1972.
323. MacKenzie DH: The Differential Diagnosis of Fibroblastic Disorders. Oxford, Blackwell Scientific Publications, 1970.
324. Stout AP: Juvenile fibromatoses. Cancer *7*:953, 1954.
325. Stout AP: Fibrous tumors of the soft tissues. Minn Med *43*:455, 1960.
326. Allen PW, Enzinger FM: Juvenile aponeurotic fibroma. Cancer *26*:857, 1970.
327. Booher RJ, McPeak CJ: Juvenile aponeurotic fibromas. Surgery *46*:924, 1959.
328. Goldman RL: The cartilage analogue of fibromatosis (aponeurotic fibroma). Further observations based on 7 new cases. Cancer *26*:1325, 1970.
329. Keasbey LE: Juvenile aponeurotic fibroma (calcifying fibroma): A distinctive tumor arising in the palms and soles of young children. Cancer *6*:338, 1953.
330. Keasbey LE, Fanselau HA: The aponeurotic fibroma. Clin Orthop Rel Res *19*:115, 1961.
331. Keller RB, Beaz-Giangreco A: Juvenile aponeurotic fibroma. Report of 3 cases and review of the literature. Clin Orthop Rel Res *106*:198, 1975.
332. Lichtenstein L, Goldman RL: The cartilage analogue of fibromatosis. A reinterpretation of the condition called "juvenile aponeurotic fibroma." Cancer *17*:810, 1964.
333. Rios-Dalenz JL, Kim JS, McDowell FW: The so-called "juvenile aponeurotic fibroma." Am J Clin Pathol *44*:632, 1965.
334. Zeide MS, Wiesel S, Terry RL: Juvenile aponeurotic fibroma, case report. Plast Reconstr Surg *61*:922, 1978.
335. Arlen M, Koven L, Frieder M: Juvenile fascial fibromatosis of the forearm with osseous involvement. J Bone Joint Surg *51A*:591, 1969.
336. Karasick D, O'Hara AE: Juvenile aponeurotic fibroma. A review and report of a case with osseous involvement. Radiology *123*:725, 1977.
337. Shapiro L: Infantile digital fibromatosis and aponeurotic fibroma. Case reports of two rare pseudosarcomas and review of the literature. Arch Dermatol *99*:37, 1969.
338. Allen PW: Recurring digital fibrous tumours of childhood. Pathology *4*:215, 1972.
339. Beckett JH, Jacobs AH: Recurring digital fibrous tumors of childhood: A review. Pediatrics *59*:401, 1977.
340. Grunnet N, Genner J, Morgensen B, Myhre-Jensen O: Recurring digital fibrous tumor of childhood, case report and survey. Acta Pathol Microbiol Scand (A) *81*:167, 1973.
341. Iwasaki H, Tsuneyoshi M, Enjoji M: Infantile digital fibromatosis histopathological and electron microscopic study with a review of the literature. Acta Pathol Jpn *24*:717, 1974.
342. O'Gorman DJ, Fairburn EA: Infantile digital fibromatosis. Proc R Soc Med *67*:880, 1974.
343. Reye RDK: Recurring digital fibrous tumors of childhood. Arch Pathol *80*:228, 1965.
344. Bloem JJ, Vuzevski VD, Huffstadt AJC: Recurring digital fibroma of infancy. J Bone Joint Surg *56B*:746, 1974.
345. Siegal A: Aggressive fibromatosis (infantile fibrosarcoma). Difficulty of diagnostic and prognostic evaluation. Clin Pediatr *17*:517, 1978.
346. Antine BE, Brown FM, Arisco MJ: Fibroma of the cornea. Report of a case associated with congenital generalized fibromatosis. Arch Ophthalmol *91*:278, 1974.
347. Beatty EC Jr: Congenital generalized fibromatosis in infancy. Am J Dis Child *103*:620, 1962.
348. Elliott DE: Congenital generalized fibromatosis. Birth Defects *11*:355, 1975.
349. Familusi JB, Nottidge VA, Antia AN, Attah EB: Congenital generalized fibromatosis. An African case with gingival hypertrophy and other unusual features. Am J Dis Child *130*:1215, 1976.
350. Kindblom LG, Termen G, Säve-Söderbergh J, Angervall L: Congenital solitary fibromatosis of soft tissues, a variant of congenital generalized fibromatosis. Two case reports. Acta Pathol Microbiol Scand (A) *85*:640, 1977.
351. Kindblom LG, Angervall L: Congenital solitary fibromatosis of the skeleton. Case report of a variant of congenital generalized fibromatosis. Cancer *41*:636, 1978.
352. Plaschkes J: Congenital fibromatosis: Localized and generalized forms. J Pediatr Surg *9*:95, 1974.
353. Shnitka TK, Asp DM, Horner RH: Congenital generalized fibromatosis. Cancer *11*:627, 1958.
354. Baer JW, Radkowski MA: Congenital multiple fibromatosis. A case report with review of the world literature. Am J Roentgenol *118*:200, 1973.
355. Schaffzin EA, Chung SMK, Kaye R: Congenital generalized fibromatosis with complete spontaneous regression. A case report. J Bone Joint Surg *54A*:657, 1972.
356. Teng P, Warden MJ, Cohn WL: Congenital generalized fibromatosis (renal and skeletal) with complete spontaneous regression. J Pediatr *62*:748, 1963.
357. Barlett RC, Otis RD, Laakso AO: Multiple congenital neoplasms of soft tissues. Report of 4 cases in one family. Cancer *14*:913, 1961.
358. Condon VR, Allen RP: Congenital generalized fibromatosis. Case report with roentgen manifestations. Radiology *76*:444, 1961.
359. Morettin LB, Mueller E, Schreiber M: Generalized hamartomatosis (congenital generalized fibromatosis). Am J Roentgenol *114*:722, 1972.
360. Schlangen JT: Congenital generalized fibromatosis: A case report with roentgen manifestations of the skeleton. Radiol Clin *45*:18, 1976.
361. Dutz W, Stout AP: The myxoma in childhood. Cancer *14*:629, 1961.
362. Enzinger FM: Intramuscular myxoma. A review and follow-up study of 34 cases. Am J Clin Pathol *43*:104, 1965.
363. Stout AP: Myxoma; the tumor of primitive mesenchyme. Ann Surg *127*:706, 1948.
364. Sponsel KH, McDonald JR, Ghormley RK: Myxoma and myxosarcoma of the soft tissues of the extremities. J Bone Joint Surg *34A*:820, 1952.
365. Fisher WC, Helwig EB: Leiomyomas of the skin. Arch Dermatol *88*:510, 1963.

366. Goodman AH, Briggs RC: Deep leiomyoma of an extremity. J Bone Joint Surg *47A*:529, 1965.
367. Stout AP: Solitary cutaneous and subcutaneous leiomyoma. Am J Cancer *29*:435, 1937.
368. Kauffman SL, Stout AP: Histiocytic tumors (fibrous xanthoma and histiocytoma) in children. Cancer *14*:469, 1961.
369. Bloom D, Kaufman SR, Stevens RA: Hereditary xanthomatosis. Familial incidence of xanthoma tuberosum associated with hypercholesteremia and cardiovascular involvement, with report of several cases of sudden death. Arch Dermatol *45*:1, 1942.
370. Montgomery H: Cutaneous xanthomatosis. Ann Intern Med *13*:671, 1939.
371. Cappell DF, Montgomery GL: On rhabdomyoma and myoblastoma. J Pathol Bacteriol *44*:517, 1937.
372. Goldman RL: Multicentric benign rhabdomyoma of skeletal muscle. Cancer *16*:1609, 1963.
373. Parsons HG, Puro HE: Rhabdomyoma of skeletal muscle; report of a case. Am J Surg *89*:1187, 1955.
374. Ackerman LV, Wheeler P: Liposarcoma. South Med J *35*:156, 1942.
375. Adair, FE, Pack GT, Farrior JH: Lipomas. Am J Cancer *16*:1104, 1932.
376. Enterline HT, Culberson JD, Rochlin DB, Brady LW: Liposarcoma: a clinical and pathological study of 53 cases. Cancer *13*:932, 1960.
377. Enzinger FM: Recent trends in soft tissue pathology. In Tumors of Bone and Soft Tissue. 8th Annual Clinical Conference on Cancer, MD Anderson Hospital and Tumor Institute, Houston, Texas, 1963. Chicago, Year Book Medical Publishers, 1965, p. 315.
378. Holtz F: Liposarcomas. Cancer *11*:1103, 1958.
379. Hutton I: Liposarcoma of the thigh: Management. Proc R Soc Med *67*:655, 1974.
380. Kelly PC, Shramowiat M: Liposarcoma of the foot: A case report. J Foot Surg *17*:27, 1978.
381. Pack GT, Pierson JC: Liposarcoma: A study of 105 cases. Surgery *36*:687, 1954.
382. Phelan JT, Perez-Mesa C: Liposarcoma of the superficial soft tissues. Surg Gynecol Obstet *115*:609, 1962.
383. Quinonez GE: Liposarcoma of the lower extremity. A review of 30 cases from Ohio State University Hospitals from 1955 to 1970. Ohio State Med J *68*:942, 1972.
384. Reszel PA, Soule EH, Coventry MB: Liposarcoma of the extremities and limb girdles. A study of two hundred twenty-two cases. J Bone Joint Surg *48A*:229, 1966.
385. Sawhney KK, McDonald JM, Jaffe HW: Liposarcoma of the hand. Am Surg *41*:117, 1975.
386. Shiu MA: Chu F, Castro EB, Hajdu SI, Fortner JG: Results of surgical and radiation therapy in the treatment of liposarcoma arising in an extremity. Am J Roentgenol *123*:577, 1975.
387. Stout AP: Liposarcoma — the malignant tumor of lipoblasts. Ann Surg *119*:86, 1944.
388. Enzinger FM, Winslow DJ: Liposarcoma. A study of 103 cases. Virchows Arch (Pathol Anat) *335*:367, 1962.
389. Kindblom LG, Angervall L, Svendsen P: Liposarcoma: A clinicopathologic, radiographic and prognostic study. Acta Pathol Microbiol Scand (A) Suppl *253*:1, 1975.
390. Cadman NL, Soule EH, Kelly PJ: Synovial sarcoma. An analysis of 134 tumors. Cancer *18*:613, 1965.
391. Cade S: Synovial sarcoma. J R Coll Surg Edinb *8*:1, 1962.
392. Galinski AW, Vlahos M: Malignant synovioma of the foot: A case report. J Am Podiatry Assoc *65*:175, 1975.
393. Gerner RE, Moore GE: Synovial sarcoma. Ann Surg *181*:22, 1975.
394. Haagensen CD, Stout AP: Synovial sarcoma. Ann Surg *120*:826, 1944.
395. Jaworek TA: Synovial sarcoma, a case report of foot involvement. J Am Podiatry Assoc *66*:544, 1976.
396. Madewell BR, Pool R: Neoplasms of joints and related structures. Vet Clin North Am *8*:511, 1978.
397. Murray JA: Synovial sarcoma. Orthop Clin North Am *8*:963, 1977.
398. Raina V: Synovial sarcoma. An analysis of 31 cases in 26 years. Indian J Cancer *15*:10, 1978.
399. Thunold J, Bang G: Synovial sarcoma: A case report. Acta Orthop Scand *47*:231, 1976.
400. Crocker DW, Stout AP: Synovial sarcoma in children. Cancer *12*:1123, 1959.
401. Lee SM, Hajdu SI, Exelby PR: Synovial sarcoma in children. Surg Gynecol Obstet *138*:701, 1974.
402. Ichinose H, Derbes VJ, Hoerner H: Cutaneous pain without tumor. A manifestation of occult synovioma. Cutis *21*:74, 1978.
403. Ichinose H, Hoerner H, Derbes VJ: Minute synovial sarcoma in the occult non-palpable phase. A ease report. J Bone Joint Surg *60A*:836, 1978.
404. Cameron HU, Kostuik JP: A long-term follow-up of synovial sarcoma. J Bone Joint Surg *56B*:613, 1974.
405. Sutro CJ: Synovial sarcoma of the soft parts in the 1st toe: recurrence after a 35 year interval. Bull Hosp Joint Dis *37*:105, 1976.
406. Dische FE, Darby AJ, Howard ER: Malignant synovioma: Electron microscopical findings in 3 patients and review of the literature. J Pathol *124*:149, 1978.
407. Fernandez BB, Hernandez FJ: Poorly differentiated synovial sarcoma. A light and electron microscopic study. Arch Pathol Lab Med *100*:221, 1976.
408. Mackenzie DH: Monophasic synovial sarcoma — a histological entity? Histopathology *1*:151, 1977.
409. deSantos LA, Lindell MM Jr, Goldman AM, Luna MA, Murray JA: Calcification within metastatic pulmonary nodules from synovial sarcoma. Orthopedics *1*:141, 1978.
410. Hale DE: Synovioma with special reference to the clinical and roentgenologic aspects. Am J Roentgenol *65*:769, 1951.
411. Lewis RW: Roentgen recognition of synovioma. Am J Roentgenol *44*:170, 1940.
412. Albores-Saavedra J, Martin RG, Smith JL, Jr: Rhabdomyosarcoma: A study of 35 cases. Ann Surg *157*:186, 1963.
413. Enterline HT, Horn RC Jr: Alveolar rhabdomyosarcoma. A distinctive tumor type. Am J Clin Pathol *29*:356, 1958.
414. Enzinger FM, Shiraki M: Alveolar rhabdomyosarcoma. An analysis of 110 cases. Cancer *24*:18, 1969.
415. Horn RC Jr, Patton RB: Rhabdomyosarcoma. Clin Orthop Rel Res *19*:99, 1961.
416. Horn RC Jr, Enterline HT: Rhabdomyosarcoma: A clinicopathological study and classification of 39 cases. Cancer *11*:181, 1958.
417. Linscheid RL, Soule EH, Henderson, ED: Pleomorphic rhabdomyosarcomata of the extremities and limb girdles. J Bone Joint Surg *47A*:715, 1965.
418. Moore O, Grossi C: Embryonal rhabdomyosarcoma of the head and neck. Cancer *12*:69, 1959.
419. Pack GT, Eberhart WF: Rhabdomyosarcoma of skeletal muscle: Report of 100 cases. Surgery *32*:1023, 1952.
420. Pinkel D, Pickren J: Rhabdomyosarcoma in children. JAMA *175*:293, 1961.
421. Stobbe GD, Dargeon HW: Embryonal rhabdomyosarcoma of head and neck in children and adolescents. Cancer *3*:826, 1950.
422. Stout AP: Rhabdomyosarcoma of skeletal muscles. Ann Surg *123*:447, 1946.
423. Mackenzie DH: Fibroma — a dangerous diagnosis. A review of 205 cases of fibrosarcoma of soft tissues. Br J Surg *51*:607, 1964.
424. Pritchard DJ, Soule EH, Taylor WF, Ivins JC: Fibrosarcoma — a clinicopathologic and statistical study of 199 tumors of the soft tissue of the extremities and trunk. Cancer *33*:888, 1974.
425. Pritchard DJ, Sim FH, Ivins JC, Soule EH, Dahlin DC: Fibrosarcoma of bone and soft tissues of the trunk and extremities. Orthop Clin North Am *8*:869, 1977.
426. Stout AP: Fibrosarcoma. The malignant tumor of fibroblasts. Cancer *1*:30, 1948.
427. van der Werf-Messing B, van Unnik JAM: Fibrosarcoma of the soft tissues. A clinicopathologic study. Cancer *18*:1113, 1965.
428. Yaghmai I: Angiographic features of fibromas and fibrosarcomas. Radiology *124*:57, 1977.
429. Chung EB, Enzinger FM: Infantile fibrosarcoma. Cancer *38*:729, 1976.
430. Soule EH, Pritchard DJ: Fibrosarcoma in infants and children. A review of 110 cases. Cancer *40*:1711, 1977.
431. Kindblom LG, Merck C, Svendsen P: Myxofibrosarcoma: A pathologico-anatomical, microangiographic and angiographic correlative study of 8 cases. Br J Radiol *50*:876, 1977.
432. Lagergren C, Lindblom A, Söderberg G: Vascularization of fibromatous and fibrosarcomatous tumors: Histopathologic, microangiographic and angiographic studies. Acta Radiol *53*:1, 1960.
433. Balsaver AM, Butler JJ, Martin RG: Congenital fibrosarcoma. Cancer *20*:1607, 1967.
434. Exelby PR, Knapper WH, Huvos AG, Beattie EJ Jr: Soft tissue fibrosarcoma in children. J Pediatr Surg *8*:415, 1973.
435. Horne CHW, Slavin G, McDonald AM: Late recurrence of juvenile fibrosarcoma. Br J Surg *55*:102, 1968.
436. Schvarcz LW: Congenital dermatofibrosarcoma protuberans of the hand. Hand *9*:182, 1977.
437. Stout AP: Fibrosarcoma in infants and children. Cancer *15*:1028, 1962.
438. Haug WA, Losli EJ: Primary leiomyosarcoma within the femoral vein. Report of a case and review of the literature. Cancer *7*:159, 1954.
439. Phelan JT, Sherer W, Mesa P: Malignant smooth-muscle tumors (leiomyosarcomas) of soft tissue origin. N Engl J Med *266*:1027, 1962.
440. Rising JA, Booth E: Primary leiomyosarcoma of the skin with lymphatic spread. Report of a case. Arch Pathol *81*:94, 1966.
441. Stout AP, Hill WT: Leiomyosarcoma of the superficial soft tissues. Cancer *11*:844, 1958.
442. Fine G, Stout AP: Osteogenic sarcoma of the extraskeletal soft tissues. Cancer *9*:1027, 1956.
443. Kauffman SL, Stout AP: Extraskeletal osteogenic sarcomas and chondrosarcomas in children. Cancer *16*:432, 1963.

444. Salm R: A case of primary osteogenic sarcoma of extraskeletal soft tissues. Br J Cancer *13*:614, 1959.
445. Enzinger FM, Shiraki M: Extraskeletal myxoid chondrosarcoma. An analysis of 34 cases. Hum Pathol *3*:421, 1972.
446. Lewis MM, Marcove RC, Bullough PG: Chondrosarcoma of the foot. A case report and review of the literature. Cancer *36*:586, 1975.
447. Marcove RC: Chondrosarcoma: Diagnosis and treatment. Orthop Clin North Am *8*:811, 1977.
448. Moore JP, Shannon E: Extraskeletal chondrosarcomas. Tex Med *70*:65, 1974.
449. Ream JR, Corson JM, Holdsworth DE, Millender LH: Chondrosarcoma of the extraskeletal soft tissue of the finger. Clin Orthop Rel Res *97*:148, 1973.
450. Smith MT, Farinacci CJ, Carpenter HA, Bannayan GA: Extraskeletal myxoid chondrosarcoma. A clinicopathological study. Cancer *37*:821, 1976.
451. Stout AP, Verner EW: Chondrosarcoma of the extraskeletal soft tissues. Cancer *6*:581, 1953.
452. Feldman F, Norman D: Intra- and extraosseous malignant histiocytoma (malignant fibrous xanthoma). Radiology *104*:497, 1972.
453. O'Brien JE, Stout AP: Malignant fibrous xanthomas. Cancer *17*:1445, 1964.
454. Soule EH, Enriquez P: Atypical fibrous histiocytoma, malignant fibrous histiocytoma, malignant histiocytoma, and epithelioid sarcoma. A comparative study of 65 tumors. Cancer *30*:128, 1972.
455. Weiss SW, Enzinger FM: Myxoid variant of malignant fibrous histiocytoma. Cancer *39*:1672, 1977.
456. Ackerman LV: Extra-osseous localized non-neoplastic bone and cartilage formation (so-called myositis ossificans). Clinical and pathological confusion with malignant neoplasms. J Bone Joint Surg *40A*:279, 1958.
457. Angervall L, Stener B, Stener, I, Ahrén C: Pseudomalignant osseous tumor of soft tissue. A clinical, radiological and pathological study of 5 cases. J Bone Joint Surg *51B*:654, 1969.
458. Chung BS: Drug-induced myositis ossificans circumscripta. Letter to Editor. JAMA *226*:469, 1973.
459. Geschickter CF, Maseritz IH: Myositis ossificans. J Bone Joint Surg *20*:661, 1938.
460. Gilmer WS Jr, Anderson LD: Reactions of soft somatic tissue which may progress to bone formation: Circumscribed (traumatic) myositis ossificans. South Med J *52*:1432, 1959.
461. Gunn DR, Young WB: Myositis ossificans as a complication of tetanus. J Bone Joint Surg *41B*:535, 1959.
462. Heilbrun N, Kuhn WG Jr: Erosive bone lesions and soft-tissue ossifications associated with spinal cord injuries (paraplegia). Radiology *48*:579, 1947.
463. Hughston JC, Whatley GS, Stone MM: Myositis ossificans traumatica (myo-osteosis). South Med J *55*:1167, 1962.
464. Jeffreys TE, Stiles PJ: Pseudomalignant osseous tumor of soft tissue. J Bone Joint Surg *48B*:488, 1966.
465. Kern WH: Proliferative myositis: A pseudosarcomatous reaction to injury. A report of 7 cases. Arch Pathol *69*:209, 1960.
466. Lewis D: Myositis ossificans. JAMA *80*:1281, 1923.
467. Skajaa T: Myositis ossificans. Acta Chir Scand *116*:68, 1958.
468. Goldman AB: Myositis ossificans circumscripta: A benign lesion with malignant differential diagnosis. Am J Roentgenol *126*:32, 1976.
469. Pack GT, Braund RR: The development of sarcoma in myositis ossificans. Report of three cases. JAMA *119*:776, 1942.
470. Shanoff LB, Spira M, Hardy SB: Myositis ossificans: Evolution to osteogenic sarcoma. Report of a histologically verified case. Am J Surg *113*:537, 1967.
471. Johnson LC: Histogenesis of myositis ossificans (Abstr). Am J Pathol *24*:681, 1948.
472. Kramer FL, Kurtz AB, Rubin C, Goldberg BB: Ultrasound appearance of myositis ossificans. Skel Radiol *4*:19, 1979.
473. Norman A, Dorfman HD: Juxtacortical circumscribed myositis ossificans: evolution and radiographic features. Radiology *96*:301, 1970.
474. Yaghmai I: Myositis ossificans: Diagnostic value of arteriography. Am J Roentgenol *128*:811, 1977.
475. Tibone J, Sakimura I, Nickel VL, Hsu JD: Heterotopic ossification around the hip in spinal cord-injured patients: A long-term follow-up study. J Bone Joint Surg *60A*:769, 1978.
476. Alguacil-Garcia A, Unni KK, Goellner JR: Giant cell tumor of tendon sheath and pigmented villonodular synovitis: An ultrastructural study. Am J Clin Pathol *69*:6, 1978.
477. Barnard JD: Pigmented villonodular synovitis in the temporomandibular joint: A case report. Br J Oral Surg *13*:183, 1975.
478. Carstens HB: Giant cell tumors of tendon sheath. An electron microscopical study of 11 cases. Arch Pathol Lab Med *102*:99, 1978.
479. Chung SMK, Janes JM: Diffuse pigmented villonodular synovitis of the hip joint. Review of the literature and report of four cases. J Bone Joint Surg *47A*:293, 1965.
480. Byers PD, Cotton RE, Deacon OW, Lowy M, Newman PH, Sissons HA, Thomson AD: The diagnosis and treatment of pigmented villonodular synovitis. J Bone Joint Surg *50B*:290, 1968.
481. Decker JP, Owen BJ: An invasive giant cell tumor of tendon sheath in the foot. Bull Ayer Clin Lab Penn Hosp *4*:43, 1954.
482. Eisenstein R: Giant-cell tumor of tendon sheath: Its histogenesis as studied in the electron microscope. J Bone Joint Surg *50A*:476, 1968.
483. Eisenberg RL, Hedgcock MW: Bilateral pigmented villonodular synovitis of the hip. Br J Radiol *51*:916, 1978.
484. Fletcher AG Jr, Horn RC Jr: Giant cell tumors of tendon sheath origin. A consideration of bone involvement and report of two cases with extensive bone destruction. Ann Surg *133*:374, 1951.
485. Granowitz SP, Mankin HJ: Localized pigmented villonodular synovitis of the knee. Report of 5 cases. J Bone Joint Surg *49A*:122, 1967.
486. Granowitz SP, D'Antonio J, Mankin HL: The pathogenesis and long-term end results of pigmented villonodular synovitis. Clin Orthop Rel Res *114*:335, 1976.
487. Jones FE, Soule EH, Coventry MB: Fibrous xanthoma of synovium (giant-cell tumor of tendon sheath, pigmented nodular synovitis). A study of 118 cases. J Bone Joint Surg *51A*:76, 1969.
488. Kindblom LG, Gunterberg B: Pigmented villonodular synovitis involving bone. J Bone Joint Surg *60A*:830, 1978.
489. Kleinstiver BJ, Rodriguez HA: Nodular fasciitis: Study of 45 cases and review of literature. J Bone Joint Surg *50A*:1204, 1968.
490. Leszczynski J, Huckell JR, Percy JS, LeRiche JC, Lentle BC: Pigmented villonodular synovitis in multiple joints. Occurrence in a child with cavernous haemangioma of lip and pulmonary stenosis. Ann Rheum Dis *34*:269, 1975.
491. Levine HA, Enrile F: Giant-cell tumor of patellar tendon coincident with Paget's disease. J Bone Joint Surg *53A*:335, 1971.
492. Lichtenstein L: Tumors of synovial joints, bursae and tendon sheaths. Cancer *8*:816, 1955.
493. Schajowicz F, Blumenfeld I: Pigmented villonodular synovitis of the wrist with penetration into bone. J Bone Joint Surg *50B*:312, 1968.
494. Shafer SJ, Larmon WA: Pigmented villonodular synovitis. A report of seven cases. Surg Gynecol Obstet *92*:574, 1951.
495. Sherry JB, Anderson W: The natural history of pigmented villonodular synovitis of tendon sheaths. J Bone Joint Surg *37A*:1005, 1055.
496. Torisu T, Iwabuchi R, Kamo Y: Pigmented villonodular synovitis of the elbow with bony erosion. Clin Orthop Rel Res *94*:275, 1973.
497. Woods C Jr, Alade CO, Anderson V, Ashby ME: Pigmented villonodular synovitis of the knee presenting as a loose body. A case report. Clin Orthop Rel Res *129*:230, 1977.
498. Yanklowitz BA: Giant cell tumor of tendon sheath: A literature review and case report. J Am Podiatry Assoc *68*:706, 1978.
499. Hoaglund FT: Experimental hemarthrosis. The response of canine knees to injections of autologous blood. J Bone Joint Surg *49A*:285, 1967.
500. McCollum DE, Musser AW, Rhangos WC: Experimental villonodular synovitis. South Med J *59*:966, 1966.
501. Roy S, Ghadially FN: Synovial membrane in experimentally-produced chronic haemarthrosis. Ann Rheum Dis *28*:402, 1969.
502. Young JM, Hudacek AG: Experimental production of pigmented villonodular synovitis in dogs. Am J Pathol *30*:799, 1954.
503. Jaffe HL, Lichtenstein L, Sutro CJ: Pigmented villonodular synovitis, bursitis and tenosynovitis. Arch Pathol *31*:731, 1941.
504. Cavanagh RC, Schwamm HA: Localized nodular synovitis. RPC of the month from the AFIP. Radiology *100*:409, 1971.
505. Johnson LC: Personal communication.
506. Byers PD, Cotton RE, Deacon OW, Lowy M, Newman PH, Sissons HA, Thomson AD: The diagnosis and treatment of pigmented villonodular synovitis. J Bone Joint Surg *50B*:290, 1968.
507. Breimer CW, Freiberger RH: Bone lesions associated with villonodular synovitis. Am J Roentgenol *79*:618, 1958.
508. Crosby EB, Inglis A, Bullough PG: Multiple joint involvement with pigmented villonodular synovitis. Radiology *122*:671, 1977.
509. Gehweiler JA, Wilson JW: Diffuse biarticular pigmented villonodular synovitis. Radiology *93*:845, 1969.
510. Greenfield MM, Wallace KM: Pigmented villonodular synovitis. Radiology *54*:350, 1950.
511. Jergesen HE, Mankin HJ, Schiller AL: Diffuse pigmented villonodular synovitis of the knee mimicking primary bone neoplasms. J Bone Joint Surg *60A*:825, 1978.
512. Lewis RW: Roentgen diagnosis of pigmented villonodular synovitis and synovial sarcoma of the knee joint: Preliminary report. Radiology *49*:26, 1947.
513. McMaster PE: Pigmented villonodular synovitis with invasion of bone. Report of six cases. J Bone Joint Surg *42A*:1170, 1960.
514. Smith JH, Pugh DG: Roentgenographic aspects of articular pigmented villonodular synovitis. Am J Roentgenol *87*:1146, 1962.
515. Scott PM: Bone lesions in pigmented villonodular synovitis. J Bone Joint Surg *50B*:306, 1968.
516. Rosenthal DI, Aronow S, Murray WT: Iron content of pigmented villo-

nodular synovitis detected by computed tomography. Radiology *133*:409, 1979.
517. Goergen IG, Resnick D, Niwayama G: Localized nodular synovitis of the knee: A report of two cases with abnormal arthrograms. Am J Roentgenol *126*:647, 1976.
518. Halpern A, Donovan TL, Horowitz B, Nagel D: Arthrographic demonstration of pigmented villonodular synovitis of the knee. Clin Orthop Rel Res *132*:193, 1978.
519. Rein BI, Bilodeau LP, Johanson P: Arthrography and arteriography in pigmented villonodular synovitis of the knee. Am J Roentgenol *92*:1322, 1964.
520. Wolfe RD, Giuliano VJ: Double-contrast arthrography in the diagnosis of pigmented villonodular synovitis of the knee. Am J Roentgenol *110*:793, 1970.
521. Chater EH: Tumoral calcinosis. Letter to Editor. Br Med J *1*:644, 1969.
522. Cooke RA: Tumoral calcinosis. Letter to Editor. Br Med J *4*:174, 1969.
523. Inclan A, Leon P, Gomez Camejo M: Tumoral calcinosis. JAMA *121*:490, 1943.
524. Maathuis JB, Koten JW: Kikuyu-bursa and tumoral calcinosis. Trop Geogr Med *21*:389, 1969.
525. McClatchie S, Bremner AD: Tumoral calcinosis — an unrecognized disease. Br Med J *1*:153, 1969.
526. Najjar SS, Farah FS, Kurban AK, Melhem RE, Khatchadourian AK: Tumoral calcinosis and pseudoxanthoma elasticum. J Pediatr *72*:243, 1968.
527. Slavin G, Klenerman L, Darby A, Bansal S: Tumoral calcinosis in England. Br Med J *1*:147, 1973.
528. Harkess JW, Peters HJ: Tumoral calcinosis. A report of six cases. J Bone Joint Surg *49A*:721, 1967.
529. Agnew CH: Tumoral calcinosis. A radiologic teaching method. J Kans Med Soc *62*:100, 1961.
530. Albright F, Reifenstein EC Jr.: Parathyroid Glands and Metabolic Bone Disease. Baltimore, Williams & Wilkins Co, 1948.
531. Baldursson H, Evans EB, Dodge WF, Jackson WT: Tumoral calcinosis with hyperphosphatemia. A report of a family with incidence in four siblings. J Bone Joint Surg *51A*:913, 1969.
532. Poppel MH, Zeitel BE: Roentgen manifestations of milk drinker's syndrome. Radiology *67*:195, 1956.
533. Hacihanefioğlu U: Tumoral calcinosis: A clinical and pathologic study of eleven unreported cases in Turkey. J Bone Joint Surg *60A*:1131, 1978.
534. Lafferty FW, Reynolds ES, Pearson OH: Tumoral calcinosis. A metabolic disease of obscure etiology. Am J Med *38*:105, 1965.
535. Reed RJ, Hunt RW: Granulomatous (tumoral) calcinosis. Clin Orthop Rel Res *43*:233, 1965.
536. Barton DL, Reeves RJ: Tumoral calcinosis. Report of three cases and review of the literature. Am J Roentgenol *86*:351, 1961.
537. Palmer PES: Tumoural calcinosis. Br J Radiol *39*:518, 1966.
538. Riemenschneider PA, Ecker A: Sciatica caused by tumoral calcinosis. J Neurosurg *9*:304, 1952.
539. Smit GG, Schmaman A: Tumoral calcinosis. J Bone Joint Surg *49B*:698, 1967.
540. Thomson JG: Calcifying collagenolysis (tumoural calcinosis). Br J Radiol *39*:526, 1966.
541. Yaghmai I, Mirbod P: Tumoral calcinosis. Am J Roentgenol *111*:573, 1971.
542. Hug I, Guncaga J: Tumoral calcinosis with sedimentation sign. Br J Radiol *47*:734, 1974.
543. Kolawole TM, Bohrer SP: Tumoral calcinosis with "fluid levels" in the tumoral masses. Am J Roentgenol *120*:461, 1974.
544. Bouhoutsos J, Martin P: Popliteal aneurysm: A review of 116 cases. Br J Surg *61*:469, 1974.
545. Gifford RW Jr, Hines EA Jr, Janes JM: An analysis and follow-up study of one hundred popliteal aneurysms. Surgery *33*:284, 1953.
546. Giustra PE, Root JA, Mason SE, Killoran PJ: Popliteal vein thrombosis secondary to popliteal artery aneurysm. Am J Roentgenol *130*:25, 1978.
547. Hardy JD, Tompkins WC Jr, Hatten LE, Chavez CM: Aneurysms of the popliteal artery. Surg Gynecol Obstet *140*:401, 1975.
548. Hunt DD: Problems in diagnosing osteoarticular tuberculosis. JAMA *190*:95, 1964.
549. Marwah V: Changing pattern of osteoarticular tuberculosis. J Indian Med Assoc *38*:18, 1962.
550. Dickson FD: Differential diagnosis of tuberculous arthritis. JAMA *107*:531, 1936.
551. Dickson FD: Differential diagnosis of tuberculous arthritis. J Lab Clin Med *22*:35, 1936.
552. Houkom SS: Tuberculosis of the ankle joint; an end result of 25 cases. Surg Gynecol Obstet *76*:438, 1943.
553. Phemister DB: Changes in the articular surfaces in tuberculosis and pyogenic infections of joints. Am J Roentgenol *12*:1, 1924.
554. Phemister DB, Hatcher CH: Correlation of pathological and roentgenological findings in diagnosis of tuberculous arthritis. Am J Roentgenol *29*:736, 1933.
555. El-Khoury GY, Bassett GS: Symptomatic bursa formation with osteochondromas. Am J Roentgenol *133*:895, 1979.
556. Smithuis T: Exostosis bursata. Report of a case. J Bone Joint Surg *46B*:544, 1964.
557. Gomez-Reino JJ, Radin A, Gorevic PD: Pseudoaneurysm of the popliteal artery as a complication of an osteochondroma. Skel Radiol *4*:26, 1979.
558. Greenway G, Resnick D, Bookstein JJ: Popliteal pseudoaneurysm as a complication of an adjacent osteochondroma: angiographic diagnosis. Am J Roentgenol *132*:294, 1979.
559. Cary GR: Juxtacortical chondroma, a case report. J Bone Joint Surg *47A*:1405, 1965.
560. Cooke GM, Pearce JG: Periosteal chondroma. Report of two cases with atypical radiologic features. J Can Assoc Radiol *27*:301, 1976.
561. Fornasier VL, McGonigal D: Periosteal chondroma. Clin Orthop Rel Res *124*:233, 1977.
562. Jaffe HL: Juxtacortical chondroma. Bull Hosp Joint Dis *17*:20, 1956.
563. Kirchner SG, Pavlov H, Heller RM, Kaye JJ: Periosteal chondromas of the anterior tibial tubercle: Two cases. Am J Roentgenol *131*:1088, 1979.
564. Lichtenstein L, Hall JE: Periosteal chondroma; a distinctive benign cartilage tumor. J Bone Joint Surg *34A*:691, 1952.
565. Nosanchuk JS, Kaufer H: Recurrent periosteal chondroma. Report of two cases and a review of the literature. J Bone Joint Surg *51A*:375, 1969.
566. Rockwell MA, Saiter ET, Enneking WF: Periosteal chondroma. J Bone Joint Surg *54A*:102, 1972.
567. Buckwalter JA, El-Khoury GY, Flatt AE: Dysplasia epiphysealis hemimelica of the ulna. Clin Orthop Rel Res *135*:36, 1978.
568. Carlson DH, Wilkinson RH: Variability of unilateral epiphyseal dysplasia (dysplasia epiphysealis hemimelica). Radiology *133*:368, 1979.
569. Fairbank TJ: Dysplasia epiphysealis hemimelica (tarso-epiphyseal aclasis). J Bone Joint Surg *38B*:237, 1956.
570. Hensinger RN, Cowell HR, Ramsey PL, Leopold RG: Familial dysplasia epiphysealis hemimelica, associated with chondromas and osteochondromas. Report of a kindred with variable presentations. J Bone Joint Surg *56A*:1513, 1974.
571. Kettelkamp DB, Campbell CJ, Bonfiglio M: Dysplasia epiphysealis hemimelica. Report of fifteen cases and a review of the literature. J Bone Joint Surg *48A*:746, 1966.
572. Trevor D: Tarso-epiphyseal aclasis: A congenital error in epiphyseal development. J Bone Joint Surg *32B*:204, 1950.
573. Freiberger RH, Loitman BS, Helpern M, Thompson TC: Osteoid osteoma, a report of 80 cases. Am J Roentgenol *82*:194, 1959.
574. Giustra PE, Freiberger RH: Severe growth disturbance with osteoid osteoma; a report of 2 cases involving the femoral neck. Radiology *96*:285, 1970.
575. Johnson GF: Osteoid osteoma of the femoral neck. Am J Roentgenol *74*:65, 1955.
576. Lawrie TR, Aterman K, Sinclair AM: Painless osteoid osteoma; a report of 2 cases. J Bone Joint Surg *52A*:1357, 1970.
577. Marcove RC, Freiberger RH: Osteoid osteoma of the elbow. A diagnostic problem: Report of 4 cases. J Bone Joint Surg *48A*:1185, 1966.
578. Sherman MS: Osteoid osteoma associated with changes in an adjacent joint. Report of two cases. J Bone Joint Surg *29*:483, 1947.
579. Snarr JW, Abell MR, Martel W: Lymphofollicular synovitis with osteoid osteoma. Radiology *106*:557, 1973.
580. Spence AJ, Lloyd-Roberts GC: Regional osteoporosis in osteoid osteoma. J Bone Joint Surg *43B*:501, 1961.
581. Lisbona R, Rosenthall L: Role of radionuclide imaging in osteoid osteoma. Am J Roentgenol *132*:77, 1979.
582. Mitnick JS, Genieser NB: Osteoid osteoma of the hip; unusual isotopic appearance. Am J Roentgenol *133*:322, 1979.
583. Winter PF, Johnson PM, Hilal SK, Feldman F: Scintigraphic detection of osteoid osteoma. Radiology *122*:177, 1978.
584. Lateur L, Baert AL: Localization and diagnosis of osteoid osteoma of the carpal area by angiography. Skel Radiol *2*:75, 1977.
585. O'Hara JP III, Tegtmeyer C, Sweet DE, McCue FC: Angiography in the diagnosis of osteoid-osteoma of the hand. J Bone Joint Surg *57A*:163, 1975.
586. Lowenstein MB, Smith JRV, Cole S: Infrapatellar pigmented villonodular synovitis: Arthrographic detection. Am J Roentgenol *135*:279, 1980.
587. Kaiser TE, Ivins JC, Unni KK: Malignant transformation of extra-articular synovial chondromatosis: Report of a case. Skel Radiol *5*:223, 1980.

75

SKELETAL METASTASES

by Donald Resnick, M.D., and Gen Niwayama, M.D.

Any primary extraskeletal malignancy can lead to changes in neighboring or distant bones and joints. Most commonly, the skeletal abnormalities result from either extension to and invasion of adjacent osseous tissue or dissemination (metastasis) of tumors to distant osseous sites, usually by the hematogenous route. The bones of the axial skeleton, especially the pelvis and the spine, are frequent sites of metastatic disease,[1-3] although virtually any bone can be affected, including those of the hands and feet[4-13, 59, 60] (Fig. 75–1). Certain malignant tumors have a propensity for skeletal metastasis; included in this group are carcinomas of the prostate, the breast, and the lung (Table 75–1). Furthermore, the osseous response to the neoplastic foci may be purely lytic (e.g., carcinoma of the thyroid gland or kidney), mixed lytic and sclerotic (e.g., carcinoma of the breast or lung), or purely sclerotic (e.g., carcinoma of the prostate, medulloblastoma, or bronchial carcinoid)[14-18] (Figs. 75–2 to 75–4).

The previous chapter has detailed the many neoplastic and pseudoneoplastic processes that can affect articular and periarticular tissue. Included in these processes are skeletal metastases. The manner in which metastatic lesions affect synovial and carti-

Text continued on page 2759

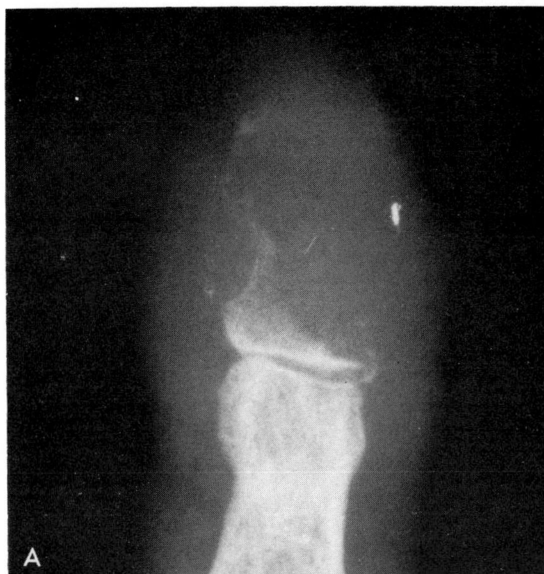

Figure 75–1. *Skeletal metastasis: Hands and feet.*

A *Bronchogenic carcinoma may metastasize to the phalanges of the hand and the foot. Extensive lysis of the terminal phalanx of the finger is associated with considerable soft tissue swelling. The articular space appears uninvolved.*

B *This patient presented to the emergency room with wrist pain. Subsequently it was learned that chest radiography had revealed a lung tumor, which proved to be carcinomatous. Note the lytic lesions of the capitate and trapezium (arrows), which are poorly defined and unassociated with sclerosis. The preservation of the joint spaces favors a diagnosis of tumor rather than pyogenic infection.*

C *The lytic lesion of the cuboid (arrows) extends to but does not violate the adjacent articular surfaces. Fragmentation and mild surrounding sclerosis with soft tissue swelling are evident. This bony defect was related to a metastatic focus of adenocarcinoma.*

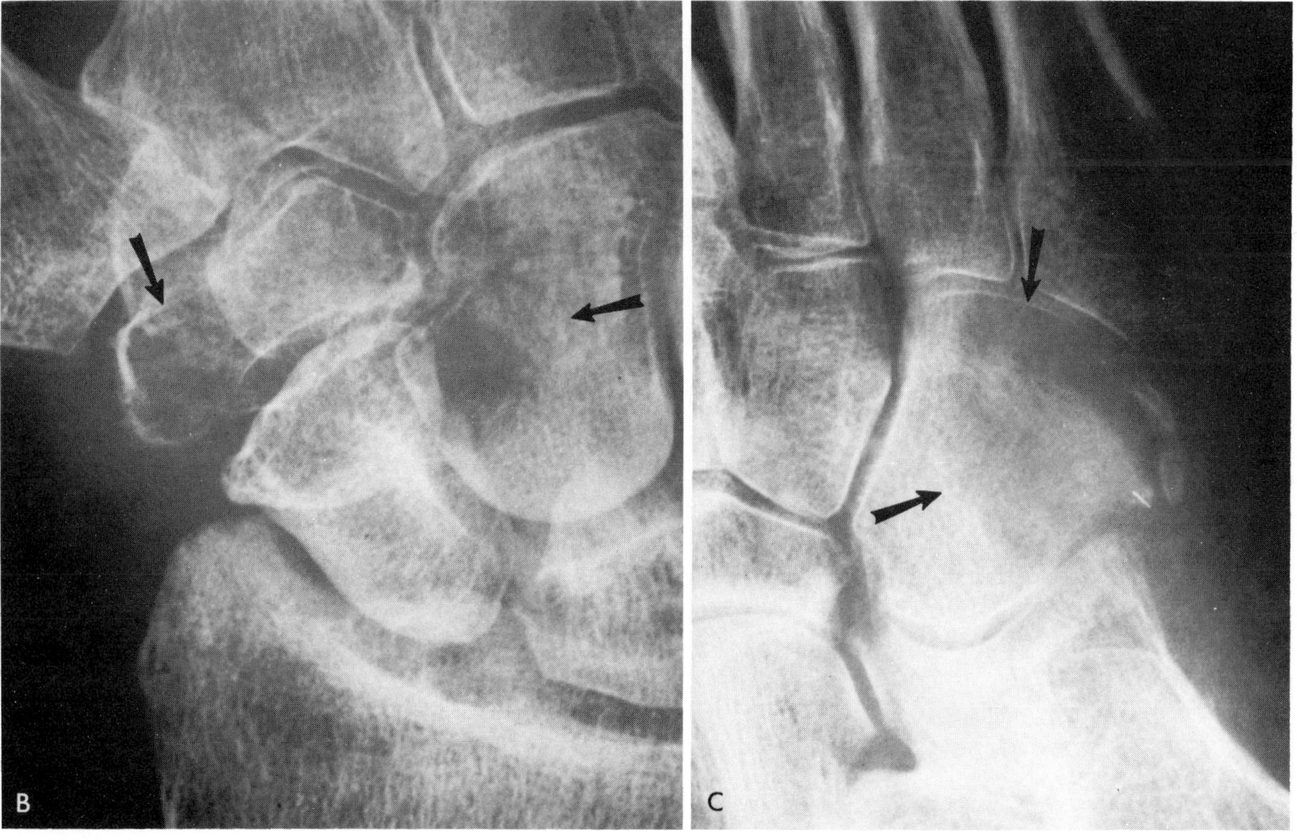

Table 75–1
SKELETAL METASTASIS*

Primary Focus	Usual Type of Skeletal Metastasis	Relative Frequency			
		VERY COMMON	*COMMON*	*INFREQUENT*	*RARE*
BREAST	Lytic and mixed	×			
LUNG					
Carcinoma	Predominantly lytic	×			
Carcinoid	Predominantly bone-forming		×		
GENITOURINARY					
Kidney					
Carcinoma	Lytic, expanding	×			
Wilms' tumor	Lytic				×
Prostate	Predominantly bone-forming; lytic in older age group	×			
Urinary bladder	Predominantly lytic; bone-forming if prostate involved			×	
Adrenal					
Pheochromocytoma	Lytic, expanding				×
Carcinoma	Lytic				×
MALE AND FEMALE REPRODUCTIVE SYSTEMS					
Uterus: Corpus	Lytic			×	
Cervix	Lytic or mixed			×	
Ovary	Predominantly lytic, occasionally bone-forming				×
Testis	Predominantly lytic, occasionally bone-forming			×	
THYROID	Lytic, expanding		×		
GASTROINTESTINAL TRACT					
Esophagus	Lytic				×
Stomach	Bone-forming or mixed			×	
Colon	Predominantly lytic; occasionally bone-forming		×		
Rectum	Predominantly lytic			×	
Biliary tree	Lytic				×
Pancreas	Lytic				×
Liver (hepatoma)	Lytic				×
HEAD, NECK, AND CENTRAL NERVOUS SYSTEM					
Brain	Lytic or bone-forming (usually after craniotomy)				×
Neuroblastoma	Lytic, mixed, or bone-forming	×			
Paranasal sinuses	Lytic				×
Nasopharynx	Lytic or bone-forming			×	
Salivary glands	Lytic				×
Chordoma	Lytic				×
SKIN					
Squamous cell carcinoma	Lytic				×
Melanoma	Lytic, expanding			×	
MALIGNANT NEOPLASMS OF BONE OR SOFT TISSUES					
Osteosarcoma	Lytic or bone-forming				×
Chondrosarcoma	Lytic or mixed				×
Ewing's tumor	Lytic, permeating	×			
Fibrosarcoma	Lytic				×
Vascular neoplasms (hemangiosarcoma, hemangiopericytoma)	Lytic			×	

*From Murray RO, Jacobsen HG: Metastatic disease of the skeleton. *In* The Radiology of Skeletal Disorders. 2nd Ed. Edinburgh, Churchill Livingstone, 1977, p 586.

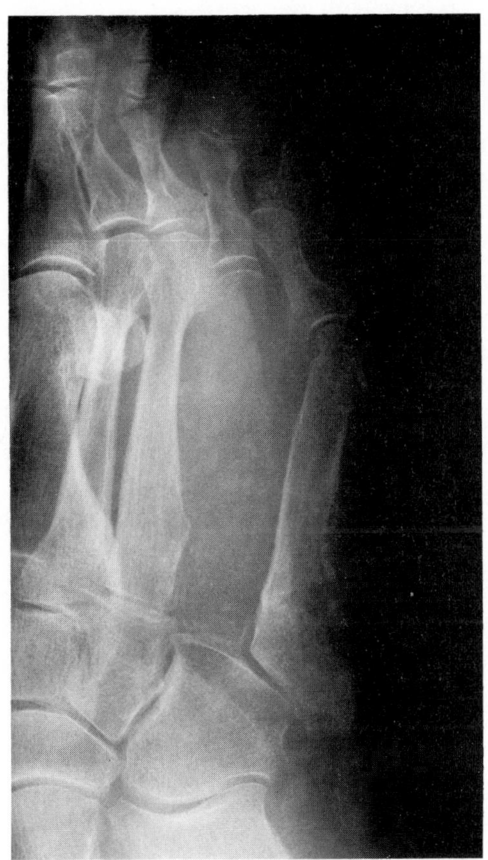

Figure 75–2. *Skeletal metastasis: Purely lytic pattern. The entire fourth metatarsal reveals lytic destruction, and a similar lesion is present at the base of the fifth metatarsal. A poorly differentiated adenocarcinoma of unknown origin was responsible for the defects.*

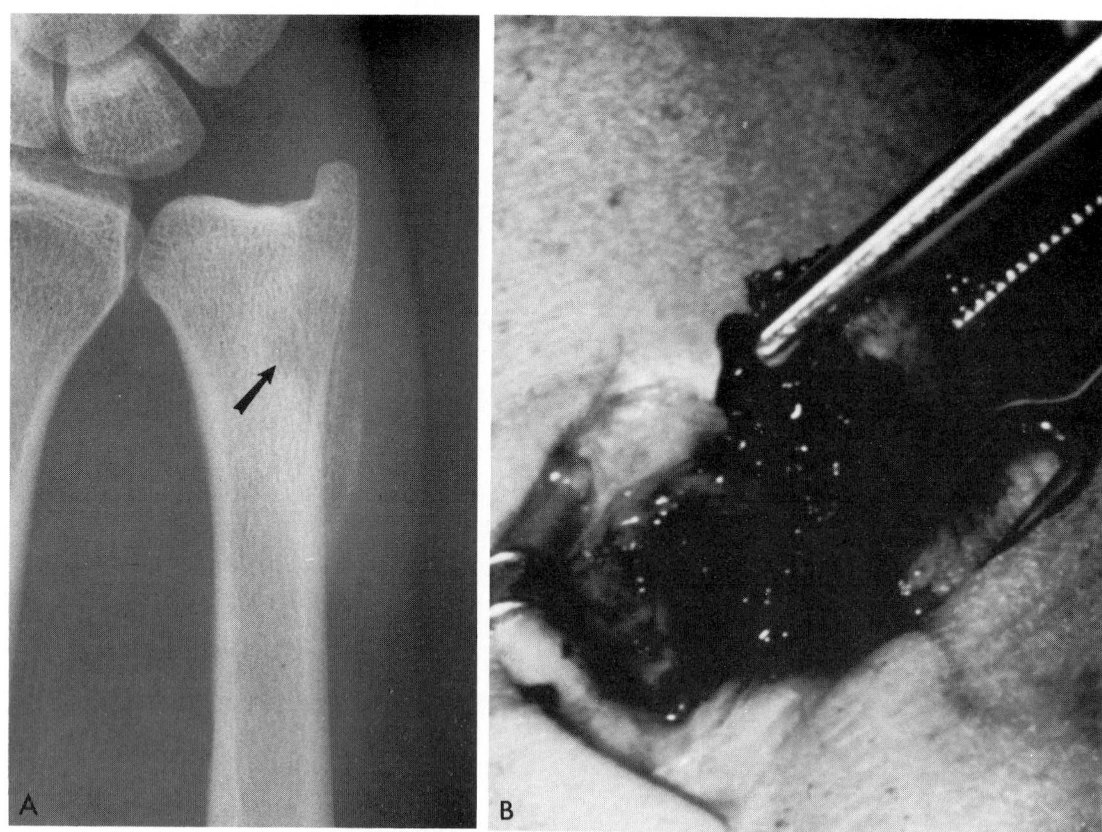

Figure 75–3. *Skeletal metastasis: Mixed lytic and sclerotic pattern. This 23 year old man presented with pain and swelling over the distal ulna. His pertinent history included the removal of a skin "cyst" several years previously.*

A *On initial evaluation, a moth-eaten or permeative destructive lesion with lysis and sclerosis of the distal ulna (arrow) is found to be associated with adjacent periosteal proliferation and soft tissue swelling. At this time, no other osseous lesions were identified, and a preoperative diagnosis of a primary malignant tumor, probably Ewing's sarcoma, was made.*

B *An operative photograph delineates a lesion of the distal ulna containing melanin (held by upper clamp), which on histologic evaluation was diagnosed as a malignant melanoma, presumably originating from the cutaneous lesion that had previously been removed. Within months, the patient developed widespread skeletal metastasis.*

Illustration continued on the opposite page

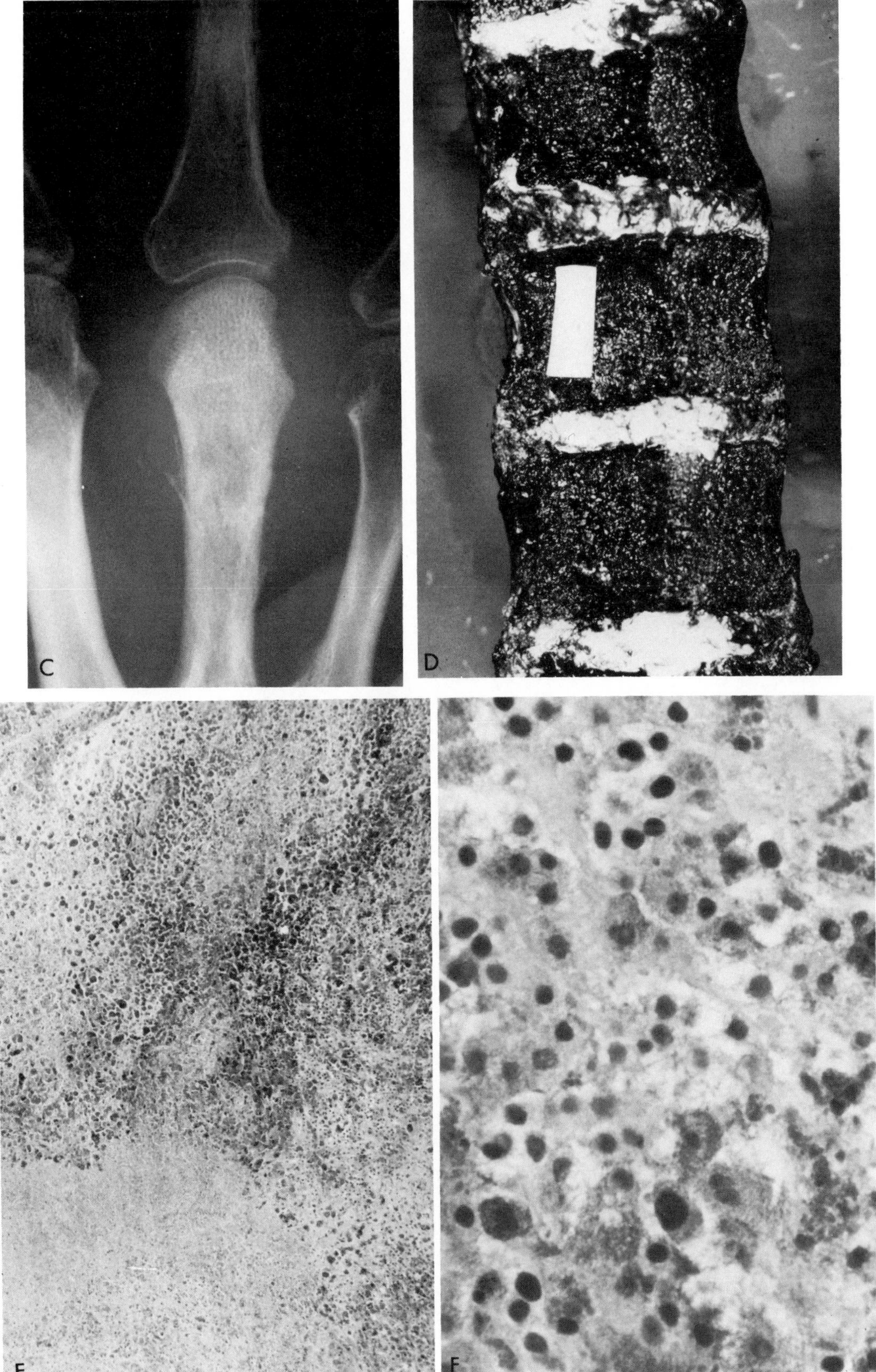

Figure 75–3. Continued

C *A subsequent skeletal survey outlined a destructive mixed lytic-sclerotic lesion of the metacarpal and proximal phalanx of the third finger, with periostitis and soft tissue swelling, as well as additional osseous metastasis.*

D *At the time of autopsy, diffuse involvement with melanotic lesions is evident on this photograph of a coronal section of the spine. Pigmentation extends into several of the intervertebral discs.*

E, F *Photomicrographs (90×, 900×) show metastatic melanoma diffusely replacing osseous and periosseous tissues. The melanoma cells vary in size and contain varying amounts of melanin pigment in the cytoplasm.*

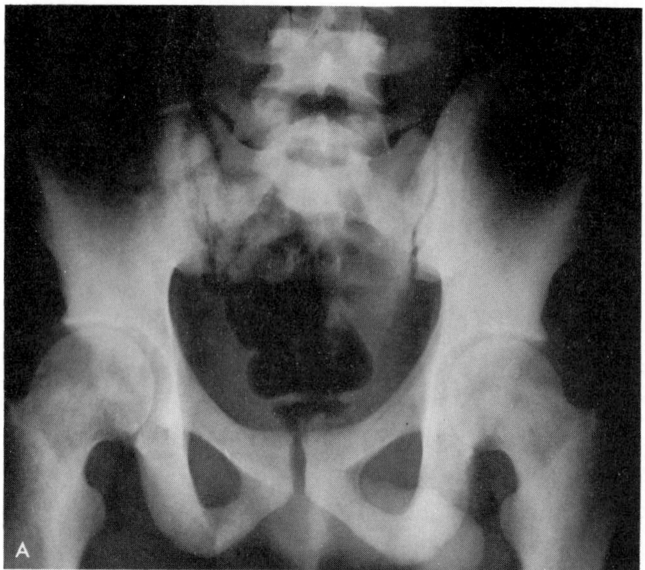

Figure 75–4. *Skeletal metastasis: Purely sclerotic pattern. This 36 year old man with gastric carcinoma developed widespread osteoblastic skeletal lesions, predominating in the axial skeleton. The radiograph of the pelvis* **(A)** *demonstrates a uniform increase in radiodensity of all the bones. A radiograph* **(B)** *and photograph* **(C)** *of a sagittal section of the spine indicate the extent of osteoblastic metastasis. A photomicrograph (***D***, 90×) shows that the marrow spaces of a vertebral body are replaced by metastatic adenocarcinoma.*

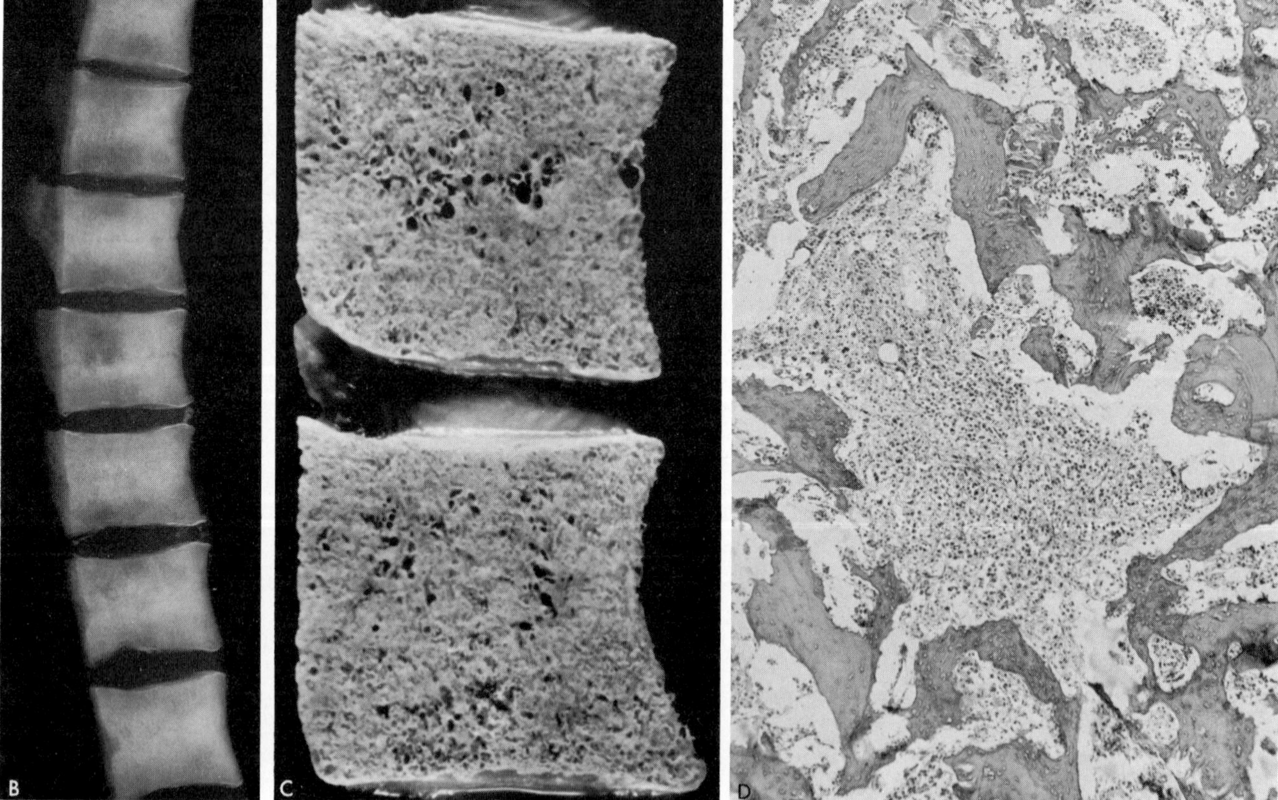

laginous joints is further delineated in the following pages. A certain degree of overlap of material contained in these two chapters is provided for emphasis.

SYNOVIAL JOINTS

Skeletal Metastasis to Periarticular Bone

Metastases to periarticular foci about synovial joints are not infrequent. Such deposits are typically encountered in the hip,[19] the shoulder,[20] and the knee[21]; at these sites and others, tumors can lead to symptoms and signs simulating arthritis.[22] The clinical manifestations may be derived from osseous foci that have not altered in any fashion the adjacent articulation, from foci that have led to disruption and collapse of the nearby articular surface, or from foci that have produced a non-neoplastic reaction within the neighboring articulation. (A fourth possibility, that of neoplastic involvement of the joint itself, is discussed later in this chapter.)

Roentgenograms reveal a lytic or sclerotic epiphyseal focus that may extend down to the subchondral bone (Figs. 75–5 to 75–7). Its appearance may be reminiscent of that of a subchondral "cyst," which may be observed in a variety of articular processes, such as rheumatoid arthritis, osteoarthritis, pigmented villonodular synovitis, and gout, a primary bone tumor such as a giant cell tumor or chondroblastoma, plasma cell myeloma, or an intraosseous ganglion. At times, weakening of bone beneath the cartilage, especially in a weight-bearing articulation, will promote osseous collapse and fragmentation identical to the findings in osteonecrosis or neuroarthropathy. Accurate clinical and radiographic diagnosis frequently depends upon the presence of a known primary tumor and the detection of additional sites of skeletal metastasis. Biopsy of the skeletal lesion may be required.

Inflammation of synovial tissue in proximity to metastatic tumor is unusual.[21] This finding should be differentiated from neoplastic involvement of the synovium and from synovial reaction in hypertrophic osteoarthropathy, although the histologic appearance of the synovial membrane in the latter condition may be identical to that associated with a neighboring skeletal metastatic site[23] (Fig. 75–8). A

Text continued on page 2765

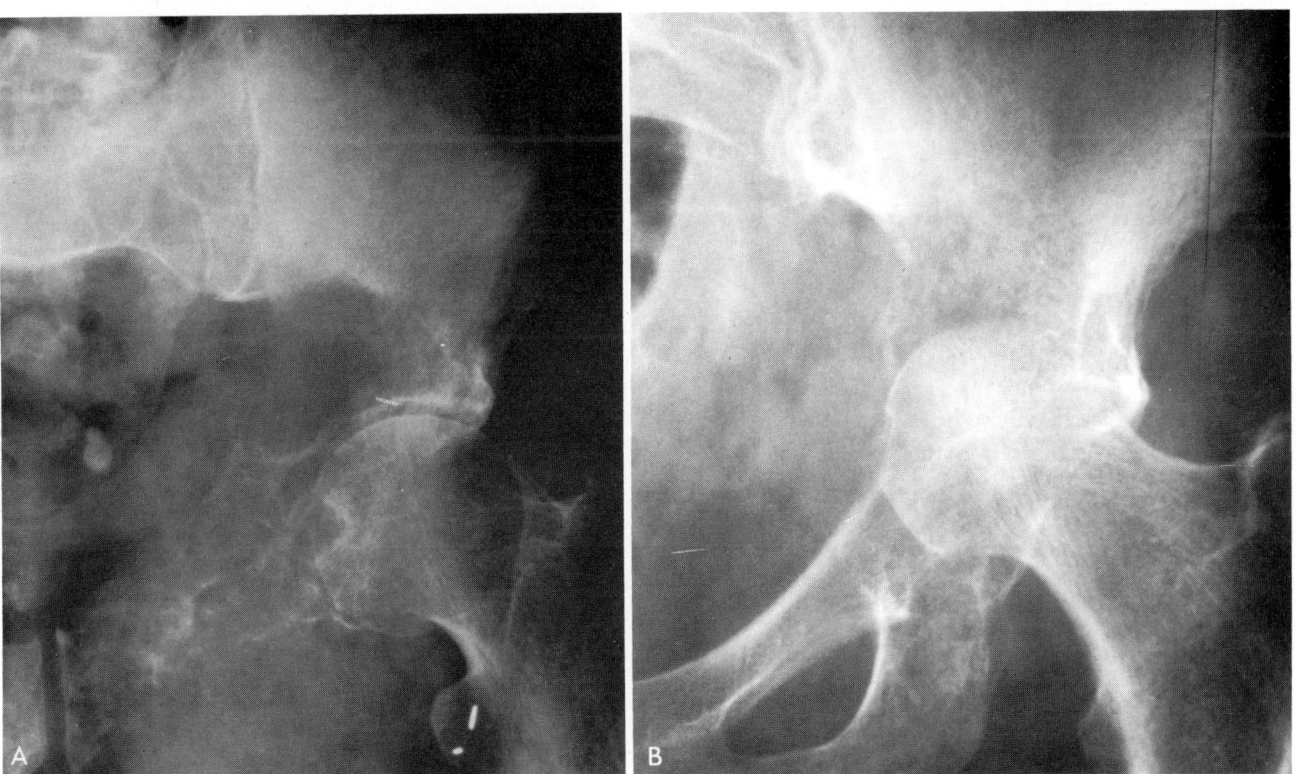

Figure 75–5. *Skeletal metastasis to periarticular bone: Hip.*

A *In this 55 year old woman, the large lytic lesion of the pelvis is related to metastasis from a renal cell carcinoma. Prominent soft tissue swelling is evident. Remarkably, the hip joint is relatively maintained.*

B *This 65 year old woman developed a destructive lesion of the left hemipelvis, which was due to metastasis (or direct invasion) from a clear cell carcinoma of the uterus. The loss of acetabular support has allowed inward protrusion of the femoral head.* (**B**, Courtesy of Dr. R. Taketa, Bauer Hospital, Long Beach, California.)

Illustration continued on the following page

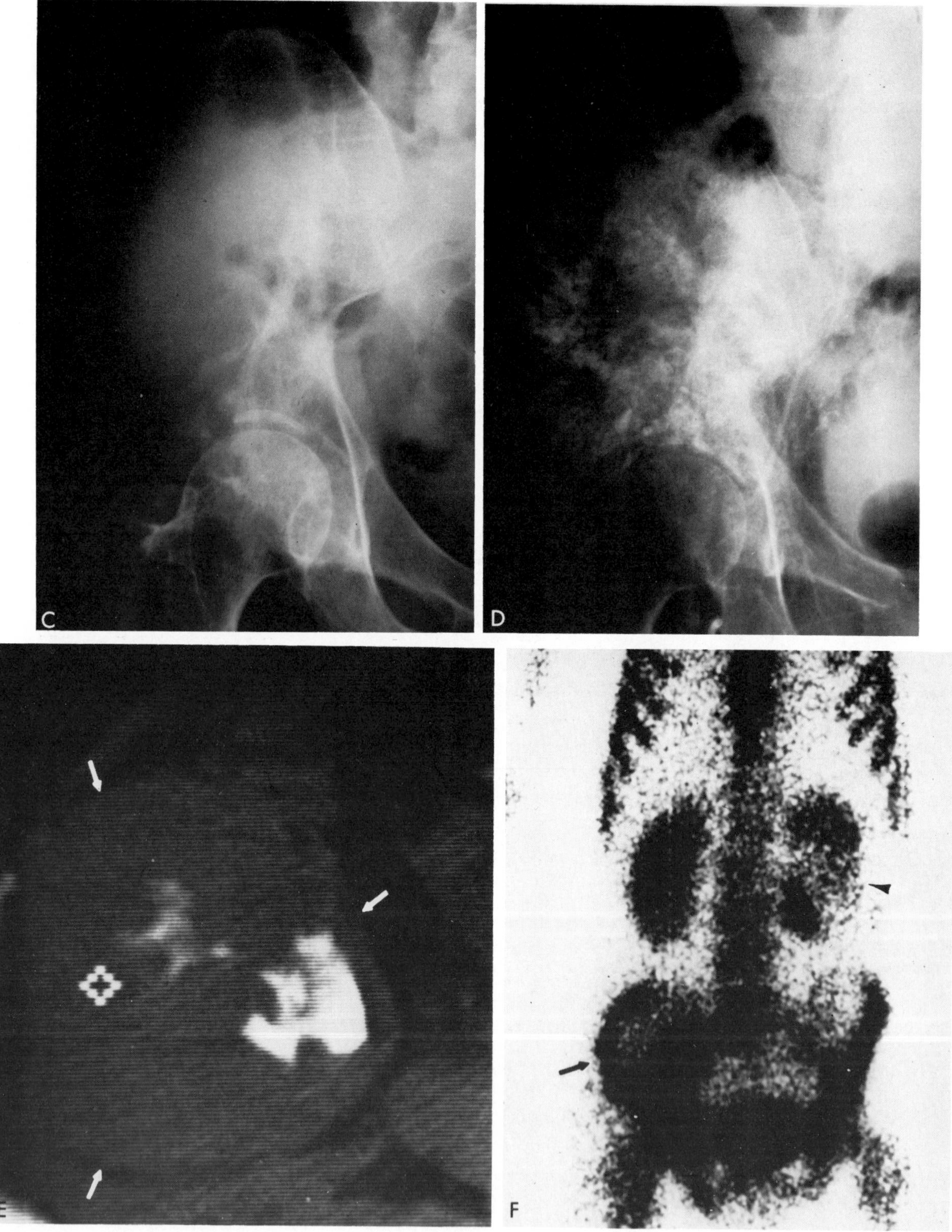

Figure 75–5. Continued

C–F *This man presented with right hip pain and a soft tissue mass. The initial radiograph* **(C)** *reveals an expansile osteolytic lesion of the right ilium extending to the subchondral acetabular bone. Angiography* **(D)** *demonstrates its vascular nature. On computed tomography* **(E)**, *the extent of iliac destruction and the size of the mass (arrows) are seen. A bone scan* **(F)** *outlines increased accumulation of radionuclide in the ilium (arrow) and a defect in the left kidney (arrowhead). Biopsy of the kidney and bone lesion documented the presence of renal carcinoma metastatic to the skeleton. Large, solitary, vascular metastatic lesions are not unusual with renal carcinoma.*

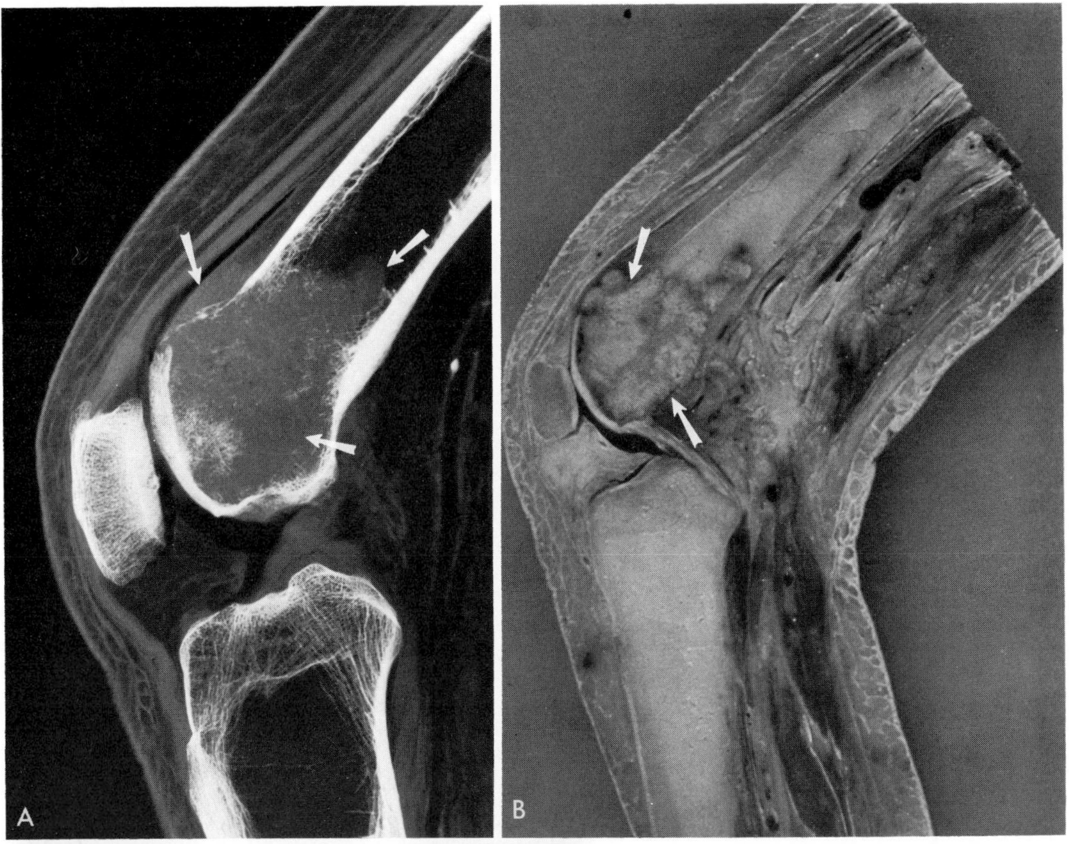

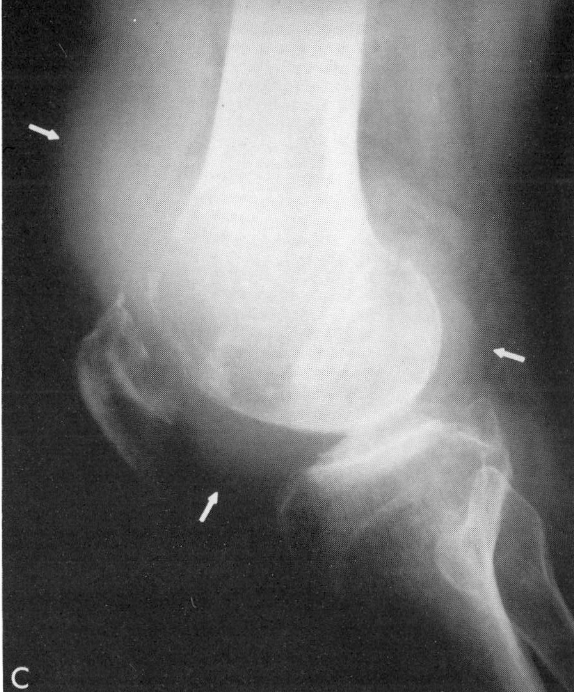

Figure 75–6. *Skeletal metastasis to periarticular bone: Knee.*

A, B *An unexpected finding in this cadaver donated to an anatomy laboratory was an adenocarcinoma of the colon metastatic to the femur. A radiograph and photograph of a sagittal section of the femur, patella, and tibia indicate the extent of the lesion (arrows). It violates the anterior femoral cortex but does not extend distally into the joint.*

(Courtesy of Dr. M, Pitt, University of Arizona, Tucson, Arizona.)

C *In another patient, a large osteolytic lesion of the distal femur is associated with a large joint effusion or mass (arrows). Biopsy indicated anaplastic carcinoma involving bone extending into the articular cavity with hemarthrosis.*

(Courtesy of Dr. V. Vint, Scripps Clinic, La Jolla, California.)

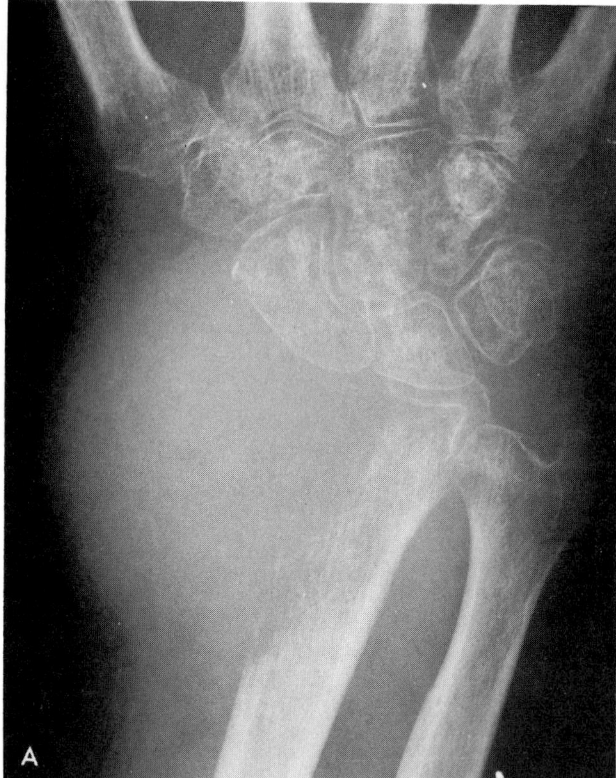

Figure 75–7. *Skeletal metastasis to periarticular bone: Wrist. This 63 year old man with known carcinoma of the lung developed left arm and wrist pain and swelling. Because of the debilitating nature of the pain, the forearm was resected following radiation therapy.*

A *An initial radiograph reveals the extent of the radial lesion. It has produced permeative bone destruction and extends into the soft tissues, with considerable mass effect. Patchy osteoporosis of the carpus is identified.*

B *A radiograph of a coronal section of the forearm delineates the permeative nature of the radial destruction.*

C *A photograph of the sectioned specimen demonstrates the extent of the radial tumor. Note that it has expanded the distal radius (solid arrow), destroyed a portion of the articular cartilage of the radius (open arrows), and enveloped surrounding tendons (arrowhead). The carpus is free of tumor.*

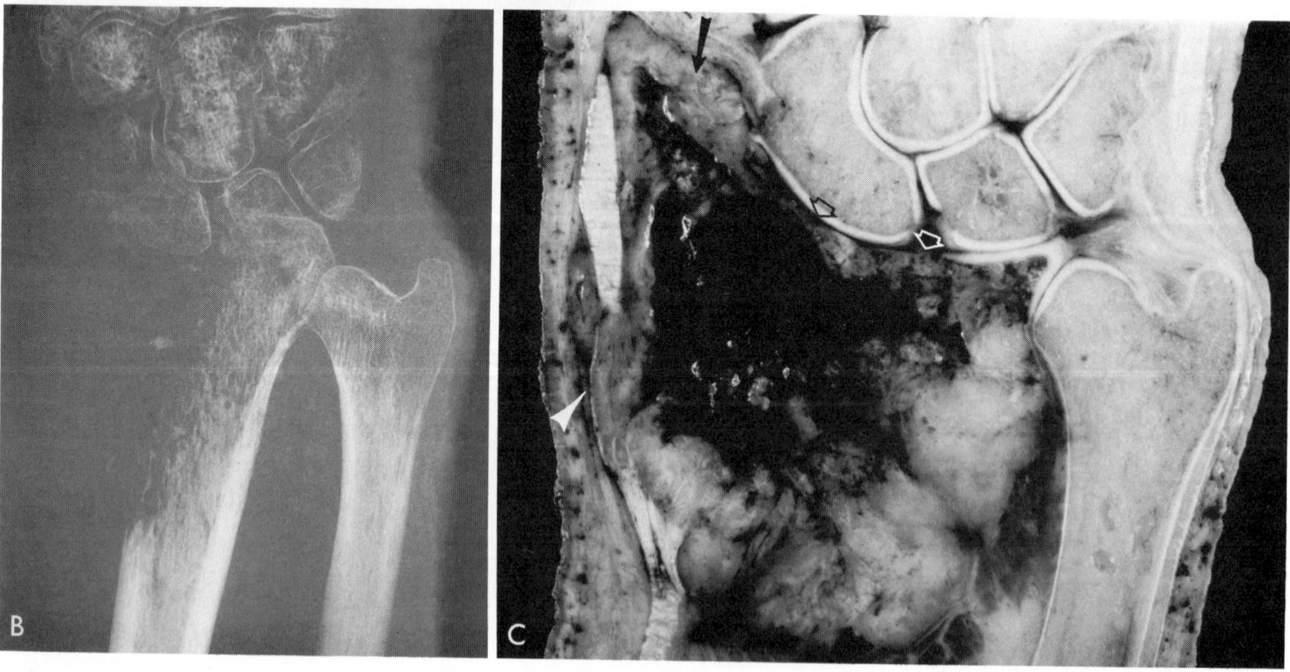

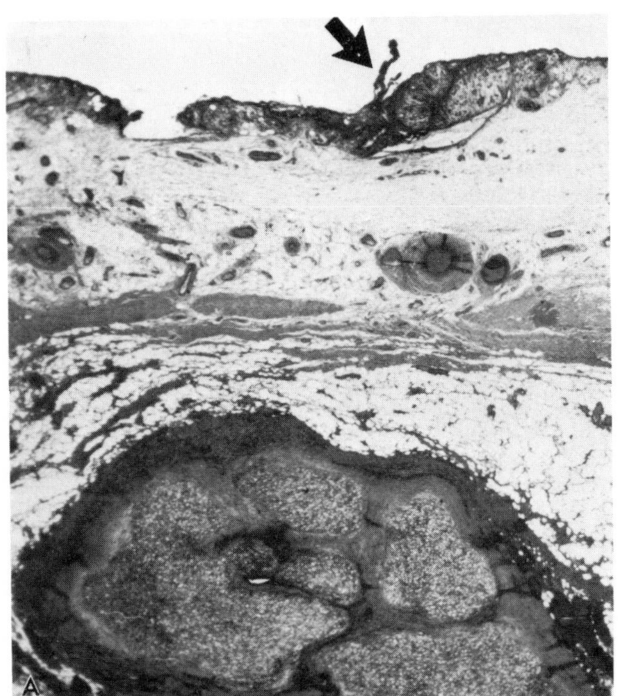

Figure 75–8. *Synovial reaction to malignant and benign tumors.*

A *Chondrosarcoma. A 70 year old man had a disarticulation for a chondrosarcoma of the inferior right femoral metaphysis. The subsynovial tissue is invaded by neoplasm, and the synovial lining is edematous with cellular hyperplasia and superficial fibrin deposits (arrow).* (**A**, *From Lagier R: J Rheumatol 4:65, 1977.*)

Illustration continued on the following page

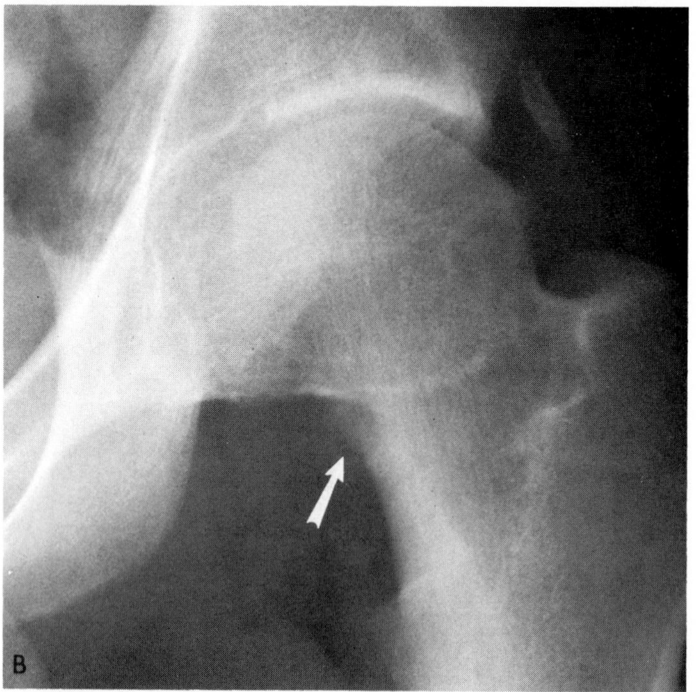

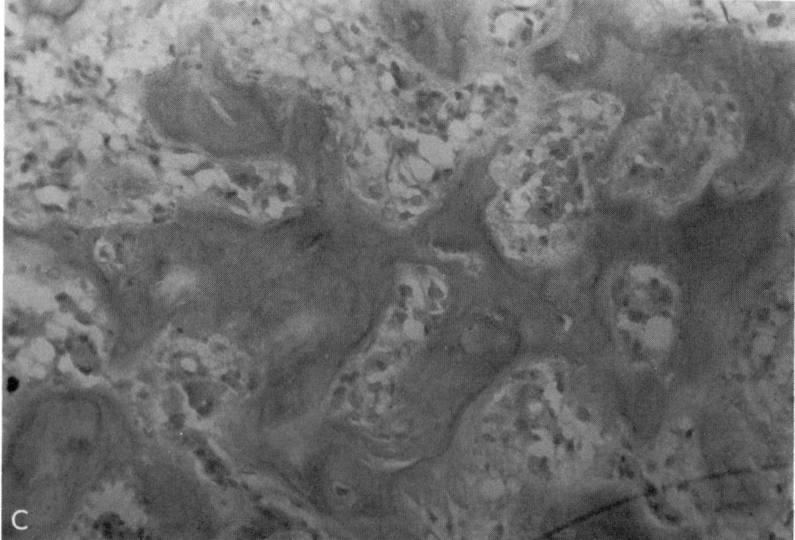

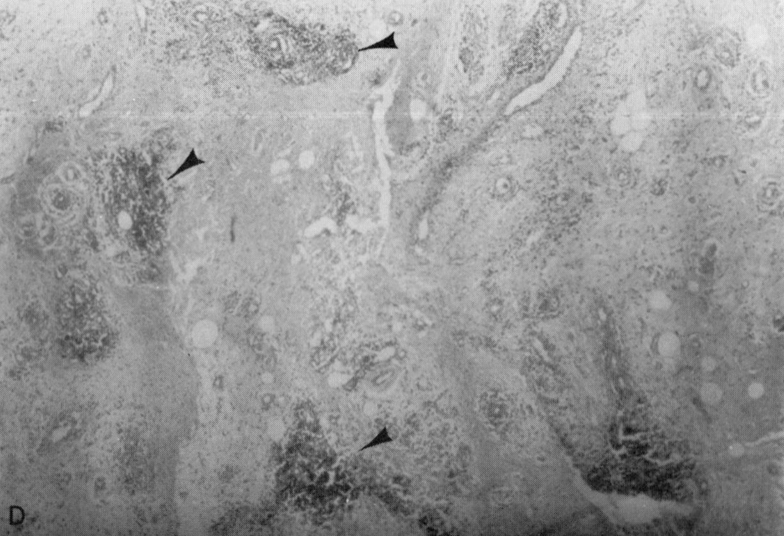

Figure 75–8. Continued

B–D *Intra-articular osteoid osteoma. The lytic lesion, eccentrically located in the medial femoral neck (arrow), is an osteoid osteoma. This neoplasm, when present within or near a joint, can evoke a synovitis. In this 21 year old man with recurrent hip pain of 2 years' duration, a synovial biopsy had been interpreted as nonspecific chronic synovitis. An additional finding in this case is the presence of osteophytosis of the femoral head, which, along with this osteoid osteoma and synovitis, was confirmed at surgery. A photomicrograph of the osteoid osteoma* **(C)** *reveals the vascular stroma of the nidus. A photomicrograph of the synovial membrane* **(D)** *shows fibrotic stroma with numerous prominent vascular channels and multiple lymphoid accumulations (arrowheads). (***B–D,** *Courtesy of Dr. H. Siegel, Mercy Hospital, San Diego, California.)*

similar synovial reaction can be encountered in conjunction with neighboring benign tumors, such as osteoid osteoma (Fig. 75–8), and malignant tumors, such as leukemia and lymphosarcoma.[24] On histologic examination, hypervascularity and cellular infiltration with lymphocytes and plasma cells are seen.[21] The synovial reaction may be related to tumor release of substances containing enzymatic or antigenic properties, a mechanism that may also be responsible for a rheumatoid arthritis–like carcinomatous polyarthritis that can be associated with a distant neoplastic focus (see discussion later in this chapter).[25]

Skeletal Metastasis to Periarticular Bone with Intra-Articular Extension

A metastatic focus in subchondral bone may extend into the nearby articulation.[19, 26-29] Although this may occur at various locations, it appears to be especially frequent about the knee. In this site, patellar, femoral, or tibial lesions can disrupt the subchondral bone plate, leading to neoplastic involvement of the synovial membrane. On radiographs, the osteolytic or osteosclerotic process is commonly combined with a joint effusion or mass. Arthroscopy may provide more direct visualization of the intra-articular extension of the tumor with nodular irregularities of the contrast-coated synovial membrane.[27] Cytologic study of the synovial fluid may detect cancer cells,[26, 30, 31] and the presence of intra-articular tumor is firmly established on histologic examination of the synovial membrane.

Metastasis to Synovial Membrane

Hematogenous spread of tumor to the synovial membrane with or without adjacent osseous involvement is occasionally encountered.[19, 32] In these instances, monoarthritis may be unaccompanied by any osseous disruption, the radiographs revealing a joint effusion or mass. Analysis of synovial fluid may show malignant cells, and tissue examination confirms the presence of metastatic synovial deposits[56-58] (Fig. 75–9). A similar pattern of synovial extension has been observed in patients with leukemia.[33] Of tumors metastasizing to the synovium, those of the breast and lung do so most frequently. In most instances the existence of a malignancy is known at the time of synovial metastasis, although the subsequent joint manifestations may be misinterpreted as those of rheumatoid arthritis, gout, or infection.

CARTILAGINOUS JOINTS

Osseous metastasis can occur in and around cartilaginous joints. Although this may be observed in relationship to the symphysis pubis or manubriosternal joint (Fig. 75–10), it is most commonly detected at the discovertebral junction. Metastatic deposits in the spine are very frequent; Fornasier and Horne[3] noted pathologic evidence of skeletal metastasis in the vertebral bodies of the thoracolumbar spine in 140 of 374 cases (38 per cent) of malignant neoplasm. The incidence of radiographically evident vertebral metastasis is lower, as it has been repeatedly emphasized that 30 to 50 per cent of bone loss in the vertebral bodies may be required before an abnormality becomes detectable on the roentgenogram.

A basic radiographic and pathologic concept in regard to vertebral metastasis is that the intervertebral disc is relatively resistant to the spread of tumor (Fig. 75–11); the presence of vertebral destruction in the absence of significant disc alteration is a reliable indication of tumor, whereas the presence of vertebral destruction and loss of intervertebral disc space suggests infection. This concept is extremely useful

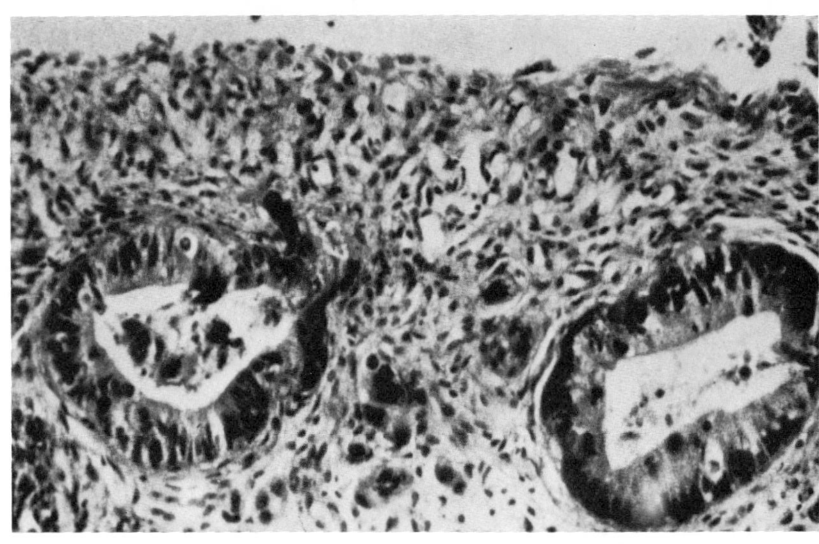

Figure 75–9. Synovial metastasis. This 62 year old man with adenocarcinoma of the sigmoid colon developed pain and swelling of the knee. Although radiographs were negative, synovial aspiration revealed malignant cells, and biopsy showed malignant invasion of the synovium with cells arranged in glandular formation (150 ×). (From Goldenberg DL, et al: Arthritis Rheum 18:107, 1975.)

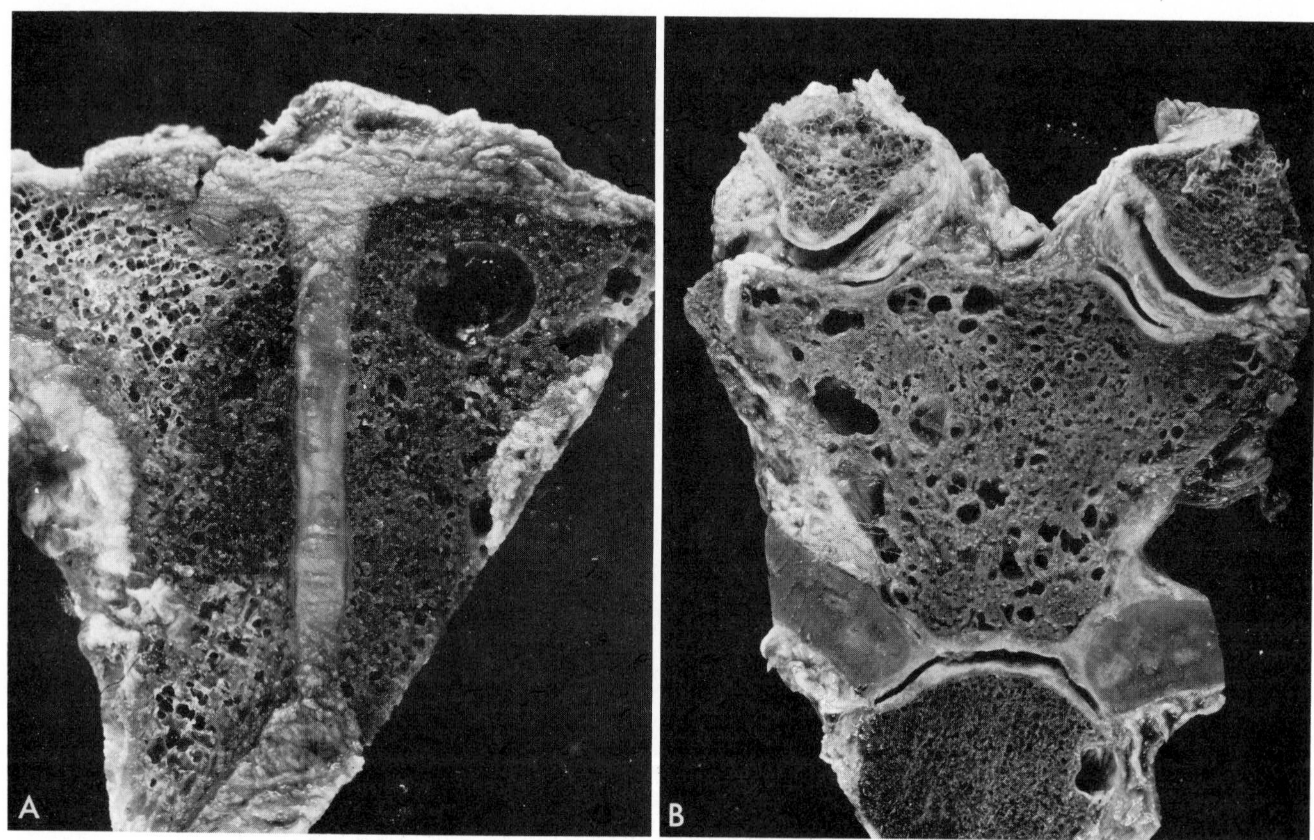

Figure 75–10. *Tumor in periarticular bone: Symphysis pubis and manubriosternal joint. Observe the focal areas of bony destruction about the symphysis pubis and proximal sternum on these coronal sections. This appearance can occur with skeletal metastasis as well as with plasma cell myeloma and other neoplasms.*

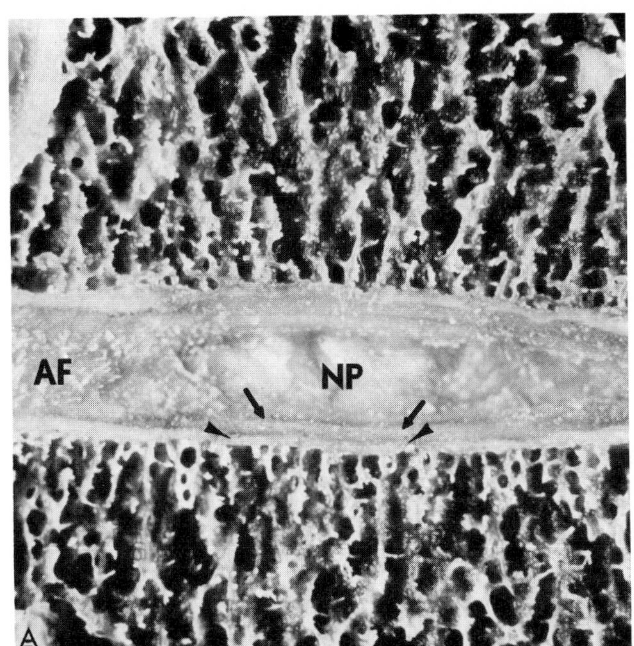

Figure 75–11. *The discovertebral junction: Anatomic considerations.*

A *A coronal section indicates the normal structures of the discovertebral junction. These include the anulus fibrosus (AF), nucleus pulposus (NP), a layer of hyaline cartilage (cartilaginous end-plate) (arrows), and a subchondral bone plate (arrowheads).*

B, C *On nonpolarized* **(B)** *and polarized* **(C)** *photomicrographs (40×), observe the interface of the cartilaginous end-plate (arrow) and subchondral bone (arrowhead). Areas of bone marrow are apposed to the undersurface of the end-plate.*

Illustration continued on the following page

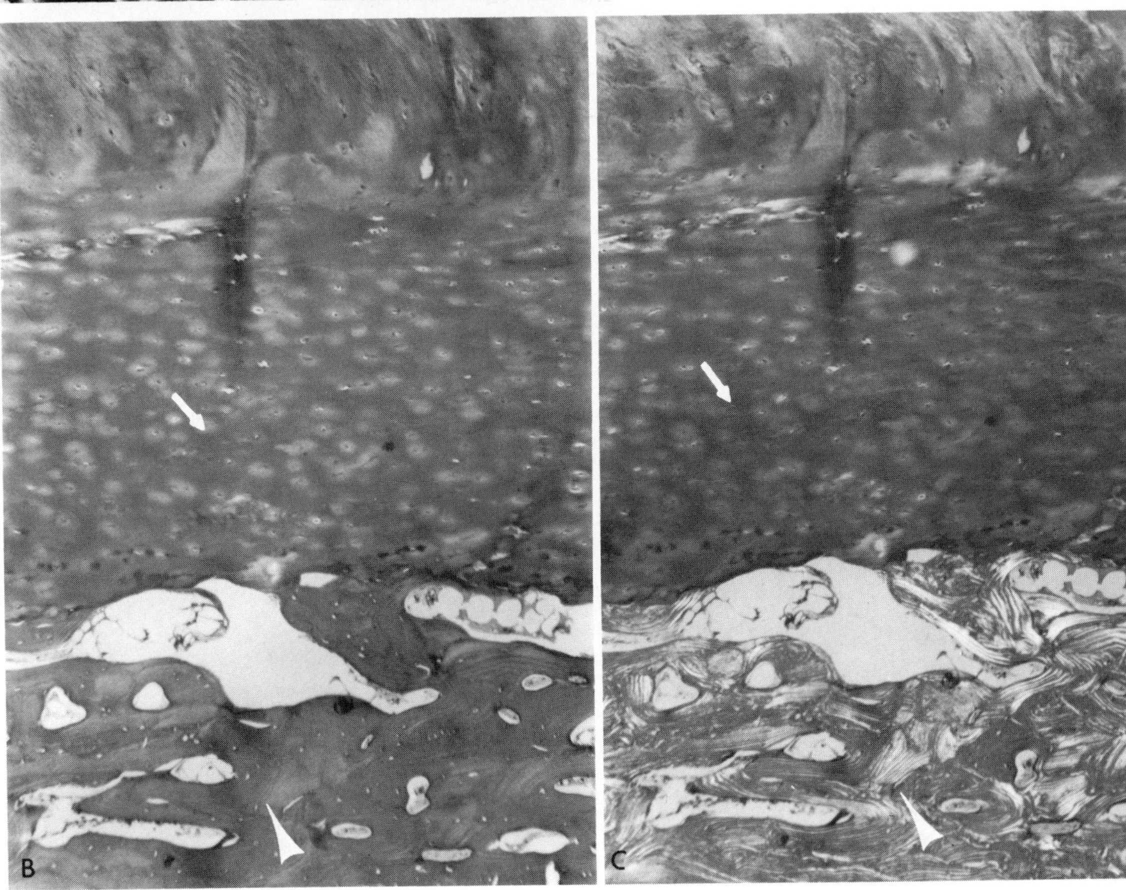

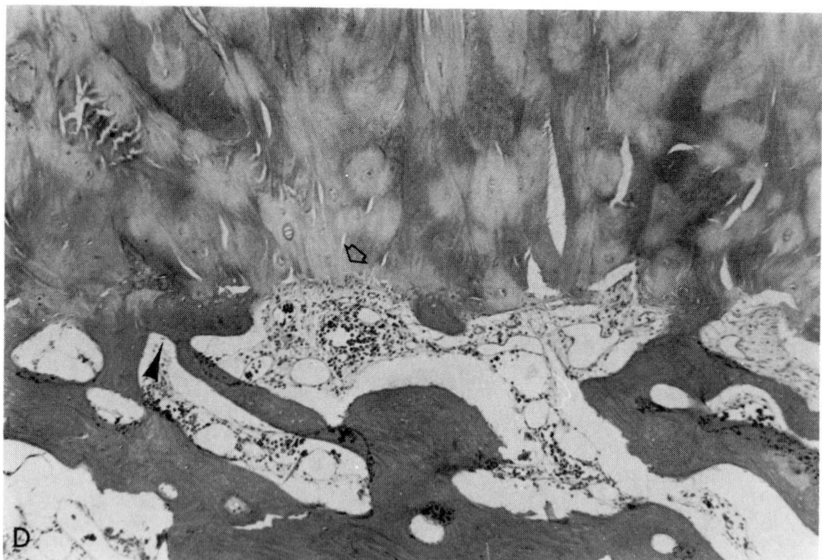

Figure 75–11. Continued

D *This photomicrograph (84×) demonstrates that the thickness of the subchondral bone plate adjacent to the cartilaginous end-plate is extremely variable. In some locations, a definite osseous layer paralleling the cartilaginous end-plate can be identified (arrowhead). In other locations, the bone is extremely thin or absent, allowing direct contact of marrow and nonmineralized cartilage (open arrow).*

but not without exception. In unusual circumstances, tumor may indeed produce abnormality of an intervertebral disc. Discal destruction has been noted in association with plasma cell myeloma, chordoma,[34] and vertebral metastases[35, 36] (Fig. 75–12).

In a radiographic and pathologic study of the vertebral column in 25 cadavers with prostatic carcinoma and spinal metastases, Resnick and Niwayama[37] noted abnormalities of the intervertebral discs in six instances. The discal changes could be classified into three types: intervertebral disc degenera-

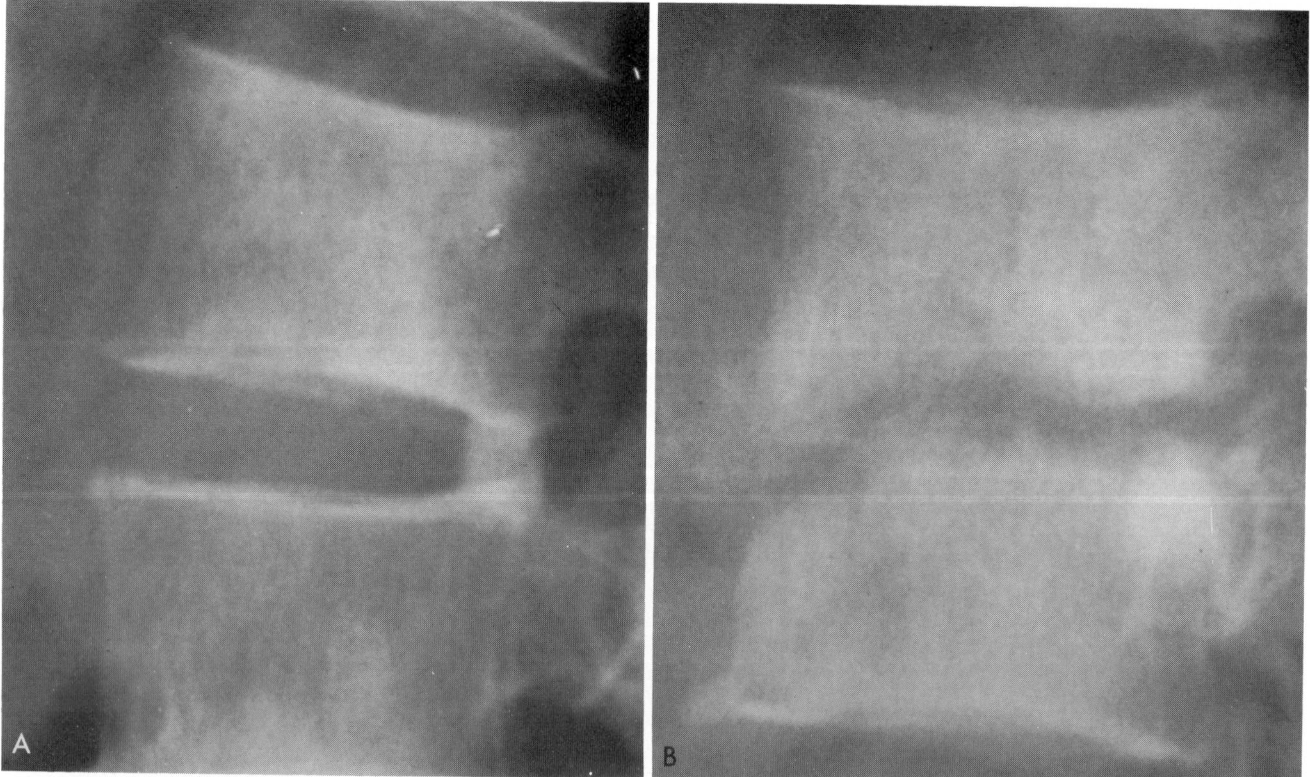

Figure 75–12. Abnormalities of the intervertebral discs in patients with skeletal metastasis.

A, B *This 58 year old man had prostatic carcinoma and metastatic disease in two adjacent vertebral bodies. On the initial radiograph* **(A)**, *sclerotic lesions are apparent within the vertebral bodies, and the intervertebral disc spaces appear normal. On a radiograph obtained 3 months later* **(B)**, *the bony outlines are extremely irregular and the disc space is narrowed. Biopsies on numerous occasions failed to document the presence of infection.*

Illustration continued on the opposite page

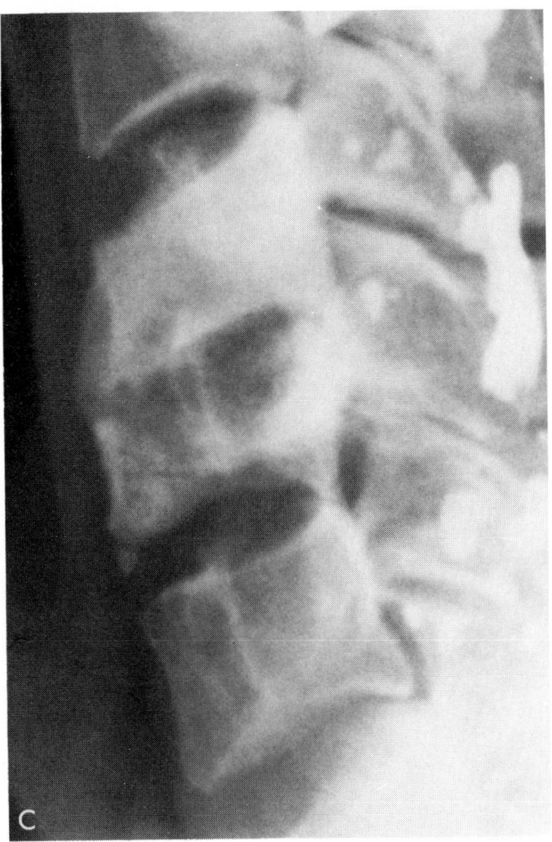

Figure 75–12. Continued

C *In another patient with carcinoma of the prostate and metastatic disease in the cervical spine, sclerotic lesions of two adjacent vertebral bodies are recognized. Both demonstrate partial collapse. The intervertebral disc space appears narrowed and focally obliterated. A myelogram had previously been obtained.*

(From Resnick D, Niwayama G: Invest Radiol 13:182, 1978.)

tion (intervertebral osteochondrosis); cartilaginous (Schmorl's) node formation; and discal invasion by tumor.

Intervertebral Disc Degeneration (Intervertebral Osteochondrosis)

Intervertebral chondrosis and osteochondrosis are terms applied to the various stages of disc degeneration that are frequent in older individuals (see Chapter 40). Disc degeneration involves predominantly the nucleus pulposus and relates to physiologic or pathologic dehydration and desiccation of the nucleus, with progressive cleft formation, discal flattening, and necrosis. Concomitant vertebral changes consist of bone eburnation or sclerosis (Fig. 75–13).

The presence of intervertebral osteochondrosis adjacent to sites of vertebral body metastasis may represent the coincidental occurrence of two not infrequent conditions. In some specimens, however, the location and prominence of disc degeneration at only one level in the spine — adjacent to a vertebral body containing metastatic deposits — are noteworthy. Furthermore, as proper nutrition of the intervertebral disc depends, at least in part, on diffusion of fluid from the marrow space of the vertebral body through the end-plates into the disc, it would appear that tumor within the vertebral body might interfere with proper disc nutrition and lead to its early degeneration. Intervertebral osteochondrosis should be particularly prominent when metastatic deposits within the vertebral body are intimate with the subchondral bone plate. The term secondary intervertebral osteochondrosis is more appropriate in these patients to distinguish this type of discal abnormality from that of primary intervertebral osteochondrosis, a process occurring as a result of gradual aging. The term secondary intervertebral osteochondrosis has already been utilized to describe abnormality of disc tissue that may accompany primary changes outside the disc, such as instability of vertebral arches and alterations in spinal curvature.[38]

Cartilaginous (Schmorl's) Node Formation

Cartilaginous (Schmorl's) nodes represent protrusions of disc material into the adjacent vertebral body, which occur when defects exist in the cartilaginous end-plate. Any disorder that weakens the osseous architecture of the vertebral body may lead to disruption of the cartilaginous end-plate and cartilaginous node formation; this disruption may be accentuated by obvious or occult trauma. Tumor metastasis to the vertebral body can lead to cartilaginous node formation (Fig. 75–14). In these instances, defects within the vertebrae contain a combination of tumor and disc material. If extensive, discal herniation can provide radiographically and pathologically evident disc space loss. It has been suggested that such discal protrusion may predispose the adjacent disc to secondary intervertebral osteochondrosis,[38, 39] which could lead to further disc space loss.

Discal Invasion by Tumor

Neoplasm can locate within the intervertebral disc by (1) tumor implantation related to direct hematogenous spread within the intervertebral disc and (2) invasion of the intervertebral disc from a contiguous source of tumor within the vertebral body. Extensive involvement of the intervertebral disc by tumor is indeed rare. Furthermore, there is rarely evidence of discal metastatic foci without contiguous neoplasm in the vertebral body. Instances of bony metastasis adjacent to the subchondral bone plate are identified with little or no alteration of the bony or cartilaginous end-plate.

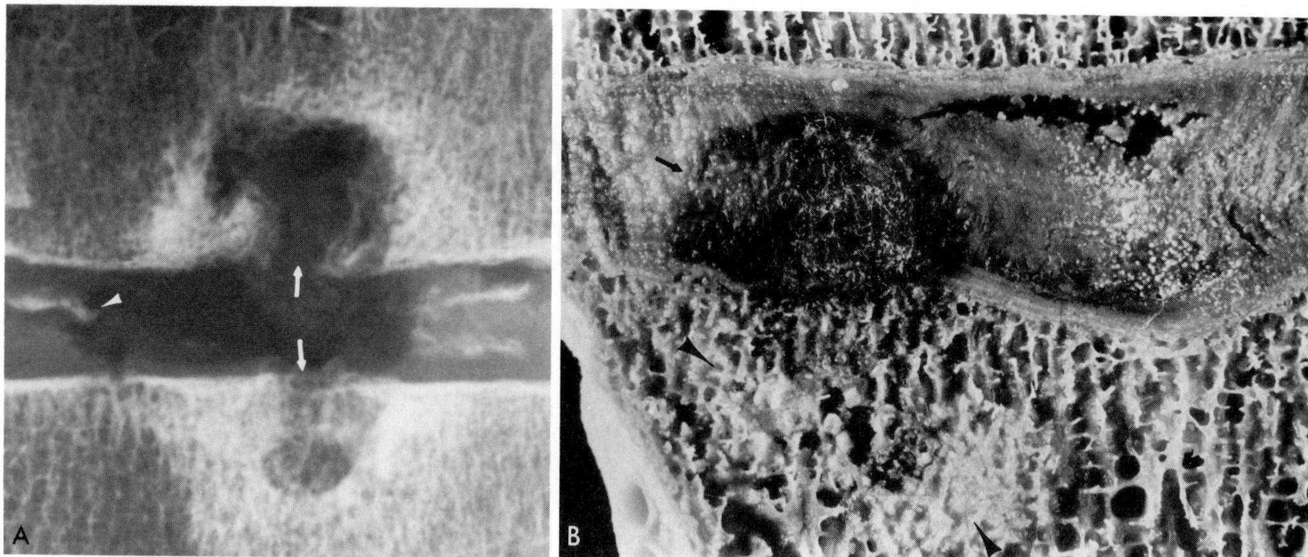

Figure 75–13. *Vertebral metastasis with intervertebral osteochondrosis.*

A *Intervertebral disc degeneration (intervertebral osteochondrosis) is evident in a cadaver with metastatic prostatic carcinoma and sclerotic lesions of two adjacent vertebral bodies. Findings include "vacuum" phenomena and disc calcification (arrowhead), disc space loss, and cartilaginous (Schmorl's) nodes (arrows). These nodes are surrounded by a thin margin of sclerosis, which merges with sclerotic metastatic foci.*

B *In another cadaver, note the sclerotic metastatic deposits (arrowheads). These extend to the subchondral bone. Discoloration and degeneration of the intervertebral disc (arrow) can be seen, presumably related to discal necrosis. No evidence of neoplasm within the disc is seen.*

(From Resnick D, Niwayama G: Invest Radiol 13:182, 1978.)

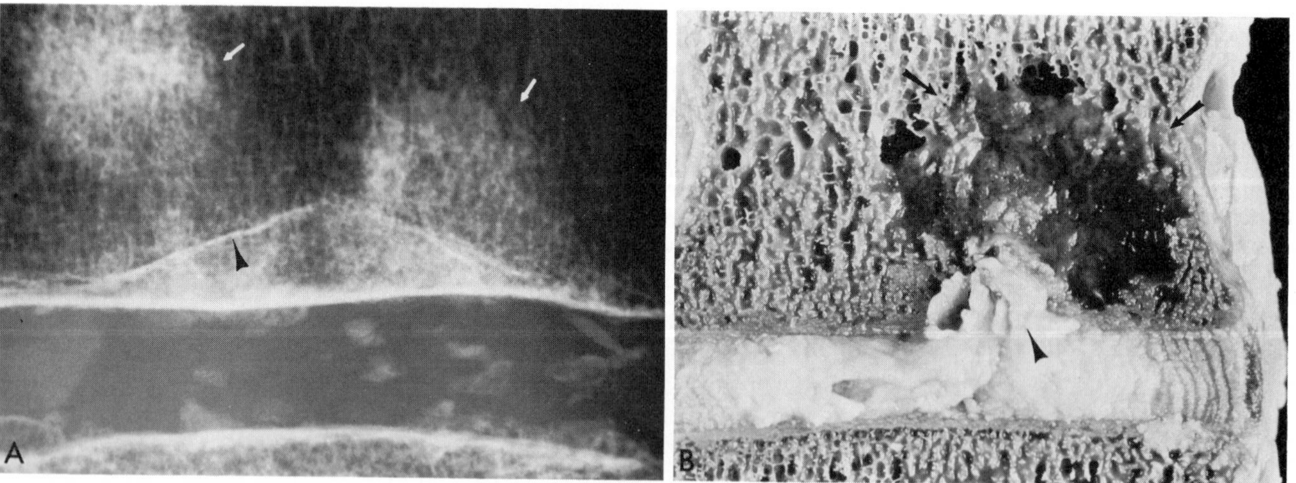

Figure 75–14. *Vertebral metastasis with cartilaginous node formation.*

A *Magnification radiograph outlines a cartilaginous node (arrowhead) producing a contour defect along the inferior surface of the vertebral body. Note the adjacent metastatic lesions (arrows).*

B *In an additional cadaver, metastasis has produced considerable destruction of a large segment of the vertebral body (arrows). Note the herniation of intervertebral disc material into the osseous defect (arrowhead).*

(From Resnick D, Niwayama G: Invest Radiol 13:182, 1978.)

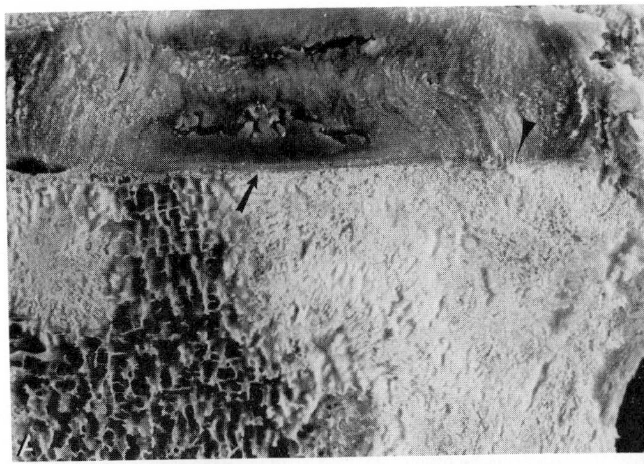

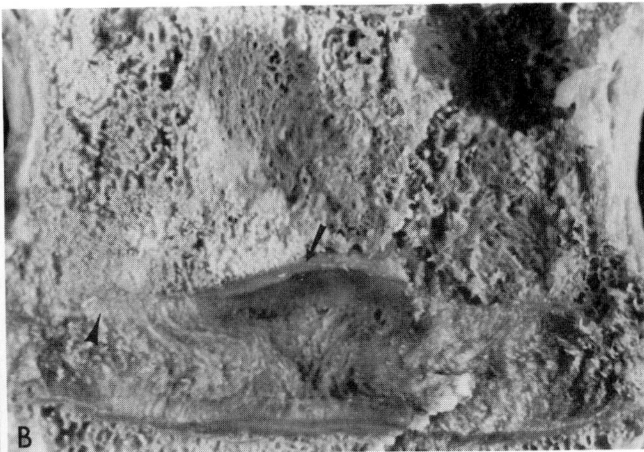

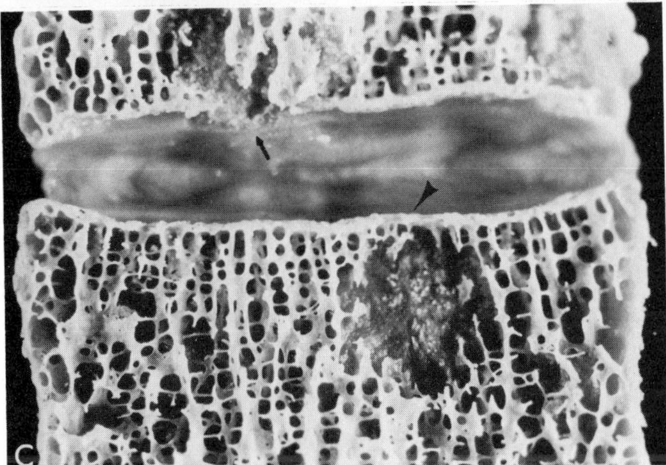

Figure 75–15. Vertebral metastasis with discal invasion by tumor.

A Sclerotic metastatic foci are apparent. Observe that these lesions extend to the cartilaginous end-plate. This latter structure appears intact in most areas (arrow). At the peripheral portion of the vertebral body, tumor has obscured the interface between intervertebral disc and bony plate (arrowhead).

B In another cadaver, widespread metastatic lesions can be seen. Portions of the cartilaginous end-plate appear intact (arrow), whereas the bone plate at the margins of the vertebra is destroyed (arrowhead).

C Metastatic lesions in two adjacent vertebral bodies are associated with varying changes in the subchondral bone plate. In some locations, the plate appears intact (arrowhead); elsewhere, it is disrupted (arrow).

Illustration continued on the following page

Additionally, examples can be noted of disruption of the bone plate (and less frequently, cartilaginous end-plate) by tumor and discal extension of tumor through normal gaps where marrow is continuous with cartilage (Fig. 75–15). Although in almost all instances neoplastic involvement of the intervertebral discs, when present, appears to result from tumor invasion from the adjacent vertebral body, isolated tumor localization at the peripheral portion of a discovertebral junction can rarely be identified.

Synopsis of the Metastatic Process

These observations indicate that mechanisms for alteration of the intervertebral disc in association with vertebral metastasis include (1) intervertebral disc degeneration (intervertebral osteochondrosis); (2) cartilaginous (Schmorl's) node formation; and (3) discal invasion by tumor. Intervertebral osteochondrosis may occur as an incidental finding, unrelated to the presence of bony metastasis in a neighboring vertebral body. However, adjacent vertebral metastatic foci may apparently interfere with proper diffusion of nutrients from the vertebral body to the intervertebral disc and thus produce extensive disc degeneration. Cartilaginous node formation associated with vertebral metastasis is not unexpected. These discal protrusions relate to weakening of osseous structure and are more prevalent with increased destruction of the vertebral body. Discal invasion by tumor is not common, a fact that may relate to avascularity of the intervertebral disc and perhaps some additional inherent quality of cartilage that inhibits tumor growth. When present within the intervertebral disc, tumor is usually associated with spread from a contiguous source within the vertebra rather than hematogenous spread directly to the intervertebral disc. Once neoplastic tissue reaches the intervertebral disc, the advancing tumor may utilize existing tears for further dissemination.

Although the study by Resnick and Niwayama was confined to an investigation of patients and cadavers with metastasis from carcinoma of the prostate, it is expected that similar abnormalities may be associated with vertebral metastasis of tumors derived from other primary sites. However, as hematogenous spread of metastasis from pelvic organs such as the prostate may relate to the peculiar anatomy of the venous plexus of the vertebral column,[40, 41] the incidence and distribution of vertebral

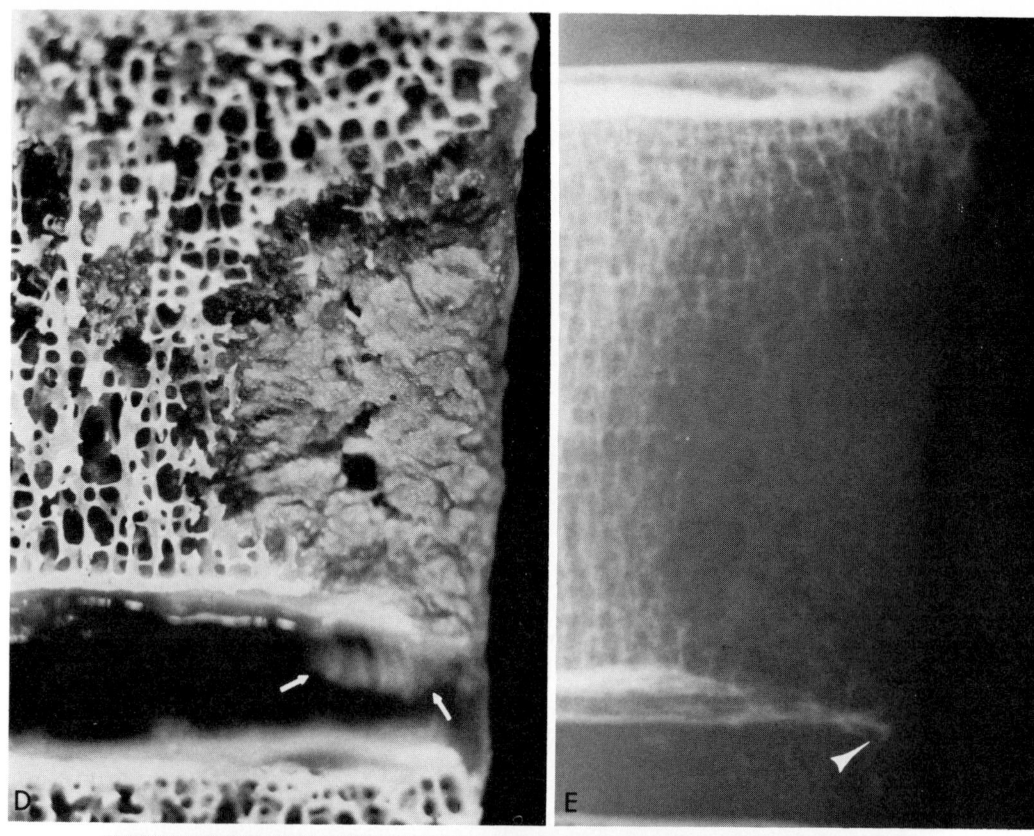

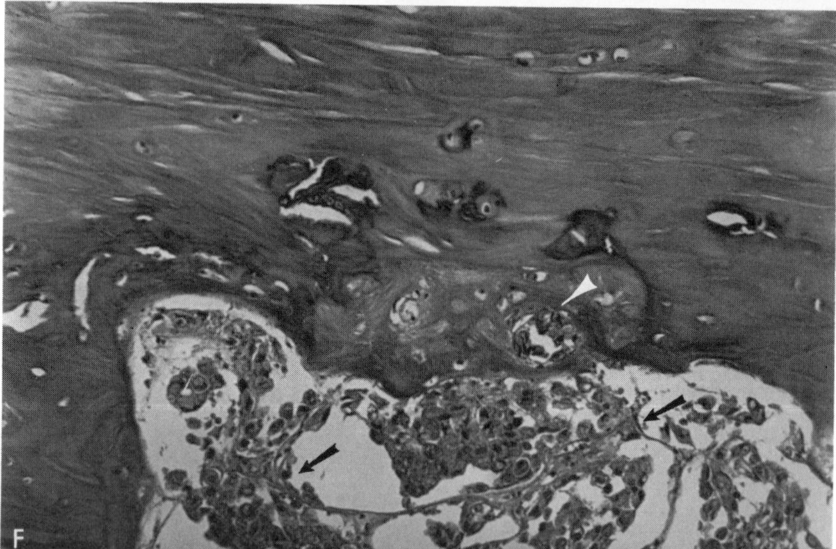

Figure 75–15. Continued

D, E *A photograph and corresponding radiograph of a section through the vertebral body demonstrate a large metastatic lesion that is extending to the discovertebral junction and into the intervertebral disc (arrows). Note on the radiograph that the bony plate has been disrupted (arrowhead).*

F *On a photomicrograph (140×), observe tumor infiltration into the junctional area between the intervertebral disc and the subchondral bone of the vertebral body. Tumor cells are readily identifiable within the bone (arrows) and extend into the cartilage (arrowhead).*

*(**A–E** From Resnick D, Niwayama G: Invest Radiol 13:182, 1978.)*

metastasis might depend upon whether the primary tumor is located within either a pelvic organ such as the prostate or a nonpelvic site. It has been suggested by Batson[40] and others[41] that tumors in nonpelvic organs such as the breast may also metastasize to the skeleton via connections with vertebral veins. In addition, although this study[37] did not concern itself with spread of tumor from adjacent soft tissues into the vertebral bodies and intervertebral discs, this pattern of tumor proliferation is well known. Metastasis in paravertebral lymph nodes or meninges and primary neoplasms of retroperitoneal tissues may advance into the vertebral structures.

DIFFERENTIAL DIAGNOSIS

The abnormalities occurring at synovial and cartilaginous articulations in patients with skeletal metastasis must be differentiated from additional joint manifestations that may accompany neoplastic disease.[42]

Secondary Hypertrophic Osteoarthropathy

Periosteal proliferation is associated with many neoplastic (and non-neoplastic) processes, principally those of the lungs and pleurae (see Chapter 81).[43] The findings are commonly bilateral and symmetric, affecting predominantly the tibiae, fibulae, radii, ulnae, metacarpals, metatarsals, phalanges, femora, and humeri (Fig. 75–16). Articular abnormalities can simulate those of rheumatoid arthritis, with clinically detectable morning stiffness, pain, warmth, and swelling, and radiographically evident soft tissue swelling, joint effusion, and osteoporosis. A nonspecific synovitis that does not require the presence of tumor within or around the involved joints may be evident.

Secondary Gout

Secondary hyperuricemia and gout may be encountered in patients with disseminated carcinoma and sarcoma (see Chapter 43). In these cases, radiographic abnormalities may be mild or absent, although occasionally asymmetric soft tissue swelling and eccentric erosion become apparent.

Carcinomatous Polyarthritis

A polyarthritis resembling rheumatoid arthritis can be an initial manifestation of malignancy.[25, 44, 45, 61] Articular findings may precede the occurrence of

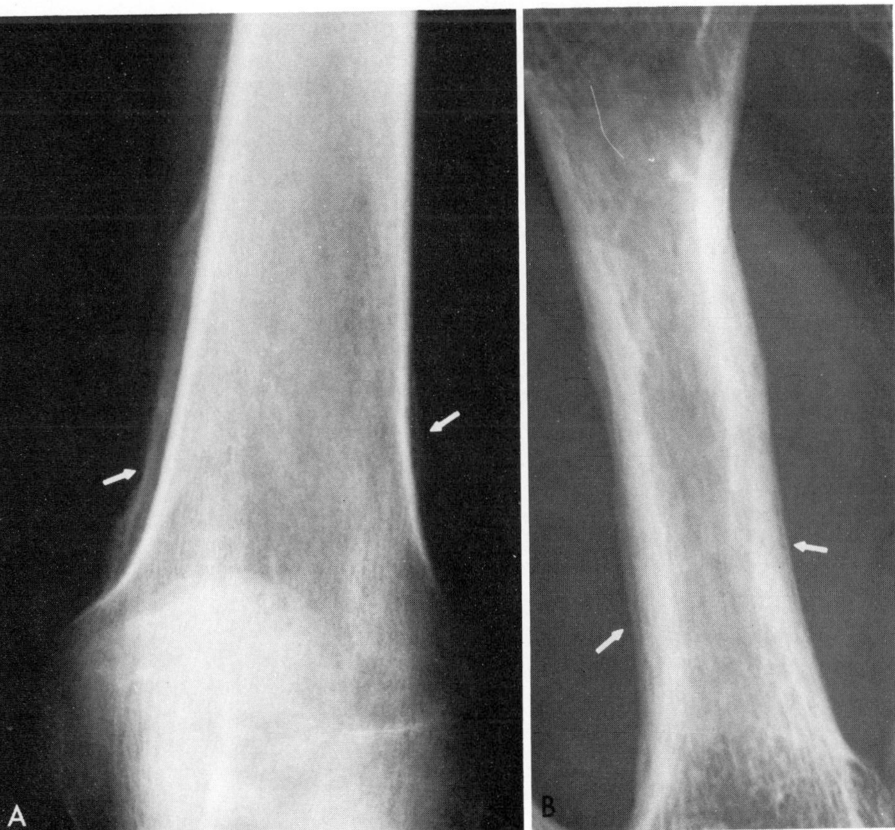

Figure 75–16. *Secondary hypertrophic osteoarthropathy: Bronchogenic carcinoma.*

A *In the femur, solid periosteal bone formation is evident in the diaphyseal and metaphyseal segments (arrows).*

B *A magnification radiograph of an affected metacarpal indicates new bone formation in the diaphysis and metaphysis (arrows).*

malignant neoplasm by a period of months to years. Differentiation from true rheumatoid arthritis may be accomplished on the basis of some unusual features: the sudden onset of symptoms and signs, asymmetric joint involvement, systemic manifestations such as fever and mental confusion, poor response to salicylates, and the absence of serum rheumatoid factor and rheumatoid nodules. Biopsy reveals a nonspecific synovitis. Rarely, a seropositive (rheumatoid factor) arthritis may accompany neoplastic disease.[61]

The etiology and pathogenesis of the process and its relationship to rheumatoid arthritis and tumor are not clear. Adjacent neoplastic osseous foci

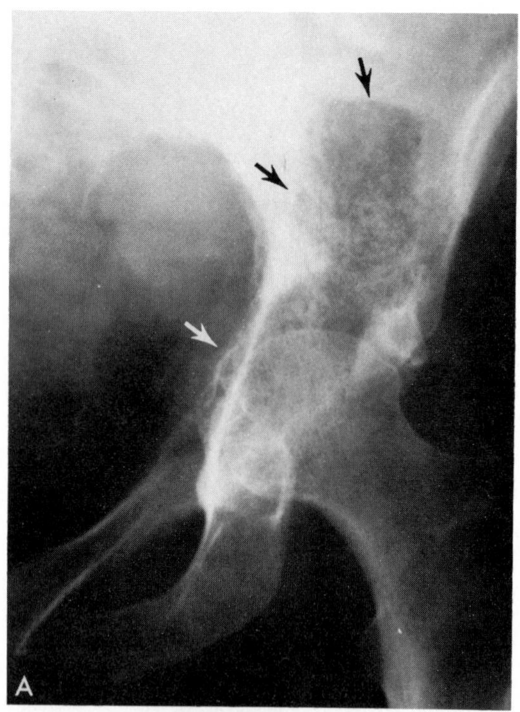

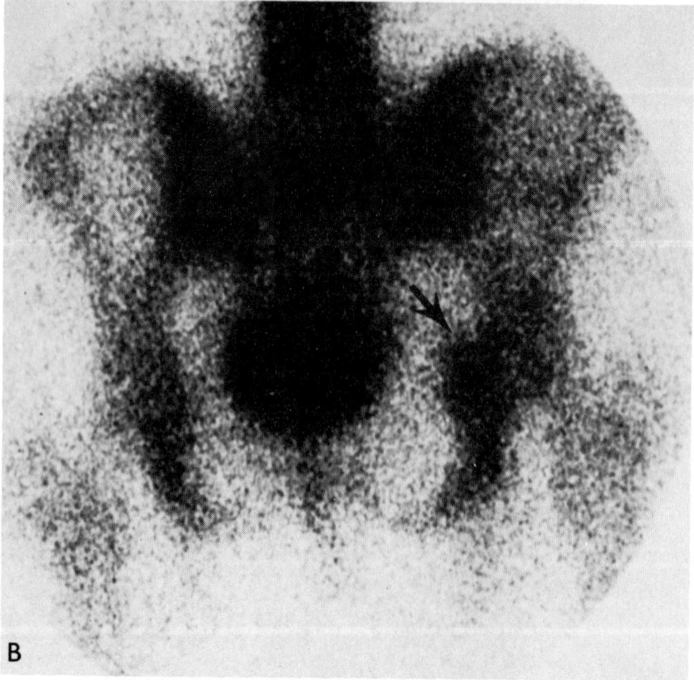

Figure 75–17. *Irradiation effect. This 46 year old woman was admitted to the hospital for investigation of left flank and left hip pain. A pelvic mass was discovered encasing the distal left ureter, producing obstructive uropathy. A lytic bone lesion was also discovered in the left acetabulum at that time. Biopsy of the pelvic mass revealed a squamous cell carcinoma of undetermined origin, most probably from the cervix. Chemotherapy and radiotherapy were administered. The calculated total dose to the ilium was 6500 rads.*

A *A radiograph obtained prior to the radiation therapy indicates neoplastic infiltration of the periacetabular region (arrows) with intrapelvic protrusion of the femoral head.*

B *A technetium bone scan reveals increased uptake of radionuclide about the left acetabulum (arrow).*

Illustration continued on the opposite page

are not required for the appearance of the polyarticular synovitis, suggesting that a generalized systemic aberration, rather than a local effect, is important. Surgical removal of the tumor may result in complete clinical remission, and regression of nodules and serum rheumatoid factor in those cases in which they are present.[46] Changes in cellular immunity and circulating immune complexes have been reported in some cases of malignancy,[47, 48] perhaps indicating a clue to the pathogenesis of carcinomatous polyarthritis.[25, 49] The roentgenographic findings, which may consist of soft tissue swelling and osteoporosis, are not related to hypertrophic osteoarthropathy, gout, or joint and bone metastasis.

Pyogenic Arthritis

Pyogenic arthritis, due to intestinal flora, has been reported as a complication of advanced neoplastic disease.[50] In fact, the presence of bacteremia due to *Streptococcus bovis* or other enteric organisms causing endocarditis[51] or arthritis[52] may be the first sign of an occult colonic neoplasm. In this

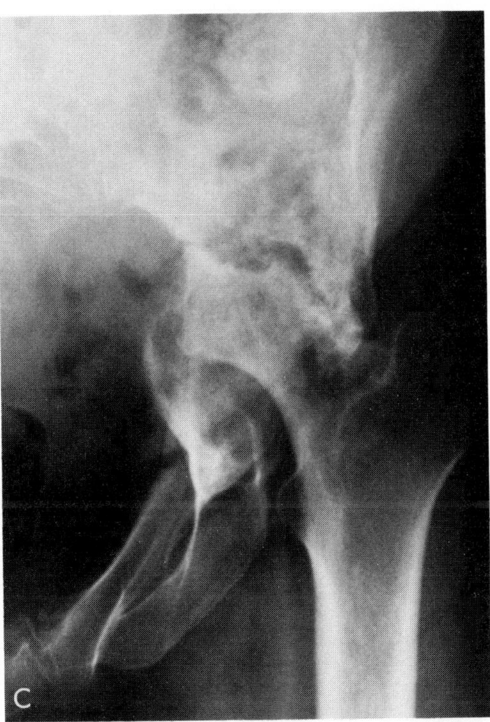

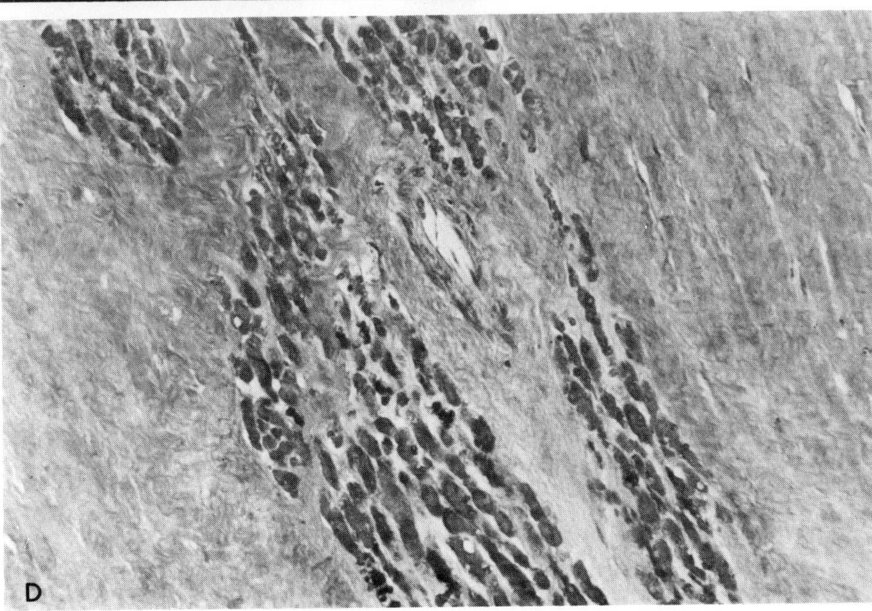

Figure 75–17. Continued

C *Two years following radiotherapy, considerable destruction of the acetabulum and femoral head with acetabular protrusion is consistent with irradiation effect. The presence of neoplasm is not required to produce this radiographic picture.*

D *A biopsy of the area indicates radiation fibrosis. Muscle bundles are surrounded by dense collagen fibers. A vessel at the center reveals intimal sclerosis (trichrome stain, 160×).*

situation, neoplastic mucosal ulceration may provide the portal of entry for the organisms.

Irradiation

Irradiation of sites of skeletal metastasis can lead to local osseous complications, including osteoporosis, osteonecrosis, and radiation-induced sarcoma (see Chapter 65). Knowledge of these complications is important so that the appearance of bony destruction following such treatment is not misinterpreted as evidence of progressive metastasis. This is especially pertinent in neoplasms about the pelvis; acetabular fracture, fragmentation, and protrusion can represent an osseous response to irradiation (Figs. 75–17 and 75–18).

Other Manifestations

Additional rheumatic disorders, such as Sjögren's syndrome, systemic lupus erythematosus,

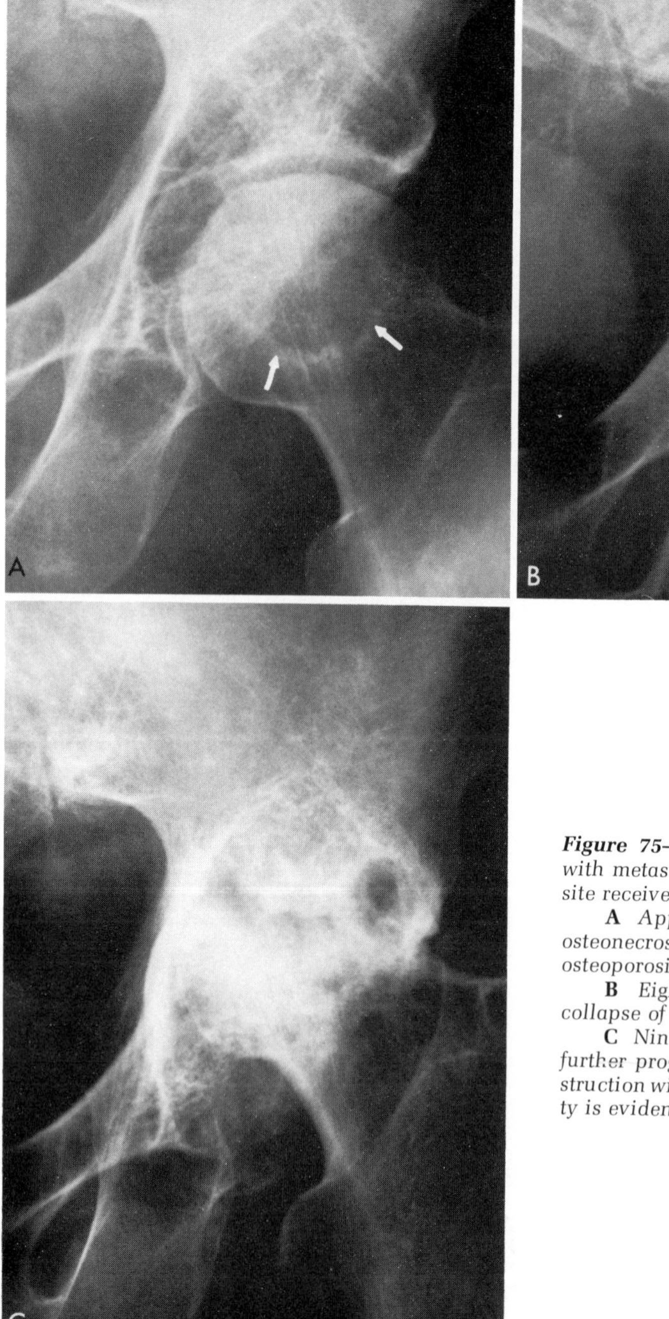

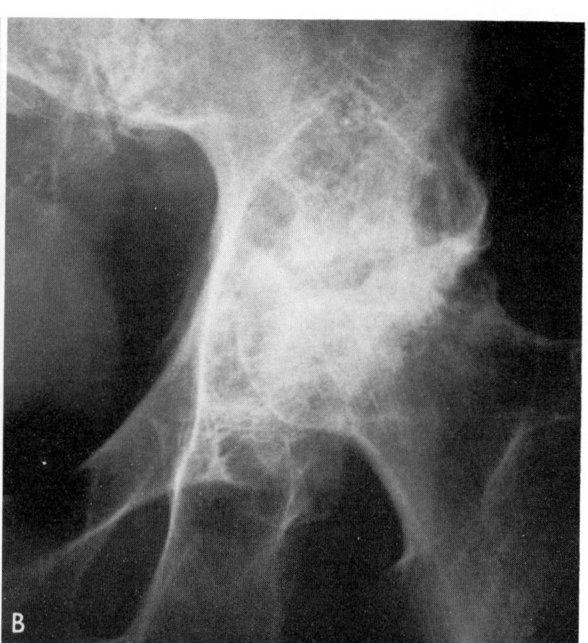

Figure 75–18. Irradiation effect. This 57 year old man with metastatic disease to the ilium from an unknown site received irradiation to the left hemipelvis.

A *Approximately 1½ years following irradiation, osteonecrosis of the femoral head (arrows) and local osteoporosis are evident.*

B *Eighteen months after the radiograph in* **A,** *the collapse of the femoral head has progressed.*

C *Nineteen months following the radiograph in* **B,** *further progression of the acetabular and femoral destruction with sclerosis and protrusio acetabuli deformity is evident.*

and dermatomyositis, may represent an initial manifestation of malignant disease.[53-55] Amyloidosis may also be associated with neoplasm, as can the reflex sympathetic dystrophy syndrome. Polymyalgia rheumatica has rarely been described in patients with underlying malignancies. Additionally, relapsing polychondritis and fat necrosis can be manifestations of neoplasms.

SUMMARY

A review of the manifestations of skeletal metastatic disease indicates that many potential mechanisms exist for articular involvement. In synovial joints, neoplastic deposits in periarticular bone can lead to collapse and fragmentation with or without intra-articular extension of a tumor. Hematogenous seeding to the synovial membrane can also occur. In cartilaginous joints (discovertebral junction), intervertebral disc space narrowing can indicate adjacent vertebral body metastatic lesions that are interfering with proper cartilage nutrition or that are associated with cartilaginous node formation or discal invasion by tumor. Additional "articular" syndromes include secondary hypertrophic osteoarthropathy, carcinomatous polyarthritis, pyogenic arthritis, irradiation effect, and associated rheumatic disorders.

REFERENCES

1. Willis RA: A review of 500 consecutive cancer autopsies. Med J Aust 2:258, 1941.
2. Young JM, Funk FJ Jr.: Incidence of tumor metastasis to the lumbar spine, a comparative study of roentgenographic changes and gross lesions. J Bone Joint Surg *35A*:55, 1953.
3. Fornasier VL, Horne JG: Metastases to the vertebral column. Cancer *36*:590, 1975.
4. Fragiadakis EG, Panayotopoulos G: Metastatic carcinoma of the hand. Hand *4*:268, 1972.
5. Kerin R: Metastatic tumors of the hand. J Bone Joint Surg *40A*:263, 1958.
6. Bryan RS, Soule EH, Dobyns JH, Pritchard DJ, Linscheid RL: Metastatic lesions of the hand and forearm. Clin Orthop Rel Res *101*:167, 1974.
7. Mulvey RB: Peripheral bone metastasis. Am J Roentgenol *91*:155, 1964.
8. Copeland MM: Bone metastases — a study of 334 cases. Radiology *16*:198, 1931.
9. Fort WA: Cancer metastatic to bone. Radiology *24*:96, 1935.
10. Gall RJ, Sim FH, Pritchard DJ: Metastatic tumors to the bones of the foot. Cancer *37*:1492, 1976.
11. Barnett LS, Morris JM: Metastases of renal-cell carcinoma simultaneously to a finger and a toe. A case report. J Bone Joint Surg *51A*:773, 1969.
12. Bouvier M, Lejeune E, Robillard J, Colombani R: Les métastases osseuses distales. Rev Lyon Med *19*:811, 1970.
13. Uriburu IJF, Morchio FJ, Marin JC: Metastases of carcinoma of the larynx and thyroid gland to the phalanges of the hand. Report of two cases. J Bone Joint Surg *58A*:134, 1976.
14. Forbes GS, McLeod RA, Hattery RR: Radiographic manifestations of bone metastases from renal carcinoma. Am J Roentgenol *129*:61, 1977.
15. Jorgens J: The radiographic characteristics of carcinoma of the prostate. Surg Clin North Am *45*:1427, 1965.
16. Peavy PW, Rogers JV Jr, Clements JL Jr, Burns JB: Unusual osteoblastic metastases from carcinoid tumors. Radiology *107*:327, 1973.
17. Napoli LD, Hansen HH, Muggia FM, Twigg HL: The incidence of osseous involvement in lung cancer, with special reference to the development of osteoblastic changes. Radiology *108*:17, 1973.
18. Debnam JW, Staple TW: Osseous metastases from cerebellar medulloblastoma. Radiology *107*:363, 1973.
19. Meals RA, Hungerford DS, Stevens MB: Malignant disease mimicking arthritis of the hip JAMA *239*:1070, 1978.
20. Kagan AR, Steckel RJ: Metastatic carcinoma presenting as shoulder arthritis. Am J Roentgenol *129*:137, 1977.
21. Lagier R: Synovial reaction caused by adjacent malignant tumors: Anatomicopathological study of three cases. J Rheumatol *4*:65, 1977.
22. Bevan DA, Ehrlich GE, Gupta VP: Metastatic carcinoma simulating gout. JAMA *237*:2746, 1977.
23. Gall EA, Bennett GA, Bauer W: Generalized hypertrophic osteoarthropathy. A pathologic study of seven cases. Am J Pathol *27*:349, 1951.
24. Hindmarsh JR, Emslie-Smith D: Monocytic leukemia presenting as polyarthritis in an adult. Br Med J *1*:593, 1953.
25. Bennett RM, Ginsberg MH, Thomsen S: Carcinomatous polyarthritis. The presenting symptom of an ovarian tumor and association with a platelet activating factor. Arthritis Rheum *19*:953, 1976.
26. Moutsopolous HM, Fye KH, Pugay PI, Shearn MA: Monarthric arthritis caused by metastatic breast carcinoma. Value of cytologic study of synovial fluid. JAMA *234*:75, 1975.
27. Stoler B, Staple TW: Metastases to the patella. Radiology *93*:853, 1969.
28. Gall EP, Didizian NA, Park Y: Acute monoarticular arthritis following patellar metastasis. A manifestation of carcinoma of the lung. JAMA *229*:188, 1974.
29. Benedek TG: Lysis of the patella due to metastatic carcinoma. Arthritis Rheum *8*:560, 1965.
30. Naib ZM: Cytology of synovial fluids. Acta Cytol *17*:299, 1973.
31. Meisels A, Berebichez M: Exfoliative cytology in orthopedics. Can Med Assoc J *84*:957, 1961.
32. Goldenberg DL, Kelley W, Gibbons RB: Metastatic adenocarcinoma of synovium presenting as an acute arthritis. Diagnosis by closed synovial biopsy. Arthritis Rheum *18*:107, 1975.
33. Spilberg I, Meyer GJ: The arthritis of leukemia. Arthritis Rheum *15*:630, 1972.
34. Firooznia H, Pinto RS, Lin JP, Baruch HH, Zausner J: Chordoma: Radiologic evaluation of 20 cases. Am J Roentgenol *127*:797, 1976.
35. Resnick D, Niwayama G: Intravertebral disk herniations: Cartilaginous (Schmorl's) nodes. Radiology *126*:57, 1978.
36. Hubbard DD, Gunn DR: Secondary carcinoma of the spine with destruction of the intervertebral disk. Clin Orthop Rel Res *88*:86, 1972.
37. Resnick D, Niwayama G: Intervertebral disc abnormalities associated with vertebral metastases: Observations in patients and cadavers with prostatic cancer. Invest Radiol *13*:182, 1978.
38. Schmorl G, Junghanns H: The Human Spine in Health and Disease. 2nd Ed. Translated by EF Besemann. New York, Grune & Stratton, 1971, p 141.
39. Hilton RC, Ball J, Benn RT: Vertebral end-plate lesions (Schmorl's nodes) in the dorsolumbar spine. Ann Rheum Dis *35*:127, 1976.
40. Batson OV: The function of the vertebral veins and their role in the spread of metastasis. Ann Surg *112*:138, 1940.
41. Coman DR, DeLong RP: The role of the vertebral venous system in the metastasis of cancer to the spinal column. Cancer *4*:610, 1951.
42. Calabro JJ: Cancer and arthritis. Arthritis Rheum *10*:553, 1967.
43. Holling HE: Pulmonary hypertrophic osteoarthropathy. Ann Intern Med *66*:232, 1967.
44. MacKenzie AH, Scherbel AL: Connective tissue syndromes associated with carcinoma. Geriatrics *18*:745, 1963.
45. Lansbury J: Collagen disease complicating malignancy. Ann Rheum Dis *12*:301, 1953.
46. Litwin SD, Allen JC, Kunkel HG: Disappearance of the clinical and serological manifestations of rheumatoid arthritis following thoracotomy for lung tumor (Abstr). Arthritis Rheum 9:865, 1966.
47. Lee JC, Yamauchi H, Hopper J Jr: The association of cancer and the nephrotic syndrome. Ann Intern Med *64*:41, 1966.
48. Wybran J, Fudenberg HH: Thymus-derived rosette forming cells in various human disease states: Cancer, lymphoma, bacterial and viral infections, and other diseases. J Clin Invest *52*:1026, 1973.
49. Friou GJ: Current knowledge and concepts of the relationship of malignancy, autoimmunity, and immunologic disease. Ann NY Acad Sci *230*:23, 1974.
50. Douglas GW, Levin RH, Sokoloff L: Infectious arthritis complicating neoplastic disease. N Engl J Med *270*:299, 1964.
51. Keusch GT: Opportunistic infections in colon carcinoma. Am J Clin Nutr *27*:1481, 1974.
52. Lyon LJ, Nevins MA: Carcinoma of the colon presenting as pyogenic arthritis. JAMA *241*:2060, 1979.
53. Williams RC Jr: Dermatomyositis and malignancy: A review of the literature. Ann Intern Med *50*:1174, 1959.

54. Curtis AC, Blaylock HC, Harrell ER Jr: Malignant lesions associated with dermatomyositis. JAMA *150*:844, 1952.
55. Talal N, Bunim JJ: The development of malignant lymphoma in the course of Sjögren's syndrome. Am J Med *36*:529, 1964.
56. Fam AG, Kolin A, Lewis AJ: Metastatic carcinomatous arthritis and carcinoma of the lung. A report of two cases diagnosed by synovial fluid cytology. J Rheumatol *7*:98, 1980.
57. Fam AG, Cross EG: Hypertrophic osteoarthropathy, phalangeal and synovial metastases associated with bronchogenic carcinoma. J Rheumatol *6*:680, 1979.
58. Murray GC, Persellin RH: Metastatic carcinoma presenting as monarticular arthritis: A case report and review of the literature. Arthritis Rheum *23*:95, 1980.
59. Nauseef W, Sundstrom WR: Lung carcinoma: Juxtaarticular disease resembling bursitis and tenosynovitis. J Rheumatol *7*:106, 1980.
60. Wu KK, Winkelman NZ, Guise ER: Metastatic bronchogenic carcinoma to the finger simulating acute osteomyelitis. Orthopedics *3*:25, 1980.
61. Simon RD Jr, Ford LE: Rheumatoid-like arthritis associated with a colonic carcinoma. Arch Intern Med *140*:698, 1980.

SECTION XVII

OSTEONECROSIS AND OSTEOCHONDROSIS

PATHOGENESIS OF OSTEONECROSIS

by Donald E. Sweet, M.D., and John E. Madewell, M.D.

76

The concepts and terminology of bone necrosis or "osteonecrosis" have undergone considerable evolution over the past two centuries.[3, 46, 54, 67, 87, 88, 102] Russell's classic essay on "disease of the bones termed necrosis," published in 1794, describes in great detail the sequestration of bone in osteomyelitis.[102] As currently used, osteonecrosis indicates that ischemic death of the cellular constituents of bone and marrow has occurred. The purpose of this chapter is to focus attention upon the sequential morphologic reparative response to the infarcted foci, primarily in the adult femoral head, and its consequences and radiographic correlation. To accomplish this, it will be helpful to discuss terminology, principles of infarction, the marrow cavity, associations and mechanisms of osteonecrosis, and the histologic-radiographic correlation of the host response.

The opinions or assertions contained herein are the private views of the authors, and are not to be construed as official, or as reflecting the views of the United States Departments of the Army, of the Air Force, of the Navy, or of Defense.

TERMINOLOGY

For most of the nineteenth century, "osteonecrosis" was regarded as septic in origin.[3, 102] Failure to appreciate the radiographic appearance of bone sequestra as of relative, rather than absolute, density resulted in almost any unexplained increased bone density on x-ray being equated with osteonecrosis. A large group of these radiographic entities known under a variety of eponyms (Fig. 76–1) were eventually brought together under the term osteochondrosis[16] despite histologic absence of dead bone in many of them.[67]

Continued negative bacteriologic studies from well-documented cases of bone necrosis led to the use of the term aseptic necrosis.[88, 89] Subsequent observations indicated the necrotic bone foci were

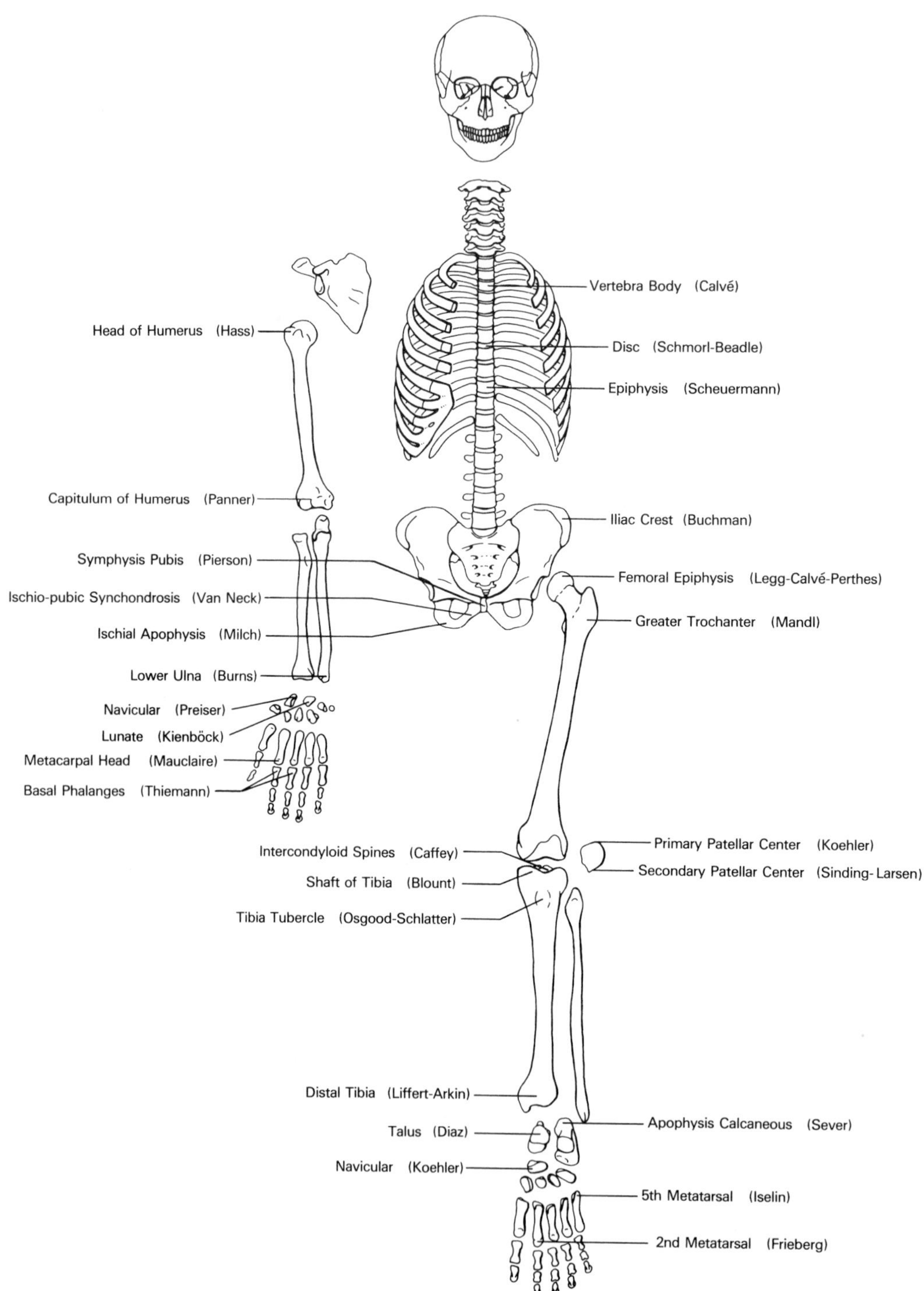

Figure 76–1. *Schematic drawing demonstrating sites of occurrence of the osteochondroses.*

not only aseptic but also avascular; hence the terms ischemic necrosis, avascular necrosis, and bone infarction. By convention, the terms "aseptic" and "avascular" necrosis are generally applied to areas of epiphyseal or subarticular involvement, whereas bone infarct is usually reserved for metaphyseal and diaphyseal involvement. However, the literature on ischemic bone necrosis indicates considerable overlap and lack of uniformity in applied terminology.

PRINCIPLES OF INFARCTION

Ischemic necrosis of bone, like infarction in other organ systems, results from a significant reduction in or obliteration of the affected area's blood supply.[98] Cessation of blood flow may be initiated in any part of the vascular network: arterial, capillary, sinusoidal, or venous. Eventually the flow of blood from the arterial side of the system will be compromised. One of the following phenomena can usually be demonstrated or inferred as impeding blood flow: (1) intraluminal obstruction (e.g., thromboembolic disorders or sludging of blood cells); (2) vascular compression (e.g., external mechanical pressure or vasospasm); or (3) physical disruption of the vessel (e.g., trauma). These factors can act alone or in combination.

The type of compromised vessel and the architectural arrangement of the involved organ's vascular network are both key factors determining the effect of blood flow interruption.[98] For example, in the absence of collateral circulation, arterial occlusion produces a bloodless infarct, as is frequently encountered in the heart, kidney, and brain. Organs with collateral circulation, such as the liver and lungs, are less susceptible to infarction by arterial occlusion; when infarction occurs, the necrotic area is frequently of relatively small size and usually hemorrhagic. Infarction resulting from venous obstruction is generally hemorrhagic, as in the small bowel following mesenteric vein thrombosis. Small arteriole or capillary blockade with microinfarction in a number of organ systems has been associated with subacute bacterial endocarditis and disseminated intravascular coagulation.[80] Organs with extensive sinusoidal vascular beds, like the spleen and medullary cavity of bone, are at particular risk for infarction without evidence of arterial or venous occlusion in such disorders as sickle cell disease.

Cell death from "anoxia" is not immediate, but rather occurs through progressive stages of ischemic injury. For the purposes of this discussion, the term "anoxia" shall be extended to include an absence or decrease in all metabolites essential for cell viability and function. Subdivision of the cellular changes of progressive ischemic injury and death into three stages is arbitrary and is done to facilitate understanding of the possible disposition of these cells. These stages are defined as follows:[96] Stage 1, alteration or interruption of intracellular enzyme systems; Stage 2, cessation of intracellular metabolic activity at a chemical level; Stage 3, disruption or dissolution of intracellular nuclear and cytoplasmic ultrastructure. Dissolution of intracellular structural integrity is irreversible and results in cell death.[96]

With reversal of anoxia, the lag period between the earliest ischemic cell change and irreversible cell death makes possible the revival and return to normal for cells in Stage 1. The more severely injured cells of Stage 2 may survive, but their rehabilitation rarely permits approximation of normal function. Once cells reach Stage 3, they cannot survive.[67] The fate of dead cells is usually progressive autolysis, with eventual removal and either restoration or reconstruction by the combined effort of the host's inflammatory and reparative responses.[97]

The production of ischemic injury or necrosis and the rapidity with which cell death can occur depend upon the sensitivity of the individual cell type as well as the degree and duration of anoxia. Neurons in the central nervous system, under normal homeostatic conditions, survive only 3 to 5 min of complete anoxia before damage becomes irreversible. The sensitivity of the cellular elements of bone and marrow to anoxia varies. The use of H_3-cytidine and H_3-thymidine studies as a measure of continued bone and marrow cell activity following anoxia under controlled circumstances seems to have produced a fairly reliable base line.[46, 73] However, there remain some unanswered questions regarding marrow fat cells. It is generally acknowledged that the hematopoietic elements are the first to undergo anoxic death (in from 6 to 12 hours), followed by bone cells (osteocytes, osteoclasts, and osteoblasts) (in 12 to 48 hours) and, subsequently, marrow fat cells (48 hours to 5 days).[53, 67, 72, 99, 125, 126] Although there are some variations in the sensitivity of osteocytes, osteoclasts, and osteoblasts to anoxia, as a group they appear to undergo cell death following 12 to 48 hours of anoxia.

The variability in cell sensitivity of the different cellular constituents of bone and marrow cavity makes it possible for temporary anoxia to result in the death of hematopoietic elements without necessarily being sufficient to cause osteocytic or marrow fat cell death. By extension, there could be foci of hematopoietic and osteocytic death without ischemic necrosis of marrow fat. Once ischemic marrow fat cell death occurs, the involved segment of bone and marrow can clearly be labeled infarcted.

Infarcts, including those in bone, are three-dimensional and can be subdivided into four zones: a central zone of cell death surrounded by successive zones of ischemic injury, active hyperemia, and finally normal tissue.[98] The ischemic zone reflects a gradation of hypoxic injury ranging from severe cell damage immediately adjacent to the central zone of cell death to marginal cellular alterations adjacent to the hyperemic zone. Once ischemic necrosis is established, the breakdown products of dying and

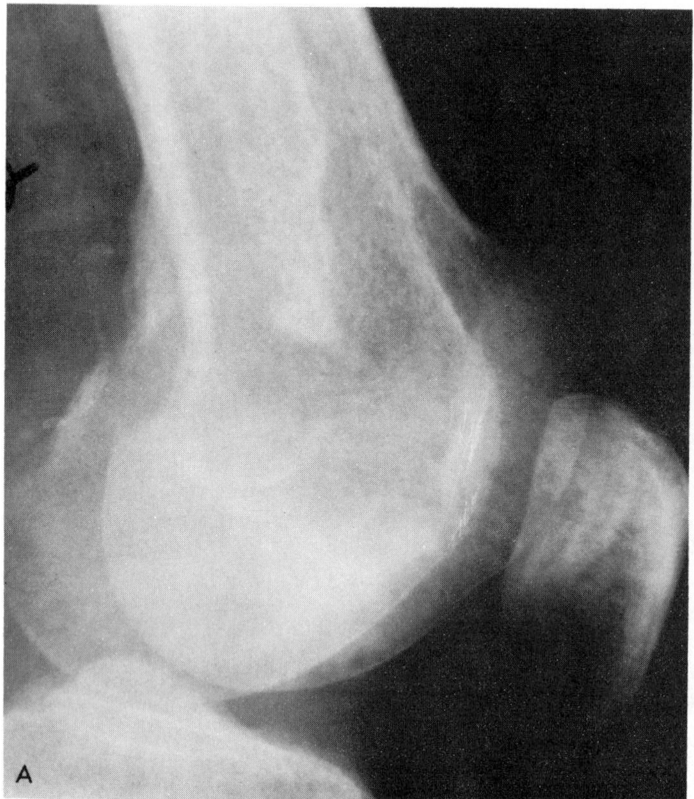

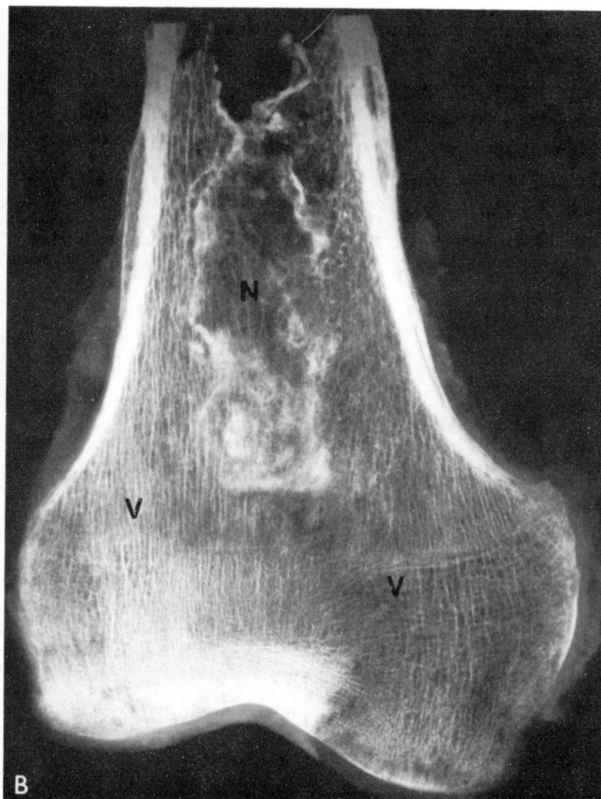

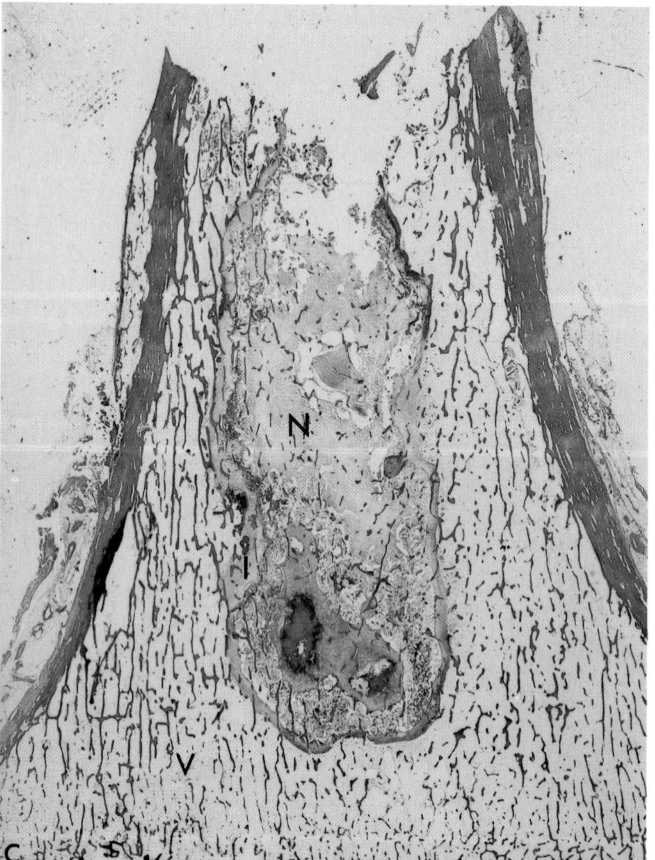

Figure 76–2. *Intramedullary bone infarct.*

A *Lateral radiographic view of the distal femur demonstrates an irregular but discrete area of increased endosteal density, which is most pronounced at the periphery of the lesion.*

B *Specimen radiograph of the coronally sectioned distal femur reveals unaltered density within the central necrotic zone (N), which is separated from the adjacent viable bone and marrow (V) by an irregular linear margin of increased density. Note the localized area of increased density that appears to be within the inferior portion of the infarct.*

C *Macroscopic section (2×, hematoxylin and eosin stain) shows the essentially unchanged but slightly opacified central necrotic zone (N) separated from the adjacent viable endosteal cavity (V) by a narrow, more darkly stained reactive ischemic zone (I). The dark-stained areas correspond to the dense areas in the specimen radiograph. The distal radiodense areas in the specimen radiograph reflect poor quality ischemic bone formation within the outer reactive fibrous zone, which appears to lie within the infarct. This is because the plane of section has cut into a portion of the posterior reactive margin. The immediately necrotic area around this region shows large numbers of cholesterol crystals due to fat breakdown.*

Illustration continued on the opposite page

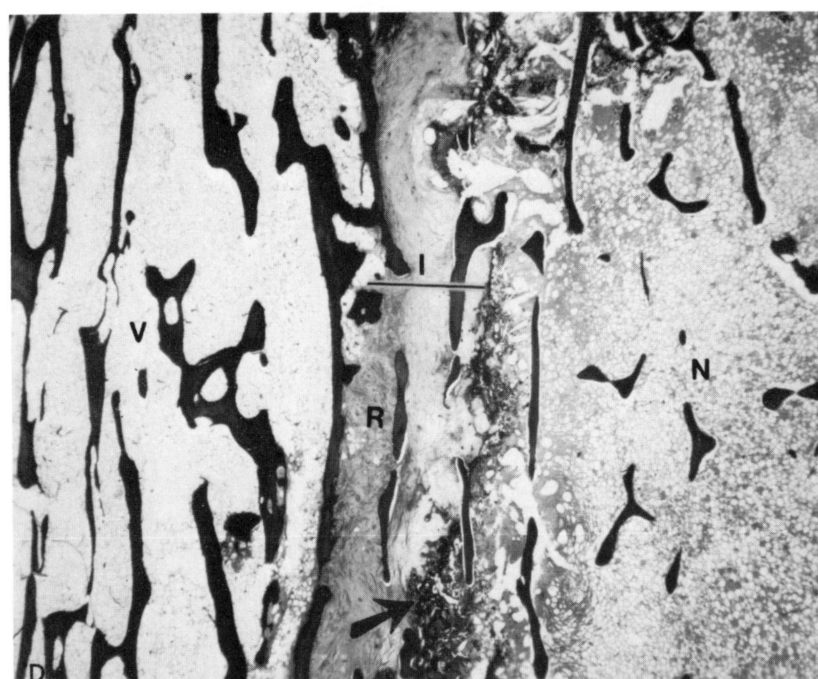

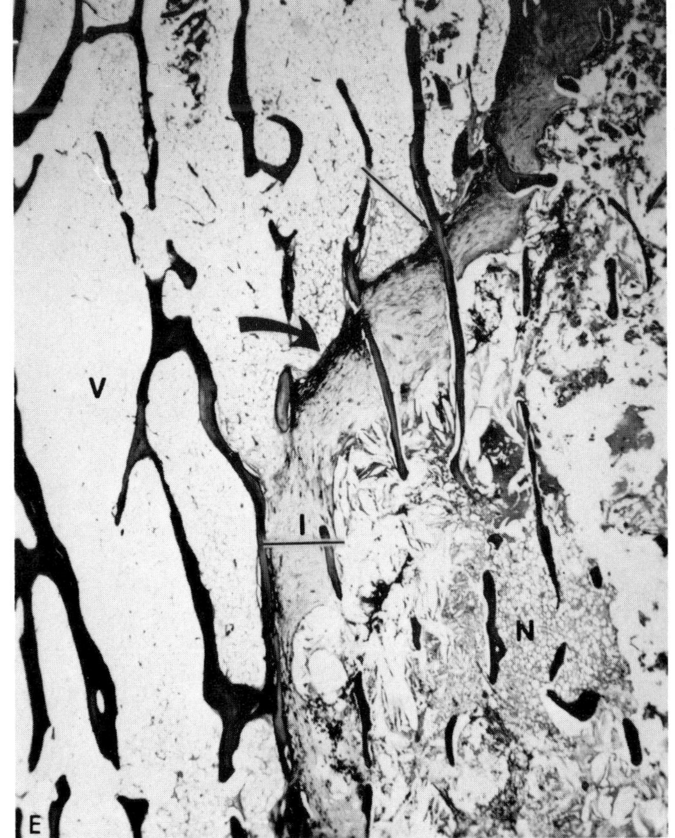

Figure 76–2. Continued

D *Photomicrograph (18×) demonstrates the ischemic zone (I, horizontal line), of which the reactive interface (R) is part, separating the slightly opacified infarcted marrow and bone (N) from the surrounding viable endosteal components (V). Dystrophic mineralization (arrow) lies just inside the reactive ischemic zone.*

E *Photomicrograph (18×) of the reactive ischemic margin (I, horizontal line) separating necrotic (N) from viable (V) bone and marrow. Atypical ischemic fiber bone formation is also seen (curved arrow). Essentially unaltered cancellous bone traverses all three zones (straight arrow).*

(Armed Forces Institute of Pathology Neg. Nos. 65-5966-3, 79-5408, 79-15021-3, 79-15021-1,2.)

severely damaged cells provoke the initial inflammatory response, characterized by vasodilatation, transudation of fluid, fibrin precipitation, and local infiltration of inflammatory cells. This response forms the basis for development of the hyperemic zone and also represents the first steps of repair, removal, and reconstruction of the infarcted area.[97]

Bone infarcts occurring in the metadiaphyseal intramedullary cavity (Fig. 76–2) will have a central core of dead marrow and bone surrounded by zones of ischemically injured marrow and bone, active hyperemia, and viable marrow and bone. Those infarcts occurring within an epiphysis or small, round bone will demonstrate a similar three-dimensional pattern, except that one surface is almost always covered by compact subchondral bone and articular cartilage. Since the articular cartilage receives the bulk of its nourishment from the synovial fluid, its viability is usually not significantly affected initially by the underlying osteonecrosis, except for the cartilage cells below the tidemark, which may die. Because the osteonecrotic segment is by definition avascular, repair can only begin along its outer perimeter at the junction between the ischemic zone surrounding the dead area and the viable area with an intact circulation (the hyperemic zone). This reparative response results in the progressive development of a reactive margin (interface) between the dead zone and adjacent viable tissues. The reactive interface generally encompasses the bulk of the ischemically injured zone and adjacent hyperemic zone.[67]

Because tissue death is essentially a cellular phenomenon, mineralized bone matrix does not appear to be materially altered directly by ischemic necrosis. What changes, if any, occur within the matrix or affect the stress-bearing capability of bone as a direct result of anoxia (in the absence of cell activity) are controversial and have yet to be fully clarified.[40, 41] From a practical point of view, bone structure is initially unaltered as a direct result of osteocyte death or osteonecrosis. The x-ray absorbing quality of bone (density) is based on attenuation of the x-ray beam by the total amount of bone matrix and mineral content (especially calcium), not on cellular viability. Therefore, any alteration in bone density — either a real increase or decrease in radiographic density — is an indication of viability requiring osteoblastic or osteoclastic cell activity, respectively, and will be initially perceived in the viable bone and marrow surrounding the osteonecrotic segment.

THE MARROW CAVITY

The medullary cavity is an admixture of cancellous trabecular bone, hematopoietic marrow, fatty marrow, and sinusoidal vascular bed confined by a nonexpandable shell of cortical bone. Radiographic observations indicate that ischemic necrosis of bone is most commonly encountered within the epiphyseal (especially the femoral and humeral heads), and metadiaphyseal marrow cavities of adult long tubular bones.[33] Occasional involvement of the small, round bones of the wrist and ankle is seen.[60]

The primary function of cancellous bone is to support the subarticular bony plate and transmit stress from the articular surface to the cortical shaft. For this reason, cancellous bone tends to be more concentrated in the epiphyseal and, to a lesser degree, the metaphyseal ends of long bones. Little cancellous bone remains in the diaphysis of long bones. The amount and architectural orientation of cancellous bone will, in large part, be determined by the changing stress requirements of each bone.

Since the femoral head is a primary area of clinical concern, the architectual arrangement of its cancellous bone will be of particular interest. For example, the stress-diffusing characteristics of the cartilaginous growth plate interposed between the articular surface and cortical shaft in a growing bone result in a tightly packed, crossing pattern of cancellous bone throughout the epiphysis (Fig. 76–3*A*). Under these circumstances, the metaphyseal cancellous bone supports the growth plate, and the growth plate in turn provides the base of support for the epiphyseal cancellous bone supporting the articular surface. Closure of the growth plate is followed by extensive architectural reorganization (remodeling) of the epiphyseal and, to a lesser extent, the metaphyseal cancellous bone such that they become a continuum (Fig. 76–3*B*). This normally results in a somewhat wedge-shaped orientation of tightly packed and thicker cancellous bone trabeculae supporting the articular surface directly beneath the anterolateral weight-bearing segment of the femoral head. Similar but less dramatic findings are encountered in the humeral head.

The arterial, sinusoidal, and venous vascular network of bone has been well demonstrated by previous anatomic studies and need not be detailed here.[116-118] The extensive arterial supply to adult long tubular bones, including the nutrient artery with its ascending and descending diaphyseal branches and the penetrating metaphyseal and epiphyseal (retinacular) arteries, as well as the superficial periosteal vessels and the diffuse intramedullary sinusoidal vascular bed, provides excellent collateral circulation. This fact is underscored by experimental data indicating the inability to produce bone infarcts by isolated occlusion of either the nutrient, metaphyseal, epiphyseal, or periosteal arterial supply.[118]

The intramedullary canal's sinusoidal vascular bed, which supplies the bulk of the marrow and cancellous bone, emanates from the terminal branches of the arterial network penetrating the

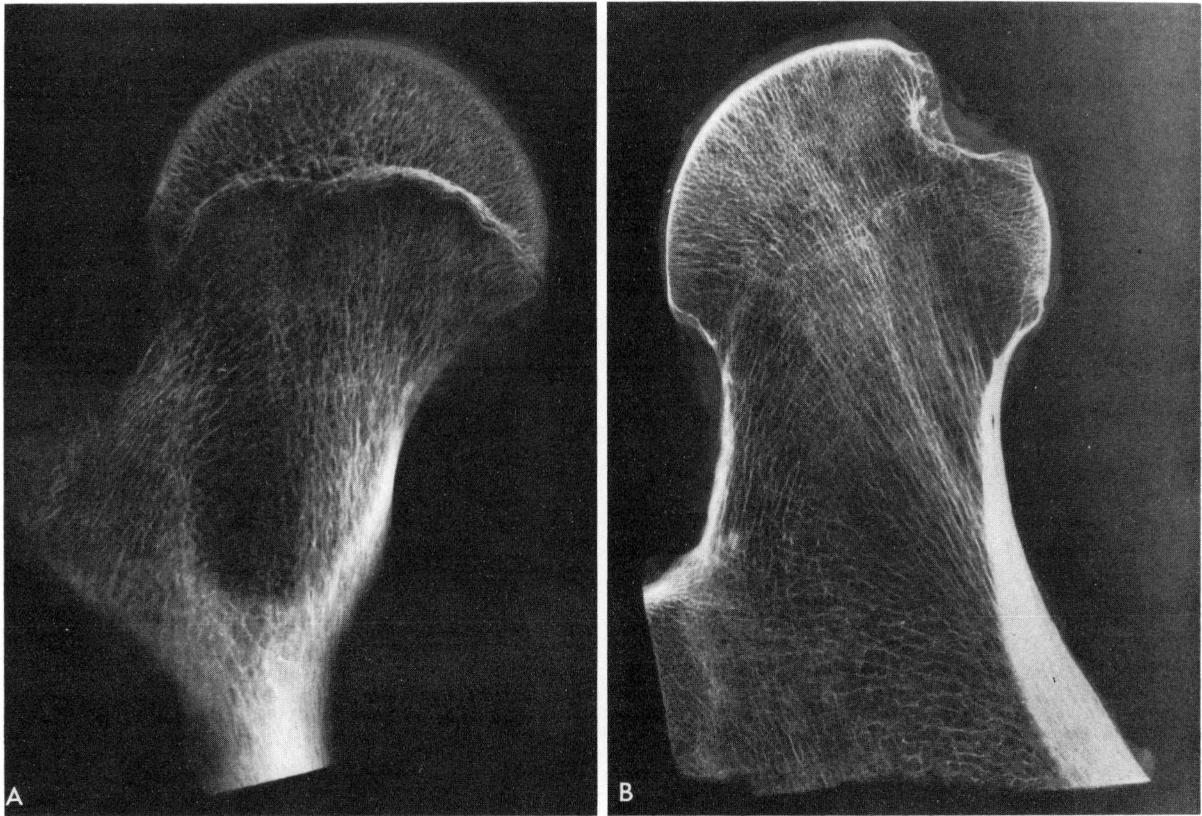

Figure 76–3. *Normal femoral heads. Specimen radiograph of the femoral head and neck from a patient with a closing capital femoral epiphysis* **(A)** *and a patient with a closed* **(B)** *capital femoral epiphyseal growth plate. Note the differing amounts and orientations of cancellous bone, especially in the epiphysis of each patient. This reflects the changing mechanical requirements as the growth plate closes. (Armed Forces Institute of Pathology Neg. Nos. 79-6007, 79-6008.)*

bony cortex. Venous outflow is also extensive, as evidenced by numerous perforating channels exiting through the cortex.[27, 50]

Despite the extensive circulation available to the metadiaphyseal cortex and intramedullary cavity, the epiphyseal ends of long bones have limited arterial access and venous outflow because much of their surface is covered by articular cartilage. This fact is reflected by reductions in both blood flow through the epiphyseal sinusoidal vascular bed and intraosseous marrow pressure (blood perfusion pressure) compared with those in the metadiaphyseal intramedullary cavity.[112] Arterial access to the epiphysis is further compromised in the growing skeleton, in which the epiphysis is separated from the metaphysis by the growth plate. Although occasional small arterioles penetrate the epiphyseal growth plate (physis), little or no significant collateral circulation exists between a developing epiphysis and its adjacent metaphysis.[116, 118] In the absence of collateral circulation, the likelihood of a single or dominant artery supplying an entire epiphysis or a significant segment of an epiphysis is increased. The small carpal and tarsal bones are also covered to a great extent by articular cartilage. In many respects, their ossification centers are analogous to the developing epiphyses of a long bone with regard to blood supply. Compromise of a dominant artery supplying a developing epiphysis or small round bone ossification center is a possible mechanism for Legg-Calvé-Perthes disease (femoral head), Köhler's disease (tarsal navicular), and Kienböck's disease (lunate bone).

Development of a sinusoidal vascular bed appears to be an important prerequisite for the emergence of normal hematopoietic activity — witness the confinement of the bulk of extramedullary hematopoiesis in the fetus (except in extreme circumstances) to the liver and spleen, both of which have well-developed sinusoidal vascular beds.

Each bone develops its own sinusoidal vascular bed and marrow cavity as it grows. The sinusoids are readily seen via the microscope in areas of active enchondral bone formation. In areas of active hematopoiesis, the sinusoids appear packed with erythroid and myeloid elements. However, the expansive sinusoidal space that is available during active hematopoiesis becomes predominantly a potential space in areas of fatty marrow. Rapid discharge of hematopoietic elements provides the abil-

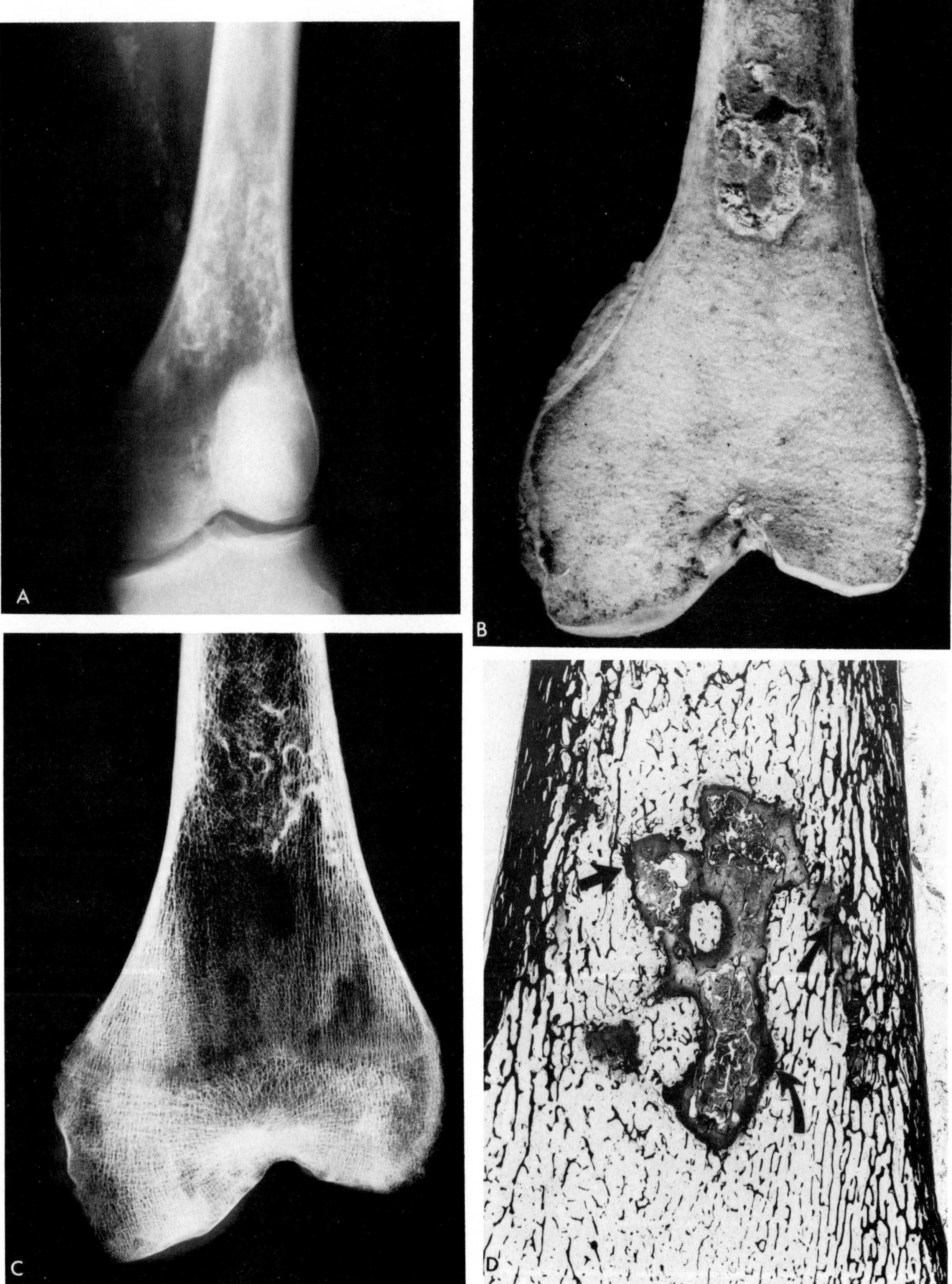

Figure 76–4. *See legend on opposite page*

ity to more quickly increase blood flow through areas of active hematopoietic marrow in comparison to fatty marrow.[67, 74] Experimental studies indicate that the rate of blood flow through fatty marrow and fatty tissue is considerably reduced per unit area over that of other tissues, such as skeletal muscle and skin.[44]

The relative amount and localization of hematopoietic or fatty marrow are primarily dependent upon hematopoietic demand. This demand is largely a function of age. The marrow cavities of all bones in the newborn and young child are actively engaged in hematopoiesis. As the total marrow volume increases with skeletal growth, normal hematopoietic demand can eventually be satisfied by the marrow capacity of the axial skeleton. Therefore, the marrow cavities of the adolescent and adult appendicular skeleton normally contain predominantly fatty marrow, unless some special circumstance requires increased hematopoiesis.

Thus, both radiographic and anatomic observations indicate that ischemic necrosis of bone, either avascular necrosis or bone infarction, almost invariably occurs within areas of predominantly fatty marrow (Figs. 76–2 and 76–4).

The converse is equally true; ischemic necrosis in areas of normal active hematopoiesis is distinctly unusual except in sickle cell disease and related hemoglobinopathies or following complete traumatic disruption of the arterial blood supply. Ischemic necrosis of cortical bone is relatively rare and occurs only when there is extensive interruption of the arterial blood supply, as in osteomyelitis (Fig. 76–5).

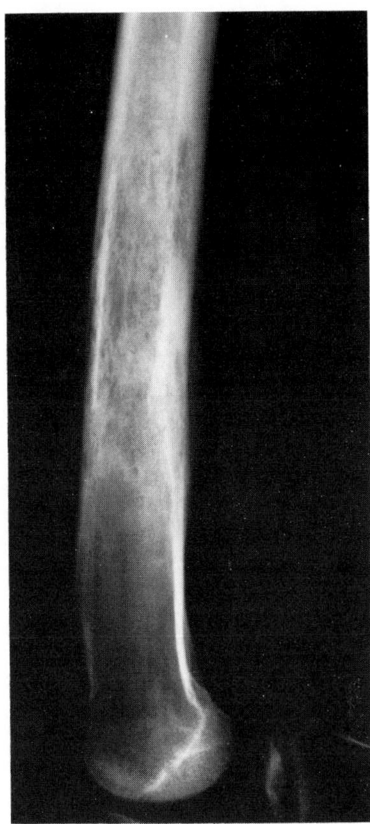

Figure 76–5. *Osteomyelitis with cortical sequestrum. Lateral view of the distal femur shows a motheaten area of bone lysis with apparent radiodensity of the inner anterior cortex. Intracortical destruction of bone just anterior to this sequestrum is also seen. (Armed Forces Institute of Pathology Neg. No. 73-11186-8.)*

ISCHEMIC BONE NECROSIS: ASSOCIATIONS AND MECHANISMS

A variable group of clinical situations are associated with the development of avascular necrosis and bone infarction. These include traumatic disruption of the blood supply (femoral head dislocation and subcapital femoral neck fracture), the hemoglobinopathies (sickle cell disease), exogenous corticosteroid therapy and Cushing's disease, alcoholism, Gaucher's disease, dysbaric disorders, and irradiation. Patients with collagen vascular disorders, such as systemic lupus erythematosus and rheumatoid arthritis, and patients who have had renal transplants are also at risk for osteonecrosis. The vast majority of patients within the latter two groups have usually received significant corticosteroid and additional immunosuppressive therapy. Patients with pancreatitis and gout have also been reported to be at risk for osteonecrosis. The incidence of chronic

Figure 76–4. *Intramedullary bone infarct.*

A *Clinical radiograph of the distal femur demonstrates an intramedullary infarct, characterized by curly, smoke-like wisps of increased density primarily at the margins.*

B *Slightly reduced gross photograph of the coronally sectioned femur shows an irregular, yellow, necrotic area of infarction within fatty marrow.*

C *Specimen radiograph of the gross section correlates the curly wisps of increased density with the margins of the infarct. The scattered radiolucent foci distal to the infarct are probably secondary to active hyperemia (reflex vascular osteoporosis).*

D *Macrosection (4 ×) reveals the dense margin of the infarct to be the result of ischemic bone formation (curved arrow), dystrophic mineralization (tapered arrow), and focal trabecular reinforcement (straight arrow). Note: The relatively small size of the infarct in* **B, C,** *and* **D** *as compared with the clinical radiograph reflects the plane of section.*

(Armed Forces Institute of Pathology Neg. Nos. 76-2218-2, 79-15023, 79-5413, 79-15024.)

alcoholism in both of these patient populations may be a significant factor.

The sequestrum of osteomyelitis, although no longer generally regarded in the context of osteonecrosis, is a manifestation of ischemic bone death occurring as a consequence of compressive and destructive suppuration that isolates a segment of bone from its blood supply (Fig. 76–5). The sequestration of cortical bone is accomplished by obliteration of the sinusoidal bed, disruption of the metaphyseal and nutrient arterial supply, and stripping of the periosteum with its penetrating periosteal arteries from the cortical surface by pus.

Finally, there is a sizeable group of patients with osteonecrosis in whom none of the above conditions are implicated, for which the term idiopathic osteonecrosis is reserved. The label "idiopathic" may reflect unknown history (e.g., "closet alcoholism") as much as unknown etiology. Interestingly, rare instances of multiple "idiopathic" bone infarcts in several members of a family in one or more generations have been encountered, suggesting a hereditary predisposition in some cases.[114]

Femoral Head Dislocation

Subluxation of the adult femoral head invariably ruptures the ligamentum teres, disrupting the arterial supply to the femoral head. In addition, the superior retinacular arteries may be partially or totally compromised.[106] Patients with dislocations[131] and delayed reductions[30] appear to be at greater risk for the development of avascular necrosis. Reduction of the femoral head returns the bone to its normal stress-bearing orientation. This will not restore blood flow through the ligamentum teres but may relieve any vascular embarrassment that had occurred as a result of twisting or stretching of the retinacular vessels.[106, 108] Whether or not avascular necrosis develops under these circumstances depends upon the availability of sufficient collateral circulation to augment the blood supply that had been reduced by the damaged extraosseous arterial vessels. Avascular necrosis of the femoral head following subluxation is usually confined to the anterolateral weight-bearing segment, although occasionally more extensive areas or the entire head will be involved[114] (see Chapters 63 and 77).

Femoral Neck Fracture

Intracapsular femoral neck fractures result in extensive interruption of blood flow to the femoral head. The sinusoidal vascular bed is interrupted[106] and the subsynovial retinacular vessels, including the lateral epiphyseal, superior metaphyseal, and inferior metaphyseal arterial extensions,[117] may also be disrupted or severely damaged.[19, 83, 105] The only remaining blood supply available to the femoral head may be within the ligamentum teres, provided that it was functional prior to fracture.[19, 91, 105]

The incidence of avascular necrosis following intracapsular femoral neck fractures will depend upon the reestablishment of adequate blood flow from the remaining intact vasculature or the revascularization (ingrowth) of new vessels in the femoral head,[19, 105] or both. Available data indicate that between 60 and 75 per cent of femoral heads removed under the previously described circumstances will demonstrate evidence of ischemic necrosis.[12, 18, 125] This is particularly true if there has been significant displacement or excessive rotation of the fractured fragments.[48] Both displacement and rotation are likely to increase the severity of damage to the retinacular vessels.

Reestablishment of blood flow to a portion of the femoral head through the ligamentum teres occurs in 50 to 60 per cent of patients, but only rarely will it supply the entire femoral head.[19, 89, 91, 103, 105, 106] Unfortunately, a small percentage of normal patients have no functional blood flow through the ligamentum teres, and in some patients the fracture disrupts the ligament.[21] Under these circumstances revascularization must occur from the femoral neck.

Close approximation of the fracture edges provides the opportunity to reestablish blood flow by local revascularization across the fracture site with ingrowth of new vessels from the retinacular group.[4, 19, 21, 105] The higher incidence of avascular necrosis that follows displaced femoral neck fractures suggests that persistent motion (instability) across the fracture site can continually rupture anastomosing vascular channels that are bridging the fracture.[19, 105] Should the fractured segment fail to unite, the reestablishment of blood flow to the femoral head will be significantly impaired.[23, 107] The extent and the distribution of necrosis within the femoral head tend to vary considerably following fracture. The majority of infarcts are localized to the anterolateral weight-bearing segment, but more extensive involvement is fairly common.[20] Not infrequently, the entire femoral head dies. The latter is most likely to occur with nonunion of the fractured neck[7, 17, 23, 48, 107, 114] (Fig. 76–6).

In the absence of a reestablished blood supply, there can be no reparative response, and the femoral head, though dead, will remain both anatomically and radiographically unchanged for a time.[46, 88, 89, 90, 107] This radiographic pattern was more frequently encountered prior to hip nailing, when patients with femoral neck fractures were treated by immobilization. The progressive disuse osteoporosis of the adjacent viable pelvis and femur resulted in a necrotic femoral head that appeared relatively dense.[103] With hip nailing and rapid weight-bearing, early radiographic identification of avascular necrosis has become more difficult.[11, 17, 48] This identification is further complicated by the cancellous bone remodeling that normally follows in response to the altered mechanics created by the fracture.[46]

Sickle Cell Disease

Sickle cell disease, sickle cell trait, and the other related hemoglobinopathies are associated with localized areas of epiphyseal and metadiaphyseal bone infarction.[5, 28, 29, 82, 84, 94] Sludging of sickled erythrocytes within the sinusoidal vascular bed results in functional occlusion. The localized anoxia further aggravates the sickling process, increasing the likelihood of additional vessel occlusion and extension of the involved area. If the process becomes sufficiently extensive, infarction will occur. Since this process frequently occurs within areas of active hematopoiesis, localized areas of intramedullary bone infarction may be found throughout the skeleton.[22, 28] However, in most cases, the foci of osteonecrosis are encountered in the epiphyseal and metadiaphyseal marrow cavities of long tubular bones.[28]

Reestablishment of the vascular supply is dependent upon stabilization of the infarcted area and reversal of the sickling phenomenon, allowing resumption of blood flow. The precise nature of the "bone-within-bone" radiographic appearance (Fig. 76–7) occasionally encountered in sickle cell disease during childhood remains uncertain, although it may possibly represent some form of cortical infarction.[8, 28] Sickle cell disease is frequently complicated by superimposed osteomyelitis (Fig. 76–8), especially due to Salmonella organisms.[56] Exclusion of cortical sequestration by infection is essential prior to ascribing the "bone-within-bone" appearance to aseptic bone necrosis.[8, 47]

Corticosteroid Therapy

The increased incidence of avascular necrosis in patients receiving corticosteroid therapy and in individuals with Cushing's disease is well established.[9, 14, 38, 45, 51, 52] Considerable experimental work has been undertaken in an attempt to explain the mechanism of osteonecrosis associated with corticosteroid therapy.[39, 70, 121] Much attention has been focused on the presence of microscopic fat emboli in the end-arteries of bone and other organ systems.[30, 39, 70, 71] It has been proposed that the fat emboli and hyperlipidemia observed in this clinical setting are derived from a fatty liver.[37, 55] Others have suggested that steroid-induced osteoporosis with subsequent microfracture causes the osteonecrosis.[40, 41, 68, 75, 95] Little attention has been paid to alterations in marrow fat cells.[67] Recent experimental evidence indicates a significant increase in individual marrow fat cell size associated with high-dose corticosteroid therapy.[121] The increasing fat cell mass is not completely accommodated by an equivalent loss of trabecular and cortical bone. Because the marrow cavity is encased by a nonexpansile shell of bone, any increase in marrow fat cell mass not accommodated by bone loss must occur at the expense of the remaining marrow constituents, especially the sinusoidal vascular bed, since hematopoietic activity is normally scant in areas of fatty marrow. The resulting mechanical infringement on the sinusoidal vascular bed will impede blood flow and theoretically increase intraosseous marrow pressure.[121]

Recent clinical and experimental studies have demonstrated significantly increased intraosseous marrow pressures within the femoral heads of patients and rabbits treated with corticosteroids.[57, 122] Perfusion of the marrow sinusoidal vascular bed is dependent upon hydrostatic pressure from the pumping action of the heart and the elastic recoil of arteries.[49] Any increase in intraosseous pressure not compensated for by an increase in hydrostatic pressure will result in the compromise of marrow sinusoidal blood flow, increasing the risk of infarction.

Alcoholism

Avascular necrosis, especially of the femoral head, in association with chronic alcoholism is fairly common.[6, 68, 85] Metadiaphyseal infarcts are rare. Similar mechanisms to those outlined for corticosteroid necrosis have been proposed for osteonecrosis in chronic alcoholism.[67] It has been suggested that the alcoholic fatty liver is associated with systemic fat emboli, which may lodge in bone.[69] Although there are no experimental data available that demonstrate an increase in marrow fat cell size, elevated intraosseous marrow pressures have been recorded in normal-appearing femoral heads of alcoholic patients who have avascular necrosis in the contralateral hip.[58]

Gaucher's Disease

Histologic examination of the bone marrow in Gaucher's disease reveals that the sinusoids are packed with lipid (glucocerebroside)-containing histiocytes termed Gaucher's cells. An increasing number of Gaucher's cells results in progressive obstruction of the flow of blood through the sinusoids, leading to osteonecrosis.[62, 67] Both avascular necrosis and metadiaphyseal infarcts are encountered in this disorder.[1, 2, 64, 101, 115]

Dysbaric Disorders

Osteonecrosis of both the epiphyseal and metadiaphyseal medullary cavities associated with dys-

Text continued on page 2795

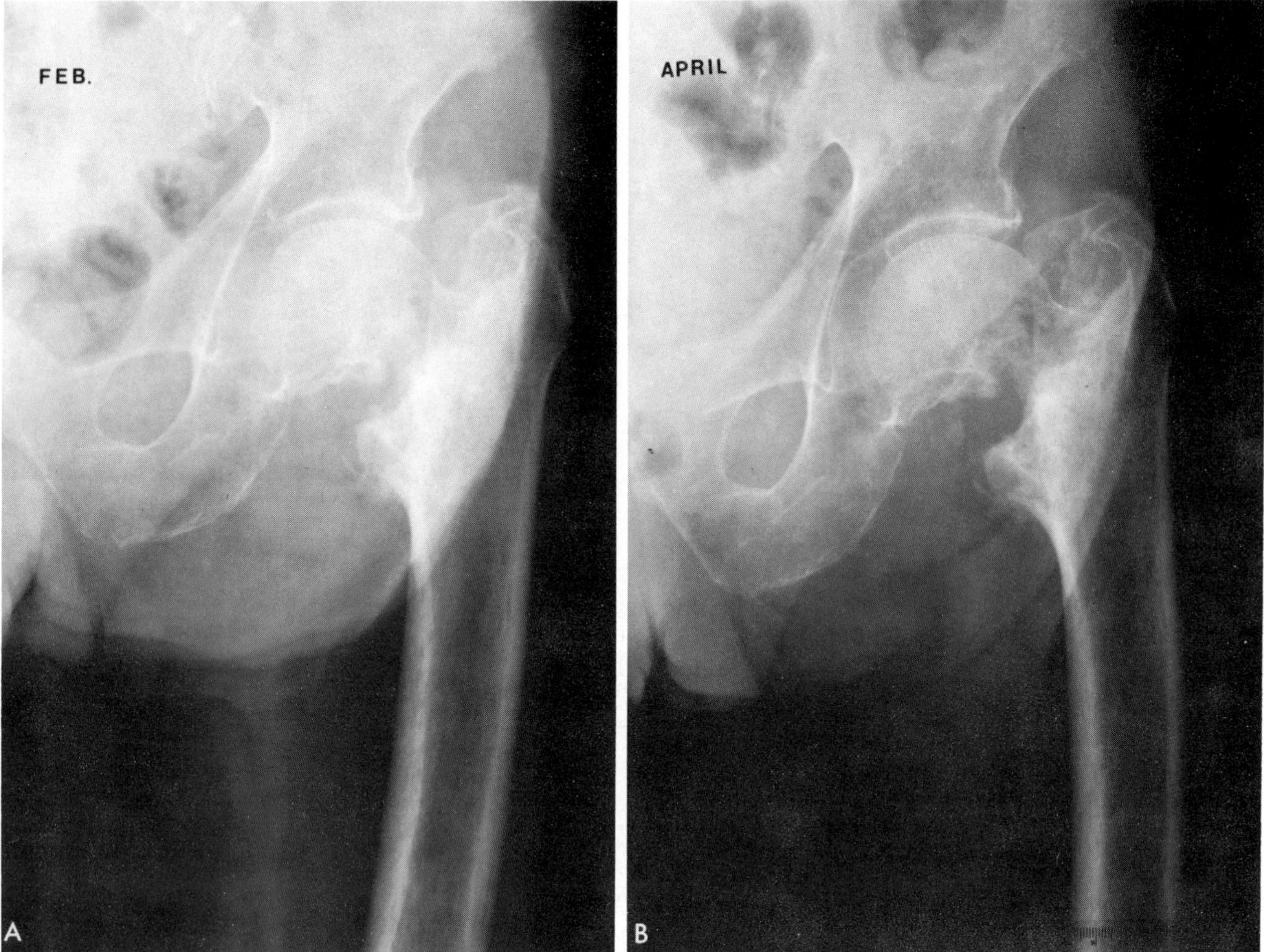

Figure 76–6. Fracture of femoral neck with fibrous nonunion.

A, B Radiographs of an ununited femoral neck fracture taken 2 months apart (February, April) with slight difference in technique. There has been no significant change over the 2 months, suggesting an impaired repair process.

C Macroscopic section (2×) of the femoral head demonstrates extensive avascular necrosis and only a partial fibrous union. Note the subchondral area of avascular necrosis (N) surrounded by a fairly well defined reactive fibrous interface (R). The remaining portion of the femoral head is an admixture of ischemic necrosis (n) and injury and revascularization (r). This suggests extension of the original infarct and is likely to have been the result of the fracture's failure to properly unite and reestablish adequate blood flow. The increased bone density at the peripheral margin adjacent to the fibrous nonunion indicates viability and mechanical reinforcement (straight arrows).

D Photomicrographic view (2×) of the subchondral area of avascular necrosis shows unaltered dead cancellous bone, lipid cysts (C) and partially opacified necrotic fat (O).

E Photomicrograph (28×) of a reactive interface demonstrates dead fat superiorly (N), the fibrous interface (R), and surrounding revitalized cancellous bone and fat (V). There is some reactive fiber bone reinforcement within the reactive interface (curved arrow).

F Photomicrograph (40×) of the outer margin of a reactive interface, showing fibrous modulation of marrow fat (R), lipid cyst formation (C), increased vascularity and new vessel formation, and revascularization surrounded by an inflammatory cell infiltrate (arrow).

(Armed Forces Institute of Pathology Neg. Nos. 64-2229-2,5; 79-15317; 79-15318-1,2; 79-15316.)

Illustration continued on the opposite page

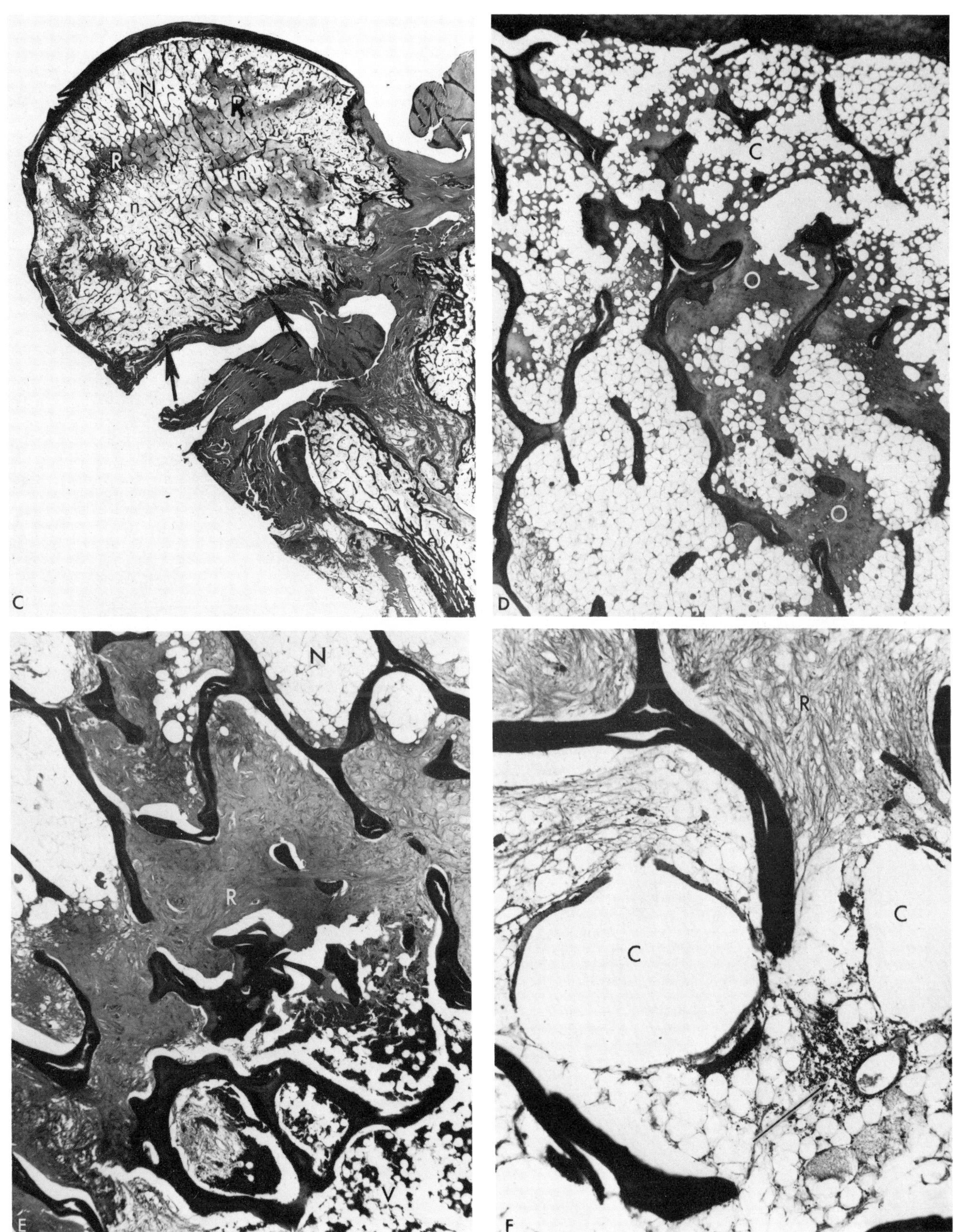

Figure 76–6. Continued

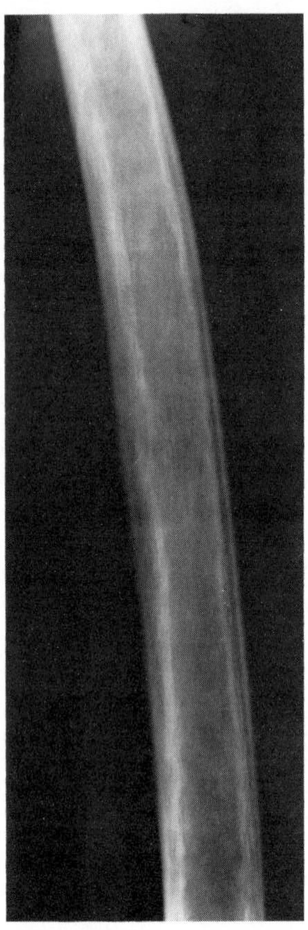

Figure 76–7. Sickle cell disease. Lateral view of midfemur demonstrates a "bone-within-bone" appearance. This is noted by the radiolucent area splitting the anterior cortex with a radiodense line on both surfaces. (Armed Forces Institute of Pathology Neg. No. 68-4951-1.)

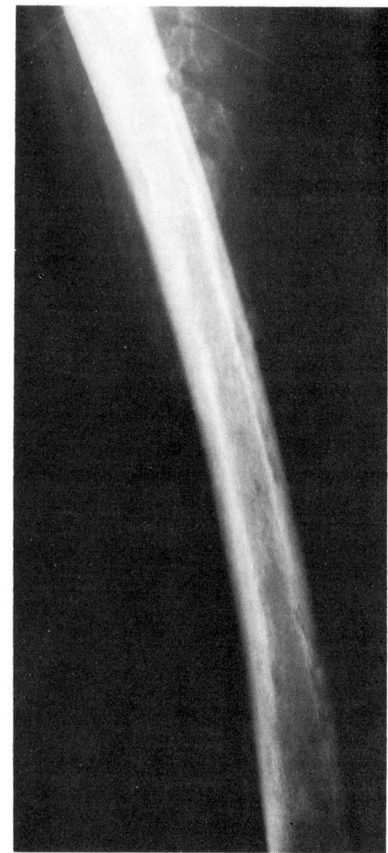

Figure 76–8. Sickle cell disease with osteomyelitis. Lateral view of femur showing a "bone-within-bone" appearance as well as patchy bone destruction in the cortex and extensive periosteal new bone formation. (Armed Forces Institute of Pathology Neg. No. 70-69023.)

baric disorders[100, 123] has been regarded as the result of air (nitrogen) embolization following rapid decompression.[26, 34, 92, 120] Partial pressures of dissolved gases demand eventual equilibrium between the atmosphere, blood, and interstitial and intracellular compartments. Invariably, there is a relative time lag in the equalization of partial pressures across vessel walls and cell membranes during both compression and decompression.[26] Experimental studies indicate that fat cells have a fivefold increased ability to absorb dissolved nitrogen.[44] Since both blood flow and the capillary–fat cell surface area are relatively reduced, the ability to transport nitrogen away from fatty tissue is only about half that of other tissues.[44] This will result in nitrogen bubbles appearing within fat cells if the rate of decompression exceeds the transporting ability of the circulation.[43] Although fat cells in soft tissue have room to expand under these circumstances, the marrow fat cells are confined by a nonexpansile shell of bone.[67] As a result, the potential for a dramatic increase in intraosseous marrow pressure during decompression is significant. Whereas the accumulation of undissolved nitrogen gas bubbles in interstitial and vascular spaces undoubtedly plays some role, failure of equalization of pressure across the marrow fat cell membrane with subsequent expansion and rupture of the fat cell may be a more significant causative factor of osteonecrosis in this condition (see Chapter 77).

Radiation-Induced Osteonecrosis

Depending upon the dosage of radiation therapy, there may be a direct cytotoxic effect, especially of the more sensitive hematopoietic marrow constituents.[21, 25, 65, 81, 124] Although the actual mechanism remains controversial, the long-term radiation effects resulting in osteonecrosis are mediated through damage to the bones' vascularity.[61, 66]

Collagen Vascular Disorders

It is likely that the relatively high incidence of ischemic bone necrosis in systemic lupus erythematosus, rheumatoid arthritis, and renal transplantation is related to corticosteroid therapy.[21, 24, 32, 110] Vasculitis with interruption of the arterial blood supply has been suggested as a possible additional mechanism[119] for at least some of the patients with collagen vascular disorders not treated with steroids who develop osteonecrosis.[109, 110, 113]

Chronic Pancreatitis and Gout

Necrosis of the peritoneal and mesenteric fat is a well-recognized complication of acute pancreatitis.[77] Similar findings have been demonstrated in the brain, kidney, subcutaneous tissue, and bone marrow at autopsy.[77] Disseminated small areas of fat necrosis in bone, presumably the result of circulating lipases,[86] have been described as a complication of acute pancreatitis.[59] However, typical patterns of femoral head and intramedullary bone infarcts are only rarely observed.[42, 78] The recognized association of pancreatitis and alcoholism requires close scrutiny to exclude the latter as a possible contributing mechanism in this patient population.

What relationship, if any, exists to explain the apparent association between gout and avascular necrosis, other than alcoholism, remains obscure.[6, 76, 79]

Circulation, Intraosseous Marrow Pressure, and Weight-Bearing

Several of the clinical situations outlined previously seem to be associated with an alteration of marrow constituents and an increase in intraosseous marrow pressure. Since the marrow cavity is encased by a rigid bony shell, any increase in one marrow component, in terms of either cell number or volume, must take place at the expense of the remaining marrow elements. Against this background, it is increasingly apparent that the cellular composition of marrow and its relationship to the sinusoidal vascular bed are fundamental to the understanding of the mechanisms of nontraumatic avascular necrosis and bone infarction. The predominance of metadiaphyseal bone infarcts in the intertrochanteric area and distal end of the femur, the proximal tibia, and the proximal humerus (all areas of fatty marrow in adults) and the relatively high incidence of avascular necrosis in the femoral head and, to a lesser extent, the humeral head and femoral condyles of adults (also areas of predominantly fatty marrow) underscore an important relationship between the fatty marrow and the sinusoidal vascular bed.

The foregoing observations leave unexplained the predominant localization of avascular necrosis of the femoral head to the anterolateral weight-bearing subchondral bony segment. This indicates that there is something unique about the weight-bearing area of the femoral head that places it at higher risk for ischemic necrosis. If increased intraosseous pressure is as significant a factor in the development of osteonecrosis as accumulating data would suggest,[57, 58] the ability to decompress the marrow space would be an equally important factor in the prevention of osteonecrosis. This ability to decompress the marrow space would depend largely on regional anatomic structure, especially bony architecture and vascular outflow.[50] Both the humeral head and the femoral head are at an anatomic disadvantage for decompression. They represent large spheres covered by articular surface, perched on narrow metaphyseal necks. Therefore, relatively few venous channels that penetrate the bony cortex are directly available for decompression. For this reason, any increase in pressure within these large spheres must be funneled through the narrow metaphyseal neck for decompression, a situation analogous to rush-hour traffic on a one lane bridge.

The subchondral weight-bearing area of the femoral head is at a special disadvantage for decompression. In response to the mechanical requirements of weight-bearing, a greater amount of more tightly packed cancellous bone is present within this area. This creates a baffle effect, which further restricts the ability to decompress the marrow space in comparison with that of the more open adjacent subchondral areas. Trabecular deformation during weight-bearing will also compress the marrow space to some degree and should result in a localized, temporary increase in intraosseous pressure. The increased intraosseous pressure tends to remain concentrated in this area because of the tightly structured bone architecture. This, coupled with a clinical situation in which the intraosseous pressure is already elevated, could transform an area of bone which is ischemic and marginally profused into an area of functional anoxia with resultant infarction.

HISTOLOGIC-RADIOGRAPHIC CORRELATION OF THE HOST RESPONSE

Once osteonecrosis or ischemic injury is an established anatomic fact, the body sets into motion the initial inflammatory host response as the first step toward revival, rehabilitation, or removal and reconstruction (repair). Anything modifying the ability of the host to generate an adequate circulatory response (e.g., increased intraosseous pressure) and inflammatory response (e.g., corticosteroids) will be a major factor affecting the morphologic, radiographic, and clinical manifestations of osteonecrosis repair. Structural disruption either prior to the development of osteonecrosis (e.g., femoral neck fracture) or during its repair will significantly alter the stress-transmitting capabilities of the involved bone. This disruption will consequently result in superimposed bone remodeling to meet the changing mechanical requirements as an addition to the inflammatory reparative process. It is the interaction of these various factors that is responsible for the relatively wide-ranging anatomic and radiographic changes observed in patients with osteonecrosis.

Within the limits of this chapter, it will not be possible to illustrate all the radiographic variations that can emerge as part of the host response to avascular necrosis of the adult femoral head. Attention will be focused on the progressive histologic changes of the host reparative response to the osteonecrotic segment and their reflection in the radiograph. The discussion will consider each of five anatomic phases, from cell death to articular collapse, stages that are not dissimilar from previously outlined radiographic and clinical stages of avascular necrosis.[35, 111]

Phase I: Cellular Death and the Initial Host Response

The recognition of cell death in osteonecrosis by light microscopy has long been a subject of considerable discussion. Proper histologic analysis can be complicated by improper fixation and decalcification of the tissue specimen, both of which can result in marked artifactual distortion of cells. Although functional cell death may have occurred, documentation of cell death is not histologically possible until sufficient cytoplasmic (coagulation) and nuclear (pyknosis, karyorrhexis, and karyolysis) changes occur to cause the cellular constituents to lose their morphologic and staining characteristics.[96] This feature is exemplified in a femoral head from a 73 year old woman that was resected 24 hours following femoral neck fracture (Fig. 76–9). Aside from the fracture (Fig. 76–9*A*) and the acute hemorrhage adjacent to the fracture site (Fig. 76–9*C*), there are no abnormal radiographic, gross pathologic, or histologic findings (Fig. 76–9*B–D*). The hematopoietic marrow, osteocytes, and marrow fat appear unremarkable. Although the clinical setting indicates that anoxia of the femoral head has been present for 24 hours, necrosis cannot be confirmed by light microscopy in this specimen. Six hours of anoxia is generally regarded as sufficient to result in death of the hematopoietic marrow.[125] However, it may be 48 to 72 hours before the degree of cell autolysis is sufficient to be recognized histologically (see Fig. 76–10*D*). Thus, in this case the time interval between the onset of anoxia and resection is not sufficient for even the most sensitive marrow elements to demonstrate anoxic damage.

Clinical and experimental studies suggest that osteocytes, osteoblasts, and osteoclasts may survive approximately 6 to 48 hours of anoxia before irreversible cell damage and death occur.[72] Because viable osteocytes within bony lacunae frequently appear pyknotic, pyknosis alone is not a reliable sign of cell death under this circumstance.[21] It has been generally accepted that empty osteocytic lacunae reflect cell death. However, as there is a normal attrition of osteocytes with age,[63] the presence of empty osteocytic lacunae does not necessarily indicate osteonecrosis. Even with functional death of osteocytes, complete autolysis, as evidenced by empty osteocytic lacunae, may take from 48 hours to 4 weeks or longer to occur.[21, 67, 72] Thus, the presence or absence of osteocytes in lacunae cannot be consid-

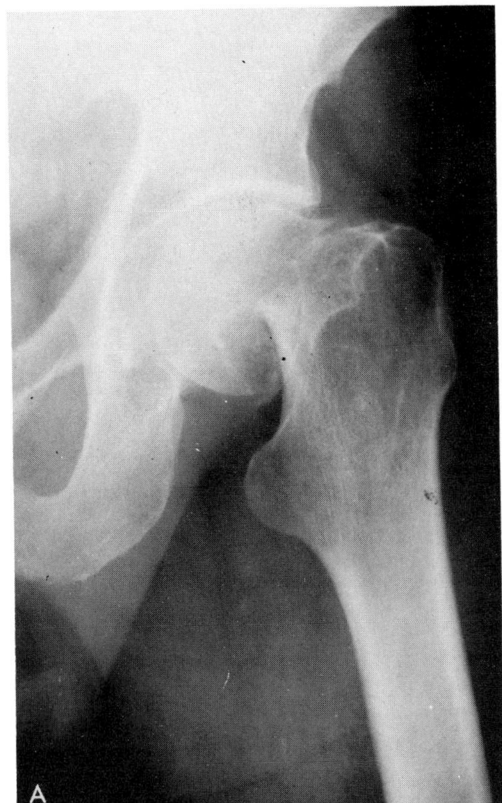

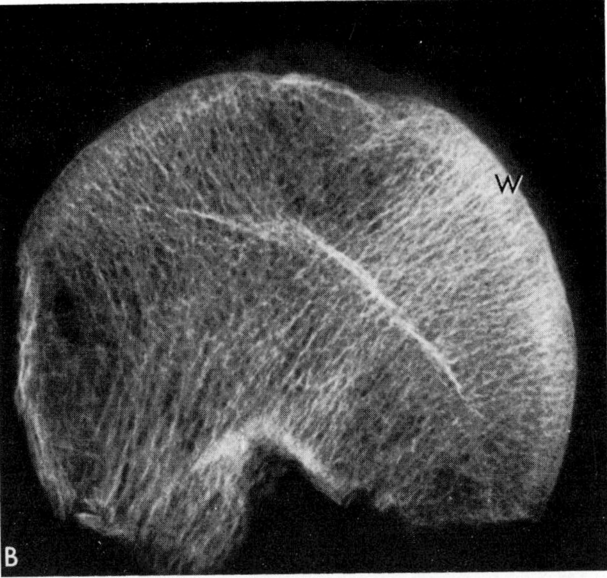

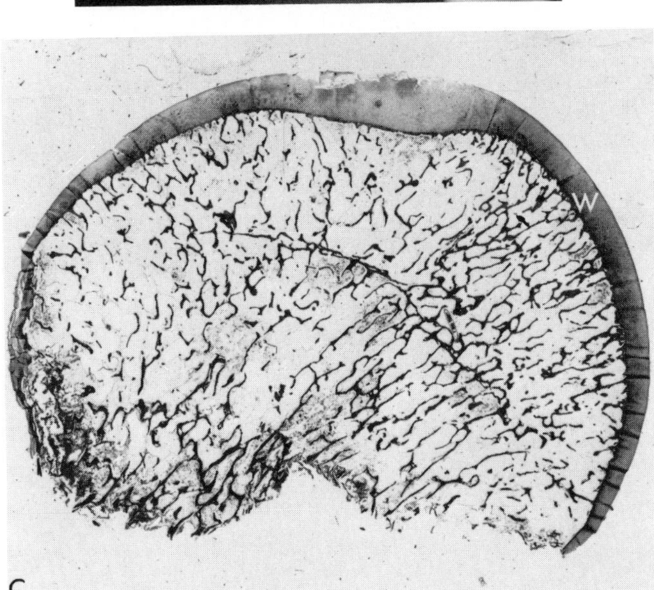

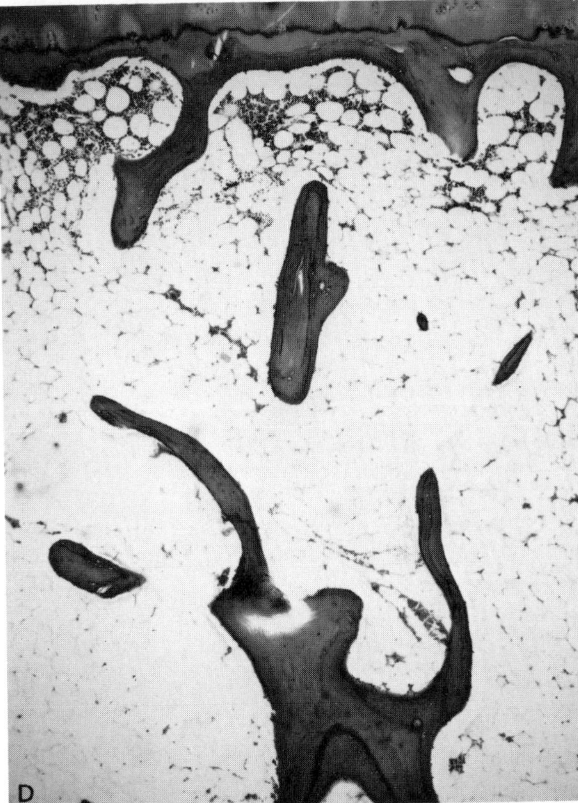

Figure 76–9. *Fracture of the femoral neck (24 hours).*

A *Clinical radiograph demonstrates a femoral neck fracture without dislocation.*

B *Specimen radiograph (2.5×) of the coronally sectioned femoral head resected 24 hours following fracture reveals a normal appearing subchondral plate and underlying cancellous bone. The concentration and orientation of the supporting trabecular bone in the weight-bearing area* (W) *are normal.*

C *Macroscopic section (2.5×) reveals an intact articular surface and subchondral plate. Note the orientation* (W) *of the cancellous bony architecture underlying the weight-bearing area. The marrow is predominantly fatty, with scattered areas of hematopoietic activity. Acute hemorrhage is present along the fracture line inferiorly.*

D *Photomicrograph (40×) shows the "tide mark" separating the articular cartilage from the subchondral bony plate as well as the underlying cancellous bone marrow. Although portions of the marrow and cancellous bone have presumably been anoxic for 24 hours, there are no histologic changes suggestive of cell death or ischemic injury. The focal areas of appositional bone formation on the preexisting cancellous trabeculae are part of normal remodeling and are not related to the fracture or ischemia.*

(Armed Forces Institute of Pathology Neg. Nos. 66-3884, 79-5414, 79-15019, 79-15020.)

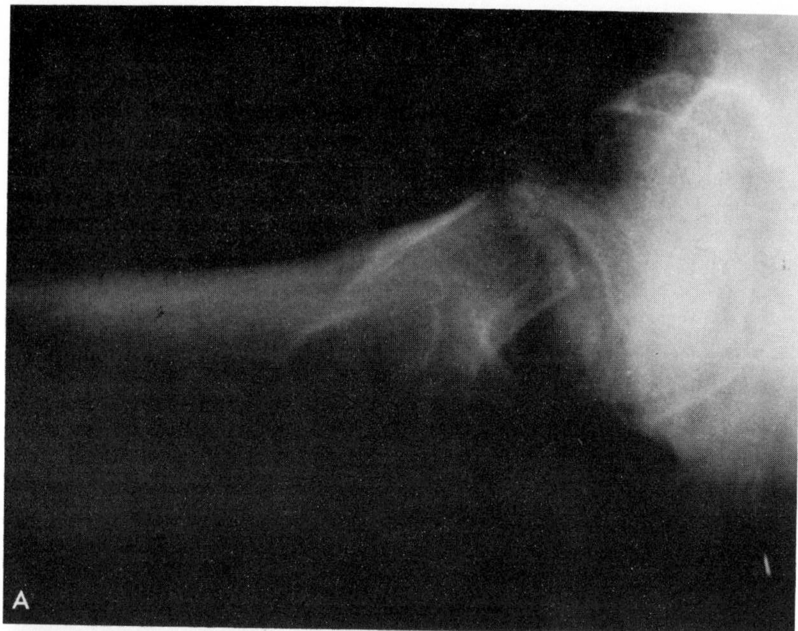

Figure 76–10. *Fracture of the femoral neck (72 hours).*

A *Clinical radiograph demonstrates a subcapital femoral neck fracture with minimal displacement of the femoral head.*

B *Specimen radiograph (2.5×) of the coronally sectioned femoral head resected 72 hours following fracture reveals an intact subchondral plate and normal appearing cancellous bone. There is some normal trabecular coarsening in the weight-bearing area (W) and a lucent area adjacent to the fovea.*

C *Macroscopic section (2.5×) from the femoral head reveals an intact and normal appearing articular surface. There is a slight artifactual buckling (A) of the articular surface inferiorly, which has resulted from processing. Although the cancellous bone appears unremarkable, there are extensive areas of altered marrow (slightly darker staining) throughout the specimen.*

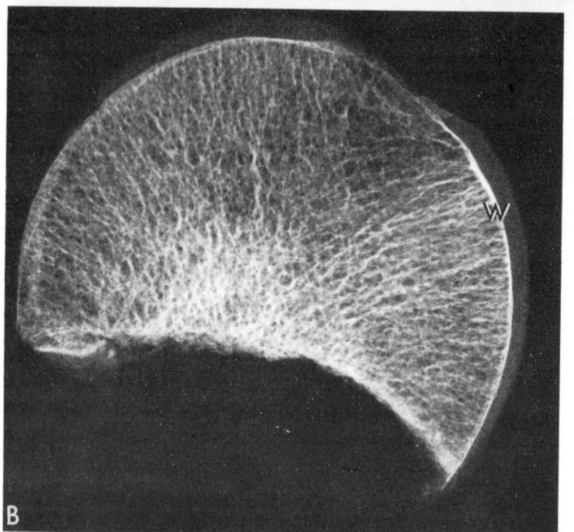

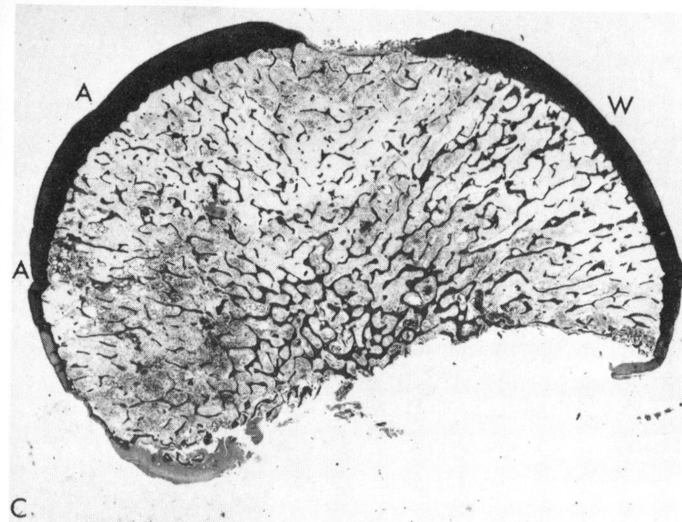

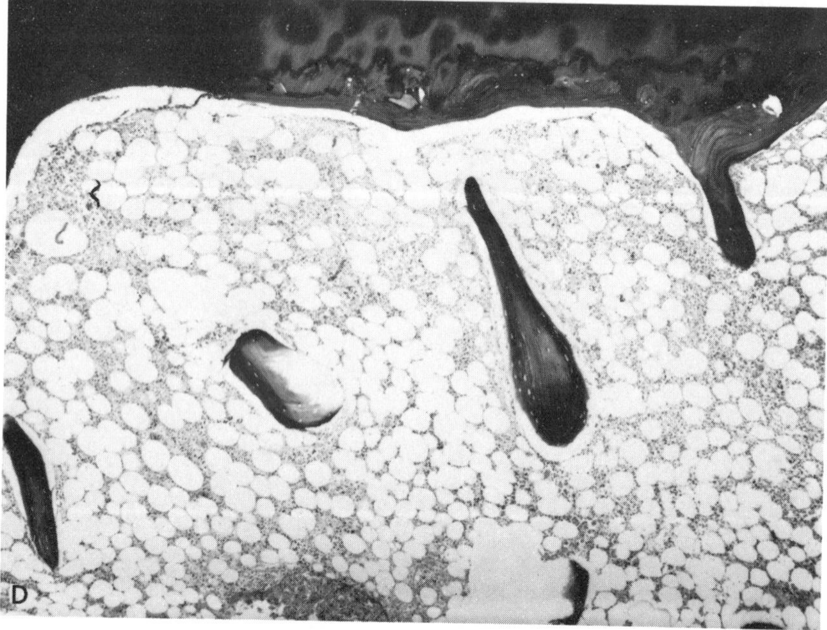

D *Photomicrograph (40×) shows essentially normal appearing articular cartilage, tide mark, and subchondral plate. The ghostlike appearance of the hematopoietic and myelopoietic marrow indicates anoxic death and accounts for the altered staining characteristics in* **C.** *Many of the osteocytic lacunae appear empty. The marrow fat cells are essentially unchanged. The recently formed appositional bone on the surface of the cancellous bone reflects remodeling that antedates the fracture.*

(Armed Forces Institute of Pathology Neg. Nos. 79-5407-1,2; 79-15017; 79-15018.)

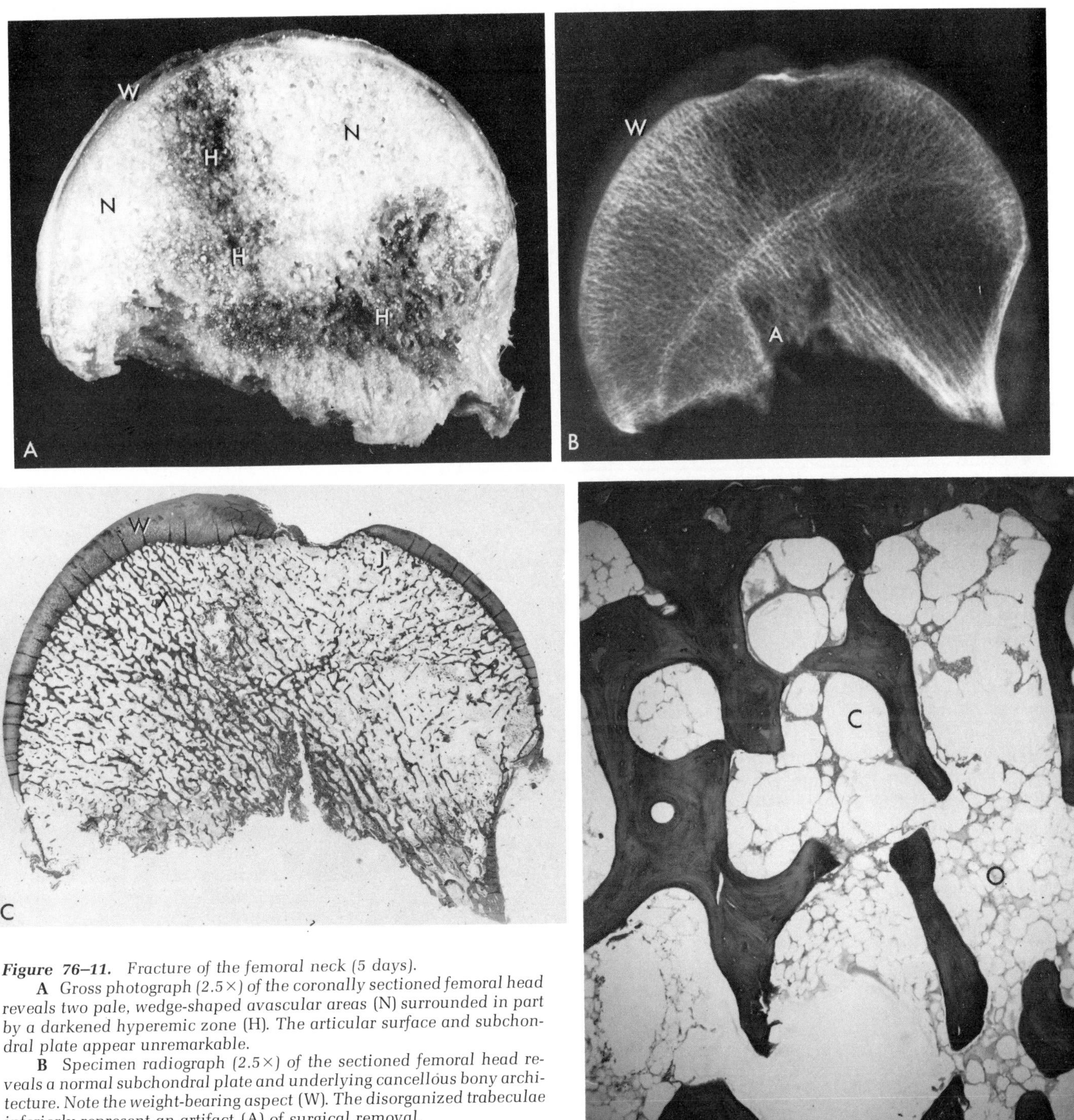

Figure 76–11. *Fracture of the femoral neck (5 days).*

A *Gross photograph (2.5×) of the coronally sectioned femoral head reveals two pale, wedge-shaped avascular areas (N) surrounded in part by a darkened hyperemic zone (H). The articular surface and subchondral plate appear unremarkable.*

B *Specimen radiograph (2.5×) of the sectioned femoral head reveals a normal subchondral plate and underlying cancellous bony architecture. Note the weight-bearing aspect (W). The disorganized trabeculae inferiorly represent an artifact (A) of surgical removal.*

C *Macroscopic section (2.5×) reveals an intact articular surface, subchondral plate and normal underlying cancellous bone with coarsening beneath the weight-bearing area (W). There is evidence of hemorrhage along the fracture line, but the remaining marrow appears unremarkable at low power.*

D *Photomicrograph (40 ×) of the subchondral area shows the tide mark, subchondral plate, and normal appearing cancellous bone. There is striking lipid cyst formation (C), opacification of marrow fat cells (O), and dissolution of hematopoietic cells, indicating ischemic death of all marrow elements. Occasional osteocytic lacunae appear empty.*

(Armed Forces Institute of Pathology Neg. Nos. 79-15016-1, 79-5217, 79-15016-2, 79-15015.)

ered as a reliable indication of either cell viability or cell death in the early stages of osteonecrosis. However, complete absence of osteocytes within localized areas of trabecular bone is a reasonably reliable indicator of previous or existing ischemic necrosis if artifactual loss can be excluded.

These considerations are exemplified in the femoral head of a 69 year old man resected 72 hours following a femoral neck fracture (Fig. 76–10). Aside from the fracture, neither the clinical nor the specimen radiographs (Fig. 76–10*A*,*B*) show any alteration in the subchondral or trabecular bone architecture. The macroscopic section shows evidence of hemorrhage along the fracture site and both hyperemic and avascular areas within the substance of the femoral head (Fig. 76–10*C*). The high power view of the microscopic section reveals an autolytic ghost-like appearance (necrosis) in the hematopoietic elements (Fig. 76–10*D*). Many of the osteocytic lacunae within the bone trabeculae also appear empty, suggesting bone death (Fig. 76–10*D*). There is no evident alteration of marrow fat cells.

Little attention has been focused on the marrow fat cells' ability to survive anoxia. Estimates of marrow fat cell survivability following complete anoxia range from 2 to 5 days or more.[67] Histologically, marrow fat cell death may be reflected by no appreciable structual change other than loss of its nucleus, a feature that is frequently difficult to identify under normal conditions because of nuclear eccentricity and section thickness relative to cell size. Loss of nuclei, disruption of a cluster of fat cells (forming lipid cysts), and partial opacification of fat cells are generally recognized as signs that reflect cell death. Such findings are exemplified in the femoral head that was resected from a 71 year old man 5 days following subcapital femoral neck fracture (Fig. 76–11). The gross photograph shows characteristic pale areas of avascularity partly surrounded by a hyperemic zone (Fig. 76–11*A*). There is no alteration observed in the specimen radiograph (Fig. 76–11*B*). The macroscopic section shows the expected hemorrhage along the fracture site, with focal areas of hyperemia but no alteration in bony architecture (Fig. 76–11*C*). The high power view of the microscopic section reveals the presence of large lipid cysts and necrotic hematopoietic elements (Fig. 76–11*D*). The lipid cysts are partially surrounded by lightly opacified but otherwise unaltered fat cells. No viable osteoblasts or osteoclasts are seen. A few osteocytic lacunae are empty, whereas others appear to contain nuclei. The findings in this case reflect unequivocal ischemic necrosis, despite the fact there is incomplete osteocyte loss.

In the early stages, histologically recognizable death of the hematopoietic elements, and especially marrow fat, is the most reliable light microscopic sign of osteonecrosis. The presence or absence of osteocytic nuclei (empty lacunae) is of lesser importance because of the wide variations in their rates of autolysis following functional death. However, uniformly empty osteocytic lacunae are important findings in the evaluation of the late stages of osteonecrosis, when they may be the only reliable histologic marker indicating the extent of the original infarcted area.

Hence, the first phase of osteonecrosis, cell death and initial host response, is characterized by microscopic changes in the hematopoietic elements, the osteocytic cellular constituents, and the marrow fat cells. Although the "central" zone of cell death is usually distinguishable from the surrounding viable

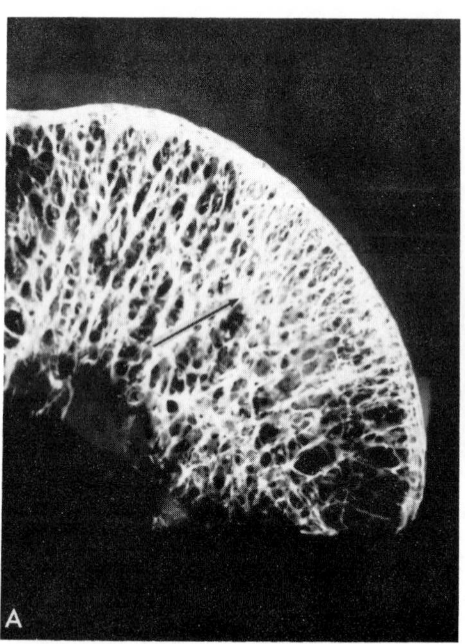

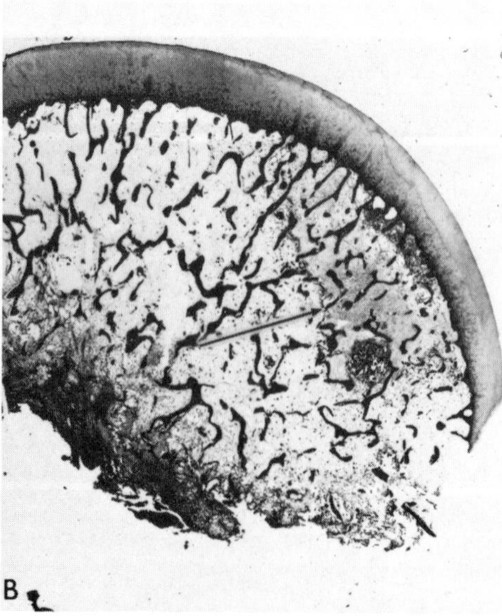

Figure 76–12. *Fracture of the subcapital femoral neck (2 months).*

A *Specimen radiograph (2.5×) of the coronally sectioned femoral head segment reveals an intact subchondral bony plate supported in part by a wedge-shaped area of apparently increased radiodensity (arrow). The surrounding cancellous bone trabeculae are coarse but considerably reduced in number.*

B *Macroscopic section (2.5×) of* **A** *indicates that the wedge-shaped focus of increased density represents an area of osteonecrosis and ischemic injury (arrow). Note the relative number and size of the cancellous trabeculae in the ischemically injured and necrotic area compared with those in the surrounding osteoporotic viable bone. There is considerable reactive change along the fracture line.*

Illustration continued on the opposite page

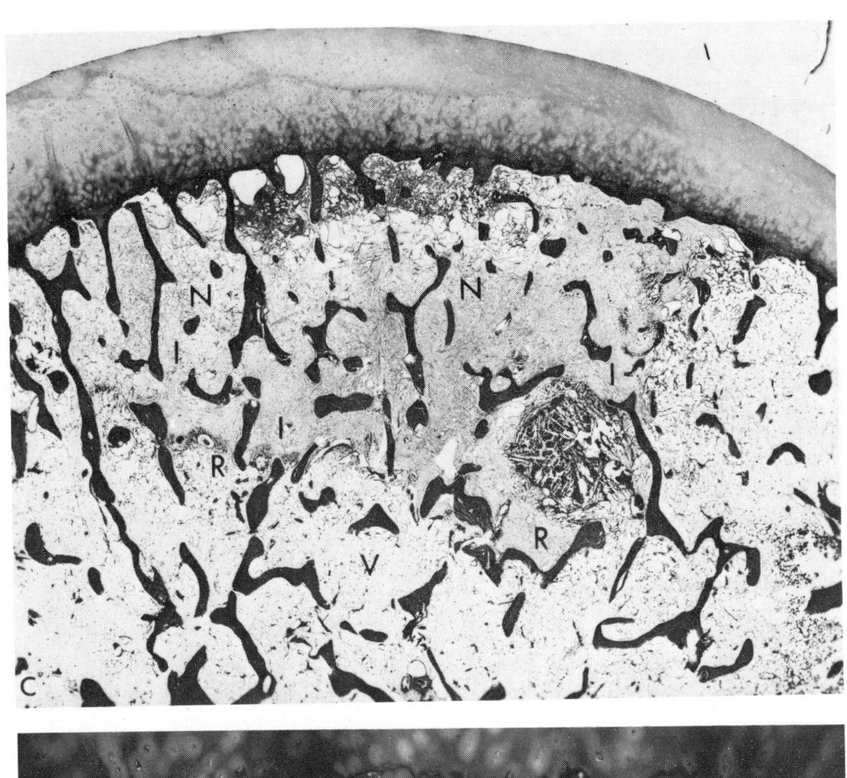

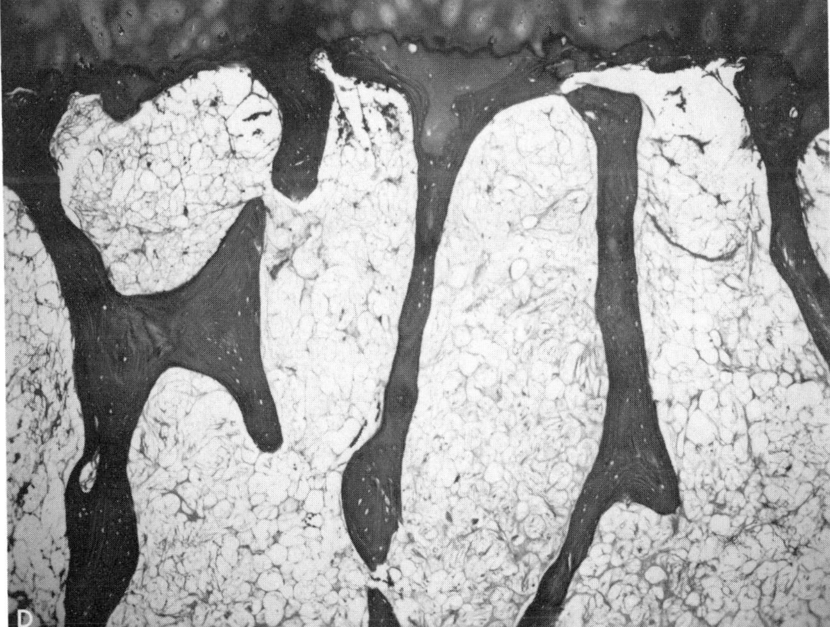

Figure 76–12. Continued

C *Photomicrograph (8×) reveals an intact articular surface and subchondral plate. Immediately beneath the subchondral plate is an area of necrosis characterized by dissolution of marrow cellular architecture, giving the appearance of basophilic debris (N). The necrotic area is surrounded by a broad area of dead and ischemically injured marrow fat (I). The hemorrhagic cyst is filled with cholesterol crystals from the breakdown of fat cells. Vascular dilatation can be seen along the reactive margin (R) between the ischemically injured fat (I) and surrounding viable marrow (V).*

D *Photomicrographic view (40×) demonstrates the crystalline appearance of ischemically dead marrow fat cells and spindling of the ischemically injured marrow fat cells. The lower portion of the articular surface above the tide mark is unremarkable. The subchondral plate and underlying cancellous bone, although architecturally intact, are devoid of osteocytic nuclei, indicating bone death. Even the cartilage below the tide mark is devoid of viable cells.*

(Armed Forces Institute of Pathology Neg. Nos. 79-5419, 79-15008, 79-15009, 79-15010.)

zone by the fifth day of complete anoxia, the ischemic zone between the zone of cell death and that of viable tissue is not histologically well defined. During this phase, the gross appearance of the unsectioned femoral head is unaltered. Sectioning of the femoral head may reveal gross areas of apparent avascularity and hyperemia. However, there are no recognizable gross architectural or radiographic changes in the cancellous and subchondral bone or overlying articular surface. Therefore, no radiographically recognizable evidence of osteonecrosis would be anticipated during Phase I.

Phase II: Cell Modulation in the Ischemic Zone and Hyperemia

Although the initial phase, cell death, is entirely a reflection of anoxia, Phase II, marked by cell modulation and hyperemia, is primarily dependent upon the availability of an adequate blood supply within the viable tissue surrounding the osteonecrotic and the ischemic zones. In the case of a femoral neck fracture, this requires either reestablishing blood flow through existing vascular spaces, or revascularization by new vessels. In the presence of adequate circulation, the breakdown products of dying and severely damaged cells initiate the host's inflammatory response, characterized by vascular dilatation, transudation of fluid, fibrin precipitation, and local infiltration of inflammatory cells. During this phase, two morphologically identifiable alterations become manifest. One is perceived radiographically (Fig. 76–12*A*), the other microscopically (Fig. 76–12*B*,*C*).

Histologically, the ischemic marrow between the central core of osteonecrosis and the surrounding viable tissue is initially characterized by modulation of ischemically injured marrow fat cells that have not undergone anoxic death (Fig. 76–12*D*). Within the immediately adjacent viable bone and marrow, evidence of increased vascularity and perivascular inflammatory cell infiltration can be identified (Fig. 76–12*C*). Radiographically, the generalized active hyperemia* in response to the injured and dying cells results in osteoporosis (mediated through osteoclastic activity) of the adjacent viable bone.

These changes are exemplified in the femoral head segment that was removed from a patient 2 months following a subcapital femoral neck fracture (Fig. 76–12). There is considerable hemorrhage and some bone loss along the fracture site (Fig. 76–12*B*). The specimen radiograph shows a small, wedge-shaped area of apparently increased bone density characterized by tightly packed but uniform-appearing cancellous bone trabeculae (Fig. 76–12*A*). The area of apparently increased radiodensity represents the zone of osteonecrosis and ischemic injury (Fig. 76–12*B*–*D*). The surrounding cancellous bone appears less radiodense and is characterized by considerable bone loss with focally coarsened trabeculae (Fig. 76–12*A*). Perception of the altered bone density is not easily appreciated in the histologic sections (Fig. 76–12*B*,*C*). The slightly opacified and spindled appearance of the marrow fat cells is characteristic of ischemically dead and injured fat tissue (Fig. 76–12*D*). The cancellous bone in the area of ischemic and dead fat is devoid of osteocytes (Fig. 76–12*D*), indicating cellular bone death. Of interest are the small tongues of cartilage below the tidemark, which are devoid of chondrocytes, indicating focal cartilage death as well (Fig. 76–12*D*). The osteonecrotic area also fails to demonstrate either osteoblastic or osteoclastic activity, which would be necessary for any radiographically perceptible changes in bone architecture (Fig. 76–12*D*). Therefore, the radiodense-appearing wedge in the specimen radiograph is relative and does not represent a true increase in bony density (Fig. 76–12*A*). The adjacent areas of less dense bone reflect a vascular induced bone loss analogous to reflex vascular osteoporosis (Fig. 76–12*A*) that is seen in other clinical situations. Hence, it is the active hyperemia within the viable tissue surrounding the ischemic and osteonecrotic segment that results in osteoporosis and represents the first recognizable radiographic alteration in osteonecrosis. The dead area remains unchanged.

Phase III: Emergence of the Reactive Interface

Phase III is characterized morphologically by the development of a reactive interface (margin) about the osteonecrotic zone. The reactive interface begins to emerge during Phase II as marrow fat cells in the ischemic zone undergo cellular alteration. Since the infarcted zone is completely avascular and the ischemic zone is sufficiently anoxic as to be unable to support osteoblasts or osteoclasts, initial repair must begin at the junction between the outer margin of the ischemic zone and the adjacent viable area. The reactive interface demonstrates an increase in vascularity associated with infiltration of inflammatory cells along the outer viable margin (Fig. 76–12*C*) and with further modulation of ischemic marrow fat toward fibroblastic cells (Fig. 76–13*D*–*F*). During this phase, atypical-appearing ischemic fiber bone may be elaborated in the modulating fibrous tissue, or even on the surface of preexisting dead bone trabeculae within the ischemic zone (Figs.

*Hyperemia means an excess of blood in a part. Active hyperemia refers to a rapidly flowing increased blood supply to an area. Active hyperemia in bone favors osteoclastic resorption of bone, whereas passive hyperemia (engorgement and slow flow) tends to favor osteoblastic activity.[67, 114]

76–13*E*,*G* and 76–14*D*). The progressive loss of mechanical support due to resorption and disruption of cancellous bone within the reactive interface stimulates compensatory reinforcement of adjacent viable cancellous bone (Fig. 76–13*D*) by osteoblastic activity. While the above changes are slowly evolving in the reactive interface, sustained active hyperemia results in progressive osteoporosis in the remaining viable portion of the femoral head.

This sequence of change is exemplified in a femoral head from a 79 year old woman that was removed 3 days following "femoral neck fracture" (Fig. 76–13*A*). The well-developed reactive interface indicates that the osteonecrotic focus dates well beyond 3 days and probably was formed somewhere between 3 and 6 months (Fig. 76–13*B–D*) ago. In this case, it is possible that the active hyperemic response to the infarcted area has sufficiently weakened the viable cancellous bone in the femoral neck to the point of fracture (Fig. 76–13*B*). The area of slightly altered density in the clinical radiograph (Fig. 76–13*A*) is more clearly

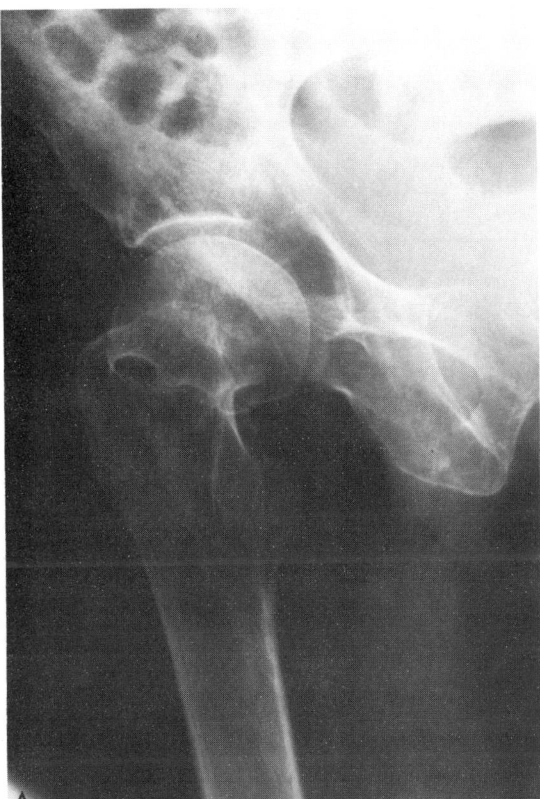

Figure 76–13. *Fracture of the femoral neck (72 hours with avascular necrosis of 3 to 6 months' duration).*

A *Clinical radiograph of a femoral neck fracture that occurred clinically 3 days prior to resection. There is a slight increase in subchondral bone density beneath the weight-bearing area. The degree of relative osteoporosis above the fracture margin indicates an active process older than 3 days.*

B *Gross photograph (2.5×) of the coronally sectioned femoral head reveals an opacified area of avascular necrosis (N). The opacified necrotic area is marginated by a rim of pale reactive tissue (R). The overlying articular surface and subchondral bone are unremarkable. Most of the remaining viable portion of the femoral head (V) has a hyperemic appearance (H). Note the weight-bearing aspect (W).*

C *Specimen radiograph (2.5×) of the sectioned femoral head reveals an area of subchondral radiodensity beneath the weight-bearing area (W), which corresponds to the area of avascular necrosis (N). The osteonecrotic segment is surrounded by a faintly perceived reactive margin of variable but focally increased density (R). The remaining viable portion of the femoral head is radiolucent (V) compared with the avascular area (N). The articular surface and subchondral plate appear intact.*

Illustration continued on the following page

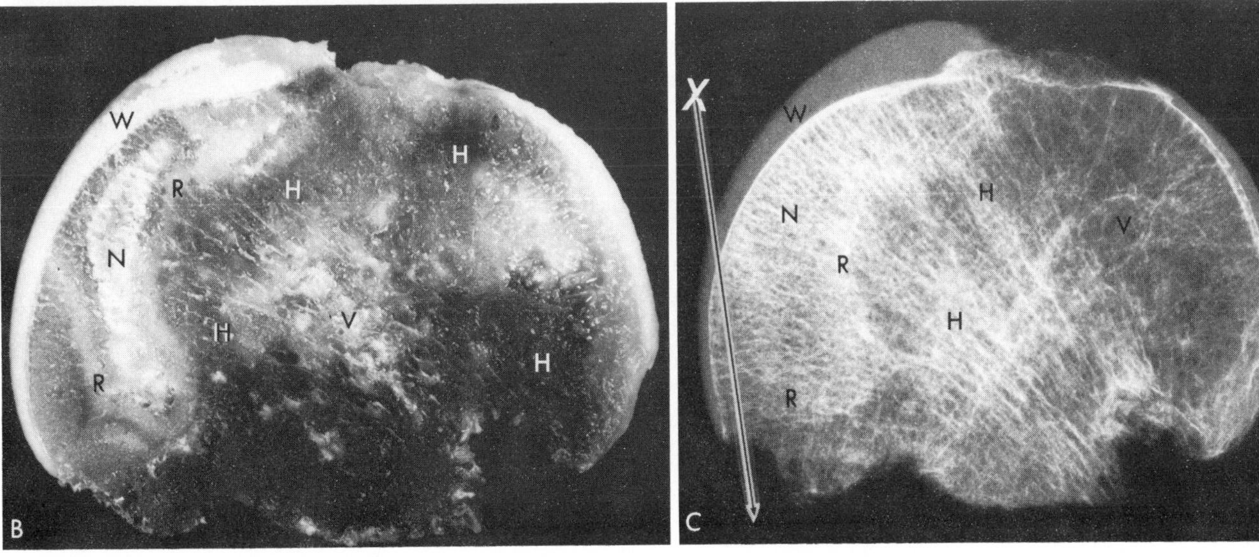

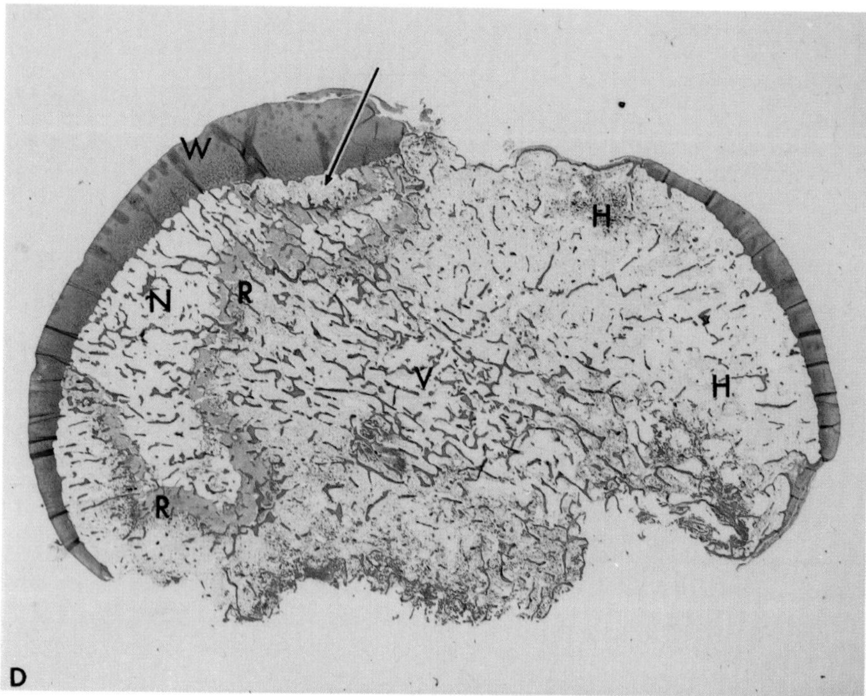

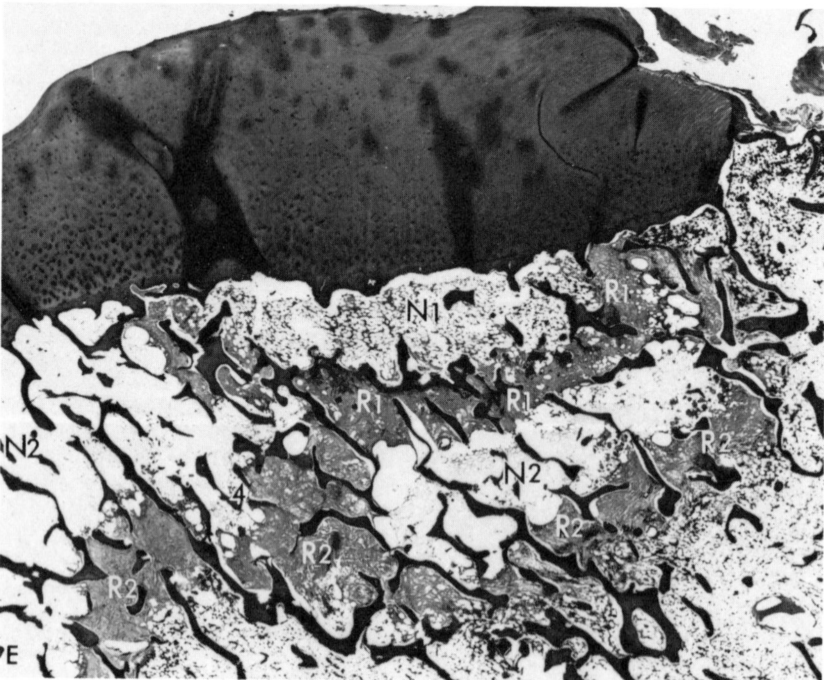

Figure 76–13. Continued

D *Macroscopic section (2.5×, hematoxylin and eosin stain) reveals the area of apparently increased subchondral radiographic density to reflect the unaltered area of avascular necrosis* (N). *The subchondral osteonecrotic bone and marrow are surrounded by and separated from the remaining viable portions of the femoral head by a reactive margin of fibrous marrow (reactive interface)* (R). *Within the reactive interface there has been some osteoclastic resorption of existing cancellous trabeculae and deposition of ischemic fiber bone. There is a small focus of previous avascular necrosis immediately superior to the foveal groove, surrounded by a fibrous reactive interface (arrow), subsequently encompassed by a more extensive zone of necrosis. The remaining viable portion of the femoral head* (V) *shows considerable reactive hyperemia.*

E *Photomicrograph (8×) of the small subchondral area of previous avascular necrosis* (N1) *and reactive margin* (R1) *surrounded by a second zone of necrosis* (N2) *and reactive margin* (R2) *(seen in* **D***) indicates extension of a repairing focus of avascular necrosis.*

Illustration continued on the opposite page

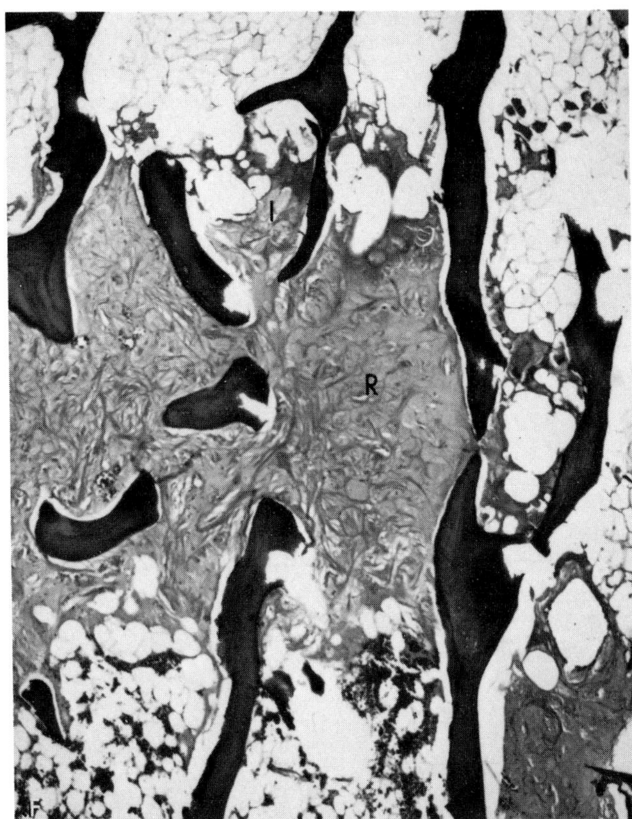

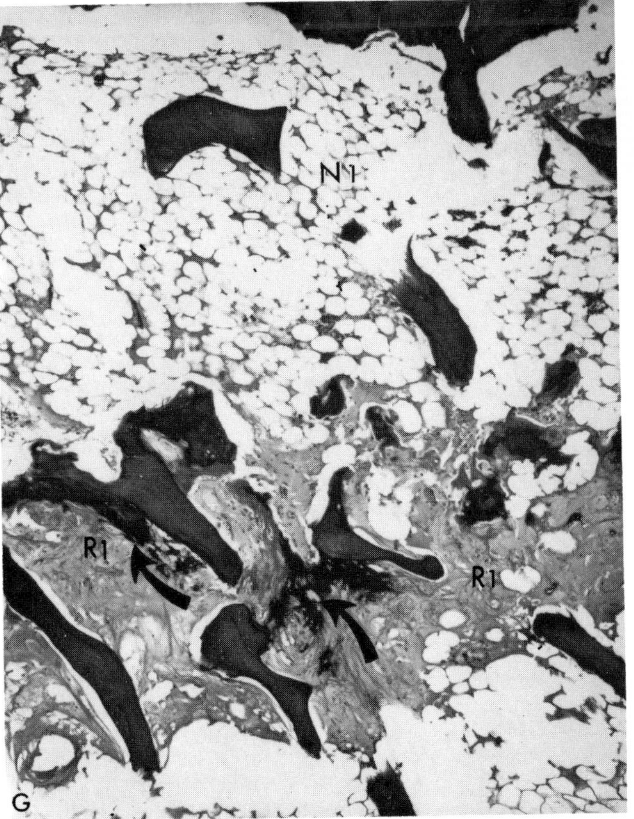

Figure 76–13. Continued

F *Photomicrograph of the reactive interface* (R) *demonstrates the hyalinized appearance of the fibrous modulation of ischemically injured marrow* (I).

G *Photomicrograph (40×) of the original area of avascular necrosis, showing the dead marrow elements and bone* (N1) *and initial reactive interface* (R1) *characterized by ischemic fibrous modulation of marrow elements and the formation of atypical ischemic fiber bone between and on the surface of dead cancellous trabeculae (curved arrows). The latter accounts for some of the focal, faintly perceived increase in density along the entire reactive interface in* **C.**

(Armed Forces Institute of Pathology Neg. Nos. 75-10099, 79-15011, 79-5411, 79-15012, 79-15013, 79-15014-1,2.)

demonstrated in the specimen radiograph (Fig. 76–13*C*) and in the macroscopic section (Fig. 76–13*D*). The infarcted zone reveals a slightly more dense appearance than the remainder of the femoral head. This appearance is due to the vascular induced osteoporosis (active hyperemia) within the viable areas (Fig. 76–13*C*). The infarcted zone is essentially unchanged histologically (Fig. 76–13*D*); therefore, the relatively dense appearance of this area (Fig. 76–13*C*) is apparent rather than real. However, the reactive interface (margin) about the infarcted zone also demonstrates a pattern of altered density on the specimen radiograph (Fig. 76–13*C*). The increase in density within the reactive interface is primarily a reflection of ischemic coarse-textured fiber bone formation between and adjacent to dead cancellous bone (Fig. 76–13*E,G*). The areas of decreased density within the reactive interface are due to osteoclastic activity that is removing injured or previously dead cancellous bone (Fig. 76–13*D*). This case also demonstrates evidence of extension of a previous area of avascular necrosis (Fig. 76–13*D,E*). In Figure 76–13*D,E*, a small zone of subchondral ischemic necrosis surrounded by a fibrous reactive interface is identified (arrow). This area has subsequently been surrounded by a second zone of ischemic necrosis and a second reactive interface. The emergence of a second reactive interface outside the old infarct indicates that the initial reactive area is now dead and will remain unchanged until repair progresses to that level.

Since the osteonecrotic (infarcted) segment during this phase is characterized by an apparent increase in radiographic density, the vascular-induced osteoporosis throughout the remaining portion of the femoral head may also be perceived as a faint subchondral lucent area (not a crescent sign). Perception of this change depends upon the geographic pattern of the osteonecrosis segment and the orientation of the x-ray beam (X arrow, Fig. 76–13*C,D*), and for this reason it cannot be demonstrated in all cases. The emergence of the reactive interface within the previously ischemic zone (with focal cancellous bone resorption, minimal trabecular bone reinforcement, and deposition of ischemic fiber bone within the reactive fibrosis) accounts for the earliest alterations of radiographic density between the infarcted and viable zones.

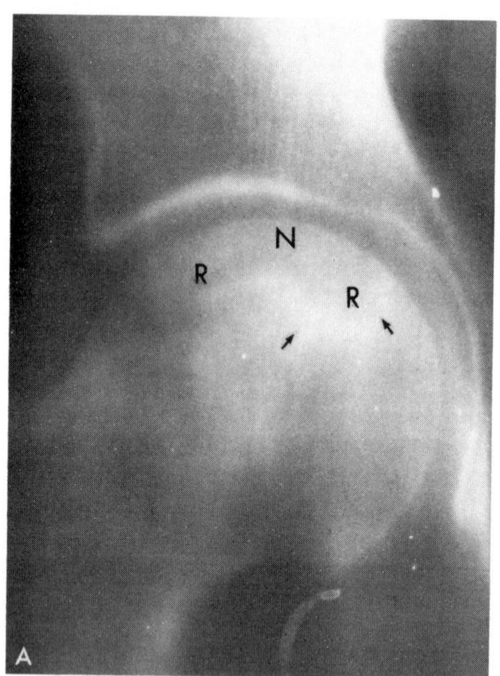

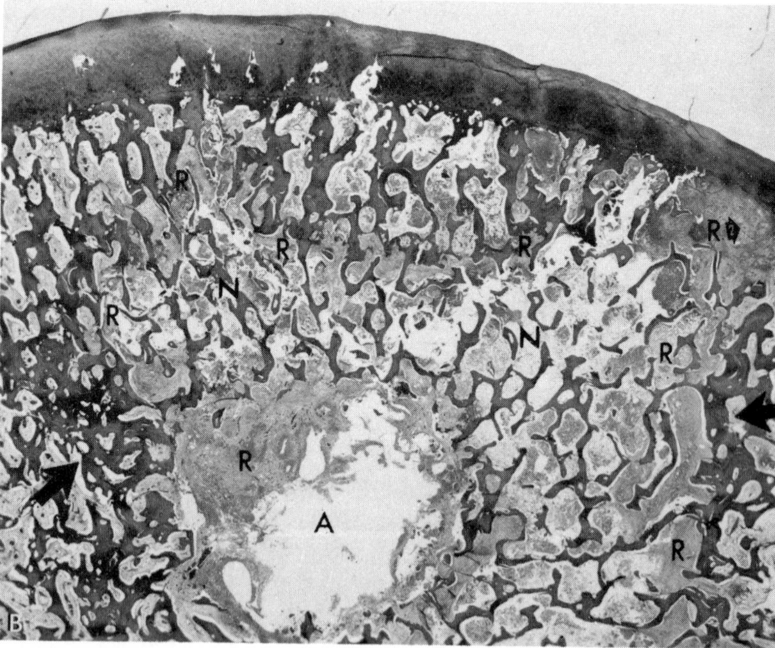

Figure 76–14. *Avascular necrosis of the femoral head (nontraumatic).*

A *Clinical tomographic view demonstrates a spherical femoral head with an unaltered zone of osteonecrosis (N) surrounded by a faint radiolucent margin (R), encompassed by a broadened rim of radiographic density (arrows). The remaining portion of the femoral head and neck show varying amounts of radiolucency.*

B *Photomicrograph (8 ×) of the articular surface and subchondral bone indicates that the radiolucent area is characterized by a broad reactive fibrous interface, within which the bulk of the cancellous bone has been, or is being, resorbed (R). The clear area represents an artifact (A) of tissue processing. The unchanged cancellous bone immediately superior and to the right of the large fibrous defect represents ischemic necrosis (N). The area of necrosis also demonstrates reactive fibrous tissue creeping in from the outer margin (R). There is considerable resorption of the subchondral bony plate where it intersects with the reactive interface (R2 arrow). Bony reinforcement of the adjacent viable trabecular bone (straight arrows) is noted (see Fig. 76–17).*

Illustration continued on the opposite page

Phase IV: Remodeling of the Reactive Interface

Phase IV is basically an extension of Phase III, with continued repair and remodeling along the entire reactive interface between the viable and osteonecrotic zones. Phase IV is exemplified by a femoral head that was resected from a 34 year old alcoholic man (Fig. 76–14*A*). The increasing resorptive activity within the reactive interface also involves the compact subchondral bone wherever the reactive interface intersects with the subchondral bone plate. Therefore, not only is the cancellous bony architecture weakened along the reactive interface because of trabecular bone resorption, but the subchondral bone plate is similarly resorbed and weakened (Fig. 76–14*B*). Weakening of the existing stress-bearing architecture results in compensatory reinforcement of the trabecular bone in the immediately adjacent viable zone (Fig. 76–14*B*). The latter response is analogous to bony reinforcement about any lytic bone defect as a mechanism to route stress around nonstress-bearing areas, and it consists primarily of lamellar bone (Fig. 76–14*B*,*D*).

Progressive remodeling in the reactive interface results in an unaltered central zone of tissue death (Fig. 76–14*A*,*B*,*D*), surrounded by a slowly inwardly expanding lucent fibroblastic reactive interface, characterized by considerable loss of cancellous bone (Fig. 76–14*B*) and some ischemic fiber bone formation (Fig. 76–14*C*). Dystrophic mineralization (deposition of mineral, especially calcium salts, in degenerating or necrotic tissue) of dead fat within the necrotic zone adjacent to the fibrous interface (Fig. 76–14*C*,*D*) is also noted. Toward the outer margin of the reactive interface, there may be partial investing of previously dead cancellous bone by either ischemic fiber or viable lamellar bone (Fig. 76–14*D*). This area is in turn surrounded by a zone of reinforcing viable trabecular bone (Fig. 76–14*B*). These latter changes in the outer reactive margin represent a true increase in radiographic density. This sequence of change has classically been re-

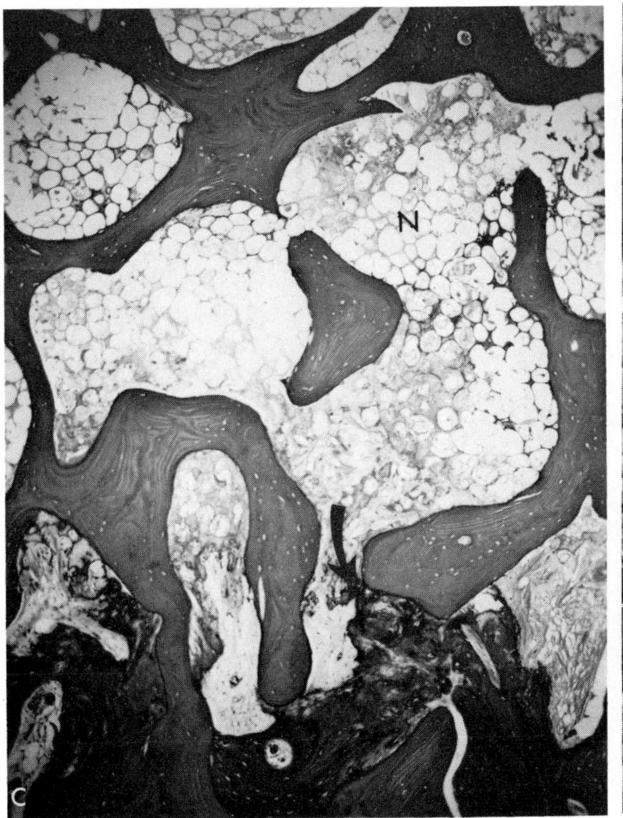

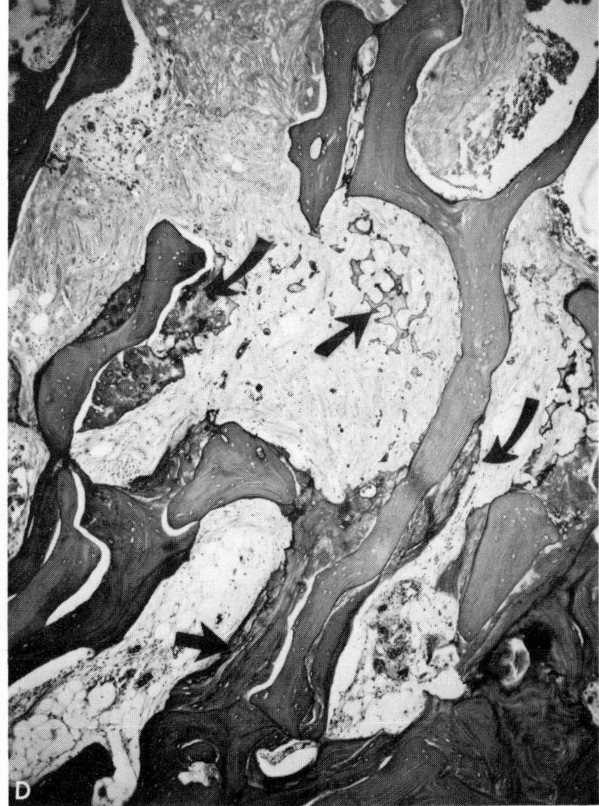

Figure 76–14. Continued

C *Photomicrograph (40×) of the osteonecrotic zone and adjacent reactive interface. Note the dead cancellous bone devoid of osteocytic nuclei and dead marrow fat with its ghost-like appearance (N). Considerable ischemic bone formation (curved arrow) is seen as an appliqué on previously dead cancellous bone trabeculae.*

D *Photomicrograph (40×) of the reactive interface is characterized by the spindled fibrous appearance of the marrow, within which ischemic fiber bone formation (curved arrows) and dystrophic mineralization (tapered arrow) can be identified. Many of the preexisting dead cancellous trabeculae within the reactive interface have been invested by an appliqué of both ischemic (curved arrows) and lamellar (straight arrow) bone. This pattern reflects a receding margin of an infarct.*

(Armed Forces Institute of Pathology Neg. Nos. 71-1553-3; 79-15005; 79-15006-1,2.)

ferred to as creeping substitution[87, 88] and more recently as creeping apposition.[46, 73]

At this stage, there is no evidence of articular buckling or collapse of the femoral head. The clinical tomogram (Fig. 76–14*A*) reveals a zone of apparently increased density (osteonecrosis), outlined by a faint radiolucent zone (the internal advancing fibrous reactive interface), and surrounded by a dense hypertrophic zone (outer reinforcing reactive margin). The lucent zone represents resorptive (osteoclastic) activity, whereas the hypertrophic zone of increased density is a combination of ischemic fiber bone formation and lamellar reinforcement (osteoblastic activity) of preexisting trabecular bone (Fig. 76–14*B–D*).

Phase V: The Crescent Sign and Articular Collapse

The supporting bony architecture may become sufficiently weakened by continued resorption of trabecular bone and subchondral bone plate along the reactive interface that the stress of weight-bearing can result in subchondral bone plate fracture with focal articular cartilage buckling and eventual collapse. Continued stress and motion across the subchondral bone plate fracture result in progressive microfracture of the adjacent dead subchondral cancellous trabeculae. Fragmentation and compaction of subchondral bony fracture debris lead to the development of a subchondral lucent area along the fracture line, the crescent sign. This sign is frequently best seen radiographically in a "frog-leg" view (Fig. 76–15*D*). In time, flattening of the articular surface becomes apparent (Fig. 76–15*A*). These findings are exemplified by a femoral head that was resected from a 62 year old man because of persistent hip pain of nine months' duration (Fig. 76–15*A–C*). The altered density and early flattening of the femoral head that are seen in the clinical radiograph (Fig. 76–15*A*) are better demonstrated in the specimen radiograph (Fig. 76–15*B*) and macroscopic section (Fig. 76–15*C*) as subchondral fracture and early articular collapse. The subchondral fracture and reactive interface are only faintly perceived in the standard clinical anteroposterior radiographic view of the hip (Fig. 76–15*A*). The primary area of collapse in this case appears just superior to the fovea centralis, about which there has been considerable resorption. The lateral extent of the reactive interface is considerably peripheral to the buckled subchondral bone plate. The remaining portion of the femoral head shows the unaltered density of the osteonecrotic zone (Fig. 76–15*B,C*) and the reactive interface (Fig. 76–15*C*).

Thus, Phase V is primarily characterized by radiographic evidence of early articular flattening (collapse) and subchondral fracture. Recognition of the crescent sign (Fig. 76–15*D*) as a radiographic indication of infraction and subarticular collapse is important, and this finding must not be confused with the faint subchondral lucent area that may occasionally be seen in the femoral head during the early stage of Phase III (X-arrow, Fig. 76–13*C,D*). Once Phase V of osteonecrosis is reached, the articular buckling and collapse will be grossly appreciable as an incongruous articular surface that will eventually result in the superimposed degenerative arthritic change.

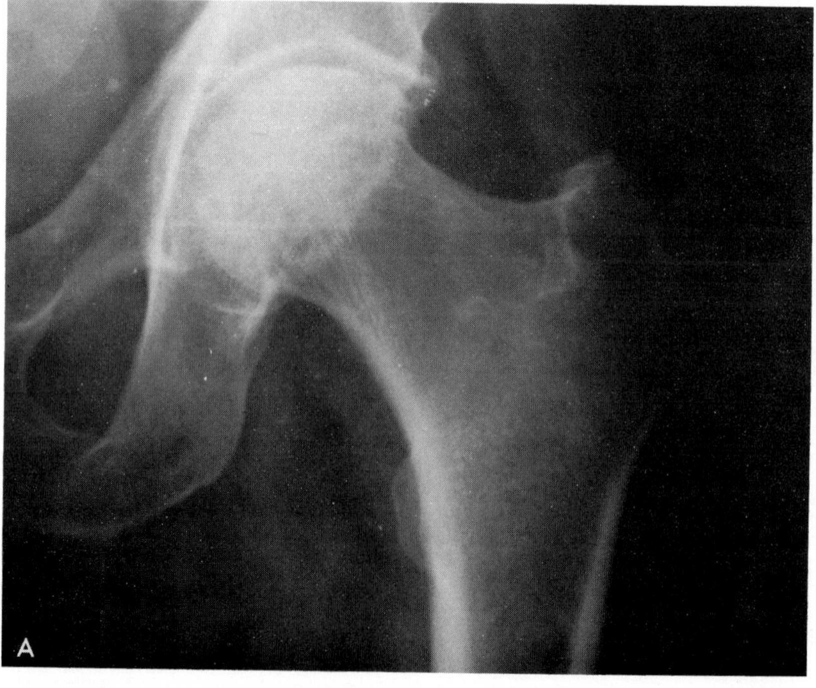

Figure 76–15. *Avascular necrosis of the femoral head with subchondral fracture (crescent sign) and early articular buckling.*

A *Clinical radiograph reveals a slightly dense femoral head with flattening and incongruity of the weight-bearing articular surface.*

Illustration continued on the opposite page

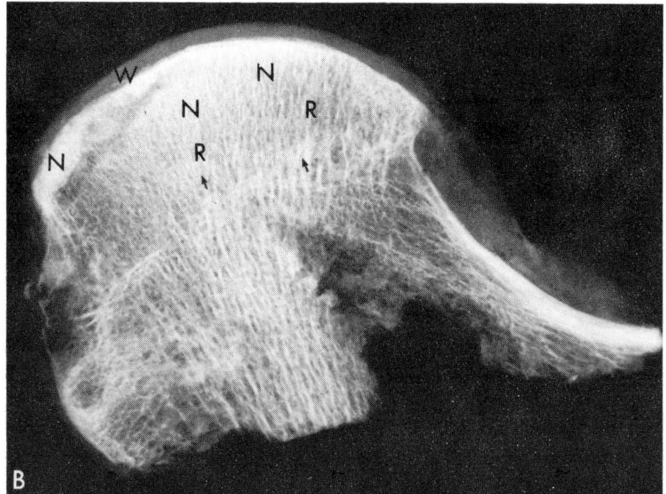

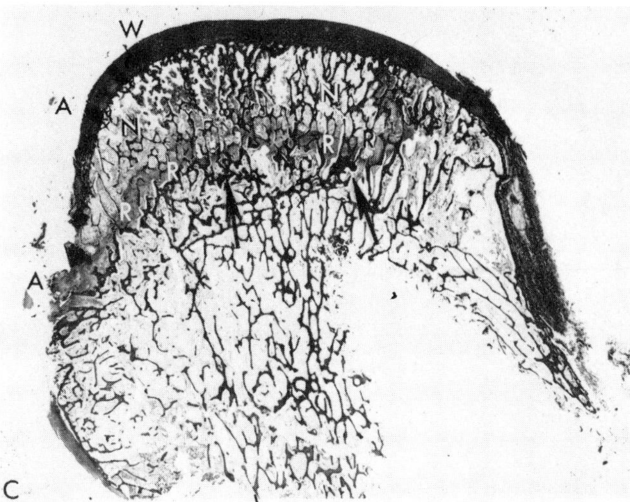

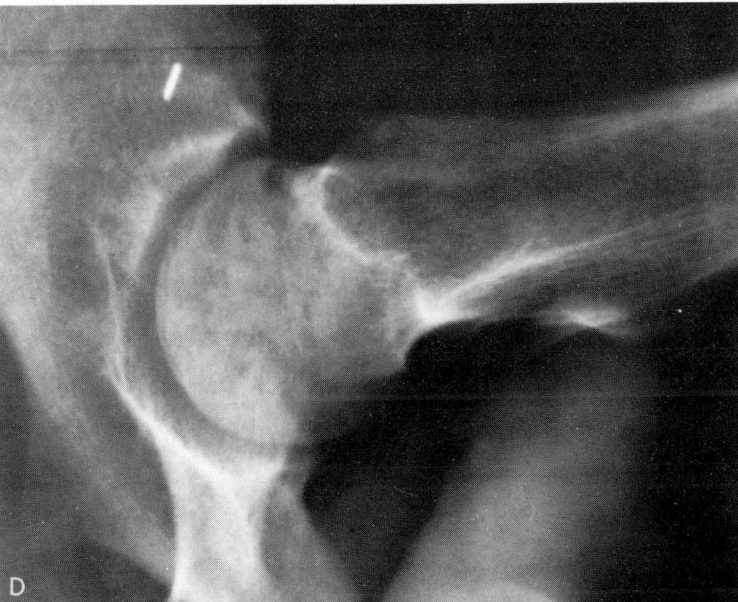

Figure 76–15. Continued

B *Specimen radiograph (2.5×) of the coronally sectioned femoral head shows subarticular bony plate fracture both inferior and superior to the fovea. This has resulted in a subchondral fracture (crescent sign) below the weight-bearing area (see* **D***). The cancellous bone immediately subjacent to the fovea shows considerable radiolucency, indicating resorption. The osteonecrotic bone (W) above the subchondral fracture is dense owing to compacted fracture debris. The remaining osteonecrotic subchondral bone demonstrates faint, relatively increased density surrounded by an ill-defined lucent area (R). An equally faint radiodense zone of bony reinforcement (arrows) is noted (see* **D***).*

C *Macroscopic section (2.5×) of the femoral head demonstrates the buckled subchondral plate and subchondral fracture (crescent sign) in the weight-bearing area (W). The subchondral fracture extends from the fovea superiorly to the weight-bearing zone but does not reach the lateral extent of the avascular segment. The appearance of the subchondral fracture is obscured by a partial artifactual collapse and loss of articular surface about the fovea. Much of the subchondral fracture debris has also been lost in processing. The remaining femoral head is characterized by the unaltered osteonecrotic zone (N), reactive interface that extends to the inferior aspect of the fovea (R), and outer reinforcing bony margin (arrows). The latter microscopic density patterns correlate well with the specimen radiographic appearance in* **B.**

D *Frog-leg radiographic view from another patient demonstrates the crescent sign, relatively dense necrotic zone, lucent reactive interface, and reinforcing margin in much greater detail.*

(Armed Forces Institute of Pathology Neg. Nos. 66-3834-2, 79-5416, 79-14989, 79-5947.)

THE TYPICAL CASE OF AVASCULAR NECROSIS

Geographic Variation in the Host Response

The cases described previously were specifically selected to illustrate the sequence of histologic and radiographic alterations in the femoral head that result from the host response to osteonecrosis. In most cases of avascular necrosis, the host response is not uniform throughout the involved area; this is especially true in the femoral head. A detailed analysis of a single resected femoral head will be used as an example. The patient was an otherwise healthy 34 year old man who complained of increasing hip pain (Figs. 76–16 to 76–20). The clinical radiograph (Fig. 76–16*A*) is characterized by a large area of apparently increased radiographic density with some marginal lucency and peripheral reinforcement. A subchondral fracture (the cresent sign) indicates articular buckling and collapse (Fig. 76–16*A*). The resected femoral head reveals severe buckling of the articular surface with partial collapse anteriorly (Fig. 76–16*B*). The femoral head was sectioned coronally at four levels (Fig. 76–16C), providing an opportunity to compare the plain, tomographic, and specimen radiographs with the gross appearance, macroscopic

Text continued on page 2823

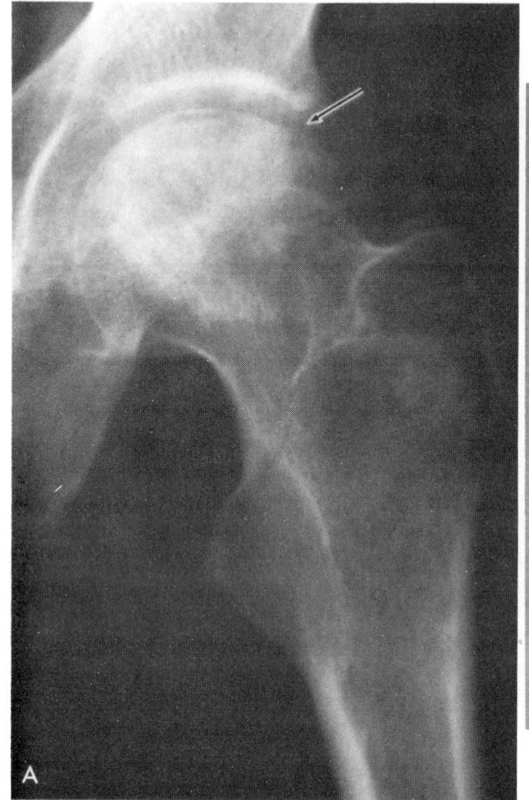

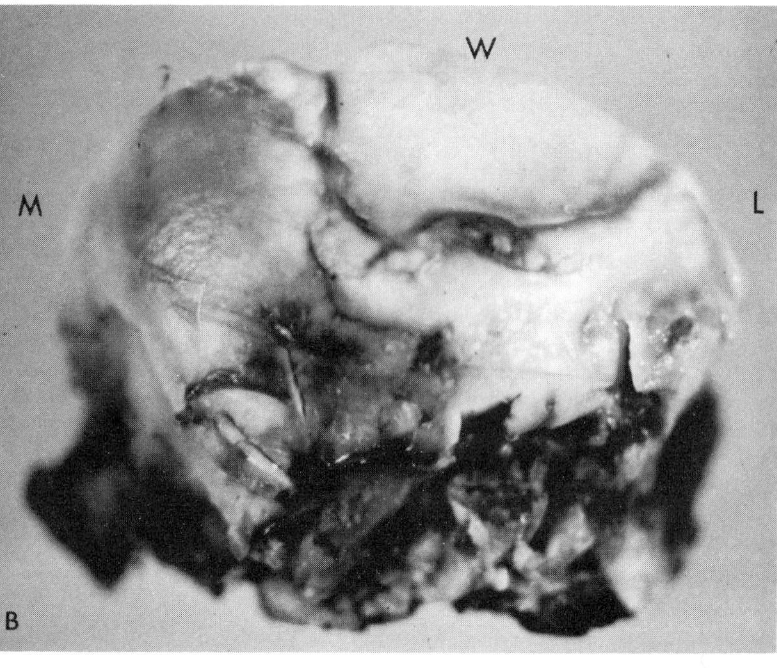

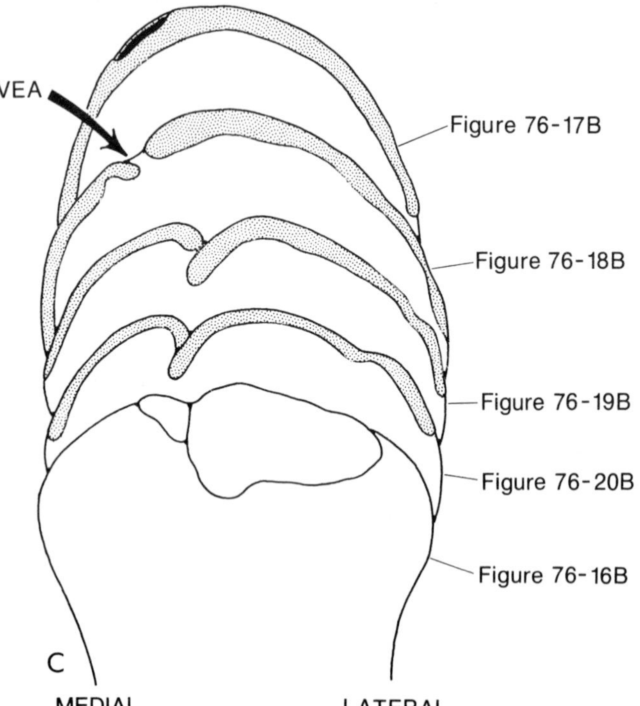

Figure 76–16. *Typical case of avascular necrosis.*

A *Clinical radiograph reveals a broad area of real and apparently increased density involving the anterolateral weight-bearing segment of the femoral head. The crescent sign indicating subchondral fracture is present. Although the joint space appears normal there is evidence of articular buckling (arrow).*

B *Gross photograph (2.5×) of the resected femoral head viewed anteriorly demonstrates severe buckling and collapse of the weight-bearing (W) articular surface. Medial (M) and lateral (L) orientation is noted.*

C *Schematic drawing indicating the level of each of the four coronal femoral head sections given in Figures 76–17 to 76–20. The most posterior (Fig. 76–17) and most anterior (Fig. 76–20) coronal sections are separated by the intermediate coronal sections (Figs. 76–18 and 76–19).*

(Armed Forces Institute of Pathology Neg. Nos. 69-7151-7, 79-14976.)

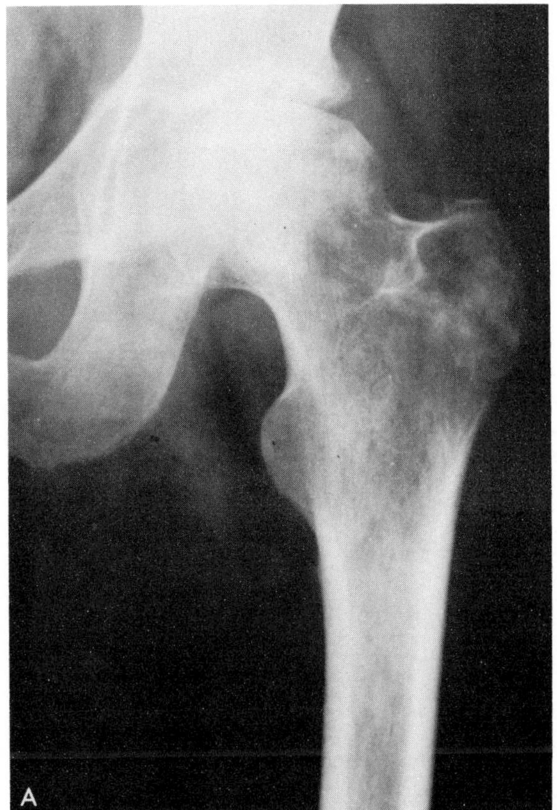

Figure 76–17. Posterior coronal section of the femoral head (see Fig. 76–16 **C**).

A Radiograph of the femoral head demonstrating both real and apparent increase in density with some faint peripheral lucency. Articular buckling is noted laterally. (Armed Forces Institute of Pathology Neg. No. 71-10417-1.)

B Gross photograph (2.5×) of posterior level of the coronally sectioned femoral head shows a normal articular surface and spherical configuration. The central osteonecrotic zone (N) appears slightly opacified and is surrounded by a faintly perceived hyperemic margin (R) encompassed by a pale rim (arrows). Note the medial (M), lateral (L), and weight-bearing (W) aspects. (AFIP Neg. No. 79-14976.)

C Radiograph (2.5×) of the gross specimen in **B** reveals an intact subchondral plate. The central necrotic zone (N) reflects an apparent increase in density surrounded by a faint lucent zone (most pronounced inferiorly) (R) and a rim of increased density (arrows). The remainder of the femoral head appears osteoporotic as a result of active hyperemia (V). (AFIP Neg. No. 79-5409.)

Illustration continued on the following page

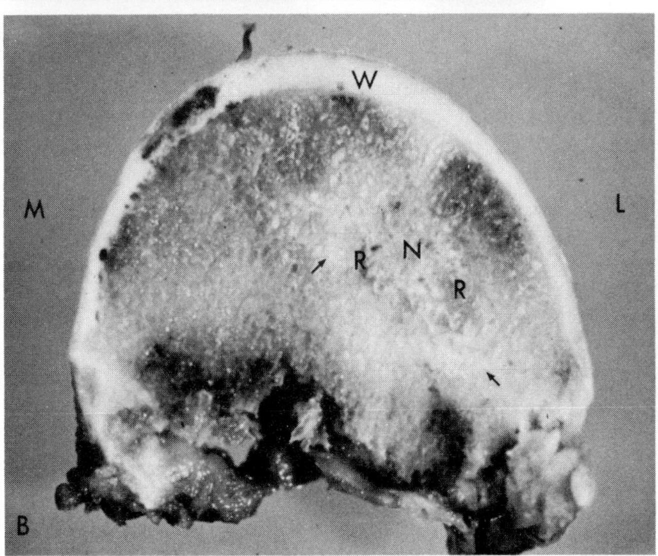

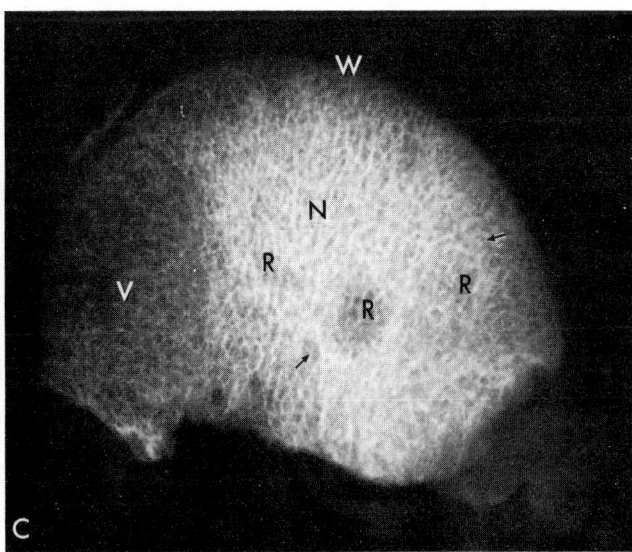

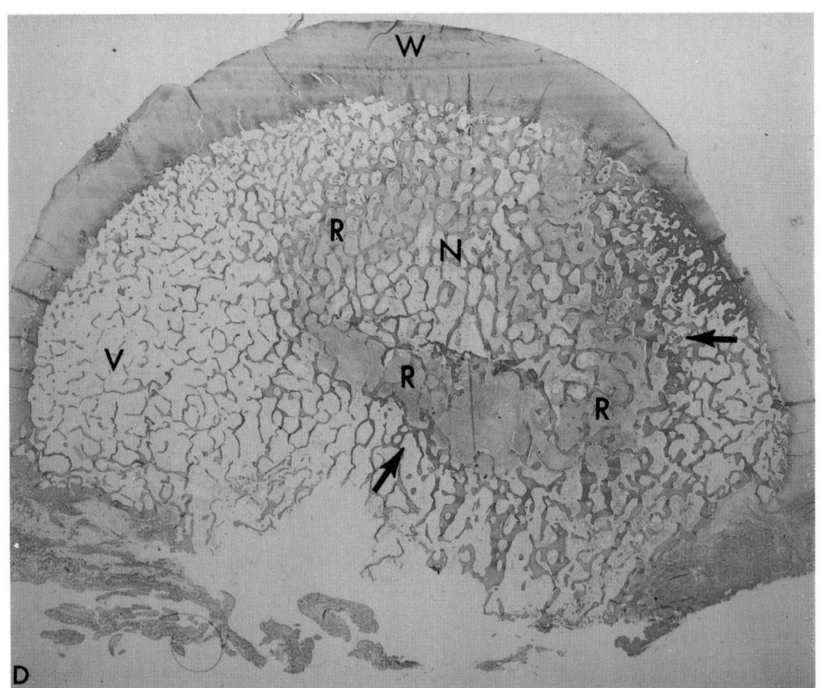

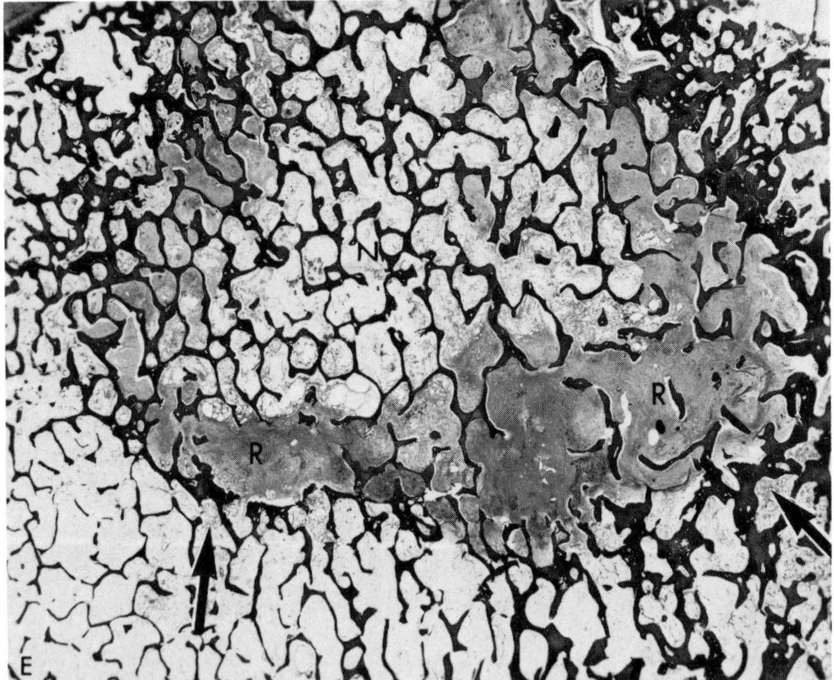

Figure 76–17. Continued

D *Macroscopic section of* **B** *reflects the essentially normal articular surface and subchondral plate. The central necrotic cancellous bone* (N) *appears unaltered and is framed by the reactive fibrous interface* (R) *and a peripheral margin of bony reinforcement (arrows). The thinned cancellous trabeculae in the nonstress-bearing areas have resulted from osteoclastic stimulation by active hyperemia* (V). *(AFIP* Neg. No. *79-14970.)*

E *Photomicrograph (8×) demonstrates the unaltered central necrotic cancellous bone* (N) *surrounded by the fibrous reactive interface* (R), *in turn surrounded by a compensatory rim of reinforced trabecular bone (arrows). Note the fairly extensive loss of cancellous trabeculae within the reactive interface. (AFIP* Neg. No. *79-14983.)*

Illustration continued on the opposite page

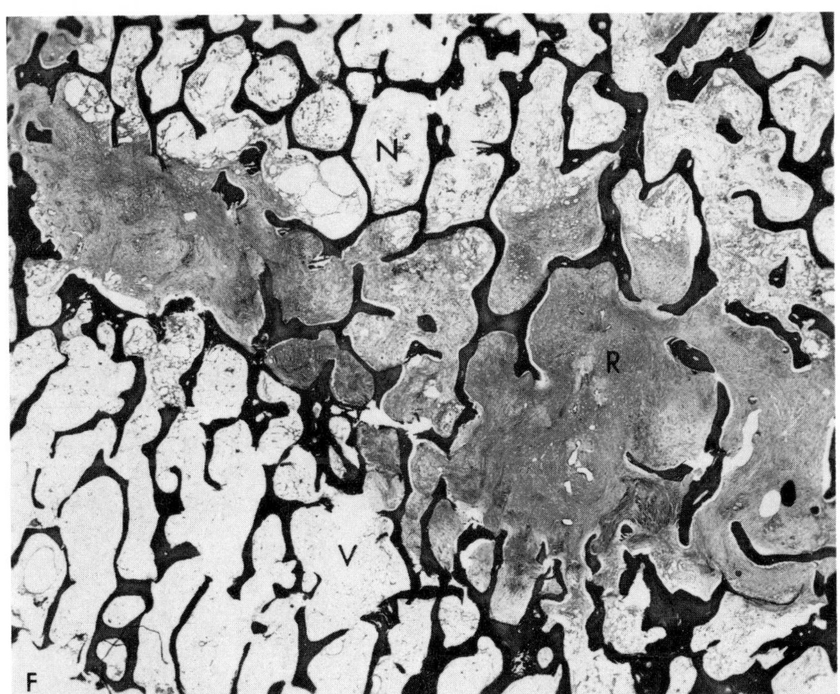

Figure 76–17. Continued

F *Photomicrograph (18×) of the reactive interface* (R) *separating the central necrotic zone* (N) *from the surrounding viable tissue* (V). *Note the loss of cancellous bone and replacement by fibrous tissue. (AFIP Neg. No. 79-14984.)*

Illustration continued on the following page

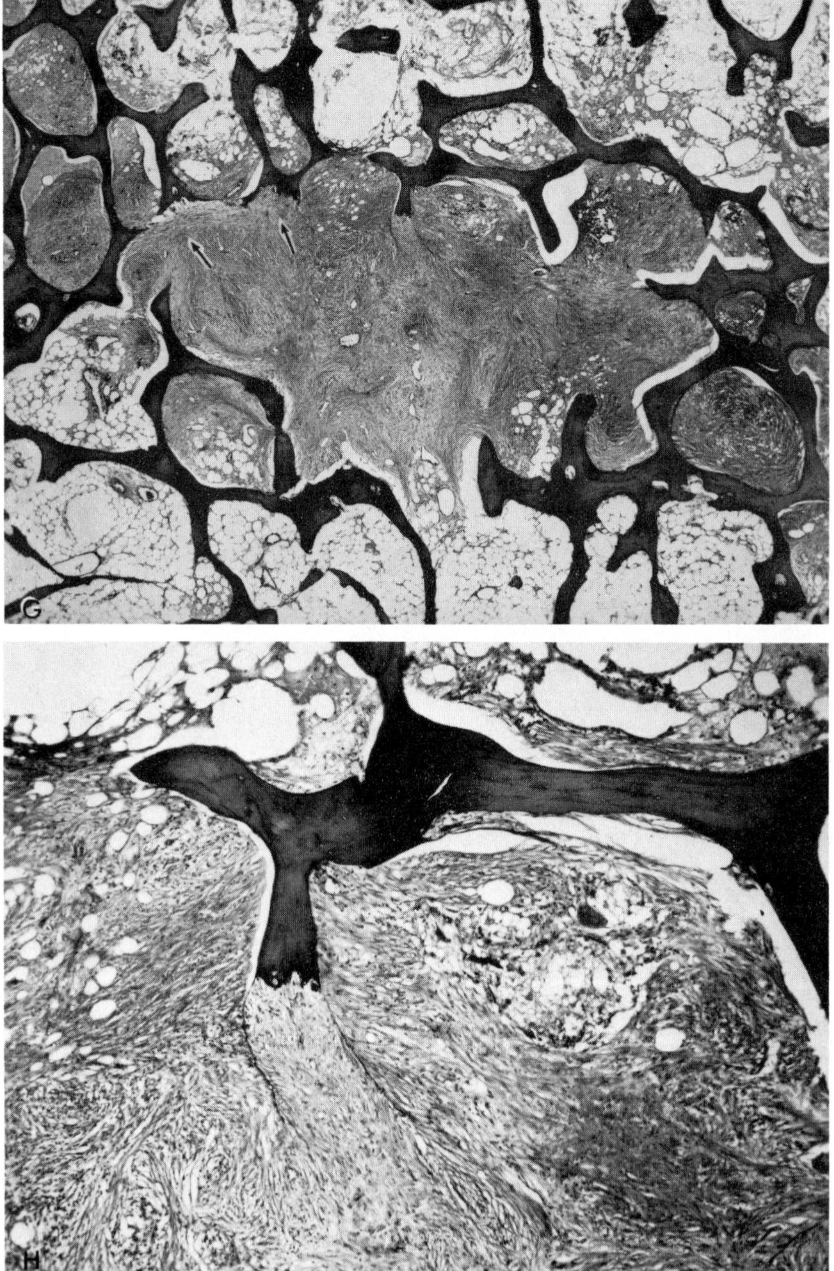

Figure 76–17. Continued

G *Photomicrograph (28×) showing the fibrous reactive interface. Witness the numerous Howship's lacunae and active osteoclastic bony resorption within the reactive fibrous interface (arrows). (AFIP Neg. No. 79-14986.)*

H *Photomicrograph (40×) shows active osteoclasts tunneling out a cancellous trabeculum within an otherwise moderately cellular reactive fibrous interface. (AFIP Neg. No. 79-14981.)*

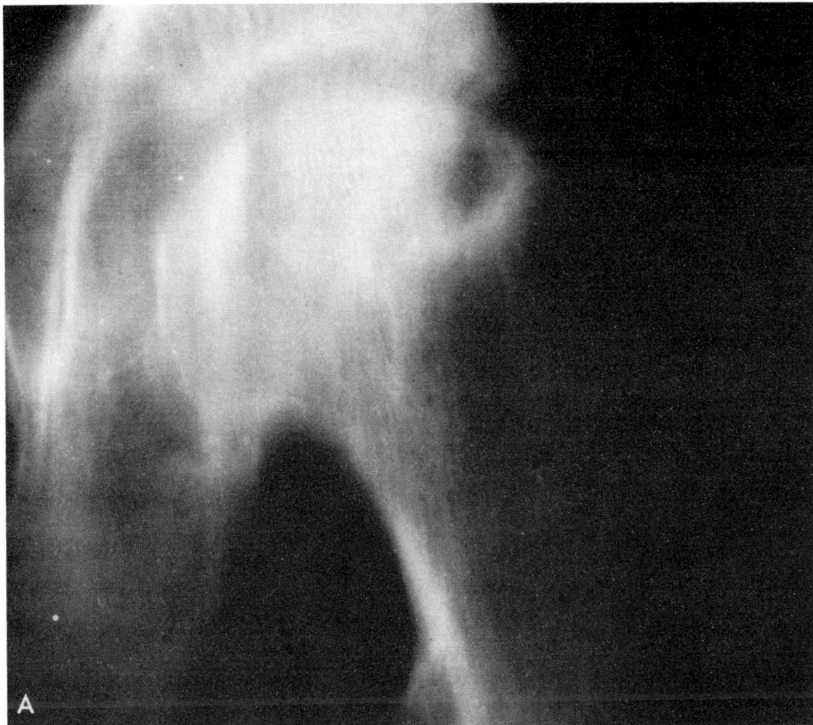

Figure 76–18. Posterior intermediate coronal section of the femoral head (see Fig. 76–16**C**).

A Clinical tomographic view reveals this level of the femoral head to be characterized by a central core of apparently increased density, surrounded by an enlarging radiolucent zone encompassed by a rim of increased density of varying degrees. Note the radiolucent appearance of the inferior medial portion of the femoral head. (Armed Forces Institute of Pathology Neg. No. 71-10417-2.)

B Gross photograph (2.5×) of the femoral head sectioned at approximately the same level and showing the same medial (M), lateral (L), and weight-bearing (W) aspects as the clinical tomogram **(A)**. There is slight articular buckling over the pale, opacified, wedge-shaped area of osteonecrosis (N), just above the subchondral fracture. Note the clearly defined hyperemic reactive margin (R) about the infarcted area. The sclerotic margin is difficult to perceive in the gross specimen (arrows). (AFIP Neg. No. 79-14976.)

C Specimen radiograph (2.5×) of the gross section reveals the relatively increased density of the unaltered osteonecrotic segment (N). The central lytic defect is an artifact (A) of surgical removal. The subchondral fracture extends laterally to the extensively resorbed area of the reactive interface. The lucent reactive interface (R1 arrow) corresponds to the hyperemic areas grossly. The peripheral bony reinforcement about the resorptive margin is well defined (straight arrows). Note the radiolucent areas of reflex vascular osteoporosis (V). (AFIP Neg. No. 79-5409.)

Illustration continued on the following page

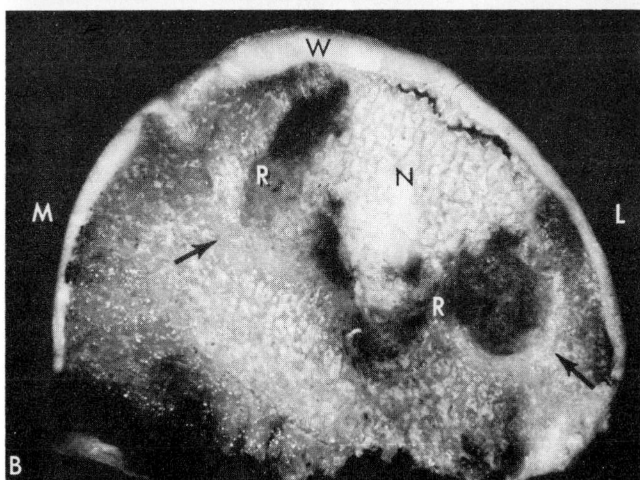

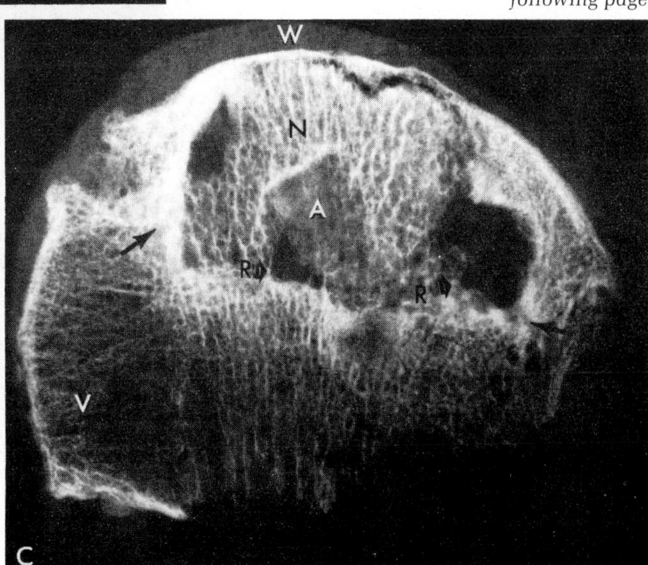

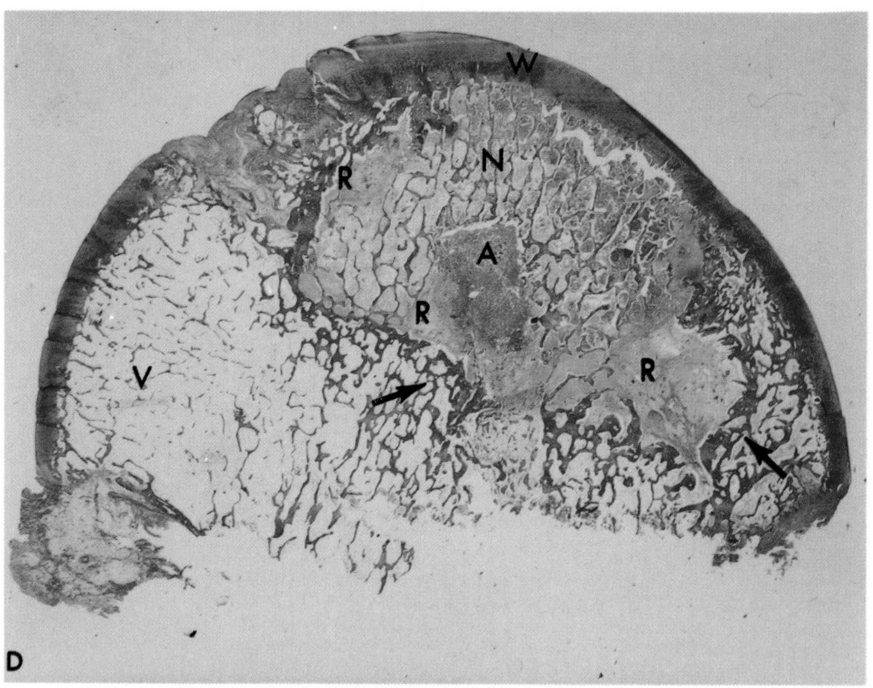

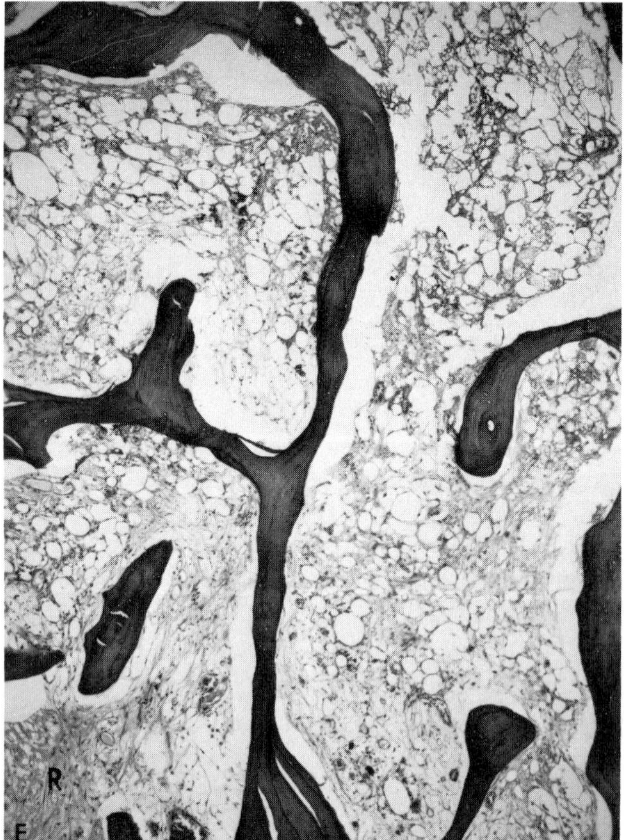

Figure 76–18. Continued

D *Macrosection (2.5×, hematoxylin and eosin stain) of the gross section* **(B)** *shows the unaltered cancellous bone in the osteonecrotic zone* (N), *extensive cancellous bone loss within the reactive fibrous interface* (R), *and marginal bony reinforcement (arrows). These findings correlate well with the radiographic appearance. Note the thinned cancellous trabeculae in the inferior medial portion of the femoral head* (V). *(AFIP Neg. No. 79-14973.)*

E *Photomicrograph (40×) of the osteonecrotic zone, characterized by the unchanged cancellous bone and marrow necrosis. Note the infiltrating margin of revascularized fibrous tissue* (R). *(AFIP Neg. No. 79-14980.)*

Illustration continued on the opposite page

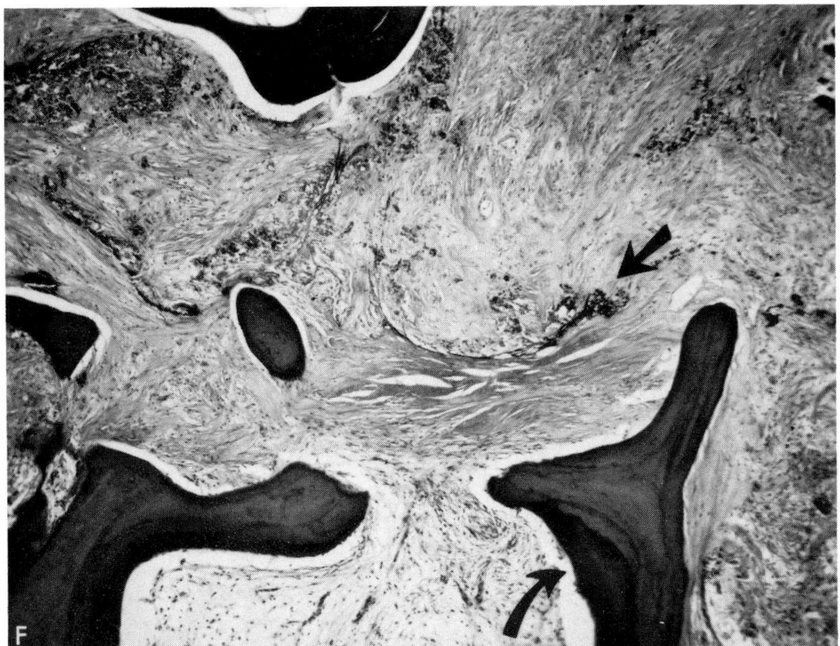

Figure 76–18. Continued

F *Photomicrograph (40×) of the fibrous reactive interface, shows dystrophic mineralization (tapered arrow) and trabecular reinforcement (curved arrow). (AFIP Neg. No. 79-14985.)*

G *Photomicrograph (40×) of the reactive margin shows active osteoclastic resorption of cancellous bone (curved arrow) within the fibrous portion of the reactive interface* (R) *and lamellar reinforcement of trabecular bone (straight arrow) in the immediately adjacent viable zone* (V).

H *Photomicrograph (40×) of the reactive margin. Note the lamellar pattern of trabecular bone reinforcement by osteoblasts (straight arrow) separating the fibrous portion of the reactive interface* (R) *from the adjacent viable marrow* (V). *(AFIP Neg. No. 79-14978.)*

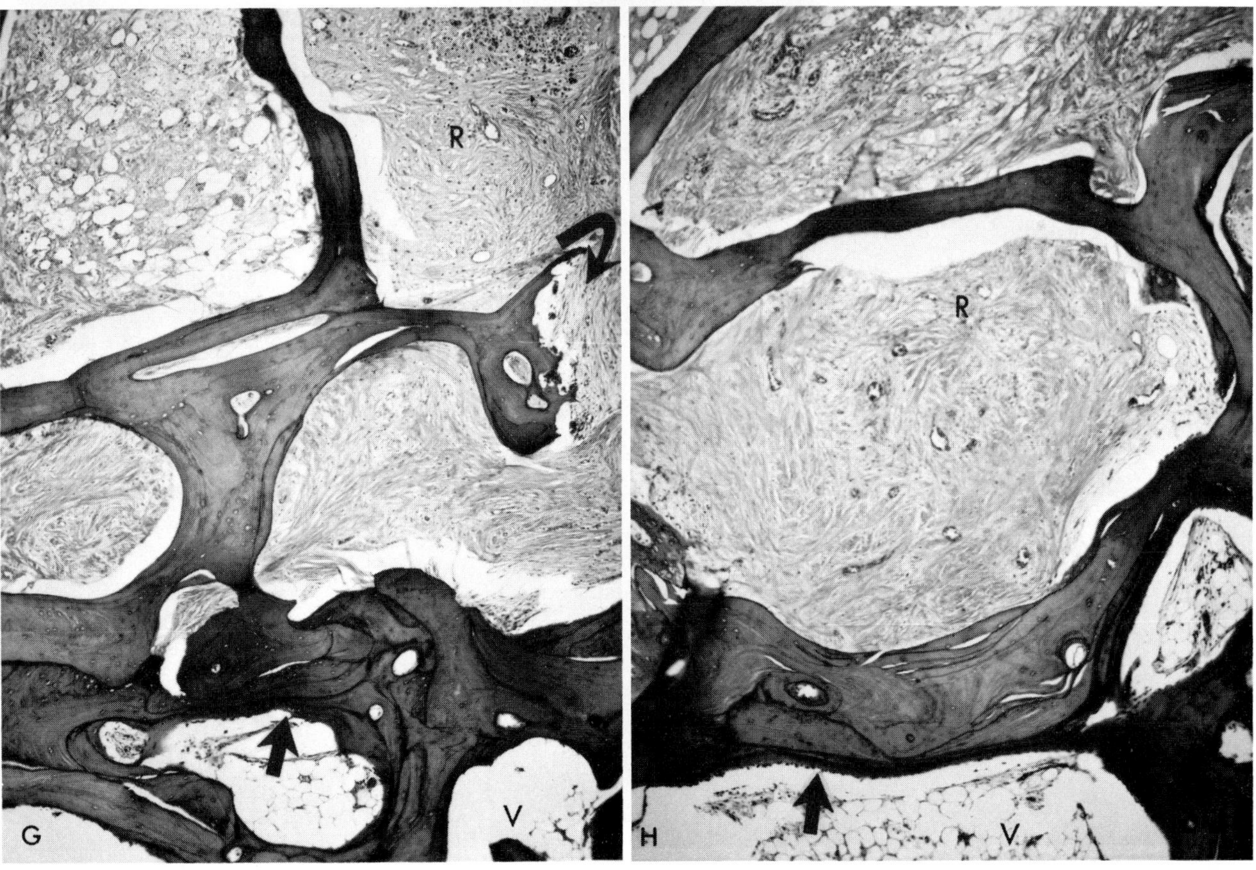

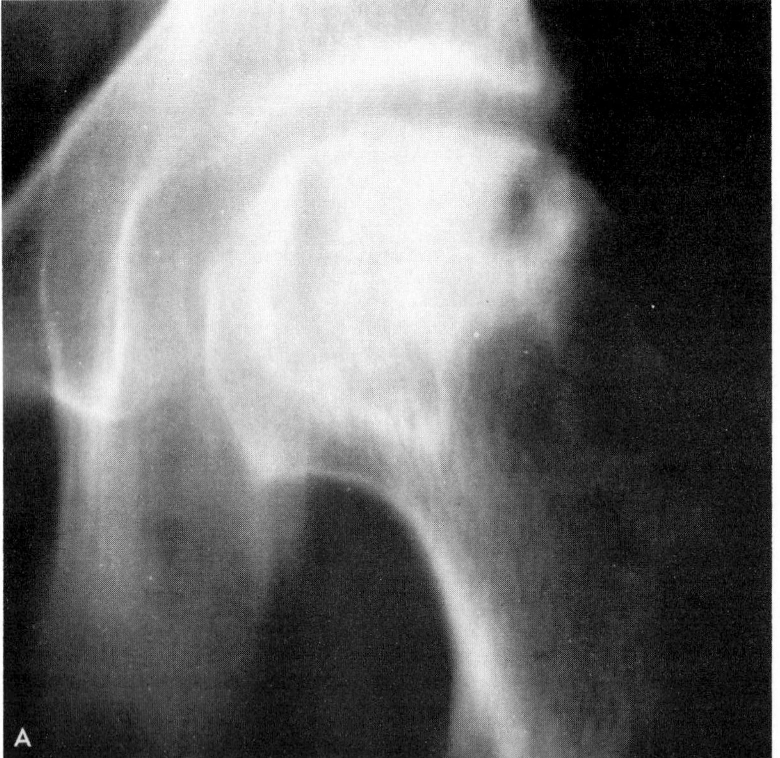

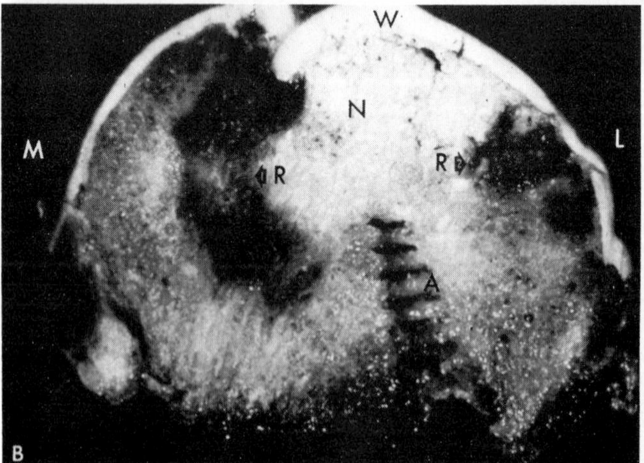

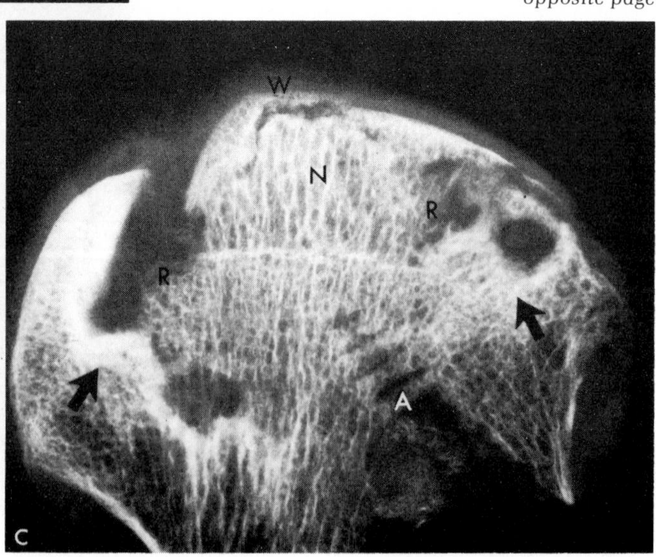

Figure 76–19. *Anterior intermediate coronal section of the femoral head (see Fig. 76–16***C***).*

A *Clinical tomogram demonstrating flattening of the femoral head. Note the reduced central area of relatively increased density and expansion of the lucent reactive margin, especially medially. The peripheral margin of increased density is well defined, but it is most prominent medially. Because of articular flattening, the subchondral fracture is difficult to see. (Armed Forces Institute of Pathology Neg. No. 79-10417-4.)*

B *Gross photograph (2.5×) of the femoral head sectioned at approximately the same level and showing medial* (M), *lateral* (L), *and weight-bearing* (W) *aspects as in the clinical tomogram* **(A)**. *The most striking feature is the extent of articular collapse into the medial reactive margin (R1 arrow). There is subchondral fracture through the pale osteonecrotic zone* (N). *Note the articular buckling and resorbed subchondral plate over the lateral reactive margin (R2 arrow). Disregard the artifactual distortion induced during removal* (A). *(AFIP Neg. No. 79-14976.)*

C *Specimen radiograph of the gross section demonstrates extensive bone loss in both the medial and lateral reactive margins* (R), *which accounts for the articular collapse and buckling, respectively. The subchondral fracture through the unaltered, but relatively dense, osteonecrotic segment* (N) *extends to both the medial and lateral resorptive margins. Note the rim of markedly increased density (arrows) peripheral to the resorptive margins, especially along the medial margin.* W, *Weight-bearing aspect;* A, *artifact. (AFIP Neg. No. 79-5409.)*

Illustration continued on the opposite page

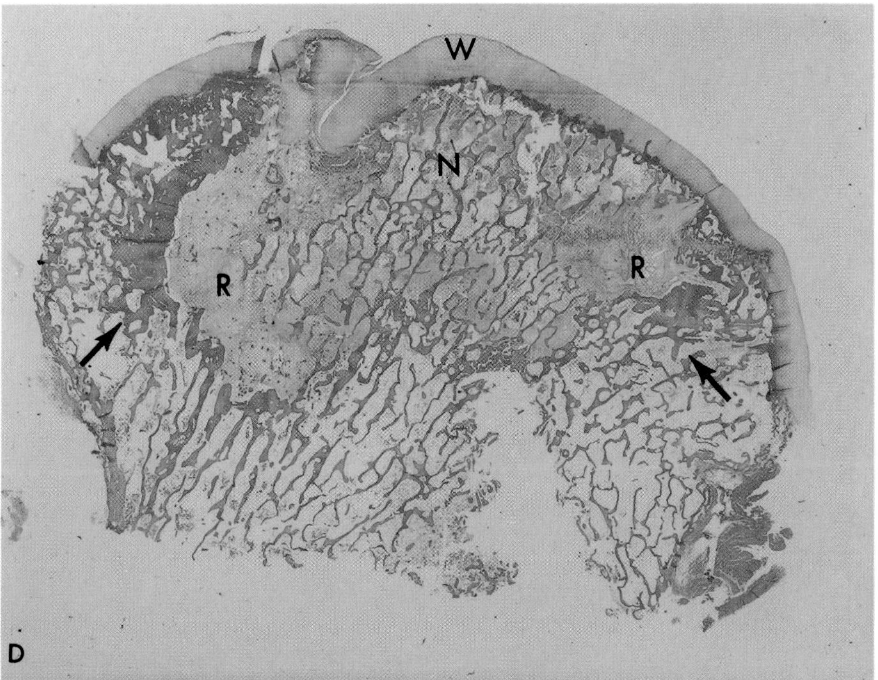

Figure 76–19. Continued

D *Macroscopic section (2.5×, hematoxylin and eosin stain) of the gross specimen in* **B** *indicates that articular collapse and buckling have occurred over areas of extensive bone loss within the fibrous reactive interface* (R). *The subchondral fracture through the unaltered cancellous bone of the osteonecrotic segment* (N) *extends from the medial to the lateral resorptive margins. Bony reinforcement (arrows) about the reactive interface is especially marked medially and accounts for the peripheral margin of increased density. (AFIP Neg. No. 79-14972.)*

Illustration continued on the following page

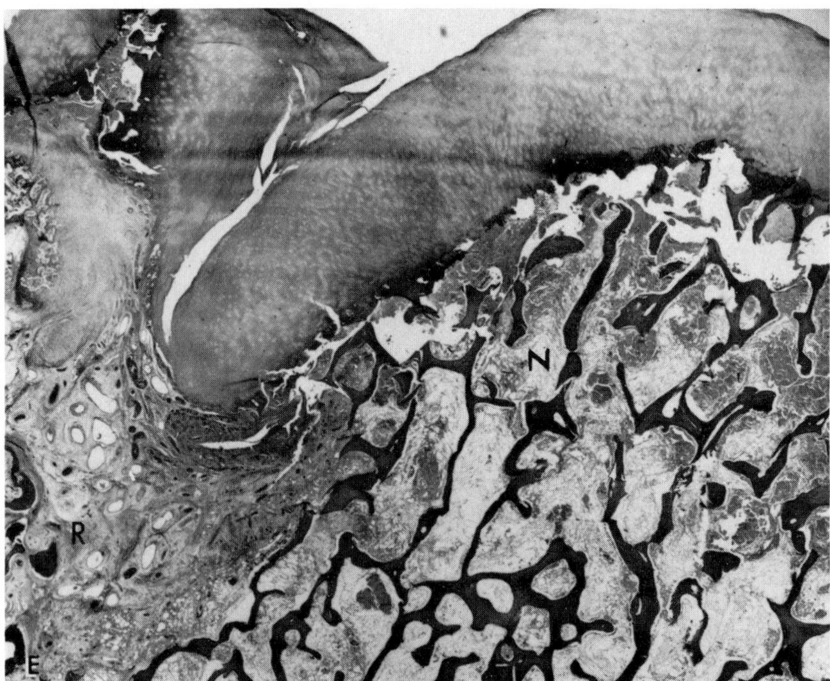

Figure 76–19. Continued

E *Photomicrograph (8×) demonstrates the area of medial articular collapse into the substance of the femoral head. Note the subchondral fracture, unaltered cancellous bone in the necrotic zone* (N), *and fibrovascular appearance of the resorbed area (reactive interface)* (R). *(AFIP Neg. No. 79-14977-1.)*

Illustration continued on the opposite page

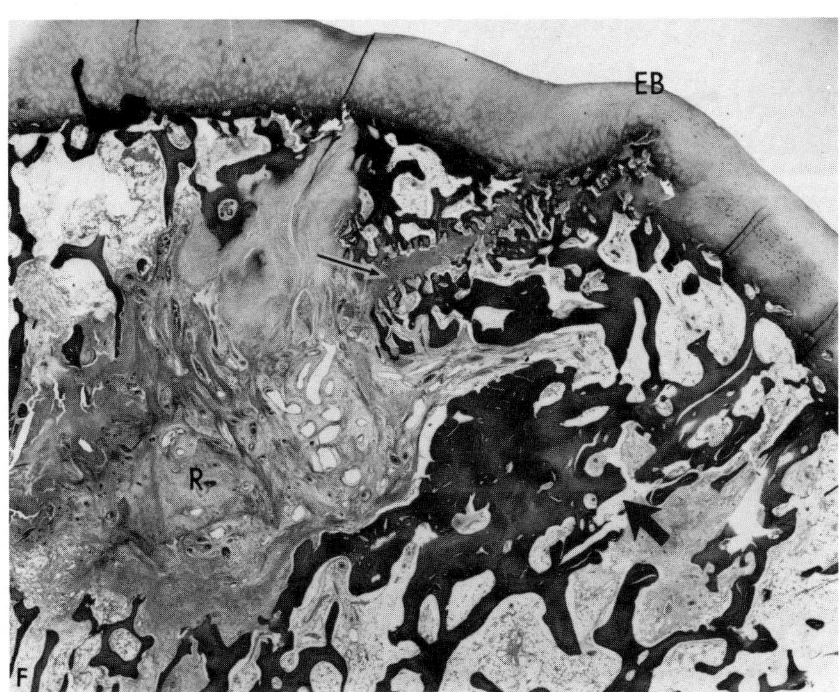

Figure 76–19. Continued

F *Photomicrograph (8×) demonstrates the lateral area of the subchondral plate fracture, and articular buckling over the fibrovascular appearing reactive interface* (R). *The linear area of cartilage metaplasia (thin arrow) along the fracture line extends into an area of endochondral new bone formation within the articular surface* (EB). *Note the marked bony reinforcement peripheral to the resorptive margin (heavy arrow). (AFIP Neg. No. 79-14977-2.)*

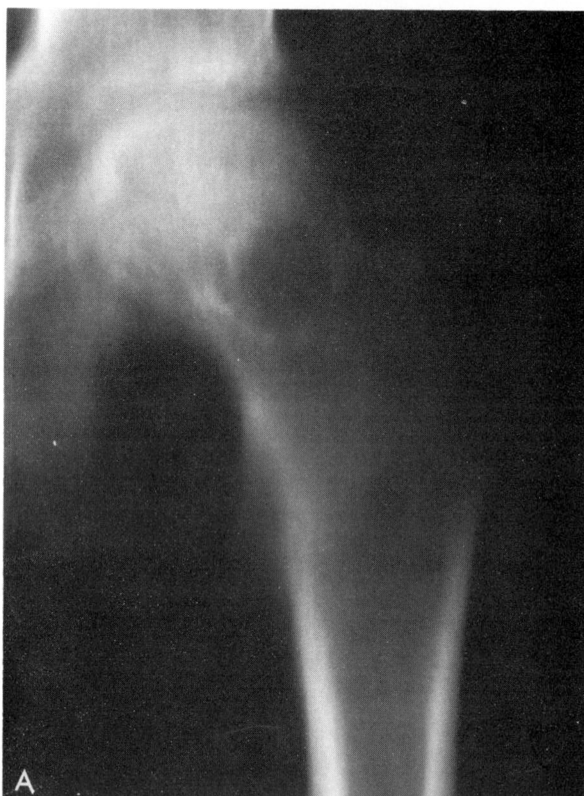

Figure 76–20. Anterior coronal section of the femoral head (see Fig. 76–16**C**).

A Clinical tomographic view reveals the anterior portion of the femoral head to be markedly distorted, with areas of both increased and decreased density. The lucent hole in the upper femoral neck below the synovial reflection represents an unusually large area of fibrovascular ingrowth from the periarticular tissues; presumably it is a part of the reparative response. (Armed Forces Institute of Pathology Neg. No. 69-7151-6.)

B Gross photograph (2.5×) of the femoral head sectioned at approximately the same level and showing the same medial (M), lateral (L), and weight-bearing (W) aspects as the clinical tomogram. There is marked flattening of the femoral head with articular buckling and collapse. The pale osteonecrotic segment (N) is reduced in size and rimmed by a hyperemic margin. (AFIP Neg. No. 79-14976.)

C Specimen radiograph (2.5×) reflects the gross distortion and shows extensive bone loss (R) partially surrounded by a sclerotic margin (arrows). The osteonecrotic segment is small and of essentially normal density (N). (AFIP Neg. No. 79-5409.)

Illustration continued on the opposite page

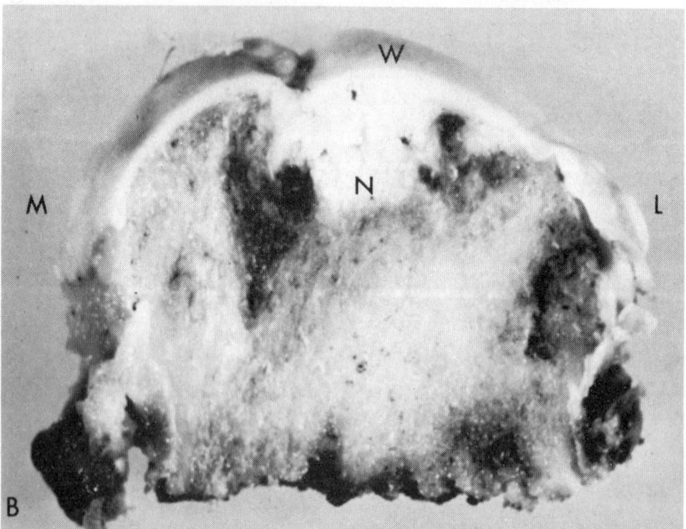

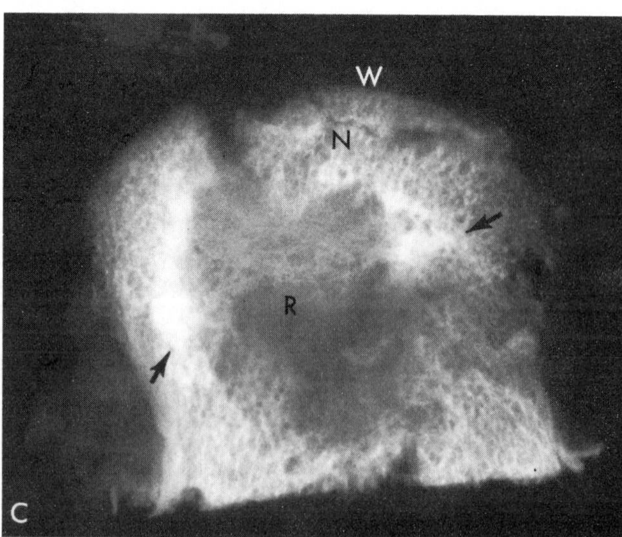

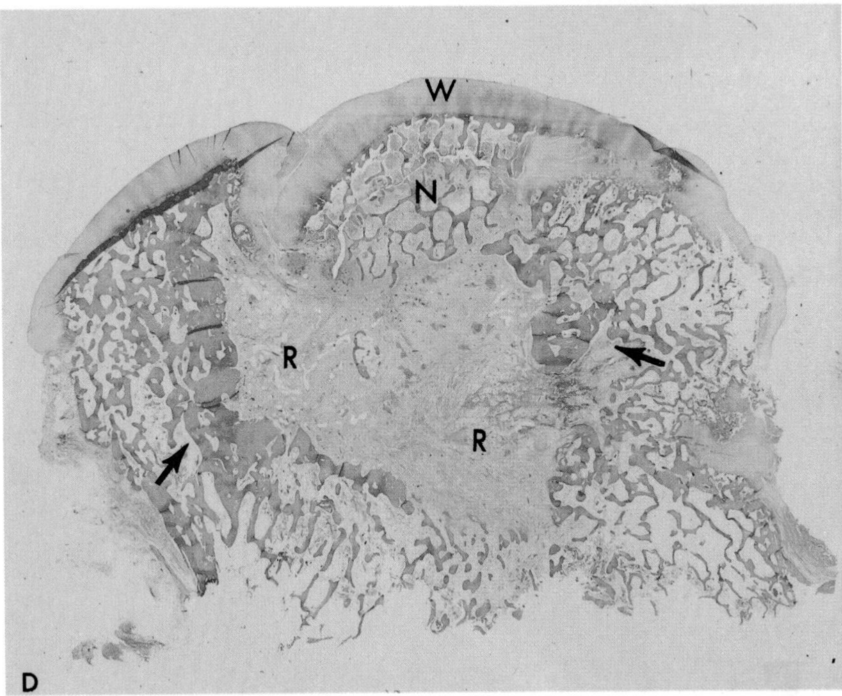

Figure 76–20. Continued
D *Macroscopic section (2.5×, hematoxylin and eosin stain) of the gross specimen in* **B** *demonstrates articular collapse into a large fibrovascular defect. The osteonecrotic zone (N) is reduced in size. The fibrous defect is an extension of the fibrous reactive interface (R) and is partially enveloped by a margin of bony reinforcement (arrows). (AFIP Neg. No. 79-14971.)*

sections, and appropriate high power microscopic views that are illustrated at each of the four successive levels (Figs. 76–17 to 76–20).

The sections (Figs. 76–17 to 76–20) portray the full medial and lateral pathologic and radiographic orientation of the osteonecrotic area and the response at each successive level, from the most posterior level (Fig. 76–17) to the most anterior level (Fig. 76–20) of involvement.

The most posterior femoral head section (Fig. 76–17) reflects primarily Phase III and Phase IV morphologic changes. The gross photograph (Fig. 76–17*B*), the specimen radiograph (Fig. 76–17*C*), and the macroscopic section (Fig. 76–17*D*) reveal an intact articular surface and a normal spherical configuration of the femoral head. The slightly opacified area in Figure 76–17*B* represents the zone of osteonecrosis and is reflected in the specimen radiograph (Fig. 76–17*C*) as a broad area of increased radiodensity with focal lucent shadows. These lucent areas represent sites of osteoclastic resorption of trabecular bone within the fibrous reactive interface and can be appreciated in the macroscopic and high-power microscopic views (Fig. 76–17*D–H*). The macroscopic section (Fig. 76–17*D*) indicates that the increased radiodensity is due to three factors: a relatively increased density of the osteonecrotic zone because of an extensive vascular-induced osteoporosis in the surrounding viable areas of the femoral head; bone formation (Fig. 76–18) and dystrophic mineralization (Fig. 76–18*F*) accounting for a small but real increase in density within the reactive interface; and the extensive loss of trabecular bone resulting from osteoclastic activity within the reactive interface, which is compensated for by reinforcement of the adjacent viable or revitalized trabecular bone along the outer margin of the reactive interface. The loss of stress-bearing capacity due to resorption of the cancellous trabeculae within the fibrous reactive interface (Figs. 76–17*D–H* and 76–18*G*) is accommodated by the adjacent intact trabecular bone. The increased mechanical stress applied to these trabeculae stimulates osteoblastic bony reinforcement by primarily lamellar bone (Figs. 76–17*E,F* and 76–18*H*). Since osteoblastic activity is only possible in areas of bone viability, the bony reinforcement is predominantly manifest along the outer margin of the reactive interface and tends to be juxtaposed to areas of maximum bone loss (Figs. 76–17*D–G*; 76–18*D,G,H*; 76–19*D,F*; 76–20*D*).

The next coronal section (Fig. 76–18) is slightly anterior to the section demonstrated in Figure 76–17 (see Fig. 76–16*C*). The clinical tomographic view demonstrates a central dense area surrounded by a lucent zone, which in turn is surrounded by another margin of increased density (Fig. 76–18*A*). This is also seen in the specimen radiograph (Fig. 76–18*C*), gross photograph (Fig. 76–18*B*), and macroscopic section (Fig. 76–18*D*). It is obvious from the specimen radiograph that the excessive vascular-induced osteoporosis of the viable areas accounts for the relatively increased density of the essentially unchanged central necrotic zone (Fig. 76–18*B,D,E*). Excessive bone resorption within the reactive interface (Fig. 76–18*G*), especially along the medial and lateral sides, has weakened the supportive bony architecture and has resulted in microfracture of the subchondral bone plate, with early articular buckling

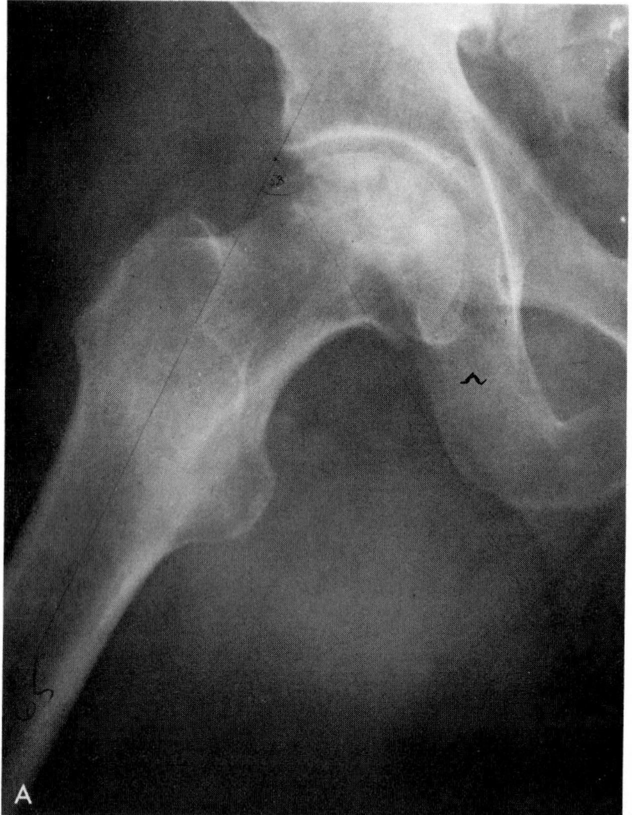

Figure 76–21. *Avascular necrosis with fragmentation.*

A *Clinical radiograph shows flattening and deformity of the femoral head without evidence of narrowing of the joint space. The altered density patterns indicate infraction through the osteonecrotic segment.*

B *Specimen radiograph (2.5×) of the coronally sectioned femoral head reveals the unaltered density of the multiple infracted osteonecrotic segments (N). There is marked bone loss along the reactive interface, characterized by a widened radiolucent zone (R). A margin of increased density (reinforced trabecular bone, arrows) is seen in the adjacent viable portion (V) of the femoral head. Circumscript foci of bone loss are also identified within the sclerotic margin (C).*

C *Macroscopic section (2.5×) of the femoral head reveals an infracted reactive interface (R) separating the partially fragmented osteonecrotic segment (N) from the remaining viable portions of the femoral head (V). The marginal sclerosis recognized in* **B** *is reflected in the macroscopic section as reinforced trabecular bone (arrows) subjacent to the infracted reactive interface. The cysts (radiolucent holes) (C) within the sclerotic margin are analogous to the subchondral cysts that form in degenerative joint disease.*

Illustration continued on the opposite page

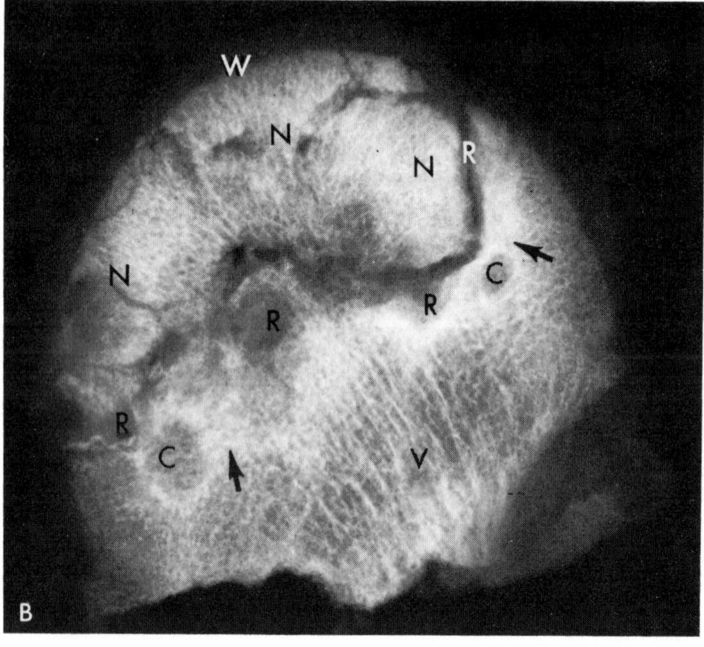

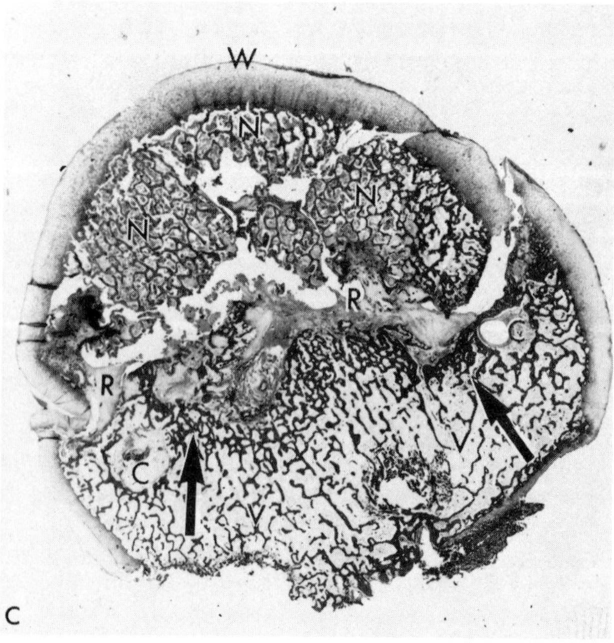

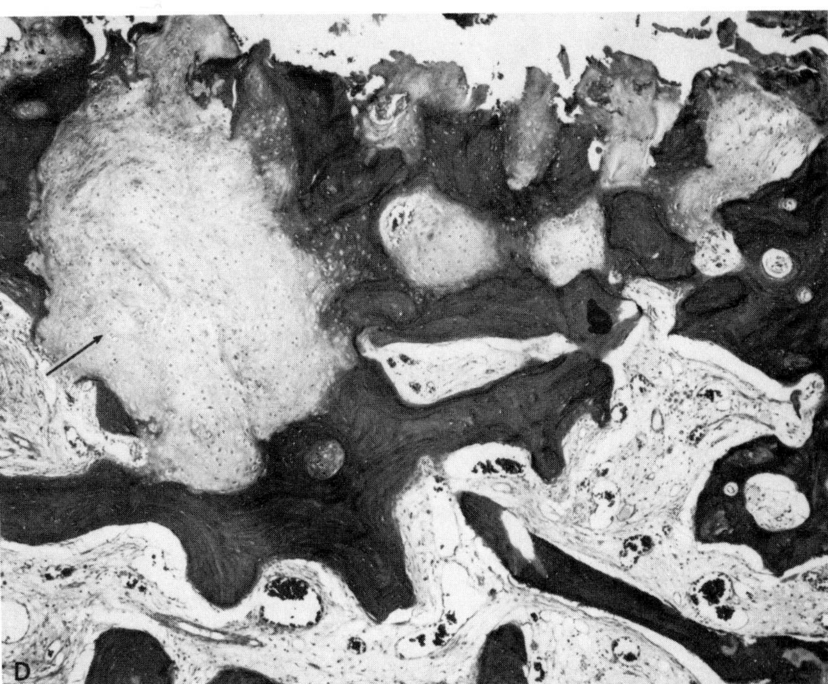

Figure 76–21. Continued

D *Photomicrographic (40×) view of the viable reinforced bony margin adjacent to the reactive interface demonstrates cartilaginous metaplasia (arrow) similar to that seen in a developing pseudoarthrosis.*

(Armed Forces Institute of Pathology Neg. Nos. 65-12798, 79-5417, 79-14990, 79-14991.)

and collapse and subchondral trabecular fracture (Fig. 76–18*B–D*). The latter occurrence produces the classic crescent sign that is well shown in the gross specimen, specimen radiograph, and macroscopic section (Fig. 76–18*B–D*). The pattern of marginal lamellar bone reinforcement (Fig. 76–18*G*,*H*) around the extent of the broadened reactive fibrous interface (Fig. 76–18*D*) is best appreciated in this level of the specimen (Fig. 76–18*C*). The dense area that is produced by the dystrophic mineralization entrapped by the slowly advancing fibrous interface (Fig. 76–18*F*) is radiographically negligible at this phase of repair.

The next slightly more anterior coronal section (Figs. 76–16*C*, 76–19) demonstrates extensive re-

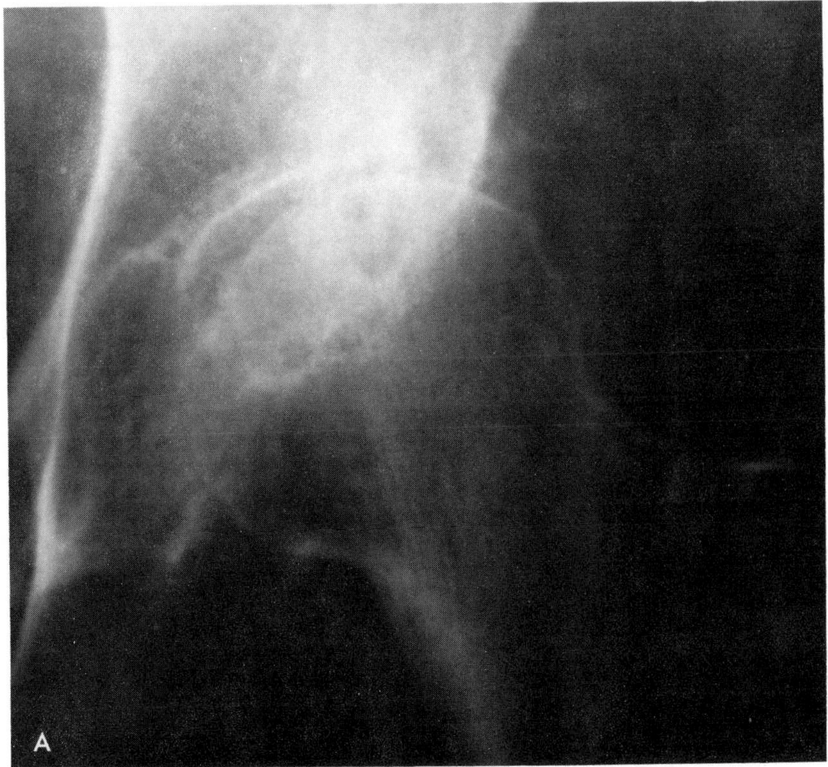

Figure 76–22. *Avascular necrosis with superimposed degenerative arthritic change.*

A *Clinical radiograph demonstrates avascular necrosis characterized by altered subchondral density and localized articular collapse. Narrowing of the joint space superiorly indicates partial loss of the articular surface.*

Illustration continued on the following page

sorption within the reactive interface, especially beneath the fovea, resulting in collapse of the articular surface into the substance of the femoral head. At this level (Fig. 76–19*A–E*), the subchondral fracture (crescent sign) is seen to extend from the lateral to the medial area of articular collapse (Fig. 76–19*C*). This zone of extensive resorption within the reactive interface is marginated by a dense reinforced bony rim. The changes in the clinical tomographic view are corroborated in the gross photograph, specimen radiograph, and macroscopic section at a comparable level (Fig. 76–19*A–D*).

In the lateral area of subchondral collapse and weakening, cartilage metaplasia along the fracture line indicates motion (Fig. 76–19*F*). With loss of the subchondral bone plate, articular cartilage proliferation and enchondral bone formation of the overlying articular surface may be seen (Fig. 76–19*F*). Repeated observations in numerous cases of avascular necrosis indicate that one end of the subchondral fracture is almost always in continuity with an area of subarticular bone plate buckling or partial collapse. This location favors the occurrence of subarticular bone plate disruption as a prior event to subchondral fracture. It is likely that continued motion across an area of subarticular bone plate fracture eventually results in extension of the fracture line into a subchondral location. The immediately peripheral reinforcing bony margin that is forming in response to the resorbing reactive interface is sufficiently thick that any extension of the subchondral fracture is usually directed through the dead cancellous bone toward another area of articular collapse (Fig. 76–19*C,D*).

The most anterior coronal section (Fig. 76–16*C*) reveals an extensive area of bone loss (resorption)

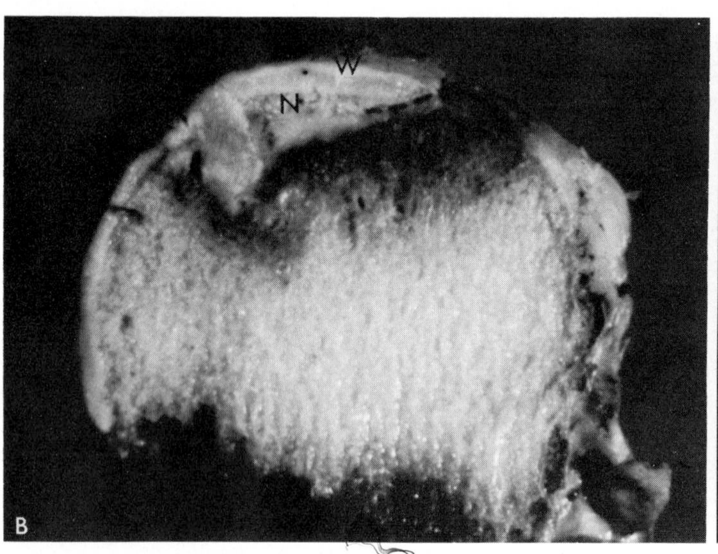

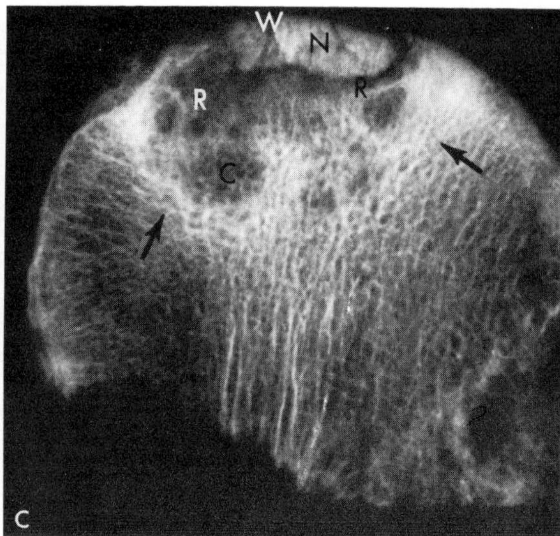

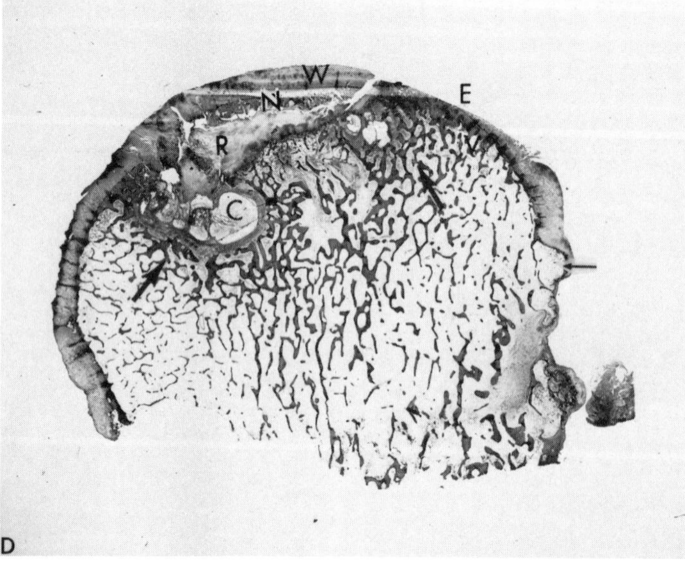

Figure 76–22. Continued

B *Gross photograph (2.5×) of an anterior coronal section of the resected femoral head shows a small zone of osteonecrosis in the weight-bearing area* (W) *covered by a partially collapsed articular surface. The pale osteonecrotic zone* (N) *is surrounded by a darkened area of hyperemic reactive tissue.*

C *Specimen radiographic view of the anterior coronal section in* **B** *indicates that the small, partially fragmented osteonecrotic zone* (N) *has collapsed into the extensively resorbed reactive interface* (R) *with cyst formation* (C). *The resorbed area is surrounded by a reinforced bony margin (arrows).*

D *Macroscopic section (2.5×) reflects the histologic basis for the altered density patterns in the specimen and clinical radiographic appearance of the femoral head. There is partial loss of the articular cartilage laterally* (E) *with early osteophyte formation (small arrow). The small residual osteonecrotic segment is surrounded by an infracted reactive interface* (R), *characterized by fibrous tissue, debris, and cyst formation* (C). *This area is framed by areas of reinforced (thickened) trabecular bone (large arrows).*

Illustration continued on the opposite page

surrounded by a sclerotic bony margin and complicated by articular collapse and fracture through the osteonecrotic segment (Fig. 76–20). These changes are amplified in the clinical tomographic view (Fig. 76–20*A*) and specimen radiograph (Fig. 76–20*C*). The medial sclerotic margin represents a rim of marked bony reinforcement within the viable portion of the femoral head Fig. 76–20*D*). The broad zone of bone loss has been replaced by an area of reactive fibrosis. A significant portion of the articular surface and osteonecrotic segment has collapsed (Fig. 76–20*B*,*D*) into the resorbed (bone-depleted) fibrous area. The degree of articular collapse has resulted in considerable flattening and buckling of the anterolateral portion of the femoral head. This change is best seen in the gross specimen (Figs. 76–16*B*, 76–20*B*).

The radiographic and pathologic features that are revealed in this sequence of coronal sections from the same femoral head demonstrate the general morphology of avascular necrosis and underscore the inequality of host response from area to area in the same bone. In this case there was no morphologic evidence to suggest secondary extension of the infarct as an explanation for the variation in host response. It seems likely that the availability of a functional circulation is a major factor modifying the repair process. Although the features of this case may be somewhat exaggerated, similar findings are usually seen in most cases of avascular necrosis if

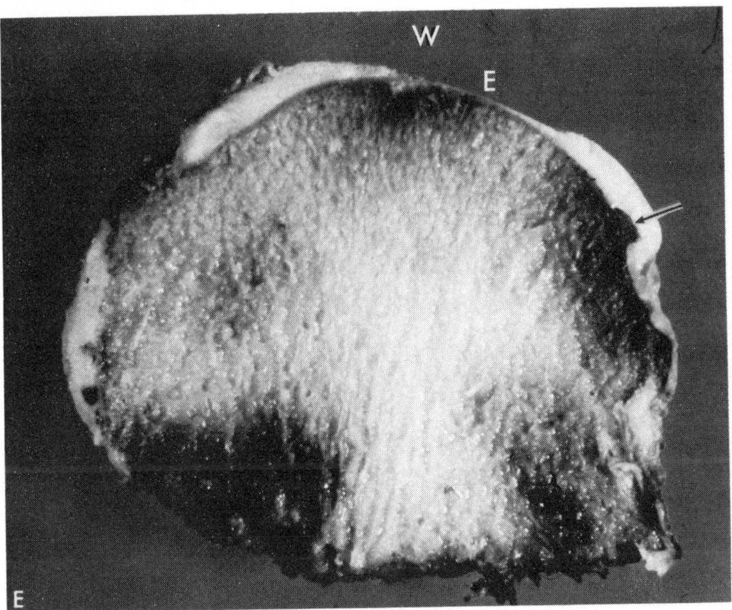

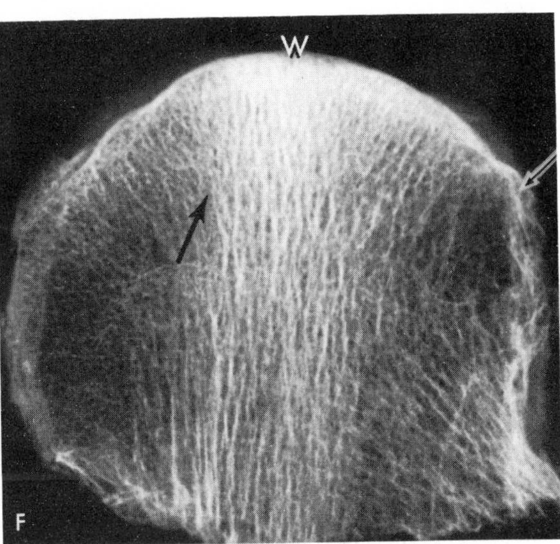

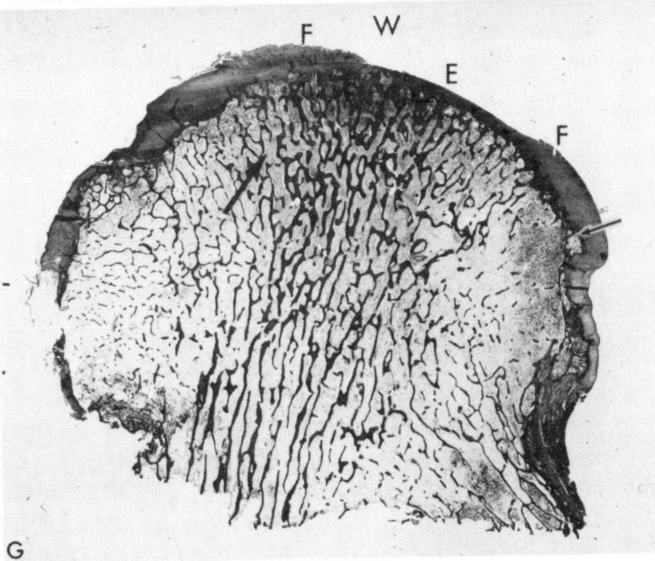

Figure 76–22. Continued

E *Gross photograph (2.5×) of a more posterior coronal section of the femoral head reveals partial loss of the articular surface (E) in the weight-bearing area (W). A minute wedge of preexisting avascular necrosis, surrounded by a hyperemic border, can be identified subchondrally. Laterally, there is early osteophyte formation (arrow).*

F *Specimen radiographic appearance (2.5×) of the gross section* **(E)** *reveals increased density characterized by thickened cancellous bony trabeculae in the subchondral weight-bearing portion of the femoral head (heavy arrow). The lateral subchondral plate appears slightly distorted by osteophyte formation (thin arrow).*

G *Macroscopic section (2.5×) of this level of the femoral head demonstrates complete loss of the articular surface in the weight-bearing area, with eburnated bone (E). Immediately adjacent to the eburnated surface there is fibrillated articular cartilage laterally and medially (F). The subchondral bone subjacent to the fibrillated cartilage and eburnated bone reveals marked mechanical reinforcement (heavy arrow) and a hyperemic-appearing reactive marrow. Laterally, the cartilage demonstrates articular endochondral bone formation (thin arrow), representing early osteophyte formation. This accounts for the irregularity of the lateral subchondral plate in the specimen radiograph* **(F)** *and gross photograph* **(E)**.

(Armed Forces Institute of Pathology Neg. Nos. 69-4218-1, 79-15003-1, 79-5410-1, 79-15002-1, 79-15003-3, 79-5410-3, 79-15002-3.)

they are examined in this fashion. In this single case of avascular necrosis, we find both histologic and radiographic evidence of a host response that ranges from Phase III through late stages of Phase V.

LATE COMPLICATIONS OF AVASCULAR NECROSIS

Fragmentation of the Osteonecrotic Segment

The case illustrated in Figures 76–16 to 76–20 demonstrates fairly extensive resorption and fibrous replacement within the reactive interface. These changes can be so excessive that infraction (i.e., incomplete fracture of bone without displacement of the fragments) may occur along the reactive interface in addition to or in place of the more typical subchondral fracture. Therefore, it is possible for a part or the entire portion of an osteonecrotic segment to become fragmented or functionally separated from the underlying viable area of the femoral head. These changes are exemplified by a femoral head that was resected from a 44 year old man with a 3 year history of hip pain (Fig 76–21). The alternating areas of radiolucency and radiodensity in association with flattening of the femoral head in the clinical radiograph (Fig. 76–21*A*) are also seen in the specimen radiograph (Fig. 76–21*B*) and macroscopic section (Fig. 76–21*C*). The prominent bony reinforcement along the outer viable margin of the reactive interface (Fig. 76–21*B,C*) indicates considerable bone loss and fibrous replacement within the reactive interface. This has resulted in an infraction along the entire reactive interface with secondary fractures through the otherwise essentially unaltered osteonecrotic area (Fig. 76–21*B,C*). The resultant motion along the infracted interface has given rise to chondroid metaplasia (Fig. 76–21*D*) similar to that seen in a pseudarthrosis.

Although the femoral head remains intact, partial microscopic fragmentation of the osteonecrotic segment forming bony debris can resemble that seen in a subchondral fracture exposed to continuous motion. Should the articular cartilage surface tear, some of the debris could escape into the joint. This type of change may account for abnormalities in a number of patients with avascular necrosis in whom the resected femoral head demonstrates partial loss of the osteonecrotic bone substance without evidence of active resorption.[114]

Superimposed Degenerative Arthritis Following Avascular Necrosis

Once patients with avascular necrosis reach Phase V (subarticular bone plate fracture of the articular surface) and exhibit buckling or partial collapse of the articular surfaces, it is usually only a matter of time until evidence of superimposed degenerative arthritis becomes manifest. The articular incongruity resulting from articular buckling or collapse exposes the cartilage surface to shear forces and rapid wear, especially of the noncollapsed portion. The resected femoral head illustrated in Figure 76–22 demonstrating a relatively small area of avascular necrosis reflects such a sequence. The clinical radiograph reveals evidence of avascular necrosis with partial loss of joint space in the weight-bearing area (Fig. 76–22*A*). The resected femoral head was cut and examined in several coronal planes (similar to those in Fig. 76–16*C*). The most anterior section (Fig. 76–22*B–D*) reveals the osteonecrotic segment with its overlying articular cartilage. There has been infraction along the reactive interface with secondary cyst formation (Fig. 76–22*D*). Much of the osteonecrotic portion has been removed by osteoclasts (Fig. 76–22*B*). Both the macroscopic section (Fig. 76–22*D*) and the specimen radiograph (Fig. 76–22*C*) indicate that the osteonecrotic segment has collapsed into the femoral head, resulting in an incongruous articular surface.

The more posterior coronal section (Fig. 76–22*E–G*) demonstrates only a minute wedge of residual avascular necrosis in the gross specimen (Fig. 76–22*E*). The remaining findings reflect a sizeable area of degenerative arthritic change readily visualized in the gross specimen, specimen radiograph, and macroscopic section (Fig. 76–22*E–G*). The articular surface shows areas of cartilage fibrillation and eburnated bone (Fig. 76–22*D,E,G*). Below these areas, the subchondral trabecular bone has been markedly reinforced and thickened (Fig. 76–22*F,G*). This change is the result of stress forces being concentrated on trabecular bone because of the absence of the stress-distributing qualities of the articular cartilage and subchondral bone plate. There is early osteophyte formation laterally (Fig. 76–22*E–G*).

SUMMARY

Although ischemic necrosis of bone results in cell death, there appears to be little or no change in bony architecture as a direct result of osteocyte death. It is the progressive reparative response of the host, both vascular and cellular, that results in the emerging altered bone density that we recognize as characteristic of osteonecrosis. The extent of resorption (removal) and reinforcement (reconstruction) associated with avascular necrosis in comparsion with those in metadiaphyseal bone infarction would seem to reflect the different mechanical requirements and the amount of bone that is involved. Because osteonecrosis is avascular and three-dimensional, the host response must initially be at the margin of the infarct rather than throughout the entire osteonecrotic segment. Why this response tends to remain relatively localized to this outer perimeter is controversial and not fully understood. Within the femoral head, the localized resorption becomes exaggerated and weakens both the cancellous and subchondral bone, resulting in eventual articular buckling or collapse in the majority of cases. Once articular buckling or collapse occurs, there is little likelihood that reconstruction can restore normal continuity or function to the joint.

The term "creeping substitution" has been used by most authors dealing with the subject to describe the repair of avascular necrosis. Unfortunately, most of the "creeping" is done along the reactive interface and most of the bony substitution is at the outer reinforcing margin, rather than throughout the entire osteonecrotic segment. In theory, the term has some basis in fact; however, from a practical point of view, it seems to be little more than wishful thinking. Were the entire infarcted segment to be uniformly repaired at the same time, as perhaps occurs occasionally in a patient with femoral neck fracture, it might be possible to circumvent the eventual articular collapse. This suggests that attention be focused not only on the prevention of osteonecrosis in the high-risk patient but also on the early detection of osteonecrosis with the hope of effecting repair without later articular collapse.

REFERENCES

1. Amstutz HA: The hip in Gaucher's disease. Clin Orthop Rel Res *90*:83, 1973.
2. Arkin AM, Schein AJ: Aseptic necrosis in Gaucher's disease. J Bone Joint Surg *30A*:631, 1948.
3. Axhausen G: Über anämische Infarkte am Knochensystem und ihre Bedeutung für dies Lehre von den primären Epiphyseonekrosen. Arch Klin Chir *151*:72, 1928.
4. Banks HH: Healing of the femoral neck fracture. *In* Proceedings of the Conference on Aseptic Necrosis of the Femoral Head. St. Louis, National Institutes of Health, 1964, p 4–65.
5. Barton CJ, Cockshott WP: Bone changes in hemoglobin SC disease. Am J Roentgenol *88*:523, 1962.
6. Boettcher WG, Bonfiglio M, Hamilton HH, Sheets RF, Smith K: Non-traumatic necrosis of the femoral head. Part I. Relation of altered hemostasis to etiology. J Bone Joint Surg *52A*:312, 1970.
7. Bohr H, Larsen EH: On necrosis of the femoral head after fracture of the neck of the femur. A microradiographic and histologic study. J Bone Joint Surg *47B*:330, 1965.
8. Bohrer SP: Acute long bone diaphyseal infarcts in sickle cell disease. Br J Radiol *43*:685, 1970.
9. Boksenbaum M, Mendelson CG: Aseptic necrosis of the femoral head associated with steroid therapy. JAMA *184*:262, 1963.
10. Bonfiglio M: Aseptic necrosis of the femoral head. Intact blood supply is of prognostic significance. *In* Proceedings of the Conference on Aseptic Necrosis of the Femoral Head. St Louis, National Institutes of Health, 1964, p 155.
11. Boyd HB: Avascular necrosis of the head of the femur. Am Acad Orthop Surg Instr Course Lect *14*:196, 1957.
12. Boyd HB, Calandruccio RA: Further observations on the use of radioactive phosphorus (P^{32}) to determine the viability of the head of the femur. Correlation of clinical and experimental data in 130 patients with fractures of the femoral neck. J Bone Joint Surg *45A*:445, 1963.
13. Brav EA: Traumatic dislocation of the hip; Army experience and results over a twelve-year period. J Bone Joint Surg *44A*:1115, 1962.
14. Bravo JF, Herman JH, Smyth CJ: Musculoskeletal disorders after renal homotransplantation. A clinical and laboratory analysis of 60 cases. Ann Intern Med *66*:87, 1967.
15. Brown JT, Abrami G: Transcervical femoral fracture. A review of 195 patients treated by sliding nail-plate fixation. J Bone Joint Surg *46B*:648, 1964.
16. Caffey J: Pediatric X-ray Diagnosis. 6th Ed. Chicago, Year Book Medical Publishers, 1972, p 1149.
17. Calandruccio RA: The use of radioactive phosphorus to determine the viability of the femoral head. *In* Proceedings of the Conference on Aseptic Necrosis of the Femoral Head. St Louis, National Institutes of Health, 1964, p 243.
18. Calandruccio RA: Comparison of specimens from non-union of neck of femur with fresh fractures and avascular necrosis specimens. J Bone Joint Surg *49A*:1471, 1967.
19. Catto M: A histological study of avascular necrosis of the femoral head after transcervical fracture. J Bone Joint Surg *47B*:749, 1965.
20. Catto M: The histological appearances of late segmental collapse of the femoral head after transcervical fracture. J Bone Joint Surg *47B*:777, 1965.
21. Catto M: Pathology of aseptic necrosis. *In* JK Davidson (Ed): Aseptic Necrosis of Bone. Amsterdam, Excerpta Medica, 1976, p 3.
22. Charache S, Page DL: Infarction of bone marrow in the sickle cell disorders. Ann Intern Med *67*:1195, 1967.
23. Coleman SS, Compere CL: Femoral neck fractures: Pathogenesis of avascular necrosis, nonunion and late degenerative changes. Clin Orthop Rel Res *20*:247, 1961.
24. Cruess RL, Blennerhassett J, MacDonald RF, MacLean LD, Dossetor J: Aseptic necrosis following renal transplantation. J Bone Joint Surg *50A*:1577, 1968.
25. Dalinka MK, Edeiken J, Finkelstein JB: Complications of radiation therapy: Adult bone. Semin Roentgenol *9*:29, 1974.
26. Davidson JK: Dysbaric osteonecrosis. *In* JK Davidson (Ed): Aseptic Necrosis of Bone. Amsterdam, Excerpta Medica, 1976, p 147.
27. Dickerson RC, Duthie RB: The diversion of arterial blood flow to bone. A preliminary report. J Bone Joint Surg *45A*:356, 1963.
28. Diggs, LW: Bone and joint lesions in sickle cell disease. Clin Orthop Rel Res *52*:119, 1967.
29. Diggs LW, Anderson LD: Aseptic necrosis of the head of the femur in sickle cell disease. *In* WM Zinn (Ed): Idiopathic Ischemic Necrosis of the Femoral Head in Adults. Stuttgart, Georg Thieme, 1971, p 107.
30. Donaldson WF Jr, Rodriguez EE, Shovron M, Gartland JJ: Traumatic dislocation of the hip joint in children. Final report by the Scientific Research Committee of the Pennsylvania Orthopedic Society. J Bone Joint Surg *50A*:79, 1968.
31. Dorfman HD, Norman A, Wolff H: Fibrosarcoma complicating bone infarction in a caisson worker. A case report. J Bone Joint Surg *48A*:528, 1966.
32. Dubois EL, Cozen L: Avascular (aseptic) bone necrosis associated with systemic lupus erythematosus. JAMA *174*:966, 1960.
33. Edeiken J, Hodes PJ, Libshitz HI, Weller MH: Bone ischemia. Radiol Clin North Am *5*:515, 1967.
34. Evans A, Barnard EEP, Walder DN: Detection of gas bubbles in man at decompression. Aerospace Med *43*:1095, 1972.
35. Arlet J, Ficat P: Diagnostic de l'ostéo-nécrose fémoro-capitale primitive au stade I (stade pré-radiologique). Rev Chir Orthop *54*:637, 1968.
36. Fisher DE: The role of fat embolism in the etiology of corticosteroid-induced avascular necrosis: Clinical and experimental results. Clin Orthop Rel Res *130*:68, 1978.
37. Fisher DE, Bickel WH, Holley KE: Histologic demonstration of fat emboli in aseptic necrosis associated with hypercortisonism. Mayo Clin Proc *44*:252, 1969.
38. Fisher DE, Bickel WH: Corticosteroid-induced avascular necrosis. A clinical study of seventy-seven patients. J Bone Joint Surg *53A*:859, 1971.
39. Fisher DE, Bickel WH, Holley KE, Ellefson RD: Corticosteroid-induced aseptic necrosis. II. Experimental study. Clin Orthop Rel Res *84*:200, 1972.
40. Frost HM: In vivo osteocyte death. J Bone Joint Surg *42A*:138, 1960.
41. Frost HM: The etiodynamics of aseptic necrosis of the femoral head. *In* Proceedings of the Conference on Aseptic Necrosis of the Femoral Head. St Louis, National Institutes of Health, 1964, p 393.
42. Gerle RD, Walker LA, Achord J, Weens HS: Osseous changes in chronic pancreatitis. Radiology *85*:330, 1965.

43. Gersh I, Hawkinson GE, Rathbun EN: Tissue and vascular bubbles after decompression from high pressure atmospheres. Correlation of specific gravity with morphological changes. J Cell Comp Physiol *24*:35, 1944.
44. Gersh I, Still MA: Blood vessels in fat tissue. Relation to problems of gas exchange. Exp Med *81*:219, 1945.
45. Ginn HE: Late medical complications of renal transplantation. Arch Intern Med *123*:537, 1969.
46. Glimcher MJ, Kenzora JE: The biology of osteonecrosis of the human femoral head and its clinical implications (3 parts). Clin Orthop Rel Res *138*:284; *139*:283; and *140*:273, 1979.
47. Golding JSR, MacIver JE, Went LN: The bone changes in sickle cell anemia and its genetic variants. J Bone Joint Surg *41B*:711, 1959.
48. Graham J, Wood SK: Aseptic necrosis of bone following trauma. *In* JK Davidson (Ed): Aseptic Necrosis of Bone. Amsterdam, Excerpta Medica, 1976, p 101.
49. Harrelson JM, Hills BA: Changes in bone marrow pressure in response to hyperbaric pressure. Aerospace Med *41*:1018, 1970.
50. Harrison RG, Gossman HH: The fate of radiopaque media injected into the cancellous bone of extremities. J Bone Joint Surg *37B*:150, 1955.
51. Harrington KD, Murray WR, Kountz SL, Belzer, FO: Avascular necrosis of bone after renal transplantation. J Bone Joint Surg *53A*:203, 1971.
52. Heimann WG, Freiberger RH: Avascular necrosis of the femoral and humeral heads after high-dosage corticosteroid therapy. N Engl J Med *263*:672, 1960.
53. Henard DC, Calandruccio RA: Experimental production of roentgenographic and histological changes in the capital femoral epiphysis following abduction, extension and internal rotation of the hip. J Bone Joint Surg *52A*:600, 1970.
54. Hesse F: Zur pathologischen Anatomie der Schenkelhalsfraktur. Arch Klin Chir *134*:141, 1925.
55. Hill RB Jr: Fatal fat embolism from steroid-induced fatty liver. N Engl J Med *265*:318, 1961.
56. Hook EW, Campbell CG, Weens HS, Cooper GR: Salmonella osteomyelitis in patients with sickle cell anemia. N Engl J Med *257*:403, 1957.
57. Hungerford DS: Bone marrow pressure, venography, and case decompression in ischemic necrosis of the femoral head. *In* The Hip, Proceedings of 7th Open Scientific Meeting of the Hip Society, 1979. St Louis, CV Mosby Co (in press).
58. Hungerford DS, Zizic TM: Alcohol associated ischemic necrosis of the femoral head. Clin Orthop Rel Res *130*:144, 1978.
59. Immelman EJ, Bank S, Krige H, Marks IN: Roentgenologic and clinical features of intramedullary fat necrosis in bones in acute and chronic pancreatitis. Am J Med *36*:96, 1964.
60. Jacobs P: Osteochondrosis (osteochondritis). *In* JK Davidson (Ed): Aseptic Necrosis of Bone. Amsterdam, Excerpta Medica, 1976, p 301.
61. Jaffe HL: Tumors and Tumorous Conditions of the Bones and Joints. Philadelphia, Lea & Febiger, 1958.
62. Jaffe HL: Metabolic, Degenerative and Inflammatory Diseases of Bones and Joints. Philadelphia, Lea & Febiger, 1972.
63. Jaffe HL, Pomeranz MM: Changes in the bones of extremities amputated because of arteriovascular disease. Arch Surg *29*:566, 1934.
64. James NE: Gaucher's disease; report of case. J Bone Joint Surg *34B*:464, 1952.
65. Jee WSS, Arnold JS: Effect of internally deposited radioisotopes upon blood vessels of cortical bones. Proc Soc Exp Biol Med *105*:351, 1960.
66. Jee WSS, Bartley MH, Dockum NL, Yee J, Kenner GH: Vascular changes in bones following bone-seeking radionuclides. *In* CW Mays, et al (Eds): Delayed Effects of Bone Seeking Radionuclides. Salt Lake City, University of Utah Press, 1969, p 437.
67. Johnson LC: Histogenesis of avascular necrosis. *In* Proceedings of the Conference on Aseptic Necrosis of the Femoral Head. St Louis, National Institutes of Health, 1964, p 55.
68. Jones JP: Alcoholism, hypercortisonism, fat embolism and osseous avascular necrosis. *In* WM Zinn (Ed): Idiopathic Ischemic Necrosis of the Femoral Head in Adults. Stuttgart, Georg Thieme, 1971, p 112.
69. Jones JP, Jr Jameson RM, Engleman EP: Alcoholism, fat embolism and avascular necrosis (Abstr). J Bone Joint Surg *50A*:1065, 1968.
70. Jones JP, Sakovich L: Fat embolism of bone. A roentgenographic and histological investigation with use of intra-arterial Lipiodol in rabbits. J Bone Joint Surg *48A*:149, 1966.
71. Kahlstrom SC, Burton CC, Phemister DB: Aseptic necrosis of bone. II. Infarction of bones of undetermined etiology resulting in encapsulated and calcified areas in diaphyses and in arthritis deformans. Surg Gynecol Obstet *68*:631, 1939.
72. Kenzora JE, Steele RE, Yosipovitch, ZH, Boyd R, Glimcher MJ: Tissue biology following experimental infarction of femoral heads. Part I. Bone studies. J Bone Joint Surg *51A*:1021, 1969.
73. Kenzora JE, Steele RE, Yosipovitch ZH, Glimcher MJ: Experimental osteonecrosis of the femoral head in adult rabbits. Clin Orthop Rel Res *130*:8, 1978.
74. Kinsell LW (Ed): Adipose Tissue as an Organ: Proceedings (Deuel Conference on Lipids). Springfield, Ill, Charles C Thomas, 1962.
75. Lagier R: Idiopathic aseptic necrosis of the femoral head. An anatomopathological concept. *In* WM Zinn (Ed). Idiopathic Ischemic Necrosis of the Femoral Head in Adults. Stuttgart, Georg Thieme, 1971, p 49.
76. Louyot P, Gaucher A: A propos de 30 observations d'ostéonécroses primitive de la tête fémorale. Rev Rhum Mal Osteoartic *29*:577, 1962.
77. Lynch MJG, Raphael SS, Dixon TP: Fat embolism in chronic alcoholism. Arch Pathol *67*:68, 1959.
78. Lucas PF, Owen TK: Subcutaneous fat necrosis, "polyarthritis" and pancreatic disease. Gut *3*:146, 1962.
79. McCollum DE, Mathews RS, Pickett PT: Gout, hyperuricemia and aseptic necrosis of the femoral head (Abstr). Arthritis Rheum *10*:295, 1967.
80. McKay DG: Disseminated Intravascular Coagulation, An Intermediary Mechanism of Disease. New York, Hoeber Medical Division, Harper & Row, 1965.
81. Marshall JH: The retention of radionuclides in bone. *In* CW Mays, et al (Eds): Delayed Effects of Bone Seeking Radionuclides. Salt Lake City, University of Utah Press, 1969, p 7.
82. Middlemiss H: Aseptic necrosis and other changes occurring in bone in the hemoglobinopathies. *In* JK Davidson (Ed): Aseptic Necrosis of Bone. Amsterdam, Excerpta Medica, 1976, p 271.
83. Müssbichler, H: Arteriographic findings in necrosis of the head of the femur after medial neck fracture. Acta Orthop Scand *41*:77, 1970.
84. Nachamie BA, Dorfman HD: Ischemic necrosis of bone in sickle cell trait. Mt Sinai J Med *41*:527, 1974.
85. Patterson RJ, Bickel WH, Dahlin DC: Idiopathic avascular necrosis of the head of the femur. A study of fifty-two cases. J Bone Joint Surg *46A*:267, 1964.
86. Perry TT III: Role of lymphatic vessels in the transmission of lipase in disseminated pancreatic fat necrosis. Arch Pathol *43*:456, 1947.
87. Phemister DB: Necrotic bone and the subsequent changes which it undergoes. JAMA *64*:211, 1915.
88. Phemister DB: Repair of bone in the presence of aseptic necrosis resulting from fractures, transplantations and vascular obstruction. J Bone Joint Surg *12*:769, 1930.
89. Phemister DB: Fractures of the neck of femur, dislocations of hip, and obscure vascular disturbances producing aseptic necrosis of head of femur. Surg Gynecol Obstet *59*:415, 1934.
90. Phemister DB: The pathology of ununited fractures of the neck of the femur with special reference to the head. J Bone Joint Surg *21*:681, 1939.
91. Phemister DB: Lesions of bones and joints arising from interruption of the circulation. Mt Sinai J Med *15*:55, 1948.
92. Philp RB, Inwood MJ, Warren BA: Interactions between gas bubbles and components of the blood. Implications in decompression sickness. Aerospace Med *43*:946, 1972.
93. Pourel J, Louyot P, Diebold P, Baumgartner J: Stéatonécrosis disséminée a déterminations articulaires, osseuses et mésentériques. J Radiol Electrol Med Nucl *51*:423, 1970.
94. Ratcliff RG, Wolf MD: Avascular necrosis of the femoral head associated with sickle cell trait (AS hemoglobin). Ann Intern Med *57*:299, 1962.
95. Riniker P, Huggler A: Idiopathic necrosis of the femoral head. (A further patho-anatomical study). *In* WM Zinn (Ed): Idiopathic Ischemic Necrosis of the Femoral Head in Adults. Stuttgart, Georg Thieme, 1971, p 67.
96. Robbins SL, Angell M: Basic Pathology. 2nd Ed. Philadelphia, WB Saunders Co, 1976, pp 7, 20.
97. Robbins SL, Angell M: Basic Pathology. 2nd Ed. Philadephia, WB Saunders Co, 1976, p 28.
98. Robbins SL, Angell M: Basic Pathology. 2nd Ed. Philadephia, WB Saunders Co, 1976, p 184.
99. Rösingh GE, James J: Early phases of avascular necrosis of the femoral head in rabbits. J Bone Joint Surg *51B*:165, 1969.
100. Royzsahegyi I: Die chronische Osteoarthropathie der Caissonarbeiter. Arch Gewerbepath Gewerbehyg *14*:483, 1956.
101. Rourke JA, Heslin DJ: Gaucher's disease. Roentgenologic bone changes over 20 year interval. Am J Roentgenol *94*:621, 1965.
102. Russell J: A Practical Essay on a Certain Disease of Bones Termed Necrosis. Edinburgh, Neill and Co, 1794.
103. Santos JV: Changes in the head of the femur after complete intracapsular fracture of the neck. Their bearing on nonunion and treatment. Arch Surg *21*:470, 1930.
104. Scarpelli DG: Fat necrosis of bone marrow in acute pancreatitis. Am J Pathol *32*:1077, 1956.
105. Sevitt S: Avascular necrosis and revascularisation of the femoral head after intracapsular fracture; a combined arteriographic and histological necropsy study. J Bone Joint Surg *46B*:270, 1964.
106. Sevitt S, Thompson RG: The distribution and anastomoses of arteries

supplying the head and neck of the femur. J Bone Joint Surg *47B*:560, 1965.
107. Sherman MS, Phemister DB: The pathology of ununited fractures of the neck of the femur. J Bone Joint Surg *29*:19, 1947.
108. Shin SS: Circulatory and vascular changes in the hip following traumatic hip dislocation. Clin Orthop Rel Res *140*:255, 1979.
109. Siemsen JK, Brook J, Meister L: Lupus erythematosus and avascular bone necrosis: A clinical study of three cases and review of the literature. Arthritis Rheum *5*:492, 1962.
110. Smith FE, Sweet DE, Brunner CM, Davis JS: Avascular necrosis in SLE. An apparent predilection for young patients. Ann Rheum Dis *35*:227, 1976.
111. Springfield DS, Enneking WJ: Surgery for aseptic necrosis of the femoral head. Clin Orthop Rel Res *130*:175, 1978.
112. Stein AH: The physiological aspects of circulation to a long bone. *In* Proceedings of the Conference on Aseptic Necrosis of the Femoral Head. St Louis, National Institutes of Health, 1964, p 41.
113. Storey GO: Bone necrosis in joint disease. Proc R Soc Med *61*:961, 1968.
114. Sweet DE: Unpublished data.
115. Todd RM, Keidan SE: Changes in the head of the femur in children suffering from Gaucher's disease. J Bone Joint Surg *34B*:447, 1952.
116. Trueta J: The normal vascular anatomy of the human femoral head during growth. J Bone Joint Surg *39B*:358, 1957.
117. Trueta J, Harrison MHM: The normal vascular anatomy of the femoral head in adult man. J Bone Joint Surg *35B*:442, 1953.
118. Trueta J: Studies of the Development and Decay of the Human Frame. Philadelphia, WB Saunders Co, 1968.
119. Velayos EE, Leidholt JD, Smyth CJ: Arthropathy associated with steroid therapy. Ann Intern Med *64*:759, 1966.
120. Walder DN: A possible explanation for some cases of severe decompression sickness in compressed-air workers. *In* DJC Cunningham and BB Lloyd (Eds): The Regulation of Human Respiration. Oxford, Blackwell, 1963, p 570.
121. Wang GJ, Sweet DE, Reger SI: Fat cell changes as a mechanism of avascular necrosis of the femoral head in cortisone treated rabbits. J Bone Joint Surg *59A*:729, 1977.
122. Wang GJ: Personal communication.
123. Werts MF, Shilling CW: Dysbaric osteonecrosis. An annotated bibliography with preliminary analyses. Washington, DC, Biological Services Communication Project, George Washington University Medical Center, 1972.
124. Woodward HQ, Coley BL: The correlation of tissue dose and clinical response in irradiation of bone tumors and of normal bone. Am J Roentgenol *57*:464, 1947.
125. Woodhouse CF: Anoxia of the femoral head. Surgery *52*:55, 1962.
126. Woodhouse CF: Dynamic influences of vascular occlusion affecting the development of avascular necrosis of the femoral head. Clin Orthop Rel Res *32*:119, 1964.

OSTEONECROSIS: DIAGNOSTIC TECHNIQUES, SPECIFIC SITUATIONS, AND COMPLICATIONS

by Donald Resnick, M.D., and Gen Niwayama, M.D.

77

Chapter 76 has described in detail the general pathologic and radiologic alterations that accompany osteonecrosis. Although specific changes are dependent, to some extent, on the precise location and cause of the bone necrosis, the morphologic findings are remarkably similar.

The causes of osteonecrosis are varied. As evidence of this fact, Greenfield[1] lists no fewer than 54 causes of a fragmented femoral head, many of which are related to osseous necrosis. Important etiologic factors include trauma (fracture or dislocation), hemoglobinopathies (sickle cell anemia, sickle "variant" states), exogeneous or endogenous hypercortisolism (corticosteroid medication, Cushing's disease), renal transplantation, alcoholism or pancreatitis, dysbaric conditions (caisson disease), small vessel disease (collagen vascular disorders), Gaucher's disease, gout and hyperuricemia, irradiation, and synovitis with elevation of intra-articular pressure (infection, hemophilia) (Fig. 77–1). In some of these conditions, the exact pathogenesis of osteonecrosis has not been defined despite the accumulation of a great deal of clinical and experimental data. There is also a group of individuals in whom no underlying causative disorder can be detected. In this situation, the term primary, idiopathic, or spontaneous osteonecrosis is utilized.

In this chapter, a review of available diagnostic modalities, specific causes or situations, and complications of osteonecrosis is provided. The reader

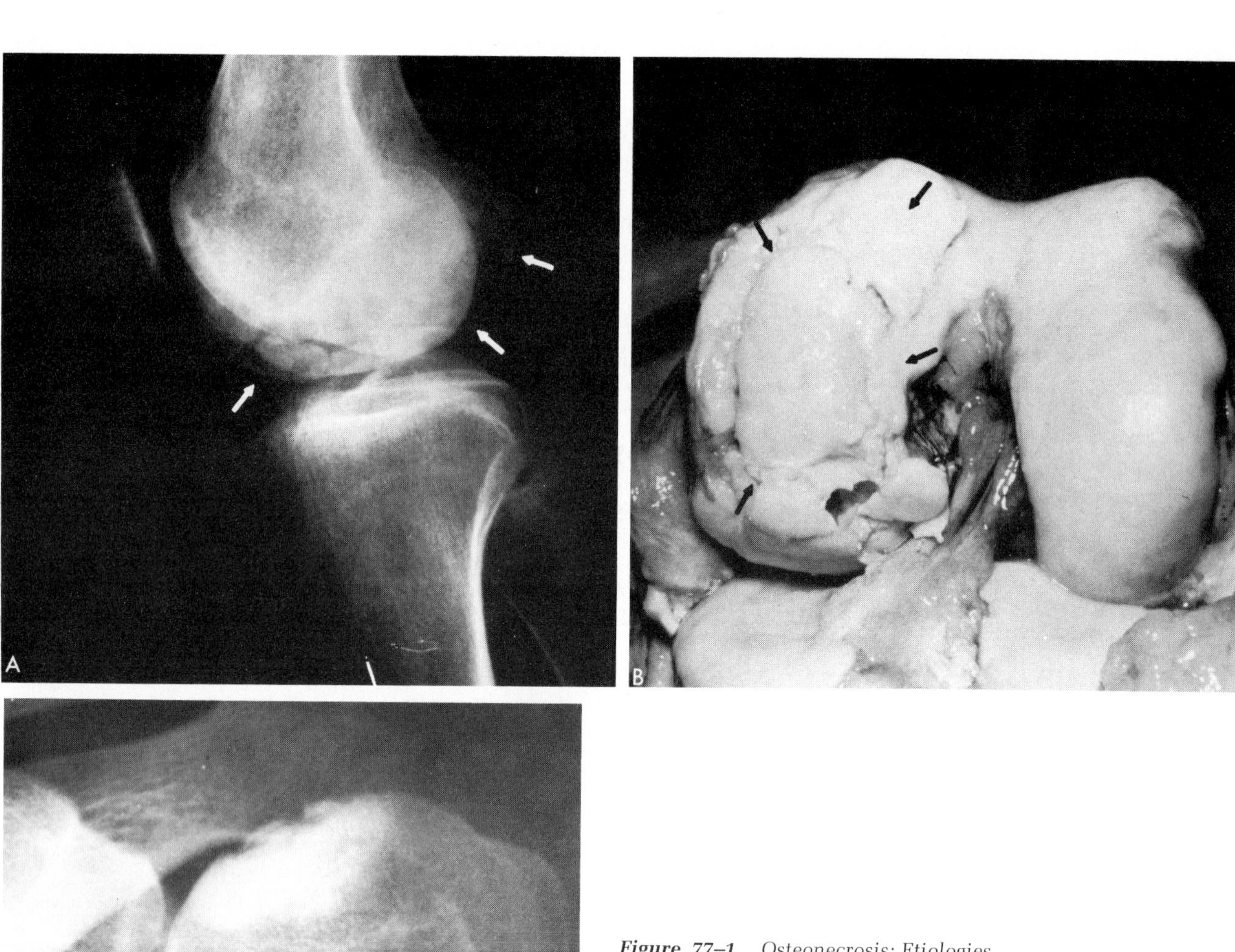

Figure 77–1. *Osteonecrosis: Etiologies.*

A, B *Exogenous hypercortisolism. Note the extensive osseous fragmentation of the medial femoral condyle (arrows).*

C *Renal transplantation. The radiodense ("snow-cap") appearance of the humeral head with associated collapse and fragmentation of bone is typical of osteonecrosis at this site. The joint space is maintained.*

Illustration continued on the opposite page

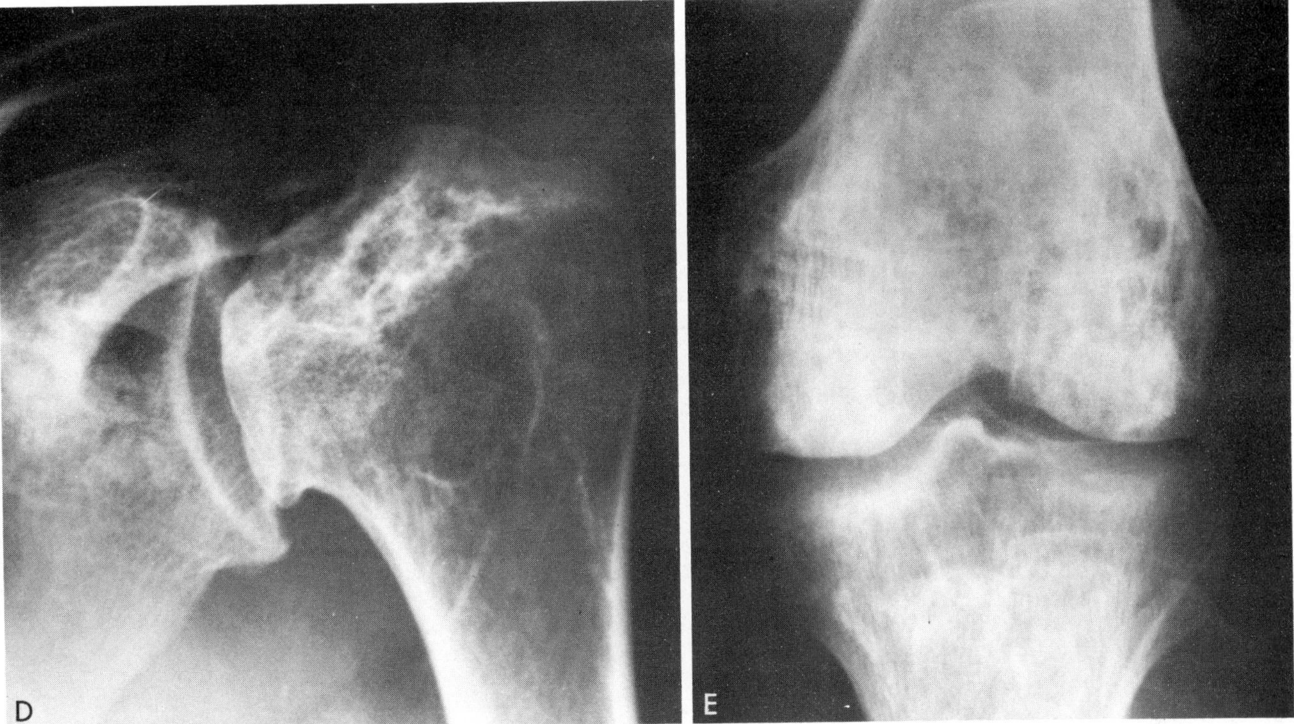

Figure 77–1. Continued
D, E *Alcoholism and pancreatitis. Examples illustrate necrosis of the humeral head with sclerosis and collapse of the articular surface and curvilinear calcification and bony eburnation of the distal femur and proximal tibia. Joint space preservation is again apparent.*

should refer to Chapter 76 as well as to additional relevant sections of the book for discussion of many of the other systemic disorders that may be associated with osseous necrosis.

DIAGNOSTIC MODALITIES

Radiography

The plain film roentgenographic findings of osteonecrosis of an epiphysis, metaphysis, or diaphysis in a tubular bone or of a flat or irregular bone are so characteristic that additional diagnostic modalities are frequently not required. Arc-like subchondral radiolucent lesions, patchy lucent areas and sclerosis, osseous collapse, and preservation of the joint space in an epiphyseal region (Fig. 77–2); lucent shadows with a peripheral rim of sclerosis and periostitis in a diametaphyseal region (Fig. 77–3); and patchy lucent areas and sclerosis with bony collapse in a flat or irregular bone are typical roentgenographic signs of osteonecrosis. Unfortunately, these abnormalities do not appear for several months following the onset of clinical manifestations in many individuals and, therefore, do not represent a sensitive indication of early disease (Fig. 77–4).

Roentgenograms obtained during the application of traction can be useful, especially about the hip.[2] This technique may accentuate the curvilinear radiolucent shadow that is evident in an osteonecrotic epiphysis, perhaps owing to the release of gas in the zone of subchondral separation with the induction of a vacuum by traction. A traction force of 30 to 50 lb can be applied manually to each leg for approximately 10 sec prior to and during the x-ray exposure. It is necessary to fix the patient's position by having him or her grasp the end of the radiographic table or by having an attendant support the patient under the arms. The failure of intra-articular gas to be released during this procedure can indicate the presence of joint fluid.[3]

Tomography is occasionally indicated for the accurate diagnosis of osteonecrosis. In this condition, a radiolucent lesion of an epiphysis with surrounding sclerosis detected on plain film radiography may simulate the appearance of a primary bone tumor, such as a giant cell tumor or chondroblastoma[4]; tomography may indicate angular or wedge-shaped lesional margins and subtle collapse of the osseous surface, allowing a precise diagnosis of bone necrosis (Fig. 77–5). Laminography of a diametaphyseal lesion or one in a flat or irregular bone may,

Text continued on page 2840

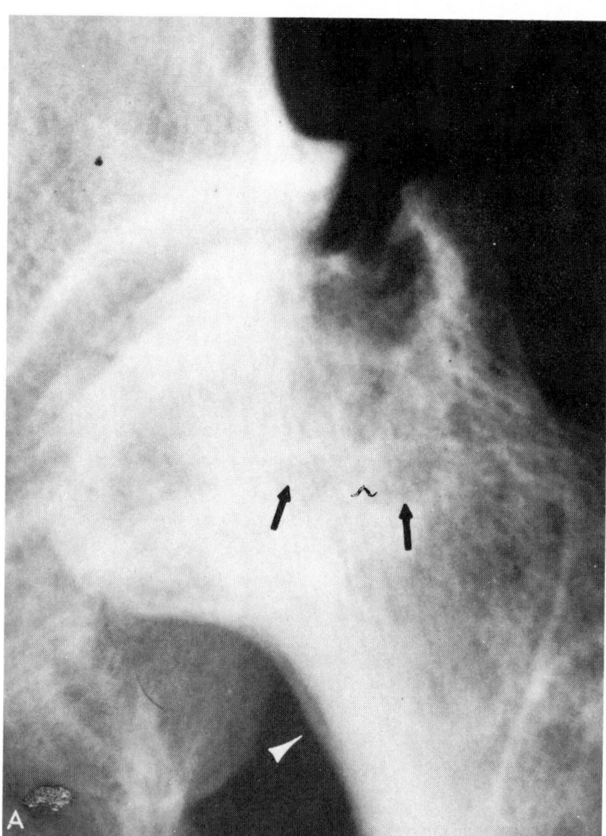

Figure 77–2. Osteonecrosis: Epiphysis —radiographic-pathologic correlation.

A *The preoperative radiograph outlines extensive collapse of the articular surface of the femoral head with cystic lucent areas (arrows), patchy sclerosis, buttressing (arrowhead), and preservation of joint space.*

B, C *Sectional radiograph and photograph show displaced cartilage and subchondral bone plate (arrowheads), subjacent osseous resorption (solid arrows), reactive bone formation, and buttressing. Osteophytic lipping is observed (open arrows).*

Illustration continued on the opposite page

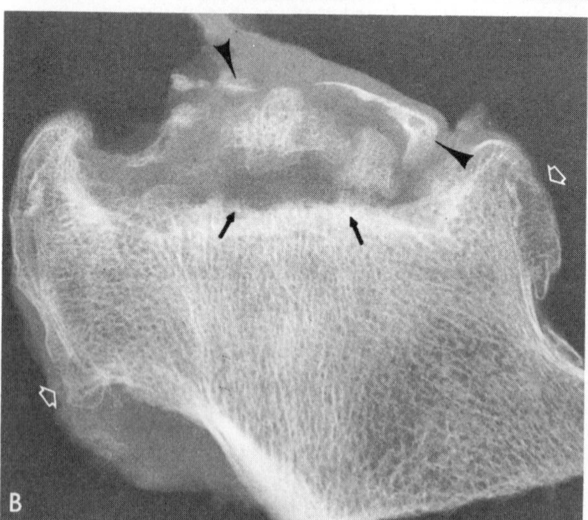

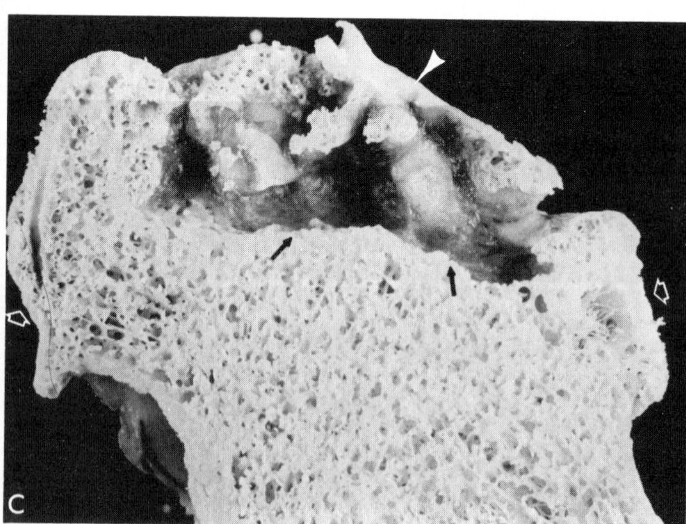

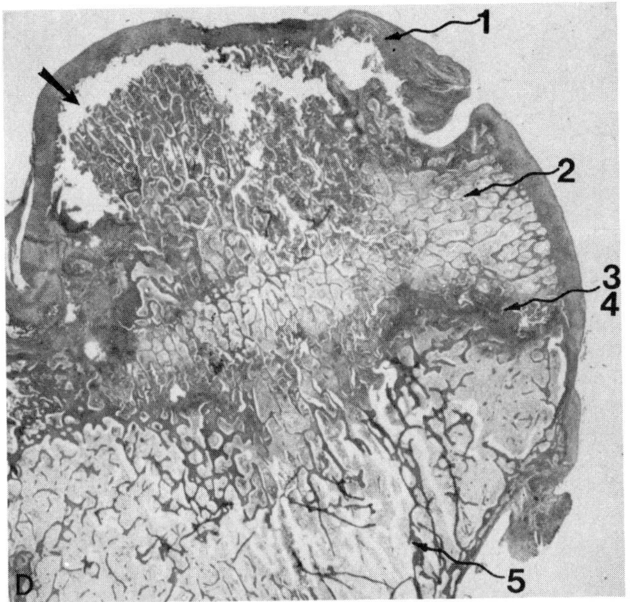

Figure 77–2. Continued

D *A photomicrograph (2 ×) shows a superficial zone of detached articular cartilage and subarticular trabeculae (1), with subjacent curvilinear area of bony separation (arrow) representing a fracture. Note also a large zone of bone necrosis (2), zones of vascular granulation tissue and new bone formation (3, 4), and deep zone of normal cancellous bone (5).*

(**A–D,** From Resnick D, et al: *Am J Roentgenol* 128:799, 1977. Copyright 1977, American Roentgen Ray Society.)

E *A photomicrograph (20×) reveals the superficial zone of detached viable articular cartilage and subarticular trabeculae (1), an area of bony separation or fracture (arrow), and a zone of bone necrosis (2).*

F *In another area, fibrosis of the marrow space and neovascularization can be identified (20×).*

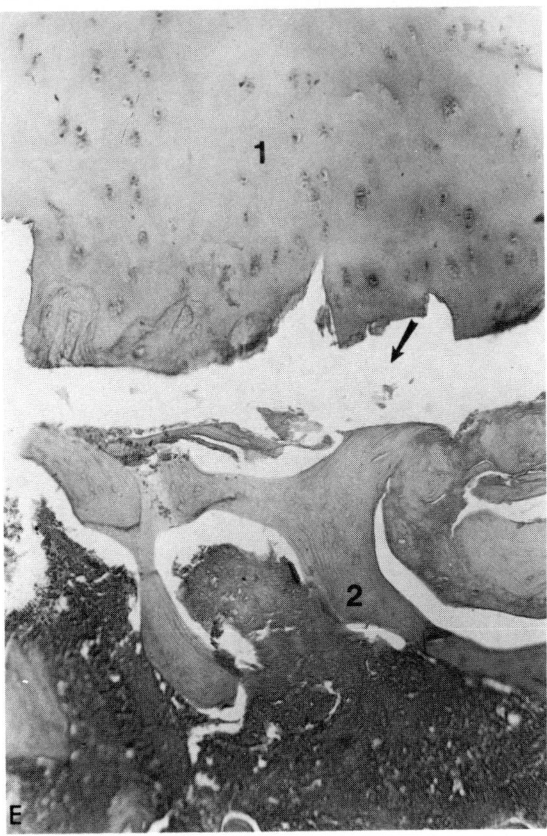

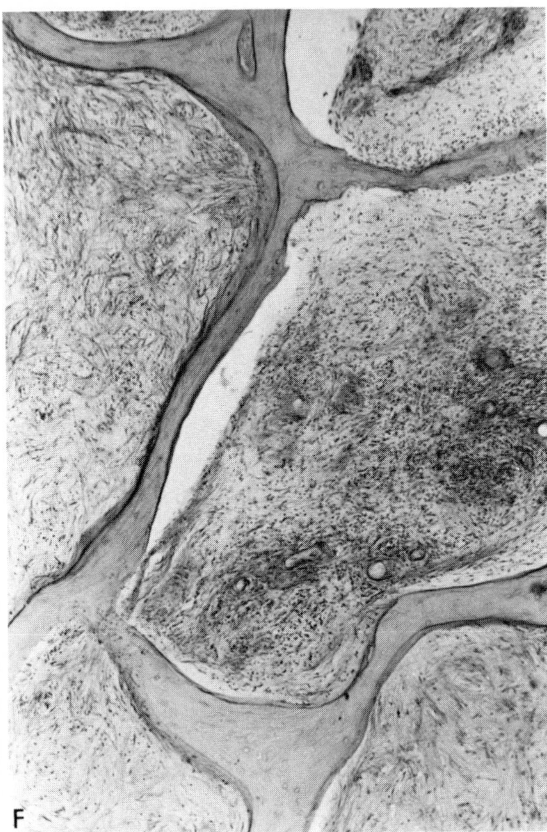

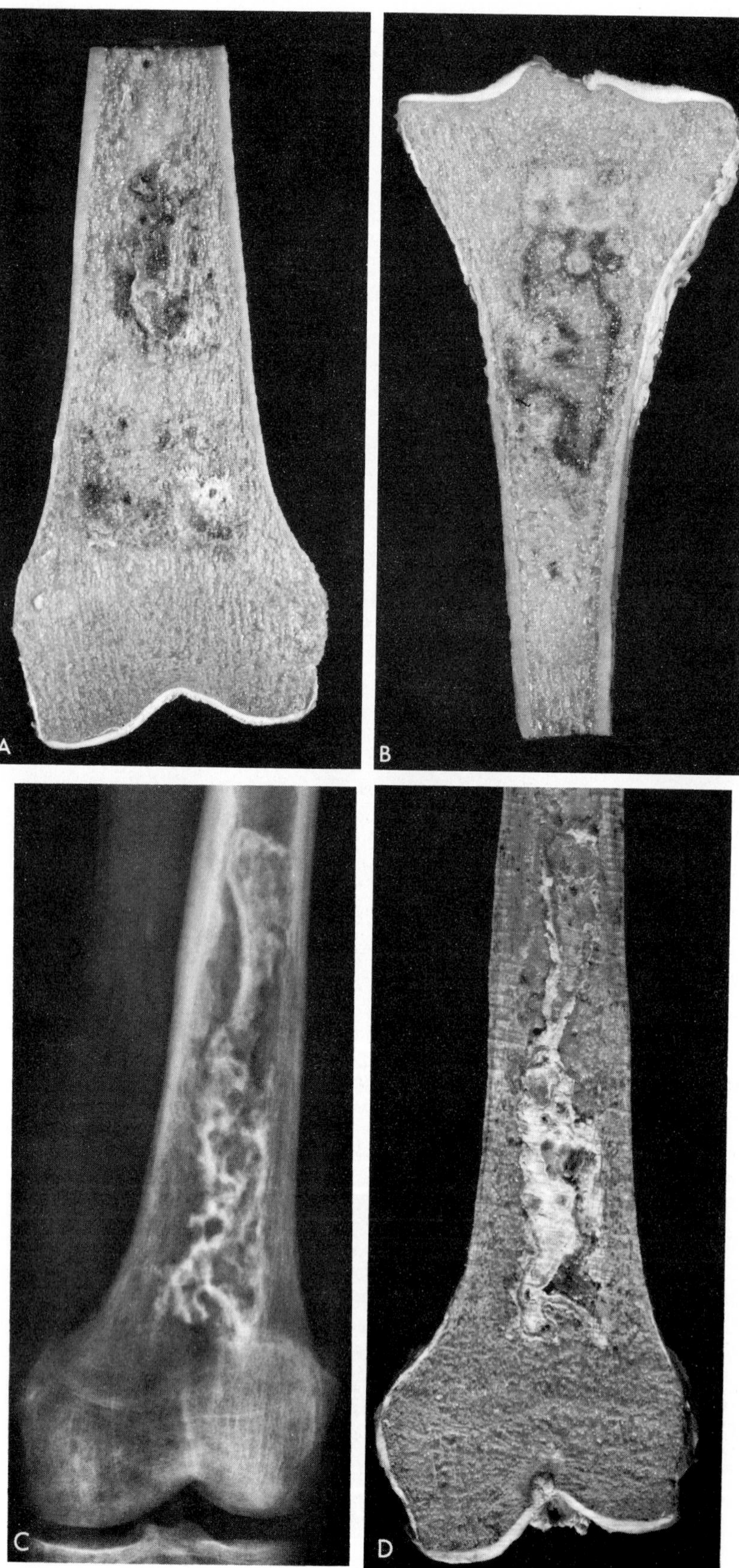

Figure 77–3. Osteonecrosis: Diametaphysis—radiographic-pathologic correlation.

A A photograph of the cut surface of the lower part of the left femur removed at autopsy from a 42 year old woman who had had clinical manifestations of systemic lupus erythematosus for about 4 years reveals a rather large and recent intramedullary infarct in the femoral shaft. This patient had received corticosteroid medications.

B A photograph of the cut surface of the upper part of the tibia shows a large irregularly contoured area of infarction in the shaft. Except in the uppermost portion, where the infarcted area appears whitish, the infarct has a dark peripheral zone of hemorrhagic discoloration.

C A roentgenogram of the lower half of the left femur of a 69 year old man with intermittent claudication of 4 years' duration demonstrates a bony infarction. Observe the typical shell-like calcification of the lesion.

D A photograph of the cut surface of the lower half of the left femur following amputation of the leg demonstrates necrotic spongy bone and marrow, which are walled off by calcified collagenous fibrous tissue, which varies in thickness from place to place and is serpentine in configuration. In some of the resultant locules, there are residual areas of necrotic spongiosa and fatty marrow.

(From Jaffe HL: Med Radiogr Photogr 45:58, 1969.)

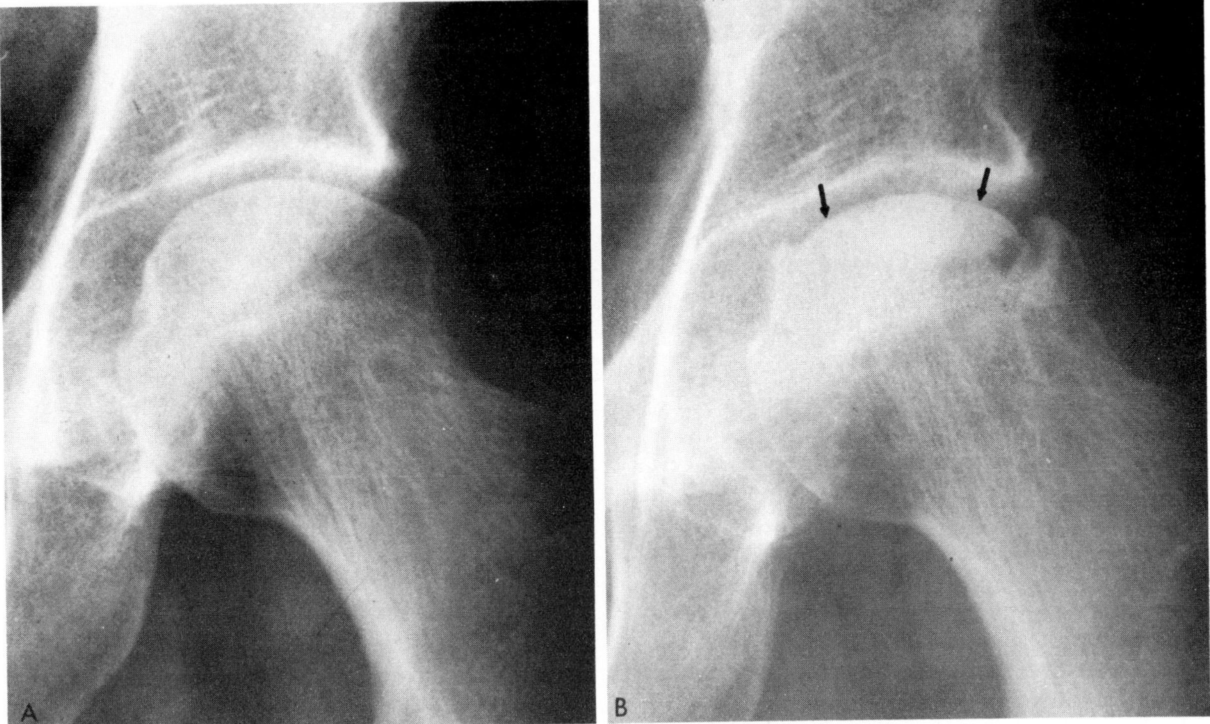

Figure 77–4. *Osteonecrosis: Inadequacy of radiographic examination. This 35 year old man had had hip pain at the time of his initial radiographic examination, which progressed over the subsequent 6 to 9 months.*

A *The initial roentgenogram was interpreted as normal. A bone scan was not accomplished.*

B *Seven months later, significant collapse of the superolateral aspect of the femoral head is identified (arrows). The joint space is not narrowed.*

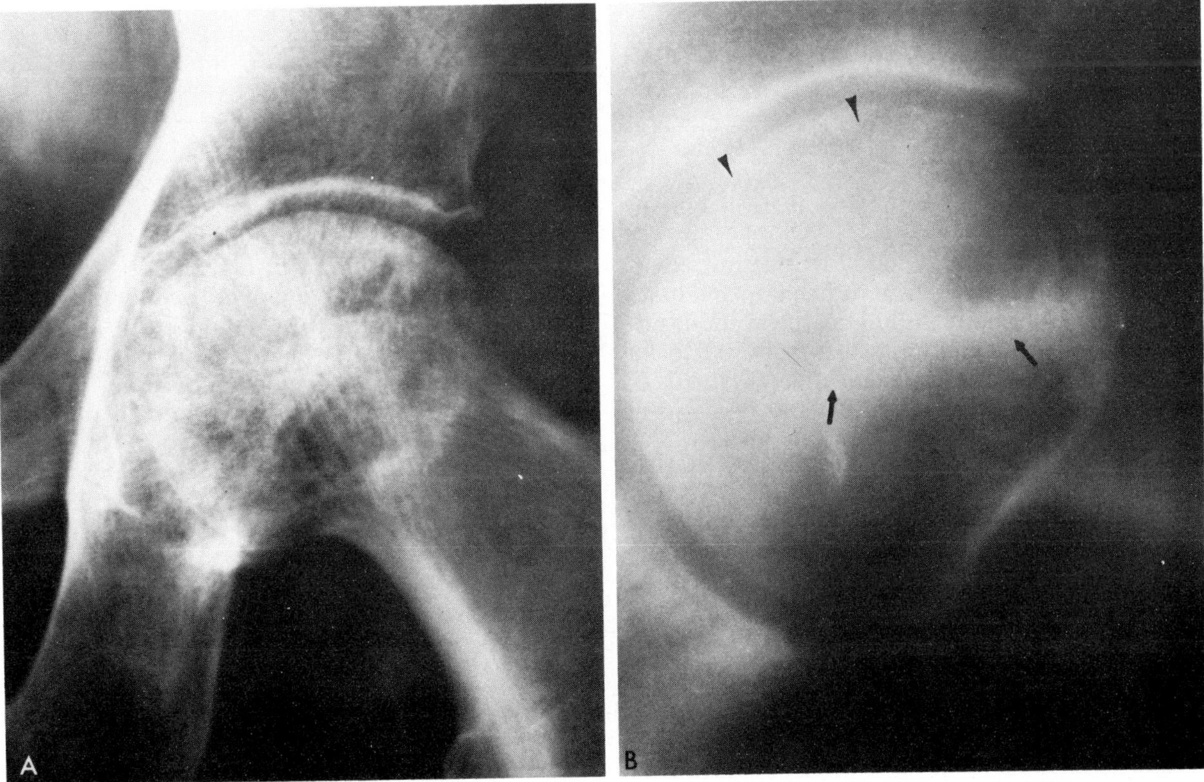

Figure 77–5. *Osteonecrosis: Role of tomography. This 47 year old man developed a dull aching pain in the hip of spontaneous onset, with stiffness and decreased range of motion.*

A *The radiograph outlines patchy lucency and sclerosis of much of the superolateral aspect of the femoral head, with subtle flattening of the osseous contour.*

B *A tomogram obtained 1 month later reveals the extent of the necrosis, surrounding new bone formation (arrows), and a subchondral curvilinear fracture line (arrowheads).*

similarly, define characteristic features of osteonecrosis in difficult cases.

Scintigraphy

The relative insensitivity of radiography in the early detection of osteonecrosis has led to the utilization of other modalities, including angiography,[5, 6] venography,[7-9] and scintigraphy.[10-12, 130, 131, 133] Although intraosseous phlebography or pressure readings may reveal elevated intraosseous pressure in the initial stages of osteonecrosis,[132] the radionuclide examination is considered the most attractive technique for early diagnosis of this disorder. Establishing a correct diagnosis at an initial stage is important, as the success of some of the proposed orthopedic procedures requires their application prior to the appearance of collapse of the articular surface (Fig. 77–6). Scintigraphy may be especially useful in studying the contralateral "silent" hip in cases of apparent unilateral osteonecrosis of the femoral head.[129]

Immediately following interruption of the osseous blood supply, scintigraphy with bone-seeking radiopharmaceuticals can reveal an area of decreased or absent uptake, a "cold" lesion. Following weeks or months, reparative processes in the surrounding bone are associated with revascularization and increased accumulation of the radioisotope, a "hot" lesion[13, 14] (Fig. 77–7). At some point between these two stages, early in the course of the process, the radionuclide examination can be normal. Even when abnormal, the study is not specific and must be interpreted with knowledge of the radiographic and clinical findings. Furthermore, the scintiscan results, reflecting the absence or presence of regional blood flow, do not evaluate the adequacy or permanency of the vascular supply.[14]

Bone marrow scans with technetium-99m-sulfur-colloid have also been utilized to evaluate osteonecrosis.[15] Normally, following intravenous administration of this agent, approximately 80 to 90 per cent of the substance is phagocytized in the liver and spleen and approximately 10 to 20 per cent is accumulated by phagocytes in the bone marrow.[16] A decrease in accumulation is suggestive of deficient or severely impaired circulation and, as such, may have predictive value regarding the likelihood of subsequent osteonecrosis and the necessity of surgical intervention. Investigation with both bone marrow–seeking and bone-seeking agents may be effective in the assessment of osteonecrosis.[13]

POSTTRAUMATIC OSTEONECROSIS

Following a fracture, bone death of variable extent on either side of the fracture line is common.[17] However, necrosis of a large segment of bone following fracture or dislocation is generally restricted to those sites that possess a vulnerable blood supply with few arterial anastomoses; the femoral head, the body of the talus, the humeral head, and the carpal scaphoid represent four such sites.[18] Other locations include the tarsal navicular and carpal lunate. In addition to the peculiarities of blood supply, characteristics common to each of these areas are an intra-articular location of necrotic bone and a limited attachment of soft tissue. In each location, the necrotic portion of the bone may appear radiodense as a result of compression of trabeculae, reactive eburnation as a consequence of the healing process, or lack of participation of the bone in the hyperemia and osteoporosis of neighboring viable bone.[19-23]

Femoral Head

Osteonecrosis of the femoral head is a well-recognized complication of femoral neck fractures and dislocations.[24, 25] Its reported incidence has varied considerably, influenced by many factors such as the age and sex of the patient, the type and severity of the injury, and the diagnostic modalities and criteria that are employed.[25, 26] Despite this variation, the importance of the local vascular anatomy in the pathogenesis of osteonecrosis of the femoral head is not questioned.

The principal blood supply to the adult femoral head is via the circumflex femoral branches of the profunda femoris artery[18, 27] (Fig. 77–8). The lateral and medial femoral circumflex arteries pass anterior and posterior to the femur to anastomose at the level of the trochanters, and from these vessels, especially the medial circumflex artery, small branches are derived that pass beneath the capsule of the hip joint and extend in folds or retinacula along the femoral neck, covered by the synovial membrane. They terminate by entering the bone at the cartilaginous margin. The superior (lateral) and the inferior retinacular vessels are the most important structures in this group. A second supply of blood is derived from the vessels of the ligamentum teres. These vascular structures enter the bone of the fovea capitis. A third vascular pathway, the nutrient artery supplying blood to the proximal femoral metaphysis, appears to have an insignificant role in perfusing the femoral head. Despite the presence of anastomoses among the major vessels of the femoral head in the adult, the connections vary from one person to another and, in many instances, are not functional.[28] It has been established that the superior (lateral) retinacular vessels represent the most important source of blood to the femoral head,[29] whereas the inferior retinacular vessels nourish only a small portion of the head and neck of the femur. A fracture of the femoral neck that traverses the entry site of the

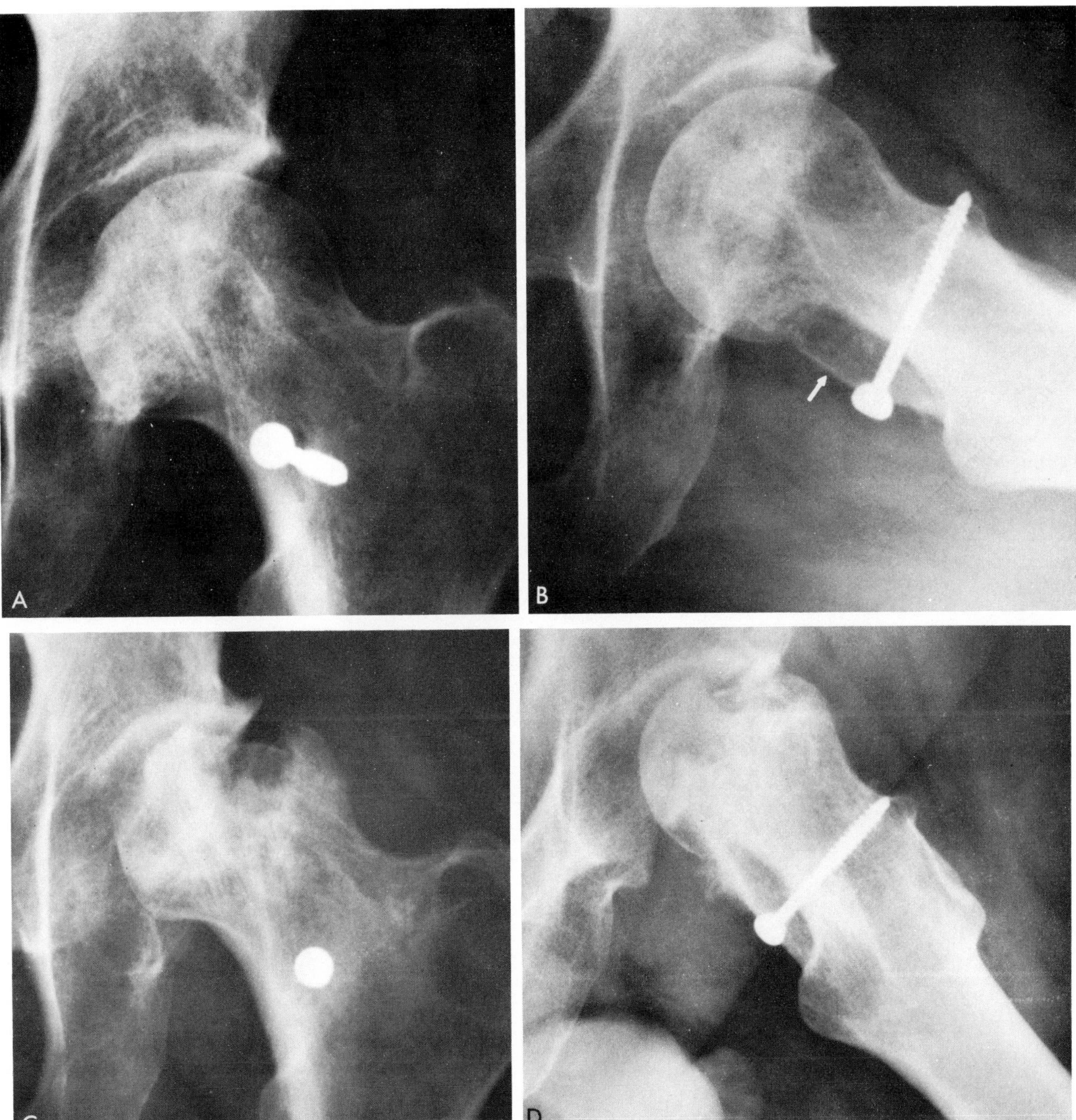

Figure 77–6. *Osteonecrosis: Various orthopedic procedures. Various procedures have been advocated in the treatment of osteonecrosis of the femoral head. Their success is largely dependent upon the early diagnosis of the condition.*

A–D *In this 41 year old man with bilateral osteonecrosis documented by radionuclide studies, a Judet bone graft was utilized. Initial anteroposterior* **(A)** *and "frog-leg"* **(B)** *projections reveal the site of the bone graft (arrow) that has been applied to the femoral neck. At this stage, collapse is not present, although patchy sclerosis and lucency are apparent. Eighteen months later, obvious collapse, lateral subluxation of the femoral head, and joint space narrowing are evident* **(C, D)**.

Illustration continued on the following page

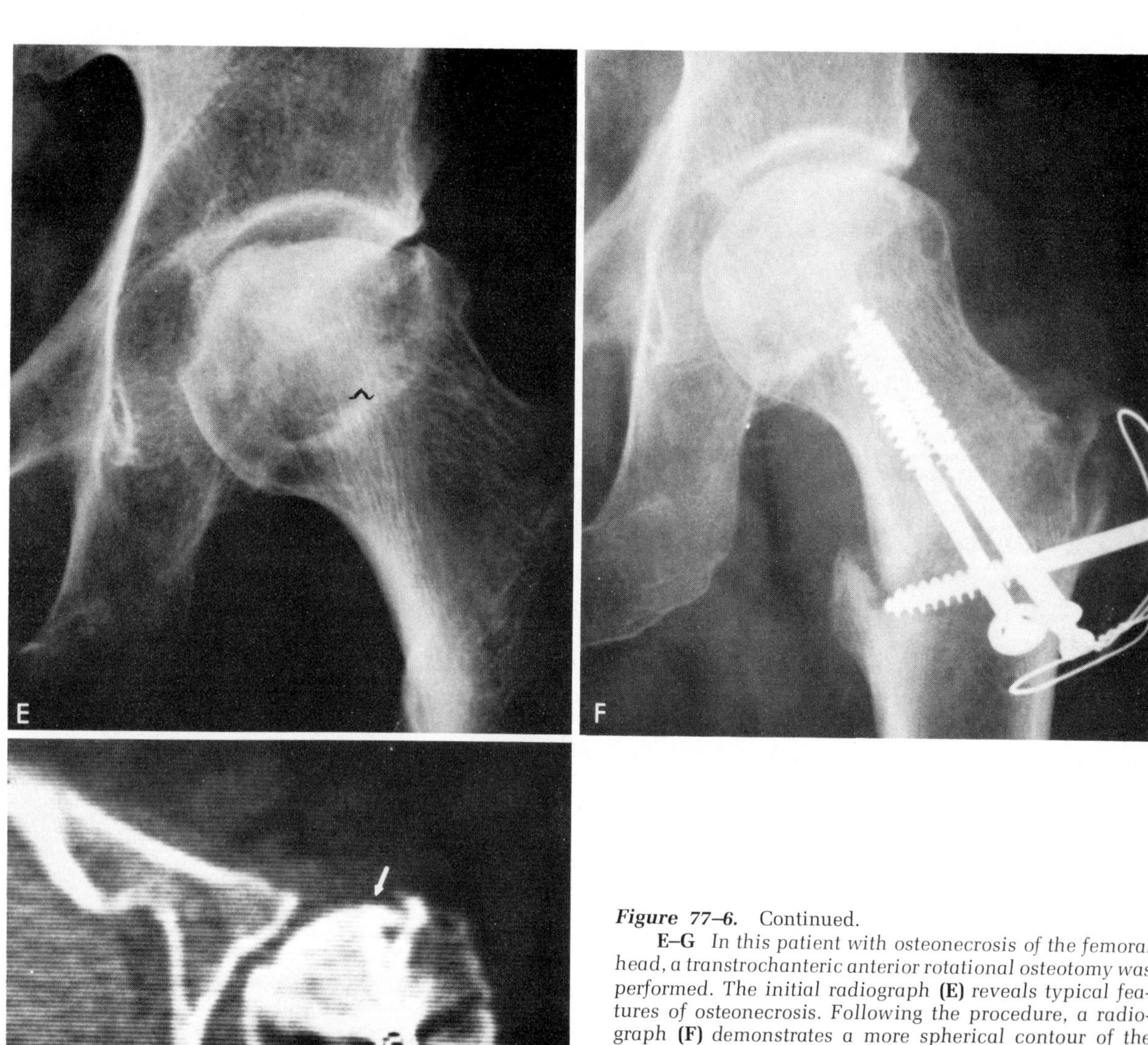

Figure 77–6. Continued.

E–G *In this patient with osteonecrosis of the femoral head, a transtrochanteric anterior rotational osteotomy was performed. The initial radiograph* **(E)** *reveals typical features of osteonecrosis. Following the procedure, a radiograph* **(F)** *demonstrates a more spherical contour of the femoral head. On computed tomography* **(G)**, *observe the anterior location of the necrotic portion of the femoral head (arrows). The screws and resulting artifacts can also be seen.*

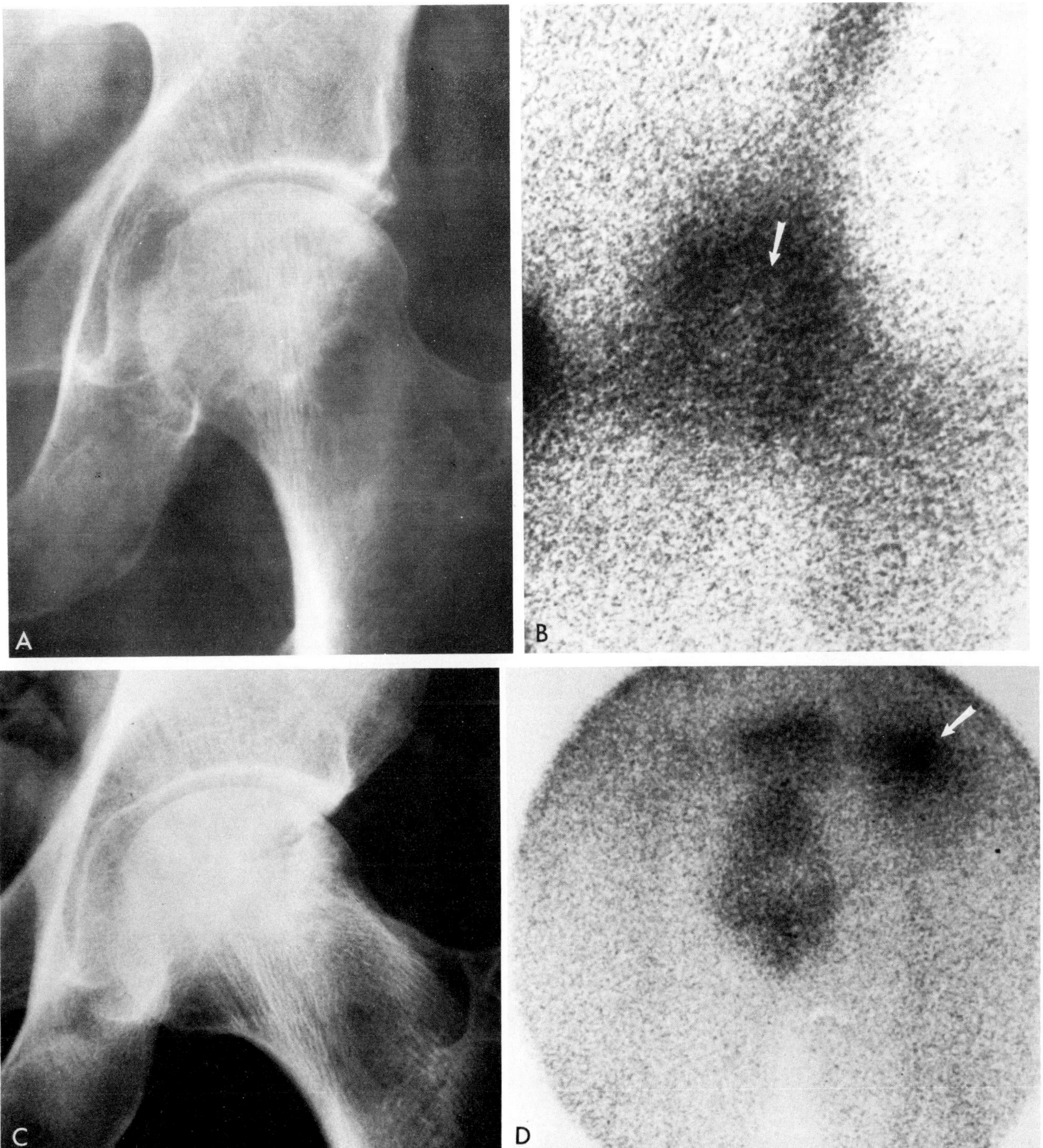

Figure 77–7. *Osteonecrosis: Value of radionuclide examination.*

A, B *A radiograph of the hip in this 55 year old man reveals a mild degree of patchy sclerosis of the femoral head without collapse of the articular surface. The scan of the hip utilizing technetium pyrophosphate depicts a central area of diminished uptake surrounded by a zone of augmented activity (arrow).*

C, D *In a different patient with osteonecrosis, the radiograph outlines subchondral resorption and cyst formation without collapse, and the scan with technetium pyrophosphate demonstrates an area of increased uptake of isotope in the left hip (arrow). Note the activity in the bladder.*

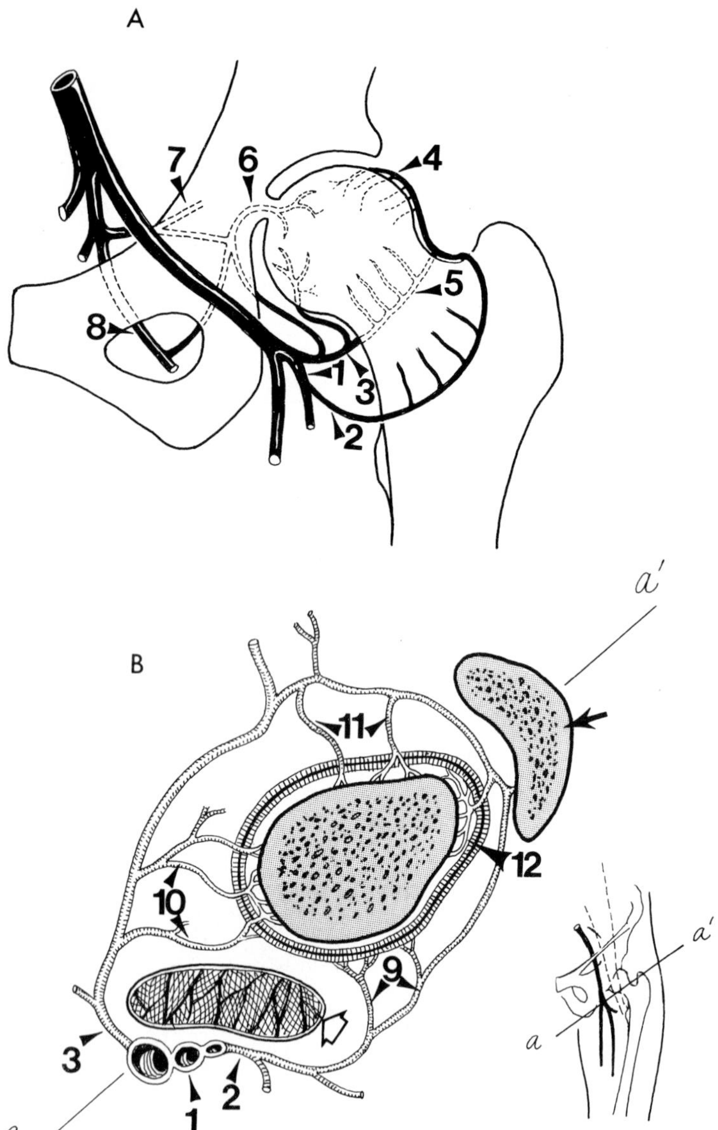

Figure 77–8. Femoral head: Vascular supply in adults.

A The major blood supply is derived from the profunda femoris artery (1), from which arise the lateral (2) and the medial (3) circumflex arteries. (The medial and lateral circumflex arteries may arise from the femoral artery rather than the profunda femoris artery in some individuals.) As these latter vessels pass anterior and posterior to the femur to anastomose at the level of the trochanters, they send off small branches beneath the capsule of the hip joint. These branches, including the superior retinacular (lateral epiphyseal) arteries (4) and the inferior retinacular (inferior metaphyseal) arteries (5), raise the synovial membrane into folds or retinacula. A second supply of blood is derived from the vessels of the ligamentum teres. Here, the foveal (medial epiphyseal) arteries (6) can be noted. Additional regional vessels are the inferior gluteal artery (7) and the obturator artery (8). (After Graham J, Wood S: In JK Davidson: Aseptic Necrosis of Bone. New York, American Elsevier Publishing Co, 1976, p. 101.)

B A cross section of the proximal femur at the base of the neck better delineates the nature of the blood supply. The greater trochanter (arrow) and iliopsoas muscle (open arrow) are indicated. Note the profunda femoris artery (1) and the lateral (2) and medial (3) circumflex arteries. From the lateral circumflex arteries are derived the anterior ascending cervical arteries (9). From the medial circumflex artery are derived the medial (10), posterior (11), and lateral (12) ascending cervical arteries, which, in combination with the anterior ascending cervical arteries, form a subsynovial anastomotic ring on the surface of the femoral neck at the margin of the articular cartilage. The inset shows the plane of section (line a-a'). (After Chung SM: J Bone Joint Surg 58A:961, 1976.)

superior retinacular vessels into the epiphysis can lead to significant disruption of blood supply and subsequent osteonecrosis.[30] The vessels within the ligamentum teres vary in diameter, and their role in the supply of blood to the femoral head is not defined.[18] Some investigators believe that a prominent vascular supply exists in this area that can anastomose with the lateral epiphyseal vessels and that does not deteriorate with age,[27, 31] whereas others maintain that this supply is of little significance.[28] Most reports indicate that the blood flow into foveal areas may provide a source of revascularization when the remainder of the femoral head has been rendered avascular.[18, 29, 32]

The adult pattern of femoral head vascularity, outlined above, usually becomes established with closure of the growth plate at approximately 18 years of age.[18] In infancy and childhood, changing vascular patterns can be noted[33] (Fig. 77–9). In the neonate, three groups of vessels are identified: a superior retinacular or lateral epiphyseal group, an inferior retinacular or inferior metaphyseal group, and a foveal or medial epiphyseal group. With the appearance of ossification, the vasculature of the ligamentum teres gradually disappears, leaving the other two groups as the major suppliers of blood to the proximal femur. Between the ages of 4 and 7 years, the importance of the lateral epiphyeal vessels is established as the metaphyseal and foveal vessels decrease in extent. After the age of 8 years, a preadolescent pattern emerges, consisting of an increased contribution of the foveal vessels. The open growth plate represents an effective barrier, preventing anastomoses between the vessels of the head and the neck. During adolescence, an increased abundance of the inferior metaphyseal vessels is recognized. As the growth plate closes, the adult pattern appears, with anastomoses between the three arterial sys-

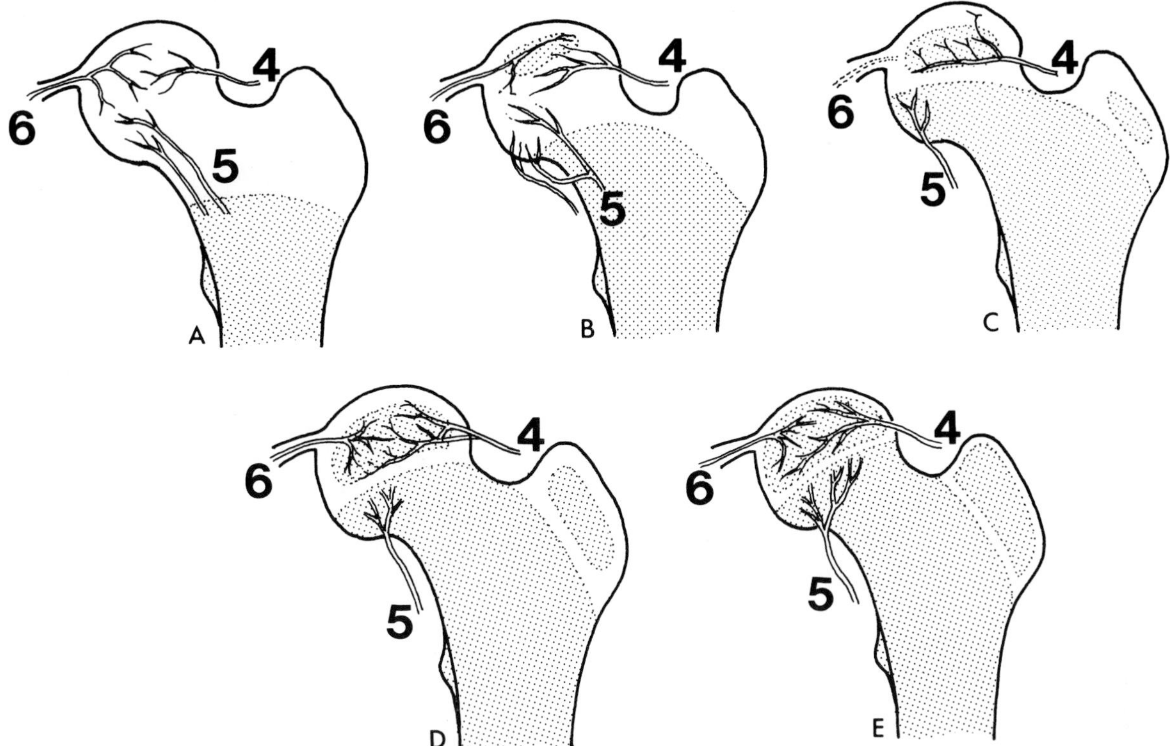

Figure 77–9. *Femoral head: Vascular supply in the infant, child, adolescent. Diagrams show the blood supply for the neonate* **(A)**, *infant and child between 4 months and 4 years of age* **(B)**, *child between 4 and 7 years of age* **(C)**, *preadolescent between 7 and 12 years of age* **(D)**, *and adolescent between 12 years and the time of closure of the growth plate* **(E)**. *Illustrated are the superior retinacular (4), inferior retinacular (5), and foveal (6) arteries. See text for details. (After Graham J, Wood S: In JK Davidson: Aseptic Necrosis of Bone. New York, American Elsevier Publishing Co, 1976, p. 101.)*

tems.[18] It is this influence of age on the pattern of femoral head blood supply that may explain the prevalence of Legg-Calvé-Perthes disease in patients between the ages of 4 and 7 years (see Chapter 78) and the high incidence of osteonecrosis following femoral neck injury in children.[34, 35]

Fractures of the femoral neck in adults (and in children) can be complicated by osteonecrosis of the femoral head (Fig. 77–10). This complication is more frequent in intracapsular fractures (subcapital, transcervical) than in extracapsular fractures (intertrochanteric). In the latter situation, the blood supply is not compromised by the fracture line, which lies distal to the capsular insertion on the proximal femur, although, rarely, osteonecrosis does follow an intertrochanteric fracture, perhaps owing to angulation or deformity of the vascular tree.[29] With transcervical or subcapital fractures, injury to the superior retinacular arteries is frequent, leading to osteonecrosis. Some investigations report that histologic examination of femoral heads following fracture of the neck may indicate necrotic foci in as many as 75 per cent of cases.[36, 37] The incidence of necrosis may increase with displacement and an exaggerated valgus position at the site of fracture, late reduction, and utilization of hardware that is positioned near the fovea, perhaps injuring the blood supply in this region.[18] The roentgenographic features may include increased density of the necrotic segment (in those cases in which immobilization leads to osteoporosis of viable bone), osseous collapse (usually delayed for a period of 9 months to 1 year following the injury in conjunction with disappearance of the fracture line), flattening, and fragmentation.

Additional traumatic causes of osteonecrosis of the femoral head include dislocation of the hip (Fig. 77–11) and slipped capital femoral epiphysis. The dislocated femoral head may be associated with tears of the vessels in the ligamentum teres and, possibly, injury to the retinacular vessels. Osteonecrosis has been reported in as many as 25 per cent of patients with dislocation, especially if it is complicated by fracture of the acetabulum, a delay in diagnosis and treatment, and early weight-bearing.[38, 39] Following a slipped capital femoral epiphysis, injury to the lateral epiphyseal vessels is more frequent in the presence of severe epiphyseal displacement and manipulative reduction[18]; thus, an incidence of osteonecrosis of less than 5 per cent in patients with minimal displacements can rise to 40 per cent in patients with severe slips in whom aggressive orthopedic manipulations have been undertaken.[40-42]

Osteonecrosis of the femoral head has also been recorded in as many as 68 per cent of patients

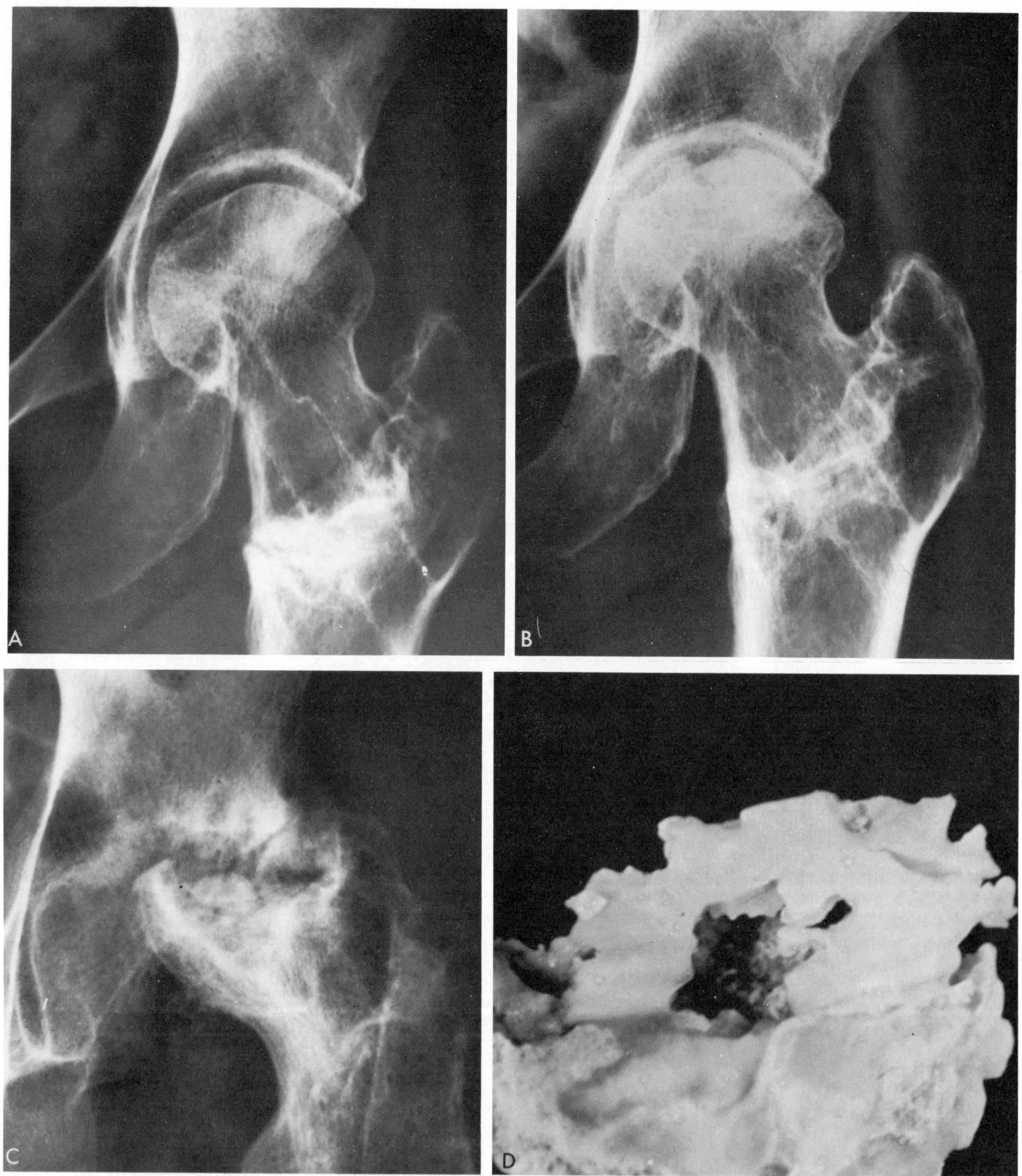

Figure 77–10. *Posttraumatic osteonecrosis: Femoral head.*

A, B *Intertrochanteric fracture. Films obtained 2½ years apart reveal evidence of a previous intertrochanteric fracture treated with a Richards nail (that has been removed) and progressive osteonecrosis of the femoral head. This complication is less frequent in intertrochanteric fractures than in subcapital fractures.*

C, D *Basicervical fracture. Following a fracture of the base of the neck, this patient developed lateral subluxation of the femur and osteonecrosis of the femoral head associated with massive collapse, well identified on the photograph of the specimen.*

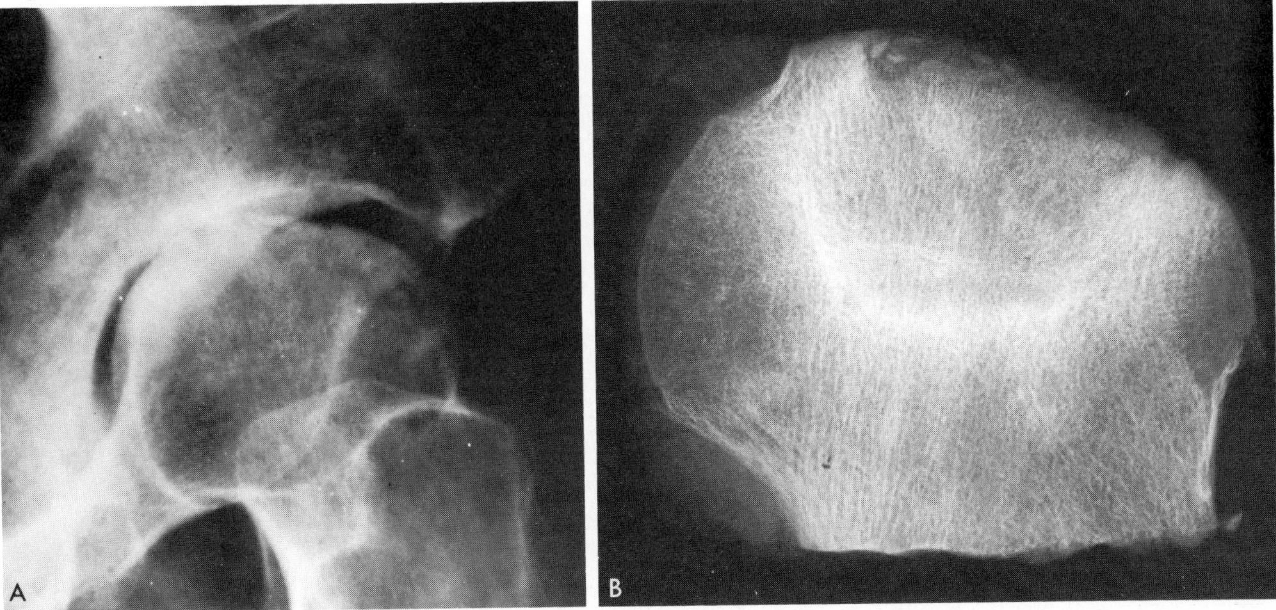

Figure 77–11. *Posttraumatic osteonecrosis: Femoral head. Posterior dislocation of the hip with acetabular rim fracture. In the period following the injury, this patient revealed collapse of the superolateral aspect of the femoral head. Note the fragmentation of the articular surface and reactive sclerosis about the area of necrosis.*

following congenital dislocation of the hip.[43] The complication appears to be influenced by the method of treatment and the position in which the hip is immobilized.[18] In this regard, it is of interest that osteonecrosis may be observed in the normal hip following immobilization of both sides in cases of unilateral congenital dislocation of the hip. Secondary osteoarthritis may later appear.[137]

Talus

Osteonecrosis of the talus is a recognized and disabling complication of various fractures and injuries. This tarsal bone is largely covered by cartilage, articulating with the tibia and fibula, the calcaneus, and the navicular through a series of joints. Graham and Wood[18] have summarized its vascular anatomy, citing the investigations of Haliburton and co-workers[44] and Mulfinger and Trueta.[45] The talar blood supply is derived mainly from branches of the posterior tibial, peroneal, and dorsalis pedis arteries; the artery of the tarsal sinus and that of the tarsal canal are the two most important branches, which, with their parent trunks, provide the major source of the blood to the bone (Fig. 77–12). The precise intraosseous vascular anatomy varies between the head of the talus and the body of the bone, but free anastomoses among the vascular branches exist. Because of these anastomosing channels, a severe soft tissue injury must occur in order to initiate osteonecrosis. The body of the talus is more prone to necrosis than the talar head and neck, and this complication is especially prevalent following fracture of the neck, in which dislocation of the subtalar or ankle joint, or both, is also evident.[46-49]

The radiographic diagnosis of osteonecrosis of the talus can be difficult, and it is usually delayed until osteoporosis of the surrounding viable bone creates a relatively increased density of the talar body. This finding can be apparent within 1 to 3 months following injury and may be combined with collapse of the articular surface (Fig. 77–13). Conversely, the participation of the entire talus in the osteoporosis of immobilization following injury is a good prognostic sign, indicating adequate blood supply to the bone. The presence of a subchondral radiolucent band in the proximal talus, the Hawkins sign, represents bony resorption and can be a useful radiographic sign of an intact vascular supply.[47] This same sign can appear during the revascularization phase after the fracture has united, combined with patchy lucency in the necrotic area of bone. Revascularization appears to be initiated on the medial aspect of the talus and proceeds in a lateral direction, underscoring the importance of the medial blood supply to the bone.[18] The healing process may take several years for completion.

Humeral Head

The blood supply of the head of the humerus is derived from three major sources: a branch of the anterior circumflex humeral artery, the arcuate artery, which enters the bone in the bicipital groove; branches of the posterior circumflex humeral artery, which enter the base of the neck; and vessels in the

Text continued on page 2851

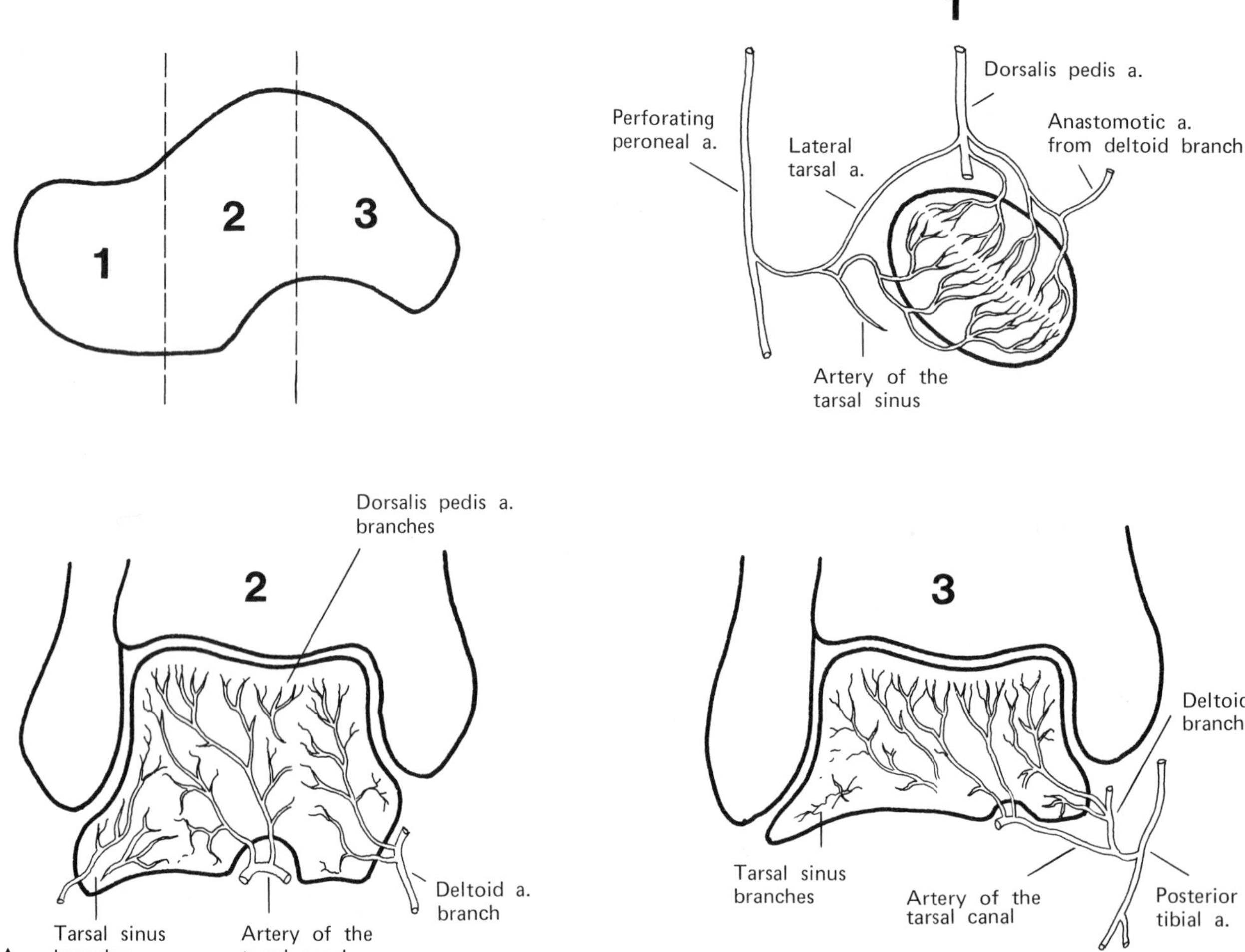

Figure 77–12. *Talus: Vascular supply.*

A *Vascular anatomy in coronal sections.* 1, *Anterior third or head of talus;* 2, *middle third of talus;* 3, *posterior third of talus. See text for details.*

Illustration continued on the opposite page

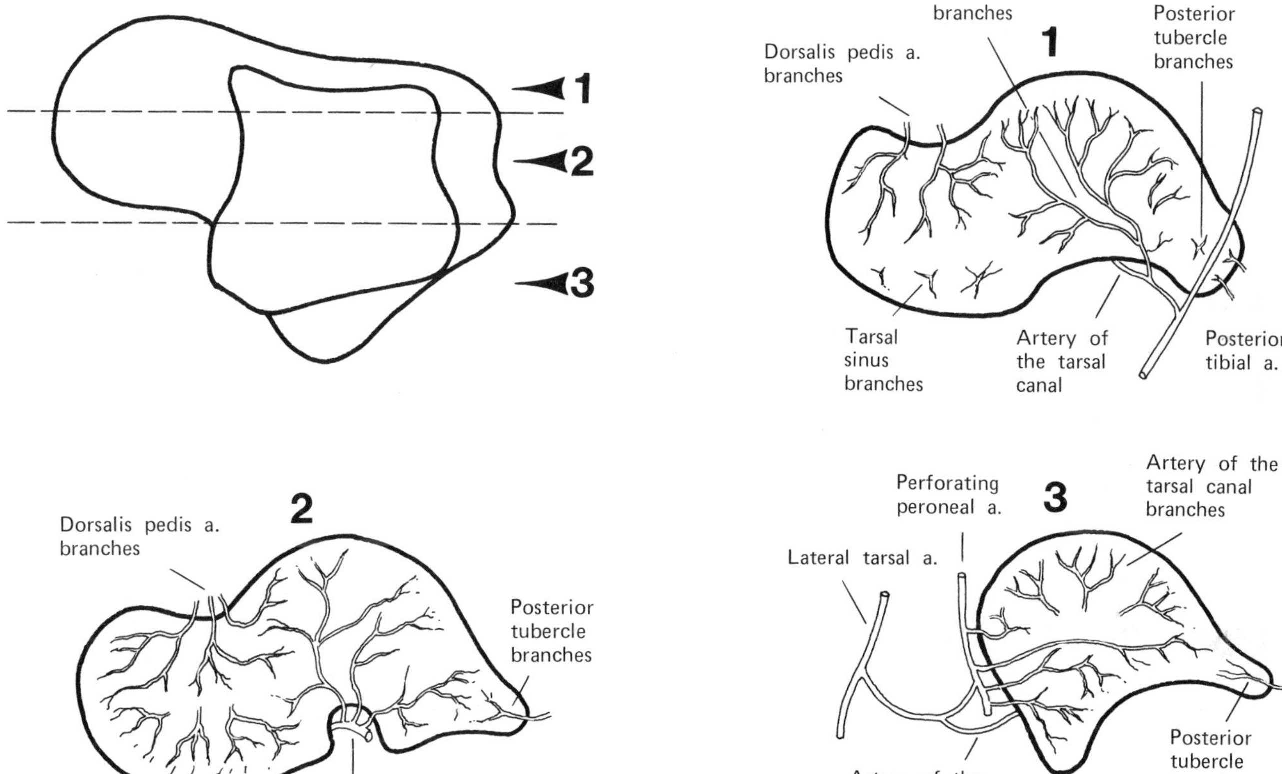

Figure 77–12. Continued

B *Vascular anatomy in parasagittal sections. 1, Medial third of talus; 2, middle third of talus; 3, lateral third of talus. See text for details.*

(After Mulfinger GL, Trueta J: J Bone Joint Surg 52B:160, 1970.)

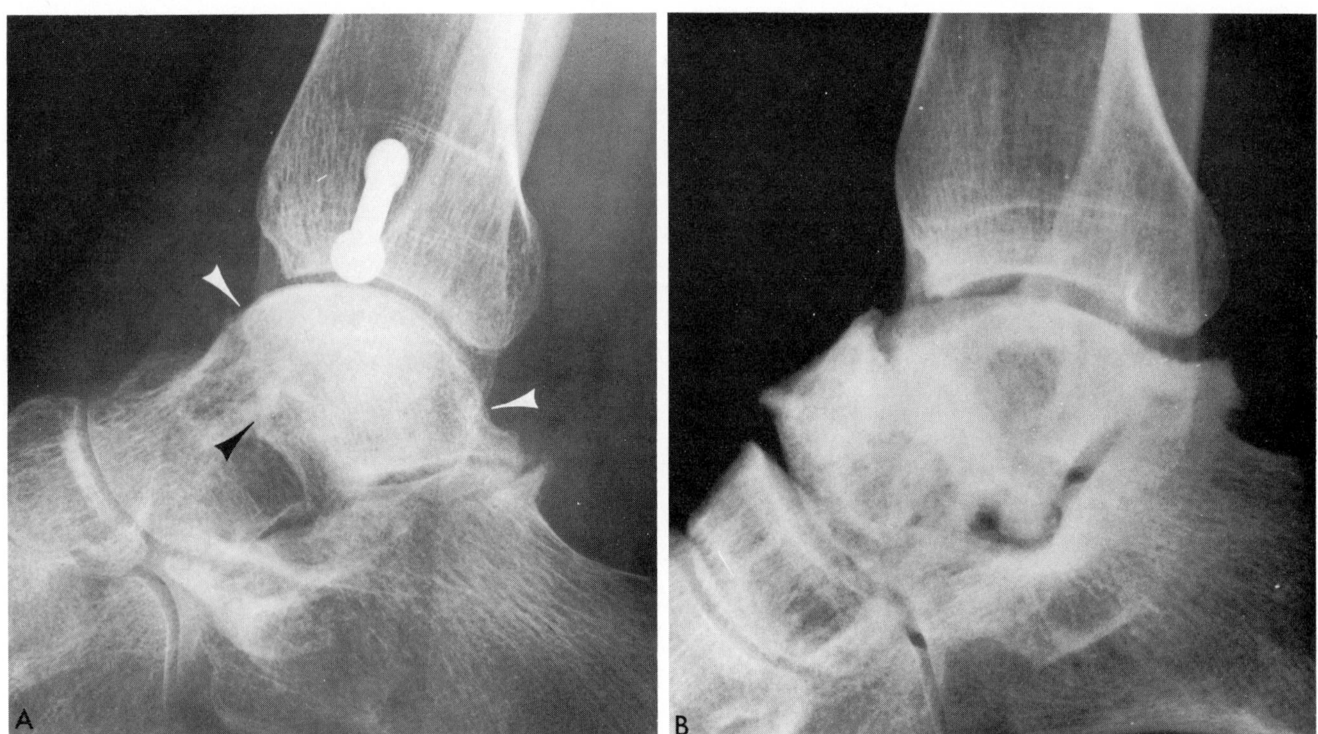

Figure 77–13. *Posttraumatic osteonecrosis: Talus.*

A *In this individual, who sustained a fracture of the body of the talus as well as of the medial malleolus (which was transfixed with a screw), note the increased radiodensity of the proximal half of the bone (arrowheads).*

B *In a different individual with a nonunion of a midtalar fracture, extensive necrosis is associated with sclerosis and cyst formation.*

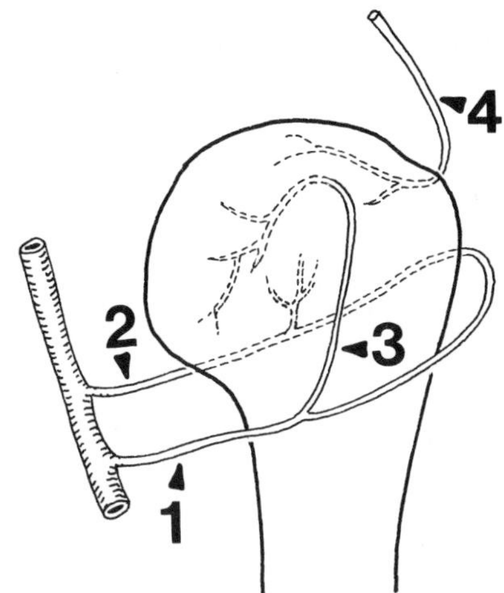

Figure 77–14. Humeral head: Vascular supply. Vessels include the anterior circumflex humeral artery (1), the posterior circumflex humeral artery (2), the arcuate artery (3), and the vessels of the rotator cuff (4). (After Graham J, Wood S: In JK Davidson: Aseptic Necrosis of Bone. New York, American Elsevier Publishing Co, 1976, p 101.)

rotator cuff, which enter at the tendinous insertion to the bone[50] (Fig. 77–14). The vascular supply pierces the bony cortex just distal to the anatomic neck. Osteonecrosis of the humeral head occurs if a fracture leads to loss of blood supply from both the muscular insertions and the arcuate branch of the anterior circumflex humeral artery[18]; this may result following a displaced fracture of the anatomic neck or a severe fracture or fracture-dislocation of the bone. The radiographic findings parallel those in the femoral head, although osseous collapse, common in the femoral "weight-bearing" area, is less prominent in the humeral head. Patchy lucent shadows and sclerosis, an arc-like subchondral radiolucent area, and depression and fragmentation of the articular surface can be seen.

Scaphoid

Osteonecrosis of the proximal pole of the carpal scaphoid is a well-documented complication following injury of this bone. Its appearance and characteristics relate to the vascular anatomy of the scaphoid, which has been outlined by Obletz and Halbstein[51] and Taleisnik and Kelly.[52] Three groups of vessels can be identified: a laterovolar group entering the bone distal to the radial articular surface on the flattened volar aspect or on the narrower lateral strip; a dorsal group entering the bone between the radial and trapezoid/trapezium articular surfaces; and a distal group entering in the region of the tubercle[18] (Fig. 77–15). The major intraosseous supply is derived from the laterovolar group of vessels.

Recently, Gelberman and Menon[139] studied the vascularity of the scaphoid in 15 fresh cadaveric specimens. They emphasized that the radial artery

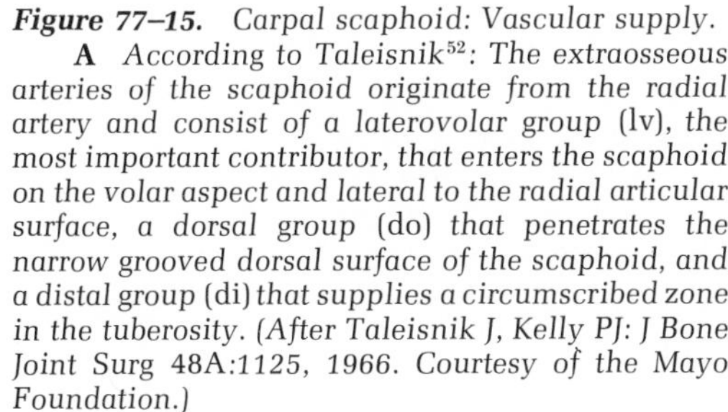

Figure 77–15. Carpal scaphoid: Vascular supply.

A According to Taleisnik[52]: The extraosseous arteries of the scaphoid originate from the radial artery and consist of a laterovolar group (lv), the most important contributor, that enters the scaphoid on the volar aspect and lateral to the radial articular surface, a dorsal group (do) that penetrates the narrow grooved dorsal surface of the scaphoid, and a distal group (di) that supplies a circumscribed zone in the tuberosity. (After Taleisnik J, Kelly PJ: J Bone Joint Surg 48A:1125, 1966. Courtesy of the Mayo Foundation.)

Illustration continued on the following page

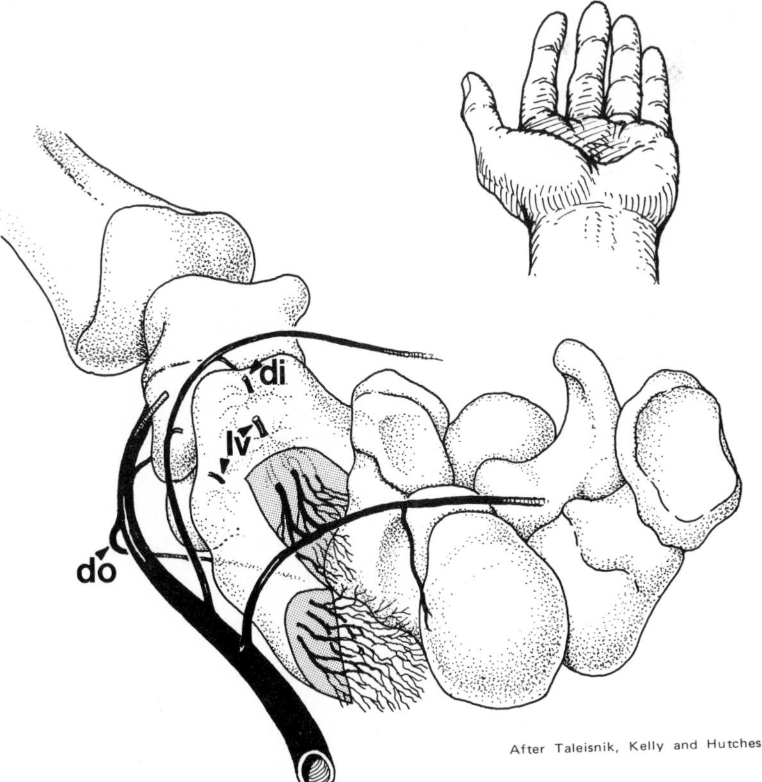

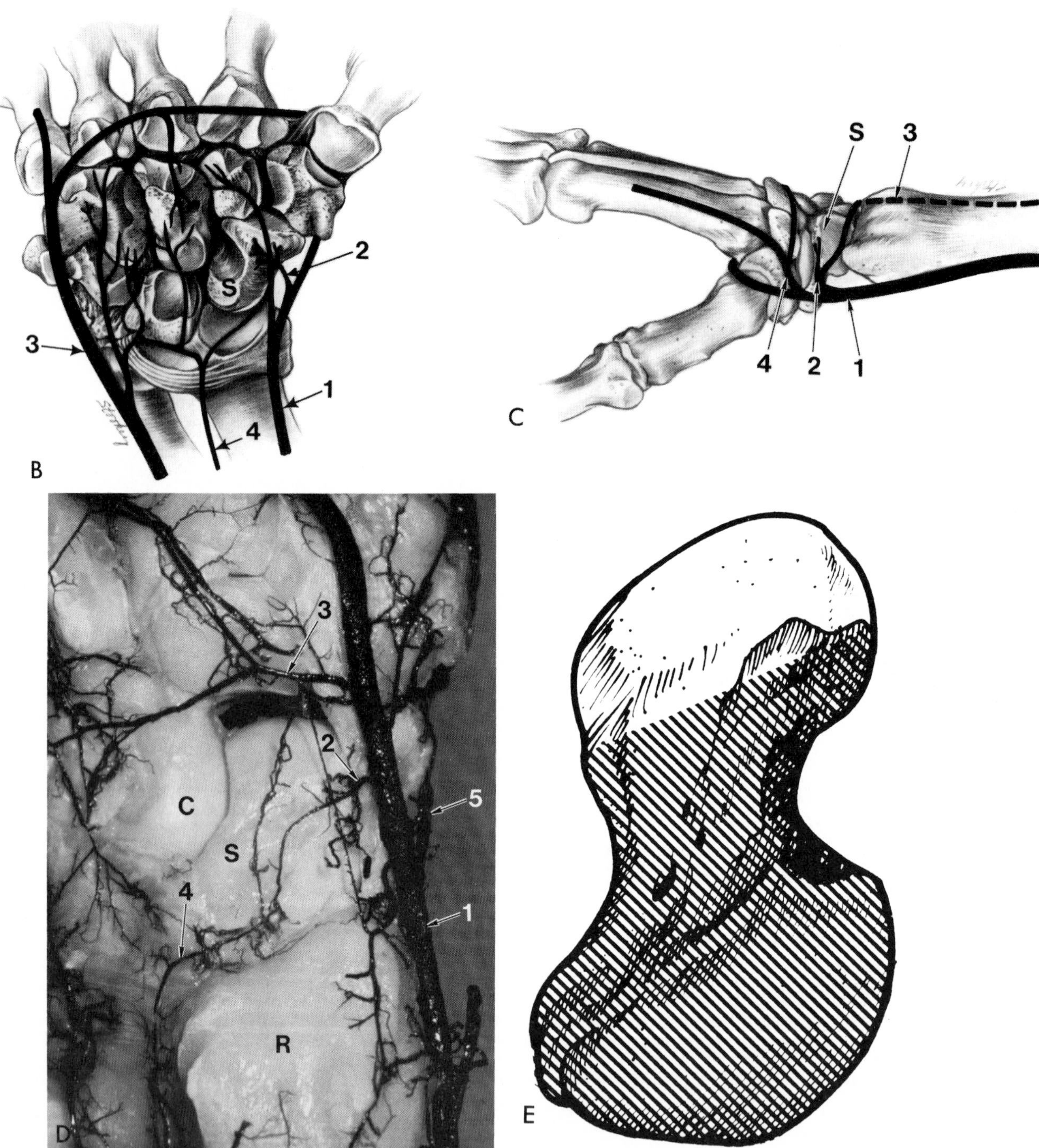

Figure 77–15. Continued

B–E *According to Gelberman and Menon*[139]: **B,** *A schematic drawing of the volar external blood supply of the scaphoid: S, scaphoid; 1, radial artery; 2, volar scaphoid branches; 3, ulnar artery; 4, anterior division of the anterior interosseous artery.* **C,** *A schematic drawing of the dorsal blood supply of the scaphoid: S, scaphoid; 1, radial artery; 2, dorsal scaphoid branch; 3, dorsal division of the anterior interosseous artery; 4, intercarpal artery.* **D,** *Dorsal external blood supply in an injected specimen: S, scaphoid; C, capitate; R, radius; 1, radial artery; 2, dorsal scaphoid branch; 3, intercarpal artery; 4, dorsal division of the anterior interosseous artery; 5, superficial palmar branch of the radial artery.* **E,** *In a drawing of the scaphoid, note that the proximal 70 to 80 per cent of the bone is supplied by dorsal vessels (shaded area), and the distal 20 to 30 per cent is supplied by volar branches of the radial artery (white area). (From Gelberman RH, Menon J: J Hand Surg 5:508, 1980.)*

supplied the major blood supply to the scaphoid, that the proximal pole and 70 to 80 per cent of the bone received its blood from vessels entering the dorsal ridge, that the tuberosity and distal 20 to 30 per cent of the bone were supplied by volar branches of the radial artery and its superficial palmar branch, and that there were no significant intraosseous anastomoses between dorsal and volar branches. These investigators also noted the excellent collateral circulation to the scaphoid that arose from the dorsal and volar branches of the anterior interosseous artery. On comparing their results with those of Taleisnik and Kelly,[52] Gelberman and Menon concluded that the laterovolar group of vessels in the former study were analogous to their dorsal ridge vessels, and that the distal group of vessels were analogous to their tuberosity vessels.

Osteonecrosis is most likely to occur when a scaphoid fracture involves the proximal pole of the bone; with more distal infractions, the interruption of blood supply is less constant or severe. It is the proximal aspect of the bone that undergoes necrosis. The reported incidence of this complication following scaphoid injuries varies with the nature and severity of the fracture or dislocation; an incidence of 11 to 65 per cent has been noted.[53, 54] Ten to 15 per cent seems to be the most common estimated incidence of this complication.[18] The radiographic diagnosis depends upon a relative increase in density of the devitalized scaphoid in comparison with the osteoporotic viable bone (Figs. 77–16 and 77–17), an appearance that is delayed for a period of 4 to 8 weeks and that may be associated with delayed union or nonunion of the fracture, collapse of the necrotic segment, and, eventually, secondary degenerative joint disease of the radiocarpal compartment of the wrist (Fig. 77–18).

Other Sites

Following significant injury avascular necrosis can appear at other sites, especially when an osseous fragment loses its soft tissue attachments. Thus, necrosis of the lunate, tarsal navicular, patella,[55] and even the metatarsal and metacarpal heads[56] can be seen (Fig. 77–19).

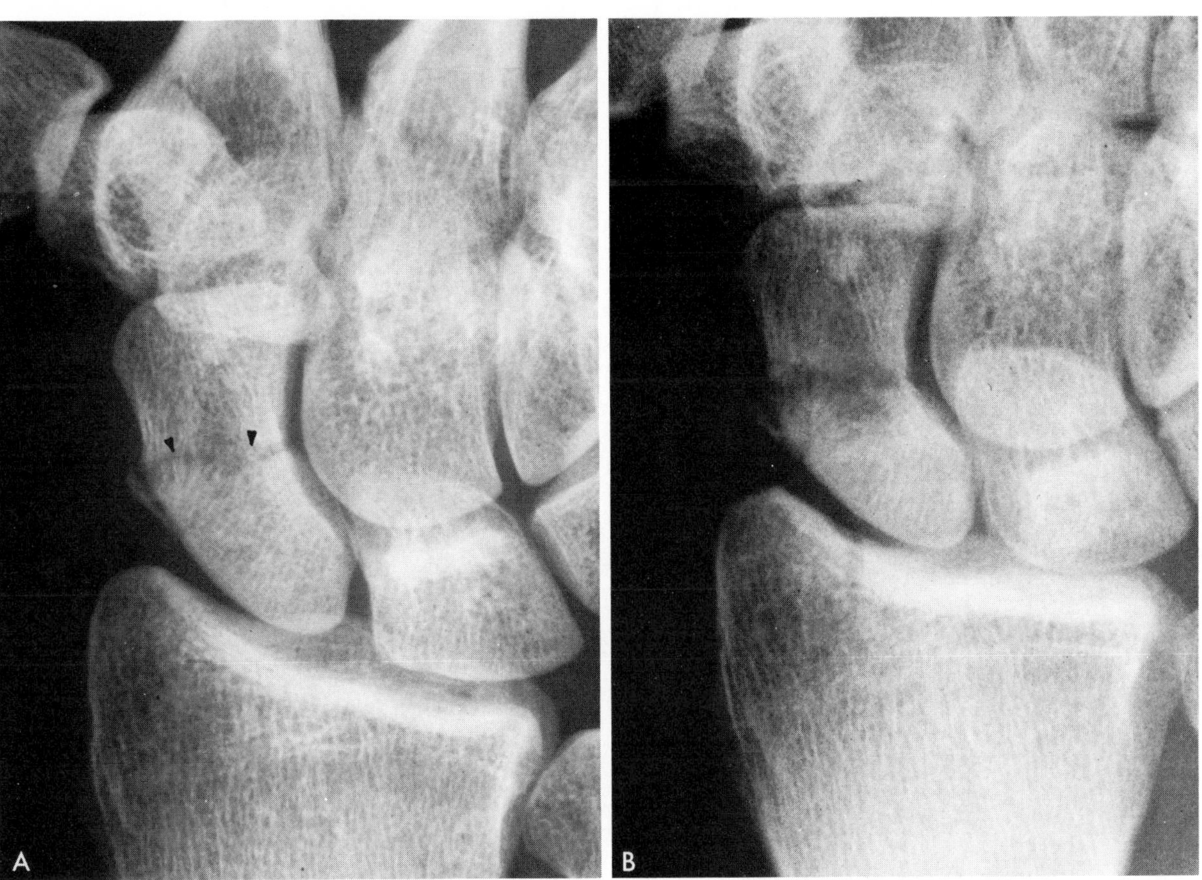

Figure 77–16. *Posttraumatic osteonecrosis: Carpal scaphoid.*

A *A film obtained 2 weeks after trauma indicates a scaphoid fracture (arrowheads).*

B *Six weeks after* **A,** *increased radiodensity of the proximal half of the scaphoid is accentuated by osteoporosis of the distal half of the bone, indicating the presence of osteonecrosis and reparative bone formation.*

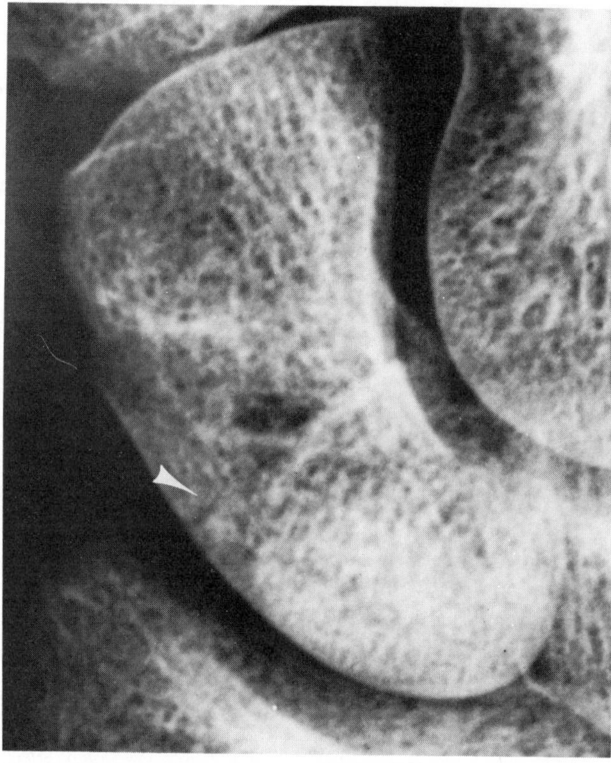

Figure 77–17. *Posttraumatic osteonecrosis: Carpal scaphoid. Role of magnification radiography. Seven weeks following a scaphoid fracture, a magnification film indicates the persistence of the fracture line (arrowhead) and increased radiodensity of the proximal portion of the scaphoid.*

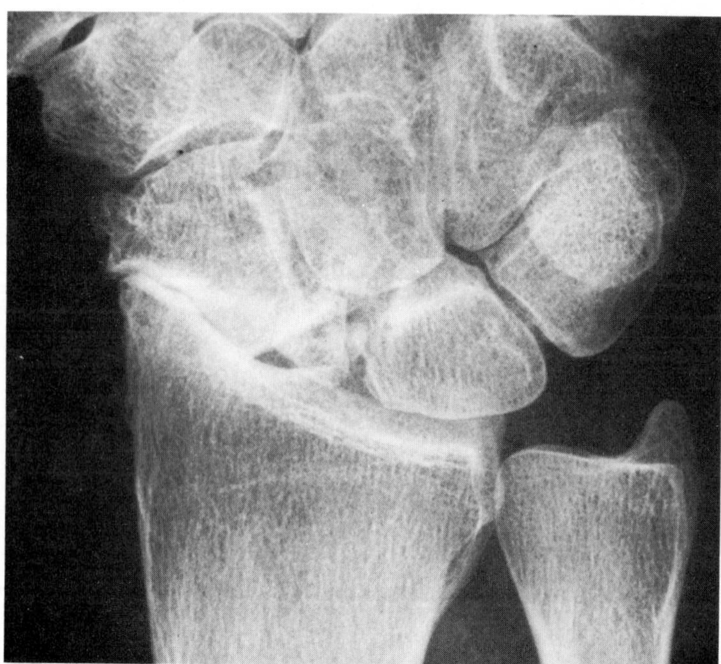

Figure 77–18. *Posttraumatic osteonecrosis: Carpal scaphoid. Nonunion and secondary degenerative joint disease. A remote fracture of the scaphoid is associated with nonunion, collapse of the necrotic proximal pole, and joint space narrowing, sclerosis, and osteophytes of the radiocarpal and midcarpal compartments.*

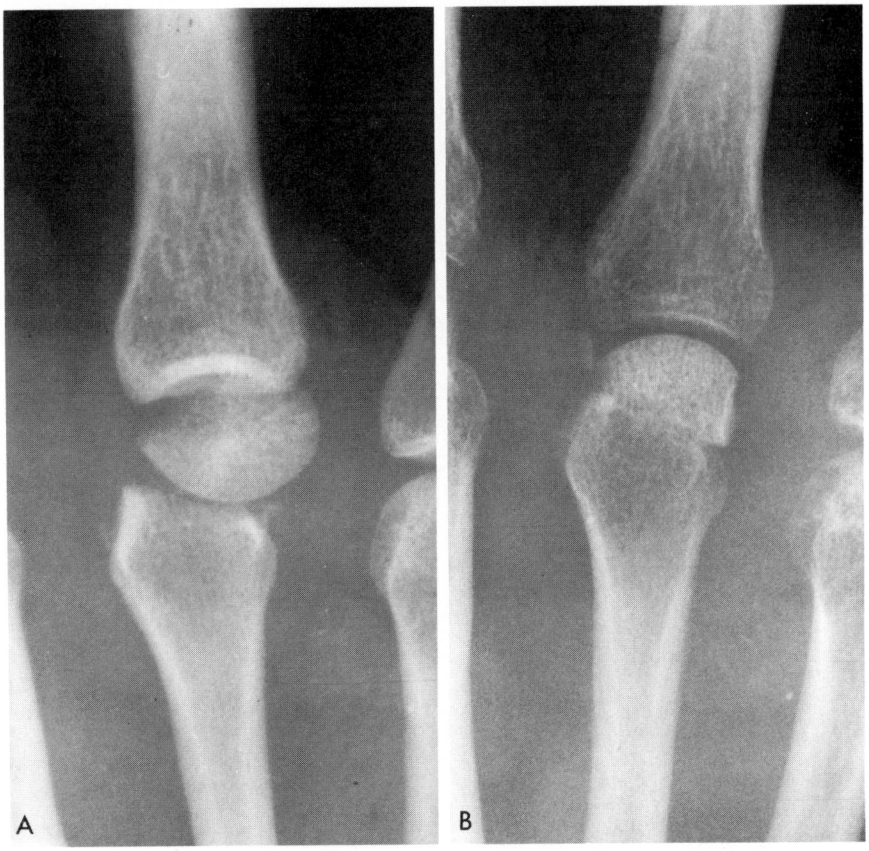

Figure 77–19. *Posttraumatic osteonecrosis: Metacarpal head.*

A *Initial radiograph reveals an unusual fracture-dislocation of the metacarpal head, in which the metacarpal fragment has rotated 180 degrees.*

B *Follow-up study several months after reduction of the fragment demonstrates increased density of the metacarpal head.*

DYSBARIC OSTEONECROSIS

General Features

Recent years have witnessed an increasing exposure of humans to high pressure environments as a result of such factors as the rising popularity of scuba diving and the expanding interest in underwater and space exploration and off-shore oil drilling. A new awareness and interest in early and late complications of this exposure have appeared. One such late complication is osteonecrosis, which has been designated as dysbaric osteonecrosis, caisson disease, pressure-induced osteoarthropathy, and barotraumatic osteoarthropathy.[57]

The term decompression sickness indicates the consequences of the liberation of gas bubbles, principally nitrogen, in the blood and the tissues of a person who has undergone decompression too rapidly following a period of exposure to a hyperbaric environment.[58] In a high pressure environment, a person's blood and tissues are saturated with the atmospheric gases, and following rapid exposure to normal atmospheric pressure, the various gases come out of solution, producing supersaturation of the tissues. Ventilation may allow dispersion of the excess of oxygen and carbon dioxide, but the released nitrogen may produce bubbles within the vascular tree, which act as air emboli that partially or completely occlude vessels at one or more sites, leading to symptoms and signs of vascular insufficiency. Nitrogen accumulation is greatest in tissues rich in fat, and the fatty marrow does not escape this accumulation. Dysbaric osteonecrosis represents one of the late complications of hyperbaric exposure; other long-term effects include paralysis and psychiatric illness.[59]

The association of decompression sickness and dysbaric osteonecrosis is controversial. In general, there appears to be a lack of correlation between these two conditions.[60, 61] Many victims of decompression sickness never develop osteonecrosis and, conversely, bony lesions are discovered in divers and workers who use compressed air who have had no earlier symptoms or signs. Despite this dissociation of findings in the two conditions, it is generally assumed that gas bubbles initiate the manifestations of decompression sickness and that they likely represent the cause of osteonecrosis as well. Experimentally, aseptic necrosis of bone can be produced in animals by exposure to dysbaric environments and artificial emboli with foreign material or lipids.[62-64] The osseous lesions in humans may develop from showers of "silent" embolic bubbles during repeated decompressions in individuals in whom the gas tension levels are below those required to produce the acute manifestations of decompression sickness.[61] The incidence of dysbaric osteonecrosis appears to be exaggerated in patients with repeated exposures,[65] exposures to greater pressures, a rapid rate of exposure,[64] and obesity.[61]

Pathogenesis

Dysbaric osteonecrosis probably represents an ischemic lesion of bone. The exact cause of the ischemia is debated, the various theories being well summarized by Chryssanthou.[61] Embolization of gas bubbles with blockage of vascular channels is considered to be the major factor by many investigators. The presence of intravascular gas bubbles even after asymptomatic decompression has been documented by ultrasound and other modalities,[61, 65, 66] as well as by light and electron microscopy of various tissues, including bone.[67] This evidence leaves little doubt about the existence of gas in the blood vessels, but the role of this gas in the production of necrosis is not clear. Ischemic changes are influenced by the type of tissue, the duration of the obstruction, the local vascular anatomy, and the size of the affected area.[61, 134] The fatty bone marrow may be especially vulnerable to infarction, particularly in the presence of repeated and sustained gas emboli, because it has an inadequate collateral circulation. Metaphyseal and subchondral regions of tubular bones possess end-arteries, which favor embolic occlusion.

An accessory role of fat embolization in the pathogenesis of dysbaric osteonecrosis has also been suggested.[68] Gas bubbles in fatty marrow and adipose tissue may cause disruption of fat cells with the introduction of potentially embolic lipid material into the circulation. This mechanism may explain the greater risk to obese patients of developing dysbaric osteonecrosis. Alternatively, it is suggested that gas bubbles within the liver may lead to local injury, with extrusion of unstable fats and embolization.[69] This process may be promoted by adhesion of plasma lipids to the blood-gas interface[70] or denaturation of plasma lipoproteins by blood-bubble interface activity, release of lipid moiety, coalescence of liberated lipid, and formation of embolic particles.[61] Thrombotic material could also contribute to embolization in dysbaric osteonecrosis.

The presence of nonembolic ischemic changes in this disorder has also been postulated. Within the rigid osseous tissue, extravascular gas collections might lead to compression of neighboring blood vessels, impairing tissue perfusion; intravascular gas accumulations could initiate injury to the vascular wall, with subsequent stenosis[67]; or release of vasoactive substances could provoke vessel narrowing, with resulting ischemia.[71]

In addition to the ischemic mechanisms that were outlined previously, other hypotheses have suggested that nonischemic changes are important in the pathogenesis of dysbaric osteonecrosis.[61] Thus, bony abnormalities may be induced by osmotic changes and fluid shifts owing to pressure alterations,[72] increased oxygen tension,[73] or altered immunity and dysproteinemia.

Incidence

The frequency of osseous lesions in patients subjected to high pressure environment depends on the number, length, and severity of exposures and the timing and method of evaluation. In compressed-air workers, the reported incidence has varied from 0 to 75 per cent,[74, 75] most estimates being in the 10 to 20 per cent range. As it has been determined that 4 to 12 months usually elapse between the time of exposure and the appearance of radiographic abnormality (an interval that is influenced by the extent of the necrotic area, the thickness of the overlying tissue, the quality of the roentgenogram, and the amount of revascularization), roentgenographic examination shortly after exposure reveals a lower incidence of osseous abnormality.[57]

The reported prevalence of osteonecrosis in divers has also varied, the pertinent literature being summarized by Davidson.[57] Cited are reports from Germany, Norway, Bulgaria, and Japan, in which the incidence of osseous lesions varied from 17 to 65 per cent. This incidence may rise substantially in studies in which long-term follow-up examinations are available. In divers in the British Royal Navy, a lower incidence (4 per cent) has been noted, perhaps owing to stricter surveillance and regulations imposed on these individuals.[76]

Radiographic and Pathologic Abnormalities

The radiographic and pathologic abnormalities of dysbaric osteonecrosis have been well outlined.[57, 77-85] A popular classification of the bone alterations recognizes two major changes: juxta-articular lesions occurring most frequently in the head of the humerus and femur (Figs. 77–20 and 77–21) and diaphyseal and metaphyseal lesions situated at a distance from the articulation (Figs. 77–22 and 77–23).[86] Juxta-articular alterations consist of radiodense areas varying between 3 and 20 mm in diameter, which are slightly less discrete than bone islands (enostoses), spherical segmental opaque areas that may eventually produce a "snow-capped" configuration, radiolucent subcortical bands ("crescent" sign), indicating a fracture of necrotic bone, and osseous collapse and fragmentation; diaphyseal and metaphyseal abnormalities con-

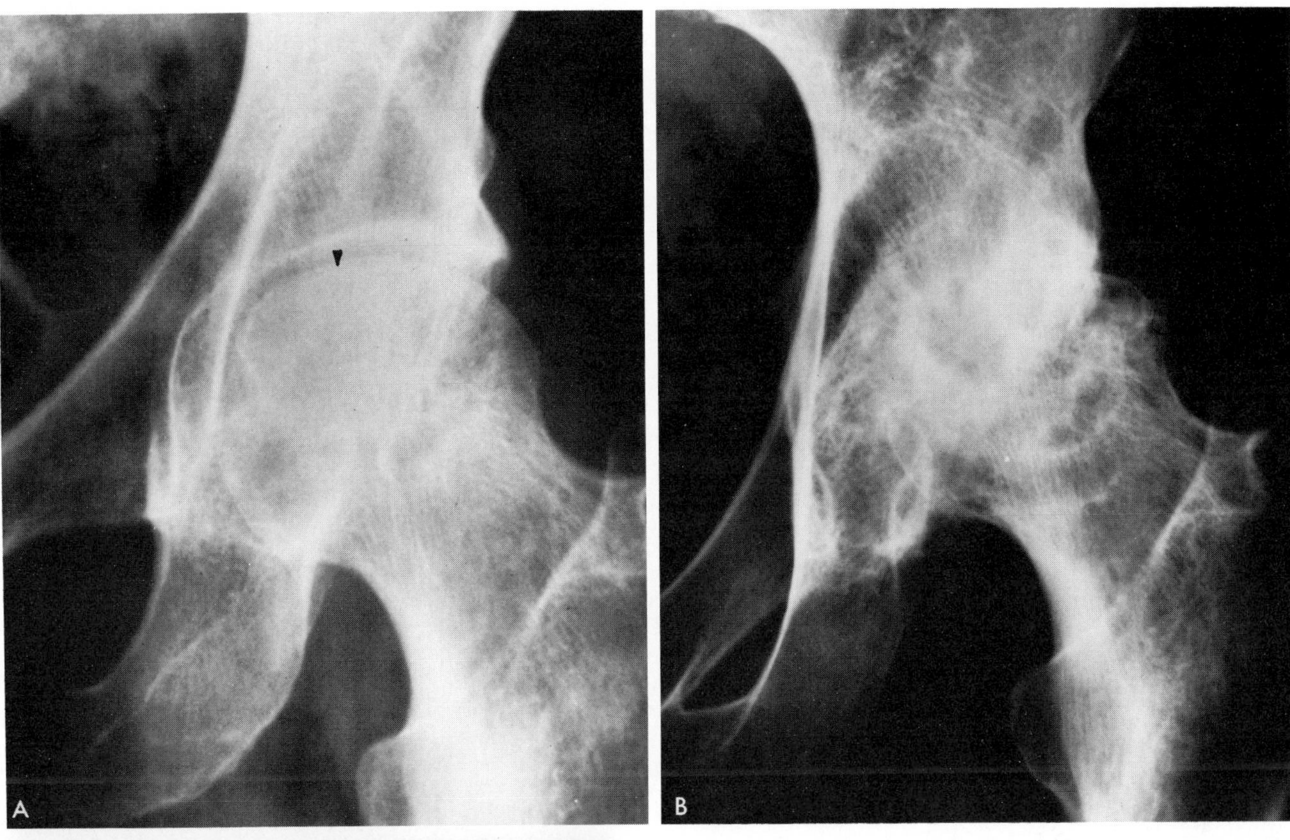

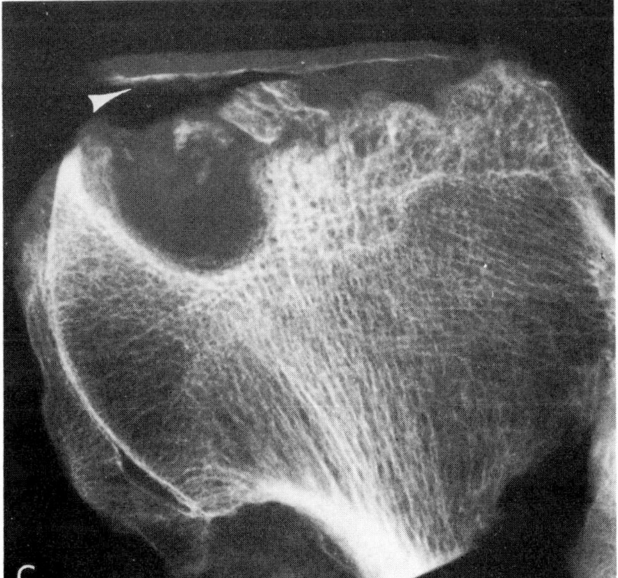

Figure 77–20. Dysbaric osteonecrosis: Juxta-articular lesions. This middle-aged man had worked in a decompression chamber for 20 years.

A *An initial film reveals patchy lucency and sclerosis of the femoral head, with subtle flattening of the articular surface, a subchondral radiolucent crescent or fracture (arrowhead), and buttressing of the femoral neck. The opposite hip was similarly affected.*

B Eighteen months after **A**, a considerable increase in the sclerosis associated with obliteration of the joint space can be identified.

C *A radiograph of a coronal section of the removed femoral head delineates depression of the subchondral bone with "viable" overlying cartilage (arrowhead) and subjacent necrosis with osseous resorption and reactive bone formation. Note osteophytosis and buttressing.*

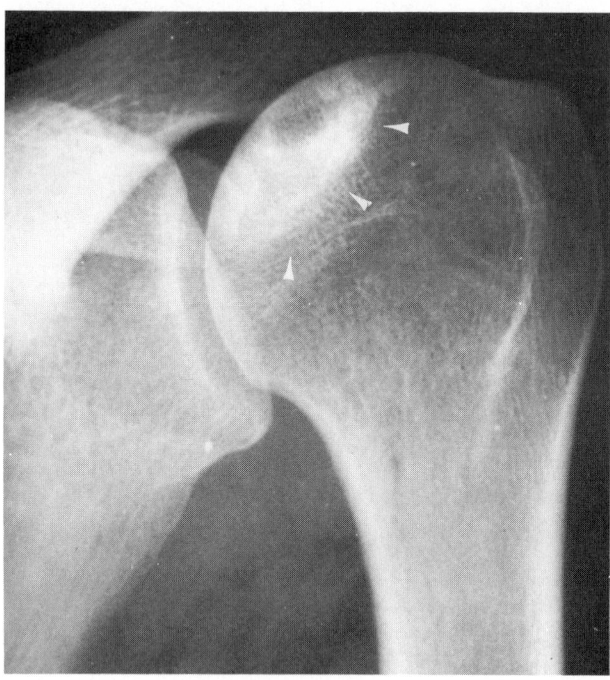

Figure 77–21. Dysbaric osteonecrosis: *Juxta-articular lesions.* *The sclerosis or "snow-cap" appearance of the humeral head (arrowheads) is typical of dysbaric osteonecrosis but may be evident in other varieties of necrosis as well.*

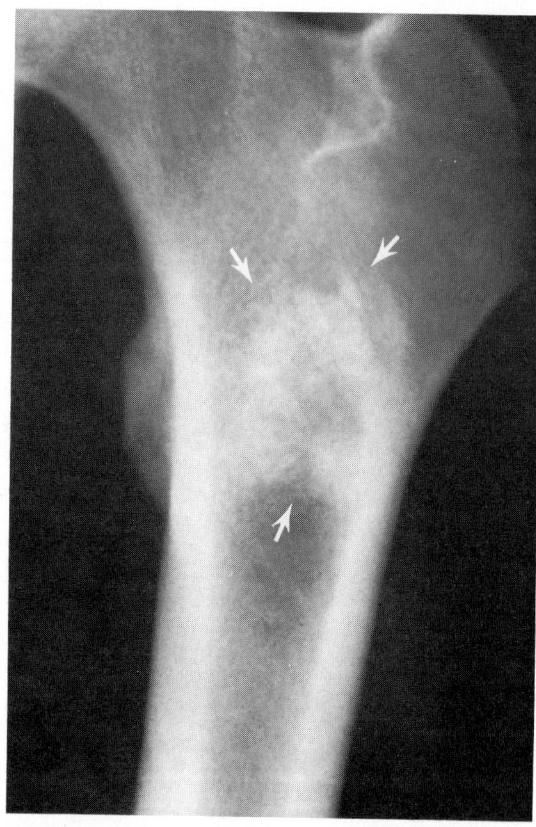

Figure 77–22. Dysbaric osteonecrosis: *Diametaphyseal lesions.* *This 28 year old man developed mild discomfort in the hip over a 3 month period without swelling. He was a scuba diver who had made dives to considerable depths. A patchy area of increased sclerosis is evident in the proximal shaft of the femur (arrows). Note the increased density of the periphery of the lesion. Biopsy with histologic evaluation indicated osseous and marrow necrosis compatible with an infarct.*

sist of indistinct, ill-defined radiodense foci, irregular calcified areas with a shell-like configuration, and, rarely, radiolucent lesions, perhaps due to sites of necrosis.[57] Debate exists regarding the significance of subtle small opaque lesions and cystic foci in this disorder; similar findings can be seen with equal or lesser frequency in "normal" individuals,[78, 87] diminishing the diagnostic importance of these changes. Thus, care must be exercised in interpreting focal sclerotic or lucent areas, especially if they are few in number and small in size. True osteonecrotic lesions may enlarge, leading to structural failure of the articular surface, or may remain stable for long periods of time.

In compressed-air workers and divers, multiple or single bilateral or unilateral alterations can be seen. The distal shaft of the femur, the humeral head, the femoral head, and the tibial shaft, in descending order of frequency, are the most typical sites of involvement. An infarct that is limited to the shaft of a tubular bone is usually not associated with clinical complaints; when involvement of an epiphysis leads to collapse of the articular surface, pain and swelling can become apparent.

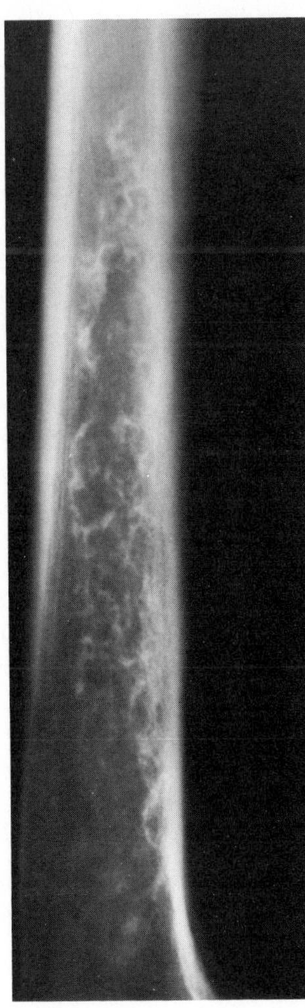

Figure 77–23. *Dysbaric osteonecrosis: Diaphyseal lesion. In this deep sea diver and astronaut, the irregular calcific deposits in the femur with a shell-like configuration are typical of a bone infarct.*

Pathologic examination reveals necrotic subchondral bone surrounded by collagenous fibrous tissue and thickened, spongy trabeculae. One or more fracture lines can extend through the cartilage, creating osteochondral fragments and an irregular bumpy or grooved articular surface.[58, 83, 88, 89] Chondral changes include brown discoloration, fibrillation, and erosion, but as in all cases of osteonecrosis, these cartilaginous abnormalities are relatively mild in comparison with the severity of the osseous alterations until secondary osteoarthritis supersedes, leading to fragmentation and dissolution of the chondral tissue, osteophytosis, sclerosis, and cyst formation.

Davidson and co-workers[87] described in detail the histologic observations related to the focal sclerotic lesions seen in dysbaric osteonecrosis. The lesions were frequently oriented in the direction of trabeculae and consisted chiefly of lamellar bone that in places was arranged concentrically in haversian systems around small blood vessels. Irregular spikes or thorns were present on the surface of the foci, and necrotic bone was not identified. These histologic observations are identical to those reported in enostoses or bone islands unassociated with dysbaric osteonecrosis, again raising doubt as to the significance of the radiodense foci.

Differential Diagnosis

The roentgenographic findings associated with dysbaric osteonecrosis are generally indistinguishable from those associated with osteonecrosis of other causes such as sickle cell anemia, Gaucher's disease, and steroid medication. Although diaphyseal calcification in an infarct may simulate that in an enchondroma, a shell-like calcific pattern in infarction differs from the punctate and central calcification in an enchondroma. Small, dense foci in dysbaric osteonecrosis are virtually identical to bone islands and only those that are larger and more numerous may allow accurate diagnosis of this condition. Small cystic areas, as seen in dysbaric osteonecrosis, can also be observed in the femoral neck of normal individuals and in periarticular locations in degenerative or posttraumatic conditions. Although tomography may aid in the differential diagnosis of the findings,[85] this technique is rarely indicated.

IDIOPATHIC (PRIMARY OR SPONTANEOUS) OSTEONECROSIS

Osteonecrosis may appear in certain locations in the absence of any recognizable underlying disorder or event. Most characteristically, it is the femoral

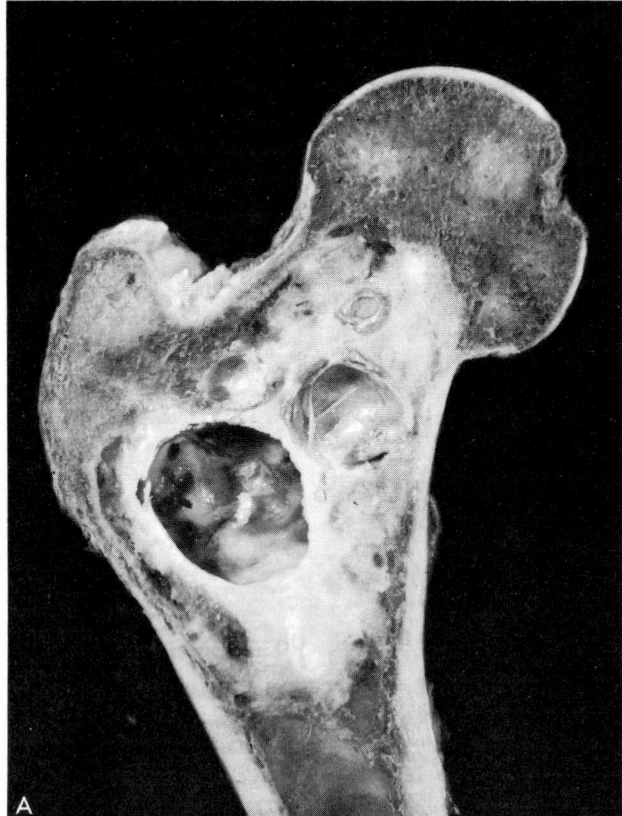

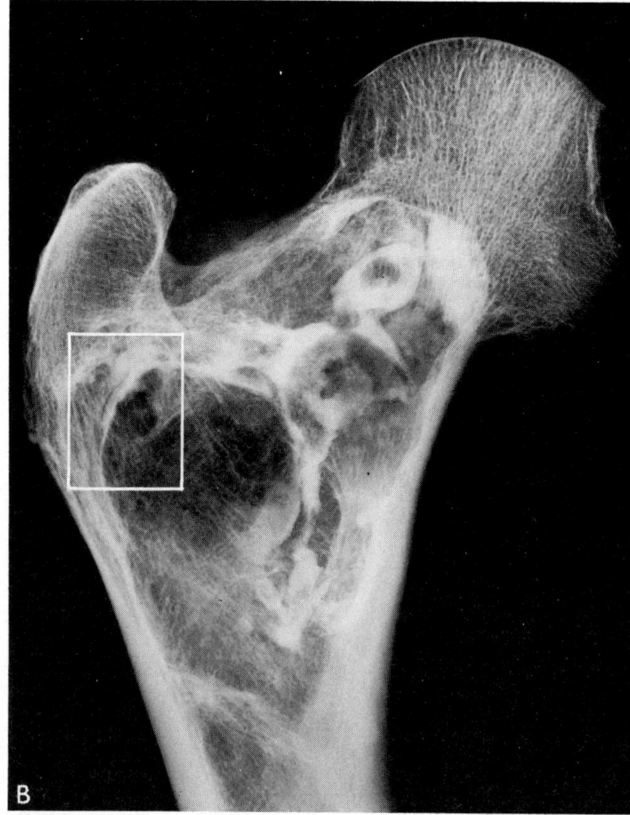

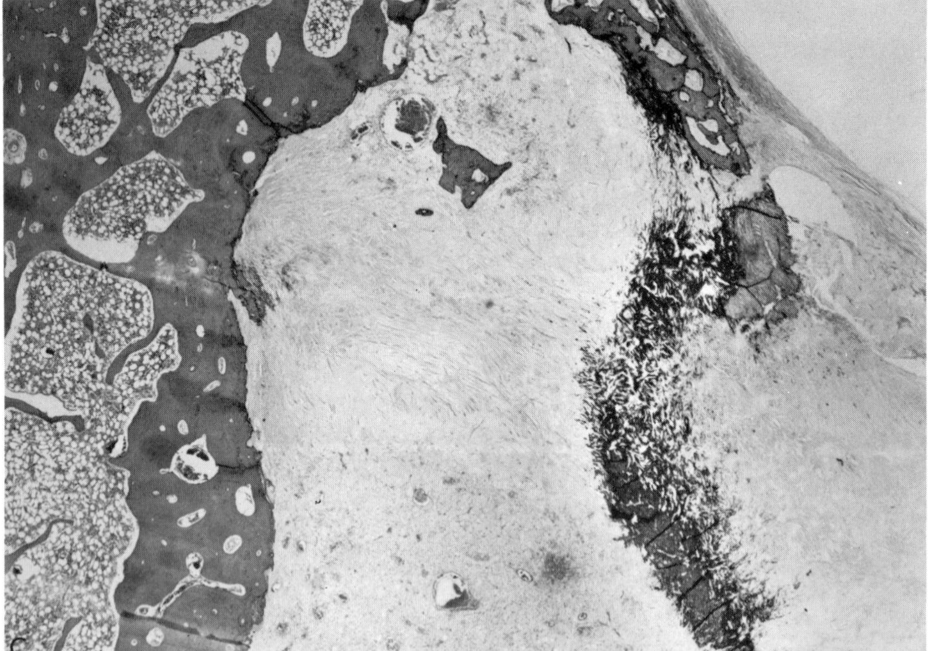

Figure 77–24. *Idiopathic (primary or spontaneous) osteonecrosis: Proximal femur.*

A *A photograph of the cut surface of the upper end of the right femur in a 72 year old man reveals a multilocular cystic area in the femoral neck and the intertrochanteric region. Detailed study of the specimen indicated that in the distant past the area must have been the site of an infarct which in the course of time underwent cystic softening. Neither the gross nor the microscopic appearance was consistent with a lesion of recent origin.*

B *Roentgenogram of the sectioned upper end of the femur delineates individual cystic areas that are surrounded by a border of radiopacity, which is thin in some places and thick in others. The radiopaque border may contain some osseous tissue but consists mainly of calcified collagenous connective tissue. The histologic appearance of a portion of the boxed area is shown in* **C.**

C *A photomicrograph (17 ×) demonstrates that the inner surface of the cyst, which is on the right side of the photograph, contains a thin lining layer that consists of acellular collagenous tissue, the deeper part of which is calcified. Immediately to the left, there is a zone of nonviable and disintegrating osseous tissue. Farther to the left, there is an area of collagenous tissue, poor in cells and heavily calcified in some places.*

(From Jaffe HL: Med Radiogr Photogr 45:58, 1969.)

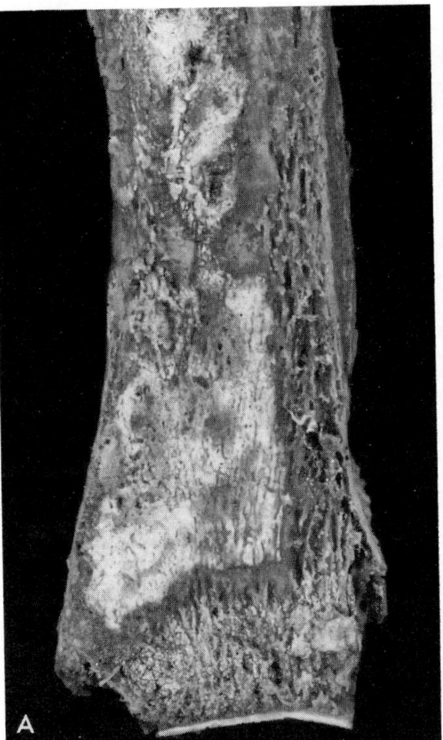

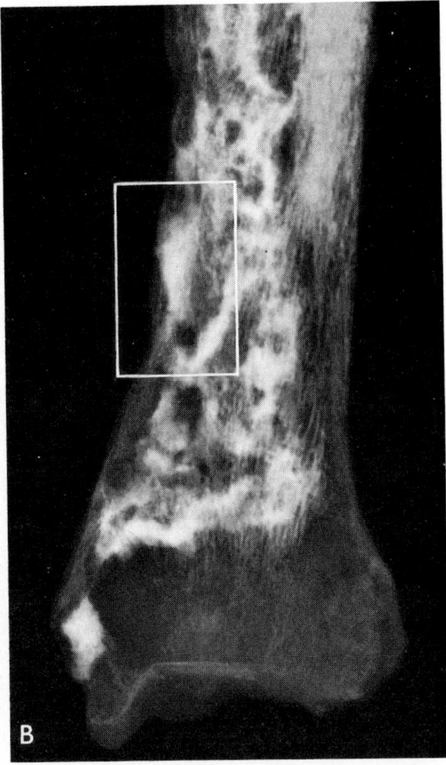

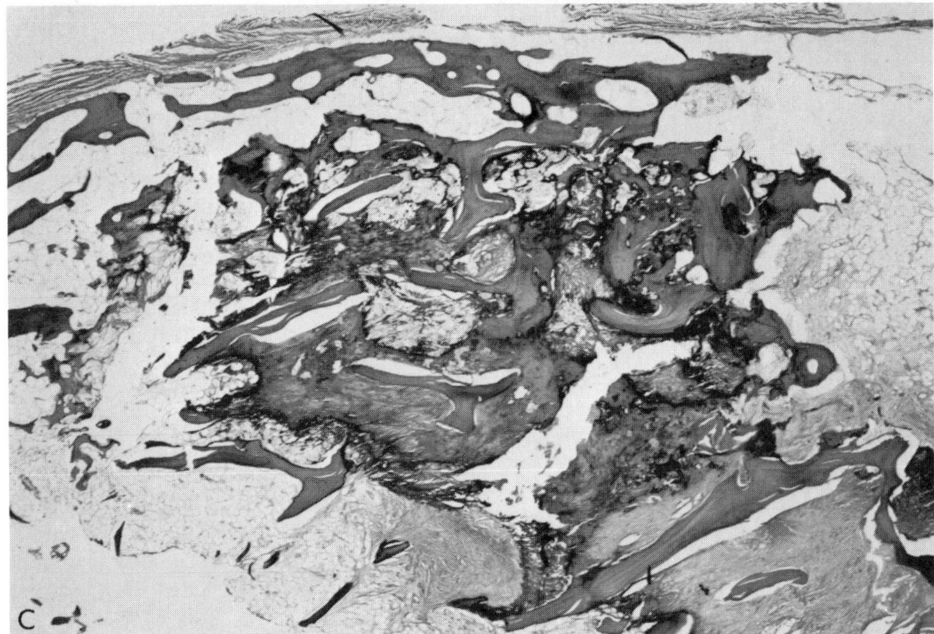

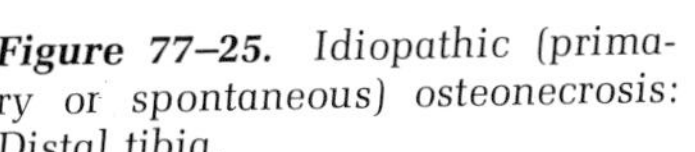

Figure 77–25. *Idiopathic (primary or spontaneous) osteonecrosis: Distal tibia.*

A *A photograph of the cut surface of the lower end of the right tibia of a 66 year old woman shows a large area of infarction. This infarct, which is more or less white, was only part of the total lesion which, indeed, occupied almost the entire shaft of the bone.*

B *A roentgenogram of the same part of the tibia indicates a vaguely loculated and variegated area of radiopacity, representing the site of infarction. The more intensely radiopaque regions correspond to those areas that are strikingly white in the photographic view.*

C *Photomicrograph of a part of the boxed area in* **B** *(25×) indicates the periosteal surface at the upper margin of the illustration. Many of the necrotic spongy trabeculae have undergone disintegration, and the intertrabecular marrow spaces are largely filled with calcified granular detritus, which stains dark.*

(From Jaffe HL: Med Radiogr Photogr 45:58, 1969.)

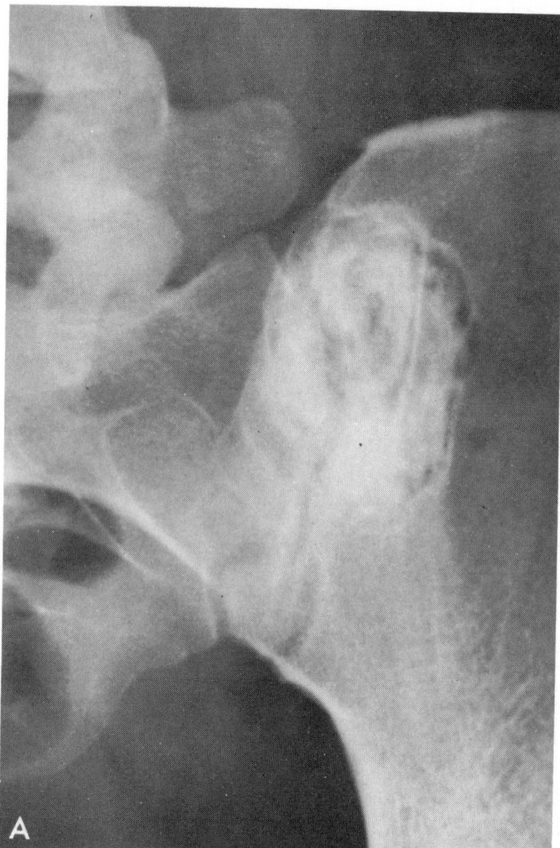

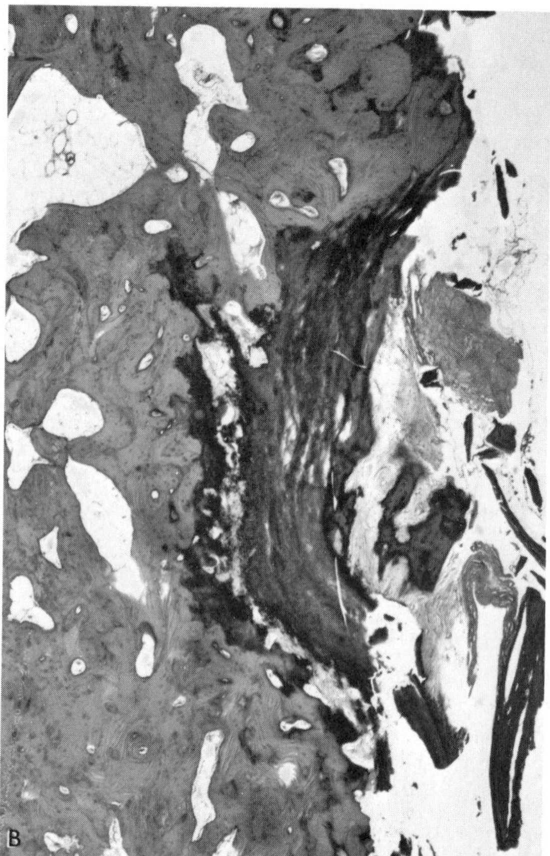

Figure 77–26. *Idiopathic (primary or spontaneous) osteonecrosis: Ilium.*

A *A roentgenogram shows an area of ischemic necrosis in the left iliac bone in the vicinity of the sacroiliac joint of a 33 year old pregnant woman with mild pain involving the lower part of her back. Observe the degree of calcification of the lesion.*

B *Photomicrograph (25×) shows a fragment of osseous tissue from the posterior or outer cortical wall of the iliac bone in the vicinity of the cyst-like space in the interior of the bone in* **A.** *The darkly discolored area represents osseous tissue that is undergoing granular disintegration. It was white or yellow-white on gross examination. Farther to the left, the disintegrating osseous tissue is lined in part by a thin layer of collagenous connective tissue.*

(From Jaffe HL: Med Radiogr Photogr 45:58, 1969.)

head or femoral condyles that are involved, although, rarely, spontaneous osteonecrosis can appear at other sites, especially in the metaphyses of long tubular bones[90-92] (Figs. 77–24 to 77–26). Here infarcts are often detected as incidental findings on radiographic examinations accomplished for unrelated reasons, appearing as peripheral rims or shells of calcification in the humerus, the femur, the tibia, or the fibula that must be distinguished from enchondromas. Once recognized, they generally remain unchanged on serial roentgenograms, although obscuration of a portion of the lesion may reflect disintegration of the central region of the necrotic tissue, liquefaction, and partial absorption.[93]

Spontaneous Osteonecrosis of the Femoral Head in Adults

The first description of idiopathic or spontaneous osteonecrosis of the femoral head in adults appears to be that of Freund in 1926.[94] Numerous publications later appeared, underscoring the continued interest in this problem, although a specific etiology has not been delineated.[95-102, 140] The condition is sometimes designated as Chandler's disease in recognition of the pertinent investigations of Chandler, who referred to spontaneous osteonecrosis of the femoral head as "coronary disease of the hip."[103]

Primary necrosis of the femoral head affects men more than women and is usually seen between the fourth and seventh decades of life. Unilateral or bilateral involvement may be detected; the reported incidence of bilateral disease has varied from 35 to 72 per cent, influenced predominantly by the method of examination and the length of follow-up.[99] Despite the frequency of bilateral involvement, the condition usually presents as a unilateral symptomatic hip related to osseous collapse in the more severely affected side. The radiographic features vary with the stage of the disorder. Initially, a femoral head of normal osseous contour may reveal mottled radiodense areas scattered throughout its anterosuperior region with a faint curvilinear band of diminished density in the anterior subchondral bone, the "crescent" sign. As the disease progresses, a focus of increased radiodensity or a lucent zone with a peripheral rim of increased radiodensity is observed. This area may be ovoid, triangular, or wedge-shaped, and although it is diagnostic of osteonecrosis, it is by no means specific for the primary or idiopathic variety. Subtle flattening of the femoral contour adjacent to the sclerotic area can be combined with increased radiodensity of the head, reflecting the presence of revascularization and an attempt at osseous repair. The eventual degree of collapse of the articular surface is variable; in some cases, severe disintegration and fragmentation of subchondral bone encourage the superimposition of osteoarthritis, with its typical roentgenographic features. A rare sequela of this condition is a synovial cyst.[135]

The pathologic findings are virtually identical to those in other varieties of osteonecrosis (see Chapter 76). On gross examination, the femoral head may appear to have a normal contour, but firm pressure will elicit segmental collapse of the articular surface, the "ping-pong ball" effect. In the area of necrosis, a wedge-shaped zone is seen, which is usually well delineated from the surrounding bone. Microscopic evaluation may reveal a zone of fibrous tissue about the necrotic bone relatively rich in blood vessels and commonly surrounded by dense sclerotic osseous tissue in the remaining spongiosa of the head and neck.

Spontaneous Osteonecrosis of the Knee in Adults

Although osteonecrosis about the knee may be observed in association with steroid therapy, sickle cell anemia, other hemoglobinopathies, and renal transplantation, it may also occur in a spontaneous or idiopathic fashion.[104-114] This disorder, which is distinct from osteochondritis dissecans occurring in adolescence (Table 77–1), is characterized by the onset, in an older patient (usually over 60 years of age) who more frequently is a woman than a man, of abrupt pain in the knee (the patient may be able to recall the exact moment in which the pain became apparent), almost always confined to the medial aspect of the joint. Localized tenderness and stiffness, an effusion, and restricted motion may be apparent. Unilateral involvement predominates over bilateral involvement. Initially radiographs are normal, and it is not until a period of weeks or months has passed that subtle flattening of the weight-bearing articular surface of the medial femoral condyle (the lateral condyle is infrequently affected) is seen (Fig. 77–27). A narrow zone of increased radiodensity adjacent to the depressed osseous surface may reflect compression of subchondral trabeculae. A radiolucent lesion in the condyle can be detected over the ensuing weeks, which at first is diffuse and irregular in outline and later is more sharply demarcated. Within the lucent area, a radiodense line consisting of cartilage and subchondral bone plate can frequently be identified (Fig. 77–27). If the affected area is small and weight-bearing is avoided, spontaneous healing can occur. However, if untreated, further depression of the bony margin, intra-articular osseous bodies, progressive sclerosis, and periostitis of the distal femur can be encountered on later examination (Fig. 77–28). Over a period of months or years, joint space narrowing, cyst formation, eburnation, and osteophytosis on apposing margins of the femur and tibia indicate the development of secondary osteoarthritis (Fig. 77–29). Bony collapse, varus deformity, and displacement can also be noted. The eventual radiographic picture may be identical to that of "medial type" osteoarthritis of the knee, and the accompanying degenerative cartilaginous and bony features may obscure the findings of osteonecrosis. In fact, the resemblance of the superimposed degenerative changes in cases of spontaneous osteonecrosis of the knee to those of typical osteoarthritis has led to speculation that a significant number of cases of degenerative joint disease of the knee have their origin in an ischemic event.

The delay in the appearance in radiographic findings in this condition has stimulated a search for more sensitive modalities. Scintigraphic examina-

Table 77–1

SPONTANEOUS OSTEONECROSIS VERSUS OSTEOCHONDRITIS DISSECANS (OF THE KNEE)

	Spontaneous Osteonecrosis	Osteochondritis Dissecans
Age of onset	Middle-aged and elderly	Adolescent
Symptomatology	Pain, tenderness, swelling, restricted motion	Variable; may be lacking
Typical location	Weight-bearing surface of medial condyle	Non-weight-bearing surface of medial condyle
Probable pathogenesis	Trauma, perhaps related to meniscal tear; or vascular insult	Trauma
Sequelae	Degenerative joint disease; intra-articular osteocartilaginous bodies	Intra-articular osteocartilaginous bodies

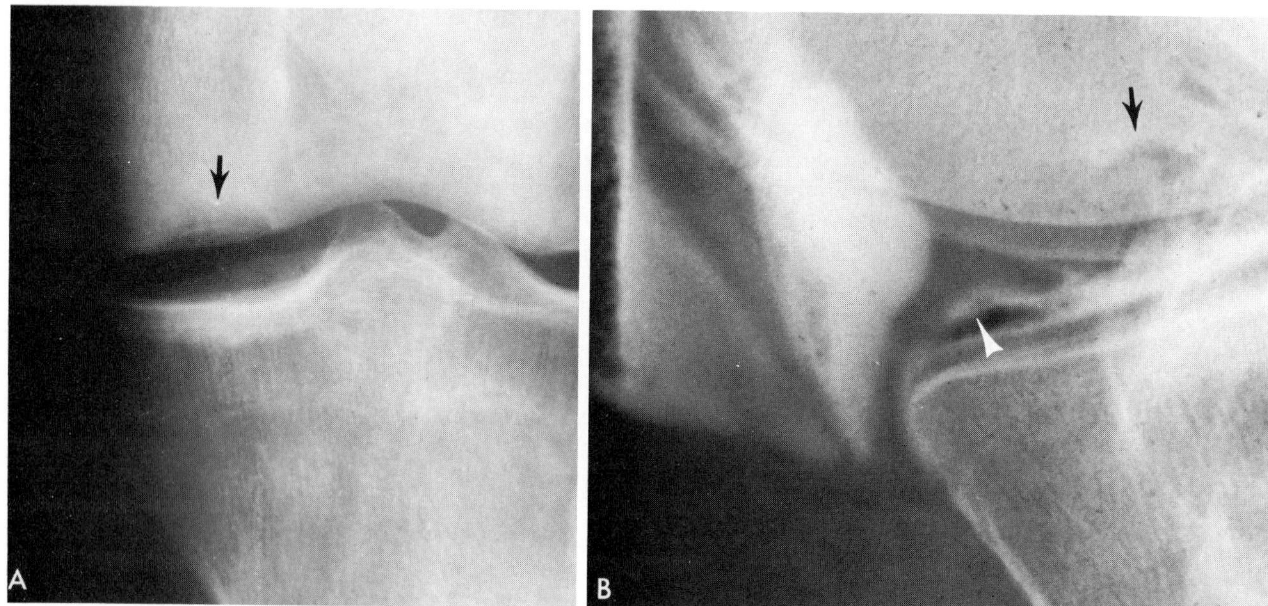

Figure 77–27. *Spontaneous osteonecrosis of the knee. This 60 year old man developed pain in the knee of acute onset, which was associated with an effusion. No history of trauma could be elicited, and the patient had not received corticosteroids.*

A *Two years following the onset of pain, a radiograph reveals flattening of the weight-bearing surface of the medial femoral condyle associated wih an osseous excavation (arrow) containing a linear radiodense shadow.*

B *An arthrogram reveals the site of necrosis (arrow), a tear on the undersurface and tip of the medial meniscus (arrowhead), and a popliteal cyst. It has been suggested that meniscal tears predispose to osteonecrosis of the adjacent femoral condyle (see text).*

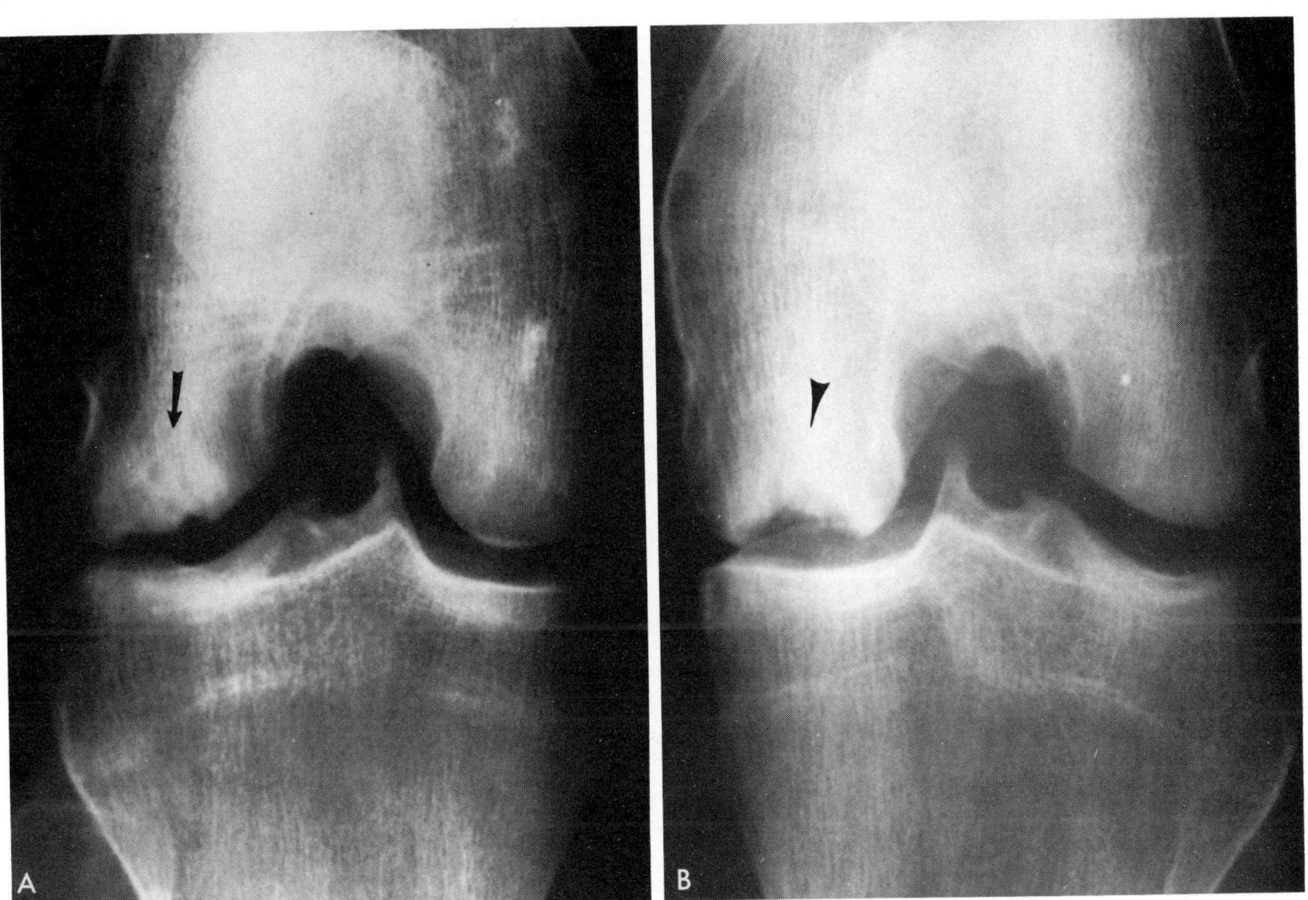

Figure 77–28. *Spontaneous osteonecrosis of the knee. This middle-aged woman developed the spontaneous onset of pain in both knees. She had not received corticosteroids. Observe osseous depression, irregularity, and sclerosis of the lateral condyle of the right femur (arrow) and the medial condyle of the left femur (arrowhead).*

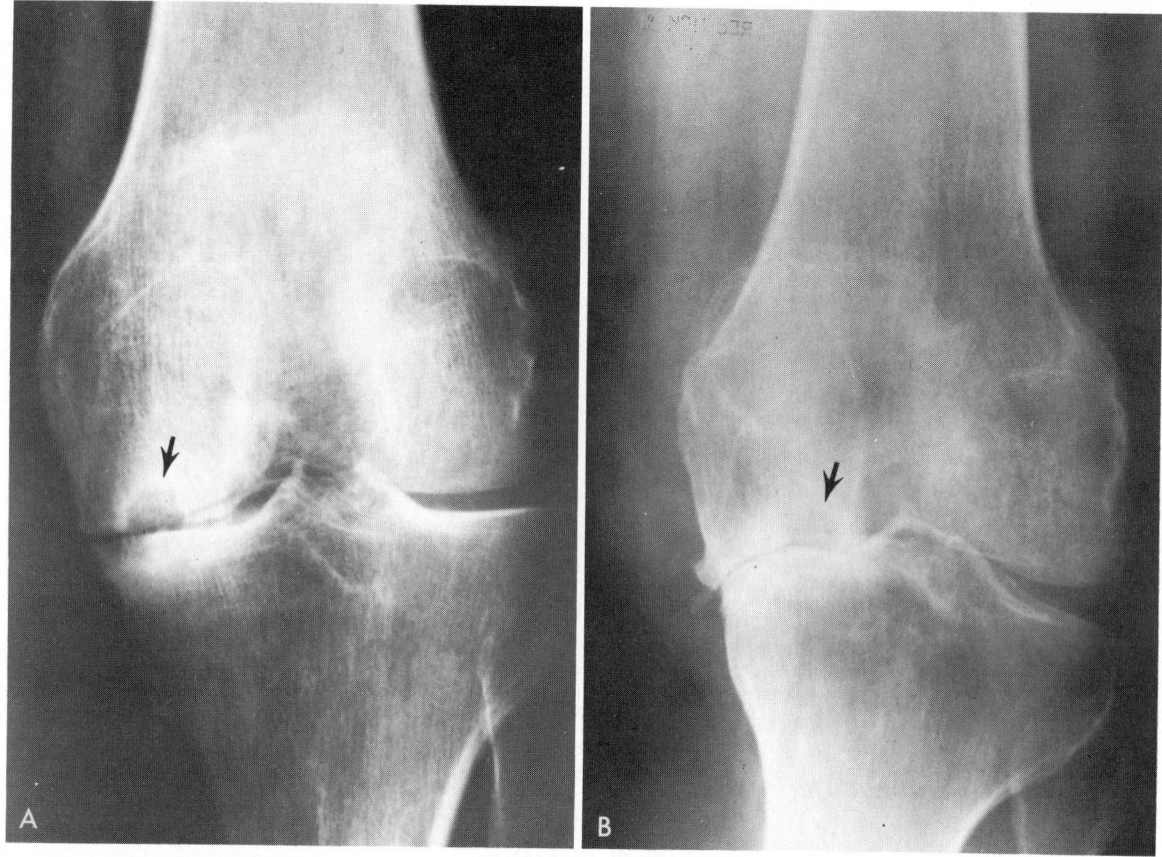

Figure 77–29. *Spontaneous osteonecrosis of the knee. Two examples of spontaneous osteonecrosis with superimposed degenerative joint disease are shown. In both cases, joint space narrowing and sclerosis are prominent. Although the appearance simulates that of uncomplicated degenerative joint disease, the degree of bony flattening and the presence of cystic lesions (arrows) in the condyle suggest that osteonecrosis has occurred.*

tion utilizing bone-seeking radiopharmaceuticals has promise in this regard, as focal accumulation of radionuclide can be identified long before roentgenographic changes appear.[105, 112, 113, 136] Lotke and coworkers[111] described a series of 12 patients with clinical and scintigraphic findings of spontaneous osteonecrosis of the knee without roentgenographic findings in whom conservative management led to amelioration of symptoms and signs and disappearance of the positive radionuclide findings and in whom roentgenographic abnormalities never appeared.

Surgical evaluation of the lesion may identify the depressed osseous surface and articular cartilage and bony fragments that can remain in situ, be slightly displaced, exist "free" in the articular cavity, or be embedded at a distant synovial site[115] (Fig. 77–30). Microscopy can delineate segmental bony necrosis with cartilaginous irregularity and collapse as well as an adjacent osseous response consisting of histiocytic resorption of necrotic material and formation of granulomatous tissue with surrounding reactive new bone formation.[106] Synovial hypertrophy and fibrosis about bony detritus can also be identified.

The etiology and pathogenesis of this condition are not clear. The dominant opinion implicates vascular insufficiency leading to infarction of bone. A traumatic insult producing microfractures in the subchondral bone plate and overlying osseous and cartilaginous collapse has also been emphasized. Traumatically induced defects in the chondral and bony coat might allow fluid from the cartilage to be expressed into the adjacent marrow space, producing an increase in marrow pressure and pain.[111] A prominent role of meniscal injury in the pathogenesis of spontaneous osteonecrosis has recently been proposed.[114] Meniscal tears have been reported in association with this condition, and the impact of the articular surface against a fragmented meniscus during everyday activity could result in local ischemia of the medial femoral condyle. Furthermore, the sudden onset of pain that characterizes spontaneous osteonecrosis of the knee could be related to an acute tear of the meniscus. However, some patients with necrosis do not reveal a torn meniscus, and in others meniscal tears demonstrated on arthrography may reflect the result rather than the cause of the osseous necrosis.[128]

The other entities that enter into the differential

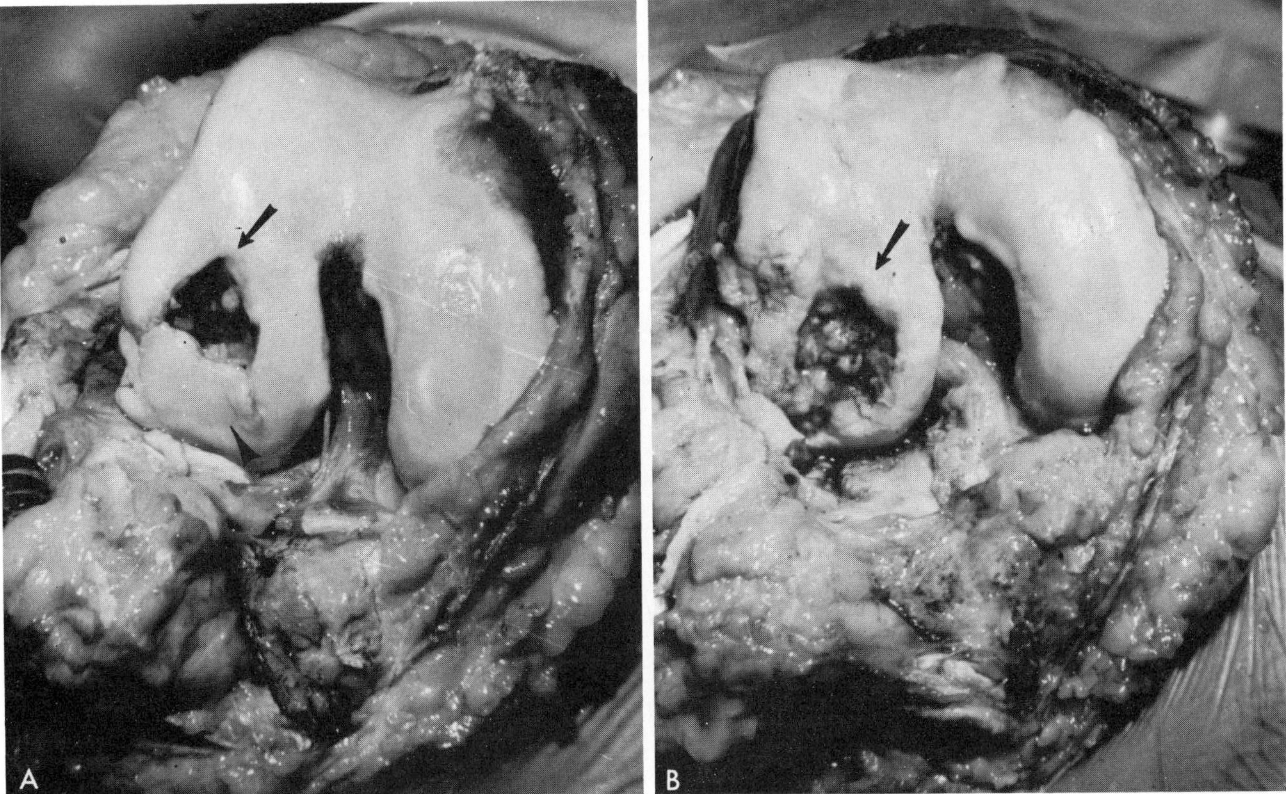

Figure 77–30. Spontaneous osteonecrosis of the knee. The surgical findings in this condition include excavation and depression of the weight-bearing osseous surface of the condyle (arrow). Note the bony fragments (arrowhead), which have been removed in **B** to reveal the size of the osseous defect. (Courtesy of Dr. R. Convery, University Hospital, University of California, San Diego, California.)

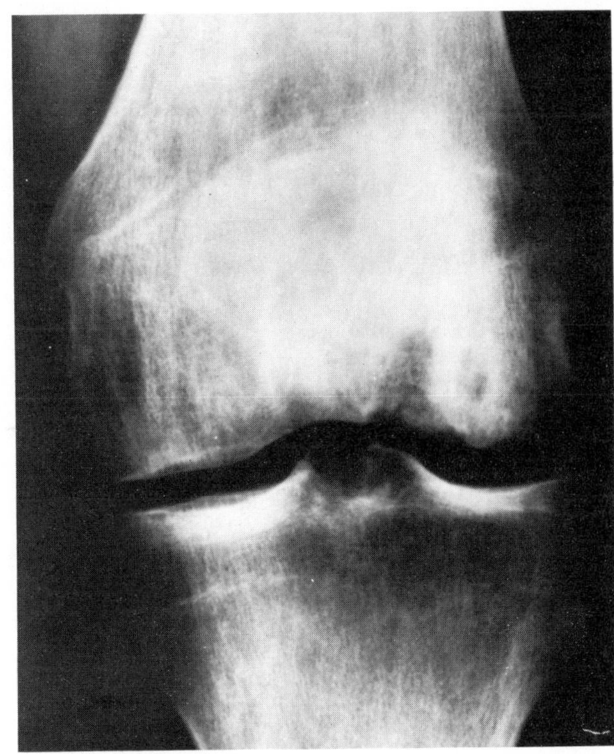

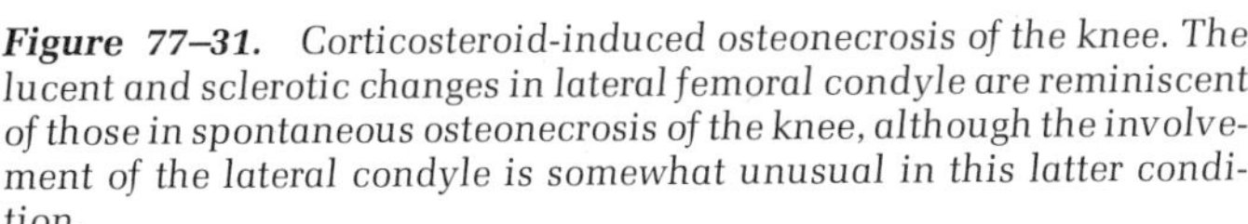

Figure 77–31. Corticosteroid-induced osteonecrosis of the knee. The lucent and sclerotic changes in lateral femoral condyle are reminiscent of those in spontaneous osteonecrosis of the knee, although the involvement of the lateral condyle is somewhat unusual in this latter condition.

diagnosis of the radiographic changes in spontaneous osteonecrosis of the knee are osteonecrosis from additional causes, osteochondritis dissecans, and neuroarthropathy. Bone necrosis due to corticosteroids or following renal transplantation produces roentgenographic features that are identical to those in spontaneous osteonecrosis (Fig. 77–31). However, historical information and involvement of multiple sites in the former two situations are helpful in the correct interpretation of the roentgenograms. Osteochondritis dissecans affects young patients and does not classically involve the weight-bearing surface of the condyle. Neuroarthropathy can produce fragmentation of the femoral condyles. Generally, the neurologic deficit is obvious, although clinical findings related to certain types of neuropathic joints, e.g., congenital insensitivity to pain, may be quite subtle.

COMPLICATIONS

Cartilaginous Abnormalities

One of the striking pathologic features of osteonecrosis is the intactness of the chondral surface despite the presence of adjacent severe osseous abnormality (Fig. 77–32*A*). This finding, which has its radiographic counterpart in preservation of the joint space, supports the commonly held impression that articular cartilage in mature adults derives most, if not all, of its nutrition from synovial fluid and is independent of the subjacent bone. It is also recognized that in those cases in which osteonecrosis leads to significant collapse of the articular surface, incongruities of apposing bony margins may lead to secondary degenerative joint disease. In this situation, cartilaginous fibrillation and erosion may be revealed on roentgenograms as diminution of the interosseous space (Fig. 77–32*B*). The possibility exists, however, that even in the presence of joint incongruity, the removal of vascular supply to the underlying bone may inhibit the development of osteoarthritic changes in the articular cartilage.[116]

An increase in metabolic activity in articular cartilage in immature animals following experimental osteonecrosis has been suggested.[117-120] In addition, roentgenograms and arthrograms of some patients with Legg-Calvé-Perthes disease have revealed an increased thickness of the chondral surface, perhaps indicating that vascular insufficiency of bone can lead to stimulation of cartilage growth in children. However, Mankin and co-workers[116] examined the cartilage from nine osteonecrotic femoral heads and were unable to detect significant alterations in histologic characteristics or biochemical and metabolic parameters. No chondrolytic changes could be discovered, although a role of chondrolysis in some cases of osteonecrosis has been proposed. Although such chondrolysis could explain the widespread or diffuse nature of the chondral loss that can be identified on serial roentgenograms in occasional patients with osteonecrosis, strong evidence for this alteration has yet to be offered. Cartilage cell necrosis is usually not a prominent feature in osteonecrosis, although regional hypocellularity can be seen.[21] Pannus-like material on the chondral surface and fibrocartilaginous replacement of hyaline articular

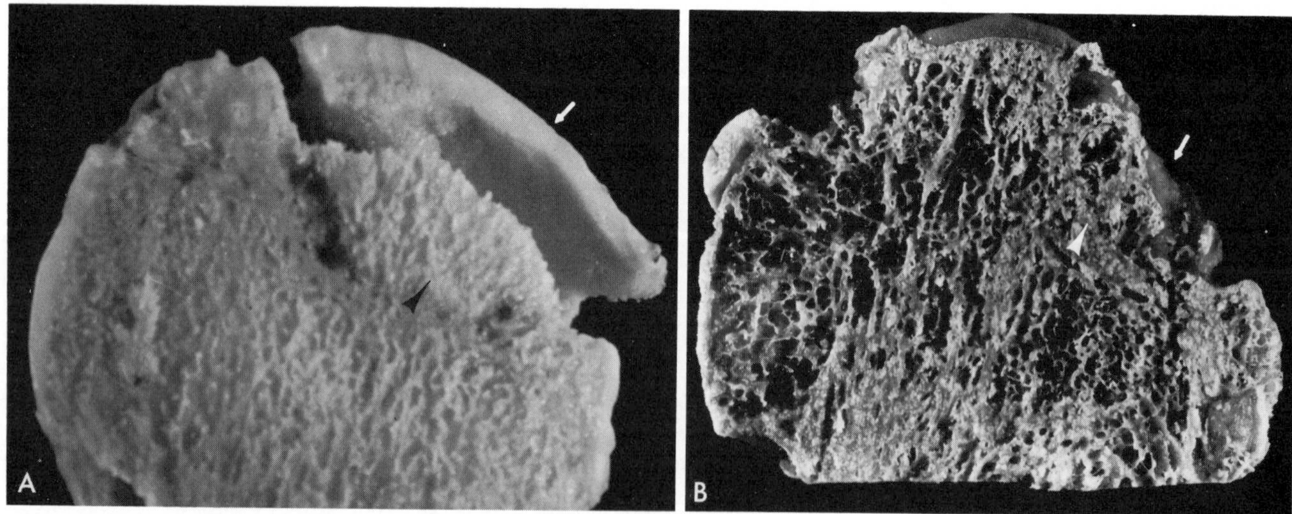

Figure 77–32. *Osteonecrosis: Complications — cartilaginous abnormalities.*

A *Cartilage preservation. The viability of the cartilage (arrow) overlying the necrotic bone (arrowhead) is a remarkable feature of osteonecrosis.*

B *In cases of severe osteonecrosis, secondary degenerative joint disease can lead to fibrillation and erosion of the chondral surface. In this case, much of the cartilaginous surface overlying the necrotic bone (arrowhead) has been eroded (arrow).*

cartilage may be apparent in advanced osteonecrosis, usually in association with osteoarthritic abnormalities.[138]

Intra-articular Osseous Bodies

Infrequently, one or more chondral or osteochondral fragments can appear in osteonecrosis.[121] They may exist free in the articular cavity, in situ in the depressed bony area, or embedded in the synovium at a distant site. In the hip, the foci may produce few or no symptoms whereas in the knee, symptoms and signs are not unusual. The histologic characteristics of the nidi are consistent with the pathology of this disease, revealing subchondral bone with trabecular reinforcement and relatively normal articular cartilage. In some cases, reattachment of the fragment to the synovial lining results in its partial or complete resorption.[122]

Malignant Degeneration

Sarcoma arising in areas of bone infarction has been documented in both idiopathic cases and those related to caisson disease or other disorders.[123-127] Men are more commonly affected, and the patient is usually in the fifth to seventh decades of life. Multiple bone infarcts are commonly present. Typically the distal femur (Fig. 77–33) or proximal tibia is the site of neoplasm, although other areas, such as the proximal femur, proximal humerus (Fig. 77–34), or distal tibia, may be altered. The lesions may be poorly differentiated, containing fibrous, osteoid, or cartilaginous tissue. They may be interpreted as fibrosarcoma, malignant fibrous histiocytoma, or, more rarely, osteogenic sarcoma. A distinct relationship between infarction and malignant transformation of bone is not accepted by all authorities, particularly because of the very few documented reports that have appeared in the literature. This apparent infrequency may relate to the fact that sarcomatous proliferation may obliterate all evidence of preexistent infarction.[125] Other investigations firmly support a real association between bone infarction and malignancy; however, a long latent period between hyperbaric exposure and malignant transformation is evident. It is possible that bone infarction results in a chronic reparative process at the revascularization margins, characterized by histiocyte proliferation. Perhaps, after many years, the histiocyte component may undergo sarcomatous transformation.[127] Although the prognosis in patients with bone infarction and sarcoma is guarded and disseminated metastasis and death commonly appear in a short period of time, the data in no way justify surgical

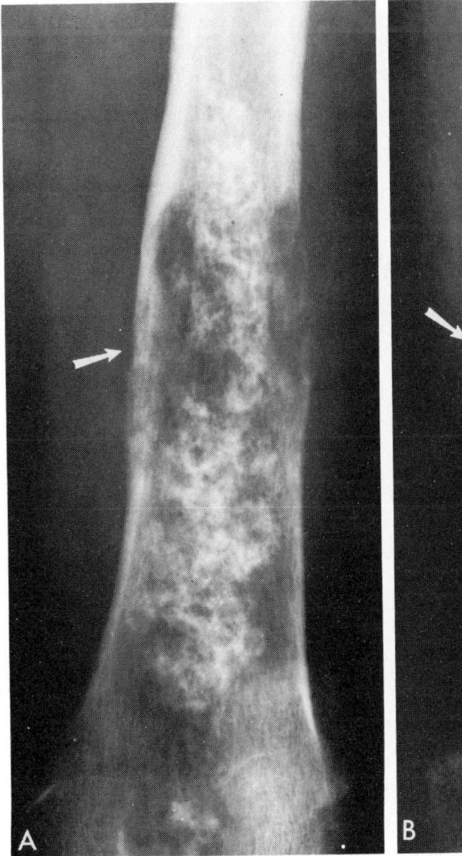

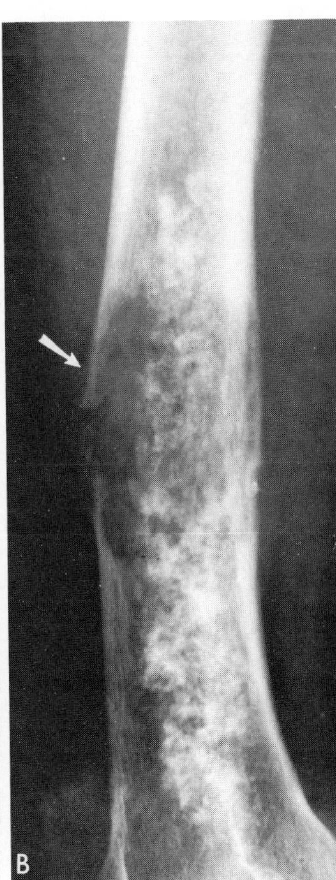

Figure 77–33. Osteonecrosis: Complications — *malignant degeneration. In this 76 year old woman with bone infarction, a fibrosarcoma developed at the site of bone necrosis in the femur. In addition to the typical calcification of a bone infarct, observe the osteolytic destruction (arrow) with a pathologic fracture representing a fibrosarcoma. (Courtesy of Dr. V. Vint, Scripps Clinic, LaJolla, California.)*

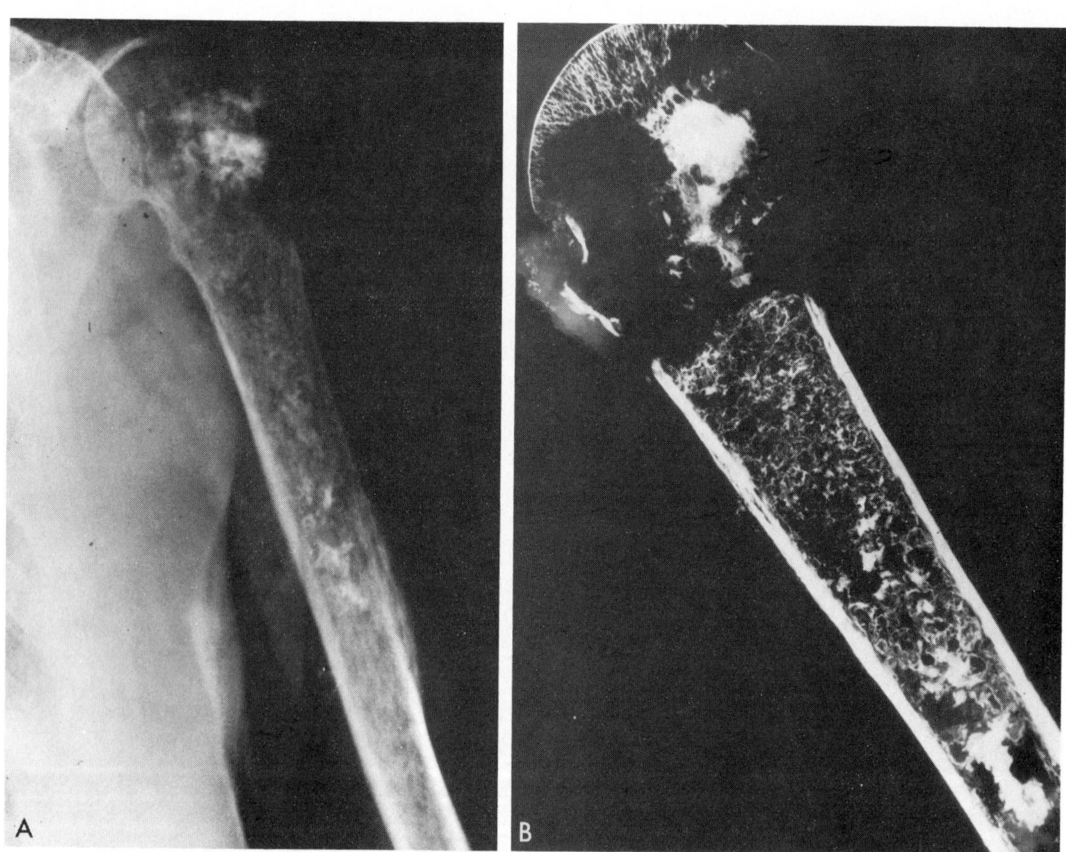

Figure 77–34. Osteonecrosis: *Complications —malignant degeneration. In a different patient, the destructive lesion of the proximal humerus containing calcification in an area of bone infarction represented a sarcoma with fibrous and cartilaginous elements. (Courtesy of Dr. R. Freiberger, Hospital for Special Surgery, New York, New York.)*

ablation of infarcts[126] because of the apparent rarity of the complication. The radiographic diagnosis is not difficult, as a soft tissue mass and osseous destruction appear at a site of obvious infarction. Occasionally, the radiographic appearance of dissolution of bone and adjacent calcification may resemble a chondrosarcoma occurring in the absence of osteonecrosis.

SUMMARY

Osteonecrosis can accompany many diverse disease processes, such as trauma, hemoglobinopathy, exogenous or endogenous hypercortisolism, alcoholism, pancreatitis, dysbaric conditions, and Gaucher's disease. It may also become evident without any recognizable disease or event (primary or spontaneous osteonecrosis). Posttraumatic osteonecrosis is most frequent in the femoral and humeral heads, scaphoid, and talus. Dysbaric osteonecrosis can produce widespread skeletal alterations of epiphyseal, metaphyseal, or diaphyseal segments of tubular bones. Spontaneous osteonecrosis is most commonly recognized about the hip and the knee. Possible complications of bone necrosis are secondary degenerative joint disease, formation of intra-articular osseous and cartilaginous bodies, and sarcomatous degeneration.

REFERENCES

1. Greenfield GB: Radiology of Bone Diseases. 2nd Ed. Philadelphia, JB Lippincott Co, 1975, p 143.
2. Martel W, Poznanski AK: The effect of traction on the hip in osteonecrosis. A comment on the "radiolucent crescent line." Radiology *94*:505, 1970.
3. Martel W, Poznanski AK: The value of traction during roentgenography of the hip. Radiology *94*:497, 1970.
4. Gohel VK, Dalinka MK, Edeiken J: Ischemic necrosis of the femoral head simulating chondroblastoma. Radiology *107*:545, 1973.
5. Müssbichler H: Arteriographic studies in fractures of the femoral neck and trochanteric region. Angiology *21*:385, 1970.
6. Hipp E: Die Gefässes des Hüftkopfes; Anatomie, Angiographie und Klinic. Stuttgart, Enke, 1962.
7. Hulth A, Johansson SH: Femoral-head venography in the prognosis of fractures of the femoral neck. Acta Chir Scand *123*:287, 1962.
8. Serre H, Simon L: L'ostéonécrose primitive de la tête fémorale chez l'adulte. Acta Rheumatol Scand *7*:265, 1961.
9. Hungerford DS: Early diagnosis of ischemic necrosis of the femoral head. Johns Hopkins Med J *137*:270, 1975.
10. Laing PG, Ferguson AB: Iodine-131 clearance-rates as an indication of the blood supply of bone. Nature *183*:1595, 1959.
11. Holmquist B, Alffram PA: Prediction of avascular necroses following cervical fractures of the femur based on clearance of radioactive iodine from the head of the femur. Acta Orthop Scand *36*:62, 1965.
12. D'Ambrosia RD, Riggins RS, DeNardo SJ, DeNardo GL: Fluoride-18 scintigraphy in avascular necrotic disorders of bone. Clin Orthop Rel Res *107*:146, 1975.
13. Alavi A, McCloskey JR, Steinberg ME: Early detection of avascular necrosis of the femoral head by 99m-technetium diphosphonate bone scan: A preliminary report. Clin Orthop Rel Res *127*:137, 1977.
14. D'Ambrosia RD, Shoji H, Riggins RS, Stadalnik RC, DeNardo GL: Scintigraphy in the diagnosis of osteonecrosis. Clin Orthop Rel Res *130*:139, 1978.
15. Meyers MH, Telfer N, Moore TM: Determination of the vascularity of the femoral head with technetium 99m-sulphur-colloid. Diagnostic and prognostic significance. J Bone Joint Surg *59A*:658, 1977.
16. Lentle BC, Russell AS, Percy JS, Scott JR, Jackson FI: Bone scintiscanning updated. Ann Intern Med *84*:297, 1976.
17. McLean FC, Urist MR: Bone. An Introduction to the Physiology of Skeletal Tissue. Chicago, University of Chicago Press, 1955.
18. Graham J, Wood SK: Aseptic necrosis of bone following trauma. *In* JK Davidson (Ed): Aseptic Necrosis of Bone. Amsterdam, Excerpta Medica, 1976, p 101.
19. Phemister DB: Necrotic bone and subsequent changes which it undergoes. JAMA *64*:211, 1915.
20. Catto M: A histological study of avascular necrosis of the femoral head after transcervical fracture. J Bone Joint Surg *47B*:749, 1965.
21. Glimcher MJ, Kenzora JE: The biology of osteonecrosis of the human femoral head and its clinical implications. I. Tissue biology. Clin Orthop Rel Res *138*:284, 1979.
22. Glimcher MJ, Kenzora JE: The biology of osteonecrosis of the human femoral head and its clinical implications. II. The pathological changes in the femoral head as an organ and in the hip joint. Clin Orthop Rel Res *139*:283, 1979.
23. Glimcher MJ, Kenzora JE: The biology of osteonecrosis of the human femoral head and its clinical implications. III. Discussion of the etiology and genesis of the pathological sequelae; comments on treatment. Clin Orthop Rel Res *140*:273, 1979.
24. Garden RS: Malreduction and avascular necrosis in subcapital fractures of the femur. J Bone Joint Surg *53B*:183, 1971.
25. Barnes R, Brown JT, Garden RS, Nicoll EA: Subcapital fractures of the femur. A prospective review. J Bone Joint Surg *58B*:2, 1976.
26. Coleman SS: Aseptic necrosis of bone due to trauma. Orthop Clin North Am *5*:819, 1974.
27. Trueta J, Harrison MHM: The normal vascular anatomy of the femoral head in adult man. J Bone Joint Surg *35B*:442, 1953.
28. Sevitt S, Thompson RG: The distribution and anastomoses of arteries supplying the head and neck of the femur. J Bone Joint Surg *47B*:560, 1965.
29. Müssbichler H: Arteriographic findings in necrosis of the head of the femur after medial neck fracture. Acta Orthop Scand *41*:77, 1970.
30. Claffey TJ: Avascular necrosis of the femoral head. J Bone Joint Surg *42B*:802, 1960.
31. Wertheimer LG, Lopes S de L: Arterial supply of the femoral head. A combined angiographic and histological study. J Bone Joint Surg *53A*:545, 1971.
32. Sevitt S: Avascular necrosis and revascularisation of the femoral head after intracapsular fractures. A combined arteriographic and histological necropsy study. J Bone Joint Surg *46B*:270, 1964.
33. Trueta J: The normal vascular anatomy of the human femoral head during growth. J Bone Joint Surg *39B*:358, 1957.
34. McDougall A: Fracture of the neck of femur in childhood. J Bone Joint Surg *43B*:16, 1961.
35. Ratliff AHC: Fractures of the neck of the femur in children. J Bone Joint Surg *44B*:528, 1962.
36. Phemister DB: Fractures of neck of femur, dislocations of hip, and obscure vascular disturbances producing aseptic necrosis of head of femur. Surg Gynecol Obstet *59*:415, 1934.
37. Catto M: A histological study of avascular necrosis of the femoral head after transcervical fracture. J Bone Joint Surg *47B*:749, 1965.
38. Brav EA: Traumatic dislocation of the hip. Army experience and results over a twelve-year period. J Bone Joint Surg *44A*:1115, 1962.
39. Epstein HC: Posterior fracture-dislocations of the hip. Long-term follow-up. J Bone Joint Surg *56A*:1103, 1974.
40. Jerre T: A study in slipped upper femoral epiphysis. With special reference to the late functional and roentgenological results and to the value of closed reduction. Acta Orthop Scand Suppl *6*:1, 1950.
41. Wilson PD, Jacobs B, Schecter L: Slipped capital femoral epiphysis: An end-result study. J Bone Joint Surg *47A*:1128, 1965.
42. Hall JE: The results of treatment of slipped femoral epiphysis. J Bone Joint Surg *39B*:659, 1957.
43. Esteve R: Congenital dislocation of the hip. A review and assessment of results of treatment with special reference to frame reduction as compared with manipulative reduction. J Bone Joint Surg *42B*:253, 1960.
44. Haliburton RA, Sullivan CR, Kelly PJ, Peterson LFA: The extraosseous and intraosseous blood supply of the talus. J Bone Joint Surg *40A*:1115, 1958.
45. Mulfinger GL, Trueta J: The blood supply of the talus. J Bone Joint Surg *52B*:160, 1970.
46. Morris HD: Aseptic necrosis of the talus following injury. Orthop Clin North Am *5*:177, 1974.

47. Hawkins LG: Fractures of the neck of the talus. J Bone Joint Surg *52A*:991, 1970.
48. Mindell ER, Cisek EE, Kartalian G, Dziob JM: Late results of injuries of the talus. Analysis of forty cases. J Bone Joint Surg *45A*:221, 1963.
49. Kenwright J, Taylor RG: Major injuries of the talus. J Bone Joint Surg *52B*:36, 1970.
50. Laing PG: The arterial supply of the adult humerus. J Bone Joint Surg *38A*:1105, 1956.
51. Obletz BE, Halbstein BM: Non-union of fractures of the carpal navicular. J Bone Joint Surg *20*:424, 1938.
52. Taleisnik J, Kelly PJ: The extraosseous and intraosseous blood supply of the scaphoid bone. J Bone Joint Surg *48A*:1125, 1966.
53. Mazet R Jr, Hohl M: Fractures of the carpal navicular. Analysis of ninety-one cases and review of the literature. J Bone Joint Surg *45A*:82, 1963.
54. Gasser H: Delayed union and pseudarthrosis of the carpal navicular: Treatment by compression-screw osteosynthesis. J Bone Joint Surg *47A*:249, 1965.
55. Scapinelli R: Blood supply of the human patella. Its relation to ischaemic necrosis after fracture. J Bone Joint Surg *49B*:563, 1967.
56. Gilsanz V, Cleveland RH, Wilkinson RH: Aseptic necrosis: A complication of dislocation of the metacarpophalangeal joint. Am J Roentgenol *129*:737, 1977.
57. Davidson JK: Dysbaric osteonecrosis. *In* JK Davidson (Ed): Aseptic Necrosis of Bone. Amsterdam, Excerpta Medica, 1976, p 147.
58. Jaffe HL: Ischemic necrosis of bone. Med Radiogr Photogr *45*:57, 1969.
59. Rószahegyi I: Neurological damage following decompression. *In* RI McCallum (Ed): Decompression of Compressed Air Workers in Civil Engineering. Proceedings of an International Working Party held at the Ciba Foundation, London, 1965. Newcastle-upon-Tyne, Oriel Press, 1967, p 127.
60. Adams GM, Parker GW: Dysbaric osteonecrosis in US Navy divers. A survey of non-random selected divers (Abstr).Undersea Biomed Res *1*:A20, 1974.
61. Chryssanthou CP: Dysbaric osteonecrosis. Etiological and pathogenetic concepts. Clin Orthop Rel Res *130*:94, 1978.
62. Reeves E, McKee AE, Stunkard JA, Schilling PW: Radiographic and pathologic studies for aseptic bone necrosis in dogs incurring decompression sickness. Aerospace Med *43*:61, 1972.
63. Jones JP Jr, Sakovich L: Fat embolism of bone. A roentgenographic and histological investigation, with the use of intra-arterial Lipiodol in rabbits. J Bone Joint Surg *48A*:149, 1966.
64. Chryssanthou CP: Dysbaric osteonecrosis in mice. Undersea Biomed Res *3*:67, 1976.
65. McCallum RI, Walder DN, Barnes R, Catto ME, Davidson JK, Fryer DI, Golding FC, Paton WDM: Bone lesions in compressed air workers. With special reference to men who worked in the Clyde tunnels 1958 to 1963. J Bone Joint Surg *48B*:207, 1966.
66. Spencer MP, Clarke HF: Precordial monitoring of pulmonary gas embolism and decompression bubbles. Aerospace Med *43*:762, 1972.
67. Stegall PJ, Huang TW, Smith KH: The etiology of experimentally induced osteonecrosis (Abstr). Undersea Biomed Res *3*:A40, 1976.
68. Amako T, Kawashima M, Torisu T, Hayashi K: Bone and joint lesions in decompression sickness. Semin Arthritis Rheum *4*:151, 1974.
69. Pauley SM, Cockett ATK: Role of lipids in decompression sickness. Aerospace Med *41*:56, 1970.
70. Philp RB, Inwood MJ, Warren BA: Interactions between gas bubbles and components of the blood: Implications in decompression sickness. Aerospace Med *43*:946, 1972.
71. Chryssanthou C, Teichner F, Goldstein G, Kalberer J Jr, Antopol W: Studies on dysbarism. III. A smooth muscle–acting factor (SMAF) in mouse lungs and its increase in decompression sickness. Aerospace Med *41*:43, 1970.
72. Hills BA: Gas-induced osmosis as an aetiologic agent for gouty arthritis and aseptic bone necrosis induced by exposure to compressed air. Rev Subaquatic Physiol Hyperbar Med *2*:3, 1970.
73. Sobel H: Oxygen-modified collagen and bone necrosis in divers. Letter to Editor. Lancet *2*:1012, 1974.
74. Lewis HE, Paton WDM: Decompression sickness during the sinking of a caisson; a study of some factors in the pathogenesis of caisson disease. Br J Indust Med *14*:5, 1957.
75. Bell ALL, Edson GN, Hornick N: Characteristic bone and joint changes in compressed air workers: A survey of symptomless cases. Radiology *38*:698, 1913.
76. Elliott DH, Harrison JAB: Bone necrosis — an occupational hazard of diving. J R Nav Med Serv *56*:140, 1970.
77. Ohta Y, Matsunaga H: Bone lesions in divers. J Bone Joint Surg *56B*:3, 1974.
78. Hauteville D, Esquirol E, Hyacinthe R, Herne N: Les lésions osseuses latentes des plongeurs. Résultats comparés d'une enquête portant sur 105 plongeurs et 105 sujets témoins. Rev Rhum Mal Osteartic *43*:635, 1976.
79. Horváth F, Rózsahegyi I: Bedeutung der Tomographie für die Diagnose der chronischen Caisson-Osteoarthropathie. Fortschr Geb Roentgenstr Nuklearmed *119*:610, 1973.
80. Williams B, Unsworth I: Skeletal changes in divers. Australas Radiol *20*:83, 1976.
81. Nellen JR, Kindwall EP: Aseptic necrosis of bone secondary to occupational exposure to compressed air: Roentgenologic findings in 59 cases. Am J Roentgenol *115*:512, 1972.
82. Heard JL, Schneider CS: Radiographic findings in commercial divers. Clin Orthop Rel Res *130*:129, 1978.
83. Kawashima M, Torisu T, Hayahi K, Kitano M: Pathological review of osteonecrosis in divers. Clin Orthop Rel Res *130*:107, 1978.
84. Weatherley CR, Gregg PJ, Walder DN, Rannie I: Aseptic necrosis of bone in a compressed air worker. J Bone Joint Surg *59B*:80, 1977.
85. Horváth F: Röntgenmorphologie des Caisson-bedingten Knochenmarkinfarktes. Fortschr Geb Roentgenstr Nuklearmed *129*:33, 1978.
86. Davidson JK, Griffiths PD: Caisson disease of bone. X-ray Focus *10*:2, 1970.
87. Davidson JK, Harrison JAB, Jacobs P, Hilditch TE, Catto M, Hendry WT: The significance of bone islands, cystic areas and sclerotic areas in dysbaric osteonecrosis. Clin Radiol *28*:381, 1977.
88. Swain VAJ: Caisson disease (compressed-air illness) of bone with a report of a case. Br J Surg *29*:365, 1942.
89. Kahlstrom SC, Phemister DB: Bone infarcts. Case report with autopsy findings. Am J Pathol *22*:947, 1946.
90. Kahlstrom SC, Burton CC, Phemister DB: Aseptic necrosis of bone. II. Infarctions of bone of undetermined etiology resulting in encapsulated and calcified areas in diaphyses and in arthritis deformans. Surg Gynecol Obstet *68*:631, 1939.
91. Bullough PG, Kambolis CP, Marcove RC, Jaffe HL: Bone infarctions not associated with caisson disease. J Bone Joint Surg *47A*:477, 1965.
92. Taylor HK: Aseptic necrosis of adults. Caisson workers and others. Radiology *42*:550, 1944.
93. Catto M: Pathology of aseptic bone necrosis. In JK Davidson (Ed): Aseptic Necrosis of Bone. Amsterdam, Excerpta Medica, 1976, p 3.
94. Freund E: Zur Frage der aseptischen Knochennekrose. Virchows Arch (Pathol Anat) *261*:287, 1926.
95. Chandler FA: Observations on circulatory changes in bone. Am J Roentgenol *44*:90, 1940.
96. Serre H, Simon L: Aspects cliniques des necroses parcellaires aseptiques primitives de la tête femorale chez l'adulte. Montpellier Med *56*:193, 1959.
97. Mankin HJ, Brower TD: Bilateral idiopathic aseptic necrosis of the femur in adults: "Chandler's disease." Bull Hosp Joint Dis *23*:42, 1962.
98. Patterson RJ, Bickel WH, Dahlin DC: Idiopathic avascular necrosis of the head of the femur. A study of fifty-two cases. J Bone Joint Surg *46A*:267, 1964.
99. Marcus ND, Enneking WF, Massam RA: The silent hip in idiopathic aseptic necrosis. Treatment by bone-grafting. J Bone Joint Surg *55A*:1351, 1973.
100. Kerboul M, Thomine J, Postel M, D'Aubigné RM: The conservative surgical treatment of idiopathic aseptic necrosis of the femoral head. J Bone Joint Surg *56B*:291, 1974.
101. Inoue A, Ono K: A histological study of idiopathic avascular necrosis of the head of the femur. J Bone Joint Surg *61B*:138, 1979.
102. Boettcher WG, Bonfiglio M, Hamilton HH, Sheets RF, Smith K: Non-traumatic necrosis of the femoral head. Part I. Relation of altered hemostasis to etiology. J Bone Joint Surg *52A*:312, 1970.
103. Chandler FA: Coronary disease of the hip. J Int Coll Surg *11*:34, 1948.
104. Rubens-Duval A, Villiaumey J, Lubetzki D, Rozenbaum H: L'ostéochondrite du genou du sujet âgé. Intérèt de la biopsie synoviale. Rev Rhum Mal Osteartic *33*:638, 1966.
105. Ahlbäck S, Bauer GCH, Bohne WH: Spontaneous osteonecrosis of the knee. Arthritis Rheum *11*:705, 1968.
106. Ahuja SC, Bullough PG: Osteonecrosis of the knee. A clinicopathological study in twenty-eight patients. J Bone Joint Surg *60A*:191, 1978.
107. Renier JC, Brégeon C, Mazaud J: L'ostéonécrose condylienne du genou de l'adulte et du sujet âgé (étude de 36 observations). Rev Rhum Mal Osteartic *43*:17, 1976.
108. Schauer A: Zur pathologischen Anatomie der spontanen Osteonekrosen. Z Orthop *115*:432, 1977.
109. Daumont A, Deplante JP, Bouvier M, Lejeune E: L'ostéonécrose des condyles fémoraux chez l'adulte. A propos de 30 cas personnels. Rev Rhum Mal Osteartic *43*:27, 1976.
110. Williams JL, Cliff MM, Bonakdarpour A: Spontaneous osteonecrosis of the knee. Radiology *107*:15, 1973.

111. Lotke PA, Ecker ML, Alavi A: Painful knees in older patients. Radionuclide diagnosis of possible osteonecrosis with spontaneous resolution. J Bone Joint Surg *59A*:617, 1977.
112. Muheim G, Bohne WH: Prognosis in spontaneous osteonecrosis of the knee. Investigation by radionuclide scintimetry and radiography. J Bone Joint Surg *52B*:605, 1970.
113. Bauer GCH: Osteonecrosis of the knee. Clin Orthop Rel Res *130*:210, 1978.
114. Norman A, Baker ND: Spontaneous osteonecrosis of the knee and medial meniscal tears. Radiology *129*:653, 1978.
115. Scaglietti O, Fineschi G: La condrite dissecante dell'eta senile. Arch Putti Chir Organi Mov *20*:1, 1965.
116. Mankin HJ, Thrasher AZ, Hall D: Biochemical and metabolic characteristics of articular cartilage from osteonecrotic human femoral heads. J Bone Joint Surg *59A*:724, 1977.
117. Sanchis M, Zahir A, Freeman MAR: The experimental simulation of Perthes disease by consecutive interruptions of the blood supply to the capital femoral epiphysis in the puppy. J Bone Joint Surg *55A*:335, 1973.
118. Rösingh GE, James J: Early phases of avascular necrosis of the femoral head in rabbits. J Bone Joint Surg *51B*:165, 1969.
119. Rösingh GE, Steendijk R, van den Hooff A, Oosterhoff J: Consequences of avascular necrosis of the femoral head in rabbits. A histological and radiological study with a statistical analysis of bone-volume ratios. J Bone Joint Surg *51B*:551, 1969.
120. Coutts RD, Bradley B, Akeson WH, Amiel D, Lavigne A: The effects of avascular necrosis on cartilage of the dog femoral head (Abstr). J Bone Joint Surg *56A*:858, 1974.
121. Milgram JW: The classification of loose bodies in human joints. Clin Orthop Rel Res *124*:282, 1977.
122. Milgram JW: The development of loose bodies in human joints. Clin Orthop Rel Res *124*:292, 1977.
123. Furey JG, Ferrer-Torells M, Reagan JW: Fibrosarcoma arising at the site of bone infarcts. A report of two cases. J Bone Joint Surg *42A*:802, 1960.
124. Johnson LC, Vetter H, Putschar WGJ: Sarcomas arising in bone cysts. Virchows Arch (Pathol Anat) *335*:428, 1962.
125. Dorfman HD, Norman A, Wolff H: Fibrosarcoma complicating bone infarction in a caisson worker. A case report. J Bone Joint Surg *48A*:528, 1966.
126. Mirra JM, Bullough PG, Marcove RC, Jacobs B, Huvos AG: Malignant fibrous histiocytoma and osteosarcoma in association with bone infarcts. Report of four cases, two in caisson workers. J Bone Joint Surg *56A*:932, 1974.
127. Mirra JM, Gold RH, Marafiote R: Malignant (fibrous) histiocytoma arising in association with a bone infarct in sickle-cell disease: Coincidence or cause-and-effect? Cancer *39*:186, 1977.
128. Hall FM: Osteonecrosis of the knee and medial meniscal tears. Radiology *133*:828, 1979.
129. Lee CK, Hansen HT, Weiss AB: The "silent hip" of idiopathic ischemic necrosis of the femoral head in adults. J Bone Joint Surg *62A*:795, 1980.
130. Greiff J: Determination of the vitality of the femoral head with ^{99m}Tc-Sn-pyrophosphate scintigraphy. Acta Orthop Scand *51*:109, 1980.
131. Greiff J, Lanng S, Høilund-Carlsen PF, Karle AK, Uhrenholdt A: Early detection by ^{99m}Tc-Sn-pyrophosphate scintigraphy of femoral head necrosis following medial femoral neck fractures. Acta Orthop Scand *51*:119, 1980.
132. Zizic TM, Hungerford DS, Stevens MB: Ischemic bone necrosis in systemic lupus erythematosus. I. The early diagnosis of ischemic necrosis of bone. Medicine *59*:134, 1980.
133. Gregg PJ, Walder DN: Scintigraphy versus radiography in the early diagnosis of experimental bone necrosis. J Bone Joint Surg *62B*:214, 1980.
134. Gregg PJ, Walder DN: Regional distribution of circulating microspheres in the femur of the rabbit. J Bone Joint Surg *62B*:222, 1980.
135. Leconte PH, Bastien J: Kyste synovial inguinal avec nécrose idiopathique de la tête fémorale. Rev Chir Orthop *65*:353, 1979.
136. Rozing PM, Insall J, Bohne W: Spontaneous osteonecrosis of the knee. J Bone Joint Surg *62A*:2, 1980.
137. Cooperman DR, Wallenstein R, Stulberg SD: Post-reduction avascular necrosis in congenital dislocations of the hip. J Bone Joint Surg *62A*:247, 1980.
138. Jacqueline F, Rabinowicz Th: Transformations de la synoviale et du cartilage dans les necroses post-traumatique et idiopathique de la hanche. *In* Ficat P, Arlet J: II Symposium International sur la Circulation Osseouse, Toulouse, 1977. Paris, Armour Montagu, 1979, p 355.
139. Gelberman RH, Menon J: The vascularity of the scaphoid bone. J Hand Surg *5*:508, 1980.
140. Lee CK, Corcoran SF, Parsons JR: Hyperlipidemia and idiopathic aseptic necrosis of the femoral head in adults. Orthopedics *3*:651, 1980.
141. Sugioka Y: Transtrochanteric anterior rotational osteotomy of the femoral head in the treatment of osteonecrosis affecting the hip: A new osteotomy procedure. Clin Orthop Rel Res *130*:191, 1978.

78

THE OSTEOCHONDROSES

by Donald Resnick, M.D.

The designation "osteochondrosis" has been traditionally utilized to describe a group of disorders that share certain features: predilection for the immature skeleton; involvement of an epiphysis, apophysis, or epiphysioid bone; and a radiographic picture that is dominated by fragmentation, collapse, sclerosis, and, frequently, reossification with reconstitution of the osseous contour. The radiologic and pathologic features of the osteochondroses were initially interpreted as evidence of a primary impairment of local arterial supply that led to osteonecrosis. With further investigation of these disorders, it became apparent that dissimilarities among them were considerable, and that the osteochondroses were a heterogeneous group of unrelated lesions (Table 78–1). In fact, it is now recognized that osteonecrosis is not apparent on histologic examination in some of the osteochondroses (e.g., Blount's tibia vara, Scheuermann's disease) and that, in others, aseptic bone necrosis is not a primary event but appears to follow a fracture or other traumatic insult (e.g., Kienböck's disease of lunate bone). Indeed, certain of the osteochondroses are not disorders at all but appear to represent variations in normal ossification (e.g., Sever's disease of the calcaneus). Therefore, it is important to put to rest finally the previously held concept that the osteochondroses are a closely related group of disorders whose basic pathogenesis is vascular insufficiency with osteonecrosis. In reality, the designations of these disorders as (juvenile) osteochondrosis, osteochondritis, osteochondropathy, epiphysitis, apophysitis, or sesamoiditis are inaccurate and should be eliminated.[1,2] In this regard, the author apologizes for the title of this chapter. To correct this deficiency, I will discuss these disorders according to their probable pathogenesis; however, in certain instances, the exact mechanisms are not yet clear and future investigation may require some adjustment in the manner in which these disorders are classified.

DISORDERS CHARACTERIZED BY PRIMARY OR SECONDARY OSTEONECROSIS

Legg-Calvé-Perthes Disease

Background. In 1910, Legg of Boston[3] described an "obscure affection of the hip joint" that clinically and radiologically simulated tuberculosis. Independently in the same year, Calvé in France[4] and Perthes in Germany[5] described the same condition, utilizing the designations pseudocoxalgia (Calvé) and arthritis deformans juvenilis (Perthes). In 1913, Perthes[6] introduced the term osteochondritis, and in 1920 Waldenström[7] recognized the flattened femoral head that might occur in this condition, designating the disorder coxa plana, and calling attention to his original description in 1909.[8] Despite the fact that some of the earlier reports falsely attributed the clinical and radiologic manifestations of this affliction to infection, the designations introduced by these investigators are still encountered today, although the term Legg-Calvé-Perthes disease is the most popular.

Clinical Abnormalities. This disorder affects children, particularly those between the ages of 4 and 8 years. Rarely, involvement of older children and adolescents is observed, although permanent sequelae are more frequent in these latter individuals. The appearance of Legg-Calvé-Perthes disease in children less than 4 years of age is usually associated with a good prognosis.[11] The disorder is more frequent in boys than in girls, in a ratio of approximately 5:1. Either hip can be altered, and bilateral abnormalities are detected in about 10 per cent of cases, rarely in girls. In those cases in which both hips are involved, the two hips are usually affected successively, not simultaneously (see discussion later in this chapter). Bilateral symmetric fragmentation of the capital femoral epiphyses should suggest the presence of other diseases, such as hypothyroidism. Legg-Calvé-Perthes disease is rare among blacks.[9] A family history of the condition may be detected in approximately 6 per cent of cases.[10]

The principal clinical signs are limping, pain, and limitation of joint motion. The pain may be localized to the region of the hip or referred to the inside of the ipsilateral knee. These clinical manifestations are neither prominent nor constant, and may persist for only a few days or weeks. At other times, more prolonged signs are detected, and atrophy of the soft tissues of the thigh, muscle spasm, and contracture are recognized. Occasionally, radiographic changes are noted in patients in whom clinical abnormalities are entirely lacking. A history of trauma can be observed in approximately 25 per cent of cases, with acute onset dating from the time of injury.

Radiographic Abnormalities. The radiographic abnormalities have been the subject of a great deal of attention.[12-20] The early changes have been summarized by Caffey[15] (Fig. 78–1).

1. *Soft tissue swelling on the lateral side of the articulation.* Capsular bulging with displacement of the "capsular" fat pad appears to be a more accurate sign of hip disease in children than in adults. Apparently, intra-articular fluid can lead to distortion and obscuration of this fat plane. It is not a specific finding, it is influenced by the position of the leg

Table 78–1
OSTEOCHONDROSES

Disorder	Site	Age (Years)	Probable Mechanism
Legg-Calvé-Perthes disease	Femoral head	4–8	Osteonecrosis, perhaps due to trauma
Freiberg's infraction	Metatarsal head	13–18	Osteonecrosis due to trauma
Kienböck's disease	Carpal lunate	20–40	Osteonecrosis due to trauma
Köhler's disease	Tarsal navicular	3–7	Osteonecrosis or altered sequence of ossification
Panner's disease	Capitellum of humerus	5–10	Osteonecrosis due to trauma
Thiemann's disease	Phalanges of hand	11–19	Osteonecrosis, perhaps due to trauma
Osgood-Schlatter's disease	Tibial tuberosity	11–15	Trauma
Blount's disease	Proximal tibial epiphysis	1–3 (infantile) 8–15 (adolescent)	Trauma
Scheuermann's disease	Discovertebral junction	13–17	Trauma
Sinding-Larsen-Johansson disease	Patella	10–14	Trauma
Sever's disease	Calcaneus	9–11	Normal variation in ossification
Van Neck's disease	Ischiopubic synchondrosis	4–11	Normal variation in ossification

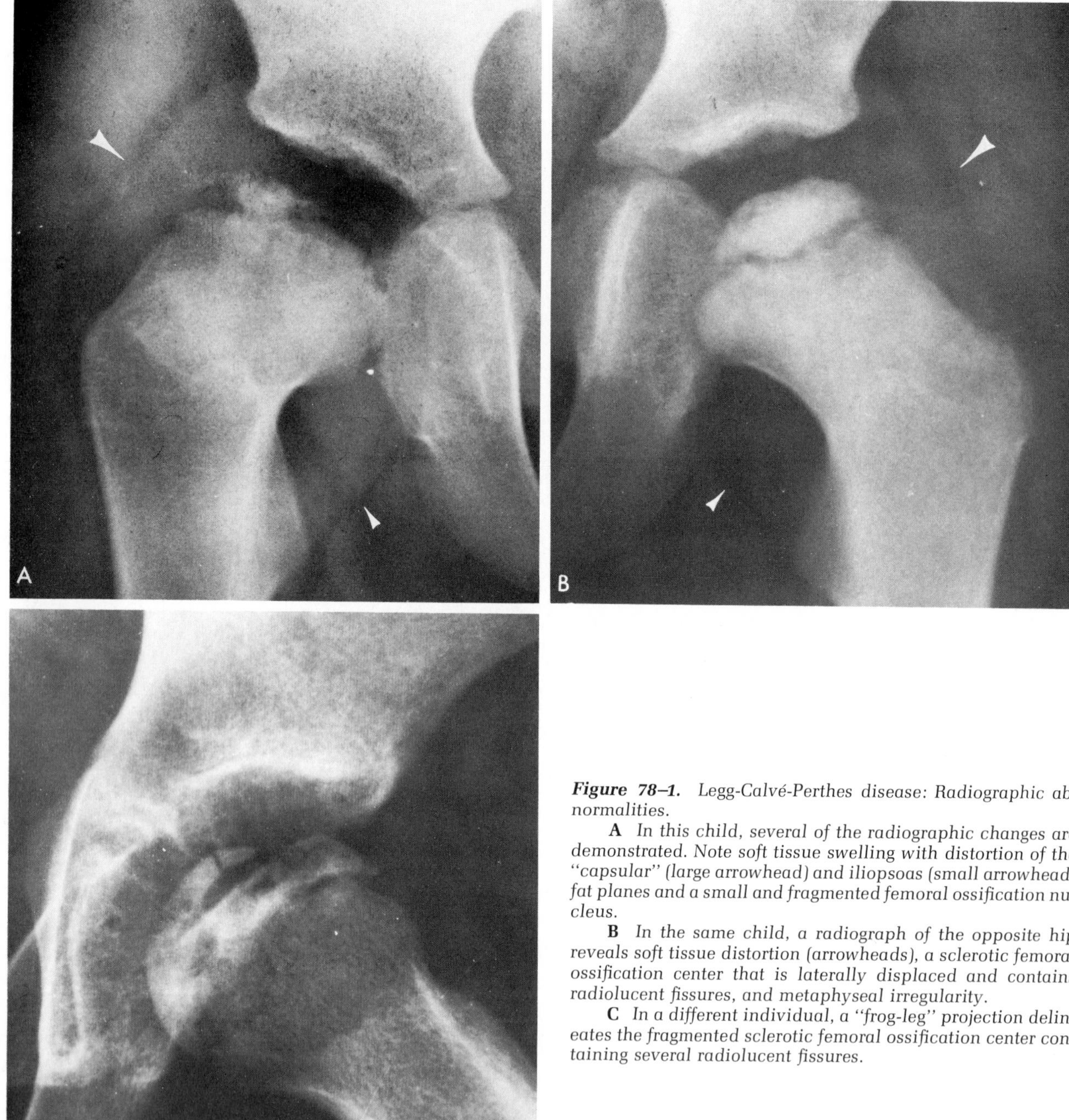

Figure 78–1. Legg-Calvé-Perthes disease: Radiographic abnormalities.

A *In this child, several of the radiographic changes are demonstrated. Note soft tissue swelling with distortion of the "capsular" (large arrowhead) and iliopsoas (small arrowhead) fat planes and a small and fragmented femoral ossification nucleus.*

B *In the same child, a radiograph of the opposite hip reveals soft tissue distortion (arrowheads), a sclerotic femoral ossification center that is laterally displaced and contains radiolucent fissures, and metaphyseal irregularity.*

C *In a different individual, a "frog-leg" projection delineates the fragmented sclerotic femoral ossification center containing several radiolucent fissures.*

during roentgenography, and it is usually accompanied by more obvious radiologic abnormalities.

2. *Smallness of the femoral ossification nucleus.* A diminutive ossification center may be apparent in as many as 50 per cent of patients. The pathogenesis of this finding is not clear. It apparently is unrelated to osseous compression, but may represent an actual retardation of bone growth. Since a decrease in the rate of ossification is not immediately associated with radiographic findings, the detection of a small ossific nucleus probably indicates that disease has been present for at least several weeks.

3. *Lateral displacement of the femoral ossification nucleus.* Calot[21] and Waldenström[22] have emphasized this early finding in Legg-Calvé-Perthes disease. The ossific nucleus may be displaced laterally 2 to 5 mm, producing an enlargement of the medial portion of the joint space.[23] This change has been regarded as an indication of a serious hip problem, and may account for overloading of the anterosuperior quadrant of the femoral head, with subsequent flattening and compression. It has been suggested that synovitis with intra-articular fluid accumulation could produce such displacement; this might explain a similar appearance seen in pyogenic and tuberculous infection and other synovial disorders.[24] Alternatively, cartilaginous hypertrophy could produce lateral displacement of the femoral head, and arthrography may outline an enlarged medial chondral surface (see discussion later in this chapter).

Lateral movement of the epiphyseal ossification center frequently precedes other radiologic evidence of disease. Fragmentation and flattening may be absent at this stage, although osteoporosis can be encountered.

4. *Fissuring and fracture of the femoral ossific nucleus.* This is a constant and well recognized roentgenographic sign of the disease. It may be detected only on radiographs obtained in the "frog-leg" position or, at least, is better delineated in this projection (Fig. 78–1C). Linear or curvilinear radiolucent shadows are seen, and the "fracture" fragment may remain in situ or be slightly displaced at its peripheral attachment. At this stage, significant displacement or separation and free fragments are not observed. A subchondral location of the infraction is preferred but not invariable, and fracture lines commonly disappear on subsequent examinations. Their appearance and characteristics are similar to those of the subchondral fractures seen in other varieties of osteonecrosis.

5. *Flattening and sclerosis of the femoral ossific nucleus.* Flattening of the epiphyseal nucleus predominates near the fracture lines on the anterolateral superior segment of the head. In almost all cases, this finding is preceded by, or occurs simultaneously with, the development of fissures in the bone, although flattening may later progress as the fissure lines disappear. The "frog-leg" position is optimal for visualizing the degree of bone flattening.

Mild to moderate sclerosis accompanies other roentgenographic signs of disease. On the anteroposterior view, the entire femoral head may appear radiodense, whereas, in the "frog-leg" position, a segmental and peripheral location is evident. The increased radiodensity of the femoral head generally follows the appearance of fracture and flattening, indicating that sclerosis is a secondary phenomenon due to compression of trabeculae and revascularization, with deposition of new bone on necrotic trabeculae.

6. *Intraepiphyseal gas.* A "vacuum" phenomenon, caused by release of gas into the clefts and gaps in the subchondral trabeculae, accentuates the exaggerated radiolucent appearance in this area. However, in most cases, this finding is not present, and the radiolucent cleft is due to the fracture line itself. Both the cleft and the "vacuum" phenomenon are better delineated in the "frog-leg" view since, in this position, stress enlarges the opening between the osteochondral fragment and the remainder of the femoral head. Gas, presumably nitrogen, flows into the enlarging space.

Although the progression and extent of disease are highly variable (see discussion later in this chapter), further compression, disintegration, fragmentation, and sclerosis of the epiphysis, together with metaphyseal changes, can be seen.

1. *Metaphyseal "cysts."* Radiolucent lesions of the metaphysis are a characteristic part of the radiographic picture of Legg-Calvé-Perthes disease, although their pathogenesis is debated (Fig. 78–2*A*). Gill[25] considered the lesions to be indicative of primary necrosis of the metaphysis that later spread to the femoral head, and the concept of metaphyseal necrosis was supported by Waldenström.[22] Mindell and Sherman[26] emphasized the late appearance of metaphyseal defects, their location opposite areas of diminished density in the epiphysis, and their ability to heal in a manner similar to that of the femoral head lesions. Ponseti[27] utilized trocar biopsies to study the metaphyseal abnormalities, and noted islands or tongues of uncalcified cartilage derived from the growth plate extending into the metaphyseal bone marrow. In a sense, the lesions represented intramedullary enchondromas composed of uncalcified cartilage. According to both Ponseti and to others,[15] the metaphyseal "cyst" was related to a distortion of normal endochondral bone formation in which a disturbance or failure of normal absorption of cartilage was detected. Caffey[15] speculated that fissuring and fibrillation of the growth plate weakened it so that the excessive compression forces on the anterior segment of the femoral head were transmitted through the cartilaginous plate to the anterior segment of the metaphysis, where they compressed capillary loops, preventing normal in-

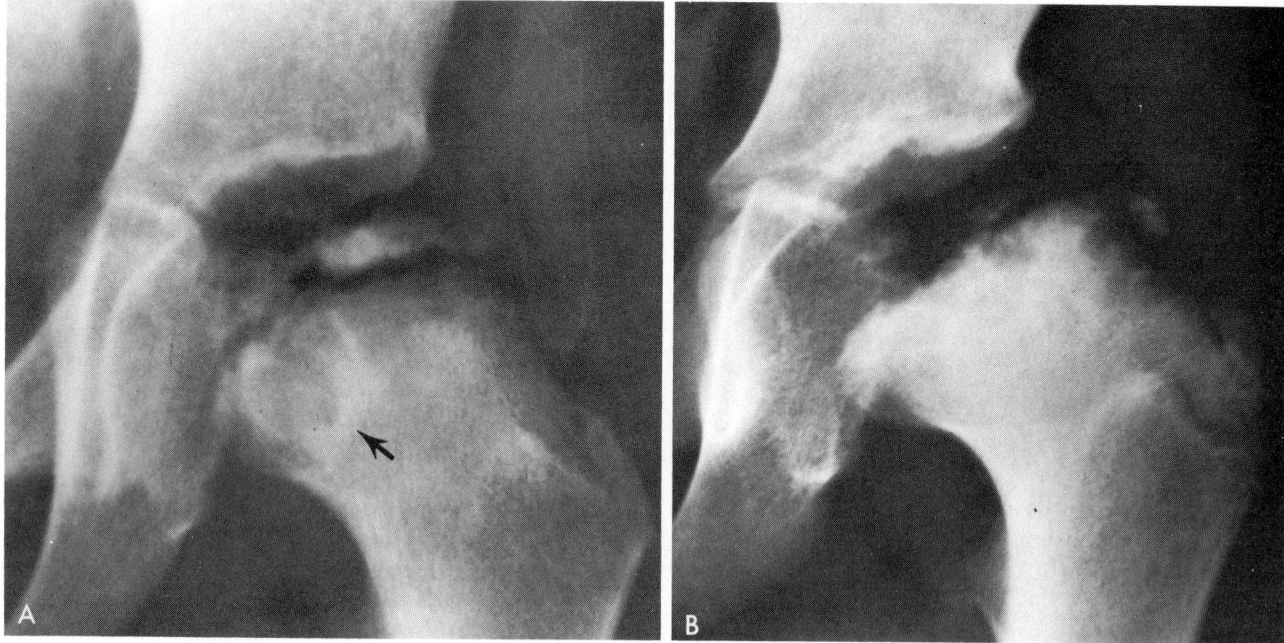

Figure 78–2. Legg-Calvé-Perthes disease: Metaphyseal abnormalities.
A *Metaphyseal "cysts." Observe the large cystic lesion of the medial metaphysis of the femur (arrow), which is associated with a fragmented, sclerotic, and laterally placed ossific nucleus.*
B *In another child, note the broad and short femoral neck containing multiple radiolucent lesions. Most of the epiphyseal ossification center is destroyed.*

flow of arterial blood. This deficiency in vascular supply then reduced the normal resorption of uncalcified cartilage, producing cartilaginous islands in the metaphysis. Caffey emphasized the relatively late appearance of the metaphyseal lesions following the detection of epiphyseal changes, and their location in the ventral segment of the metaphysis directly beneath the area of epiphyseal fracture and flattening. Despite this evidence underscoring a disturbance of endochondral bone formation in the development of metaphyseal lucent areas, support for a necrotic process in the metaphysis still appears.[18] In either case, alterations of vascular supply may represent the primary event, initiating either necrosis or disturbed osseous development. The resulting lucency of the metaphysis, which is detected on radiographic examination,[215] may simulate an abscess or tumor. However, biopsy is unnecessary if the observer recognizes that such lesions are a definite part of the radiographic appearance in Legg-Calvé-Perthes disease.

2. *Widening and shortening of the femoral neck.* Widening and irregularity of the growth plate and broadening of the metaphysis are additional manifestations of this disorder (Fig. 78–2*B*). Ponseti and Cotton[28] described increased apposition of bone throughout the length of the femoral neck. Edgren[10] attributed the widening of the neck to metaphyseal alterations as well as appositional growth. Robichon and co-workers[19] cited experimental work in animals that indicated that diminished blood supply to the femoral head caused not only epiphyseal necrosis, but also a decrease in cartilage cell production in the germinal layer of the growth plate, producing a diminution in longitudinal bone growth; appositional growth continued in the metaphysis because of its intact vascular supply. This combination of factors created the short, wide neck that was evident in Legg-Calvé-Perthes disease. Measurements by Robichon and colleagues of the length and width of the femoral neck on radiographs of patients with this disease documented that the degree of shortening and widening of the neck was related to the extent of structural change in the head.

The greater trochanter possesses a separate blood supply, and can continue to develop despite growth disturbance in the adjacent bone. Eventually, it may appear disproportionately large in comparison to the shortened femoral neck.[227]

Pathologic Abnormalities. The fundamental pathologic aberration of the femoral head in this disease is osteonecrosis.[29-33] Necrosis of trabeculae and marrow is observed, which is eventually accompanied by structural failure of the femoral head, resulting in flattening and collapse. In the area of collapse, compression of trabeculae and intertrabecular, amorphous detritus are seen. As in other varieties of osteonecrosis, the chondral surfaces are remarkably well preserved during the early and intermediate stages of Legg-Calvé-Perthes disease. As opposed to the situation in other forms of osteonecrosis, however, separation of articular cartilage and underlying necrotic bone even in late stages of Legg-Calvé-Perthes disease is unusual.[224]

Healing is characterized by revascularization of the necrotic portion of the femoral head. Vessels that contribute to an increase in blood supply to the bone are the periosteal and marrow vessels of the neck, and the vessels in the ligamentum teres. Viable bone is deposited on dead trabeculae. Reconstitution of intertrabecular marrow may be accompanied by phagocytic and giant cell activity. Cystic areas containing necrotic trabeculae and detritus can be seen. In some cases, reconstitution of the femoral head is almost complete, although some degree of flattening of the head and shortening and broadening of the femoral neck is not unusual. The healing process appears to be more prominent in those cases in which the disorder begins at a young age,[1] although this is not a constant feature of early-onset Legg-Calvé-Perthes disease.[33]

Course of Disease. The course of Legg-Calvé-Perthes disease is variable. The degree of reconstitution of the ossific nucleus and the ultimate shape of the femoral head are dependent on the amount of necrosis, its exact location, and the magnitude of forces across the joint. In some instances, the eventual radiographic appearance of the involved head may be indistinguishable from its uninvolved counterpart (Fig. 78–3), whereas in others, coxa plana, shortening and widening of the femoral neck, degenerative joint disease, and intra-articular osseous bodies may be identified (Figs. 78–4 to 78–6).

In most cases of Legg-Calvé-Perthes disease, changes are isolated to or predominantly involve one

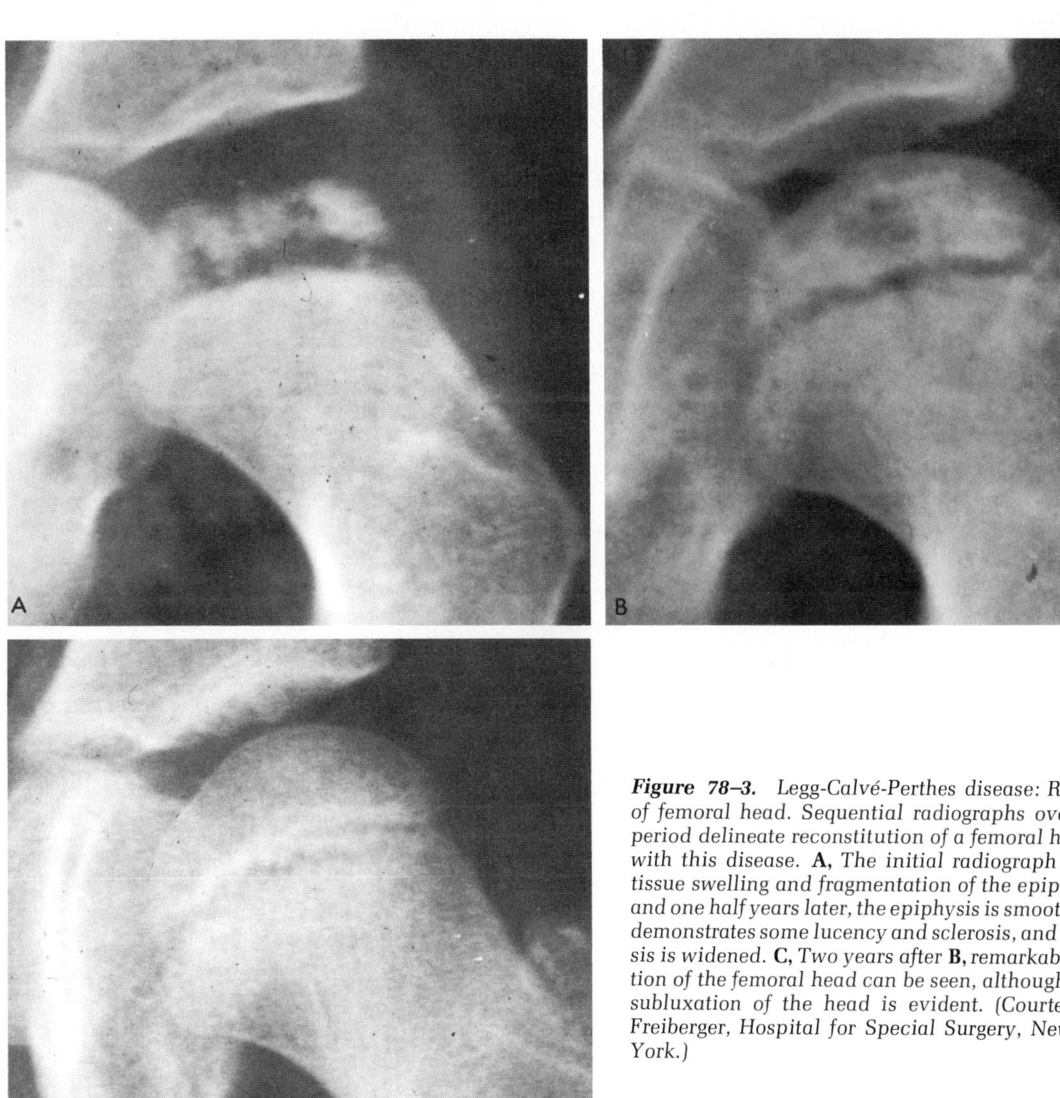

Figure 78–3. *Legg-Calvé-Perthes disease: Reconstitution of femoral head. Sequential radiographs over a 3½ year period delineate reconstitution of a femoral head involved with this disease.* **A,** *The initial radiograph outlines soft tissue swelling and fragmentation of the epiphysis.* **B,** *One and one half years later, the epiphysis is smooth, although it demonstrates some lucency and sclerosis, and the metaphysis is widened.* **C,** *Two years after* **B,** *remarkable reconstitution of the femoral head can be seen, although mild lateral subluxation of the head is evident. (Courtesy of Dr. R. Freiberger, Hospital for Special Surgery, New York, New York.)*

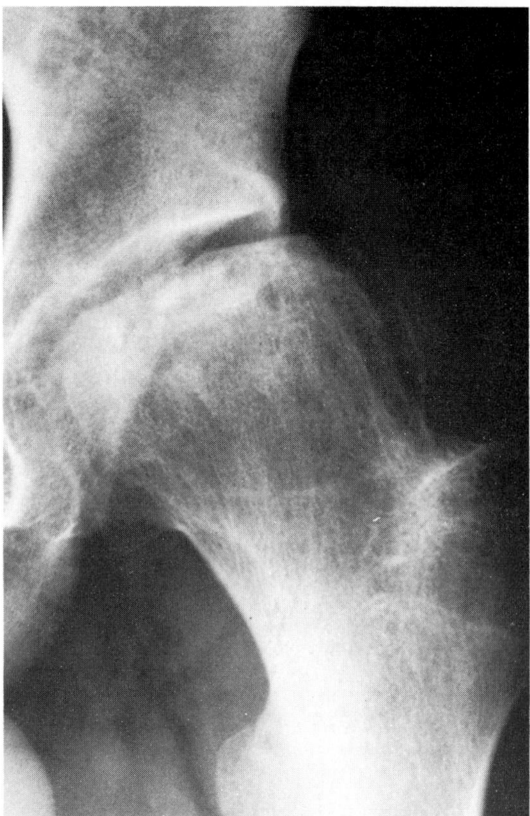

Figure 78–4. Legg-Calvé-Perthes disease: *Coxa plana and coxa magna. This 14 year old boy with known Legg-Calvé-Perthes disease reveals residual flattening and enlargement of the femoral head with surface irregularity and widening of the femoral neck. The acetabulum is mildly flattened.*

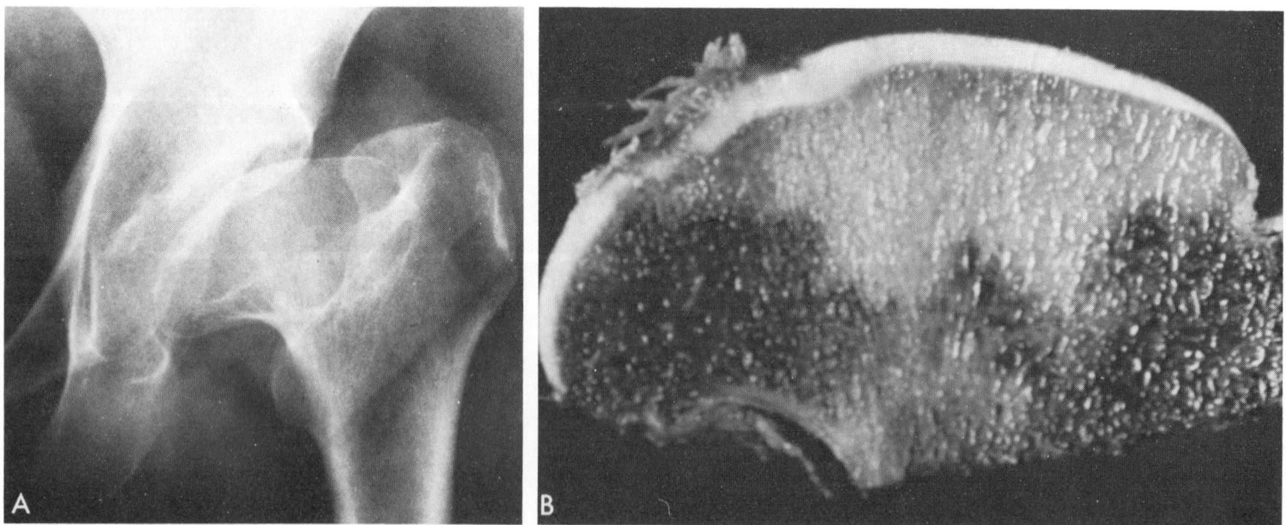

Figure 78–5. Legg-Calvé-Perthes disease: *Coxa plana and coxa magna. This 53 year old man had had Legg-Calvé-Perthes disease as a child and had experienced pain and tenderness in the left hip.*

A *Note the smoothly flattened femoral head, the prominent greater trochanter, and the flattened acetabular margin.*

B *A coronal section of the femoral head following total hip replacement reveals the flattened osseous contour and the remarkable preservation of the chondral surface.*

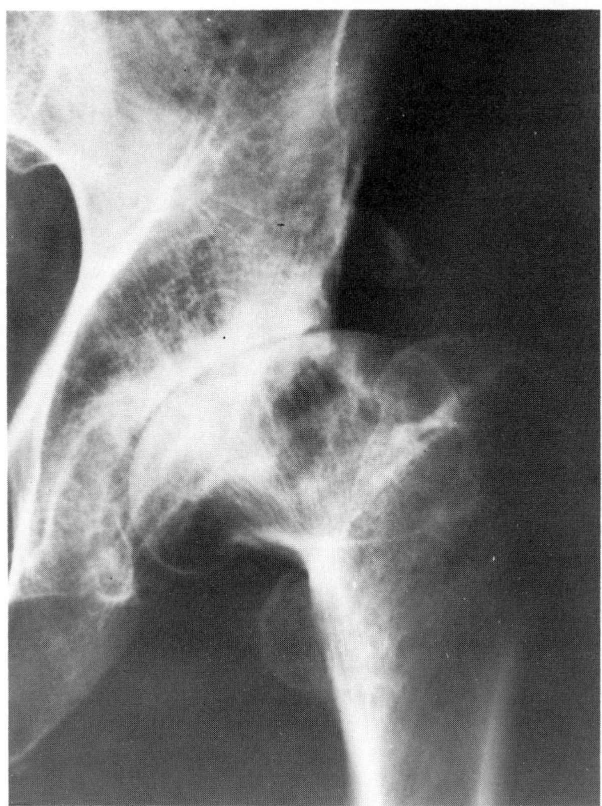

Figure 78–6. Legg-Calvé-Perthes disease: Secondary degenerative joint disease. This 60 year old man with a history of Legg-Calvé-Perthes disease developed secondary degenerative joint disease, characterized by articular space narrowing, and sclerosis. Note lateral subluxation and cystic lesions of the femoral head and buttressing of the medial portion of the femoral neck.

hip. In an extensive review of 147 patients with this disease, Nevelös[221] noted the simultaneous onset of changes in both hips that progressed concurrently in only two patients (approximately 1 per cent of cases). Additionally he observed six patients (approximately 4 per cent) who had simultaneous involvement of both sides but in whom only one side revealed fragmentation. Sixty-two patients (42 per cent) had "unilateral" disease with minimal radiographic changes in the opposite hip (irregularities in density or outline of epiphysis or metaphysis); nine patients (6 per cent) had "unilateral" disease affecting first one hip and then, after a clear interval, the other hip; and 68 patients (46 per cent) had purely unilateral disease. Other investigators have noted mild radiographic changes in the "normal" hip in children with "unilateral" Legg-Calvé-Perthes disease.[222] The nature of these changes is unknown, although clinical findings are generally lacking. Their relationship to findings in "minimal" Legg-Calvé-Perthes disease[223] is unclear.

Although the chondral surface is relatively uninvolved in this disease, joint incongruity can lead to secondary osteoarthritis with cartilaginous fibrillation and erosion.[34] This complication may be more prominent in patients with irregularly healed femoral heads than in those with normal or smoothly flattened heads.

A detached osteochondral fragment (osteochondritis dissecans) can be seen in this disease.[14, 16, 35, 36, 219, 220] The reported incidence of this complication is approximately 2 to 4 per cent, and it is observed almost exclusively in male patients. The risk of developing a persistent, ununited osteocartilaginous fragment appears to increase in patients with a late clinical presentation.[14] Furthermore, the incidence of osteochondritis dissecans in Legg-Calvé-Perthes disease is greater in individuals with bilateral involvement. This incidence does not correlate with the degree of deformity of the head nor with the length or time of therapy. The average interval between the diagnosis of Legg-Calvé-Perthes disease and the presentation of an intra-articular osteocartilaginous body is about 8 years.

The pathogenesis of osteochondritis dissecans in this condition is not clear; it may be due to persistence of an ununited fragment or to fragmentation of a femoral head that is weakened by revascularization during the healing process. The superolateral aspect of the head is the typical location of the fragment. Usually, the osteocartilaginous body remains at its site of origin or becomes depressed into the parent bone. "Loose" bodies are unusual, but when present may account for symptoms and signs, including pain, limp, limitation of motion, and secondary degenerative joint disease. Although this complication may be diagnosed on plain roentgenograms, especially those obtained in a "frog-leg" position, arthrography (with or without tomography) may further delineate the nature and position of the fragment and the integrity of the overlying cartilage.[14] Furthermore, contrast opacification of the joint can identify purely cartilaginous fragments that cannot be recognized on plain films or tomograms.

Although recurrent episodes of infarction may be essential to the development of Legg-Calvé-Perthes disease, cases demonstrating clinical and radiographic evidence of recurrent disease are unusual.[37-39] In such cases, a second episode of disease occurs 3 to 6 years after the initial attack when the patients are between 6 and 11 years of age. Boys are more commonly affected. Clinical findings of increasing pain, restricted motion, and limp are associated with fragmentation of an epiphysis that had partially or completely healed from a previous episode of disease. It is possible that the initial alterations of the proximal capital femoral epiphysis in patients with recurrent disease represent not Legg-Calvé-Perthes disease but Meyer's dysplasia of the femoral head (see discussion later in this chapter).

Prognosis. It is the variability in the course of Legg-Calvé-Perthes disease that has led to investigations into the predictive value of certain radiographic or clinical signs in the eventual outcome of the disorder. In general, a better prognosis is observed in younger patients, perhaps indicating that a longer elapsed time prior to skeletal maturity allows more extensive remodeling and healing. Other prognostic signs related to the radiographic characteristics of the affected hip have been emphasized by Catterall,[40] who has utilized four classes or grades of involvement.

Group I. The anterior part of the epiphysis is the only affected site. Collapse and sequestration are not evident. Metaphyseal changes are unusual in the early stage of the disease, but may occur in later stages. Radiographically, the course of the disease is characterized by absorption of the involved segment, followed by regeneration commencing from the periphery.

Group II. Greater involvement is apparent. Collapse and sequestration are followed by absorption and healing. A viable medial and lateral bony segment provides osseous support and maintains epiphyseal height.

Group III. Only a small portion of the epiphysis is not sequestered. Anteroposterior radiographs reveal a "head-within-a-head" appearance, and collapse of a centrally placed sequestrum is identified. The lateral fragment is often small and osteoporotic, appearing as specks of calcification. From the onset of collapse, this osteoporotic segment and its associated growth plate are displaced in an anterolateral direction, accounting for subsequent broadening of the femoral neck. A small, viable posterior segment may be evident. The course of the disease is similar to that in Group II, although metaphyseal changes are more generalized.

Group IV. The whole epiphysis is affected. Total collapse is associated with loss of height between the growth plate and acetabular roof. Epiphyseal displacement can occur anteriorly or posteriorly, and a mushroom-like appearance of the head can be identified. Metaphyseal changes may be extensive.

The purpose of this classification system is to allow identification of the degree of epiphyseal involvement and to relate this involvement to the prognosis of the disease. In general, patients in Groups III and IV have a relatively poor prognosis, whereas those in Groups I and II do better.[198] These generalizations are not without exception, as some patients in Groups III and IV have an unexpectedly good result, whereas others in Group II have a poor result. An additional limitation of this classification system is a difficulty in recognizing which pattern is present at an early phase of the disease;[226] at times, patients initially placed in one category will shift to another class on follow-up roentgenograms.[216] Catterall attempted to improve the predictive value of early radiographic changes by identifying four radiologic signs that indicated a capital femoral epiphysis "at risk" for collapse. These findings are: (1) Gage's sign (a small, osteoporotic segment that forms a transradiant "V" on the lateral side of the epiphysis); (2) calcification lateral to the epiphysis (reflecting the presence of extruded cartilage); (3) lateral subluxation of the head; and (4) a transverse epiphyseal line. Murphy and Marsh[41] found that these four "head-at-risk" signs and a fifth, diffuse metaphyseal reaction, correlated better with a poor radiologic result than did the degree of epiphyseal involvement. Dickens and Menelaus[42] observed that the most reliable radiologic factors indicating the prognosis of the disease were the Catterall grouping, the extent of uncovering of the femoral head, the presence of calcification lateral to the outer limit of the acetabulum, and the lateral displacement of the femoral head.

It is evident that no simple radiologic observation is indicative of a good or poor result, and that a combination of findings must be utilized for prognostic accuracy. Most patients are symptom-free 30 to 40 years later, although persistent roentgenographic alterations are usually evident. Mild limp, leg shortening, and pain can be seen.[43]

OTHER DIAGNOSTIC MODALITIES. *Arthrography* may be utilized in the evaluation of Legg-Calvé-Perthes disease.[44] In the early stages, contrast opacification of the joint can reveal subtle flattening of the chondral surface at the site of osseous fissuring, and an increase in width of both the femoral and acetabular cartilage. Synovial and soft tissue thickening may[45] or may not[44] be seen. In later stages, arthrography frequently indicates a smooth cartilaginous surface despite the presence of considerable ossific fragmentation (Fig. 78–7). Flattening and lateral extrusion of the chondral coat can be identified in some instances. In late stages of remodeling, the cartilaginous shape generally parallels that of the reconstituted ossification center. A detached or attached osteochondral fragment may be outlined. As arthrography more accurately identifies the actual size and shape of the abnormal femoral head than does plain film radiography and, in fact, will commonly define a marked enlarged osteochondral femoral head, it is a useful guide for the orthopedic surgeon who is interested in knowing what percentage of the head is contained within the acetabulum.[208]

Radionuclide examination with bone-seeking radiopharmaceuticals can identify an area of deficient uptake in the early phase of the disease, due to varying degrees of impairment of the blood supply.[46-48, 210] This defect is seen most frequently in the anterolateral aspect of a femoral head with partial necrosis and across the entire width of the epiphysis in a head with total necrosis. The scintigraphic abnormality antedates radiographic alterations and coincides with the onset of clinical manifestations (Fig. 78–8). It has been suggested that the size and pattern of the radionuclide defect in early stages of the disease may be correlated with the ultimate prognosis of the disease,[212] especially if computer processing of the scintigraphic data is utilized.[211, 218] With the appearance

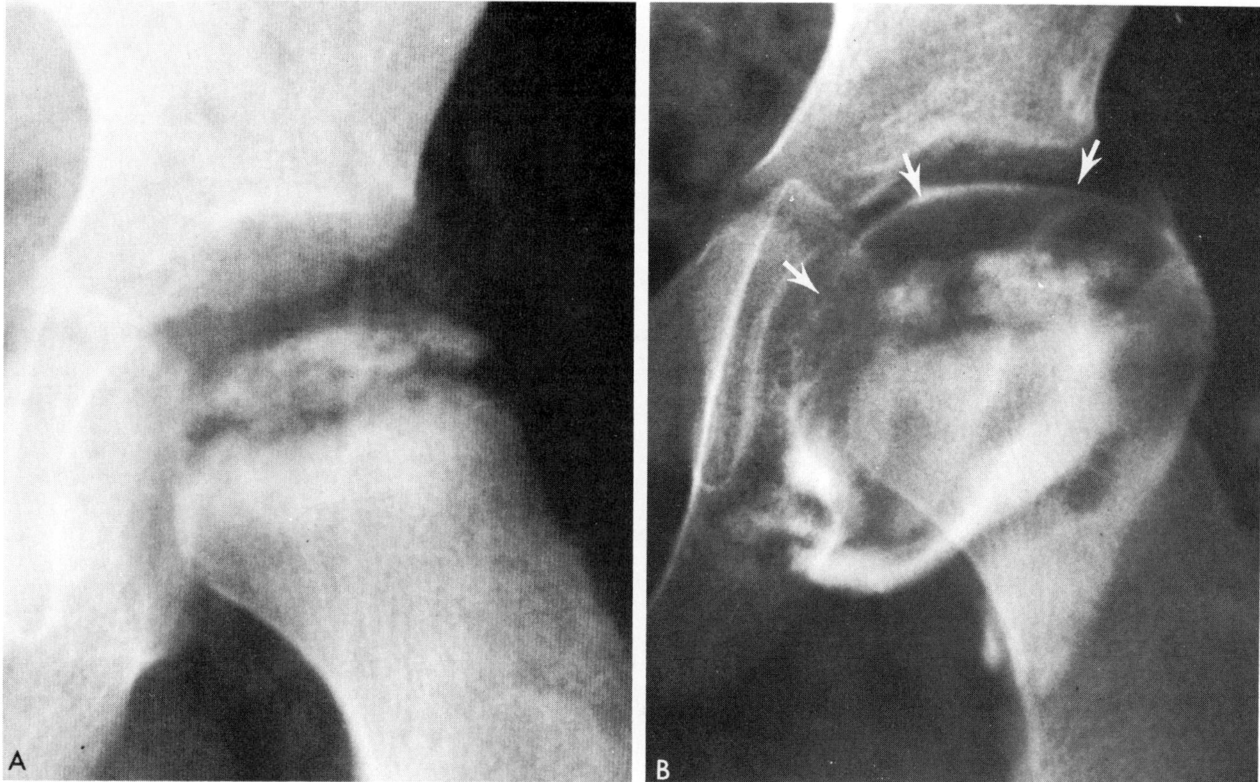

Figure 78–7. *Legg-Calvé-Perthes disease: Arthrographic abnormalities. This 5 year old boy developed Legg-Calvé-Perthes disease of the left hip.*

A *The radiograph reveals fragmentation and increased density of the epiphysis, with mild lateral subluxation.*

B *One month later, an arthrogram reveals a relatively smooth cartilaginous surface (arrows) despite the presence of extensive ossific irregularity. There is some thickening of the medial chondral surface of the femoral head.*

(Courtesy of Dr. T. Goergen, Palomar Hospital, Escondido, California.)

of regeneration and increased vascularity, the photodeficient areas may return to normal or be replaced by areas of augmented activity.[213] A follow-up scan that outlines a focus of deficient activity at a site that was previously normal may indicate a second episode of infarction.

Angiography has been employed as an investigative modality in some patients with Legg-Calvé-Perthes disease.[209] In the early phases of the disease, angiography is not especially useful, although it may demonstrate an interruption of the superior capsular arteries. Subsequently the procedure may allow identification of the size and the position of sequestered fragments of bone as well as of the distribution of revascularized osseous segments.

Intraosseous venography has also been utilized as a means of evaluating the prognosis in patients with this disease.[214]

Etiology and Pathogenesis. It is generally held that vascular insufficiency to the femoral head triggers the radiographic and pathologic findings in Legg-Calvé-Perthes disease, although the factors leading to deficiency of blood supply have not been precisely identified. Trueta's investigations of blood supply to the femoral head during growth identified a vulnerable period between the ages of 4 and 8 years in which the retinacular arteries represented the only important vascular route to the epiphysis, whereas a double vascular supply existed at younger (metaphyseal and retinacular arteries) and older (foveal and retinacular arteries) ages.[49] In adolescence and adulthood, three groups of vessels supply the proximal femur (foveal, retinacular, and metaphyseal arteries). This analysis is interesting, but does not account for those cases in which infants are affected, nor for the predilection of the disease for boys. Trueta did suggest that a more abundant foveal vascular supply in blacks might explain the relative infrequency of Legg-Calvé-Perthes disease in black individuals.

Caffey[15] favored a traumatic etiology in which direct compression of the femoral head by the adjacent acetabular roof led to the characteristic radiographic features of the disease, including fracture, flattening, and sclerosis. He emphasized the general retardation of bone development that can be identified in patients with this disease, a finding that has been confirmed by other investigators,[50–52, 199] and

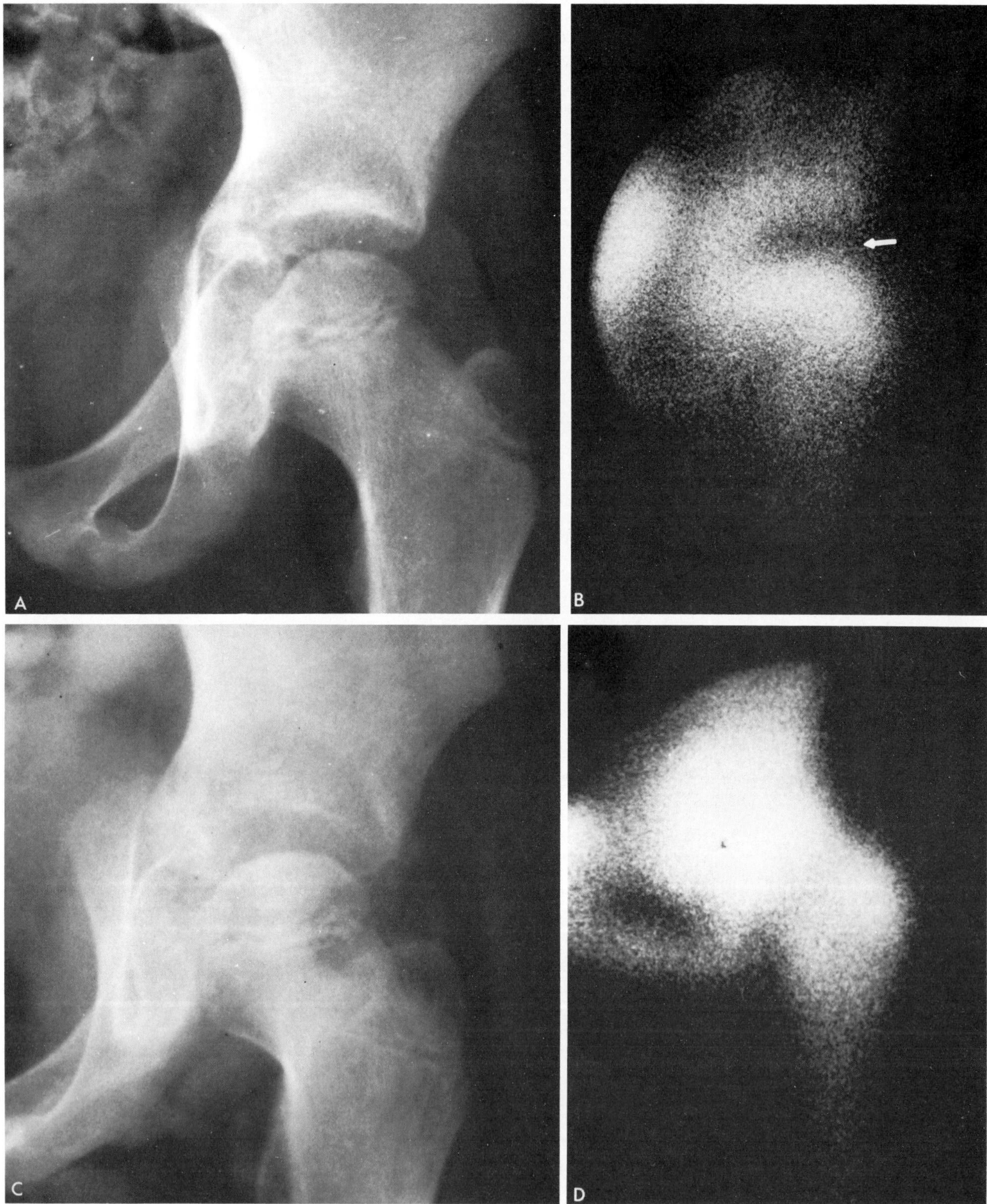

Figure 78–8. Legg-Calvé-Perthes disease: Radionuclide abnormalities.

A, B *An initial radiograph of a painful left hip in this young girl is equivocally abnormal, but the corresponding bone scan utilizing technetium pyrophosphate reveals a definite area of decreased activity in the left hip (arrow) consistent with early Legg-Calvé-Perthes disease.*

C, D *Three months later, the capital femoral epiphysis is slightly dense and flattened, and a metaphyseal lucent area is evident. At a slightly later time, a repeat scan reveals increased radionuclide activity in the hip.*

(Courtesy of Dr. John Wilcox, Naval Hospital, San Diego, California.)

suggested that concomitantly retarded supporting connective tissues about the hip might not be able to provide adequate support for the normal heavy stresses in this location. Primary traumatic events producing osseous collapse or traumatic synovitis could lead to compression of adjacent vasculature and secondary osteonecrosis of the head. In addition to arterial insufficiency, disturbed patterns of venous drainage have been identified.[57]

There is experimental evidence that suggests that more than one episode of ischemia and infarction is required for the development of osteonecrosis of the proximal capital femoral epiphysis.[54, 55] Pathologic data in humans underscore the importance of multiple infarctions.[31, 32, 56] The requirement of repeated vascular insults in the production of the disease could explain the chronicity of the disorder, the occurrence of recurrent clinical and radiographic findings, and the eventual appearance of significant growth disturbance.

The role of synovitis and raised intra-articular pressure in the pathogenesis of Legg-Calvé-Perthes disease has also been emphasized. Kemp[58] produced changes in the femoral heads of puppies that simulated those in osteonecrosis by artifically raising the intracapsular pressure for various lengths of time. Legg-Calvé-Perthes disease has been identified in as many as 12 per cent of patients with transient synovitis of the hip.[53] A history of synovitis or the presence of thickening and sclerosis of the capsular and synovial tissues on pathologic examination in individuals with this disease could indicate that the obliteration of blood supply to the femoral head is caused by vascular compression from accumulation of intra-articular fluid.

Finally, the delayed skeletal maturation of individuals with this disease and the reported higher frequency of congenital anomalies in extraskeletal sites have suggested to some investigators that genetic and developmental factors may be important. The possibility must be considered that congenital alterations in the blood vessels supplying the femoral capital epiphysis or in the normal development of the acetabulum and femur may lead to vascular or mechanical factors that predispose the individual to subsequent osseous collapse. It is obvious that further experimental and clinical data need to be collected before the true etiology and pathogenesis of this disease can be identified.[217]

Differential Diagnosis. Fragmentation and collapse of the femoral head can be seen in hypothyroidism and in osteonecrosis due to other causes (sickle cell anemia, Gaucher's disease, corticosteroid medication). The appearance of femoral head necrosis in a black patient should lead to hemoglobin analysis before the changes are ascribed to Legg-Calvé-Perthes disease. Similarly, bilateral symmetric alterations should be interpreted cautiously, as they are uncommon in the latter disease.

Meyer's dysplasia of the femoral head[59] is characterized by retarded skeletal maturation, mild or absent clinical signs, and femoral bony nuclei that appear late and are small and granular. The abnormal femoral head epiphyses are usually apparent by the age of 2 years, and are gradually transformed over the ensuing 2 to 4 years by growth and coalescence into enlarging, normal-appearing ossification centers. Sclerosis and metaphyseal changes are not evident in Meyer's dysplasia, and bilaterality is seen in almost 50 per cent of cases. Residua are unusual, although slight or moderate coxa plana is occasionally recognized. The earlier age of onset, the bilateral nature of the changes, the absence of prominent radiographic abnormalities, and the lack of progression are all features that allow differentiation of Meyer's dysplasia from Legg-Calvé-Perthes disease.

Freiberg's Infraction

In 1914, Freiberg[60] described a series of patients with metatarsalgia in whom the metatarsal head appeared to be crushed or collapsed, terming the condition an infraction of bone. Despite the attention that an additional early investigator, Köhler, paid to this condition, Freiberg is usually credited with the first analysis. Both of these men emphasized the typical involvement of the head of the second metatarsal, although it is now recognized that the third and fourth metatarsal heads can also be affected and, in rare instances, perhaps the first metatarsal head as well (see *Hallux rigidus*, Chapter 39).[1, 61-66] Unilateral changes are characteristic, although bilateral involvement and alterations of more than one digit can be encountered (Fig. 78–9).

Women predominate among patients affected with this disease, the ratio of women to men being approximately 3 or 4:1. The disease is usually seen in adolescents between the ages of 13 and 18 years; rare examples of younger or older patients can be uncovered in a review of available literature, and even adults in the fourth to sixth decades of life occasionally first present with evidence of Freiberg's infraction. Clinical manifestations consist of local pain, tenderness, and swelling, and limitation of motion of the corresponding metatarsophalangeal joint. Disabling symptoms and signs can be evident and may require surgical intervention.

Roentgenographic abnormalities include, initially, subtle flattening, increased radiodensity, and cystic lucent lesions of the metatarsal head and widening of the metatarsophalangeal articulation (Fig. 78–10); and, subsequently, an osteochondral fragment with progressive flattening and sclerosis of the metatarsal head, and periostitis with increased cortical thickening of the adjacent metaphysis and diaphysis of the bone (Fig. 78–11). Premature closure of the growth plate, intra-articular osseous

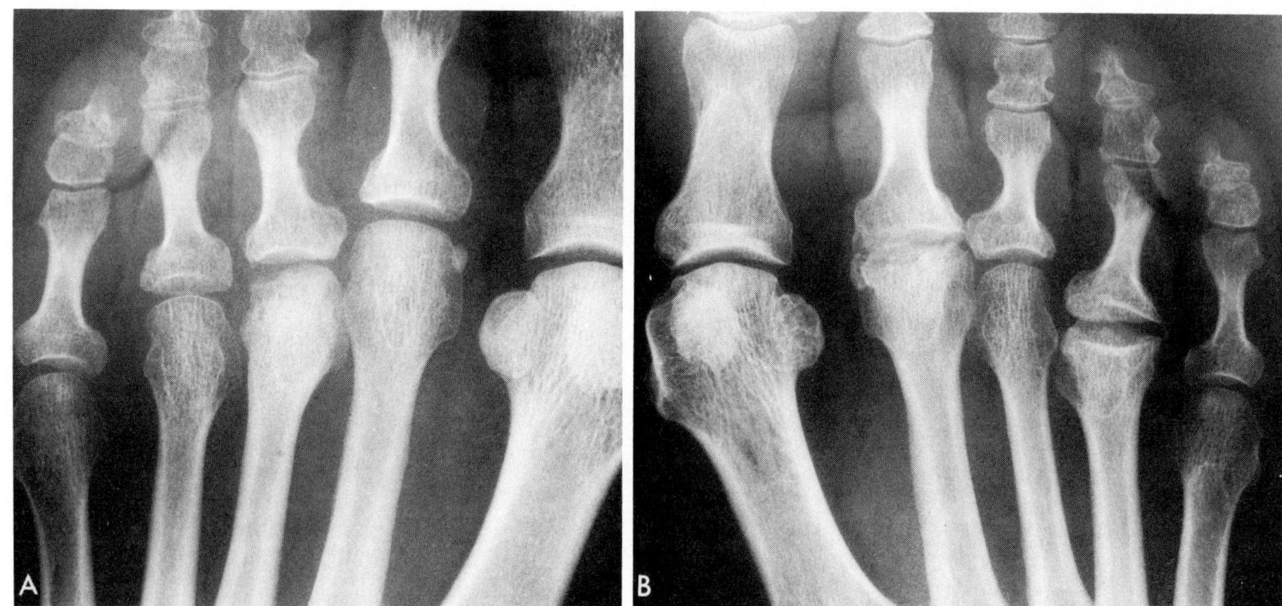

Figure 78–9. *Freiberg's infraction: Bilateral involvement. This 48 year old woman complained of pain and tenderness about several metatarsal heads in both feet.*

A *Note the sclerosis and collapse of the third metatarsal head, with narrowing of the adjacent metatarsophalangeal joint. There is equivocal increased density of the second metatarsal head as well. Adjacent phalangeal new bone formation is seen.*

B *On the opposite foot, the heads of the second and fourth metatarsals are fragmented and flattened. Note the expansion of the corresponding phalangeal bases.*

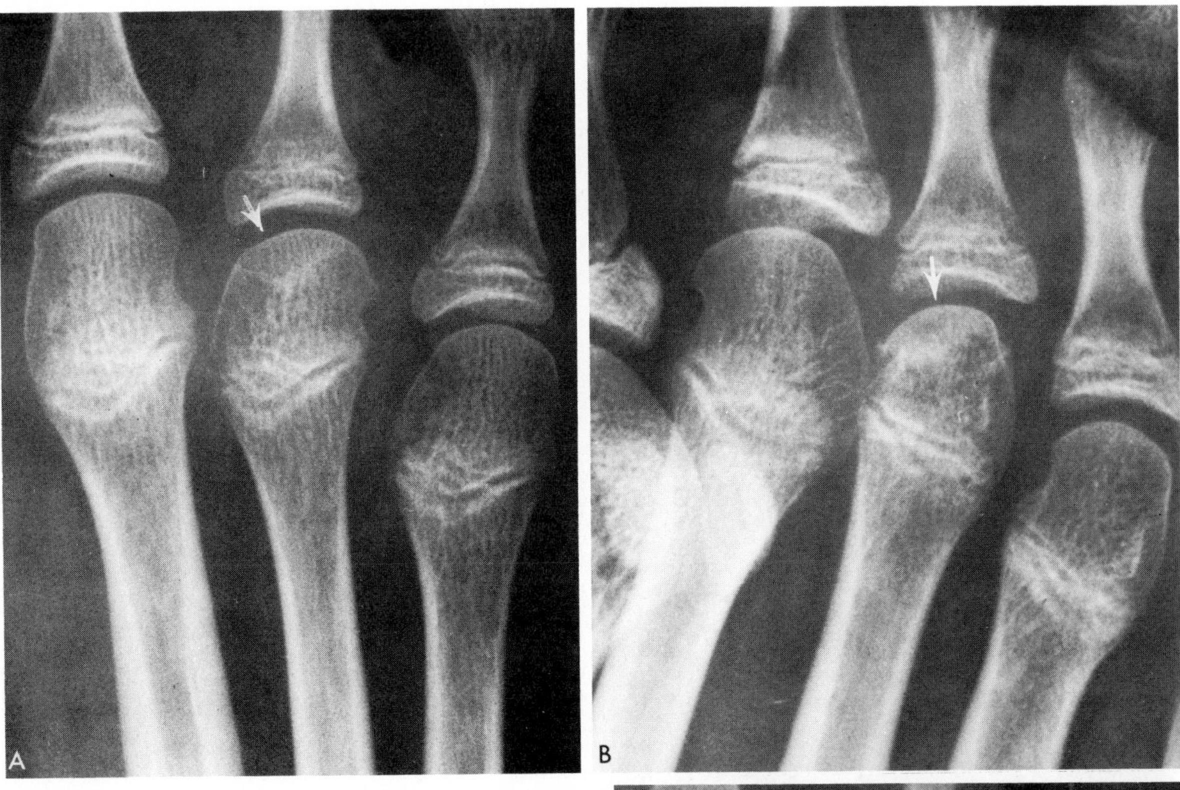

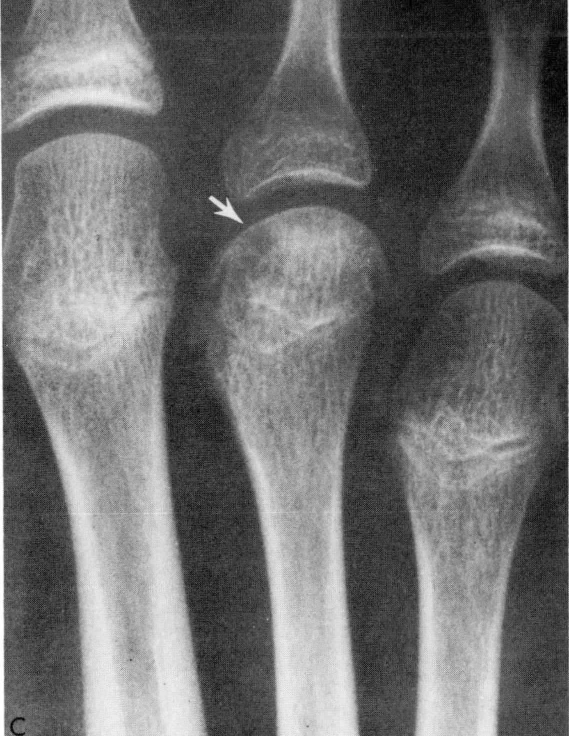

Figure 78–10. Freiberg's infraction: Early radiographic abnormalities. A 14 year old girl developed pain and swelling over the metatarsophalangeal joint. She denied a history of trauma.

A *An initial radiograph reveals minimal increased radiodensity of the head of the third metatarsal (arrow).*

B *Two weeks later, the depression of the articular surface of the metatarsal head and the sclerosis are more apparent (arrow).*

C *Four months after* **B,** *considerable collapse with shortening of the metatarsal is evident (arrow).*

bodies, deformity and enlargement of the metatarsal head, and secondary degenerative joint disease are recognized complications of the process (Fig. 78–12). The nearby phalangeal base may enlarge and appear irregular.

Pathologic aberrations have been well summarized.[1] Microscopic evidence of necrosis of trabeculae and marrow can be seen at a stage in which the radiographs are entirely normal. Comminution of subchondral trabeculae can be associated with

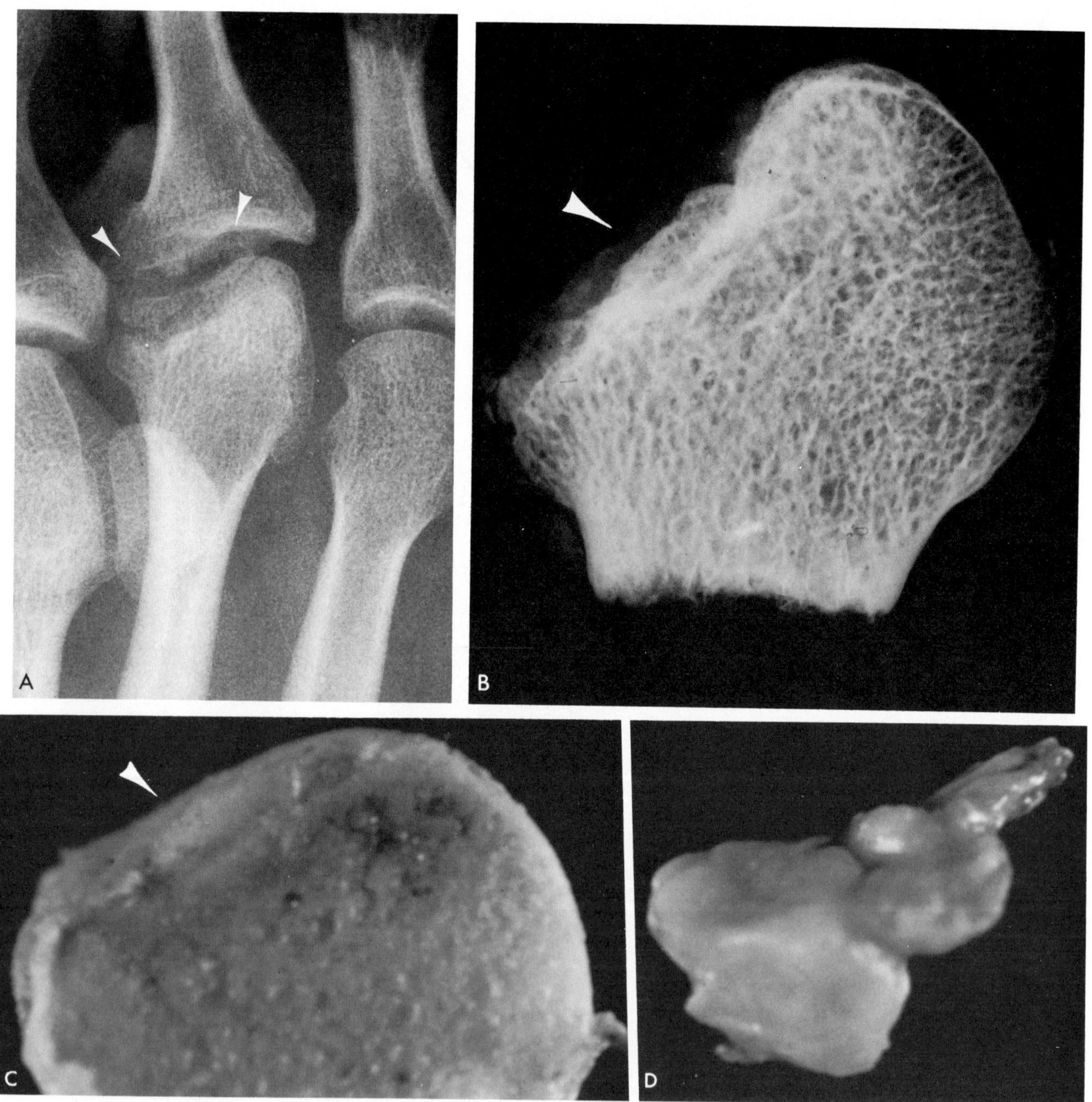

Figure 78–11. *Freiberg's infraction: Later radiographic abnormalities. This 36 year old man had had pain in his second toe for 12 years. A "loose" body had been removed from the second metatarsophalangeal joint 2 years prior to his current evaluation.*

A *Note the flattened metatarsal head with two osteochondral fragments (arrowheads), osteophytosis, joint space narrowing, and widening of the phalangeal base.*

B, C *A radiograph and photograph of a section of the metatarsal head delineate the collapse and irregularity of the bone (arrowhead).*

D *Photograph of the removed intra-articular bodies.*

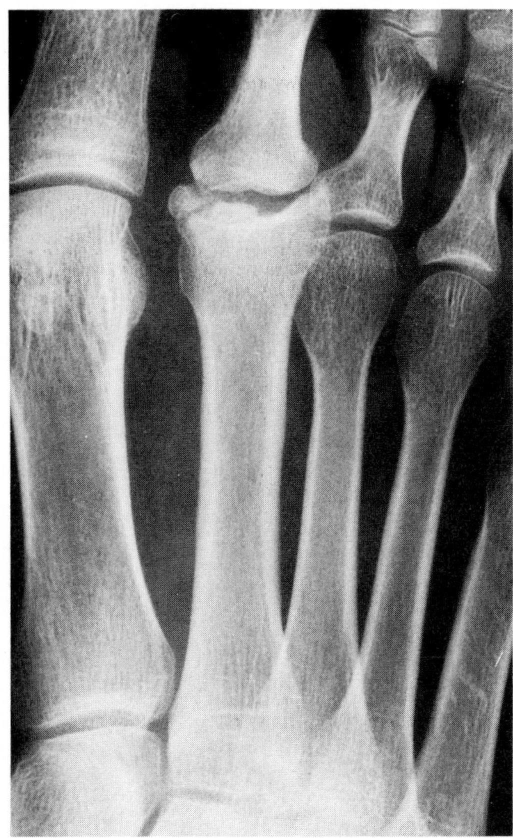

Figure 78–12. Freiberg's infraction: Residual deformities. In this 41 year old man, note residual flattening of the second metatarsal head, narrowing of the adjacent joint space, intra-articular osseous bodies, expansion of the phalangeal base, and widening of the second metatarsal with cortical thickening.

collapse and compression of the articular surface. Revascularization occurs through vascular invasion from the periosteum and metaphyseal regions. Resorption of necrotic trabeculae, osseous regeneration, highly vascular intertrabecular marrow, and cortical thickening related to subperiosteal bony apposition are observed. Complete healing is not usually seen, and even after many years, evidence of previous osteonecrosis exists. Other long-term effects can include osteocartilaginous fragments that remain in situ or are displaced, secondary degenerative joint disease, and proliferative alterations of the base of the neighboring phalanx.

The pathogenesis of the disease process remains speculative. Prevailing opinion suggests that single or multiple episodes of trauma represent the primary event in Freiberg's infraction.[62] Experimental studies have indicated that the epiphysis of the second metatarsal is most vulnerable to injury owing to its relative length and firm fixation.[64] The high incidence of the disorder in women could conceivably be related to the wearing of high heeled shoes, which creates increased stress on the second metatarsal. Repeated injury at this site may then lead to disruption of the articular cartilage, ischemic necrosis of subchondral bone, compression fracture, collapse, and fragmentation.[200]

The radiographic features of Freiberg's infraction are virtually pathognomonic, as they indicate osteonecrosis at a characteristic site, the metatarsal head. Occasionally, other disorders, such as systemic lupus erythematosus, can produce bone necrosis at this location. Additional diseases leading to fragmentation of metatarsal heads with articular abnormality include rheumatoid arthritis, calcium pyrophosphate dihydrate crystal deposition disease, and gout, but other radiographic features allow accurate diagnosis. In some individuals, a mild degree of normal flattening of the articular surface of the metatarsal head, especially the second, in association with apparent widening of the joint space, can resemble Freiberg's infraction.

Kienböck's Disease

A peculiar affliction of the carpal lunate was described by Peste in 1843[67] and by Kienböck in 1910.[68] Because of the detailed description of the clinical and radiologic features of the disorder offered by the latter investigator, the designation of Kienböck's disease is most frequently utilized for this condition, although the term lunatomalacia is also encountered.[69-76] In regard to its incidence, Kienböck's disease is most commonly observed between the ages of 20 and 40 years, and has a predilection for the right hand in individuals engaged in manual labor; this latter characteristic may indicate that exaggerated use in the dominant hand produces the trauma necessary for the initiation of this condition (see discussion later in this chapter). Bilateral abnormalities occur but are less frequent than unilateral changes.[77]

A history of trauma may be elicited, but this is not a constant feature. Progressive pain, swelling, and disability can be apparent. Radiographic changes are distinctive. Initially, the lunate may have a normal architecture and density, but a linear or compression fracture can be delineated, especially on tomograms.[69, 78, 79, 201] Subsequently, an increased density of the lunate relative to the other carpal bones is noted, followed by evidence of altered shape and diminished size of the bone (Fig. 78–13). Eventually the entire lunate may collapse and fragment; the degree of fragmentation, particularly that of the posterior surface, can be well shown on lateral tomograms.[72] Complications include disruption of the carpal architecture, scapholunate separation or dissociation, ulnar deviation of the triquetrum, and secondary degenerative joint disease in the radiocarpal and midcarpal compartments of the wrist with articular space narrowing, sclerosis, osteophytosis, and cyst formation.

Pathologic descriptions emphasize the occur-

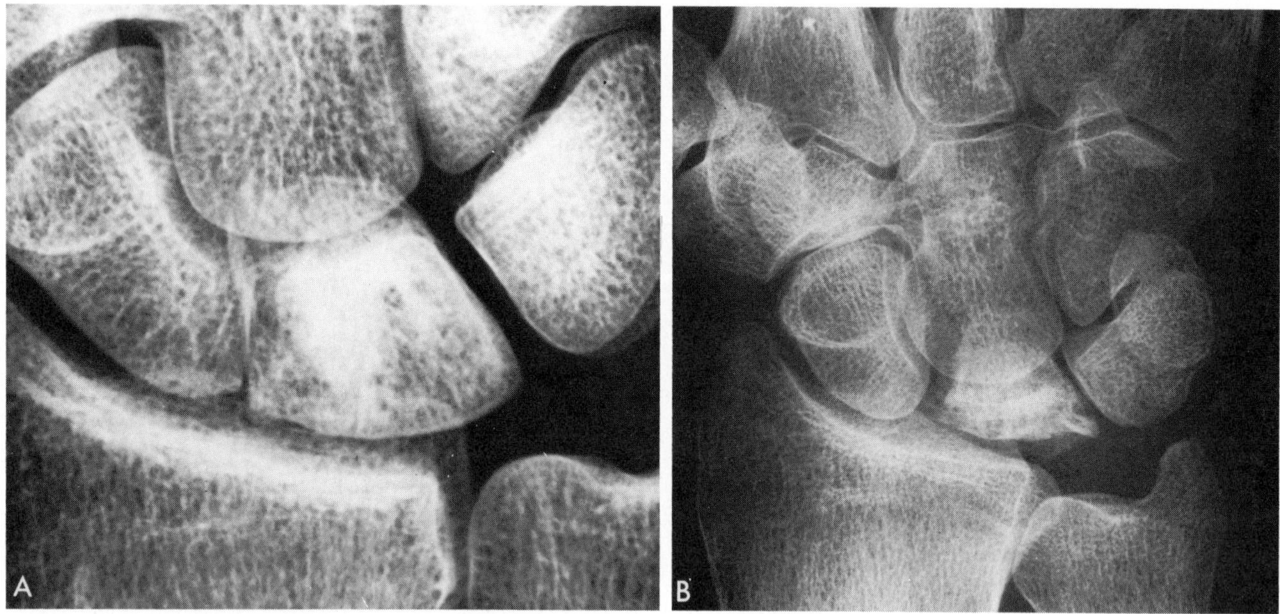

Figure 78–13. Kienböck's disease.
A *A magnification radiograph demonstrates patchy increased density of the lunate without alterations in the shape of the bone.*
B *In a different patient, observe the collapse of a sclerotic lunate bone.*

rence of both fracture and osteonecrosis.[1] An incomplete fracture line can be evident in the subchondral spongiosa of the proximal portion of the lunate associated with osteoclastic resorption, trabecular disintegration and granular detritus, and scar tissue in the intertrabecular marrow. Additional fractures appear, some of which violate the articular cartilage, and necrosis of adjacent trabeculae can be observed. Repair and regeneration are characterized by vascular proliferation and deposition of new bone. Secondary

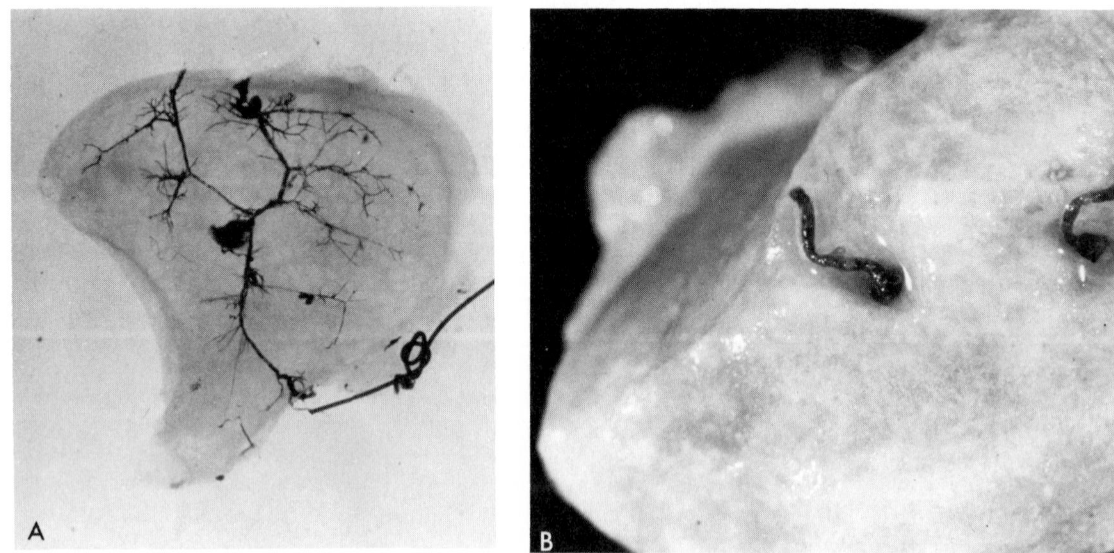

Figure 78–14. Lunate bone: Vascular supply.
A *A lateral view of a preparation of a lunate bone following vascular injection with latex reveals two dorsal vessels and one volar vessel that are anastomosing within the bone. In some cases, two vessels enter the volar aspect of the bone and one vessel enters the dorsal aspect (see B). In either case, a "Y" pattern of vascularity within the bone is seen, as anastomoses occur in the midportion of the lunate just distal to its center.*
B *A photograph of the volar surface of a different specimen demonstrates the anatomy of the two nutrient vessels.*
(From Gelberman RH, Menon J: J Hand Surg 5:272, 1980.)

degenerative joint disease is manifested as fibrillation and erosion of cartilage.

The etiology and pathogenesis of the condition are not clear. Its occurrence following single or repeated episodes of trauma is a prominent feature in many cases. Certain anatomic and biomechanical features of the lunate exist that may predispose this bone to injury and subsequent osteonecrosis.[1] These features include the following: (1) a vulnerable blood supply arising from vessels that enter the bone on its dorsal or volar aspect, anastomosing within its substance[80, 86, 202] (Fig. 78–14), and (2) a fixed position in the wrist, resulting in substantial forces of various orders of magnitude that may be greater than those on neighboring carpal bones.[81] Mechanical forces may be accentuated by the presence of a short ulna (ulna minus variant), a finding that can be encountered in as many as 75 per cent of cases.[82-84] This anatomic arrangement, which might be expected to produce exaggerated contact between the lunate and radius, is not uniformly considered an important finding in patients with Kienböck's disease[85]; furthermore, as Kienböck's disease is rare and ulna minus variance is not infrequent, other factors must be important in the pathogenesis of the disease.

Many methods have been utilized for the treatment of Kienböck's disease. Their success is influenced positively by early diagnosis prior to collapse of bone. In this regard, tomography and scintigraphy may be indicated in some instances. Furthermore, immobilization in equivocal cases may lead to osteoporosis of normal carpal bones, producing exaggerated radiodensity of an avascular lunate and allowing accurate diagnosis[69] (Fig. 78–15).

In cases in which increased radiodensity and collapse of the lunate are observed, the radiographic features are easily differentiated from other conditions affecting the wrist.

Köhler's Disease

The relationship of Köhler's disease of the tarsal navicular and osteonecrosis is not defined. Although some investigators regard the condition as a manifestation of normal or altered ossification, the discussion of this disorder is placed here because the predominant theory of its pathogenesis is still one of vascular insufficiency. The disease was first described in 1908 by Köhler[87] as a self-limited condi-

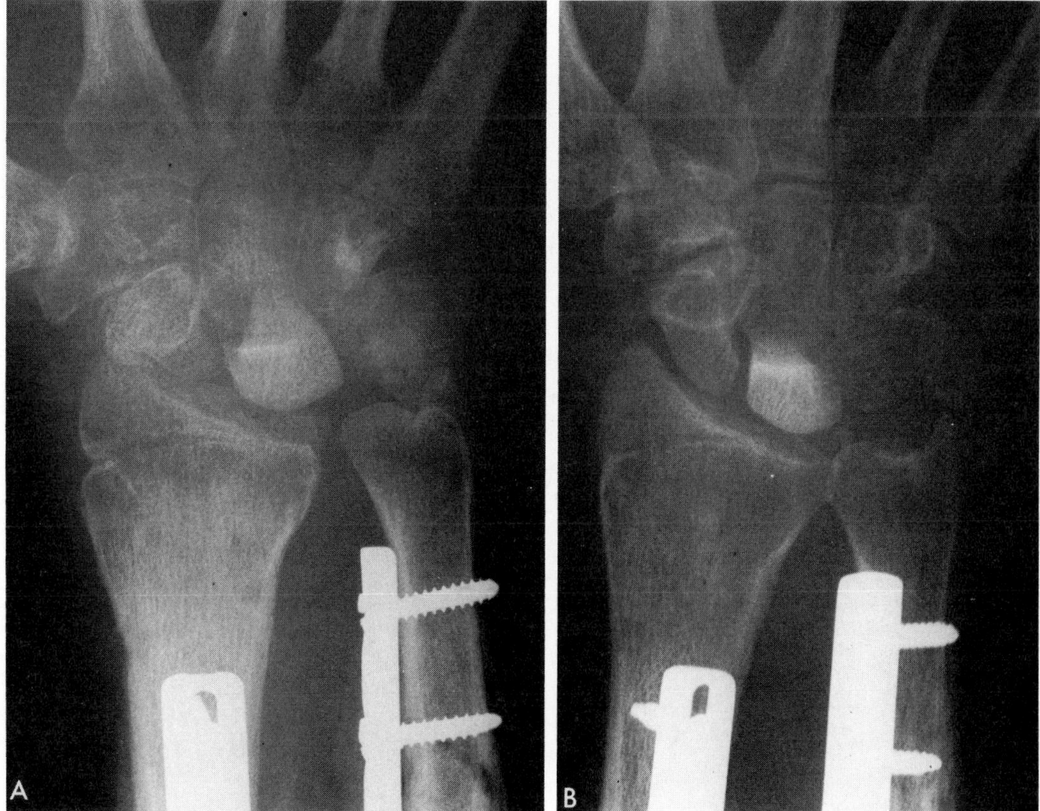

Figure 78–15. *Osteonecrosis of the lunate. This patient revealed multiple fractures of the distal radius and ulna with lunate dislocation following an injury. Two radiographs obtained several months apart reveal progressive osteoporosis of the distal radius and distal ulna and carpus, with increased radiodensity of the lunate. This indicates that the injury has disrupted the normal blood supply to the lunate. (Courtesy of Dr. V. Vint, Scripps Clinic, La Jolla, California.)*

tion of the tarsal navicular characterized by flattening, sclerosis, and irregular rarefaction. Köhler's disease is relatively rare, although its exact incidence is difficult to determine because the symptoms and signs may not be of sufficient magnitude to require radiography, and it is impossible to distinguish the radiographic abnormalities from those that occur as a normal variation of growth.

The disorder is more frequent in boys, the ratio of affected boys to affected girls being approximately

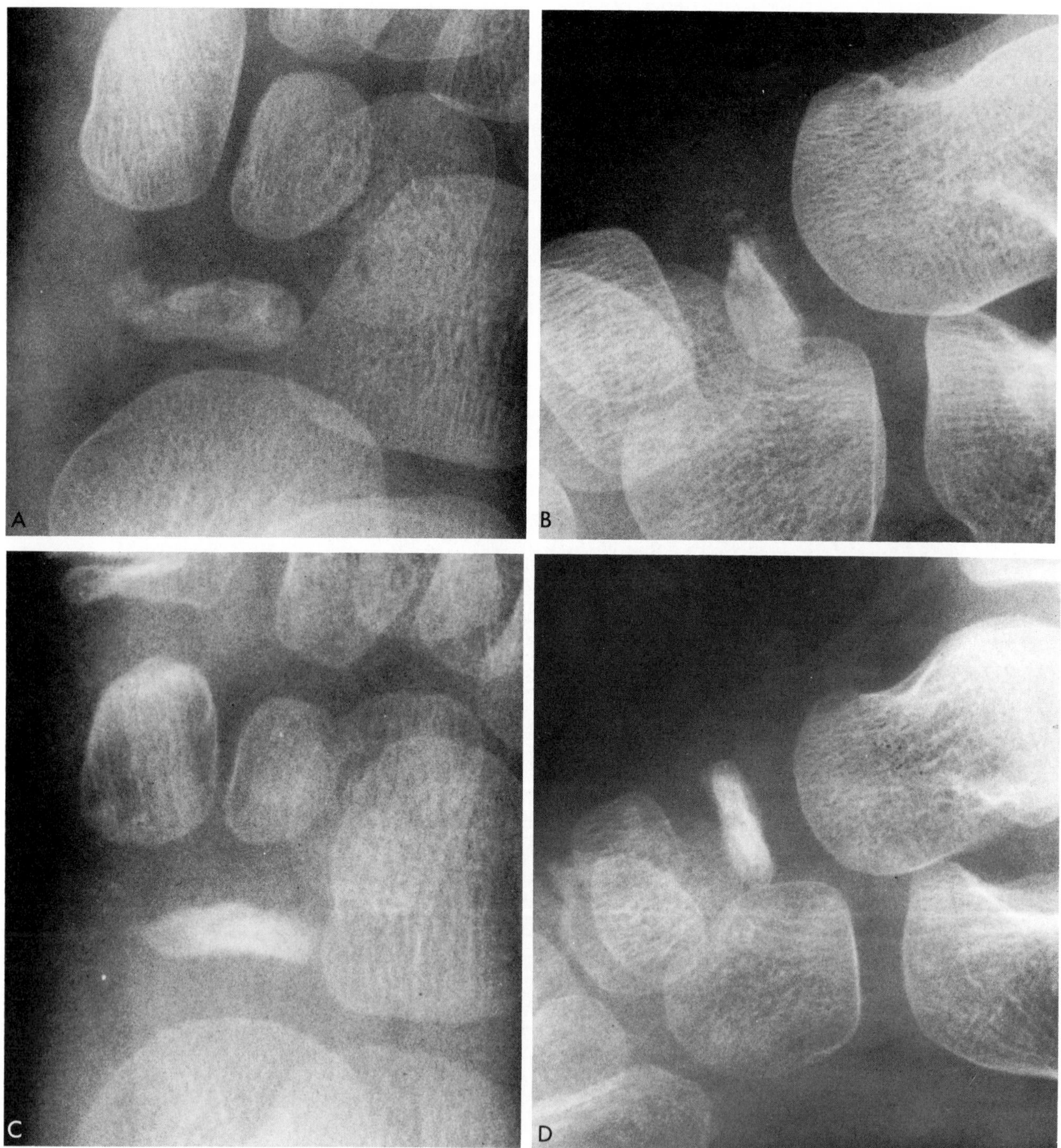

Figure 78–16. *Köhler's disease.*

A, B *In this 7 year old boy, anteroposterior and lateral radiographs reveal the small fragmented and slightly dense tarsal navicular bone. The interosseous spaces of the tarsus are not disturbed.*

C, D *In a 4 year old boy, a wafer-like radiodense tarsal navicular bone is identified. Again, the neighboring joint spaces are not diminished in width.*

4 to 6:1. Complaints are most commonly observed between the ages of 3 and 7 years, occurring at a younger age in girls. Unilateral involvement is evident in approximately 75 to 80 per cent of cases. Clinical manifestations may be quite mild, consisting of local pain, tenderness, swelling, and decreased range of motion.[88-90] The foot may be held in slight varus position so that the patient walks on the outer side of the foot.[1] A history of trauma can be elicited in about 35 per cent of cases. Köhler's disease may occur simultaneously with Legg-Calvé-Perthes disease.[91]

Roentgenograms at an early stage can reveal patchy increase in density, nodularity, and fragmentation with multiple ossific nuclei (Fig. 78–16*A*, *B*). Soft tissue swelling may be evident.[203] The bone may be diminished in size and flattened or wafer-like in appearance, yet the interosseous space between the navicular and neighboring bones can be normal, indicating an integrity of the chondral surface (Fig. 78–16*C*, *D*). Over a period of 2 to 4 years the bone may regain its normal size, density, and trabecular structure. It is the self-limited and reversible nature of the process that has led to speculation that the "disease" is, in reality, an altered sequence of tarsal ossification. Differences in the time of appearance, the degree of maturity, and the size, shape, and radiodensity of the ossifying navicular are common in many children, and even in cases of apparent unilateral disease the changes in the asymptomatic extremity may be remarkably similar to those on the symptomatic side. This apparent "overlap" with normal patterns of ossification leads to considerable difficulty in diagnosis, and certain criteria must be utilized in establishing the presence of Köhler's disease: (1) changes are detected in a previously normal navicular bone; (2) alterations consisting of resorption and reossification must be compatible with those of osteonecrosis.[92] Radionuclide examination can further substantiate the diagnosis by revealing diminished uptake of bone-seeking radiopharmaceuticals during the early stages of the process and accentuated uptake during revascularization.[90]

Pathologic data are meager.[1] A disturbance in endochondral ossification is suggested by the presence of a thickened zone of cartilage about the ossific nucleus.[93, 94] The latter structure may reveal signs of necrosis of both spongiosa and marrow.

There is evidence that Köhler's disease may have a mechanical basis. The location of the tarsal navicular at the apex of the longitudinal arch of the foot may lead to concentration of forces on this bone during normal locomotion. The forces may be further concentrated by the existence of a small space between the distal end of the talus and the first cuneiform, with resulting crowding of the navicular bone.[95] Compression of the bony nucleus at a critical phase of growth could result in altered ossification.[88] Compression forces may occlude vessels in the spongiosa of the bone, producing osteonecrosis.

The only major differential diagnostic consideration in this disease is that of a normal pattern of ossification of the navicular bone in some patients that may result in a fragmented and sclerotic appearance. Differentiation of the normal and abnormal states is discussed above.

Panner's Disease

Panner's disease, or osteochondrosis of the capitellum of the humerus, is a rare disease described in 1927 by Panner,[96] who was impressed by its resemblance to Legg-Calvé-Perthes disease. Further descriptions of this disorder have documented that it usually appears between the ages of 5 and 10 years, although it may be seen as early as 4 years and as late as 16 years.[97-102] Boys are almost exclusively affected, and the condition is commonly linked to a history of trauma. It is sometimes termed "little-leaguer's elbow" because of its frequency in young baseball pitchers.[103] Bilateral involvement is rare.

The clinical manifestations are typically mild, and complete recovery is frequent. Pain and stiffness, with restricted range of motion of the elbow (particularly extension), are seen. Local tenderness over the capitellum, synovial thickening and effusion, and flexion contracture can be detected on physical examination. Radiographs reveal fissuring and increased density of the capitellum, decreased size and condensation of bone with increase in the radiohumeral space, fragmentation, and resorption (Fig. 78–17*A*). These findings are usually more evident if comparison radiographs of the contralateral, uninvolved side are obtained. Regeneration and reconstitution of the capitellum are subsequently observed, and in most cases no residual deformity or disability is seen. Hyperemia can lead to abnormal skeletal maturation of the radial head.

The detection of a subchondral radiolucent band in the capitellum in the early stages of the disorder is reminiscent of findings in Legg-Calvé-Perthes disease.[104] This abnormality apparently relates to a fracture that in some cases is accompanied by accumulation of gas in the fissure. It probably indicates that osteonecrosis has occurred as a secondary event related to a traumatic insult, with disruption of blood supply to the bone. Panner's disease should be differentiated from osteochondritis dissecans of the elbow, which may occur in children or adults as a result of trauma, and which may lead to osteochondral fragments (Fig. 78–17*B*).

Thiemann's Disease

In 1909, Thiemann[105] described a teenaged boy with progressive enlargement of the proximal interphalangeal joints of the fingers. Additional re-

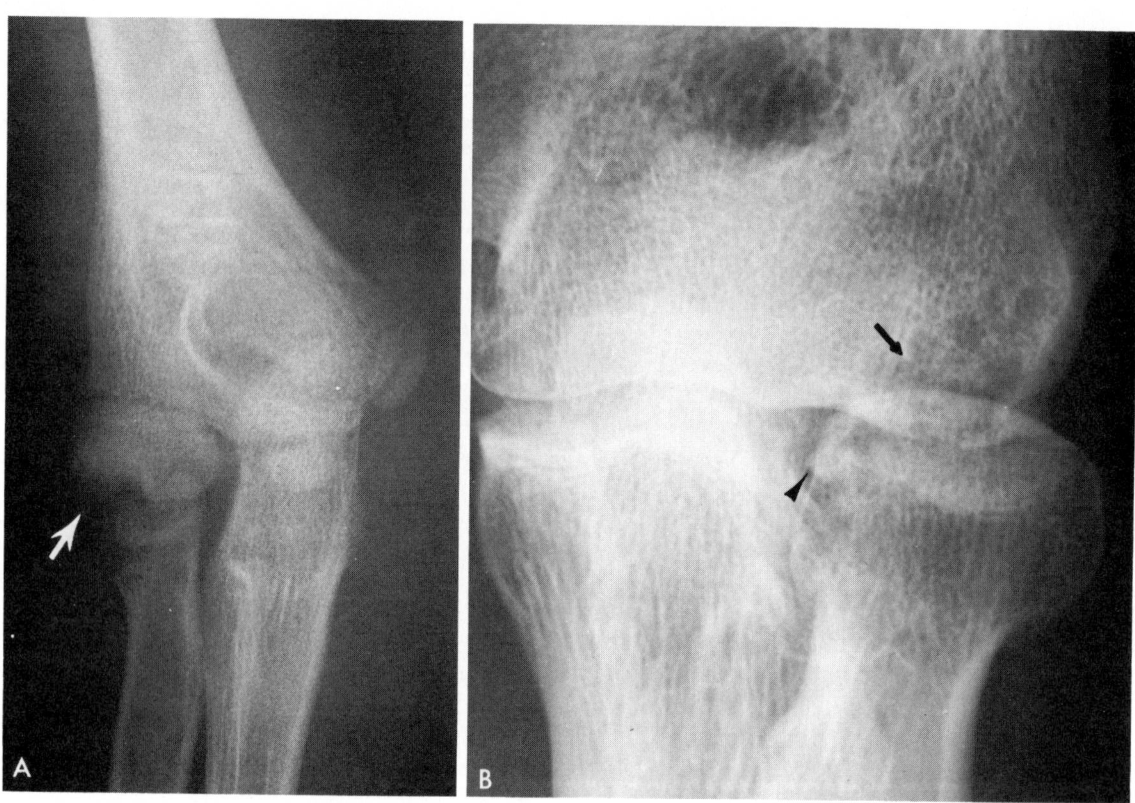

Figure 78–17. *Panner's disease.*

A *Findings include fissuring and fragmentation of the capitellum (arrow) and deformity of the adjacent radial head in this child with elbow pain and swelling. (Courtesy of Dr. V. Vint, Scripps Clinic, La Jolla, California.)*

B *Included in the differential diagnosis of Panner's disease is osteochondritis dissecans, as illustrated here. Observe the radiolucent lesion of the capitulum (arrow). Osteochondritis dissecans of the elbow can be observed in adults. Osteochondral fragments are not unusual (arrowhead).*

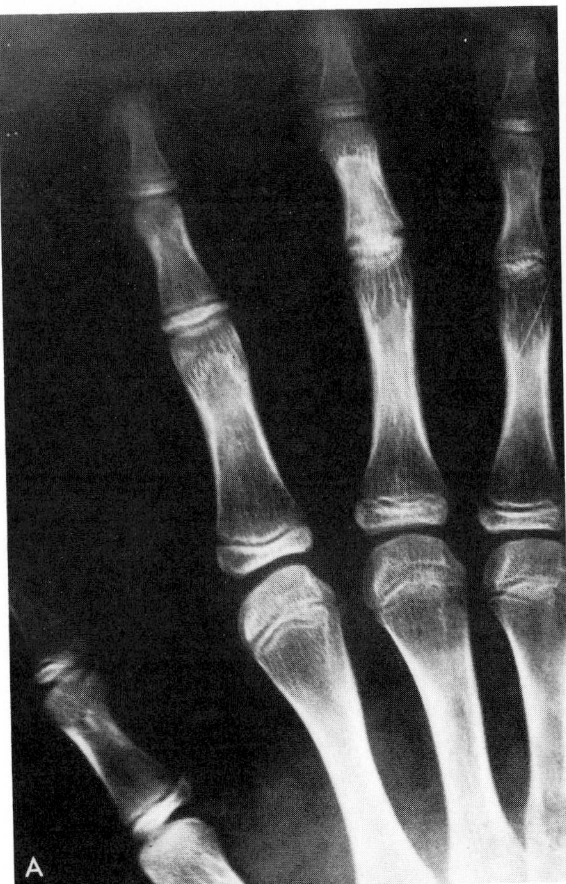

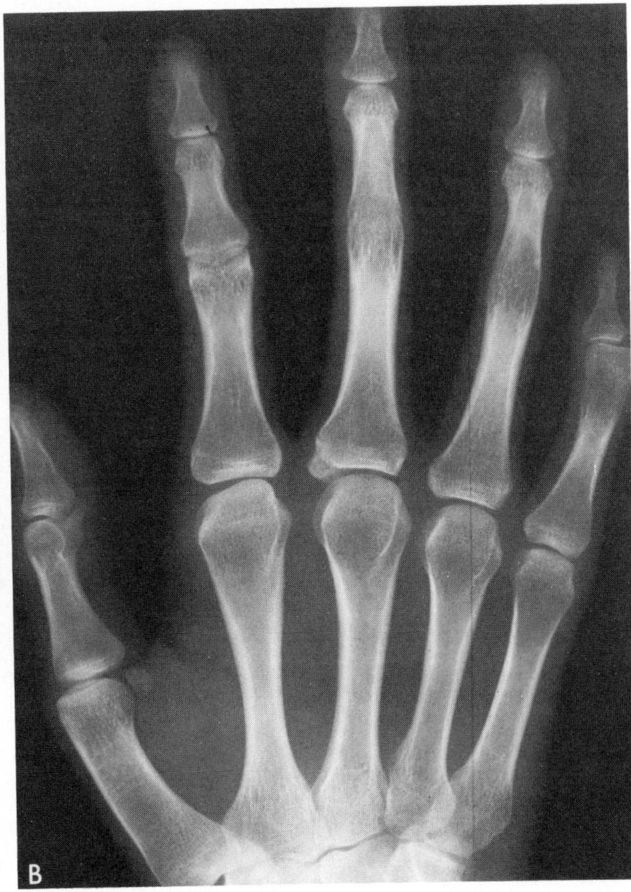

Figure 78–18. *Possible Thiemann's disease. This 10 year old girl developed pain and swelling of the proximal interphalangeal and metacarpophalangeal joints of the hands. Several family members had had similar abnormalities. Although the diagnosis is not proved and some features are atypical, Thiemann's disease is a prime consideration; juvenile chronic arthritis is another diagnostic possibility, as is familial coalition of joints (Shrewsbury mark).*

A *Note flattening and increased sclerosis of epiphyses of several metacarpals and phalanges, with expansion of the adjacent bony contour. Early fusion of the third and fourth proximal interphalangeal joints can be seen.*

B *Six years later, bony ankylosis of several proximal interphalangeal joints is observed. The metacarpal heads are irregular.*

(Courtesy of Dr. L. Goldberger, Scripps Clinic, La Jolla, California.)

ports of this disease have indicated that its principal clinical manifestations are an onset in the second decade of life, a predilection for boys, painless swelling of proximal interphalangeal articulations, digital shortening, and deformity.[106-109] Involvement of the metacarpophalangeal and tarsometatarsal joints and the interphalangeal articulations of the toes has also been noted in some cases. The disease is familial, probably transmitted as a dominant trait with virtually complete penetrance. A relationship to trauma has also been suggested. Although not fully delineated, the pathogenesis of the disease appears to be an osteonecrosis. Dessecker's description of the histology of an involved epiphysis of a proximal interphalangeal joint indicated features of necrosis, with normal vessels and absent inflammation.[106]

Radiographs reveal irregularity of the epiphyses of the phalanges, especially in the middle fingers. The epiphyses appear sclerotic and fragmented, and may contain medial and lateral osseous excrescences[110] (Fig. 78–18). Eventually, the joint space becomes narrowed, the base of the phalanx thickens, and phalangeal shortening is seen.

Additional alterations that may accompany Thiemann's disease are Legg-Calvé-Perthes disease, bipartite patella, pterygium colli, thyroid enlargement, and diabetes mellitus, but a definite association of this interesting disorder with any of these latter conditions has not been verified.[109]

DISORDERS RELATED TO TRAUMA OR ABNORMAL STRESS WITHOUT EVIDENCE OF OSTEONECROSIS

Osgood-Schlatter's Disease

In 1903, Osgood of Boston[111] and Schlatter of Zurich[112] each described a disorder of the developing tibial tuberosity that they considered to represent a manifestation of trauma. This interpretation was accurate but some subsequent reports incorrectly emphasized the occurrence of "apophysitis" or osteonecrosis in the pathogenesis of this condition.

Osgood-Schlatter's disease occurs in adolescents, usually between the ages of 11 and 15 years, with a younger age of onset in girls than in boys. Boys are affected more frequently than girls, and a history of participation in sports and a rapid growth spurt prior to the onset of symptoms and signs is typical. Although the disease is generally unilateral in distribution, bilateral alterations are detected in approximately 25 per cent of cases.

Clinically, patients usually present with local pain and tenderness of variable severity.[1, 113, 114] The pain may be aggravated during activity and ameliorated with rest. Soft tissue swelling and firm masses can be palpated in the involved region, and there is no synovial effusion in the knee.

Although radiographic abnormalities are well known in Osgood-Schlatter's disease,[115, 116] technical difficulties may prevent adequate visualization of the region in some cases. Lateral films should not be overpenetrated as subtle soft tissue alterations may be missed.[116, 117] In this regard, low KV and xeroradiography may be helpful. Furthermore, as the tibial tuberosity lies slightly lateral to the midline, a lateral projection with the knee in slight internal rotation should be utilized.[92] Two radiographs obtained in this position, one with bone technique and one with soft tissue technique, should be added to the routine knee roentgenograms in the evaluation of patients with this disorder.

Interpretation of the roentgenograms requires knowledge of the normal pattern of ossification of the tibial tuberosity[92, 118] (Fig. 78–19). During initial stages of fetal development, no discrete tuberosity is present and the growth plate of the proximal tibia is transversely oriented. In subsequent stages, an anterior outgrowth occurs from the tibial chondroepiphysis concomitant with fibrovascular ingrowth and vascularization of the chondroepiphysis, and the developing tuberosity is displaced distally by longi-

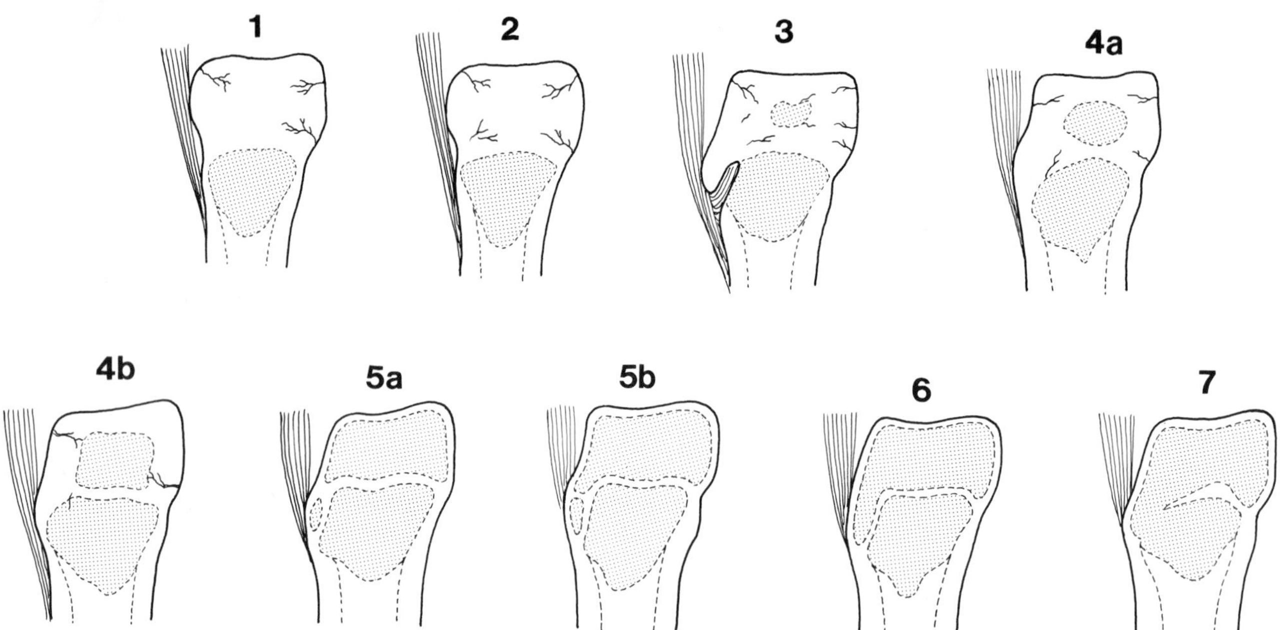

Figure 78–19. *Tibial tuberosity and proximal tibia: Normal sequence of ossification.*

1 *Stage 1: Prenatal phase. No tibial tuberosity is present. The growth plate of the proximal tibia is transversely oriented.*

2 *Stage 2: Prenatal phase. An anterior outgrowth develops from the tibial chondroepiphysis concomitant with fibrovascular ingrowth and vascularization of the chondroepiphysis.*

3 *Stage 3: Prenatal phase. There is relative distal displacement of the tuberosity by longitudinal growth at the proximal tibial physis, and anatomic separation from the proximal tibial physis takes place by continued fibromesenchymal-vascular ingrowth.*

4a,b *Stage 4: Postnatal phase. Development of a separate growth plate associated with the tibial tuberosity occurs, and there is subsequent coalescence with the primary proximal tibial growth plate.*

5a,b *Stage 5: Postnatal phase. A secondary ossification center develops in the distal portion of the tuberosity.*

6 *Stage 6: Postnatal phase. Coalescence of the ossification center of the tuberosity and the proximal tibial epiphysis occurs.*

7 *Stage 7: Postnatal phase. Closure of the contiguous growth plates of the proximal tibia and tuberosity takes place.*

(After Ogden JA, Southwick WO: Clin Orthop Rel Res 116:180, 1976.)

tudinal growth at the proximal tibial physis. Postnatally, a separate growth plate of the tibial tuberosity develops and coalesces with the primary proximal tibial growth plate. A secondary ossification center develops in the distal portion of the tuberosity and later coalesces with the ossification center of the proximal tibial epiphysis. Finally, closure of the contiguous growth plates of the proximal tibia and tuberosity is seen. On the radiograph, one or more osseous centers in the cartilaginous extension of the tuberosity are normally recognized in girls between the ages of 8 and 12 years and in boys between 9 and 14 years. Thus, the detection of several ossific nodules anterior to the tibial metaphysis must not be misinterpreted as abnormal fragmentation of bone. Also, bony fusion of the tuberosity and tibial metaphysis normally does not occur before the age of 15 years in girls and 17 years in boys.[115]

Roentgenographic abnormalities in this disease are influenced by the age of the patient. Initially, soft tissue swelling in front of the tuberosity results from edema of the skin and subcutaneous tissue (Fig. 78–20). The margins of the patellar tendon, which attaches to the cartilage of the tibial tuberosity in the child and to the periosteum in the adult, may be indistinct, and increased radiodensity of the infrapatellar fat pad may be identified. If the tuberosity is entirely cartilaginous in structure, no change will be detected in it initially, but examination 3 or 4 weeks later may show single or multiple ossific collections in the avulsed fragment (see discussion later in this chapter)[92] (Fig. 78–21). In the older child in whom the ossification center has begun to develop, one or more foci of radiopacity can be recognized in the vicinity of the tubercle, and the latter protuberance may have surface irregularities marking the sites from which fragments of cartilage and bone have been avulsed.[1]

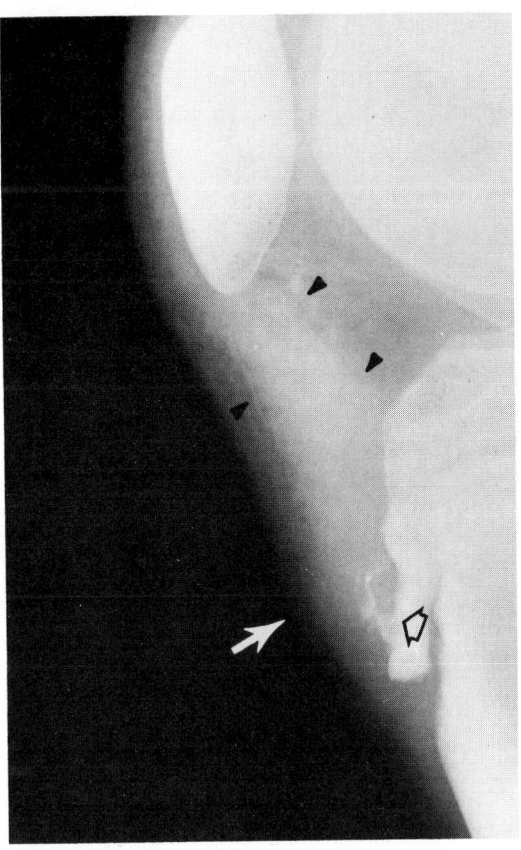

Figure 78–20. Osgood-Schlatter's disease: Soft tissue abnormalities. Low KV radiography indicates soft tissue edema over the tibial tuberosity (solid arrow). Note indistinctness of the infrapatellar tendon (arrowheads) and osseous irregularity of the tuberosity (open arrow). (Courtesy of Dr. J. Weston, Hutt Hospital, Lower Hutt, New Zealand.)

Following the acute stage, soft-tissue swelling diminishes and displaced pieces of bone may increase in size owing to endochondral bone formation and callus formation or may reunite with each other and the underlying tibial tuberosity. Eventually, the radiographic appearance may revert to normal, although persistent ossific fragments frequently mark the site of previous disease. It has recently been suggested that the radiographic demonstration of a persistent ossicle at the proximal aspect of the tibial tuberosity may indicate "unresolved" Osgood-Schlatter's disease with significant pain and swelling related to bursitis about the mobile ossicle.[204] In addition to a bursa between the ossicle and tibial tuberosity, histologic evaluation may reveal a thin band of scar tissue in these patients with unresolved disease.

The accurate diagnosis of this condition is based on both the radiographic and the clinical findings. A fragmented tuberosity can occur in other conditions,[119] and, in the absence of current or previous symptomatology, may indicate only a normal ossification pattern. Soft tissue swelling is fundamental to the roentgenographic diagnosis of Osgood-Schlatter's disease. In equivocal cases, comparison views of the opposite, uninvolved side may be helpful.

In the past, Osgood-Schlatter's disease was considered by some investigators to be an osteonecrosis.[120] However, more recent studies have indicated that the tibial tuberosity possesses an excellent blood supply,[118, 121] and that the pathologic findings in this condition are most consistent with a traumatically induced disruption somewhere along the site of attachment of the patellar ligament to the tibial tuberosity.[1, 122, 123] The mechanical weakness of the patellar ligament-cartilage attachment on the tibial tuberosity favors the occurrence of avulsion of fragments of cartilage and underlying bone.[1] This avulsion can appear either at a cartilaginous stage, a chondro-osseous stage, or an osseous stage in the developing ossification center. The normal tuberosity growth plate is not affected because it is well adapted to tensile stress.[118] Thus, premature closure of the physis of the tibial tuberosity with genu recurvatum is rare in this disease.[124, 125] Delayed distal displacement of the developing tuberosity

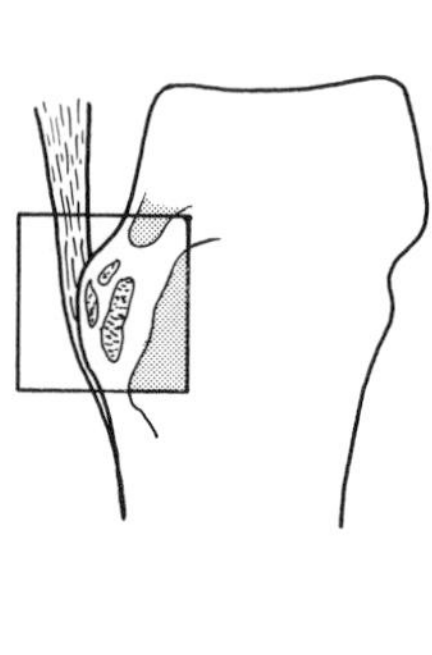

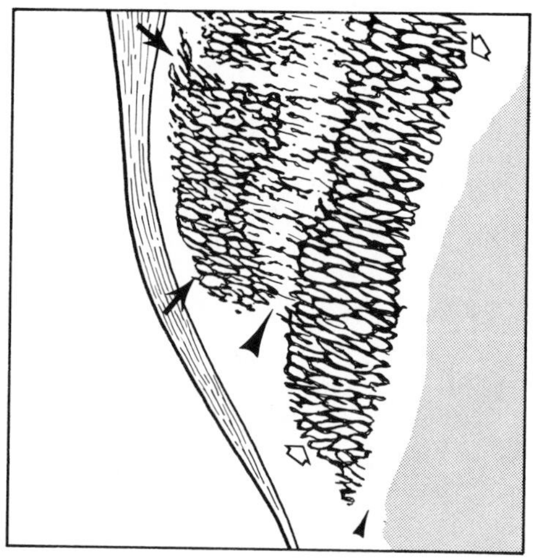

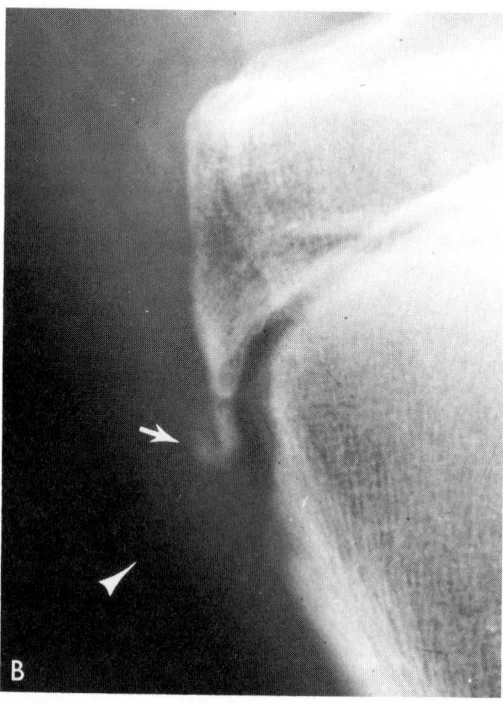

Figure 78–21. *Osgood-Schlatter's disease: Osseous abnormalities.*

A *A schematic representation of the bony changes in Osgood-Schlatter's disease is shown. Inset shows area of bony changes. Avulsion with separation (large arrowhead) of small ossicles (solid arrows) of the developing ossification center of the tibial tuberosity (open arrows) is observed. Note the physis (small arrowhead) and underlying tibia. (**A,** After Ogden JA, Southwick WO: Clin Orthop Rel Res 116:180, 1976.)*

B *Observe soft tissue swelling (arrowhead) and an avulsed osseous fragment of the tibial tuberosity (arrow).*

could result in patella alta, whereas excessive displacement could lead to patella baja.[118] Although a relationship between Osgood-Schlatter's disease and patella alta has been emphasized in some reports, this has been questioned by other investigators, who cite the difficulty in accurately measuring patellar position in patients with this disease.[204]

Blount's Disease

Blount's disease, tibia vara, or osteochondrosis deformans tibiae is a local disturbance of growth of the medial aspect of the proximal tibial epiphysis, described in 1937 by Blount.[126] The condition is classified into two types, an infantile type in which deformity is noted in the first few years of life, and an adolescent type in which deformity appears in children between the ages of 8 and 15 years (Table 78–2). The infantile type is approximately five to eight times more frequent than the adolescent variety.

Infantile Tibia Vara. Infantile tibia vara appears to develop when normal physiologic bowing, rather than disappearing progressively to a straight leg or slight valgus position, persists and worsens when the growing child becomes heavier and begins to put weight on the knee joint.[127] In Jamaica, children walk at a relatively early age and have an increased incidence in the degree of physiologic bowing, which persists longer than in English children. These two factors apparently contribute to create an unusually high incidence of tibia

Table 78–2
INFANTILE VERSUS ADOLESCENT TIBIA VARA

	Infantile	Adolescent
Age of onset	1–3 years	8–15 years
Distribution	Bilateral: 50–75%	Unilateral: 90%
Clinical findings	Obesity Absent pain, tenderness Prominent deformity Slight leg shortening	Normal body weight Pain and tenderness Mild deformity Moderate, severe leg shortening
Etiology/pathogenesis	Trauma Growth arrest or dysplasia	Trauma Growth arrest

vara.[128, 130] Other factors leading to increased stress on the medial aspect of the proximal tibia may also be important, as an affinity of this disease with individuals of black African stock cannot always be traced to a propensity of affected children to walk at an earlier age.[131] Additional mechanical factors that may contribute to infantile tibia vara include excessive body weight, peculiarities in the manner in which children are carried on their mothers' backs, and abnormal articular laxity, but these factors, although possibly important, are not constantly present.[131] Sibert and Bray[132] stressed an autosomal dominant pattern of inheritance with variable penetrance in this condition, and it is possible that infantile tibia vara results from specific environmental agents acting upon a genetically predisposed individual.

Altered mechanical forces in the proximal tibia from various primary causes could increase the mobility of the tibia on the femur, resulting in a change of direction of weight-bearing forces on the upper tibial epiphysis from perpendicular to oblique. This obliquity tends to displace the tibial epiphysis in a lateral direction, overloading the mediodorsal segment of the bone, bending it in a mediad and caudad direction. With further longitudinal growth, a vicious circle of events ensues that culminates in progressive varus deformity.[225]

Histologic examination confirms the absence of changes of infection or osteonecrosis. The microscopic findings are consistent with the effects of persistent abnormal pressure on the growth plate; changes predominate in the zone of resting cartilage in the medial part of the proximal tibial growth plate and consist of islands of densely packed and hypertrophied cells, acellular fibrous cartilage, and abnormal groups of capillaries.[129, 133]

Clinically, affected children may be early walkers. Progressive bilateral (60 per cent) or unilateral (40 per cent) bowing of the leg during the first year of life is difficult to differentiate from physiologic changes. The tibia may be acutely angulated inward just below the knee, and a nontender bony protuberance can be palpated along the medial aspect of the proximal tibia. The fibular head may also be prominent. Pain is not evident. Associated findings are obesity, shortening of the leg, tibial torsion, and pronated feet.

Radiographic abnormalities simulate those of physiologic bowing, but are more severe and can be unilateral or asymmetric in distribution. The tibia is in varus position owing to angulation of the metaphysis, and the tibial shaft is adducted without intrinsic curvature.[92, 205] A depressed medial tibial metaphysis with an osseous excrescence or spur is seen. The nature and severity of the osseous changes are highly variable. Six stages have been recognized on the roentgenogram[133-135] (Figs. 78–22, 78–23).

Stage I (2 to 3 Years). A progressive increase in the degree of varus deformity of the tibia is associat-

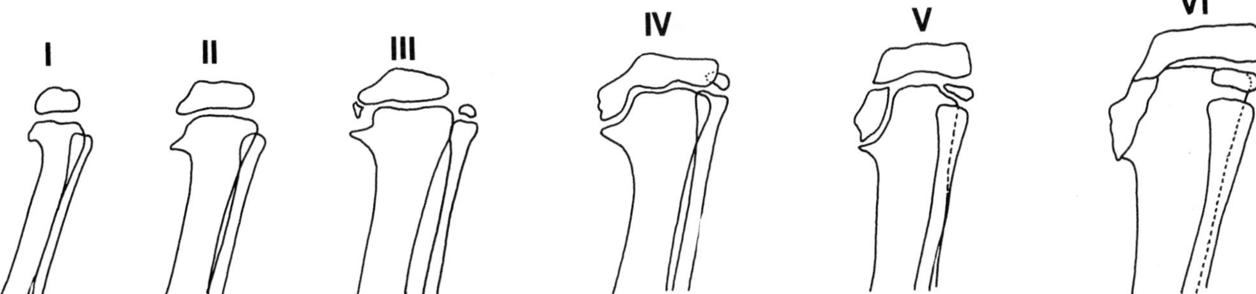

Figure 78–22. *Blount's disease: Infantile tibia vara. Six stages of the disease (see text for details). (After Langenskiold A: Acta Chir Scand 103:1, 1952.)*

ed with irregularity of the entire growth plate. The medial part of the metaphysis is protruded, with a medial and distal beak.

Stage II ($2^1/_2$ to 4 Years). A lateromedial depression of the ossification line of the medial portion of the metaphysis and a wedge-shaped medial end of the epiphysis are observed. Complete healing of the lesion is possible at this stage.

Stage III (4 to 6 Years). The cartilage-filled depression in the metaphyseal beak deepens. The

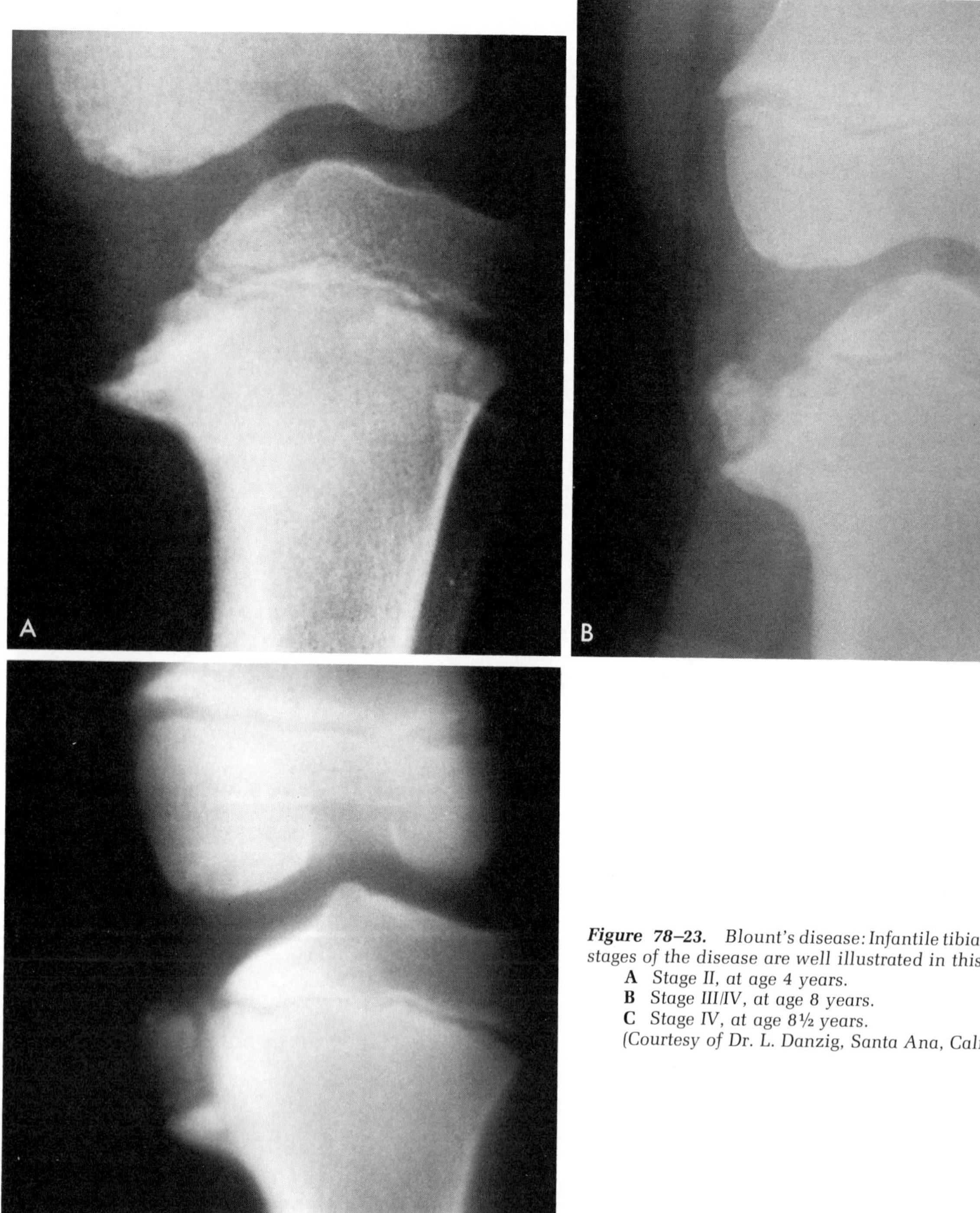

Figure 78–23. Blount's disease: *Infantile tibia vara. The various stages of the disease are well illustrated in this child.*
A *Stage II, at age 4 years.*
B *Stage III/IV, at age 8 years.*
C *Stage IV, at age 8½ years.*
(Courtesy of Dr. L. Danzig, Santa Ana, California.)

medial part of the bony epiphysis remains wedge-shaped and is less distinct. Small calcific foci may be evident beneath the medial border.

Stage IV (5 to 10 Years). With increasing bone maturation, the cartilaginous growth plate is reduced to a narrow plate, and the bony epiphysis occupies an increasing part of the end of the bone. The medial margin of the epiphysis shows definite irregularity. Even at this stage, restoration of a relatively normal epiphysis can occur. In the presence of partial restoration, the resulting radiographic abnormalities may resemble those in the late stages of the adolescent type of tibia vara.

Stage V (9 to 11 Years). The bony epiphysis and the corresponding articular surface are greatly deformed. A "partial double epiphyseal plate" results as the bony epiphysis is separated in two portions by a clear band, extending medially from the lateral portion of the growth plate to the articular cartilage. The triangular area of bone lying between the two branches of the plate is generally considered to be a part of the epiphysis because it possesses a considerable amount of articular cartilage.

Stage VI (10 to 13 Years). The branches of the medially located double growth plate ossify, whereas growth continues in the normal lateral part. Stages V and VI represent phases of irreparable structural damage.

Recently, lateral widening of the growth plate of the proximal tibia and, less frequently, the distal femur has been identified in infantile tibia vara as well as in other conditions associated with bow-leg

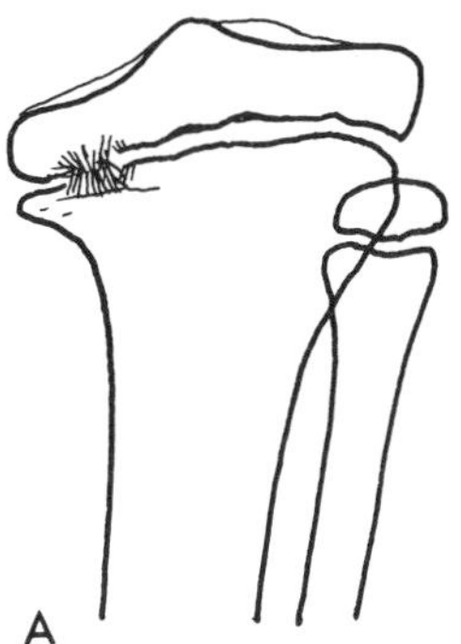

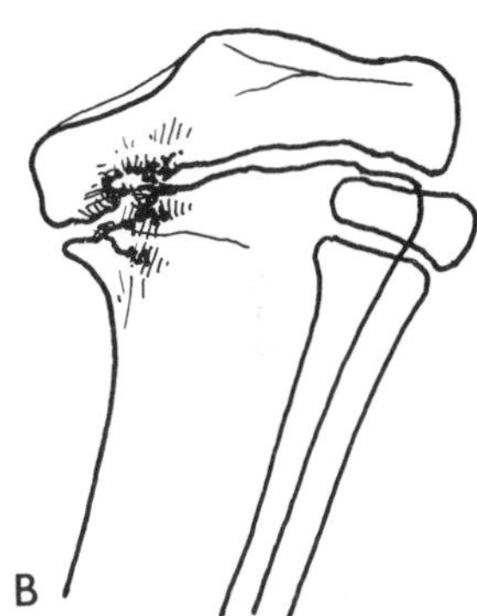

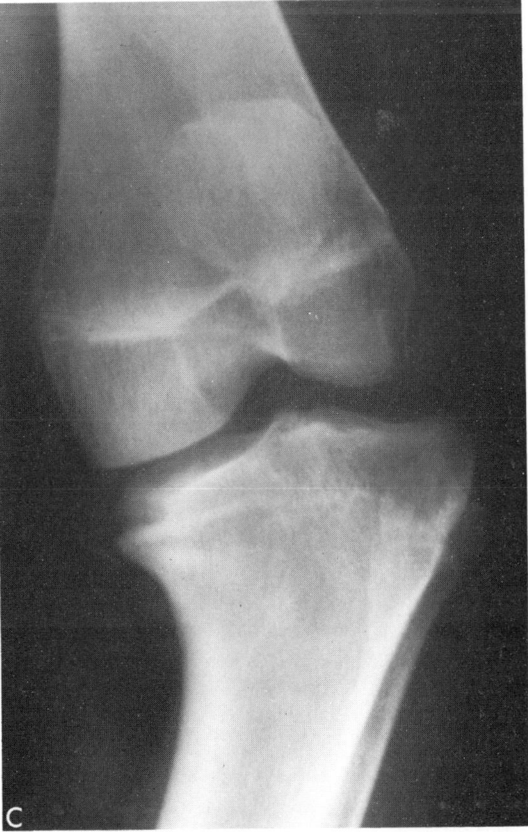

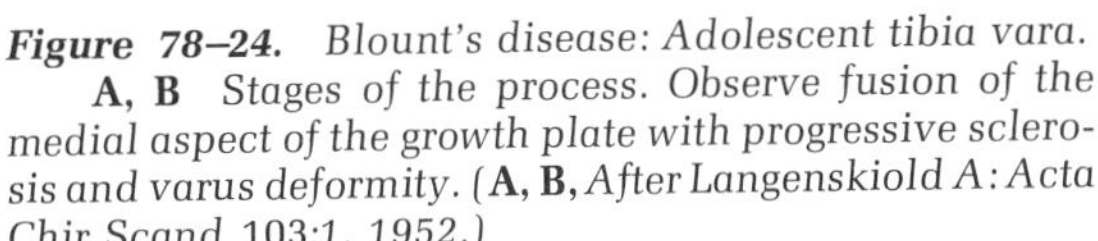

Figure 78–24. *Blount's disease: Adolescent tibia vara.*

A, B *Stages of the process. Observe fusion of the medial aspect of the growth plate with progressive sclerosis and varus deformity. (**A, B,** After Langenskiold A: Acta Chir Scand 103:1, 1952.)*

C *An example of adolescent tibia vara. Note varus deformity, depression of the articular surface of the medial tibial plateau, sclerosis, and osteophyte formation.*

deformity.[136] This diastasis may result from the chronic stress of the genu varum upon the growth plates in the area of the knee; most stress during weight-bearing on the bowed leg is projected medially, producing distraction or tension force on the lateral aspect of the joint.[137] Similar distraction changes on the medial portion of the growth plate have been noted in association with genu valgum.[138]

Arthrography may be utilized to investigate infantile tibia vara[92] (see Chapter 15). Findings in initial stages include hypertrophy of the articular cartilage, creating a horizontal joint line despite the presence of angular osseous deformity, and a hypermobile and enlarged medial meniscus. In later stages, angulation of the articular surface may be noted.

Adolescent Tibia Vara. This condition, which is much less frequent than infantile tibia vara, develops in children between the ages of 8 and 15 years. The cause is not clear, although an arrest of epiphyseal growth is suspected. A history of trauma or infection is occasionally elicited, and tomography may indicate an osseous bridge between the epiphysis and metaphysis.[133] Irregularities of the growth zone may be demonstrated on examination of biopsy specimens.[139]

Unilateral alterations occur in approximately 90 per cent of cases. Leg shortening and mild to moderate varus deformity may be associated with pain and tenderness over the medial prominence of the proximal tibia. Radiographs outline a proximal tibia that is angled about 10 to 20 degrees. The proximal tibial epiphysis reveals medial wedging, and the medial tibial growth plate is diminished in height, but a sharp step-off in the tibial plateau usually is not apparent[92] (Fig. 78–24). Sclerosis on either side of the growth plate, and segmental widening of the lateral portion of the plate of the proximal tibia or distal femur, can be seen.

Differential Diagnosis. The radiographic abnormalities in infantile and adolescent tibia vara are usually diagnostic. Some difficulty is occasionally encountered in differentiating the infantile type from physiologic bowed legs, and serial roentgenograms may be necessary (Fig. 78–25). The sharply angular appearance of infantile tibia vara differs from the gradual curve in physiologic bowed legs. Metaphyseal alterations and bowing in Blount's disease may also simulate findings in mild or healing rickets. Additional differential diagnostic possibilities include fractures of the proximal tibial growth plate, osteomyelitis, and Ollier's disease.

Scheuermann's Disease

Background. In 1921, Scheuermann[140] described a disorder that led to lower thoracic kyphosis, designating the condition "kyphosis dorsalis juvenilis." On the basis of irregularities involving the rims of the vertebral bodies, this investigator concluded that pathologic aberrations had occurred in the region of the growth areas between the vertebral bodies and the ring-like epiphyses, that these changes differed from those in other kyphotic condi-

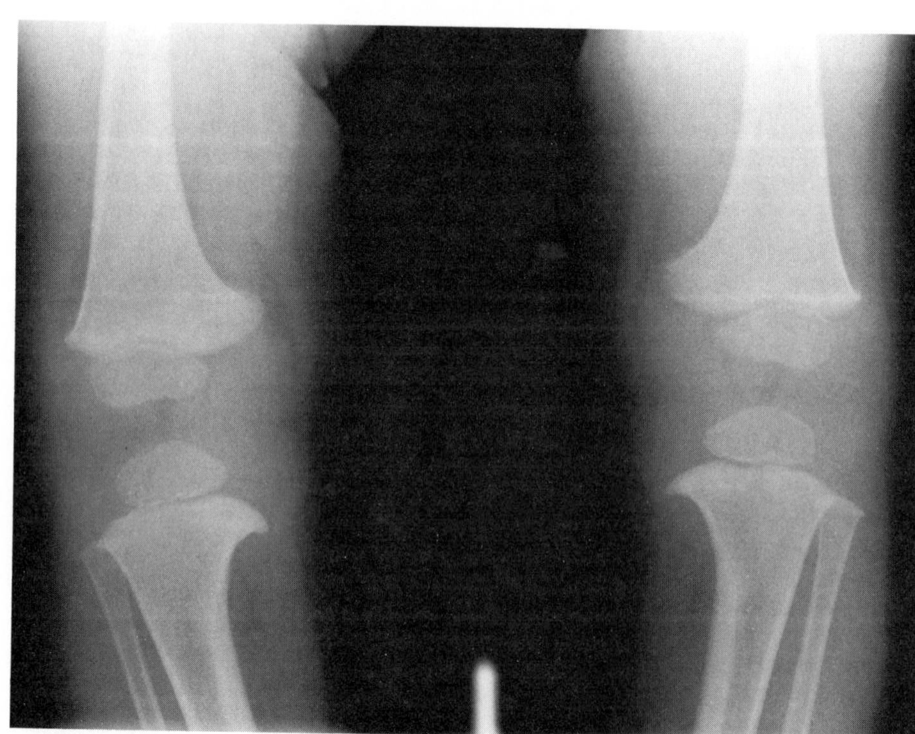

Figure 78–25. *Physiologic bowed legs. Note the gradual varus curvature of the knees in this child. There is no evidence of a proximal tibial step-off or varus deformity.*

tions, and that this disease had a close relationship to Legg-Calvé-Perthes disease. Numerous descriptions of juvenile kyphosis followed, and additional terms were introduced, such as vertebral epiphysitis, osteochondrosis juvenilis dorsi, and preadolescent and adolescent kyphosis.[1] Although the predominant involvement of the epiphysis of the vertebral rim was initially interpreted as evidence of osteonecrosis, considerable disagreement as to the etiology and pathogenesis of this disorder subsequently developed. Debate also existed regarding the criteria necessary for the diagnosis of Scheuermann's disease. Scheuermann suggested that the roentgenographic findings were indispensable in establishing the presence of this disorder; in most of his cases, he detected three abnormal vertebrae, but later he reported that the number of altered vertebrae might vary from one to five.[141] Currently utilized criteria frequently require the presence of abnormalities of at least three contiguous vertebrae, each with wedging of 5 degrees or more.[142] Such criteria are not ideal, as they exclude those cases of Scheuermann's disease that are associated predominantly with vertebral irregularity without wedging.[143] Diagnostic criteria based on the presence of clinical findings are inadequate, since many patients with this disorder are entirely asymptomatic.

Because of the discrepancies in the criteria used to diagnose juvenile kyphosis, a precise incidence is difficult to define. The reported frequency in military personnel is approximately 4 to 6 per cent,[144, 145] and in industrial workers, approximately 8 per cent.[142] Most affected individuals are between the ages of 13 and 17 years, and the disorder is unusual before the age of 10 years.[146, 147] There is slight predominance of male patients in many series of Scheuermann's disease, although this sex preference is not constant.

Clinical Abnormalities. Clinical manifestations are highly variable. In some individuals the disease is totally asymptomatic, being discovered as an incidental finding on lateral radiographs of the chest. In others, prominent symptoms and signs can be seen. Most typically, these relate to the middle and lower thoracic spine, although isolated alterations of the lumbar or, more rarely, the cervical spine can be noted.[148-151] Fatigue, defective posture, aching pain aggravated by physical exertion, and tenderness to palpation are encountered. Kyphotic deformity, which may be associated with mild scoliosis, predominates in the thoracic region (75 per cent of patients), although it may be observed in the thoracolumbar (20 to 25 per cent) or lumbar (0 to 5 per cent) segments. A dorsal kyphosis is frequently combined with an exaggerated lumbar and cervical lordosis and a protuberant abdomen. The deformity may be initially correctable, but may become progressively more fixed in position. An angular gibbus deformity is unusual in Scheuermann's disease. Neurologic complaints are not common. Herniation of thoracic intervertebral discs can lead to neurologic manifestations and even paraparesis in occasional cases.[155] Extradural spinal cysts and cord compression at the apex of the abnormal spinal curvature have also been noted.[156-159]

Radiographic and Pathologic Abnormalities. On radiographs, irregularity of vertebral contours is identified. An undulant superior and inferior surface of affected vertebral bodies is associated with intraosseous radiolucent zones of variable size (cartilaginous or Schmorl's nodes), with surrounding sclerosis (Figs. 78–26 and 78–27). The degree of osseous irregularity is variable, but when severe can be accompanied by loss of intervertebral disc height, particularly in the midportion of the kyphotic curvature. In this same region, wedging or reduction of height of the anterior portion of the vertebral bodies may be seen, a phenomenon that is less striking at the upper and lower limits of the spinal curvature. Small or moderate-sized hyper-

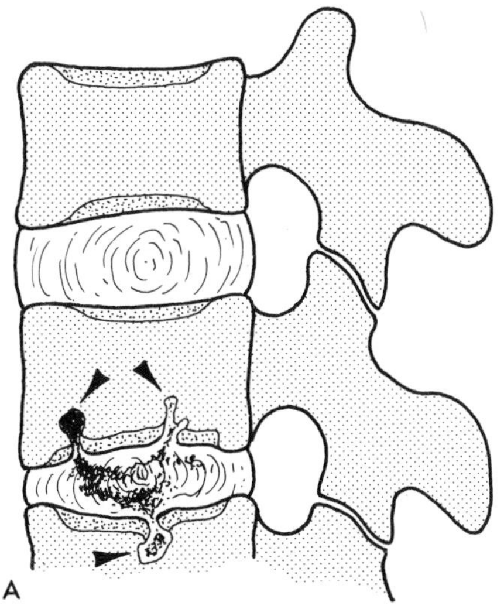

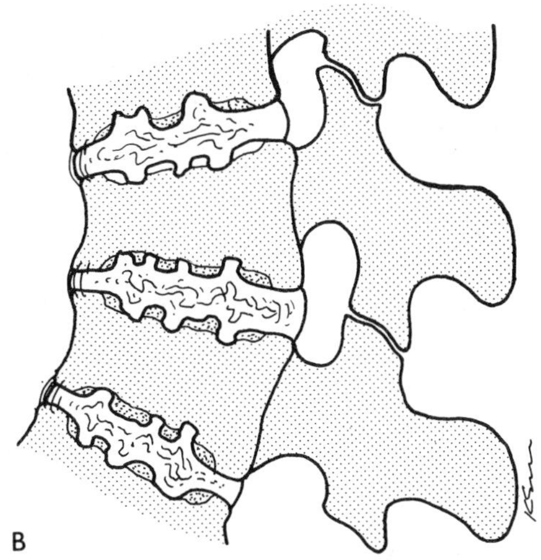

Figure 78–26. Scheuermann's disease. The underlying abnormality relates to intraosseous herniation of disc material (cartilaginous nodes) through the cartilaginous end-plates (arrowheads). This produces radiolucent lesions of the vertebral bodies with surrounding sclerosis, intervertebral disc space narrowing, and irregularity of vertebral contour. Kyphosis may appear.

trophic spurs may be evident about the narrowed intervertebral discs and wedge-shaped vertebrae, identical in appearance to the osteophytes of spondylosis deformans.

The degree of thoracic kyphosis is also variable; a kyphotic index can be calculated on a lateral radiograph by measuring the angle at the intersection of two lines, one through the upper end-plate of the most craniad vertebra that is involved in the kyphosis, and a second through the lower end-plate of the most caudad vertebra. In general, the kyphotic curvature develops slowly unless aggravated by severe physical stress, a factor that may lead to sudden intraosseous herniation of discal material and rapid onset of kyphosis.[152]

Prolapse of large foci of intervertebral disc tissue may be observed anteriorly, and the extruded discal material may extend beneath the apophyseal centers of ossification, appearing submarginally behind the anterior longitudinal ligament.[1] Under

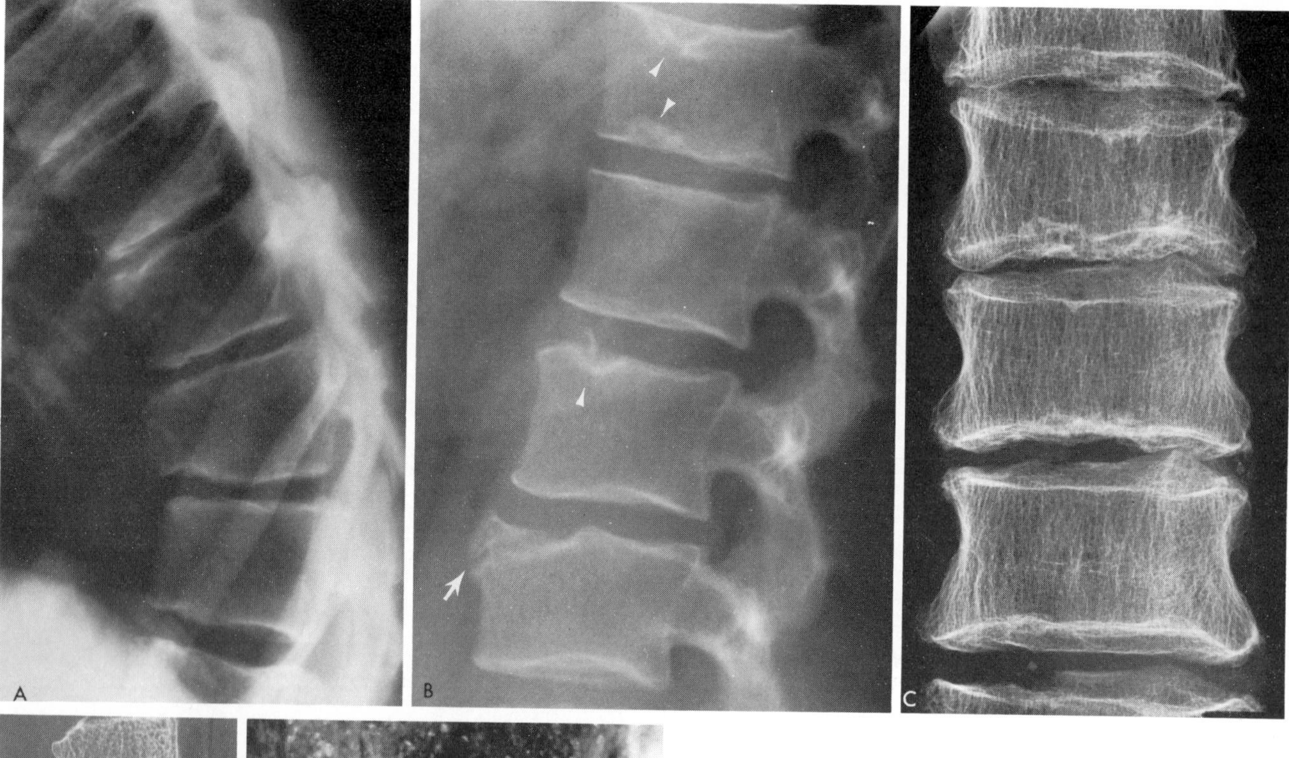

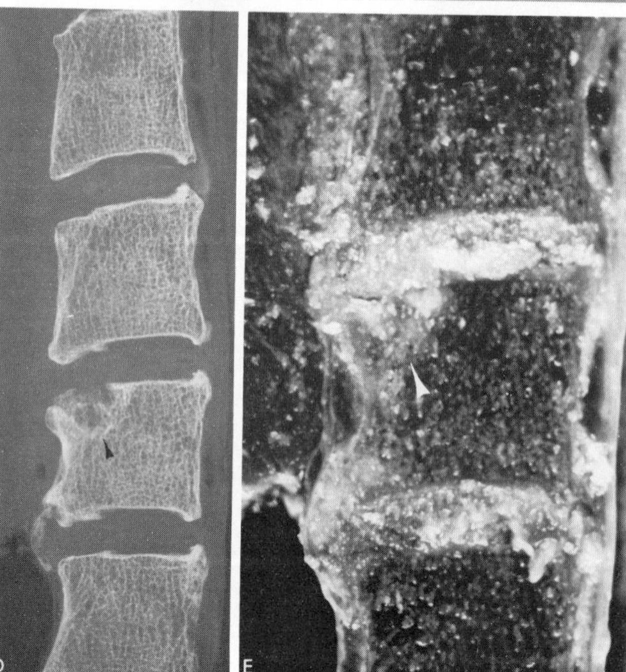

Figure 78–27. *Scheuermann's disease.*

A *Thoracic spine. Findings include irregularity of vertebral contour, reactive sclerosis, intervertebral disc space narrowing, anterior vertebral wedging, and kyphosis.*

B *Lumbar spine. Observe the cartilaginous nodes (arrowheads) creating surface irregularity, lucent areas, and reactive sclerosis. An anterior discal herniation (arrow) has produced an irregular anterosuperior corner of a vertebral body, the limbus vertebra.*

C *Thoracolumbar spine. A radiograph of a coronal section of a spine delineates the extent of the irregular vertebral contour and intervertebral disc space narrowing.*

D, E *Cervical spine. A sagittal sectional radiograph and photograph of the cervical spine demonstrate cartilaginous node formation (arrowhead).*

these circumstances, a portion of the proximal or distal ring-like apophyseal centers of ossification may be separated from the vertebral body, producing a "limbus" vertebra (Fig. 78–27*B*). The subsequent development and ossification of the apophysis can be irregular, creating fragmented ossific radiodense areas that were initially interpreted as evidence of an osteonecrosis of the apophyseal centers. Furthermore, the discal tissue beneath the anterior longitudinal ligament can produce pressure erosion on the adjacent anterior surface of the vertebral body.

Radiographic evidence of healing of the lesions can take several forms. Ossification of the anterior portions of the intervertebral disc can lead to synostosis of one vertebral body with its neighbor[153] (Fig. 78–28). The fusion between the anterior parts of the vertebral bodies may be associated with an unossified but narrowed posterior discal space. This phenomenon can be unaccompanied by symptoms and signs, although a period of discomfort may occur during the ossifying process. If fusion occurs at an early age, persistence of growth of the posterior portions of the vertebrae can accentuate the kyphotic deformity.[153, 154] The resulting anterior contour of the spine can be relatively smooth, although accompanying osteophytes can create surface irregularities.

The pathologic alterations in Scheuermann's disease involve the intervertebral discs and the vertebral bodies, including the cartilaginous end-plates.[1, 152, 160] The intervertebral discs may appear bulged or biconvex in shape, and the neighboring cartilaginous end-plates may appear thinner than normal, presumably owing to the pressure of the discal tissue, which deforms the plate, preventing normal endochondral ossification. The cartilaginous end-plate may then degenerate, with fissuring, ulceration, and microscopic focal areas of "necrosis."[161] Intraosseous nuclear protrusions occur through the weakened end-plates, and the prolapsed disc material becomes surrounded first by a cartilaginous casing, and later by an osseous one.[152] The cartilaginous nodes eventually consist of both nucleus pulposus and anulus fibrosus, and in some cases even the cartilaginous plate itself may be displaced into the vertebral body. Fibrovascular proliferation and narrowing of the intervertebral disc can ensue. This narrowing is maximal on the anterior aspect of the disc, and the resultant pressure on the vertebral bodies in this area may impede normal growth and accentuate the kyphosis. Healing of the discal alterations can result in ossification, with synostosis of vertebral bodies.

Etiology and Pathogenesis. Many concepts of the etiology of Scheuermann's disease have been developed and are well summarized by Alexander.[143] Scheuermann's initial assessment stressed the importance of the apophyseal changes, which he attributed to necrosis. This theory has not withstood the test of time, and it is not consistent with the pathologic abnormalities (which do not reveal osteonecrosis) or with the absence of these changes in patients with known ischemic disorders, such as

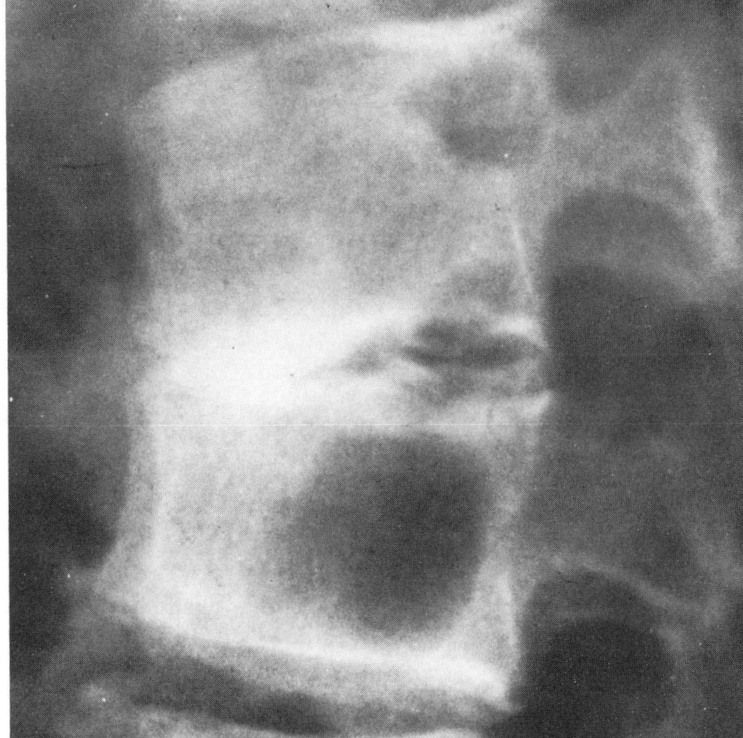

Figure 78–28. *Scheuermann's disease. Note synostosis of two vertebral bodies owing to ossification of the intervening intervertebral disc. The disc space is narrowed and osteophytosis is present.*

sickle cell anemia. Similarly, the concept that the disorder relates to osteomyelitis, tuberculosis, disproportionate growth between the spine and the sternum, rickets, or endocrine dysfunction has not been verified.[152, 162-164] The possibility that Scheuermann's disease is the product of osteoporosis or some other alteration in bone metabolism has received some support,[165-167] although the absence of osteoporosis in some patients with this disorder and the absence of Scheuermann's disease in some varieties of osteoporosis suggest that other factors are important in the initiation and progression of the spinal deformity.

The importance of genetic factors in the pathogenesis of juvenile kyphosis is supported by the reports of its familial occurrence.[142, 168, 206] Bradford and associates[146] noted a positive family history in approximately one fourth of cases, and Kewalramani and co-workers[169] described the coexistence of Scheuermann's disease and Charcot-Marie-Tooth syndrome in three men of a single family. Halal and colleagues,[168] in a study of five families with juvenile kyphosis, postulated an autosomal dominant pattern of inheritance. These results indicate that hereditable factors could be important in this disease, perhaps as a result of genetic influences on the osseous strength of vertebral bodies.

Schmorl[170] and Beadle[171] concluded that cartilaginous node formation is fundamental to the disease process, and that these nodes occurred through congenital indentations of the intervertebral disc in the region of an expanded nucleus pulposus, at which site the cartilaginous end-plates were thinner than normal. It was suggested that congenital weakness of the end-plates predisposed certain individuals to intraosseous discal prolapse during periods of excessive physical stress. This theory is attractive because it is consistent with many of the histologic findings in the disease, although the precise nature of the weakened cartilaginous areas has not been clarified. Defects due to vascular channels and notochordal remnants have been emphasized, but such sites do not always correspond to areas of node formation, and, in fact, the precise location of discal herniations varies from one individual to another.

Alexander[143] has postulated that nuclear expansion represents a traumatically induced growth arrest with secondary nuclear degeneration, and that the cartilaginous node is simply an end-plate fracture resulting from failure under dynamic load in compression or shear, at a time when the plate and the metaphysis are vulnerable as a result of rapid growth. This investigator introduced the terms "adolescent end-plate injury" and "traumatic spondylodystrophy." In support of this theory, Alexander listed the following observations: (1) Scheuermann's disease and cartilaginous nodes are infrequent in children whose illnesses (e.g., Cushing's disease) preclude normal activity and a normal growth spurt; (2) in the presence of normal activity and growth, osteoporosis appears to predispose the spine to cartilaginous node formation; (3) irregular ossification occurs in conditions in which defects in mucopolysaccharide or other matrix components impair vectoring of chondrocytes (e.g., mucopolysaccharidosis IV, multiple epiphyseal dysplasia); (4) a familial occurrence of the disease may reflect genetically determined defects in vertebral strength; and (5) Scheuermann's disease appears to correlate with other spinal disorders indicative of failure under compression (e.g., intervertebral disc degeneration, spondylolysis).

Analysis of the previously outlined hypotheses and of others[172, 173] indicates that this disorder is most likely a manifestation of cartilaginous node formation. The basis for the nodes is not clear, although stress-induced intraosseous herniations through congenitally or traumatically weakened portions of the cartilaginous end-plate appear probable. The radiographic findings reflect the presence of discal material within the vertebral bodies (intraosseous lucent areas) and arrested or abnormal vertebral growth (irregularity of osseous contour), either or both of which can be evident in any one patient with the disease.

Differential Diagnosis. Cartilaginous nodes can accompany any disease process that weakens the cartilaginous end-plate or subchondral bone of the vertebral body, allowing intraosseous discal herniation. A partial list of such processes includes trauma, neoplasm, metabolic disorders (hyperparathyroidism, osteoporosis, Paget's disease), infection, intervertebral osteochondrosis, and articular disorders (rheumatoid arthritis). Accurate roentgenographic diagnosis of these conditions is based on additional spinal and extraspinal manifestations. The combination of kyphosis, cartilaginous nodes, and irregular vertebral outlines is virtually pathognomonic of Scheuermann's disease. Other causes of kyphosis, such as tuberculosis, and postural, osteoporotic, and senile kyphosis can be eliminated by the absence of these characteristic radiologic findings. Occasionally the spinal abnormalities in certain congenital or inherited disorders, such as the mucopolysaccharidoses and Turner's syndrome, can simulate those of Scheuermann's disease, but additional skeletal alterations ensure accurate diagnosis.

Sinding-Larsen-Johansson Disease

In 1921 and 1922, Sinding-Larsen[174] and Johansson[175] independently described a syndrome that occurred most commonly in the adolescent between 10 and 14 years of age, consisting of tenderness and soft tissue swelling over the lower pole of the patella, accompanied by radiographic evidence of osseous

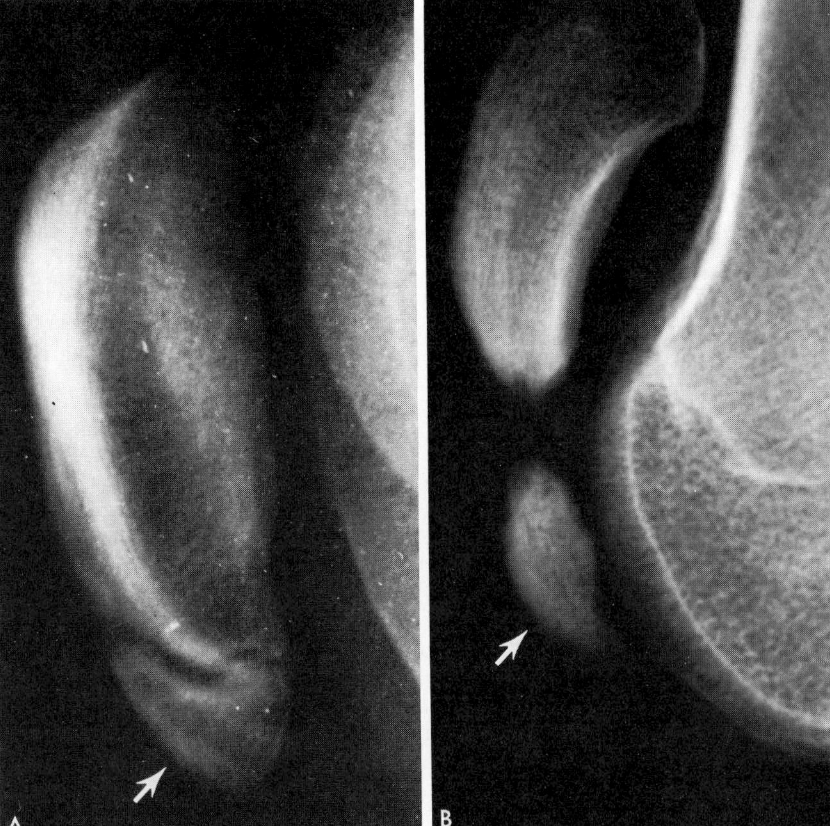

Figure 78–29. Sinding-Larsen-Johansson disease.

A *In this teen-age boy with painful swelling of the knee, note the extraossific dense area (arrow) adjacent to the inferior pole of the patella.*

B *In this patient with spastic paralysis, observe fragmentation of the lower pole of the patella (arrow) related to abnormal stress.*

fragmentation. Early reports suggested that the disorder was an "epiphysitis," "apophysitis," or "osteochondritis." It is now recognized that inflammatory changes and osteonecrosis are not fundamental to this condition, but rather that it is traumatic in etiology. Its pathogenesis appears to be very similar to that of Osgood-Schlatter's disease, and in fact a coexistence of the two disorders has been noted.[176] The lesion is probably related to a traction phenomenon in which contusion or tendinitis in the proximal attachment of the patellar tendon can be followed by calcification and ossification,[177] or in which patellar fracture or avulsion produces one or more distinct ossification sites. The association of fragmentation of the inferior portion of the patella with spastic paralysis[178, 179] is consistent with this traction phenomenon. Clinically, pain and tenderness can be aggravated by activity. The roentgenogram reveals small bony fragments adjacent to the distal surface of the patella with overlying soft tissue swelling (Fig. 78–29). The radiodense areas may subsequently coalesce and become incorporated into the patella, eventually yielding a normal radiographic appearance. The natural duration of the disease is approximately 3 to 12 months.

Patellar "fragmentation" may also represent a normal variation of ossification or the presence of accessory ossification centers.[180]

"DISORDERS" DUE TO VARIATIONS IN OSSIFICATION

Sever's Disease

Irregularity of the secondary calcaneal ossification center was emphasized in 1912 by Sever,[181] who related the change to an apophysitis of the os calcis that might produce pain and tenderness of the heel. Further support for this concept appeared in subsequent publications[182-184] until, in 1948, Hughes[185] proposed that the condition was a normal variation unrelated to the painful heels of adolescents. It is now generally accepted that fragmentation and sclerosis of the secondary ossification center of the calcaneus can be entirely normal (Fig. 78–30) and, in fact, are the result of proper weight-bearing.[186] Such osseous changes may be absent in patients who are immobilized as a result of neurogenic disease or fracture, and may appear with resumption of normal levels of activity.

Ischiopubic Osteochondrosis

A lesion consisting of rarefaction and swelling of the ischiopubic synchondrosis and the neighbor-

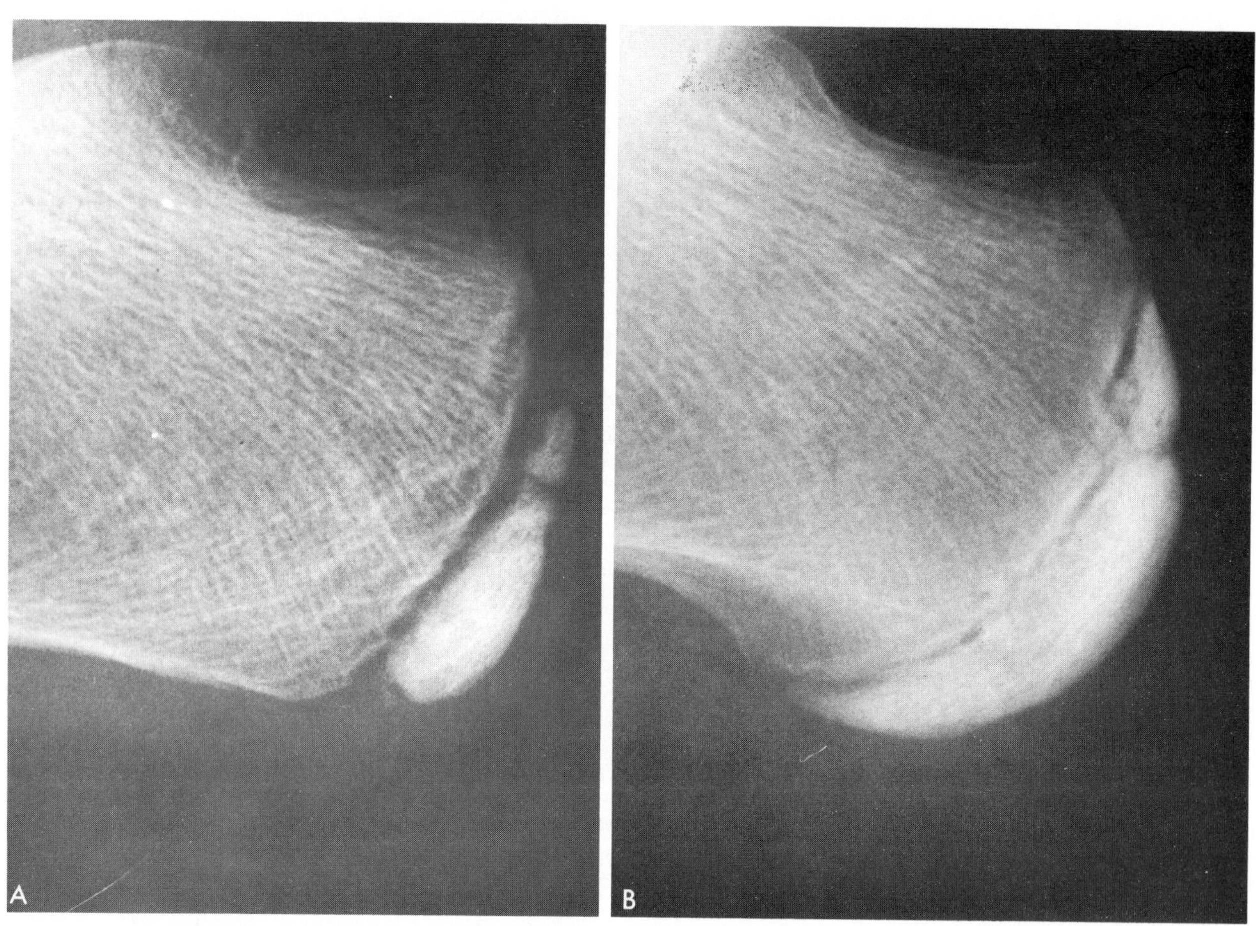

Figure 78–30. *Sever's disease. Two examples of sclerosis of the secondary calcaneal ossification center are illustrated. This is a normal consequence of weight-bearing.*

ing bone was described as an osteochondritis by Van Neck.[187] On the basis of clinical, radiologic, and pathologic observations, this condition is now regarded as a very common, normal pattern of ossification.[188] The time of closure of the synchondrosis is somewhat variable: it usually takes place between the ages of 9 and 11 years.

MISCELLANEOUS DISORDERS

Osteochondroses have been described in almost every epiphysis and apophysis in the body. In most cases, boys are affected more frequently than girls, alterations rarely develop before the age of 3 years or after the age of 12 years, and developmental irregularities in ossification can be encountered at many of the same skeletal sites. Other sites of osteochondroses include the primary ossification center of the patella,[189] greater trochanter,[190] proximal tibial epiphysis,[191] distal tibial epiphysis,[192] talus, os tibiale externum, cuneiforms,[193] epiphysis of the fifth metatarsal,[194] humeral head, distal ulnar epiphysis,[195] carpal scaphoid,[207] heads of the metacarpals,[196] radial head,[197] iliac crest, ischial apophysis, and symphysis pubis. In many instances, the pathogenesis of the osseous fragmentation and sclerosis is not clear, although alterations due to stress or variations of normal ossification appear likely at certain locations. "Osteochondrosis" of the vertebral body, termed Calvé's disease, leading to flattening and collapse, is almost invariably the result of an eosinophilic granuloma.

SUMMARY

The osteochondroses are a heterogeneous group of disorders that are usually characterized by fragmentation and sclerosis of an epiphyseal or apophyseal center in the immature skeleton. Reossification and reconstitution of osseous contour can be evident in some cases. These disorders can be divided into three major categories: (1) conditions characterized by primary or secondary osteonecrosis; (2) conditions related to trauma or abnormal stress, without evidence of osteonecrosis; and (3) conditions that represent variations in normal patterns of ossification. In some cases, a definite pathogenesis has not been identified.

REFERENCES

1. Jaffe HL: Metabolic, Degenerative and Inflammatory Diseases of Bones and Joints. Philadelphia, Lea & Febiger, 1972, p 565.
2. Jacobs P: Osteochondrosis (osteochondritis). *In* JK Davidson (Ed): Aseptic Necrosis of Bone. Amsterdam, Excerpta Medica, 1976, p 301.
3. Legg AT: An obscure affection of the hip joint. Boston Med Surg J *162*:202, 1910.
4. Calvé J: Sur une forme particulière de pseudo-coxalgie greffée sur des déformations caractéristiques de l'extrémité supérieure du fémur. Rev Chir *30*:54, 1910.
5. Perthes GC: Über Arthritis deformans juvenilis. Dtsch Z Chir *107*:111, 1910.
6. Perthes GC: Über osteochondritis deformans juvenilis. Arch Klin Chir *101*:779, 1913.
7. Waldenström H: Coxa plana. Osteochondritis deformans coxae, Calvé-Perthes'sche Krankheit. Legg's disease. Zentralbl Chir *47*:539, 1930.
8. Waldenström H: Der obere tuberkulöse Collumherd. Z Orthop Chir *24*:487, 1909.
9. Sutro CJ, Pomeranz MM: Perthes' disease. Arch Surg *34*:360, 1937.
10. Edgren W: Cox plana: A clinical and radiological investigation with particular reference to the importance of the metaphyseal changes for the final shape of the proximal part of the femur. Acta Orthop Scand Suppl *84*:1, 1965.
11. Clarke TE, Finnegan TL, Fisher RL, Bunch WH, Gossling HR: Legg-Perthes disease in children less than four years old. J Bone Joint Surg *60A*:166, 1978.
12. Spragge JW: Legg-Calvé-Perthes disease. *In* RH Freiberger, et al (Eds): Hip Disease of Infancy and Childhood. Curr Probl Radiol *3*:30, 1973.
13. Nevelös AB, Colton CL, Burch PRJ, Woodward PM: Perthes' disease. A study of radiological features. Acta Orthop Scand *48*:411, 1977.
14. Goldman AB, Hallel T, Salvati EM, Freiberger RH: Osteochondritis dissecans complicating Legg-Perthes disease. A report of four cases. Radiology *121*:561, 1976.
15. Caffey J: The early roentgenographic changes in essential coxa plana; their significance in pathogenesis. Am J Roentgenol *103*:620, 1968.
16. Kamhi E, MacEwen GD: Osteochondritis dissecans in Legg-Calvé-Perthes disease. J Bone Joint Surg *57A*:506, 1975.
17. Somerville EW: Perthes' disease of the hip. J Bone Joint Surg *53B*:639, 1971.
18. Katz JF, Siffert RS: Capital necrosis, metaphyseal cyst, and subluxation in coxa plana. Clin Orthop Rel Res *106*:75, 1975.
19. Robichon J, Desjardins JP, Koch M, Hooper CE: The femoral neck in Legg-Perthes' disease. Its relationship to epiphyseal change and its importance in early prognosis. J Bone Joint Surg *56B*:62, 1974.
20. Zweymüller K, and Wicke B: Zur Lateralisation der Oberschenkelkopfes beim M. Perthes. Arch Orthop Unfallchir *75*:239, 1973.
21. Calot F: L'orthopédie Indispensable aux Praticiens. 9th ed. Paris, Maloine, 1926, p 833.
22. Waldenström H: The first stages of coxa plana. J Bone Joint Surg *20*:559, 1938.
23. Kemp HS, Boldero JL: Radiological changes in Perthes' disease. Br J Radiol *39*:744, 1966.
24. Anderson J, Stewart AM: The significance of the magnitude of the medial hip joint space. Br J Radiol *43*:238, 1970.
25. Gill AB: Legg-Perthes disease of the hip: Its early roentgenographic manifestations and its cyclical course. J Bone Joint Surg *22*:1013, 1940.
26. Mindell ER, Sherman MS: Late results in Legg-Perthes disease. J Bone Joint Surg *33A*:1, 1951.
27. Ponseti IV: Legg-Perthes' disease: Observations on pathological changes in two cases. J Bone Joint Surg *38A*:739, 1956.
28. Ponseti IV, Cotton RL: Legg-Calvé-Perthes disease — pathogenesis and evaluation. Failure of treatment with L-triiodothyronine. J Bone Joint Surg *43A*:261, 1961.
29. Ferguson AB Jr: The pathology of Legg-Perthes disease and its comparison with aseptic necrosis. Clin Orthop Rel Res *106*:7, 1975.
30. Dolman CL, Bell HM: The pathology of Legg-Calvé-Perthes disease. A case report. J Bone Joint Surg *55A*:184, 1973.
31. McKibbin B, Ráliš Z: Pathological changes in a case of Perthes' disease. J Bone Joint Surg *56B*:438, 1974.
32. Jensen OM, Lauritzen J: Legg-Calvé-Perthes' disease. Morphological studies in two cases examined at necropsy. J Bone Joint Surg *58B*:332, 1976.
33. Snyder CR: Legg-Perthes disease in the young hip — does it necessarily do well? J Bone Joint Surg *57A*:751, 1975.
34. Mose K, Hjorth L, Ulfeldt M, Christensen ER, Jensen A: Legg Calvé Perthes disease. The late occurrence of coxarthrosis. Acta Orthop Scand Suppl *169*:1, 1977.
35. Stillman BC: Osteochondritis dissecans and coxa plana. Review of the literature with a personal case report. J Bone Joint Surg *48B*:64, 1966.
36. Ratliff AHC: Osteochondritis dissecans following Legg-Calvé-Perthes' disease. J Bone Joint Surg *49B*:108, 1967.

37. Katz JF: Recurrent Legg-Calvé-Perthes disease. J Bone Joint Surg *55A*:833, 1973.
38. Bjerkreim I, Hauge MF: So-called recurrent Perthes' disease. Acta Orthop Scand *47*:181, 1976.
39. Axer A, Hendel D: Recurrent Legg-Calvé-Perthes' disease. A case report. Clin Orthop Rel Res *126*:170, 1977.
40. Catterall A: The natural history of Perthes' disease. J Bone Joint Surg *53B*:37, 1971.
41. Murphy RP, Marsh HO: Incidence and natural history of "head at risk" factors in Perthes' disease. Clin Orthop Rel Res *132*:102, 1978.
42. Dickens DRV, Menelaus MB: The assessment of prognosis in Perthes' disease. J Bone Joint Surg *60B*:189, 1978.
43. Gower WE, Johnston RC: Legg-Perthes disease. Long-term follow-up of thirty-six patients. J Bone Joint Surg *53A*:759, 1971.
44. Ozonoff MB: Pediatric Orthopedic Radiology. Philadelphia, WB Saunders Co, 1979.
45. Jonsäter S: Coxa plana. A histo-pathologic and arthrographic study. Acta Orthop Scand Suppl *12*:7, 1953.
46. Danigelis JA: Pinhole imaging in Legg-Perthes disease: Further observations. Semin Nucl Med *6*:69, 1976.
47. Danigelis JA, Fisher RL, Ozonoff MB, Sziklas JJ: ^{99m}Tc-polyphosphate bone imaging in Legg-Perthes disease. Radiology *115*:407, 1975.
48. Fasting OJ, Langeland N, Bjerkreim I, Hertzenberg L, Nakken K: Bone scintigraphy in early diagnosis of Perthes' disease. Acta Orthop Scand *49*:169, 1978.
49. Trueta J: Normal vascular anatomy of the human femoral head during growth. J Bone Joint Surg *39B*:358, 1957.
50. Girdany BR, Osman MZ: Longitudinal growth and skeletal maturation in Perthes' disease. Radiol Clin North Am *6*:245, 1968.
51. Harrison MHM, Turner MH, Jacobs P: Skeletal immaturity in Perthes' disease. J Bone Joint Surg *58B*:37, 1976.
52. Wynne-Davies R, Gormley J: The aetiology of Perthes' disease. Genetic, epidemiological and growth factors in 310 Edinburgh and Glasgow patients. J Bone Joint Surg *60B*:6, 1978.
53. Jacobs BW: Early recognition of osteochondrosis of the capital epiphysis of the femur. JAMA *172*:527, 1960.
54. Zahir A, Freeman MAR: Cartilage changes following a single episode of infarction of the capital femoral epiphysis in the dog. J Bone Joint Surg *54A*:125, 1972.
55. Sanchis M, Zahir A, Freeman MAR: The experimental simulation of Perthes disease by consecutive interruptions of the blood supply to the capital femoral epiphysis in the puppy. J Bone Joint Surg *55A*:335, 1973.
56. Inoue A, Freeman MAR, Vernon-Roberts B, Mizuno S: The pathogenesis of Perthes' disease. J Bone Joint Surg *58B*:453, 1976.
57. Suramo I, Puranen J, Heikkinen E, Vuorinen P: Disturbed patterns of venous drainage of the femoral neck in Perthes' disease. J Bone Joint Surg *56B*:448, 1974.
58. Kemp HBS: Perthes disease: An experimental and clinical study. Ann R Coll Surg Engl *52*:18, 1973.
59. Meyer J: Dysplasia epiphysealis capitis femoris. A clinical-radiological syndrome and its relationship to Legg-Calvé-Perthes disease. Acta Orthop Scand *34*:183, 1964.
60. Freiberg AH: Infraction of the second metatarsal bone; a typical injury. Surg Gynecol Obstet *19*:191, 1914.
61. Panner HJ: A peculiar characteristic metatarsal disease. Acta Radiol *1*:319, 1921–1922.
62. Smillie IS: Freiberg's infraction (Koehler's second disease). J bone Joint Surg *39B*:580, 1955.
63. Freiberg AH: The so-called infraction of the second metatarsal bone. J Bone Joint Surg *8*:257, 1926.
64. Braddock GTF: Experimental epiphyseal injury and Freiberg's disease. J Bone Joint Surg *41B*:154, 1959.
65. Wagner A: Isolated aseptic necrosis in the epiphysis of the first metatarsal bone. Acta Radiol *11*:80, 1930.
66. Hoskinson J: Freiberg's disease: a review of long-term results. Proc R Soc Med *67*:106, 1974.
67. Peste: Discussion. Bull Soc Anat Paris *18*:169, 1843.
68. Kienböck R: Über traumatische Malazie des Mondbeins und ihre Folgezustände: Entartungsformen und Kompressionsfrakturen. Fortschr Geb Roentgenstr Nuklearmed *16*:77, 1910–1911.
69. Lichtman DM, Mack GR, MacDonald RI, Gunther SF, Wilson JN: Kienböck's disease: The role of silicone replacement arthroplasty. J Bone Joint Surg *59A*:899, 1977.
70. Cave EF: Kienböck's disease of the lunate. J Bone Joint Surg *21*:858, 1939.
71. Therkelsen F, Andersen K: Lunatomalacia. Acta Chir Scand *97*:503, 1949.
72. Gentaz R, Lespargot J, Levame JH, Poli P: La maladie de Kienböck. Approche tomographique. Analyse de 5 cas. Nouv Presse Med *1*:1207, 1972.
73. Simmons EH, Dommisse I: The pathogenesis and treatment of Kienböck's disease (Abstr). Clin Orthop Rel Res *105*:300, 1974.
74. Roca J, Beltran JE, Fairen MF, Alvarez A: Treatment of Kienböck's disease using a silicone rubber implant. J Bone Joint Surg *58A*:373, 1976.
75. Rooker GD, Goodfellow JW: Kienböck's disease in cerebral palsy. J Bone Joint Surg *59B*:363, 1977.
76. Rosemeyer B, Artmann M, Viernstein K: Lunatum-malacie. Nachuntersuchungsergebnisse und therapeutische Erwägungen. Arch Orthop Unfallchir *85*:119, 1976.
77. Sobel A, Sobel P: Un cas de maladie de Kienboeck bilatérale. J Radiol Electrol Med Nucl *31*:13, 1950.
78. Ståhl F: On lunatomalacia (Kienböck's disease). A clinical and roentgenological study, especially on its pathogenesis and the late results of immobilization treatment. Acta Chir Scand Suppl *126*:1, 1947.
79. Mouat TB, Wilkie J, Harding HE: Isolated fracture of the carpal semilunar and Kienböck's disease. Br J Surg *19*:577, 1932.
80. Lee MLH: The intraosseous arterial pattern of the carpal lunate bone and its relation to avascular necrosis. Acta Orthop Scand *33*:43, 1963.
81. Cordes E: Über die Entstehung der subchondralen Osteonekrosen. A. Die Lunatumnekrose. Bruns Beitr Klin Chir *149*:28, 1930.
82. Hultén O: Über anatomische Variationen der Handgelenkknochen. Acta Radiol *9*:155, 1928.
83. Hultén O: Über die Entstehung und Behandlung der Lunatummalazaie (Morbus Kienböck). Acta Chir Scand *76*:121, 1935.
84. Gelberman RH, Salamon PB, Jurist JM, Posch JL: Ulnar variance in Kienböck's disease. J Bone Joint Surg *57A*:674, 1975.
85. Chan KP, Huang P: Anatomic variations in radial and ulnar lengths in the wrists of Chinese. Clin Orthop Rel Res *80*:17, 1971.
86. Koken E-W: Anatomische Untersuchungen zum Problem der Blutversorgung des Os lunatum. Z Orthop *113*:1022, 1975.
87. Köhler A: Ueber eine häufige bisher anscheinend unbekannte Erkrankung einzelner Kindlicherknochen. Munchen Med Wochnschr *55*:1923, 1908.
88. Waugh W: The ossification and vascularisation of the tarsal navicular and their relation to Köhler's disease. J Bone Joint Surg *40B*:765, 1958.
89. Karp MG: Köhler's disease of the tarsal scaphoid. An end-result study. J Bone Joint Surg *19*:84, 1937.
90. McCauley RGK, Kahn PC: Osteochondritis of the tarsal navicula. Radioisotopic appearances. Radiology *123*:705, 1977.
91. Froelich R: Des apophysites de croissance. Paris Med *37*:430, 1929.
92. Ozonoff MB: Pediatric Orthopedic Radiology. Philadelphia, WB Saunders Co, 1979.
93. Lecène P, Mouchet A: La scaphoidite tarsienne (anatomie pathologique et pathogénie). Rev Orthop *11*:105, 1924.
94. Kidner FC, Muro F: Köhler's disease of the tarsal scaphoid or os naviculare pedis retardatum. JAMA *83*:1650, 1924.
95. Scaglietti O, Stringu G, Mizzau M: Plus-variant of the astragalus and subnormal scaphoid space, two important findings in Koehler's scaphoid necrosis. Acta Orthop Scand *32*:499, 1962.
96. Panner HJ: An affection of the capitulum humeri resembling Calvé-Perthes disease of the hip. Acta Radiol *8*:617, 1927.
97. Smith MGH: Osteochondritis of the humerus capitulum. J Bone Joint Surg *46B*:50, 1964.
98. Elward JF: Epiphysitis of the capitellum of the humerus. JAMA *112*:705, 1939.
99. Klein EW: Osteochondrosis of the capitulum (Panner's disease). Report of a case. Am J Roentgenol *88*:466, 1952.
100. Laurent LE, Lindström BL: Osteochondrosis of the capitulum humeri (Panner's disease). Acta Orthop Scand *26*:111, 1957.
101. Heller CJ, Wiltse LL: Avascular necrosis of the capitellum humeri (Panner's disease) A report of a case. J Bone Joint Surg *42A*:513, 1960.
102. March HC: Osteochondritis of the capitellum (Panner's disease). Am J Roentgenol *51*:682, 1944.
103. Adams JE: Injury to the throwing arm. A study of traumatic changes in the elbow joints of boy baseball players. Calif Med J *102*:127, 1965.
104. Jacobs P: Osteochondritis dissecans of the hip. Clin Radiol *13*:316, 1962.
105. Thiemann H: Juvenile Epiphysenstörungen. Fortschr Geb Roentgenstr Nuklearmed *14*:79, 1909.
106. Dessecker C: Zur Epiphyseonekrose der Mittelphalangen beider Hände. Dtsch Z Chir *229*:327, 1930.
107. Allison AC, Blumberg BS: Familial osteoarthropathy of the fingers. J Bone Joint Surg *40B*:538, 1958.
108. Cullen JC: Thiemann's disease. Osteochondrosis juvenilis of the basal epiphyses of the phalanges of the hand. Report of two cases. J Bone Joint Surg *52B*:532, 1970.
109. Rubinstein HM: Thiemann's disease. A brief reminder. Arthritis Rheum *18*:357, 1975.

110. Giedion A: Acrodysplasias, cone-shaped epiphyses, peripheral dysostosis, Thiemann's disease, and acrodysostosis. Progr Pediatr Radiol *4*:325, 1973.
111. Osgood RB: Lesions of the tibial tubercle occurring during adolescence. Boston Med Surg J *148*:114, 1903.
112. Schlatter C: Verletzungen des schnabelförmigen Fortsatzes der oberen Tibiaepiphyse. Bruns Beitr Klin Chir *38*:874, 1903.
113. Woolfrey BF, Chandler EF: Manifestations of Osgood-Schlatter's disease in late teenage and early adulthood. J Bone Joint Surg *42A*:327, 1960.
114. Stinchfield AJ: The tenosynovitis of Osgood-Schlatter disease. J Bone Joint Surg *45A*:1335, 1963.
115. Hulting B: Roentgenologic features of fracture of the tibial tuberosity (Osgood-Schlatter's disease). Acta Radiol *48*:161, 1957.
116. Ehrenborg G, Lagergren C: Roentgenologic changes in the Osgood-Schlatter lesion. Acta Chir Scand *121*:315, 1961.
117. Scotti DM, Sadhu, VK, Heimberg F, O'Hara AE: Osgood-Schlatter's disease, an emphasis on soft tissue changes in roentgen diagnosis. Skel Radiol *4*:21, 1979.
118. Odgen JA, Southwick WO: Osgood-Schlatter's disease and tibial tuberosity development. Clin Orthop Rel Res *116*:180, 1976.
119. D'Ambrosia RD, MacDonald GL: Pitfalls in the diagnosis of Osgood-Schlatter disease. Clin Orthop Rel Res *110*:206, 1975.
120. Lutterotti M: Beitrag zur Genese der Schlatterschen Krankheit. Z Orthop *77*:160, 1947.
121. Ogden JA, Hempton RF, Southwick WO: Development of the tibial tuberosity. Anat Rec *182*:431, 1975.
122. Uhry E Jr: Osgood-Schlatter disease. Arch Surg *48*:406, 1944.
123. LaZerte GD, Rapp IH: Pathogenesis of Osgood-Schlatter's disease. Am J Pathol *34*:803, 1958.
124. Jeffreys TE: Genu recurvatum after Osgood-Schlatter's disease Report of a case. J Bone Joint Surg *47B*:298, 1965.
125. Stirling RI: Complications of Osgood-Schlatter's disease. J Bone Joint Surg *34B*:149, 1952.
126. Blount WP: Tibia vara. Osteochondrosis deformans tibiae. J Bone Joint Surg *19*:1, 1937.
127. Shopfner CE, Coin CG: Genu varus and valgus in children. Radiology *92*:723, 1969.
128. Bateson EM: Non-rachitic bowleg and knock-knee deformities in young Jamaican children. Br J Radiol *39*:92, 1966.
129. Golding JSR, McNeil-Smith JDG: Observations on the etiology of tibia vara. J Bone Joint Surg *45B*:320, 1963.
130. Bateson EM: The relationship between Blount's disease and bow legs. Br J Radiol *41*:107, 1968.
131. Bathfield CA, Beighton PH: Blount disease. A review of etiological factors in 110 patients. Clin Orthop Rel Res *135*:29, 1978.
132. Sibert JR, Bray PT: Probable dominant inheritance in Blount's disease. Clin Genet *11*:394, 1977.
133. Langenskiöld A: Tibia vara. Osteochondrosis deformans tibiae. A survey of 23 cases. Acta Chir Scand *103*:1, 1952.
134. Langenskiöld A, Riska EB: Tibia vara (Osteochondrosis deformans tibiae). J Bone Joint Surg *46A*:1405, 1964.
135. Tachdjian MO: Pediatric Orthopedics. Philadelphia, WB Saunders Co, 1972.
136. Currarino G, Kirks DR: Lateral widening of epiphyseal plates in knees of children with bowed legs. Am J Roentgenol *129*:309, 1977.
137. Kettelkamp DB, Chao EY: A method for quantitative analysis of medial and lateral compression forces at the knee during standing. Clin Orthop Rel Res *83*:202, 1972.
138. Kilburn P: A metaphysial abnormality: Report of a case with features of metaphysial dysostosis. J Bone Joint Surg *55B*:643, 1973.
139. Pitzen P, Marquardt W: O-Beinbildung durch umschriebene Epiphysenwachstumsstörung (Tibia-vara-Bildung). Z Orthop *69*:174, 1939.
140. Scheuermann HW: Kyphosis dorsalis juvenilis. Z Orthop Chir *41*:305, 1921.
141. Scheuermann H: Kyphosis juvenilis (Scheuermann's Krankheit). Fortschr Geb Roentgenstr Nuklearmed *53*:1, 1936.
142. Sørensen KH: Scheuermann's Juvenile Kyphosis. Copenhagen, Munksgaard, 1964.
143. Alexander CJ: Scheuermann's disease. A traumatic spondylodystrophy? Skel Radiol *1*:209, 1977.
144. Wassman K: Kyphosis juvenilis Scheuermann — an occupational disorder. Acta Orthop Scand *21*:65, 1951.
145. Dameron TE Jr, Gulledge WH: Adolescent kyphosis. US Armed Forces Med J *4*:871, 1953.
146. Bradford DS, Moe JH, Montalvo FJ, Winter RB: Scheuermann's kyphosis and roundback deformity. Results of Milwaukee brace treatment. J Bone Joint Surg *56A*:740, 1974.
147. Bradford DS, Moe JH, Montalvo FJ, Winter RB: Scheuermann's kyphosis. Results of surgical treatment by posterior spine arthrodesis in twenty-two patients. J Bone Joint Surg *57A*:439, 1975.
148. Butler RW: The nature and significance of vertebral osteochondritis. Proc R Soc Med *48*:895, 1955.
149. Edgren W, Vainio S: Osteochondrosis juvenilis lumbalis. Acta Chir Scand Suppl *227*:1, 1957.
150. Fried K: Die zervikale juvenile Osteochondrose (Scheuermannsche Krankheit). Fortschr Geb Roentgenstr Nuklearmed *105*:69, 1966.
151. Lamb DW: Localised osteochondritis of the lumbar spine. J Bone Joint Surg *36B*:591, 1954.
152. Schmorl G, Junghanns H: The Human Spine in Health and Disease. Translated by EF Besemann. 2nd Ed. New York, Grune & Stratton, 1971.
153. Butler RW: Spontaneous anterior fusion of vertebral bodies. J Bone Joint Surg *53B*:230, 1971.
154. Knutsson F: Fusion of vertebrae following non-infectious disturbance in the zone of growth. Acta Radiol *32*:404, 1949.
155. Bradford DS, Garcia A: Neurological complications in Scheuermann's disease. A case report and review of the literature. J Bone Joint Surg *51A*:567, 1969.
156. Wise BL, Foster JJ: Congenital spinal extradural cyst. Case report and review of the literature. J Neurosurg *12*:421, 1955.
157. Van Landingham JH: Herniation of thoracic intervertebral discs with spinal cord compression in kyphosis dorsalis juvenilis (Scheuermann's disease). Case report. J Neurosurg *11*:327, 1954.
158. Adelstein LJ: Spinal extradural cyst associated with kyphosis dorsalis juvenilis. J Bone Joint Surg *23*:93, 1941.
159. Cloward RB, Bucy PC: Spinal extradural cyst and kyphosis dorsalis juvenilis. Am J Roentgenol *38*:681, 1937.
160. Bradford DS, Moe JH: Scheuermann's juvenile kyphosis. A histologic study. Clin Orthop Rel Res *110*:45, 1975.
161. Laederer R: La dégénérescence juvénile du disque inter-vertebral. (Contribution à la pathogénèse de la maladie de Scheuermann). Schweiz Z Pathol *11*:590, 1948.
162. Müller G, Gschwend N: Endokrine Störungen und Morbus Scheuermann. Arch Orthop Unfallchir *65*:357, 1969.
163. Simon RS: The diagonosis and treatment of kyphosis dorsalis juvenilis (Scheuermann's kyphosis) in the early stage. J Bone Joint Surg *24*:681, 1942.
164. Kemp FH, Wilson DC, Emrys-Roberts E: Social and nutritional factors in adolescent osteochondritis of the spine. Br J Soc Med *2*:66, 1948.
165. Mühlbach R, Hähnel H, Cohn H: Zur Bedeutung biochemischer Parameter bei der Beurteilung der Scheuermannschen Krankheit. Med Sport *10*:331, 1970.
166. Gardemin H, Herbst W: Wirbeldeformierung bei der Adoleszentenkyphose und Osteoporose. Arch Orthop Unfallchir *59*:134, 1966.
167. Bradford DS, Brown DM, Moe JH, Winter RB, Jowsey J: Scheuermann's kyphosis. A form of osteoporosis? Clin Orthop Rel Res *118*:10, 1976.
168. Halal F, Gledhill RB, Fraser FC: Dominant inheritance of Scheuermann's juvenile kyphosis. Am J Dis Child *132*:1105, 1978.
169. Kewalramani LS, Riggins RS, Fowler WM Jr: Scheuermann's Kyphoscoliosis associated with Charcot-Marie-Tooth syndrome. Arch Phys Med Rehabil *57*:391, 1976.
170. Schmorl G: Die Pathogenese der juvenilen Kyphose. Fortschr Geb Roentgenstr Nuklearmed *41*:359, 1930.
171. Beadle O: The intervertebral disc. Med Res Council Spec Rep Series *161*:1, 1931.
172. Aufdermaur M: Zur Pathogenese der Scheuermannschen Krankheit. Dtsch Med Wochenschr *89*:73, 1964.
173. Aufdermaur M: Die Scheuermannsche Adoleszentenkyphose. Orthopaede *2*:153, 1973.
174. Sinding-Larsen MF: A hitherto unknown affection of the patella in children. Acta Radiol *1*:171, 1921.
175. Johansson S: En forut icke beskriven sjukdom i patella. Hygiea *84*:161, 1922.
176. Wolf J: Larsen-Johansson disease of the patella. Seven new case records. Its relationship to other forms of osteochondritis. Use of male sex hormones as a new form of treatment. Br J Radiol *23*:335, 1950.
177. Medlar RC, Lyne ED: Sinding-Larsen-Johansson disease. Its etiology and natural history. J Bone Joint Surg *60A*:1113, 1978.
178. Kay JJ, Freiberger RH: Fragmentation of the lower pole of the patella in spastic lower extremities. Radiology *101*:97, 1971.
179. Rosenthal RK, Levine DB: Fragmentation of the distal pole of the patella in spastic cerebral palsy. J Bone Joint Surg *59A*:934, 1977.
180. Green WT: Painful bipartite patella. A report of three cases. Clin Orthop Rel Res *110*:197, 1975.
181. Sever JW: Apophysitis of the os calcis. N Y Med J *95*:1025, 1912.
182. Allison N: Apophysitis of the os calcis. A clinical report. J Bone Joint Surg *6*:91, 1924.
183. Christie AC: Osteochondritis, or epiphysitis: A review. JAMA *87*:291, 1926.

184. Lewin P: Apophysitis of the os calcis. Surg Gynecol Obstet *41*:579, 1925.
185. Hughes ESR: Painful heels in children. Surg Gynecol Obstet *86*:64, 1948.
186. Shopfner CE, Coin CG: Effect of weight-bearing on the appearance and development of the secondary calcaneal epiphysis. Radiology *86*:201, 1966.
187. Van Neck M: Ostéochondrite du pubis. Arch Franco-Belges Chir *27*:238, 1924.
188. Caffey J, Ross SE: The ischiopubic synchondrosis in healthy children: Some normal roentgenologic findings. Am J Roentgenol *76*:488, 1956.
189. Köhler A: Ueber eine häufige, bisher anscheinend unbekannte Erkrankung einzelner kindlicher Knochen. Munch Med Wochenschr *55*:1923, 1908.
190. Mandl F: Die "Schlatter'sche Krankheit" als "Systemerkrankung." Bruns Beitr Klin Chir *126*:707, 1922.
191. Boldero JL, Mitchell GP: Osteochondritis of the superior tibial epiphysis. J Bone Joint Surg *36B*:114, 1954.
192. Siffert RS, Arkin AM: Post-traumatic aseptic necrosis of the distal tibial epiphysis. J Bone Joint Surg *32A*:691, 1950.
193. Meilstrup DB: Osteochondritis of the internal cuneiform, bilateral. Case report. Am J Roentgenol *58*:329, 1947.
194. Iselin H: Wachstumsbeschwerden zur Zeit der Knöchernen Entwicklung der Tuberositas metatarsi quinti. Dtsch Z Chir *117*:529, 1912.
195. Burns BH: Osteochondritis juvenilis of the lower ulnar epiphysis. Proc R Soc Med *24*:912, 1931.
196. Mauclaire P: Epiphysitis der Metakarpusköpfchen mit Hohlbildung der Hand. Fortschr Geb Roentgenstr Nuklearmed *37*:425, 1928.
197. Ellman H: Unusual affections of the preadolescent elbow. J Bone Joint Surg *49A*:203, 1967.
198. Blakemore ME, Harrison MHM: A prospective study of children with untreated Catterall Group I Perthes' disease. J Bone Joint Surg *61B*:329, 1979.
199. Bohr HH: Skeletal maturation in Legg-Calvé-Perthes' disease. Int Orthop (SICOT) *2*:277, 1979.
200. Gauthier G, Elbaz R: Freiberg's infraction: A subchondral bone fatigue fracture. A new surgical treatment. Clin Orthop Rel Res *142*:93, 1979.
201. Beckenbaugh RD, Shives TC, Dobyns JH, Linscheid RL: Kienböck's disease: The natural history of Kienböck's disease and consideration of lunate fractures. Clin Orthop Rel Res *149*:98, 1980.
202. Gelberman RH, Bauman TD, Menon J, Akeson WH: The vascularity of the lunate bone and Kienböck's disease. J Hand Surg *5*:272, 1980.
203. Weston WJ: Kohler's disease of the tarsal scaphoid. Australas Radiol *22*:332, 1978.
204. Mital MA, Matza RA, Cohen J: The so-called unresolved Osgood-Schlatter lesion. J Bone Joint Surg *62A*:732, 1980.
205. Catonné Y, Pacault C, Azaloux H, Tiré J, Ridarch A, Blanchard P: Aspects radiologiques de la maladie de Blount. J Radiol *61*:171, 1980.
206. Bjersand AJ: Juvenile kyphosis in identical twins. Am J Roentgenol *134*: 598, 1980.
207. Guelpa G, Chamay A, Lagier R: Bilateral osteochondritis dissecans of the carpal scaphoid. Internat Orthop (SICOT) *4*:25, 1980.
208. Gershuni DH, Axer A, Hendel D: Arthrography as an aid to diagnosis, prognosis, and therapy in Legg-Calvé-Perthes' disease. Acta Orthop Scand *51*:505, 1980.
209. Théron J: Angiography in Legg-Calvé-Perthes disease. Radiology *135*:81, 1980.
210. Murray IPC: Bone scanning in the child and young adult. Part II. Skel Radiol *5*:65, 1980.
211. Morley TR, Short MD, Dowsett DJ: Femoral head activity in Perthes' disease: Clinical evaluation of a quantitative technique for estimating tracer uptake. J Nucl Med *19*:884, 1978.
212. Fisher RL, Roderique JW, Brown DC, Danigelis JA, Ozonoff MB, Sziklas JJ: The relationship of isotopic bone imaging findings to prognosis in Legg-Perthes disease. Clin Orthop Rel Res *150*:23, 1980.
213. Sutherland AD, Savage JP, Paterson DC, Foster BK: The nuclide bonescan in the diagnosis and management of Perthes' disease. J Bone Joint Surg *62B*:300, 1980.
214. Heikkinen E, Lanning P, Suramo I, Puranen J: The venous drainage of the femoral neck as a prognostic sign in Perthes' disease. Acta Orthop Scand *51*:501, 1980.
215. Langenskiöld A: Changes in the capital growth plate and the proximal femoral metaphysis in Legg-Calvé-Perthes disease. Clin Orthop Rel Res *150*:110, 1980.
216. Kelly FB Jr, Canale ST, Jones RR: Legg-Calvé-Perthes disease. J Bone Joint Surg *62A*:400, 1980.
217. Wynne-Davies R: Some etiologic factors in Perthes' disease. Clin Orthop Rel Res *150*:12, 1980.
218. Fasting OJ, Bjerkreim I, Langeland N, Hertzenberg L, Nakken K: Scintigraphic evaluation of the severity of Perthes' disease in the initial stage. Acta Orthop Scand *51*:655, 1980.
219. Katz JF, Siffert RS: Osteochondritis dissecans in association with Legg-Calvé-Perthes disease. International Orthop (SICOT) *3*:189, 1979.
220. Milgram JW: Synovial osteochondromatosis in association with Legg-Calvé-Perthes disease. Clin Orthop Rel Res *145*:179, 1979.
221. Nevelös AB: Bilateral Perthes' disease. Acta Orthop Scand *51*:649, 1980.
222. Harrison MHM, Blakemore ME: A study of the "normal" hip in children with unilateral Perthes' disease. J Bone Joint Surg *62B*:31, 1980.
223. Herring JA, Lundeen MA, Wenger DR: Minimal Perthes' disease. J Bone Joint Surg *62B*:25, 1980.
224. Inoue A, Ono K, Takaoka K, Yoshioka T, Hosoya T: A comparative study of histology in Perthes' disease and idiopathic avascular necrosis of the femoral head in adults (IANF). Internat Orthop (SICOT) *4*:39, 1980.
225. Zayer M: Osteoarthritis following Blount's disease. International Orthopaedics (SICOT) *4*:63, 1980.
226. Hardcastle PH, Ross R, Hamalainen M, Mata A: Catterall grouping of Perthes' disease. J Bone Joint Surg *62B*:428, 1980.
227. Barnes, JM: Premature epiphysial closure in Perthes' disease. J Bone Joint Surg *62B*:432, 1980.

SECTION XVIII

MISCELLANEOUS DISEASES

79

SARCOIDOSIS

by Donald Resnick, M.D., and Gen Niwayama, M.D.

Sarcoidosis is a granulomatous disorder of unknown etiology affecting multiple organ systems, especially in young adults, and leading principally to bilateral hilar adenopathy, pulmonary infiltrates, and skin or eye lesions.[1] The diagnosis of the disease is substantiated by a combination of clinical, radiologic, and histologic features, the latter consisting predominantly of widespread, noncaseating epithelioid cell granulomas. The course of the disease is variable, and it may be associated with significant musculoskeletal abnormalities.

ETIOLOGY AND PATHOGENESIS

Theories of the etiology of this disorder abound, yet none has been confirmed. Many of its features, such as the disseminated distribution, the presence of granulomas that morphologically resemble those associated with infection, and the familial and geographic clustering, suggest that sarcoidosis is an infectious disorder.[2] *Mycobacterium tuberculosis* and other mycobacteria, fungi, and viruses have been offered as possible etiologic agents. However, typical or atypical mycobacteria are not consistently recovered from the granulomatous lesions of sarcoidosis. Similarly, isolation of fungal or viral agents has not been accomplished.[3] Although elevation of antibody titers to viruses such as Epstein-Barr, herpes simplex, rubella, measles, and parainfluenza is recorded, the finding is not consistent, nor does it correlate with the clinical activity or stage of the disease.[2] Evidence has existed that an agent from human sarcoid tissue can be transmitted into the foot pads of mice much more consistently than from normal lymph node tissue; autoclaved or irradiated sarcoid tissue does not induce granuloma formation.[2]

The occasional reports of sarcoidosis occurring in families suggest that hereditary influences may also be important in the etiology or pathogenesis of this disease;[3] the clinical and radiologic features of familial sarcoidosis are generally similar to those of sporadic sarcoidosis. However, no significant association between sarcoidosis and either serologically defined or lymphocyte-defined transplantation antigens has been demonstrated, although there may be a higher frequency of HLA B8 in patients with erythema nodosum and polyarthralgias.[2]

Although immunologic abnormalities are well recognized manifestations of the disease, they are not fully understood, they vary from one individual to another, and they occur in patients with a variety of other disorders. The immune mechanisms influence the clinical symptoms and signs associated with the various forms of the disease, but the abnormal immune reactivity per se does not cause sarcoidosis.[2]

CLINICAL ABNORMALITIES

Sarcoidosis has a worldwide distribution and is by no means rare in the United States, where the highest concentration of cases occurs in the Southeast. The disease affects men and women equally, although it is particularly common in women of childbearing age. It usually becomes apparent between 20 and 40 years of age. Blacks are more frequently affected than whites; in the United States, the disease is ten times more common in black patients. Sarcoidosis appears to be rare in Chinese individuals.

The clinical manifestations are highly variable. In some patients, radiographic evidence of hilar adenopathy may appear in the absence of any symptoms and signs.[4] In others, an acute or chronic form of the disease becomes evident.[3] Pulmonary manifestations are frequent, and include cough, chest pain, and dyspnea. Ocular abnormalities include a granulomatous uveitis, iritis, and iridocyclitis. Discrete, agglomerated, reddish skin nodules that are flat or slightly raised are seen, which upon histologic examination are found to consist of typical granulomas. Also, in acute sarcoidosis, erythema nodosum is common, which, when combined with hilar adenopathy and arthralgia, indicates a favorable prognosis. Malaise, anorexia, weight loss, fever, hepatosplenomegaly, and lymphadenopathy are also detected in many cases. Additional findings relate to involvement of other organs, including those of the central or peripheral nervous system, the heart, and the musculoskeletal system.

Laboratory analysis may indicate anemia, leukopenia, eosinophilia, a reduction in serum albumin concentration, and an elevation of serum globulin level. Hypercalcemia can be seen in approximately 25 per cent of cases, reflecting increased sensitivity to vitamin D and increased intestinal absorption of calcium. It is usually mild, and may be associated with normal or slightly elevated serum phosphate levels and hypercalciuria. The administration of cortisone reduces the hypercalcemia.[5]

In 60 to 80 per cent of patients with sarcoidosis, especially those with early disease and prominent adenopathy,[6] an intradermal injection of 0.2 ml of a 10 per cent saline suspension of sarcoid tissue produces a nodule containing noncaseating granulomas. This represents a positive Kveim test,[7] a reaction that is present in only 3 to 4 per cent of patients with other granulomatous disorders.[2] However, the general lack of availability of Kveim antigen and the occasional positivity of the test in other diseases such as regional enteritis[8] limit the usefulness of this reaction. Furthermore, as hypergammaglobulinemia and cutaneous anergy[9] represent nonspecific findings of sarcoidosis, a search for more diagnostic laboratory tests has been undertaken. Recently, the demonstration that circulating levels of angiotensin-converting enzyme (ACE) are elevated in approximately 80 per cent of patients with acute pulmonary sarcoidosis, perhaps related to increased synthesis of the enzyme by epithelioid cells in the granuloma, may indicate that a more specific test for the disorder is available, although elevations of ACE have also been recorded in Gaucher's disease and leprosy.[10]

GENERAL PATHOLOGIC ABNORMALITIES

The accurate diagnosis of sarcoidosis is based on compatible clinical and radiologic findings, the presence of supporting laboratory data such as a positive reaction to Kveim antigen, anergy, and elevated serum gamma globulins, and the demonstration of typical noncaseating granulomas in the absence of other identifiable causes for such lesions. Although the histologic features of sarcoidosis are well known, it must be recognized that noncaseating granulomas can be evident in additional neoplastic and infectious disorders. The granuloma is composed of discrete hyperplastic tubercles consisting predominant-

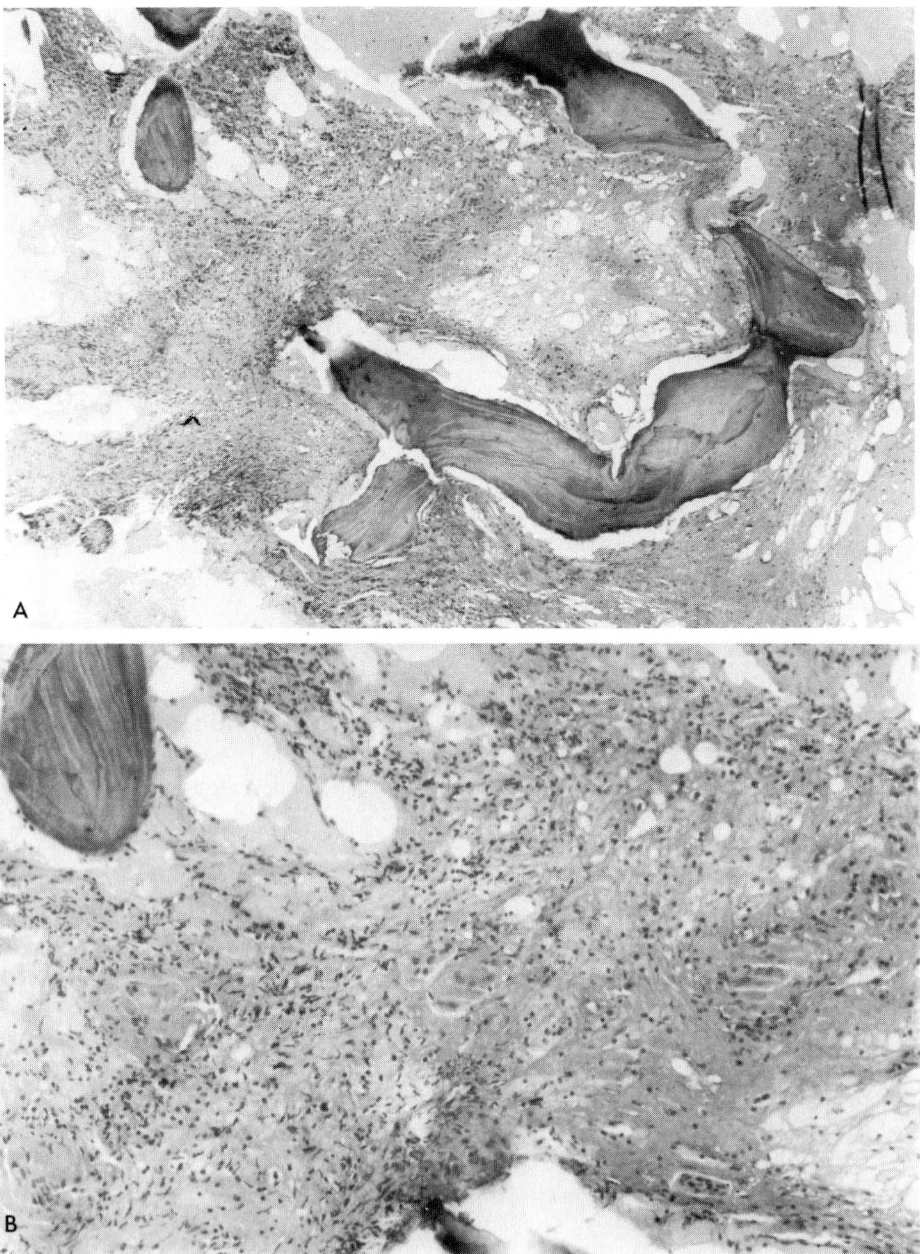

Figure 79–1. Sarcoidosis: Pathologic abnormalities.

A The bone marrow spaces are replaced by granulomatous lesions (72×).

B At higher power (180×), epithelioid cells and multiple Langhans' giant cells are observed.

Illustration continued on the opposite page

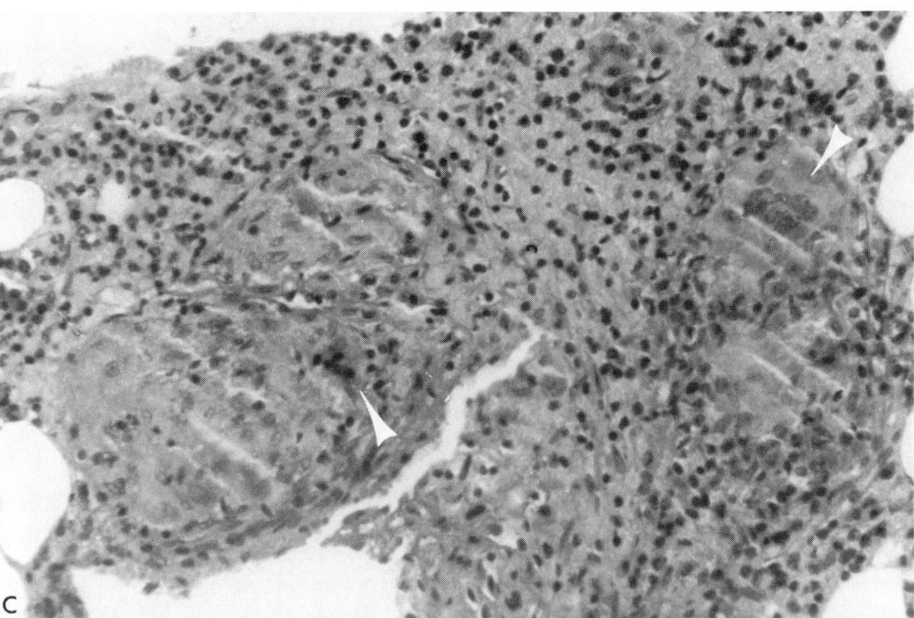

Figure 79–1. Continued
C *In this photomicrograph, note the epithelioid cells, multiple Langhans' giant cells (arrowheads), lymphocytes, and fibroblasts. No caseation is present. Special stains and culture for acid-fast bacilli and fungi gave negative results (360 ×).*

ly of epithelioid cells[11, 12] (Fig. 79–1). Additional cell types that are present are lymphocytes, giant cells, and plasma cells. Caseation is characteristically absent. Granulomas can be apparent in almost any organ but are most often present in the lung, lymph nodes, liver, and spleen.[11] They can grow slowly or rapidly, but in many cases they remain relatively unchanged in both size and number. As they resolve, the granulomas are frequently replaced with fibrous elements. It is this fibrosis, in addition to the mechanical compression of the adjacent tissue by the granuloma itself, that accounts for the clinically apparent organ dysfunction in many systems of the body that characterizes sarcoidosis.[2]

MUSCULOSKELETAL ABNORMALITIES

Sarcoidosis can involve muscles, bones, and joints and results in prominent clinical, radiologic, and pathologic findings.

Muscle Involvement

Granulomatous involvement of muscular tissues in sarcoidosis can be symptomatic or asymptomatic. Pain, tenderness, and nodular swelling are typical clinical findings. A true symmetric proximal sarcoid myopathy can occur with or without evidence of disease in other locations.[13] The myopathy, which can cause weakness, elevated muscle enzyme levels, and abnormal electromyograms, may respond favorably to corticosteroid treatment and is associated with noncaseating granulomatous, lymphocytic infiltration, and muscle necrosis and regeneration.

Osseous Involvement

Incidence. Clinical evidence of bone involvement was noted before the discovery of X rays. Pronounced chronic swelling about affected fingers and toes in association with lupus pernio (Boeck's sarcoid) was recognized by Besnier in 1898[14] and further described by Kreibich in 1904.[15] Rieder in 1910[16] and Jüngling in 1928[17] noted radiographic findings in lupus pernio, although accurate differentiation of the sarcoid lesions from tuberculosis was not accomplished until later. Although there now are innumerable reports of osseous involvement in sarcoidosis that define its radiographic characteristics,[18-22] there has been much disagreement about the incidence of skeletal involvement in the disease. In a review of reports of sarcoidosis throughout the world, the incidence of radiographic evidence of osseous involvement varied from 1 to 13 per cent, averaging 5 per cent[3] (Table 79–1). It is obvious that variations in these reports and others are related to differences in patient selection and method of examination. As many of the skeletal lesions of sarcoidosis are asymptomatic, an accurate appraisal of the incidence of osseous involvement in this disease would require complete skeletal surveys of patients with all forms of sarcoidosis, regardless of their clinical manifestations. Furthermore, as minor cystic bone changes in this disorder may resemble findings in "normal" individuals,[23] an age- and sex-matched control population must also be evaluated. As this type of comprehensive investigation has not been accomplished to

Table 79–1

FREQUENCY OF BONE LESIONS IN LARGE SERIES OF SARCOIDOSIS PATIENTS FROM 10 CITIES*

	Number of Patients		Bone Lesions	
City	*WITH SARCOIDOSIS*	*UNDERGOING SKELETAL RADIOGRAPHY*	*NUMBER*	*PER CENT*
London	537	475	19	4
New York	311	139	13	9
Paris	329	165	6	3.5
Los Angeles	150	60	3	4
Tokyo	282	282	5	2
Reading	425	425	5	1
Lisbon	89	89	12	13
Edinburgh	502	502	6	1.2
Novi Sad	285	225	25	11
Geneva	121	121	4	3
Total	3031	2483	98	5

*Used by permission from James DG, Neville E, Carstairs LS: Bone and joint sarcoidosis. Semin Arthritis Rheum 6:53–81, 1976.

date, the quoted figure of 5 per cent must be viewed with caution.

Osseous sarcoidosis is rarely detected in the absence of skin lesions,[24] although the skeletal abnormalities can be prominent even when cutaneous alterations are quite subtle. It has been estimated that 80 to 90 per cent of patients with sarcoidosis involving bone have radiographic evidence of pulmonary disease.[2] Bone changes in this disease, in the absence of additional clinical or radiologic manifestations, are distinctly unusual.

Clinical Manifestations. Although bone changes often are entirely asymptomatic,[11, 18, 25, 26] clinical manifestations in some cases may be prominent. Soft tissue swelling and cutaneous lesions of the hands and, less typically, the feet can accompany osseous disease. These clinical findings are frequently symmetric in distribution, and are most prominent over the proximal and middle phalanges of the digits. Less often, the areas of the metacarpals, metatarsals, terminal phalanges, wrists, and midfeet are affected.[12] Tenderness, stiffness, and restricted motion can be seen. Soft tissue swelling and deformity may be apparent also at other sites, including the nose,[27-29] face and sinuses,[30-34] skull, and extremities. Pathologic fractures of tubular bones of the extremities[35] and spinal cord compression[36-38] due to sarcoidosis can also lead to prominent clinical manifestations.

Radiographic Manifestations. The roentgenographic manifestations of sarcoidosis vary with the region of the skeleton that is affected. Certain specific patterns can be recognized, especially in the bones of the hand.

Osteoporosis producing generalized osteopenia, a decrease in cortical thickness, and striations of the cortex has been observed in sarcoidosis, perhaps related to granulomatous destruction and displacement of spongy trabeculae and perivascular infiltration of the haversian systems. A coarsened, reticulated, or lacework trabecular pattern becomes evident. Localized rarefactions or cystic lesions may lead to a "punched-out" appearance that can simulate that which is encountered in a variety of benign or malignant processes. These cysts can be centrally or eccentrically located, sharply marginated, and round or ovoid, and are frequently combined with alterations in the adjacent trabecular structure. At times, osseous destruction can appear rapidly, associated with a permeative pattern, cortical violation, and sequestration. Remarkably, even in the presence of this aggressive dissolution of bone, periostitis is distinctly unusual. Furthermore, osteosclerosis about these rarefactions is absent or mild.

Less typically, localized or generalized osteosclerosis is evident (Fig. 79–2). Nodular opacities can appear in the medullary cavities of the tubular bones of the hands and feet, or about the terminal phalanges (acro-osteosclerosis) (see discussion later in this chapter). In unusual circumstances, a widespread increase in skeletal radiodensity may be seen.[39-42] The latter osteosclerotic changes are most frequent in the spine, pelvis, skull, ribs, and proximal long bones; they can be diffuse or focal in nature, resembling changes in Paget's disease, skeletal metastasis, lymphoma, myelofibrosis, mastocytosis, hemoglobinopathies, renal osteodystrophy, and fluorosis. Skeletal biopsy has revealed typical granulomas, confirming the diagnosis of sarcoidosis as the cause of the increased radiodensity.

Hands and Feet. The hand is the predominant site of skeletal sarcoidosis.[18-21, 43, 44, 109] Involvement of the wrist and foot is less frequent. Unilateral or bilateral changes can be encountered, but close symmetry between lesions on the two sides of the body is unusual. In the hand, abnormalities are found in the middle and distal phalanges, and, less often, the proximal phalanges and metacarpals. Several types of lesions are seen (Fig. 79–3). Diffuse trabecular alterations are especially characteristic, leading to a

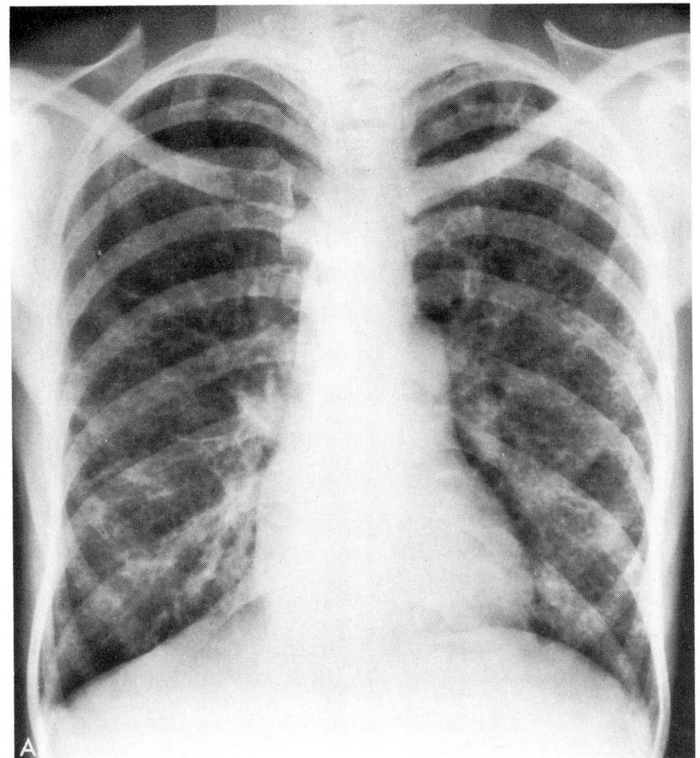

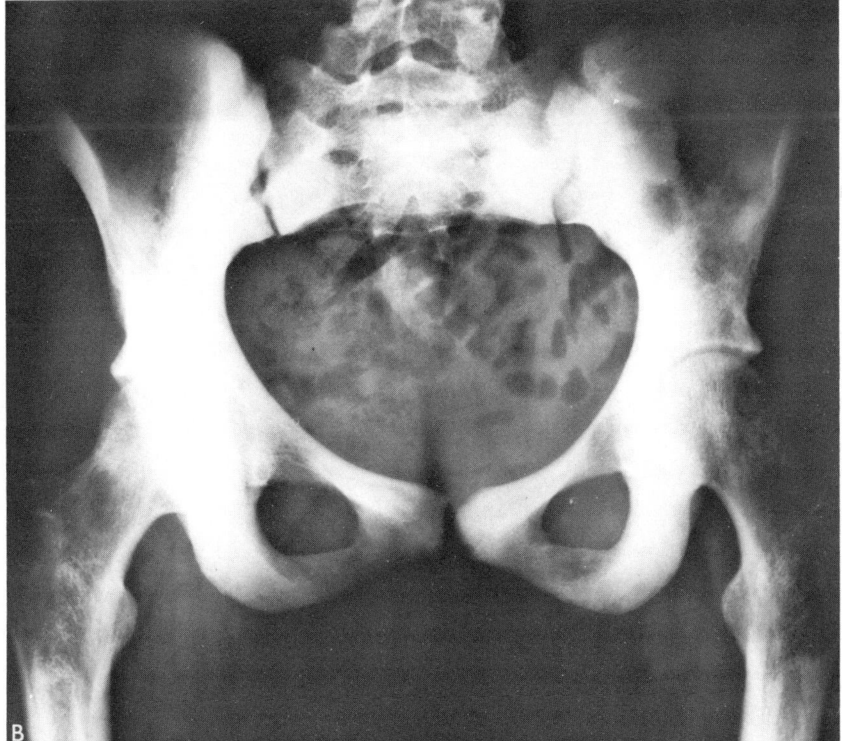

Figure 79–2. *Sarcoidosis: Osteosclerosis. This 29 year old black woman had an established diagnosis of sarcoidosis of 13 years' duration with involvement of lungs, lymph nodes, and liver.*

A *A chest roentgenogram reveals diffuse pulmonary fibrosis compatible with sarcoidosis.*

B *In the pelvis, there is uniform increased bone density, especially in the iliac bones, ischii, and superior pubic rami.*

Illustration continued on the following page

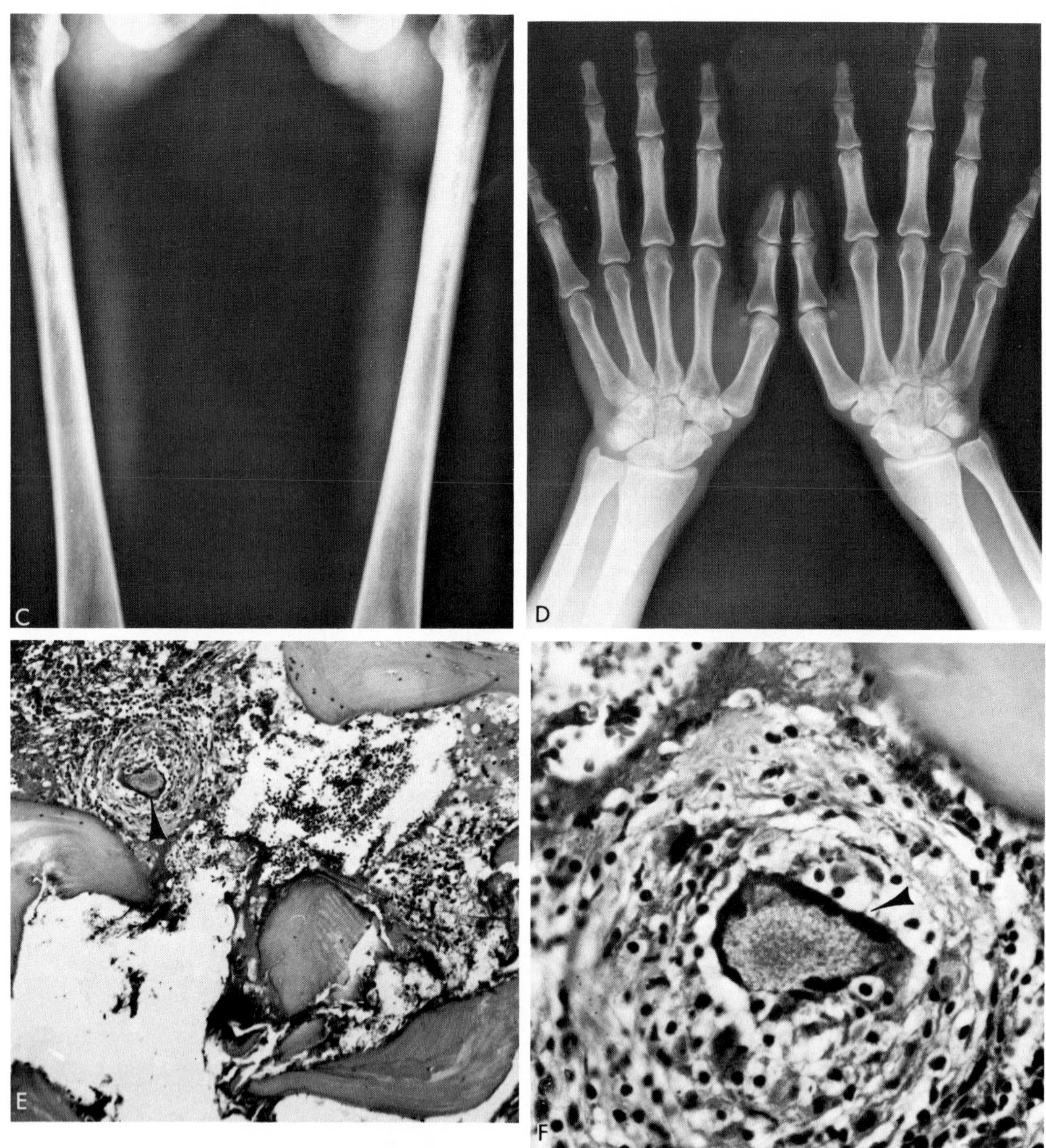

Figure 79–2. Continued

C *A "bone-within-bone" appearance in the femora is evident. Observe the increased density in the proximal two thirds of the bones.*

D *In the hands, small foci of increased density can be seen in the terminal phalanges.*

E, F *Following an iliac crest biopsy, low* **(E)** *and high* **(F)** *power views reveal thickened, cancellous bone with a noncaseating granuloma containing a characteristic giant cell (arrowhead).*

Illustration continued on the opposite page

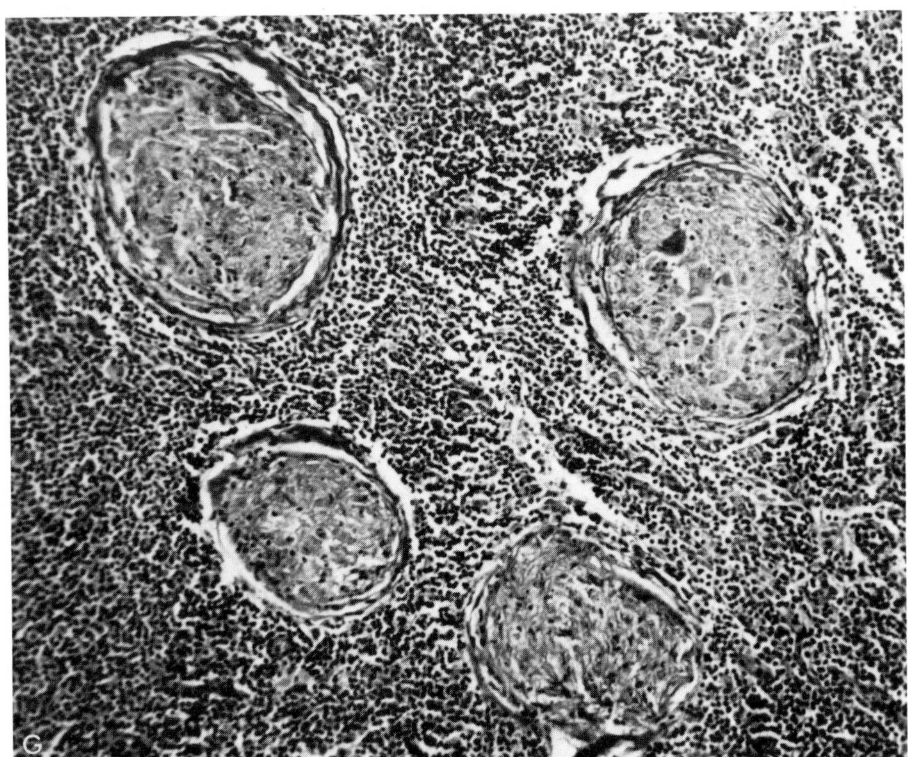

Figure 79–2. Continued

G *Following an axillary lymph node biopsy, a photomicrograph reveals a lymph node containing four well-defined noncaseating granulomas.*

(From Bonakdarpour A, et al: Am J Roentgenol 113:646, 1971. Copyright 1971, American Roentgen Ray Society.)

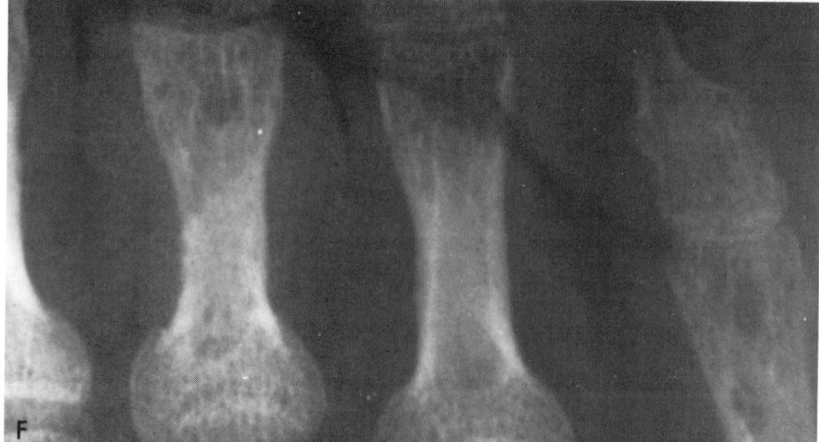

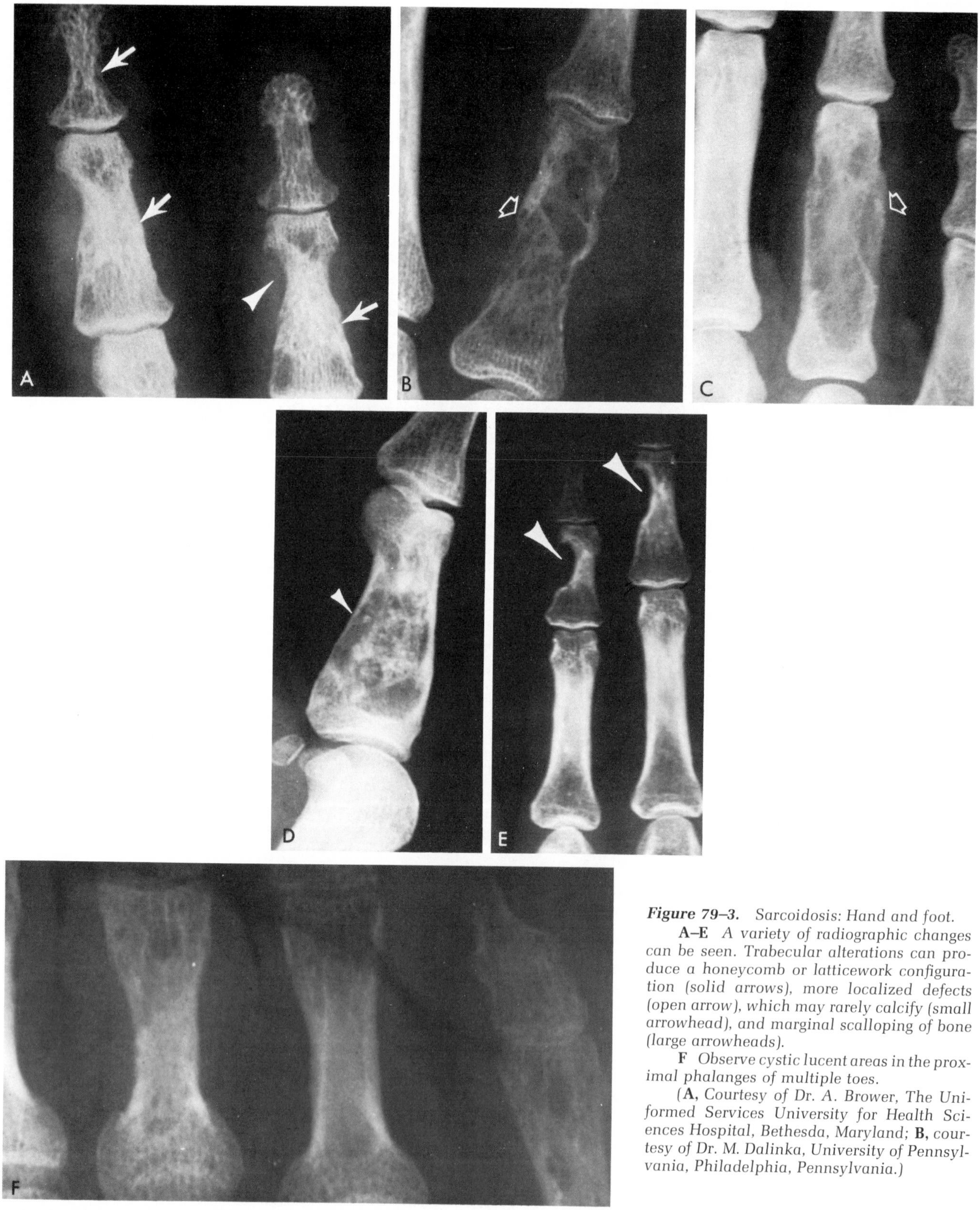

Figure 79–3. *Sarcoidosis: Hand and foot.*

A–E *A variety of radiographic changes can be seen. Trabecular alterations can produce a honeycomb or latticework configuration (solid arrows), more localized defects (open arrow), which may rarely calcify (small arrowhead), and marginal scalloping of bone (large arrowheads).*

F *Observe cystic lucent areas in the proximal phalanges of multiple toes.*

*(**A,** Courtesy of Dr. A. Brower, The Uniformed Services University for Health Sciences Hospital, Bethesda, Maryland; **B,** courtesy of Dr. M. Dalinka, University of Pennsylvania, Philadelphia, Pennsylvania.)*

honeycomb or latticework configuration. More localized lytic lesions produce cystic defects that, as they heal, may become surrounded by a thin rim of sclerosis. These lesions can appear centrally in the spongiosa or eccentrically, leading to marginal scalloping of the bone. An entire phalanx can be affected in association with pathologic fracture, fragmentation, soft tissue swelling, and "telescoping" of a digit. Periostitis is uncommon.

The circumscribed areas need not be homogeneously lucent. Residual trabeculae or small nodular opacities can produce recognizable radiodense shadows. In some instances, calcification of the lesion may simulate the appearance of one or more enchondromas.

Acro-osteosclerosis has been reported as a sign of sarcoidosis of the hands (Fig. 79–4). This was emphasized by McBrine and Fisher in 1975[45] as well as by other investigators,[46, 47] although earlier reports of the roentgenographic appearance in sarcoidosis had dismissed acro-osteosclerosis as an incidental finding.[18] The appearance is characterized by focal opacities, frequently of the terminal phalanges, and endosteal thickening. The finding is not specific, having been noted in scleroderma,[48] rheumatoid arthritis, systemic lupus erythematosus,[49] Hodgkin's disease, and hematologic disorders.[46] Its usefulness as a diagnostic sign of sarcoidosis is further limited by the appearance of one or more nodular opacities in phalanges of "normal" individuals. However, sclerosis of the digits has been observed in 31 per cent[47] and 54 per cent[45] of sarcoid patients, statistics that underscore the fact that osteolysis should not be regarded as the sole skeletal manifestation of the disease.

Changes in the wrist can include cystic or marginal lucent shadows, whereas those in the feet parallel the findings in the hand, with a coarsened trabecular pattern, localized lesions, and opaque areas (Fig. 79–3).

Long Tubular Bones. Examples of destructive lesions of the long tubular bones of the extremities are rare.[35, 50, 51] Single or multiple lytic foci can lead to cortical erosion and violation, with pathologic fracture. Periostitis usually is not observed.

Skull and Face. Calvarial destruction in sarcoidosis is unusual.[52-57] When present, such destruction may be asymptomatic and is characterized by single or multiple lytic lesions of varying size, usually without adjacent eburnation. These defects, which are nearly always associated with evidence of sarcoidosis elsewhere in the body, must be differentiated from eosinophilic granuloma, chronic infections, and tumors such as metastases, plasma cell myeloma, lymphoma, and meningioma.

Osseous destruction of the facial bones can reflect the presence of granulomatous lesions in adjacent structures, such as the nasal skin, paranasal sinuses, nasal mucosa, optic nerve and canal, and lacrimal sac. Nasal bone destruction is especially characteristic,[27-29, 58, 59] although dissolution of the walls of the paranasal sinuses[32, 60, 61] and orbit[30, 34, 62] and enlargement of one or both optic canals[63, 64] have been noted, simulating the changes associated with other granulomatous processes such as leprosy or Wegener's granulomatosis.

Spine and Spinal Cord. Although vertebral sarcoidosis is uncommon, postmortem[65, 66] and antemortem[67-72] studies have verified the localization of granulomas within vertebral marrow. Clinical findings include pain, tenderness, deformity, and neurologic dysfunction. On radiographs, bone lysis with marginal sclerosis can involve one or more contiguous or noncontiguous vertebral bodies, with preservation of the intervening intervertebral disc spaces.[67-74] Predilection for the lower thoracic and upper lumbar vertebrae is noted, although cervical involvement,[51, 72] including a pathologic fracture of the odontoid process,[57] has been recorded. Extension into the pedicles can be observed, although isolated

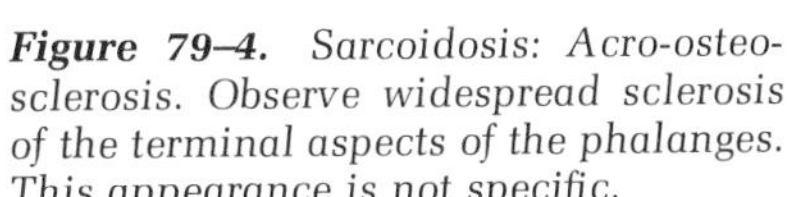

Figure 79–4. *Sarcoidosis: Acro-osteosclerosis. Observe widespread sclerosis of the terminal aspects of the phalanges. This appearance is not specific.*

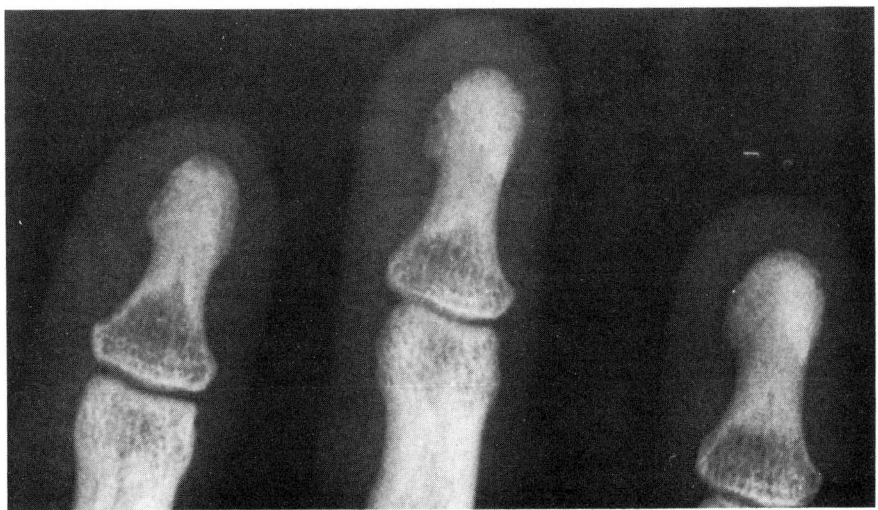

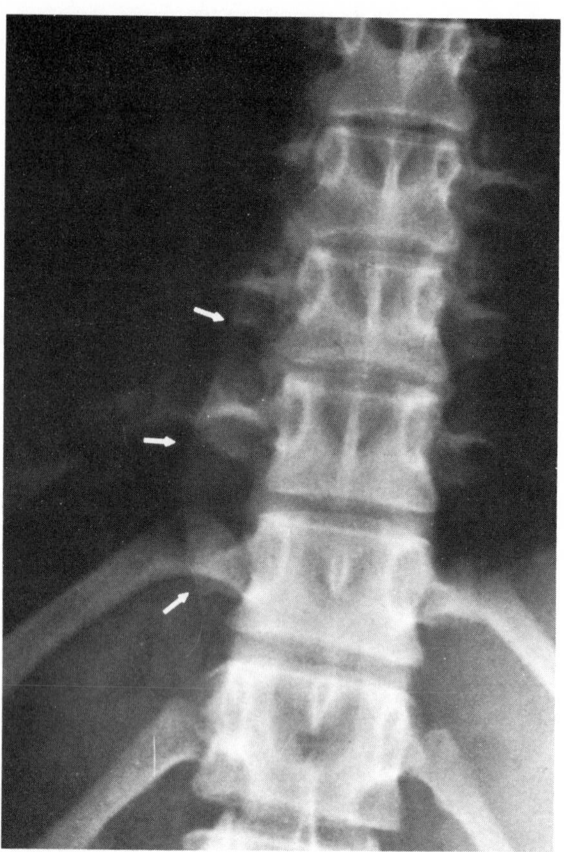

Figure 79–5. *Sarcoidosis: Paraspinal swelling. Observe a large paraspinal mass (arrows) in the thoracic spine of this patient with sarcoidosis. Such a finding can accompany vertebral involvement or represent a manifestation of posterior lymphadenopathy.*

involvement of the posterior elements of the spine is apparently rare. Paraspinal swelling is also evident in some cases (Fig. 79–5); occasionally, such swelling may accompany posterior lymphadenopathy without osseous involvement.[75] The roentgenographic appearance can simulate osteomyelitis and neoplasm. The involvement of multiple levels and the absence of intervertebral disc space narrowing in some cases are helpful clues to the correct diagnosis.

Spinal cord and cauda equina involvement in sarcoidosis is rare.[36-38, 76-81] Such involvement can occur from intramedullary granulomas (a rare manifestation), or granulomatous infiltration of the meninges or peripheral nerves. Myelography may reveal an intramedullary or intradural mass or evidence of arachnoiditis and meningeal thickening. Prominent neurologic findings are usually associated with other evidence of the disease.

Articular Involvement

Joint symptoms and signs appear in 10 to 35 per cent of patients with sarcoidosis, more frequently in women than in men.[6, 19, 22, 82-89, 111, 114] There are two fundamental patterns of articular disease: acute polyarthritis and chronic polyarthritis (Fig. 79–6). Rarely, other patterns are seen.

Acute Polyarthritis. Peripheral symmetric polyarthralgia or polyarthritis affects small and medium-sized joints, especially the ankles, knees, elbows, wrists, and articulations of the hands, appearing early in the course of the disease in association with erythema nodosum, hilar lymph node enlargement, fever, uveitis, and typical skin lesions. This pattern of joint disease, which is virtually identical to that in uncomplicated erythema nodosum, leads to soft tissue swelling, joint effusion, pain, tenderness, limitation of motion, and stiffness, findings that disappear in 4 to 6 weeks. Radiographs generally reveal soft tissue swelling and, perhaps, osteoporosis, and histologic examination of the synovial membrane confirms a nonspecific inflammatory response. Laboratory analysis may indicate elevation of the erythrocyte sedimentation rate and C-reactive protein.

Chronic Polyarthritis. A second variety of joint disease, which occurs in cases of sarcoidosis that have persisted for months to years, is a chronic polyarthritis that subsides and recurs, and that may eventually lead to permanent disability and irreversible joint damage. On initial evaluation some of the patients who have chronic disease have had acute episodes of polyarthritis. A gradual transition ensues in which symptoms and signs wax and wane over a period of years. The articulations most typically affected are the ankles, knees, shoulders, wrists, and small joints of the hands. Rarely, monoarticular arthritis rather than polyarticular arthritis is evident. Cutaneous and pulmonary alterations are frequent. Analysis of synovial fluid may indicate an elevated total protein, with white blood cell counts in the range of 15,000 to 20,000 cells per cu mm and a predominance of lymphocytes.[2]

On roentgenograms, osseous sarcoidosis may or may not be present.[90, 91] In those cases in which adjacent bony involvement is evident, articular destruction and collapse may occur secondary to extension of the osseous disease into the subchondral bone. Without such extension, radiologic changes related to the joint disease are unusual. Soft tissue swelling may be evident, in combination with periarticular osteoporosis. Mild diffuse joint space loss and eccentric and well-defined erosive alterations can also be noted. Without detection of characteristic changes in periarticular osseous tissues, the radiographic findings related to the chronic polyarthritis of sarcoidosis are not diagnostic.

Histologic examination of the synovium in either situation can indicate the presence of noncaseating granulomas[91, 92] (Fig. 79–7). These lesions are not specific, resembling the findings in tuberculosis, mycotic infections, berylliosis, and certain

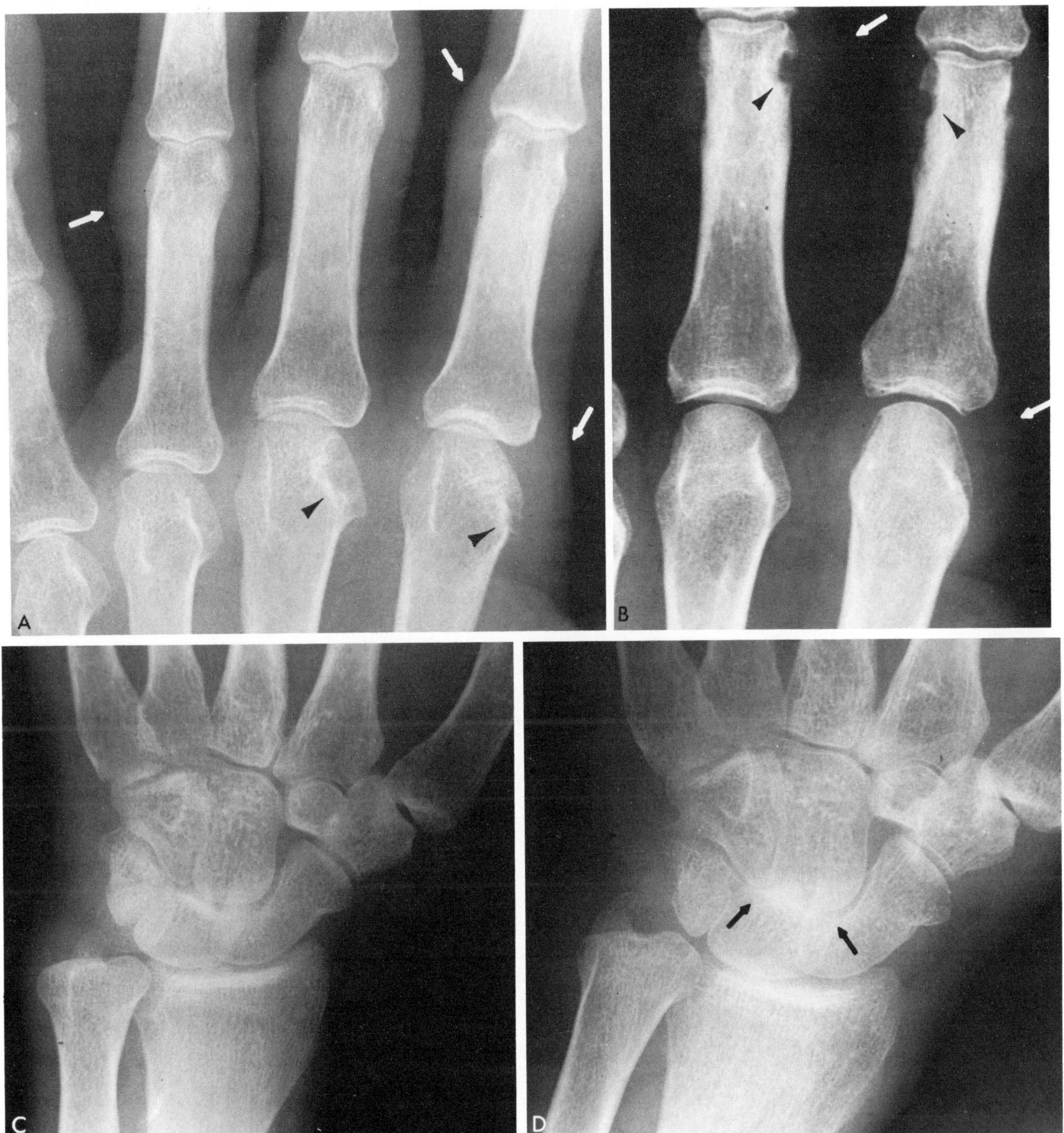

Figure 79–6. *Sarcoidosis: Articular involvement (radiographic abnormalities).*

A *Observe soft tissue swelling of multiple proximal interphalangeal and metacarpophalangeal joints (arrows) with articular space narrowing and small osseous defects (arrowheads). The absence of obvious osseous sarcoid is unusual in patients with such joint alteration.*

B *In another patient, prominent soft tissue swelling is evident about the proximal interphalangeal and metacarpophalangeal joints (arrows), and osseous defects (arrowheads) are again seen.*

C, D *Radiographs obtained over a 3 year period in a 30 year old black woman with sarcoidosis show soft tissue swelling and progressive joint space narrowing (arrows), mainly confined to the midcarpal compartment of the wrist. Osteoporosis and marginal osseous erosions are not evident. The appearance is not diagnostic, resembling that in rheumatoid arthritis and other disorders.*

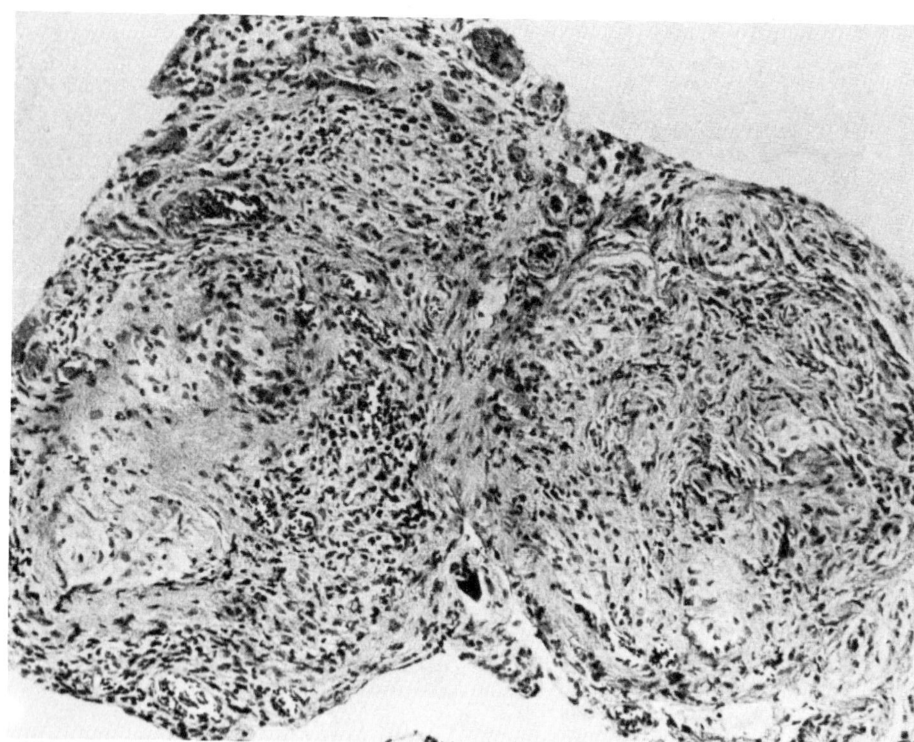

Figure 79–7. *Sarcoidosis: Articular involvement (pathologic abnormalities). A 51 year old black woman with sarcoidosis developed bilateral knee effusions and stiffness. Radiographs revealed lytic lesions of the subchondral bone in both femurs. The photomicrograph of the synovium of one knee following biopsy reveals noncaseating granulomas and scattered chronic inflammatory cells (75×). Cultures for bacteria and fungi were negative. (From Bjarnason DJ et al: J Bone Joint Surg 55A:618, 1973.)*

foreign body reactions,[93] although no fungi or acid-fast organisms are recovered from the granuloma.[92]

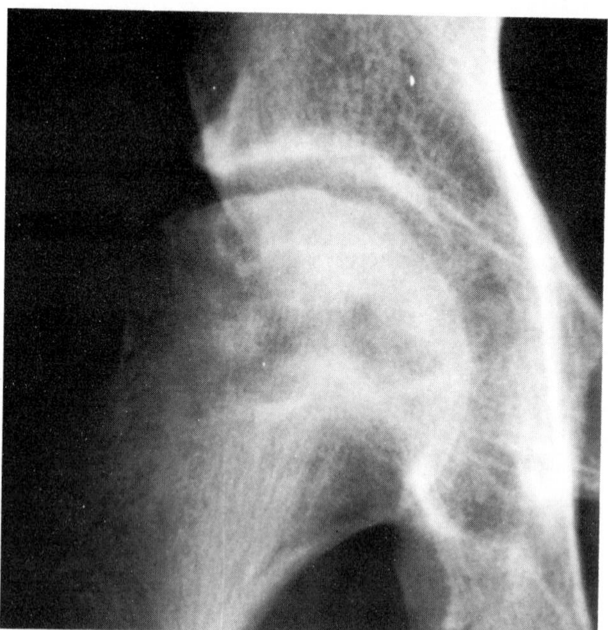

Figure 79–8. *Sarcoidosis: Osteonecrosis. This 47 year old man had a systemic granulomatous process that appeared to represent sarcoidosis. He had not received corticosteroid therapy. The radiograph of the hip reveals osteonecrosis of the femoral head with cyst formation, sclerosis, and osseous collapse. The relationship of the osseous findings to sarcoidosis and, in fact, the presence of sarcoidosis in this patient remain speculative. (Courtesy of Dr. S. Shaul, Yakima, Washington.)*

An additional inflammatory component is also evident, characterized by infiltration of leukocytes and plasma cells, and proliferation of fibroblasts. The synovial lining of tendon sheaths may be similarly affected.

Other Patterns. Pelvic and spinal changes resembling those in ankylosing spondylitis or other seronegative spondyloarthropathies are rarely observed in sarcoidosis.[84, 94-98] Sacroiliac joint erosions, sclerosis, and bony ankylosis with or without spinal changes have been described, although the pathogenesis is unknown. Perlman and co-workers[99] noted a young black man with granulomatous disease of the vertebrae who developed quadriplegia after a fall. Destructive osseous spinal lesions were combined with anterior and lateral paravertebral ossification in the cervical, thoracic, and lumbar regions, resembling changes in psoriasis or Reiter's syndrome. The sacroiliac joints were normal. The authors postulated that the bony outgrowths represented a reparative response to the extensive vertebral granulomatous process.

Sarcoidosis has also been reported in association with psoriasis, hyperuricemia and pseudopodagra, rheumatoid arthritis, and elevation of serum rheumatoid factor.[2, 100-102] Steroid therapy in patients with sarcoidosis can be complicated by osteonecrosis. The presence of this complication in sarcoid patients not receiving such medication is extremely rare and may not be related to the disease process itself (Fig. 79–8).

Rarely, sarcoidosis may be associated with large periosseous or periarticular soft tissue masses with or without calcification.[112] An association of sarcoidosis and hyperparathyroidism has also been suggested.[113]

Other Diagnostic Modalities

Scintigraphy has been employed to delineate the extent of skeletal involvement in sarcoidosis.[103] Abnormalities following administration of ^{99m}Tc pyrophosphate are more extensive than those depicted on corresponding radiographic studies, and appear to relate to sites of histologically evident noncaseating granulomas. Further utilization of this sensitive diagnostic modality may lead to identification of bone involvement in a high percentage of patients with sarcoidosis.[110]

Differential Diagnosis

The skeletal alterations in sarcoidosis are sufficiently characteristic in most cases to allow an accurate radiographic diagnosis. Occasionally, the trabecular and cystic changes in the hand may be confused with abnormalities in other disorders (Table 79–2). In *tuberous sclerosis,* cyst-like foci in the phalanges and metacarpals are usually associated with a distinctive variety of periosteal proliferation, leading to nodular excrescences attached to the outer aspect of the bones.[104] Adjacent eburnation is frequently evident, and periostitis of metatarsal shafts and intracranial calcification substantiate the correct diagnosis (see Chapter 80).

Fibrous dysplasia can produce monostotic or polyostotic abnormalities. A widened medullary space of phalanges and metacarpals with a diffuse ground-glass appearance is typical, commonly combined with focal areas of lucency or sclerosis and more widespread skeletal abnormalities[105] (Fig. 79–9) (see Chapter 80).

Table 79–2

MULTIPLE CYST-LIKE LESIONS OF THE METACARPALS AND PHALANGES*

Sarcoidosis
Gout
Rheumatoid arthritis
Xanthomatosis
Tuberous sclerosis
Fibrous dysplasia
Enchondromatosis (Ollier's disease)
Tuberculosis
Fungal disease
Metastasis (r)
Plasma cell myeloma (r)
Hyperparathyroidism (r)
Basal cell nevus syndrome (r)
Hemangiomas (r)

*r = Rare manifestation of the disease.

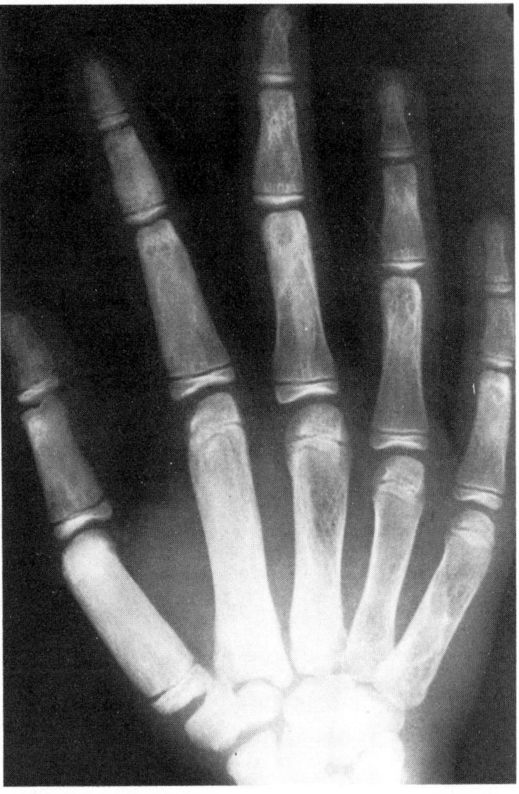

Figure 79–9. *Fibrous dysplasia. In this child with polyostotic fibrous dysplasia, note the diffuse ground-glass appearance of the metacarpals and phalanges. Cortical thinning and osseous expansion are seen.*

Enchondromas are benign tumors composed of cartilage that are often identified in the hands of asymptomatic individuals. Here, the tumor commonly produces a central rarefied area with or without calcification, and scalloping of the endosteal margin of the cortex.[106] Occasionally, enchondromas are eccentric or parosteal in location, producing an altered radiographic picture. Although the appearance of a lucent lesion containing calcification in sarcoidosis can exactly simulate an enchondroma, other skeletal findings ensure accurate diagnosis.

Enchondromatosis or *Ollier's disease* is a syndrome of multiple enchondromas that lead to soft tissue swelling in one or more extremities.[107] This nonfamilial disorder is related to the persistence of cartilaginous islands in the metaphyses and diaphyses of tubular bones that can lead to disturbances in skeletal growth and deformity. Although the clinical findings can be mistaken for arthritis, the soft tissue prominences are hard. Furthermore, radiographs reveal multiple lucent and calcified lesions, although a more diffuse and bizarre appearance can be seen (Fig. 79–10). When enchondromatosis is combined with cavernous hemangiomas, the *Maffucci syndrome* is diagnosed.[108]

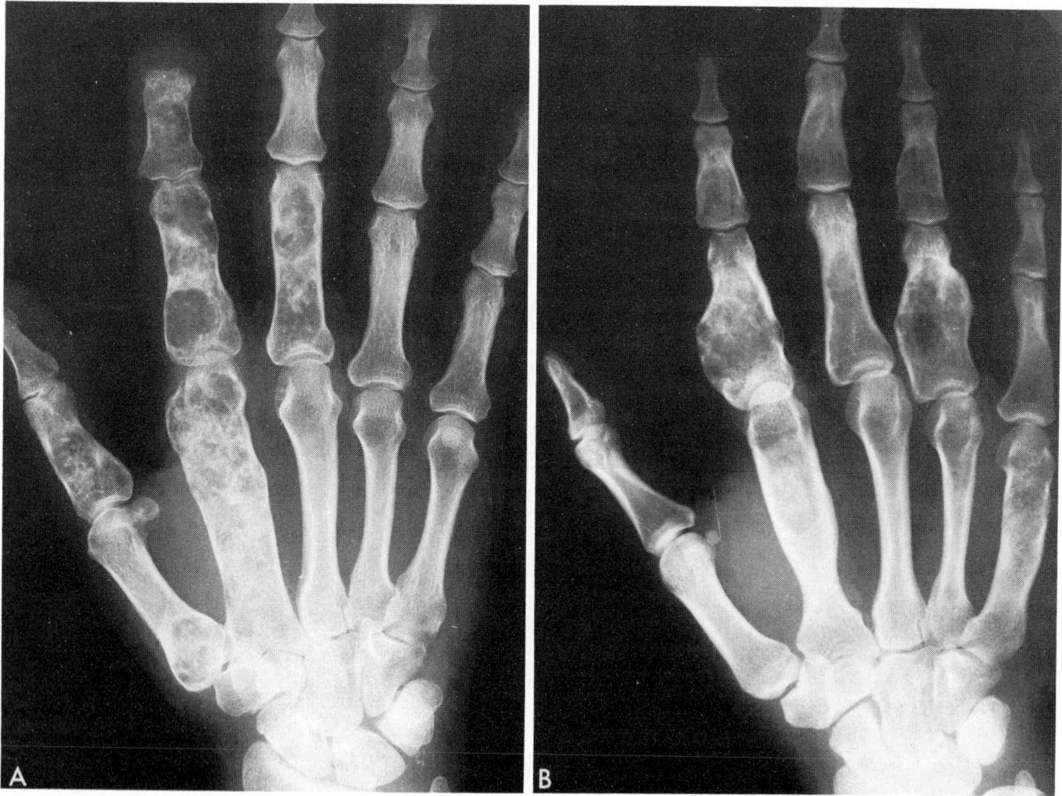

Figure 79–10. Enchondromatosis (Ollier's disease). In one patient **(A)**, observe radiolucent foci containing calcification in the first, second, and third digits. Note endosteal scalloping, cortical diminution, and osseous expansion. The distal phalanx of the second finger had been removed surgically. In a second patient **(B)**, lesions are present in the second, third, fourth, and fifth digits. They are associated with a coarsened trabecular pattern, endosteal scalloping, and localized osseous expansion.

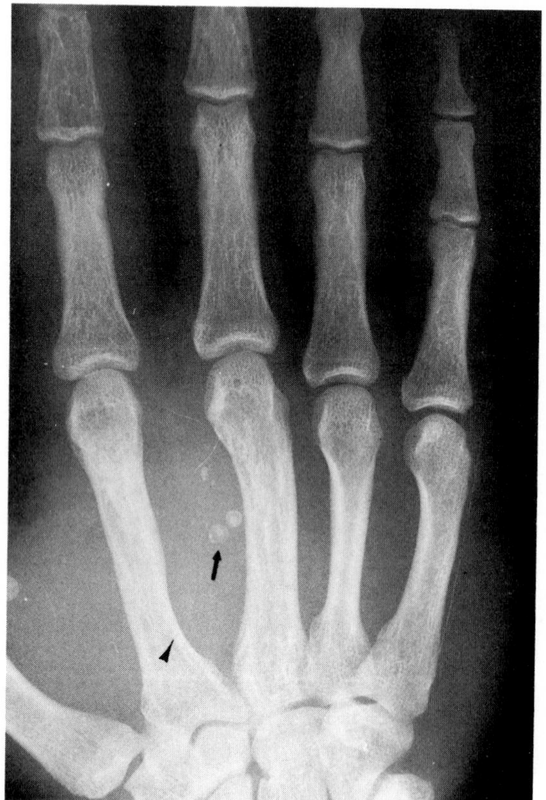

Figure 79–11. Hemangiomatosis. Observe a coarsened trabecular pattern, most evident in the middle phalanges and metacarpals of the second and third digits, and a soft tissue mass containing phleboliths (arrow), which has led to pressure erosion of the second metacarpal (arrowhead). The findings are diagnostic of osseous and soft tissue hemangiomatosis.

Considerable malignant potential of the cartilaginous lesions exists in this latter syndrome, which is less striking in multiple enchondromatosis alone and rare in the solitary enchondroma. In all three of these disorders, the radiographic features are easily differentiated from those of sarcoidosis.

Multiple lucent lesions of phalanges, metacarpals, and metatarsals can also accompany tuberculosis and other granulomatous infections (see Chapter 62), hemangiomatosis (Fig. 79–11), xanthomatosis, hyperparathyroidism, plasma cell myeloma, and skeletal metastasis.

Nasal and facial bone destruction is encountered in sarcoidosis, syphilis, fungal and other infections, Wegener's granulomatosis, and neoplasms.

The articular findings in sarcoidosis are not specific. Acute arthritis with soft tissue swelling and osteoporosis is seen in numerous processes. Chronic changes with joint space narrowing and osseous destruction simulate alterations in many infections, particularly tuberculosis. The absence of periostitis in sarcoid skeletal lesions is a helpful sign.

SUMMARY

Skeletal abnormalities in sarcoidosis are most frequently encountered in the hand; in this location, a coarsened trabecular pattern, cystic and marginal bone defects, and sclerosis are virtually diagnostic. Although findings can be encountered in other skeletal sites, such as the skull, facial bones, spine, and long tubular bones, as well as various articulations, these latter alterations usually are not specific. Thus, skull abnormalities can simulate eosinophilic granuloma and various neoplasms, spinal changes can mimic infection, and articular alterations can resemble rheumatoid arthritis, gout, and infectious arthritis.

REFERENCES

1. Siltzbach LE (Ed): Seventh International Congress on Sarcoidosis and Other Granulomatous Disorders. Ann, NY Acad Sci *278*:1, 1976.
2. Stobo JD: Sarcoidosis. *In* AS Cohen (Ed). The Science and Practice of Clinical Medicine. Vol. 4. Rheumatology and Immunology. New York, Grune & Stratton, 1979, p 290.
3. James DG, Neville E, Carstairs LS: Bone and joint sarcoidosis. Semin Arthritis Rheum *6*:53, 1976.
4. Bacharach T: Sarcoidosis. A clinical review of 111 cases. Am Rev Respir Dis *84*:12, 1961.
5. Goetz AA: Effect of cortisone on hypercalcemia in sarcoidosis. Relief of gastrointestinal, dermatological, and renal symptoms with steroid therapy. JAMA *174*:380, 1960.
6. Israel HL, Sones M: Selection of biopsy procedures for sarcoidosis diagnosis. Arch Intern Med *113*:255, 1964.
7. Kveim A: En ny og spesifikk kutan-reaksjon ved Boecks sarcoid. Nord Med *9*:169, 1941.
8. Mitchell DN, Cannon P, Dyer NH, Hinson KFW, Willoughby JMT: The Kveim test in Crohn's disease. Lancet *2*:571, 1969.
9. Sulzberger MB: Sarcoid of Boeck (benign miliary lupoid) and tuberculin anergy. Am Rev Tuberc *28*:734, 1933.
10. Lieberman J: Elevated serum angiotensin-converting-enzyme (ACE) levels in sarcoidosis. Am J Med *59*:365, 1975.
11. Longcope WT, Freiman DG: A study of sarcoidosis based on a combined investigation of 160 cases including 30 autopsies from Johns Hopkins and Massachusetts General Hospitals. Medicine *31*:1, 1952.
12. Jaffe HL: Metabolic Degenerative and Inflammatory Diseases of Bones and Joints. Philadelphia, Lea & Febiger, 1972, p 1004.
13. Talbot PS: Sarcoid myopathy. Br Med J *4*:465, 1967.
14. Besnier E: Lupus pernio de la face. Ann Dermatol Syph *10*:333, 1898.
15. Kreibich K: Über-Lupus pernio. Arch Dermatol Syphilol *71*:3, 1904.
16. Rieder H: Über Kombination von chronischer Osteomyelitis (Spina ventosa) mit Lupus-Pernio. Fortschr Geb Roentgenstr Nuklearmed *15*:125, 1910.
17. Jüngling O: Über Ostitis tuberculosa multiplex cystoides, Zugleich ein Beitrag zur Lehre von der Tuberkuliden des Knochens. Beitr Klin Chir *143*:401, 1928.
18. Holt JF, Owens WI: The osseous lesions of sarcoidosis. Radiology *53*:11, 1949.
19. Israel HL, Sones M: Sarcoidosis. Clinical observation on one hundred sixty cases. Arch Intern Med *102*:766, 1958.
20. Stein GN, Israel HL, Sones M: A roentgenographic study of skeletal lesions in sarcoidosis. Arch Intern Med *97*:532, 1956.
21. FitzGerald P, Meenan FOC: Sarcoidosis of the hands. J Bone Joint Surg *40B*:256, 1958.
22. Mayock RL, Bertrand P, Morrison CE, Scott JH: Manifestations of sarcoidosis: Analysis of 145 patients with a review of 9 series selected from the literature. Am J Med *35*:67, 1963.
23. Baltzer G, Behrend H, Behrend T, Dombrowski H: Zur Häufigkeit zystischer Knochenveränderungen (Ostitis cystoides multiplex Jüngling) bei der Sarkoidose. Dtsch Med Wochenschr *95*:1926, 1970.
24. James DG: Dermatological aspects of sarcoidosis. Q J Med *28*:109, 1959.
25. Reisner D: Boeck's sarcoid and systemic sarcoidosis (Besnier-Boeck-Schaumann disease). A study of thirty-five cases. I. Clinical observations. Am Rev Tuberc *49*:289, 1944.
26. Mather G: Calcium metabolism and bone changes in sarcoidosis. Br Med J *1*:248, 1957.
27. Bridgman JF, Mistry PK: Sarcoidosis of the nose. Practitioner *208*:393, 1972.
28. Fletcher R: Sarcoid of the nose. Arch Otolaryngol *39*:470, 1949.
29. O'Brien P: Sarcoidosis of the nose. Br J Plast Surg *23*:242, 1970.
30. Stein HA, Henderson JW: Sarcoidosis of the orbit. Survey of the literature and report of a case. Am J Ophthalmol *41*:1054, 1956.
31. Neault RW, Riley FC: Report of a case of dacrocystitis secondary to Boeck's sarcoid. Am J Ophthalmol *70*:1011, 1970.
32. Livingstone G: Sarcoidosis of maxillary antrum. J Laryngol Otol *70*:426, 1956.
33. Fischer OE, Burton GG, Bryan WF: Sarcoidosis involving the lacrimal sac. Am Rev Respir Dis *103*:708, 1971.
34. Bodian M, Lasky MA: Sarcoidosis of the orbit. Am J Ophthalmol *33*:343, 1950.
35. Watson RC, Cahen I: Pathological fracture in long bone sarcoidosis. Report of a case. J Bone Joint Surg *55A*:613, 1973.
36. Nathan MPR, Chase PH, Elguezabel A, Weinstein M: Spinal cord sarcoidosis. NY State J Med *76*:748, 1976.
37. Snyder R, Towfighi J, Gonatas NK: Sarcoidosis of the spinal cord. Case report. J Neurosurg *44*:740, 1976.
38. Bernstein J, Rival J: Sarcoidosis of the spinal cord as the presenting manifestation of the disease. South Med J *71*:1571, 1978.
39. Bonakdarpour A, Levy W, Aergerter EE: Osteosclerotic changes in sarcoidosis. Am J Roentgenol *113*:646, 1971.
40. Lin S-R, Levy W, Go EB, Lee I, Wong WK: Unusual osteosclerotic changes in sarcoidosis simulating osteoblastic metastases. Radiology *106*:311, 1973.
41. Young DA, Laman ML: Radiodense skeletal lesions in Boeck's sarcoid. Am J Roentgenol *114*:553, 1972.
42. Smith J, Farr GH Jr: An unusual case of dense bones. Clin Bull Memorial Sloan-Kettering Cancer Center *7*:40, 1977.
43. Knutsson F: Skeletal changes in sarcoidosis. Acta Radiol *51*:429, 1959.
44. Centea A, Gherman E: Knochenveränderungen bei Sarkoidose. Z Orthop *111*:321, 1973.
45. McBrine CS, Fisher MS: Acrosclerosis in sarcoidosis. Radiology *115*:279, 1975.
46. Godin E, Capesius P, Kempf F: Acro-ostéosclérose au course de la maladie de Besnier-Boeck-Schaumann. J Radiol Electrol Med Nucl *58*:115, 1977.
47. Pavlica P, Stasi G, Tonti R, Veneziano S, Viglietta G: L'ostéosclérose phalangienne dans la sarcoïdose. J. Radiol Electrol Med Nucl *58*:603, 1977.

48. Edeikin L: Scleroderma with sclerodactylia. Report of 3 cases with roentgen findings. Am J Roentgenol *22*:42, 1929.
49. Goodman N: The significance of terminal phalangeal osteosclerosis. Radiology *89*:709, 1967.
50. Robert F: Les manifestations osseuses de la maladie de Besnier-Boeck-Schaumann (la maladie de Perthes-Jüngling) Sem Hôp *25*:2327, 1944.
51. Toomey F, Bautista A: Rare manifestations of sarcoidosis in children. Radiology *94*:569, 1970.
52. Nielsen J: Recherches radiologiques sur les lésions des os et des poumons dans les sarcoïdes de Boeck. Bull Soc Fr Dermatol Syphiligr *41*:1187, 1934.
53. Posner I: Sarcoidosis: Case report. J Pediatr *20*:486, 1942.
54. Teirstein AS, Wolf BS, Siltzbach LE: Sarcoidosis of the skull. N Engl J Med *265*:65, 1961.
55. Olsen TG: Sarcoidosis of the skull. Radiology *80*:232, 1963.
56. Turner OA, Weiss SR: Sarcoidosis of the skull. Report of a case. Am J Roentgenol *105*:322, 1969.
57. Zimmerman R, Leeds NE: Calvarial and vertebral sarcoidosis. Case report and review of the literature. Radiology *119*:384, 1976.
58. Curtis GT: Sarcoidosis of the nasal bones. Br J Radiol *37*:68, 1964.
59. Trachtenberg SB, Wilkinson EE, Jacobson G: Sarcoidosis of the nose and paranasal sinuses. Radiology *113*:619, 1974.
60. Hoggins, GS, Allan D: Sarcoidosis of the maxillary region. Oral Surg *28*:623, 1969.
61. Bordley JE, Proctor DF: Destructive lesion in the paranasal sinuses associated with Boeck's sarcoid. Arch Otolaryngol *36*:740, 1942.
62. Rider JA, Dodson JW: Sarcoidoses. Report of a case manifested by retrobulbar mass, proptosis, destruction of the orbit, and infiltration of the paranasal sinuses. Am J Ophthalmol *33*:117, 1950.
63. Goodman SS, Margulies ME: Boeck's sarcoid simulating a brain tumor. Arch Neurol Psychiatry *81*:419, 1959.
64. Anderson WB, Parker JJ, Sondheimer FK: Optic foramen enlargement caused by sarcoid granuloma. Radiology *86*:319, 1966.
65. Nickerson DA: Boeck's sarcoid. Report of six cases in which autopsies were made. Arch Pathol *24*:19, 1937.
66. Rubin EH, Pinner M: Sarcoidosis. One case report and literature review of autopsied cases. Am Rev Tuberc *49*:146, 1944.
67. Rodman T, Funderburk EE Jr, Myerson RM: Sarcoidosis with vertebral involvement. Ann Intern Med *50*:213, 1959.
68. Goodbar JE, Gilmer WS Jr, Carroll DS, Clark GM: Vertebral sarcoidosis. JAMA *178*:1162, 1961.
69. Zener JC, Alpert M, Klainer LM: Vertebral sarcoidosis. Arch Intern Med *111*:696, 1963.
70. Berk RN, Brower TD: Vertebral sarcoidosis. Radiology *82*:660, 1964.
71. Brodey PA, Pripstein S, Strange G, Kohout ND: Vertebral sarcoidosis. A case report and review of the literature. Am J Roentgenol *126*:900, 1976.
72. Stump D, Spock A, Grossman H: Vertebral sarcoidosis in adolescents. Radiology *121*:153, 1976.
73. Baldwin DM, Roberts JG, Croft HE: Vertebral sarcoidosis. A case report. J Bone Joint Surg *56A*:629, 1974.
74. Bloch S, Movson IJ, Seedat YK: Unusual skeletal manifestations in a case of sarcoidosis. Clin Radiol *19*:226, 1968.
75. Schabel SI, Foote GA, McKee KA: Posterior lymphadenopathy in sarcoidosis. Radiology *129*:591, 1978.
76. Wood EH, Bream CA: Spinal sarcoidosis. Radiology *73*:226, 1959.
77. Banerjee T, Hunt WE: Spinal cord sarcoidosis. Case report. J Neurosurg *36*:490, 1972.
78. Semins H, Nugent GR, Chou SM: Intramedullary spinal cord sarcoidosis. Case report. J Neurosurg *37*:233, 1972.
79. Walker AG: Sarcoidosis of the brain and spinal cord. Postgrad Med J *37*:431, 1961.
80. Moldover A: Sarcoidosis of the spinal cord. Report of a case with remission associated with cortisone therapy. Arch Intern Med *102*:414, 1958.
81. Wiederholt WC, Siekert RG: Neurological manifestations of sarcoidosis. Neurology *15*:1147, 1965.
82. Siltzbach LE, Duberstein JL: Arthritis in sarcoidosis. Clin Orthop Rel Res *57*:31, 1968.
83. Gumpel JM, Johns CJ, Shulman LE: The joint disease of sarcoidosis. Ann Rheum Dis *26*:194, 1967.
84. Cabanel G, Jacquot F, Phelip X, Gras J-P, Mouries D: Les formes articulaires de la sarcoïdose. Sem Hôp Paris *49*:3051, 1973.
85. Gayrard M, Bouteiller G, Durroux R, Pujol M, Gourdou JF, Arlet-Suau E, Arlet J: Le rhumatisme sarcoïdosique. A propos de 2 observations. Rev Med Toul *14*:543, 1978.
86. Kaplan H: Sarcoid arthritis: A review. Arch Intern Med *112*:924, 1963.
87. Kitridou RC, Schumacher HR: Arthritis of acute sarcoidosis (Abstr). Arthritis Rheum *13*:328, 1970.
88. Lebacq E, Ruelle M: Les manifestations articulaires de la sarcoïdose. Rev Rhum Mal Osteoartic *33*:611, 1966.
89. Sèze S de, Caroit M, Leonetti P: Les manifestations articulaires de la sarcoïdose. Rev Rhum Mal Osteoartic *35*:571, 1968.
90. Turek SL: Sarcoid disease of bone at the ankle joint. J Bone Joint Surg *35A*:465, 1953.
91. Bjarnason DF, Forrester DM, Swezey RL: Destructive arthritis of the large joints. A rare manifestation of sarcoidosis. J Bone Joint Surg *55A*:618, 1973.
92. Sokoloff L, Bunim JJ: Clinical and pathological studies of joint involvement in sarcoidosis. N Engl J Med *260*:841, 1959.
93. Grier RS, Nash P, Freiman DG: Skin lesions in persons exposed to beryllium compounds. J Indust Hyg Toxicol *30*:228, 1948.
94. Blanchon P, Paillas J, Lauriat H, Tominez G: Localisations pelvi-rachidiennes et rachidiennes de la sarcoïdose de B.B.S. Ann Med Interne (Paris) *127*:843, 1976.
95. Deshayes P, Desseauve J, Hubert J, Lemercier JP, Geoffroy Y: Un cas de polyarthrite au cours d'une sarcoïdose. Un cas de spondylarthrite ankylosante au cours d'une sarcoïdose. Rev Rhum Mal Osteoartic *32*:671, 1965.
96. Verstraetten JM, Bekaert J: Association de spondylite ankylosante et de sarcoïdose. Acta Tuberc Belg *42*:149, 1951.
97. Martin E, Fallet GH: Pneumopathies chroniques et rhumatisme. Schweiz Med Wochenschr *83*:776, 1953.
98. Brun J, Pozzetto H, Buffat JJ, Soustelle J, Vauzelle JL, Patin R: Sarcoïdose vertébrale et sacro-iliaque avec image de pseudo-abcès pottique. Guérison par corticothérapie. Presse Med *74*:511, 1966.
99. Perlman SG, Damergis J, Witorsch P, Cooney FD, Gunther SF, Barth WF: Vertebral sarcoidosis with paravertebral ossification. Arthritis Rheum *21*:271, 1978.
100. Putkonen T, Virkkunen M, Wager O: Joint involvement in sarcoidosis with special reference to the coexistence of sarcoidosis and rheumatoid arthritis. Acta Rheum Scand *11*:53, 1965.
101. Kaplan H, Klatskin G: Sarcoidosis, psoriasis, and gout: Syndrome or coincidence. Yale J Biol Med *32*:335, 1960.
102. Loefgren S, Norberg R: Metabolic aspect of sarcoidosis. Acta Tuberc Scand Suppl *45*:40, 1959.
103. Reginato AJ, Schiappaccasse V, Guzman L, Claure H: ^{99m}Technetium-pyrophosphate scintiphotography in bone sarcoidosis. J Rheumatol *3*:426, 1976.
104. Holt JF, Dickerson WW: The osseous lesions of tuberous sclerosis. Radiology *58*:1, 1952.
105. Pritchard JE: Fibrous dysplasia of the bones. Am J Med Sci *222*:313, 1951.
106. Takigawa K: Chondroma of the bones of the hand. A review of 110 cases. J Bone Joint Surg *53A*:1591, 1971.
107. Mainzer F, Minagi H, Steinbach HL: The variable manifestations of multiple enchondromatosis. Radiology *99*:377, 1971.
108. Andrén L, Dymling JF, Elner A, Hogeman KE: Maffucci's syndrome. Report of 4 cases. Acta Chir Scand *126*:397, 1963.
109. Forouzesh S, Fan PT, Bluestone R: Universal sarcoid dactylitis: A case report. Arthritis Rheum *22*:1403, 1979.
110. Rohatgi PK: Radioisotope scanning in osseous sarcoidosis. Am J Roentgenol *134*:189, 1980.
111. Prier A, Camus J-P: Les manifestations rhumatologiques de la sarcoïdose. Rev Méd *22*:1109, 1980.
112. Schwartz JM: Sarcoid tumor of knee. NY State Journal Med *80*:806, 1980.
113. Lavalard JF, Philippe JM, Preux MC, Vorhauer W, Veyssier P: Sarcoïdose hypercalcémique révélée par une biopsie osseuse. Ann Méd Interne *131*:35, 1980.
114. Müller W, Wurm K: Rheumatische syndrome bei der Sarcoidose. Akt Rheumatol *5*:39, 1980.

80

TUBEROUS SCLEROSIS, NEUROFIBROMATOSIS, AND FIBROUS DYSPLASIA

by Frieda Feldman, M.D.

Tuberous sclerosis, neurofibromatosis, and polyostotic fibrous dysplasia involve multiple systems in multiple ways and they may, therefore, be associated with a variety of seemingly unrelated radiographic stigmata. Familiarity with fragmented aspects of these entities is further fostered by their diverse clinical presentations, which are usually attended to by a variety of physicians. Each specialist, though readily recognizing the particular expression of the disease to which he or she is most attuned, is often unaware of its relationship to a larger mosaic, which may be assuming larger and larger proportions as finer facets of these entities become appreciated and explored.

Prior to a discussion of the distinctions among these three conditions however, it is important to note that tuberous sclerosis, neurofibromatosis, and fibrous dysplasia share certain common characteristics. Although they are grouped with the neuroectodermal and mesodermal dysplasias, body tissues not derived from ectoderm may also be affected and at present it is theorized that all germ layers are involved in the development of each of these entities. They have all been associated with certain classic clinical triads, which reflect their particular underlying dysplasias, and which are sought as aids in their identification. They are, furthermore, all hereditary or familial diseases in the majority of cases. Although mutations do occur, greater knowledge of the history and more detailed examinations of such patients and their relatives often reveal incomplete, unfamiliar, or atypical expressions of these syndromes, which, when recognized, serve to reclassify many so-called "sporadic" cases as hereditary or familial.

TUBEROUS SCLEROSIS

General Features

Tuberous sclerosis or Bourneville's disease[8] (or "epiloia," which combines the words epilepsy and anoia, i.e., "mindless") is a disease of dominant autosomal inheritance. New mutations have been cited as occurring in 25 to 90 per cent of cases,[10, 56] and incidence has ranged from 1 in every 100,000[14] to 1 in every 30,000 births.[76]

Cutaneous and Cranial Abnormalities

This disorder is classically characterized by a clinical triad of epileptic seizures, mental retardation, and skin lesions, which have been considered to be hamartomas of the skin and brain. However, similar lesions in other sites — e.g., eyes, kidneys, heart, lungs, liver, spleen, and bones — result in varied presentations whose recognition as a part of the complex disorder is of prime importance since components of the triad may not always appear simultaneously or may not even appear at all owing to the occurrence of formes frustes. Seizures, although observed in the first decade of life, are nonspecific; mental retardation is difficult to appreciate at birth; and adenoma sebaceum (Fig. 80–1), the most familiar cutaneous stigma, although present in 80 to 90 per cent of cases, occurs only in 13 per cent of cases during the first year of life, usually appears between 2 to 5 years of age, and often is not manifest until puberty or pregnancy.[47, 56]

Other cutaneous stigmata include shagreen patches, periungual and gingival fibromas, and café au lait and white macules (Figs. 80–2 and 80–3). Shagreen patches (or shagreen skin), present in 20 to 50 per cent of patients, are flat, slightly elevated plaques with a flesh-colored, wrinkled appearance and a time of onset akin to that of adenoma sebaceum.[40] Periungual (Fig. 80–2) and gingival fibromas usually appear at puberty.[47] However, hypopigmented macules (leukoderma) have received recent emphasis as the earliest cutaneous sign of tuberous sclerosis and may be noted at birth or in the neonatal

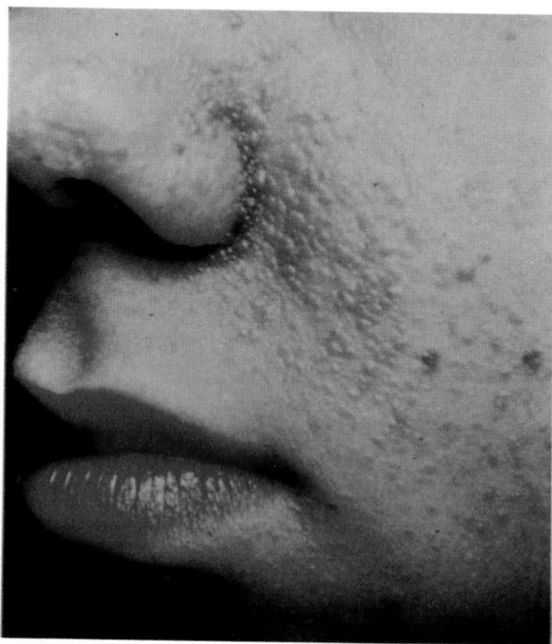

Figure 80–1. *Tuberous sclerosis: Adenoma sebaceum. This 15 year old girl had had seizures since birth. These skin lesions usually develop in the first 5 years of life but most commonly occur after the onset of seizures. (Courtesy of Dr. L. Shapiro.)*

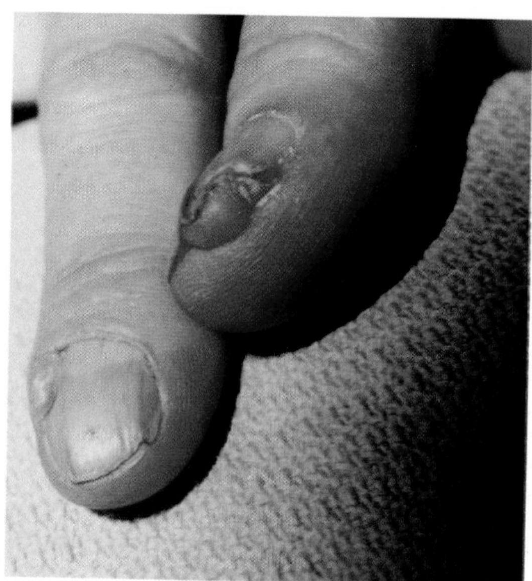

Figure 80–2. *Tuberous sclerosis: Periungual fibromas. Such fibromas occur in about 20 per cent of patients and usually appear at puberty. They may be solitary or multiple and affect the toes as well as the digits. (Courtesy of Dr. L. Shapiro.)*

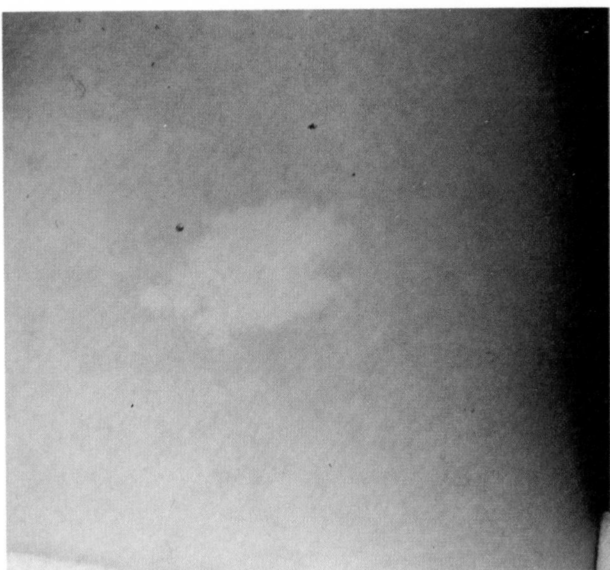

Figure 80–3. Tuberous sclerosis. The hypopigmented macule is usually oval or leaf-shaped with irregular margins, has an average diameter of 10 to 15 cm, and most commonly occurs on the abdomen and legs. (Courtesy of Dr. L. Shapiro.)

period.[10, 25, 27, 40] Erroneously called vitiligo or depigmented nevi, they are not as milk-white in color, since they are not completely lacking in melanin pigmentation, and may be overlooked in fair-skinned patients. A Wood's ultraviolet lamp is helpful in enhancing their contrast with normal skin.[25] They usually have oval, lanceolate, or ash-leaf configurations, irregular margins, and an average diameter of 1.3 cm and are concentrated on the abdomen (Fig. 80–3) and legs. It is claimed that the presence of tuberous sclerosis is probable in infants with typical white macules and highly probable when the macules occur in conjunction with seizures.[25]

Of 71 Mayo Clinic patients, 38 per cent were of average intelligence, 93 per cent had seizures, and 87 per cent had abnormal findings on electroencephalograms.[47, 56] Such nonspecific neurologic findings may, in addition to cutaneous stigmata, be supported by neuroradiologic evidence of calvarial or intracerebral calcifications. Routine skull films may show focal, calvarial sclerotic patches due to hyperostosis of the inner table and trabeculae of the diploic spaces (Fig. 80–4). Generalized thickening and increased density of both tables of the vault may also be noted. Intracerebral calcification occurs in 50 to 80 per cent of cases; however, its absence does not exclude the diagnosis (Fig. 80–4). Its incidence increases with age, but it is infrequently detected on routine films of the very young. A recent neuroradiologic survey of 45 children with tuberous sclerosis[24] noted 21 with intracranial calcifications on routine skull films. Incidence ranged from 14 per cent in infants under 1 year old to 60 per cent in 10 to 14 year old children. Only three patients were under 2 years old; one was 7 months old.

Calcifications may assume several forms. Multiple nodular discrete calcific deposits, several millimeters in diameter, are common in the basal ganglia and paraventricularly. Occasionally linear or single

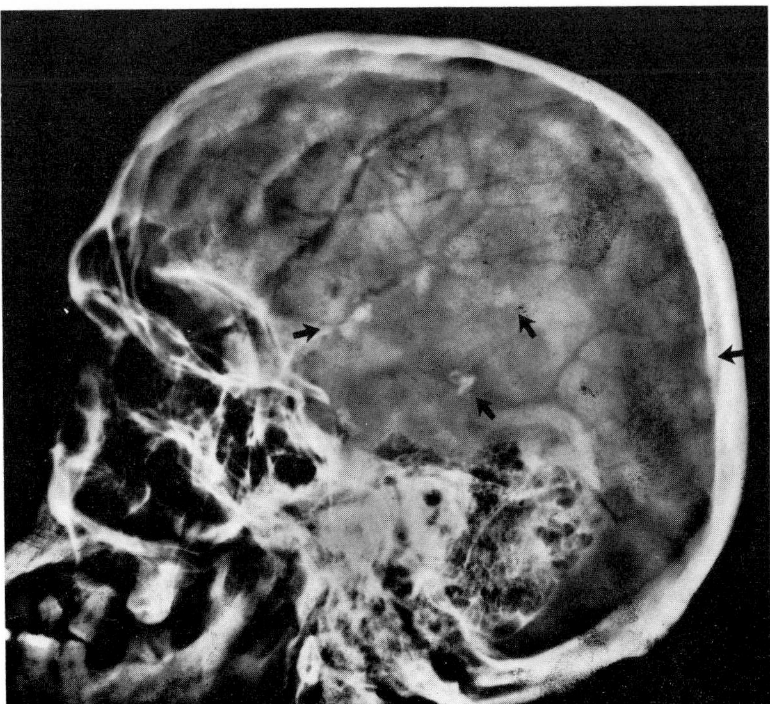

Figure 80–4. Tuberous sclerosis: Lateral view of the skull. Multiple intracerebral calcific deposits are noted, together with several scattered areas of calvarial sclerosis (arrows).

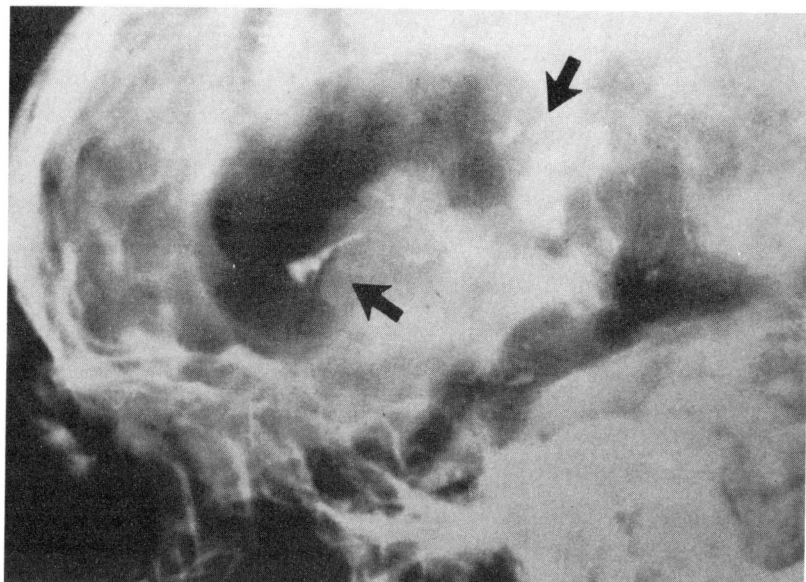

Figure 80–5. Tuberous sclerosis: Pneumoencephalogram. The multiple calcified paraventricular subependymal nodules or "tubers" are well outlined by air, so-called "candle guttering" (arrows).

calcified conglomerates 2 to 3 cm in diameter may be noted (Fig. 80–5).

Hamartomatous foci, which may or may not calcify and which vary in size and number, may be found in the cerebrum, cerebellum, medulla, and spinal cord. The majority lie adjacent to the cerebrospinal fluid pathways and are of two types: cortical foci or tubers and subependymal nodules located about the ventricular system (Fig. 80–5). The subependymal nodules arise within the basal ganglia and are as characteristic as cortical lesions. Cortical tubers were so named by Bourneville[8] because of their potato-like appearance; they may involve any portion of the cerebral cortex.

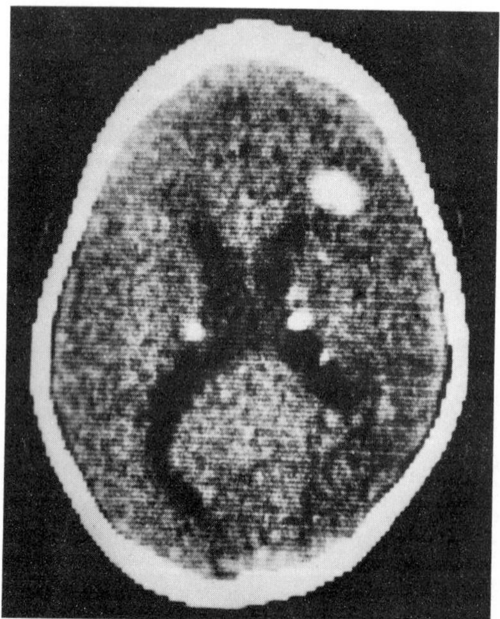

Figure 80–6. Tuberous sclerosis: Computed tomography. CT scan of a 9 year old boy taken at the level of the ventricles shows numerous subependymal and intracerebral calcifications.

Tuberous sclerosis literally means hard humps—i.e., tuber is from the Latin and may be translated as "hump" and sklero from the Greek as "hard." The majority of intracranial lesions containing small amounts of calcium have not been detectable on routine films and have, in the past, been identified by pneumoencephalography (Fig. 80–5) and ventriculography owing to their proximity to cerebrospinal fluid pathways. Recently, computed tomographic (CT) scanning or computer assisted tomography, a relatively less invasive technique, has demonstrated its superiority to standard roentgenography by delineating intracranial calcifications at an earlier and heretofore undetectable stage. CT scan evidence of appropriate intracranial calcification (Fig. 80–6), combined with dermatologic evidence of white macules (Fig. 80–3) and a clinical history of seizures, with or without mental deficiency, assures the diagnosis of tuberous sclerosis.

Extracranial Skeletal Abnormalities

In addition to the skull, osseous abnormalities, focal or diffuse, may involve the remainder of the skeleton with medullary or cortical cyst-like radiolucent areas or dense sclerotic deposits.[29] Cortical lesions in the form of localized concretions or nodules of bone, defects or pits, or depressions, as well as irregular subperiosteal new bone deposition, which results in a thickened, undulating cortical contour, most often involve the tubular bones of the hands and feet[9, 86] (Figs. 80–7 and 80–8). A thickened, undulating cortex may also be noted about the long bones, whereas rounded, sharply demarcated lucent areas microscopically identified as nonspe-

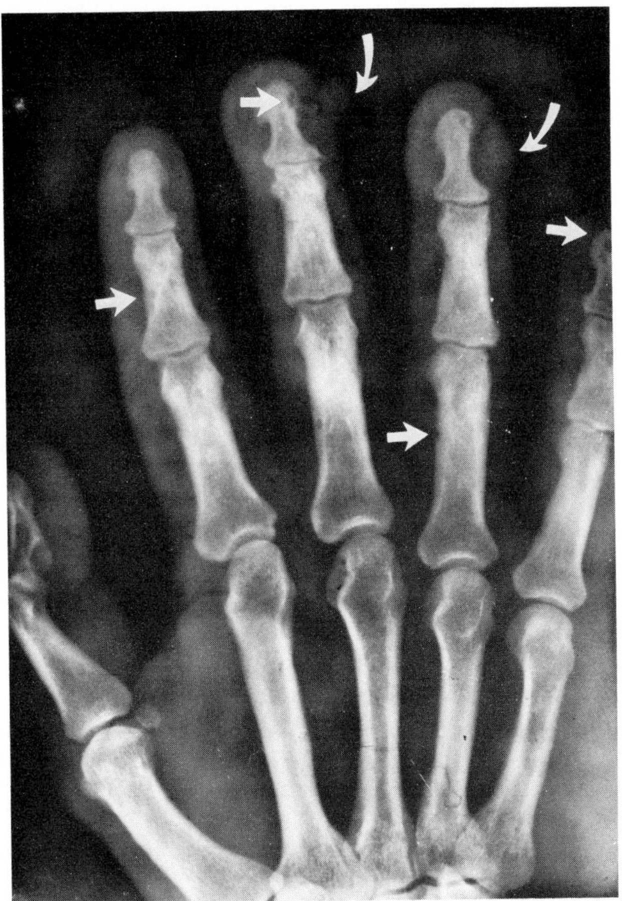

Figure 80–7. *Tuberous sclerosis: Posteroanterior view of the hand. Numerous rounded intramedullary radiolucent lesions are seen in several phalanges of various digits, together with cortical pitting (straight arrows). Note neighboring periungual fibromas in the third and fourth digits (curved arrows).*

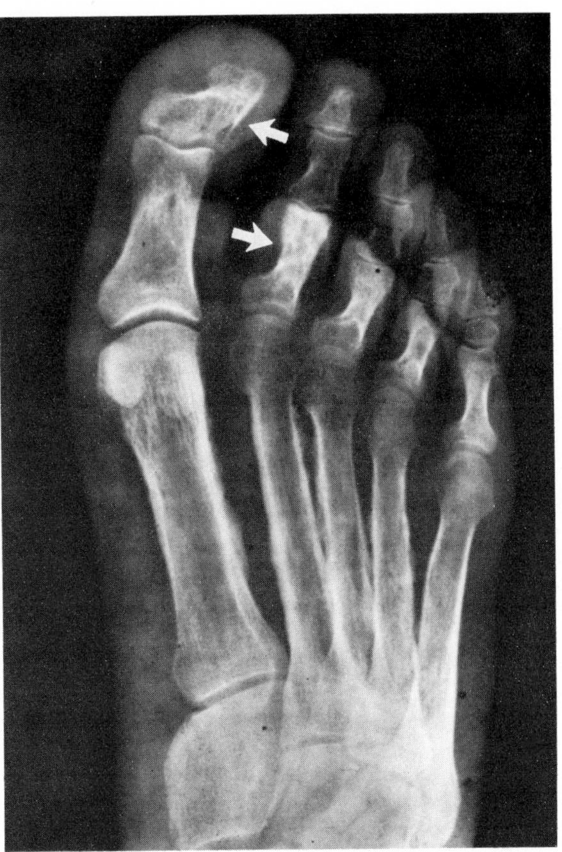

Figure 80–8. *Tuberous sclerosis: Frontal view of the foot. A thickened, undulating cortex with well-defined external contours cloaks the first four metatarsals. Several small, rounded intramedullary radiolucent areas are seen in the distal phalanx of the first toe and the proximal phalanx of the second toe (arrows).*

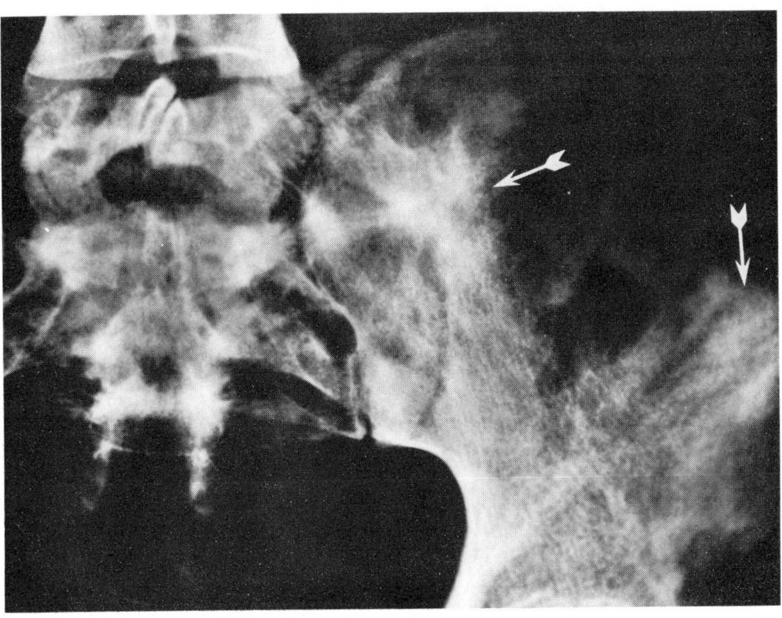

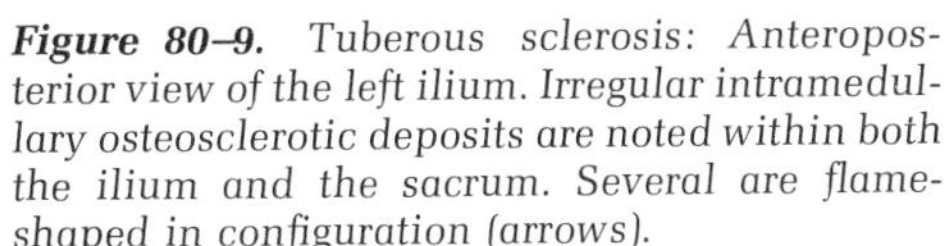

Figure 80–9. *Tuberous sclerosis: Anteroposterior view of the left ilium. Irregular intramedullary osteosclerotic deposits are noted within both the ilium and the sacrum. Several are flame-shaped in configuration (arrows).*

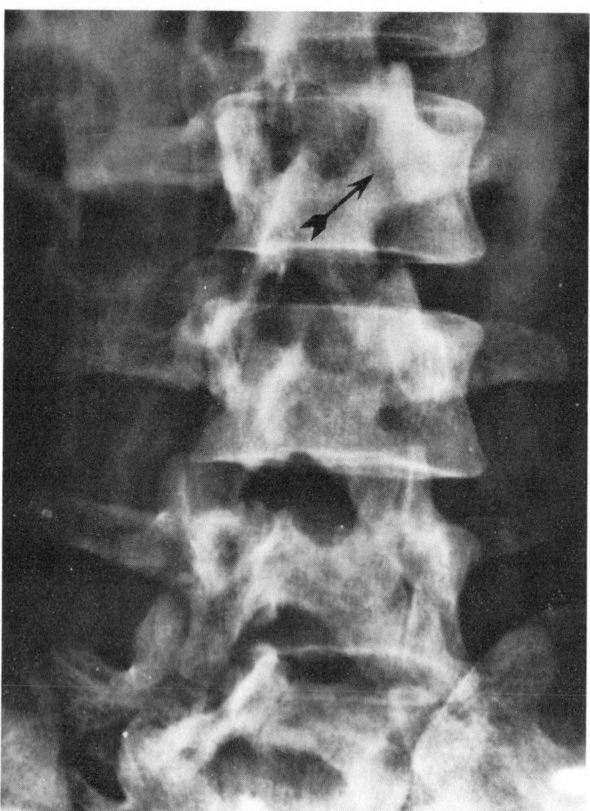

Figure 80–10. *Tuberous sclerosis: Left oblique view of lumbar spine. The left pedicle and superior articular facet of a lumbar vertebral body of a 32 year old man are homogeneously dense (arrow). This was an incidental finding on intravenous pyelography.*

cific fibrous replacement of bone show predilection for the distal phalanges of the hand. Rarely, the distal phalanges may be eroded by associated subungual fibromas (Figs 80–2 and 80–7).

The spine and pelvis are additional sites for medullary osteoblastic deposits, a few millimeters to centimeters in diameter, which may be discrete and round, ovoid, or flame-shaped in contour[45] (Fig. 80–9). Ill-defined, patchy areas of increased density have also been observed (Fig. 80–10).The intraosseous lesions are usually homogeneously dense but may have a somewhat mottled appearance. However, they do not produce coarsening of the local trabecular pattern, nor do they produce bone expansion. Such lesions, rarely reported prior to puberty,[3, 58] occur as later manifestations of the disease. They are most commonly asymptomatic and may, therefore, be overlooked. However, they have been noted to show considerable, albeit slow, progression over a period of years when comparison studies were available. An awareness of their association with tuberous sclerosis as well as correlation with other clinical information should eliminate their confusion with osteoblastic metastases.

Visceral Abnormalities

The viscera, as well as skin, brain, and bones, serve as silent sites of tumor-like formations containing varying proportions of vascular, smooth muscle, fatty, and fibrous tissue. Depending on the predominant elements, a lesion may be variously identified as an angiomyoma, angiofibroma, myolipoma, or sarcoma if histologic pleomorphism is prominent. These hamartomas are rarely shown to be initiated in embryonic life[76] or in neonates. Their incidence increases with age and in addition to appearing as nodular masses in the brain and skin or phakomas in the eyes, they may involve the kidneys, heart, liver, lungs, spleen, or gastrointestinal tract. Radiographs may then again assume a dominant role in their identification.

Clinically, palpable abdominal masses, painless hematuria, and episodic flank pain are features shared by renal neoplasms and renal polycystic disease as well as renal tuberous sclerosis. Bilaterality serves as a distinguishing feature of tuberous sclerosis, since more than 90 per cent of renal cell carcinomas, Wilms' tumors, or transitional carcinomas are unilateral. Age of onset of symptoms, i.e., usually 35 to 50 years, and proteinuria are distinguishing features of adult polycystic disease, whereas in infants uremia and poor prognosis are commonly associated. A rare instance of polycystic kidneys and seizures in an infant[85] and the occurrence of polycystic kidneys alone or in combination with angiomyolipomas in patients with tuberous sclerosis have been noted. A difference in the microscopic appearance of cysts associated with tuberous sclerosis has been alleged.[63]

Hamartomas may enlarge slowly. However, progressive renal failure and other renal complications due to parenchymal replacement, previously thought to be unusual, have received recent emphasis and have been related to longer survival resulting from more effective anticonvulsant drugs and neurosurgical techniques.[60]

Renal hamartomas occur in 40 to 80 per cent of patients and may be detected on routine radiographs as a result of their high fat content,[15] as intraparenchymal radiolucent shadows and by unilateral or bilateral enlargement or contour irregularities. Retrograde or intravenous pyelograms further reveal pelvocalyceal distortion or displacement by masses mimicking neoplastic or polycystic disease. The bilaterality of the hamartomas distinguishes them from neoplasms, whereas the radiolucency of their fatty components contrasts with the relative radiopacity of the fluid-filled cysts in polycystic disease.

Arteriography, by delineating an increased and abnormal vasculature with tortuous vessels and puddling of contrast material, distinguishes tuberous sclerosis from polycystic disease, but not from neoplasia, which depends for its distinction on unilaterality. The specificity of angiography is controversial, since similar vascular patterns have been observed in renal neoplasms and angiomyolipomas. The latter have been noted to have a whorled or onion-peel appearance in the nephrographic or venous phase, small or berry aneurysms in the arterial stage, lack of arteriovenous shunting, and no arterial response to epinephrine, as in renal carcinoma.[79] Hamartomas tend to bleed as a result of their rich and abnormal vascularity, making percutaneous needle biopsy hazardous. Shock secondary to spontaneous retroperitoneal or intra-abdominal hemorrhage has been reported.[32]

Therefore, a patient may present with urologic problems. A history of epilepsy in any form, in any patient with "cystic" renal enlargement, should arouse suspicion of tuberous sclerosis. Rarely polycystic kidney and renal angiomyolipoma may coexist. Approximately 50 per cent of patients with renal angiomyolipomas have no other manifestations of tuberous sclerosis. However, multiple hamartomas are more likely to be associated with tuberous sclerosis than are solitary hamartomas. A detailed family history as well as careful scrutiny of the skin is essential.

Cardiac involvement is rare, but in a series of 69 cardiac rhabdomyomas, 49 per cent of patients had tuberous sclerosis.[43] Rhabdomyoma is the second most common cardiac tumor after myxoma. As with renal hamartomas, multiplicity is more likely to be associated with other manifestations of tuberous sclerosis. Any cardiac chamber may be involved. An irregular cardiac contour may suggest the tumor on routine chest films, but more commonly the films are normal or show nonspecific cardiac or main artery or central pulmonary artery prominence, with a normal peripheral vascular pattern.

Pulmonary lesions occur in fewer than 1 per cent of patients with tuberous sclerosis, and unlike other manifestations, which predominate in women, these lesions have no sex predilection. Pulmonary lesions are associated with a low incidence of epilepsy (20 per cent) and mental retardation (46 per cent) and occur later in the course. Pulmonary symptoms develop at an average age of 24 years and not before 20 years. Dyspnea, which is most common, has been reported in 58 per cent of cases; it may be secondary to spontaneous pneumothorax, which occurs in 50 per cent of cases, subpleural blebs, or cor pulmonale.[29] Chest films may show a uniform and diffuse or basilar interstitial infiltrative process.[22, 55]

Endocrine Abnormalities

Endocrine and metabolic abnormalities are less well appreciated associations of tuberous sclerosis. Hepatic, thyroid, and pancreatic adenomas have been noted.[13] Pituitary, adrenal, and thyroid dysfunctions as well as abnormal intravenous glucose tolerance test results were recently noted in seven patients with high serum alkaline phosphatase levels. Abnormalities in sella turcica size were included among the multiple skeletal defects noted.[68]

Therefore, tuberous sclerosis, although its pathogenesis is still unknown, represents a widespread dysplasia, which begins during embryonic life and which may involve all germ layers.

NEUROFIBROMATOSIS

General Features

Neurofibromatosis is also a congenital and hereditary dysplasia. It is inherited as an autosomal mendelian dominant trait with no sex predilection. It has an estimated incidence of 1 in 3000 births.[16] Spontaneous mutations account for 50 per cent of cases. Reports by Tiresius[77] (1793), Smith[74] (1849), Virchow[80] (1863), and Payne[61] (1887) antedated that of von Recklinghausen,[66] (1882) who first associated the neural and the fibrous elements in neurofibromatosis. This disorder was most commonly considered to be a neuroectodermal dysplasia, but it is now recognized as a mesodermal dysplasia with diffuse systemic expressions. However, regional or limited involvement, formes frustes, shared characteristics, and a lack of specific diagnostic laboratory aids make a knowledge of its numerous manifestations essential for diagnosis.

Cutaneous Abnormalities

Neurofibromatosis may also be characterized by a classic clinical triad, which includes cutaneous lesions, mental deficiency, and skeletal deformities. In addition to its characteristic skin tumors, which histologically are neurofibromas, plexiform neurofibromas, and schwannomas, neurofibromatosis is most commonly associated with café au lait spots (Fig. 80–11). Therefore, the skin lesions of neurofibromatosis themselves constitute a triad — i.e., pedunculated lesions, multiple fibrous neural tumors, and café au lait spots. Café au lait spots are an excellent example of a shared characteristic, since they are not specific for or pathognomonic of neurofibromatosis. However, differences in their distribution, configuration, and number as compared with those associated with tuberous sclerosis and fibrous dysplasia make them useful indicators of neurofibromatosis. Six or more macules 1.5 cm or greater in diameter are unusual in tuberous sclerosis and are

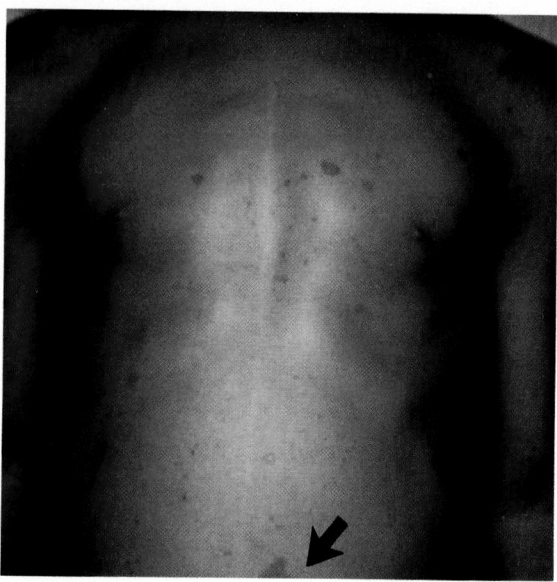

Figure 80–11. *Neurofibromatosis in a 16 year old boy. Café au lait pigmentations are scattered over the anterior chest and abdominal wall. They may vary in size from freckles to larger macules (arrow) with smooth edges. Any patient with six or more café au lait spots measuring 1.5 cm or more in diameter may be presumed to have neurofibromatosis.*

considered as reliable evidence of neurofibromatosis.[16] More than two such macules are present in fewer than 1 per cent of normal children (Fig. 80–11). However, café au lait spots are age-related since they are not uniformly present at birth but tend to increase in number, size, and pigmentation until the middle of the third decade of life. They may then begin to fade.

The flat, elevated, or pedunculated lesions of molluscum fibrosum are another associated cutaneous stigma. They are soft, elevated, nipple-like lesions that may be pedunculated (Fig. 80–12). Localized or diffuse plexiform neurofibromas of peripheral nerves also occur and may lead to elephantiasis neuromatosa, with massive enlargement of the skin, soft tissues, and underlying skeleton of an affected extremity. The etiology of this overgrowth is unknown. An increase in serum nerve-growth-stimulating activity has been noted in some patients.[70] The incidence of sarcomatous change in neurofibromas has been variously quoted as occurring in from 2 to 13 per cent of patients. It is likely, however, that this is an exaggerated estimate, since inclusion of less severely affected or more subtle cases would tend to lower the incidence.[4]

Cranial and Skeletal Abnormalities

Neurofibromatosis may frequently be diagnosed by means of skull and skeletal radiographs. Bony hypoplasia of the posterosuperior orbital wall[73] of the skull may be associated with herniation of the temporal lobe and subarachnoid space into the posterior orbit via the bone defect. This eventually may be clinically manifested by a pulsating exophthalmos.[11, 38] Neurofibromatous tissue is usually not identified in the vicinity of the defect. The defect results from either the complete absence of bone or the formation of abnormal bone (Fig. 80–13). Another bony deficiency in the skull, again primarily due to the underlying mesodermal dysplasia, favors the left side and the lambdoid suture just posterior to the junction of the parietomastoid and occipitomastoid sutures (Fig. 80–14). An underdeveloped ipsilateral mastoid may be associated.[44, 73]

Other stigmata noted on routine skull films include aggregated granular calcifications in the temporal lobe area.[88] Though similar to those commonly seen in the choroid plexus glomus, they usually spare the glomus, may be unilateral or bilateral, and seem to extend along part of the wall of the temporal horn choroid plexus. Such calcifications with an atypical relationship to the choroid plexuses in a young person with tumor symptoms should lead to the consideration of neurofibromatosis.[88]

The spinal column as well as its contents is frequently involved.[48, 50, 57] Kyphoscoliosis, the most common skeletal abnormality in neurofibromatosis, is classically of the short-segment and angular type (Fig. 80–15). The T3 to T7 segment is most commonly involved when scoliosis or meningoceles accompany neurofibromatosis[4] (Fig. 80–16*A–C*). The kyphoscoliosis may not be present at birth, but it may be rapidly progressive[71] after its initial presentation (Fig. 80–17). The development of kyphoscoliosis has been attributed to the primary mesodermal dysplasia of bone, as have the generalized vertebral body alterations. Posterocentral vertebral body scalloping with erosion of the pedicles is frequently evident and may also be progressive (Fig. 80–18). A congenitally weak dural sac that progressively enlarges in response to CSF pulsations has been blamed (Fig. 80–19). Intraspinal or paraspinal tumors or neighboring neurofibromas may also be responsible, particularly for localized vertebral body destruction or deformity. The deformity or erosion associated with an adjacent neurofibroma is most commonly eccentric and is occasionally accompanied by vertebral body enlargement whereas the scalloping seen in association with dural ectasia is usually central (Fig. 80–20*A,B*)). Myelography or CT scanning will aid in defining the cause. Myelograms will serve to outline meninges protruding from enlarged neural foramina (Fig. 80–21). When these protrude laterally they may create posterior mediastinal or posterior intrathoracic masses, which may be visible on routine films. Thoracic meningoceles are most often found in conjunction with neurofibromas. These lesions occasionally are present at birth and may cause shortness of breath as the initial symptom (Fig. 80–16*A–C*).

Text continued on page 2944

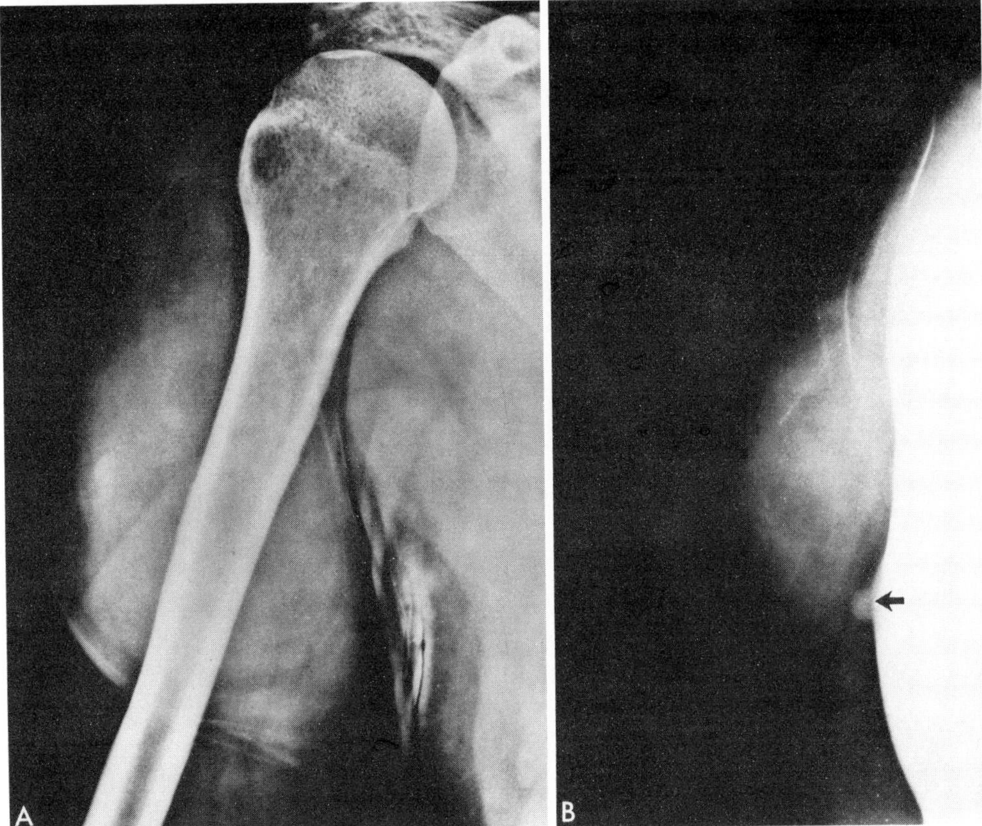

Figure 80–12. *Neurofibromatosis in a 50 year old man: Fibroma molluscum.*

A *Anteroposterior view of the right arm. These soft tissue nodules or masses may be single or multiple and may grow under, be flush with, or be raised above skin level. Larger lesions may be pedunculated.*

B *Tangential view of the right arm. Note second lesion with nipple-like configuration (arrow). These lesions have a tendency to invaginate on digital compression. Tumors involving nerves are designated as neurofibromas or neurilemomas depending on their relationship with the nerve fibers. Diffuse neoplastic involvement of a nerve and its branches is termed a plexiform neuroma.*

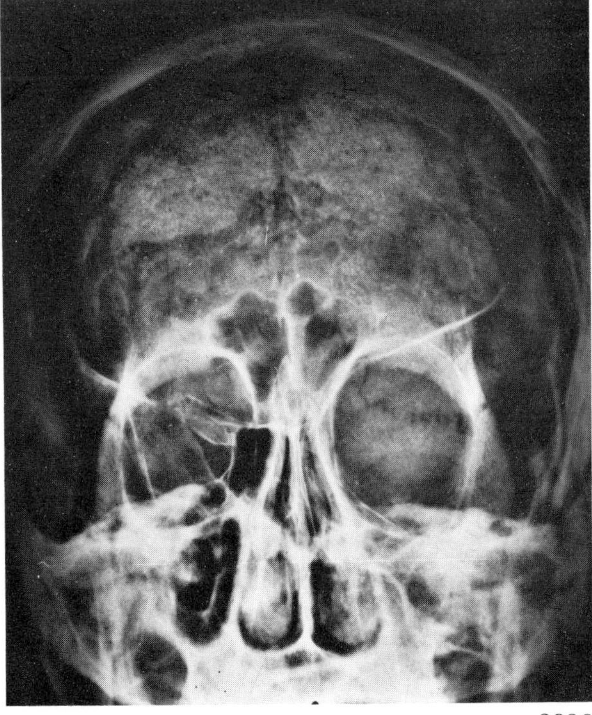

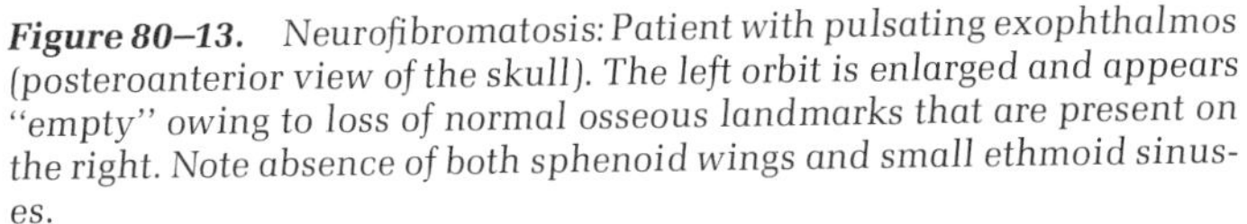

Figure 80–13. *Neurofibromatosis: Patient with pulsating exophthalmos (posteroanterior view of the skull). The left orbit is enlarged and appears "empty" owing to loss of normal osseous landmarks that are present on the right. Note absence of both sphenoid wings and small ethmoid sinuses.*

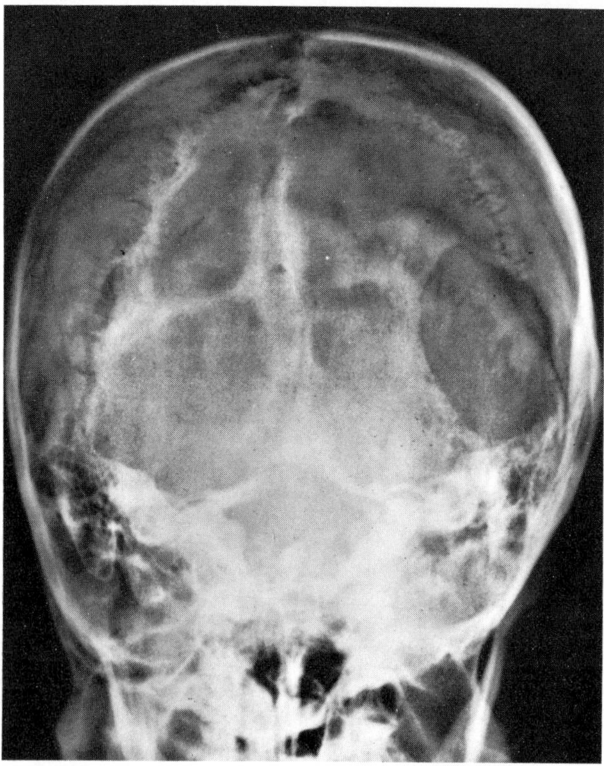

Figure 80–14. Neurofibromatosis: Posteroanterior (Towne) view of the skull. An oval calvarial defect involves the left lambdoid suture and extends towards the midline. This defect occurs predominantly on the left.

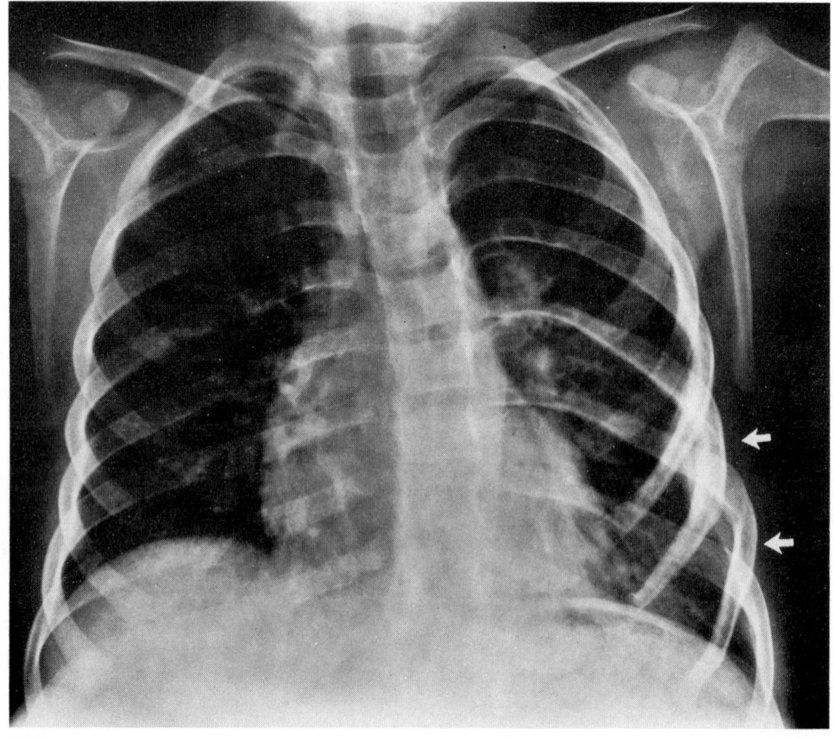

Figure 80–15. Neurofibromatosis: Posteroanterior view of the chest. A moderate degree of thoracic spine scoliosis is associated with widened interpedicular distances of the thoracic vertebrae and deformed, widely spaced, overconstricted, and irregularly contoured ribs on the left side (arrows).

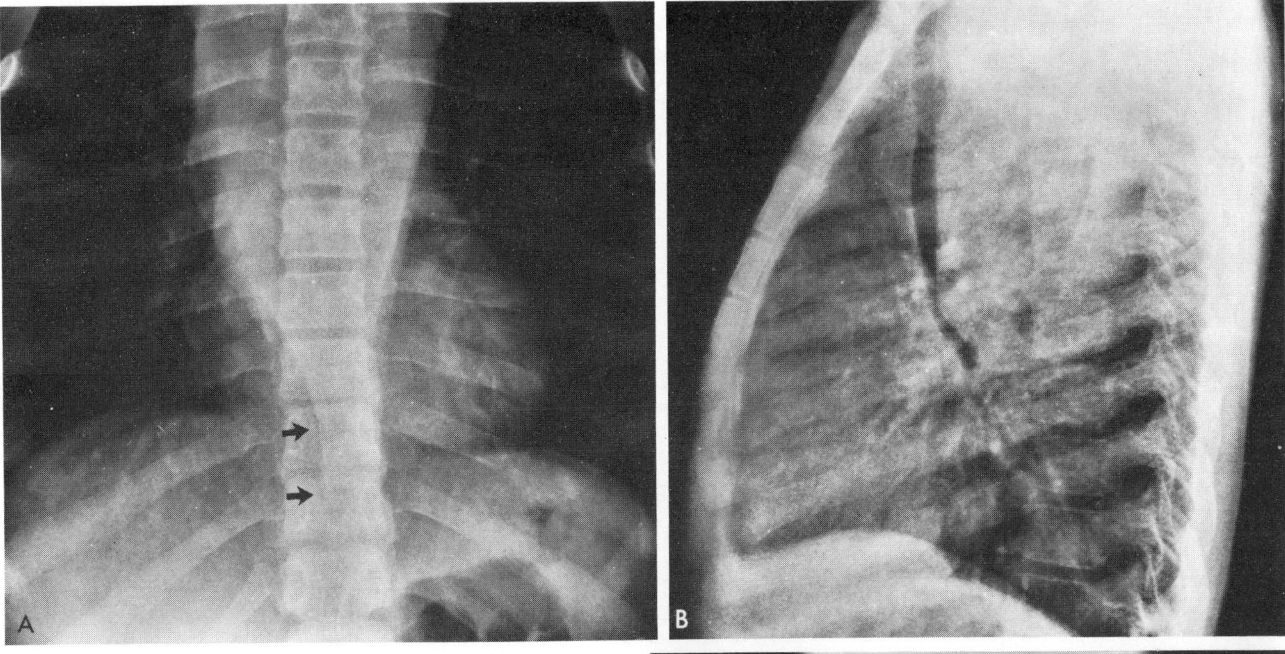

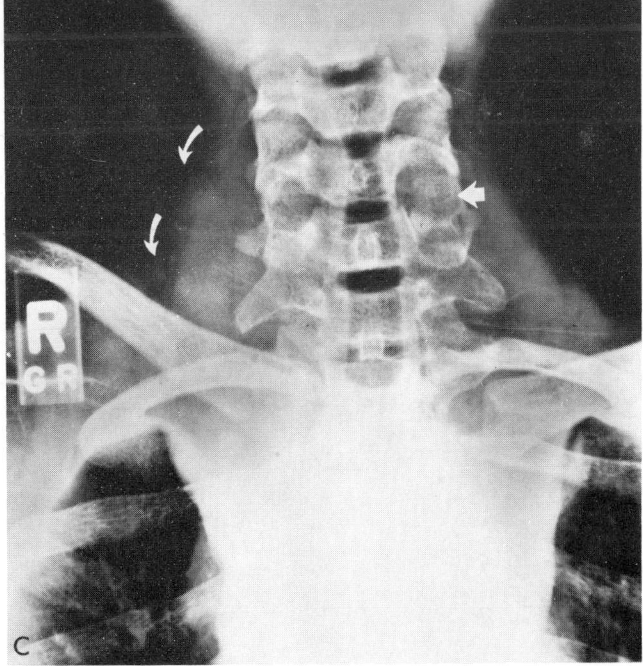

Figure 80–16. *Neurofibromatosis: Intrathoracic plexiform neurofibroma in an 8 year old girl with multiple skin nodules.*

A *Posteroanterior view of the chest. The extensive triangular tumor was broadly based at both apices but descended to involve the entire mediastinum. Note apex at the T10-T11 level (arrows) and slightly lobulated contours of the right side of the mass.*

B *Lateral view of the chest. The tumor impinged on the trachea and left main-stem bronchus. Note that the mass is entirely posterior to the trachea. At surgery extensive tumor mass was found to be fixed along the posterior gutter. The lungs were uninvolved. The vertebrae, foramina, and ribs appear normal.*

C *Anteroposterior view of the chest — apical lordotic view at 14 years of age. The tumor has grown proportionately. Enlarging neurofibroma at the base of the right side of the neck (curved arrows) necessitated readmission. Note the markedly enlarged left cervical spine foramen (straight arrow).*

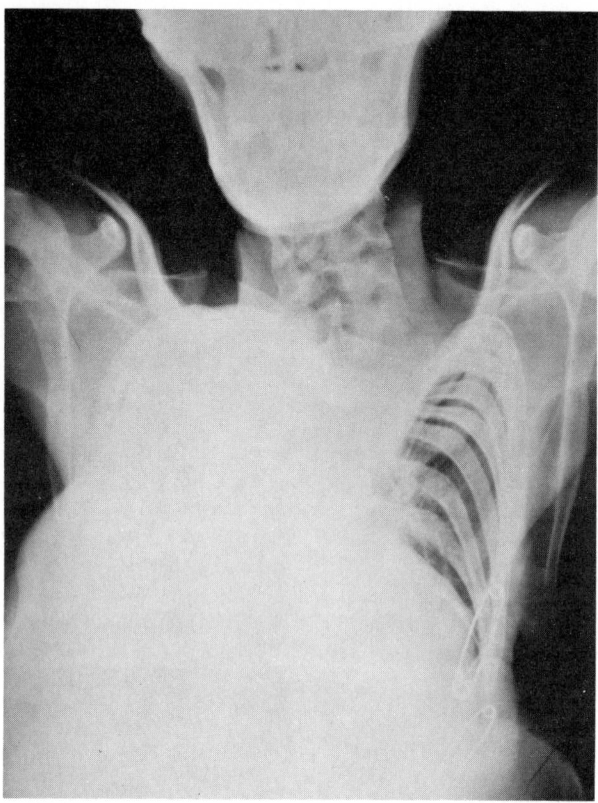

Figure 80–17. Neurofibromatosis. Severe midthoracic kyphoscoliosis is present owing to acute angulation of the midthoracic spine over a relatively short distance. A large intrathoracic neurofibroma contributed to the severe distortion, with resultant progressive pulmonary and cardiovascular compromise.

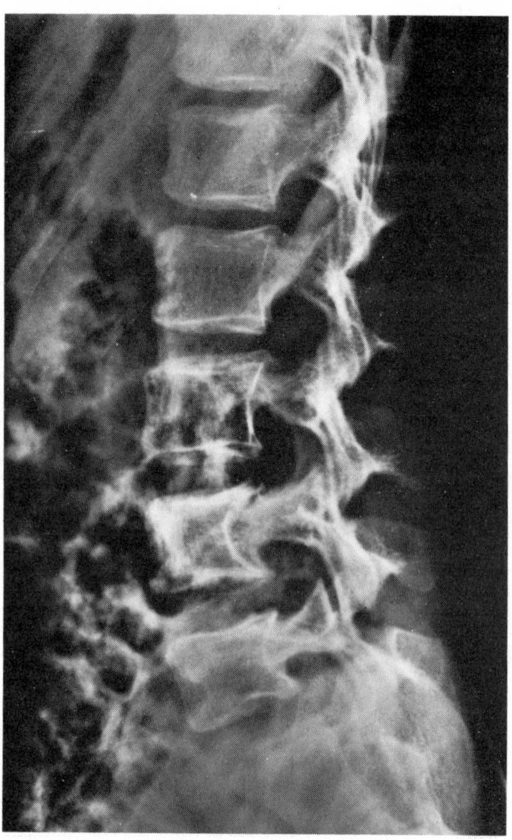

Figure 80–18. Neurofibromatosis. Marked posterior vertebral body scalloping is localized to the L3, L4, and L5 levels. There is no associated scoliosis and no change in the intervertebral disc spaces. Scalloping may result from the intrinsic dysplastic change within bone as well as from neighboring dural ectasia (see Fig. 80–20**B**) rather than from mechanical pressure exerted by a local neurofibroma.

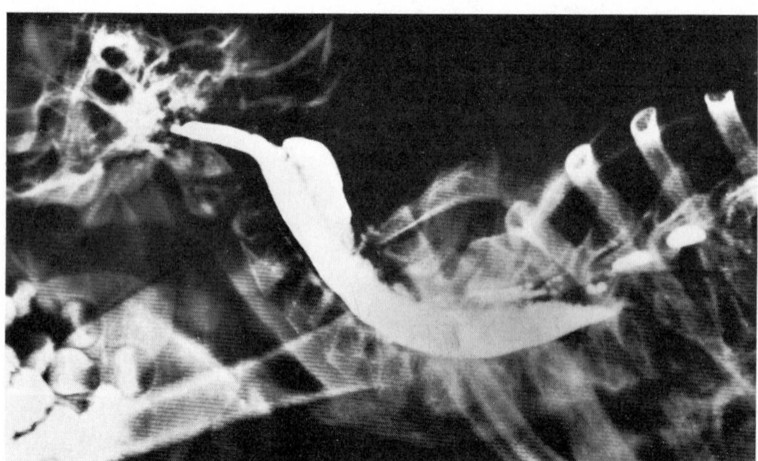

Figure 80–19. Neurofibromatosis. Prone cervical-thoracic myelogram demonstrates gross enlargement of the spinal canal with posterolateral dural ectasia.

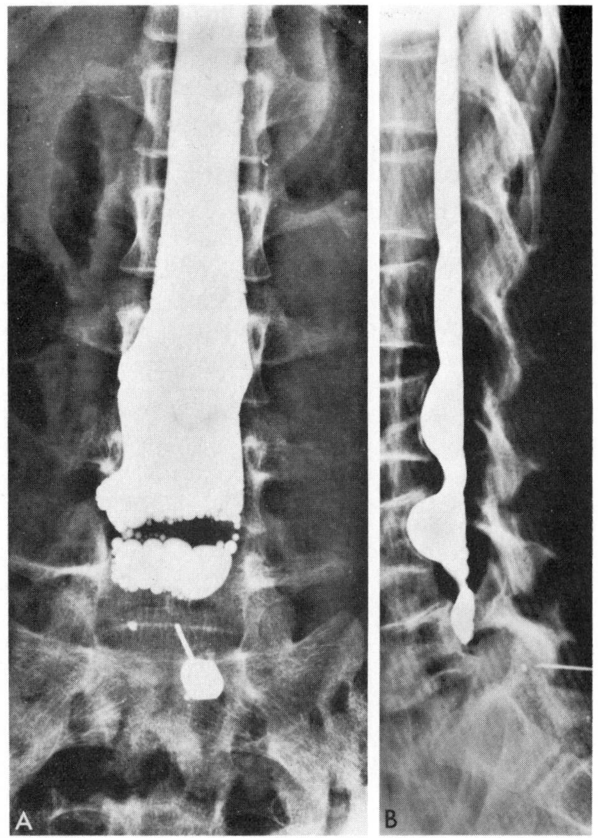

Figure 80–20. Neurofibromatosis: Lumbar myelogram.

A Posteroanterior view. The grossly enlarged subarachnoid space has uniform lateral boundaries outlined by the iophendylate column. Note widened interpedicular distances.

B Prone lateral view reveals evidence of localized pooling of the contrast medium at the L3, L4, and L5 levels owing to dural ectasia. Scalloping usually occurs earlier than interpediculate widening, since the spongy bone of vertebral bodies offers less resistance to local pressure than the compact bone of pedicles.

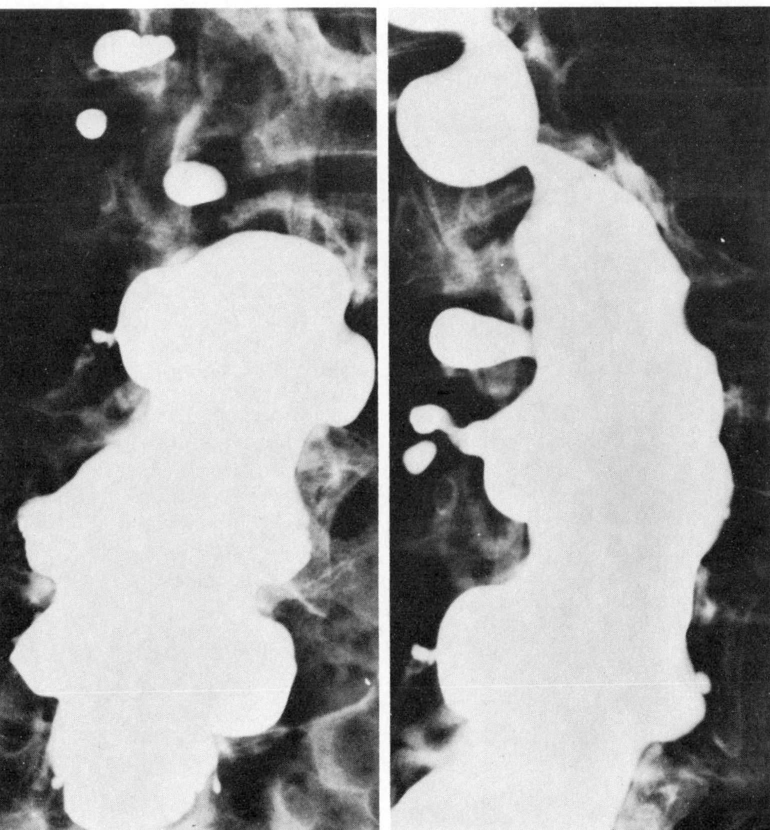

Figure 80–21. Neurofibromatosis: Lumbar myelogram. This patient had severe lumbar scoliosis and widespread vertebral body dysplasia. Note marked dural ectasia with involvement of multiple nerve root sleeves.

However, usually no neurologic symptoms are present. Paraplegia may complicate neurofibromatosis and may be secondary to severe kyphoscoliosis, to bony dysplasia per se, or to spinal cord pathology in the form of meningoceles or tumors. Patients with spinal cord pathology should also be evaluated for the presence of other central nervous system tumors as well as visceral tumors.

Many types of central nervous system (CNS) lesions are known to accompany neurofibromatosis, including those of the cervical and spinal nerves and of the brain and spinal cord. Usually, however, CNS lesions are found in the presence of a minimal number of peripheral nerve lesions. Most types of glial tumors, which may be single or multiple, have been encountered, including glioblastoma multiforme. Meningeal tumors may be solitary (Fig. 80–22) but are often multiple and may be found in either the cranial or spinal region. The finding of multiple meningiomas in association with acoustic neuromas, which may also be multiple, is highly suggestive of neurofibromatosis. Neuromas of the acoustic (eighth cranial) nerves are the most frequent intracranial tumors. Therefore, in addition to erosion of pedicles and enlargement of spinal foramina, the enlargement of the cranial foramina is frequently the first radiographic sign of these lesions. Likewise, the bony orbit, in addition to being dysplastic and in addition to showing evidence of a deficient or absent sphenoid wing, may also reveal evidence of concentric enlargement of the optic foramina indicative of an optic glioma (Fig. 80–23). Over 20 per cent of patients with optic gliomas also have neurofibromatosis.[4]

Additional but less familiar expressions of neurofibromatosis are macrocranium and macrencephaly. These are not isolated or incidental findings. Weichert and co-workers[84] found that 75 per cent of 24 children with neurofibromatosis had macrocranium (increased skull size), which may well be due to macrencephaly (increased brain size). In a review by Holt and Kuhns,[37] 44 per cent of 52 patients had cranial capacities above the ninety-fifth percentile, whereas 70 per cent were above the fiftieth percentile. The presence of intracranial tumors or hydrocephalus did not influence skull size. In addition, volumetric measurements of the sella turcica in 27 patients suggested that idiopathic sellar enlargement in patients with neurofibromatosis is uncommon. There is no correlation between sellar volume and cranial capacity in neurofibromatosis. Therefore, if sellar enlargement is noted, a diligent search should be made for a specific cause. It is of interest that patients with tuberous sclerosis do not have a significant degree of macrocranium. Fewer than 47 per cent of patients with tuberous sclerosis are above the ninety-fifth percentile in this respect and fewer than 50 per cent are at or above the fiftieth percentile. As Holt and Kuhns point out,[37] more than 2000 articles have been written on the subject of neurofibromatosis, yet only a few isolated references to macrocranium are found in them. This sign was, in fact, the most prominent feature in one of the earliest documented cases of

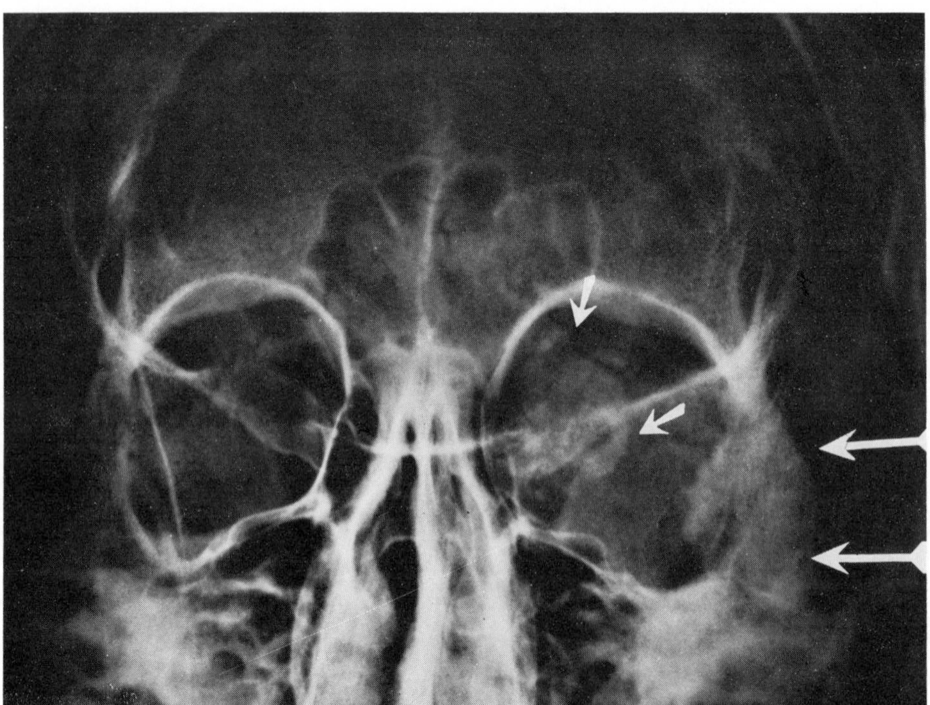

Figure 80–22. *Neurofibromatosis with meningioma: Posteroanterior view of the skull. Note intraorbital calcification and sclerosis and expansion of the left lesser sphenoid wing, which was the site of a meningioma (small arrows). Note also the dysplastic zygoma (large arrows).*

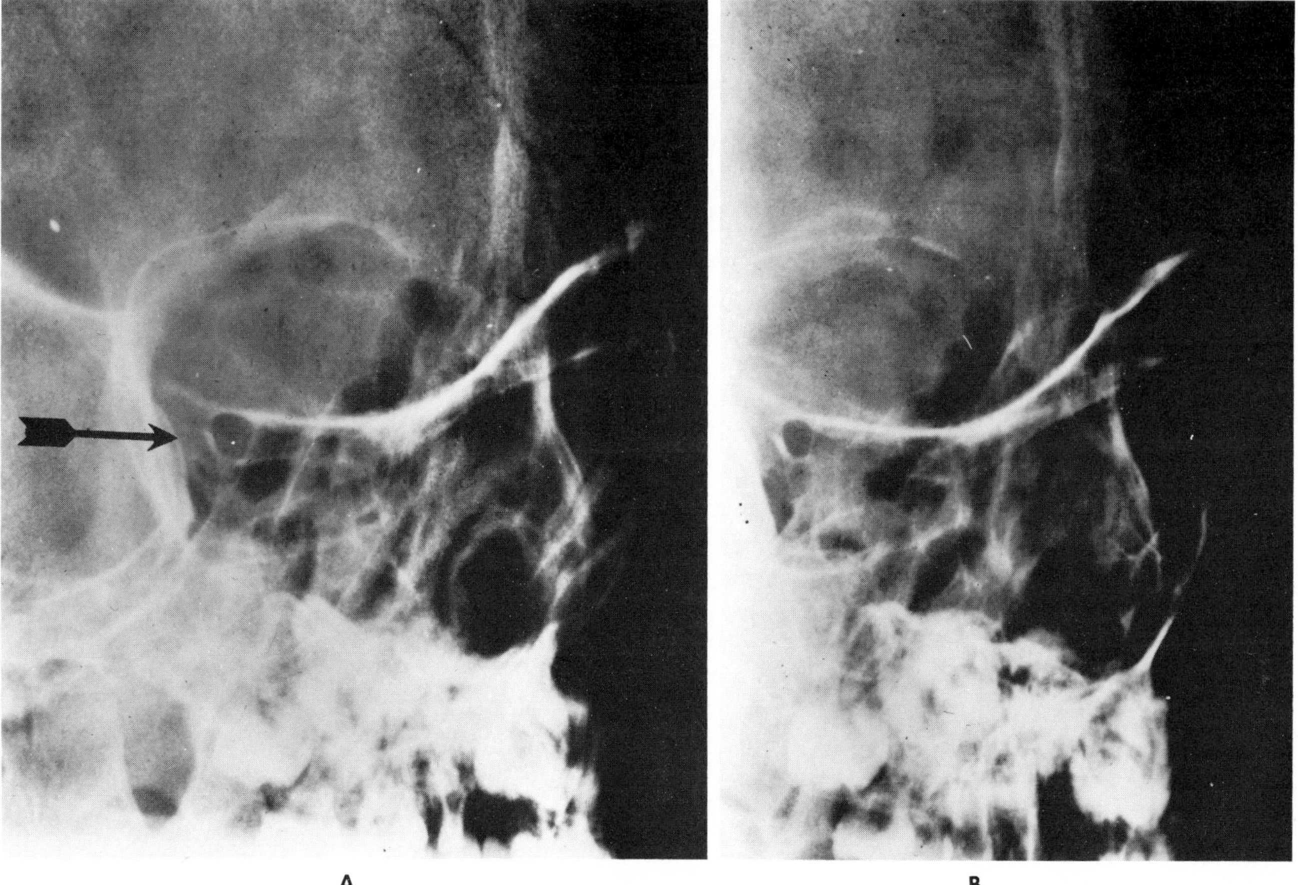

Figure 80–23. *Neurofibromatosis: Optic foramina. A 4 year old boy has a normal right optic foramen* **(B)** *with concentric enlargement of the left owing to an optic nerve glioma (arrow)* **(A).** *Neurofibromas of the orbital nerve and meningiomas of the optic nerve sheath are other orbital lesions that may be encountered in association with neurofibromatosis.*

this disease, the so-called "elephant man," whose large and misshapen head was repeatedly referred to by Treves.[78] It took a century for macrocranium and macrencephaly to be appreciated as a frequent and significant skeletal manifestation of the disease.

Mental deficiency, occasionally seen in these patients, is usually mild. Therefore, changes in intelligence or in orientation that occur later in the life of patients with neurofibromatosis should initiate a search for CNS involvement and particularly for a brain tumor or hydrocephalus.

Other skeletal loci, in addition to the skull and spine, may exhibit abnormal or deficient bone formation, which also reflects the basic mesodermal dysplasia. Microscopically a monotonous pattern of fibrocytes without neurofibromatous tissue may be seen. Bowing and pseudarthrosis of the tibia and fibula (Fig. 80–24) occur, together with bending, pathologic fracture, and inability to form normal callus in healing. An abnormally formed, deficient, or gracile fibula is a frequent accompaniment of a pseudarthrosis of the tibia (Fig. 80–24). Irregular, notched, scalloped, and twisted ribbon-like configurations of the ribs are another expression of dysplastic bone formation (Figs. 80–15 and 80–25). However, rib deformities, though most often related to the primary bone dysplasia, may also be secondary to mechanical pressure caused by neighboring intercostal neurofibromas. Generally, rib deformities only superficially resemble those seen in conjunction with coarctation. It is of interest, however, that coarctation has, in fact, also been documented in association with neurofibromatosis.

Miscellaneous Abnormalities

Deficient growth and overgrowth of bones as well as of the soft tissues are additional stigmata of neurofibromatosis; these may occur separately or together and in various permutations and combinations[36] (Figs 80–26*A*,*B*). Elephantoid soft tissue hypertrophy of a limb and even part of a limb — e.g., gigantism of a finger — may be associated with a normal-appearing, hypertrophied, or underdeveloped underlying skeleton.

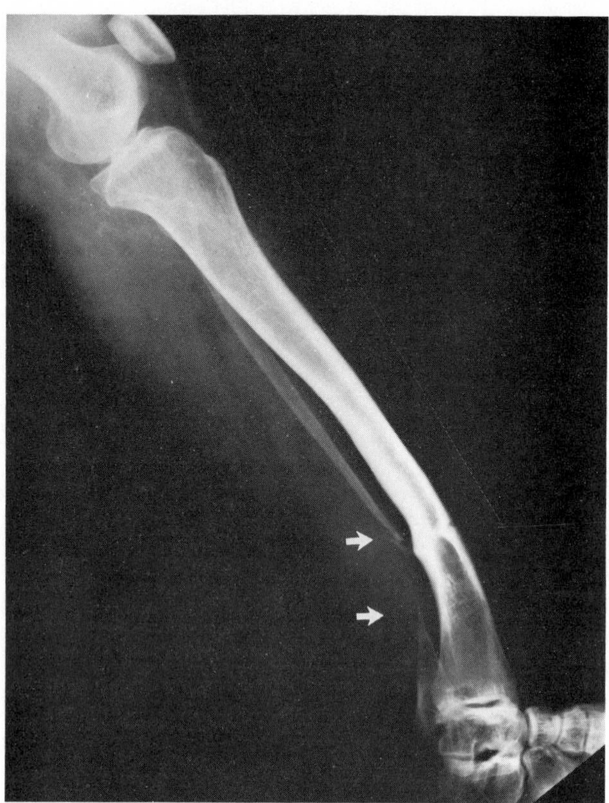

Figure 80–24. Neurofibromatosis: *Lateral view of the tibia and fibula. Note pseudoarthrosis at the most common site — i.e., junction of the middle and lower thirds of the tibia or fibula (or both) with attenuation and "pencil-pointing" of the neighboring fibular segments (arrows), disuse osteoporosis distal to the pseudoarthrosis, and secondary deformities of the talus and calcaneus. Anterior bowing of the leg is characteristic and is usually evident in the first years of life. Pseudoarthrosis may develop spontaneously, after fracture, or following an osteotomy done to correct bowing.*

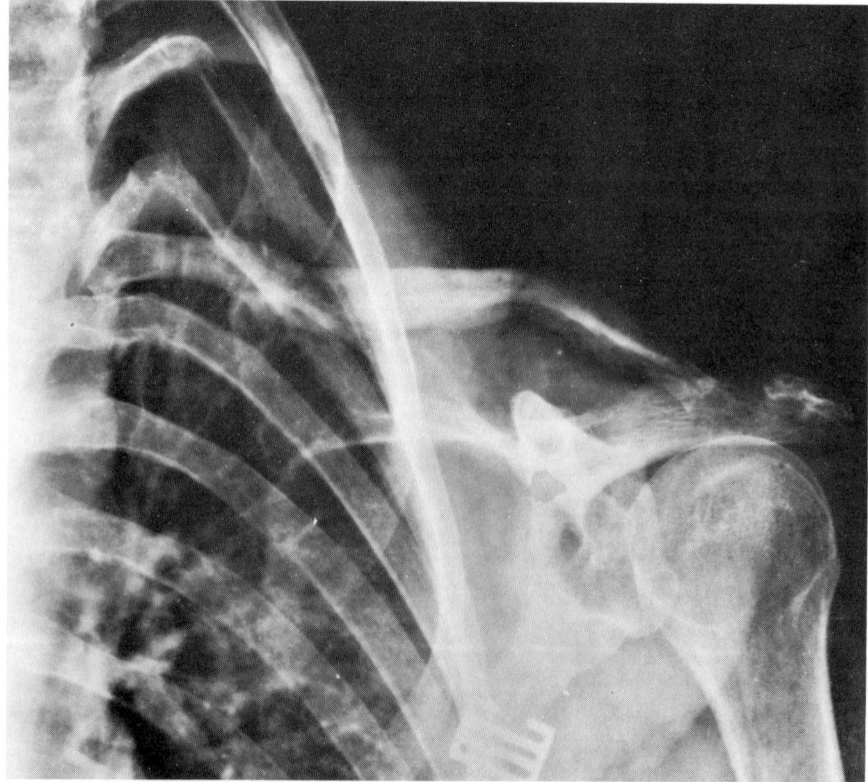

Figure 80–25. Neurofibromatosis: *Left upper hemithorax. Typical appearing ribs are angulated and overconstricted. Some have wavy, undulating, ribbon-like configurations. The upper ribs are widely separated. A pseudoarthrosis of the left clavicle is another associated abnormality.*

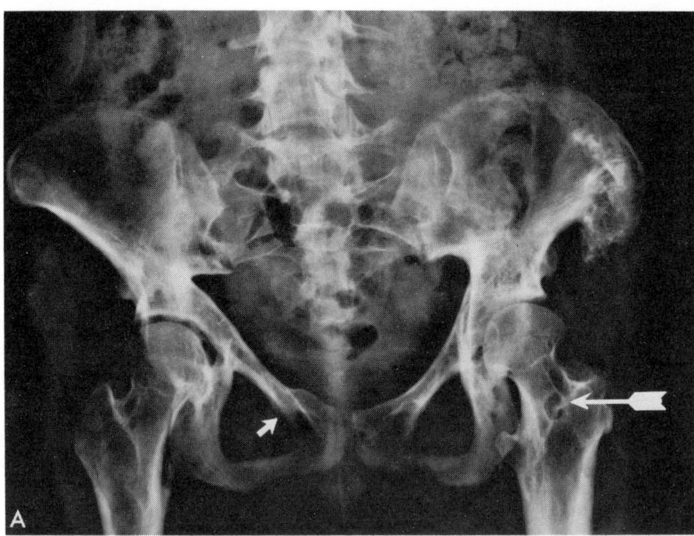

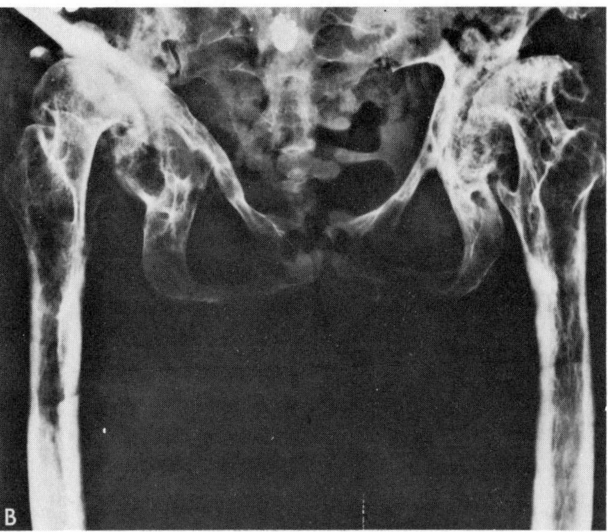

Figure 80–26. *Neurofibromatosis: Anteroposterior view of the pelvis (13 year follow-up).*

A *Radiograph of 5/17/65. There is marked pelvic asymmetry and hypertrophy accentuated by irregular mineralization and beak-like projections of the left inferior and superior iliac spines and proximal left femur. Note the elongated and partially detached right lesser tuberosity and deformed right pubis (small arrow) owing to previously fractured dysplastic bone. The involved acetabula still have a cup-like configuration. Note associated spinal involvement, relatively enlarged, flattened femoral heads, and the rounded, sharply circumscribed radiolucent area in the left femoral neck (large arrow). Intraosseous defects that are considered as characteristically associated abnormalities and commonly attributed to intraosseous neurofibromas are controversial. Superficial cortical depressions when not radiographed in profile may simulate intraosseous lesions. They may, in fact, be due to incidental causes unrelated to the basic disease. There is particular disagreement among authorities who dispute the existence of intramedullary or intracortical nerve fibers. Some defects result from periosteal proliferations that have formed a shell of bone enclosing a previous subperiosteal hemorrhage or an originally external neurofibroma.*

B *Radiograph of 7/18/78. All deformities have progressed markedly. Severe bilateral acetabular distortion and thinning and overconstriction of the ischial and pubic bones have resulted in a triradiate pelvis. Note overgrowth, flattening, and cephalad subluxation of the femoral head. The left femoral neck defect appears relatively large. However, larger, less well defined radiolucent lesions now involve the left pubis, ischium, and acetabulum. Intermittent fractures and osteomalacia had intervened.*

A predilection for hemorrhage, commonly unappreciated in patients with neurofibromatosis,[46, 62, 87] may be massive or fatal, whereas bleeding about bones and surrounding soft tissues is frequent, even after minor insults (Fig. 80–27*A*,*B*). An inherent abnormality of the periosteum, which is a mesodermal derivative, as well as its loose adherence to the underlying cortex has been incriminated. Subperiosteal hemorrhage has also been blamed for the twisted, ribbon-like appearance of the ribs and for the overtubulation and irregularity of the bone shafts.

Neurofibromatosis, like tuberous sclerosis, has therefore been classically identified on the basis of skin, soft tissue, CNS, and skeletal manifestations. However, other dysfunctions of multiple organ systems have been recognized with increasing frequency, and a variety of genitourinary, endocrine, and cardiovascular abnormalities have been documented.

Arterial lesions are common, and in addition to the known association of pheochromocytoma, renal artery stenosis constitutes another underlying cause of hypertension in neurofibromatosis[31] (Fig. 80–28). In a hypertensive child with neurofibromatosis, renal artery stenosis is the most common cause, whereas in an adult hypertensive patient with neurofibromatosis, pheochromocytoma is the more common culprit.[44] Approximately 1 per cent of patients with neurofibromatosis have pheochromocytomas, but 20 per cent of patients with pheochromocytomas have neurofibromatosis. Therefore, a hypertensive adult patient should be carefully evaluated for both pheochromocytoma and renal artery stenosis.

Vascular lesions are found at autopsy in approximately 50 per cent of cases of neurofibromatosis, but most have apparently been asymptomatic. Although they most commonly occur in the kidney, vascular abnormalities consisting of arterial wall thickening, stenoses, and aneurysm formation have been found in the heart, spleen, gastrointestinal tract, and pancreas and other endocrine glands. Stenoses of the mesenteric, iliac, and pulmonary arteries have also been reported.[42]

Coexistent aortic coarctations at the abdominal and thoracic levels have also been described.[65] (Fig. 80–28). Rib notching may therefore reflect associated coarctation rather than or as well as the underlying

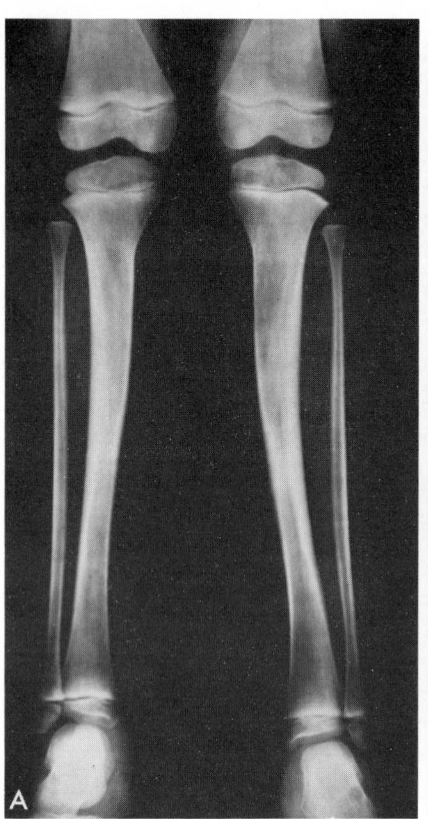

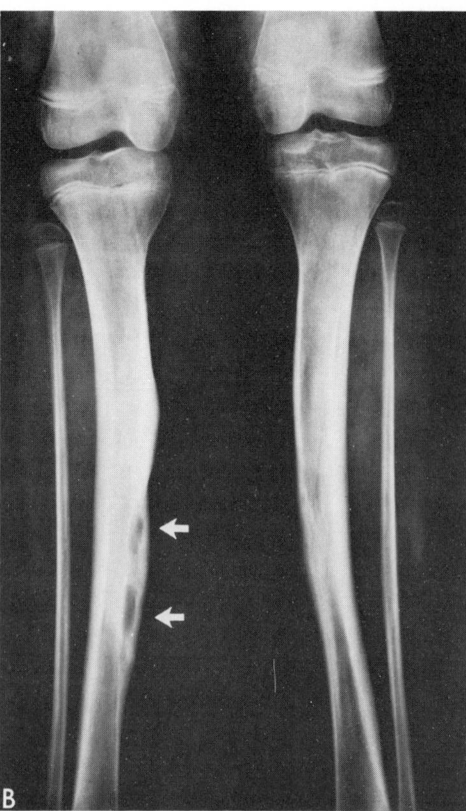

Figure 80–27. *Neurofibromatosis: Anteroposterior view of tibias and fibulas.*

A *Radiograph of 7/16/53. Dysplastic changes in both lower legs include bilateral bowing, most marked on the left, overgrowth and increased leg length on the left, distal femoral modeling deformities resulting in Ehrlenmeyer flask configurations, and genu valgum.*

B *Radiograph of 2/19/59. Progression of the deformities in* **A** *has occurred, particularly along the medial aspect of right midtibial shaft. Cortical thickening and hypertrophy have resulted in the development of two intracortical radiolucent lesions (arrows). These cyst-like, apparently intraosseous lesions may result from subperiosteal hemorrhage, with subsequent periosteal proliferation and repair, or from the incorporation or overgrowth of the periosteum around a previously external soft tissue lesion, such as a neurofibroma.*

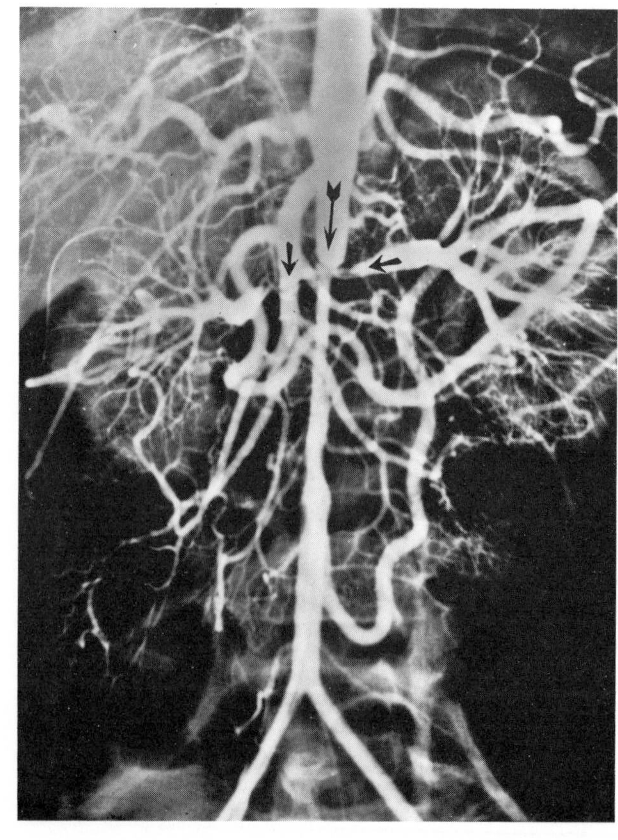

FIgure 80–28. *Neurofibromatosis: Abdominal aortogram in a 10 year old girl with neurofibromatosis and a 4 month history of hypertension. Severe coarctation of the abdominal aorta as well as bilateral renal artery stenoses with poststenotic dilatations are defined (arrows). Both kidneys were normal in size and were normally perfused. Note rich collateral network. Concomitant stenoses or coarctation of the abdominal aorta occurs in approximately 25 per cent of patients with neurofibromatosis and renal artery stenosis.*

bone dysplasia. However, the rib notching associated with coarctation has distinctive roentgenographic features in that it appears as a localized pit or depression, which most commonly involves the undersurface of the rib. The generalized deformities, many of which are ribbon-like in configuration, that are typical of the involved ribs in neurofibromatosis (Figs. 80–15 and 80–25) are not seen in association with isolated coarctation. An increased incidence of congenital heart disease in neurofibromatosis, e.g., ventricular and atrial septal defects and pulmonary valvular stenosis, has also been reported.[44, 59] Another less well appreciated vascular abnormality is that of stenosis or occlusion of arteries at the base of the brain.[35] The type of arterial abnormality differs according to the size of the artery. Generally, the microscopic pattern is one of internal hypertrophy, disorganization of the muscular and elastic fibers of the tunica media, and true *aneurysm* formation. Neurofibromatous changes occurring solely in the adventitia of arteries have also been noted so that hypertension may occasionally be related to compression of a renal artery or other artery by a neurofibroma instead of or in addition to intrinsic arterial disease.

Neurofibromas have also involved the urinary bladder as well as the gastrointestinal tract, where they usually arise from subserosal nerves and from the Auerbach and submucosal plexuses. Patients may present with symptoms related to pressure, intussusception, or bleeding from ulceration or obstruction. Anemia may be a clue to gastrointestinal involvement in a patient with neurofibromatosis. Sarcomatous degeneration is no more common in these lesions than in those found in other areas.[17, 67]

Pulmonary Kerley's B lines, cystic bullae, and infiltrates arranged in a honeycomb pattern reminiscent of the roentgenographic changes in tuberous sclerosis have been described. Severe interstitial fibrosis, indistinguishable from end-stage fibrosing alveolitis, has also been noted.[56, 83] The pathogenesis of pulmonary changes remains unknown.

Associated endocrine abnormalities include small bowel carcinoid tumors,[44] multiple endocrine adenomatosis, hyperparathyroidism,[18] and Sipple's syndrome. The latter is a hereditary disorder consisting of medullary thyroid carcinoma, pheochromocytoma, and multiple mucosal neuromas involving the lips, tongue, eyes, or gastrointestinal tract.[39] Precocious sexual development, which more frequently is linked with fibrous dysplasia, has also been reported.[69]

When the classic cutaneous triad is present or the triad of cutaneous, mental, and skeletal deformities is noted, diagnosis is not difficult. Neither is diagnosis difficult when patients with classic neurofibromatosis have a variety of other lesions in addition to the triad. Less familiar lesions, however, although individually recognized, may not be recognized as "part and parcel" of the neurofibromatosis complex, particularly when they may constitute the patient's initial or major complaint. This is particularly true when the classic triads are absent or are not obvious. Therefore, familiarity with and the identification of the presumably more unusual manifestations are of the utmost importance. Some of these lesions or combinations of lesions are, in fact, as pathognomonic as the more classic stigmata and may certainly be more life-threatening.

FIBROUS DYSPLASIA

General Features

Fibrous dysplasia, a disorder of expanding fibro-osseous lesions, was the designation coined by Lichtenstein[51] in 1938 to describe a skeletal developmental anomaly of bone-forming mesenchyme of unknown etiology, which is not hereditary, which may exist independently,[52] and which may affect one or many bones. However, the polyostotic variety, and rarely the monostotic type,[81] when associated with endocrine dysfunction and cutaneous pigmentation has been known as the McCune-Albright syndrome.[2, 54] Fibrous dysplasia may, therefore, like tuberous sclerosis and neurofibromatosis, also be associated with skin, skeletal, CNS, and endocrine abnormalities, a fact that generated controversy between Thannhauser[75] and Albright as to whether neurofibromatosis and fibrous dysplasia were one and the same disease.[82]

The classic clinical triad associated with Albright's syndrome includes polyostotic fibrous dysplasia, which tends to be unilateral, café au lait spots, which favor the side of the bone lesions, and endocrine dysfunction, most commonly manifested by precocious female sexual development.

Cutaneous Abnormalities

The pigmented skin macules or café au lait spots of fibrous dysplasia have been a prime source of confusion with neurofibromatosis. Although they are brown and widely distributed in both diseases, those associated with Albright's syndrome have serrated, irregular contours, are often darker in color (i.e., flat melanotic areas), and are usually fewer in number, although they may cover an area of several centimeters. They may be arranged in a linear or segmental pattern, or they may be isolated, but they often tend to appear on either side of the midline. The skin texture of the pigmented area is exactly the same as that of the surrounding normal skin. The most frequent locations of the pigmented areas are over the sacrum, buttocks, and upper spine; however, they often parallel the distribution of the skeletal lesions. Pigmentation may date from birth or infancy, but the appearance of new lesions and the enlargement of preexisting ones, even after puberty, are not unusual. The most common extraskeletal manifestation of fibrous dysplasia is abnormal cutaneous pigmentation.

In contrast, the macules of neurofibromatosis have a lighter brown hue, have smoother borders, are more numerous (i.e., there are usually more than six in number), and tend to be generalized and irregularly distributed. Differences in pigment granules based on microscopic studies utilizing histochemical dopa reactions have been noted.[7] White freckle-like axillary macules, molluscum fibrosum, and cutaneous and plexiform neurofibromas are other distinguishing cutaneous features of neurofibromatosis.

Cranial and Skeletal Abnormalities

Skeletal lesions commonly underlie the clinical complaints associated with fibrous dysplasia, whereas fracture and deformity constitute its cardinal roentgenographic features. Radiologic findings depend on the anatomic sites affected and the pathologic stage of the disease. The monostotic lesion is the most common form of fibrous dysplasia. Any bone may be involved, although vertebral lesions are particularly uncommon. The most frequently encountered loci are in the proximal femur, tibia, rib cage, and facial bones. Fibrous dysplasia is the most common benign lesion of the rib cage, and it is usually asymptomatic (Fig. 80–29).

Skull involvement occurs in 50 per cent of patients with polyostotic fibrous dysplasia and in 10 to 25 per cent of patients with the monostotic form; it is responsible for the grossly appreciated asymmetry and deformity of the head and face.

Common sites of skull involvement include the frontal, sphenoid, maxillary, and ethmoid bones (Fig. 80–30*A*,*B*). Occipital and temporal bone involvement is less frequent[49] (Fig. 80–31). Lucent and sclerotic lesions are noted (Fig. 80–32*A*,*B*), with the latter predominating in the skull and most commonly involving the base and sphenoid wings (Fig. 80–30*A*). Radiolucent lesions may be associated with widening of the diploic spaces, which may be localized. Expansion is almost always in an outward direction with the inner table remaining undisturbed (Fig. 80–32*A*,*B*).

Initially silent or asymptomatic cranial lesions may progress slowly, with gradual visual impairment and hearing loss, which are related to compromise of the optic nerve in the optic canal or of the middle ear by temporal bone changes. Downward

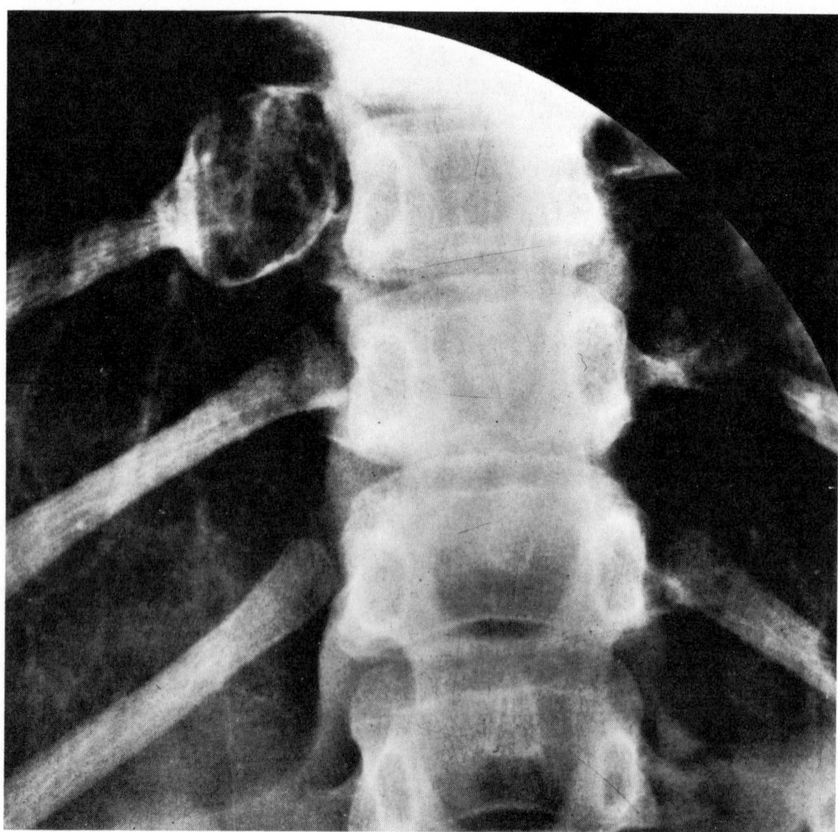

Figure 80–29. *Fibrous dysplasia: Anteroposterior view of the rib. This solitary, expansile, multilocular-appearing lesion with an intact cortex was an incidental finding on a chest film of a teen-aged boy. The likeliest cause of such a focal rib lesion is fibrous dysplasia. Rib lesions are more commonly associated with prominent fibrous replacement of bone and therefore are commonly radiolucent.*

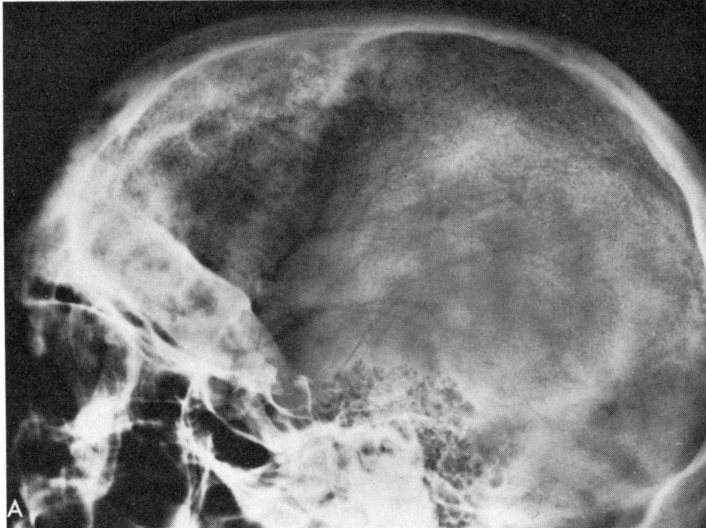

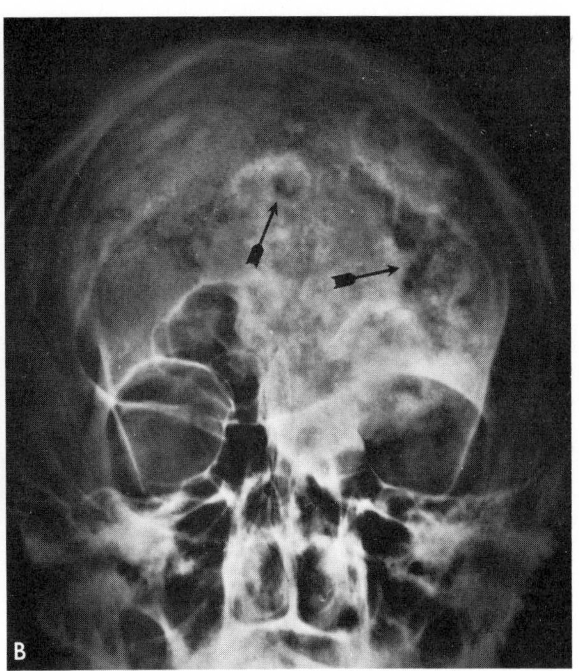

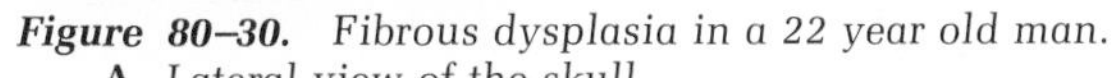

Figure 80–30. *Fibrous dysplasia in a 22 year old man.*

A *Lateral view of the skull.*

B *Posteroanterior view of the skull. The frontal bone and anterior fossa are predominantly affected. The sphenoid and orbital portions of the frontal bone are markedly involved by the hyperostotic, sharply defined productive process, which also partially obliterates the left frontal and ethmoid sinuses. Several patchy, well-marginated radiolucent lesions (arrows) are evident within the area of sclerosis.*

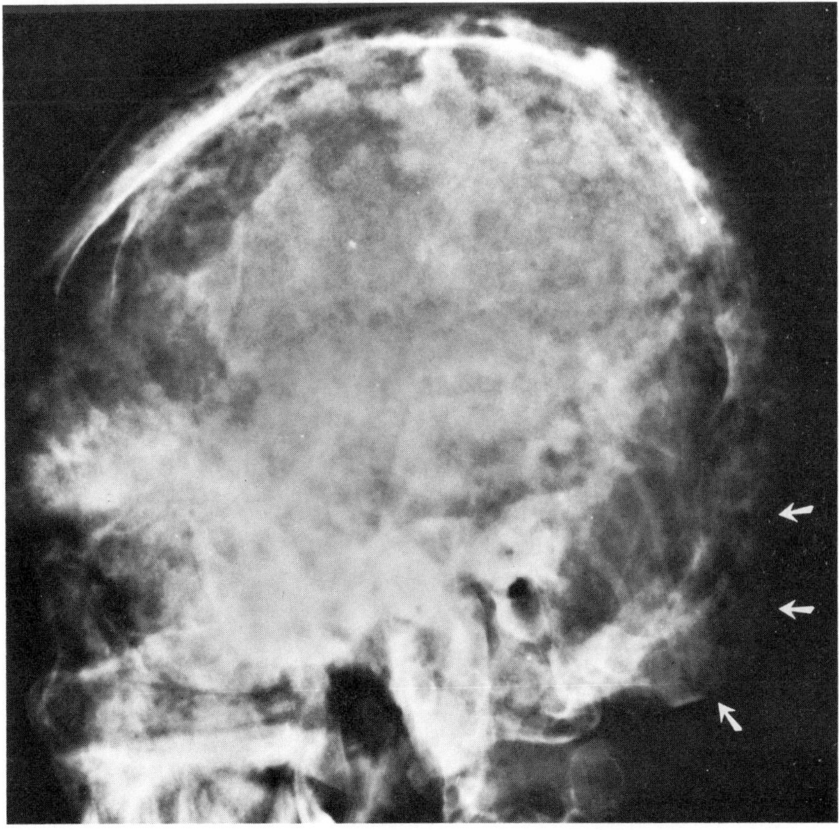

Figure 80–31. *Fibrous dysplasia: Twenty year old woman with polyostotic fibrous dysplasia and McCune-Albright syndrome admitted to hospital for investigation of an enlarging thyroid gland. Lateral view of the skull shows that the skull vault, base, and facial bones are extensively involved. Note involvement of less frequent sites, such as the temporal and occipital portions of the calvarium, with particularly marked thickening and expansion of the occipital outer table (arrows).*

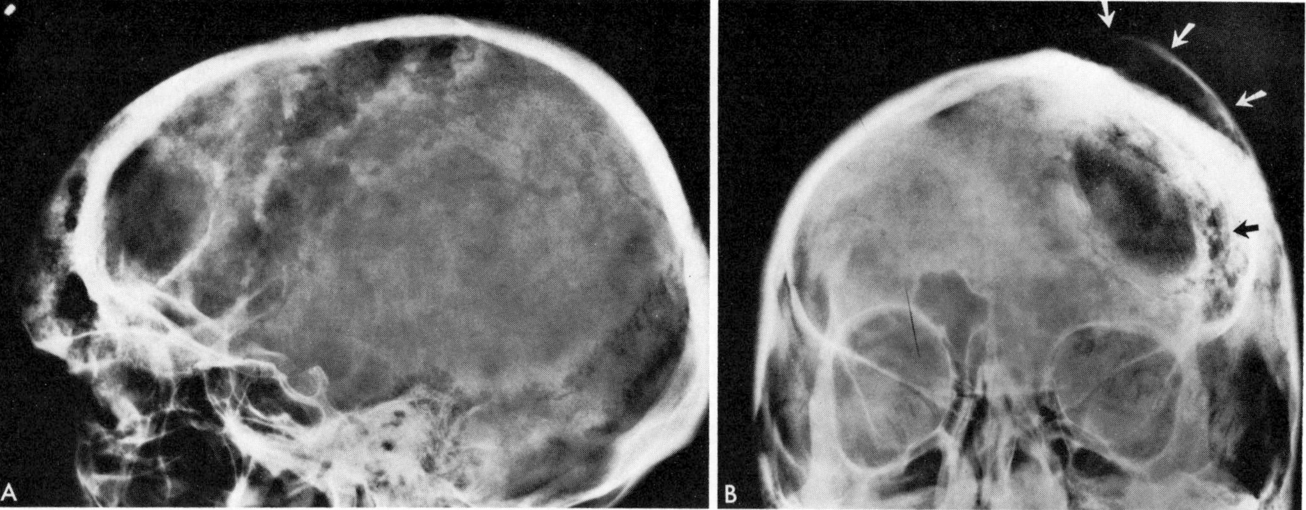

Figure 80–32. Fibrous dysplasia in 30 year old woman.

A Lateral view. The frontal bone is involved by a mixed sclerotic and lytic process. The multiple irregular radiolucent areas are all bounded by sclerotic rims. Note the relative preservation of the inner table, with expansion of the outer frontal table.

B Posteroanterior view. The large ovoid radiolucent lesion in the left frontal bone is marginated by a sclerotic rim or "rind." Faint, punctate radiodense areas within the confines of the lesion (black arrow) represent calcified osteoid. Note the marked expansion and attenuation of the outer table, which is now a thin bony shell (white arrows). Although the lesions of fibrous dysplasia tend to stabilize with adulthood, some may enlarge after puberty owing to "cystification" rather than malignant change.

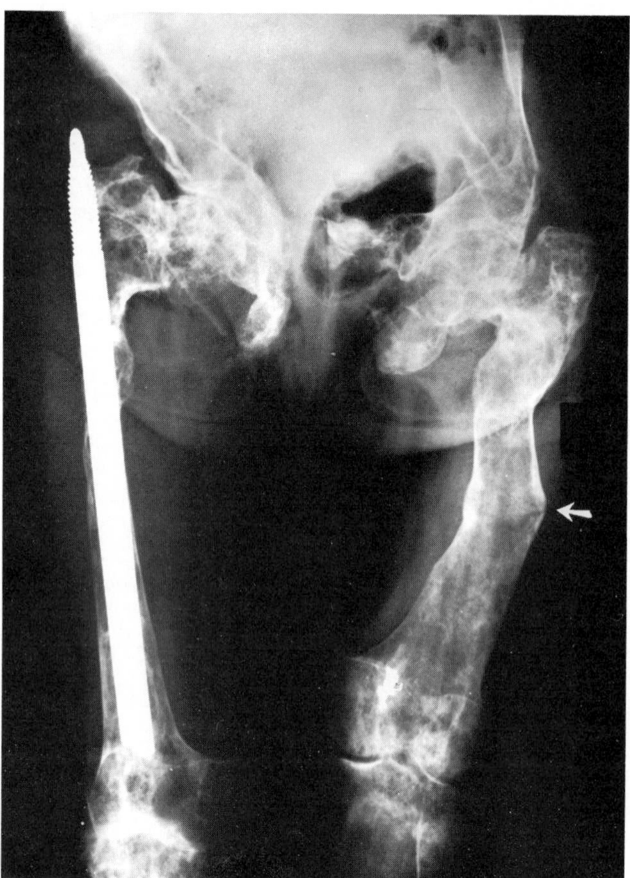

Figure 80–33. Fibrous dysplasia: Anteroposterior view of the pelvis and femurs. Polyostotic involvement is seen in a 20 year old woman with McCune-Albright syndrome and a history of multiple fractures and surgical interventions. Note the severe pelvic distortion and bilateral proximal femoral varus deformities, the so-called "shepherd's crook" deformities. The femoral shafts are poorly modeled, with an intrinsic hazy, lucent appearance, and little sclerosis or lesional calcification. The entire shafts, including the bone ends, are affected. There is an acute angulation at the site of a previously healed fracture (arrow).

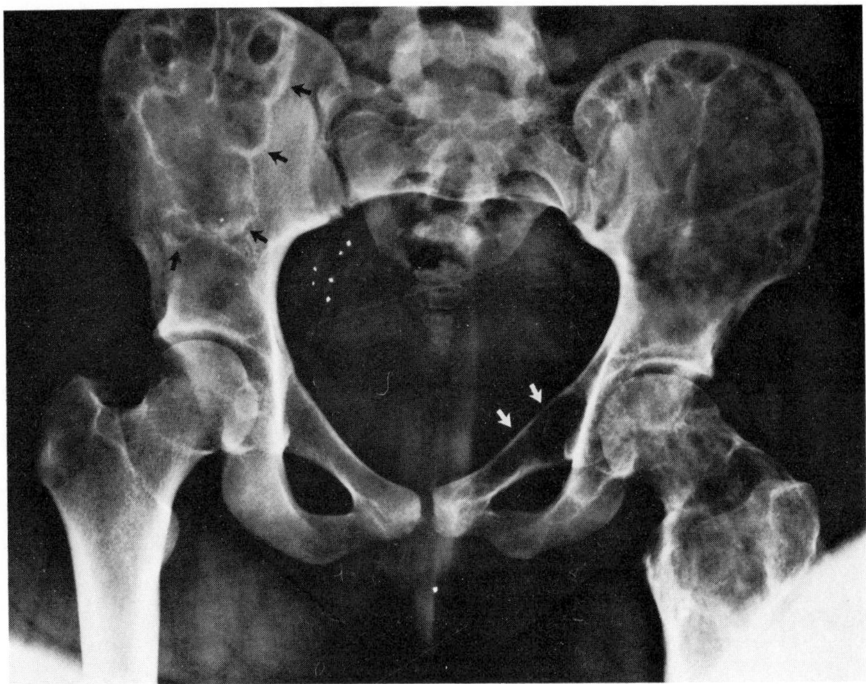

Figure 80–34. *Fibrous dysplasia: Anteroposterior view of the pelvis in a 16 year old girl with polyostotic fibrous dysplasia and McCune-Albright syndrome. The dysplasia has resulted in a thickened, foreshortened femoral neck and shaft held in varus position, i.e., a "shepherd's crook" deformity. Note the hazy, ground-glass appearance of the involved left femur, with relative sparing of the femoral head. The left pubis and both ilia are also involved by roentgenographically typical lesions of fibrous dysplasia. The purely radiolucent pubic lesion is expansile and nonmineralized (white arrows). The central segments of the right iliac locus are hazy and smoky in appearance owing to a high proportion of osteoid and are well demarcated by an almost continuous curvilinear sclerotic rim (black arrows).*

displacement of the orbital contents may also result from the gross deformity and asymmetry of the skull and may be clinically confused with the exophthalmus of neurofibromatosis. Roentgenographic evidence of concomitant facial bone involvement helps to differentiate fibrous dysplasia of the skull from neurofibromatosis as well as from meningioma. An increased incidence of seizure disorders has also been noted.

Other skeletal lesions and deformities, though asymptomatic, are, like the facial and cranial asymmetry, frequently obvious. The major effect of fibrous dysplasia is to weaken the structural integrity of the involved bone. Weight-bearing bones, in particular, bow under stress, resulting in deformity and fracture (Fig. 80–33). Leg length discrepancies reflect abnormalities in shape and modeling, such as the shepherd's crook or varus configurations caused by intrinsic femoral neck lesions, as well as angular deformities secondary to fracture (Figs. 80–33 and 80–34). Overgrowth or undergrowth of bones and adjacent soft tissues may also occur and roentgenographically may superficially resemble the changes seen in association with neurofibromatosis (Fig. 80–35).

Growth discrepancies and gross deformities such as bowed limbs are more commonly associated with polyostotic fibrous dysplasia and are predominantly unilateral. Skin lesions, too, tend to favor the side of bony involvement. Pain in an extremity associated with a limp or spontaneous fracture, or both, often constitutes the initial symptom complex.

The age range affected in the monostotic variety is from 10 to 70 years, but recognition is most frequent in the second and third decades of life. The age distribution is younger in the polyostotic form, since more severe manifestations lead to earlier clinical and roentgenographic recognition. Two thirds of patients with polyostotic fibrous dysplasia are symptomatic before the age of 10 years.[34]

In 25 per cent of patients with polyostotic fibrous dysplasia more than 50 per cent of the skeleton is reported to be involved at the time of initial presentation (Figs. 80–31 and 80–33). In a series by Harris and co-workers,[34] 85 per cent of patients with polyostotic fibrous dysplasia had sustained fractures and 40 per cent had three or more fractures.

The only significant laboratory abnormality associated with fibrous dysplasia is an elevation of the serum alkaline phosphatase level. This was present in one third of the 90 patients reviewed by Harris and associates.[34] The highest value was 96 Bodansky units. It is of interest that there was no correlation between the alkaline phosphatase level and the extent of bone involvement. The serum alkaline phosphatase level may be elevated in the absence of fractures in adults as well as in children.

Radiographically, the long bone lesions of fibrous dysplasia are predominantly diametaphyseal, with only occasional epiphyseal or end of bone involvement (Fig. 80–36). They are relatively radiolucent and often have a hazy quality reminiscent of ground glass. They are usually well defined within the medullary cavity and are frequently bordered by a sclerotic rim or margin (Figs. 80–34 and 80–36). They may have a loculated or trabeculated appearance as well as a partially calcified or ossified matrix with radiopaque areas within the confines of the lesion. Eccentric lesions are often accompanied by a

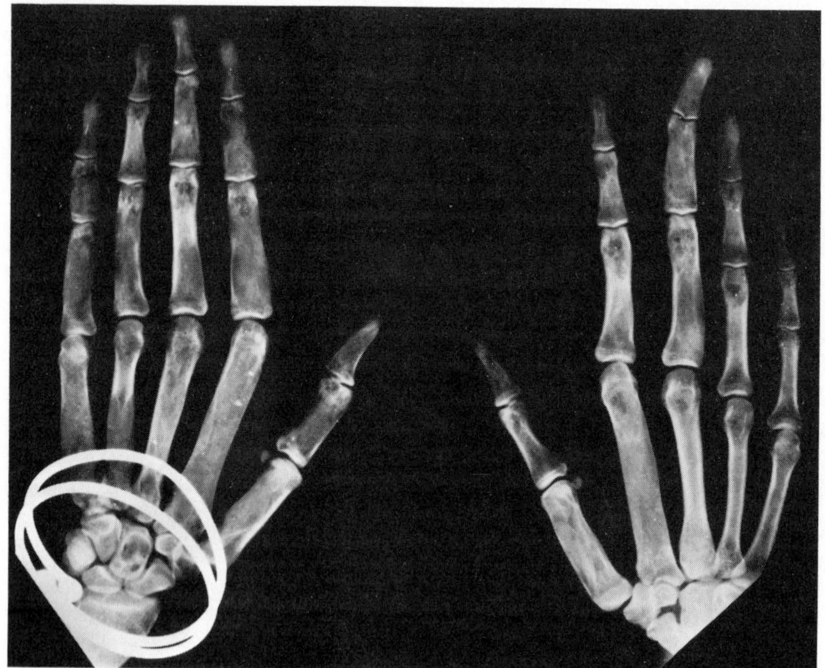

Figure 80–35. *Fibrous dysplasia: Posteroanterior view of the hands. Expansion of the spongiosa, cortical thinning, and alteration of bone texture are common roentgenographic findings in affected tubular bones. This 16 year old girl had widespread failure of modeling with abnormal angulation and localized overgrowth of bones and soft tissues. Several metacarpals and phalanges have rectangular or fusiform shapes, with a loss of definition between medullary and cortical bone. The hazy or ground-glass appearance is particularly uniform in the second metacarpals. Localized radiolucent lesions with endosteal scalloping and areas of medullary sclerosis are also seen in several phalanges.*

Figure 80–36. *Fibrous dysplasia: Anteroposterior view of the femur. The hazy, irregularly contoured, but well-defined lesion is typically situated in the diametaphysis. Note the partially calcified osseous matrix and the sclerotic rim of the proximal portion of the lesion. Its lowermost extension has an entirely lucent blade-like configuration, which is not as well demarcated (arrow).*

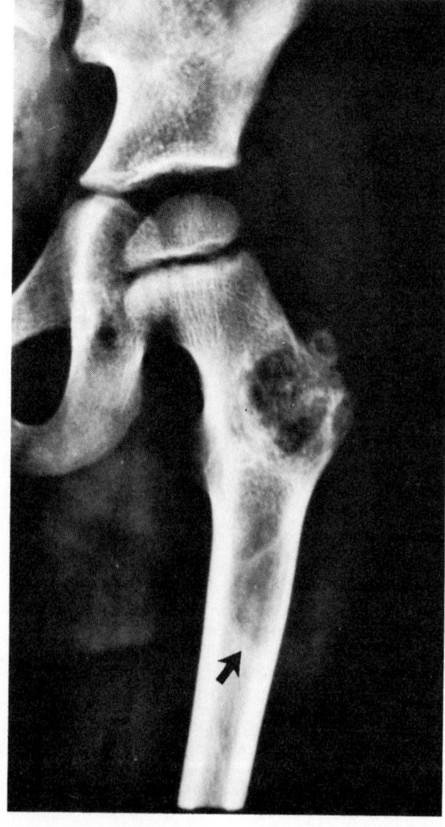

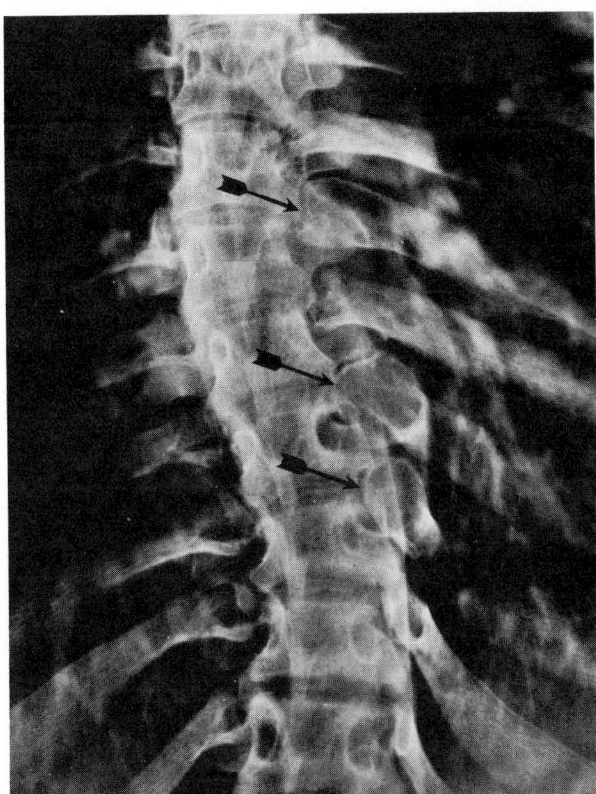

Figure 80–37. *Fibrous dysplasia: Anteroposterior view of the thoracic spine in a 14 year old boy. The vertebral column is more likely to be involved in polyostotic rather than in monostotic fibrous dysplasia. The dysplastic bone per se, as well as multiple fractures due to poorly tolerated mechanical stresses, results in both primary and secondary scolioses. Note several lucent expansile lesions involving the left posterior ribs at the costovertebral junctions (arrows).*

thickened or hypertrophied adjacent cortex, with occasional endosteal scalloping or erosion. Cortical thinning may also be noted with focally expansile lesions. These changes may involve a limited segment or a major portion of a bone. The periosteal surface may have an undulating appearance but is usually smooth and intact unless fractured. Fractures in fibrous dysplasia are frequently produced by mild trauma. They seldom become displaced and heal within a normal period of time with identifiable callus formation. Stress or fissure fractures, however, are often not readily identifiable and may be difficult to diagnose despite the presence of symptoms. The osseous lesions of fibrous dysplasia may be intrinsically vascular, so that increased concentrations of radionuclide on bone scans may occur. However, the finding is nonspecific. Osteomyelitis and a variety of tumors, both benign and malignant, could have a similar appearance on bone scan. Diagnosis depends on correlation with routine radiographs as well as on clinical findings.

The hazy, radiolucent or radiopaque areas seen on roentgenograms directly reflect the relative amounts of fibrous and osseous tissue present in a particular lesion at a particular time. Mature fibrous collagenous tissue loosely arranged in a whorled pattern often contains haphazardly placed trabeculae of woven bone within its confines. The trabeculae, which may be well mineralized although irregular in size and shape, are responsible for the radiopaque areas within the lesion. The alternate areas, which are predominantly fibrous, are relatively radiolucent. Grossly, the masses of dysplastic tissue often appear solid and gritty, and they feel sandy to the touch. They may additionally contain small, degenerated, fluid-filled areas, which are associated with cellular necrosis. If large enough, they appear markedly radiolucent, clear, and cystic rather than hazy or like ground glass on roentgenograms.

The spine is infrequently affected. Rarely associated sequelae have included angular deformity, vertebral collapse, and spinal cord compression (Fig. 80–37). Vertebral collapse most commonly occurs in the lumbar spine, but collapse per se is not necessarily associated with cord compression (Fig. 80–38). The latter finding may occur primarily as a result of posteriorly expanding fibrous tissue masses rather than on the basis of bony impingement.

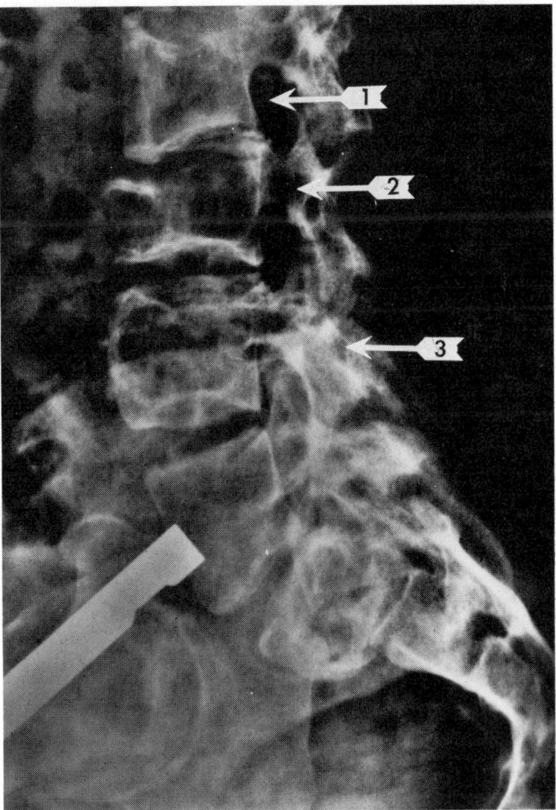

Figure 80–38. *Fibrous dysplasia: Lateral view of the lumbar spine. Vertebral involvement may take the form of deformed vertebral bodies or posterior elements having a ground-glass appearance (arrow 1) or clearer, purely radiolucent lesions having a "cystic" appearance. The latter most frequently contain a rubbery, fibrous tissue that does not weaken bone (arrow 3) as much as actual cystic, fluid-filled cavities, which have also been noted. The latter "cysts" have been presumed to be related to hemorrhage or ischemia and are more prone to compression and collapse (arrow 2).*

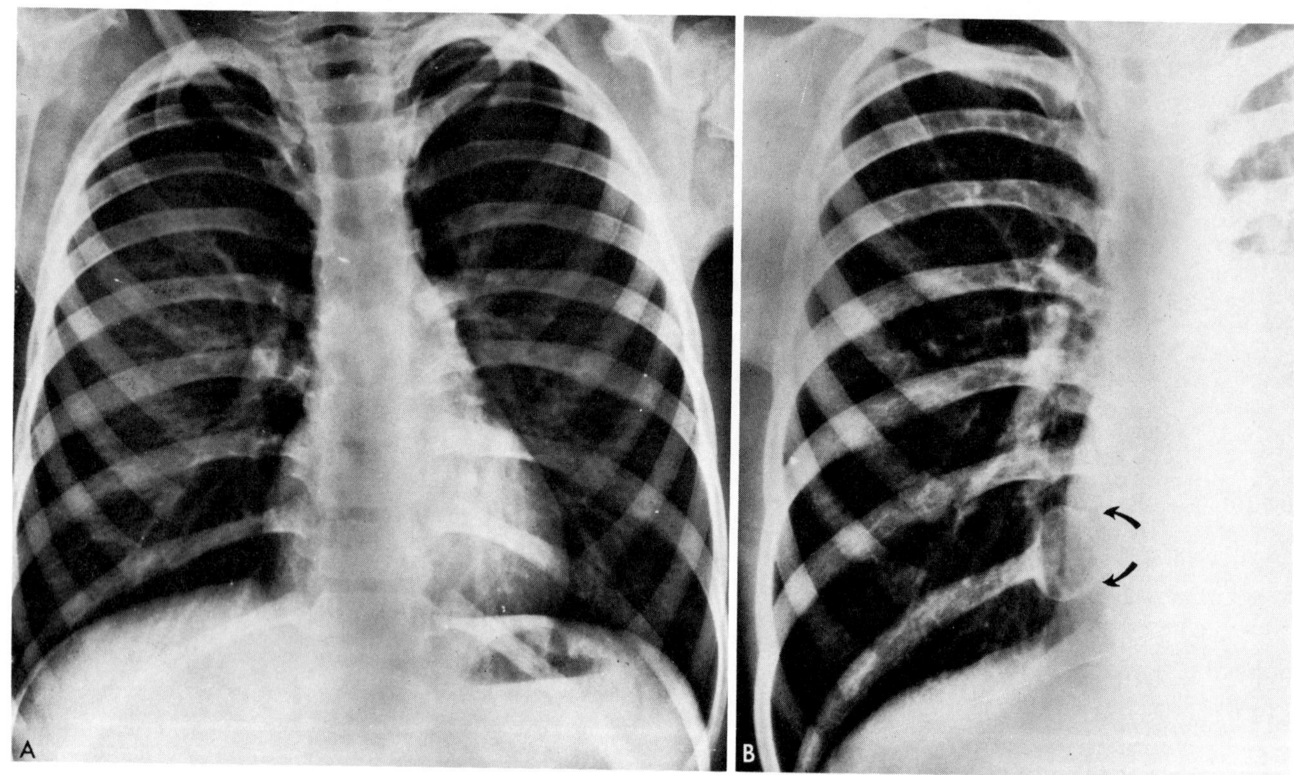

Figure 80–39. Fibrous dysplasia: *De novo appearance in the rib of an asymptomatic patient.*

A *Posteroanterior view of the chest — 1/24/55. Note normal rib cage at 8 years of age.*

B *Posteroanterior view of the chest — 12/15/59. Note the expansile lesion of the right tenth rib, discovered as an incidental finding at 13 years of age. The lesion is hazy in appearance and sharply outlined by an attenuated but intact cortex (arrows).*

(Courtesy of Dr. W. B. Seaman.)

Most patients show no evidence of spontaneous improvement or resolution of individual lesions. Conversely, the evolution of skeletal lesions may occur by extension of existing lesions or by the appearance of new lesions. One case of monostotic fibrous dysplasia was observed by the author to have arisen de novo (Fig. 80–39*A*,*B*). However, after initial roentgenographic documentation, most monostotic lesions remain quiescent throughout life. In a series of 46 cases of monostotic fibrous dysplasia reviewed at the Bristol Bone Tumor Registry, "no further lesion was demonstrated subsequent to the original investigation."[26] However, it is not clear whether skeletal surveys were initially obtained or for what period of time individual cases were followed. New lesions and progressive deformity more commonly occur in patients with severe involvement and early onset of symptoms. In general, when extensive fibrous dysplasia appears early in life, fractures are common, deformity is severe, progression is pronounced, and prognosis is poor. Lesions do not necessarily cease to be active after puberty, and some have been known to be reactivated by pregnancy. However, initial moderate or sparse involvement is usually associated with slow progression and connotes a favorable prognosis regardless of the age of onset.[34] The most common reason for symptoms in either the monostotic or the polyostotic form is that of spontaneous fracture. Small stress or fissure fractures may be particularly problematic, since they are frequently symptomatic but not readily detectable on routine radiographs.

Fibrous dysplasia appears histologically benign with no evidence of mitoses or cellular atypism. However, malignant transformation has been rarely reported. Its spontaneous occurrence has not been accurately evaluated chiefly because of the lack of adequate pathologic documentation of many of the reported cases and because radiotherapy was employed in the treatment of several of these cases. Radiation rather than prior surgical intervention has been incriminated as a factor in precipitating malignancy in previously presumably benign lesions. The incidence of malignant transformation has been estimated at less than 1 per cent on the basis of fewer than 50 reported cases. Less than half occurred in patients with polyostotic fibrous dysplasia. Malignant tumors most often described in association with fibrous dysplasia have included osteosarcoma, fibrosarcoma, chondrosarcoma, and giant cell tumor. The facial bones and femurs have constituted the most commonly affected sites. Therefore, a painful lesion may rarely herald the occurrence of malignant change rather than fracture or progressive enlargement.[64]

Although many of the features described are common to both forms of fibrous dysplasia, some are more typically associated with the solitary lesion than with multiple lesions. Generally most monostotic long bone lesions are "silent" until the occurrence of an obvious pathologic fracture or of an occult stress fracture. Severe deformities as in the polyostotic form are exceptional. Bowing is usually slight, and deformity is most commonly limited to local expansion of bone with focal cortical thinning or hypertrophy. The monostotic lesion is most commonly situated in the diametaphysis of the medullary cavity of a long bone, where it may be eccentrically or centrally placed and where it may be further characterized by having a translucent and trabeculated center.

The polyostotic lesion is more often of "ground glass" appearance and commonly causes a fusiform expansion over a larger segment of affected bone, which gradually tapers to merge with neighboring normal bone (Fig. 80–35). Commonly, the whole bone may be involved, and although the bone ends are usually spared, gross bending and bowing deformities invariably occur. Although polyostotic fibrous dysplasia favors one side[51, 52] extensive disease is usually associated with generalized bilateral involvement (Fig. 80–33). Biopsy of the polyostotic form is rarely necessary, but it may be called for in order to confirm the diagnosis in a monostotic lesion. Polyostotic fibrous dysplasia is much less frequent than the monostotic form, while a still rarer eventuality is the association of the polyostotic form with nonskeletal or endocrine manifestations.[23, 28]

The majority of cases involve one or a few bones. A surprising relationship between lesions in the ilium and in the femur, in particular, has been noted. In the Bristol series, the femur was involved in all patients who had had involvement of the ilium. However, the converse was not true — i.e., not all patients with femoral involvement had concomitant involvement of the ilium.[26] In our experience, although solitary involvement of the ilium is not as frequent as solitary involvement of the femur it does occur, with the lesion occasionally attaining dramatic proportions.

Endocrine Abnormalities

There is no sexual predominance in fibrous dysplasia, although in one series of monostotic lesions, men outnumbered women 27 to 19. However, female to male ratios as high as 3:1 have been reported. Usually, the greater the number of polyostotic cases included in a review, the more likely a female bias will be present. Not all patients with polyostotic fibrous dysplasia and cutaneous pigmentation exhibit precocious puberty or other endocrine changes. Likewise, the osseous lesions can occur together with precocious puberty and without associated cutaneous pigmentation. Precocious puberty, rare in boys, occurs in 30 to 50 per cent of girls and is characterized by the early appearance of vaginal bleeding and of axillary and pubic hair as well as of breast development. Gynecomastia has been reported[5, 6] in the male; however, its etiology is uncertain. The term sexual precocity is preferred by some over precocious puberty, since puberty implies mature gonadal function.[5, 6, 19, 41, 81, 82] In the past, few cases have warranted the designation of true precocious puberty specifically on the basis of circulating ovulatory leutinizing hormone (LH) levels or on the basis of testicular biopsies yielding mature spermatozoa. Rarely reported cases of gonadal examinations of sexually precocious girls yielded no evidence of ovulation,[12] and true precocious puberty has been argued not to exist in these cases.

The fact that many patients had normal gonadotropin and estrogen levels with obvious clinical changes suggested the possibility of increased sensitivity of target glands (i.e., gonads and breast tissue) to normal prepubertal or minimally elevated levels of circulating pituitary hormone. Particularly in the face of unmeasurable LH levels, vaginal bleeding has been presumed to reflect an early release or an ovarian oversensitivity to follicle stimulating hormone (FSH). Others[6, 7, 12] suggest that low gonadotropin levels reflect their suppression by estrogen and testosterone. However, elevated levels of estrogen and testosterone were not uniformly found. Cell membrane alteration with increased binding of trophic hormones to target cells and increased intracellular concentration of cyclic AMP are other explanations for end-organ sensitivity. Furthermore, tumors had not been well documented in any of these organs. In recent years, continuing technical advances in the measurement of gonadotropins, radioimmunoprotein binding and radioreceptor assays, and the isolation and synthesis of GNRH (hypothalamic gonadotropin releasing hormone) have provided more accurate tools for the study of the pubertal process. It is now possible to determine with greater accuracy if the sexual precocity is or is not central in origin. This is also feasible when the syndrome includes Cushing's syndrome or hyperthyroidism.[1]

The reports of Danon and co-workers[19, 20] are of special importance in view of the arrest of sexual precocity (presence of vaginal bleeding in one patient at the age of 6 months) after the removal of a functioning luteinized ovarian cyst. Three of the patients had elevated levels of estradiol and estrone at the same time that plasma concentrations of FSH and LH were at or below the lowest detectable level of the assay. The 6 month old patient also had Cushing's syndrome secondary to nodular hyperplasia of the adrenal glands with strong evidence that the adrenal glands were not under pituitary control, e.g., corticotropin levels were low, large doses of dexamethasone failed to decrease plasma levels of cortisol, and administration of metyrapone did not result in a large increase in the concentration of plasma deoxycortisol. These observations established the occurrence of both adrenal and gonadal autonomy in this one case. These authors also suggested that autonomy of the endocrine glands may not be rare in this syndrome and that their hyperfunction may not be mediated by hypothalamic pituitary mechanisms. Another documented case[21] was of further interest in this regard since the patient was found to have not only a solid tumor of the ovary in association with Albright's syndrome but rickets as well.

Pleuriglandular disturbances in addition to precocious sexual development have long been appreciated, particularly as reflected in accelerated linear growth and advanced skeletal age and maturation even in the absence of overt sexual precocity. Albright, too, in noting other associated endocrinopathies initially stressed increased end-organ sensitivity as a cause.

As recently as 1972 Hall and Warrick[30] presented cogent arguments supporting the thesis that all of the endocrine manifestations, i.e., precocious puberty, Cushing's syndrome, acromegaly, and hyperthyroidism — probably result from hypersecretion of hypothalamic releasing hormones.

Although thyroid abnormalities, predominantly hyperthyroidism with toxic multinodular goiter, occur in 5 to 30 per cent of patients, the prediction that the hyperthyroidism may be caused by hypersecretion of hypothalamic-releasing hormones has not been supported.[33] Levels of thyroid-stimulating hormone (TSH) in serum have been measured in at least three adults with Albright's syndrome and hyperthyroidism; one patient had the complete triad and the other two had only the osseous and skin lesions. In all instances the low levels of TSH failed to support the suggestions that excessive pituitary secretion of TSH is the cause of the hyperthyroidism in this syndrome. Other unusual features of the hyperthyroidism associated with Albright's syndrome include an absence of the characteristic lymphocyte infiltration of Graves' disease and the observations that the goiters tend to be multinodular, with an average age of onset of 23 years and an almost equal distribution between men and women. Under usual circumstances, the onset of toxic multinodular goiter occurs later in life, with an average age of onset between the fourth and fifth decades and with a female to male ratio of 3:1. In addition, the exophthalmos occurring in some patients with hyperthyroidism and Albright's syndrome is an additional finding simulating Graves' disease. However, frontal and orbital bone involvement by fibrous dysplasia may explain the cause of proptosis in many cases. The definitive cause of the hyperthyroidism, however, remains undetermined, although a previously undescribed form of thyroid autonomy is a current suggestion.

Likewise, few of the early reported cases of associated "acromegaly" have been acceptable as such by modern endocrinologic criteria.[72] Clinical diagnoses must similarly be regarded with caution since acromegaly may be mimicked by the facial and skeletal involvement of fibrous dysplasia. Optic foramina so involved may produce visual defects superficially suggestive of a pituitary tumor.

Pituitary lesions or lesions in higher centers, such as the hypothalamus, leading to overproduction of releasing hormone and multiple endocrine dysfunctions have been postulated.[30]

The hypothalamus controls anterior lobe pituitary function by producing releasing hormones. These independent releasing hormones which stimulate release of TSH, corticotropin, LH, FSH, and diuretic hormone (DH) and inhibit release of melanocyte stimulating hormone and prolactin, are well known. They reach the anterior lobe via the portal venous circulation. There they affect the synthesis and release of trophic hormones. Hall and Warrick[30] subsequently proposed that the endocrine manifestations are due to hypersecretion of hypothalamic releasing hormones. However, lesions of the hypothalamus have not been documented, although its anatomic and functional complexities are only now being elucidated with the application of modern histologic and histochemical methods. Recent suggestions include the possibility that Albright's syndrome may represent initial or subsequent function of multiple organs in an autonomous fashion. Until recently, pituitary nodularity and hyperplasia but no frank pituitary tumors have been noted. In recent years, however, in addition to hyperplasia of target organs, single or multiple adenomas have been found in the pituitary, adrenal, thyroid, and parathyroid glands.[53] This has led some investigators to speculate that the disease might be a variety of multiple endocrine adenomas.

Prior to Lichtenstein's paper (1938), the lesion with which monostotic and polyostotic fibrous dysplasia was most confused, particularly on the basis of bone biopsy, was hyperparathyroidism. With subsequent advances in biochemical techniques and an improved understanding of hyperparathyroidism, its distinction from fibrous dysplasia became more clearly established.

However, recently this distinction is once again becoming unsharp. Not only has the association of hyperparathyroidism and Albright's syndrome been documented, but in addition new combinations and permutations, including fibrous dysplasia, have been reported. Hypophosphatemic osteomalacia and rickets in association with both monostotic and polyostotic fibrous dysplasia have also been noted. Furthermore, not all cases of fibrous dysplasia and osteomalacia or rickets were associated with Albright's syndrome.[21, 53] Some of these cases suggest a syndrome analogous to "tumor rickets," in which the hypophosphatemic rickets or osteomalacia appears to be due to the presence of a mesenchymal lesion or tumor. The endocrinopathy has been shown to regress or to be alleviated when the associated tumor is removed. Fibrous dysplasia has been incriminated as such a "mesenchymal lesion" in some cases in which surgical excision resulted in an alleviation of symptoms, including bone pain, as well as partial or total return of serum chemistry values to normal. It has been postulated that the dysplastic bone in fibrous dysplasia, as well as the abnormal tissue in other lesions could either be elaborating a phosphaturic hormone or consuming some compound that is antiphosphaturic.

Furthermore, not only has the polyostotic form been associated with nonskeletal manifestations in general and with endocrinopathy in particular, but also very recently monostotic lesions have likewise been found to have such an association. Therefore, as far as the skeleton is concerned, fibrous dysplasia represents a continuum of involvement, the etiology of which continues to remain obscure. No consistent familial or hereditary factor has been established, and most recently the possibility has been raised that a number of diseases may have been grouped together largely on histologic grounds.

SUMMARY

In view of the many ramifications of all of these syndromes, the prompt and proper identification of tuberous sclerosis, neurofibromatosis, and fibrous dysplasia cannot be overemphasized. The advantages which accrue from early recognition include not only the anticipation, prevention, and treatment of some of their associated corollaries and complications but also the privilege of genetic planning where applicable.

Radiologists, in particular, are often in an advantageous position to either initially suggest or corroborate the diagnosis made by primary care physicians or by any one of a host of specialists who may be involved in the early care of these patients.

REFERENCES

1. Aarskog D, Tveteraas E: McCune-Albright's syndrome following adrenalectomy for Cushing's syndrome in infancy. J Pediatr *73*:89, 1968.
2. Albright F, Butler AM, Hampton AO, Smith P: Syndrome characterized by osteitis fibrosa disseminata, areas of pigmentation and endocrine dysfunction with precocious puberty in females. N Engl J Med *216*:727, 1937.
3. Ashby DW, Ramage D: Lesions of the vertebrae and innominate bones in tuberose sclerosis. Br J Radiol *30*:274, 1957.
4. Baltzell JW, Davis DO, Condon VR: Unusual manifestations of neurofibromatosis. Med Radiogr Photogr *50*:2, 1974.
5. Benedict PH: Endocrine features in Albright's syndrome (fibrous dysplasia of bone). Metabolism *11*:30, 1962.

6. Benedict PH: Sex precocity and polyostotic fibrous dysplasia. Report of a case in a boy with testicular biopsy. Am J Dis Child *111*:426, 1966.
7. Benedict PH, Szabo G, Fitzpatrick TB, Sinesi SJ: Melanotic macules in Albright's syndrome and in neurofibromatosis. JAMA *205*:618, 1968.
8. Bourneville DM: Contribution à l'étude de l'idiotie. Arch Neurol *1*:69, 1880.
9. Brown B: The radiologic features of bone changes in tuberous sclerosis with a case report. J Can Assoc Radiol *12*:1, 1961.
10. Bunde S: The significance of a white macule on the skin of a child. Dev Med Child Neurol *12*:805, 1970.
11. Burrows EH: Bone changes in orbital neurofibromatosis. Br J Radiol *36*:549, 1963.
12. Senior B, Robboy SH: Sexual precocity with polyostotic fibrous dysplasia. N Engl J Med *292*:199, 1975.
13. Charlot-Charles J, Jones GW: Renal angiomyolipoma associated with tuberous sclerosis. Review of the literature. Urology *3*:465, 1974.
14. Critchley M, Earl CJC: Tuberose sclerosis and allied conditions. Brain *55*:311, 1932.
15. Crosett AD Jr: Roentgenographic findings in the renal lesion of tuberous sclerosis. Am J Roentgenol *98*:739, 1966.
16. Crowe FW, Schull WJ, Neel JV: A Clinical, Pathological and Genetic Study of Multiple Neurofibromatosis. Springfield, Ill, Charles C Thomas, 1956.
17. D'Agostino AN, Soule EH, Miller RH: Sarcomas of the peripheral nerves and somatic soft tissues associated with multiple neurofibromatosis (von Recklinghausen's disease). Cancer *16*:1015, 1963.
18. Daly D, Kaye M, Estrada RL: Neurofibromatosis and hyperparathyroidism — a new syndrome? Can Med Assoc J *103*:258, 1970.
19. Danon M, Crawford JD: Peripheral endocrinopathy causing sexual precocity in Albright's syndrome. Pediatr Res *8*:368, 1974.
20. Danon M, Robboy SJ, Kim S, Scully R, Crawford JD: Cushing syndrome, sexual precocity and polyostotic fibrous dysplasia (Albright syndrome) in infancy. J Pediatr *87*:917, 1975.
21. Dent CE, Gertner JM: Hypophosphatemic osteomalacia in fibrous dysplasia. Q J Med *45*:411, 1976.
22. Dwyer JM, Hickie JB, Gravan J: Pulmonary tuberous sclerosis: report of three patients and a review of the literature. Q J Med *40*:115, 1971.
23. Firat D, Stutzman L: Fibrous dysplasia of the bone. Review of 24 cases. Am J Med *44*:421, 1968.
24. Fitz CR, Harwood-Nash DCF, Thompson JR: Neuroradiology of tuberous sclerosis in children. Radiology *110*:635, 1974.
25. Fitzpatrick TB, Szabó G, Hori Y, Simone A, Reed W, Greenberg M: White leaf-shaped macules: earliest visible signs of tuberous sclerosis. Arch Dermatol *98*:1, 1968.
26. Gibson MJ, Middlemiss JH: Fibrous dysplasia of bone. Br J Radiol *44*:1, 1971.
27. Gold AP, Freeman JM: Depigmented nevi: The earliest sign of tuberous sclerosis. Pediatrics *35*:1003, 1965.
28. Grabias SL, Campbell CJ: Fibrous dysplasia. Orthop Clin North Am *8*:771, 1977.
29. Green GJ: The radiology of tuberose sclerosis. Clin Radiol *19*:135, 1968.
30. Hall R, Warrick CK: Hypersecretion of hypothalamic releasing hormones. A possible explanation of the endocrine manifestations of polyostotic fibrous dysplasia (Albright's syndrome). Lancet *1*:1313, 1972.
31. Halpern M, Currarino G: Vascular lesions causing hypertension in neurofibromatosis. N Engl J Med *273*:248, 1965.
32. Hamburger RJ, Clark JE, Moran JJ, Cohn HE, Wilkerson JL: Symptomatic benign renal mesenchymoma. A case necessitating bilateral nephrectomy. Arch Intern Med *120*:78, 1967.
33. Hamilton CRJ, Maloof F: Unusual types of hyperthyroidism. Medicine *52*:195, 1973.
34. Harris WH, Dudy HR Jr, Barry RJ: The natural history of fibrous dysplasia. J Bone Joint Surg *44A*:207, 1962.
35. Hilal SK, Solomon GE, Gold AP, Carter S: Primary cerebral arterial occlusive disease in children. II. Neurocutaneous syndromes. Radiology *99*:87, 1971.
36. Holt JF, Dickerson WW: The osseous lesions of tuberous sclerosis. Radiology *58*:1, 1952.
37. Holt JF, Kuhns LR: Macrocranium and macrencephaly in neurofibromatosis. Skel Radiol *1*:25, 1976.
38. Hunt JC, Pugh DG: Skeletal lesions in neurofibromatosis. Radiology *76*:1, 1961.
39. Hurwitz S: Sipple syndrome. Arch Dermatol *110*:139, 1974.
40. Hurwitz S, Braverman IM: White spots in tuberous sclerosis. J Pediatr *77*:587, 1970.
41. Husband P, Graeme JAI, Snodgrass AI: McCune-Albright syndrome with endocrinological investigations. Report of a case. Am J Dis Child *119*:164, 1970.
42. Itzchak Y, Katznelson D, Boichis H, Jonas A, Deutsch V: Angiographic features of arterial lesions in neurofibromatosis. Am J Roentgenol *122*:643, 1974.
43. Kidder LA: Congenital glycogenic tumors of the heart. Arch Pathol *49*:55, 1950.
44. Klatte EC, Franken EA, Smith JA: The radiographic spectrum in neurofibromatosis. Semin Roentgenol *11*:17, 1976.
45. Komar NN, Gabrielsen TO, Holt JF: Roentgenographic appearance of lumbosacral spine and pelvis in tuberous sclerosis. Radiology *89*:701, 1967.
46. Kullmann L, Wouters HW: Neurofibromatosis, gigantism, and subperiosteal haematoma. Report of two children with extensive subperiosteal bone formation. J Bone Joint Surg *54B*:130, 1972.
47. Lagos JC, Holman CB, Gomez MR: Tuberous sclerosis: Neuroroentgenologic observations. Am J Roentgenol *104*:171, 1968.
48. Leeds NE, Jacobson HG: Spinal neurofibromatosis. Am J Roentgenol *126*:617, 1976.
49. Leeds N, Seaman WB: Fibrous dysplasia of the skull and its differential diagnosis. A clinical and roentgenographic study of 46 cases. Radiology *78*:570, 1962.
50. Levin B: Neurofibromatosis: clinical and roentgen manifestations. Radiology *71*:48, 1958.
51. Lichtenstein L: Polyostotic fibrous dysplasia. Arch Surg *36*:874, 1938.
52. Lichtenstein L, Jaffe HL: Fibrous dysplasia of bone: A condition affecting one, several or many bones, the graver cases of which may present abnormal pigmentation of skin, premature sexual development, hyperthyroidism or still other extraskeletal abnormalities. Arch Pathol *33*:777, 1942.
53. McArthur RG, Hayles AB, Lambert PW: Albright's syndrome with rickets. Mayo Clin Proc *54*:313, 1979.
54. McCune DJ: Osteitis fibrosa cystica; the case of a 9-year-old girl who also exhibits precocious puberty, multiple pigmentation of the skin and hyperthyroidism. Transaction of the Society for Pediatric Research, Annual Meeting, May 5, 1936. Am J Dis Child *52*:743, 1936.
55. Malik SK, Pardee N, Martin CJ: Involvement of the lungs in tuberous sclerosis. Chest *58*:538, 1970.
56. Medley BE, McLeod RA, Houser OW: Tuberous sclerosis. Semin Roentgenol *11*:35, 1976.
57. Meszaros WT, Guzzo F, Schorsch H: Neurofibromatosis. Am J Roentgenol *98*:557, 1966.
58. Nathanson N, Avnet NL: An unusual x-ray finding in tuberous sclerosis. Br J Radiol *39*:786, 1966.
59. Nieman HL, Mena E, Holt JF, Stern Am, Perry BL: Neurofibromatosis and congenital heart disease. Am J Roentgenol *122*:146, 1974.
60. O'Callaghan TJ, Edwards JA, Tobin M, Mookerjee BK: Tuberous sclerosis with striking renal involvement in a family. Arch Intern Med *135*:1082, 1975.
61. Payne JF: Multiple neurofibromata in connection with molluscum fibrosum. Trans Pathol Soc Lond *38*:69, 1887.
62. Pitt MJ, Mosher JF, Edeiken J: Abnormal periosteum and bone in neurofibromatosis. Radiology *103*:143, 1972.
63. Potter EL: Pathology of the Fetus and the Infant. 2nd Ed. Chicago, Year Book Medical Publishers, 1961, p 441.
64. Riddell DH: Malignant change in fibrous dysplasia. J Bone Joint Surg *46B*:251, 1964.
65. Rowen M, Dorsey TJ, Kegel SM, Ostermiller WE Jr: Thoracic coarctation associated with neurofibromatosis. Am J Dis Child *129*:113, 1975.
66. von Recklinghausen K: Über die multiplen Fibrome der Haut und ihre Beziehung zu den multiplen Neuromen. Berlin, A. Hirschwald, 1882.
67. Sands MJ, McDonough MT, Cohen AM, Rutenberg HL, Eisner JW: Fatal malignant degeneration in multiple neurofibromatosis. JAMA *233*:1381, 1975.
68. Sareen CK, Ruvalcaba RHA, Scotvold MJ, Mahoney CP, Kelley VC: Tuberous sclerosis. Am J Dis Child *123*:34, 1972.
69. Saxena KM: Endocrine manifestations of neurofibromatosis in children. Am J Dis Child *120*:265, 1970.
70. Schenkein I, Bueker ED, Helson L, Axelrod F, Dancis J: Increased nerve-growth-stimulating activity in disseminated neurofibromatosis. N Engl J Med *290*:613, 1974.
71. Scott JC: Scoliosis and neurofibromatosis. J Bone Joint Surg *47B*:240, 1965.
72. Scurry MT, Bicknell JM, Fajans SS: Polyostotic fibrous dysplasia and acromegaly. Arch Intern Med *114*:40, 1964.
73. Seaman WB, Furlow LT: Anomalies of the bony orbit. Am J Roentgenol *71*:51, 1954.
74. Smith RW: A Treatise on the Pathology, Diagnosis and Treatment of Neuroma. Dublin, Hodges & Smith, 1849.
75. Thannhauser SJ: Neurofibromatosis (von Recklinghausen) and osteitis fibrosa cystica localisata et disseminata (von Recklinghausen). Medicine *23*:105, 1944.
76. Thibault JH, Manuelidis EE: Tuberous sclerosis in a premature infant. Report of a case and review of the literature. Neurology *20*:139, 1970.
77. Tiresius TWC: Historia Pathologica Singularis Cutis Turpitudinis. Leipzig, SL Crusius, 1793.
78. Treves F: Congenital deformity. Br Med J *2*:1140, 1884.

79. Viamonte M Jr, Ravel R, Politano V, Bridges B: Angiographic findings in a patient with tuberous sclerosis. Am J Roentgenol *98*:723, 1966.
80. Virchow R: Die krankhaften Geschwülste. Berlin, A Hirschwald, 1863, Vol 3, p 233.
81. Warrick CK: Polyostotic fibrous dysplasia — Albright's syndrome. A review of the literature and report of four male cases, two of which were associated with precocious puberty. J Bone Joint Surg *31B*:175, 1949.
82. Warrick CK: Some aspects of polyostotic fibrous dysplasia: possible hypothesis to account for the associated endocrinological changes. Clin Radiol *24*:125, 1973.
83. Webb WR, Goodman PC: Fibrosing alveolitis in patient with neurofibromatosis. Radiology *122*:289, 1977.
84. Weichert KA, Dine MS, Benton C, Silverman, FN: Macrocranium and neurofibromatosis. Radiology *107*:163, 1973.
85. Wenzl JE, Lagos JC, Albers DD: Tuberous sclerosis presenting as polycystic kidneys and seizures in an infant. J Pediatr *77*:673, 1970.
86. Whitaker PH: Radiological manifestations in tuberose sclerosis. Br J Radiol *32*:152, 1959.
87. Yaghmai I, Tafazoli M: Massive subperiosteal hemorrhage in neurofibromatosis. Radiology *122*:439, 1977.
88. Zatz LM: Atypical choroid plexus calcifications associated with neurofibromatosis. Radiology *91*:1135, 1968.

ENOSTOSIS, HYPEROSTOSIS, AND PERIOSTITIS

by Donald Resnick, M.D., and Gen Niwayama, M.D.

81

Single or multiple areas of increased radiodensity are commonly detected on skeletal roentgenograms. These may appear as discrete foci within the spongiosa (enostosis) or on the surface of the cortex (osteoma), or as more diffuse and widespread areas of cortical hyperostosis or periostitis. In some cases, the detection of such osseous alterations indicates the presence of a distant (and significant) extraskeletal lesion or an underlying systemic disorder.

ENOSTOSIS (BONE ISLAND)

Since the initial report of bone islands by Stieda in 1905[1] in which the name "kompakten Knochenkerne" was utilized, numerous terms have been applied to these lesions, including bone nucleus, compact island,[2] focal sclerosis,[3] calcified island in bone,[4] sclerotic bone island,[5] and enostosis.[6] The considerable attention devoted to a description of enostoses is not surprising in view of their common appearance on skeletal roentgenograms.[7,8] Although the true incidence of these lesions is not known, Onitsuka,[9] in a review of roentgenograms of 189 subjects, noted that the prevalence of rib and pelvic bone islands was 0.43 and 1.08 per cent, respectively. There appears to be no significant sex preference in the incidence of these lesions, and they are encountered in all age groups, with perhaps a decreasing frequency in pediatric patients.[7] Any osseous site can be affected, but the lesions have a predilection for the pelvis, proximal femur, and ribs.[7-9] Involvement of the skull is distinctly unusual. In the tubular bones, an epiphyseal location is common.

Enostoses or bone islands appear radiographically as single or multiple intraosseous sclerotic areas with discrete margins in asymptomatic individuals. They may be ovoid, round, or oblong in shape, and are usually aligned with the long axis of the trabecular architecture. Thorny, radiating bony spicules extend from the center of the lesion, intermingling with the surrounding trabeculae of the

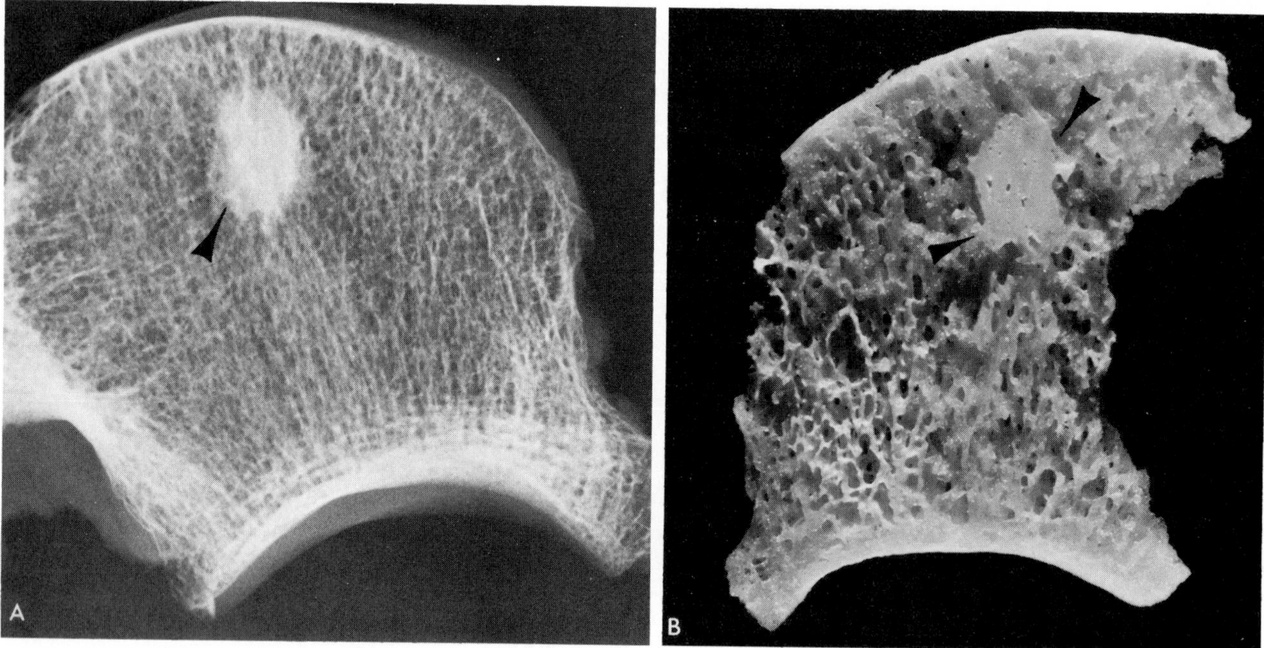

Figure 81–1. Enostosis: Talus. Observe the single osteosclerotic focus in the superior portion of the talus, possessing thorny radiating spicules that extend from the lesion into the surrounding spongiosa trabeculae (arrowheads).

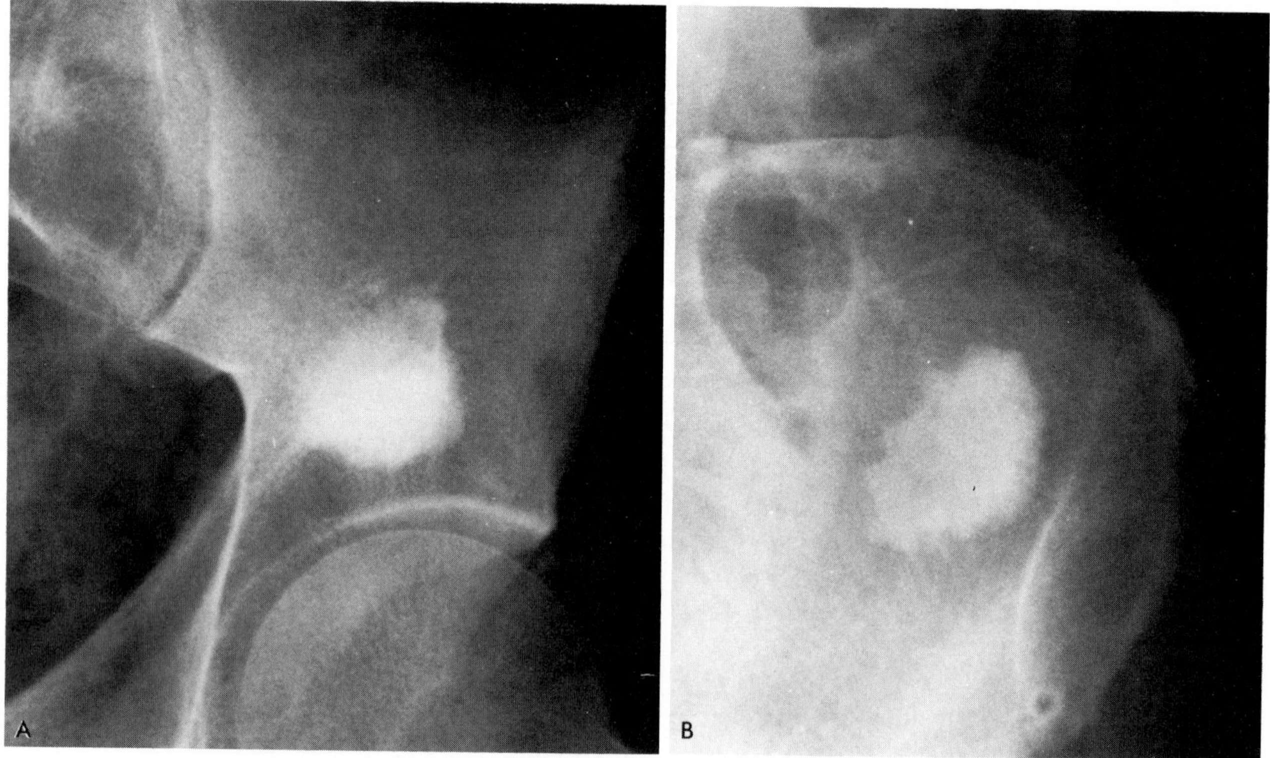

Figure 81–2. Enostosis: Pelvis.

A, B Two examples of large enostoses of the pelvis. In this location, such lesions are commonly of this size. Note the homogeneous nature of the dense area and the radiating spicules extending into the adjacent bone.

Illustration continued on the opposite page

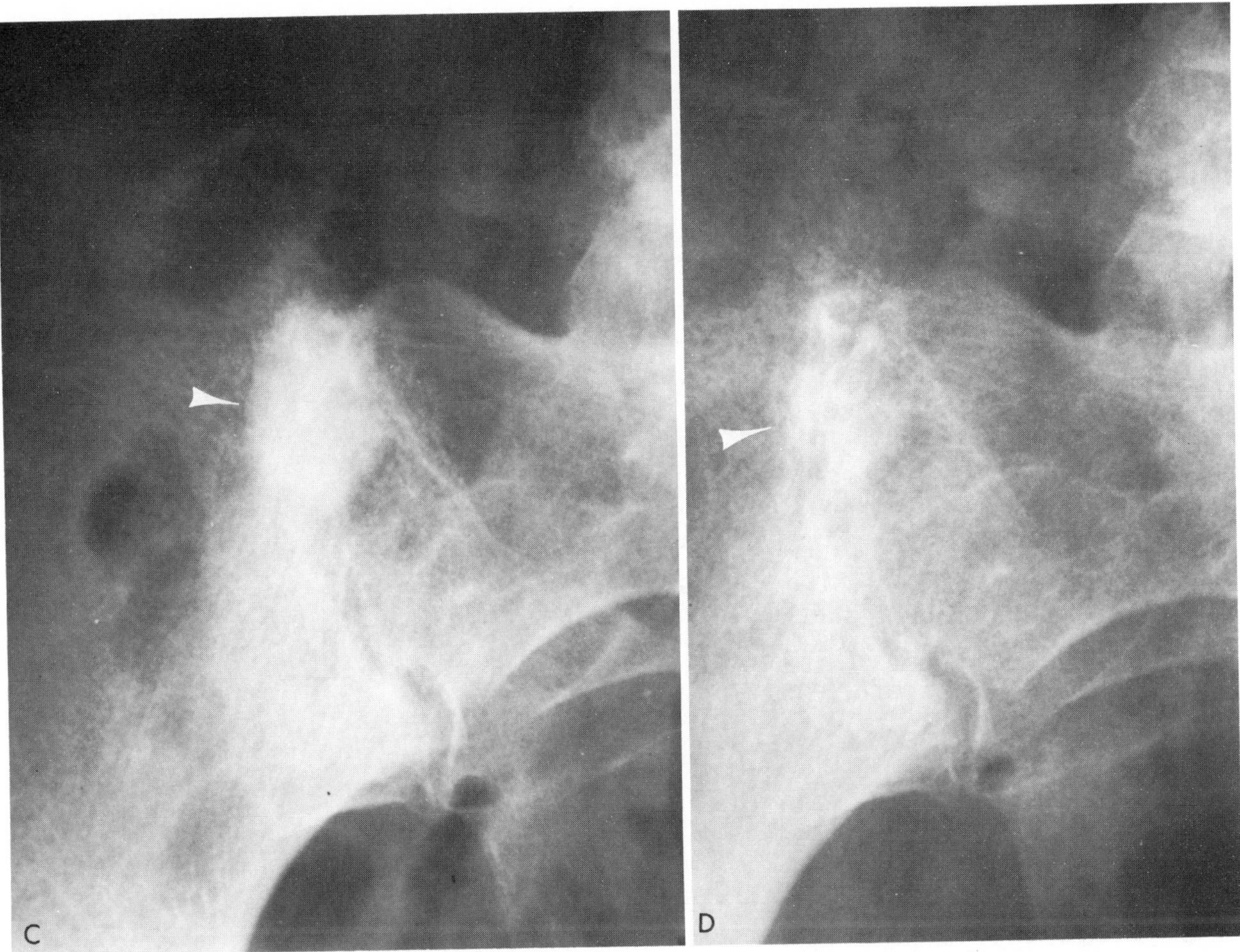

Figure 81–2. Continued
C, D *Radiographs of the pelvis obtained several years apart reveal an enostosis of the ilium that has decreased in size (arrowhead).*

spongiosa (Fig. 81–1). The lesions do not protrude from the cortical surface of the involved bone. Their size is variable; some are less than 1 × 1 mm, whereas others, especially in the pelvis, may reach proportions greater than 40 × 40 mm[10] (Fig. 81–2).

Initially, it was generally considered that bone islands were stable lesions representing no more than a radiographic curiosity, but recent evidence suggests that the sclerotic areas may be more dynamic in nature.[7, 8, 11] They may increase or decrease in size or disappear completely. During periods of observation in adolescents, enostoses may appear for the first time and enlarge in proportion to bone growth.[9] Even in adult patients, such enlargement can be encountered, simulating the appearance of an osteoblastic skeletal metastasis. Ngan[12] has suggested that enostoses can be differentiated from metastatic foci by the absence of clinical findings. Furthermore, bone imaging in cases of bone islands is usually normal, although a patient has been described with a large bone island of the ilium and a positive bone scan.[13] Other reports have also indicated positive bone scans in areas of enostoses.[288, 290, 291] Such radionuclide uptake may indicate an increased regional blood flow associated with new bone formation during the appearance and growth of the lesion.

Nonetheless, the detection of one or more areas of increased bone density in an elderly patient, especially in one suspected of having a prostatic carcinoma, can lead to difficulty in differential diagnosis. This is especially true when bone islands appear in the axial skeleton. In the spine, enostoses may be apparent in approximately 1 per cent of individuals.[14] At this location, they have been termed endosteomas, and they create circular or triangular areas of increased density in the vertebral body that may reach 20 × 30 mm in size[6, 15, 16]; occasionally, they are seen in the posterior elements (Fig. 81–3). The lesions are usually homogeneous in density, with a well defined margin and occasional radiating spicules. They may border on the intervertebral discs or anterior or posterior surface of the vertebral body without expanding the vertebral contour. Radionuclide bone imaging of such lesions of the spine is usually normal,[6] serving to distinguish them from skeletal metastasis, infection, cartilaginous node formation, or intervertebral osteochondrosis. The absence of intervertebral disc space narrowing, irregularity of the vertebral surface, and radiolucent foci are radiographic characteristics of spinal bone islands that aid in their differentiation from more significant processes.

Histologically, enostoses are composed of normal-appearing compact bone (Fig. 81–4). The haversian structure may be more remodeled than that of normal bone, but coarse fibrillar bone, cartilage remnants, and fibrous tissue are not usually apparent.[7, 11, 17] The peripheral lamellar bone is connected to the thickened, spongy trabeculae, and their regular arrangement may be associated with slow bone formation not compensated for by bone resorption. The central core of the lesion can be irregular, suggesting the existence of a previous, more active site of bone remodeling.[17] These latter histologic

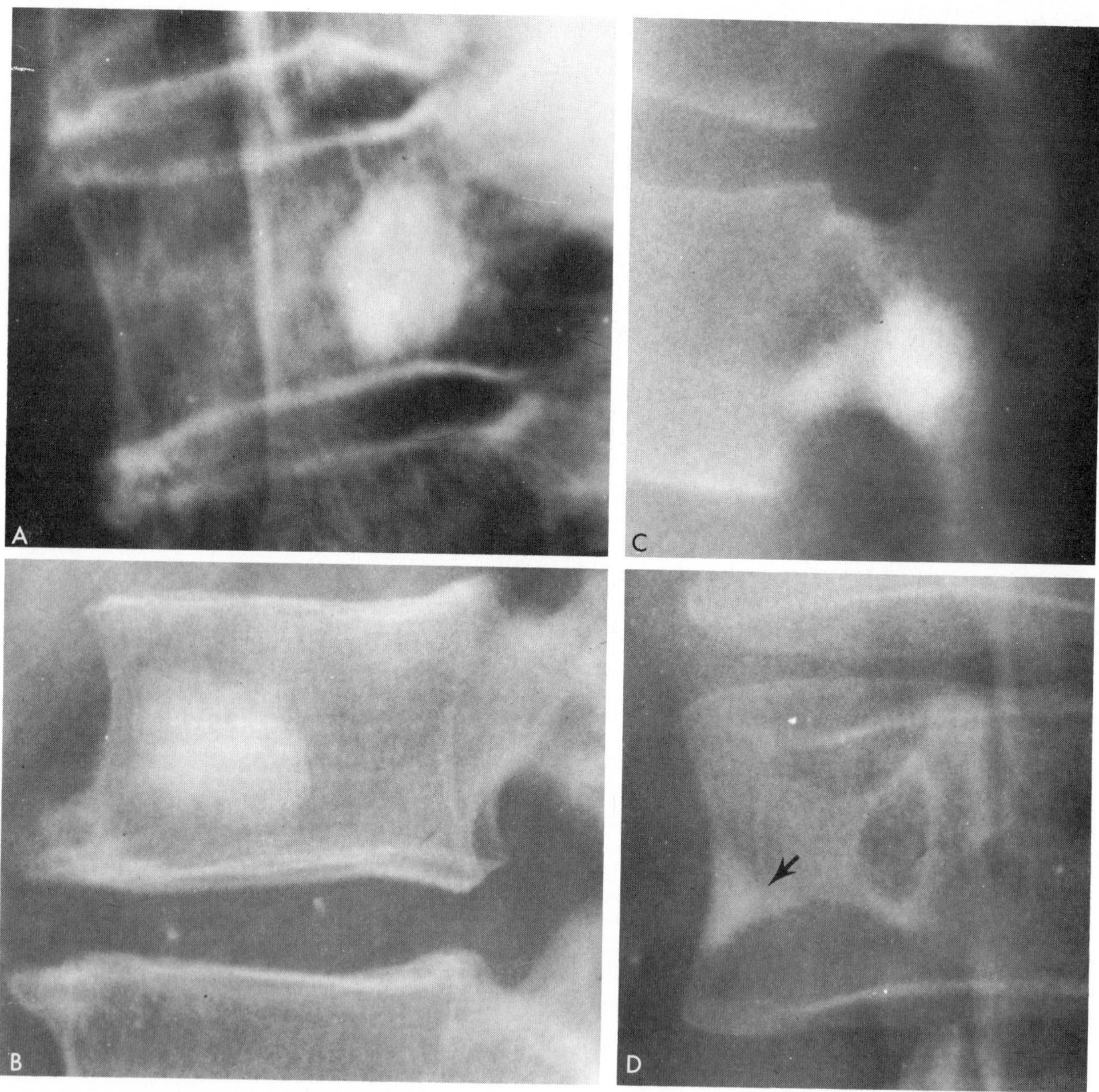

Figure 81–3. *Enostosis: Spine.*

A, B *Two examples of enostoses of the vertebral body are presented. They are relatively homogeneous and well defined, circular, and of differing size.*

C *This lesion extends from the pedicle and lamina into the posterior surface of the vertebral body. There is no expansion of osseous contour.*

D *A right posterior oblique projection outlines the border-forming triangular enostosis (arrow).*

*(***A, B, D,** *From Broderick TW, et al: Spine 3:167, 1978.)*

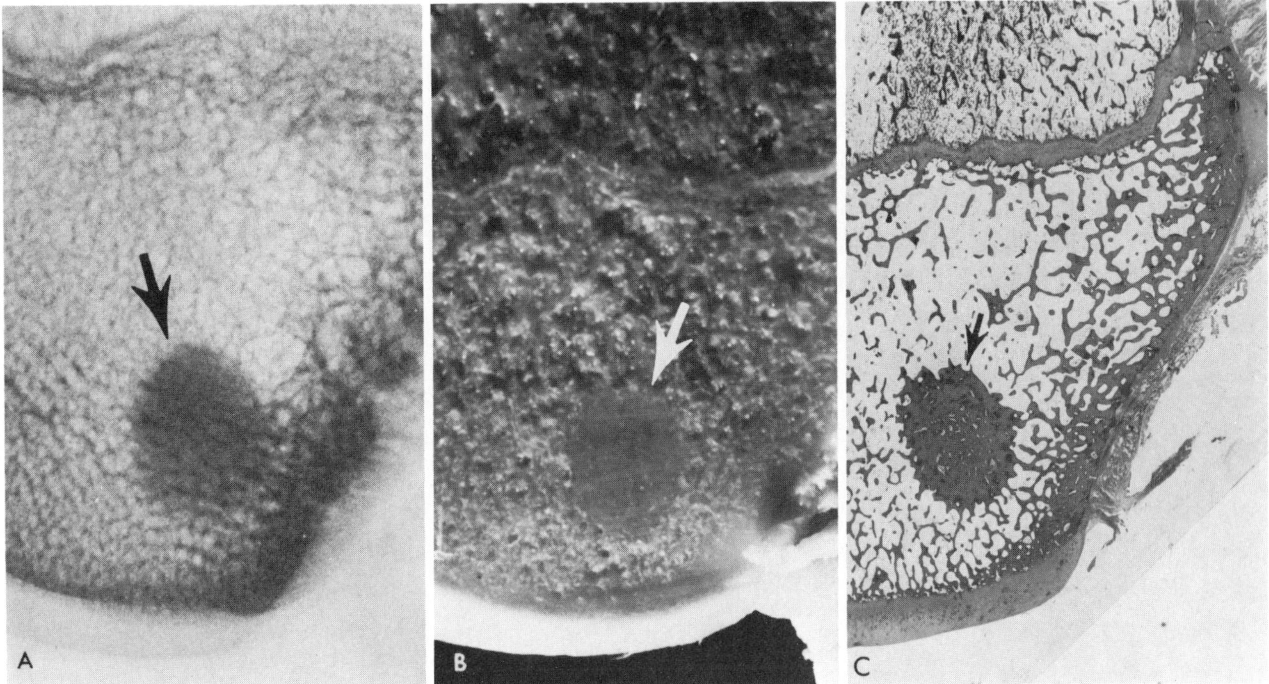

Figure 81–4. Enostosis: Histologic abnormalities. Note the bone island within the epiphysis (arrow). It is connected to surrounding trabeculae by thorny excrescences. (From Lagier R, Nussle D: Fortschr Röntgenstr 128:261, 1978. Courtesy of Georg Thieme Verlag, Stuttgart, Germany.)

observations suggest that active, albeit slight, remodeling capabilities exist in these lesions, explaining their occasional growth or disappearance, and their "participation" in any coexistent systemic disorder, such as hyperparathyroidism.[18]

The exact nature of enostoses is not clear. Their pathologic characteristics can be readily differentiated from those associated with bone infarction, infection, or neoplasms, such as osteoid osteoma or osteosarcoma. A traumatic etiology appears unlikely. The lesions are probably developmental in nature, although a minimal ossification disorder may also be instrumental in their appearance.[9] Thus, a disturbance of the normal sequence of bone formation and resorption could lead to a localized excess of bone formation and the development of a bone island.[8]

In addition to skeletal metastases, the differential diagnosis of enostoses includes osteomas, osteoid osteomas, enchondromas, bone infarcts, fibrous dysplasia, and osteopoikilosis (Table 81–1). Osteomas protrude from the surface of the bone, a feature not present with enostoses. Osteoid osteomas, when located in the cortex, consist of lucent

Table 81–1
LOCALIZED RADIODENSE LESIONS

Lesion	Location	Appearance
Enostosis (bone island)	Medullary	Round or oblong, thorny radiating spicules
Osteoma	Cortical protrusion	Homogeneous, smooth or lobular, extend from osseous surface
Osteochondroma	Cortical and medullary protrusion	Cortical and spongiosa are continuous with parent bone, calcified cap
Enchondroma	Medullary	Lucent, well-circumscribed, central calcifications
Bone infarct	Medullary	Lucent, well or poorly circumscribed, peripheral shell of calcification
Osteoid osteoma	Cortical, medullary, or subperiosteal	Cortical: Lucent with or without calcification surrounded by sclerotic bone Medullary: Lucent or calcified, with little sclerosis Subperiosteal: Scalloped excavation with or without calcification and sclerosis

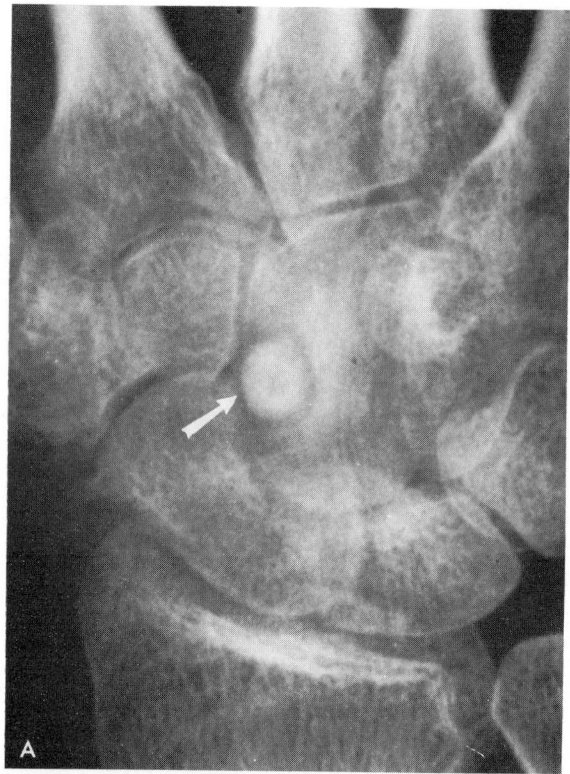

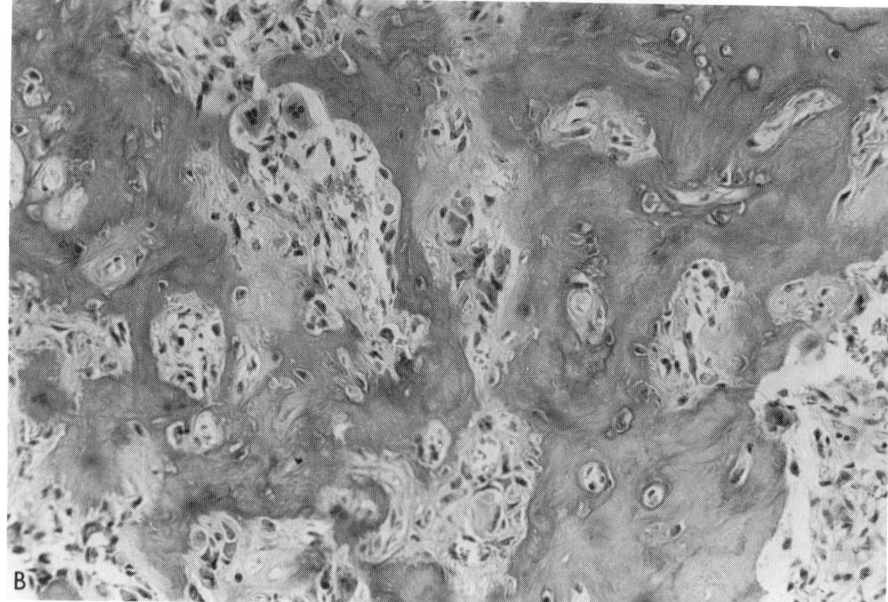

Figure 81–5. *Osteoid osteoma.*

A *Observe the lesion of the capitate (arrow) with a partially calcified nidus and surrounding sclerosis. Soft tissue swelling and osteoporosis are evident.*

B *The center of the nidus of an osteoid osteoma contains irregular abnormal bone, cement lines, and vascular stroma (50×).*

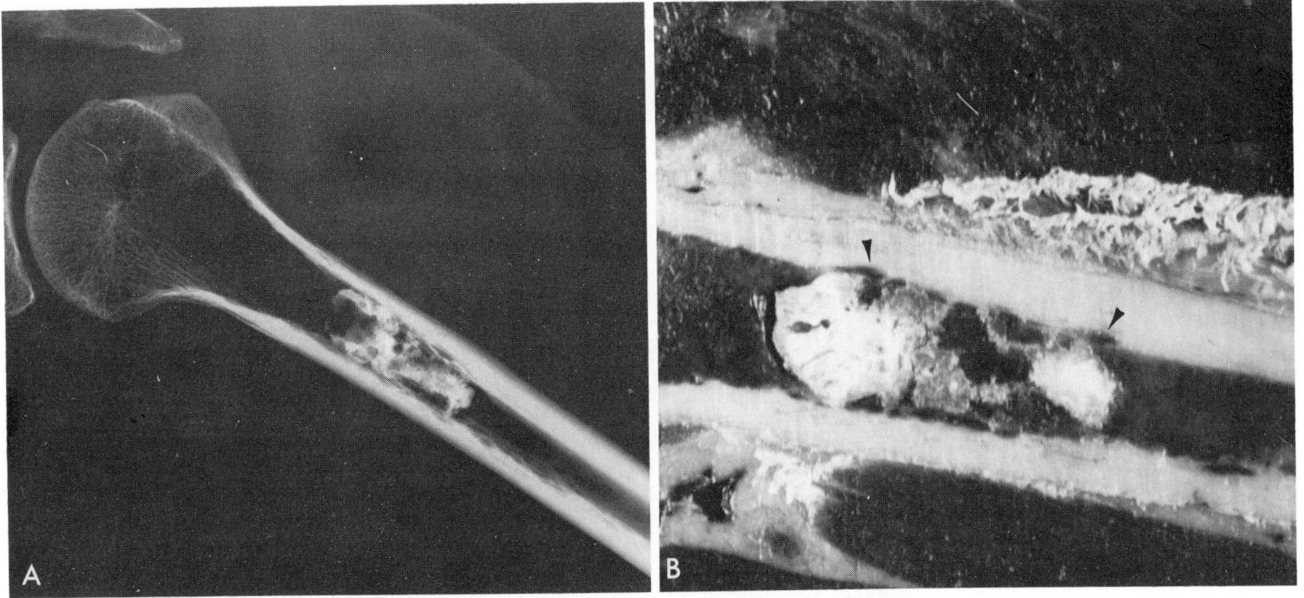

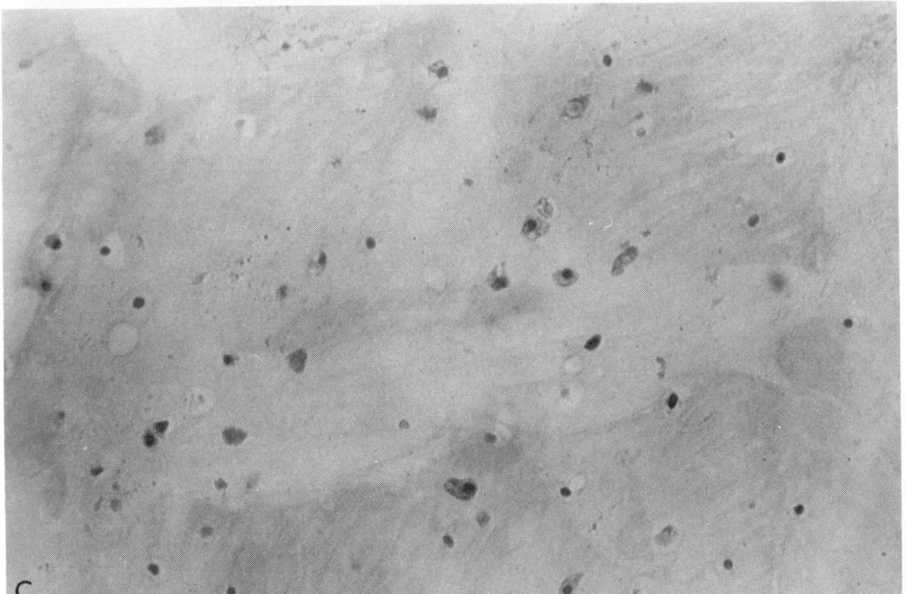

Figure 81–6. Enchondroma.

A, B *A radiograph and photograph of a coronal section of the humerus reveal a calcified medullary lesion of the diaphysis of the bone. Note the "popcorn" appearance of the calcified deposits and the scalloping (arrowheads) of the endosteal margin of the cortex.*

C *The cartilage cells reveal only slight variation of the nuclei (430×).*

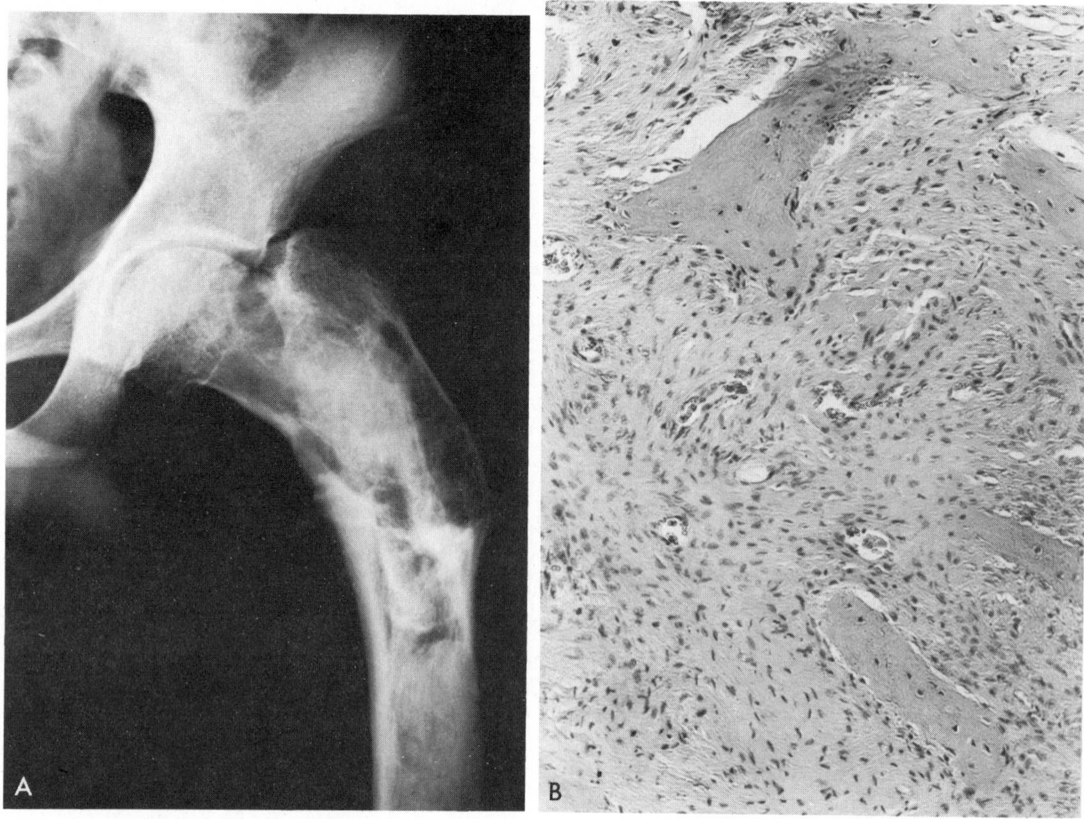

Figure 81–7. *Fibrous dysplasia.*

A *The classic radiographic picture of fibrous dysplasia consists of an elongated lesion of the metaphysis and diaphysis of the proximal femur and a matrix that is alternately radiodense and of ground-glass appearance. Observe the varus "shepherd's crook" deformity.*

B *Note irregular bone formation resulting in osseous tissue that is poorly oriented and not lined with osteoblasts. The fibrous stroma is cellular and vascular (50×).*

nidi, with or without calcification, and surrounding sclerosis. In a medullary location, a calcified nidus of an osteoid osteoma can create problems in differential diagnosis (Fig. 81–5). Enchondromas are characterized by lucent areas of variable size containing typical central calcification (Fig. 81–6), whereas bone infarcts are associated with sclerotic margins. In fibrous dysplasia, single or multiple lesions of variable density can be observed that have a predilection for the proximal femur (Fig. 81–7). Osteopoikilosis leads to formation of multiple radiodense foci, each one of which resembles an enostosis radiographically and histologically.

OSTEOMA

An osteoma is a protruding mass composed of abnormally dense but otherwise normal bone that is formed in the periosteum.[19] Thus, the lesion represents no more than a localized exaggeration of intramembranous bone formation, and it is confined to areas of the bone that are normally produced by the periosteal membrane. Osteomas predominate in the skull and facial bones, although they may occasionally arise at other sites, including the tubular bones of the extremities. In the latter locations, osteochondromas containing cartilaginous caps are much more frequent and represent a different lesion.

Osteomas are very frequent in the sinuses, especially the frontal sinus, but they also are found in the ethmoid sinus and, rarely, in the sphenoid or maxillary sinuses.[20, 21] Their incidence has been estimated to be 0.42 per cent in patients who have had sinus radiographs. Osteomas also arise from the inner and outer tables of the cranial vault, the mandible, and the maxilla. They have been detected in individuals of all ages, although the lesions predominate in patients in the fourth and fifth decades of life. Men are more commonly affected. Osteomas are asymptomatic unless they protrude significantly into the sinus cavity (interfering with normal drainage), encroach on the orbital contents, extend into the cranial cavity, or prohibit normal dental formation or tongue movement.

Osteomas are hard, nodular, or granular masses

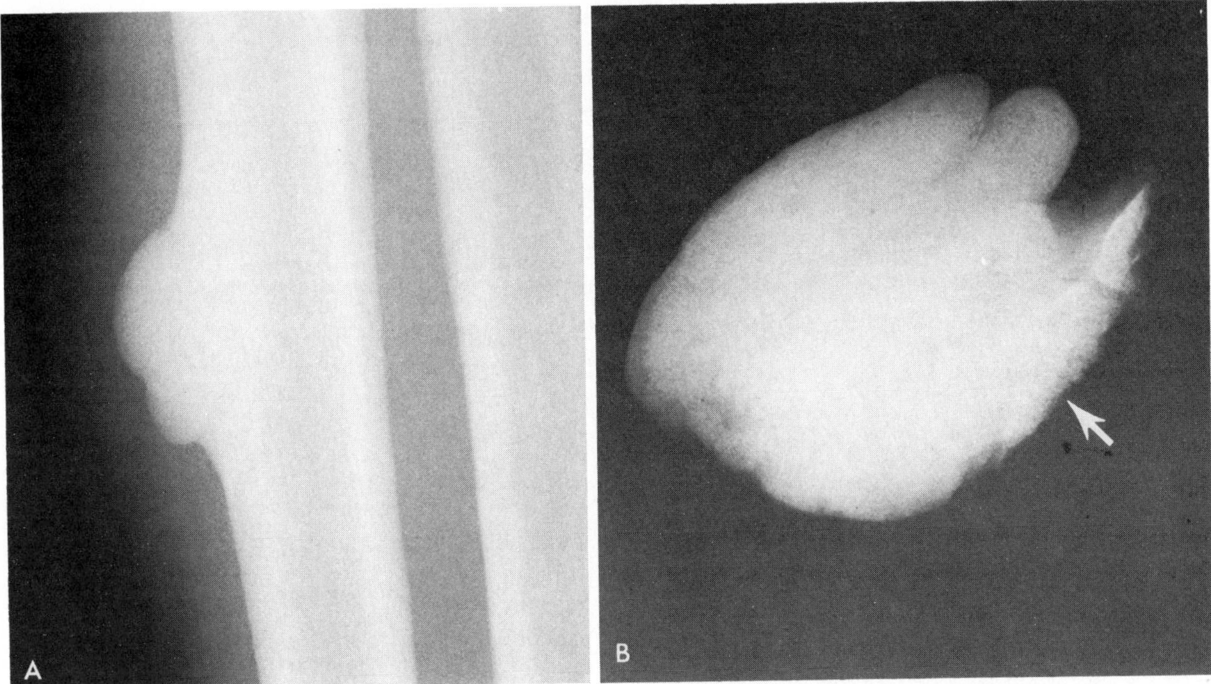

Figure 81–8. *Osteoma.*

A *A protruding, homogeneously dense mass of the ulna is evident. It is of the same radiodensity and appearance as the underlying cortex. Note that there is no connection between the medullary bone of the ulna and the lesion.*

B *A radiograph of a removed osteoma delineates its homogeneous nature, extending from the parent bone (arrow).*

Illustration continued on the following page

of bone that, on histologic examination, are found to consist of wide, irregularly arranged trabeculae of mature bone.[19] Prominent osteoid seams and osteoblasts may be evident. The intertrabecular tissue is sparse and may be highly vascular, with fibrous, fatty, and hematopoietic elements. The outer surface of the lesions is covered by a periosteal membrane, and a cartilaginous cap is not present.

On roentgenograms, the lesions appear as single or multiple radiodense foci that protrude into a sinus or extend from the surface of a parent bone (Fig. 81–8). Their outline is smooth or lobular, and they are frequently homogeneous in appearance. Once discovered, osteomas usually remain unchanged on serial studies. These radiographic characteristics differ from those of an enostosis, which is contained within a bone, and an osteochondroma, which is continuous with the spongiosa and cortex of the underlying bone and may contain calcific foci.

Table 81–2

MAJOR RADIOGRAPHIC ABNORMALITIES IN GARDNER'S SYNDROME

Colonic polyposis
Osteomas
Soft tissue tumors
Dental lesions

There are several opinions regarding the pathogenesis of osteomas. Jaffe[22] suggests that they are the sclerotized end-stage of fibrous dysplasia, whereas Aegerter and Kirkpatrick[23] consider osteomas to be hamartomas of bone.

Multiple osteomas of the mandible, calvarium, or tubular bones can accompany Gardner's syndrome[24-28] (Table 81–2). This is a familial disease consisting of colonic polyposis, osteomatosis, and soft tissue tumors.[292, 293] The osseous lesions frequently precede the appearance of clinical and radiographic evidence of intestinal polyposis, so that their accurate recognition is important. Weary and colleagues,[29] reported that 50 per cent of patients with Gardner's syndrome had osteomas, especially in the skull, sinuses, and mandible. The lesions may also be detected in the ribs and long bones, but in the latter sites the outgrowths may not be well defined, but instead appear as localized, wavy cortical thickening, especially in the femur, tibia, and ulna. In fact, any tubular bone, including those of the hands and feet, can reveal osseous protuberances or, more rarely, enostoses in this syndrome.[28] The vertebrae are rarely affected. Dental abnormalities include hypercementosis, supernumerary and unerupted teeth, odontomas, and dentigerous cysts.[311] The major differential diagnostic possibility is tuberous sclerosis, which can lead to similar bony excrescences, particularly in the metacarpals and metatarsals.

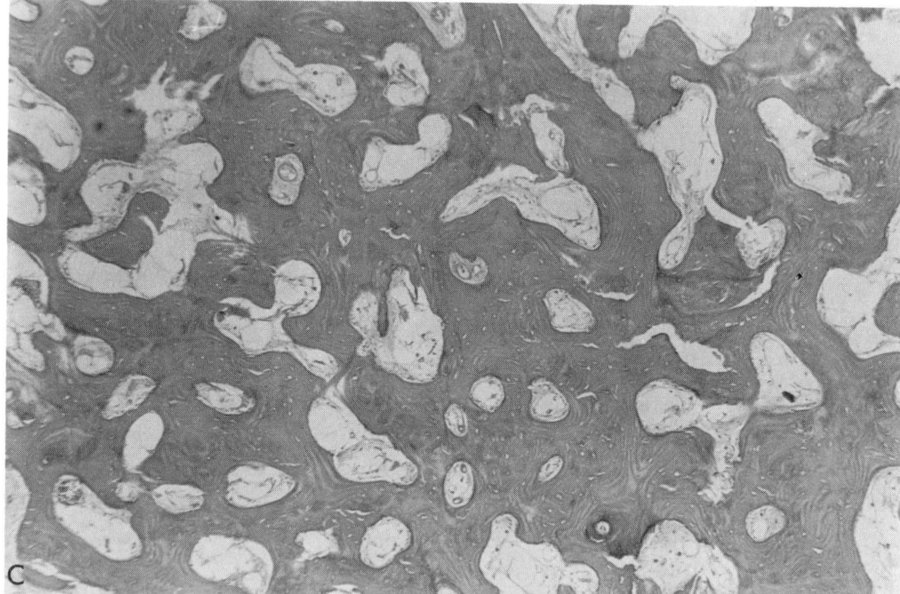

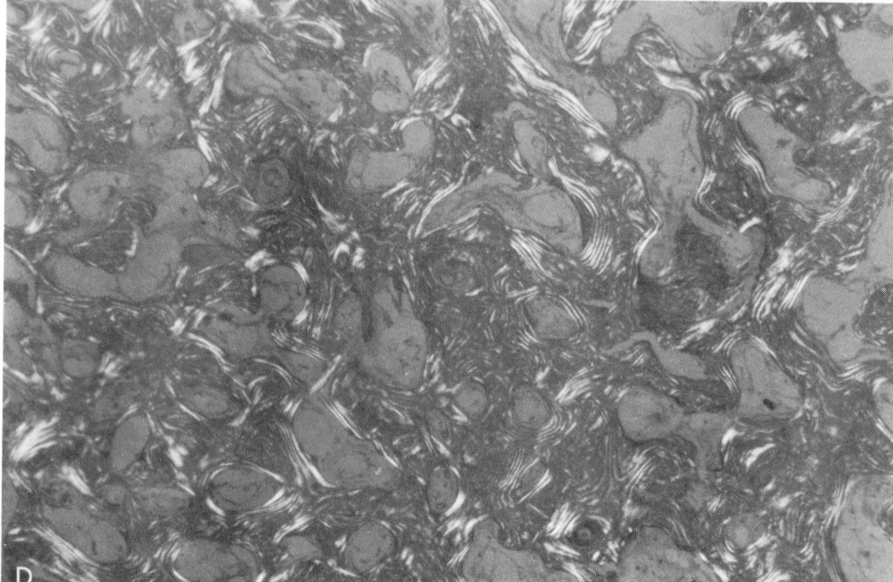

Figure 81–8. Continued

C, D *Nonpolarized and polarized photomicrographs (86×) reveal numerous osseous trabeculae with increased width and sparse intertrabecular space.*

OSTEOPOIKILOSIS

Osteopoikilosis (osteopathia condensans disseminata; spotted bones) is an asymptomatic osteosclerotic dysplasia initially described by Albers-Schönberg[30] and Ledoux-Lebard and associates[31] in the early twentieth century. Although the disorder is described as extremely rare,[32] the experience of many radiologists (including one of the authors) suggests that osteopoikilosis is more common than previous reports have indicated. The disorder is seen in both men and women and may become evident at any age, although its appearance below the age of 3 years is distinctly uncommon.[33] Inherited and sporadic cases of osteopoikilosis have both been reported. Studies of the familial occurrence indicate an autosomal dominant pattern of genetic transmission that may become more prominent in each succeeding generation.[34-37]

Clinical manifestations are usually absent or mild. Cutaneous lesions may be evident in approximately 25 per cent of cases, consisting of closely situated, elevated, whitish fibrocollagenous infiltrations (dermatofibrosis lenticularis disseminata),[38-40] a predisposition to keloid formation,[41, 42] and scleroderma-like lesions.[43, 44] Osteopoikilosis has also been associated with dwarfism,[40, 45] dystocia,[42] and, in 15 to 20 per cent of patients, mild articular pain with or without joint effusion.[46]

Roentgenographic findings are diagnostic.[294] Numerous small, well defined, homogeneous circular or ovoid foci of increased radiodensity are clustered in periarticular osseous regions. A symmetric distribution is observed, with a predilection for the epiphyses and metaphyses of long tubular bones, carpus, tarsus, pelvis, and scapulae; involvement of the ribs, clavicles, spine, and skull is rare and, when present, is less marked (Fig. 81–9). On serial roentgenograms, the radiopaque areas can increase or decrease in size and number or disappear.[37, 47] The dynamic nature of the lesions is more marked in children and adolescents than in adults, in whom the radiodense areas may change slowly or not at all.

Radionuclide examination with bone-seeking radiopharmaceuticals usually reveals no evidence of increased activity about the skeletal lesions.[48, 49]

Pathologically, the lesions of osteopoikilosis appear as oval or round foci of compact bone within the spongiosa.[50] In the epiphyses of the tubular bones the foci rarely are in contact with the subchondral bone plate, whereas in the metaphyses they may be located eccentrically, abutting on the endosteal surface of the cortex. On histologic examination, the lesions are found to be composed of lamellar osseous tissue containing haversian systems. Although osteoblasts, osteocytes, and even osteoclasts may be evident, residual calcified cartilage matrix is not seen, indicating that the foci probably are not formed via endochondral ossification of cartilage rests. The microscopic features of the lesion are identical to those encountered in bone islands.

The etiology and pathogenesis of osteopoikilosis are not known. Some evidence suggests a relationship between this condition and other osteosclerotic skeletal disorders, especially osteopathia striata and melorheostosis[50-52] (Table 81–3). Thus, round and linear areas of increased radiodensity can be encountered in multiple skeletal sites in the same patient, combined with flowing or undulating periosteal bone formation and even calvarial hyperostosis (hyperostosis frontalis interna) (Fig. 81–10). Osteopoikilosis (and these related disorders) may represent a hereditary failure to form normal trabeculae along lines of stress, in which small or large bony foci appear.[53] As such, the lesions may arise as a consequence of altered osteogenesis. In this regard, a report of a patient with both osteopoikilosis and osteosarcoma is of interest[54] (Fig. 81–11). It has been

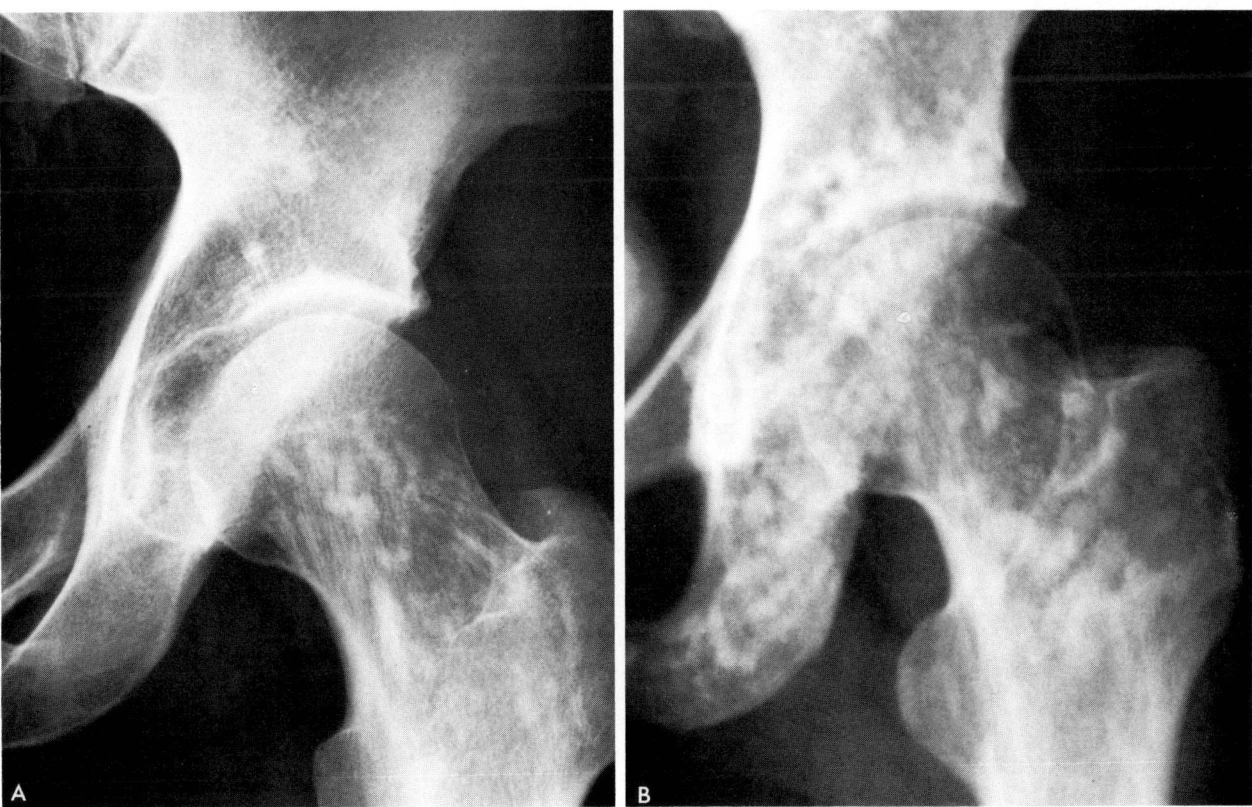

Figure 81–9. *Osteopoikilosis.*

A, B *Hip. Two examples of mild and severe changes are shown. Note the circular or ovoid radiodense foci of the femur and pelvis without abnormality of the intervening joint space.*

Illustration continued on the following page

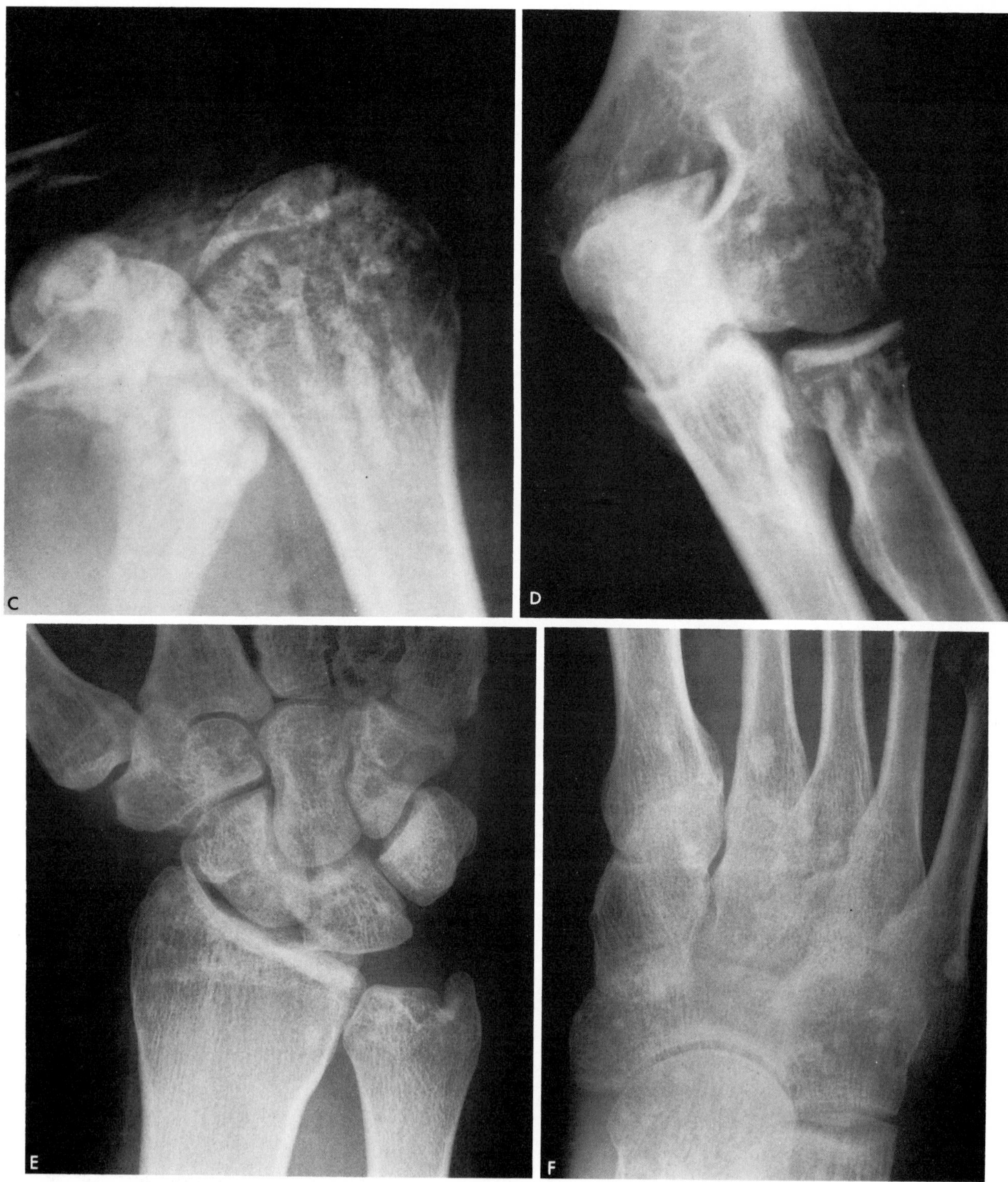

Figure 81–9. Continued

C, D *Shoulder and elbow. The same radiographic characteristics are evident. Although epiphyses can be affected, metaphyseal foci commonly predominate.*

E, F *Carpus and tarsus. In these areas, foci are less numerous and less prominent.*

Illustration continued on the opposite page

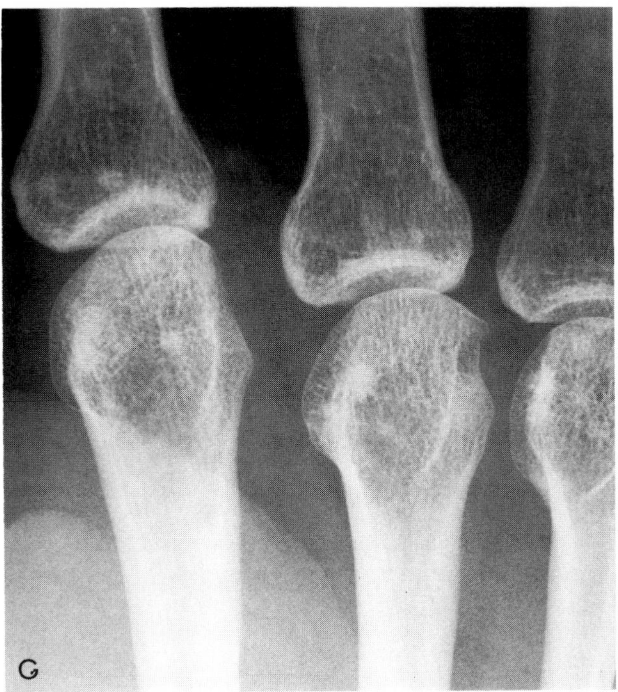

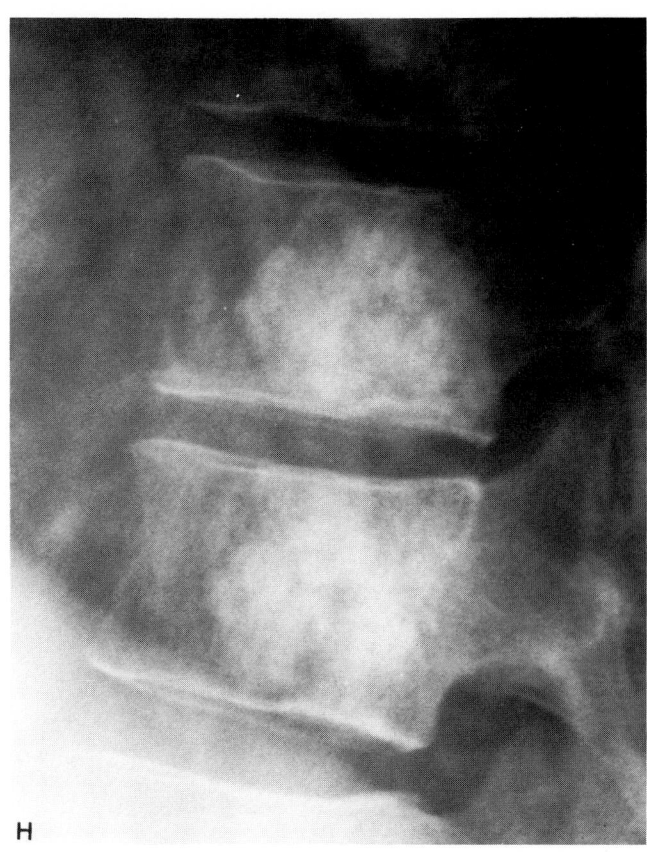

Figure 81–9. Continued

G *Hand. Note several lesions in the metacarpal heads and proximal phalanges of the second, third, and fouth digits.*

H *Spine. This is an unusual case, in which multiple, centrally located foci of the vertebral bodies were associated with widespread involvement of other skeletal sites.*

suggested that this latter tumor may be related to active osteogenesis;[55] perhaps the chronic abnormal remodeling of bone that is evident in patients with osteopoikilosis can be associated with malignant transformation.[54]

The major differential diagnostic considerations in cases of widespread focal round or oval radiodense lesions are osteopoikilosis, osteoblastic metastases, mastocytosis, and tuberous sclerosis. The symmetric distribution, the propensity for epiphyseal and metaphyseal involvement, and the uniform size of the foci are features that suggest osteopoikilosis, a diagnosis that is supported by a normal-appearing bone scan. Asymmetry, common involvement of the axial skeleton, including the spine, osseous destruction, variation in size, and positive scintigraphic findings characterize skeletal metastases. In both mastocytosis and tuberous sclerosis, symmetry, metaphyseal and epiphyseal preference, and uniform, well defined foci are less striking than in osteopoikilosis.

Table 81–3

DISEASES ASSOCIATED WITH VARIOUS HYPEROSTOTIC LESIONS

Lesion	Possible Associated Diseases
Osteoma	Gardner's syndrome
Osteopoikilosis	Osteopathia striata Melorheostosis Hyperostosis frontalis interna
Osteopathia striata	Osteopoikilosis Melorheostosis Osteopetrosis Focal dermal hypoplasia
Melorheostosis	Linear scleroderma Osteopoikilosis Osteopathia striata Neurofibromatosis Tuberous sclerosis Hemangiomas

OSTEOPATHIA STRIATA

Osteopathia striata (Voorhoeve's disease) was first described in 1924 by Voorhoeve[56] as a variant of osteopoikilosis. Subsequent reports of the disease have been few, verifying its very rare occurrence.[57-64, 296] Men and women of any age can be affected, and a genetic transmission, probably an autosomal dominant one, has been suggested, but is

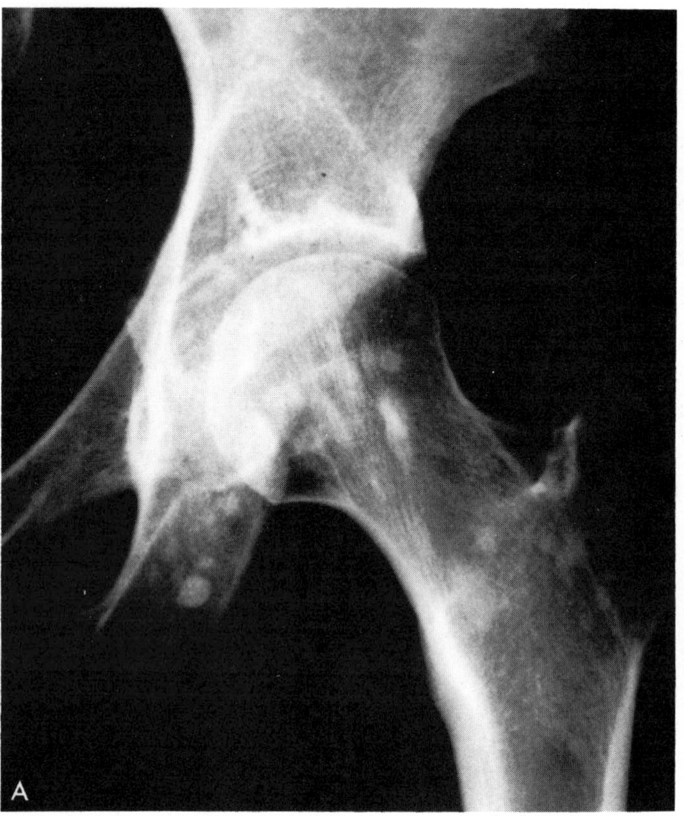

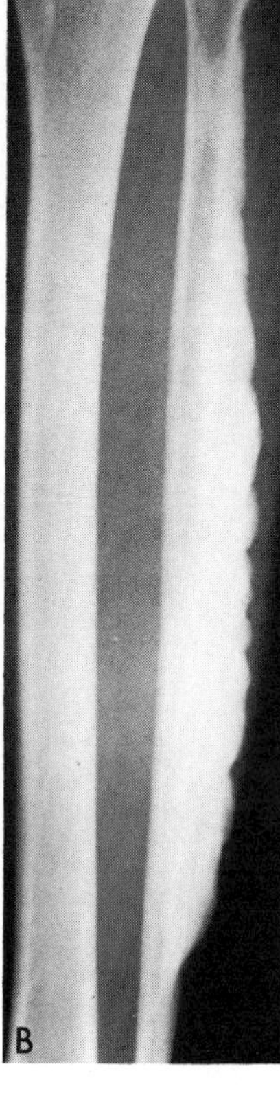

Figure 81–10. *Osteopoikilosis and melorheostosis.*

A *The changes in the hip are diagnostic of osteopoikilosis, although some of the foci are elongated or linear in shape.*

B *Involvement of the fibula in the same patient consists of flowing, eccentrically located ossification, an appearance that is typical of melorheostosis.*

(Courtesy of Dr. A. Brower, The Uniformed Services University for Health Sciences, Bethesda, Maryland.)

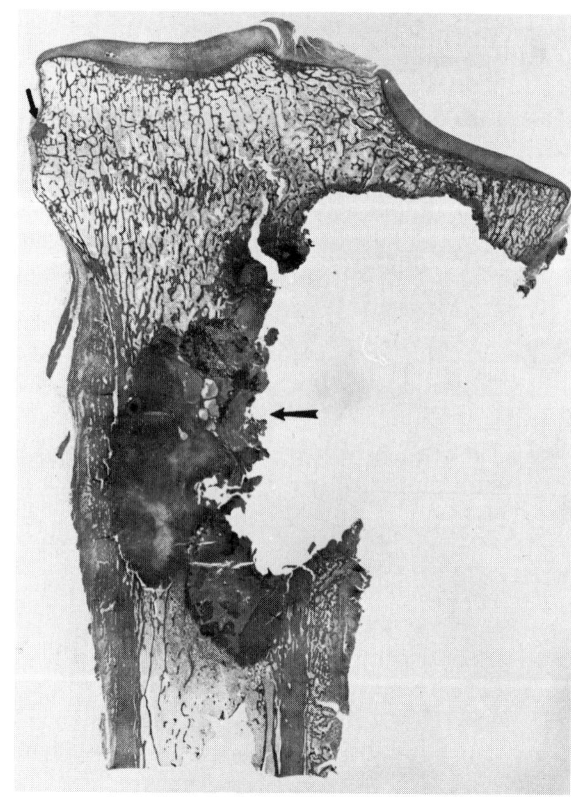

Figure 81–11. *Osteopoikilosis and osteosarcoma. A histologic section of the proximal end of the tibia in a 48 year old man with both osteopoikilosis and osteosarcoma reveals a sarcomatous lesion containing a bone island (large arrow) and an additional subchondral bone island (small arrow). (From Mindell ER, et al: J Bone Joint Surg 60A:406, 1978.)*

not definite. Clinical manifestations are usually absent, although joint discomfort has been encountered in some individuals.[57] Facial deformity may be apparent.

Radiography reveals linear, regular bands of increased radiodensity that extend from the metaphyses of tubular bones for variable distances into the diaphyses, and which are interspersed with areas of rarefaction. The length of the striations may be related to the growth rate of the involved bone; the longest lesions are frequently found in the femora.[59] In the flat bones, especially the ilium, a fan-like arrangement of radiodense striations radiates toward the iliac crests. Involvement of the small bones of the hands and feet, the skull, and the spine is unusual (Fig. 81–12). Rarely, small exostoses are seen. The skeletal abnormalities are usually bilateral in distribution, but may also be unilateral.[60, 65]

Scintigraphy with bone-seeking radiopharmaceuticals fails to reveal significant abnormalities.[49, 60]

Histologic findings are rarely recorded, although Willert and Zichner[61] noted abnormalities in biopsy specimens of two patients that suggested osteonecrosis.

Osteopathia striata may coexist with osteopoikilosis, melorheostosis, or osteopetrosis[50, 52, 63] (Table 81–3). Metaphyseal flaring in some cases of osteopathia striata resembles the findings in Pyle's disease.[66] Recently, a relationship between osteopathia striata and focal dermal hypoplasia (Goltz syndrome) has been noted.[58, 295] This syndrome includes areas of skin atrophy, digital abnormalities, scoliosis, tooth, eye, and ear anomalies, and mental retardation.[60, 67] In a group of 11 patients with focal dermal hypoplasia, nine demonstrated features of osteopathia striata.[58]

The etiology and pathogenesis of this skeletal disorder are not known. Its differential diagnosis includes a prominent vertical trabecular formation that may be a normal variant;[60] the adult form of osteopetrosis, in which linear striations of long bones and pelvis may be encountered; enchondromatosis (Ollier's disease), in which oval-shaped lesions may produce metaphyseal bands of diminished density; and osteopoikilosis, in which oval or circular radiodense foci are seen.

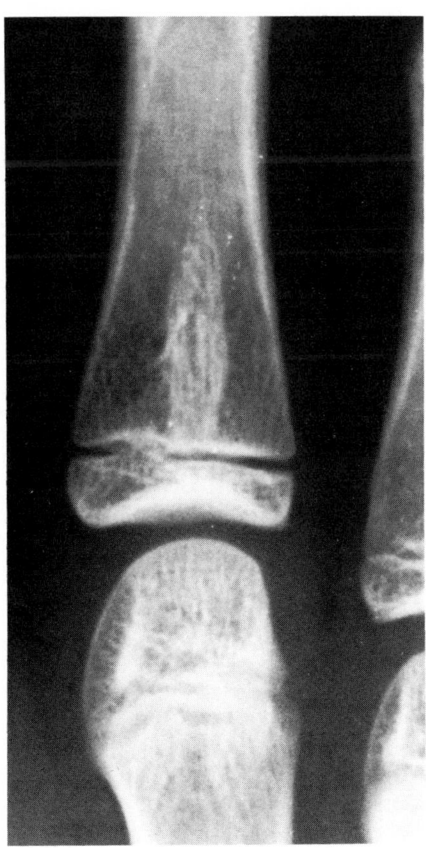

Figure 81–12. *Possible osteopathia striata. An elongated linear radiodense lesion in the proximal metaphysis and diaphysis of a phalanx is compatible with osteopathia striata. One cannot exclude the possibility that such lesions can also represent fibrous dysplasia or benign sclerosis of unknown etiology.*

MELORHEOSTOSIS

Melorheostosis is a rare bone disorder first described by Léri and Joanny in 1922.[68] It generally becomes manifest after early childhood, rarely in the first days of life,[68, 70] and in approximately 40 to 50 per cent of cases, the disease is evident by the age of 20 years.[71] Occasionally, patients in the fourth and fifth decades of life may reveal evidence of melorheostosis.[69, 72] Men and women are affected equally, and no hereditary features have been established.

The clinical alterations of the disorder have been well documented[73-76] and are summarized in a recent review of the subject.[77] Initial manifestations are variable. Intermittent swelling of joints can be evident. Pain and limitation of motion are more frequent in adults than in children,[299] and, with increasing muscle contractures, tendon and ligament shortening, and soft tissue involvement, these findings may become profound. Growth disturbances include increased circumference and angulation of affected limbs and an inequality of limb length. Such disturbances can be severe and can lead to scoliosis, joint contracture and rigidity, and pes valgus, varus, or equinus. Soft tissue changes include tense, erythematous, and shiny skin, anomalous pigmentation, induration and edema of subcutaneous tissues, fibrosis, weakness and atrophy of muscles, and linear scleroderma (see discussion later in this chapter). These changes, which have been demonstrated with thermography,[72] may precede the osseous abnormalities for an extended period and may be evident at birth. The clinical manifestations may progress rapidly during childhood and more slowly during adult life. Although life expectancy is not shortened, the disease can result in considerable deformity and disability, and may require one or more orthopedic operations, including capsulotomy, fasciotomy, and even amputation.

Radiographic alterations are highly characteristic. Changes are commonly limited to a single limb, in which one or more bones may be affected. The lower extremity is more frequently involved than the upper extremity. Abnormalities may also be encountered in the skull and facial bones,[69] ribs,[69, 73] and vertebrae.[78] Changes in the scapulae, clavicles, and pelvis are frequently combined with alterations in the corresponding limb.

Peripherally located (cortical) hyperostosis is evident in one bone or a series of bones (Figs. 81–13 and 81–14). The appearance of the osseous excrescences extending along the length of the bone simulates that of candle wax flowing down the side of a lit candle. A wavy and sclerotic bony contour is produced that may involve one side of the tubular bones of the upper or lower extremity, reaching the carpus and tarsus as well as the metacarpals, metatarsals, or phalanges. Endosteal hyperostosis is an associated feature that may partially or completely obliterate the medullary cavity. In the carpal and tarsal areas, more discrete round foci may resemble the findings of osteopoikilosis, whereas in the flat bones, such as the pelvis or scapula, radiating or localized sclerotic patches are seen (Fig. 81–15). Bone masses may protrude into adjacent articulations, appearing as osteochondromas. Soft tissue calcification and ossification are not infrequent, having a predilection for para-articular regions, and may lead to complete ankylosis of the joint[297, 298] (Fig. 81–16).

As opposed to the situation in osteopoikilosis and osteopathia striata, scintigraphy in cases of melorheostosis can reveal areas of increased skeletal accumulation of radionuclide,[49, 72, 79] and the resulting scintigraphic image may simulate Paget's disease. This positivity, when compared to the negativity of scintigraphy in the former two disorders, may indicate the cortical location or greater size of the bony deposits or the presence of more metabolic activity.

On pathologic examination, thickened and enlarged bony trabeculae are found to contain normal-appearing haversian systems that may be irregularly arranged[71, 72] (Fig. 81–17). Within the marrow space, cellular fibrous tissue is apparent. Occasionally, cartilage islands revealing endochondral ossification and cellular fibrous tissue revealing intramembra-

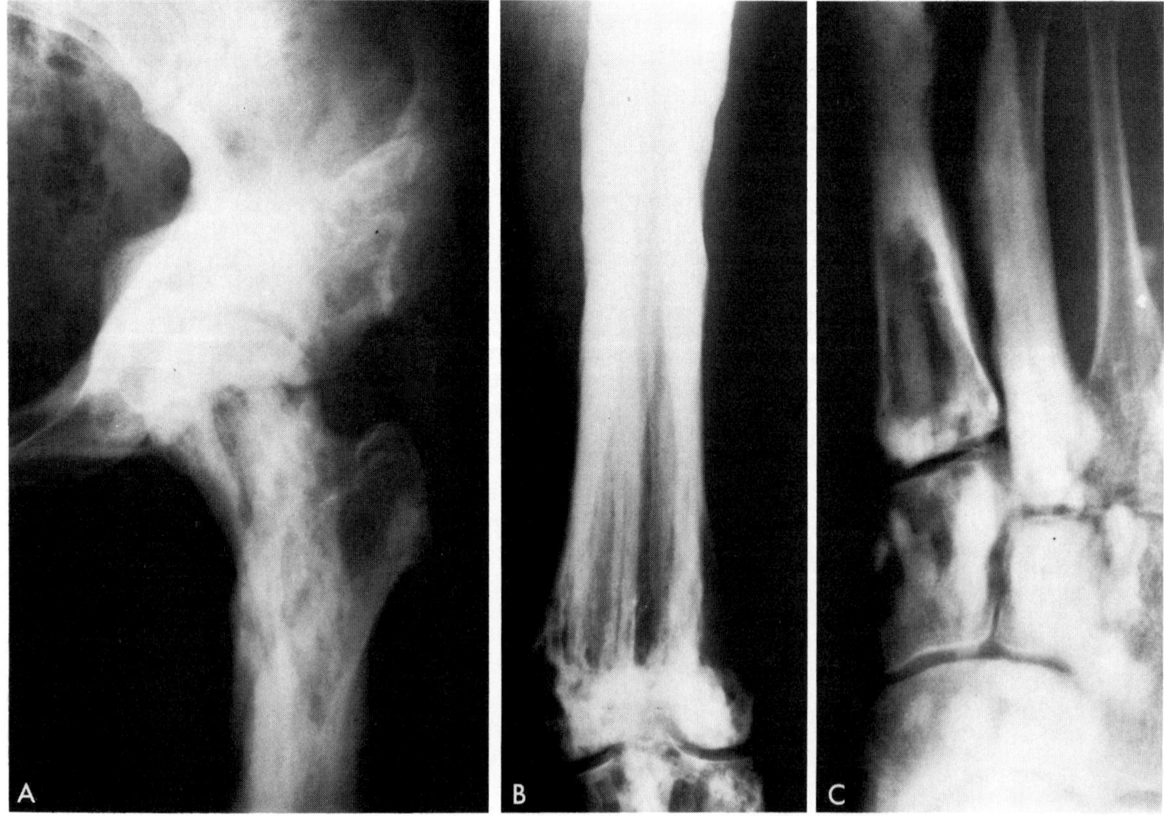

Figure 81–13. *Melorheostosis. In this patient, characteristic radiographic abnormalities are evident throughout a single extremity. Note the hyperostosis of the left hemipelvis, para-acetabular region, and medial aspect of the proximal femur. In the distal femur, a peculiar linear radiodense pattern extends across the knee joint. Involvement of the medial rays of the foot is also seen. (Courtesy of Dr. R. Freiberger, Hospital for Special Surgery, New York, New York.)*

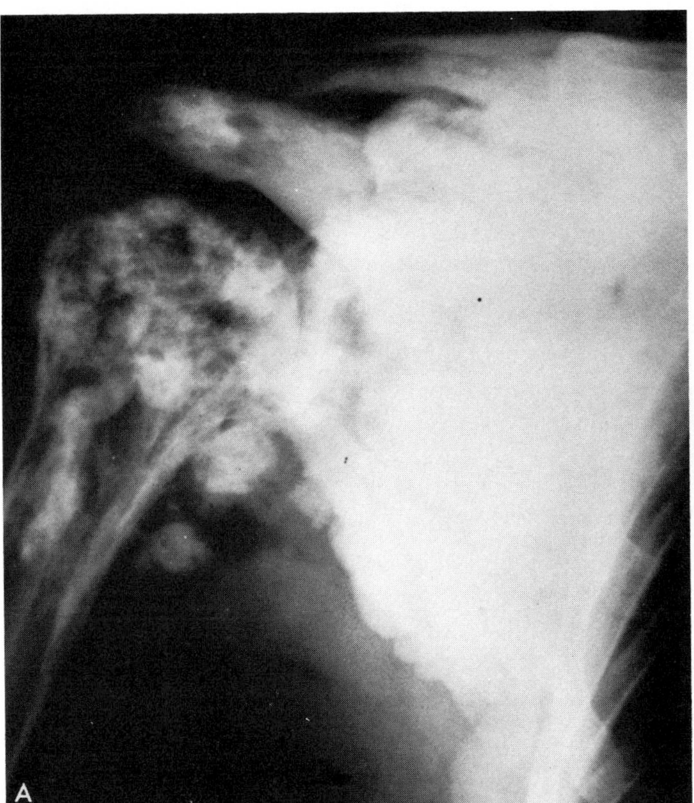

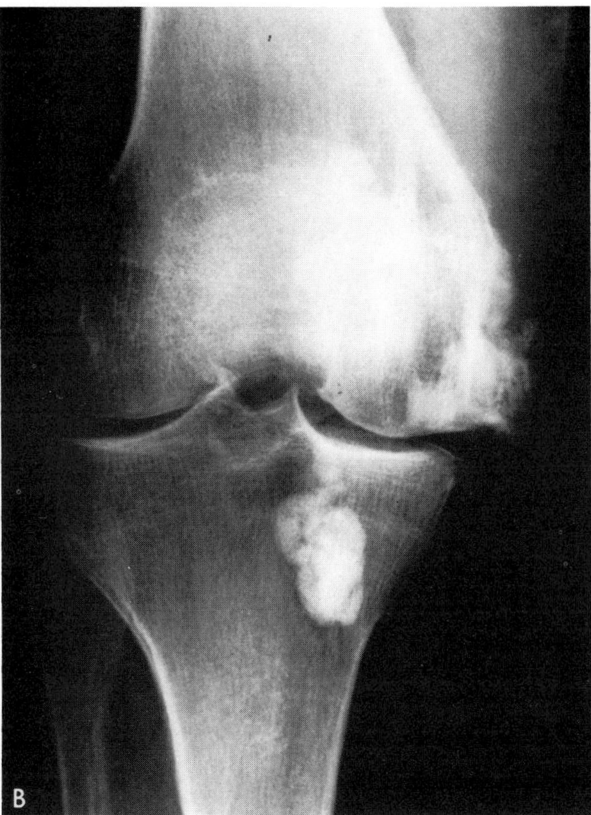

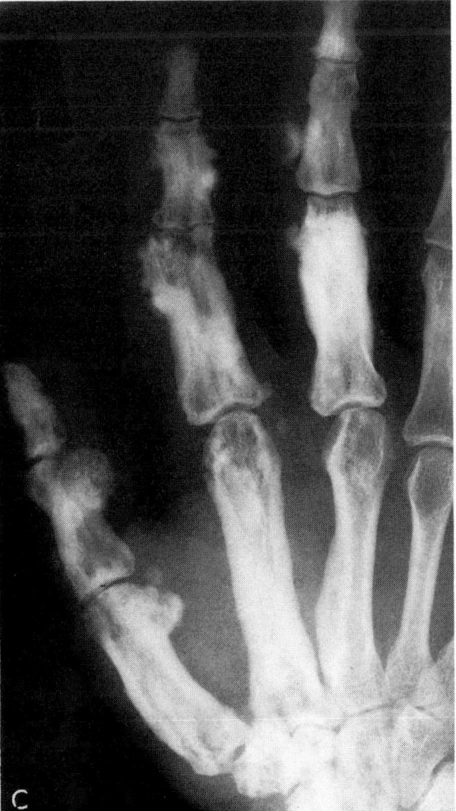

Figure 81–14. Melorheostosis. *In another patient, observe the bizarre osseous overgrowth of the scapula, the hyperostosis of the proximal humerus, soft tissue ossification about the shoulder, bony enlargement and increased radiodensity of the distal medial femur, and enlargement, deformity, and hyperostosis of the radial rays of the hand. The undulating irregular bony contours are typical of this condition. (Courtesy of Drs. J. Mink and R. Gold, Los Angeles, California.)*

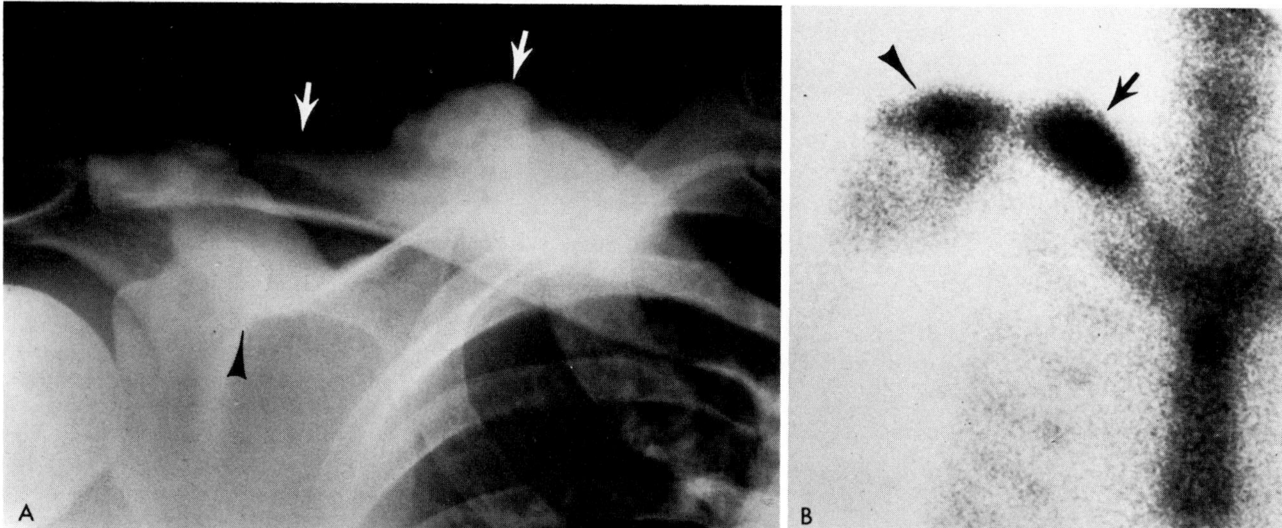

Figure 81–15. Melorheostosis. *This 29 year old man presented with a painful swelling of the right clavicle. A biopsy of the clavicle revealed findings of melorheostosis.*

A *Observe localized hyperostosis of the middle and distal clavicle (arrows) and scapula (arrowhead). The process extended down the proximal aspect of the humerus.*

B *A technetium bone scan delineates increased activity in the clavicle (arrow) and scapula (arrowhead).*

(Courtesy of Dr. W. Pogue, Grossmont Hospital, San Diego, California.)

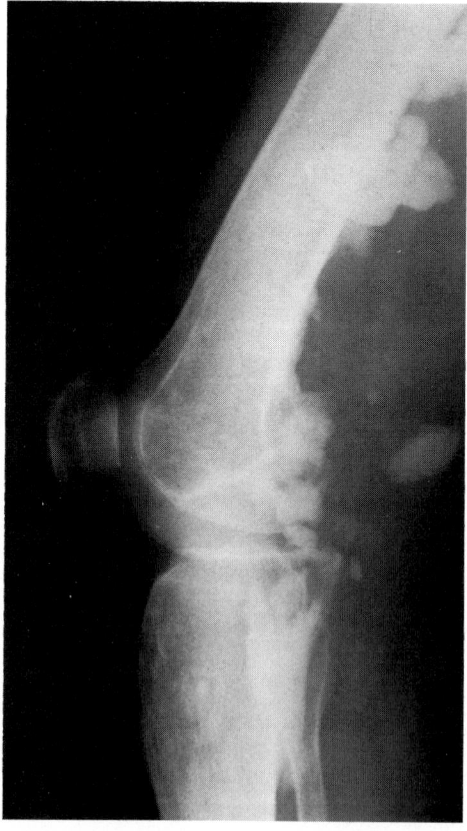

Figure 81–16. Melorheostosis. *Prominent soft tissue calcification and ossification are noted along the posterior aspect of the thigh and the knee. Minor hyperostosis of the underlying cortex is evident.*

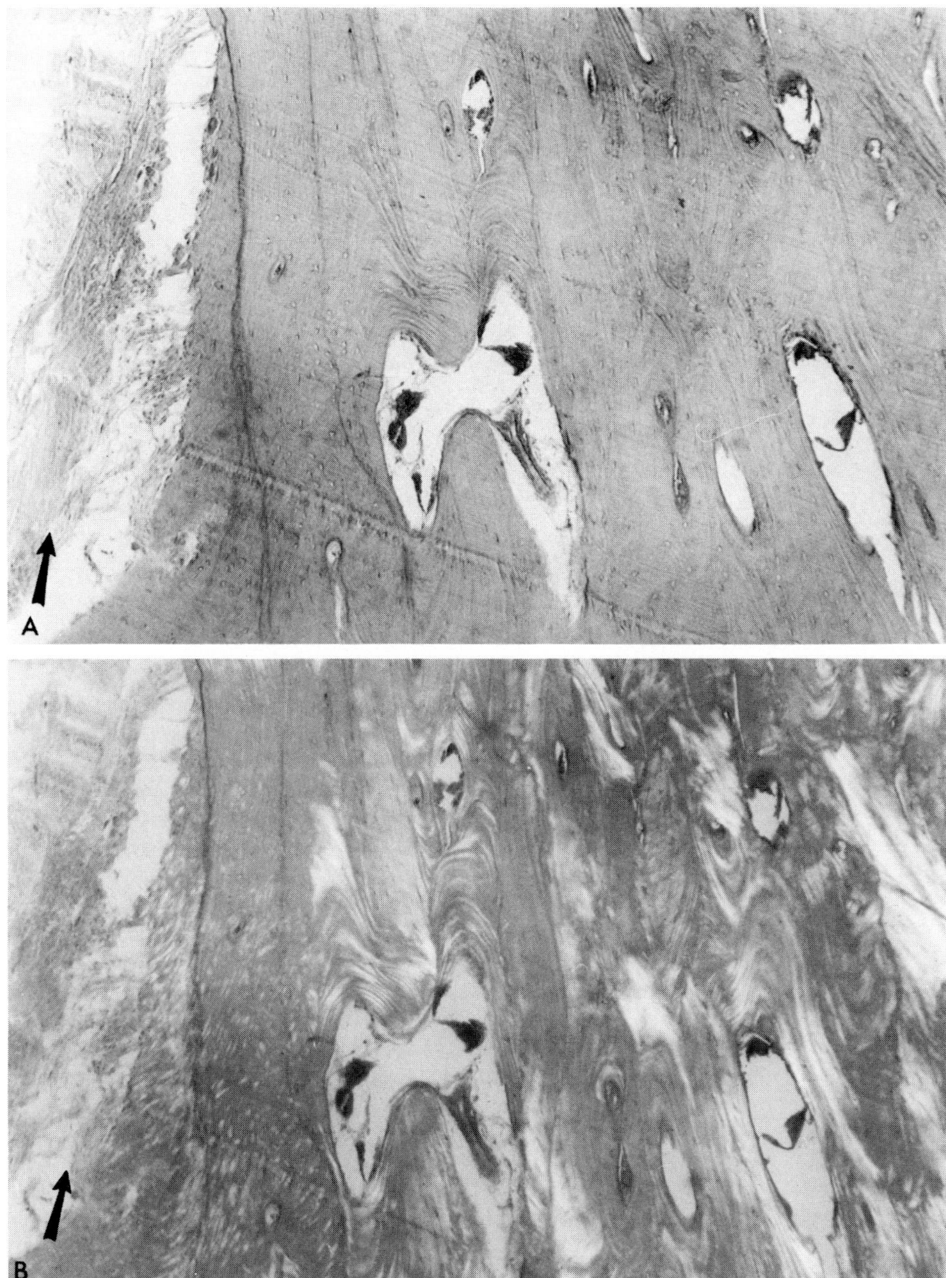

Figure 81–17. Melorheostosis.

A, B *A nonpolarized* **(A)** *and polarized* **(B)** *photomicrograph reveal the hypertrophic bony trabeculae and periosteal fibrous tissue (arrow) (68×).*

Illustration continued on the following page

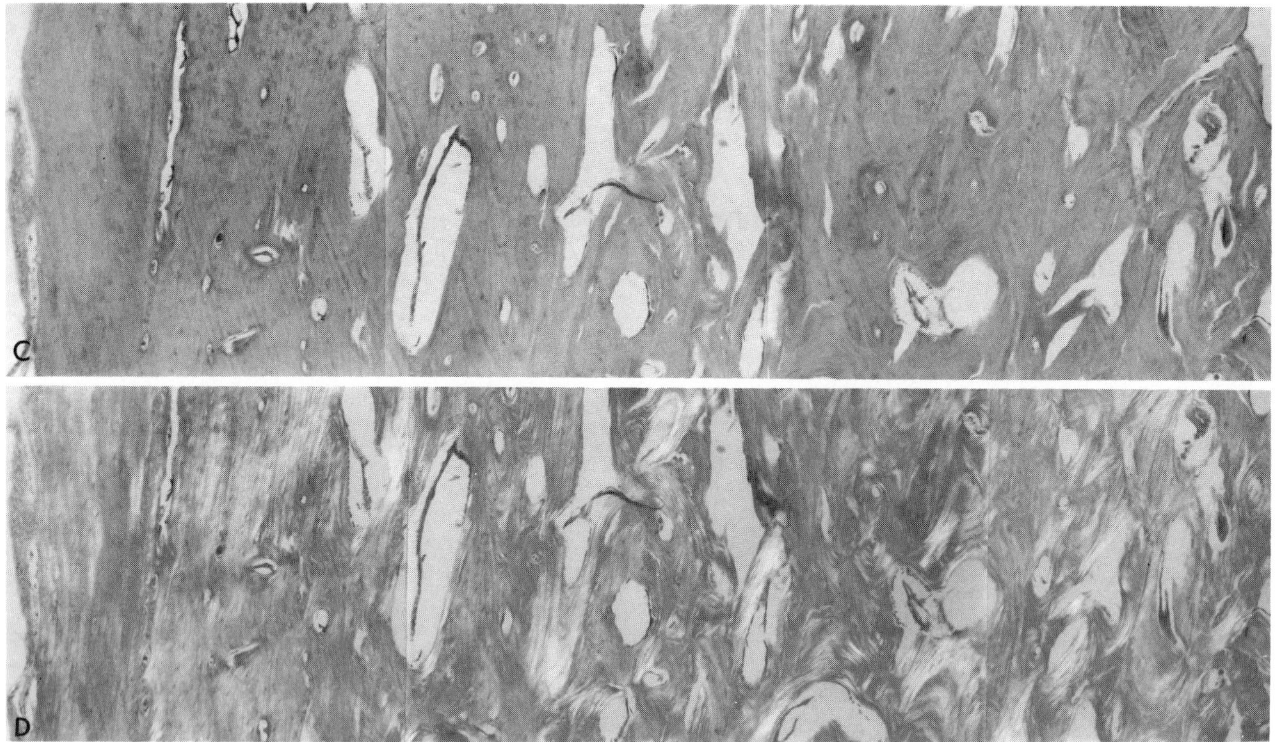

Figure 81–17. Continued
C, D *Additional nonpolarized* **(C)** *and polarized* **(D)** *photomicrographs reveal the extent of the sclerotic bone (68×).*

nous bone formation are encountered. However, osteoblastic or osteoclastic activity usually is not prominent, and inflammatory lesions are lacking.[298]

Melorheostosis has been reported in association with other disorders[77] (Table 81–3). Band-like linear scleroderma overlying osseous excrescences has been noted.[73, 80-85] The histologic characteristics of the soft tissue involvement in these cases suggest that cutaneous abnormalities are secondary to the same proliferative disorder that produces the bony hyperostosis.[82] The association of melorheostosis with osteopoikilosis and osteopathia striata has also been reported;[52, 86, 87] in some cases of melorheostosis, the sclerotic foci in the carpus and tarsus that form part of the disease process itself may have been misinterpreted as evidence of osteopoikilosis.[77] Additional investigations have indicated possible associations between melorheostosis and neurofibromatosis,[88] tuberous sclerosis,[89] and hemangiomas or other vascular lesions.[89, 90]

The etiology and pathogenesis of melorheostosis are not known. Putti[91] postulated that vascular disturbances represented the primary cause of the disorder, and the role of vascular insufficiency has been emphasized by other investigators.[89, 90] An inflammatory process,[71] a degenerative disorder of connective tissue,[90, 92] an abnormality of innervation, and a defect in embryogenesis[73] have each been offered at one time or another as a possible etiologic factor.[77]

Since one of the most striking characteristics of the disease is a peculiar pattern of distribution, clues to the pathogenesis of melorheostosis may be uncovered by analyzing this characteristic.[93] The segmental distribution of the lesions does not correspond to the anatomic course of blood vessels or mixed nerve roots of the limbs,[94] although it might result from a congenital disturbance initiated early in embryonic life prior to formation of the limb buds.[73, 95] Recently, Murray and McCredie[93] have emphasized the role of sclerotomes in the distribution of hyperostosis in melorheostosis. Sclerotomes represent zones of the skeleton supplied by individual spinal sensory nerves;[96] sclerotome maps can be constructed indicating patterns of skeletal innervation. In many cases of melorheostosis, skeletal alterations correspond to a single sclerotome or a part thereof, suggesting that the disease may represent the late result of a segmental sensory nerve lesion. The accompanying cutaneous lesions, including linear scleroderma, may be related to the same nerve segment, whereas para-articular ossification could result from involvement of the corresponding myotome.[93]

The radiographic abnormalities of melorheostosis are sufficiently characteristic to allow accurate diagnosis in most cases. Although hyperostosis can accompany tuberous sclerosis, neurofibromatosis, Gardner's syndrome, infantile cortical hyperostosis, and fibrous dysplasia, the distribution of bone deposition in these disorders does not reveal the unusual segmental features that appear in melorheostosis. In some patients with the latter disease, soft tissue calcification and ossification in para-articular regions may resemble the findings of idiopathic synovial osteochondromatosis, heterotopic ossification following burns or paralysis, or soft tissue sarcomas.

PRIMARY HYPERTROPHIC OSTEOARTHROPATHY (PACHYDERMOPERIOSTOSIS)

Hypertrophic osteoarthropathy represents a clinical syndrome consisting of clubbing of the digits of the hands and feet, enlargement of the extremities secondary to periarticular and osseous proliferation, and painful and swollen joints. The syndrome may be divided into two categories: primary (hereditary or idiopathic) hypertrophic osteoarthropathy and secondary hypertrophic osteoarthropathy. The primary form represents approximately 3 to 5 per cent of all cases of hypertrophic osteoarthropathy. In either primary or secondary varieties, the syndrome may be incomplete, or additional features, such as thickening of skin on the face and scalp (pachydermia), may become prominent.

Primary hypertrophic osteoarthropathy has also been called pachydermoperiostosis, idiopathic hypertrophic osteoarthropathy, generalized hyperostosis with pachydermia, pachydermohyperostosis, idiopathic familial generalized osteophytosis, and Touraine-Solente-Golé syndrome. It was first described by Friedreich in 1868[97] and Marie in 1890.[98] In 1907, Unna[99] delineated the condition of cutis verticis gyrata, and in 1927 Grönberg[100] associated the latter condition with the one previously described by Friedreich.[101] Additional accounts of this entity followed,[102-111] which, when combined with more recent reports,[101, 112-119] delineate in great detail the clinical and radiologic aspects of pachydermoperiostosis.

Clinical Abnormalities

This rare disease demonstrates an autosomal dominant genetic transmission with marked variability of expression. It predominates in men, is more severe in men than in women, and shows a predilection for blacks. An adolescent onset is typical, although cases appearing before puberty or in adult life have been recorded.[112, 113, 120] The clinical manifestations are somewhat variable, depending on whether the patient demonstrates the complete syndrome (pachydermia, periostitis, cutis verticis gyrata), the incomplete form (sparing of the scalp), or the forme fruste (pachydermia with minimal or absent periostitis).[113, 116]

There is an insidious onset of enlargement of the hands and feet producing a paw-like appearance, clubbing of the distal ends of the fingers and toes, and convexity of the nails. Coarsening of the skin of the face and scalp with ptosis, furrowing and oiliness of the cutaneous tissue, excessive sweating, enlargement and disruption of the normal contour of the extremities, fatigability, and vague pains in the bones and joints are also encountered. Pachydermoperiostosis generally progresses for approximately 10 years before arresting spontaneously. However, chronic disabling complications may appear, with stiffness and restricted motion in the axial and appendicular skeleton, kyphosis, and neurologic manifestations due to osseous compression of the spinal cord or nerve roots as well as the cranial nerves (conductive and sensory hearing loss, vestibular dysfunction). Life expectancy is normal.

These clinical features are not constant in all individuals with the disease. Pachydermia may be limited or absent,[120-125] or periostitis may not be apparent.[116] In some cases, the appearance resembles that of acromegaly, with thickened and coarsened cutaneous features,[126, 127] but macroglossia, mandibular and sellar enlargement, and visual defects are not evident.[50, 128] Furthermore, laboratory analysis fails to document the findings of acromegaly since growth hormone levels are normal.[116]

Of interest in some patients is the appearance of bone marrow failure and extramedullary hematopoiesis, due to encroachment on the marrow space by the thickened cortex.[129, 130] Hepatosplenomegaly and anemia in these individuals may be associated with endocrine abnormalities,[129] although the latter findings have also been noted in patients with pachydermoperiostosis who do not have bone marrow failure.[131]

Radiographic Abnormalities

The predominant radiographic feature of pachydermoperiostosis is periostitis (Figs. 81–18 and 81–19). Widespread and symmetric findings occur, although osseous thickening is most pronounced in the tubular bones of the extremities, especially the tibia, fibula, radius, and ulna. Involvement of the carpus, tarsus, metacarpals, metatarsals, phalanges, and pelvis is also frequent. Thickening of the calvarium and base of the skull can be detected;[111] however, changes in the spine are unusual.

Superficially, the periosteal proliferation of the tubular bones resembles that in secondary hypertrophic osteoarthropathy, but careful evaluation reveals definite and significant differences (Table 81–4). Although the diaphyses and metaphyses can be affected in both conditions, periostitis commonly

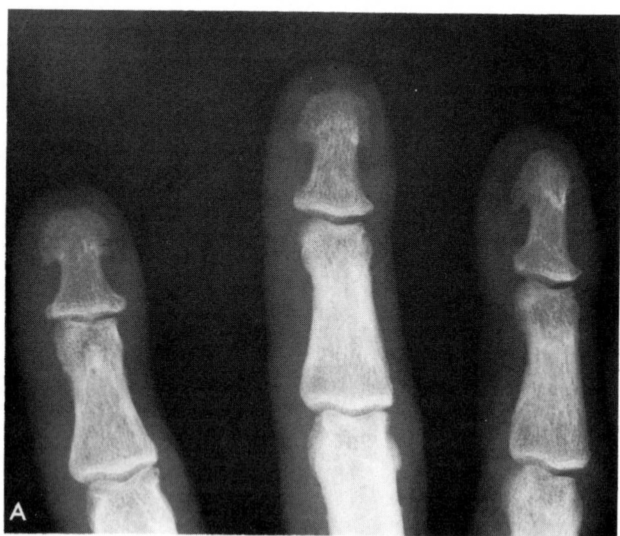

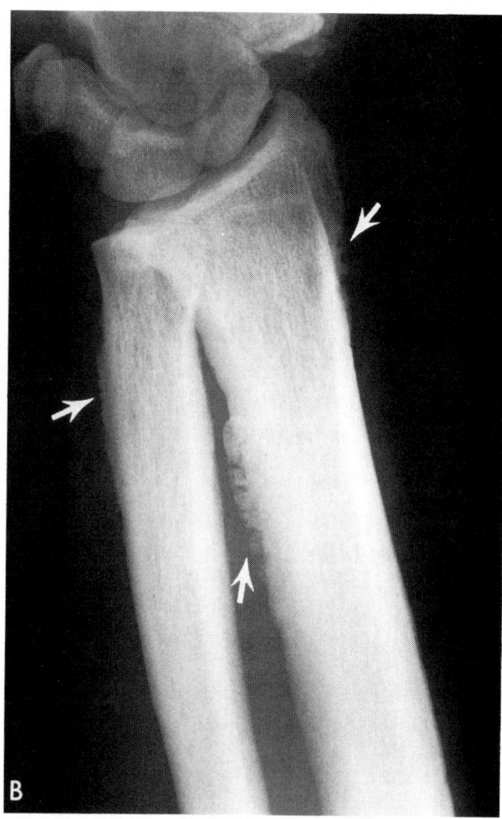

Figure 81–18. *Primary hypertrophic osteoarthropathy (pachydermoperiostosis). A 55 year old black man had coarse facial features, clubbed digits, and painful but nontender bones; other family members had similar problems.*

A *A radiograph of the fingers delineates soft tissue enlargement and some broadening of the terminal phalangeal tufts.*

B *A semisupinated oblique roentgenogram of the forearm delineates the peculiar variety of periosteal proliferation (arrows), which extends into the epiphyses.*

C *Fluffy new bone formation is also evident about the ischial and pubic rami (arrows).*

Illustration continued on the opposite page

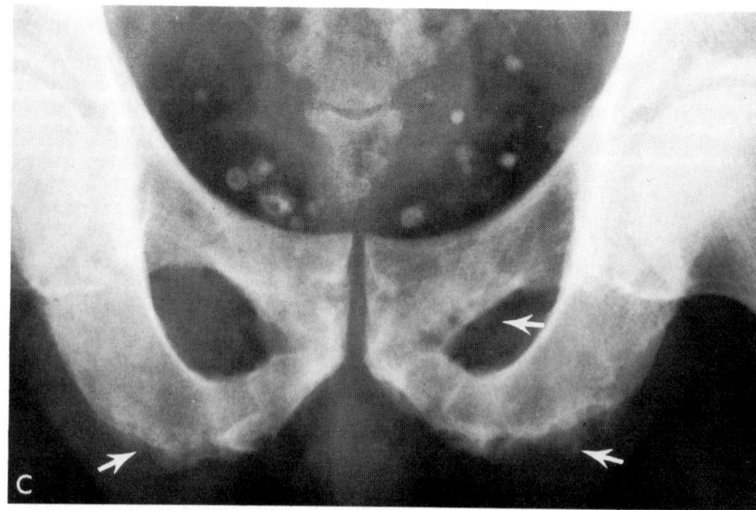

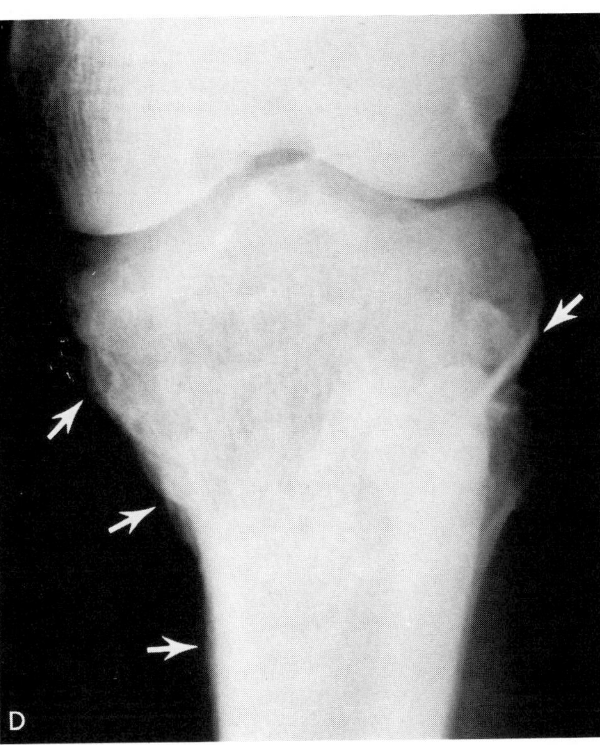

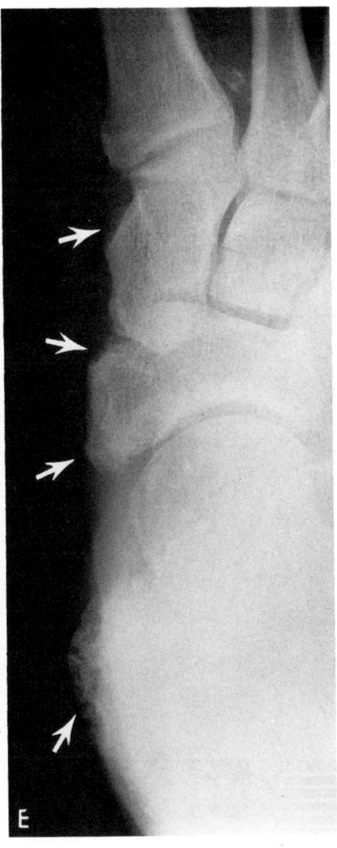

Figure 81–18. Continued

D *Observe the periosteal proliferation in the proximal tibial epiphysis, metaphysis, and diaphysis (arrows).*

E *An irregular osseous surface on the medial malleolus and tarsus can be seen (arrows).*

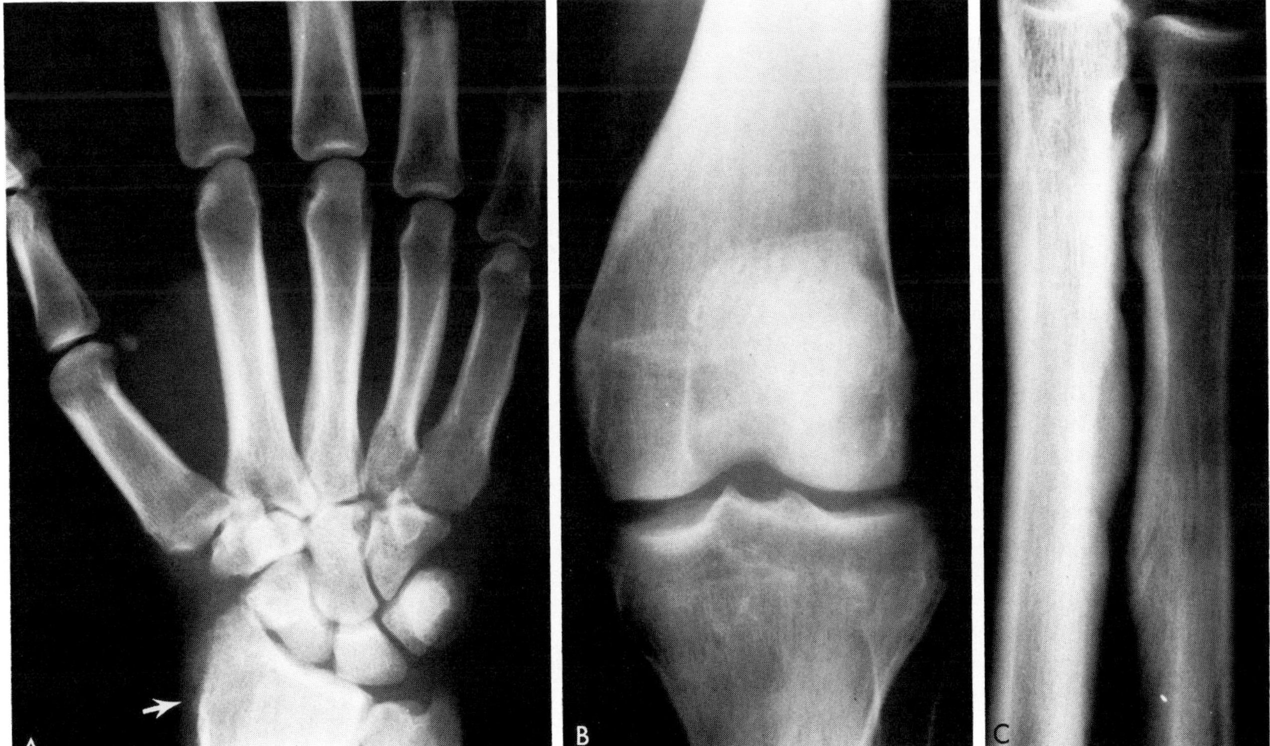

Figure 81–19. *Primary hypertrophic osteoarthropathy (pachydermoperiostosis). A 26 year old man developed acromegalic features and cutaneous abnormalities.*

A *In addition to periosteal proliferation of the distal radius (arrow), note the widened metacarpals and phalanges.*

B *An expanded contour of the distal femur is associated with cortical thickening.*

C *Exuberant osseous proliferation is evident along apposing surfaces of radius and ulna.*

Table 81–4
SOME CAUSES OF DIFFUSE PERIOSTITIS

Disease	Location	Characteristics
Primary hypertrophic osteoarthropathy (pachydermoperiostosis)	Tibia, fibula, radius, ulna (less commonly, carpus, tarsus, metacarpals, metatarsals, phalanges, pelvis, ribs, clavicle)	Diaphyseal, metaphyseal, and epiphyseal involvement Shaggy, irregular excrescences Diaphyseal expansion Clubbing Ligamentous ossification Cranial and facial changes
Secondary hypertrophic osteoarthropathy	Tibia, fibula, radius, ulna (less commonly, femur, humerus, metacarpals, metatarsals, phalanges)	Diaphyseal and metaphyseal involvement Single or laminated, regular or irregular proliferation Clubbing Periarticular osteoporosis, soft tissue swelling Underlying primary lesion
Thyroid acropachy	Metacarpals, metatarsals, phalanges (less commonly, other tubular bones)	Diaphyseal involvement Radial side predilection Dense, solid, and spiculated proliferation Clubbing Soft tissue swelling Thyroid gland abnormalities
Venous stasis	Tibia, fibula, femur, metatarsals, phalanges	Diaphyseal and metaphyseal involvement Undulating osseous contour Cortical thickening Soft tissue swelling, ulceration, ossification Phleboliths
Hypervitaminosis A	Ulna, metatarsals, clavicle, tibia, fibula	Diaphyseal involvement Undulating contour Epiphyseal deformities Soft tissue nodules Intracranial hypertension
Infantile cortical hyperostosis (Caffey's disease)	Mandible, clavicle, scapula, ribs, tubular bones	Periostitis and cortical hyperostosis May become extreme Cranial destruction Soft tissue nodules Deformities

extends into the epiphyseal region in pachydermoperiostosis, producing shaggy excrescences about various articulations. In fact, ill-defined bony outgrowths are especially characteristic of this disease, differing from the linear deposits that most typically accompany secondary hypertrophic osteoarthropathy. These outgrowths are also encountered in the pelvis, particularly about the ischium, symphysis pubis, acetabulum, and iliac crest.

In more advanced cases, expansion of the diaphyses of the tubular bones and sclerosis of the spongiosa in both appendicular and axial skeletal sites are evident. The ribs and clavicles may be diffusely expanded, with coarsened trabeculae and prominent sclerotic islands. In addition to osseous thickening, the skull may reveal prominent sinuses, especially in the frontal and sphenoid regions, and moderate enlargement of the mandible (alveolar portions). Intervertebral disc space and foraminal narrowing, vertical or horizontal osseous ridges in the vertebral bodies, and ligamentous ossification are spinal manifestations of the disease. Soft tissue prominence of the distal digits may rarely be associated with tuftal osteolysis.[101] The bony resorption produces tapering, pointing, or disappearance of terminal phalanges.

Ligamentous calcification and ossification may appear in portions of the appendicular skeleton, including the calcaneus, the ulnar olecranon, the patella, and the interosseous regions between radius and ulna and between tibia and fibula. Osseous bridges may also appear in the scapulae and sternum and may lead to bony ankylosis of articulations, particularly the joints of the hands and feet.

Pathologic Abnormalities

Inspection of involved bones delineates a roughened surface due to periosteal deposition of bone.[50, 102, 112, 132] On cross section, the delineation between the original cortical bone and the periosteal new bone is less distinct in this condition than in secondary hypertrophic osteoarthropathy.[50] This difference may be related to the longer survival period encountered in patients with pachydermoperiostosis, allowing enough time for incomplete or complete incorporation of the periosteal deposits into the subjacent cortex.

Articular Abnormalities

Articular inflammation is less prominent in pachydermoperiostosis than in secondary hypertrophic osteoarthropathy. Pain and swelling are uncommon and, when present, are of only moderate severity. Joint effusions may be encountered.[114, 115] Aspiration of joint contents reveals noninflammatory synovial fluid, although in one patient calcium pyrophosphate dihydrate crystals were detected.[133] Histologic examination of the synovial membrane outlines mild cellular hyperplasia of the lining and thickening of the subsynovial blood vessels[134] (Fig. 81–20). With electron microscopy, multilayered basement laminae can be detected about small blood vessels in the subsynovial tissue.

In long-standing cases, increased rigidity and limitation of joint motion reflect mechanical interference due to periarticular osseous excrescences and intra-articular bony masses.[50] Carpal and tarsal ankylosis is particularly characteristic.

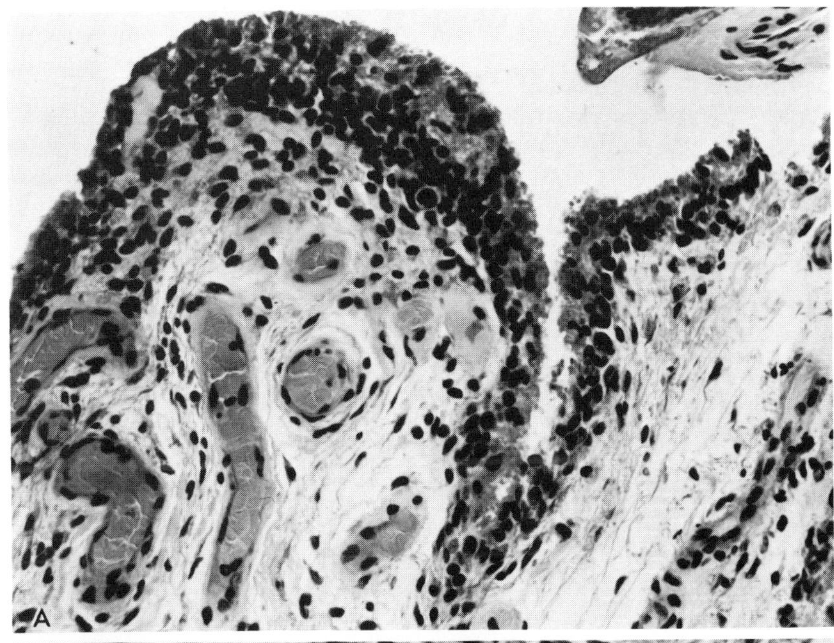

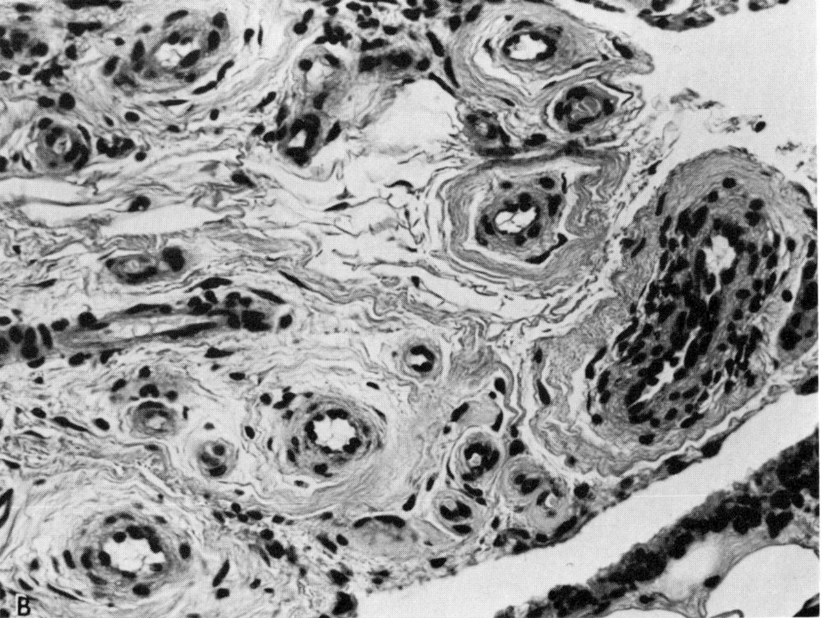

Figure 81–20. *Primary hypertrophic osteoarthropathy (pachydermoperiostosis): Synovial abnormalities. A 40 year old man with pachydermoperiostosis and chronic articular symptoms underwent synovial biopsy of the right knee.*

A *Cellular hyperplasia of the synovial lining is evident (40×).*

B *Thickening of subsynovial blood vessels is also apparent (40×).*

(From Lauter SA, et al: J Rheum 5:85, 1978.)

Etiology and Pathogenesis

A definite etiology and pathogenesis of pachydermoperiostosis have not been unraveled. Although increased peripheral blood flow appears to be significant in the pathogenesis of secondary hypertrophic osteoarthropathy, measurements in patients with long-standing pachydermoperiostosis reveal diminished blood flow.[135] The cause and significance of this finding are not clear; it has been postulated that diminished peripheral blood flow may indicate secondary thickening of the arterial wall, as has been described in cases of secondary hypertrophic osteoarthropathy,[136] or massive connective tissue overgrowth, in the process of which small and medium-sized arteries are compressed or obliterated.[135] Whether or not a similar decrease in peripheral circulation accompanies the early active phase of the disease is not known. Perhaps, in early stages, an increase in peripheral blood flow through arteriovenous shunts bypasses the capillary beds, producing capillary stasis, local hypoxia, and connective tissue proliferation.[112]

Differential Diagnosis

The irregular periosteal deposits that appear about metaphyses and epiphyses of tubular bones as well as axial skeletal sites in this condition are distinctive, and they are not encountered in secondary hypertrophic osteoarthropathy. The early age of onset, a family history of disease, and the absence of significant joint pain are clinical characteristics of pachydermoperiostosis that differ from those of secondary hypertrophic osteoarthropathy. In thyroid acropachy, fluffy, spiculated periosteal bone is encountered in the hands and feet. It is rarely observed elsewhere, a fact that, taken in combination with typical clinical characteristics such as exophthalmos and pretibial myxedema, ensures accurate diagnosis of thyroid acropachy. Some of the clinical and radiologic manifestations of acromegaly are observed in pachydermoperiostosis, but radiographic and laboratory signs of a pituitary tumor differentiate acromegaly from pachydermoperiostosis. In endosteal hyperostosis (van Buchem's disease), thickening of the cranial vault and cortices of the tubular bones are not combined with digital clubbing, skin changes, enlargement of paranasal sinuses, and irregular para-articular osseous excrescences. Similarly, in diaphyseal dysplasia (Camurati-Engelmann disease), endosteal and periosteal proliferation of the diaphyses of the tubular bones is characteristic. Other disorders, such as Paget's disease, fibrous dysplasia, and fluorosis, are easily differentiated from pachydermoperiostosis.

SECONDARY HYPERTROPHIC OSTEOARTHROPATHY

A description of clubbing of the digits was first provided by Hippocrates in the fifth century BC.[137] Following the descriptions of Bamberger in 1889[138] and Marie in 1890,[98] the entire syndrome of clubbing, arthritis, and periostitis became known. Currently, an extensive literature is available that describes the features of secondary hypertrophic osteoarthropathy.[139-144] In many of the reports, the condition is termed hypertrophic pulmonary osteoarthropathy, emphasizing the fact that pulmonary problems represent a major cause of the periostitis. It has been estimated that between 1 per cent[145, 146] and 12 per cent[147, 148] of patients with bronchogenic carcinoma develop hypertrophic osteoarthropathy, although estimates as high as 25 to 50 per cent have been recorded.[149] A 5 per cent incidence appears to be a typical approximation of the frequency of this complication in cases of bronchogenic carcinoma. Hypertrophic osteoarthropathy is also common in patients with pleural mesothelioma, and may be apparent in as many as 50 per cent of these patients.[141, 150] Other intrathoracic diseases associated with this complication include pulmonary abscess, bronchiectasis, emphysema, Hodgkin's disease,[151-154] diaphragmatic tumors, and metastasis[155-160, 312] (Table 81–5). Hypertrophic osteoarthropathy is rarely, if ever, encountered in cases of pulmonary tuberculosis. Of all these potential intrathoracic causes, bronchogenic carcinoma is by far the most common underlying lesion. The incidence of hypertrophic osteoarthropathy is greater in those lung tumors that are peripherally situated, of squamous origin, and cavitary in nature. There is no relationship between

Table 81–5

SOME CAUSES OF SECONDARY HYPERTROPHIC OSTEOARTHROPATHY

Pulmonary	Bronchogenic carcinoma Abscess Bronchiectasis Emphysema Hodgkin's disease Metastasis Cystic fibrosis
Pleural/diaphragmatic	Mesothelioma
Cardiac	Cyanotic congenital heart disease
Abdominal	Portal/biliary cirrhosis Ulcerative colitis Crohn's disease Dysentery Neoplasms Biliary atresia
Miscellaneous	Nasopharyngeal carcinoma Esophageal carcinoma

tumor size and the incidence and severity of hypertrophic osteoarthropathy.

Hypertrophic osteoarthropathy has also been associated with cyanotic congenital heart disease (tetralogy of Fallot, transposition of the great vessels, Eisenmenger's complex, patent ductus arteriosus with flow reversal, and others),[161-166] and such extrathoracic conditions as portal and biliary cirrhosis[167, 214] ulcerative colitis,[220] Crohn's disease,[221, 222] and amebic and bacillary dysentery. In addition, nasopharyngeal,[168-171] esophageal,[172] gastric,[215] and pancreatic[173] neoplasms[216] can produce hypertrophic osteoarthropathy even in the absence of pulmonary metastasis.

Hypertrophic osteoarthropathy is infrequent in childhood. In this age group, potential causes include pulmonary suppuration,[306] cystic fibrosis,[301] congenital cyanotic heart disease, Hodgkin's disease, and metastasis,[174-179] as well as Crohn's disease, biliary atresia, or primary pulmonary neoplasms.

Clinical Abnormalities

Digital clubbing is a frequent but not invariable feature of hypertrophic osteoarthropathy; however, the manifestation should not be equated with the full syndrome, since patients with diverse disorders can reveal clubbing without any associated findings of hypertrophic osteoarthropathy.[180] The initial alteration is thickening of the fibroelastic tissue at the base of the nail bed followed by increased fluctuance of the bed, and prominence, striations, shininess, and increased curvature of the nail itself. Skin thickening and swelling of the limbs can also be evident.

Articular symptoms and signs are apparent at some time in approximately 30 to 40 per cent of patients and may be the presenting manifestation of hypertrophic osteoarthropathy. Typically, pain and tenderness appear about one or more articulations. The discomfort is aggravated by motion and is more pronounced at night. Neighboring subcutaneous tissues become swollen, and the overlying skin may appear warm and dusky red. The knees, ankles, wrists, elbows, and metacarpophalangeal articulations are most commonly involved, occasionally in an asymmetric fashion.[181] Synovial effusions are frequent, and the character of the fluid is noninflammatory.[181, 182] The fluid is clear and viscous, mucin clot is good to fair, and low leukocyte counts and few neutrophils are seen.[182, 183] Elevated synovial fluid fibrinogen levels have been reported.[184]

These clinical manifestations are not uniform in all patients with hypertrophic osteoarthropathy and are dependent to some extent on the nature of the underlying lesion. Hypertrophic osteoarthropathy due to pulmonary neoplasm is commonly associated with an acute onset of digital clubbing, warmth and burning of the fingertips, and occasionally skin thickening and hyperhidrosis. Joint findings appear in approximately 30 to 35 per cent of cases, and may precede pulmonary symptoms and signs. Hypertrophic osteoarthropathy associated with other disorders may be characterized by an insidious onset of digital clubbing; arthritis, skin thickening, and hyperhidrosis may be mild or absent.

In cases of hypertrophic osteoarthropathy secondary to intrathoracic causes, thoracotomy frequently leads to prominent remission of the joint symptoms and signs within 24 hours, although radiographic findings may recede more slowly, requiring a period of months to years for complete resolution. Even patients with nonresectable tumors may benefit from thoracotomy. Other surgical procedures that can lead to a regression of the clinical manifestations include hilar neurectomy, vagotomy, and ipsilateral occlusion of the pulmonary artery.[217] Radiotherapy or chemotherapy[300] may be associated with similar improvement.[185, 289] Additionally, clinical relief has been recorded utilizing intercostal nerve section, hypophysectomy, and even laparotomy.[186, 187, 218, 219] Chemical vagotomy may also have beneficial results.[304, 305] Regrowth of the neoplasm is commonly associated with exacerbation of the clinical and radiographic findings.[148, 188]

Radiographic Abnormalities

Periosteal bone deposition initially appears in the proximal and distal diaphyses of the tibiae, fibulae, radii, ulnae, and (less frequently) the femora, humeri, metacarpals, metatarsals, and phalanges (with the exception of the terminal phalanges) (Fig. 81–21). With progression, periostitis becomes prominent in the metaphyseal regions as well as at musculotendinous insertions, but does not extend into the epiphyses. Furthermore, a more widespread skeletal distribution can become apparent that is generally symmetric in nature. Rarely, radiographic abnormalities may be detected in the scapulae, clavicles, ribs, spine, and even the cranium and facial bones, although involvement at these latter sites is more obvious on scintigraphic examination (see discussion later in this chapter).

Various types of periostitis are seen: simple elevation of the periosteum with a radiolucent area between the periosteal bone and subjacent cortex; laminated or "onion-skin" appearance, with smooth layers of new bone formation; irregular areas of periosteal elevation; irregular, solid areas of periosteal cloaking with a wavy contour; and cortical thickening, with application of the periosteal bone to the outer surface of the cortex.[142] In fact, the appearance of the periostitis changes during the course of the process. Initially, it may present as a single layer of new bone that is separate from the

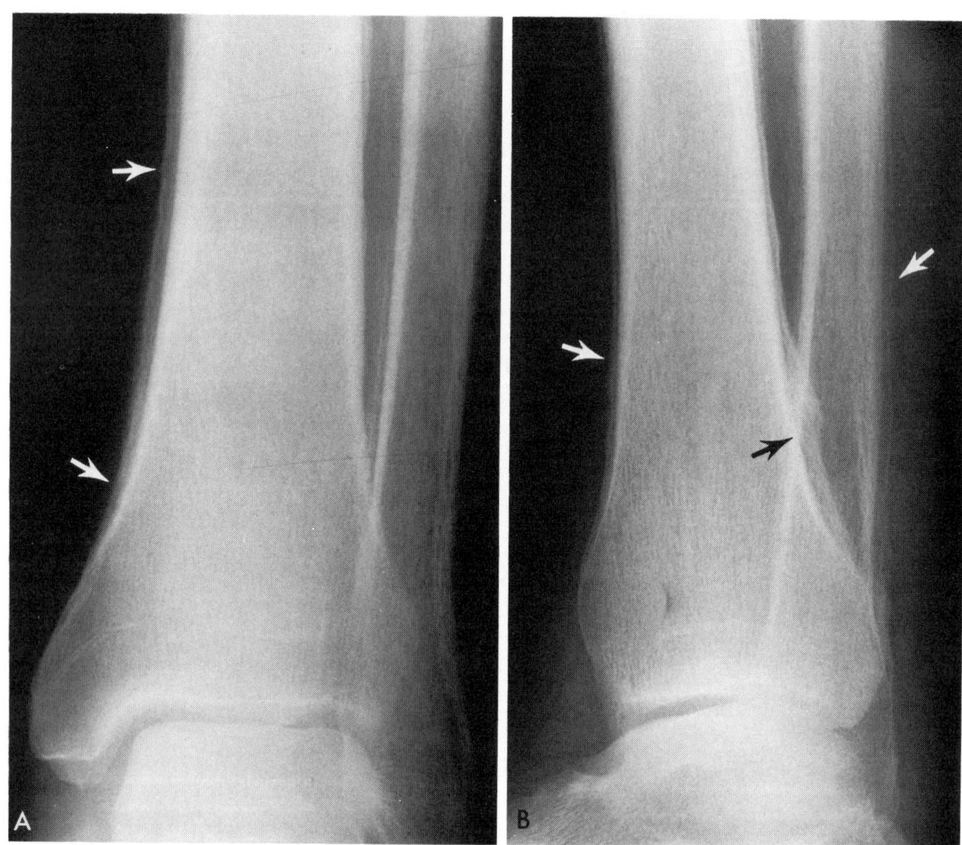

Figure 81–21. Secondary hypertrophic osteoarthropathy: Periostitis.

A, B *Distal tibia and fibula. Elevation of the periosteal membrane in the diaphyses of these bones has resulted in linear deposition of new bone (arrows). Involvement ends at the metaphyses.*

Illustration continued on the opposite page

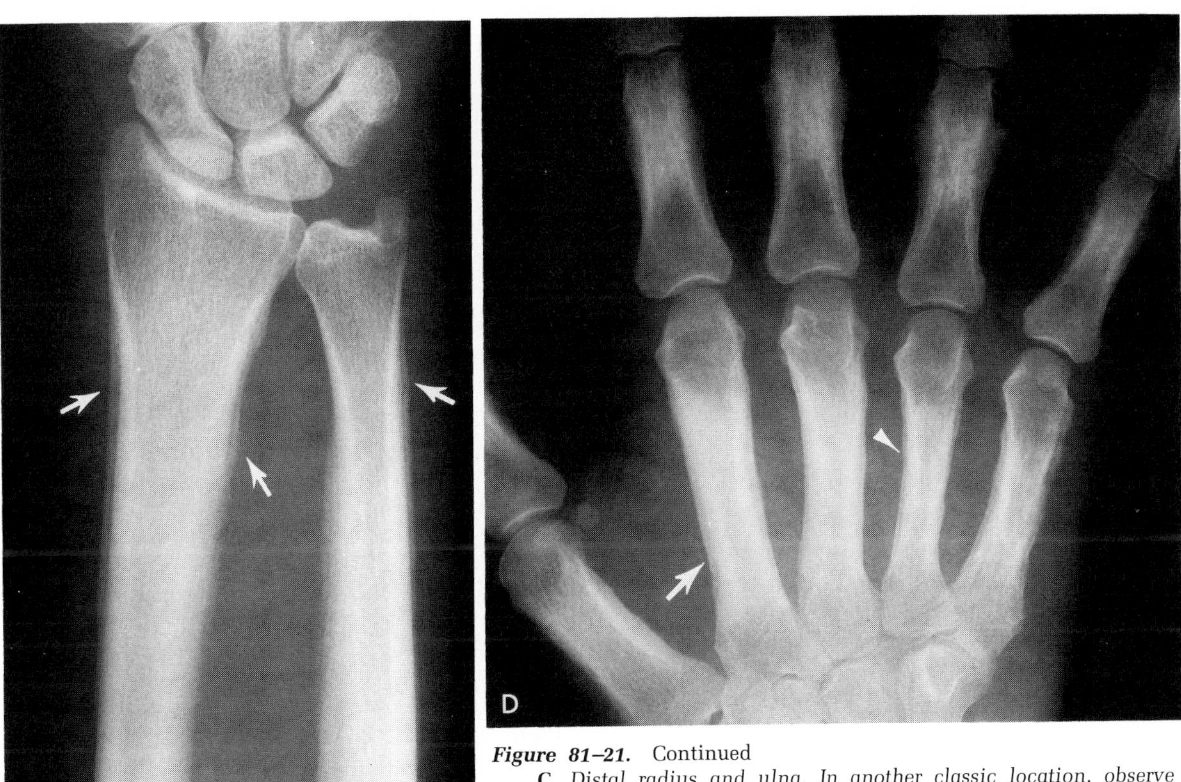

Figure 81–21. Continued

C *Distal radius and ulna. In another classic location, observe linear periostitis of the diaphysis extending to the metaphysis of both bones (arrows).*

D *Metacarpals and phalanges. Linear periostitis of the metacarpals has produced bone that is either separated from (arrowhead) or firmly merged with (arrow) the underlying osseous tissue. Bony proliferation at muscular insertions of the phalanges is also seen. Note some degree of periarticular osteoporosis.*

Illustration continued on the following page

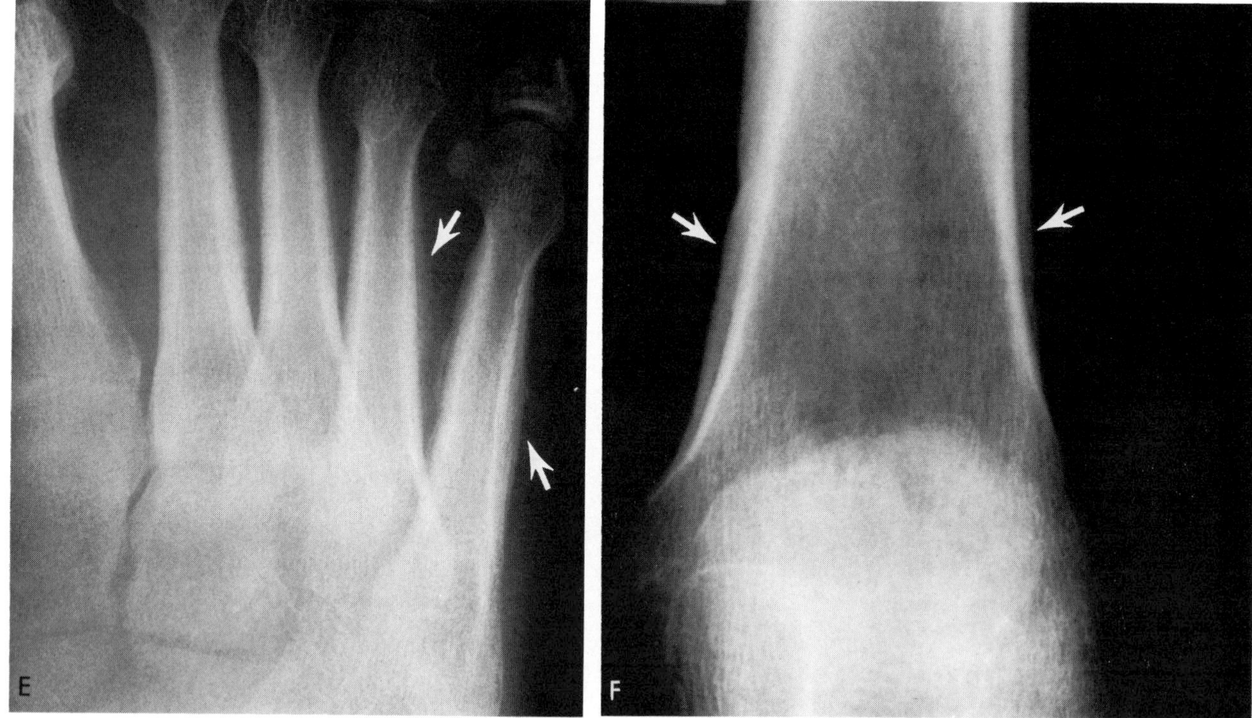

Figure 81–21. Continued

E *Metatarsals. New bone is evident along the diaphyses of multiple metatarsals (arrows).*

F *Femur. Observe thick linear periosteal bone formation on the medial and lateral aspects of the femur (arrows). The endosteal surface of the cortex is not affected.*

subjacent osseous structures. Subsequently, with exacerbations and remissions of the underlying disease, layered new bone formation can be evident, eventually merging with the cortical bone.

Digital clubbing leading to radiographically detectable soft tissue swelling is also evident. The finding is nonspecific, and on rare occasions may be associated with focal areas of tuftal resorption (Fig. 81–22).

Pathologic Abnormalities

Prior to the deposition of new bone by the periosteum, its outer or fibrous layer is the site of round cell infiltration.[50, 136, 189] Proliferation of the inner or cambium layer follows, leading to deposition of new bone on the original cortex (Fig. 81–23). Initially, the osseous deposits are separated from the

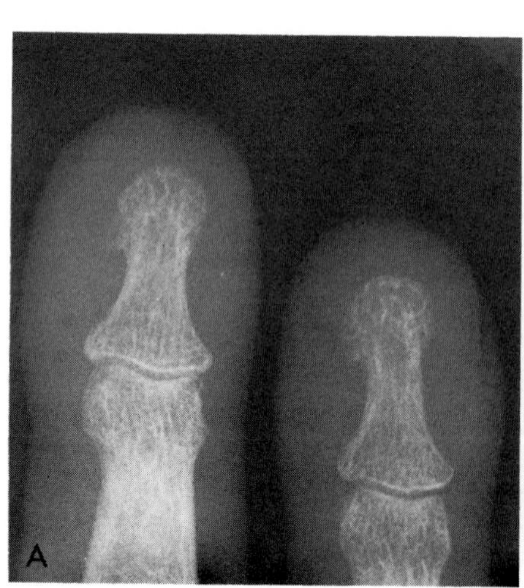

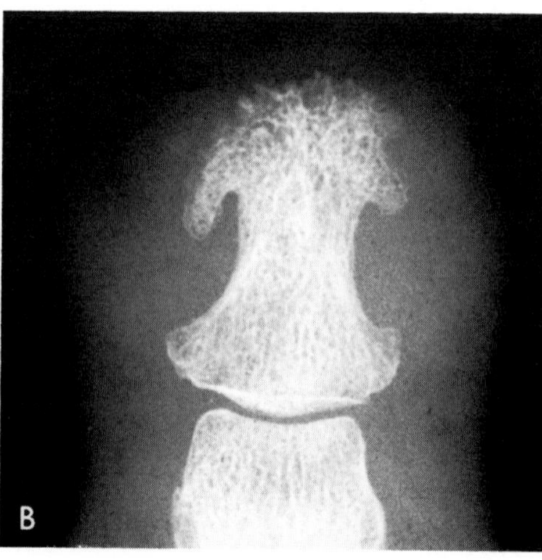

Figure 81–22. *Secondary hypertrophic osteoarthropathy: Digital clubbing.*

A *Soft tissue prominence represents the radiographic counterpart of clinically evident clubbing. Minor resorption of the tuft of the third digit is seen.*

B *In another patient, the soft tissue swelling and osseous resorption are more prominent.*

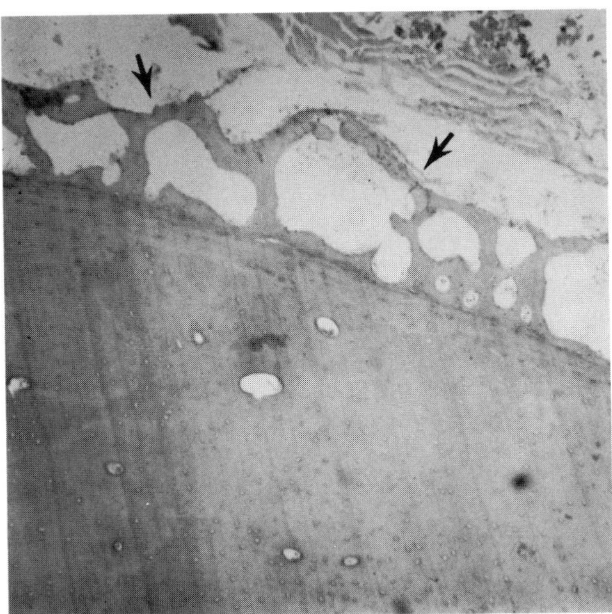

Figure 81–23. *Secondary hypertrophic osteoarthropathy: Pathologic abnormalities. Note the lace-like deposition of bone (arrows) beneath the periosteum, which is uniting with the underlying cortex.*

cortex and are composed predominantly of meshy trabeculae or coarse-fibered tissue.[50] As the deposits become more extensive, their deeper part becomes lamellar in character and the cortical bone may reveal focal areas of porosity. Eventually a clear demarcation between the periosteal and cortical bone is no longer identifiable. Endosteal deposition of bone is not apparent, a fact that is helpful in the accurate diagnosis of the radiographic and pathologic findings.

Holling and Brodey[144] have argued that descriptions of pathologic abnormalities in hypertrophic osteoarthropathy concentrate too heavily on the bone lesions. These investigators cite experimental studies in dogs in which exuberant new bone formation is preceded by an intense overgrowth of vascular connective tissue in portions of the affected limbs. This newly formed tissue surrounds tendons, bones, and even joints. Studies in humans reveal similar findings of newly formed vascular tissue investing osseous and periarticular structures; this tissue is composed of collagenous bundles supplied with many thick-walled blood vessels, often containing perivascular collections of lymphocytes.[136]

Articular Abnormalities

Pain and swelling about the knees, ankles, wrists, and even the fingers may be the presenting manifestation of hypertrophic osteoarthropathy,[182] simulating the clinical presentation of rheumatoid arthritis.[190, 191] This clinical dilemma is accentuated by the presence of soft tissue swelling, joint effusions, and periarticular osteoporosis on radiographic examination, and (rarely) by the simultaneous occurrence of true rheumatoid disease.[192] In hypertrophic osteoarthropathy, the predilection for large joint involvement with relative sparing of the interphalangeal articulations[193] as well as the absence of inflammatory synovial fluid on aspiration and an inflammatory synovial membrane on biopsy permits its differentiation from rheumatoid arthritis. However, early reports of synovial membrane histology cited evidence of chronic synovitis with fibrinoid degeneration, subsynovial congestion, cellular infiltration with lymphocytes, plasma cells, and histiocytes, and some degree of hyperplasia of synovial lining cells.[136] Even pannus formation and fibrous and bony ankylosis were noted in some specimens.[180] In hypertrophic osteoarthropathy secondary to congenital heart disease and cirrhosis, synovial biopsies have also demonstrated mild chronic inflammation[162] as well as synovial calcification.[194] Despite these reports, many investigators agree that considerable synovial inflammation is not a feature of hypertrophic osteoarthropathy, although increased inflammation could perhaps develop in disease of long duration[150, 182] (Fig. 81–24). Schumacher,[182] utilizing electron microscopic examination of the synovial membrane, detected electron-dense deposits in the vessel walls and prominent, fibrin-like material on the synovial surface, in the interstitium, and in some of the dense deposits. He speculated that the dense material arrived at the joint via the circulation, and that the prominent fibrin collections could have resulted from a microvascular injury to the synovial membrane allowing leakage of molecular weight proteins from the injured vessels.

In any case, it is generally regarded that the joint manifestations of hypertrophic osteoarthropathy are not specific, nor are they as inflammatory in nature as the changes in rheumatoid arthritis. In experimental hypertrophic osteoarthropathy, specific articular findings also are not detectable.[195] Articular space narrowing, marginal and central erosions (as noted in patients with rheumatoid arthritis), and osseous excrescences and bony ankylosis (seen in patients with primary hypertrophic osteoarthropathy) are not found in individuals with secondary hypertrophic osteoarthropathy.

Radionuclide Abnormalities

Radionuclide bone imaging represents a highly sensitive method of detecting abnormalities of hypertrophic osteoarthropathy.[196-203] A diffuse, symmetric increased uptake in the diaphyses and metaphyses of tubular bones along their cortical margins creates a distinctive "double stripe" or

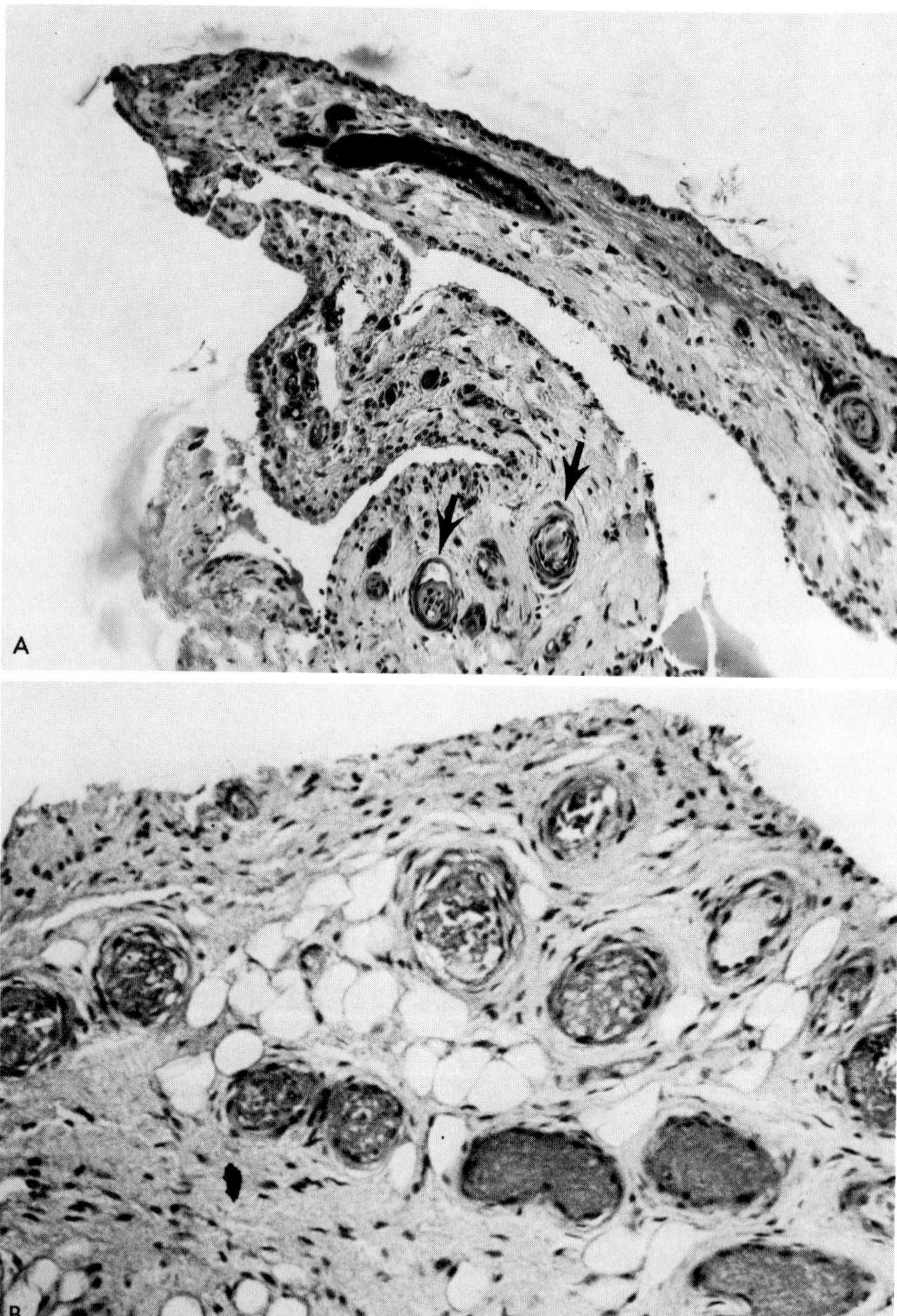

Figure 81–24. *Secondary hypertrophic osteoarthropathy: Articular abnormalities.*

A *Observe old thrombi (arrows) in several small vessels of the synovial villi (90×).*

B *Marked congestion of small synovial vessels is unassociated with inflammatory cellular infiltration (180×).*

(From Schumacher HR Jr: Arthritis Rheum 19:629, 1976.)

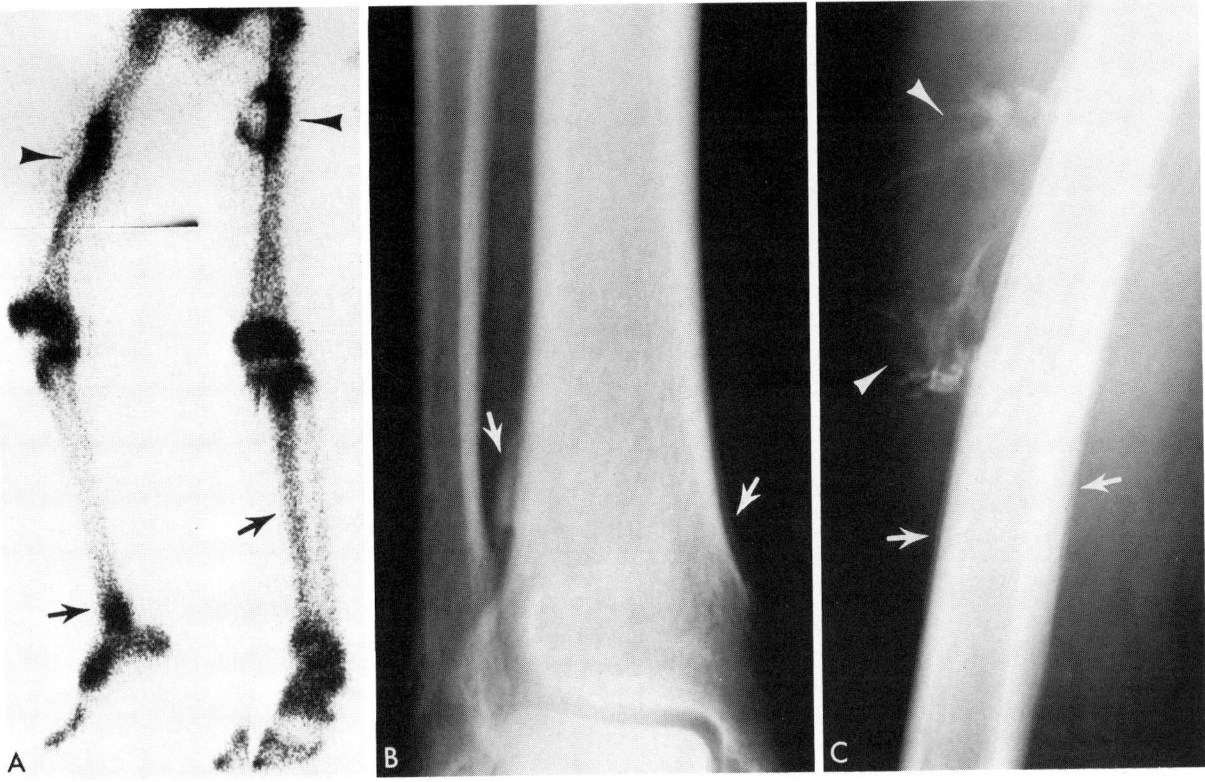

Figure 81–25. Secondary hypertrophic osteoarthropathy: Radionuclide abnormalities. This man presented with bilateral painful masses of the thigh and an abnormal chest x-ray. Biopsy of both the pulmonary and appendicular skeletal lesions confirmed the presence of bronchogenic carcinoma with metastasis.

A The radionuclide study utilizing technetium indicates diffuse uptake in the diaphyses and metaphyses of the tubular bones, most marked about the ankles and in the tibiae (arrows). Focal accumulations are evident in both femora (arrowheads).

B A radiograph of the distal right leg reveals periosteal proliferation (arrows) indicative of hypertrophic osteoarthropathy.

C The bizarre lesion of the left midfemur (arrowheads) consisting of soft tissue swelling and ossification represents the site of a metastatic focus. A similar lesion was evident on the other side. Note periostitis (arrows) compatible with hypertrophic osteoarthropathy.

"parallel track" sign. Associated synovitis can lead to increased radionuclide uptake in periarticular regions also. Unusual alterations include accumulation of radiopharmaceuticals in the clavicles, scapulae, pelvis, and bones of the face, asymmetric uptake, and digital accumulation related to clubbing.[199, 204, 302]

The scintigraphic abnormalities frequently appear before the roentgenographic findings, correspond well with clinical manifestations, and decrease following appropriate therapeutic regimens, such as surgery and radiation therapy. Occasionally, they may disappear without any treatment.[203] Recurrence of a tumor is followed by the return of an abnormal radionuclide pattern. Although an accumulation of radiopharmaceuticals in the patient with malignant tumor can also represent evidence of skeletal metastasis, differentiation of the scintigraphic patterns in hypertrophic osteoarthropathy and in metastasis is not difficult (Fig. 81–25). Asymmetry, focal areas of increased activity, and prominent involvement of the axial skeleton and medullary spaces characterize the radionuclide abnormalities of metastatic disease involving the skeleton.[197, 198]

Pathogenesis

Since the early description of hypertrophic osteoarthropathy by Bamberger[138] and Marie,[98] numerous theories have been proposed to explain the pathogenesis of the condition, none of which is entirely adequate. Marie[98] believed that the primary disease elaborated a chemical irritant that, when absorbed, led to the osseous lesions. Other investigators also postulated the presence of a toxic substance that initiated a periosteal response.[205, 206] The humoral theory has been further developed through the years, and has been encouraged by the detection of high urinary output of certain steroid metabolites in patients with hypertrophic osteoarthopathy.[211, 212]

However, some evidence, including the inability to produce hypertrophic osteoarthropathy in normal dogs following cross-circulation with affected dogs, has suggested that other factors are more important.[144]

A neurogenic mechanism in this condition has gained increasing support from the observation that prompt relief of symptoms and signs can follow surgical disruption of the vagus nerve.[187, 207] Vagal nerve interruption apparently reduces the increased blood flow that is present in cases of secondary hypertrophic osteoarthropathy.[208] It is postulated that neural impulses arise in the pulmonary or pleural lesion and pass as afferent impulses in the vagus nerve. Similar afferent pathways may exist when the causative lesion is located in certain additional viscera; in fact, many of the organs in which primary diseases lead to secondary hypertrophic osteoarthropathy are supplied by fibers from either the ninth or tenth cranial nerves.[213] The efferent pathways have not been delineated; denervation of affected limbs or high spinal anesthesia are without significant effect, either on clinical manifestations or limb blood flow. Sympathetic nerve activity appears to be unimportant, since sympathectomy produces little effect. Anticholinergic medication also has no effect, suggesting that vagal or other parasympathetic efferent nerves are not involved. If and when the efferent limb of the arc can be fully delineated, the attractiveness of the neurogenic theory will increase dramatically.

The importance of increased blood flow in the pathogenesis of periostitis in hypertrophic osteoarthropathy has been emphasized. Pathologic studies of clubbed digits have outlined dilatation of vessels and dense neovascularity. The newly formed vascular channels envelop bones and joints, consisting of wide, thick-walled vessels, collagenous bundles, and cellular infiltration. Capillary flow studies that have utilized isotope washout rates have indicated increased vascular perfusion of affected areas in secondary hypertrophic osteoarthropathy.[209] Experimentally, periosteal changes can be produced in the dog by establishing a permanent fistula between the left auricle and pulmonary arteries; perhaps these changes are related to constantly excessive peripheral blood volume that increases periosteal nutrition and promotes bone proliferation.[210] A similar increase in blood flow could be expected in humans with cyanotic congenital heart disease and accounts for the clinical findings of warmth and burning that accompany hypertrophic osteoarthropathy. This type of flow consists of excessive blood that is poorly oxygenated and might produce local passive congestion and poor tissue oxygenation, with resulting stimulation of various connective tissues, including the periosteal membrane.[50] However, in most cases of hypertrophic osteoarthropathy, no evidence of arteriovenous shunting in the pulmonary circulation is demonstrated, and the appearance of periostitis in these situations may require the presence of some factor other than deoxygenated blood.

Differential Diagnosis

Periostitis (and clubbing) can also be observed in primary hypertrophic osteoarthropathy (pachydermoperiostosis) and thyroid acropachy (Table 81–4) (Fig. 81–26). In the former condition, the osseous excrescences are more irregular and extend into the epiphyses of the tubular bones. A family history of disease is also evident. In thyroid acropachy, periosteal proliferation has a predilection for the small bones of the hands and feet; significant or isolated abnormalities of the major tubular bones are distinctly unusual. Pretibial myxedema and a history of dysfunction of the thyroid gland are evident.

Chronic venous stasis can produce periostitis, usually confined to the lower extremities (see discussion later in this chapter). Cases of hypertrophic osteoarthropathy involving one or both lower extremities, without involving the upper extremity, have been reported but are very rare.[204, 223-225, 303] Furthermore, the nature of periosteal proliferation in the presence of venous insufficiency is unique.

Additional causes of diffuse periostitis or bone proliferation, such as hypervitaminosis A, infantile cortical hyperostosis, diffuse idiopathic skeletal hyperostosis, or fluorosis are not usually confused with hypertrophic osteoarthropathy.

VASCULAR INSUFFICIENCY

Periosteal bone formation has been noted in association with chronic venous insufficiency.[226-230] The lower extremities are almost exclusively affected, with involvement of the tibia, fibula, femur, metatarsals, and phalanges (Table 81–4). The diaphyseal and metaphyseal segments are predominantly altered, and an undulating osseous contour is produced, with considerable new bone appearing on the outer aspect of the cortex (Figs. 81–27 and 81–28). Although initially separated from the underlying bone, the periosteal deposits soon merge with the cortex.

The incidence of periostitis increases with the severity and duration of the venous insufficiency and may be detected in 10 to 60 per cent of patients with chronic disabling venous stasis.[227, 229, 231, 232] Although many patients also reveal soft tissue ulcerations, these cutaneous abnormalities are not always present in patients with venous periostitis, and the periostitis may be more severe in locations distant from the ulcerations. These observations indicate that infection is not fundamental to the appearance

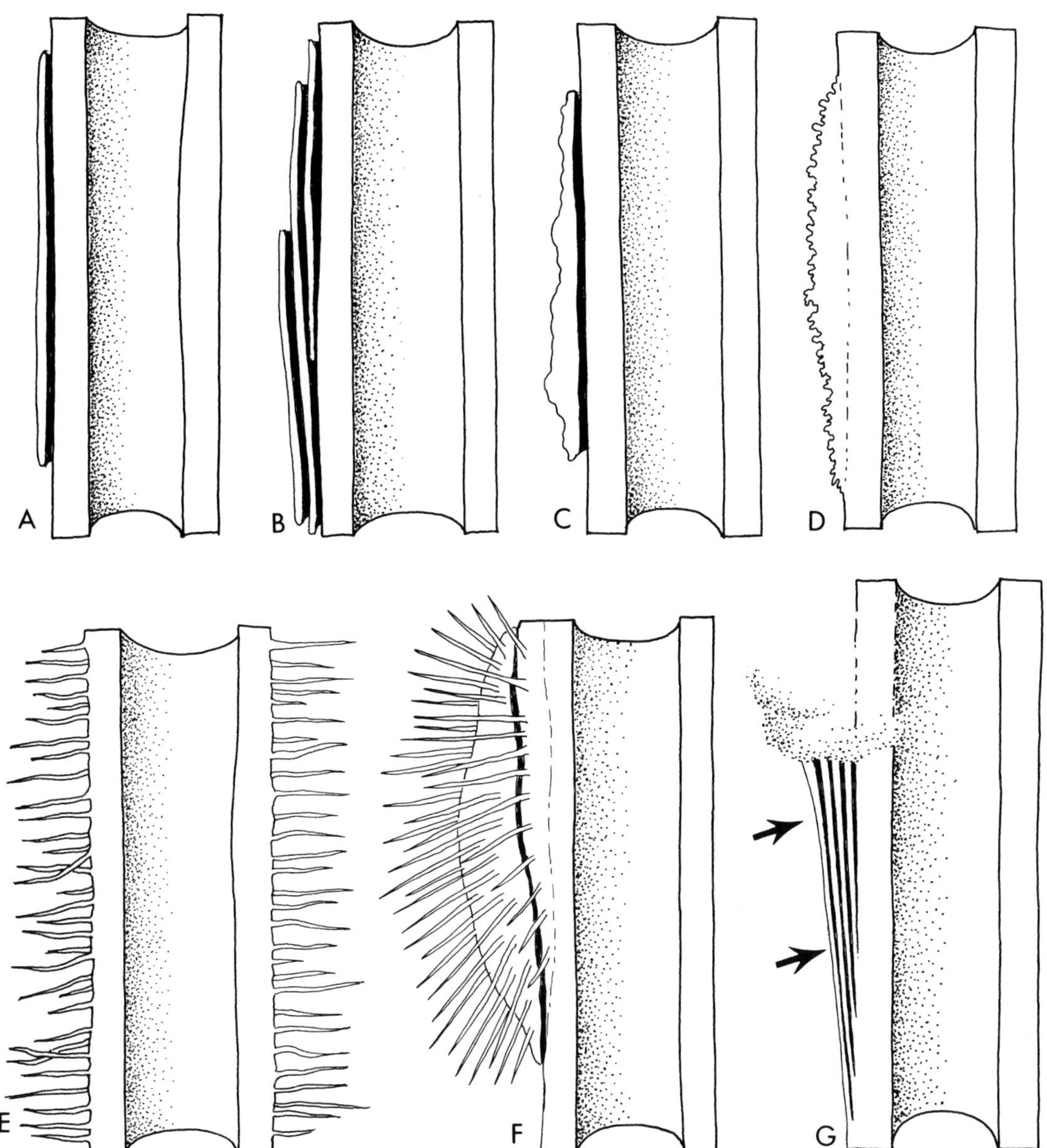

Figure 81–26. *Differential diagnosis of periosteal new bone formation.*

A–G *Various types of periostitis are identified.* **A,** *Single layer of new bone, which may be observed in benign or malignant tumors, infection, and secondary hypertrophic osteoarthropathy.* **B,** *Multiple layers of new bone or "onion-skinning," which can be evident in infection, malignant tumors such as Ewing's sarcoma, hypertrophic osteoarthropathy, and other conditions.* **C,** *A thick linear osseous deposit, which can be separate from (as indicated here) or mixed with the underlying bone. This pattern is common in hypertrophic osteoarthropathy and venous stasis.* **D,** *An irregular osseous excrescence with spiculated contour that merges with the underlying cortex. This pattern can be observed in thyroid acropachy or primary hypertrophic osteoarthropathy (pachydermoperiostosis).* **E,** *Thin, linear osseous deposits that extend in a direction perpendicular to the underlying cortex, a pattern that is highly characteristic of Ewing's sarcoma.* **F,** *A "sunburst" pattern, in which linear deposits fan out from a single focus, an appearance that can be evident in osteogenic sarcoma.* **G,** *A Codman's triangle, consisting of triangular elevation of the periosteum with one or more layers of new bone (arrows), a pattern that is suggestive but not diagnostic of malignancy.*

Illustration continued on the following page

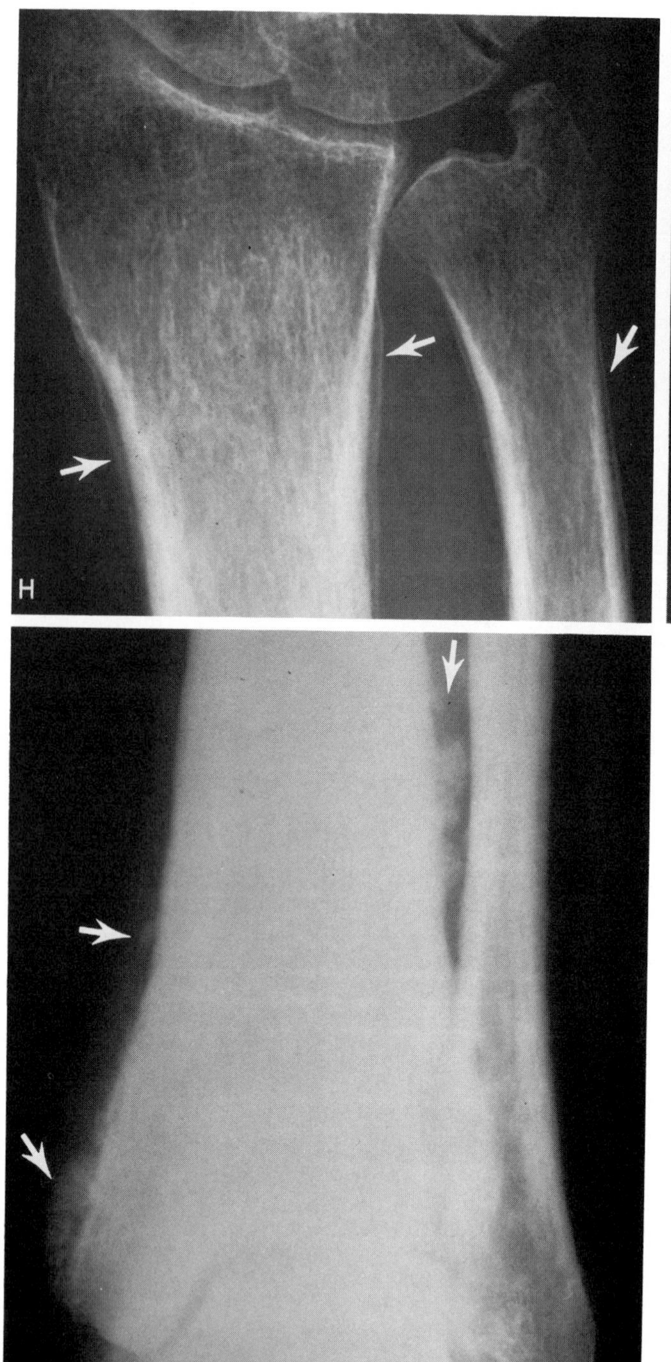

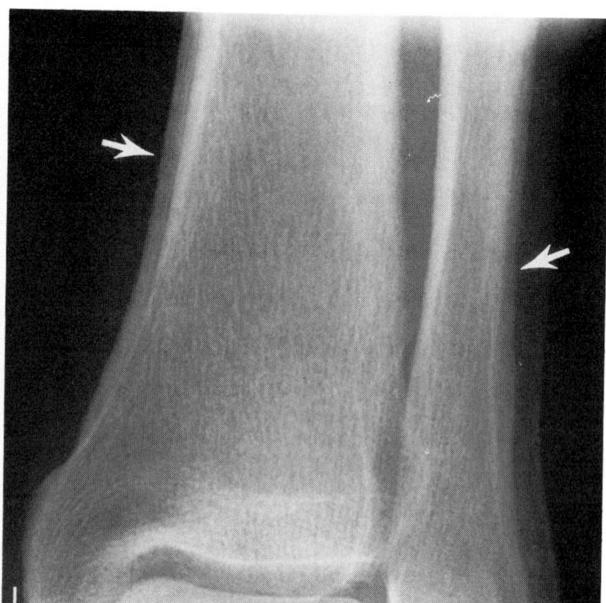

Figure 81–26. Continued

H *A single layer of periosteal bone (arrows), corresponding to pattern* **A**, *is evident in this patient with secondary hypertrophic osteoarthropathy.*

I *A thick single layer of new bone (arrows) that is merging with the subjacent tibia and fibula, corresponding to pattern* **C**, *is seen in this patient with secondary hypertrophic osteoarthropathy.*

J *Irregular osseous excrescences (arrows) merging with the underlying bone, corresponding to pattern* **D**, *is apparent in this patient with primary hypertrophic osteoarthropathy (pachydermoperiostosis).*

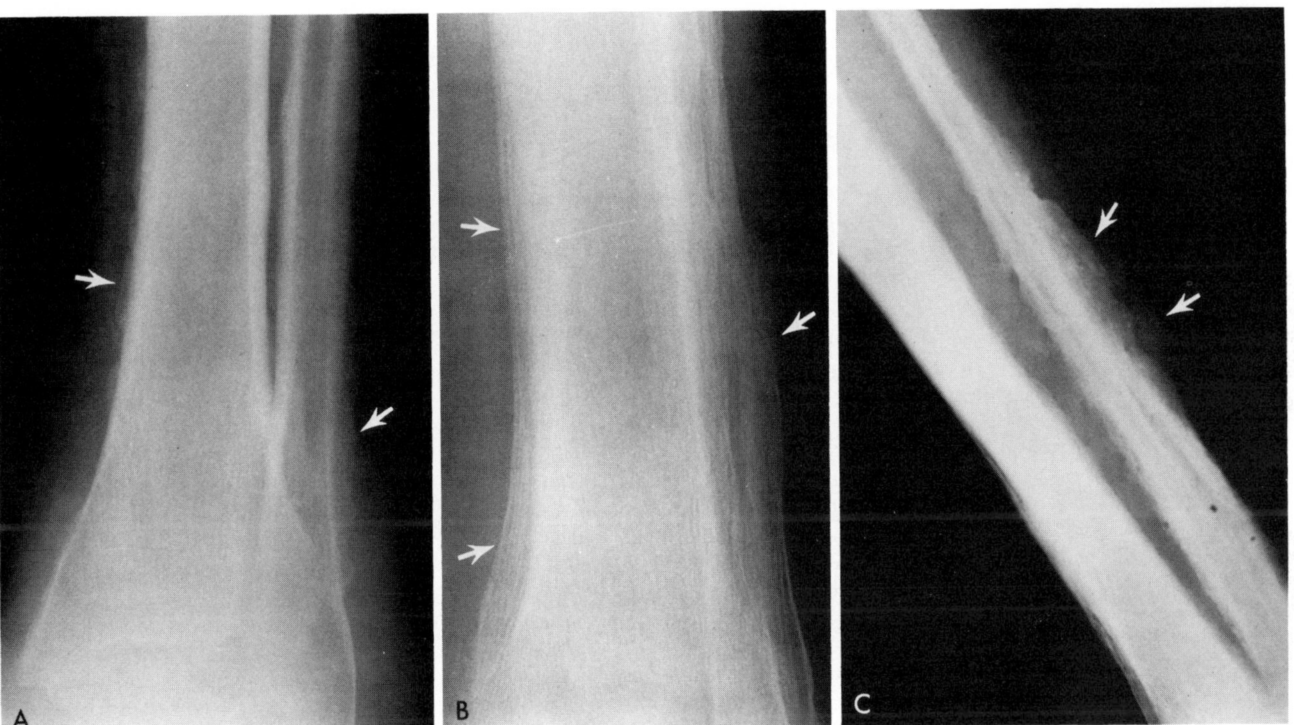

Figure 81–27. Chronic venous stasis: Periostitis.

A *Observe undulating periosteal new bone on the diaphyses and metaphyses of the distal tibia and fibula (arrows). Soft tissue edema is present.*

B *In this individual, a laminated or solid coat of periosteal bone surrounds the distal tibia and fibula (arrows).*

C *A more nodular and irregular appearance of periosteal bone formation (arrows) characterizes the situation in this patient with chronic venous stasis and soft tissue infection.*

of periosteal proliferation. Similarly, although lymphatic insufficiency may also be noted in some patients with venous periostitis, it, too, does not appear to be a necessary component of the process. The pathogenesis of the periostitis may relate to hypoxia created by vascular stasis or hypertension, but a single mechanism has yet to be substantiated.

Soft tissue edema and ossification represent roentgenographic findings that are commonly associated with venous insufficiency and periostitis (Fig. 81–29). Single or multiple phleboliths may be apparent, and in some cases a diffuse reticular ossific pattern is evident.

Arterial insufficiency has also been associated with periosteal bone proliferation. This may occur in polyarteritis nodosa or other arteritides.[233] Any bone can be affected, but most cases are confined to the lower extremity. The degree of bone formation is

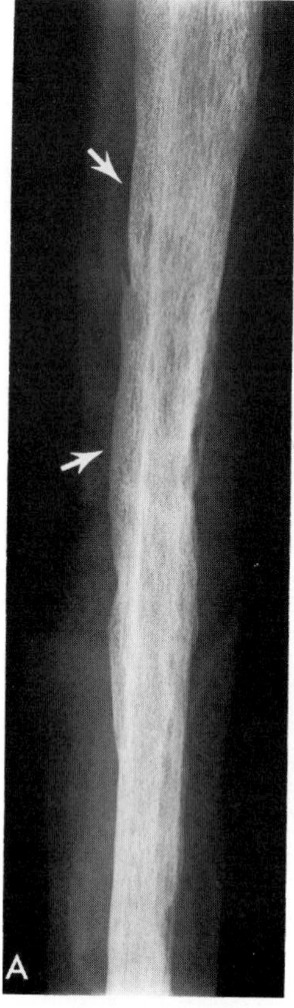

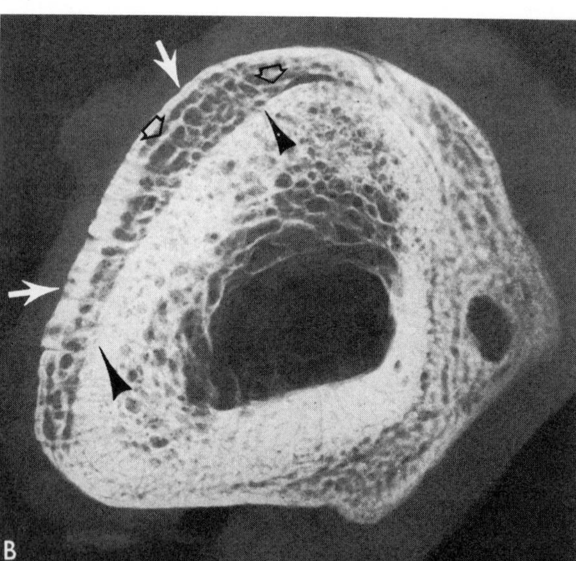

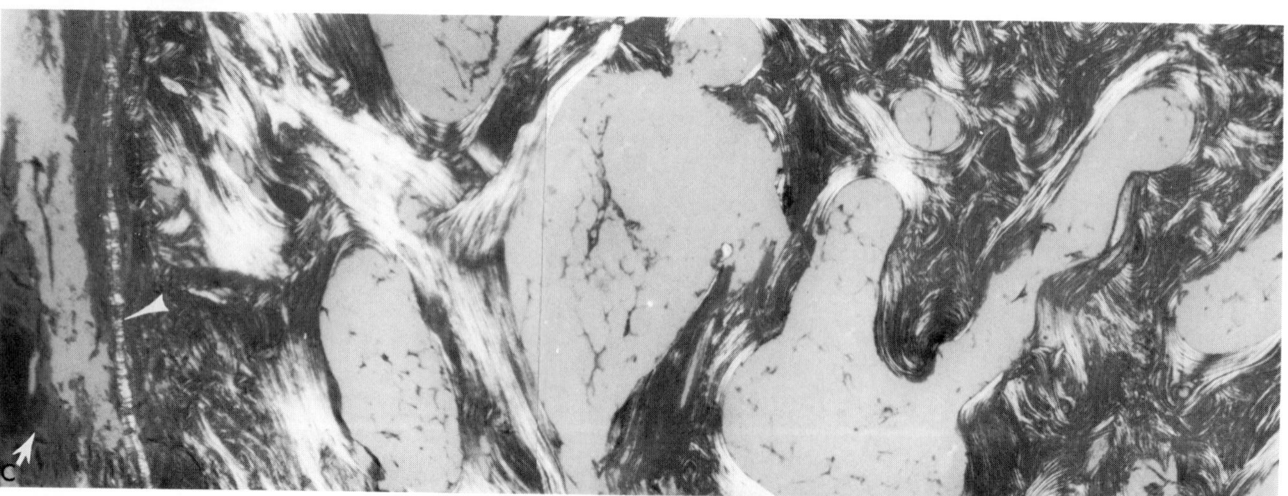

Figure 81–28. Chronic venous stasis: Periostitis.

A *A radiograph of a removed fibula in a patient with venous insufficiency reveals the undulating nature of the periosteal bony deposition (arrows).*

B *A radiograph of a cross section through the upper fibular shaft outlines a ring of new bone (arrows) that has buried the original cortical surface (arrowheads). Note the laminated nature of the bony deposits (open arrows).*

C *On a polarized photomicrograph of the section (72×), note the periosteal fibrous tissue (arrow), periosteum with polarized collagen fibers (arrowhead), and hypertrophic polarized osseous trabeculae.*

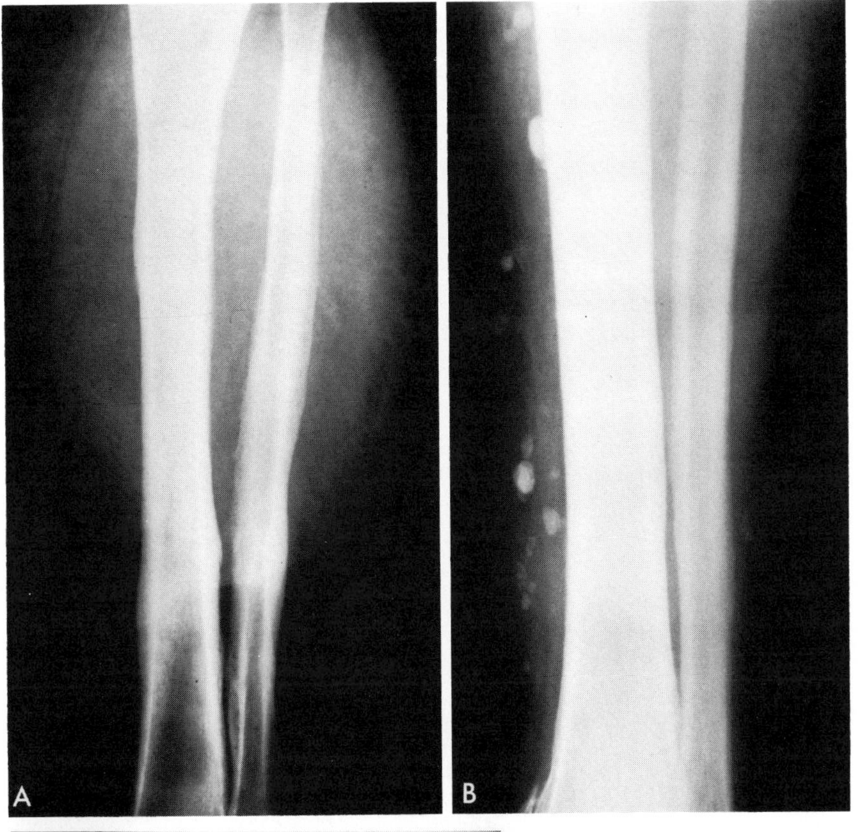

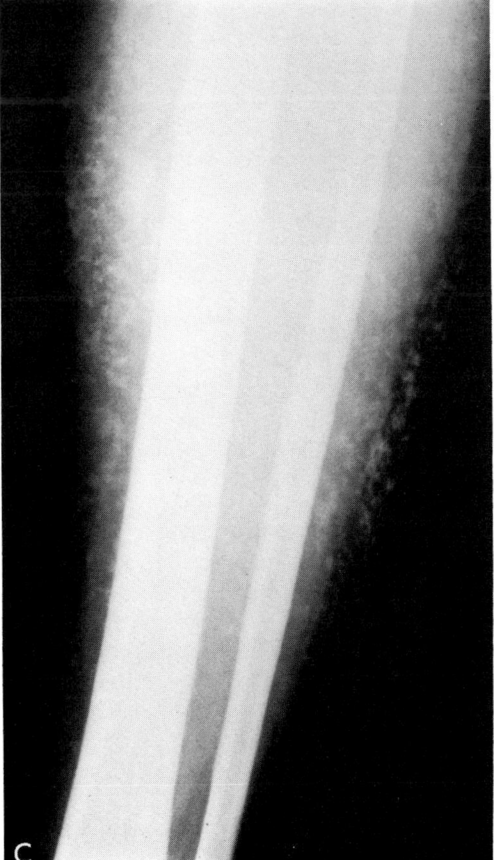

Figure 81–29. *Chronic venous stasis: Soft tissue abnormalities. Examples of soft tissue edema* **(A)**, *phlebolith calcification* **(B)**, *and reticular ossification* **(C)** *are given.*

usually mild, but cases with exuberant periostitis have been reported.

INFANTILE CORTICAL HYPEROSTOSIS

Infantile cortical hyperostosis (Caffey's disease) is an uncommon disease, usually commencing in infancy, that affects predominantly the skeleton and adjacent fascial, muscular, and connective tissues.[234] It was first reported as a distinct entity in 1945 by Caffey and Silverman[235] and in 1946 by Smyth and co-workers.[236] Infantile cortical hyperostosis has a worldwide distribution, is evident in all racial strains, and affects boys and girls with approximately equal frequency.

Clinical Abnormalities

Almost without exception, the disease becomes evident in an infant less than 5 months of age; it may be apparent in the first days or weeks of life, and has even been recognized in utero.[237, 238] The average age of onset is 9 to 10 weeks. Familial instances of the disease are recognized,[239-243] although most cases are sporadic. Fever of abrupt onset, hyperirritability, and soft tissue swelling are typical. The swelling is especially prominent over the mandible, but can also appear at other sites. On palpation, indurated, hard, and tender soft tissue masses are noted, and these may be attached to the underlying bones. Such swelling reflects the soft tissue extension of periosteal reaction in the underlying bone, although it may antedate radiographic evidence of osseous abnormality. Discoloration and warmth are not evident. Subsidence of the soft tissue process is slow, and at any time it may recur at the original site or at a new location.

Additional clinical features may include pallor, painful pseudoparalysis, and pleurisy.[234] Laboratory analysis may indicate an elevated erythrocyte sedimentation rate and an elevated serum level of alkaline phosphatase, a moderate leukocytosis, and anemia.

The clinical course is extremely variable. In many instances, clinical and radiographic features subside slowly over a period of a few months to a few years, but this self-limited quality is not uniform. Occasionally, active disease may persist, recurring intermittently for years, and leading to a marked delay in musculoskeletal development and crippling deformities.[234] Thus, residua of the disease may be evident even in the third and fourth decades of life.[234-248] In these instances, mandibular asymmetry,[235, 249] interosseous bony bridges,[247, 250, 251] and bowing of the limbs[239-240] can be observed.[242] Rarely, a severely affected infant will die, usually as a result of a secondary infection.[50, 252-254]

Radiographic Abnormalities

In any one patient, a single bone or many bones can be involved (Table 81–4). Sequential involvement is typical, with one area being affected initially, followed in later stages of the disease by changes in other sites. The mandible, clavicles, and ribs are more often involved, and changes in these bones may be symmetric[255] (Fig. 81–30). Thoracic cage abnormalities can be combined with pleural effusions. The scapulae are altered in approximately 10 per cent of cases, and involvement at this site may be monostotic or unilateral, exuberant, and associated with neurologic deficit and diaphragmatic elevation[256-258, 307] (Fig. 81–31). Changes in the ilia, cranial vault (parietal and frontal regions), and tubular bones are also encountered.[259] In the tubular bones, asymmetry predominates, and the ulnae are most frequently involved, although changes in the tibiae, fibulae, humeri, femora, radii, metacarpals, and metatarsals may be seen[234, 260] (Fig. 81–32). Alterations of the vertebrae, carpus, tarsus, and phalanges are unusual.

Cortical hyperostosis is the hallmark of the disease. New bone formation begins in the soft tissue swelling directly contiguous to the original cortex, becomes progressively more dense, and may reach profound proportions. Thus, the deposits of bone merge with the underlying osseous tissue, doubling or tripling the normal width of the parent bone. Predilection for the lateral arches of the ribs and the diaphyses and metaphyses of tubular bones is evident. The epiphyseal ossification centers are generally spared. The endosteal surfaces can also undergo new bone formation, resulting in diminution of the medullary cavity.

Destructive lesions of the skull have been identified in some cases.[234, 262, 263] These may be single or multiple, unilateral or bilateral; they may have a predilection for the frontal squamosa, and may simulate histiocytosis or metastatic neuroblastoma. The lesions probably relate to focal resorption of peripheral layers of the cortex.

Radiographic improvement can occur in a period of weeks to months, to an extent that evidence of hyperostosis may be entirely lacking on follow-up examinations after 6 months to 1 year. During healing, the cortical thickening may become lamellated with increased porosity, and the medullary canal can widen. Residual changes can be encountered, such as diaphyseal expansion, longitudinal overgrowth and bowing deformities, osseous bridging between adjacent bones such as the radius and ulna, tibia and fibula, and ribs, exophthalmos, and facial asymmetry[261] (Fig. 81–33).

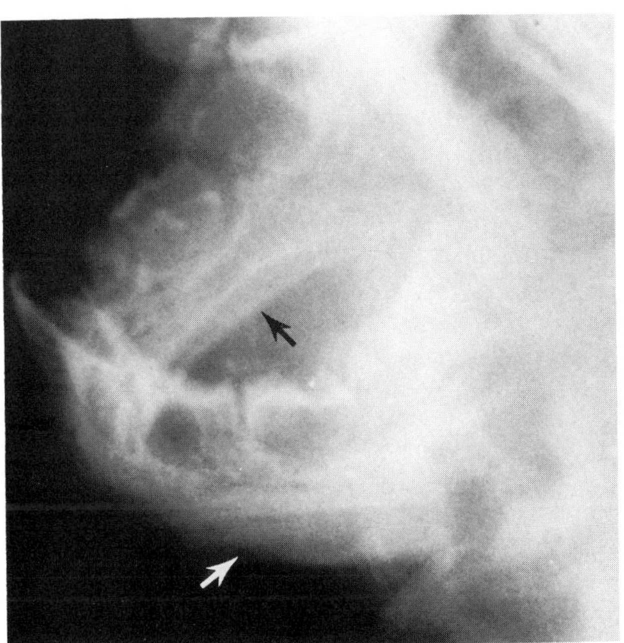

Figure 81–30. *Infantile cortical hyperostosis: Mandible. Observe diffuse periosteal proliferation of the mandible (arrows).*

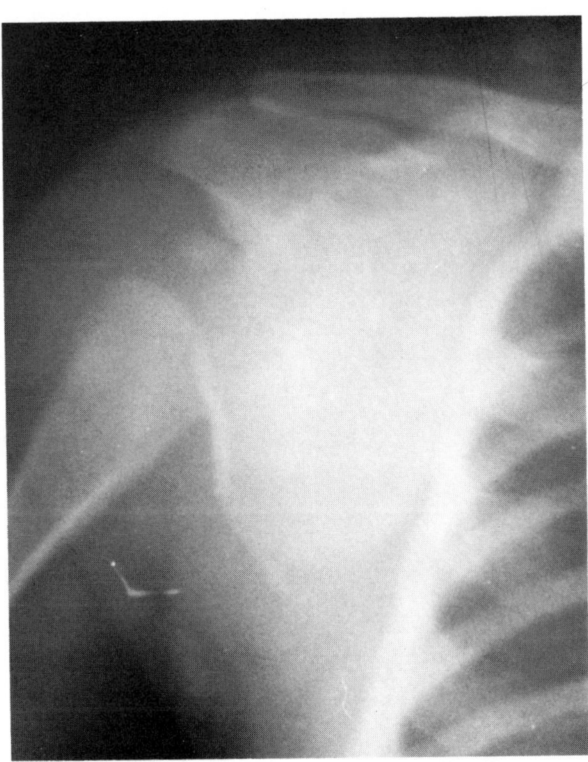

Figure 81–31. *Infantile cortical hyperostosis: Scapula. Monostotic scapular disease has resulted in exuberant bone formation and considerable deformity and enlargement.*

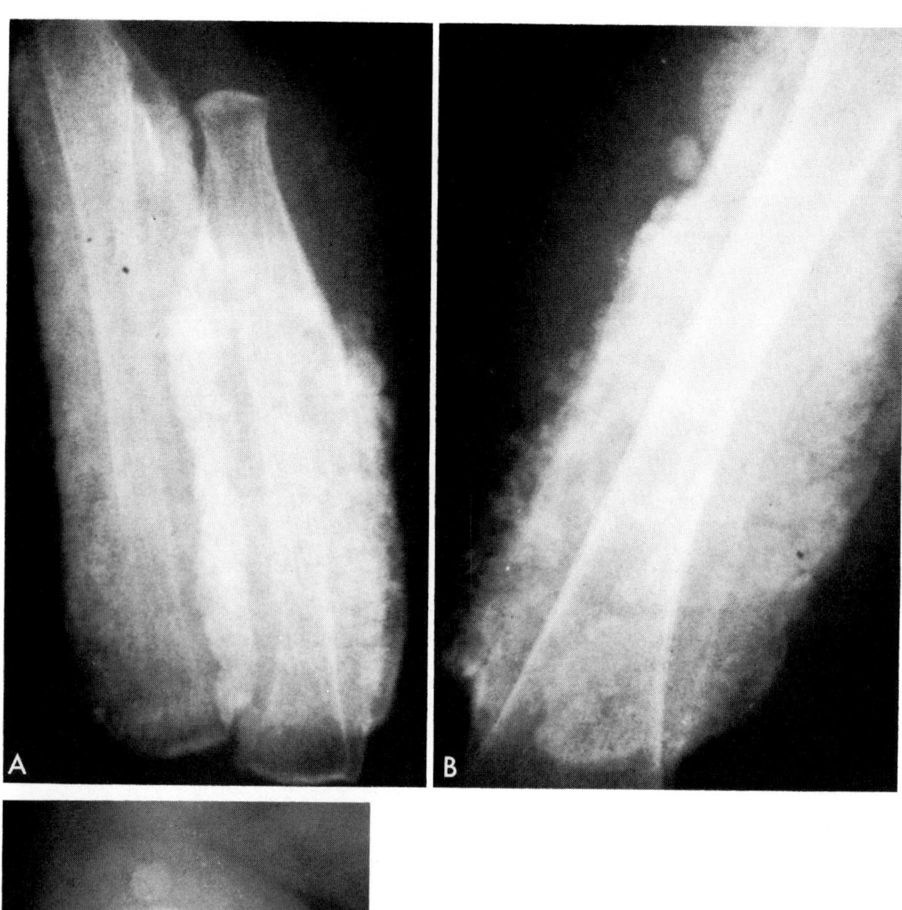

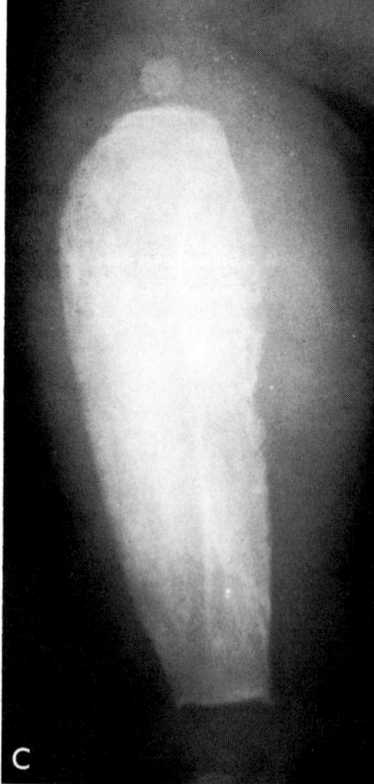

Figure 81–32. *Infantile cortical hyperostosis: Tubular bones. Examples of radial and ulnar* **(A)**, *femoral* **(B)**, *and tibial* **(C)** *involvement are shown. The extent of new bone formation is remarkable. These deposits are initially evident in the soft tissues and later merge with the underlying bone.*

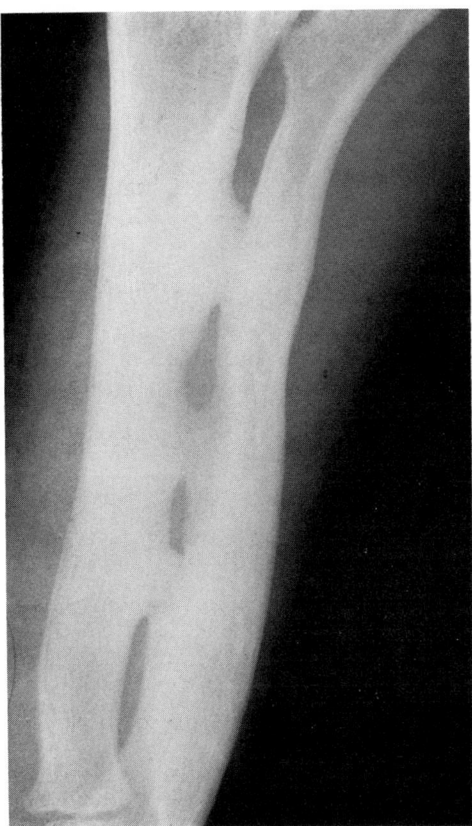

Figure 81–33. *Infantile cortical hyperostosis: Residual changes. In this child, residual enlargement and deformity of the radius and ulna with interosseous bridging are apparent.*

Pathologic Abnormalities

Caffey[234] has reviewed in detail the pathologic data contained in previous descriptions of this disease[264] (Fig. 81–34). In the early stage, acute inflammatory changes appear in the periosteal membrane, consisting of edema and cellular infiltration with polymorphonuclear leukocytes. The thickened and inflamed membrane loses its peripheral limiting fibrous layer, blending with the adjacent fasciae, tendons, and muscles. Proliferation of connective tissue cells and of osteoblasts indicates considerable activity. Cortical resorption and porosity can be identified in this phase. In the subacute phase, inflammatory changes diminish. Beneath the periosteum, a layer of immature, coarse-fibered trabeculae of variable thickness becomes identifiable[50]; between trabeculae, vascularized connective tissue appears. In the late phases, the peripheral bone is removed, beginning in the interior and extending peripherally. Thus, dilatation of the medullary cavity is seen, with subsequent remodeling and shrinkage of the dilated, thin-walled bone shaft.

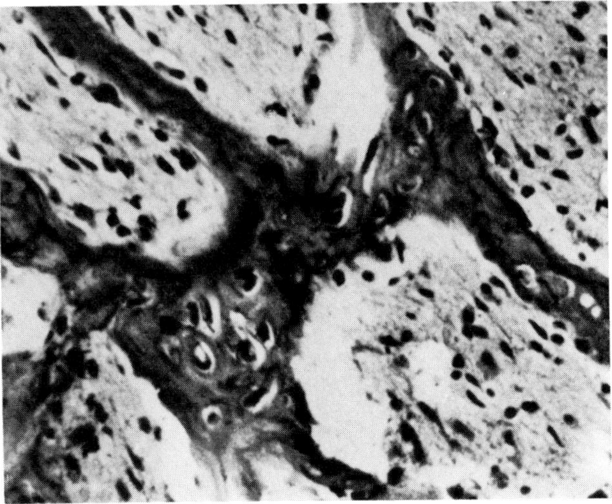

Figure 81–34. *Infantile cortical hyperostosis: Pathologic abnormalities. A photomicrograph (270×) of a biopsy of an involved bone indicates striking new bone formation and an inflammatory reaction characterized by acute and chronic cellular infiltration. (From Kaufmann HJ, Skel Radiol 2:109, 1977.)*

The involvement of adjacent soft tissue has been emphasized in these early reports. The presence of intimal proliferation of the small arteries in both the fascial and osseous lesions has suggested to some investigators that hypoxia may be an initial event that stimulates soft tissue and bone proliferation.[253]

Etiology and Pathogenesis

Although there has been considerable speculation regarding the etiology of infantile cortical hyperostosis, it remains unknown. There are many clinical and pathologic features suggesting that an infectious agent is responsible for the disease. The presence of severe and protracted fever, an elevated erythrocyte sedimentation rate, an occasional pleural exudate in association with thoracic cage lesions, and clustering of cases, both in time and in location, are clinical findings consistent with an infection.[265] The identification of acute inflammatory changes in the periosteum also raises the possibility of an infectious agent. The apparent immunity to recurrence after the initial course of the disease is not unlike that which is evident in certain viral diseases. A viral etiology is also suggested by the demonstration of a virus in the hamster that has affinity for bones, including the mandible,[266] the lack of response to antibiotic therapy and sulfonamides, the alterations in serum proteins that resemble responses to known infections, and the elevation of gamma globulins that is consistent with an in utero viral infection. However, no bacterial or viral agents have yet been identified in the disease, and serologic tests for such agents have also been unsuccessful.

Abnormalities of serum proteins in infantile cortical hyperostosis may also indicate the importance of an altered immune status.[265] This possibility may explain the occurrence of the disease in patients with immunodeficient disorders,[267] although this association could also reflect the proclivity of such individuals to develop infections. Further speculation exists that infantile cortical hyperostosis represents an allergic response to altered collagen tissue.[268] Hyperplasia and fibrinoid degeneration of collagen fibers can be prominent in this disorder, and may promote alterations in the surrounding osseous, muscular, soft tissue, and vascular tissues.

The appearance of infantile cortical hyperostosis in many members of a single family over one or more generations underscores the importance of genetic factors in the pathogenesis of the disease. An autosomal recessive or dominant inheritance may be operational in these patients, and sporadic cases may indicate spontaneous dominant mutation.

Differential Diagnosis

Although periostitis and hyperostosis in an infant can also be observed in rickets and scurvy, the absence of epiphyseal or metaphyseal alterations and the resolution of clinical and roentgenographic features over a period of months in patients with infantile cortical hyperostosis allow its differentiation from these other disorders. Similarly, trauma, including that in the abused child, can lead to calcifying subperiosteal hematomas, but additional findings, such as microfractures and metaphyseal irregularity, are evident. In hypervitaminosis A, clinical and radiographic manifestations initially appear toward the end of the first year of life, metatarsal predilection is apparent, facial swelling and mandibular involvement are rare, and serologic testing indicates an elevation of vitamin A levels. The findings in osteomyelitis, leukemia, neuroblastoma, the kinky hair syndrome, and Camurati-Engelmann disease usually are not hard to differentiate from those of infantile cortical hyperostosis.

HYPEROSTOSIS FRONTALIS INTERNA

Hyperostosis frontalis interna is a descriptive term that is applied to hyperostosis involving predominantly the inner table of the frontal squama. Originally emphasized by Morgagni over 200 years ago,[50] this condition has been further delineated in numerous reports.[269, 270] It is of interest that Morgagni's original patient was an elderly woman with obesity and virulism, and these findings, combined with hyperostosis of the cranial vault, are sometimes referred to as the "Morgagni syndrome" or "metabolic craniopathy."[50] However, this association is neither constant nor frequent, as most individuals with this cranial abnormality fail to reveal significant systemic manifestations.

Hyperostosis frontalis interna is usually observed in patients over the age of 40 years. Women predominate over men,[271] and many of the women are postmenopausal. In fact, Henschen[272] observed some degree of cranial hyperostosis in approximately 40 per cent of postmenopausal women. In these patients, rhizomelic obesity, facial hirsutism, hypertension, headache, depression, anxiety, and historical evidence of menstrual irregularity are common but inconstant findings.[50] Hyperostosis has also been considered a roentgenographic finding in insane patients[273] or an indication of brain loss.[274, 275]

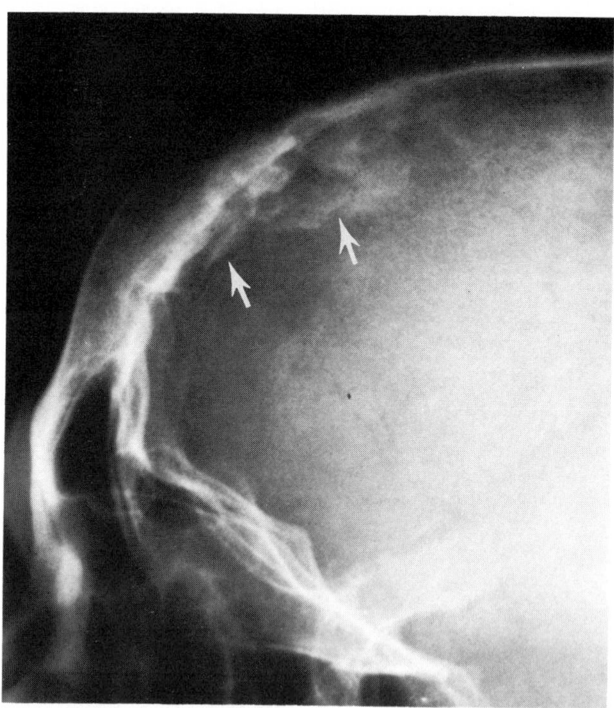

Figure 81–35. *Hyperostosis frontalis interna. Note nodular hyperostosis of the inner table of the frontal bone (arrows).*

Radiographically, the disorder leads to mild to moderate thickening of the inner table that is sessile or nodular in outline (Fig. 81–35). Single or multiple sclerotic patches can progress slowly over a period of many years. The outer cranial contour is not altered, and the position of the superficial veins and longitudinal sinus is not affected. Pathologic examination frequently demonstrates excessive diploic bone, with thinning of either or both of the tables.[50] Bone deposition occurs on the inner table in association with spongy transformation. The roentgenographic findings are virtually diagnostic, although in some cases they may be misinterpreted as evidence of a meningioma, skeletal metastasis, or acromegaly.

OTHER DISORDERS

Numerous additional congenital disorders can lead to hyperostosis and increased skeletal density.[314]

These include osteopetrosis, pyknodysostosis, sclerosteosis, endosteal hyperostosis (van Buchem's disease, hyperostosis corticalis generalisata), hereditary hyperphosphatasia (juvenile Paget's disease), diaphyseal dysplasia (Camurati-Engelmann disease), and idiopathic hypercalcemia (Williams' syndrome), some of which are discussed elsewhere in this book.

Idiopathic Periosteal Hyperostosis with Dysproteinemia

In 1966, Goldbloom and colleagues[276] reported two unrelated children who developed severe limb pain without edema, clubbing, or joint symptoms following an upper respiratory infection and acute febrile illness. Neither patient had an intrathoracic lesion. Roentgenograms outlined marked periosteal bone formation involving the mandible, humeri, ulnae, metacarpals, femora, tibiae, fibulae, and metatarsals. A biopsy revealed subperiosteal bone deposition without inflammatory cells. Analysis of the serum from both patients showed decreased albumin with an increase in the alpha-2 gamma globulins. With resolution of the fever over a period of weeks or months, the bone pain decreased and the radiographic findings improved. The etiology of the changes remained unexplained, although the possibility of an infectious agent, perhaps viral, may be significant.[265]

Plasma Cell Dyscrasia with Polyneuropathy, Organomegaly, Endocrinopathy, M-Protein, and Skin Changes

In 1968, Shimpo[277] first described a unique syndrome characterized by severe progressive sensorimotor polyneuropathy that might be associated with a plasma cell dyscrasia, osteosclerotic bone lesions, production of M-protein, hepatosplenomegaly, lymphadenopathy, endocrine dysfunction (diabetes mellitus, amenorrhea, gynecomastia, impotence, hypothyroidism), skin thickening and hyperpigmentation, papilledema, and episodes of anasarca. Additional reports of this syndrome soon appeared.[278-280] Although some of its radiographic features, including single or multiple solid or "bull's eye" osteosclerotic lesions, resemble findings in skeletal metastasis, plasma cell myeloma, cystic angiomatosis, or tuberous sclerosis, a peculiar pattern of bone proliferation appears to be unique to this condition. It consists of fluffy, spiculated, hyperostotic areas that show a predilection for the sites of ligamentous attachment in the spine (apophyseal joints, transverse processes, laminae), as well as other axial and extra-axial locations[281] (Fig. 81–36) (see Chapter 56). The genesis of the osteosclerotic lesions and bone proliferation is obscure. The abnormalities conceivably could result from the elaboration of an osteoblastic principle by the cells in the plasmacytoma or from osteoclast dysfunction. To facilitate recognition of the most constant and important features of the syndrome, the acronym POEMS has been suggested as appropriate:[281] polyneuropathy(P), organomegaly (O), endocrinopathy (E), M-protein (M), and skin changes (S).

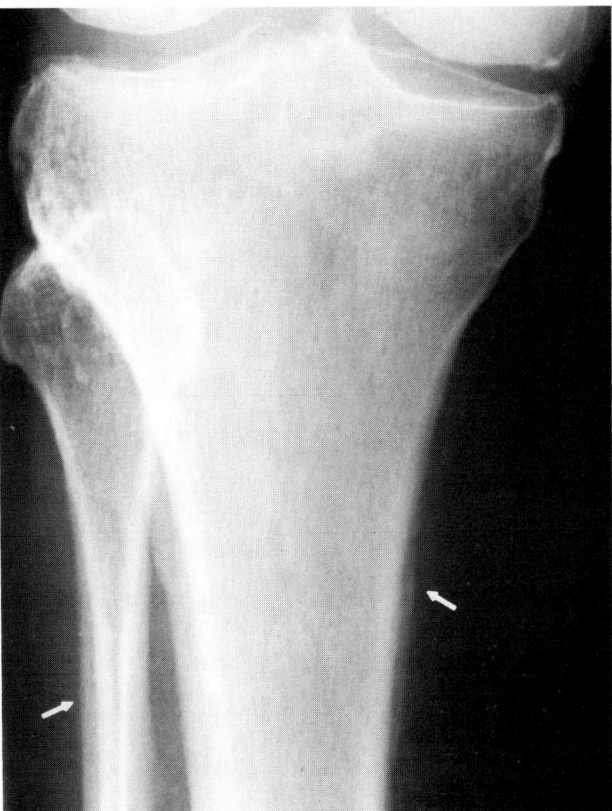

Figure 81–36. *Plasma cell dyscrasia with polyneuropathy, organomegaly, endocrinopathy, M-protein, and skin changes — the POEMS syndrome. Observe periostitis of the proximal tibia and fibula (arrows).*

Periostitis Deformans

In 1952, Soriano[282] described a group of six patients, as young as 16 years of age, who developed a disorder characterized by outbreaks and remissions lasting for a period up to 20 years. Attacks were accompanied by toxic symptoms, pain, and anorexia lasting 2 to 12 months. Nodular subcutaneous tumors appeared rapidly. Osseous lesions developed, particularly in the forearms, hands, and legs, characterized by exuberant periosteal reaction. Histologic examination documented periosteal proliferation and osteoporosis. Spontaneous recovery occurred but residual bone deformities were encountered.

The clinical and radiologic manifestations in

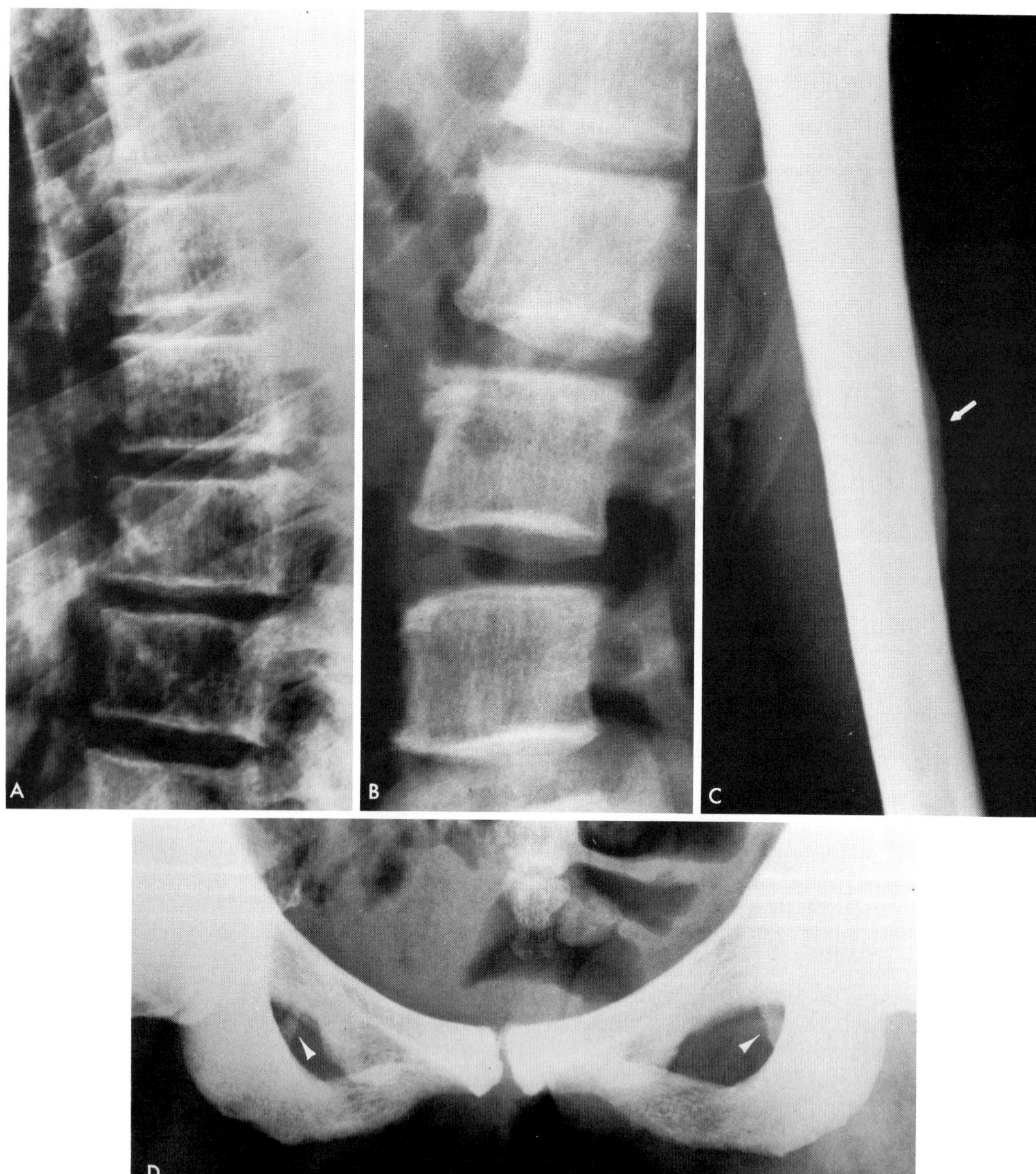

Figure 81–37. *Fluorosis. Findings include a coarsened trabecular pattern in the thoracic and lumbar spine with osteophytosis* **(A, B)**, *periosteal proliferation about the deltoid tuberosity of the humerus (arrow)* **(C)**, *and sacrotuberous ligament ossification (arrowheads)* **(D)**.

these individuals resembled the findings in two additional patients described by Melhem and coworkers.[283] In these latter cases, soft tissue swelling and cortical hyperostosis of the tubular bones were associated with hyperphosphatemia. Other laboratory parameters were unremarkable, and biopsy in one patient showed vascular connective tissue, periosteal bone formation, and cellular infiltration.

These unusual forms of cortical hyperostosis may represent the sequelae of an infectious disorder.[265]

Fluorosis

Exuberant periosteal proliferation in the appendicular skeleton is encountered in patients with fluorosis, usually in combination with more well known axial skeletal alterations (see Chapter 66). These latter changes include osteosclerosis, osteophytosis, and ligamentous calcification and ossification (Fig. 81–37).

Neurofibromatosis

Massive subperiosteal proliferation is seen in patients with neurofibromatosis.[284-287] Involvement of the tubular bones of the lower extremity is characterized by bizarre, undulating periosteal deposits of varying size (Fig. 81–38). The pathogenesis of the changes is not clear; hypotheses include vascular abnormalities with subperiosteal hemorrhage, neurofibromatous infiltration of subperiosteal tissue, and abnormally loose periosteum as a primary manifestation of the mesoderm dysplasia (see Chapter 80).

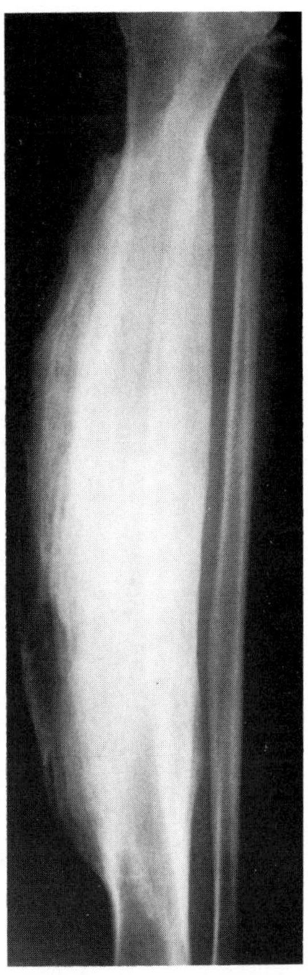

Figure 81–38. *Neurofibromatosis. Exuberant subperiosteal bony deposition on the diaphysis of the tibia has resulted in an enlarged and bowed bone. (Courtesy of Dr. D. MacEwan, Winnipeg, Manitoba, Canada.)*

Diffuse Idiopathic Skeletal Hyperostosis

Hyperostosis is a common manifestation of this disorder (see Chapter 41). Such hyperostosis affects spinal and extraspinal sites, leading to diagnostic flowing ossification of the spine, bony excrescences at sites of tendinous and ligamentous attachment, para-articular osteophytes, and ligamentous calcification and ossification (Fig. 81–39).

Sternocostoclavicular Hyperostosis

This represents a recently described disorder that is characterized by hyperostosis and soft tissue ossification between the clavicle and anterior portion of the upper ribs.[308-310] Patients are usually in the fourth to sixth decades of life; men are affected more frequently than women. Bilateral alterations predominate. Clinical findings include pain, swelling, and local heat in the anterior upper chest. Osseous overgrowth may lead to occlusion of the subclavian veins, leading to considerable edema. In some patients, pustulosis palmaris and plantaris can be evident. The erythrocyte sedimentation rate may be elevated.

The radiographic appearance is characteristic.[313] Ossification of various degrees involves the region of the costoclavicular ligament, inferior margin of the clavicle, and superior margin of the first rib (Fig. 81–40*A*,*B*). Additional changes in the vertebral column may include spondylitis, diffuse idiopathic skeletal hyperostosis, and sacroiliac joint abnormalities (Fig. 81–40*C*–*F*). Pathologic examination of the ossified mass may demonstrate considerable fibrosis and bone formation, with mild granulation tissue accumulation and round cell infiltration. The histologic changes resemble those of Paget's disease.

The pathogenesis of this condition is unknown. Its relation to other ossifying diatheses is unclear.

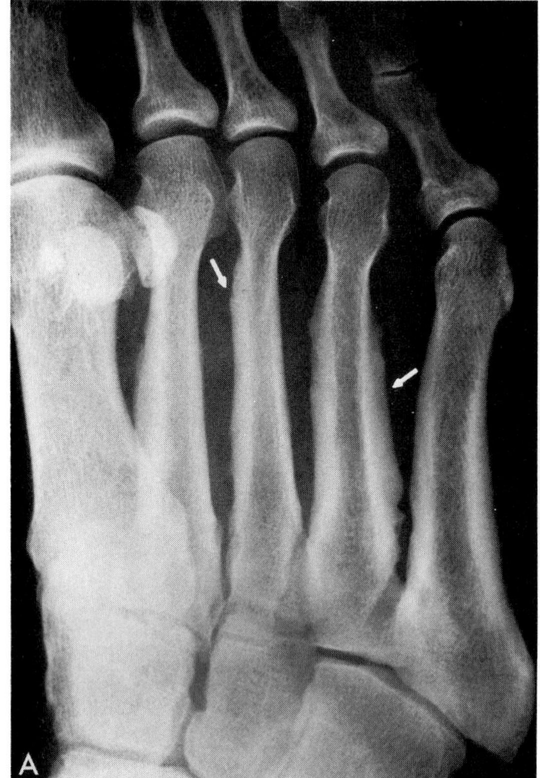

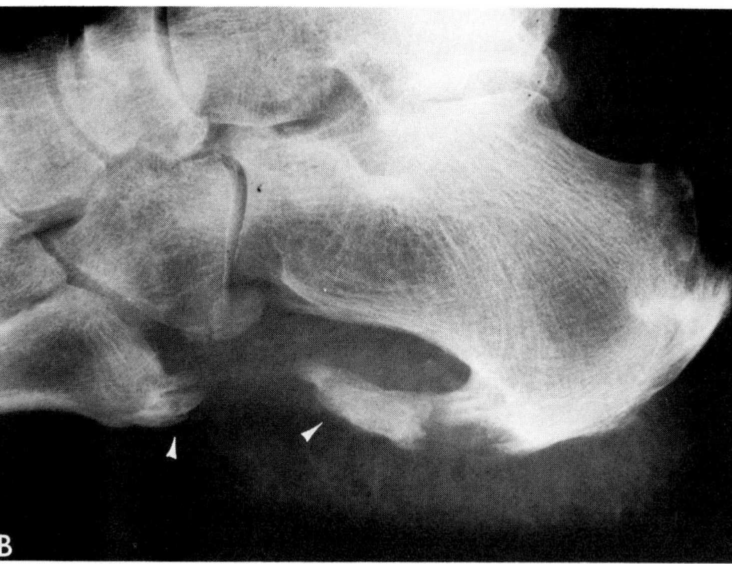

Figure 81–39. *Diffuse idiopathic skeletal hyperostosis. In extraspinal sites, this disorder may be associated with periostitis (arrows)* **(A)** *and bony excrescences at tendinous attachments (arrowheads)* **(B)**.

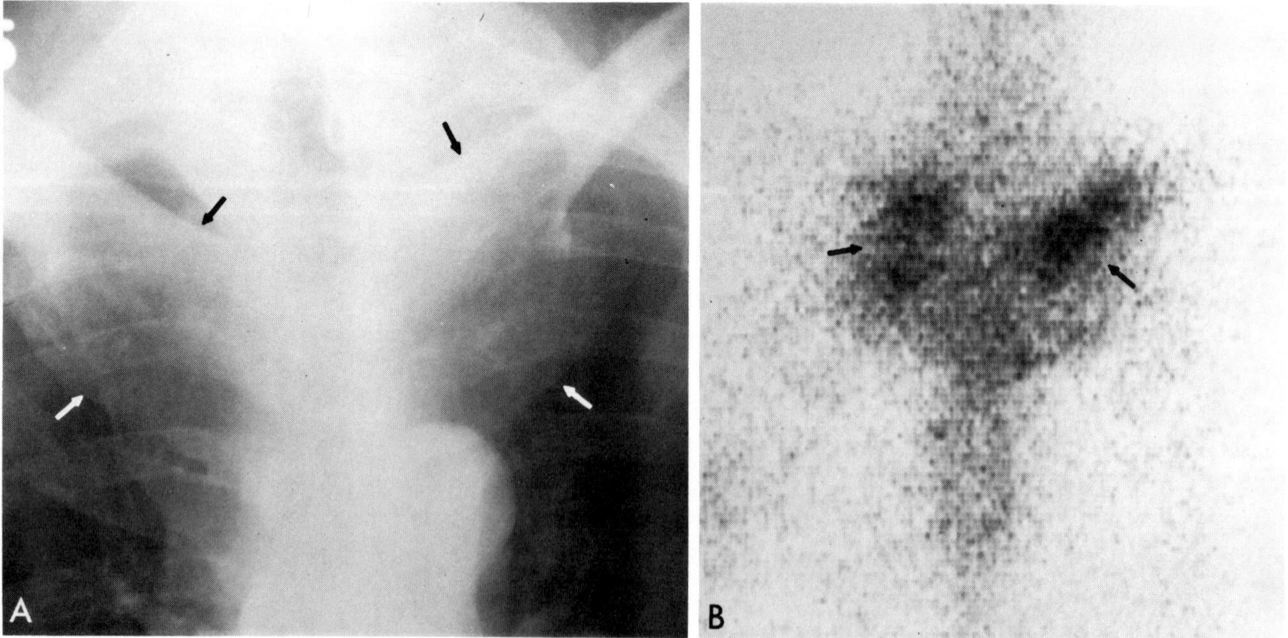

Figure 81–40. *Sternocostoclavicular hyperostosis. This 72 year old man developed soft tissue swelling over the medial end of both clavicles.*

A, B *A radiograph* **(A)** *outlines considerable osseous overgrowth about the clavicles (arrows) with bony expansion and sclerosis. A bone scan* **(B)** *reveals bilateral accumulation of the radionuclide (arrows) in the areas of bony overgrowth.*

Illustration continued on the opposite page

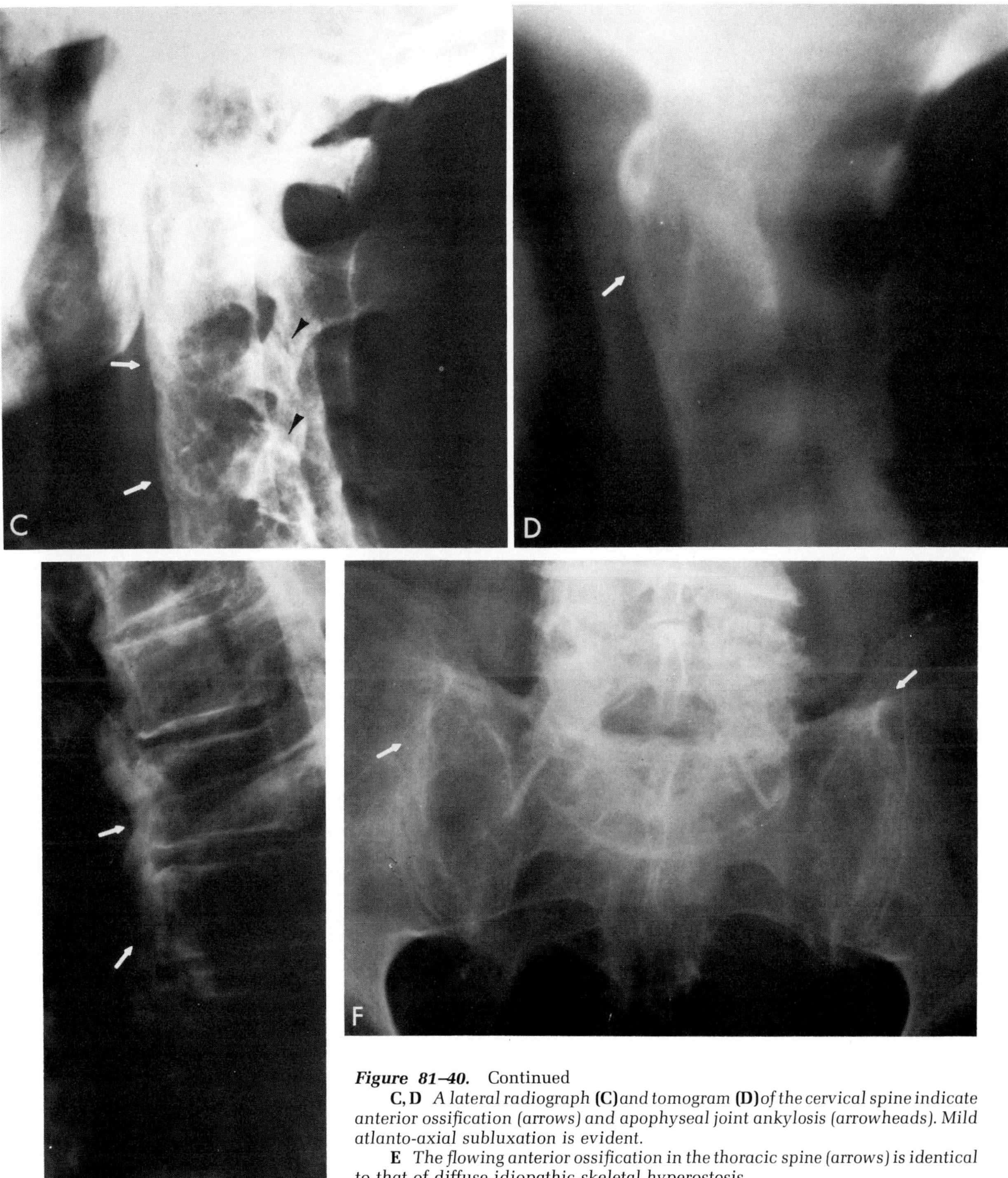

Figure 81–40. Continued

C, D *A lateral radiograph* **(C)** *and tomogram* **(D)** *of the cervical spine indicate anterior ossification (arrows) and apophyseal joint ankylosis (arrowheads). Mild atlanto-axial subluxation is evident.*

E *The flowing anterior ossification in the thoracic spine (arrows) is identical to that of diffuse idiopathic skeletal hyperostosis.*

F *Ligamentous ossification (arrows) between sacrum and ilium is seen. There is no evidence of sacroiliitis.*

Serologic testing for the histocompatibility antigen HLA B27 usually yields negative results.

SUMMARY

Certain disorders are associated with localized or generalized cortical hyperostosis or periostitis. These include enostoses (bone islands), osteomas with or without associated Gardner's syndrome, osteopoikilosis, osteopathia striata, melorheostosis, pachydermoperiostosis, secondary hypertrophic osteoarthropathy, vascular insufficiency, infantile cortical hyperostosis, hyperostosis frontalis interna, diffuse idiopathic skeletal hyperostosis, fluorosis, plasma cell dyscrasias, neurofibromatosis, and several rare and poorly defined syndromes. The changes must be distinguished from periostitis that occurs as a response to an adjacent osseous process (neoplasm, infection, trauma) and from hyperostosis accompanying additional congenital disorders.

REFERENCES

1. Stieda A: Ueber umschriebene Knochenverdichtungen im Bereich der Substantia spongiosa im Röntgenbilde. Bruns Beitr Klin Chir *45*:700, 1905.
2. Fischer H: Beitrag zur Kenntnis der Skelettvarietäten (überzählige Karpalia und Tarsalia, Sesambeine, Kompaktainseln). Fortzchr Geb Roentgenstr Nuklearmed *19*:43, 1912.
3. Caffey J: Focal scleroses of the spongiosa (bone islands). *In* Pediatric X-ray Diagnosis. 6th Ed. Chicago, Year Book Publishers, 1972, Vol. 2, p 961.
4. Steel HH: Calcified islands in medullary bone. J Bone Joint Surg *32A*:405, 1950.
5. Meschan I: Roentgen Signs in Clinical Practice. Philadelphia, WB Saunders Co, 1966, Vol 1, p. 372.
6. Broderick TW, Resnick D, Goergen TG, Alazraki N: Enostosis of the spine. Spine *3*:167, 1978.
7. Kim SK, Barry WF Jr: Bone island. Am J Roentgenol *92*:1301, 1964.
8. Kim SK, Barry WF Jr: Bone islands. Radiology *90*:77, 1968.
9. Onitsuka H: Roentgenologic aspects of bone islands. Radiology *123*:607, 1977.
10. Smith J: Giant bone islands. Radiology *107*:35, 1973.
11. Blank N, Lieber A: The significance of growing bone islands. Radiology *85*:508, 1965.
12. Ngan H: Growing bone islands. Clin Radiol *23*:199, 1972.
13. Sickles EA, Genant HK, Hoffer PB: Increased localization of ^{99m}Tc-pyrophosphate in a bone island: Case report. J Nucl Med *17*:113, 1976.
14. Schmorl G, Junghanns H: The Human Spine in Health and Disease. Translated by EF Besemann. 2nd Ed. New York, Grune & Stratton, 1971, p. 327.
15. Ackermann W, Schwarz GS: Non-neoplastic sclerosis in vertebral bodies. Cancer *11*:703, 1958.
16. Epstein BS: The Spine. A Radiological Text and Atlas. 3rd Ed. Philadelphia, Lea & Febiger, 1969.
17. Lagier R, Nussle D: Anatomy and radiology of a bone island. Fortschr Geb Roentgenstr Nuklearmed *128*:261, 1978.
18. Hoffman RR Jr, Campbell RE: Roentgenologic bone-island instability in hyperparathyroidism. Case report. Radiology *103*:307, 1972.
19. Spjut HJ, Dorfman HD, Fechner RE, Ackerman LV: Tumors of bone and cartilage. *In* Atlas of Tumor Pathology. Washington, DC, Armed Forces Institute of Pathology, 1971, Second Series, Fascicle 5, p. 117.
20. Childrey JH: Osteoma of the sinuses, the frontal and the sphenoid bone. Report of fifteen cases. Arch Otolaryngol *30*:63, 1939.
21. Hallberg OE, Begley JW Jr: Origin and treatment of osteomas of the paranasal sinuses. Arch Otolaryngol *51*:750, 1950.
22. Jaffe HL: Tumors and Tumorous Conditions of the Bones and Joints. Philadelphia, Lea & Febiger, 1958, p. 138.
23. Aegerter EE, Kirkpatrick JA Jr: Orthopedic Diseases: Physiology, Pathology, Radiology. 4th Ed. Philadelphia, WB Saunders Co, 1975, p. 496.
24. Dolan KD, Seibert J, Seibert RW: Gardner's syndrome. A model for correlative radiology. Am J Roentgenol *119*:359, 1973.
25. Gardner EJ, Plenk HP: Hereditary pattern for multiple osteomas in a family group. Am J Hum Genet *4*:31, 1952.
26. Gardner EJ, Richards RC: Multiple cutaneous and subcutaneous lesions occurring simultaneously with hereditary polyposis and osteomatosis. Am J Hum Genet *5*:139, 1953.
27. Shiffman MA: Familial multiple polyposis associated with soft tissue and hard tissue tumors. JAMA *179*:514, 1962.
28. Chang CHJ, Piatt ED, Thomas KE, Watne AL: Bone abnormalities in Gardner's syndrome. Am J Roentgenol *103*:645, 1968.
29. Weary PE, Linthicum A, Cawley EP, Coleman CC Jr, Graham GF: Gardner's syndrome: A family group study and review. Arch Dermatol *90*:20, 1964.
30. Albers-Schönberg H: Eine seltene, bisher nicht bekannte Strukturanomalie des Skelettes. Fortschr Geb Roentgenstr Nuklearmed *23*:174, 1915–1916.
31. Ledoux-Lebard R, Chabaneix, Dessane: L'ostéopoecilie forme nouvelle d'ostéite condensante généralisée sans symptomes cliniques. J Radiol Electrol Med Nucl *2*:133, 1916–1917.
32. Jonasch E: 12 Fälle von Osteopoikilie. Fortschr Geb Roentgenstr Nuklearmed *82*:344, 1955.
33. Busch KFB: Familial disseminated osteosclerosis. Acta Radiol *18*:693, 1937.
34. Szabo AD: Osteopoikilosis in a twin. Clin Orthop Rel Res *79*:156, 1971.
35. Wilcox LF: Osteopoikilosis. Am J Roentgenol *30*:615, 1933.
36. Risseeuw J: Familiaire osteopoikilie. Ned Tijdschr Geneeskd *80*:3827, 1936.
37. Melnick JC: Osteopathia condensans disseminata (osteopoikilosis). Study of a family of 4 generations. Am J Roentgenol *82*:229, 1959.
38. Sutherland CG: Osteopoikilosis. Radiology *25*:470, 1935.
39. Windholz F: Über familiäre Osteopoikilie und Dermatofibrosis lenticularis disseminata. Fortschr Geb Roentgenstr Nuklearmed *45*:566, 1932.
40. Berlin R, Hedensiö B, Lilja B, Linder L: Osteopoikilosis — a clinical and genetic study. Acta Med Scand *181*:305, 1967.
41. Buschke A, Ollendorff H: Ein Fall von Dermatofibrosis lenticularis disseminata und Osteopathia condensans disseminata. Dermatol Wochenschr *86*:257, 1928.
42. Raskin MM: Osteopoikilosis. Possible association with dystocia and keloid. South Med J *68*:270, 1975.
43. Windholz F: Systemerkrankung des Skeleta (Osteopoikilie) kombiniert mit einer Affektion der Haut (Dermatofibrosis lenticularis disseminata). Wien Klin Wochnschr *44*:1611, 1931.
44. Weissmann G: Scleroderma associated with osteopoikilosis. Arch Intern Med *101*:108, 1958.
45. Pastinszky J, Csató Z: Uber Hautveränderungen bei Osteopoikilie (Buschke-Ollendorff Syndrom). Z. Hautkr *43*:313, 1968.
46. Bethge JFJ, Ridderbusch KE: Über Osteopoikilie und das neue Krankheitsbild Hyperostose bei Osteopoikilie. Ergeb Chir Orthop *49*:138, 1967.
47. Holly LE: Osteopoikilosis. Five year study. Am J Roentgenol *36*:512, 1936.
48. Grassberger A, Seyss R: Knochenszintigramm bei Osteopoikilosis familiaris. Radiol Clin *44*:372, 1975.
49. Whyte MP, Murphy WA, Siegel BA: ^{99m}Tc-pyrophosphate bone imaging in osteopoikilosis, osteopathia striata, and melorheostosis. Radiology *127*:439, 1978.
50. Jaffe HL: Metabolic, Degenerative and Inflammatory Diseases of Bones and Joints. Philadelphia, Lea & Febiger, 1972.
51. Walker GF: Mixed sclerosing bone dystrophies. Two case reports. J Bone Joint Surg *46B*:546, 1964.
52. Abrahamson MN: Disseminated asymptomatic osteosclerosis with features resembling melorheostosis, osteopoikilosis, and osteopathia striata. Case report. J Bone Joint Surg *50A*:991, 1968.
53. Jancu J: Osteopoikilosis. A case report and a suggestion of its pathogenesis. Acta Orthop Belg *37*:284, 1971.
54. Mindell ER, Northup CS, Douglass HO Jr: Osteosarcoma associated with osteopoikilosis. Case report. J Bone Joint Surg *60A*:406, 1978.
55. Dahlin DC: Pathology of osteosarcoma. Clin Orthop Rel Res *111*:23, 1975.

56. Voorhoeve N: L'image radiologique non encore décrite d'une anomalie du squelette. Ses rapports avec la dyschondroplasie et l'osteopathia condensans disseminata. Acta Radiol *3*:407, 1924.
57. Fairbank HAT: Osteopathia striata. J Bone Joint Surg *32B*:117, 1950.
58. Larrègue M, Maroteaux P, Michey Y, Faure C: L'osteopathie striée, symptome radiologique de l'hypoplasia dermique en aires. Ann Radiol *15*:287, 1972.
59. Gehweiler JA, Bland WR, Carden TS Jr, Daffner RH: Osteopathia striata — Voorhoeve's disease. Review of the roentgen manifestations. Am J Roentgenol *118*:450, 1973.
60. Carlson DH: Osteopathia striata revisited. J Can Assoc Radiol *28*:190, 1977.
61. Willert HG, Zichner L: Osteopathia striata — juvenile metaphysäre Knochennekrosen. Z Orthop *111*:836, 1973.
62. Bloor DU: A case of osteopathia striata. J Bone Joint Surg *36B*:261, 1954.
63. Hurt RL: Osteopathia striata — Voorhoeve's disease. Report of a case presenting the features of osteopathia striata and osteopetrosis. J Bone Joint Surg *35B*:89, 1953.
64. Fermin HEA: Osteorabdotose. Een voor het eerst door N. Voorhoeve beschreven bijzondere vorm van osteopathia condensans disseminata. Ned Tijdschr Geneeskd *106*:1188, 1962.
65. Fairbank HAT: A case of unilateral affection of the skeleton of unknown origin. Br J Surg *12*:594, 1925.
66. Culver GJ, Thumasathit C: Osseous changes of osteopathic striata and Pyle's disease occurring in a patient with a 11-year follow-up. A case report. Am J Roentgenol *116*:640, 1972.
67. Ginsburg LD, Sedano HP, Gorlin RJ: Focal dermal hypoplasia syndrome. Am J Roentgenol *110*:561, 1970.
68. Léri A, Joanny J: Une affection non décrite des os. Hyperostose "en coulée" sur toute la longueur d'un membre ou "melorhéostose." Bull Mem Soc Hop Paris *46*:1141, 1922.
69. Widmann BP, Stecher WR: Rhizomonomelorheostosis. Radiology *24*:651, 1935.
70. Walker GF: Mixed sclerosing bone dystrophies: Two case reports. J Bone Joint Surg *46B*:546, 1964.
71. Morris JM, Samilson RL, Corley CL: Melorheostosis: review of the literature and report of an interesting case with a nineteen-year follow-up. J Bone Joint Surg *45*:1191, 1963.
72. Bied JC, Malsh C, Meunier P: La mélorhéostose chez l'adulte. A propos de deux cas dont l'un traité par un diphosphonate. Rev Rhum Mal Osteoartic *43*:193, 1976.
73. Campbell CJ, Papademetriou T, Bonfiglio M: Melorheostosis: A report of the clinical, roentgenographic, and pathological findings in fourteen cases. J Bone Joint Surg *50A*:1281, 1968.
74. Hove E, Sury B: Melorheostosis. Report on 5 cases with follow-up. Acta Orthop Scand *42*:315, 1971.
75. Gold RH, Mirra JM: Case report 35. Skel Radiol *2*:57, 1977.
76. Léri A, Lièvre JA: La mélorhéostose (hyperostose d'un membre en coulée). Presse Med *36*:801, 1928.
77. Beauvais P, Fauré C, Montagne JP, Chigot PL, Maroteaux P: Leri's melorheostosis: Three pediatric cases and a review of the literature. Pediatr Radiol *6*:153, 1977.
78. Masserini A: Sul morbo de Léri: Revisione della literatura e contributo casistico. Radiol Med Torino *31*:183, 1944.
79. Janousek J, Preston DF, Martin NL, Robinson RG: Bone scan in melorheostosis. Letters to the editor. J Nucl Med *17*:1106, 1976.
80. Dillehunt RB, Chuinard EG: Melorheostosis Léri: A case report. J Bone Joint Surg *18*:991, 1936.
81. Gillespie JB, Siegling JA: Melorheostosis Léri. Am J Dis Child *55*:1273, 1938.
82. Wagers LT, Young AW Jr, Ryan SF: Linear melorheostotic scleroderma. Br J Dermatol *86*:297, 1972.
83. Muller SA, Henderson ED: Melorheostosis with linear scleroderma. Arch Dermatol *88*:142, 1963.
84. Thompson NM, Allen CEL, Andrews GS, Gillwald FN: Scleroderma and melorheostosis. Report of a case. J Bone Joint Surg *33B*:430, 1951.
85. Soffa DJ, Sire DJ, Dodson JH: Melorheostosis with linear sclerodermatous skin changes. Radiology *114*:577, 1975.
86. Buchmann J: Osteopoikilie und Melorheostose. Beitr Orthop Traumatol *15*:641, 1968.
87. Wellmitz G: Ein Beitrag zum Krankheitsbild der Melorheostose und Osteopoikilie. Beitr Orthop Traumatol *19*:117, 1972.
88. McCarroll HR: Clinical manifestations of congenital neurofibromatosis. J Bone Joint Surg *32A*:601, 1950.
89. Hall GS: A contribution to the study of melorheostosis: Unusual bone changes associated with tuberous sclerosis. Q J Med *12*:77, 1943.
90. Patrick JH: Melorheostosis associated with arteriovenous aneurysms of the left arm and trunk: Report of a case with long follow-up. J Bone Joint Surg *51B*:126, 1969.
91. Putti V: L'osteosi eburneizzante monomelica (una nuova sindrome osteopatical). Chir Organi Mov *11*:335, 1927.
92. Valentin B: Über einen Fall von Mélorhéostose (Osteosclerosis, Osteosis eburnisans monomelica, Osteopathica hyperostotica). Fortschr Geb Roentgenstr Nuklearmed *37*:884, 1924.
93. Murray RO, McCredie J: Melorheostosis and the sclerotomes: A radiological correlation. Skel Radiol *4*:57, 1979.
94. Murray RO: Melorheostosis associated with congenital arteriovenous aneurysms. Proc R Soc Med *44*:473, 1951.
95. Zimmer P: Über einen Fall einer eigenartigen seltenen Knochenerkrankung, Osteopathia hyperostotica — Mélorhéostose. Beitr Klin Chir *140*:75, 1927.
96. Inman VT, Saunders JB: Referred pain from skeletal structures. J Nerv Ment Dis *99*:660, 1944.
97. Friedreich N: Hyperostose des gesammten Skelettes. Virchous Arch [Pathol Anat] *43*:83, 1868.
98. Marie P: De l'osteo-arthropathie hypertrophiante pneumique. Rev Med *10*:1, 1890.
99. Unna PG: Cutis verticis gyrata. Monatsschr Praktische Dermatol *45*:227, 1907.
100. Grönberg A: Is cutis verticis gyrata a symptom in an endocrine syndrome which has so far received little attention? Acta Med Scand *67*:24, 1927.
101. Guyer PB, Brunton FJ, Wren MWG: Pachydermoperiostosis with acro-osteolysis. A report of five cases. J Bone Joint Surg *60B*:219, 1978.
102. Uehlinger E: Hyperostosis generalisata mit Pachydermie. Virchows Arch [Pathol Anat] *308*:396, 1941.
103. Vague J: La pachydermopériostose; pachydermie plicaturée avec pachypériostose des extrémités (syndrome de Touraine, Solente et Golé) Rev Rhum Mal Osteoartic *15*:201, 1948.
104. Touraine A, Solente G, Golé L: Un syndrome osteó-dermopathique: La pachydermie plicaturée avec pachypériostose des extrémitiés. Presse Med *43*:1820, 1935.
105. Langston HH: Bone dystrophy of unknown etiology (presented for diagnosis). Proc R Soc Med *43*:299, 1950.
106. Angel JH: Pachydermo-periostosis (idiopathic osteo-arthropathy). Br Med J *2*:789, 1957.
107. Brugsch HG: Acropachyderma with pachyperiostitis. Arch Intern Med *68*:687, 1941.
108. Camp JD, Scanlan R: Chronic idiopathic hypertrophic osteoarthropathy. Radiology *50*:581, 1948.
109. Sèze S de, Jurmand S-H: Pachydermopériostose. Bull Mem Soc Hop Paris *66*:860, 1950.
110. Findlay GH, Oosthuizen WJ: Pachydermoperiostosis. The syndrome of Touraine, Solente and Golé. S Afr Med J *25*:747, 1951.
111. Schönenberg H: Zum Krankheitsbild der Osteo-Arthropathie hypertrophiante (Pierre-Bamberger). Z Kinderheilkd *74*:388, 1954.
112. Vogl A, Goldfischer S: Pachydermoperiostosis. Primary or idiopathic hypertrophic osteoarthropathy. Am J Med *33*:166, 1962.
113. Ursing B: Pachydermoperiostosis. Acta Med Scand *188*:157, 1970.
114. Herman MA, Massaro D, Katz S, Sachs M: Pachydermoperiostosis: Clinical spectrum. Arch Intern Med *116*:918, 1965.
115. Shawarby K, Ibrahim MS: Pachydermoperiostosis. A review of the literature and report on four cases. Br Med J *1*:763, 1962.
116. Harbison JB, Nice CM Jr: Familial pachydermoperiostosis presenting as an acromegaly-like syndrome. Am J Roentgenol *112*:532, 1971.
117. Fournier A-M, Mourou M: Pachydermopériostose. J Radiol Electrol Med Nucl *54*:417, 1973.
118. Lazarus JH, Galloway JK: Pachydermoperiostosis. An unusual cause of finger clubbing. Am J Roentgenol *118*:308, 1973.
119. Katoh T: Pachydermoperiostosis (syndrome of Touraine, Solente, and Golé). Jap J Clin Dermatol *23*:275, 1969.
120. Currarino G, Tierney RC, Giesel RG, Weihl, C: Familial idiopathic osteoarthropathy. Am J Roentgenol *85*:633, 1961.
121. Keats TE, Bagnall WS: Chronic idiopathic osteoarthropathy. Radiology *62*:841, 1954.
122. Berk M: Chronic idiopathic hypertrophic osteoarthropathy. Report of a case and review of the literature. N Engl J Med *247*:123, 1952.
123. Cremin BJ: Familial idiopathic osteoarthropathy of children: A case report and progress. Br J Radiol *43*:568, 1970.
124. Bartolozzi G, Bernini G, Maggini M: Hypertrophic osteoarthropathy without pachydermia. Idiopathic form. Am J Dis Child *129*:849, 1975.
125. Bhate DV, Pizarro AJ, Greenfield GB: Idiopathic hypertrophic osteoarthropathy without pachyderma. Radiology *129*:379, 1978.
126. Rimoin DL: Pachydermoperiostosis (idiopathic clubbing and periostosis): Genetic and physiologic considerations. N Engl J Med *272*:923, 1965.
127. Bruwer A, Holman CB, Kierland RR: Roetngenologic recognition of cutis verticis gyrata. Mayo Clin Proc *28*:63, 1953.
128. Roy JN: Hypertrophy of the palpebral tarsus, the facial integument and

the extremities of the limbs associated with widespread osteo-periostitis: A new syndrome. Can Med Assoc J *34*:615, 1936.
129. Metz EN, Dowell A: Bone marrow failure in hypertrophic osteoarthropathy. Arch Intern Med *116*:759, 1965.
130. Neiman HL, Gompels BM, Martel W: Pachydermoperiostosis with bone marrow failure and gross extramedullary hematopoiesis. Report of a case. Radiology *110*:553, 1974.
131. Chamberlain DS, Whitaker J, Silverman FN: Idiopathic osteoarthropathy and cranial defects in children (familial idiopathic osteoarthropathy). Am J Roentgenol *93*:408, 1965.
132. Arnold J: Acromegalie, Pachyacrie oder Ostitis? Ein anatomischer Bericht über den Fall Hagner I. Beitr Pathol Anat *10*:1, 1891.
133. Appelboom T, Busscher H, Famaey JP: Chondrocalcinosis as a possible cause of arthritis in pachydermoperiostosis? Letter to Editor. Arthritis Rheum *21*:174, 1978.
134. Lauter SA, Vasey FB, Hüttner I. Osterland CK: Pachydermoperiostosis: Studies on the synovium. J Rheumatol *5*:85, 1978.
135. Kerber RE, Vogl A: Pachydermoperiostosis. Peripheral circulatory studies. Arch Intern Med *132*:245, 1973.
136. Gall E, Bennett GA, Bauer W: Generalized hypertrophic osteoarthropathy: Pathologic study of seven cases. Am J Pathol *27*:349, 1951.
137. Hippocrates: The Book of Prognostics. *In* The Genuine Works of Hippocrates. Translated by F Adams. London, Syndenham Society, 1849.
138. Bamberger E: Protokoll der Kaisereiche und Koenigliche. Koenigliche Gesselschaft der Aertz in Wien. Sitzung vom 8 Marz, 1889. Wien Klin Wochenschr *2*:225, 1889.
139. Vogl A, Blumenfeld S, Gutner LB: Diagnostic significance of pulmonary hypertrophic osteoarthropathy. Am J Med *18*:51, 1955.
140. Berman B: Pulmonary hypertrophic osteoarthropathy. Arch Intern Med *112*:947, 1963.
141. Temple HL, Jaspin G: Hypertrophic osteoarthropathy. Am J Roentgenol *60*:232, 1948.
142. Greenfield GB, Schorsch HA, Shkolnik A: The various roentgen appearances of pulmonary hypertrophic osteoarthropathy. Am J Roentgenol *101*:927, 1967.
143. Holling HE, Brodey RS, Boland C: Pulmonary hypertrophic osteoarthropathy. Lancet *2*:1269, 1961.
144. Holling HE, Brodey RS: Pulmonary hypertrophic osteoarthropathy. JAMA *178*:977, 1961.
145. Aufses AH: Primary carcinoma of the lung. 14 year survey. J Mt Sinai Hosp *20*:212, 1953.
146. Jack GD: Bronchogenic carcinoma. Trans Med Chir Soc Edinb *132*:75, 1952–1953.
147. Hansen JL: Bronchial carcinoma presenting as arthralgia. Acta Med Scand Suppl *266*:467, 1952.
148. Wierman WH, Clagett OT, McDonald JR: Articular manifestations in pulmonary diseases. An analysis of their occurrence in 1024 cases in which pulmonary resection was performed. JAMA *155*:1459, 1954.
149. Alvarez GH: Clinica del cáncer de pulmón. Rev Assoc Med Argent *62*:690, 1948.
150. Berg R Jr: Arthralgia as a first symptom of pulmonary lesions. Dis Chest *16*:483, 1949.
151. Peck B: Hypertrophic osteoarthropathy with Hodgkin's disease in the mediastinum. JAMA *238*:1400, 1977.
152. Adler JJ, Sharma OP: Hypertrophic osteoarthropathy with intrathoracic Hodgkin's disease. Am Rev Respir Dis *102*:83, 1970.
153. Kay CJ, Rosenberg MA, Burd R: Hypertrophic osteoarthropathy and childhood Hodgkin's disease. Radiology *112*:177, 1974.
154. Shapiro RF, Zvaifler NJ: Concurrent intrathoracic Hodgkin's disease and hypertrophic osteoarthropathy. Chest *63*:912, 1973.
155. Aufses AH, Aufses BH: Hypertrophic osteoarthropathy in association with pulmonary metastases from extrathoracic malignancies. Dis Chest *38*:399, 1960.
156. Gibbs DD, Schiller KF, Stovin PG: Lung metastases heralded by hypertrophic pulmonary osteoarthropathy. Lancet *1*:623, 1960.
157. Coury C: Hippocratic fingers and hypertrophic osteoarthropathy: Study of 350 cases. Br J Dis Chest *54*:202, 1960.
158. Yacoub MH, Simon G, Ohnsorge J: Hypertrophic pulmonary osteoarthropathy in association with pulmonary metastases from extrathoracic tumors. Thorax *22*:226, 1967.
159. Firooznia H, Seliger G, Genieser NB, Barasch E: Hypertrophic pulmonary osteoarthropathy in pulmonary metastases. Radiology *115*:269, 1975.
160. Sethi SM, Saxton GD: Osteoarthropathy associated with solitary pulmonary metastases from melanoma. Can J Surg *17*:221, 1974.
161. Fellows KE Jr, Rosenthal A: Extracardiac roentgenographic abnormalities in cyanotic congenital heart disease. Am J Roentgenol *114*:371, 1972.
162. McLaughlin GE, McCarty DJ Jr, Downing DF: Hypertrophic osteoarthropathy associated with cyanotic congenital heart disease. A report of two cases. Ann Intern Med *67*:579, 1967.
163. Means MG, Brown NW: Secondary hypertrophic osteoarthropathy in congenital heart disease. Am Heart J *34*:262, 1947.
164. Trevor RW: Hypertrophic osteoarthropathy in association with congenital cyanotic heart disease: Report of two cases. Ann Intern Med *48*:660, 1958.
165. Shaw HB, Cooper RH: Pulmonary hypertrophic osteoarthropathy occurring in a case of congenital heart disease. Lancet *1*:880, 1907.
166. Shaffer HA Jr, Heckman JD: Hypertrophic osteoarthropathy associated with cyanotic congenital heart disease. J Can Assoc Radiol *24*:265, 1973.
167. Han SY, Collins LC: Hypertrophic osteoarthropathy in cirrhosis of the liver. Report of two cases. Radiology *91*:795, 1968.
168. Martin CL: Complications produced by malignant tumors of the nasopharynx. Am J Roentgenol *41*:377, 1939.
169. Diner WC: Hypertrophic osteoarthropathy. Relief of symptoms by vagotomy in a patient with pulmonary metastases from a lymphoepithelioma of the nasopharynx. JAMA *181*:555, 1962.
170. Papavasiliou CG: Pulmonary metastases from cancer of the nasopharynx associated with hypertrophic osteoarthropathy. Br J Radiol *36*:680, 1963.
171. Zornoza J, Cangir A, Green B: Hypertrophic osteoarthropathy associated with nasopharyngeal carcinoma. Am J Roentgenol *128*:679, 1977.
172. Peirce TH, Weir DG: Hypertrophic osteoarthropathy associated with a non-metastasising carcinoma of the oesophagus. Ir Med J Assoc *66*:160, 1973.
173. Heylen W, Baert AL: Hypertrophic osteoarthropathy secondary to malignant islet-cell tumor of the pancreas. J Belge Radiol *62*:79, 1979.
174. Grossman H, Denning CR, Baker DH: Hypertrophic osteoarthropathy in cystic fibrosis. Am J Dis Child *107*:1, 1964.
175. Cavanaugh JJA, Holman GH: Hypertrophic osteo-arthropathy in childhood. J Pediatr. *66*:27, 1965.
176. Kay CJ, Rosenberg MA, Burd R: Hypertrophic osteoarthropathy and childhood Hodgkin's disease. Radiology *112*:177, 1974.
177. Petty RE, Cassidy JT, Heyn R, Kenien AG, Washburn RL: Secondary hypertrophic osteoarthropathy. An unusual cause of arthritis in childhood. Arthritis Rheum *19*:902. 1976.
178. Ameri MR, Alebouyeh M, Donner MW: Hypertrophic osteoarthropathy in childhood malignancy. Am J Roentgenol *130*:992, 1978.
179. Howard CP, Telander RL, Hoffman AD, Burgert EO Jr: Hypertrophic osteoarthropathy in association with pulmonary metastasis from osteogenic sarcoma. Mayo Clin Proc *53*:538, 1978.
180. Mendlowitz M: Clubbing and hypertrophic osteoarthropathy. Medicine *21*:269, 1942.
181. Calabro JJ: Cancer and arthritis. Arthritis Rheum *10*:553, 1967.
182. Schumacher HR Jr: Articular manifestations of hypertrophic pulmonary osteoarthropathy in bronchogenic carcinoma. A clinical and pathological study. Arthritis Rheum *19*:629, 1976.
183. Ropes MW, Bauer W: Synovial Fluid Changes in Joint Disease. Cambridge Mass, Harvard University Press, 1963, p 88.
184. Caughey D: Quoted by HR Schumacher. Arthritis Rheum *19*:629, 1976.
185. Steinfeld AD, Munzenrider JE: The response of hypertrophic pulmonary osteoarthropathy to radiotherapy. Radiology *113*:709, 1974.
186. Greco FA, Kushner I: Loss of symptoms of pulmonary hypertrophic osteoarthropathy after laparotomy. Letter to Editor. Ann Intern Med *81*:555, 1974.
187. Holman CW: Osteoarthropathy in lung cancer: Disappearance after section of intercostal nerves. J Thorac Cardiovasc Surg *45*:679, 1963.
188. Polley HF, Clagett OT, McDonald JR, Schmidt HW: Articular reactions associated with localized fibrous mesothelioma of the pleura. Ann Rheum Dis *11*:314, 1952.
189. Crump C: Histologie der allgemeinen Osteophytose. (Ostéoarthropathie hypertrophiante pneumique). Virchows Arch (Pathol Anat) *271*:467, 1929.
190. Ginsburg J: Hypertrophic pulmonary osteoarthropathy. Postgrad Med J *39*:639, 1963.
191. Mills JA: The connective tissue disease associated with malignant neoplastic disease. J Chronic Dis *16*:797, 1963.
192. Schechter SL, Bole GG: Hypertrophic osteoarthropathy and rheumatoid arthritis. Simultaneous occurrence in association with diffuse interstitial fibrosis. Arthritis Rheum *19*:639, 1976.
193. Hammarsten JF, O'Leary J: The features and significance of hypertrophic osteoarthropathy. Arch Intern Med *99*:431, 1957.
194. Kieff ED, McCarty DJ Jr: Hypertrophic osteoarthropathy with arthritis and synovial calcification in a patient with alcoholic cirrhosis. Arthritis Rheum *12*:261, 1969.
195. Holmes JR, Price CH: Hypertrophic pulmonary osteoarthropathy with osteophytosis in a dog. Br J Radiol *31*:412, 1958.
196. Rosenthal L, Kirsh J: Observations on the radionuclide imaging in hypertrophic pulmonary osteoarthropathy. Radiology *120*:359, 1976.
197. Terry DW Jr, Isitman AT, Holmes RA: Radionuclide bone images in

hypertrophic pulmonary osteoarthropathy. Am J Roentgenol *124*:571, 1975.

198. Donnelly B, Johnson PM: Detection of hypertrophic pulmonary osteoarthropathy by skeletal imaging with ^{99m}Tc-labeled diphosphate. Radiology *114*:389, 1975.
199. Freeman MH, Tonkin AK: Manifestations of hypertrophic pulmonary osteoarthropathy in patients with carcinoma of the lung. Demonstration by ^{99m}Tc-pyrophosphate bone scans. Radiology *120*:363, 1976.
200. Kay CJ, Rosenberg MA: Positive ^{99m}Tc-polyphosphate bone scan in a case of secondary hypertrophic osteoarthropathy. J Nucl Med *15*:312, 1973.
201. Brower AC, Teates CD: Positive ^{99m}Tc-polyphosphate scan in case of metastatic osteogenic sarcoma and hypertrophic pulmonary osteoarthropathy. J Nucl Med *15*:53, 1974.
202. Costello P, Gramm HF, Likich J: Detection of hypertrophic pulmonary osteoarthropathy associated with pulmonary metastatic disease. Clin Nucl Med *2*:397, 1977.
203. Sagar VV, Meckelnburg RL, Piccone JM: Resolution of bone scan changes in hypertrophic pulmonary osteoarthropathy in untreated carcinoma of the lung. Clin Nucl Med *3*:472, 1978.
204. Rosenthall L, Hawkings D, Chuang S: Radionuclide demonstration of relative increased blood flow in uniappendicular secondary hypertrophic osteoarthropathy. Clin Nucl Med *3*:278, 1978.
205. Davis NJ Jr: Pulmonary hypertrophic osteoarthropathy. JAMA *24*:845, 1895.
206. Kessel L: Relation of hypertrophic osteoarthropathy to pulmonary tuberculosis. Arch Intern Med *19*:239, 1917.
207. Flavell G: Reversal of pulmonary hypertrophic osteoarthropathy by vagotomy. Lancet *1*:260, 1956.
208. Rutherford RB, Rhodes BA, Wagner HN: The distribution of extremity blood flow before and after vagectomy in a patient with hypertrophic pulmonary osteoarthropathy. Dis Chest *56*:19, 1969.
209. Racoceanu SN, Mendlowitz M, Suck AF, Wolf RL, Naftchi NE: Digital capillary blood flow in clubbing: ^{85}Kr studies in hereditary and acquired cases. Ann Intern Med *75*:933, 1971.
210. Mendlowitz M, Leslie A: Experimental simulation in the dog of cyanosis and hypertrophic osteoarthropathy which are associated with congenital heart disease. Am Heart J *24*:141, 1942.
211. Jao JY, Barlow JJ, Krant MJ: Pulmonary hypertrophic osteoarthropathy, spider angiomata, and estrogen hyperexcretion in neoplasia. Ann Intern Med *70*:581, 1969.
212. Ginsburg J, Brown JB: Increased oestrogen excretion in hypertrophic pulmonary osteoarthropathy. Lancet *2*:1274, 1961.
213. Carroll KB, Doyle L: A common factor in hypertrophic osteoarthropathy. Thorax *29*:262, 1974.
214. Buchan DJ, Mitchell DM: Hypertrophic osteoarthropathy in portal cirrhosis. Ann Intern Med *66*:130, 1967.
215. Singh A, Jolly SS, Bansal BB: Hypertrophic osteoarthropathy associated with carcinoma of the stomach. Br Med J *2*:581, 1960.
216. Hollis WC: Hypertrophic osteoarthropathy secondary to upper gastrointestinal tract neoplasm. Case report and review. Ann Intern Med *66*:125, 1967.
217. Wyburn-Mason R: Bronchial carcinoma presenting as polyneuritis. Lancet *1*:203, 1948.
218. Kourilsky R, Pieron R, Bonnet JL, Jacquillat C, Demay C, Levy G, Hivet M, Verley JM: Bilateral vagotomy and hypophysectomy in a case of hypertrophic pulmonary osteoarthropathy caused by a secondary cancer of the lungs. Bull Mem Soc Med Hop Paris *77*:113, 1961.
219. Holman CW: Osteoarthropathy in lung cancer: Disappearance after section of intercostal nerves. J Thorac Cardiovasc Surg *45*:679, 1963.
220. Honska WL Jr, Strenge H, Hammarsten J: Hypertrophic osteoarthropathy and chronic ulcerative colitis. Gastroenterology *33*:489, 1967.
221. Neale G, Kelsall AR, Doyle FH: Crohn's disease and diffuse symmetrical periostitis. Gut *9*:383, 1968.
222. Pastershank SP, Tchang SPK: Regional enteritis and hypertrophic osteoarthropathy. J Can Assoc Radiol *23*:35, 1972.
223. Dailey FH, Genovese PD, Behnke RH: Patent ductus arteriosus with reversal of flow in adults. Ann Intern Med *56*:865, 1962.
224. King JO: Localized clubbing and hypertrophic osteoarthropathy due to infection in an aortic prosthesis. Br Med J *4*:404, 1972.
225. Gibson T, Joye J, Schumacher HR, Agarwal B: Localized hypertrophic osteoarthropathy with abdominal aortic prosthesis and infection. Letter to Editor. Ann Intern Med *81*:556, 1974.
226. Pearse HE Jr, Morton JJ: The stimulation of bone growth by venous stasis. J Bone Joint Surg *12*:97, 1930.
227. Gally L, Arvay N: Les lésions osseuses dans les troubles circulatoires et trophiques des membres. J Radiol Electrol Med Nucl *31*:690, 1950.
228. Horvath F, Hajos A: Altérations des os de la jambe dues aux troubles des circulations veineuse et lymphatique. J Radiol Electrol Med Nucl *40*:257, 1959.
229. Fontaine R, Warter P, Weill F, Tuchmann L, Suhler A: Les altérations morphologiques des os de la jambe déclenchées par les troubles circulatoires veineux des membres inférieurs. J Radiol Electrol Med Nucl *45*:219, 1964.
230. Daumont A, Queneau P, Deplante JP, Bouvier M: Périostose hypertrophique et varices des membres inférieurs. Lyon Med *233*:1261, 1975.
231. Melcore G, Chiarotte F: Quadro radiologico della gambe nell' insufficienza chronica venosa. Radiol Med (Torino) *58*:867, 1972.
232. Graumann W, Braband H: Über periostveränderungen bei peripheren Durchblutungsstörungen. Fortschr Geb Roentgenstr Nuklearmed *92*:337, 1960.
233. Lovell RRH, Scott GBD: Hypertrophic osteoarthropathy in polyarteritis. Ann Rheum Dis *15*:46, 1956.
234. Caffey J: Pediatric X-ray Diagnosis. 7th Ed. Chicago, Year Book Medical Publishers, 1978, p 1430.
235. Caffey J, Silverman WA: Infantile cortical hyperostoses. Preliminary report on a new syndrome. Am J Roentgenol *54*:1, 1945.
236. Smyth FS, Potter A, Silverman W: Periosteal reaction, fever and irritability in young infants. A new syndrome? Am J Dis Child *71*:333, 1946.
237. Bennett HS, Nelson TR: Prenatal cortical hyperostosis. Br J Radiol *26*:47, 1953.
238. Barba WP II, Freriks DJ: The familial occurrence of infantile cortical hyperostosis in utero. J Pediatr *42*:141, 1953.
239. Van Buskirk FW, Tampas JP, Peterson OS Jr: Infantile cortical hyperostosis: Inquiry into its familial aspects. Am J Roentgenol *85*:613, 1961.
240. Clemett AR, Williams JH: Familial occurrence of infantile cortical hyperostosis. Radiology *80*:409, 1963.
241. Gerrard JW, Holman GH, Gorman AA, Morrow IH: Familial infantile cortical hyperostosis. J Pediatr. *59*:543, 1961.
242. Fráña L, Sekanina M: Infantile cortical hyperostosis. Arch Dis Child *51*:589, 1976.
243. Zeben W Van: Infantile cortical hyperostosis. Acta Paediatr *35*:10, 1948.
244. Pajewski M, Vure E: Late manifestations of infantile cortical hyperostosis (Caffey's disease). Br J Radiol *40*:90, 1967.
245. Taj-Eldin S, Al-Jawad J: Cortical hyperostosis. Infantile and juvenile manifestations in a boy. Arch Dis Child *46*:565, 1971.
246. Swerdloff BA, Ozonoff MB, Gyepes MT: Late recurrence of infantile cortical hyperostosis (Caffey's disease). Am J Roentgenol *108*:461, 1970.
247. Staheli LT, Church CC, Ward BH: Infantile cortical hyperostosis (Caffey's disease). Sixteen cases with a late follow-up of eight. JAMA *203*:384, 1968.
248. Blank E: Recurrent Caffey's cortical hyperostosis and persistent deformity. Pediatrics *55*:856, 1975.
249. Burbank PM, Lovestedt SA, Kennedy RLJ: The dental aspects of infantile cortical hyperostosis. Oral Surg *11*:1126, 1958.
250. Caffey J: On some late skeletal changes in chronic infantile cortical hyperostosis. Radiology *59*:651, 1952.
251. Scott EP: Infantile cortical hyperostosis. Report of an unusual complication. J Pediatr *62*:782, 1963.
252. Holman GH: Infantile cortical hyperostosis. A review. Q Rev Pediatr *17*:24, 1962.
253. Sherman MS, Hellyer DT: Infantile cortical hyperostosis. Review of the literature and report of five cases. Am J Roentgenol *63*:212, 1950.
254. Matheson WJ, Markham M: Infantile cortical hyperostosis. Br Med J *1*:742, 1952.
255. Kaufmann HJ, Mahboubi S, Mandell GA: Case report 39. Skel Radiol *2*:109, 1977.
256. Holtzman D: Infantile cortical hyperostosis of the scapula presenting as an ipsilateral Erb's palsy. J Pediatr *81*:785, 1972.
257. Padfield E, Hicken P: Cortical hyperostosis in infants: A radiological study of sixteen patients. Br J Radiol *43*:231, 1970.
258. Marquis JR: Infantile cortical hyperostosis. A report of an unusual case. Radiology *89*:282, 1967.
259. Jackson DR, Lyne ED: Infantile cortical hyperostosis. Case report. J Bone Joint Surg *61A*:770, 1979.
260. Harris VJ, Ramilo J: Caffey's disease: A case originating in the first metatarsal and review of a 12 year experience. Am J Roentgenol *130*:335, 1978.
261. Minton LR, Elliott JH: Ocular manifestations of infantile cortical hyperostosis. Am J Ophthalmol *64*:902, 1967.
262. Neuhauser EBD: Infantile cortical hyperostosis and skull defects. Postgrad Med *48*(b):57, 1970.
263. Boyd RDH, Shaw DG, Thomas BM: Infantile cortical hyperostosis with lytic lesions in the skull. Arch Dis Child *47*:471, 1972.
264. Eversole SL Jr, Holman GH, Robinson RA: Hitherto undescribed characteristics of the pathology of infantile cortical hyperostosis (Caffey's disease). Bull Johns Hopkins Hosp *101*:80, 1957.

265. Silverman FN: Virus diseases of bone. Do they exist? Am J Roentgenol *126*:677, 1976.
266. Dalldorf G: Viruses and human cancer. Bull NY Acad Med *36*:795, 1960.
267. McEnery G, Nash FW: Wiskott-Aldrich syndrome associated with idiopathic infantile cortical hyperostosis (Caffey's disease). Arch Dis Child *48*:818, 1973.
268. Sauterel L, Rabinowicz T: Contribution to the study of a new etiological aspect of infantile cortical hyperostosis. Ann Radiol *4*:211, 1961.
269. Moore S: Hyperostosis Cranii. Springfield, Ill, Charles C Thomas, 1955.
270. Salmi A, Voutilainen A, Holsti LR, Unnérus CE: Hyperostosis cranii in a normal population. Am J Roentgenol *87*:1032, 1962.
271. Gershon-Cohen J, Schraer H, Blumberg N: Hyperostosis frontalis interna among the aged. Am J Roentgenol *73*:396, 1955.
272. Henschen F: Über die verschiedenen Formen von Hyperostose des Schädeldachs. Acta Pathol Microbiol Scand Suppl *37*:236, 1938.
273. Stewart RM: Localized cranial hyperostosis in the insane. J Neurol Psychopathol *8*:321, 1928.
274. Dorst JP: Functional craniology: An aid in interpreting roentgenograms of the skull. Radiol Clin North Am *2*:347, 1964.
275. Stewart RM: Hyperostosis frontalis interna: Its relationship to cerebral atrophy. J Ment Sci *87*:600, 1941.
276. Goldbloom RB, Stein PB, Eisen A, McSheffrey JB, Brown BS, Wiglesworth FW: Idiopathic periosteal hyperostosis with dysproteinemia. A new clinical entity. N Engl J Med *274*:873, 1966.
277. Shimpo S: Solitary myeloma causing polyneuritis and endocrine disorders. Nihon Rinsho (Jap J Clin Med) *26*:2444, 1968.
278. Meshkinpour H, Myung CG, Kramer LS: A unique multisystemic syndrome of unknown origin. Arch Intern Med *137*:1719, 1977.
279. Trentham DE, Masi AT, Marker HW: Polyneuropathy and anasarca: Evidence in a new connective-tissue syndrome and vasculopathic condition. Ann Intern Med *84*:271, 1976.
280. Waldenström JG, Adner A, Gydell K, Zettervall O: Osteosclerotic "plasmacytoma" with polyneuropathy, hypertrichosis and diabetes. Acta Med Scand *203*:297, 1978.
281. Bardwick P, Zvaifler NJ, Gill G, Newman D, Greenway G, Resnick D: Plasma cell dyscrasia with polyneuropathy, organomegaly, endocrinopathy, M protein, and skin changes. The POEMS syndrome. Report of two cases and a review of the literature. Medicine *59*:311, 1980.
282. Soriano M: Periostitis deformans. Ann Rheum Dis *11*:154, 1952.
283. Melhem RE, Najjar SS, Knachadurian AK: Cortical hyperostosis with hyperphosphatemia: A new syndrome? J Pediatr *77*:986, 1970.
284. Hooper G, McMaster MJ: Neurofibromatosis with tibial cysts caused by recurrent hemorrhage. A case report. J Bone Joint Surg *61A*:274, 1979.
285. Yaghmai I, Tafazoli M: Massive subperiosteal hemorrhage in neurofibromatosis. Radiology *122*:439, 1977.
286. Kullmann L, Wouters HW: Neurofibromatosis, gigantism, and subperiosteal haematoma. Report of two children with extensive subperiosteal bone formation. J Bone Joint Surg *54B*:130, 1972.
287. Pitt MJ, Mosher JF, Edeiken J: Abnormal periosteum and bone in neurofibromatosis. Radiology *103*:143, 1972.
288. Davies JAK, Hall FM, Goldberg RP, Kasdon EJ: Positive bone scan in a bone island. Case report. J Bone Joint Surg *61A*:943, 1979.
289. Rao GM, Guruprakash GH, Poulose KP, Bhaskar G: Improvement in hypertrophic pulmonary osteoarthropathy after radiotherapy to metastasis. Am J Roentgenol *133*:944, 1979.
290. Roback DL: Tc-99m-MDP bone scintigraphy and "growing" bone islands: A report of two cases. Clin Nucl Med *5*:98, 1980.
291. Hall FM, Goldberg RP, Davies JAK, Fainsinger MH: Scintigraphic assessment of bone islands. Radiology *135*:737, 1980.
292. Small IA, Shandler H, Husain M, David H: Gardner's syndrome with an unusual fibro-osseous lesion of the mandible. Oral Surg *49*:477, 1980.
293. Rödl W: Das Gardner-syndrom — drei eigene Beobachtungen mit unterschiedlicher organmanifestation. Fortschr Geb Roentgenstr Nuklearmed *130*:558, 1979.
294. Young LW: Radiological case of the month. Am J Dis Child *134*:415, 1980.
295. Knockaert D, Dequecker J: Osteopathia striata and focal dermal hypoplasia. Skel Radiol *4*:223, 1979.
296. Bass HN, Weiner JR, Goldman A, Smith LE, Sparkes RS, Crandall BF: Osteopathia striata syndrome. Clinical, genetic and radiologic considerations. Clin Pediatr *19*:369, 1980.
297. Dissing I, Zafirovski G: Para-articular ossifications associated with melorheostosis Léri. Acta Orthop Scand *50*:717, 1979.
298. Kinzinger H, Blaimont P, Wollast R: Un cas de mélorhéostose. Internat Orthop (SICOT) *3*:55, 1979.
299. Younge D, Drummond D, Herring J, Cruess AL: Melorheostosis in children. Clinical features and natural history. J Bone Joint Surg *61B*:415, 1979.
300. Evans WK: Reversal of hypertrophic osteoarthropathy after chemotherapy for bronchogenic carcinoma. J Rheumatol *7*:93, 1980.
301. Nathanson I, Riddlesberger MM Jr: Pulmonary hypertrophic osteoarthopathy in cystic fibrosis. Radiology *135*:649, 1980.
302. Ali A, Tetalman MR, Fordham EW, Turner DA, Chiles JT, Patel SL, Schmidt KD: Distribution of hypertrophic pulmonary osteoarthropathy. Am J Roentgenol *134*:771, 1980.
303. Sorin SB, Askari A, Rhodes RS: Hypertrophic osteoarthropathy of the lower extremities as a manifestation of arterial graft sepsis. Arthritis Rheum *23*:768, 1980.
304. López-Enriquez E, Morales AR, Robert F: Effect of atropine sulfate in pulmonary hypertrophic osteoarthropathy. Arthritis Rheum *23*:822, 1980.
305. d'Eshougues JR, Gille C, Smadja A: Interet du sulfate d'atropine dans les formes "rheumatoides" de la maladie de Pierre Marie: a propos du proies-verbal. Bull Soc Med Hôp Paris *113*:343, 1962.
306. Hamza M, Janier M, Moalla M, Hamza R, Ayed HB: Ostéo-arthropathie hypertrophiante de l'enfant. J Radiol *61*:369, 1980.
307. Finsterbush A, Husseini N: Infantile cortical hyperostosis with unusual clinical manifestations. Clin Orthop Rel Res *144*:276, 1979.
308. Köhler H, Uehlinger E, Kutzner J, West TB: Sternocostoclavicular hyperostosis: Painful swelling of the sternum, clavicles, and upper ribs. Ann Intern Med *87*:192, 1977.
309. Sonozaki H., Azuma A, Okai K, Nakamura K, Fukuoka S, Tateishi A, Kurosawa H, Mannoji T, Kabata K, Mitsui H, Seki H, Abe I, Furusawa S, Matsuura M, Kudo A, Hoshino T: Clinical features of 22 cases with "inter-sterno-costo-clavicular ossification." Arch Orthop Traumat Surg *95*:13, 1979.
310. Camus JP, Prier A, Cassou B: L'hyperostose sterno-costo-claviculaire. Rev Rhum Mal Osteoartic *47*:361, 1980.
311. Scott RL, Pinstein ML, Sebes JI: Case report 129. Skel Radiol *5*:270, 1980.
312. Bhate DV, Chandraskhar H, Greenfield GB, Vedantham KS, Lo MC: Case report 126. Skel Radiol *5*:258, 1980.
313. Resnick D: Sternocostoclavicular hyperostosis. Am J Roentgenol *135*:1278, 1980.
314. Amendola MA, Brower AC, Tisnado J: Weismann-Netter-Stuhl syndrome: Toxopachyostéose diaphysaire tibio-péronière. Am J Roentgenol *135*:1211, 1980.

82

OSTEOLYSIS AND CHONDROLYSIS

by Donald Resnick, M.D., and Gen Niwayama, M.D.

Destruction of bone (osteolysis) or cartilage (chondrolysis) can become evident in innumerable neoplastic, infectious, metabolic, traumatic, vascular, congenital, and articular disorders. In fact, severe and progressive cartilaginous or osseous dissolution at multiple sites can lead to considerable clinical deformity in some of these disorders, such as rheumatoid arthritis, psoriatic arthritis, juvenile chronic arthritis, systemic lupus erythematosus, scleroderma, mixed connective tissue disease, multicentric reticulohistiocytosis, gout, calcium pyrophosphate dihydrate crystal deposition disease, neuroarthropathy, osteonecrosis, hyperparathyroidism, plasma cell myeloma, skeletal metastasis, tuberculosis, fungal infections, and sarcoidosis as well as following irradiation, frostbite and thermal and electrical burns.[1, 130] These conditions are discussed in detail elsewhere in this book. There remains a group of heterogeneous conditions in which significant and severe osteolysis and chondrolysis may become manifest, and these are described in this chapter.

OSTEOLYSIS

Occupational Acro-osteolysis

The 1950 report by Harnasch[2] focused attention on a new form of acro-osteolysis that appeared to represent an occupational hazard. This investigator noted shortened, thickened, and deformed fingers and widespread eczema in a blacksmith who had been handling oil and tar over a period of years. Subsequent reports by Suciu and co-workers[3] in 1963 and Cordier and colleagues[4] in 1966 implicated exposure to vinyl chloride monomer in the pathogenesis of acro-osteolysis, an observation that has been confirmed in numerous other investigations.[5-11] Routine radiographic surveys of individuals in certain industrial plants have revealed that as many as 1 to 2 per cent of workers involved in the polymerization of vinyl chloride may develop acro-osteolysis.[10] Occasionally, exposure to vapors of other synthetic materials used in the manufacture of plastic products may produce similar abnormalities.[12] Initial clinical manifestations include fatigue, asthenia, nervousness, and insomnia.[10] A Raynaud's phenomenon–like disorder ensues, with digital pain, numbness, and tingling followed by the appearance of "drumstick" fingers and "watch-glass" nails. Some individuals with these latter manifestations may not develop radiographically evident changes, although arteriography can outline alterations in the palmar arches and digital arteries.[13, 137] Additional clinical findings can include scleroderma-like plaques on the hands, wrists, and forearms, soft tissue nodules, hyperhidrosis and discoloration, and medial nerve compression in the carpal tunnel.[10] Further complications of vinyl chloride disease may include hepatic fibrosis or tumor, splenomegaly, portal hypertension, thrombocytopenia, and pulmonary changes.[136]

The roentgenographic hallmark of the disorder is osteolysis that predominates in the terminal phalanges of the hands, although it may also affect other phalanges, the sacroiliac joints,[7, 8] the foot,[4,7] and, rarely, additional skeletal structures,[10] including the mandible. Band-like radiolucent areas across the waist of one or more terminal phalanges may be combined with tuftal resorption and beveling, and osseous fragmentation (Fig. 82–1). The thumb is affected more commonly than the other digits. Similar changes may appear in the foot, and bone erosion and sclerosis about one or both sacroiliac articulations resemble the changes of sacroiliitis found in association with the seronegative spondyloarthropathies. If the exposure to polyvinylchloride is halted, the patient may reveal slow improvement of the radiographic abnormalities. Consolidation and coalescence of phalangeal fragments can be evident, although some residue usually persists, associated with shortening and clubbing of the digits. Elsewhere, roentgenographic improvement may also be recognized, and even the sacroiliac joint changes may regress. These improvements can be verified by scintigraphy, during which the accumulation of bone-seeking radiopharmaceuticals in one or more skeletal sites can be seen to diminish following the elimination of contact with polyvinylchloride.[14]

The etiology and pathogenesis of the condition

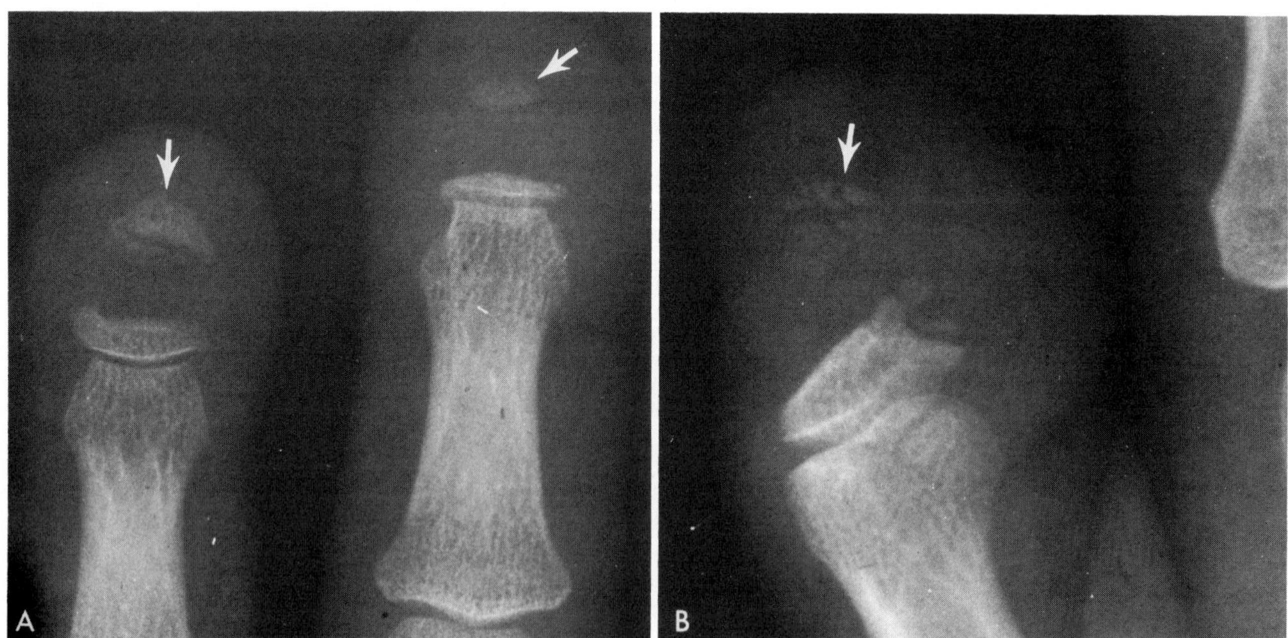

Figure 82–1. *Occupational acro-osteolysis.*

A *Note band-like resorption of the terminal phalanges of two digits, isolating small osseous fragments in the terminal tufts (arrows). Observe that the distal interphalangeal articulations are intact.*

B *In the thumb, involvement is especially marked. The proximal portion of the terminal phalanx is tapered and small bony foci (arrow) are located distally.*

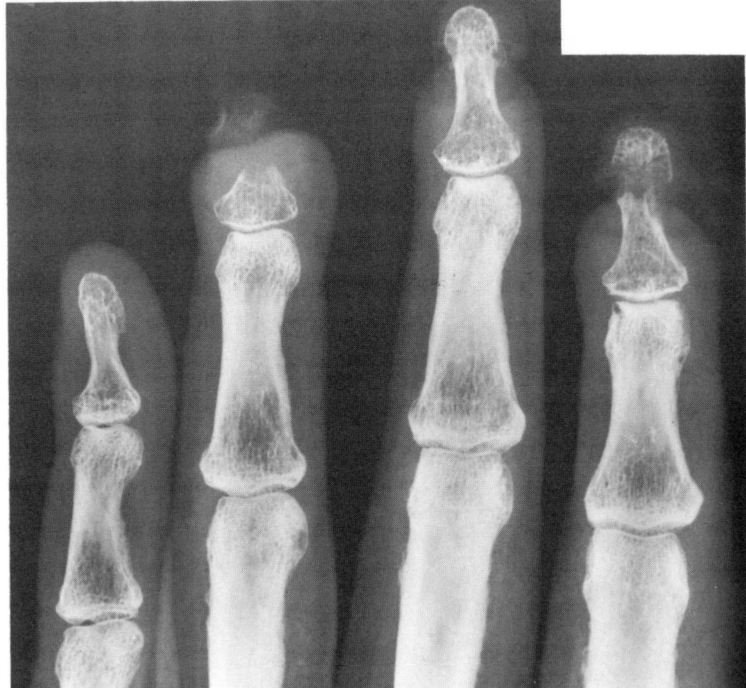

Figure 82–2. Rheumatoid vasculitis with acro-osteolysis. A 47 year old woman with classic rheumatoid arthritis and no evidence of another collagen vascular disorder developed digital gangrene, which eventually required distal phalangectomy. A radiograph of the left fingers reveals marked resorption and atrophy of distal soft tissues with self-amputation of the tufts of several digits. Note the absence of erosive arthritis. (From Rohlfing BM, et al: Br J Radiol 50:830, 1977.)

are unclear. Wilson and associates[5] postulated that three factors were important, all of which were required for the development of the syndrome: a chemical insult, a physical insult, and a personal idiosyncrasy. The role of chemical or physical trauma would explain the predilection for involvement of the hand, the appearance of symmetric areas of osteopenia at skeletal sites of major muscle insertions, and the improvement in the clinical, radiographic, and scintigraphic alterations following cessation of the exposure to polyvinylchloride.[14] A disturbance in circulation, especially in the small peripheral arteries of the hands, may be attributable to a toxic chemical substance. The substance may act on the central or peripheral nervous system or directly on the walls of the arterioles and capillaries.[10] The lack of correlation between the duration of the exposure or the concentration of the toxic substances and the severity of the osteolysis, as well as the appearance of Raynaud's phenomenon without osteolysis in some individuals, suggests that host factors are also important in the clinical expression of this disease.

The incidence of acro-osteolysis in workers involved in the polymerization of vinyl chloride has diminished in recent years.[10] This is due to an increase in the preventive measures currently being employed in this industry in view of the well-known skeletal and extraskeletal (angiosarcoma of the liver) complications of polyvinylchloride exposure.[15]

Band-like resorption of the terminal phalanges in this condition differs from the pattern of osteolysis that may accompany vasculitis (Fig. 82–2), collagen vascular disorders (e.g., scleroderma) (Fig. 82–3), psoriasis, epidermolysis bullosa, frostbite, thermal and electrical burns, and neuroarthropathy. Similar band-like resorption can be seen in hyperparathyroidism (in association with more characteristic alterations) and in certain familial conditions (see discussion later in this chapter).

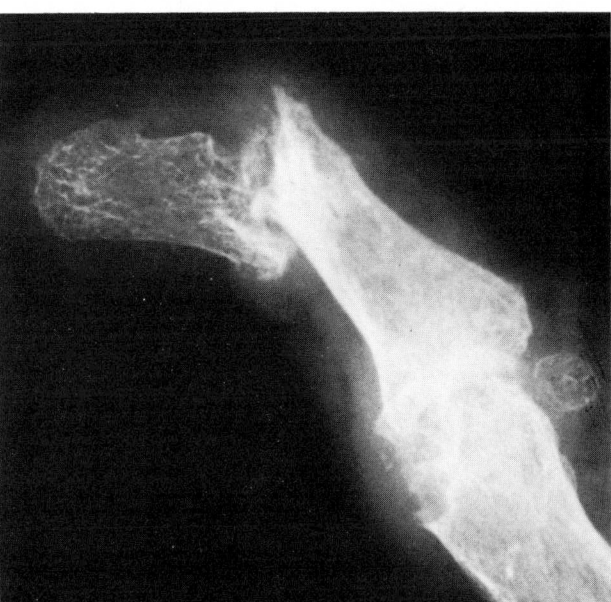

Figure 82–3. Scleroderma. Considerable destruction of the interphalangeal and metacarpophalangeal articulations of the thumb is observed in this patient with scleroderma. This is an unusual manifestation of the disease. A similar pattern of joint destruction may accompany psoriatic arthritis and multicentric reticulohistiocytosis.

Posttraumatic Osteolysis

Although some degree of bone loss is common following traumatic insult, particularly when complicated by fracture, there exist certain situations and sites in which the degree of posttraumatic osteolysis may appear excessive (Table 82–1). Knowledge of the existence and appearance of such osteolysis is important so that the resorption of bone that accompanies a traumatic insult is not mistaken for an inflammatory or neoplastic process.

Posttraumatic osteolysis can lead to progressive resorption of the outer end of the clavicle. According to Strauch,[16] this complication was first reported by Dupas in 1936. Numerous accounts of posttraumatic osteolysis of the clavicle have now appeared.[17-28] The process becomes apparent after single or repeated episodes of local trauma. Frequently, the traumatic insult is minor in nature and unassociated with obvious fracture or dislocation. The osteolytic process begins as early as 2 to 3 weeks and as late as several years after the injury. When untreated, it leads to lysis of 0.5 to 3 cm of bony substance from the distal clavicle over a period of 12 to 18 months, which may be associated with erosion and cupping of the acromion, soft tissue swelling, and dystrophic calcification[22] (Fig. 82–4). Pain, diminished strength, local crepitation, and restricted mobility may be evident at this stage. After the lytic phase stabilizes, reparative changes occur over a period of 4 to 6 months, emphasizing the self-limited nature of the process. Eventually, the subchondral bone becomes reconstituted, although the acromioclavicular joint can remain permanently widened.[22]

Careful analysis of roentgenograms in the early posttraumatic period may allow identification of prominent soft tissues, osteoporosis, and small gaps in the subchondral bone plate of the clavicle that, when recognized and treated with immobilization, can shorten the course of the process.

Table 82–1
COMMON SITES OF POSTTRAUMATIC OSTEOLYSIS

Distal clavicle[16–28]
Pubic/ischial rami[29]
Distal ulna[21, 31]
Distal radius[21, 31]
Carpus[21, 31]
Femoral neck[132]

The pathogenesis of posttraumatic osteolysis of the clavicle is not certain. Osteoclastic resorption, autonomic nervous system dysfunction, and catabolic hyperemia have been suggested as possible important factors.[17] Levine and co-workers[22] postulated that a slowly progressive, posttraumatic synovial reaction in the acromioclavicular articulation could account for the osteolysis, citing such supporting evidence as acromial involvement, the presence of villous hyperplasia and marked vascular proliferation of the synovium following biopsy or resection, and the osseous reconstitution following synovectomy.

The differential diagnosis of osteolysis about the acromioclavicular articulation includes, in addition to trauma, hyperparathyroidism, collagen vascular disorders, infection, rheumatoid arthritis, and other articular processes.

Posttraumatic osteolysis can become prominent at other skeletal sites as well. In the pubic or ischial rami, exaggerated resorption of bone about a fracture, with or without associated sclerosis, can simulate the appearance of a malignant process[29] (Figs. 82–5 and 82–6). Furthermore, the pathologist may misinterpret the exuberant cartilage and disorderly

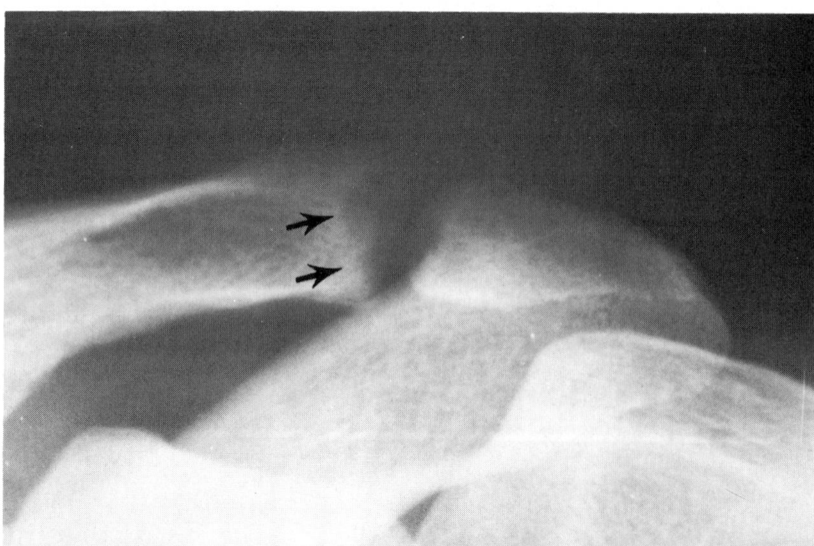

Figure 82–4. Posttraumatic osteolysis: Clavicle. Several weeks following local trauma, marked resorption of the distal end of the clavicle is seen (arrows). Similar but less extensive findings are evident in the acromion. The resulting radiographic picture, consisting of ill-defined osseous margins and a widened acromioclavicular joint, resembles that in septic arthritis, rheumatoid arthritis, and hyperparathyroidism.

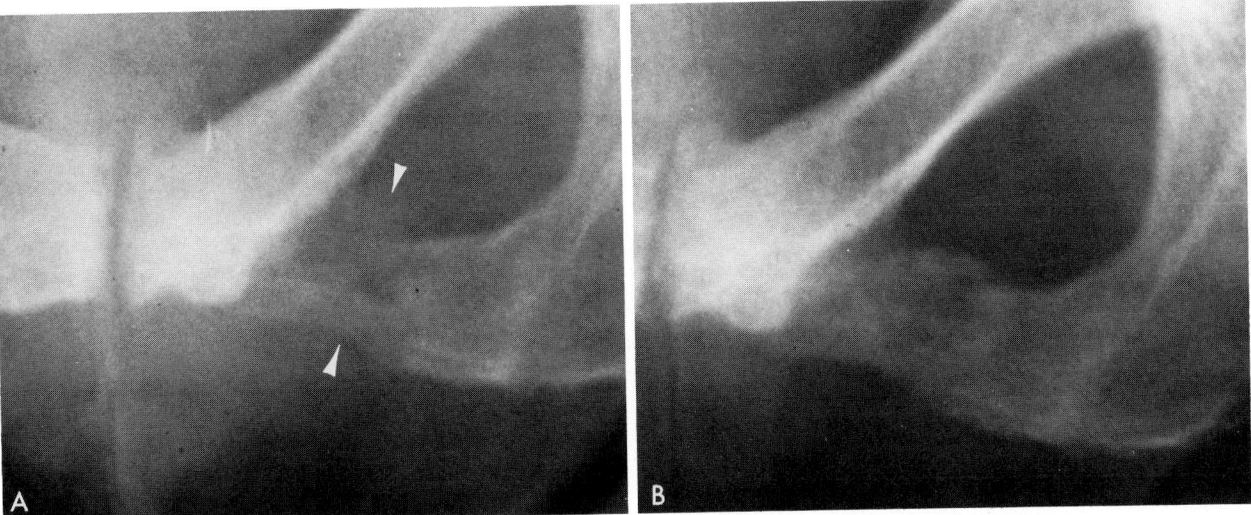

Figure 82–5. Posttraumatic osteolysis: Inferior pubic ramus. *A 44 year old woman presented with pelvic pain following a fall. The initial film revealed an undisplaced fracture of the left inferior pubic ramus. The patient continued to experience pain.*

A *A radiograph obtained 4 weeks after the fracture reveals significant osteolysis about the fracture site (arrowheads). At this stage, the appearance resembles that of a pathologic fracture.*

B *Four weeks later, considerable healing at the fracture site is evident, indicating the true nature of the radiographic findings.*

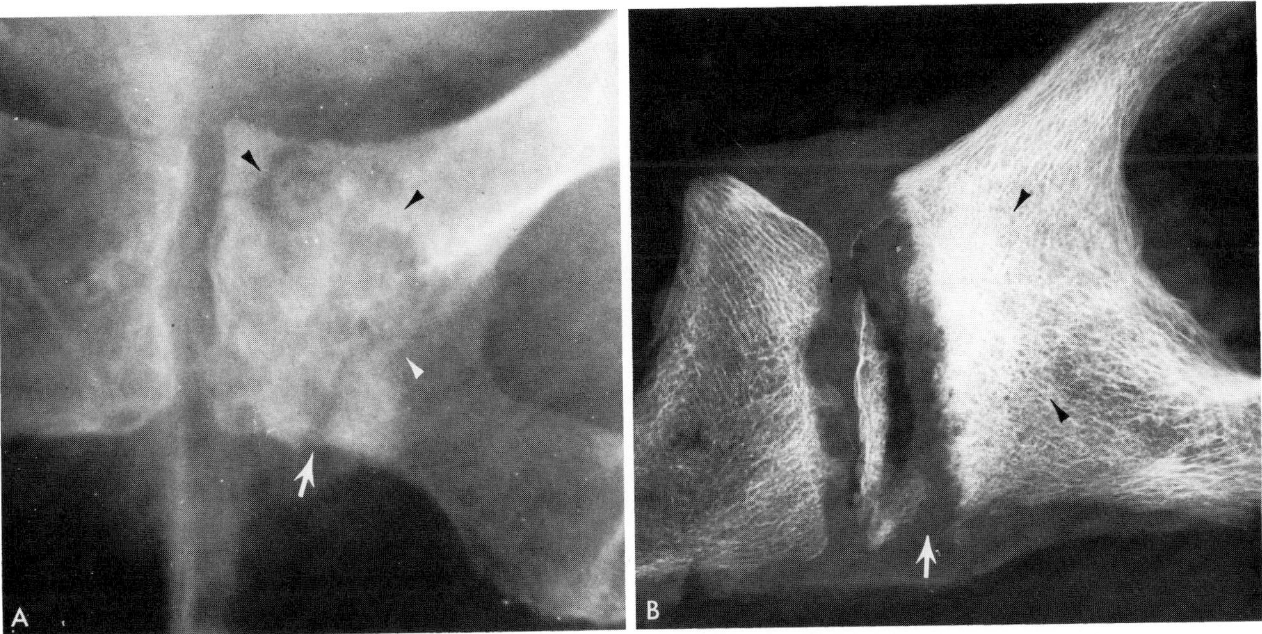

Figure 82–6. Posttraumatic osteolysis: Pubic bone. *This 54 year old alcoholic woman complained of a dull left groin ache of 4 months' duration and weight loss of 30 pounds. A history of trauma was denied. Because of the radiographic findings, which suggested a neoplastic process, an extensive search for other osseous or extraosseous lesions was undertaken and was unrewarding. A biopsy demonstrated areas of atypical cartilage, suggestive but not diagnostic of chondrosarcoma. A radical excision of the left pubic bone was performed. Histologic material was examined by five experienced bone pathologists, the diagnoses including chronic osteomyelitis, a benign cartilage tumor, and a reactive fibro-osseous proliferation most consistent with an ununited fracture. The patient later developed fractures of the sternum and ribs, although she continued to deny any significant trauma.*

A *A preoperative radiograph reveals a mixed lytic and sclerotic lesion of the left pubis (arrowheads) with a fracture (arrow).*

B *A radiograph of the removed bone indicates the probable "benign" nature of the lesion. The fracture line (arrow) is seen with surrounding bony eburnation (arrowheads).*

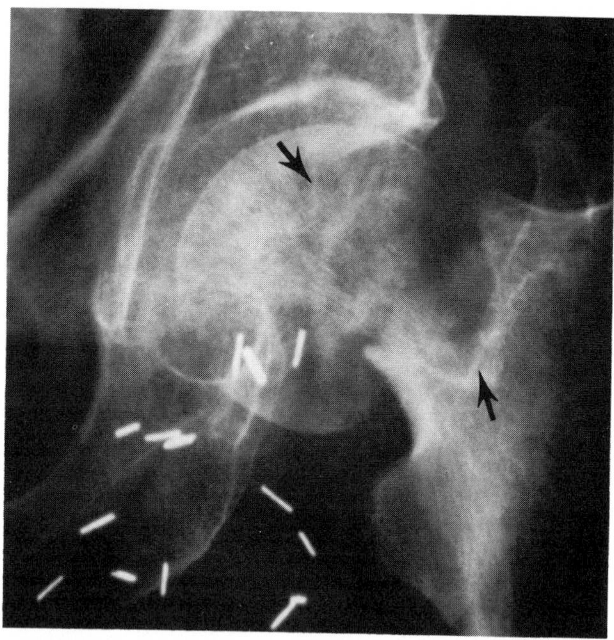

Figure 82–7. Posttraumatic osteolysis: Femoral neck. Following a fracture of the femoral neck, resorption and rotation at the fracture site (arrows) can produce a radiographic picture resembling that of a malignant process.

membranous bone formation of a rapidly forming primary callus as evidence of a chondrosarcoma or other malignancy, thus compounding the diagnostic dilemma.[30] The cause of osteolysis about these ramus fractures is not known, although instability, particularly in single ramus fractures, should not be a factor. As there is no impaction of bone in these latter fractures, perhaps a lack of sound, direct bone contact is an explanation for the excessive osteolysis and delayed union.[29]

Prominent posttraumatic osteolysis has also been noted in the ulna, radius, and carpal bones.[21, 31] In the femoral neck, resorption and rotation at a fracture site can produce a radiographic picture that may be misinterpreted as a malignant process[132, 139] (Fig. 82–7). Osteolysis following odontoid fracture[133] or atlanto-axial subluxation[134] can produce a separate bone at the tip of the dens, resembling or identical to the os odontoideum.

Primary Osteolysis Syndromes

A diverse group of idiopathic disorders can lead to significant skeletal lysis. They differ in the presence or absence of genetic transmission, the associated clinical manifestations, and the major locations of osteolysis[32] (Table 82–2).

Acro-osteolysis Syndrome of Hajdu and Cheney. An unusual variety of cranioskeletal dysplasia was described by Hajdu and Kauntze in a sporadic case in 1948[33] and by Cheney in a family in 1965.[34] Further reports of this syndrome have

Table 82–2

OSTEOLYSIS SYNDROMES

Syndrome	Age of Onset	Major Site of Osteolysis	Patterns of Inheritance	Associated Features
Acro-osteolysis of Hajdu/Cheney[32–46]	Second decade	Distal phalanges; rarely tubular bones, mandible, acromio-clavicular joints	Dominant or sporadic	Generalized bone dysplasia, fractures, osteoporosis
Massive osteolysis of Gorham[47–68]	Young adult	Variable; pelvic or shoulder girdles	Sporadic	Slowly progressive, extreme dissolution
Carpotarsal osteolysis:				
Multicentric osteolysis with nephropathy[77–84]	Infant, child	Carpal and tarsal areas, elbows	Sporadic; occasionally dominant	Osteoporosis, deformity, hypertension, renal failure, death
Hereditary multicentric osteolysis[85-90]	1–5 years	Carpal and tarsal areas, elbows, digits	Dominant; occasionally recessive or sporadic	Progressive deformity
Neurogenic osteolysis[97, 98]	Childhood	Phalanges	Dominant or recessive	Sensory neuropathy, skin ulcerations
Acro-osteolysis of Joseph[101]	Childhood	Distal phalanges	Recessive	Otherwise healthy
Acro-osteolysis of Shinz[102]	Second decade	Phalanges	Dominant	Skin ulcerations, no neurologic defect
Farber's disease[95, 103]	Infancy	Elbows, wrists, knees, ankles	Sporadic	Subcutaneous nodules
Winchester syndrome[104]	Infancy	Carpal and tarsal areas, elbows	Recessive	Osteoporosis, joint contractures, thick skin, corneal opacities
Osteolysis with detritic synovitis[105]	Adulthood	Widespread	Sporadic	Progressive

appeared,[32, 35-45, 129, 135] allowing delineation of its clinical and radiologic manifestations. The disorder may be familial, with a dominant mode of inheritance, or sporadic in nature, and is manifested by short stature, low-set ears, recessed mandible, malocclusion and early loss of teeth, coarse hairs, pseudoclubbing of the digits, joint laxity, conductive hearing loss, and speech impairment. Radiographic features include osteolysis of distal phalanges of the hands and feet; a bizarre-shaped dolichocephalic skull with basilar impression, delayed closure of cranial sutures, multiple wormian bones, hypoplastic or absent frontal sinuses, prominent occipital ridge, and enlarged sella turcica; diminutive mandible and maxilla with poor dentition; generalized osteoporosis with vertebral compressions and deformities, and fractures of tubular bones; valgus deformities of the knees; and hypoplasia and subluxation of the proximal radius. Laboratory analysis is usually unremarkable, and renal function, which is altered in other osteolysis syndromes, is normal in this condition.

Osteolysis is especially characteristic (Figs. 82–8 and 82–9). Changes in the phalanges, which consist of resorption of tufts and band-like areas of lucency, simulate abnormalities in occupation-induced (polyvinylchloride) acro-osteolysis, pyknodysostosis, Rothmund's syndrome, and collagen vascular disorders. Osteolysis can also be apparent in the tubular bones, mandibular rami, and acromioclavicular joints.[46] The pathogenesis is unknown. It may represent a manifestation of a generalized osseous dysplasia, since an abnormality of bone mineral and metabolism has not been documented. Bone and skin collagen appear normal on electron microscopy, although iliac crest biopsies demonstrate a decrease in skeletal mass.[44] The percentage of endosteal bone surfaces characteristic of bone formation may be diminished, and resorptive surfaces may be increased. Brown and colleagues[44] concluded, on the basis of their morphologic studies, that an abnormality of osteoblast function may be the cause of an alteration of structural protein. Their findings differed from those in hyperparathyroidism and hyperthyroidism. Elias and associates[32] obtained biopsy specimens of an area of active osteolysis in a phalanx and noted active replacement of central medullary bone by a fibrous and angiomatous process, characterized by the presence of small, thick-walled vessels and an unusual number of interspersed nerve fibers and mast cells. They suggested that a neurovascular dysfunction with local release of osteolytic mediators might be involved in the pathogenesis of the disorder.

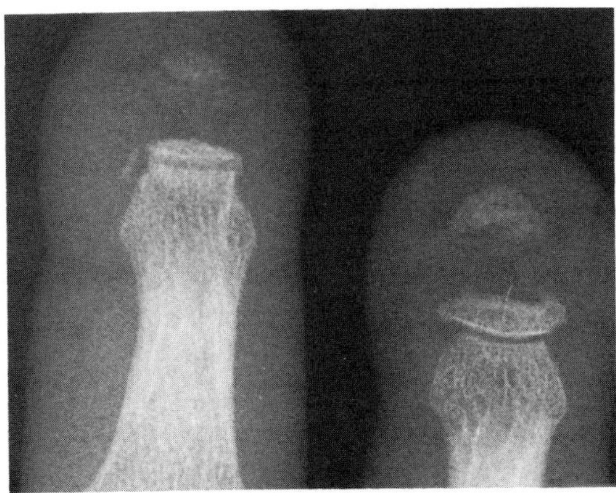

Figure 82–8. *Acro-osteolysis of Hajdu and Cheney. The typical pattern of osteolysis of the digits is demonstrated. Note that resorption occurs in a band-like fashion across the waist of the terminal phalanges, isolating one or more phalangeal fragments. Soft tissue swelling is also evident. The appearance is identical to that in occupational acro-osteolysis. (Courtesy of Dr. M. Dalinka, University of Pennsylvania, Philadelphia, Pennsylvania.)*

Massive Osteolysis of Gorham. In 1954, Gorham and collaborators[47] reported two patients with a peculiar variety of massive osteolysis. One year later, Gorham and Stout,[48] in a more comprehensive report, detailed the previous descriptions of this entity in the literature,[49-55] and proposed the term hemangiomatosis for this condition. Subsequently, numerous other descriptions have appeared, some of which have introduced additional names such as massive osteolysis, disappearing bone disease, vanishing bone disease, and Gorham disease.[56-68, 140]

The disease can become evident in men and women of all ages, although most cases are discovered before the age of 40 years. A family history is not apparent. The process may affect either the axial or the appendicular skeleton; numerous cases document the frequency of changes in the pelvic or shoulder regions. Clinical manifestations vary; some patients have a relatively abrupt onset of pain and swelling, whereas others describe an insidious onset of soft tissue atrophy and limitation of motion that is without pain unless an associated pathologic fracture develops. Of interest, some individuals note the onset of the disorder following significant trauma. Laboratory analysis may show unremarkable results, with slight elevation of the serum alkaline phosphatase level.

The most dramatic aspect of massive osteolysis is its radiographic appearance (Fig. 82–10). Initially, radiolucent foci appear in the intramedullary or subcortical regions, which resemble findings in patchy osteoporosis. Slowly progressive atrophy, dissolution, fracture, fragmentation, and disappearance of a portion of the bone then occur, with tapering or "pointing" of the remaining osseous tissue and atrophy of soft tissue. The process subsequently extends to contiguous bones, the intervening articulations affording no protection. Thus, osteolysis of the ilium may be associated with resorption of the proximal femur, whereas changes in the scapula may later be combined with osteolysis of the proximal humerus, clavicle, and ribs. This

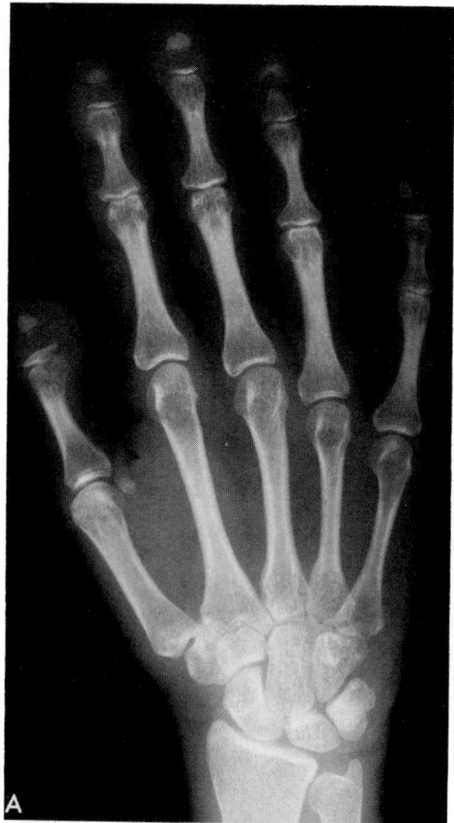

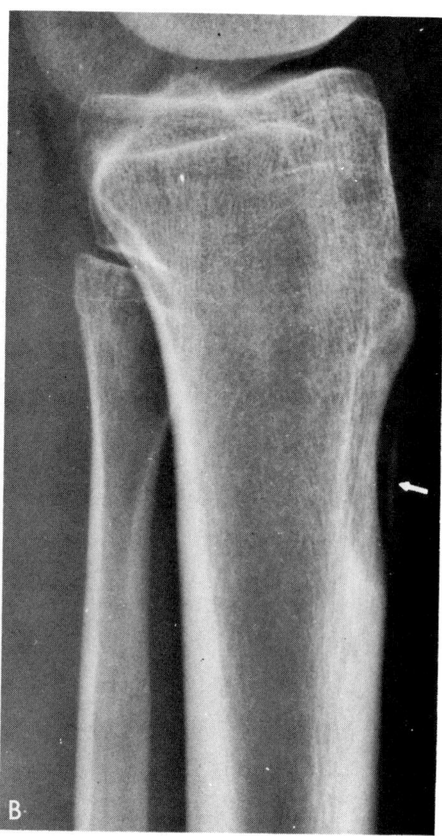

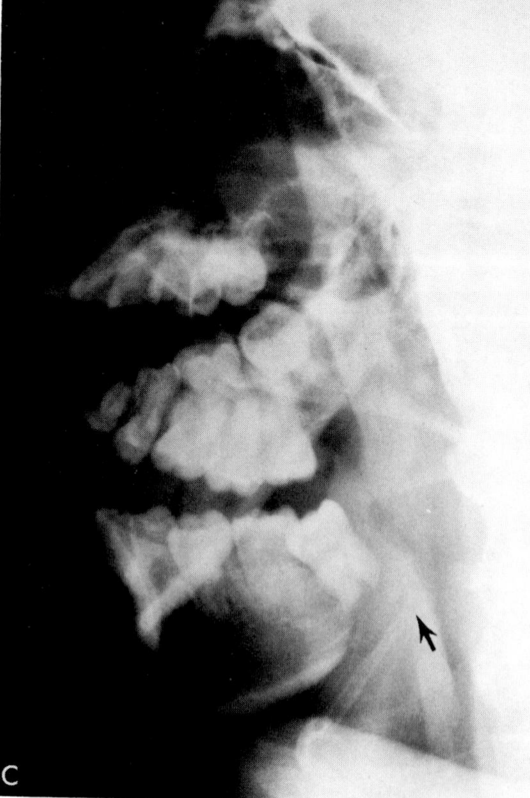

Figure 82–9. *Acro-osteolysis of Hajdu and Cheney. A 20 year old woman developed progressive acro-osteolysis of the hands as well as of other skeletal sites. A family history of similar problems was not apparent.*

A *Note osteolysis of the terminal phalanges in all of the digits. The opposite hand was equally affected.*

B *A 5 cm long cortical defect containing a linear piece of bone (arrow) involves the anterior aspect of the proximal tibia just inferior to the tibial tuberosity. The opposite knee was also affected.*

C *The right mandibular ramus is completely absent (arrow).*

Illustration continued on the opposite page

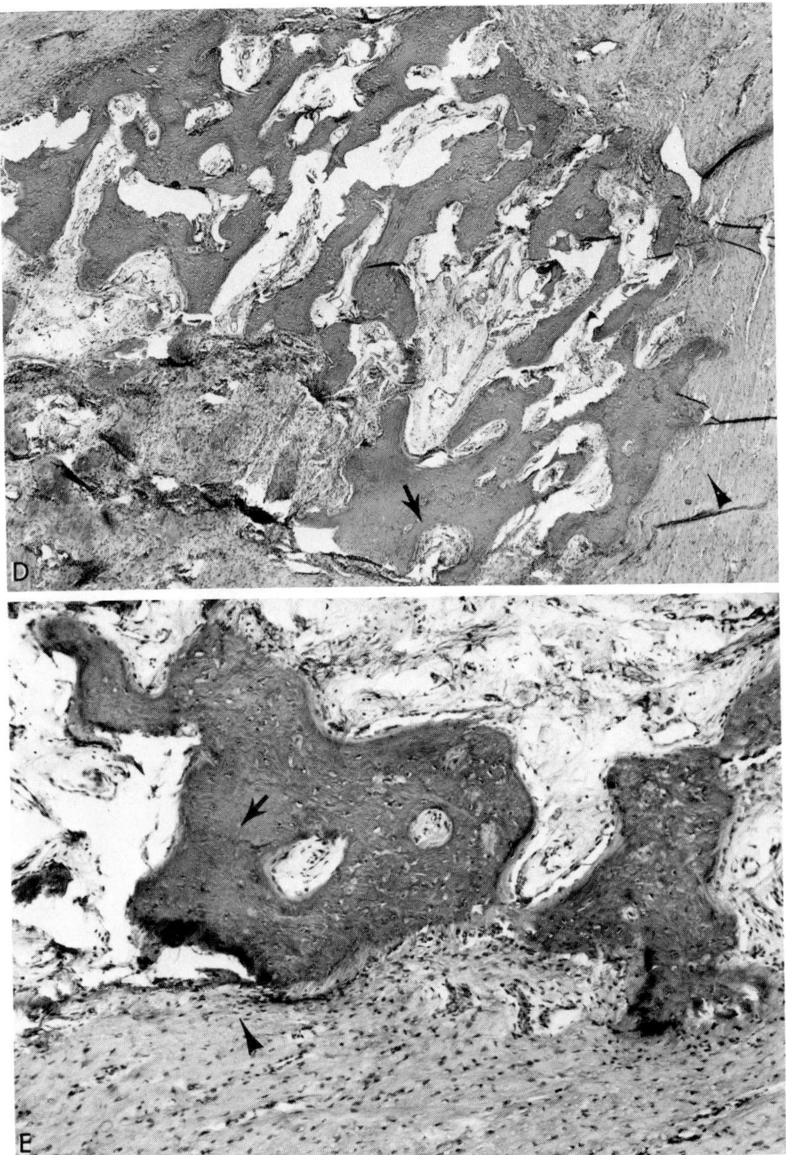

Figure 82–9. Continued

D *A section of the lesion in the anterior proximal tibia shows erosion of bony trabeculae (arrow) by fibrous connective tissue. The periosteum (arrowhead) is indicated (40×).*

E *Bony trabeculae (arrow) have a woven appearance. Osteoclasts are not seen. The periosteum (arrowhead) is again labeled (90×).*

Illustration continued on the following page

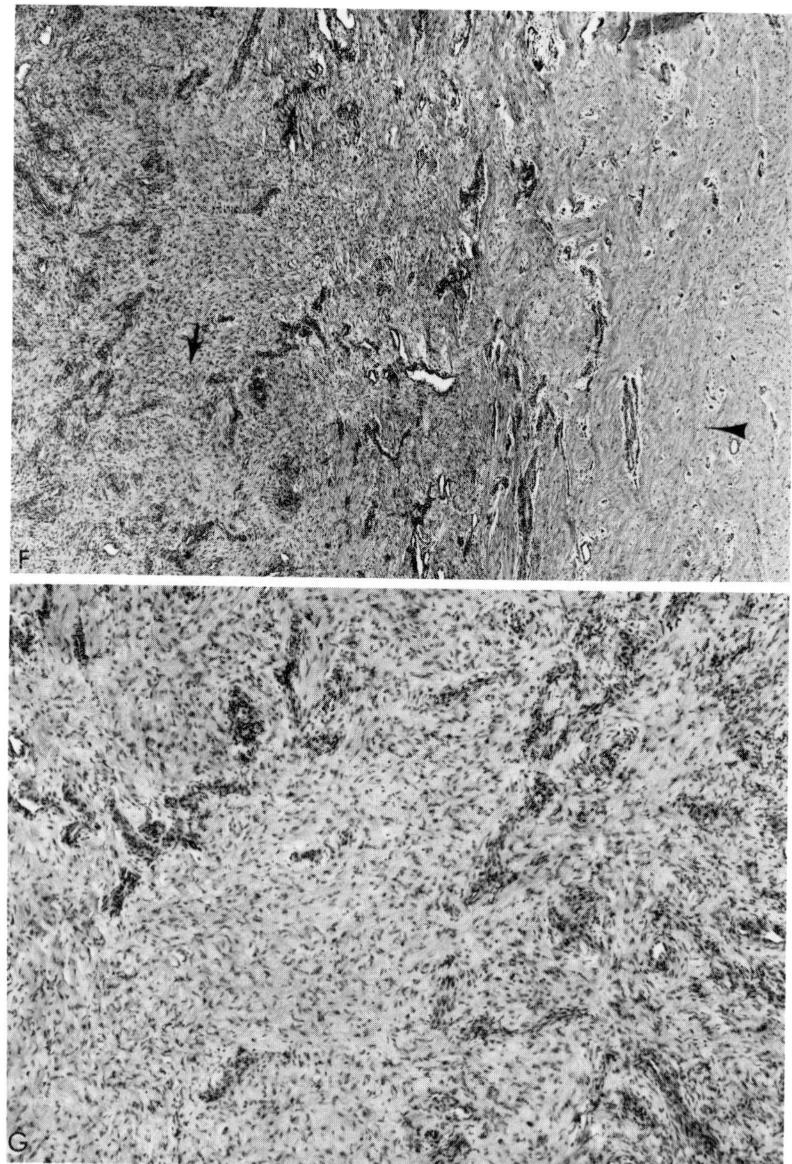

Figure 82–9. Continued

F *Note the proliferating fibrovascular connective tissue (arrow). The periosteum (arrowhead) is at the right (40×).*

G *At higher magnification (90×), the proliferating fibrovascular connective tissue demonstrates a loose stellate cellular configuration with a mixture of capillaries. Chronic inflammatory cells surround the vessels.*

(From Gilula LA, et al: Radiology 121:63, 1976.)

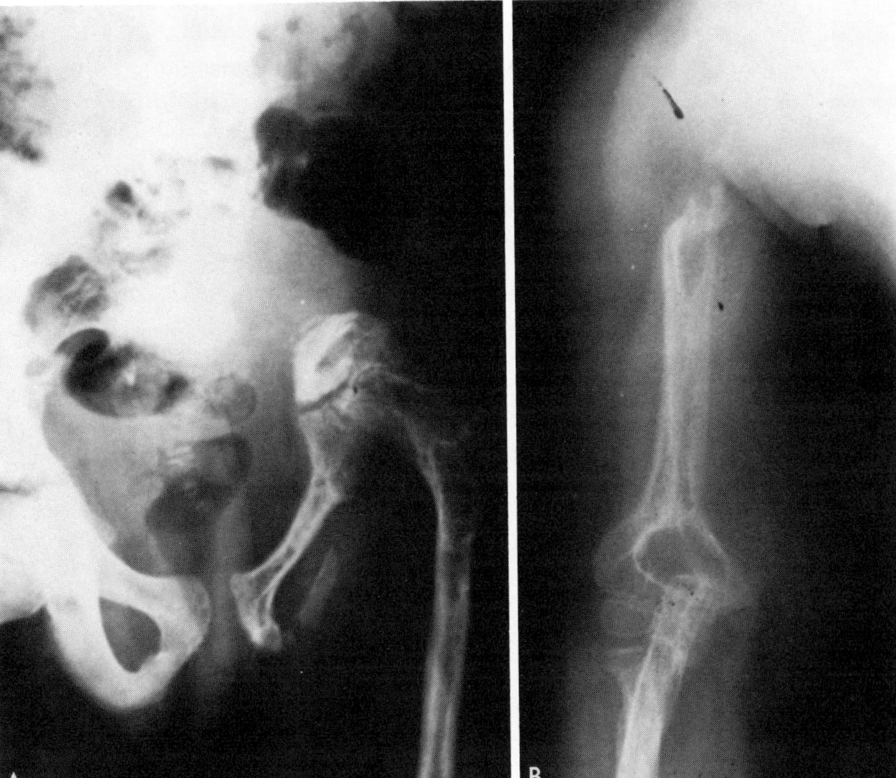

Figure 82–10. *Massive osteolysis of Gorham.*

A *In this 14 year old boy, observe the dissolution of most of the left hemipelvis and the narrowed and tapered left femur. Radiolucent foci and a coarsened trabecular pattern are seen in the femur and pubic bone.*

B *In a 6 year old girl, resorption of the proximal half of the humerus is evident. The remaining bone is osteoporotic, with lucent lesions.*

pattern of regional destruction is dramatic and should suggest the correct diagnosis. Rarely, two or more anatomic regions are affected, separated by normal osseous structures. Apparently, any bone can be involved, including the small tubular bones of the hands and feet, the spine, the skull, and the mandible.[62, 64, 68, 69] The degree of osseous destruction generally increases relentlessly over a period of years, although it may eventually stabilize. Occasional reports of massive osteolysis describe spontaneous recovery of some of the lost bone tissue.[65]

Arteriography may indicate stretching of vessels in the area of lysis.[59, 60] Prominent vascularity usually is not evident during this study, although direct injection of contrast medium into the lesion will result in opacification of the involved area.[66] As one main structural feature of the lesion is the presence of unusually wide capillary-like vessels (see discussion later in this chapter), it appears likely that the blood flow through these vessels is very slow. It has been suggested that the slow circulation produces local hypoxia and lowering of the pH, favoring the activity of various hydrolytic enzymes.[64]

Scintigraphy utilizing bone-seeking radiopharmaceuticals may demonstrate an area of decreased uptake corresponding to the site of diminished or absent bone tissue.[59]

In the early stages of the disorder, the pathologic features resemble those of skeletal hemangioma. In later stages, vascular fibrous tissue replaces the angiomatous tissue. Irregular wide spaces in cortical bone and enlarged marrow spaces in spongy bone contain numerous thin-walled, capillary-like vessels, most of them wider than normal capillaries and filled with blood cells.[64] Many of the abnormal vessels are situated in, and in direct contact with, osseous depressions. Inflammatory infiltrates generally are not evident.

The exact nature of the process is unknown. The resemblance of the pathologic characteristics to those of hemangiomas, coupled with the presence of soft tissue hemangiomatous or lymphangiomatous tissue and, occasionally, pleural effusions containing chyle, has suggested to some investigators, including Gorham and Stout,[48] that massive osteolysis represents a vascular derangement or a diffuse hemangiomatosis; this perhaps is due to a congenital condition in which hyperplastic vascular components form arteriovenous fistulae. Gorham and Stout[48] maintained that active hyperemia, changes in local pH, and mechanical forces promote bone resorption, that trauma might trigger the process by stimulating the production of vascular granulation tissue, and that osteoclastosis is not necessary. The virtual absence of multinucleated osteoclasts in areas of excessive bone resorption has been noted in other reports. Heyden and co-workers[64] observed strong activity of both acid phosphatase and leucine aminopeptidase in mononuclear perivascular cells that were in contact with remaining bone, perhaps indicating that these cells are important in the process of osseous resorption. As the perivascular cells may represent pericytes, the observation that pericytes may be precursors of mononuclear and multinuclear cells with osteolytic capacity is important.[64]

The possibility that massive osteolysis may represent a neoplastic proliferation of hemangiomatous (or lymphangiomatous) tissue has also been suggested in the past. It should be noted, however, that the process does not closely resemble ordinary hemangioma or lymphangioma of bone, or even cystic angiomatosis.[70-75]

Although the degree of osseous deformity in the disease may become severe, serious complications are not frequent. Paraplegia due to spinal cord involvement may occur in cases of vertebral osteolysis.[66] Death can result from thoracic cage, pulmonary, or pleural involvement that leads to compromise of respiratory function. Infection of bone and septic shock appear to be rare.[58]

Idiopathic Multicentric Osteolysis (Carpal-Tarsal Osteolysis). In 1976, Tyler and Rosenbaum[76] proposed the term idiopathic multicentric osteolysis for a rare disorder associated with extensive osteolysis, usually in the carpal or tarsal areas, that had been previously described under a variety of names; these included idiopathic osteolysis, essential osteolysis, progressive essential osteolysis, essential acro-osteolysis, familial osteolysis, hereditary osteolysis, carpal and tarsal agenesis, familial dysostosis carpi, and bilateral carpal necrosis. Idiopathic multicentric osteolysis was further classified into two basic types: multicentric osteolysis with nephropathy and hereditary multicentric osteolysis. Not all cases fit neatly into one of these two categories, so that a third designation, miscellaneous patterns, is required.

Multicentric Osteolysis with Nephropathy. This entity, which has been recognized in only a handful of cases, is characterized by an early age of onset (first few years of life) of osteolysis, associated with progressive renal failure that is commonly fatal by the third decade.[77-84] There is no family history of either osteolysis or renal disease. Presenting clinical manifestations include swollen, painful wrists with the presence or absence of foot deformities. Roentgenograms reveal progressive disappearance of the carpus and, less strikingly, the tarsus, with tapering of the adjacent tubular bones (Fig. 82–11). Osteolysis and subluxation about the elbow, and congenital foot deformities, can also be apparent. Rarely, other sites are affected. Renal alterations accompany the onset of osteolysis. Chronic glomerulonephritis results in hypertension, azotemia, and death in early adult life.

Hereditary Multicentric Osteolysis. This condition reveals a familial distribution, with most cases exhibiting a dominant mode of transmission, although the trait is occasionally recessive.[76, 85-90] In the dominant variety, the onset of disease usually occurs at the age of 3 to 4 years, with articular complaints involving the wrists and ankles. Following this, an asymptomatic period arises in adolescence in which a varying amount of carpal and tarsal osteolysis is associated with progressive deformity. In the recessive variety, the clinical course is basically similar.

Radiographs in both dominant and recessive forms outline dissolution of carpus and tarsus that, in most cases, is not associated with tapering of the adjacent tubular bones (Figs. 82–12 to 82–14). This latter characteristic, which differs from the "penciling" of tubular bones that is evident in multicentric osteolysis with nephropathy, is not constant, and patients with hereditary multicentric osteolysis can reveal such tapering of metacarpals, distal radius, and ulna. Rarely, osteolysis at additional sites can be encountered, including the elbows, shoulders, clavicles, and ribs.[76]

Miscellaneous Patterns. Some cases of idiopathic multicentric osteolysis may not fall precisely into one of these two groups. Thus, nonfamilial cases of carpal and tarsal osteolysis may be discovered that do not reveal renal disease.[85, 91, 92] Conversely, examples of carpal-tarsal osteolysis with evidence of renal involvement may demonstrate familial patterns (dominant mode of inheritance), although the nephropathy may differ in type and degree from that in the sporadic (nonfamilial) cases[93, 94] Erickson and colleagues[94] speculated that a child of a patient with a mild form of multicentric osteolysis with nephropathy could conceivably demonstrate features of the disease, revealing a dominant form of inheritance.

An extensive classification of the types of carpal and tarsal osteolysis was recently proposed by Beals and Bird,[95] who addressed themselves to the difficulty of separating cases of such osteolysis on the basis of absence or presence of recognizable modes of inheritance, and absence or presence of renal disease. It is apparent that dominant and recessive genetic patterns can be identified, that renal disease is not confined to nonhereditary cases, that the presence of so-called sporadic cases may not rule out a genetic transmission, and that other syndromes can reveal similar radiographic patterns.

Pathology and Pathogenesis. The involved tissues in idiopathic multicentric osteolysis usually reveal an increased content of fibrous elements and increased vascularity, with little evidence of inflammation.[95] Osteolysis is accompanied by osteoclastic activity. Bone formation appears normal, and reparative changes may be evidenced by the presence of woven bone formation.[85] Biopsies of involved joints may reveal no significant abnormalities of the synovial membrane, and encroachment on cartilage by fibrocellular tissue.

The pathogenesis of the process is unknown. A primary defect may occur in the osseous and carti-

Text continued on page 3034

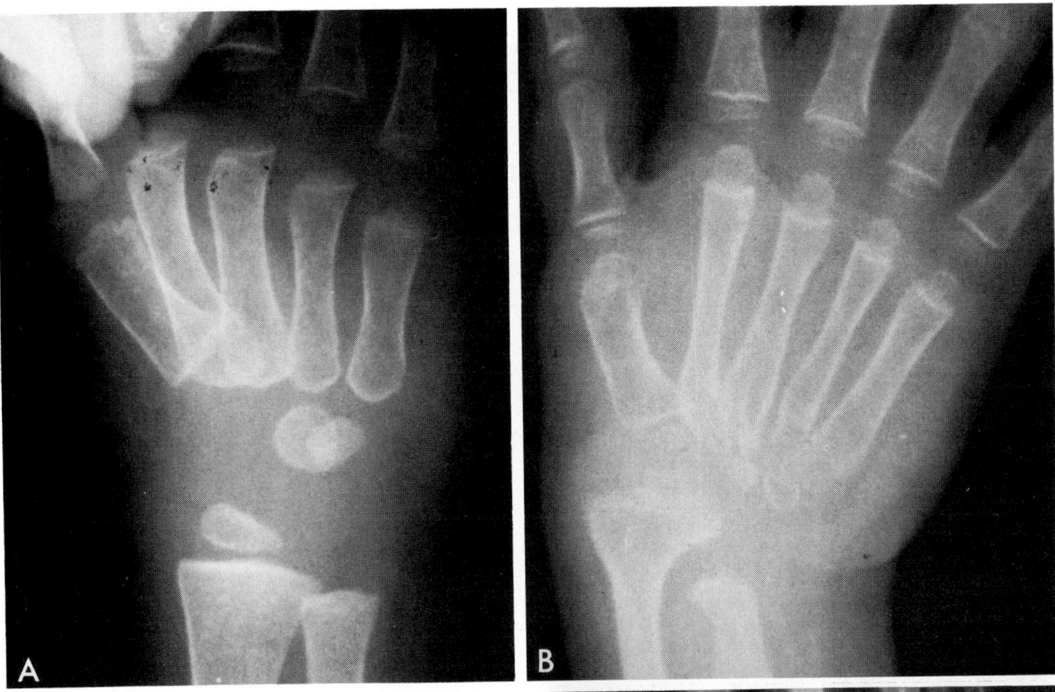

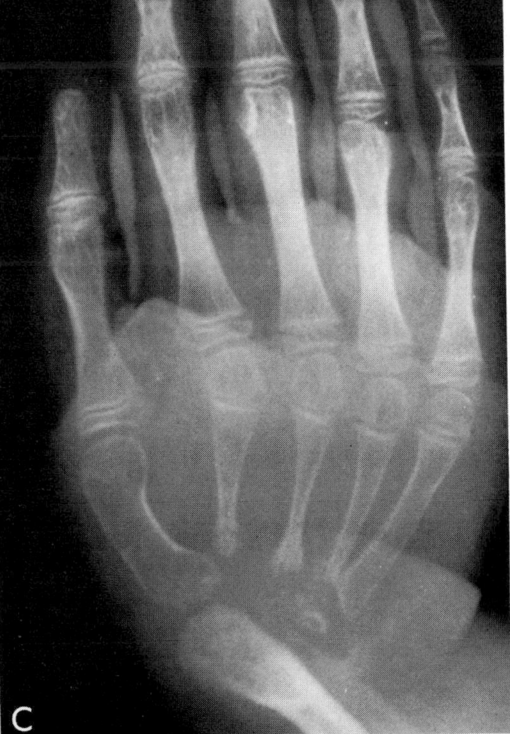

Figure 82–11. *Multicentric osteolysis with nephropathy. A 14 year old boy developed progressive symmetric osteolysis involving hands, wrists, elbows, and feet, with associated renal failure and hypertension. Family history was not contributory.*

A *Radiograph obtained in the second year of life fails to reveal osseous resorption.*

B *At approximately 4 years of age, a radiograph shows ulnar deviation of the hands on the wrists, principally due to shortening of the distal ulna. The two visible carpal bones are small and irregular, and the bases of the second, third, fourth, and fifth metacarpals are tapered.*

C *At 14 years of age, progression of the osteolysis of the carpal bones, metacarpal bases, radius, and ulna is seen. The opposite side was similarly affected.*

(**B, C,** From MacPherson RI, et al: J Can Assoc Radiol 24:98, 1973.)

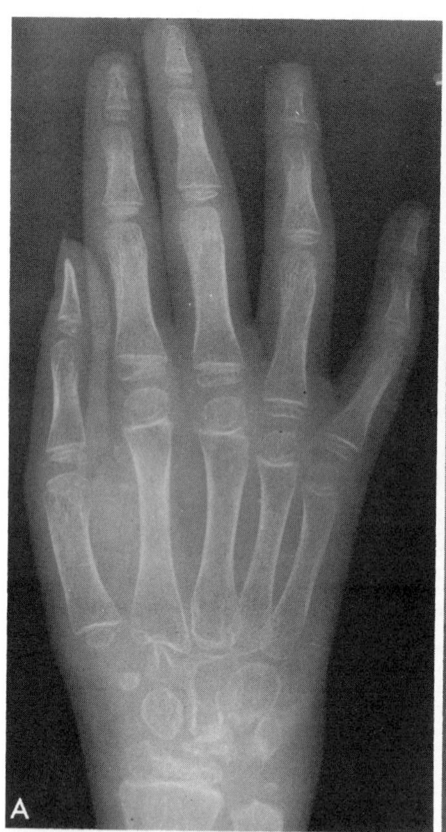

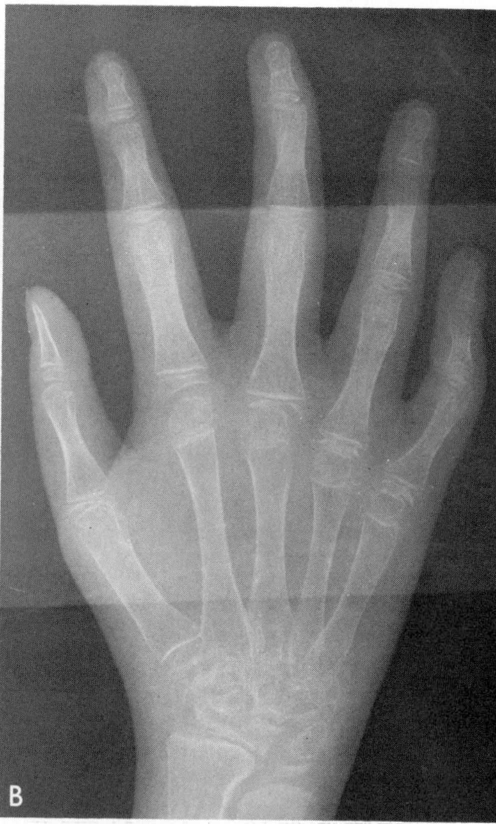

Figure 82–12. Hereditary multicentric osteolysis. This 6 year old boy developed pain, swelling, and stiffness of his right wrist that progressed over the next 2 years, with involvement of both wrists and feet. His father had had a similar disorder.

A *A radiograph of the right hand at age 6 years 9 months reveals osteopenia and carpal bones that are irregular in outline.*

B *At 8½ years of age, carpal osteolysis has progressed, and epiphyseal dissolution has developed at the bases of the second to fifth proximal phalanges.*

C *The roentgenogram of the right foot at 6 years 9 months outlines early erosion of the tarsal navicular (arrow).*

D *Twenty months after* **C**, *the navicular erosion has progressed, the talonavicular cartilage space has disappeared, and the talus shows erosive changes (arrows).*

Illustration continued on the opposite page

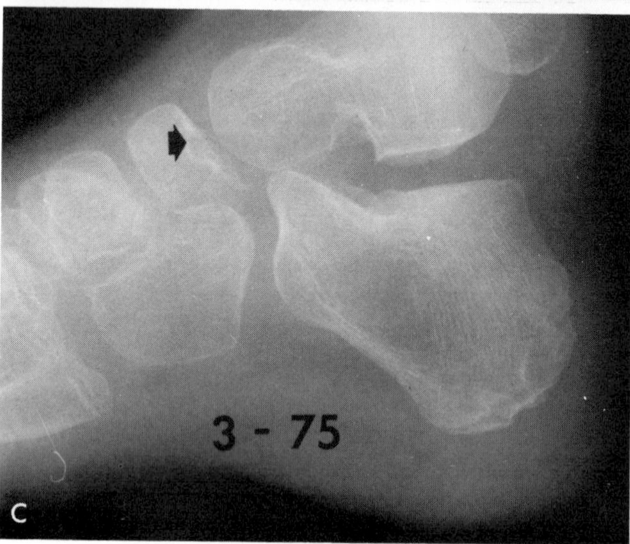

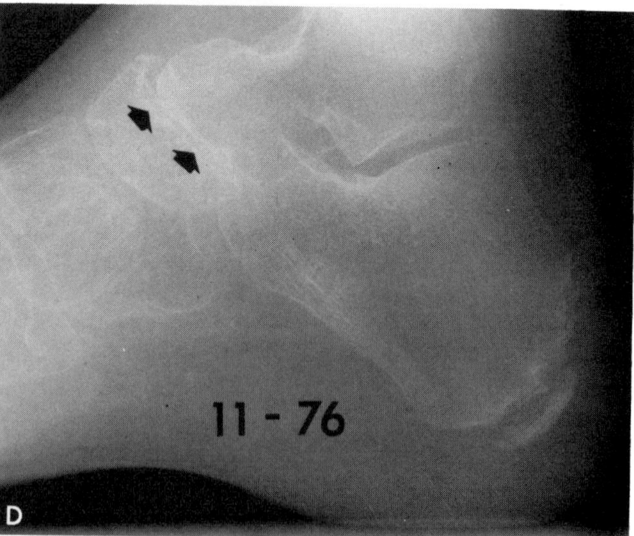

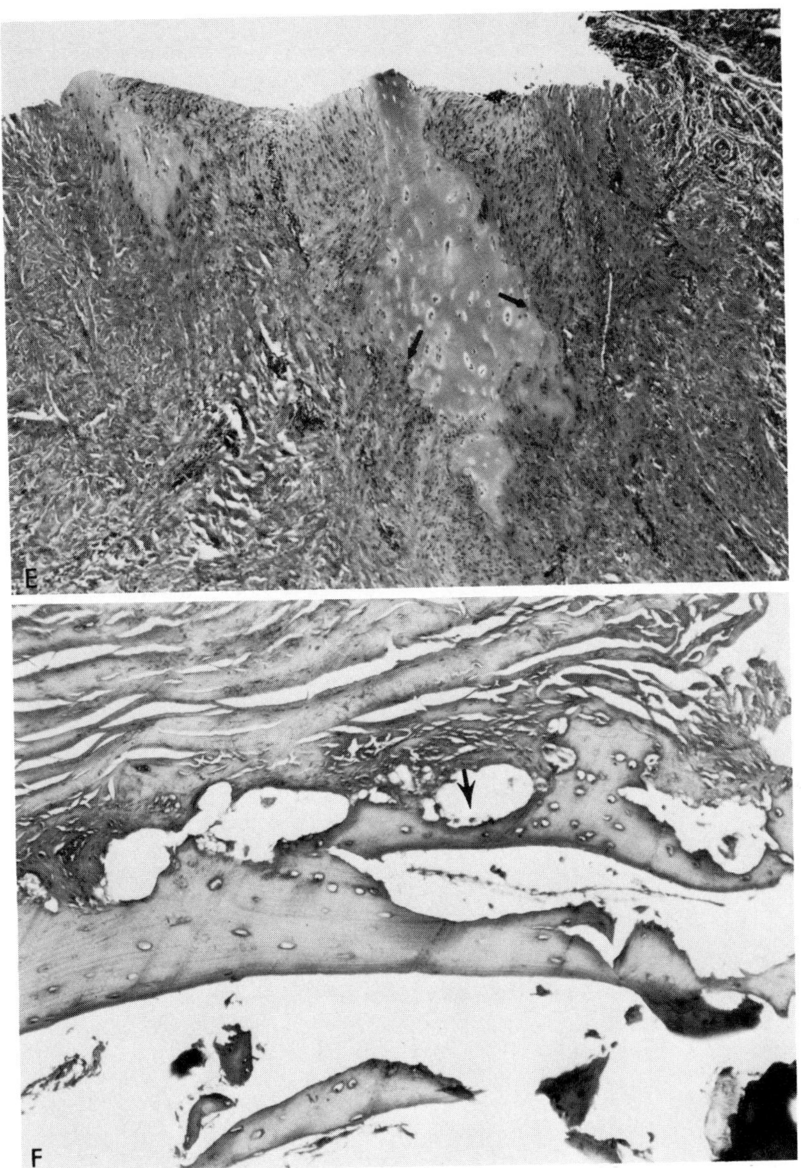

Figure 82–12. Continued

E *A biopsy of the left wrist of the patient at 5 years of age delineates fibrocellular tissue encroaching upon the cartilage (arrows) (120×).*

F *Two years later, biopsy of the same wrist demonstrates a thin rim of cortical bone beneath the periosteum with subperiosteal resorption (arrow) (120 ×). (From Whyte MP, et al: Arthritis Rheum 21:367, 1978.)*

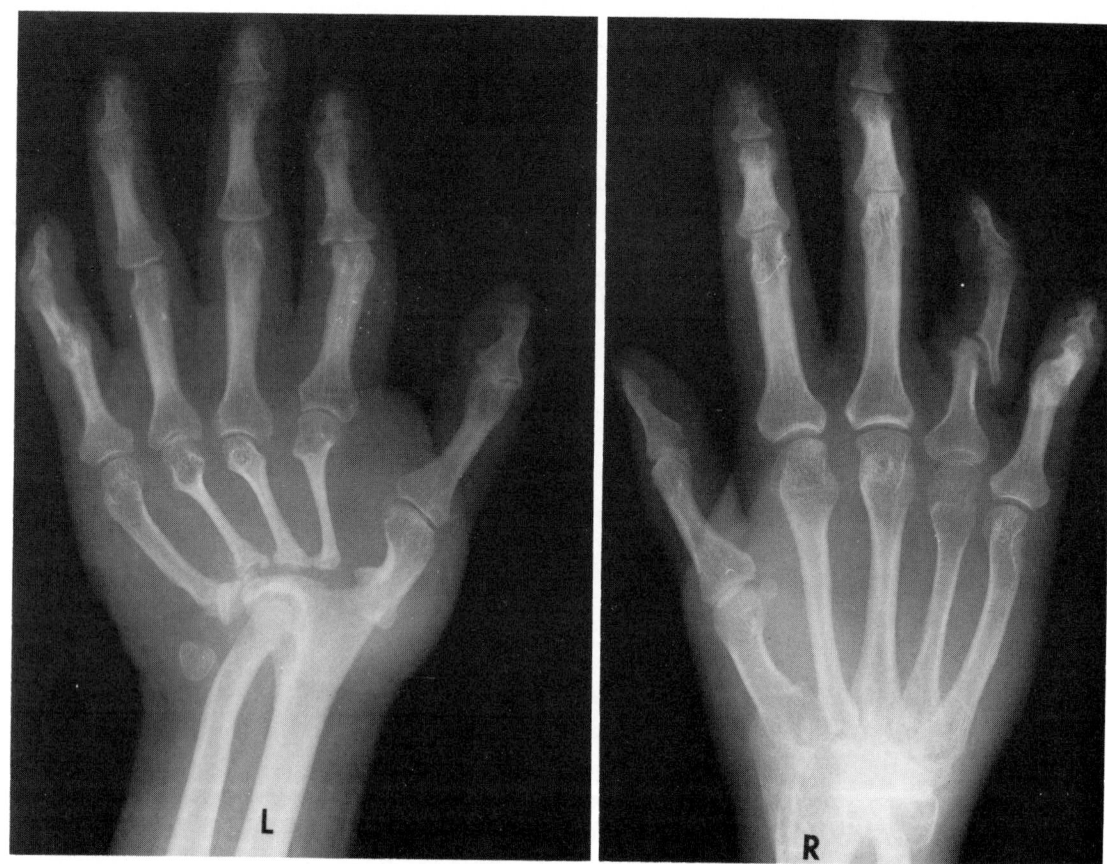

Figure 82–13. *Hereditary multicentric osteolysis. The father of the patient described in Figure 82–12 developed wrist symptoms and signs when he was an infant. A radiograph of the left wrist at age 40 years outlines absence of all but one of the carpal bones, hypoplasia of the metacarpals, and fusion of the fifth proximal interphalangeal joint. The right carpus is resorbed and fused, and there is destruction of the fourth proximal interphalangeal joint and fusion of the fifth. Osteolysis of portions of the metacarpal heads is evident. (From Whyte MP, et al: Arthritis Rheum 21:367, 1978.)*

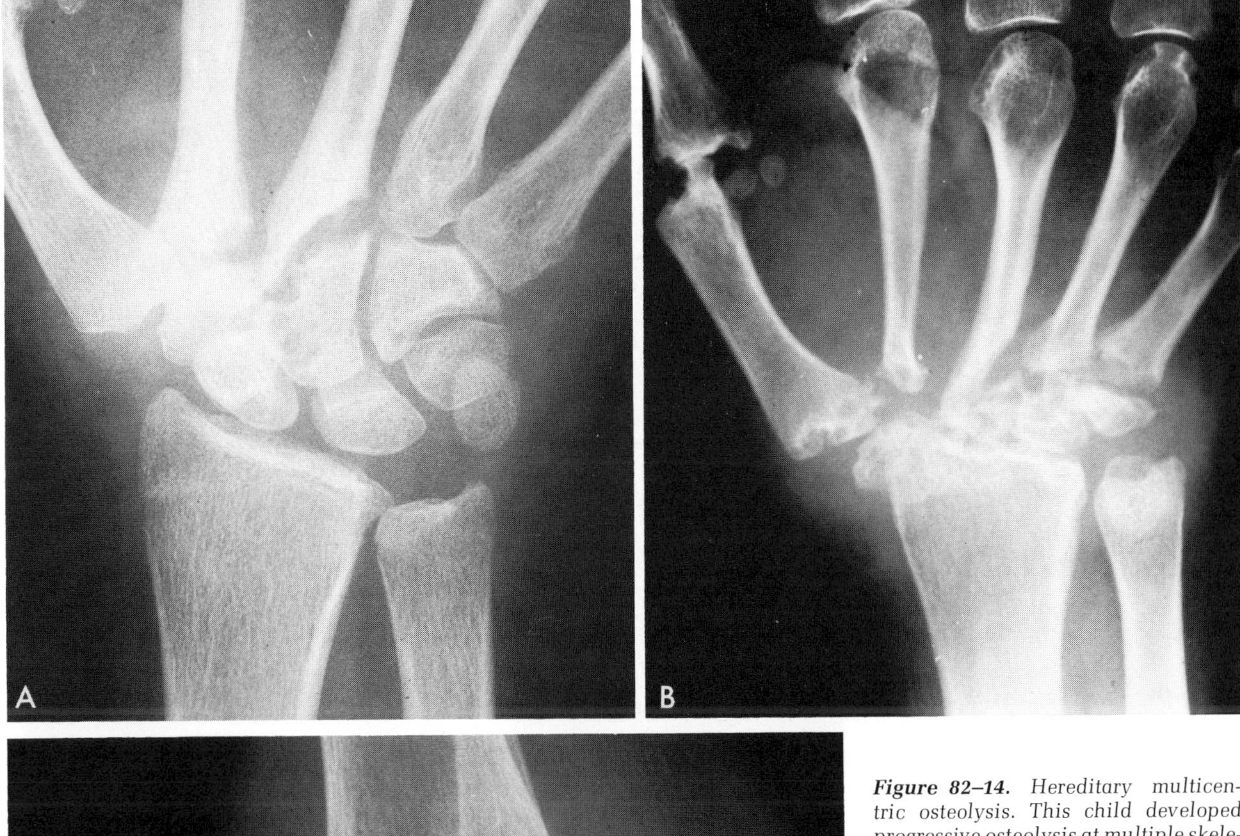

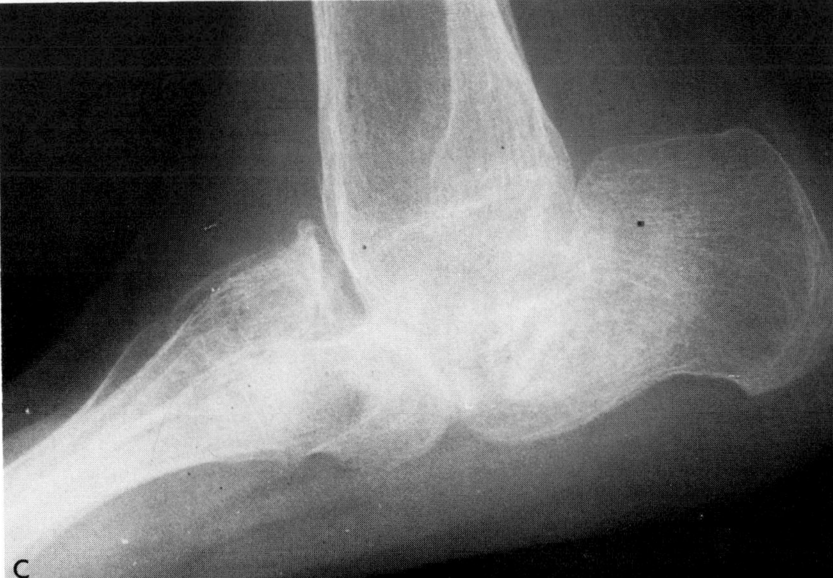

Figure 82–14. *Hereditary multicentric osteolysis. This child developed progressive osteolysis at multiple skeletal sites without evidence of renal disease.*

A, B *Radiographs of the wrists obtained at the ages of 16 and 22 years reveal progressive resorption of the carpus and metacarpal bases, with soft tissue swelling. The tapered appearance of the proximal metacarpals and the osseous erosions at several metacarpophalangeal joints are readily apparent.*

C *A radiograph of the foot at age 16 years demonstrates the great degree of lysis of most of the tarsal bones. The tibia is articulating with the calcaneus.*

Illustration continued on the following page

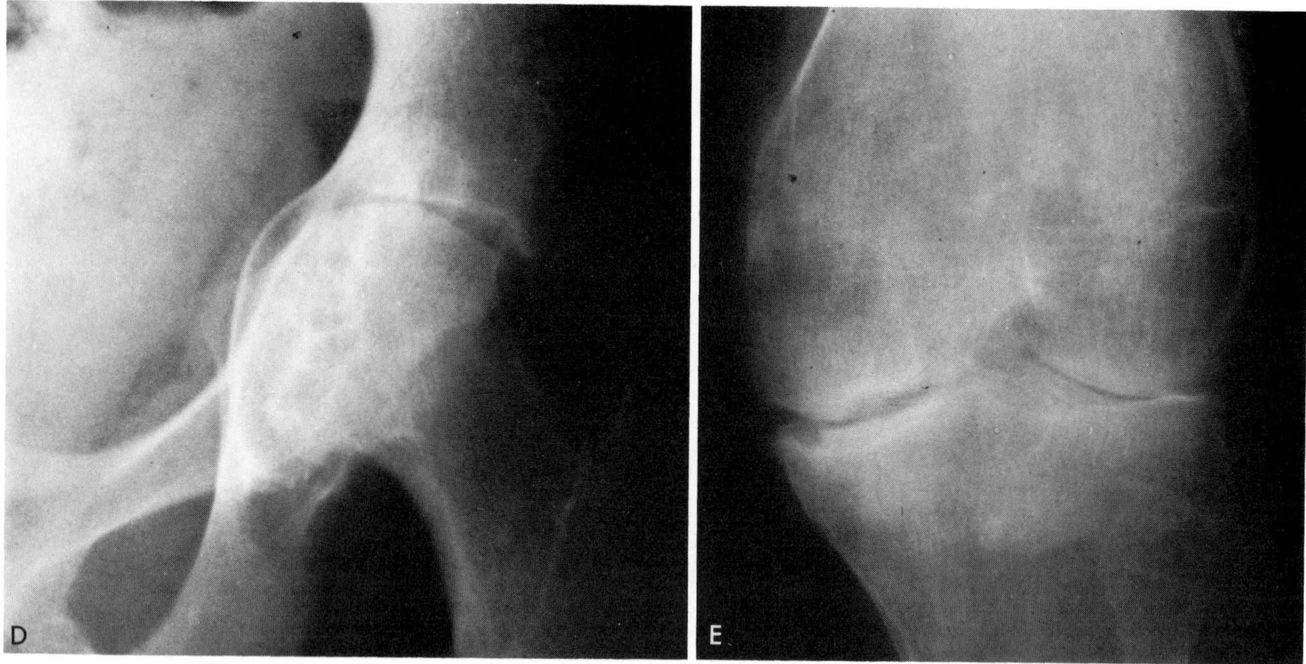

Figure 82–14. Continued

D, E *Unusual aspects of this case are the joint space narrowing, osseous erosion, and acetabular protrusion of the left hip and the loss of articular space in the knee.*

(Courtesy of Dr. A. Brower, The Uniformed Services University for Health Sciences, Bethesda, Maryland.)

laginous tissues, or these latter sites may be secondarily affected as a result of primary involvement and proliferation of articular fibrous tissue. Occasional reports of increased urinary hydroxyproline excretion[85] and elevated serum phosphatase levels may indicate the progressive destruction of bone or the presence of an underlying metabolic disorder characterized by increased bone turnover; however, the evidence of increased collagen turnover is inconstant.[95]

Differential Diagnosis. The major radiographic characteristic of the various forms of idio-

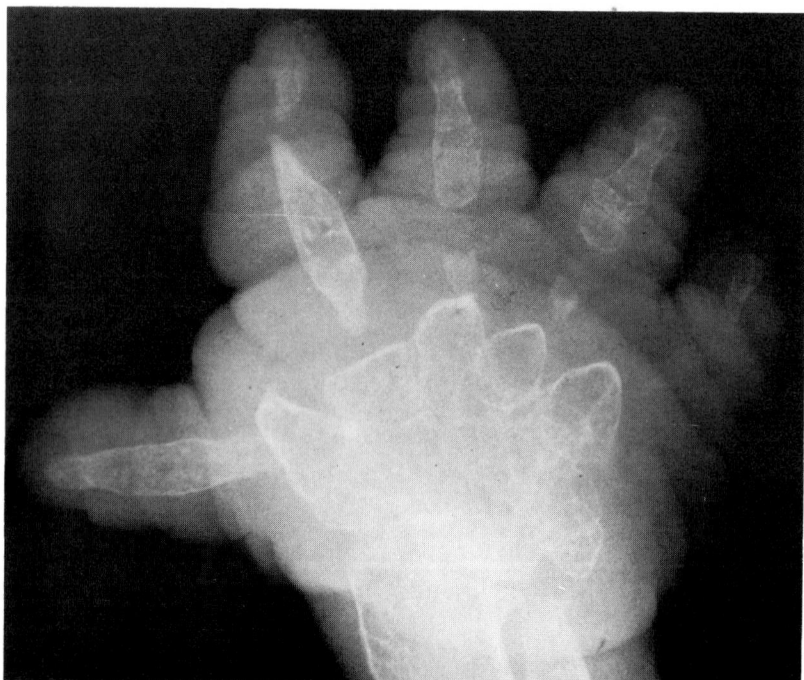

Figure 82–15. *Multicentric reticulohistiocytosis. The degree of osteolysis of metacarpals and phalanges is striking. Carpal fusion and resorption of the distal radius and ulna are evident. (Courtesy of Dr. D. Chambers, Norfolk, Virginia.)*

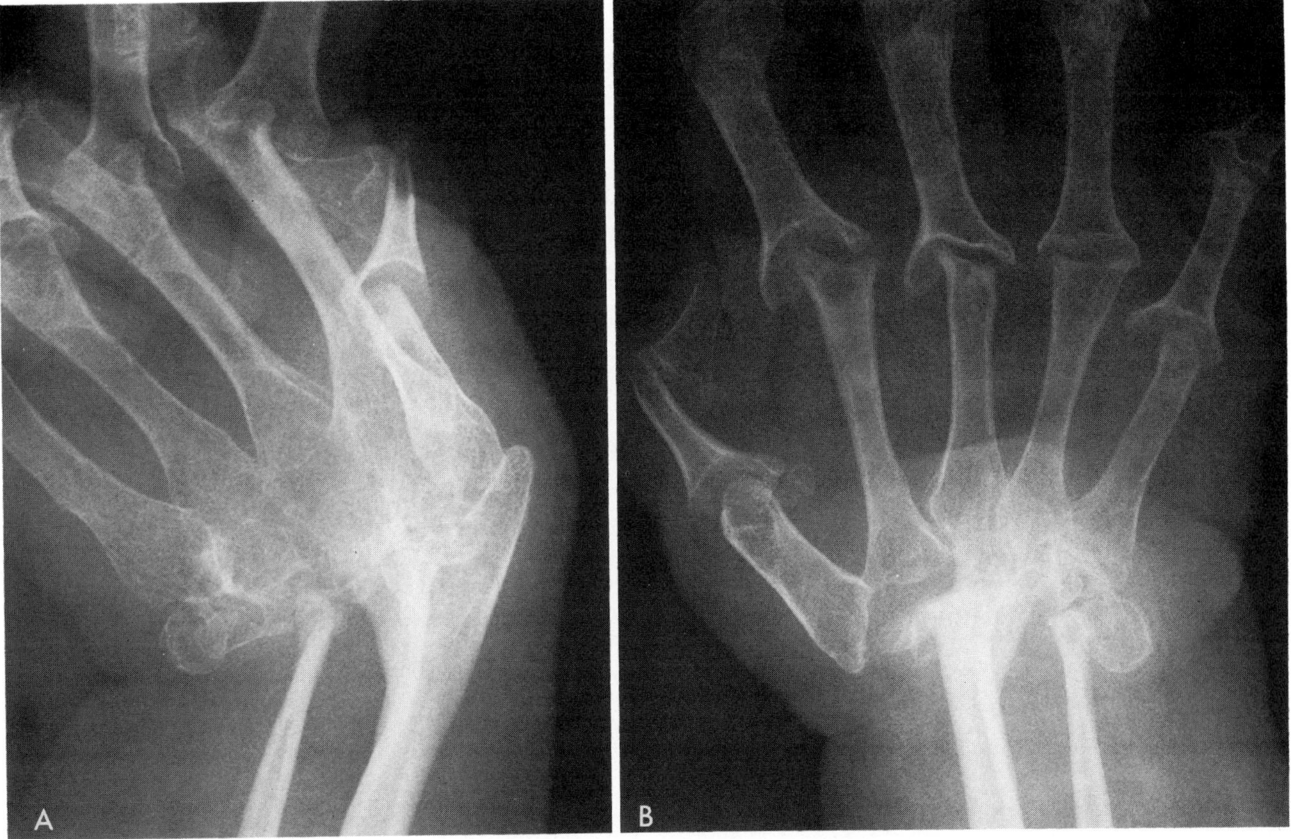

Figure 82–16. *Still's disease. Observe the extreme destruction and resorption of carpus, radii, ulnae, metacarpals, and phalanges. The findings are not unlike those of carpal-tarsal osteolysis syndromes. (Courtesy of Dr. V. Vint, Scripps Clinic, LaJolla, California.)*

pathic multicentric osteolysis is the striking resorption of bone that predominates in the carpal and tarsal areas (and occasionally in the elbows). This distribution differs from that typically associated with other varieties of osteolysis, such as occupational acro-osteolysis (phalanges), posttraumatic osteolysis (distal clavicle, pubic and ischial rami, femoral neck, ulna, radius), acro-osteolysis syndrome of Hajdu and Cheney (phalanges), massive osteolysis of Gorham (variable distribution with predilection for pelvic and shoulder girdles), multicentric reticulohistiocytosis (hands, feet, wrists, ankles) (Fig. 82–15), acro-osteolysis syndrome of Joseph or Shinz (phalanges), and neurogenic acro-osteolysis (phalanges). The changes may resemble those in juvenile chronic arthritis (Fig. 82–16) (see Chapter 28), the Winchester syndrome, and Farber's disease. Accurate diagnosis requires knowledge of the associated clinical manifestations, including the presence and mode of inheritance and the appearance of renal disease.

OTHER OSTEOLYSIS SYNDROMES

Neurogenic Acro-Osteolysis. Both recessive and dominant forms of progressive peripheral bone destruction associated with sensory neuropathy have been described.[96] The disease becomes clinically apparent in childhood and is associated with skin ulcerations and progressive resorption of phalanges of the hands and feet.[97, 98] Vitamin B_{12} determinations in the spinal fluid of some patients have indicated abnormalities that suggest vitamin B_{12} hypovitaminosis as a possible direct cause of the disease.[99] A somewhat similar pattern of osteolysis, with more widespread bone destruction, has been noted in Vietnamese patients who revealed severe scarring of the skin, no neurologic alterations, and positive serologic tests for syphilis.[100] Some of these latter patients may have had the acro-osteolysis syndrome of Shinz (see below).

Acro-Osteolysis of Joseph and Shinz. Joseph and associates[101] described a single sibship of recessive inheritance of osteolysis of the distal phalanges in otherwise normal boys. Shinz[102] observed a form of peripheral osteolysis characterized by a dominant inheritance, onset in the second decade of life, destruction of phalanges of the hands and feet, and ulcerating skin lesions, without neurologic abnormalities.

Farber's Disease. This disease is characterized by an onset in infancy of progressive, painful periarticular swelling, joint rigidity and contracture, osteolysis, and subcutaneous nodules.[95] It may represent a disorder of mucopolysaccharide metabolism of the fibroblast.[103]

Winchester Syndrome. Winchester and associates[104] described a disorder with recessive inheritance manifested as extensive and progressive destruction of the carpus, tarsus, and elbows beginning in infancy and associated with increased acid mucopolysaccharides in cell cultures, but not in the urine.[95] Additional findings include dwarfism, coarsened facial features, peripheral corneal opacities, arthralgias and joint stiffening, progressive deformities of the trunk and limbs, and generalized and profound osteoporosis. Although originally classified as a form of mucopolysaccharidosis, the Winchester syndrome may be more accurately regarded as a nonlysosomal connective tissue disease.[95]

Osteolysis with Detritic Synovitis. In 1978, Resnick and co-workers[105] described a new pattern of osteolysis in both the appendicular and the axial skeleton in a 71 year old woman without a family history of similar abnormalities. A severely destructive and mutilating arthropathy of the hands was associated with bone resorption of the phalanges, metacarpals, metatarsals, clavicles, tubular bones, and spine (Fig. 82–17). Pathologic examination documented the presence of superficial ulceration and necrosis of the synovium, fibrosis of deeper connective tissue, subsynovial fibrin deposition, focal areas of palisaded synovial cells, infrequent inflammatory cells, and numerous shards of necrotic bone embedded within fibrotic synovium and periarticular fibrous tissue. The roentgenographic characteristics resembled, in part, the findings of hyperparathyroidism; however, the absence of more classic features of subperiosteal and subchondral resorption, the presence of severe digital deformities, and the normal values for serum calcium, phosphorus, and parathyroid hormone made this latter diagnosis untenable.

CHONDROLYSIS

Cartilage loss or destruction is an important complication of many articular disorders, including rheumatoid arthritis, seronegative spondyloarthropathies, septic arthritis, degenerative joint disease, and relapsing polychondritis (see Chapters 26 to 30, 39, and 83). In addition, cartilage atrophy can appear following disuse, immobilization, or paralysis, perhaps related to interruption of normal patterns of

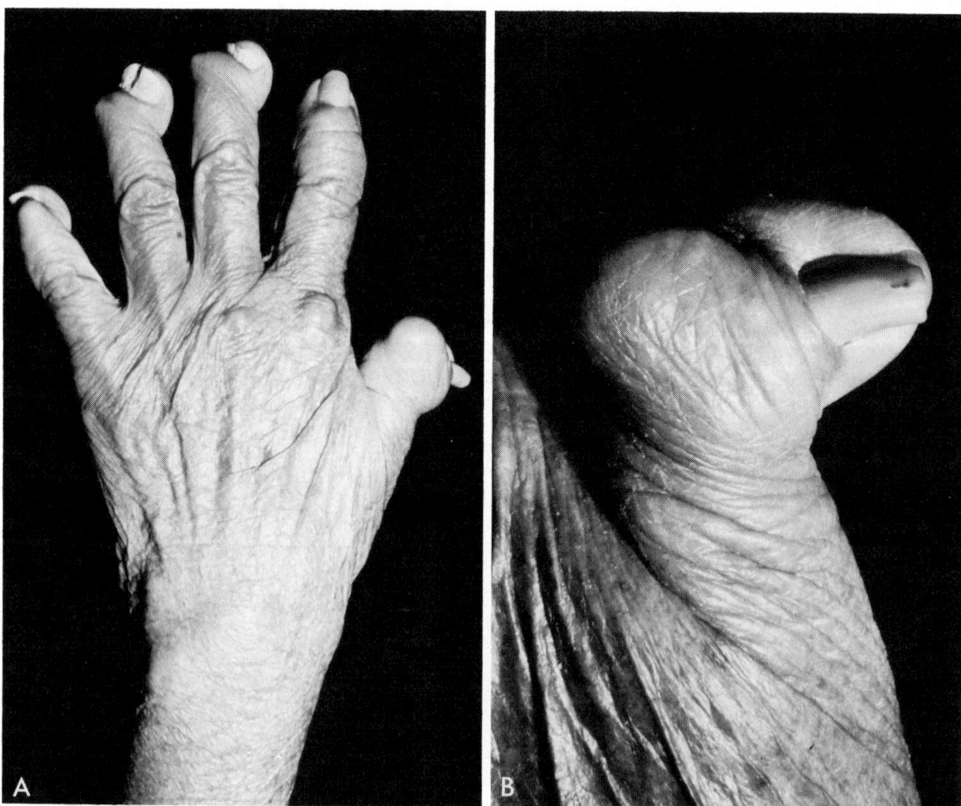

Figure 82–17. *Osteolysis with detritic synovitis. A 71 year old woman developed a severely destructive and mutilating arthropathy of her hands. There was no pertinent family, occupational, or traumatic history.*

A, B *Note deformities of the terminal phalanges of each digit. Similar changes were apparent on the opposite side.*

Illustration continued on the opposite page

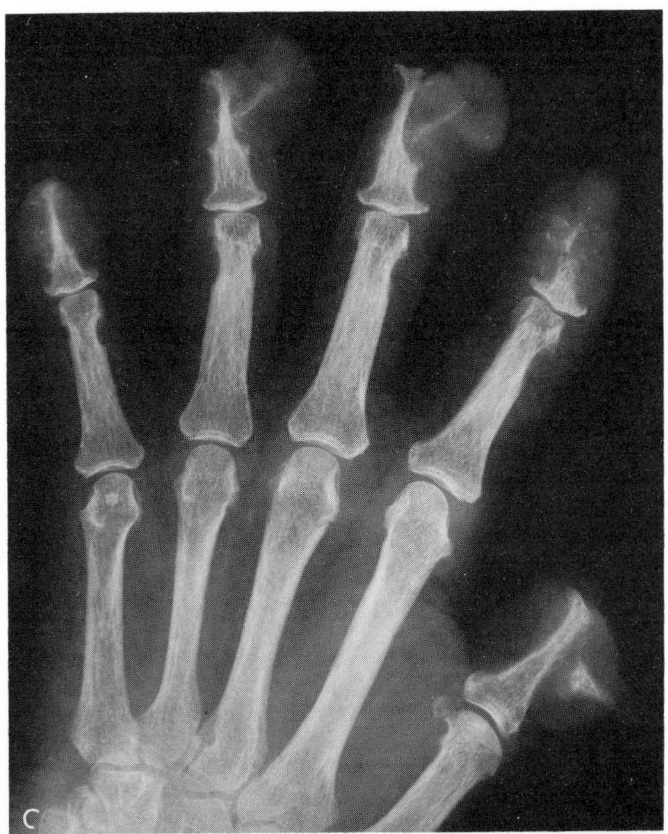

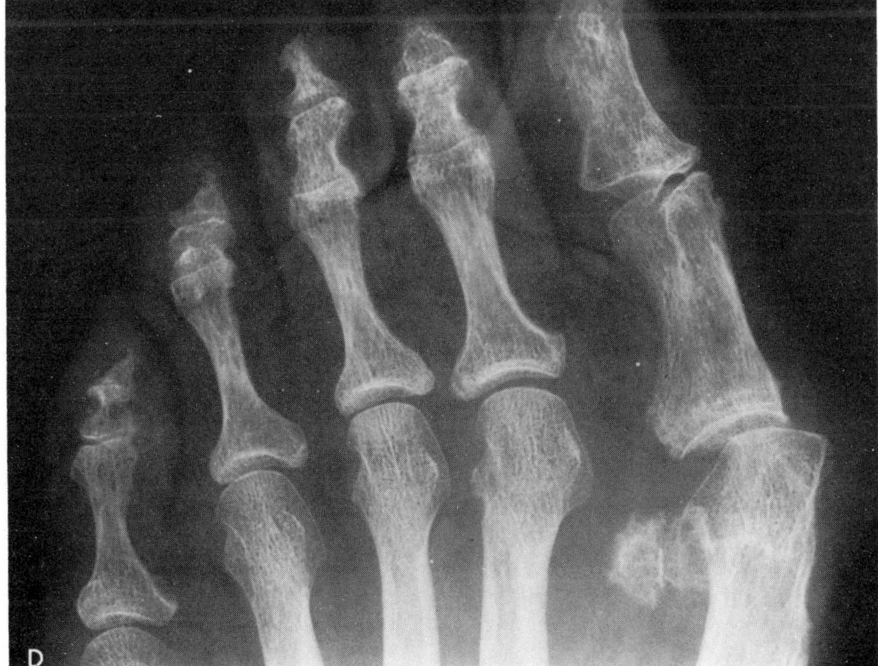

Figure 82–17. Continued

C *Note almost complete resorption of all terminal phalanges with proximal subluxation of the remaining bone, resorption along both radial and ulnar aspects of the phalanges and metacarpals, and articular spaces that appear unremarkable.*

D *Resorption of the medial aspect of the proximal and middle phalanges, tufts, and sesamoids is seen.*

Illustration continued on the following page

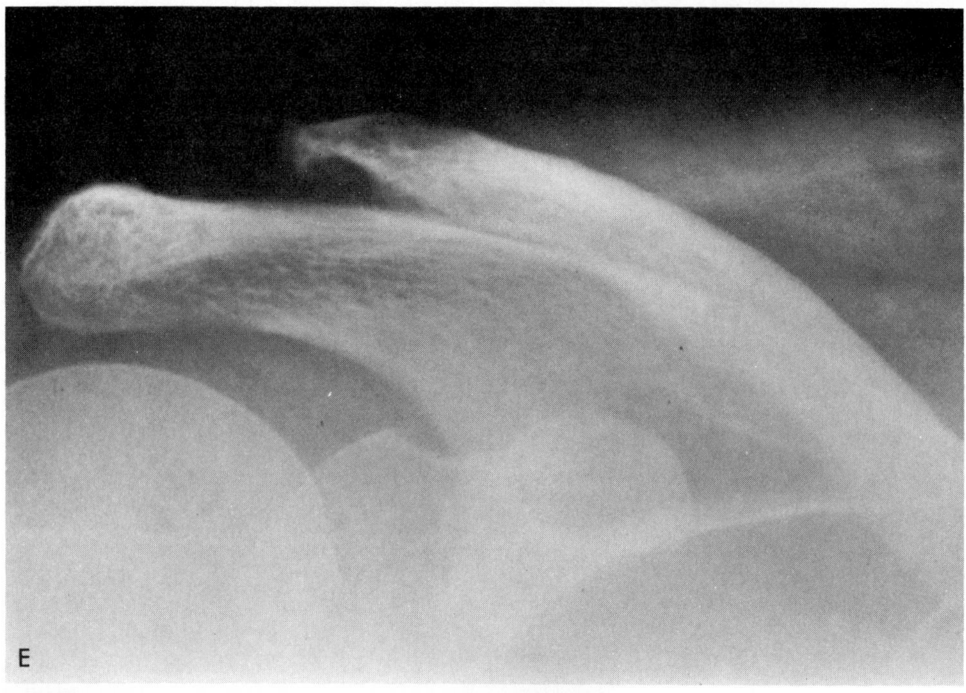

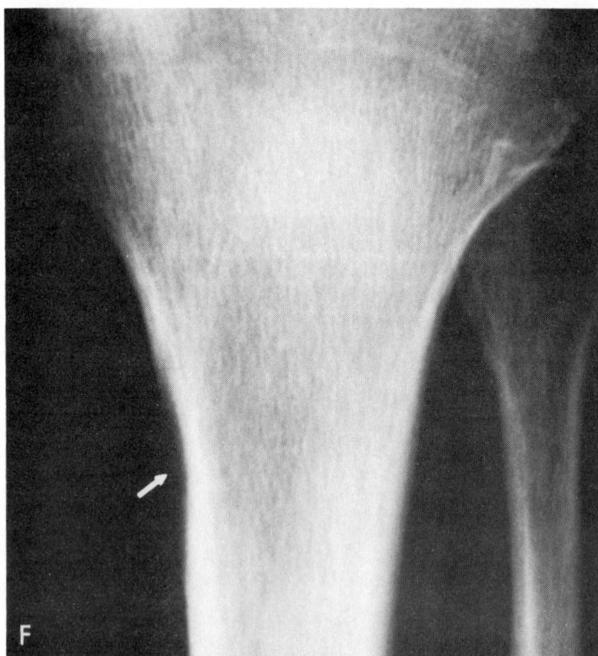

Figure 82–17. Continued

E *Lysis of the distal clavicle has produced a shortened and tapered osseous contour.*

F *Bony lysis of the medial tibia (arrow) is identical to that which occurs in hyperparathyroidism.*

Illustration continued on the opposite page

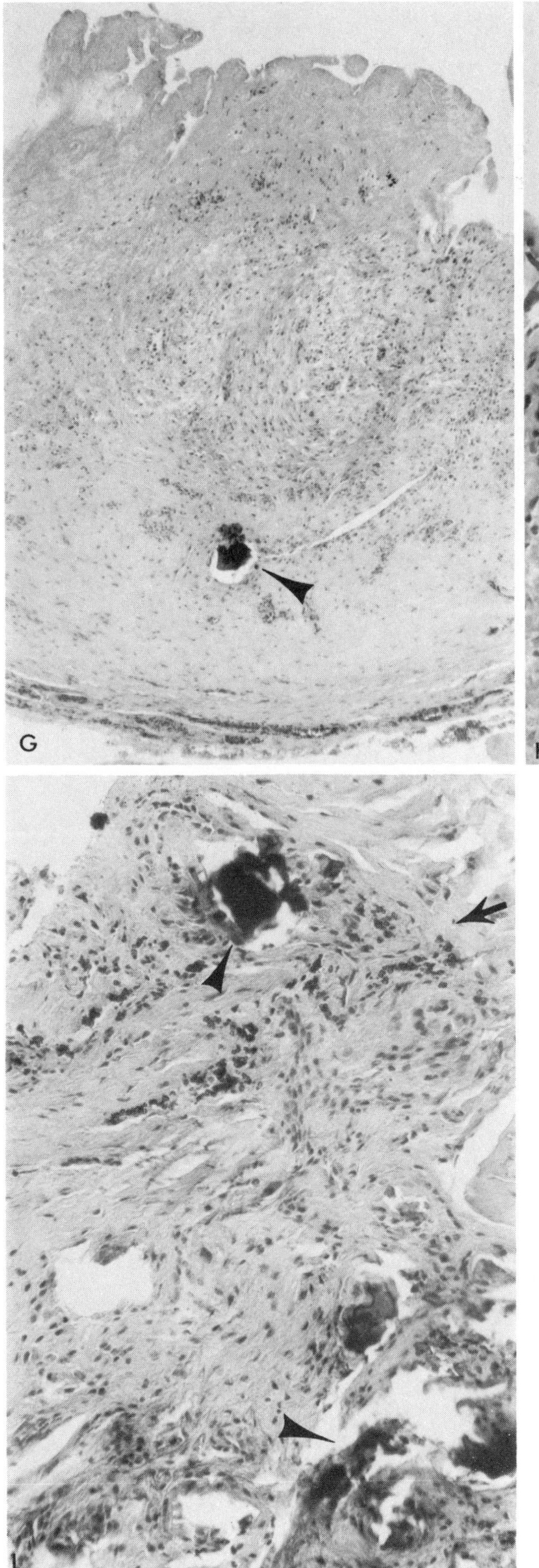

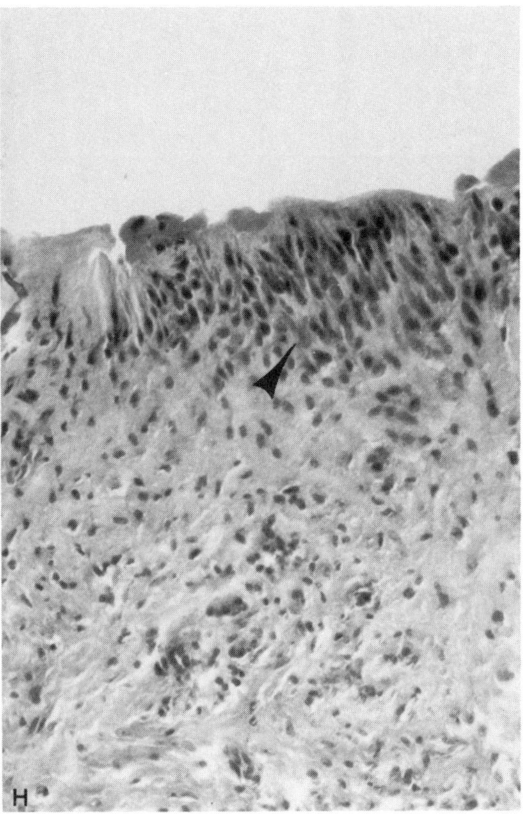

Figure 82–17. Continued

G *Biopsy specimen from an involved distal interphalangeal articulation reveals chronic synovitis with surface ulceration, deeper fibroblastic proliferation and fibrosis, and a bony fragment (arrowhead) embedded in the subsynovial tissue (64 ×).*

H *At higher magnification (100×), palisading of synovial lining cells (arrowhead) and infrequent inflammatory cells are observed.*

I *Note multiple bony fragments in the synovial and subsynovial tissue (arrowheads) and hemosiderin deposition (arrow) (160 ×).*

*(**A, C, E,** From Resnick D, et al: Arch Intern Med 138:1003, 1978, Copyright 1978, American Medical Association.)*

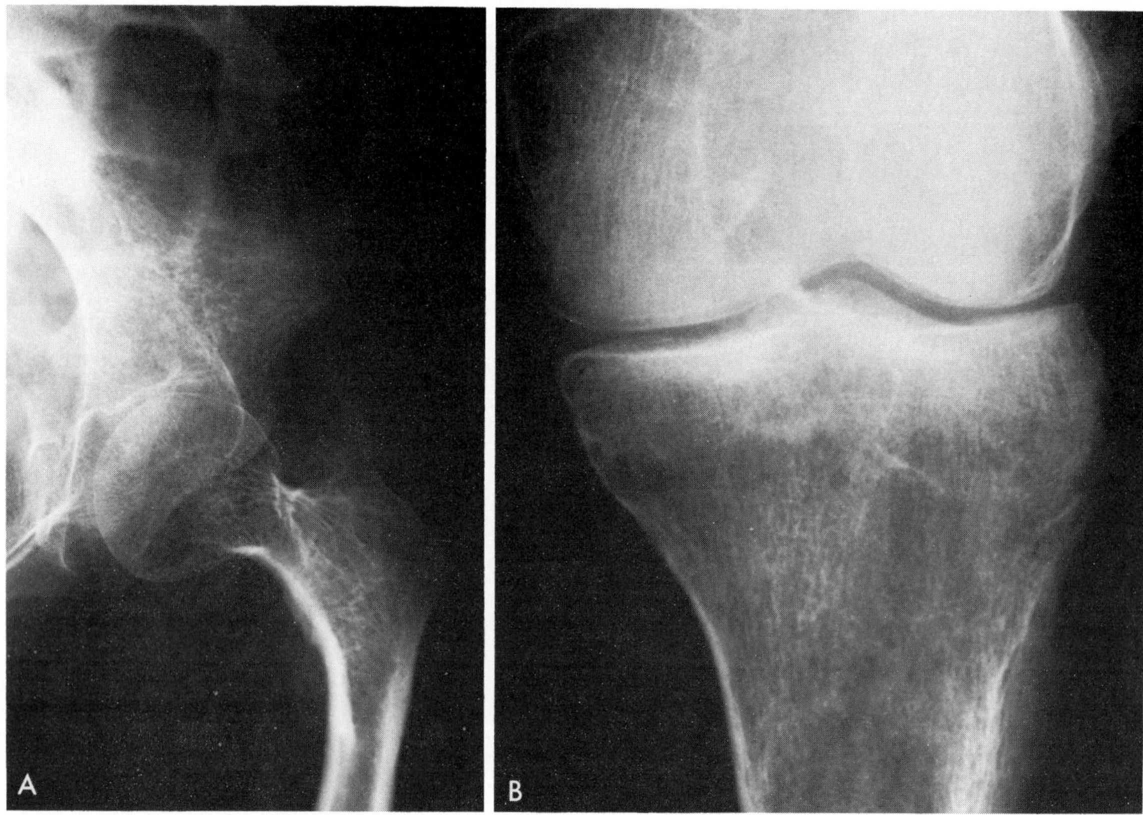

Figure 82–18. *Cartilage atrophy. Following paralysis* **(A)** *or disuse* **(B)**, *cartilage atrophy can lead to diffuse loss of joint space.*

chondral nutrition (Fig. 82–18) (see Chapter 69). Finally, chondrolysis may appear during the course of a slipped capital femoral epiphysis or on an idiopathic basis.

Chondrolysis Following Slipped Capital Femoral Epiphysis

This association of chondrolysis was first recognized by Waldenström in 1930.[106] Subsequent reports are numerous,[107-115] and chondrolysis currently is recognized as a definite and important complication of slipping of the capital femoral epiphysis. An excellent review of the subject is provided in an article by Goldman and associates.[116]

The reported incidence of chondrolysis appearing during the course of slipped femoral capital epiphyses varies from approximately 1 per cent[110] to 40 per cent,[117] much of the variation being related to differences in patient selection and the clinical and radiographic criteria utilized for diagnosis. A high incidence is recorded in black, Hawaiian, and Hispanic patients.[108, 110, 113, 118] Men and women are both affected, and the incidence of chondrolysis in women is relatively high in view of the male predominance in cases of uncomplicated slipped epiphyses.[116] The age of the patient, the acuteness and extent of the epiphyseal separation, and the method of treatment are probably of minor importance in influencing the incidence of this complication, although chondrolysis may be more frequent in individuals treated by long-term immobilization or by surgical procedures other than in situ fixations.

Clinical manifestations of chondrolysis generally appear within a year of the epiphyseal separation and, occasionally, are observed simultaneously with the slipping itself. Pain, tenderness, limitation of motion, and flexion contracture are noted in the affected hip or, very rarely, in the hip that is contralateral to that with the slipped capital femoral epiphysis. These findings may not allow precise or early diagnosis, since similar manifestations can accompany the slipping process itself, the severity of the clinical abnormalities is extremely variable, and additional complications of epiphyseal slipping may produce almost identical clinical alterations.[116] The diagnostic dilemma is further accentuated by the absence of characteristic laboratory abnormalities. Thus, correct interpretation of radiographic findings becomes important in establishing a specific diagnosis.

Goldman and co-workers[116] emphasized three roentgenographic features of chondrolysis (Fig. 82–19). Initially, periarticular osteoporosis appears that may persist for variable amounts of time, probably

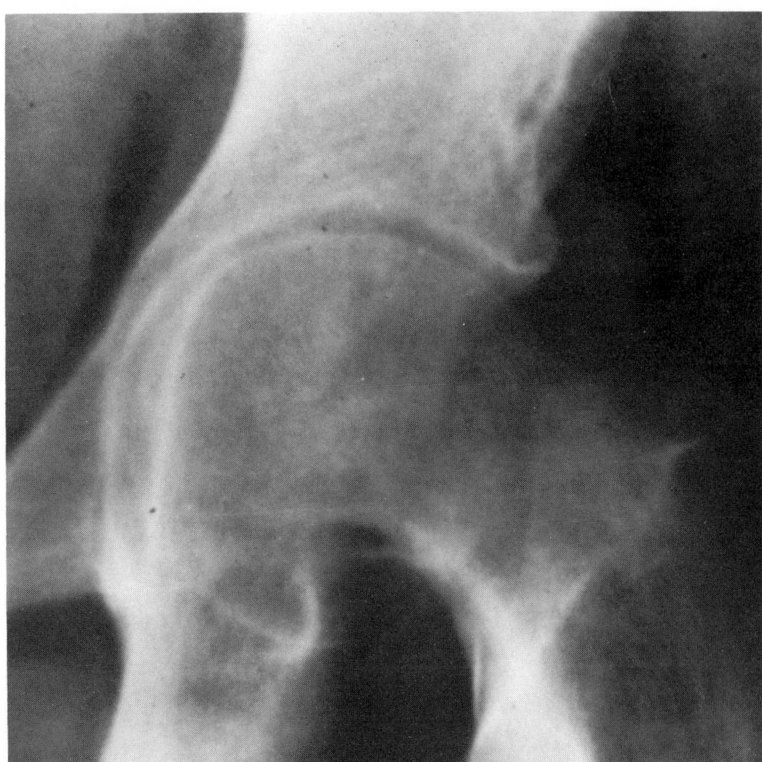

Figure 82–19. *Chondrolysis following slipped capital femoral epiphysis: Radiographic abnormalities. Note osteoporosis, concentric joint space narrowing, protrusio acetabuli deformity, and an abnormal alignment of the femoral head and femoral neck.*

reflecting the pathologically evident increased vascularity of the subchondral osseous tissue.[107, 109] The second finding is rapid narrowing of the joint space that most typically affects the entire articulation, or is isolated to the superior aspect of the joint. Superior joint space diminution is especially common when osteonecrosis is also present (7 to 25 per cent of cases),[109, 113] or when osteotomies have been utilized in the treatment of the epiphyseal slipping.[116] Third, thinning and disappearance of the subchondral bone plate, osseous erosion, and flattening can be seen, particularly at sites of chondral destruction, about the fovea, and on both femoral and acetabular surfaces. Acetabular protrusion (which generally is mild), subchondral cysts (which usually are small or moderate in size), and premature fusion of adjacent growth plates may be apparent.

The radiographic findings appear in a relatively short time, and can subsequently stabilize, to be followed by changes of cartilaginous and osseous repair characterized by partial or complete "recovery" of the articular space, bony eburnation or sclerosis, and osteophytosis. At other times, especially in the presence of osteonecrosis, progressive deterioration of the joint is seen.

Pathologic alterations include thinning and pitting of the articular cartilage of the acetabulum and femoral head, replacement of portions of the cartilaginous surface with fibrous tissue or fibrocartilage, and capsular thickening[108, 110, 119] (Fig. 82–20). The synovium initially undergoes proliferation with hypervascularity,[116] and is later replaced by fibrous tissue and a chronic inflammatory infiltrate.[107, 109]

The etiology and pathogenesis of chondrolysis in slipped capital femoral epiphyses are not clear. The presence of sparse synovial tissue has led to speculation that chondral loss relates to poor cartilage nutrition from inadequate synovial fluid production,[106, 107] perhaps accentuated by prolonged immobilization that prevents appropriate diffusion of nutrients into the cartilage. This theory is supported by the similarity of the radiographic and pathologic findings to those related to cartilage atrophy following extended periods of inactivity, and the occasional presence of chondrolysis of both hips following bilateral immobilization for a unilateral slipped capital epiphysis.[108, 120] Other investigators have emphasized the role of compromise of the subchondral vascular supply in the appearance of cartilage necrosis.[121-123] Evidence for this theory includes the occasional coexistence of chondrolysis and osteonecrosis in the patient with a slipped femoral epiphysis, and the appearance of similar cartilage loss accompanying osteonecrosis in patients without slipped capital femoral epiphyses.

Currently, it is believed that chondrolysis is a primary articular disorder distinct from osteonecrosis, although the basis for the cartilage loss has not been identified. In this regard, the study by Eisenstein and Rothschild is of interest.[115] These investigators noted biochemical abnormalities in patients with slipped capital femoral epiphyses, which included significant elevations of the serum immunoglobulins and C^3 component of complement, the highest values being recorded for IgA, and with a greater elevation of the IgM fraction in those patients

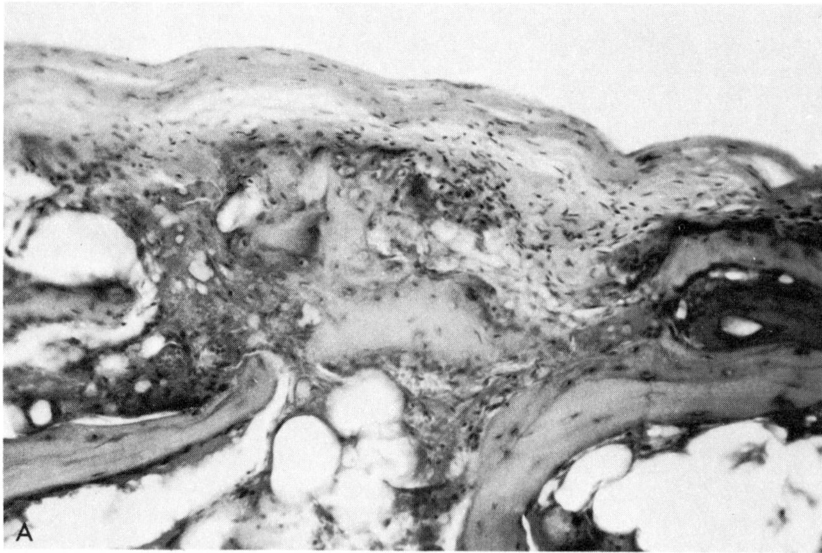

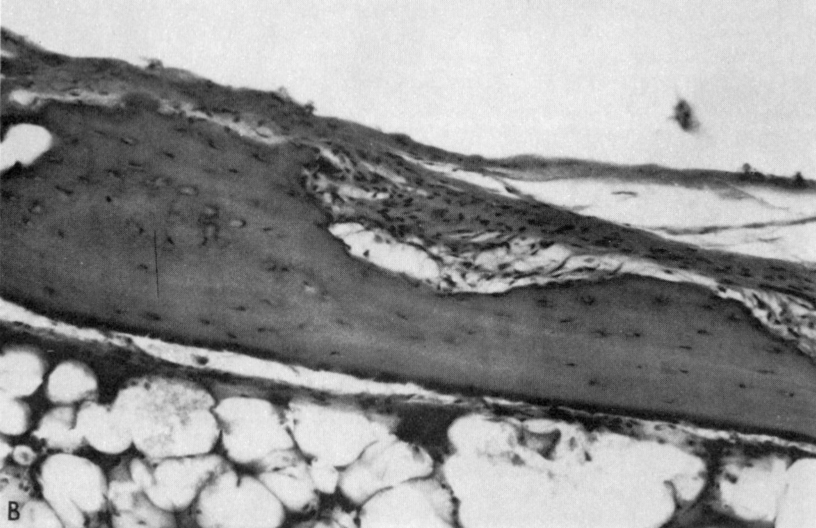

Figure 82–20. Chondrolysis following slipped capital femoral epiphysis: Pathologic abnormalities.

A *Observe cartilage and subchondral bone erosions with an attempt at fibrous repair.*

B *In another photomicrograph, an attempt at fibrous repair in an area of cartilage erosion is seen.*

(**A, B,** From Heppenstall RB, et al: Clin Orthop Rel Res 103:136, 1974.)

C, D *A photograph and photomicrograph of a different femoral head indicate the severity of chondrolysis and subchondral bone erosion.*

(**C, D,** Courtesy of Dr. R. B. Heppenstall, University of Pennsylvania, Philadelphia, Pennsylvania.)

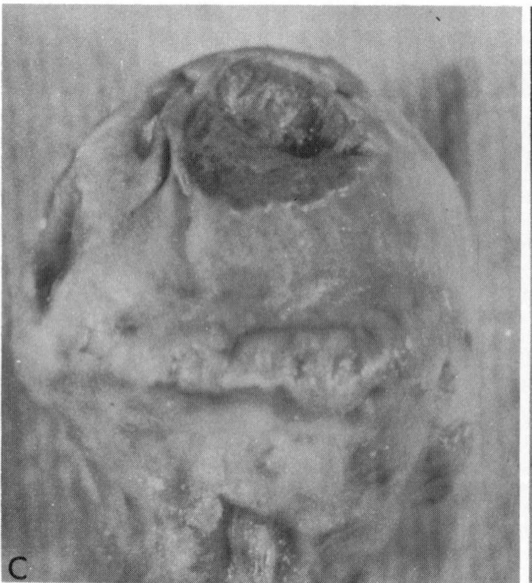

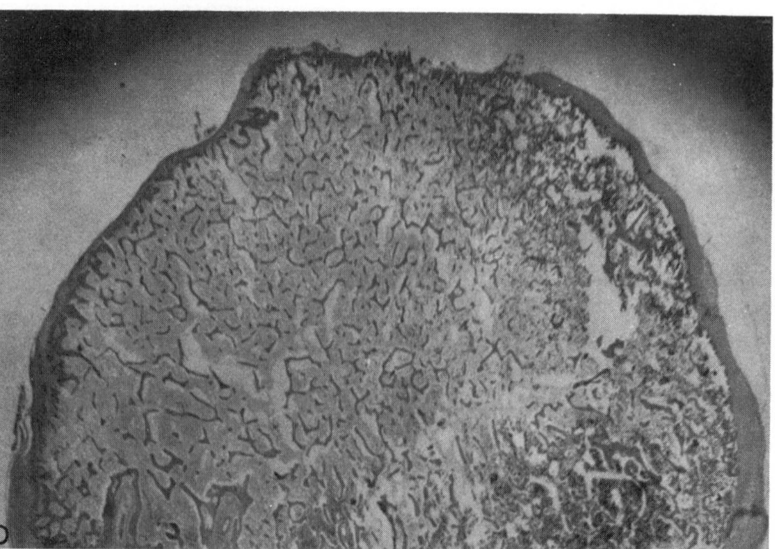

demonstrating chondrolysis. They suggested that slipping of an epiphysis either produces an antigen that induces an autoimmune state, or is a localized manifestation of a generalized process resembling a connective tissue disorder or inflammatory state; and that a genetically determined subgroup of patients with slipped capital femoral epiphyses developed chondrolysis caused by the autoimmune-induced release of lysosomal enzymes, and interference with synthetic processes of the articular cartilage.

The differential diagnosis of the roentgenographic features of chondrolysis accompanying slipped capital femoral epiphyses varies with the stage of the process.[116] Initially, the osteoporosis observed in chondrolysis is identical to that seen in various inflammatory synovial disorders such as rheumatoid arthritis and infection, and in regional forms of osteoporosis such as the reflex sympathetic dystrophy syndrome, transient osteoporosis of the hip, and regional migratory osteoporosis. At this stage, aspiration of joint contents is mandatory to exclude the possibility of infection, and subsequent contrast opacification of the joint may be useful in confirming the presence of acute cartilage loss prior to diminution of the interosseous space. In the later stages of chondrolysis, loss of the articular space and subchondral osseous thinning and erosion simulate changes in infection, rheumatoid arthritis and other inflammatory disorders, but differ from the typical findings of the reflex sympathetic dystrophy syndrome, regional migratory osteoporosis and transient osteoporosis of the hip. The absence of systemic symptoms, of elevation of the erythrocyte sedimentation rate, and of leukocytosis in chondrolysis is a clinical clue that helps to exclude a septic process. In advanced stages of chondrolysis, differential diagnosis includes other disorders such as pigmented villonodular synovitis and idiopathic synovial osteochondromatosis. At all stages, the history and clinical and radiographic manifestations of a slipped capital femoral epiphysis itself should serve as important indicators of the possible presence of chondrolysis to those physicians who are aware of this potential complication.

Idiopathic Chondrolysis of the Hip

The reports of Jones in 1971[124] and Moule and Golding in 1974[125] focused attention on the occurrence of chondrolysis of the hip joint in adolescent girls, particularly blacks, who did not have slipped capital femoral epiphyses. Subsequent investigators confirmed the presence of this entity, noting its occasional appearance not only in black female

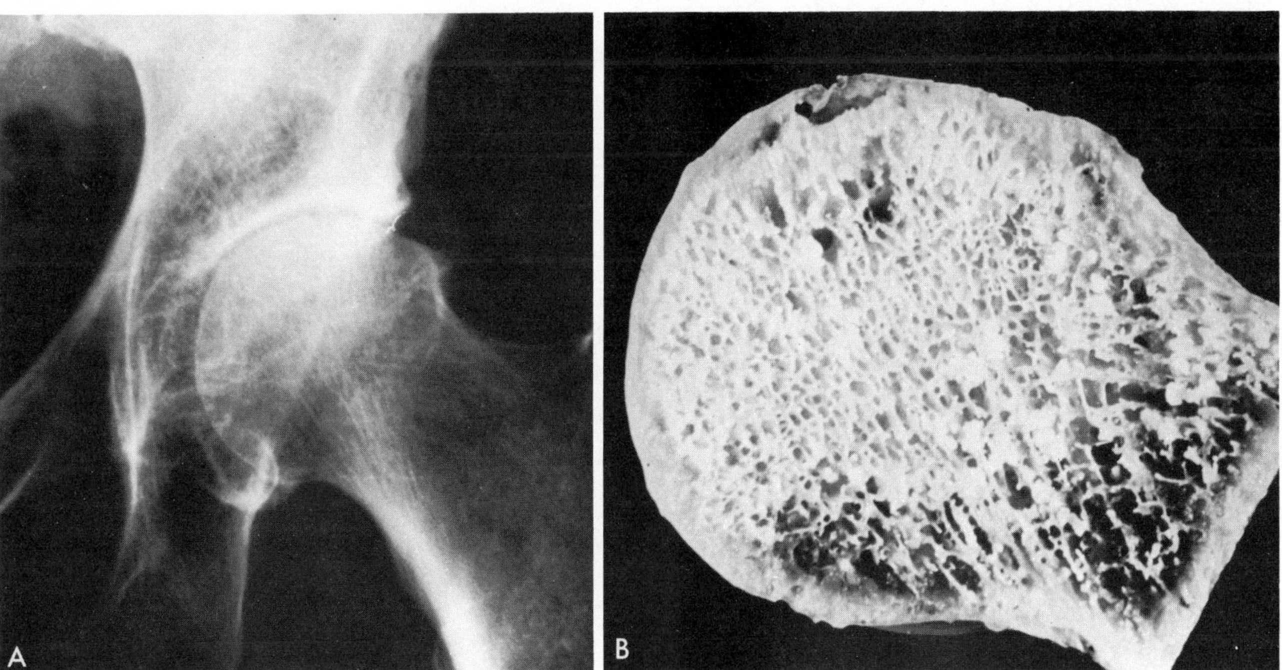

Figure 82–21. *Idiopathic chondrolysis of the hip. A 67 year old woman developed spontaneous hip pain and stiffness with loss of joint space over a period of 1 year. Idiopathic chondrolysis must be considered a prime potential diagnosis.*

A *A radiograph outlines diffuse loss of joint space, a small lateral femoral osteophyte, and "buttressing" of the medial femoral neck.*

B *At surgery, some degree of cartilage lysis was found to be present. A macerated section of the femoral head reveals essentially normal osseous structures. There was no evidence of inflammatory pannus, infection, or osteonecrosis.*

(Courtesy of Dr. S. Shaul, Yakima, Washington.)

adolescents, but also in men, in Caucasians and Indians, and in individuals over the age of 20 years.[126-128, 131, 138] Monoarticular disease of the hip is typical, and clinical findings include pain, stiffness, restriction of motion, and the absence of a history of trauma. Radiographs outline periarticular osteoporosis, joint space narrowing that is usually diffuse or maximal on the weight-bearing surface, and irregularity and erosion of the subchondral bone (Fig. 82–21). In addition, slight enlargement and alteration in shape of the femoral head, an increase in width and periosteal bone formation of the femoral neck, narrowing of the growth plate, and mild protrusio acetabuli may be evident. Joint aspiration usually confirms the absence of an effusion or organisms, and arthrography may demonstrate the irregularity and narrowing of the chondral surface. Pathologic examination outlines changes in cartilage that are identical to those that occur in chondrolysis complicating slipped capital femoral epiphysis, including replacement of the deep layers of the articular cartilage, thinning of the superficial layers, and absence of widespread synovial inflammation. Some degree of villous formation, nodular lymphoid hyperplasia in the subsynovial areas, and perivascular infiltrates of lymphocytes, plasma cells, and monocytes may be noted. Fibrinoid necrosis and granulomas are not seen. The adjacent bone is osteoporotic, and cystic areas may be filled with synovium. Osteonecrosis has also been reported.[128]

Later stages of the process can be associated with obliteration of the articular space, cysts, osteophytes, and deformity.

Major alternatives in differential diagnosis include juvenile chronic arthritis and infection. Monoarticular involvement of the hip is somewhat unusual in juvenile chronic arthritis, although its clinical and radiologic features can simulate those in idiopathic chondrolysis of the hip. Similarly, infection can lead to an identical radiographic picture, necessitating joint aspiration and culture of the fluid in all suspected cases of chondrolysis.

SUMMARY

A variety of disorders can lead to osteolysis and chondrolysis. In some, bone resorption is especially evident in the phalanges of the hand and foot, and may be related to occupational or inherited factors. Posttraumatic osteolysis can be evident at many sites, particularly the distal clavicle, pubic and ischial rami, and femoral neck. Massive osteolysis of Gorham can lead to regional destruction and disappearance of bone. Idiopathic multicentric osteolysis shows a predilection for the carpal and tarsal areas, and must be differentiated from juvenile chronic arthritis, the Winchester syndrome, and Farber's disease. Additional osteolysis syndromes include neurogenic acro-osteolysis, acro-osteolysis of Joseph and of Shinz, and osteolysis with detritic synovitis. Chondrolysis of the hip can accompany a slipped capital femoral epiphysis or can appear on an idiopathic basis. It must be differentiated from juvenile chronic arthritis, infection, and regional osteoporosis.

REFERENCES

1. Swezey RL, Bjarnason DM, Alexander SJ, Forrester DB: Resorptive arthropathy and the opera-glass hand syndrome. Semin Arthritis Rheum *2*:1972–1973.
2. Harnasch H: Die Akroosteolysis ein neues Krankheitsbild. Fortschr Geb Roentgenstr Nuklearmed *72*:352, 1950.
3. Suciu I, Drejman I, Valaskai M: Contributii la studiul imbolnavirilor produse de clorura de vinil. Med Interna *15*:967, 1963.
4. Cordier JM, Fievez C, Lefevre MJ, Sevrin A: Acroosteolyse et lesides cutanées associées chez deux ouvriers affectes au nettoyage d'autodaves. Cah Med Travail *4*:3, 1966.
5. Wilson RH, McCormick WE, Tatum CF, Creech JL: Occupational acroosteolysis. Report of 31 cases. JAMA *201*:577, 1967.
6. Markowitz SS, McDonald CJ, Fethiere W, Kerzner MS: Occupational acroosteolysis. Arch Dermatol *106*:219, 1972.
7. Dodson VN, Dinman BD, Whitehouse WM, Nasr ANM, Magnuson HJ: Occupational acroosteolysis. III. A clinical study. Arch Environ Health *22*:83, 1971.
8. Harris DK, Adams WGF: Acro-osteolysis occurring in men engaged in the polymerization of vinyl chloride. Br Med J *3*:712, 1967.
9. Stein G, Jühe S, Lange CE, Veltman G: Bandförmige Osteolysen in den Endphalangen des Handskeletts. Fortsch Geb Roentgenstr Nuklearmed *118*:60, 1973.
10. Gama C, Meira JBB: Occupational acro-osteolysis. J Bone Joint Surg *60A*:86, 1975.
11. Ross JA: An unusual occupational bone change. *In* AM Jelliffe, B Strickland (Eds): Symposium Ossium. Edinburgh, E & S Livingstone, 1970, p 321.
12. Kind R, Hornstein OP: Akroosteopathia ulcero-mutilans bei einem Kunststoffarbeiter. Dtsch Med Wochenschr *100*:1001, 1975.
13. Bookstein JJ: Arteriography. *In* AK Poznanski (Ed): The Hand in Radiologic Diagnosis. Philadelphia, WB Saunders Co, 1974, p 75.
14. Murray IPC: Bone scanning in occupational acro-osteolysis. Skel Radiol *3*:149, 1978.
15. Creech JL Jr, Johnson MN: Angiosarcoma of the liver in the manufacture of polyvinyl chloride. J Occup Med *16*:150, 1974.
16. Strauch W: Posttraumatische Osteolysen des lateralen Klavikulaendes. Radiol Diagn *11*:221, 1970.
17. Werder H: Posttraumatische Osteolyse des Schlüsselbeinendes. Schweiz Med Wochenschr *34*:912, 1950.
18. Madsen B: Osteolysis of the acromial end of the clavicle following trauma. Br J Radiol *36*:822, 1963.
19. Smart MJ: Traumatic osteolysis of the distal ends of the clavicles. J Can Assoc Radiol *23*:264, 1972.
20. Jacobs P: Post-traumatic osteolysis of the outer end of the clavicle. J Bone Joint Surg *46B*:705, 1964.
21. Halaby FA, DiSalvo EI: Osteolysis: A complication of trauma. Am J Roentgenol *94*:590, 1965.
22. Levine AH, Pais MJ, Schwartz EE: Posttraumatic osteolysis of the distal clavicle with emphasis on early radiologic changes. Am J Roentgenol *127*:781, 1976.
23. Seymour EQ: Osteolysis of the clavicular tip associated with repeated minor trauma to the shoulder. Radiology *123*:56, 1977.
24. Zsernaviczky J, Horst M: Kasuistischer Beitrag zur Osteolyse am distalen Klavikulaende. Arch Orthop Unfallchir *89*:163, 1977.
25. Alnor P: Die posttraumatische Osteolyse des lateralen Claviculaendes. Fortschr Geb Roentgenstr Nuklearmed *75*:364, 1951.
26. Hasselmann W: Die sog. posttraumatische Osteolyse des lateralen Claviculaendes. Monatsschr Unfallheilkd *58*:242, 1955.

27. Ehricht HG: Die Osteolyse im lateralen Claviculaende nach Pressluftschaden. Arch Orthop Unfallchir *50*:576, 1959.
28. Murphy OB, Bellamy R, Wheeler W, Brower TD: Post-traumatic osteolysis of the distal clavicle. Clin Orthop Rel Res *109*:108, 1975.
29. Goergen TG, Resnick D, Riley RR: Post-traumatic abnormalities of the pubic bone simulating malignancy. Radiology *126*:85, 1978.
30. Ackerman LV, Rosai J: Surgical Pathology. 5th Ed. St Louis, CV Mosby Co, 1974, p 1018.
31. Fischer E: Posttraumatische karpale Osteolysen nach isolierter Fraktur am distalen Radius. Fortsch Geb Roentgenstr Nuklearmed *112*:541, 1970.
32. Elias AN, Pinals RS, Anderson HC, Gould LV, Streeten DHP: Hereditary osteodysplasia with acro-osteolysis (the Hajdu-Cheney syndrome). Am J Med *65*:627, 1978.
33. Hajdu N, Kauntze R: Cranio-skeletal dysplasia. Br J Radiol *21*:42, 1948.
34. Cheney WD: Acro-osteolysis. Am J Roentgenol *94*:595, 1965.
35. Schulze R, Gulbin O: Beitrag zum Problem der Akroosteolyse (gleichzeitig ein Beitrag zur Kenntner der Patella profunda). Fortschr Geb Roentgenstr Nuklearmed *109*:209, 1968.
36. Matisonn A, Ziady F: Familial acro-osteolysis. S Afr Med J *47*:2060, 1973.
37. Harnasch H: Die Akroosteolysis, ein neues Krankheitsbild. Fortschr Geb Roentgenstr Nuklearmed *72*:352, 1950.
38. Greenberg BE, Street DM: Idiopathic non-familial acro-osteolysis. Report of a case observed for five years. Radiology *69*:259, 1957.
39. Papavasiliou CG, Gargano FP, Walls WL: Idiopathic nonfamilial acro-osteolysis associated with other bone abnormalities. Am J Roentgenol *83*:687, 1960.
40. Chawla S: Cranio-skeletal dysplasia with acro-osteolysis. Br J Radiol *37*:702, 1964.
41. Dorst JP, McKusick VA: Acro-osteolysis (Cheney syndrome). Birth Defects *5*(3):215, 1969.
42. Weleber RG, Beals RK: The Hajdu-Cheney syndrome. Report of two cases and review of the literature. J Pediatr *88*:243, 1976.
43. Silverman FN, Dorst JP, Hajdu N: Acro-osteolysis (Hajdu-Cheney syndrome). Birth Defects *10*(12):106, 1974.
44. Brown DM, Bradford DS, Gorlin RJ, Desnick RJ, Langer LO Jr, Jowsey J, Sauk JL Jr: The acro-osteolysis syndrome: Morphologic and biochemical studies. J Pediatr *88*:573, 1976.
45. Shaw DG: Acro-osteolysis and bone fragility. Br J Radiol *42*:934, 1969.
46. Gilula LA, Bliznak J, Staple TW: Idiopathic nonfamilial acro-osteolysis with cortical defects and mandibular ramus osteolysis. Radiology *121*:63, 1976.
47. Gorham LW, Wright AW, Shultz HH, Maxon FC Jr: Disappearing bones: A rare form of massive osteolysis. Report of two cases, one with autopsy findings. Am J Med *17*:674, 1954.
48. Gorham LW, Stout AP: Massive osteolysis (acute spontaneous absorption of bone, phantom bone, disappearing bone). J Bone Joint Surg *37A*:985, 1955.
49. Branch HE: Acute spontaneous absorption of bone. Report of a case involving a clavicle and a scapula. J Bone Joint Surg *27*:706, 1945.
50. Dupas J, Baldelon P, Dayde G: Sur un cas d'ostéolyse progressive de la main gauche d'origine indéterminée. Rev Orthop *23*:333, 1936.
51. Henderson MS: Acute atrophy of bone: Report of an unusual case involving the radius and ulna. Minn Med *19*:214, 1936.
52. Simpson BS: An unusual case of post-traumatic decalcification of the bones of the foot. J Bone Joint Surg *19*:223, 1937.
53. King DJ: A case resembling hemangiomatosis of the lower extremity. J Bone Joint Surg *28*:623, 1946.
54. Leriche R: A propos des ostéolyses d'origine indéterminée. Mem Acad Chir *63*:418, 1937.
55. Jackman WA: A case of spontaneous absorption of bone. Br J Surg *26*:944, 1939.
56. Fornasier VL: Haemangiomatosis with massive osteolysis. J Bone Joint Surg *52B*:444, 1970.
57. Torg JS, Steel HH: Sequential roentgenographic changes occurring in massive osteolysis. J Bone Joint Surg *51A*:1649, 1969.
58. Kery L, Wouters HW: Massive osteolysis. Report of two cases. J Bone Joint Surg *52B*:452, 1970.
59. Thompson JS, Schuman DJ: Massive osteolysis. Case report and review of literature. Clin Orthop Rel Res *103*:206, 1974.
60. Imbert J-C, Picault C: Ostéolyse massive idiopathique ou maladie de Jackson-Gorham. Rev Chir Orthop *60*:73, 1974.
61. Sage MR, Allen PW: Massive osteolysis. Report of a case. J Bone Joint Surg *56B*:130, 1974.
62. Iyer GV, Nayar A: Massive osteolysis of the skull. Case report. J Neurosurg *43*:92, 1975.
63. Patrick JH: Massive osteolysis complicated by chylothorax successfully treated by pleurodesis. J Bone Joint Surg *58B*:347, 1976.
64. Heyden G, Kindblom L-G, Nielsen JM: Disappearing bone disease. A clinical and histological study. J Bone Joint Surg *59A*:57, 1977.
65. Campbell J, Almond HGA, Johnson R: Massive osteolysis of the humerus with spontaneous recovery. Report of a case. J Bone Joint Surg *57B*:238, 1975.
66. Halliday DR, Dahlin DC, Pugh DG, Young HH: Massive osteolysis and angiomatosis. Radiology *82*:637, 1964.
67. Hambach R, Pujman J, Malý V: Massive osteolysis due to hemangiomatosis. Report of a case of Gorham's disease with autopsy. Radiology *71*:43, 1958.
68. Heuck F: Case report 78. Skel Radiol *3*:241, 1979.
69. Cadenat H, Combelles R, Fabert G, Clouet M: Ostéolyse cryptogénétique de la mandibule. J Radiol Electrol Med Nucl *59*:509, 1978.
70. Graham DY, Gonzales J, Kothari SM: Diffuse skeletal angiomatosis. Skel Radiol *2*:131, 1978.
71. Schajowicz F, Aiello CL, Francone MV, Giannini RE: Cystic angiomatosis (hamartous haemolymphangiomatosis) of bone. A clinicopathological study of three cases. J Bone Joint Surg *60B*:100, 1978.
72. Rosenquist CJ, Wolfe DC: Lymphangioma of bone. J Bone Joint Surg *50A*:158, 1968.
73. Boyle WJ: Cystic angiomatosis of bone. A report of three cases and review of the literature. J Bone Joint Surg *54B*:626, 1972.
74. Singh R, Grewal DS, Bannerjee AK, Bansal VP: Haemangiomatosis of the skeleton. Report of a case. J Bone Joint Surg *56B*:136, 1974.
75. Brower AC, Culver JE Jr, Keats TE: Diffuse cystic angiomatosis of bone. Report of two cases. Am J Roentgenol *118*:456, 1973.
76. Tyler T, Rosenbaum HD: Idiopathic multicentric osteolysis. Am J Roentgenol *126*:23, 1976.
77. Derot M, Rathery M, Rosselin G, Catellier C: Acroosteolyse du carpe, pied creus, scoliose et strabisme chez une jeune fille atteinte d'une insuffisance renale. Bull Mem Soc Med Hop Paris *77*:223, 1961.
78. MacPherson RI, Walker RD, Kowall MH: Essential osteolysis with nephropathy. J Can Assoc Radiol *24*:98, 1973.
79. Torg JS, Steel HH: Essential osteolysis with nephropathy. A review of the literature and case report of an unusual syndrome. J Bone Joint Surg *50A*:1629, 1968.
80. Mahoudeau D, Dubrisay J, Elissalde B, Sraër C: Ostéolyse essentielle et néphrite. Bull Mem Soc Med Hop Paris *77*:229, 1961.
81. Lagier R, Rutishauser E: Osteoarticular changes in a case of essential osteolysis. J Bone Joint Surg *47B*:339, 1965.
82. Marie J, Lévêque B, Lyon G, Bêbe M, Watchi JM: Acro-ostéolyse essentielle compliquée d'insuffisance rénal d'évolution fatale. Presse Med *71*:249, 1963.
83. Marie J, Salet J, Lévêque B: Polydystrophies sequelettiques avec ostéolyse progressive. Arch Fr Pediatr *8*:752, 1951.
84. Marie J, Salet J, Lévêque B, Sauvegrain J: Syndrome ostéodystrophique de nature congénitale probable. Presse Med *64*:2173, 1956.
85. Whyte MP, Murphy WA, Kleerekoper M, Teitelbaum SL, Avioli LV: Idiopathic multicentric osteolysis. Report of an affected father and son. Arthritis Rheum *21*:367, 1978.
86. Thieffry S, Sorrel-Dejerine J: D'ostéolyse essentielle héréditaire et familiale. Presse Med *66*:1858, 1958.
87. Kohler E, Babbit D, Huizenga B, Good TA: Hereditary osteolysis: A clinical, radiological and chemical study. Radiology *108*:99, 1973.
88. Torg JS, DiGeorge AM, Kirkpatrick JA Jr, Trujillo MM: Hereditary multicentric osteolysis with recessive transmission: A new syndrome. J Pediatr *75*:243, 1969.
89. Coleman SS, Litton RJ, Christensen WR: Familial dysostosis carpi. J Bone Joint Surg *47A*:850, 1965.
90. Gluck J, Miller JJ: Familial osteolysis of the carpal and tarsal bones. J Pediatr *81*:506, 1972.
91. Amin PH, Evans ANW: Essential osteolysis of carpal and tarsal bones. Br J Radiol *51*:539, 1978.
92. Beals RK, Bird CB: Carpal and tarsal osteolysis. Birth Defects *11*(6):107, 1973.
93. Shurtleff DB, Sparkes RS, Clawson DK, Guntheroth WE, Mottet NK: Hereditary osteolysis with hypertension and nephropathy. JAMA *188*:363, 1964.
94. Erickson CM, Hirschberger M, Stickler GB: Carpal-tarsal osteolysis. J Pediatr *93*:779, 1978.
95. Beals RK, Bird CB: Carpal and tarsal osteolysis. A case report and review of the literature. J Bone Joint Surg *57A*:681, 1975.
96. McKusick VA: Mendelian Inheritance in Man, 3rd Ed. Baltimore, Johns Hopkins University Press, 1971.
97. Thévenard MA: L'acropathie ulcéro-mutilante familiale. Acta Neurol Psych Belg *53*:1, 1953.
98. Thévenard MA: L'acropathie ulcéro-multilante familiale. Rev Neurol *74*:193, 1942.
99. Kozlowski K, Hanicka M, Garapich M: Neurogene ulcerierende Akropathie (Akroosteolyse-Syndrom). Monatsschr Kinderheilkd *119*:169, 1971.

100. White AA III: Disappearing bone disease with arthropathy and severe scarring of the skin. A report of four cases seen in South Vietnam. J Bone Joint Surg *53B*:303, 1971.
101. Joseph R, Nézelof C, Guéraud L, Job JC: Acro-ostéolyse idiopathique familiale; renseignements fournis par la biopsie. Sem Hop Paris *35*:622, 1959.
102. Shinz HR: Roentgen-Diagnostics. New York, Grune & Stratton, 1951, Vol 1, p 734.
103. Bierman SM, Edgington T, Newcomer VD, Pearson CM: Farber's disease: A disorder of mucopolysaccharide metabolism with articular, respiratory, and neurologic manifestations. Arthritis Rheum *9*:620, 1966.
104. Winchester P, Grossman H, Lim WN, Danes BS: A new acid mucopolysaccharidosis with skeletal deformities simulating rheumatoid arthritis. Am J Roentgenol *106*:121, 1969.
105. Resnick D, Weisman M, Goergen TG, Feldman PS: Osteolysis with detritic synovitis. A new syndrome. Arch Intern Med *138*:1003, 1978.
106. Waldenström H: On necrosis of the joint cartilage by epiphyseolysis capitis femoris. Acta Chir Scand *67*:936, 1930.
107. Cruess RL: The pathology of acute necrosis of cartilage in slipping of the capital femoral epiphysis. A report of two cases with pathological sections. J Bone Joint Surg *45A*:1013, 1963.
108. Lowe HG: Necrosis of the articular cartilage after slipping of the capital femoral epiphysis. Report of six cases with recovery. J Bone Joint Surg *52B*:108, 1970.
109. Heppenstall RM, Marvel JP Jr, Chung SMK, Brighton CT: Chondrolysis of the hip. Clin Orthop Rel Res *103*:136, 1974.
110. Tillema DA, Golding JSR: Chondrolysis following slipped capital femoral epiphysis in Jamaica. J Bone Joint Surg *53A*:1528, 1971.
111. El-Khoury GY, Mickelson MR: Chondrolysis following slipped capital femoral epiphysis. Radiology *123*:327, 1977.
112. Ogden JA, Simon TR, Southwick WO: Cartilage space width in slipped capital femoral epiphysis: The relationship to cartilage necrosis. Yale J Biol Med *50*:17, 1977.
113. Mauer RC, Larsen IJ: Acute necrosis of cartilage in slipped capital femoral epiphysis. J Bone Joint Surg *52A*:39, 1970.
114. Frymoyer JW: Chondrolysis of the hip following Southwick osteotomy for severe slipped capital femoral epiphysis. Clin Orthop Rel Res *99*:120, 1974.
115. Eisenstein A, Rothschild S: Biochemical abnormalities in patients with slipped capital femoral epiphysis and chondrolysis. J Bone Joint Surg *58A*:459, 1976.
116. Goldman AB, Schneider R, Martel W: Acute chondrolysis complicating slipped capital femoral epiphysis. Am J Roentgenol *130*:945, 1978.
117. Wiberg G: Considerations on surgical treatment of slipped epiphysis with special reference to nail fixation. J Bone Joint Surg *41A*:253, 1959.
118. Orofino C, Innis JJ, Lowrey CW: Slipped capital femoral epiphysis in Negroes. A study of ninety-five cases. J Bone Joint Surg *42A*:1079, 1960.
119. Ponseti I, Barta CK: Evalulation of treatment of slipping of the capital femoral epiphysis. Surg Gynecol Obstet *86*:87, 1948.
120. Jerre T: A study in slipped upper femoral epiphysis. With special reference to the late functional and roentgenological results and to the value of closed reduction. Acta Orthop Scand Suppl *6*:1, 1950.
121. Hall JE: The results of treatment of slipped femoral epiphysis. J Bone Joint Surg *39B*:659, 1957.
122. Wilson PD: Discussion. Roentgenographic changes in nailed slipped epiphysis. J Bone Joint Surg *31A*:21, 1949.
123. Moore RD: Conservative management of adolescent slipping of the capital femoral epiphysis. Surg Gynecol Obstet *80*:324, 1945.
124. Jones BS: Adolescent chondrolysis of the hip joint. S Afr Med J *45*:196, 1971.
125. Moule NJ, Golding JSR: Idiopathic chondrolysis of the hip. Clin Radiol *25*:247, 1974.
126. Wenger DR, Mickelson MR, Ponseti IV: Idiopathic chondrolysis of the hip. Report of two cases. J Bone Joint Surg *57A*:268, 1975.
127. Duncan JW, Schrantz JL, Nasca RJ: The bizarre stiff hip. Possible idiopathic chondrolysis. JAMA *231*:382, 1975.
128. Sivanantham M, Kutty MK: Idiopathic chondrolysis of the hip: Case report with a review of the literature. Aust NZ J Surg *47*:229, 1977.
129. Kozlowski K, Barylak A, Eftekhari F, Pasyk K, Wislocka E: Acroosteolysis. Problems of diagnosis — report of four cases. Pediatr Radiol *8*:79, 1979.
130. Bauer F, Lagier R, Wettstein P, Cox JN: Anatomo-radiological study of a case of post-radiotherapeutic osteolysis of the hip. Strahlentherapie *155*:396, 1979.
131. Duncan JW, Nasca R, Schrantz J: Idiopathic chondrolysis of the hip. J Bone Joint Surg *61A*:1024, 1979.
132. Roback DL: Posttraumatic osteolysis of the femoral neck. Am J Roentgenol *134*:1243, 1980.
133. Fielding JW, Hensinger RN, Hawkins RJ: Os odontoideum. J Bone Joint Surg *62A*:376, 1980.
134. Hukuda S, Ota H, Okabe N, Tazima K: Traumatic atlantoaxial dislocation causing os odontoideum in infants. Spine *5*:207, 1980.
135. Iwaya T, Taniguchi K, Watanabe J, Iinuma K, Hamazaki Y: Hajdu-Cheney syndrome. Arch Orthop Traumat Surg *95*:293, 1979.
136. Binns CHB: Vinyl chloride: A review. J Soc Occup Med *29*:134, 1979.
137. Koischwitz D, Marsteller HJ, Lackner K, Brecht G, Brecht Th: Veränderungen der Hand- und Fingerarterien bei der Vinylchloridkrankheit. Fortschr geb Roentgenstr Nuklearmed *132*:62, 1980.
138. Herman JH, Herzig EB, Crissman JD, Dennis MV, Hess EV: Idiopathic chondrolysis — an immunopathologic study. J Rheumatol *7*:694, 1980.
139. Newberg AH, Howe JG: Posttraumatic osteolysis vs. fracture. Am J Roentgenol *135*:1317, 1980.
140. Abrahams J, Ganick D, Gilbert E, Wolfson J: Massive osteolysis in an infant. Am J Roentgenol *135*:1084, 1980.

83

PERIODIC, RELAPSING, AND RECURRENT DISORDERS

by Donald Resnick, M.D.

Included in this chapter are three diseases that are characterized clinically by intermittent periods of activity separated by disease-free intercritical periods.[1] The grouping of these disorders into a single section does not imply that other diseases might not be associated with similar periodicity, nor does it indicate that they are etiologically related. In fact, their etiologies are generally unclear or unknown. These diseases are relatively uncommon and are associated with nonspecific or unremarkable roentgenograms.

FAMILIAL MEDITERRANEAN FEVER

Clinical Abnormalities

Familial Mediterranean fever (familial recurrent polyserositis) is an uncommon disease that predominantly affects Sephardic (non-Ashkenazi) Jews, Armenians, and Arabs.[2-6] It is inherited as an autosomal recessive trait with complete penetrance. Men are more commonly affected than women. Symptoms and signs of the disorder usually appear in childhood or adolescence, and subsequently recur throughout the remainder of life. The typical manifestations include episodes of fever with abdominal, thoracic, or joint pain due to inflammation of the peritoneum, pleura, and synovial membrane. Attacks occur at irregular intervals without periodicity, with widely varying breaks between episodes that may last for years. Amyloidosis, which is a recognized complication of the disease, is genetically determined, and may affect as many as 35 to 45 per cent of Sephardic Jews who have familial Mediterranean fever. It is rare in other groups with the disease. Amyloidosis can produce the nephrotic syndrome and renal failure, resulting in early death.[74]

Attacks of familial Mediterranean fever are usually brief in duration. They are characterized by the rapid onset of fever, with or without abdominal or thoracic pain. The abdominal pain, which may be evident in 80 to 95 per cent of patients, varies in severity and persists for 12 to 24 hours or, rarely, longer. Chest discomfort is of short duration, may involve only one hemithorax, and is commonly accompanied by pleuritis or pericarditis, or both.

Musculoskeletal manifestations can occur in 60 to 70 per cent of patients.[7-13] Asymmetric arthritis in the larger joints of the lower extremity is most typical; the affected articulations, in order of decreasing frequency, are the knees, ankles, hips, shoulders, feet, elbows, and hands and wrists.[1] The sacroiliac, temporomandibular, and other articulations can also be involved. Monoarticular arthritis is more common than polyarticular arthritis. Joint attacks vary in severity, reach a peak in 1 to 2 days, and generally resolve in 1 to 2 weeks. Occasionally, more prolonged attacks are encountered.[74] Following repeated bouts, a chronic destructive arthritis may develop, especially in the hip.[11]

Pain, tenderness, and swelling accompany the arthritis of familial Mediterranean fever. Muscle spasm, restriction of joint motion, and bursitis are also encountered. An effusion is present, and the synovial fluid may be noninflammatory in type, with a paucity of cells, or inflammatory in type, with cell counts greater than 100,000 cells per cu mm, predominantly polymorphonuclear leukocytes. Viscosity is poor but the mucin clot is adequate. Glucose levels in the synovial fluid are normal or depressed, and bacteria are not found.

An erysipelas-like erythema is frequently evident on the lower extremities.[14] Histologically it is similar to that noted in the synovium or peritoneum during attacks, with acute inflammation characterized by edema, vasodilatation, and perivascular collections of neutrophils.

Radiographic Abnormalities

Osteoporosis can develop rapidly and become profound.[9] In children, hyperemia can lead to epiphyseal overgrowth that, when combined with soft tissue swelling and an effusion, can simulate the findings in juvenile chronic arthritis or hemophilia. Chronicity leads to joint space narrowing and juxta-articular erosions. Rarely, more extensive alterations are encountered. These include bony ankylosis,[11, 15-17] productive osseous changes with sclerosis and osteophytosis, and osteonecrosis. These latter changes are most evident in the hip and the knee and may require arthroplasty (Fig. 83–1). The pathogenesis of the femoral capital epiphyseal necrosis and collapse is not clear, although vascular compromise due to joint distention has been cited.[11]

Sacroiliac joint abnormalities have also been described in familial Mediterranean fever[18-20, 75] (Table 83–1). The reported incidence of these abnormalities has varied. Shahin and co-workers[19] observed sacroiliac joint changes in one of 40 cases (2.5 per cent), whereas Heller and colleagues[7] noted similar changes in three of 34 cases (9 per cent), and Brodey and Wolff[18] detected sacroiliac joint abnormalities in six of 43 patients (14 per cent). Widening of the articular space, loss of the normal subchondral bone definition, sclerosis with or without erosions, predominantly on the ilium, and bony ankylosis can appear in one or both sacroiliac articulations; asymmetric abnormalities predominate (Fig. 83–1). The absence of HLA B27 antigen in patients with familial Mediterranean fever and sacroiliitis[20-22] may indicate that the pathogenesis of the articular changes is different from that in classic ankylosing spondylitis, although it is of interest that patchy calcified and ossified bridges between lumbar vertebrae have been identified in individuals with familial Mediterranean fever.[7]

Pathologic Abnormalities

Nonspecific synovitis is evident on biopsies of inflamed joints.[1] Perivascular round cell aggregates, increased vascularity, and the accumulation of stromal fibroblasts and polymorphonuclear leukocytes are evident.[7] Fibrous tissue is contained within lytic lesions of bones.

Differential Diagnosis

The roentgenographic findings in familial Mediterranean fever are not diagnostic. In children, soft tissue swelling, osteoporosis, and epiphyseal overgrowth are evident in other articular disorders, such as juvenile chronic arthritis and hemophilia. In children and adults, joint space narrowing and os-

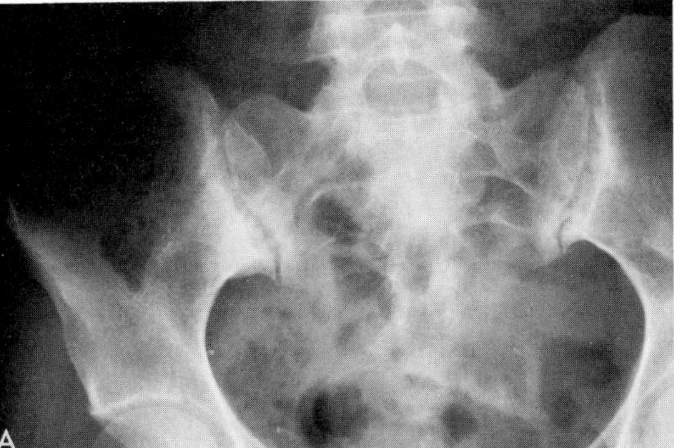

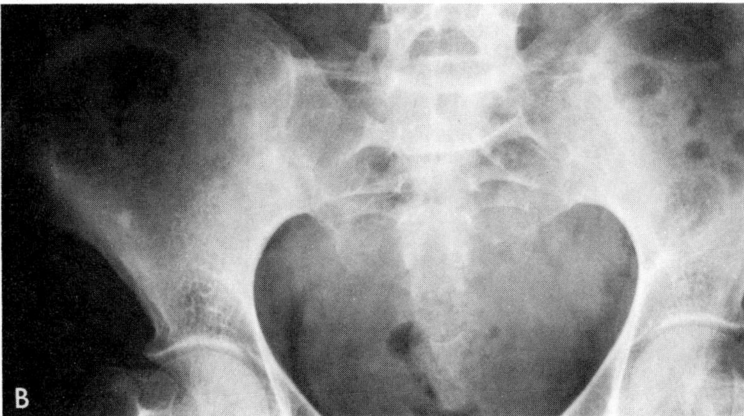

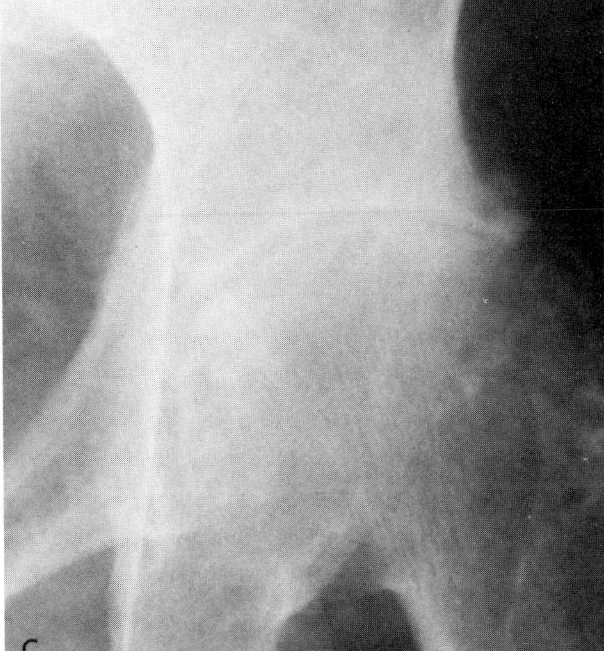

Figure 83–1. *Familial Mediterranean fever: Sacroiliitis; hip involvement.*

A *Bilateral asymmetric sacroiliac joint disease is characterized by osseous erosions and reactive sclerosis, predominantly in the ilium.*

B *Bony ankylosis of the sacroiliac joints is seen.*

*(**A**, **B**, From Brodey PA, Wolff SM: Radiology 114:331, 1975.)*

C *This 41 year old man with episodic hip and knee pain reveals symmetric loss of joint space and osteophytosis.*

*(**C**, Courtesy of Dr. D. Gershuni, Veterans Administration Hospital, San Diego, California.)*

seous erosion can simulate the findings of arthritides associated with synovial inflammation, such as rheumatoid arthritis and septic arthritis. Sacroiliitis in familial Mediterranean fever simulates that of ankylosing spondylitis and other seronegative spondyloarthropathies; the absence of symmetry in the sacroiliac joint changes in some cases of familial Mediterranean fever may allow its differentiation from classic ankylosing spondylitis and the sacroiliitis of inflammatory bowel disease. Although a relatively specific pattern of femoral osteoporosis has been noted in some patients with familial Mediterranean fever,[7] further documentation of this finding is necessary.

Table 83–1

SACROILIAC JOINT ABNORMALITIES

Disorder	Distribution: *BILATERAL SYMMETRIC*	*BILATERAL ASYMMETRIC*	*UNILATERAL*
Familial Mediterranean fever	X	X[1]	X
Relapsing polychondritis	X	X[1]	X
Behçet's syndrome[2]	X	X	X

[1]Probably the predominant pattern of involvement.
[2]Questionable association with sacroiliitis.

RELAPSING POLYCHONDRITIS

Clinical Abnormalities

Relapsing polychondritis is an uncommon disorder characterized by episodic inflammation of cartilaginous tissue and special sense organs; abnormalities are especially prominent in the external ear, nose, trachea, larynx, sclera, ribs, and articular cartilage. The term "relapsing polychondritis" was introduced in 1960 by Pearson and associates,[23] although the entity was recognized initially in 1923[24] and was known by such names as systemic chondromalacia, panchondritis, chronic atrophic polychondritis, rheumatic chondritis, and diffuse perichondritis.[25] In the last two decades, numerous reviews of relapsing polychondritis have appeared.[26-28] McAdam and co-workers[29] empirically established the following diagnostic criteria: recurrent chondritis of both auricles; nonerosive inflammatory polyarthritis; chondritis of nasal cartilage; inflammation of ocular structures, including conjunctivitis, keratitis, scleritis, episcleritis, and uveitis; chondritis of the respiratory tract involving laryngeal or tracheal cartilages; and cochlear or vestibular damage manifested by neurosensory hearing loss, tinnitus, or vertigo.

Relapsing polychondritis appears in all age groups, with a maximal frequency in the fourth decade of life. Men and women are affected in equal numbers. The initial clinical findings usually are auricular chondritis and arthritis; less typically, respiratory tract involvement, nasal chondritis, and ocular involvement are evident at the outset of the disease. Auricular chondritis leads to painful erythematous swelling of one or both ears lasting from 5 to 10 days[29] (Fig. 83–2). This finding is limited to the cartilaginous portion of the external ears (helix, antihelix, tragus, and external auditory canal).

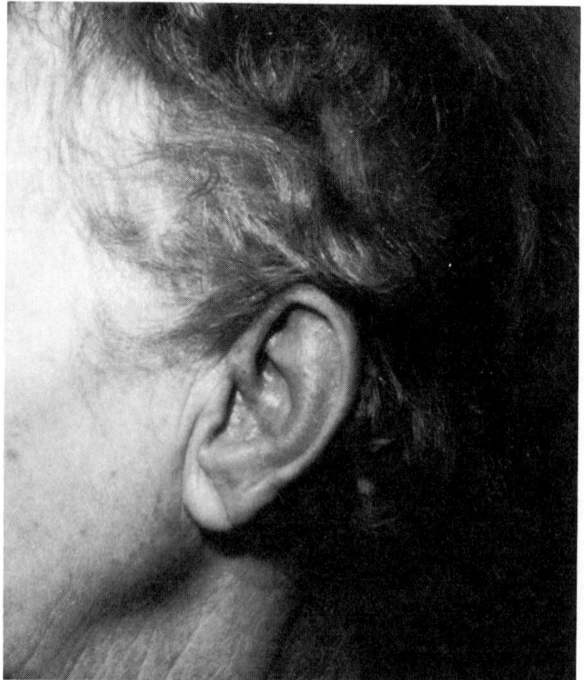

Figure 83–2. Relapsing polychondritis: Auricular chondritis. Observe the erythematous swelling on most of the external ear. (Courtesy of Dr. N. Zvaifler, University of California, San Diego, California.)

Arthralgia and arthritis generally affect more than one joint, including the hips, knees, manubriosternal and sternoclavicular articulations, costochondral junctions, and small and large joints of the upper extremity. Less frequently, the feet, ankles, and spine are involved. Migratory polyarthritis can simulate rheumatoid arthritis or a seronegative spondyloarthropathy, although occasionally monoarticular arthritis appears that mimics infection or crystal-induced arthritis. Although commonly nonerosive in type, the arthritis may produce considerable deformity and mutilation in some individuals. Tendinitis can appear. Relapsing polychondritis can also be superimposed on a preexisting polyarthritis, such as rheumatoid arthritis, juvenile chronic polyarthritis, collagen vascular disorders,[76] or Reiter's syndrome.[29-31]

Respiratory tract involvement is a potentially serious manifestation of the disease that may require tracheostomy. Laryngeal and tracheal tenderness, cough, hoarseness, and dyspnea secondary to collapse of the tracheal rings, edema, or granulomatous tissue proliferation within the respiratory tree can be evident. Nasal chondritis may be sudden in onset, painful, and associated with a feeling of fullness in the bridge of the nose and surrounding tissue.[29] Although these latter manifestations may disappear in a few days, chronic involvement can lead to characteristic saddle nose deformity. Episcleritis is the most common ocular abnormality, although any tissue in the eye can be affected in this disorder.

Additional manifestations include back pain due to spinal alterations, chest pain related to costochondritis, hearing loss attributable to obstruction of the external auditory meatus, fever, anorexia and weight loss, and cardiovascular abnormalities. McAdam and colleagues[29] have tabulated the clinical manifestations in approximate order of frequency: auricular chondritis (89 per cent); polyarthritis (81 per cent); nasal chondritis (72 per cent); ocular inflammation (65 per cent); respiratory tract chondritis (56 per cent); audiovestibular damage (46 per cent); cardiovascular involvement (24 per cent); and cutaneous lesions (17 per cent).

Laboratory findings are not specific. During the active phases of the disease, anemia, leukocytosis, elevated erythrocyte sedimentation rate, moderate serum protein alterations, and, occasionally, a low serum titer positivity for rheumatoid factor may be detected. Synovial fluid is usually noninflammatory in type.

Radiographic Abnormalities

In most cases, radiographic features of joint involvement in relapsing polychondritis are not striking, although there may be extra-articular findings, such as tracheal narrowing or stenosis, calcification of the auricular cartilage, and aortic alter-

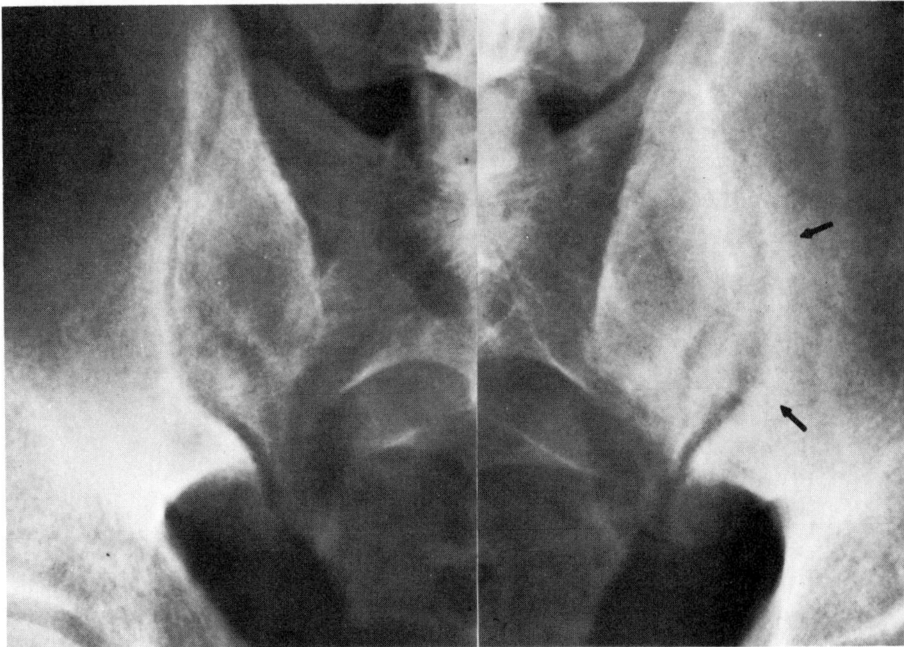

Figure 83–3. Relapsing polychondritis: Sacroiliac joint abnormalities. A 37 year old man with relapsing polychondritis of 4 years' duration reveals bilateral asymmetric abnormalities of the sacroiliac joints. On the right side **(A)**, the changes are minimal; on the left side **(B)**, moderate osseous erosions and reactive sclerosis are seen (arrows). (From Braunstein EM, et al: Clin Radiol 30:441, 1979.)

ations after repeated attacks.[32, 33] Periarticular osteoporosis may or may not be evident.[34] Joint space narrowing and osseous erosions of the metacarpophalangeal and metatarsophalangeal articulations, identical to those of rheumatoid arthritis,[33] and "arthritis mutilans"[28, 35, 36] have been encountered, but in some of these cases, changes may have been due to an underlying articular disorder. Typically, a nonerosive, nondeforming arthropathy appears.[37, 38]

Sacroiliitis has been evident in some patients with relapsing polychondritis,[38] although the incidence probably is not high[29, 37] (Table 83–1). Unilateral or bilateral abnormalities characterized by the presence of joint space loss, erosion, and eburnation, and the absence of spinal alterations predominate[38] (Fig. 83–3). Of interest in this regard, HLA B27 antigens do not appear to be associated with the arthropathy of relapsing polychondritis.[37]

Pathologic Abnormalities

Synovial membrane biopsy can reveal a synovitis characterized by chronic inflammation with preponderance of plasma cells[39] (Fig. 83–4). The lining layer of the synovium may have an increase of cells not unlike that in rheumatoid arthritis or other types of chronic synovitis. An accumulation of lipid and lysosomes in all the superficial cells of the articular cartilage in this disease is also like that in rheumatoid arthritis. The findings in the middle and deeper layers of the cartilage may be unique, with large, perichondrocytic clear spaces containing one or more multivesicular bodies.[39]

Light microscopic histochemical studies of involved cartilage at other sites, including the ear, suggest that there is a loss of acid mucopolysaccharide early in the process of cartilage destruction.[40, 41] In the ear, inflammatory reaction predominates in superficial areas of the cartilage[42] (Fig. 83–5). Deeper areas appear normal in most cases, although, occasionally, necrotic chondrocytes are seen. Typical pathologic changes also appear in vascular structures, including the aortic ring and ascending aorta, at which sites prominent abnormalities are seen in the media consisting of loss of elastic tissue, a decrease in basophilia, collagenous replacement, and focal accumulation of chronic inflammatory cells.

Etiology and Pathogenesis

The etiology of relapsing polychondritis is unknown. It is generally considered a connective tissue disorder with an immunologic mediation.[43] Despite the low antigenicity of cartilage proteoglycans, antibodies and delayed hypersensitivity have been demonstrated in this disease. Hughes and co-workers,[27] Rogers and colleagues,[44] and Shaul and Schumacher[42] observed anticartilage antibodies, using indirect immunofluorescent tests. Others could not confirm the presence of these antibodies, but did detect delayed hypersensitivity to cartilage proteoglycan.[45, 46] The focal perichondrial chronic inflammatory collections that are observed during active phases of the disease, and that lead to matrix depletion of proteoglycans, could be caused by release of lysosomal enzymes either from chondrocytes or ad-

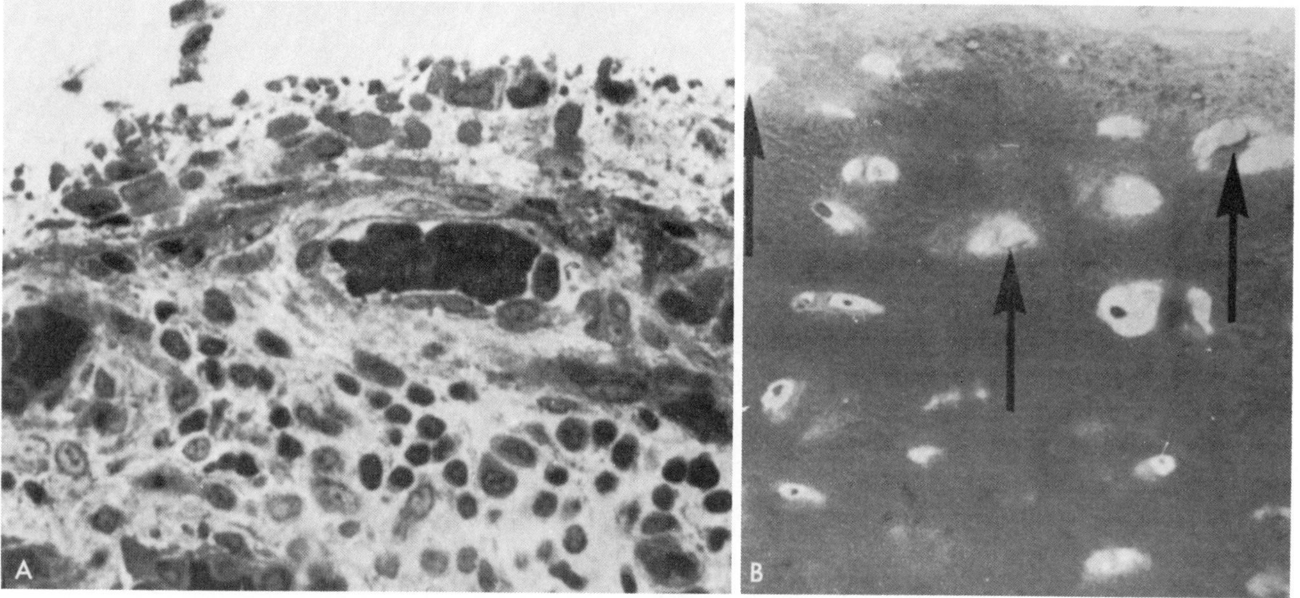

Figure 83–4. *Relapsing polychondritis: Synovial and articular cartilage abnormalities.*

A *A biopsy of a swollen, tender right third metacarpophalangeal joint in a 26 year old man with relapsing polychondritis reveals synovial inflammation with hypertrophy of the lining layer, cellular infiltration and dilatation of blood vessels (300×).*

B *Evaluation of the articular cartilage from the same joint reveals an irregular chondral surface, decreased uptake of stain, and fat droplets (arrows) (340×).*

(From Mitchell N, Shepard N: J Bone Joint Surg 54A:1235, 1972.)

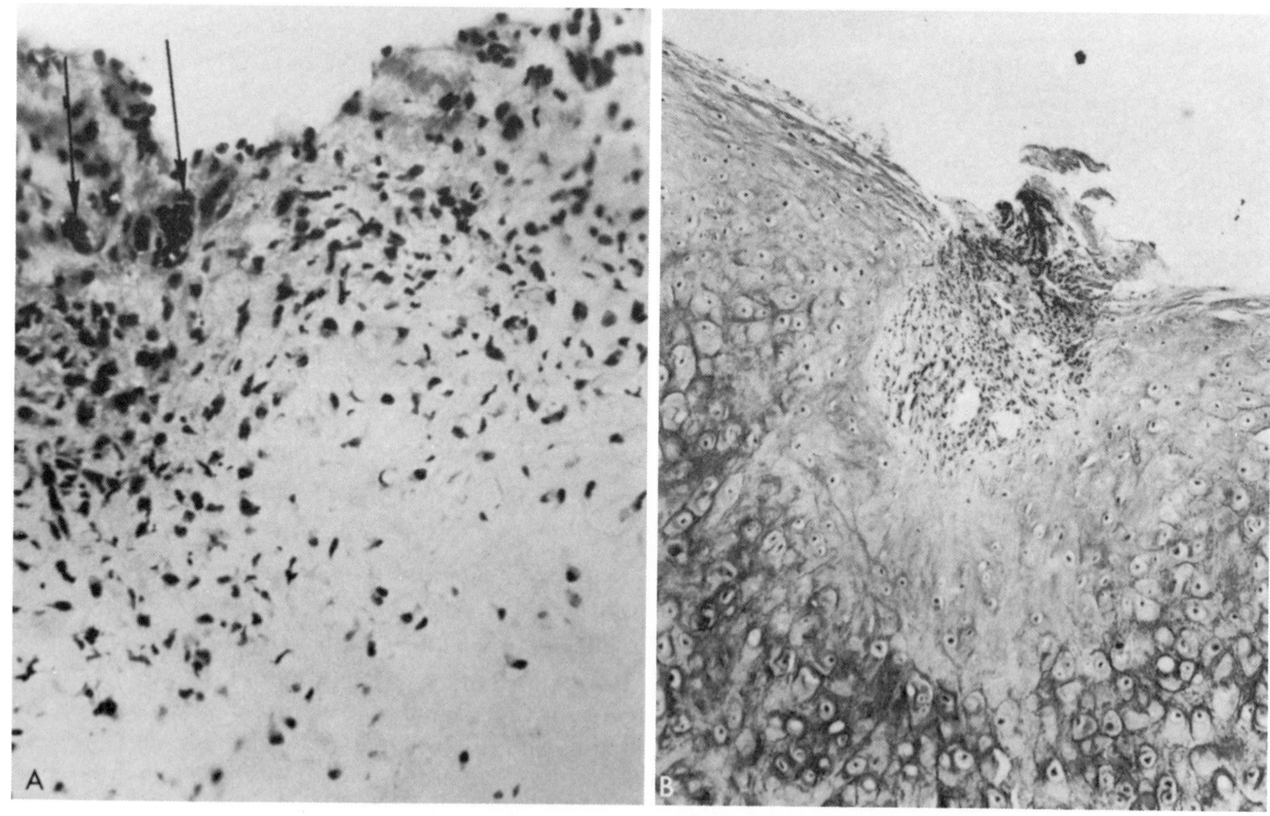

Figure 83–5. *Relapsing polychondritis: Auricular cartilage abnormalities.*

A *Superficial inflammatory cell reaction with infiltration of neutrophils and lymphocytes can be identified. Basophilic staining is lost. Blood vessels can be seen (arrows) (180 ×). (From Shaul SR, Schumacher HR: Arthritis Rheum 18:617, 1975.)*

B *In another patient, an area of focal chondritis with a proliferative infiltrate is seen. There is significant damage of cartilage in the area of infiltrate (100×). (From McAdam LP, et al: Medicine 55:193, 1976. Copyright 1976, The Williams & Wilkins Co, Baltimore.)*

jacent tissues.[42] Similar enzymatic release could be responsible for the aortic lesions that characterize relapsing polychondritis.

Differential Diagnosis

The radiographic features of articular involvement in this disease lack specificity. Periarticular osteoporosis and soft tissue swelling about synovial articulations simulate changes in a variety of disorders. With the occurrence of diffuse joint space narrowing and osseous erosions in these sites, the radiographic picture is almost identical to that of rheumatoid arthritis, although symmetry and more extensive cartilaginous and osseous destruction with deformities are more characteristic of the latter disease. Sacroiliitis in relapsing polychondritis is similar to that in ankylosing spondylitis or other seronegative spondyloarthropathies. In some cases, the appearance may also resemble osteitis condensans ilii.

BEHÇET'S SYNDROME

Clinical Abnormalities

This syndrome was initially described as a triad of painful, recurrent oral and genital ulcerations and ocular inflammation.[47] It is now recognized that many additional systems can be affected, including the skin, joints, and cardiovascular, neurologic, and gastrointestinal organs.[48-52] Original cases of Behçet's syndrome were evident in Mediterranean countries, but the disorder has also been noted in individuals throughout Europe, the Middle East and Far East, and the United States. The age of onset varies from 5 to 70 years, with a mean age of approximately 25 to 30 years; men are affected more commonly than women.

Over 90 per cent of patients reveal ulcerations in portions of the mouth or pharynx. Single or multiple and of varying size, the ulcerations appear rapidly, resolve in a period of 1 to 2 weeks, and recur. Biopsy of the mucosal lesions may reveal cellular infiltration, predominantly of mononuclear cells, and no vasculitis.

Ophthalmic lesions are evident in approximately 80 per cent of patients. Typically, iritis is seen, although episcleritis, conjunctivitis, keratitis, iridocyclitis, retinothrombophlebitis, optic neuritis and atrophy, and papilledema can be encountered. Late complications include glaucoma, cataracts, and blindness. Genital lesions appear in approximately 60 per cent of cases. In men, these include painful ulcerations of the penis and scrotum; in women, similar ulcerations of the vulva and vagina may produce few symptoms. Skin lesions may be observed in approximately 75 per cent of cases, consisting of pyoderma with pustules of varying size, and erythema nodosum–like abnormalities of the lower extremity. Cutaneous induration at sites of trauma (e.g., needle puncture) is common.

Additional manifestations include venous thrombosis and thrombophlebitis; gastrointestinal inflammation leading to abdominal pain, distention, and diarrhea; and central nervous system findings, such as meningitis, transverse myelitis, and psychiatric disorders.[53] Myositis has also been noted.[79]

Articular alterations appear in more than 50 per cent of patients. Monoarticular or oligoarticular involvement predominates, affecting principally the knees, but also other joints, including the ankles, wrists, and elbows. The sacroiliac and manubriosternal articulations[54] may also be involved. An insidious onset, a variable duration, and recurrence following disappearance of the findings typify the bouts of arthralgia or arthritis. Joint effusion, stiffness, warmth, and tenderness are observed, but permanent changes are rare.

Laboratory analysis may reveal an elevated erythrocyte sedimentation rate, a strongly positive C-reactive protein, and elevation of alpha-2 globulins during the acute phase of the disease.[1] Low grade anemia and mild leukocytosis are also observed. Many patients reveal high titers of serum antibodies directed against human oral mucosa, and some have peripheral lymphocytes that are stimulated by mucosal antigen, abnormalities that are not specific.[55]

An increased frequency of the tissue typing antigen HLA B5 has been found in some series,[56] although this has not been confirmed by other investigators. A modest increase in incidence of HLA B27 has also been identified in some reports,[52] but this association, too, must await further documentation.

Evaluation of synovial fluid reveals poor mucin clot, elevation in complement levels, and a polymorphonuclear leukocytosis.[57]

Radiographic Abnormalities

Roentgenographic findings in the skeleton are usually mild. Osteoporosis and soft tissue swelling can be seen, but joint space narrowing and osseous erosions are only rarely encountered[58] (Fig. 83–6). When present, these latter findings resemble changes in rheumatoid arthritis or other disorders characterized by synovial inflammation. One report has also noted a patient with spontaneous atlantoaxial subluxation (Fig. 83–7).[77] Some reports have indicated the occurrence of sacroiliitis in Behçet's syndrome,[59, 60] although others have failed to identify such an association[52] (Table 83–1, Fig. 83–8). It has been suggested that patients with Behçet's disease who are HLA B27–positive are at risk of devel-

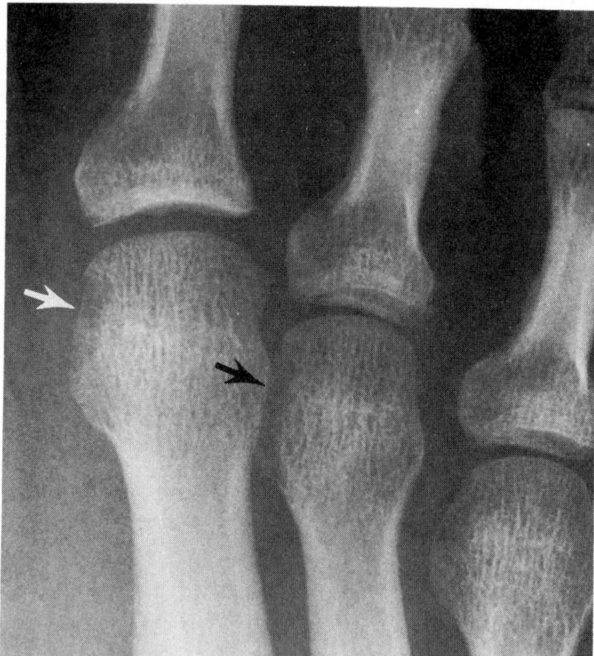

Figure 83–6. Behçet's syndrome: Peripheral joint abnormalities. Observe small osseous erosions of metatarsal heads (arrows) and osteoporosis. (Courtesy of Dr. A. Brower, The Uniformed Services University for Health Sciences, Bethesda, Maryland.)

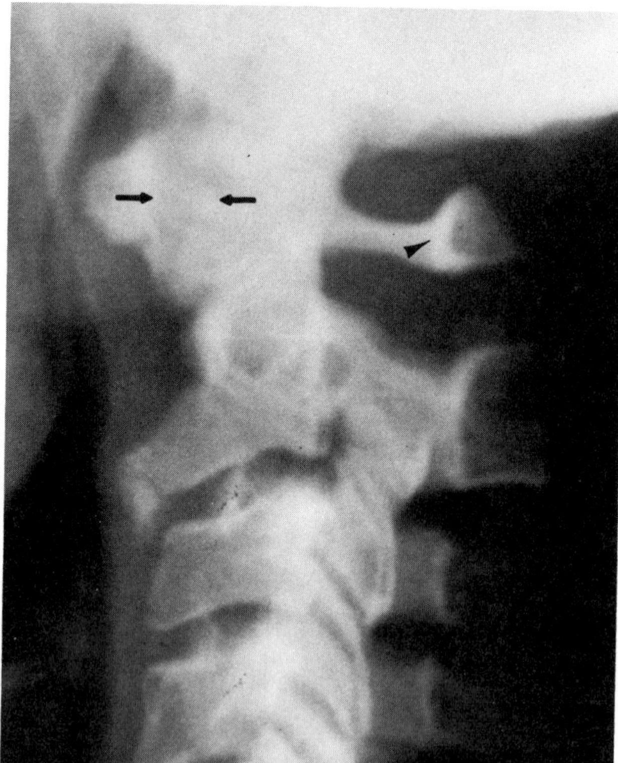

Figure 83–7. Behçet's syndrome: Atlanto-axial subluxation. Note the increased distance between the posterior surface of the anterior arch of the atlas and the odontoid process (between arrows), as well as an anterior position of the spinolaminar line (arrowhead). (Courtesy of Dr. M. Dalinka, University of Pennsylvania, Philadelphia, Pennsylvania.)

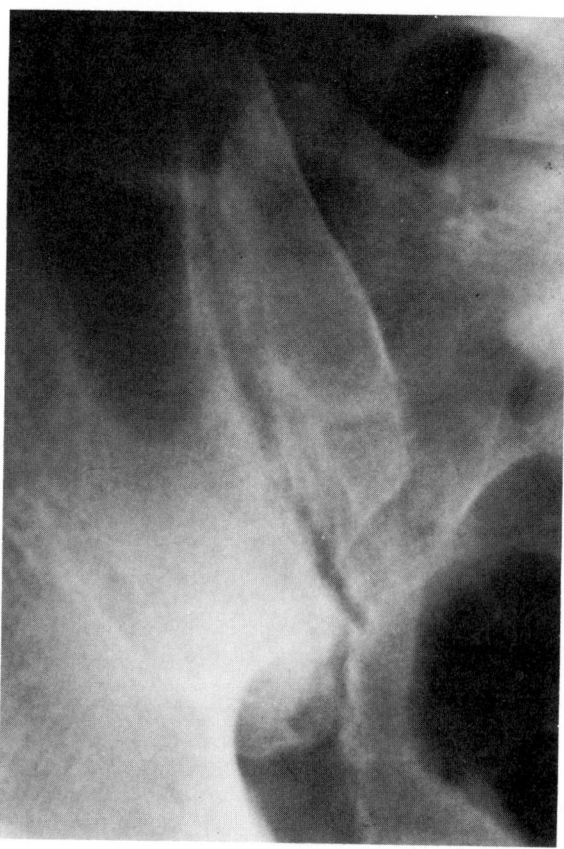

Figure 83–8. Behçet's syndrome: Sacroiliitis. In this patient, unilateral sacroiliitis is characterized by subchondral erosions and reactive sclerosis, predominantly in the ilium. (Courtesy of Dr. A. Brower, The Uniformed Services University for Health Sciences, Bethesda, Maryland.)

oping a mild sacroiliitis and spondylitis.[61] In addition, a possible relationship between Behçet's syndrome and inflammatory bowel disorders such as ulcerative colitis and Crohn's disease could account for a link with sacroiliitis in the former disease.[52, 62, 63]

Pathologic Abnormalities

Histologic examination shows replacement of the superficial zones of the synovial membrane by dense, inflamed granulation tissue composed of lymphocytes, macrophages, fibroblasts, neutrophils, and vascular elements[58] (Fig. 83–9). Pannus, with erosion of cartilaginous and osseous surfaces, can be noted, and organisms cannot be recovered.

At sites of ulceration in the skin and mucosa, vasculitis is generally prominent. It may also be evident about ocular and gastrointestinal lesions, as well as in other locations. Aneurysms in the aorta and elsewhere may reveal acute and chronic cellular infiltration in the vessel walls, with an endarteritis of the vasa vasorum.[64, 65]

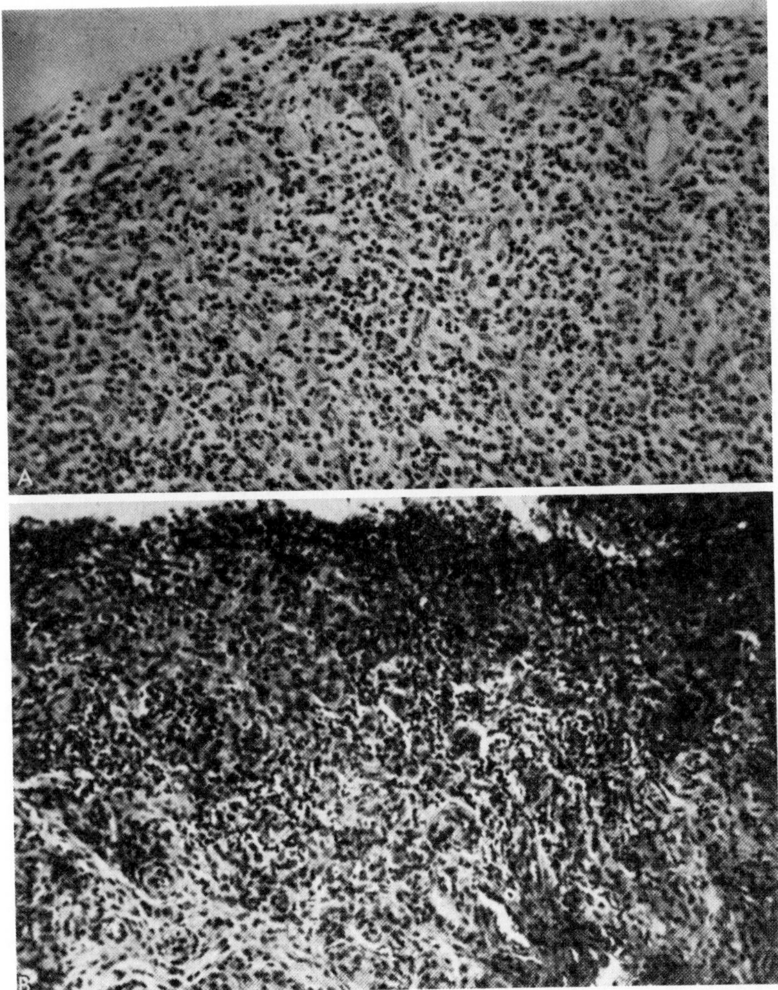

Figure 83–9. *Behçet's syndrome: Pathologic abnormalities of synovial and cartilaginous joints.*

A *Following a biopsy of the synovial membrane from an inflamed wrist joint, note the absence of lining cells and the presence of heavily inflamed granulation tissue (150×).*

B *The synovial membrane from an involved knee reveals heavy inflammation and marked macrophage proliferation in the superficial zone (150×).*

Illustration continued on the following page

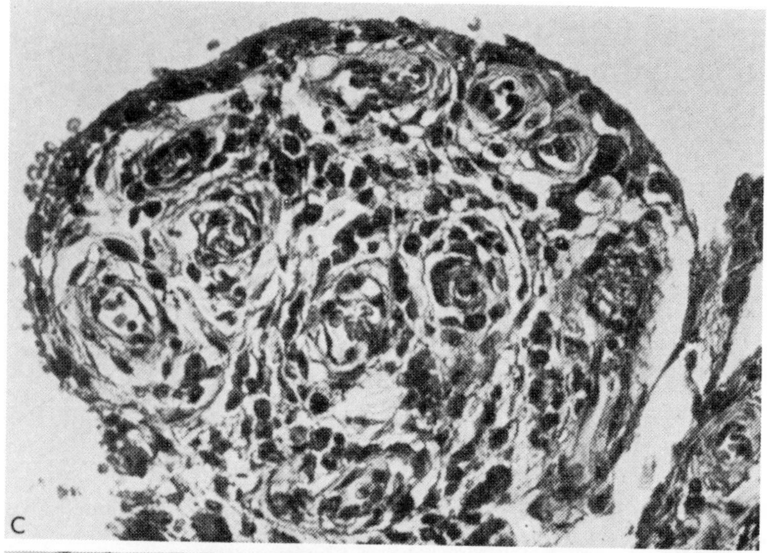

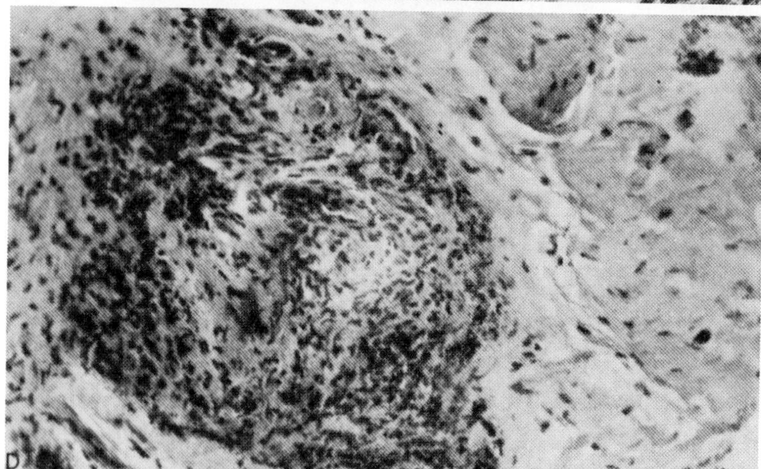

Figure 83–9. Continued

C *A high-power view of a synovial villous process reveals numerous small vessels, some fibrosis, and a moderate plasma cell infiltrate (550×).*

D *Tissue obtained from the manubriosternal joint indicates that the fibrocartilage (right) is being replaced by inflammatory pannus containing many macrophages and polymorphonuclear neutrophils (left) (150 ×).*

(From Vernon-Roberts B, et al: Ann Rheum Dis 37:139, 1978.)

Etiology and Pathogenesis

The etiology of Behçet's syndrome is unknown. Although there has been considerable speculation about the role of infection in this disorder,[47] particularly a viral disease[66, 67] or tuberculosis, this possibility has been discounted by some investigators.[68] Environmental pollutants have been stressed as etiologic factors in other reports.[61] The known geographic concentration of cases, the familial clustering,[69-71] and the recognition of the association of the disease with HLA B5 in Japanese patients suggest that host factors are important.[55, 78] An immunologic disturbance is implicated by the detection of antibodies against buccal mucosa.[72, 73]

Differential Diagnosis

When evident, radiologic alterations of joints in Behçet's syndrome may resemble those of rheumatoid arthritis or related disorders. Sacroiliitis can simulate the changes in ankylosing spondylitis or other seronegative spondyloarthropathies.

SUMMARY

Familial Mediterranean fever, relapsing polychondritis, and Behçet's syndrome represent three uncommon disorders that may be associated with periodic, relapsing, or recurrent clinical manifestations. In each disease, synovitis can occasionally lead to soft tissue swelling and periarticular osteoporosis, and in rare instances cartilaginous and osseous destruction can become evident. Furthermore, each of these three disorders has been associated with sacroiliitis, although this association is not frequent, nor is it without controversy in some cases.

REFERENCES

1. Ehrlich GE: Intermittent and periodic arthritis syndromes. *In* JL Hollander, DJ McCarty Jr (Eds): Arthritis and Allied Conditions, 8th Ed. Philadelphia, Lea & Febiger, 1972, p 821.
2. Heller H, Sohar E, Sherf L: Familial Mediterranean fever. Arch Intern Med *102*:50, 1958.
3. Priest RJ, Nixon RK: Familial recurring polyserositis: A disease entity. Ann Intern Med *51*:1253, 1959.
4. Sohar E, Gafni J, Pras M, Heller H: Familial Mediterranean fever. A survey of 470 cases and review of the literature. Am J Med *43*:227, 1967.
5. Siegal S: Familial paroxysmal polyserositis. Analysis of 50 cases. Am J Med *36*:893, 1964.
6. Schwabe AD, Peters RS: Familial Mediterranean fever in Armenians. Analysis of 100 cases. Medicine *53*:453, 1974.
7. Heller H, Gafni J, Michaeli D, Shahin N, Sohar E, Ehrlich G, Karten I, Sokoloff L: The arthritis of familial Mediterranean fever. Arthritis Rheum 9:1, 1966.
8. Makin M, Levin S: The articular manifestations of periodic disease (familial Mediterranean fever). J Bone Jont Surg *47A*:1615, 1965.
9. Herness D, Makin M: Articular damage in familial Mediterranean fever. J Bone Joint Surg *57A*:265, 1975.
10. Simon G, Marbach JJ: Familial Mediterranean fever with temporomandibular joint arthritis. Pediatrics *57*:810, 1976.
11. Sneh E, Pras M, Michaeli D, Shahin N, Gafni J: Protracted arthritis in familial Mediterranean fever. Rheumatol Rehabil *16*:102, 1977.
12. Sohar E, Pras M, Gafni J: Familial Mediterranean fever and its articular manifestations. Clin Rheum Dis *1*:195, 1975.
13. Dinarello CA, Wolff SM, Goldfinger SE, Dale DC, Alling DW: Colchicine therapy for familial Mediterranean fever. N Engl J Med *291*:934, 1974.
14. Azizi E, Fisher BK: Cutaneous manifestations of familial Mediterranean fever. Arch Dermatol *112*:364, 1976.
15. Mamou H, Cattan R: La maladie périodique (sur 14 cas personnels dont 8 compliqués de néphropathies). Sem Hôp Paris *28*:1062, 1952.
16. Siguier F: Maladies — Vedettes; Maladies d'Avenir, Maladies Quotidiennes, Maladies d'Exception. Paris, Masson, 1957, p 279.
17. Gumpel JM: Familial Mediterranean fever. Proc R Soc Med *65*:977, 1972.
18. Brodey PA, Wolff SM: Radiographic changes in the sacroiliac joints in familial Mediterranean fever. Radiology *114*:331, 1975.
19. Shahin N, Sohar E, Dalith F: Roentgenologic findings in familial Mediterranean fever. Am J Rotentgenol *84*:269, 1960.
20. Lehman TJA, Hanson V, Kornreich H, Peters RS, Schwabe AD: HLA-B27 negative sacroiliitis: A manifestation of familial Mediterranean fever in childhood. Pediatrics *61*:423, 1978.
21. Schwabe AD, Terasaki PI, Barnett EV, Territo MC, Klinenberg JR, Peters RS: Familial Mediterranean fever: Recent advances in pathogenesis and management. West J Med *127*:15, 1977.
22. Lehman TJA, Peters RS, Hanson V, Schwabe AD: Diagnosis and treatment of familial Mediterranean fever (FMF) in childhood (Abstr). Arthritis Rheum *21*:573, 1978.
23. Pearson CM, Kline HM, Newcomer VD: Relapsing polychondritis. N Engl J Med *263*:51, 1960.
24. Jaksch-Wartenhorst R: Polychondropathia. Wien Arch Inn Med *6*:93, 1923.
25. Harders H: Panchondritis. Verh Dtsch Ges Rheumatol *3*:71, 1974.
26. Kaye RL, Sones DA: Relapsing polychondritis. Clinical and pathological features in fourteen cases. Ann Intern Med *60*:653, 1964.
27. Hughes RAC, Berry CL, Seifert M, Lessof MH: Relapsing polychondritis. Three cases with a clinico-pathologic study and literature review. Q J Med *41*:363, 1972.
28. Dolan DL, Lemmon GB, Teitelbaum SL: Relapsing polychondritis: Analytical literature review and studies on pathogenesis. Am J Med *41*:285, 1966.
29. McAdam LP, O'Hanlan MA, Bluestone R, Pearson CM: Relapsing polychondritis: Prospective study of 23 patients and a review of the literature. Medicine *55*:193, 1976.
30. Barth WF, Berson EL: Relapsing polychondritis, rheumatoid arthritis and blindness. Am J Ophthalmol *66*:890, 1969.
31. Anderson B Sr: Ocular lesions in relapsing polychondritis and other rheumatoid syndromes. Am J Ophthalmol *64*:35, 1967.
32. Rabuzzi DD: Relapsing polychondritis. Arch Otolaryngol *91*:188, 1970.
33. Owen DS Jr, Irby R, Toone E: Relapsing polychondritis with aortic involvement. Arthritis Rheum *13*:877, 1970.
34. Johnson TH, Mital N, Rodnan GP, Wilson RJ: Relapsing polychondritis. Radiology *106*:313, 1973.
35. Butcher RB II, Tabb HG, Dunlap CE: Relapsing polychondritis. South Med J *67*:1443, 1974.
36. Rogers FB, Lansbury J: Atrophy of auricular and nasal cartilages following administration of chorionic gonodotrophins in a case of arthritis mutilans with the sicca syndrome. Am J Med Sci *229*:55, 1955.
37. O'Hanlan M, McAdam LP, Bluestone R, Pearson CM: The arthropathy of relapsing polychondritis. Arthritis Rheum *19*:191, 1976.
38. Braunstein EM, Martel W, Stillwill E, Kay D: Radiological aspects of the arthropathy of relapsing polychondritis. Clin Radiol *30*:441, 1979.
39. Mitchell N, Shepard N: Relapsing polychondritis. An electron microscopic study of synovium and articular cartilage. J Bone Joint Surg *54A*:1235, 1972.
40. Verity MA, Larson WM, Madden SC: Relapsing polychondritis: Report of two necropsied cases with histochemical investigations of the cartilage lesion. Am J Pathol *42*:251, 1963.
41. Feinerman LK, Johnson WC, Weiner J, Graham JH: Relapsing polychondritis: A histopathologic and histochemical study. Dermatologica *140*:369, 1970.
42. Shaul SR, Schumacher HR: Relapsing polychondritis. Electron microscopic study of ear cartilage. Arthritis Rheum *18*:617, 1975.
43. Tourtellotte CD: Relapsing polychondritis. *In* AS Cohen (Ed): The Science and Practice of Clinical Medicine. Vol. 4, Rheumatology and Immunology. New York, Grune & Stratton, 1979, p 350.
44. Rogers PH, Boden G, Tourtellotte CD: Relapsing polychondritis with insulin resistance and antibodies to cartilage. Am J Med *55*:243, 1973.
45. Herman JH, Dennis MV: Immunopathologic studies in relapsing polychondritis. J Clin Invest *52*:549, 1973.
46. Rajapakse DA, Bywaters EGL: Cell mediated immunity to cartilage proteoglycan in relapsing polychondritis. Clin Exp Immunol *16*:497, 1974.
47. Behçet H: Some observations on the clinical picture of the so-called triple symptom complex. Dermatologica *81*:73, 1940.
48. Mason RM, Barnes CG: Behçet's syndrome with arthritis. Ann Rheum Dis *28*:95, 1969.
49. Chajek T, Fairnaru M: Behçet's disease. Report of 41 cases and review of the literature. Medicine *54*:179, 1975.
50. O'Duffy JD, Carney JA, Deodar S: Behçet's disease: Report of 10 cases, 3 with new manifestations. Ann Intern Med *75*:561, 1971.
51. Oshima Y, Shimizu T, Yokohari R, Matsumoto T, Kano K, Kagami T, Nagaya H: Clinical studies on Behçet's syndrome. Ann Rheum Dis *22*:36, 1973.
52. Chamberlain MA: Behçet's syndrome in 32 patients in Yorkshire. Ann Rheum Dis *36*:491, 1977.
53. O'Duffy JD, Goldstein NP: Neurologic involvement in seven patients with Behçet's disease. Am J Med *61*:170, 1976.
54. Currey HLF, Elson RA, Mason RM: Surgical treatment of manubriosternal pain in Behçet's syndrome. Report of a case. J Bone Joint Surg *50B*:836, 1968.
55. Medsger TA Jr: Behçet's disease. In AS Cohen (Ed): The Science and Practice of Clinical Medicine. Vol. 4, Rheumatology and Immunology. New York, Grune & Stratton, 1979, p 233.
56. Ohno S, Aoki K, Sugiura S, Nakayama E, Itakura K, Aizawa M: HL-A 5 and Behçet's disease. Lancet *2*:1383, 1973.
57. Zizic TM, Stevens MB: The arthropathy of Behçet's disease. Johns Hopkins Med J *136*:243, 1975.
58. Vernon-Roberts B, Barnes CG, Revell PA: Synovial pathology in Behçet's syndrome. Ann Rheum Dis *37*:139, 1978.
59. Cooper DA, Penny R: Behçet's syndrome: Clinical, immunological and therapeutic evaluation of 17 patients. Aust NZ J Med *4*:585, 1974.
60. Dilşen AN: Sacroiliitis and ankylosing spondylitis in Behçet's disease (Abstr). Scand J Rheum Suppl *8*:20-08, 1975.
61. O'Duffy JD: Summary of international symposium on Behçet's disease. Istanbul, September 29–30, 1977. J Rheumatol *5*:229, 1978.
62. Bøe J, Dalgaard JB, Scott D: Mucocutaneous-ocular syndrome with intestinal involvement. A clinical and pathological study of four fatal cases. Am J Med *25*:857, 1958.
63. Empey DW, Hale JE: Rectal and colonic ulceration in Behçet's disease. Proc R Soc Med *65*:163, 1972.
64. Enoch BA, Castillo-Olivares JL, Khoo TCL, Grainger RG, Henry L: Major vascular complications in Behçet's syndrome. Postgrad Med J *44*:453, 1968.
65. Hills EA: Behçet's syndrome with aortic aneurysm. Br Med J *4*:152, 1967.
66. Sezer FN: The isolation of a virus as the cause of Behçet's disease. Am J Ophthalmol *36*:301, 1953.
67. Sezer FN: Further investigation on the virus of Behçet's disease. Am J Ophthalmol *41*:41, 1956.
68. Dugeon JA: Virological aspects of Behçet's disease. Proc R Soc Med *54*:104, 1961.
69. Goolamali SK, Comaish JS, Hassanyek F, Stephens A: Familial Behçet's syndrome. Br J Dermatol *95*:637, 1976.
70. Fowler TJ, Humpston DJ, Nussey AM, Small M: Behçet's syndrome with neurological manifestations in two sisters. Br Med J *2*:473, 1968.

71. Berman L, Trappler B, Jenkins T: Behçet's syndrome: A family study and the elucidation of a genetic role. Ann Rheum Dis *38*:118, 1979.
72. Jensen T: Rückfällige apthöse Geschwürsbildung an Mundscheleimhaut und Geschlechtsteilen nebst rückfälliger Regenbogenhautenzündung und Sehnervenschwund (Behçet's Syndrom) (Abstr). Zentralbl Ges Ophthalmol *46*:446, 1941.
73. Shimizu T, Katsuta Y, Oshimo Y: Immunological studies on Behçet's syndrome. Ann Rheum Dis *24*:494, 1965.
74. Meyerhoff J: Familial Mediterranean fever: Report of a large family, review of the literature, and discussion of the frequency of amyloidosis. Medicine *59*:66, 1980.
75. Gilsanz V, Stanley P: Pediatric case of the day. Am J Roentgenol *134*:1293, 1980.
76. Small P, Frenkiel S: Relapsing polychondritis. A feature of systemic lupus erythematosus. Arthritis Rheum *23*:361, 1980.
77. Koss JC, Dalinka MK: Atlantoaxial subluxation in Behçet's syndrome. Am J Roentgenol *134*:392, 1980.
78. Yazici H, Tuzun Y, Pazarli H, Yalcin B, Yurdakul S, Muftuoglu A: The combined use of HLA-B5 and the pathergy test as diagnostic markers of Behçet's disease in Turkey. J Rheumatol *7*:206, 1980.
79. Arkin CR, Rothschild BM, Florendo NT, Popoff N: Behçet's syndrome with myositis. A case report with pathologic findings. Arthritis Rheum *23*:600, 1980.

SECTION XIX

TEMPORO-MANDIBULAR, SOFT TISSUE, AND SYSTEMIC MANIFESTA-TIONS OF SKELETAL DISEASES

84

THE TEMPOROMANDIBULAR JOINT*

by William A. Murphy, M.D., and Roger J. Adams, D.M.D., M.S.

Among the joints of the body, the temporomandibular joint (TMJ) has long been considered an "orphan," both clinically and radiologically. Its diseases, organic or functional, and therapies are less well understood than those of the other joints, and a broad spectrum of professionals is involved in its care. Although dentists most commonly encounter TMJ problems, oral surgeons, neurologists, rheumatologists, otolaryngologists, and family practitioners are often consulted. Unfortunately, there is no single source of currently accepted knowledge to guide these professionals regarding radiologic diagnosis.

Radiographic examination is an important adjunct for evaluation of TMJ afflictions. If effective, this examination should provide the clinician with documentation of normal or pathologic anatomy. However, conventional radiography has not proved satisfactory for a variety of reasons, including the small size of the joint, its complex anatomic structure, and its unique location among the many bones

*To facilitate interpretation, all illustrations of the temporomandibular joint are oriented similarly: Lateral radiographs are viewed facing the left; Towne radiographs are displayed as a left joint seen from the front.

of the skull. Difficulty in producing well-positioned radiographs has made interpretation doubly difficult. As a result, many radiologists are unsure of themselves when they encounter TMJ films. Recent technologic advancements (conventional tomography, microfocus magnification radiography, and arthrography) have greatly improved radiography and diagnosis.

RADIOGRAPHY

As with many areas of the body, TMJ radiographic techniques have developed to meet clinical and imaging needs. The various atlases of radiographic technique present a multitude of positions that might be used to obtain conventional films, but none illustrates the techniques necessary for modern TMJ imaging and diagnosis.

Conventional Lateral Views

Atlases describing these views contain a particular abundance of positions for a lateral projection, the most important view for general diagnostic purposes. They all share the same aim, to project a profiled joint free of surrounding structures. All are transfacial or transcranial and all require angling of the head, tube, or both. All suffer from the same inability to guarantee initial or reproducible profile from patient to patient or from time to time. When centering and profile are optimal, conventional lateral films do provide an acceptable image for study of anatomy and function (Fig. 84–1). However, many suboptimal films are obtained, which nevertheless are deemed acceptable and interpreted (Fig. 84–2). Even if all conventional lateral films were as good as those in Figure 84–1, they would still have some weaknesses. In particular, the part of interest makes up only a small percentage (less than 10 per cent) of the total image. Furthermore, tight coning might altogether exclude the TMJ from the image.

Updegrave* Positioned Lateral Views

A logical way to improve lateral radiography was to standardize positioning of the TMJ. This has been accomplished with several positioning devices,[9, 46, 51] including that described by Updegrave,[43] which we believe is one of the most convenient and reliable instruments available (Fig. 84–3) for contact radiography. This device standardizes location of the central beam at the TMJ and inclines the head 15 degrees with respect to the incident x-ray beam. In

*The UPRAD Corporation, Fort Lauderdale, Florida.

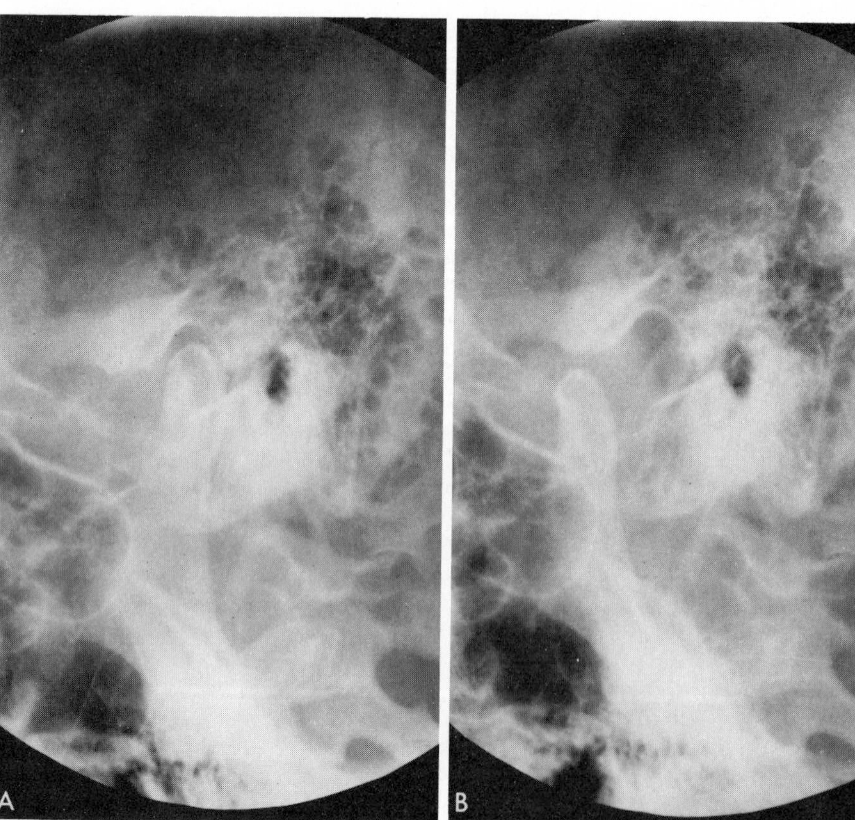

Figure 84–1. *Temporomandibular joint.*

A *Optimal transcranial lateral view. The closed temporomandibular joint (TMJ) is projected free of other cranial structures. The condylar head and mandibular fossa are profiled.*

B *The open mouth view shows normal motion, and the bone structures remain profiled. The TMJ makes up less than 10 per cent of this image.*

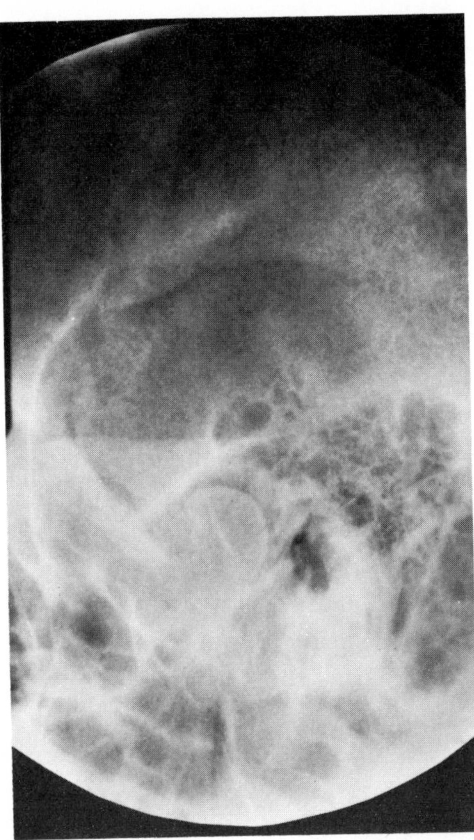

Figure 84–2. Suboptimal transcranial lateral view. The TMJ is no longer centered and because the head (or tube) angle is not precise, neither the condylar head nor the mandibular fossa is in profile.

addition to ensuring a reproducibly accurate TMJ profile (Fig. 84–4), this device permits tight coning of the beam. Such coning allows six exposures on an 8 × 10 in film and improves detail by decreasing scatter. Finally, sequential studies, often necessary during several years of therapy, are sufficiently similar for accurate comparison. Still, positioning units have not gained general acceptance.

Microfocus Magnification Lateral Views

The most recent advancement in TMJ imaging was the marriage of a positioning device to magnification capability.[32] A positioning unit (Fig. 84–5) based on principles similar to the Updegrave device was designed to replace the standard object tray of the RSI* Microfocus Magnification System (Fig. 84–6). This technique solved the need for both minute radiologic detail and dependable positioning of a small anatomic part (Fig. 84–7). The positioning unit ensured a reproducible quality image, permitted tight coning of the radiation field, and allowed precise correction of technical malposition. Geometric magnification with the microfocus tube resulted in an image with improved resolution, decreased noise, enhanced visual appreciation, and greater diagnostic value (Fig. 84–8). A rare-earth screen,

*Radiologic Sciences Incorporated, a subsidiary of Pfizer, Inc., Santa Clara, California 95051.

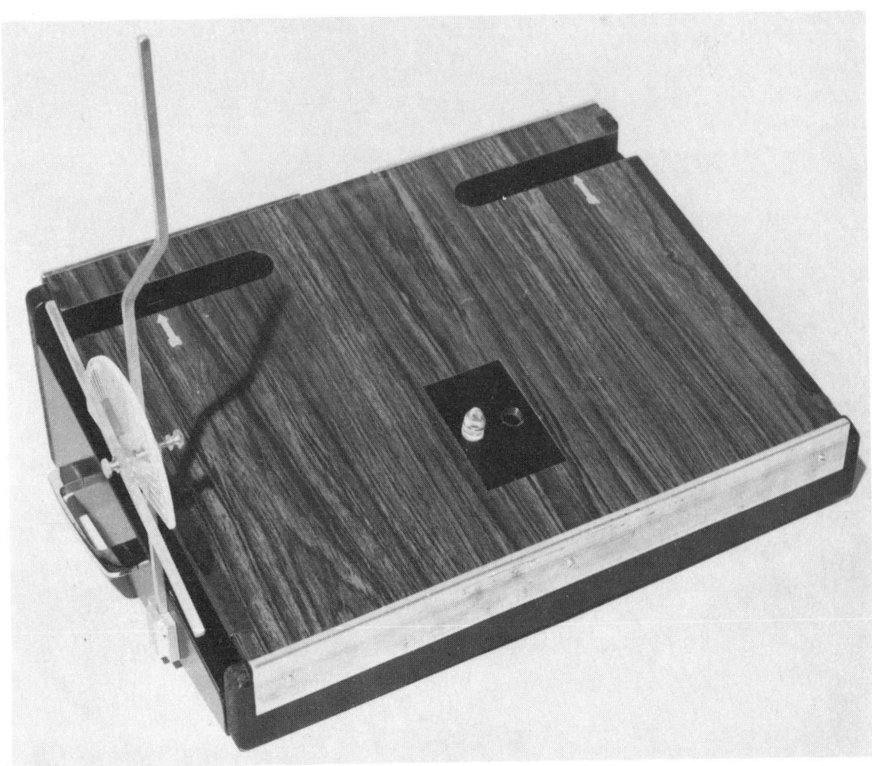

Figure 84–3. Updegrave Positioning Unit for lateral radiography. The ear plug in the central portion of the device serves to locate the external auditory canal and hence the TMJ for the central beam, which is coned to the limits of the central rectangle. The entire device is inclined 15 degrees and a standard 8 × 10 in screened cassette is slid into the slot just below the textured head support surface. The vertical bar and protractor also document head position for reproducibility.

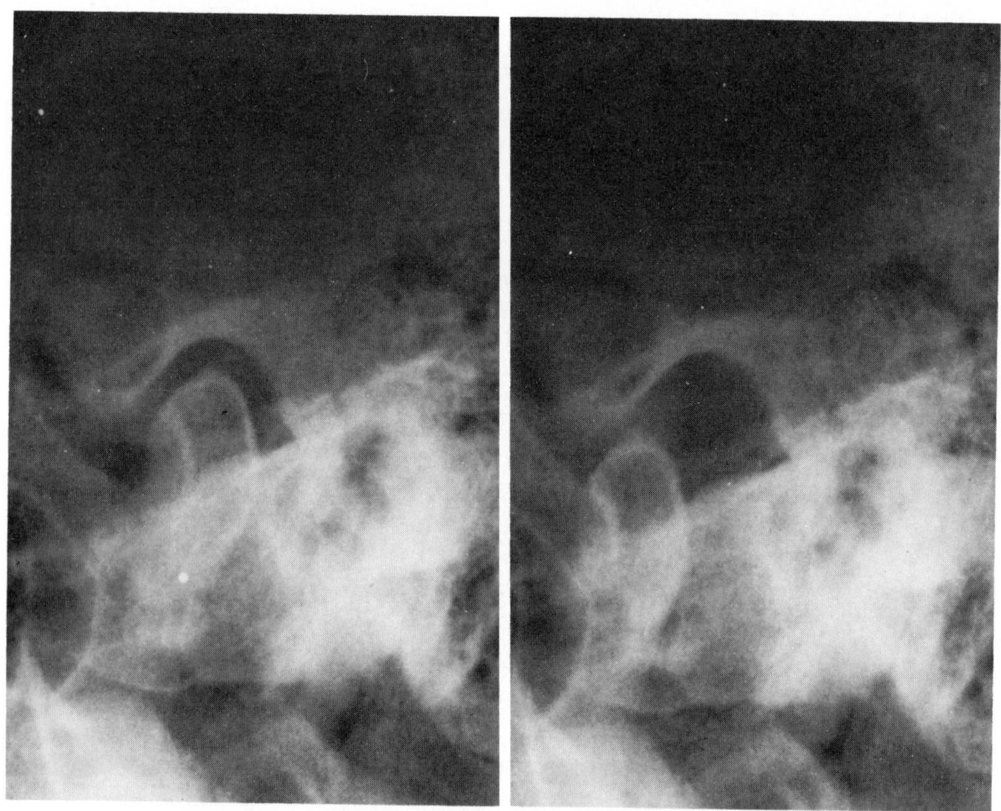

Figure 84–4. *Updegrave lateral images of the TMJ are usually centered and profiled (~ 15 per cent of the area). Variable shape of facial structures and rotation of the head about the longitudinal axis will cause loss of profile, but such profile problems are easily corrected.*

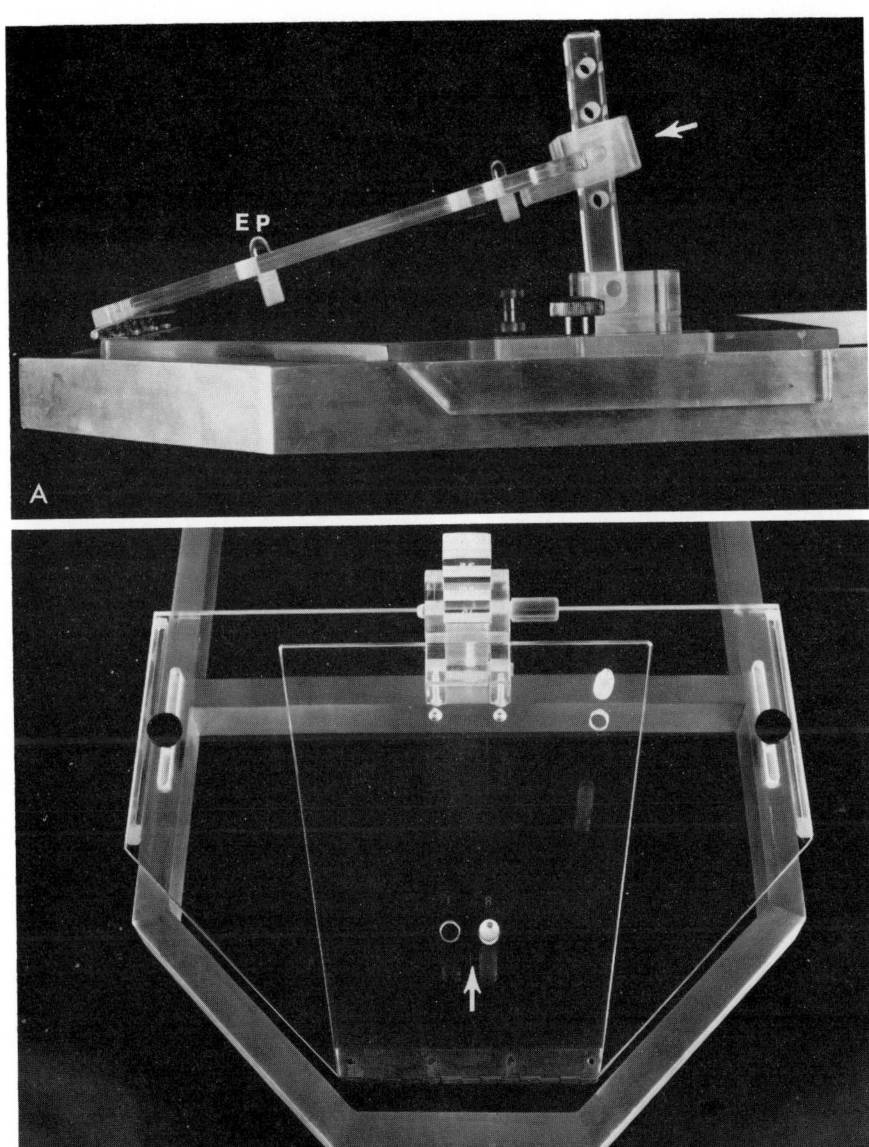

Figure 84–5. *Microfocus Magnification Positioning Unit.*

A *Lateral view of magnification positioning unit. The Plexiglas head support surface is hinged along the front edge to allow 5 degree changes in inclination along the coronal axis of the skull, accomplished by a simple peg-in-hole device (arrow). An ear plug (EP) stabilizes the head and locates the TMJ for the central beam.*

B *Surface view. The Plexiglas unit can slide along the arms of its metal frame to accommodate all head sizes. A cross hatch (arrow) is provided for localization of the central beam to the TMJ. Right and left ear plug positions are marked, and the threaded plug can be interchanged quickly.*

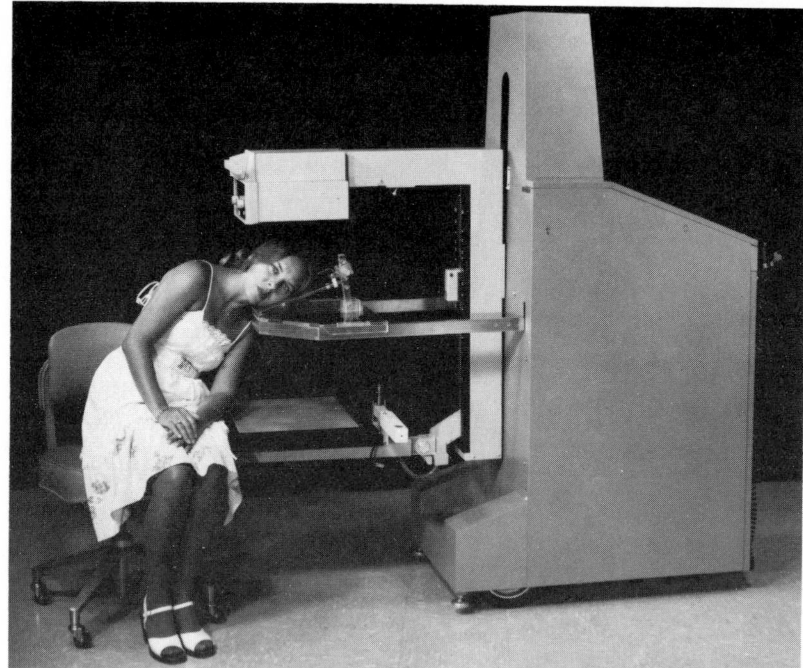

Figure 84–6. RSI Microfocus system adapted for geometric magnification of the TMJ in the lateral position; model demonstrates ease of access and positioning. (From Murphy WA, et al: Radiology 133:524, 1979.)

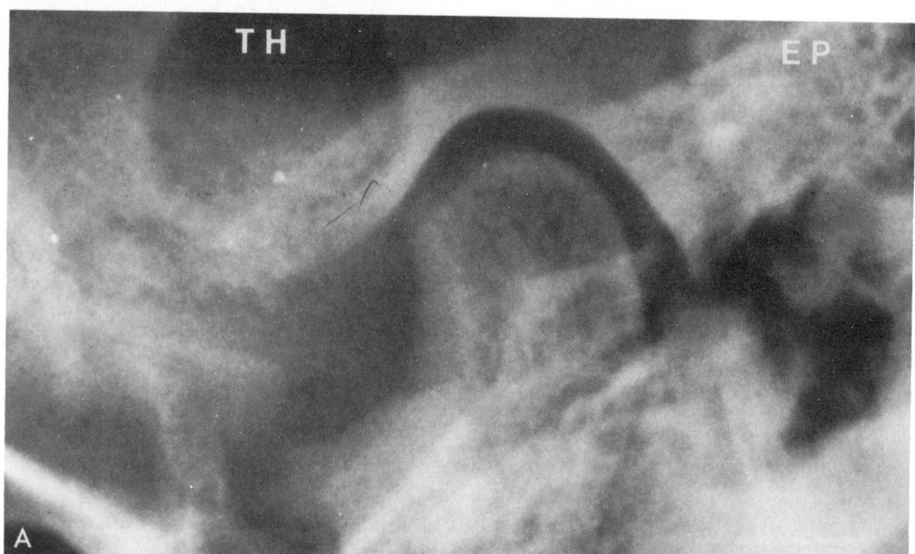

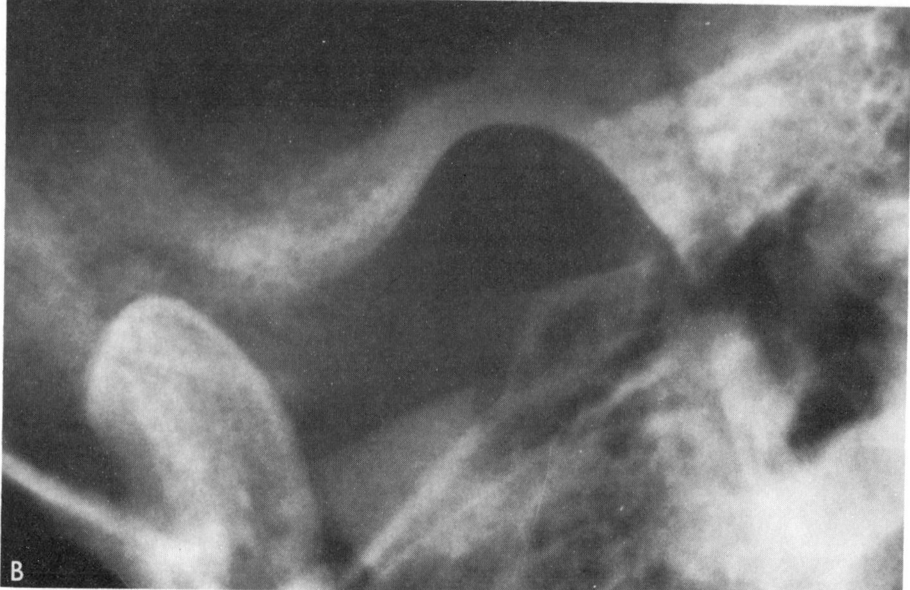

Figure 84–7. Magnification lateral image of a normal TMJ in closed **(A)** and open **(B)** positions. Bone detail is exquisite, and the TMJ constitutes about 50 per cent of the overall image. Side-by-side round artifacts result from the positioning device; the lucent area is the threaded ear plug hole (TH) and the dense area is the ear plug (EP) itself.

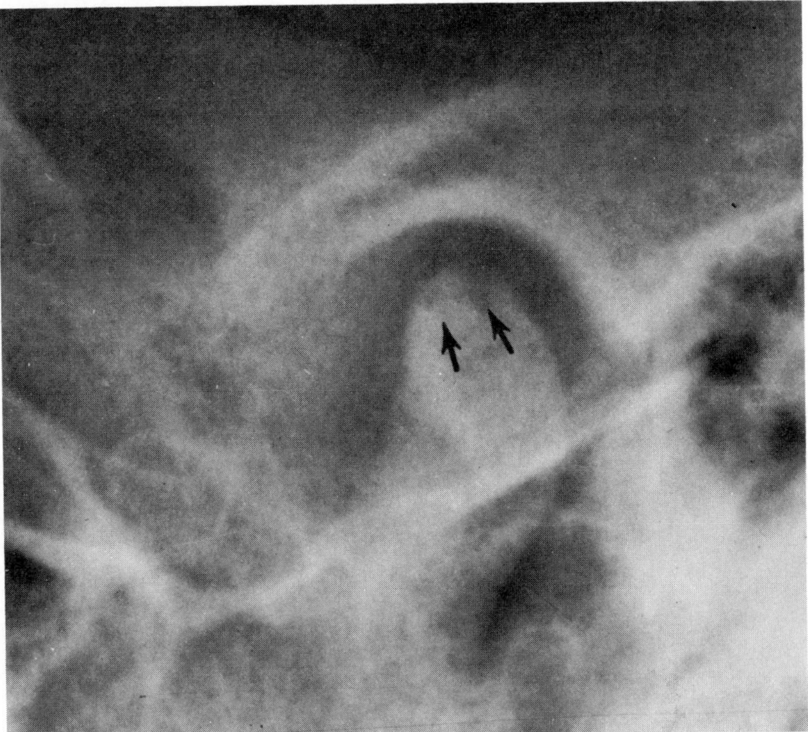

Figure 84–8. Subtle erosions of the condylar head (arrows) are easily appreciated in this microfocus magnification image, but were not seen on conventional or tomographic images obtained several days before.

fast-film recording system complemented the technique and held radiation exposure within an acceptable range.

The majority of lateral and Towne TMJ images in this chapter were obtained with the microfocus magnification system.

Tomographic Lateral Views

Tomography in the radiologic diagnosis of TMJ problems was introduced in the late 1930s [28, 36] and gained considerable popularity among clinicians and radiologists. It required careful positioning of the patient and review of the images as they were obtained. As a result, the tomographic images were generally better than conventional lateral images (Fig. 84–9). In fact, tomography became the recommended primary radiographic technique for TMJ evaluation.[15, 39, 40, 49] In addition to the disadvantage of being more time consuming for technologist and radiologist, multiple exposures were necessary for complete examination. Since the introduction and rapid clinical acceptance of magnification radiography in our hospital, we have performed TMJ tomography only rarely. Substitution of the magnification study for tomography has resulted in a reduced radiation exposure per patient.[32]

Towne Projection

Because of the complex shape of the condylar head of the mandible, lateral views alone are insufficient for complete evaluation. The condylar head and adjacent mandibular fossa of the temporal bone have considerable depth in the coronal plane. The Towne projection provides an image of medial and lateral poles of the condylar head as well as its posterosuperior cortical surface and neck. An angle of approximately 30 degrees is optimal for TMJ images, because at this angle, the TMJ is projected free of mastoid air cells. Conventional contact Towne projections (Fig. 84–10) must be relatively underexposed or the TMJ is badly overpenetrated. Microfocus magnification images in the Towne projection provide more radiological detail (see Fig. 84–16).

Submental-Vertical (Base) Projection

In this view, medial and lateral condylar poles are again imaged, but a different cortex is tangent to the incident beam. Anterior and posterior cortical surfaces are profiled, and information about adjacent bone structures at the base of the skull is provided (Fig. 84–11).

Panoramic Radiography

Since the temporomandibular joints are at opposite ends of the mandible, they may reflect disease processes of mandibular bone or its dental components. The standard panoramic radiograph (Fig. 84–12) provides an excellent survey of the mandible and dentition.[44] Furthermore, it provides a relatively

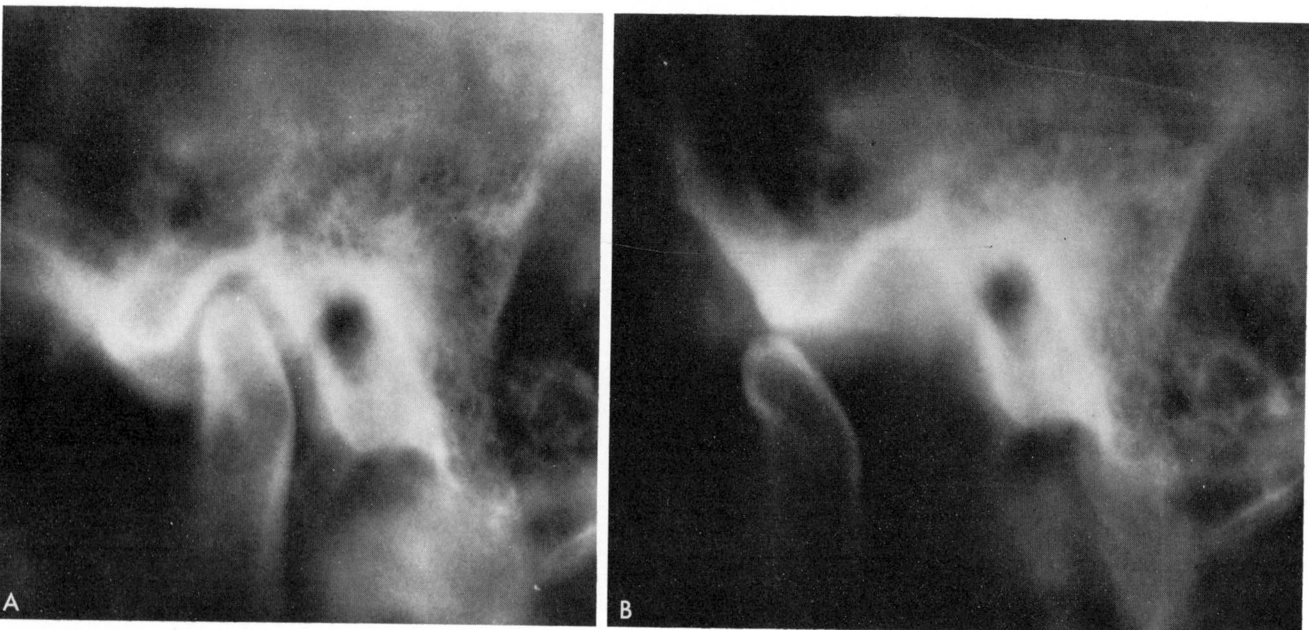

Figure 84–9. *Tomographic lateral images provide sharp detail of a 5 mm section of a normal TMJ in closed* **(A)** *and open* **(B)** *positions.*

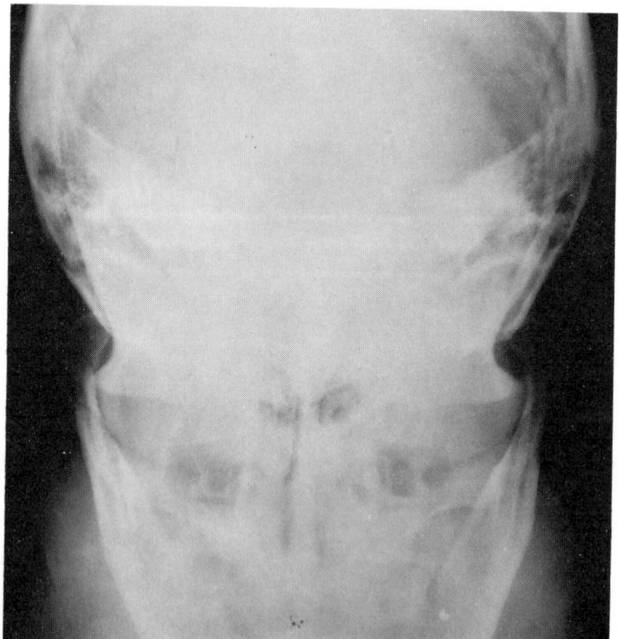

Figure 84–10. *Contact Towne projection at 30 degrees provides a survey of cranial anatomy about the TMJ as well as a view of the temporal fossa and the condylar head and neck.*

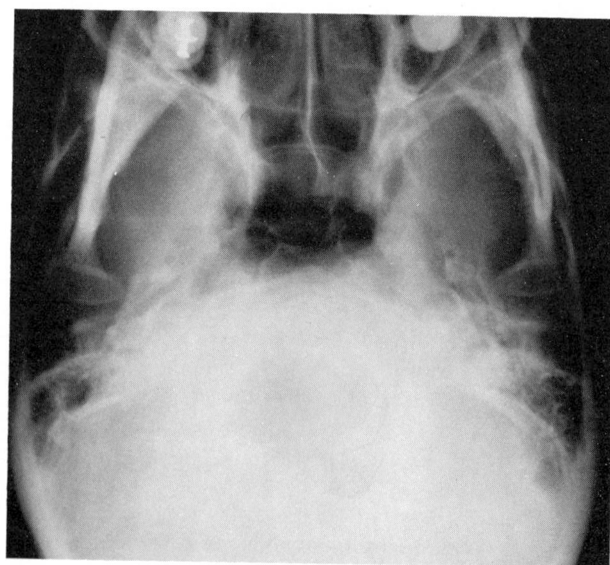

Figure 84–11. *Contact submental vertical (base) projection also surveys cranial anatomy surrounding the TMJ. Medial and lateral poles and anterior and posterior cortices of the condylar heads are well shown.*

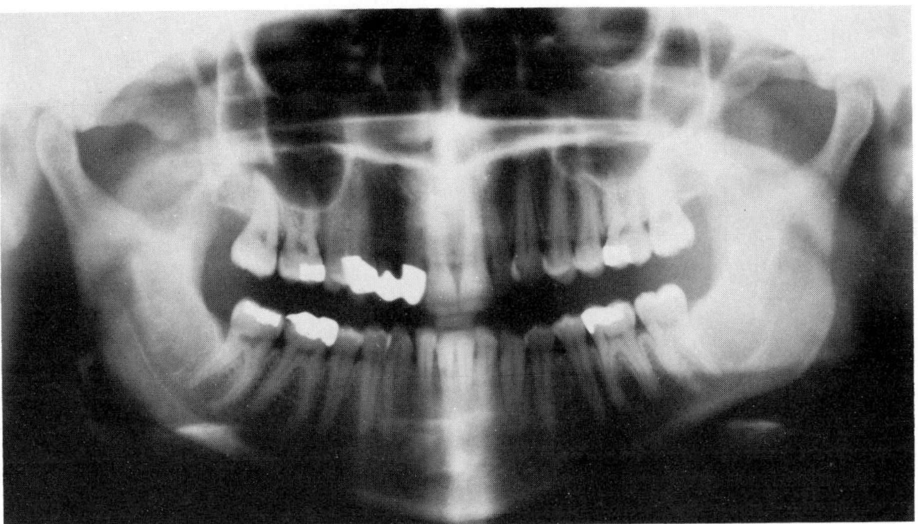

Figure 84–12. *Panoramic radiograph shows mandible, dental structures, and temporomandibular joint in a single image, a useful survey for periarticular diseases, which might present as TMJ pain.*

lateral projection of both temporomandibular joints on the same image. This is particularly useful for evaluation of symmetry. By changing patient positioning within most panoramic units, a thick section lateral tomogram may be obtained (Fig. 84–13).

Standard Series

Because of the complex anatomic structure, small size, and obscure location of the TMJ, a selected series of radiographs is obtained that provides both a detailed examination of the TMJ and a survey of surrounding bone anatomy. Detailed evaluation of the TMJ is provided by microfocus magnification images in lateral and Towne projections with the mouth opened and closed. Surrounding cranial anatomy is surveyed with contact Towne and base views. Mandibular and dental anatomy is evaluated with a single panoramic radiograph.

EMBRYOLOGY

Temporomandibular joints develop relatively later than the large joints. Although the shoulders, hips, and knees are well formed at 7 weeks' gestation, the temporomandibular joints are as yet undifferentiated.

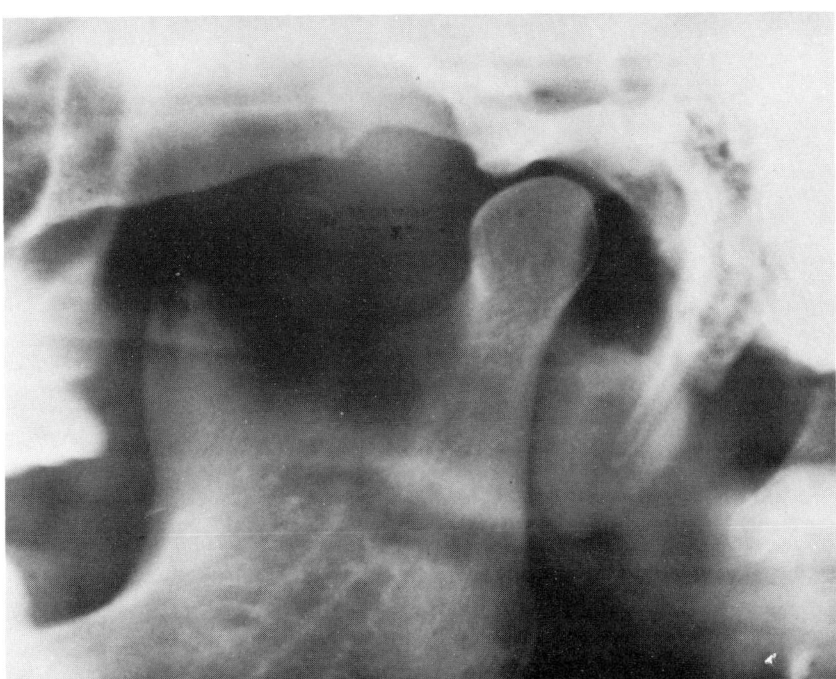

Figure 84–13. *With appropriate positioning, panoramic radiography can provide a thick section tomogram in a lateral projection.*

During development of the pharynx from the cranial end of the foregut, four endodermal pouches form and then expand into the surrounding mesenchymal tissue. Similarly, superficial branchial grooves form in the ectoderm. When these pharyngeal pouches and branchial grooves meet, they fuse and entrap mesenchymal tissue. Each such region is called a branchial arch. The mesenchymal cells become closely packed, and rapid differentiation begins.

Mesenchymal condensation in each arch forms an internal skeleton. In the first arch, the most distal portion of the skeletal core is Meckel's cartilage, about which the mandible forms as membrane bone. At the opposite end of the first arch skeleton, the incus and malleus of the middle ear form.

Between the sixth and eighth weeks of gestation, the mandible begins to ossify just lateral to Meckel's cartilage. About the tenth week, the condylar growth center develops and thereafter is responsible for mandible size and shape. By the twelfth week, the temporal center has appeared, and the two centers grow toward one another.

As early as the eighth week of gestation, a primordial articular disc (meniscus) is present in the form of a band of fibrous cells. About the tenth week, as the condylar growth center becomes well defined, the inferior joint space develops and defines the

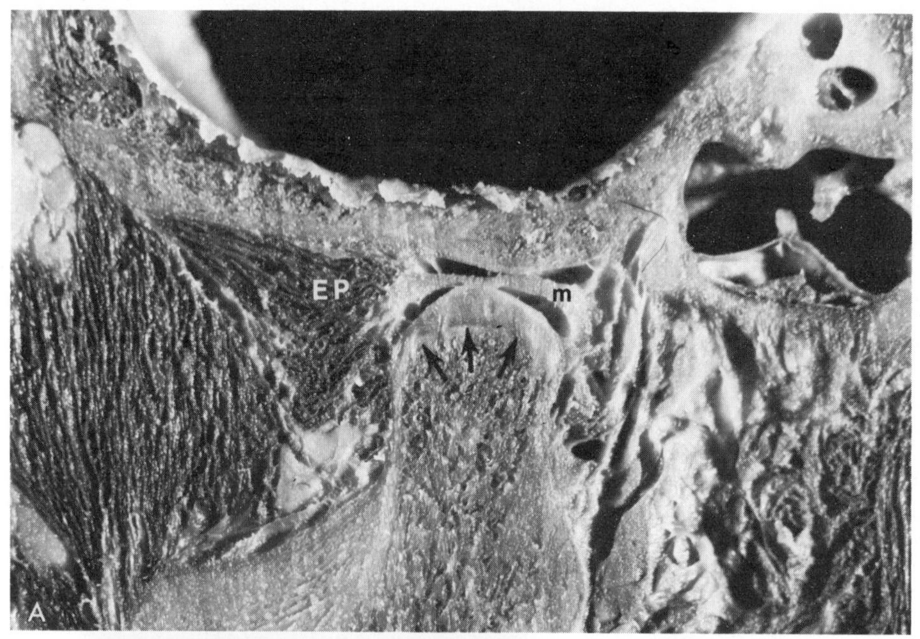

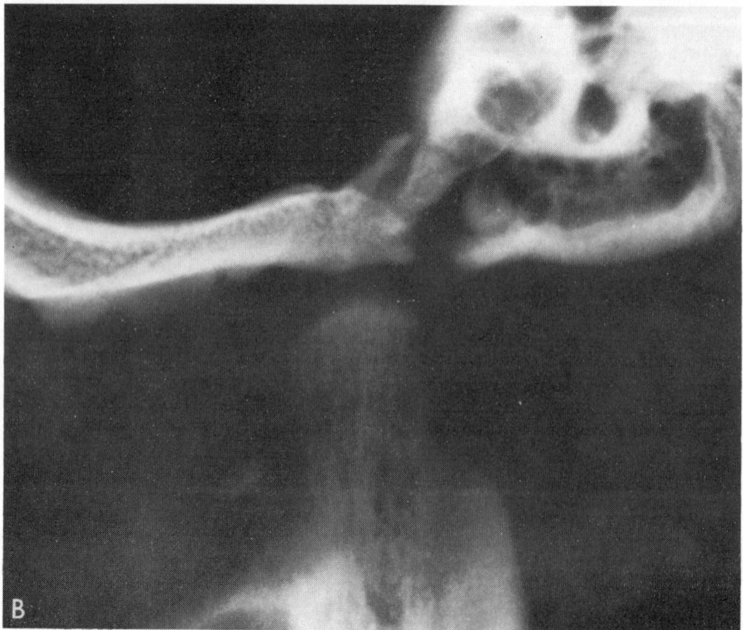

Figure 84–14. *Early development of the temporomandibular joint.*

A *Sagittal section of a 28 week fetus demonstrates a well-formed temporomandibular joint with a thin meniscus (m) separating superior and inferior joint cavities. The condylar head growth cartilage (arrows) is very thick and is responsible for growth and shape of the mandible. Note that fibers of the external pterygoid (EP) muscle attach to the anterior aspect of the meniscus.*

B *Specimen radiograph of sagittal section shows early ossification. Adult shape of the articular eminence will not develop for several years.*

inferior surface of the meniscus. Within the next several weeks, the superior joint cavity forms and temporal bone maturation approaches that of the mandibular condyle. Although there is undoubtedly some variation from the above timetable, the TMJ is always fully developed before the fourth fetal month (Fig. 84–14).[4, 5, 27, 50]

ADULT ANATOMY

The temporomandibular joint is an articulation of the condyle of the mandible with the mandibular fossa and articular eminence of the temporal bone. The capsule attaches about the joint margins and is reinforced laterally by a strong temporomandibular ligament and medially by two weaker ligaments. Branches of the mandibular division of the trigeminal nerve innervate the joint. Similarly, branches of the superficial temporal and maxillary arteries provide the blood supply.

Mandibular motion is governed by a pair (left and right) of small, anatomically complex diarthrodial joints that must function synchronously. Each joint is divided into two synovial spaces (one inferior and one superior) by an interposed articular disc or meniscus. This design permits the complex gliding, hinged, and rotary motions necessary for mastication. Normal TMJ function depends on balanced forces from both sides of the body. The

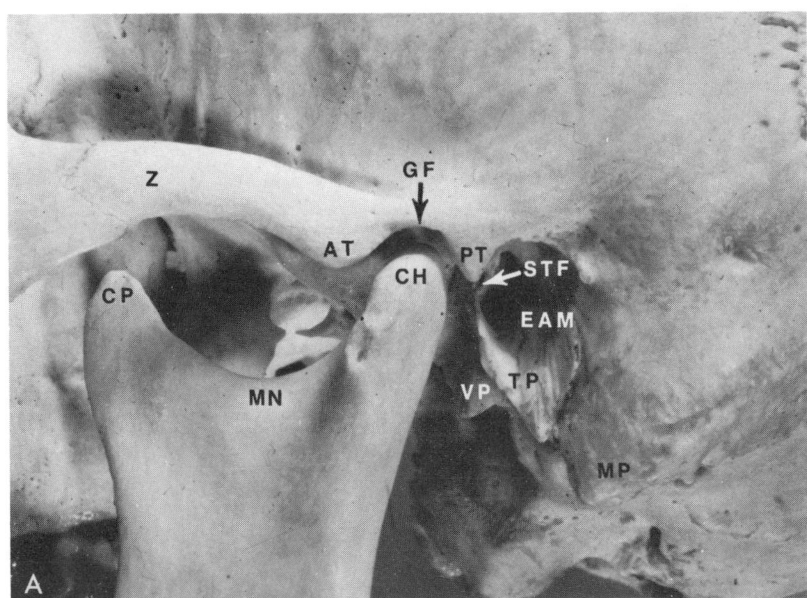

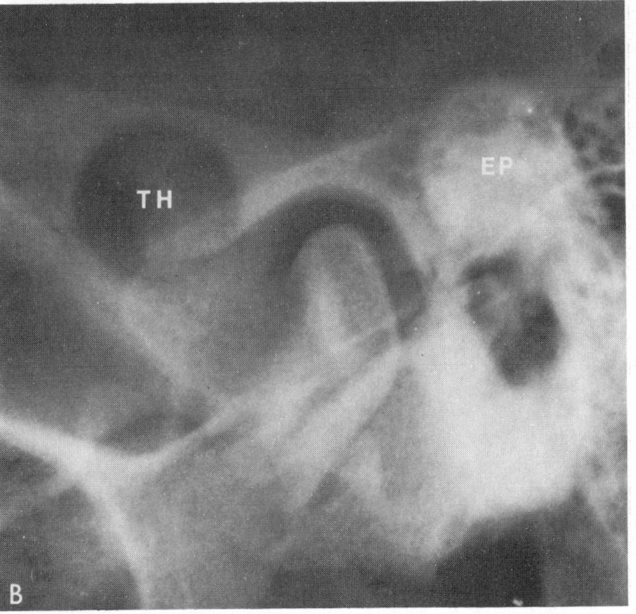

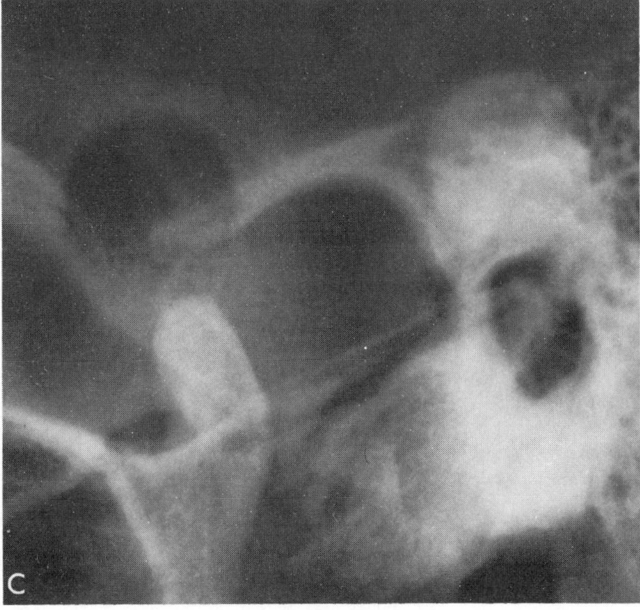

Figure 84–15. *External bone anatomy in the lateral projection.* **A,** *Surface of the skull.* **B,** *magnified lateral projection (closed), 22 year old woman;* **C,** *magnified lateral projection (open). Utilizing photographs and radiographs, the following anatomic landmarks can be identified and compared: Z, zygoma; GF, glenoid (mandibular) fossa; AT, anterior glenoid tubercle (articular eminence); PT, posterior glenoid tubercle; CH, condylar head; CP, coronoid process; STF, squamotympanic fissure; EAM, external auditory meatus; VP, vaginal process; TP, tympanic process; MP, mastoid process; TH, threaded hole; EP, ear plug.*

joints themselves must be symmetric; muscles of mastication must act simultaneously, and teeth must have proper occlusion.

Understanding of radiologic anatomy is aided by dividing it into three categories — external, internal, and functional. External or surface bone anatomy will be considered in this section. Internal and functional anatomy, which are closely interrelated, will be discussed in the arthrography section.

In the lateral projection (Fig. 84–15A), many

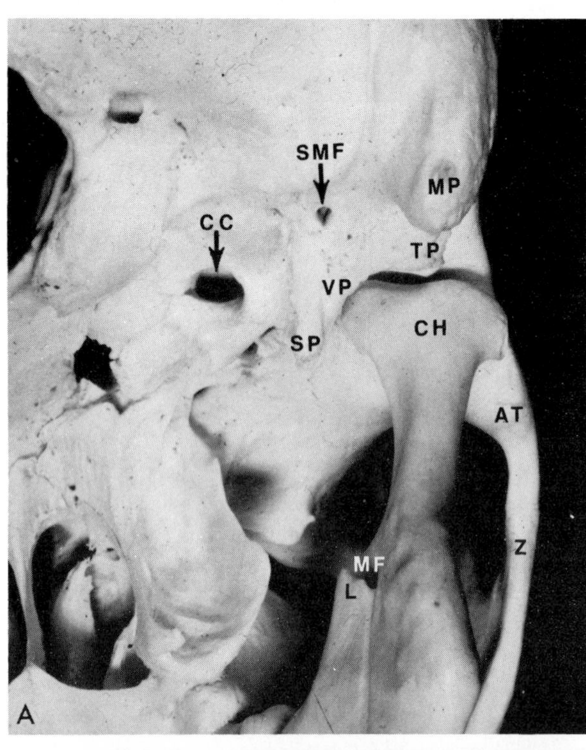

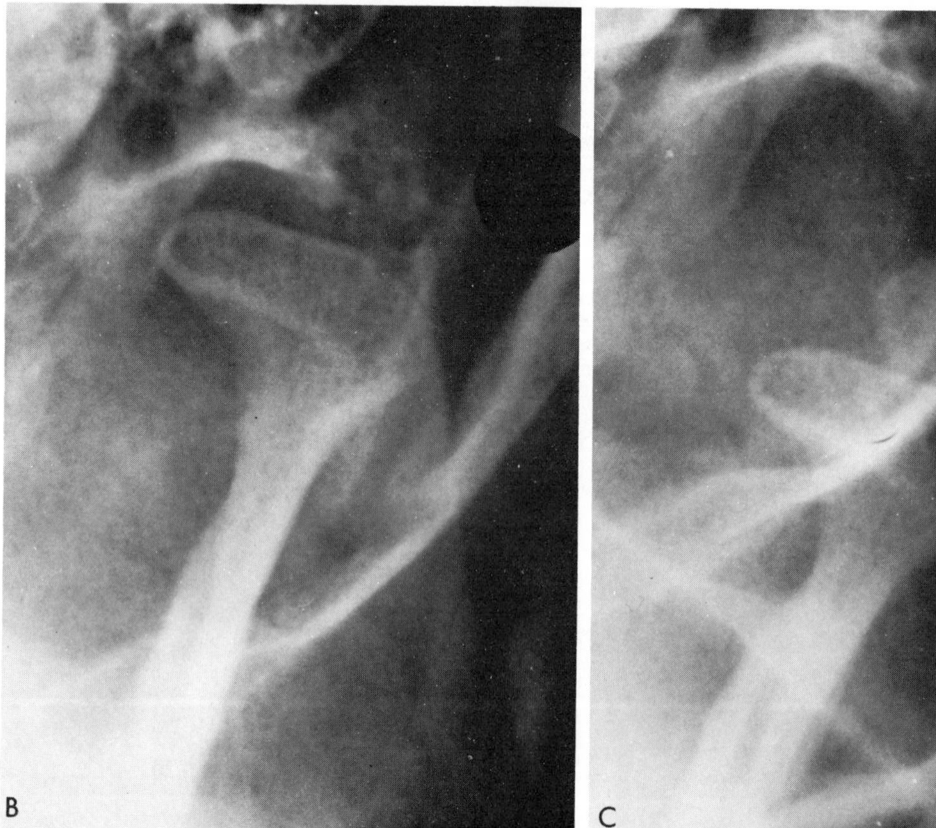

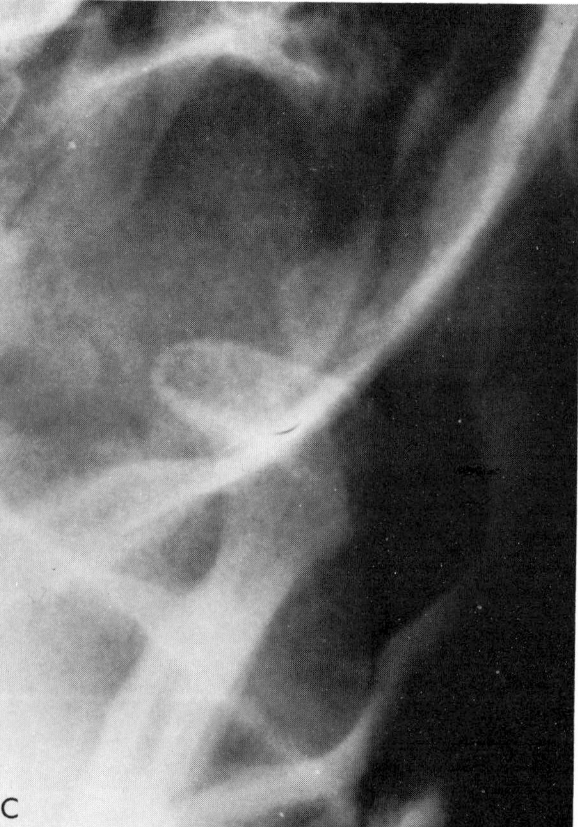

Figure 84–16. *External bone anatomy in the Towne projection.* **A,** *Surface of skull;* **B,** *magnified Towne projection (closed), 23 year old woman;* **C,** *magnified Towne projection (open). Utilizing photographs and radiographs, the following anatomic landmarks can be identified and compared:* CC, *Carotid canal;* SMF, *stylomastoid foramen;* SP, *styloid process;* VP, *vaginal process;* MP, *mastoid process;* TP, *tympanic process;* CH, *condylar head;* AT, *anterior glenoid tubercle;* MF, *mandibular foramen;* L, *lingula;* Z, *zygoma.*

bone landmarks can be identified, and most of these have occasional diagnostic importance. For example, the squamotympanic fissure has often been mistaken for a fracture. More important is evaluation of joint space width and cortical margin. The cartilage space of a normal TMJ is symmetric between articulating parts of the condylar head and mandibular fossa (Fig. 84–15*B*). The temporal bone describes a smooth sigmoid curve, and the cortex is of homogeneous radiodensity. Likewise, the condylar head is smooth and marginated by a distinct cortex of uniform thickness. In the open position, it should be possible to translocate the condylar head at least to the apex of the anterior tubercle, if not beyond (Fig. 84–15*C*). Since the meniscus is interposed, the condylar head and anterior tubercle should not touch.

Many landmarks can be identified in the Towne projection as well (Fig. 84–16*A*). Careful attention should be directed at the medial and lateral poles, the articular cortex, and the neck of the mandibular condyle (Fig. 84–16*B*). The entire condylar head is uniformly corticated, and well-developed trabeculae are usually seen. Again, the joint space should be of uniform thickness. In the open position, the joint space widens considerably and the posterior aspect of the glenoid fossa is uncovered (Fig. 84–16*C*).

DISORDERS

In recent years, there has been renewed interest in temporomandibular joint disorders.[19, 20, 30, 31, 53, 55] Combined clinical and radiologic investigations[10, 47] have expanded basic knowledge and shown that a simple division of TMJ complaints into organic and functional is not sufficient. Where one ends and the other begins cannot be defined. More likely, both functional and organic elements are active simultaneously. Alderman's differentiation of TMJ disorders into intracapsular and extracapsular[2] is a useful framework for discussion and further investigation (Table 84–1). Importantly, symptoms of pain, joint noise, and limitation of motion are common to both categories. Radiographic studies are often part of the evaluation regardless of the presumptive diagnosis.

Table 84–1

ALDERMAN'S CLASSIFICATION OF TMJ DISORDERS

EXTRACAPSULAR DISORDERS

1. Psychophysiologic: Tension, anxiety, oral habits
2. Iatrogenic: Misdirected mandibular nerve block, excessive depression of the mandible during anesthesia or oral procedures
3. Traumatic: Blow to the face not involving fractures
4. Dental: Occlusal abnormalities; periapical or periodontal lesions; mobile, sensitive or damaged teeth; ulcerations
5. Infectious: Secondary, outside the joint
6. Otologic: Otitis media or external ear infection
7. Neoplastic: Parotid gland, nasopharyngeal tumor, etc.

INTRACAPSULAR DISORDERS

1. Congenital: Agenesis, hyperplastic or hypoplastic condyle
2. Infectious: Primary bacterial infection within the joint
3. Arthritic: Rheumatoid arthritis, osteoarthritis, psoriatic arthritis, juvenile chronic arthritis
4. Traumatic: Fractures, disc tears
5. Functional: Subluxation, dislocation, disc derangement, hypermobility, ankylosis
6. Neoplastic: Benign or malignant tumors

Extracapsular Disorders

These are probably the most common group seen by clinicians and are often diagnosed as a myofascial pain–dysfunction syndrome (MPDS).[2, 17, 25] The patients usually complain of some combination of neck and masticatory muscle pain, headache, joint noise, tinnitus, malocclusion, deviation of the mandible, loss of motion, and stress or anxiety. Many pathophysiologic theories are currently extant, with proponents at one end of the spectrum supporting psychosomatic mechanisms and others, at the opposite end, supporting organic causes. Similarly, therapeutic interventions are not standardized. Whatever the cause, conventional or magnification TMJ radiographs should be normal among the extracapsular disorders. If structural changes are identified, an organic diagnosis must be considered.

Intracapsular Disorders

Intracapsular disorders, although presenting with similar symptoms, are commonly accompanied by radiologic changes. These findings are often sufficiently characteristic to allow formation of a radiologic diagnosis. The following discussion considers these entities in an order roughly proportional to their frequency in our practice. Meniscal derangements are described in the arthrography section.

ARTHRITIDES. Osteoarthritis (degenerative joint disease) of the TMJ[22, 41] is similar to osteoarthritis of other joints in its radiologic appearance. It is more common in older persons, a fact that suggests that osteoarthritis is often a primary disease of aging. However, similar clinical and radiologic patterns are found in younger persons following various insults. Perhaps, at all ages, osteoarthritis results from an imbalance between the natural integrity of the joint and the forces applied across it. With aging, cartilage is no longer able to withstand normal forces, and primary osteoarthritis develops. In other patients, normal cartilage cannot withstand abnormal forces, and secondary osteoarthritis develops. In MPDS, secondary osteoarthritis seems to develop as a result of unnatural forces across the TMJ. Current therapies are devoted to relief of symptoms, restoration of

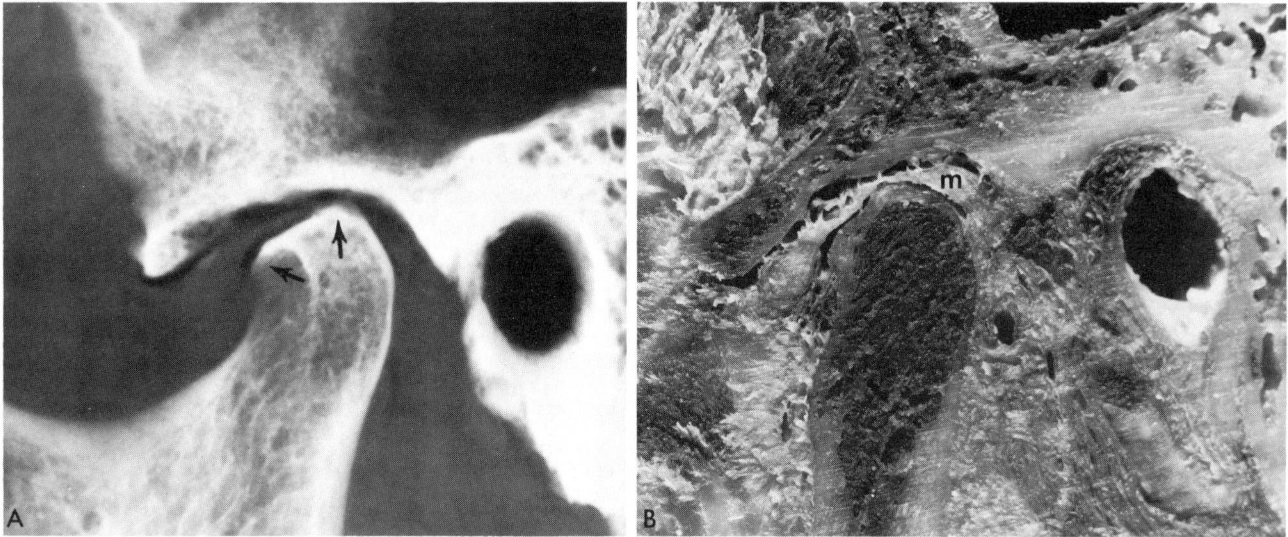

Figure 84–17. Osteoarthritis compared in a radiograph **(A)** and photograph **(B)** of a sagittally sectioned specimen. The joint space is narrow and the meniscus (m) is thin and frayed. The condylar head cortex is thickened, with small spurs (arrows). The mandibular fossa is sclerotic and reshaped, with a resultant shallow concavity where the articular eminence once was.

balance across the TMJ and prevention of osteoarthritis.

Radiologic findings in osteoarthritis are variations of cartilage loss and bone production (Fig. 84–17). Cartilage loss may be the predominant finding (Fig. 84–18), or it may be associated with a wide range of spur formation and structural joint changes. Early spur formation usually begins at the margins of the condylar head (Figs. 84–19 and 84–20). When the spurs become large, the new condylar head shape causes re-formation of the mandibular fossa (Fig. 84–21). A variable amount of sclerosis may accompany cartilage loss and spur formation (Fig. 84–22). Even with advanced osteoarthritic changes, considerable joint motion is retained (Fig. 84–23), and fibrous or bony ankylosis rarely occurs.

Rheumatoid arthritis (RA)[11, 30, 35] and its related arthropathies, juvenile chronic arthritis,[38] psoriatic arthritis,[7, 26] ankylosing spondylitis,[18, 37] and so forth, may all affect the TMJ. In fact, these patients may have their first arthritic complaint isolated to the TMJ, and may first present to a dentist.

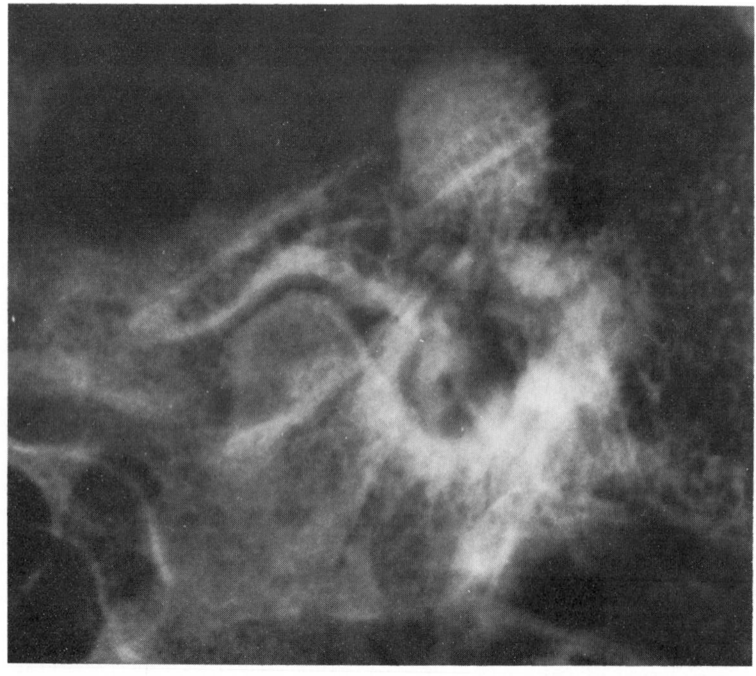

Figure 84–18. Osteoarthritis in a 70 year old woman, in whom the predominant findings are joint space narrowing, indicative of cartilage loss, and mild cortical thickening, indicative of reinforcement of the subchondral bone.

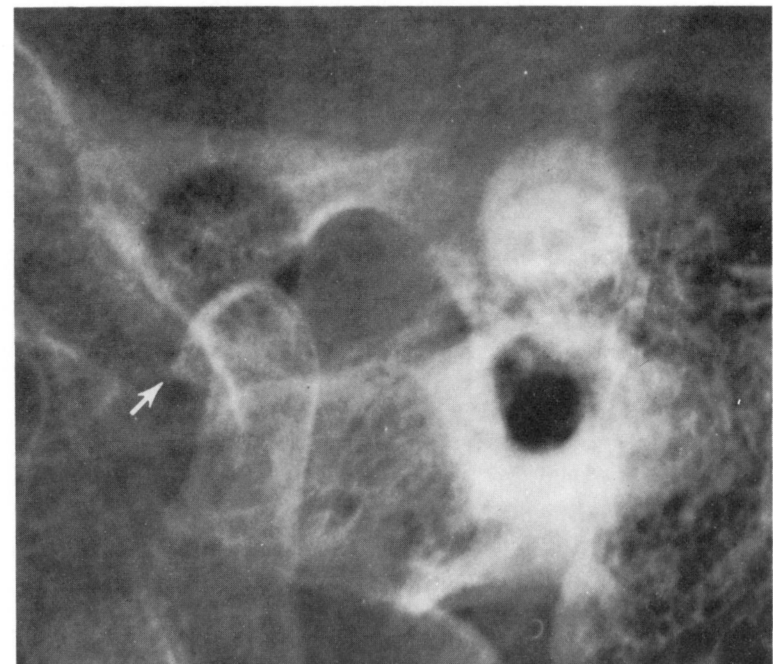

Figure 84–19. *Osteoarthritis in a 64 year old woman. With the TMJ in the open position, a single small spur (arrow) is shown at the anterior margin of the condylar head.*

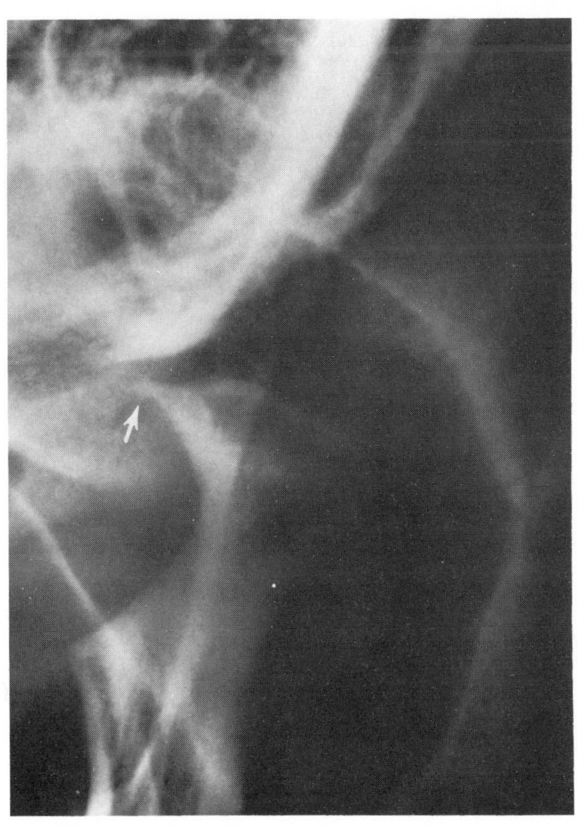

Figure 84–20. *Osteoarthritis in a 22 year old woman. Small spur (arrow) on the medial pole of the condylar head was obvious only on the Towne projection.*

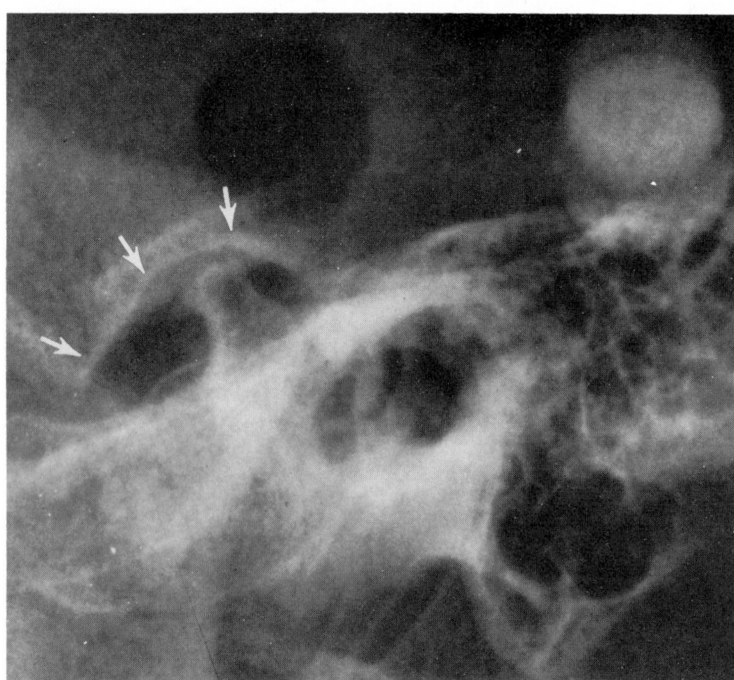

Figure 84–21. Osteoarthritis in a 72 year old woman is manifested as a huge spur arising from the anterosuperior aspect of the condylar head, with resultant erosion and reformation of the mandibular fossa (arrows).

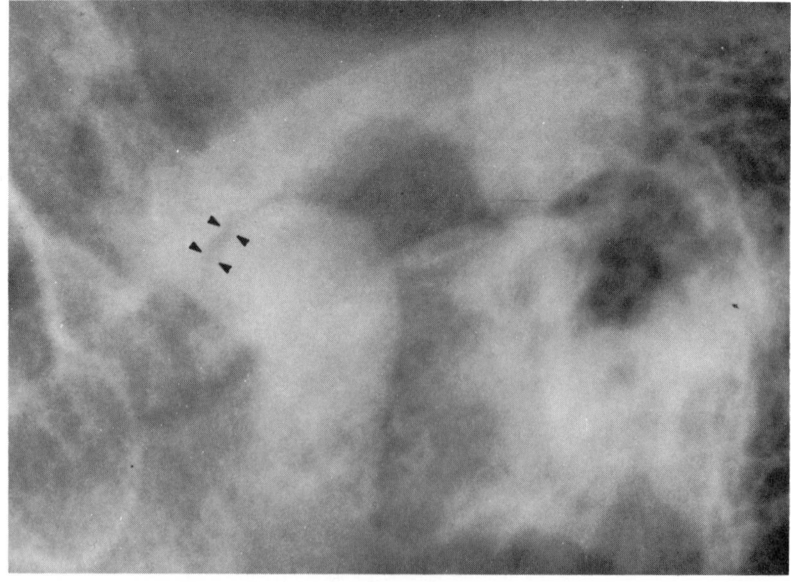

Figure 84–22. Osteoarthritis in a 55 year old woman imaged in the open position is associated with diffuse osteosclerosis of condylar head and mandibular fossa. The fact that the head abuts the articular eminence (arrowheads) indicates that the meniscus is absent.

Because the rheumatoid arthropathies share similar pathophysiologic mechanisms, they may be indistinguishable both clinically and radiologically, especially if the TMJ is the only joint involved. These inflammatory or granulomatous arthritides have an inflammatory response as their common pathway. All have some degree of immune reaction, periarticular hyperemia, and pannus formation. Similarly, all may show a spectrum of radiologic change, including demineralization, joint space narrowing, and bone erosion or production. Function may be impaired.

Demineralization is often difficult to document (Fig. 84–24) until it is advanced (Fig. 84–25). However, bone erosions are much easier to document. They may be diffuse (Fig. 84–25) or focal (Fig. 84–26). Furthermore, they may become apparent only on analysis of projections other than the standard lateral views. The reason for this is that the synovial reflections of the two joint compartments are extensive and wrap around the condylar head. Synovial proliferation and pannus formation often begin in these recesses, and the earliest bone erosions may not be across articular cartilage but rather about the margins of bone not covered by cartilage. Accessory views such as the Towne projection are very important for early diagnosis of erosions (Fig. 84–27).

Arthropathies similar to rheumatoid arthritis may produce joint changes identical to those of RA at various stages in their natural histories, but especially when the joints are inflamed. However, most

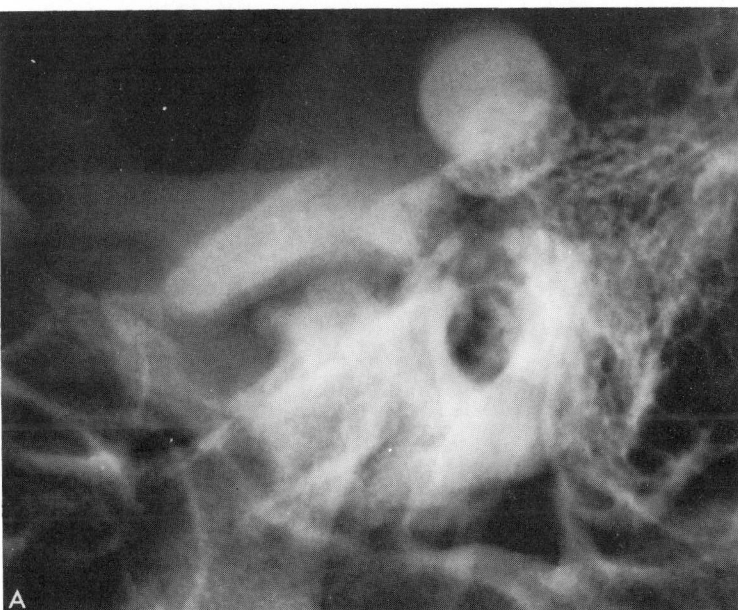

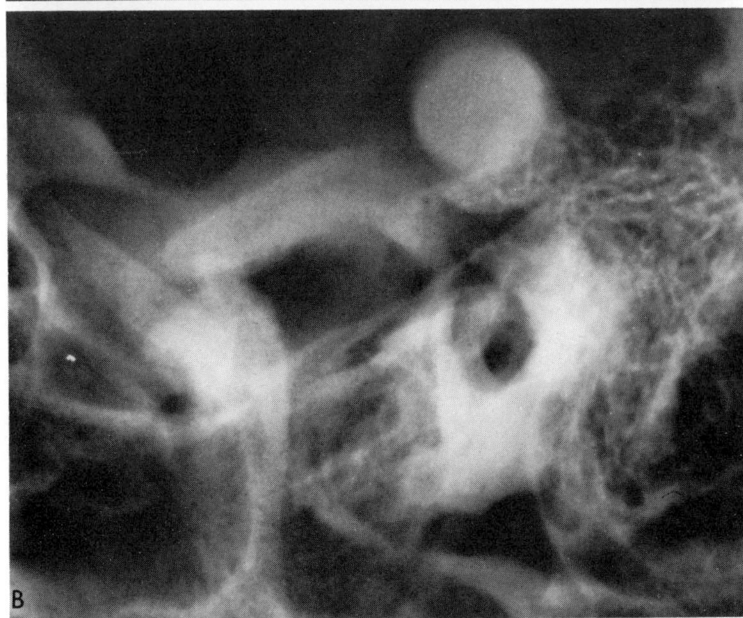

Figure 84–23. *Osteoarthritis in a 41 year old woman in both closed* **(A)** *and open* **(B)** *positions. Despite advanced joint space loss, large spur formation, remarkable re-formation of the mandibular fossa, and dense osteosclerosis, functional motion is relatively maintained.*

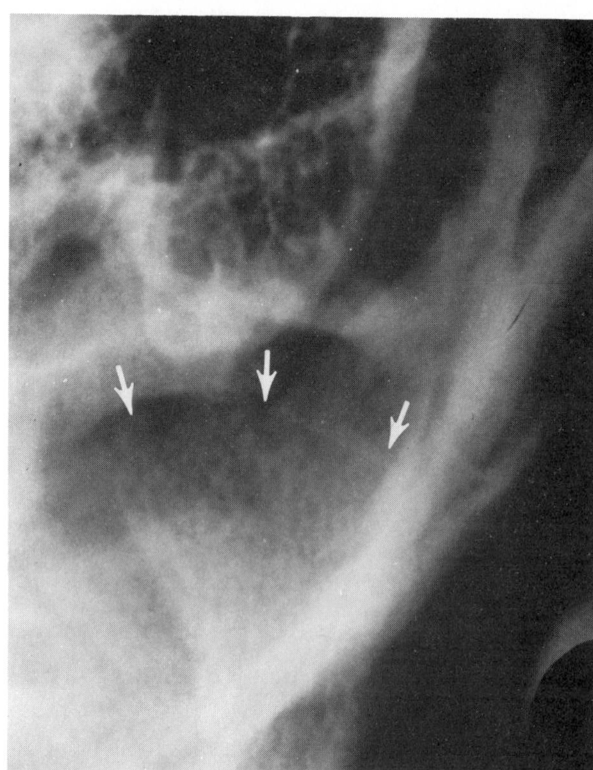

Figure 84–24. Seronegative rheumatoid arthritis in an 18 year old woman with recent onset of polyarticular inflammatory arthritis. Towne view shows demineralization of condylar head, with loss of distinct subchondral cortex (arrows).

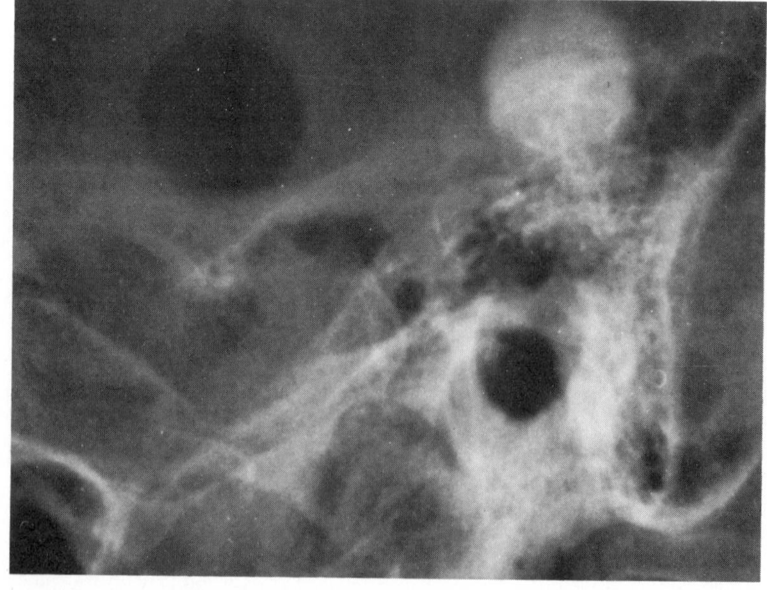

Figure 84–25. Seropositive rheumatoid arthritis in a 46 year old woman. The joint space is very narrow, periarticular demineralization is advanced, and bone erosions are large and diffuse.

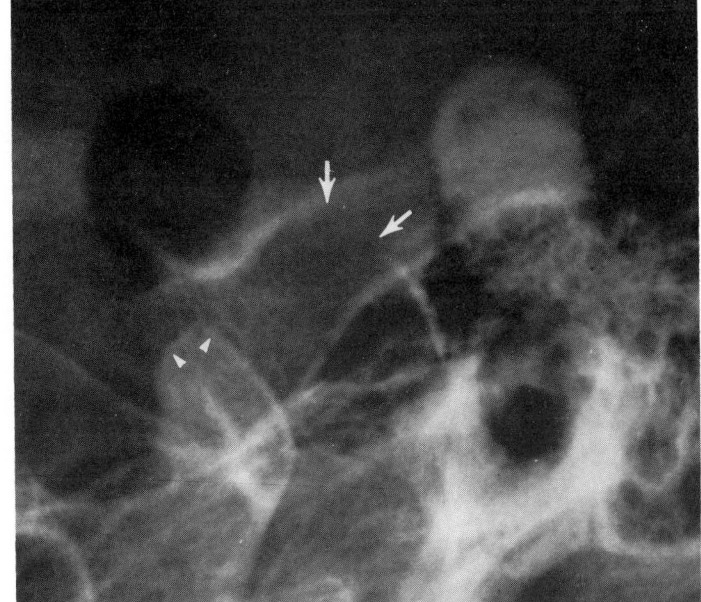

Figure 84–26. Seropositive rheumatoid arthritis in a 46 year old woman. The open view shows early bone changes, with subtle loss of condylar cortex (arrowheads) and focal erosion of the mandibular fossa (arrows). Note that the space between the head and eminence is maintained, indicating an intact meniscus.

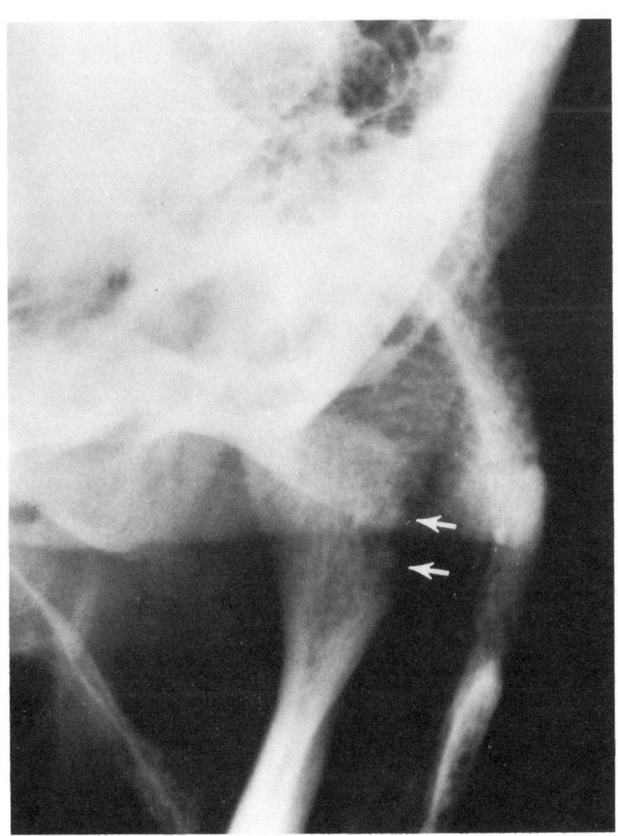

Figure 84–27. Seropositive rheumatoid arthritis in a 53 year old woman. Towne view showed the only erosion, located on the lateral pole of the condylar head (arrows).

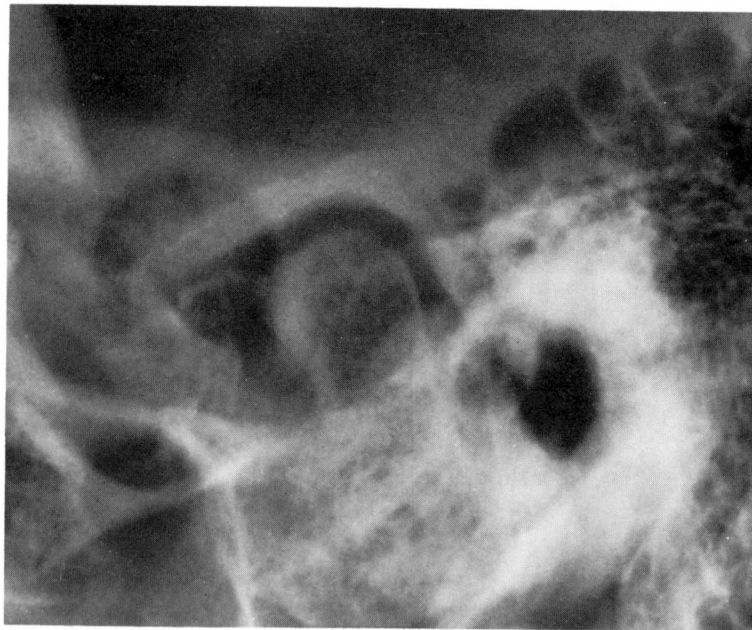

Figure 84–28. Juvenile chronic arthritis, now quiescent, in a 24 year old woman. Although symptomatic, the TMJ shows only mild narrowing of the joint space and slight osteosclerosis of the subchondral cortex.

of these related arthropathies are active intermittently, which permits bone formation during quiescent periods. Therefore, juvenile chronic arthritis (Fig. 84–28), psoriatic arthritis (Fig. 84–29), and ankylosing spondylitis may be expected to show some amount of bone formation. When they do, they may be more easily separated from RA, which seldom shows productive changes. History and clinical and laboratory studies are usually more important than radiologic findings for differentiation among these diseases.

Other arthritides may affect the TMJ, but very rarely in our experience. Apparently, in certain ethnic populations, attacks of gout may affect the TMJ.[14]

Trauma. Injury to the mandible or a direct blow to the temporomandibular joint is a common cause of TMJ pain and dysfunction.[31] The trauma may result in soft tissue injury, a fracture, or a combination of both. Whatever the trauma, detailed radiographs are necessary and must be carefully studied. The panoramic radiograph has been particularly useful, since it provides a survey of the entire mandible as well as a nearly lateral view of each condyle.

The vast majority of mandibular fractures involve the condyle and can be classified according to anato-

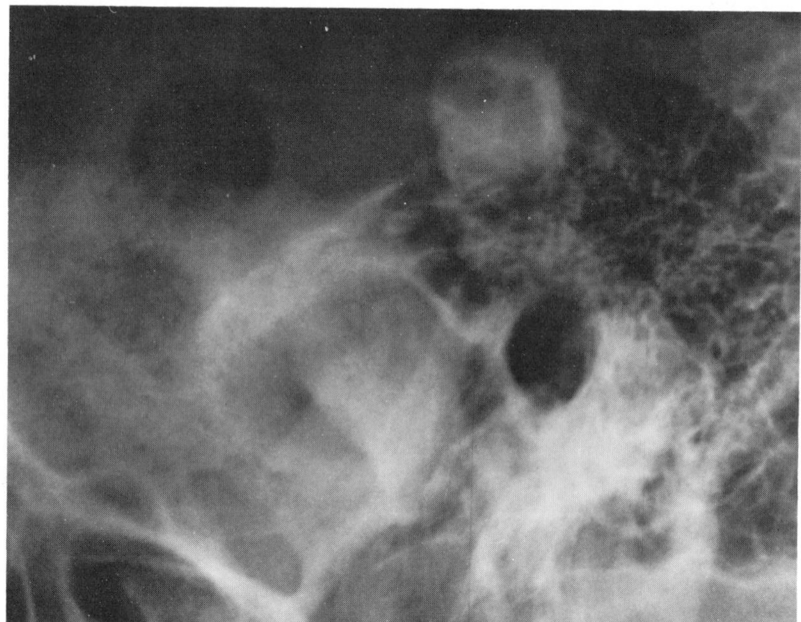

Figure 84–29. Psoriatic arthritis in a 40 year old woman had presented in this TMJ 14 years previously. More recently several joints in the hands became abnormal. The TMJ shows advanced cartilage loss and both bone erosion and production, involving the condylar head, mandibular fossa, and articular eminence.

Table 84–2
FRACTURES OF THE MANDIBULAR CONDYLE

I. Intracapsular Head Fracture
  A. Nondisplaced
  B. Displaced
II. Extracapsular Neck Fracture
  A. Nondisplaced
  B. Displaced—head located
  C. Displaced—head dislocated
III. Extracapsular Subcondylar Fracture
  A. Nondisplaced
  B. Displaced

my (Table 84–2). Those that directly affect the TMJ are intracapsular fractures of the condylar head (Fig. 84–30) and extracapsular fractures of the condylar neck. Each of these may be nondisplaced (Fig. 84–31) or displaced (Fig. 84–32). Fractures that are initially in anatomic position may heal with a malalignment that affects function. When this occurs, surgical intervention may be necessary (Fig. 84–33).

In our institution, a condylar head and neck replacement (Fig. 84–34) may be implanted in selected cases of fracture (Fig. 84–33) or in advanced arthritis with ankylosis (Fig. 84–35). The prosthesis usually relieves pain and improves function. However, joint mobility is generally restricted to hinge motion, with little, if any, translation of the condylar head across the articular eminence (Fig. 84–36).

Many other surgical interventions exist for a wide variety of indications.[1, 3, 12, 19, 21, 23, 29, 31] Each of these may result in a bone change visible radiographically. Among these are condylar shaving (Fig. 84–37), condylectomy (Fig. 84–38) and eminectomy (Fig. 84–39).

A final form of trauma follows local radiotherapy. Radiation vasculitis induces inflammatory reaction and scar formation, with resultant fibrous ankylosis (Fig. 84–40).

CONGENITAL DISORDERS. Congenital TMJ disturbances generally result from abnormalities of development in the first branchial arch. This may result in agenesis, hypoplasia, or hyperplasia of the mandible. The defects may be focal, diffuse, unilateral, or bilateral. Agenesis is rare, and because of multiple anomalies, affected individuals usually do not survive. Mandibular hypoplasia[6, 8, 16] is often associated with other craniofacial deformities. Because of the relationship with Meckel's cartilage, middle ear anomalies are particularly common. The degree of microsomia is quite variable. Similarly, there is a spectrum of mandibular hyperplasia.[45] Radiologic findings include condylar head enlargement, elongation of the condylar neck, flattening of the mandibular fossa, and enlargement of the mandible (Fig. 84–41).

Many other congenital or developmental diseases may affect the mandible and temporomandibular joints. They may cause functional (Fig. 84–42) or arthritic (Fig. 84–43) disturbances. Far too many congenital, developmental, or dysplastic diseases with variants of TMJ afflictions exist for discussion here.

TUMORS. Fortunately, tumors are rarely found in the temporomandibular joints.[34] However, most bone or joint tumors have been described in this joint and may be encountered by clinicians and radiologists. Of the malignant bone tumors, osteosarcoma (Fig. 84–44) and metastases from other sites (Fig. 84–45) are more common. Benign bone tumors, including exostoses, osteomas, and giant cell tumors,

Text continued on page 3087

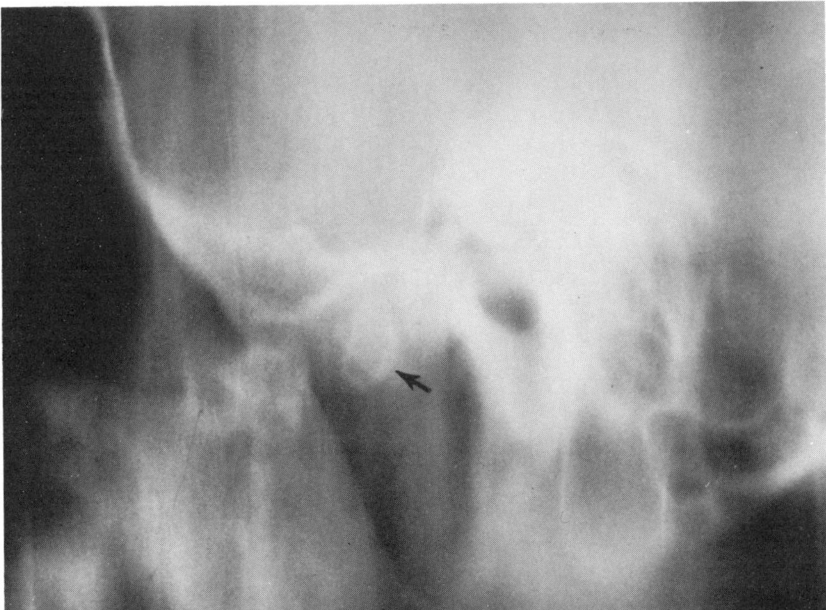

Figure 84–30. *Intracapsular condylar head fracture with fragmentation and displacement shown by linear tomography. The main condylar head fragment (arrow) remains in the mandibular fossa.*

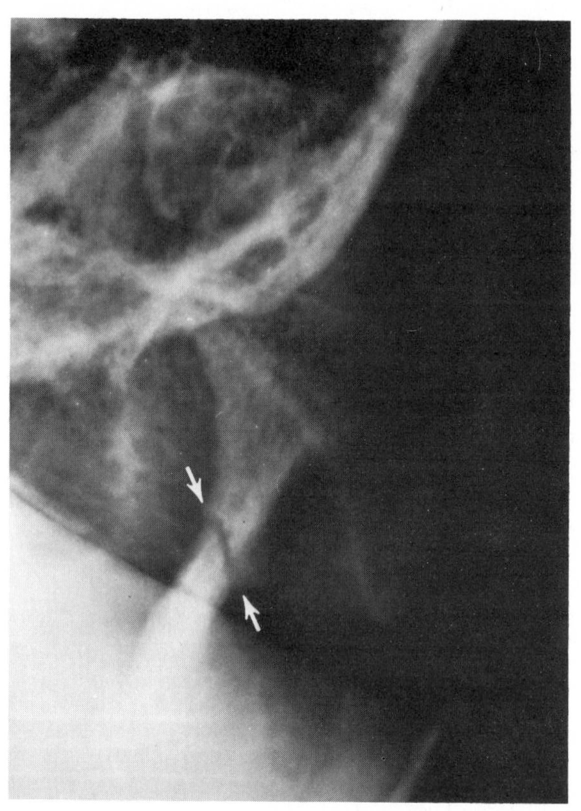

Figure 84–31. Extracapsular nondisplaced condylar neck fracture (arrows) with early callus formation was shown only on this magnification Towne image.

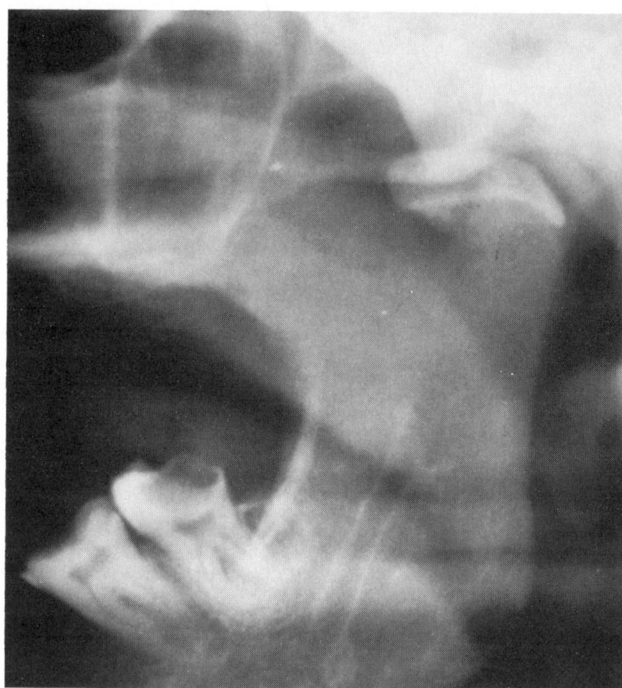

Figure 84–32. Extracapsular condylar neck fracture with dislocation of the condylar head as shown on a panoramic radiograph.

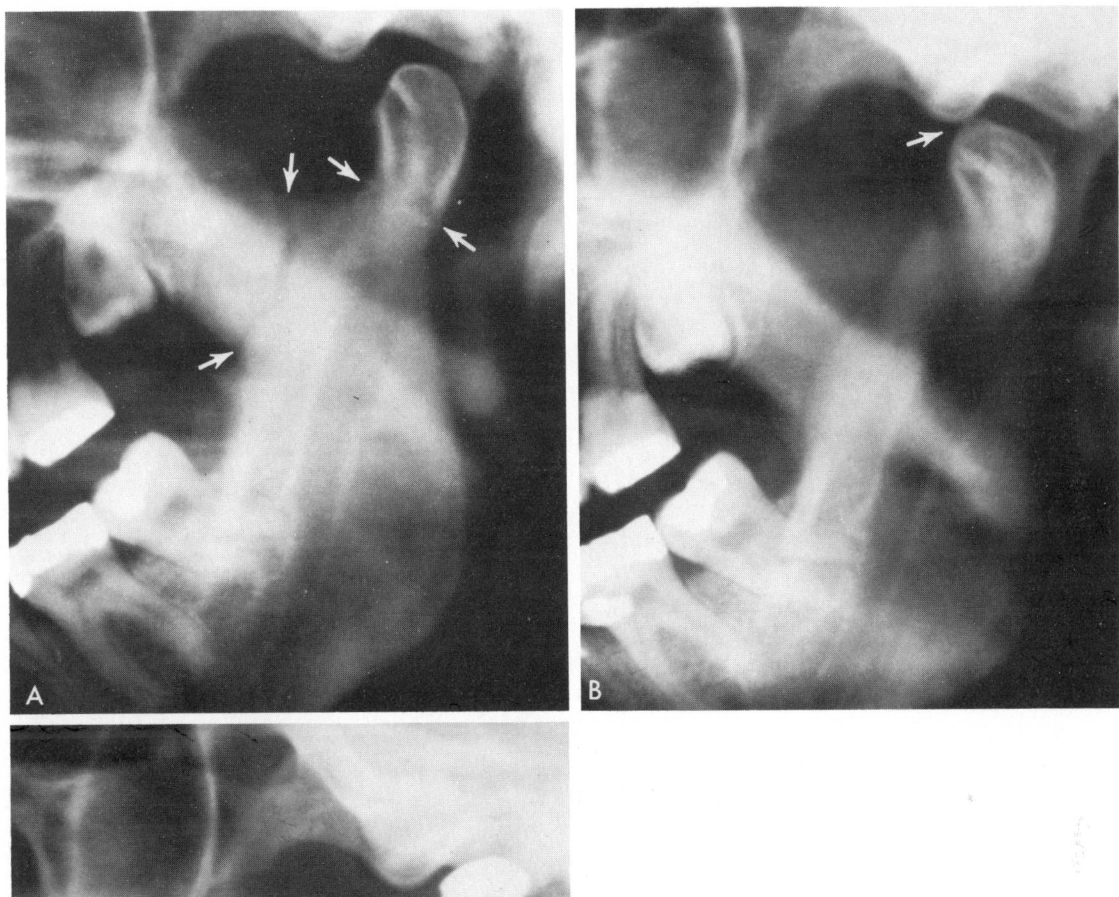

Figure 84–33. Fracture with malalignment. Panoramic radiographs from a 34 year old man with extracapsular fractures **(A)** of the condylar neck and coronoid process (arrows), which healed with the condylar head dislocated and juxtaposed to the articular eminence (arrow) **(B)**. Because of persistent pain and loss of joint function, a condylar head and neck prosthesis was implanted **(C)**. Note that the prosthetic head is well seated in the mandibular fossa and that occlusion is restored.

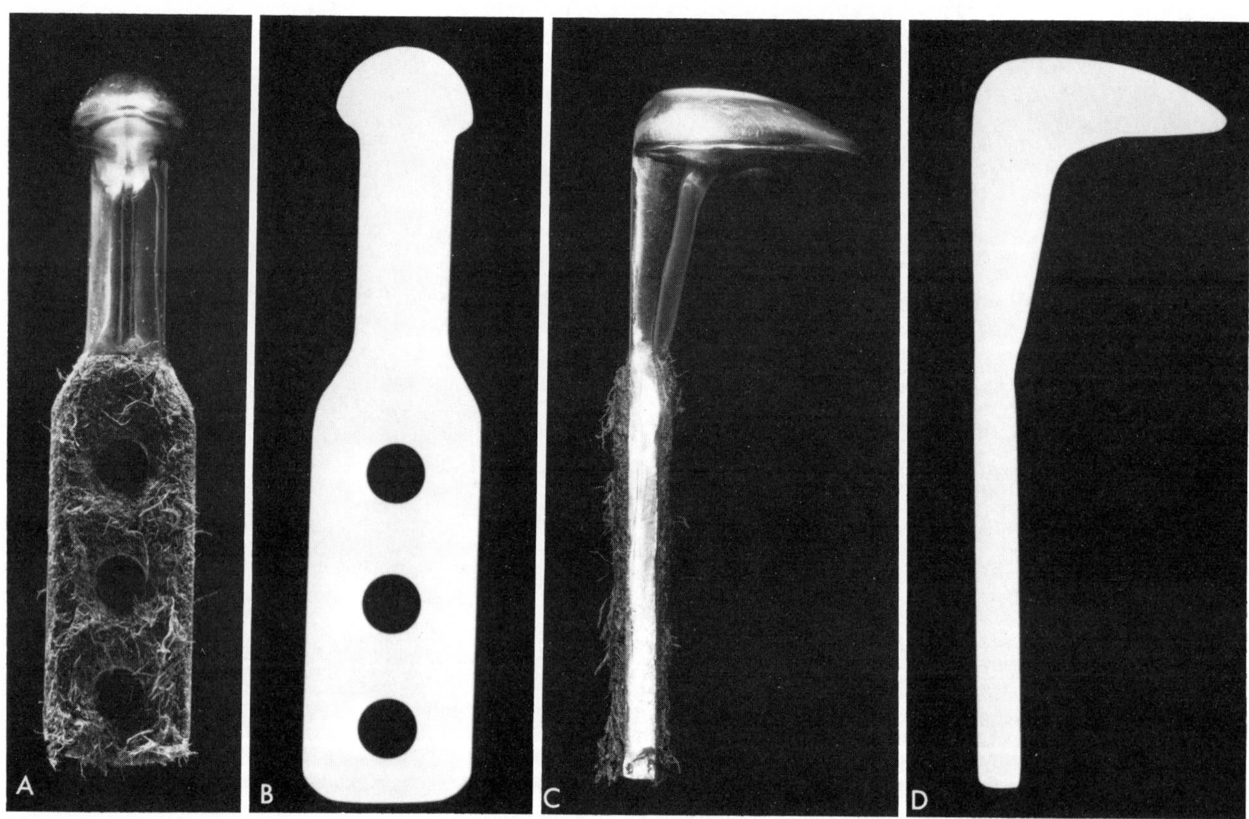

Figure 84–34. *The prosthetic condylar head and neck (Proplast) currently used at our institution are shown in frontal and lateral photographs* **(A, C)** *and radiographs* **(B, D)**. *This prosthesis is manufactured by Dow-Corning Corporation, Midland, Michigan.*

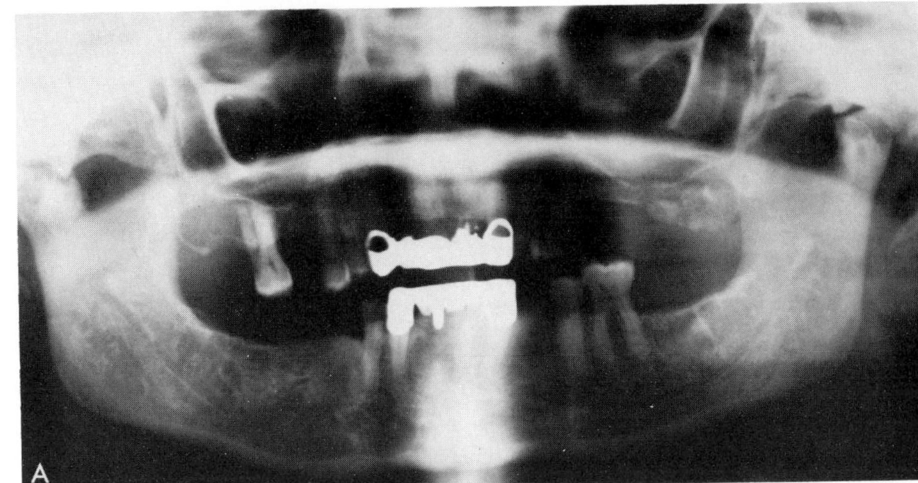

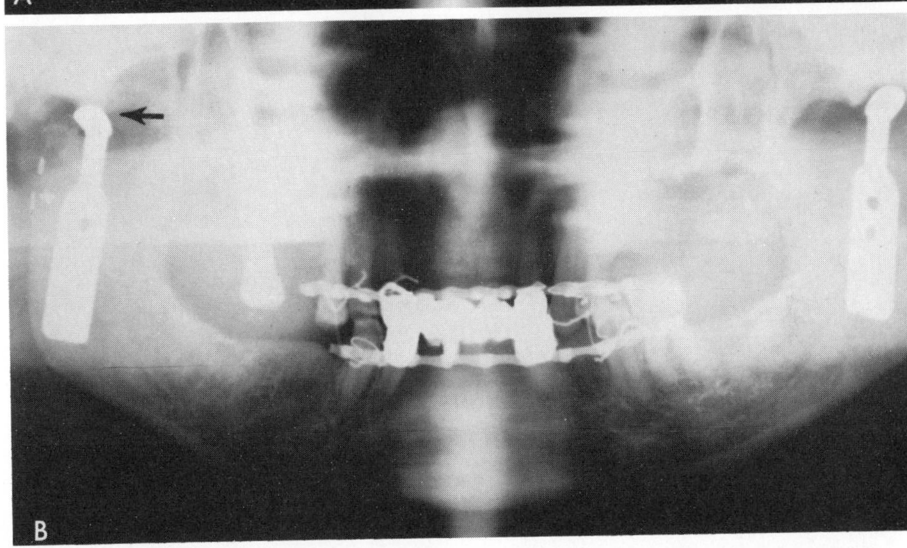

Figure 84–35. *Osteoarthritis requiring surgical intervention. Panoramic radiographs show a 50 year old woman with severe bilateral TMJ osteoarthritis* **(A)**, *which was very painful and which limited motion* **(B)**. *A bilateral prosthesis implantation was performed; the dislocated right prosthesis (arrow) was later reimplanted.*

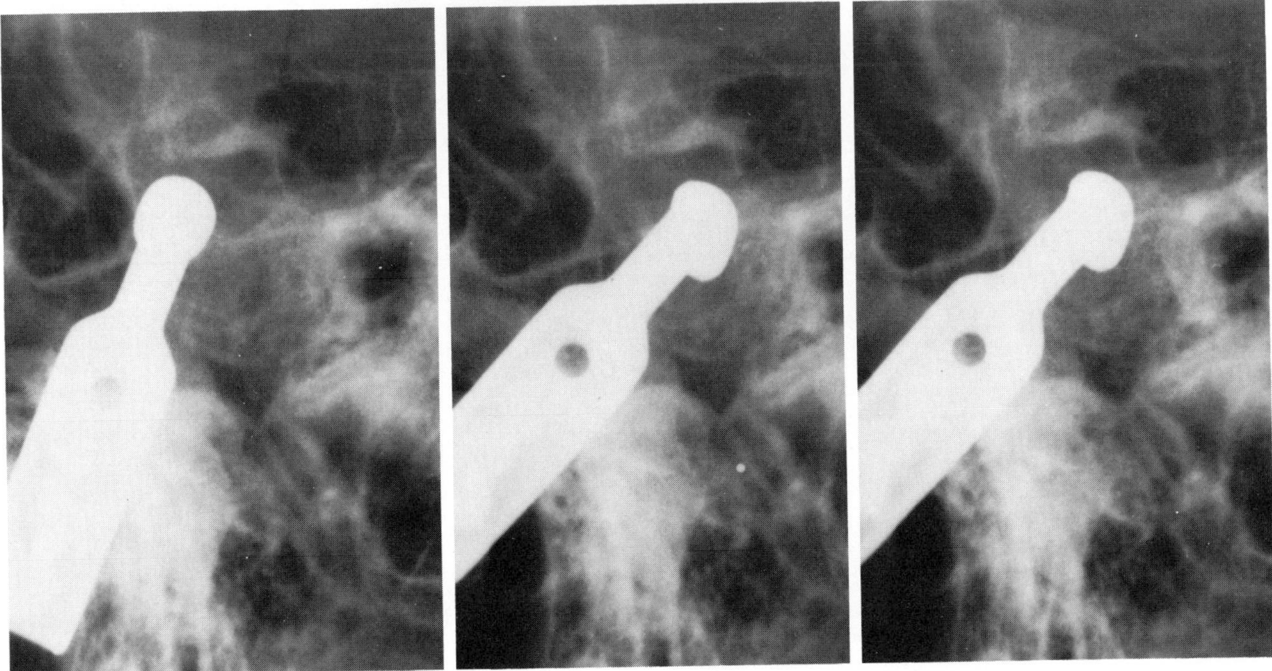

Figure 84–36. *Joint motion following prosthetic replacement. A series of Updegrave lateral images shows that between full open (left), resting (middle), and closed (right) positions, this patient is able to attain a moderate translatory motion. In fact, this individual demonstrates an unusually good excursion of the prosthetic head across the articular eminence.*

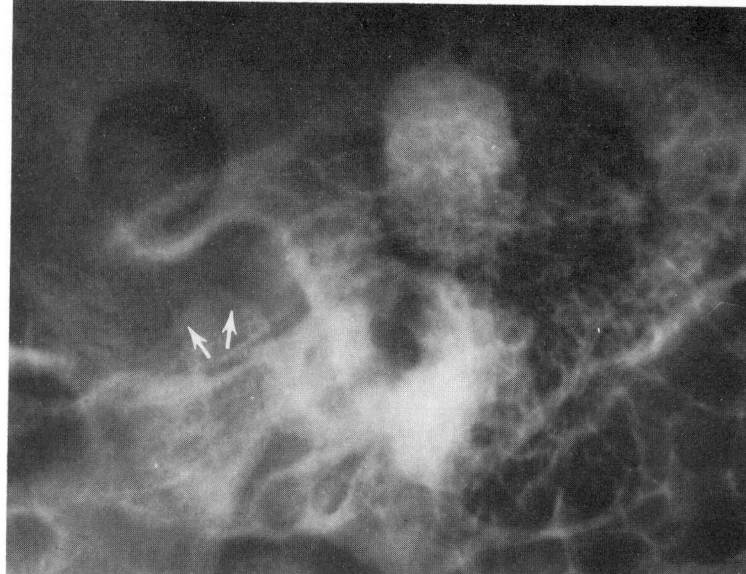

Figure 84–37. Surgical condylar shaving is manifested as loss of the articular cortex (arrows).

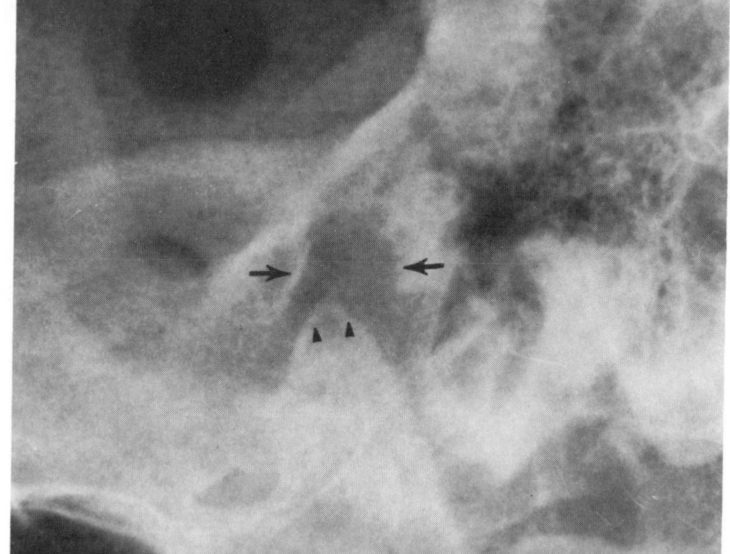

Figure 84–38. Surgical condylectomy is manifested as an absent condylar head (arrowheads) and an empty mandibular fossa (arrows).

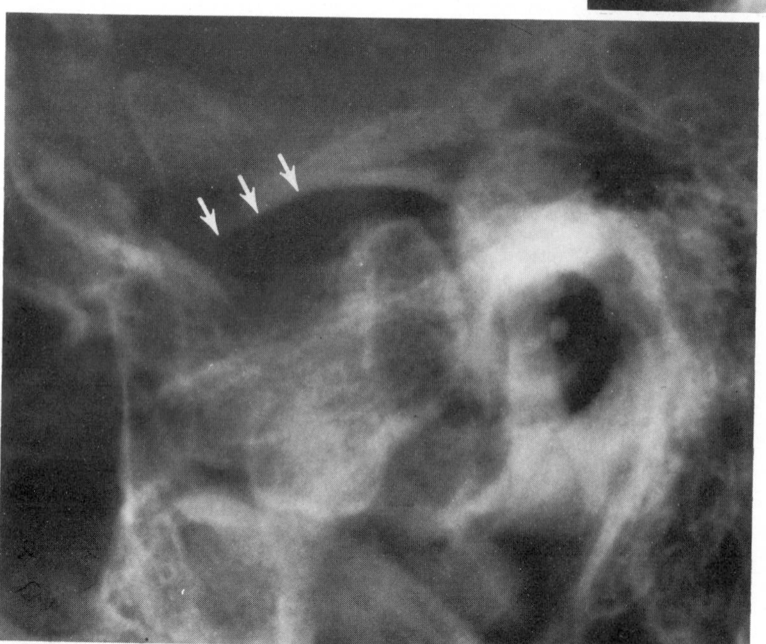

Figure 84–39. Surgical eminectomy is manifested as absence of the articular eminence and flattening of the mandibular fossa (arrows).

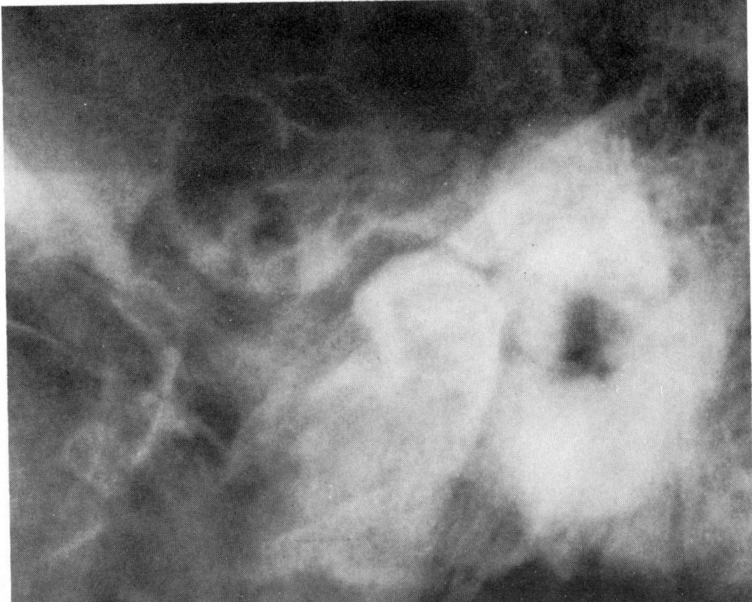

Figure 84–40. *Radiation injury. Following 7000 rads of radiotherapy delivered in two courses several years apart for a salivary gland tumor, cartilage atrophy, osteosclerosis, and fibrous ankylosis developed.*

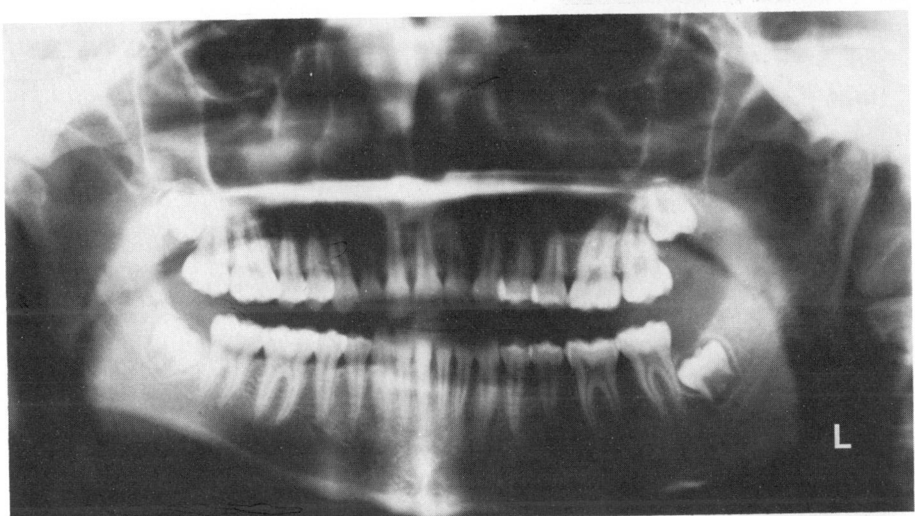

Figure 84–41. *Mandibular hyperplasia. Panoramic image in this 16 year old girl shows left hemifacial mandibular hypertrophy manifested by enlargement of the condylar head, elongation of the condylar neck, and hypertrophy of the hemimandible.*

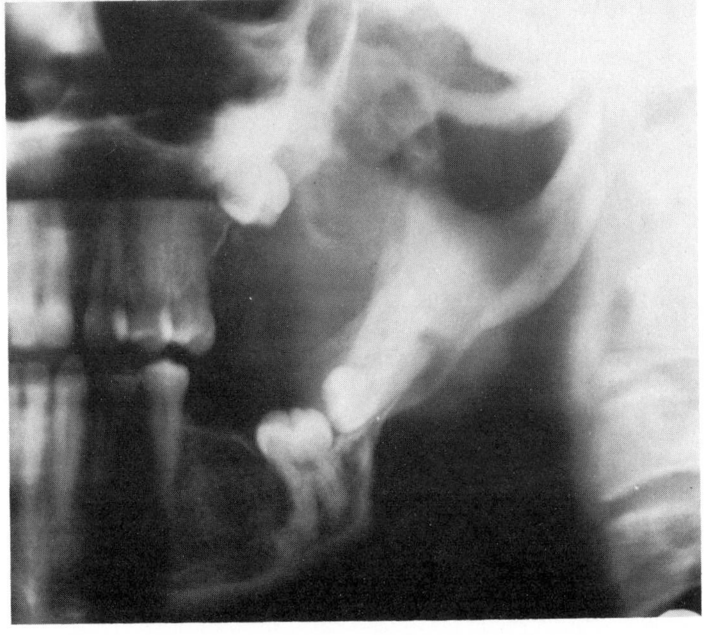

Figure 84–42. *Mandibular dysplasia from neurofibromatosis caused left TMJ pain and dysfunction for this 32 year old woman.*

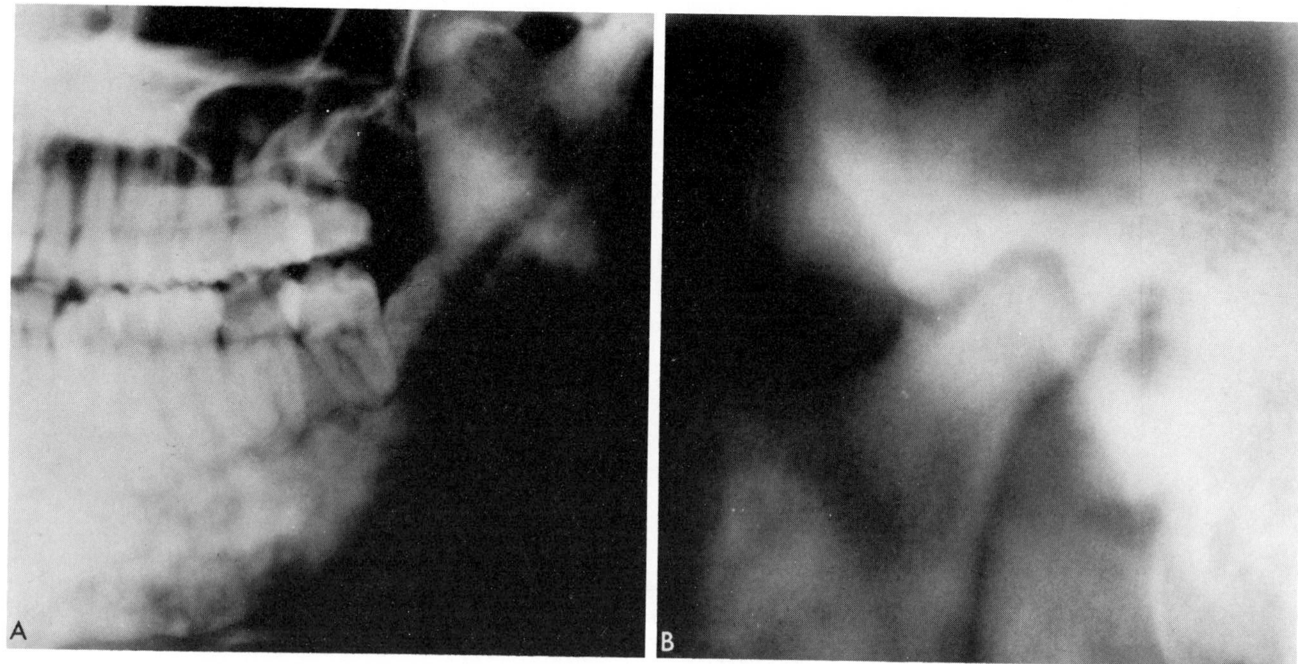

Figure 84–43. Fibrous dysplasia (**A**) enlarged the entire mandible including the condylar head (**B**), causing secondary osteoarthritis, pain, and dysfunction for this 25 year old man.

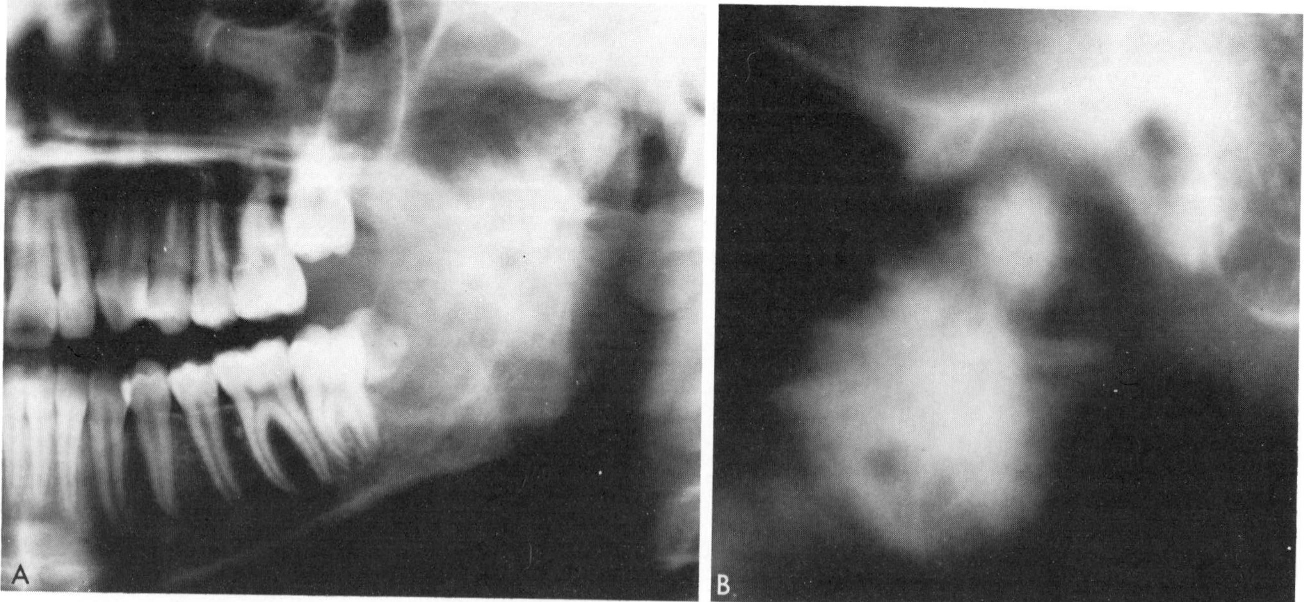

Figure 84–44. Osteosarcoma of the mandible (**A**) and the condylar head and neck (**B**) in a 12 year old girl.

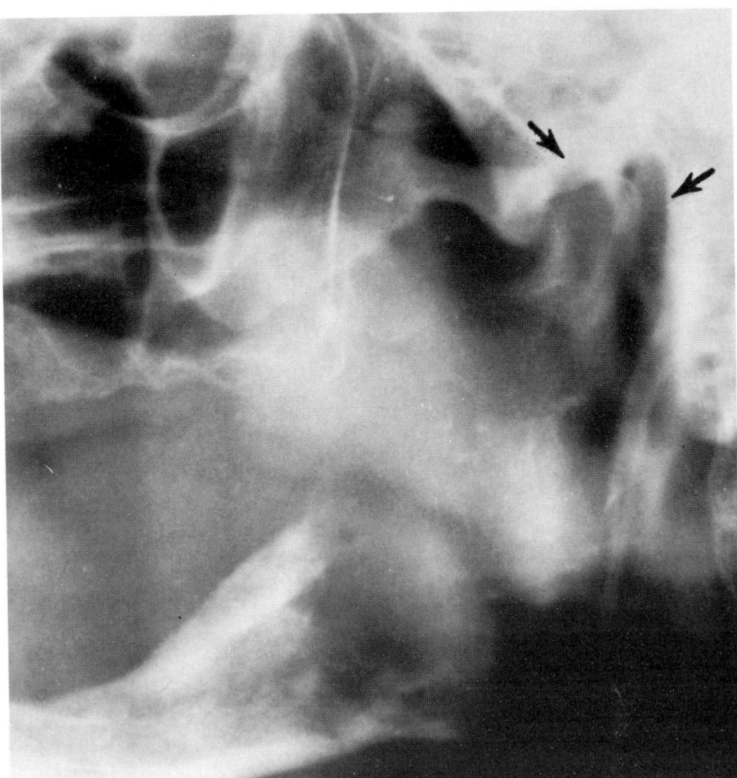

Figure 84–45. Metastatic lung carcinoma to ascending ramus of mandible leaves the condylar head floating freely (arrows) in the mandibular fossa.

have been described. Benign intra-articular soft tissue neoplasms such as osteochondromatosis are rare.

INFECTIONS. Pyogenic[13] or granulomatous infections are uncommon in our experience. They may develop as a result of hematogenous seeding from a distant infection. More commonly, they develop as a direct extension of other oral infections or following TMJ surgery. The radiologic findings are similar to those of rheumatoid arthritis, but the clinical course is much more rapid. History and physical examination should suggest the diagnosis. Radiography may document both treatment success and various complications of infection.

ARTHROGRAPHY

Thus far, only diseases with abnormal bony anatomy have been considered. However, there remains a large group of symptomatic patients in whom standard studies yield normal results. These individuals have been given the general diagnosis of myofascial pain–dysfunction syndrome,[2, 25] previously called TMJ pain–dysfunction syndrome[30] or Costen's syndrome.[17] The majority of these patients are young women with regional pain, headaches, joint noises, and intermittent limitation of mandibular motion.

The justification for TMJ arthrography in this group of patients is to document an abnormality of meniscal anatomy or function and, on the basis of these findings, to design a conservative or surgical therapeutic plan that will correct the abnormality. Based on the premise that meniscal dysfunction leads to structural abnormality, the long-range goal is to prevent the development of osteoarthritis.

Technique

Currently, there is no universally accepted method for TMJ arthrography.[10, 24, 33, 42, 48, 52, 54, 56-58] The method we use combines fluoroscopy and microfocus magnification radiography.

A cotton ball is placed in the external auditory canal to prevent fluids from reaching the tympanic membrane; hair is retracted from the preauricular region to avoid continuous contamination. With the patient lying on either side, the head can be positioned so that the TMJ of interest is exposed. Since the opposite side of the head rests against the table top and the cervical spine is laterally flexed, the TMJ to be studied is fluoroscopically projected free of other bone structures, which might cause obscuration. In fact, the fluoroscopic appearance is identical to that of the transcranial lateral image.

Following sterile preparation, the preauricular region is anesthetized locally and a 23 gauge disposable needle is inserted into the inferior joint space. The needle is positioned with fluoroscopic control so that its tip touches the mandible posteriorly at the junction of the head and neck. It is easier to attain this position if the mouth is slightly open. If correctly placed, the needle tip will move precisely with the mandible as the mouth is opened and closed.

With another needle and syringe, the hub of the percutaneous needle is evacuated of residual local anesthetic or blood and then filled with contrast medium (Renografin-76 with 1 ml. of 1:1000 epinephrine per 10 ml of contrast medium), taking care to provide a bubble-free system. If the needle is positioned correctly, the first drop of contrast medium will flow into the joint without resistance and will immediately outline the inferior joint space. Following fluoroscopic confirmation of intra-articular position, contrast medium is injected until the patient experiences a sense of fullness. No more than 1 ml of contrast medium is necessary.

Although the inferior joint space is more difficult to cannulate, it is necessary to study this space first because the superior space is much larger and, when filled with contrast, obscures the inferior space. Second, if the superior space fills when the inferior space is injected, a diagnosis of meniscal tear can be made. Third, it is important to visualize the relationship between the condylar head and the meniscus, which can only be accomplished from the inferior space. Finally, if indicated, the superior

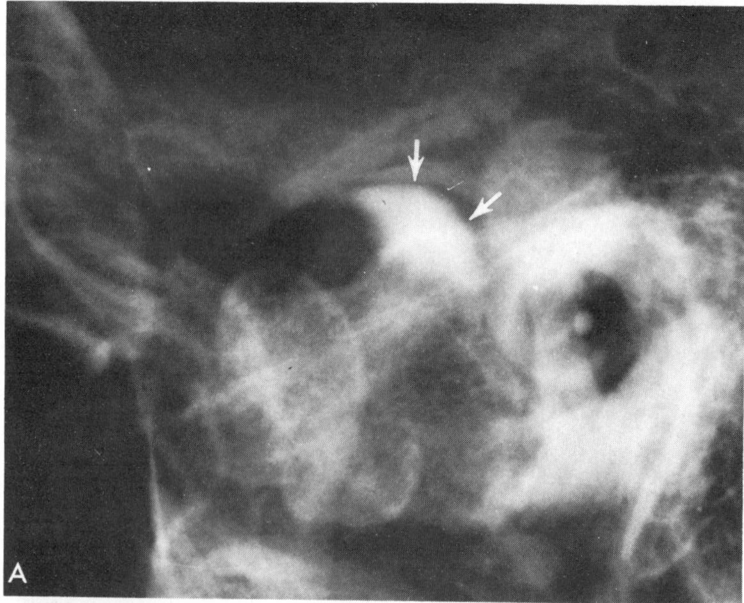

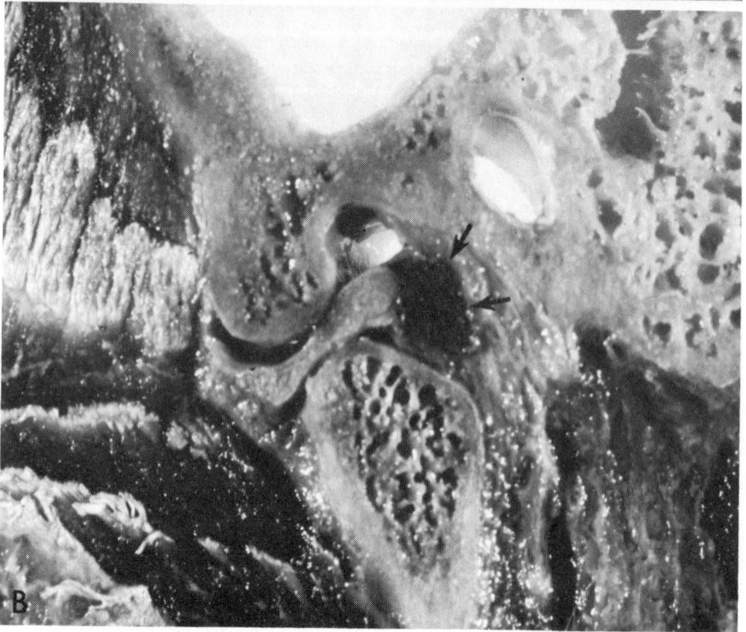

Figure 84–46. *Technical difficulties with TMJ arthrography.*

A *Extravasated contrast medium (arrows) does not conform to one of the joint spaces and stays distant from the condylar head in the open mouth position.*

B *Specimen shows extravasated latex (arrows) located in the posterior attachment of the meniscus.*

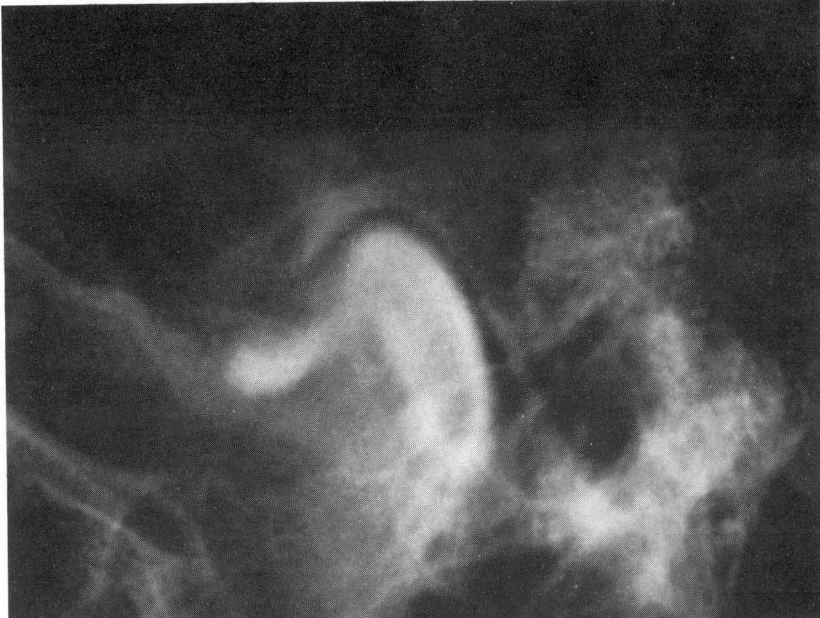

Figure 84–47. *Technical difficulties with TMJ arthrography. As shown in this inferior space arthrogram taken less than 10 minutes after injection, positive contrast agents resorb or dilute rapidly, with resultant unsharpness.*

space can be studied immediately following study of the inferior space.

Prior to obtaining any permanent films, it is of utmost importance to evaluate joint motion fluoroscopically and to direct particular attention to meniscal function. If the patient has complained of noise or limited motion, the symptoms should be reproduced as nearly as possible and studied. Unfortunately, it is not always possible to document functional abnormalities by film techniques, unless videotape or 105 mm rapid-sequence spot films are available. Conventional transcranial lateral films should be obtained in two to four mandibular positions from mouth closed to fully open. Open and closed Towne projections are also useful. Conventional transcranial lateral views may be tailored to include a film or films in the symptomatic position.

There are three common technical difficulties. First, malposition of the needle leads to extravasation of contrast medium beyond the articular space (Fig. 84–46*A*). This is commonly into the posterior attachment of the meniscus (Fig. 84–46*B*), which is very vascular and well innervated. Second, nearly every patient has some degree of pain on TMJ arthrography, which varies from minimal to severe. Immediate pain can be caused by contrast extravasation, overdistention of the joint space, or idiosyncratic sensitivity to the contrast agent. Most patients experience a delayed, mild aching that lasts 24 to 48 hours. Finally, the positive contrast agent, even with epinephrine added, diffuses rapidly into the very vascular periarticular tissues, with resultant image unsharpness (Fig. 84–47). Carefully performed studies, filmed with dispatch, will result in uniformly good TMJ arthrograms and minimal patient discomfort.

Normal Anatomy

The TMJ is divided into two diarthrodial spaces by a fibrocartilaginous meniscus or disc (Fig. 84–48*A*). The condylar head and mandibular fossa of the temporal bone are devoid of the hyaline cartilage usually found in synovial joints, but instead are covered by fibrocartilaginous articular cartilage. The oval meniscal plate is thick peripherally, thin and avascular centrally, and attached to both bone and joint capsule. Anteriorly and posteriorly the meniscus flares and attaches to the capsule as the capsule inserts at articular cartilage margins. Medially and laterally, the meniscus attaches to the condylar head (Fig. 84–48*B*). Although the meniscus is restrained by its attachments, it also accommodates specific movements. Its anterior and posterior attachments are particularly broad, permitting a redundancy that forms sulci in both superior and inferior joint cavities. Without these sulci, joint and meniscal motion would be severely restricted.

The inferior joint space (Fig. 84–49*A*) forms a helmet over the condylar head, with the meniscus and its attachments establishing joint space limits. The superior articular space is like a second helmet covering the meniscus, inferior space, and condylar head. This space is larger than the inferior space and in lateral radiographs has a sigmoid shape (Fig. 84–49*B*).

A complex dynamic relationship exists among the condylar head, meniscus, and temporal articular

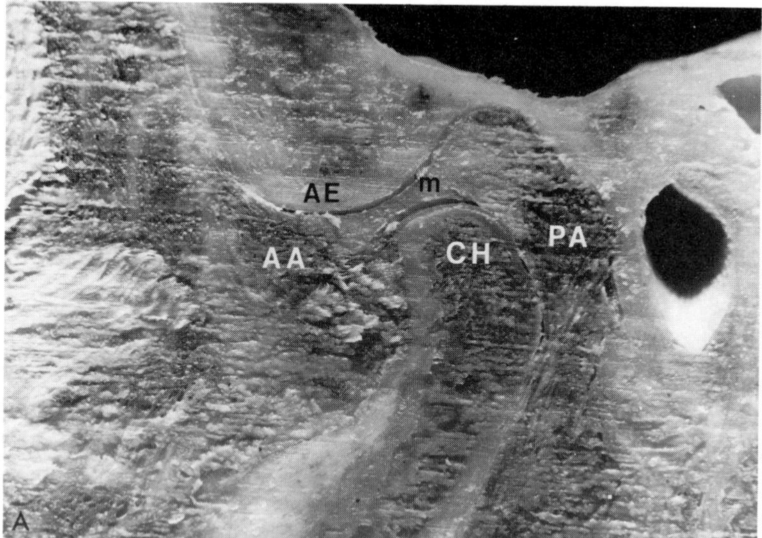

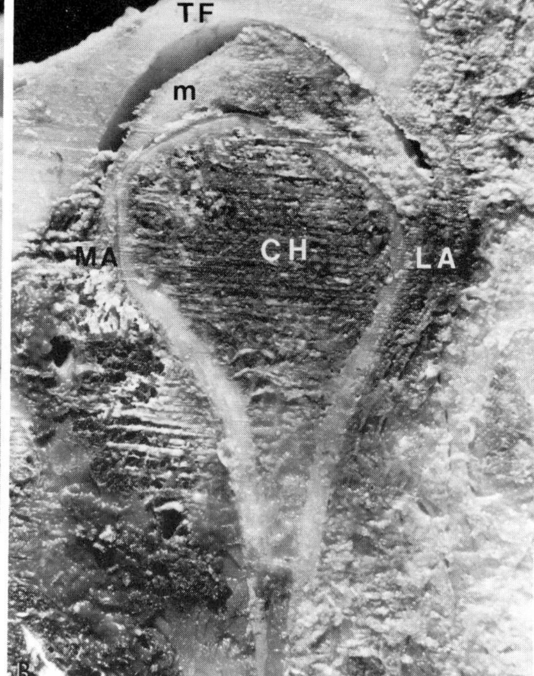

Figure 84–48. *Normal internal anatomy of the temporomandibular joint.*

A *Sagittal section shows meniscus (m) separating articular eminence (AE) from condylar head (CH). Anterior (AA) and posterior (PA) meniscal attachments are broadly based in the adjacent soft tissues.*

B *Coronal section shows meniscus (m) separating temporal fossa (TF) from condylar head (CH). Meniscal attachments to the condylar head are thin medially (MA) and thick laterally (LA).*

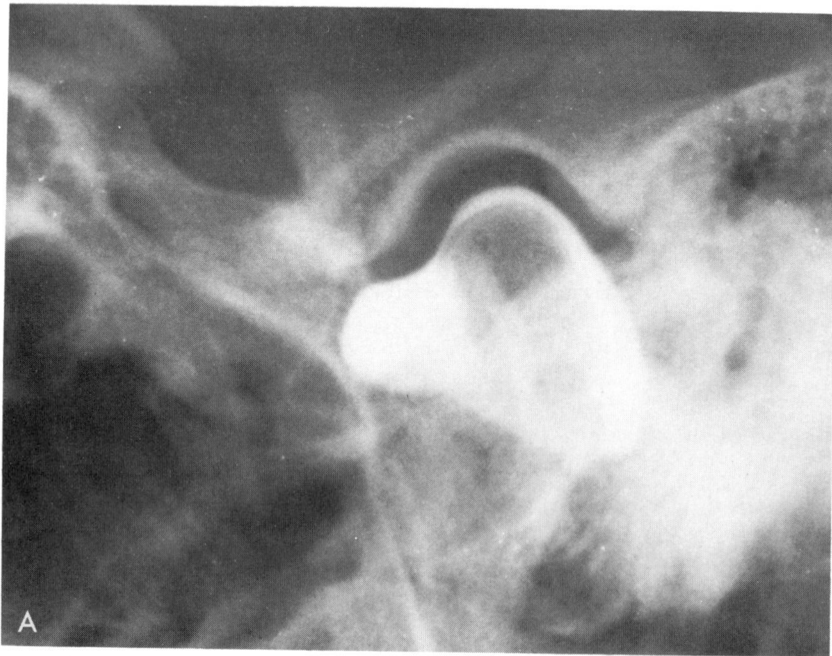

Figure 84–49. *Normal TMJ arthrography.*

A *Inferior joint space arthrogram in closed position shows contrast medium closely surrounding the condylar head and neck.*

Illustration continued on the opposite page

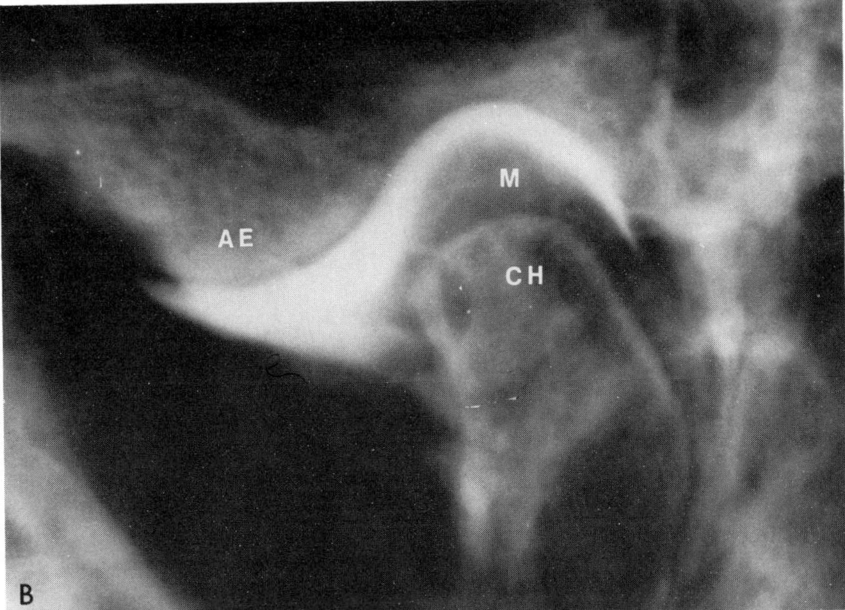

Figure 84–49. Continued
B *Superior joint space arthrogram in closed position shows long sigma-shaped superior space separating temporal fossa and articular eminence* (AE) *from meniscus* (M) *and condylar head* (CH).

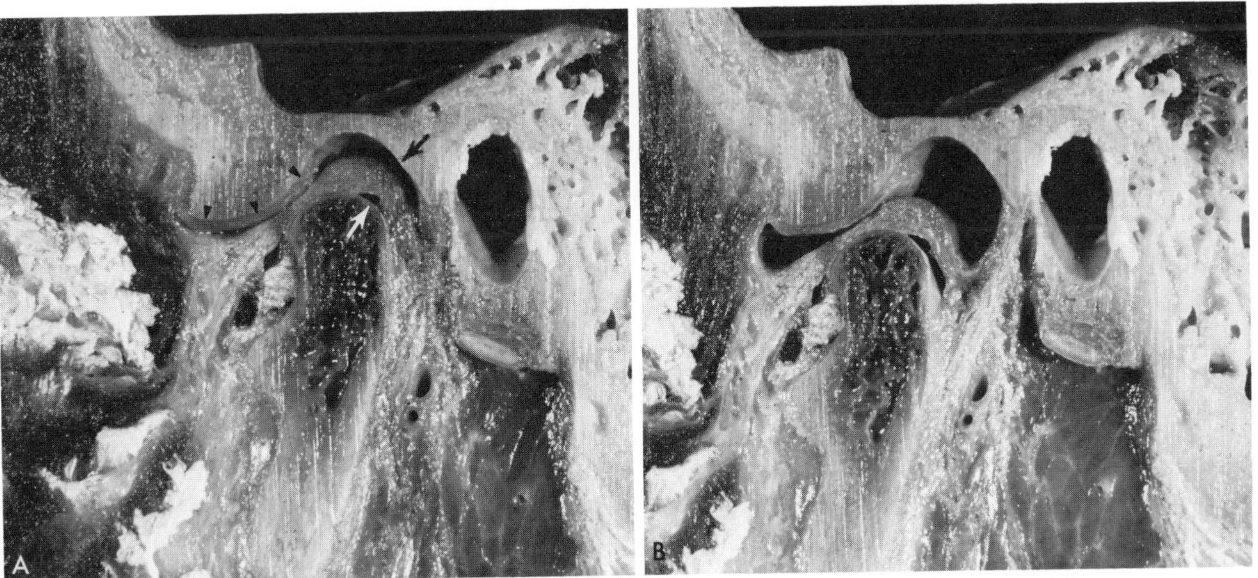

Figure 84–50. *Functional anatomy of the temporomandibular joint.*
A *Sagittal section of a fresh specimen in a slightly open position shows posterior sulci (arrows) beginning to open. Note articular cartilage (arrowheads) covering the articular eminence.*
B *The intermediate open position shows open posterior and anterior superior sulci. Note that the thin region of the meniscus stays between the articular surfaces and that changes in the joint shape are primarily a result of changes in the soft tissues about the sulci.*

eminence. To date, this interrelationship is incompletely described or understood. Throughout all phases of joint mobility, meniscal motion is coordinated with mandibular motion. Although the meniscus is pliable and changes shape somewhat with opening and closing of the mouth, most of the necessary soft tissue deformation occurs in the periarticular soft tissues and articular sulci.

With the mouth closed, the meniscus is situated deep in the mandibular fossa, and the posterior sulci of both joint cavities are collapsed (Fig. 84–50*A*). Initial opening of the mouth is a hinge action that takes place in the inferior space as the condylar head rotates on the meniscus. With each increment of opening, the posterior superior and inferior sulci become larger (Fig. 84–50*B*), as does the anterior superior sulcus. Just the opposite happens to the anterior inferior sulcus, which becomes progressively smaller with incremental opening. Intermediate steps in opening of the mouth require coordination of the meniscus's posterior rotation on the condylar head with gliding of the menisco-condylar complex along the articular eminence. Normally, the thinnest part of the meniscus lies between the condylar head and articular eminence during all phases of joint motion. Terminal opening of the mouth requires additional anterior movement of the condylar head on the meniscus as well as additional anterior gliding of the meniscus on the articular eminence. Between the extremes of fully open and

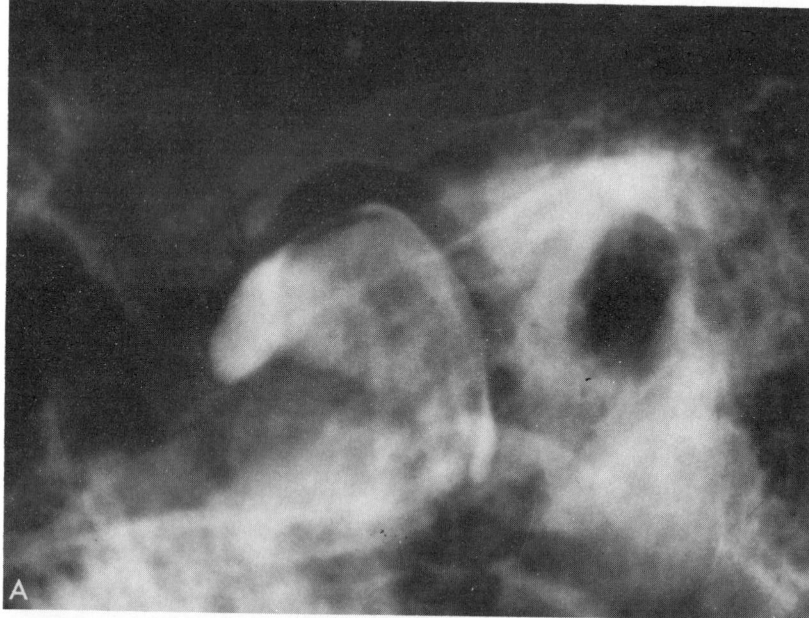

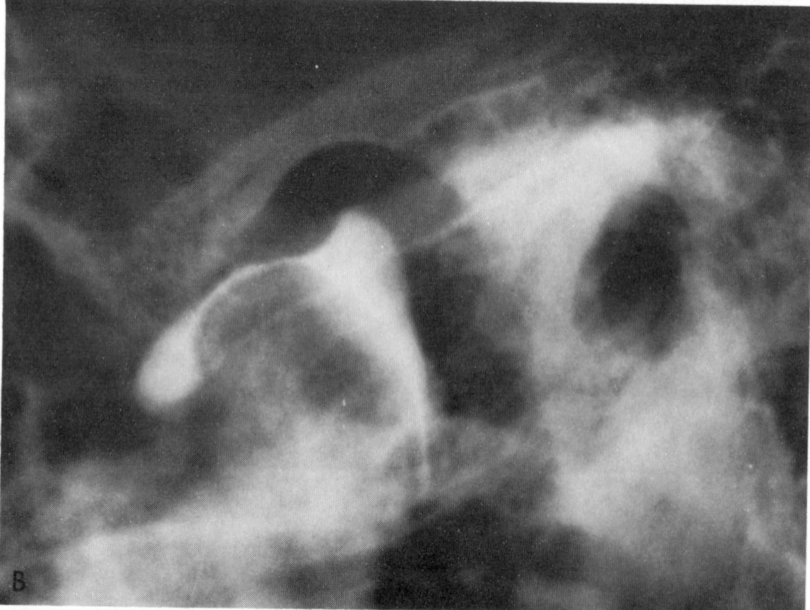

Figure 84–51. *Normal inferior space arthrogram.* ***A,*** *Closed;* ***B,*** *Intermediate open.*

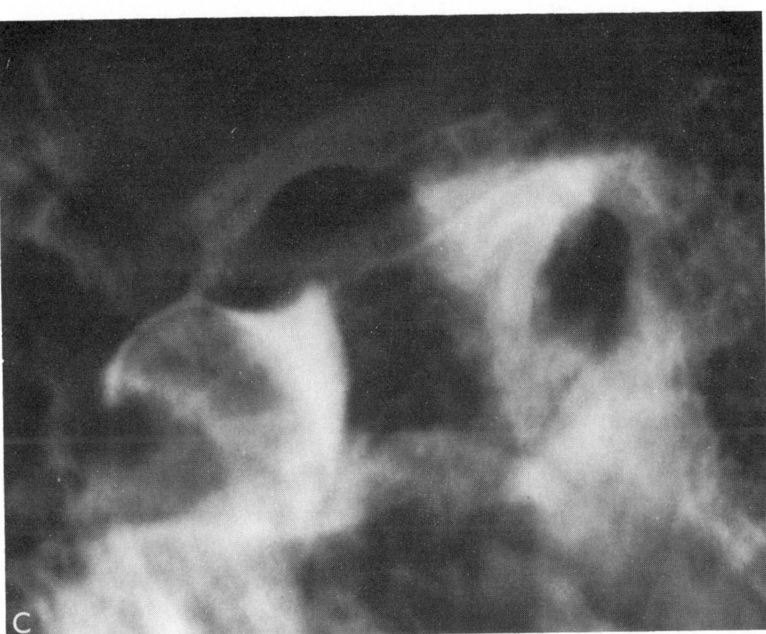

Figure 84–51. Continued
C, *Terminal open. The posterior sulcus is compressed in the closed position, but it becomes progressively larger with wider opening. Similarly, the anterior sulcus is largest in the closed position and smallest in the open position. The inferior surface of the meniscus remains smooth during all phases of mandibular motion.*

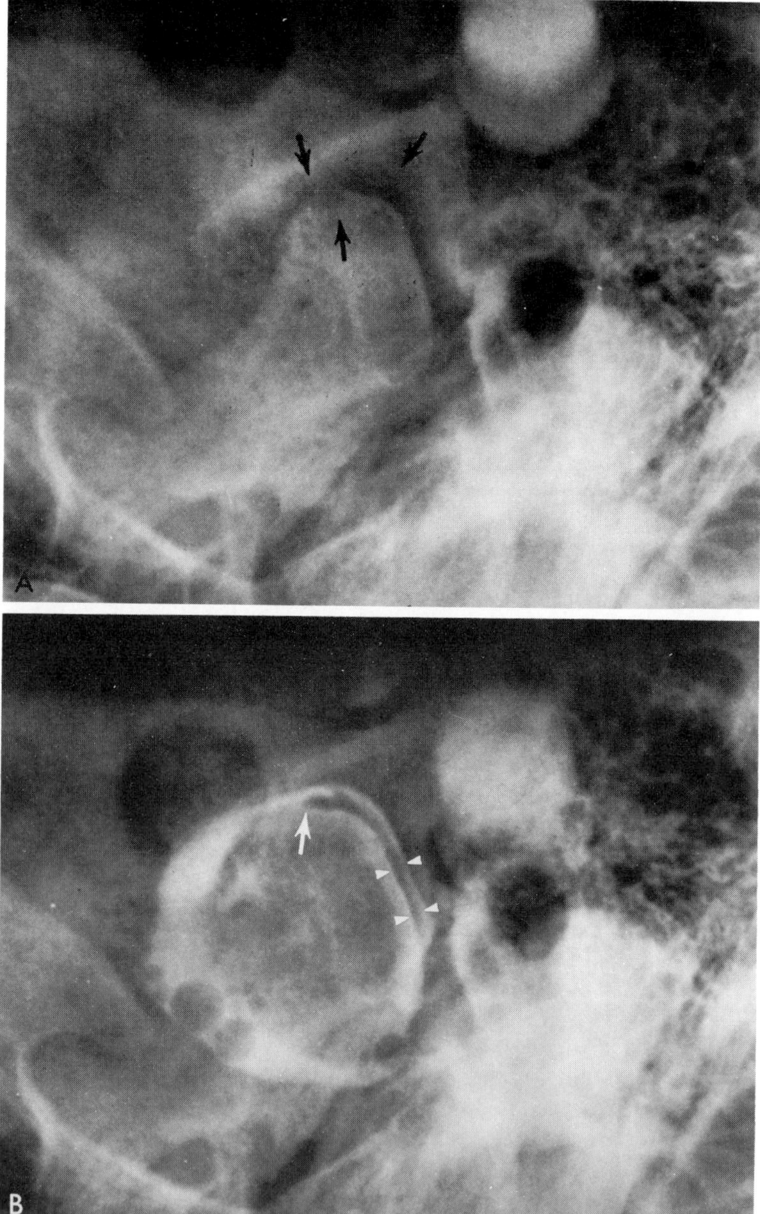

Figure 84–52. Arthrography in inflammatory arthritis.

A Inflammatory arthritis with advanced demineralization and erosion (arrows) of condylar head and temporal fossa is seen.

B Arthrogram shows filling of both superior and inferior spaces, indicating a torn meniscus (arrow). The residual meniscus (between arrowheads) is very thin.

closed positions, the meniscus deforms just enough to maintain smooth, straight joint surfaces (Fig. 84–51).

Disorders

Since conventional radiography can only show abnormalities of bone contour and condylar head position, arthrography is necessary to evaluate meniscal integrity and functional derangement.

Meniscal tears, erosions, and atrophy may accompany inflammatory or degenerative arthritides (Fig. 84–52). When bone destruction is advanced, such abnormalities are no surprise. However, meniscal abnormalities may occur much earlier in the natural history of an arthritic TMJ. More importantly, meniscal tears may be isolated abnormalities following trauma or may arise de novo (Fig. 84–53). These usually have a history of acute onset and yield perfectly normal conventional radiographs.

Causes of joint locking in either the open or the closed position can be evaluated by arthrography. Only a few patients present with fixed "open lock," a dislocation of the condylar head anterior to the articular eminence. This is usually caused when the condylar head impacts against the articular eminence, but it may also be due to a torn meniscus that has rolled up behind the condylar head and acts as a block to closure.

A chronic fixed "closed lock" is often due to

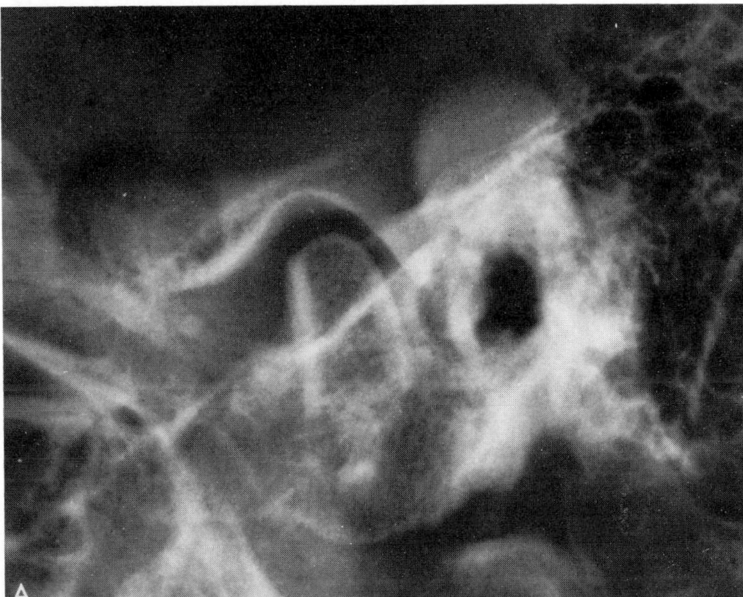

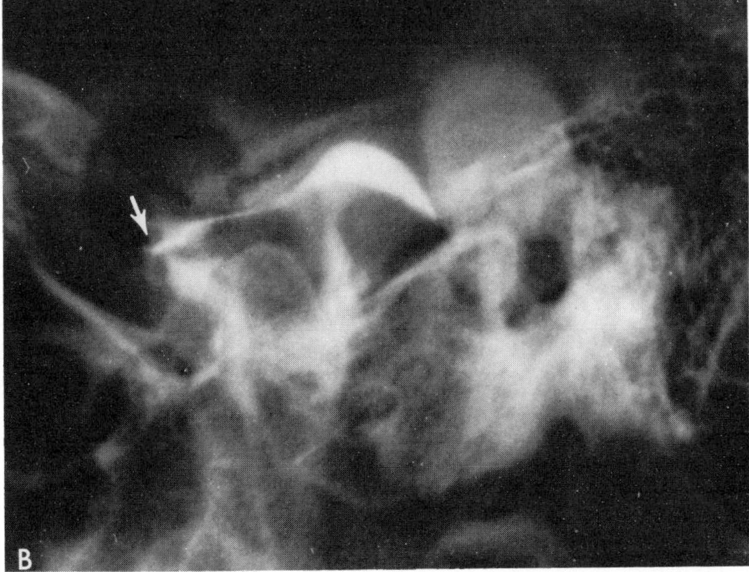

Figure 84–53. *Arthrography in meniscal tears. A 28 year old woman with TMJ pain and intermittent popping and locking.*

A *Magnification radiograph is normal.*

B *Arthrogram shows filling of both spaces, indicating a torn meniscus, in this example rupture of the anterior attachment (arrow). The meniscus still has normal thickness and nearly normal motion.*

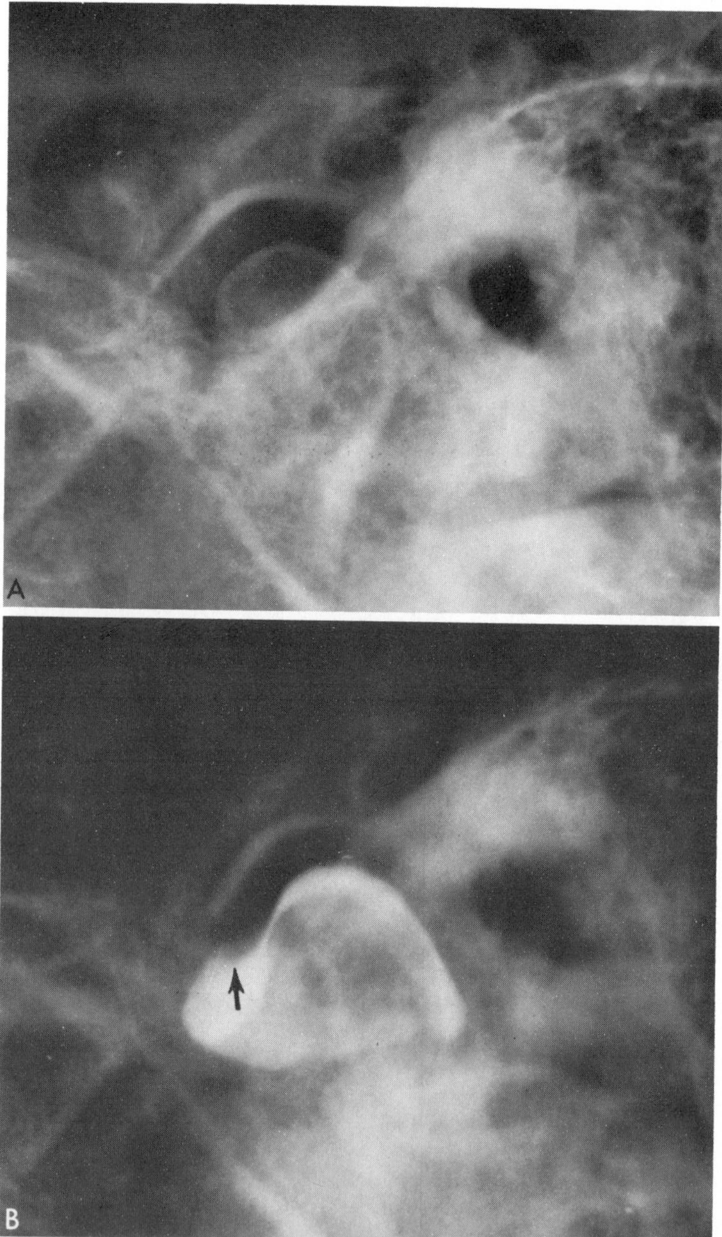

Figure 84–54. *Meniscal derangement. A 20 year old woman with popping and intermittent pain.*

A *Magnification radiograph is normal.*

B *Inferior space arthrogram in nearly closed position shows prominent meniscal ridge just anterior to condylar head (arrow).*

Illustration continued on the opposite page

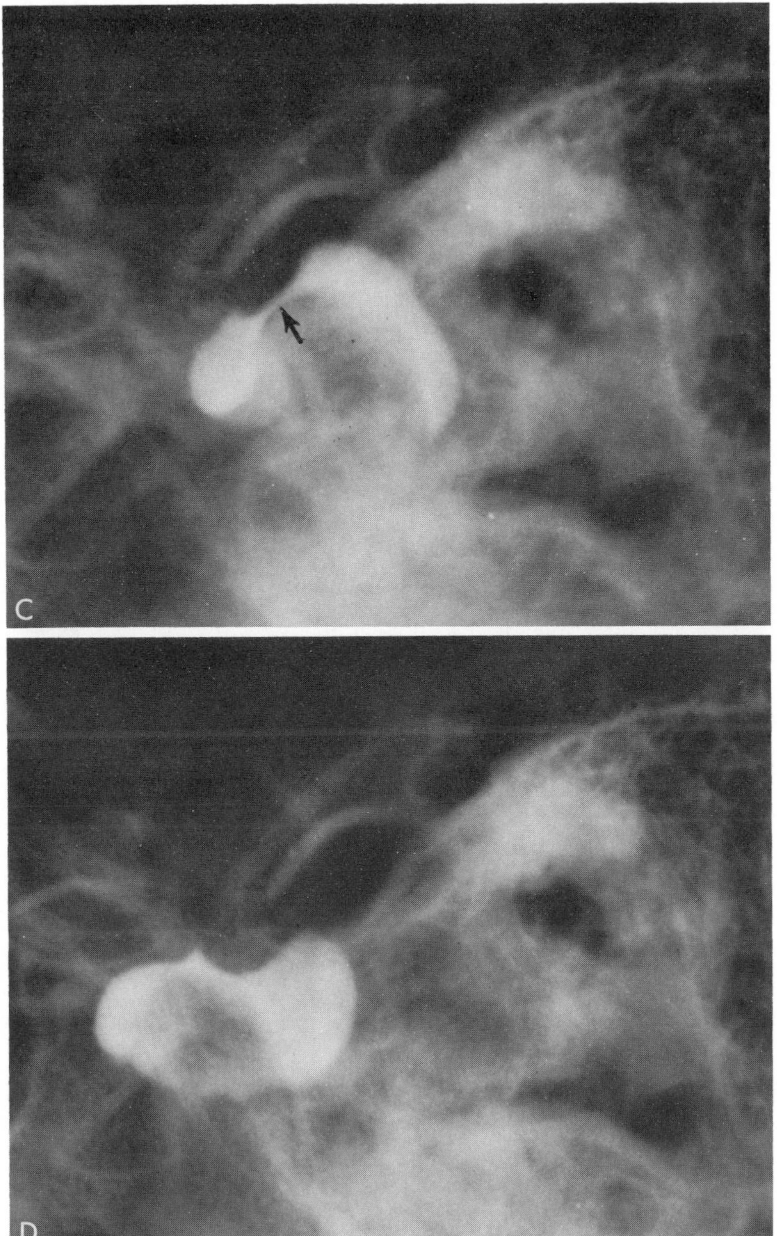

Figure 84–54. Continued

C *With intermediate opening, the meniscal bulge is compressed and deformed by the condylar head (arrow).*

D *With terminal opening, the condylar head translocates beyond the articular eminence, and the meniscus snaps back into a more relaxed position, with an audible and palpable pop.*

fibrous ankylosis or adhesive capsulitis following one of several insults. Immobilization of the jaw, either voluntarily or with external fixation following facial fracture or surgery, is a common cause. Inflammation (i.e., arthritis, infection, radiation therapy) is another common agent producing scar formation and joint immobility. Arthrography in these cases has a spectrum of appearances from complete obliteration of joint spaces to decreased volume of the individual spaces with obliteration of the sulci.

Intermittent locking accompanied by clicking or popping sounds is very common and is probably caused by a meniscal derangement. Once a tear is excluded, meniscal motion must be evaluated. Inferior joint arthrography permits examination of condylar head action across the undersurface of the meniscus. When symptoms are reproduced for fluoroscopic observation and conventional film documentation, uncoordinated meniscal movement is generally found. Often the meniscus is caught between the condylar head and articular eminence so that the anterior portion of the meniscus bulges as the head translocates across the eminence. With further opening, the meniscus is released and snaps back into a more natural position, accompanied by an audible pop (Fig. 84–54). This common meniscocondylar dysfunction seems to be caused by subluxation of the meniscus. Variations of meniscal subluxation may be associated with clicks at several stages of jaw opening or closing. Anterior meniscal subluxation eventually results in anterior dislocation and clinically a "closed lock." No universally accepted therapy has developed for this common meniscal abnormality. However, conservative and surgical trials are under way.

SUMMARY

Temporomandibular joint pain and dysfunction are important clinical problems, which present in many disciplines. Causes, diagnoses, and therapies are complex and to some degree still uncertain. An understanding of joint dysfunction rests on a firm foundation in embryology and adult anatomy. Radiographic evaluation deserves the best techniques possible and close radiologic scrutiny of the images obtained. Arthrography is in its infancy, and its findings should further advance our understanding of joint function and malfunction.

REFERENCES

1. Agerberg G, Lundberg M: Changes in the temporomandibular joint after surgical treatment: A radiologic follow-up study. Oral Surg *32*:865, 1971.
2. Alderman MM: Disorders of the temporomandibular joint and related structures: Rationale for diagnosis, etiology, management. Alpha Omegan, p 12, December 1976.
3. Anastassov K: Surgery of the temporomandibular joint. Int Dent J *18*:79, 1968.
4. Baume LJ: Ontogenesis of the human temporomandibular joint. I. Development of the condyles. J Dent Res *41*:1327, 1962.
5. Baume LJ, Holz J: Ontogenesis of the human temporomandibular joint. II. Development of the temporal components. J Dent Res *49*:864, 1970.
6. Berger SS, Stewart RE: Mandibular hypoplasia secondary to perinatal trauma: Report of case. J Oral Surg *35*:578, 1977.
7. Blair GS: Psoriatic arthritis and the temporomandibular joint. J Dent *4*:123, 1976.
8. Bowden CM Jr, Kohn MW: Mandibular deformity associated with unilateral absence of the condyle. J Oral Surg *31*:469, 1973.
9. Buhner WA: A headholder for oriented temporomandibular joint radiographs. J Prosthet Dent *29*:113, 1973.
10. Campbell W: Clinical radiological investigations of the mandibular joints. Br J Radiol *38*:401, 1965.
11. Chalmers IM, Blair GS: Rheumatoid arthritis of the temporomandibular joint: A clinical and radiologic study using circular tomography. Q J Med *42*:369, 1973.
12. Cherry CQ, Frew AL Jr: Bilateral reductions of articular eminence for chronic dislocation: Review of eight cases. J Oral Surg *35*:598, 1977.
13. Chue PWY: Gonococcal arthritis of the temporomandibular joint. Oral Surg *39*:572, 1975.
14. Chun HH: Temporomandibular joint gout. Letter to Editor. JAMA *226*:353, 1973.
15. Coin CG: Tomography of the temporomandibular joint. Med Radiogr Photogr *50*:26, 1974.
16. Converse JM, Coccaro PJ, Becker M, Wood-Smith D: On hemifacial microsomia: The first and second branchial arch syndrome. Plast Reconstr Surg *51*:268, 1973.
17. Costen JB: A syndrome of ear and sinus symptoms dependent upon disturbed function of the temporomandibular joint. Ann Otol Rhinol Laryngol *43*:1, 1934.
18. Davidson C, Wojtulewski JA, Bacon PA, Winstock D: Temporomandibular joint disease in ankylosing spondylitis. Ann Rheum Dis *34*:87, 1975.
19. Gelb H: Clinical Management of Head, Neck and TMJ Pain and Dysfunction: A Multi-Disciplinary Approach to Diagnosis and Treatment. Philadelphia, WB Saunders Co, 1977.
20. Guralnick W, Kaban LB, Merrill RG: Temporomandibular-joint afflictions. New Engl J Med *299*:123, 1978.
21. Hatzifotiadis D, Haralambous M, Elefteriadis I: Meniscectomy. Acta Stomatol Belg *73*:307, 1976.
22. Hecker R, Eversole LR, Packard HR, Kramer HS Jr: Symptomatic osteoarthritis of the temporomandibular joint: Report of a case. J Oral Surg *33*:780, 1975.
23. Husted E: Surgical methods. In L Schwartz, CM Chayes (Eds): Facial Pain and Mandibular Dysfunction. Philadelphia, WB Saunders Co, 1968, p 289.
24. Katzberg RW, Dolwick MF, Bales DJ, Helms CA: Arthrotomography of the temporomandibular joint: New technique and preliminary observations. Am J Roentgenol *132*:949, 1979.
25. Laskin DM: Etiology of the pain-dysfunction syndrome. J Am Dent Assoc *79*:147, 1969.
26. Lowry JC: Psoriatic arthritis involving the temporomandibular joint. J Oral Surg *33*:206, 1975.
27. MacAlister AD: The development of the human temporomandibular joint. Aust J Dent *59*:21, 1955.
28. Moore S: Body section roentgenography with the laminagraph. Am J Roentgenol *39*:514, 1938.
29. Morgan DH: Surgical correction of temporomandibular joint arthritis. J Oral Surg *33*:766, 1975.
30. Morgan DH: The great imposter: Diseases of the temporomandibular joint. JAMA *235*:2395, 1976.
31. Morgan DH, Hall WP, Vamvas SJ: Diseases of the Temporomandibular Apparatus: A Multidisciplinary Approach. St Louis, CV Mosby Co, 1977.
32. Murphy WA, Adams RJ, Gilula LA, Barbier JY: Magnification radiography of the temporomandibular joint: Technical considerations. Radiology, *133*:524, 1979.
33. Nørgaard F: Temporomandibular Arthrography. Copenhagen, Munksgaard, 1947.

34. Nwoku ALN, Koch H: The temporomandibular joint: A rare localisation for bone tumours. J Maxillofac Surg *2*:113, 1974.
35. Ogus H: Rheumatoid arthritis of the temporomandibular joint. Br J Oral Surg *12*:275, 1975.
36. Petrilli A, Gurley JE: Tomography of the temporomandibular joint. J Am Dent Assoc *26*:218, 1939.
37. Resnick D: Temporomandibular joint involvement in ankylosing spondylitis: Comparison with rheumatoid arthritis and psoriasis. Radiology *112*:587, 1974.
38. Rönning O, Väliaho ML, Laaksonen AL: The involvement of the temporomandibular joint in juvenile rheumatoid arthritis. Scand J Rheumatol *3*:89, 1974.
39. Rozencweiz D: Three-dimensional tomographic study of the temporomandibular articulation. J Periodontal *46*:348, 1975.
40. Stanson AW, Baker HL Jr: Routine tomography of the temporomandibular joint. Radiol Clin North Am *14*:105, 1976.
41. Toller PA: Osteoarthrosis of the mandibular condyle. Br Dent J *134*:223, 1973.
42. Toller PA: Opaque arthrography of the temporomandibular joint. Int J Oral Surg *3*:17, 1974.
43. Updegrave WJ: An evaluation of temporomandibular joint roentgenography. J Am Dent Assoc *46*:408, 1953.
44. Updegrave WJ: Visualizing the mandibular ramus in panoramic radiography. Oral Surg *31*:422, 1971.
45. Wang-Norderud R, Ragab RR: Unilateral condylar hyperplasia and the associated deformity of facial asymmetry. Scand J Plast Reconstr Surg *11*:91, 1977.
46. Weinberg LA: Technique for temporomandibular joint radiographs. J Prosthet Dent *28*:284, 1972.
47. Weinberg LA: Correlation of temporomandibular dysfunction with radiographic findings. J Prosthet Dent *28*:519, 1972.
48. Wilkes CH: Arthrography of the temporomandibular joint in patients with the TMJ pain-dysfunction syndrome. Minn Med *61*:645, 1978.
49. Yune HY, Hall JR, Hutton CE, Klatte EC: Roentgenologic diagnosis in chronic temporomandibular joint dysfunction syndrome. Am J Roentgenol *118*:401, 1973.
50. Yuodelis RA: The morphogenesis of the human temporomandibular joint and its associated structures. J Dent Res *45*:182, 1966.
51. Zech JM: A comparison and analysis of three technics of taking roentgenograms of the temporomandibular joint. J Am Dent Assoc *59*:725, 1959.
52. Dolwick MF, Katzberg RW, Helms CA, Bales DJ: Arthrotomographic evaluation of the temporomandibular joint. J Oral Surg *37*:793, 1979.
53. Farrar WB: Characteristics of the condylar path in internal derangements of the TMJ. J Prosthet Dent *39*:319, 1978.
54. Farrar WB, McCarty WL Jr: Inferior joint space arthrography and characteristics of condylar paths in internal derangements of the TMJ. J Prosthet Dent *41*:548, 1979.
55. Farrar WB, McCarty WL Jr: The TMJ dilemma. J Ala Dent Assoc *63*:19, 1979.
56. Katzberg RW, Dolwick MF, Helms CA, Hopens T, Bales DJ, Coggs GC: Arthrotomography of the temporomandibular joint. Am J Roentgenol *134*:995, 1980.
57. Lynch TP, Chase DC: Arthrography in the evaluation of the temporomandibular joint. Radiology *126*:667, 1978.
58. Murphy WA: Temporomandibular joint arthrography. Radiol Clin North Am (in press).

SOFT TISSUES

by Donald Resnick, M.D., and Gen Niwayama, M.D.

85

Both localized and generalized processes can affect the soft tissues. The prominent soft tissue abnormalities that may accompany many rheumatologic and related disorders have received considerable attention throughout this textbook. In this chapter, a generalized radiographic approach to the differential diagnosis of such abnormalities is presented. Although note is made of changes accompanying some of the rheumatologic disorders that are discussed elsewhere in the book, the interested reader should refer to the appropriate sections for more detailed discussion. Instead, additional entities are included that are important to physicians engaged in the diagnosis and treatment of articular diseases. By design, the analysis is direct and abbreviated, as a complete discussion of the multitude of soft tissue processes is beyond the scope of this textbook.

Abnormalities of the skin are much more amenable to clinical than radiologic examination and are the subject of an entire medical subspecialty, dermatology. Conversely, processes of the subcutaneous and muscular tissues are frequently better evaluated by radiography and related modalities than by palpation, percussion, or auscultation. Roentgenographic manifestations of such processes may include mass formation, alteration in radiodensity, including exaggerated lucency, calcification and ossification, and resorption and contracture.

SOFT TISSUE MASSES

Available Diagnostic Modalities

The etiology of soft tissue masses is diverse. Only a partial list of the causes of soft tissue "tumors" would include the following: primary and secondary neoplasms; articular diseases leading to tophi (gout) (Fig. 85–1), nodules (rheumatoid arthritis), xanthomas (Fig. 85–2), and synovial cysts; collagen, metabolic, and endocrine disorders producing calcific collections (scleroderma, dermatomyositis, mixed connective tissue disease, hyperparathyroidism, renal osteodystrophy, hypervitaminosis D, milk-alkali syndrome); neurologic and traumatic

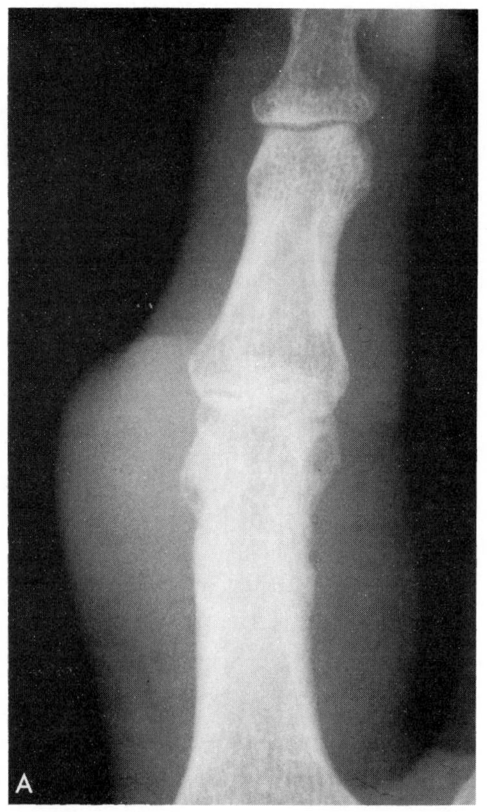

Figure 85–1. Gouty tophi.

A *A bulky mass about the proximal phalanx and proximal interphalangeal joint represents a tophus. Observe subjacent osseous erosion and flexion of the digit.*

Illustration continued on the opposite page

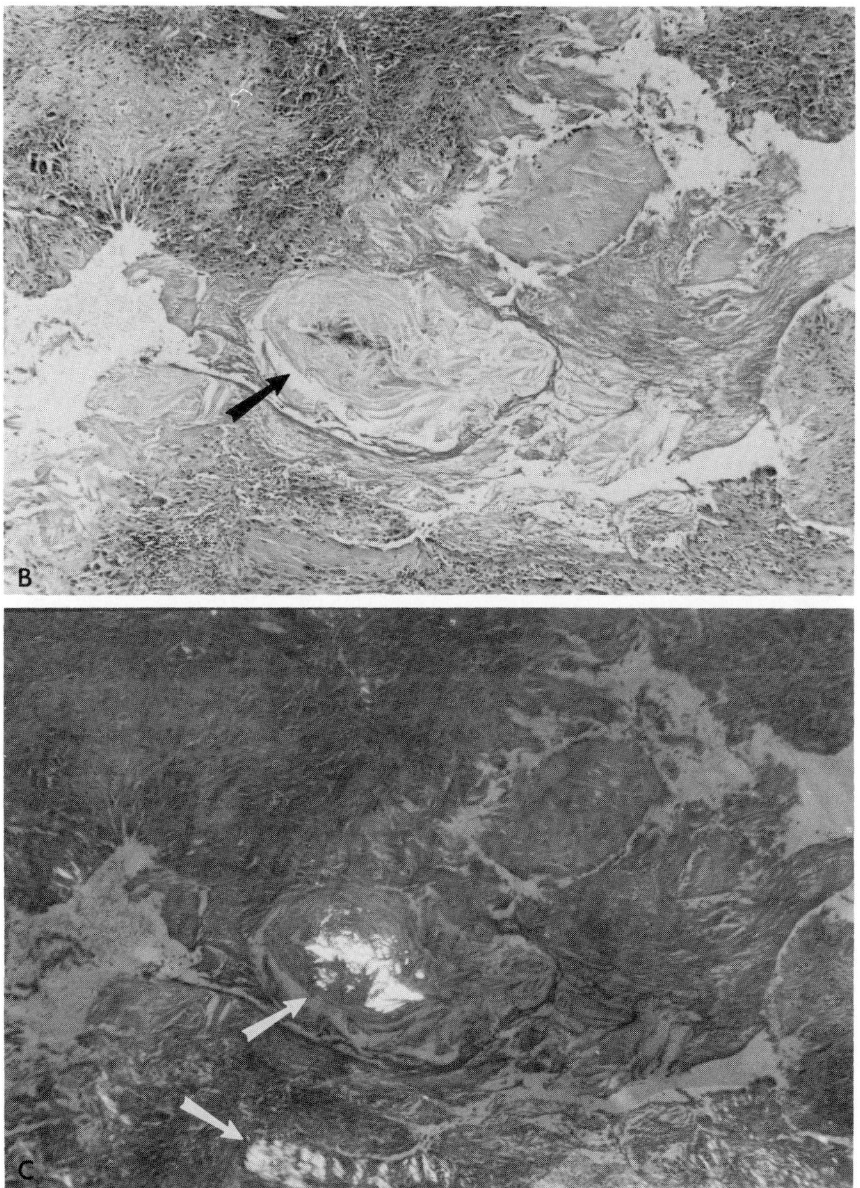

Figure 85–1. Continued
B, C *Nonpolarized* **(B)** *and polarized* **(C)** *photomicrographs (250×) indicate urate crystal deposition (arrows) in a nodular fibrous lesion of the synovial tissue.*

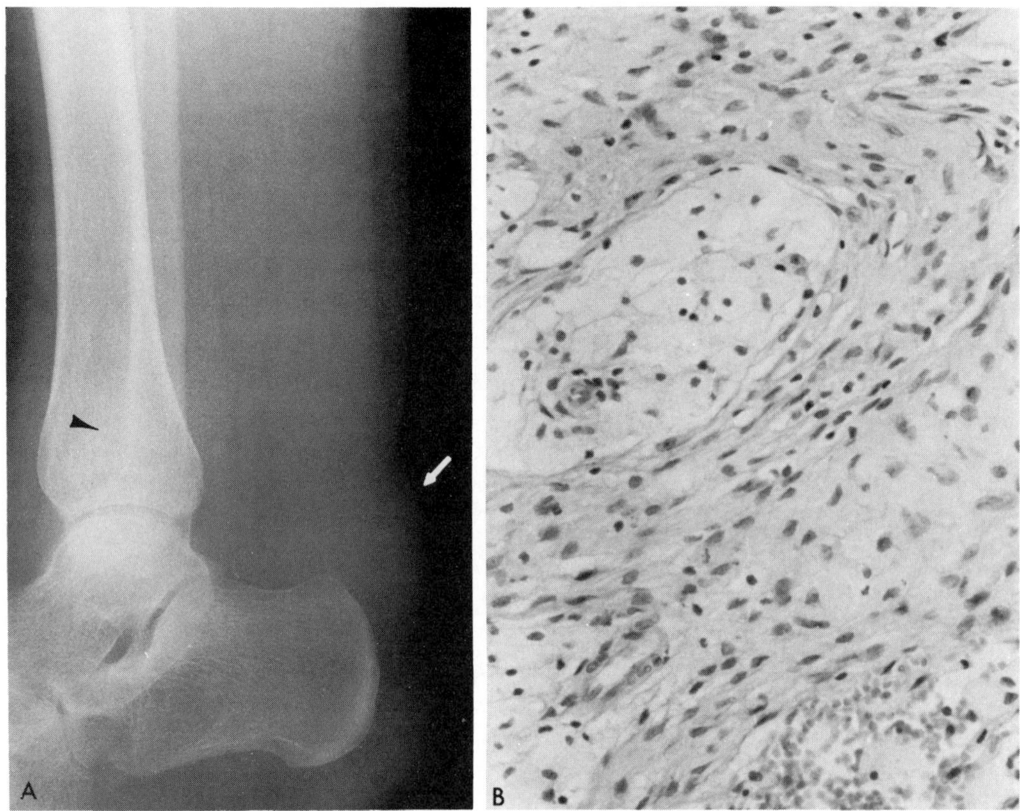

Figure 85–2. *Xanthoma.*

A *Observe xanthomatous infiltration in and around the Achilles tendon, producing lobulated soft tissue swelling (arrow). The anterior aspect of the distal fibula is eroded (arrowhead).*

B *The photomicrograph (100×) demonstrates the typical appearance of a xanthoma.*

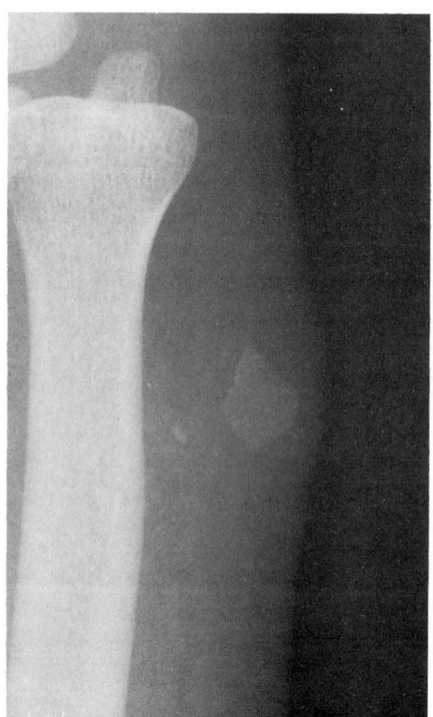

Figure 85–3. *Foreign body: glass shards. Several radiopaque areas in the distal forearm represent pieces of glass. Note soft tissue swelling.*

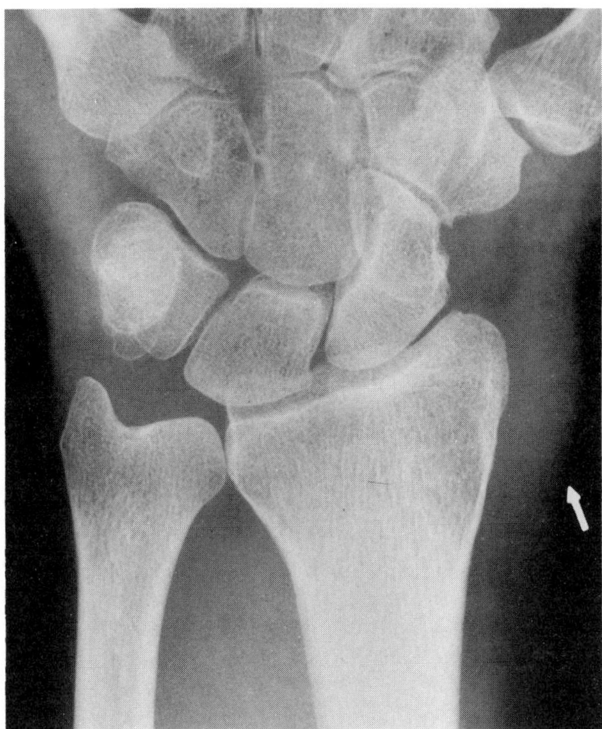

Figure 85–4. *De Quervain's tenosynovitis. In this patient, localized soft tissue swelling adjacent to the radial styloid process (arrow) is a result of tenosynovitis. (Courtesy of Dr. J. Weston, Hutt Hospital, Lower Hutt, New Zealand.)*

conditions causing ossification (paralysis, immobilization, thermal burns); infections with abscess formation; hematomas; foreign bodies (Fig. 85–3); tendinitis (Fig. 85–4); and hyperostotic processes of bone. In many instances, local or distant clinical findings provide important clues in the differential diagnosis of the various processes. Supplementary plain film radiography commonly adds useful information that, although not diagnostic, indicates whether a neoplasm is present and, if so, whether that neoplasm is benign or malignant. It is frequently necessary to alter the radiographic technique to maximize the information on the soft tissues that is obtained from the roentgenogram. Low kilovoltage (below 50 kVp), by exaggerating the differences in radiographic density of fat and muscle,[1] can be useful (see Chapter 10), although the adjacent osseous tissue is poorly evaluated with this technique. A fine-grain x-ray film is essential for anatomic detail,[2] and the utilization of a small focal spot x-ray tube allows radiographic magnification (see Chapter 9). These procedures increase local radiation exposure but are justified in many cases because of the additional data that are supplied.

The role of conventional tomography in the evaluation of soft tissue masses is limited. The interface between the process and the subjacent bone may be better visualized with this technique, and subtle changes in the osseous tissue may indicate the nature and aggressiveness of the soft tissue lesion.

Xeroradiography with its edge contrast enhancement and great latitude is better suited for delineating soft tissue changes than is conventional radiography[3-5] (see Chapter 11). This modality may define the characteristics of a tumor contour and the presence and extent of internal calcification or ossification. The expansile nature of a neoplasm can occasionally be differentiated from the retractile appearance of an organizing hematoma by xeroradiography.[5] Furthermore, both osseous and soft tissue structures can be evaluated on a single exposure, an advantage that cannot be obtained with conventional roentgenograms. Disadvantages of xeroradiography include the requirement for special equipment, limitation in field size, and high radiation exposure.

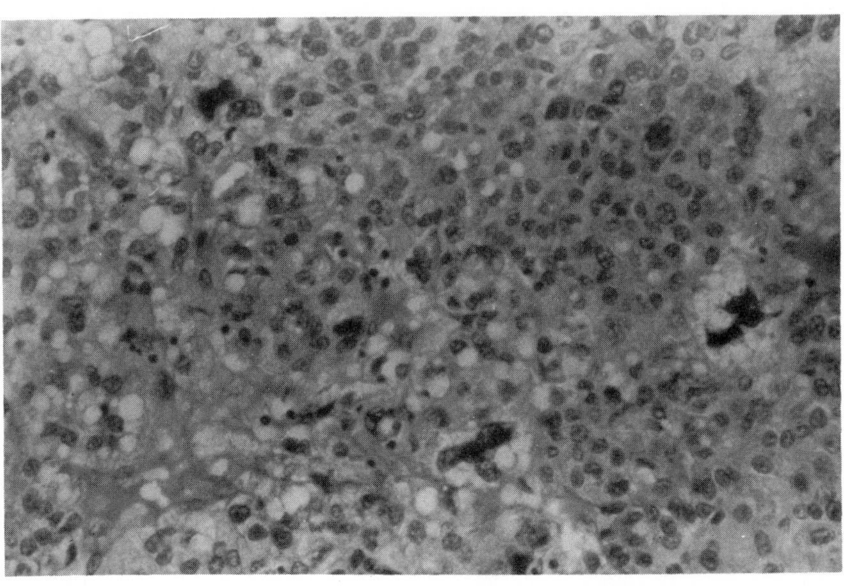

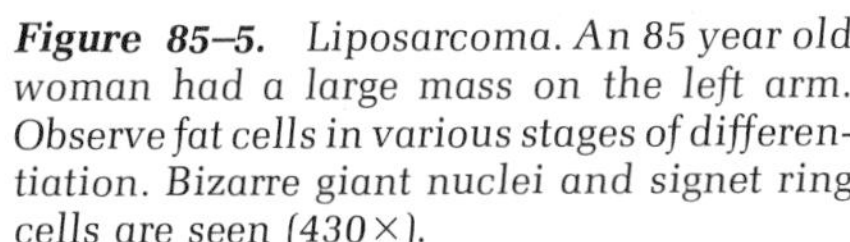

Figure 85–5. *Liposarcoma. An 85 year old woman had a large mass on the left arm. Observe fat cells in various stages of differentiation. Bizarre giant nuclei and signet ring cells are seen (430×).*

Computed tomography has recently been emphasized as a useful technique in evaluating soft tissue masses, especially about the pelvis[6-10] (see Chapter 12). The ability of this modality to define the exact dimension of a lesion, the relationship of the tumor to nearby bone structures, and the density characteristics of the affected tissue is important, both in correct diagnosis and in proper therapy.[302, 308]

Angiography may be utilized to define the extent and vascular supply of a tumor and to differentiate a benign from a malignant neoplasm[11-14] (see Chapter 16). Differentiation of malignancy and hypervascular inflammatory masses may be more difficult,[2, 14] although evaluation of hemangiomas and vascular malformations can be accomplished with this technique.[15-17] Selective arterial injections, magnification and subtraction films, and administration of pharmacologic agents potentiate the role of angiography.[277]

Scintigraphy with technetium (or other radiopharmaceuticals) may delineate the presence and extent of soft tissue tumors[18, 19] (see Chapter 17). The mechanism of such uptake is incompletely understood, although increased blood flow, microcalcification, or a binding of the compounds by enzymes released in response to tissue damage may be important. Many of the tumors in which bone-seeking radioisotopes localize reveal radiographic or histologic evidence of calcification, although this is not invariable. Because of the diverse nature of the process that may produce accumulation of technetium (and other agents), the diagnostic capabilities of this modality are limited. Positive scans can accompany soft tissue neoplasm, infection, and diseases associated with local or widespread calcification. Although gallium was initially regarded as a tumor-localizing agent, it too may accumulate in inflamed or infarcted soft tissues.[29]

Types of Tumors

Tumors of soft tissues can arise from the epidermis and the ectodermal structures of the skin, from the lymph nodes, and from two additional primitive tissue sources: the mesoderm and the neuroectodermal tissues of the peripheral nervous system.[20] From the primitive mesenchyme are derived the supportive and reticuloendothelial tissues and their corresponding tumors; from the neuroectoderm are formed the schwann sheath and possibly the endoneurium and perineurium and their corresponding tumors. The result is an overwhelming list of potential primary soft tissue neoplasms. Several additional factors complicate the characterization and recognition of histologic patterns of soft tissue tumors. The histology of a neoplasm may be altered through a process of differentiation or dedifferentiation of the primary cell type or as a result of proliferation of fibroblast cells due to local tissue injury. Admixtures and conglomerations of various neoplastic cells can result, typical examples of which are the malignant mesenchymoma, synovioma, and teratoma. Furthermore, although tumors of certain types generally arise at sites where corresponding varieties of tissue are normally found, this is not a constant rule.[20] Thus, not only are the types of neoplasm frequently difficult to classify, but in addition their locations are quite variable, and one is left with an endless list of tumor types and sites. However, certain characteristics of relative frequency and distribution allow probable preoperative diagnoses, and typical histologic patterns in certain neoplasms allow a specific pathologic appraisal.

In general, benign tumors or tumor-like processes are more frequent than malignant processes. At Columbia University, the ratio of benign to malignant "tumors" detected on pathologic examination over a 45 year period was approximately 5.5:1.[20] Primary benign tumors can be classified as fibroblastic processes (fibroma, various forms of fibromatosis), myxomatoses, fibrous histiocytomas, lipomatoses, xanthomatoses, myomatoses, angiomatoses, lymphangiomatoses, and muscular types; primary malignant tumors can be regarded as fibrosarcomas, malignant histiocytomas, liposarcomas, lipomyosarcomas, rhabdomyosarcomas, angiosarcomatoses, lymphoid and reticuloendothelial tumors, extraskeletal osteogenic sarcomas and chondrosarcomas, synovial sarcomas, malignant mesenchymomas, and miscellaneous types.[20] If to this list are added the neurogenic tumors, metastatic deposits, and non-neoplastic masses, the diverse nature of soft tissue masses is readily apparent.

Of the primary malignant soft tissue tumors, liposarcoma, fibrosarcoma, rhabdomyosarcoma, unclassified sarcomas, leiomyosarcoma, and synovial sarcoma, in descending order of frequency, are most commonly encountered. However, the incidence of the specific types of malignant tumors varies with the age of the patient. Of the benign neoplasms, lipomas and hemangiomas are relatively common.

Tumors of Fat

Liposarcoma is a frequent malignant neoplasm of soft tissues that is usually encountered in middle-aged and elderly patients[10, 21, 22, 287] (Fig. 85–5). It is common in the thigh, gluteal region, retroperitoneum, and leg. It does not usually arise from a preexisting lipoma. On radiographs, an ill-defined mass of both water density and fat density may be observed. In general, more malignant lesions reveal increasing radiodensity, whereas less aggressive tumors have a greater fat content and increased lucency. One type of lipoma, the infiltrating angiolipoma, is composed of mature lipocytes with foci of angiomatous prolifera-

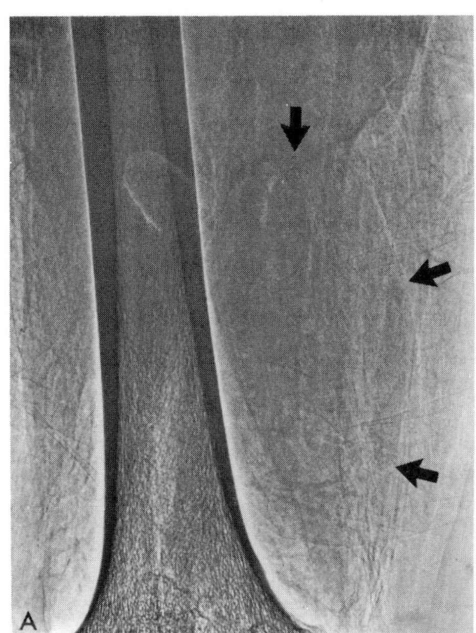

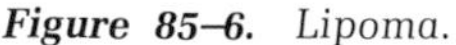

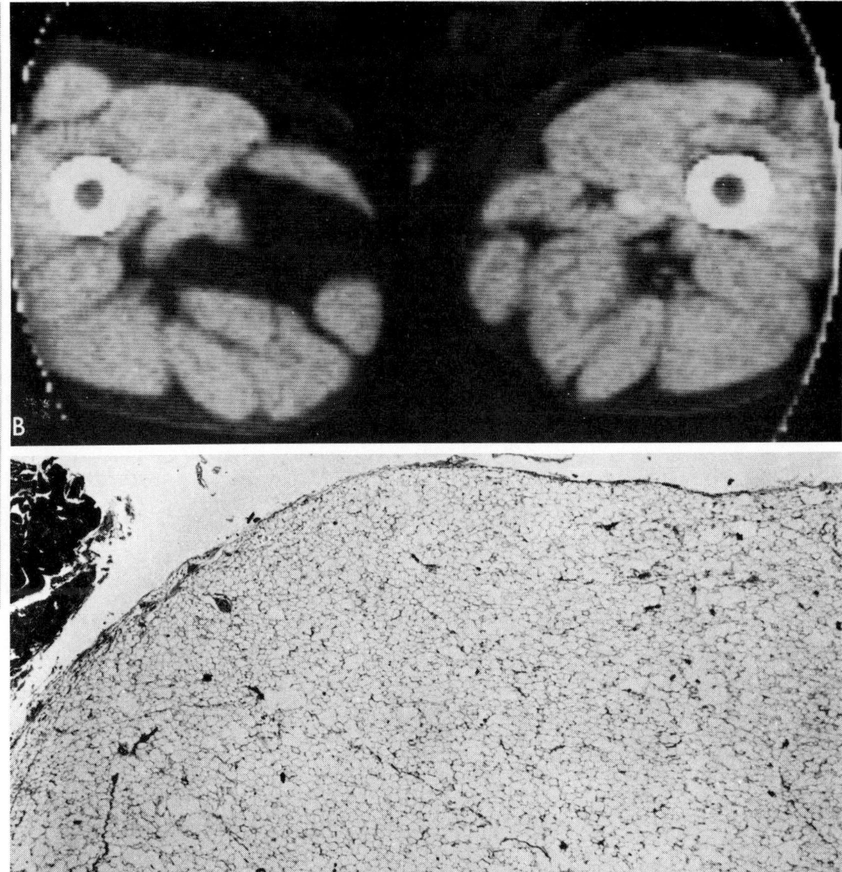

Figure 85–6. *Lipoma.*

A–C *A 57 year old man presented with a 2 × 5 cm soft, nontender, movable but ill-defined mass overlying the anteromedial aspect of the thigh. Xeroradiography* **(A)** *demonstrates a poorly defined mass (arrows). Computed tomography* **(B)** *following administration of intravenous contrast material shows an area of low density medially, which extends from the subcutaneous fat to the area beneath the vastus medialis muscle. The CT number is −52 (normal fat is −51). Photomicrograph* **(C)** *demonstrates adipose tissue containing a thin fibrous capsule (13.5×).*

*(**A–C,** From Hunter JC et al: Skel Radiol 4:79, 1979.)*

Illustration continued on the following page

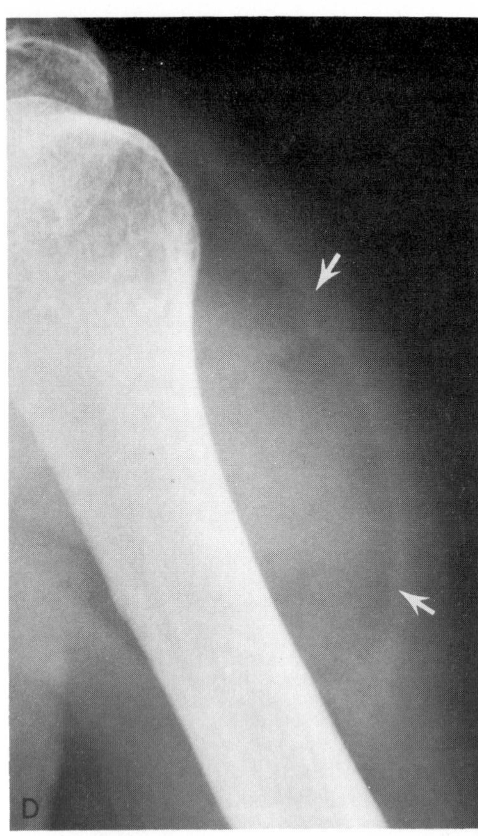

Figure 85–6. Continued
D *In a different patient with a lipoma about the shoulder, a well-defined and radiolucent mass (arrows) is seen, which contains trabeculation. The bone is normal.*

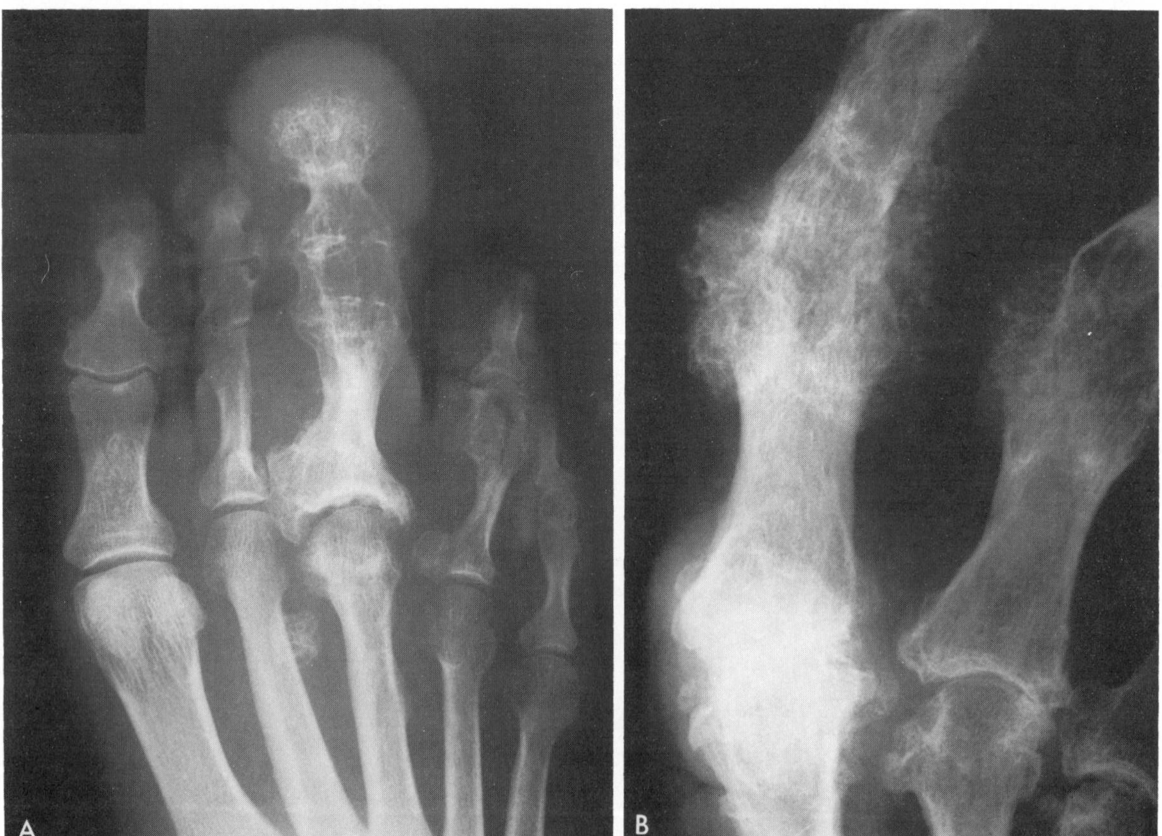

Figure 85–7. *Macrodystrophia lipomatosa. Two examples reveal the massive enlargement of soft tissue and osseous tissue that can accompany this condition. Observe the degree of joint space narrowing, bony ankylosis, and proliferative alterations. (Courtesy of Dr. L. Ginsburg, Long Beach, California.)*

tion and is locally aggressive. A distinctive radiographic appearance is evident, characterized by serpiginous densities intermixed with fat.[288]

Lipomas are common lesions which are typically encountered in patients who are 30 to 50 years of age.[23, 24] Women are more frequently affected, and solitary lesions predominate. The tumors may be located throughout the body, although they show predilection for the subcutaneous tissues of the back, extremities, and thorax. A well-defined radiolucent mass is detected on the roentgenogram (Fig. 85–6). Histologically and chemically, the tumor tissue is similar to ordinary body fat. Of interest, the fat of the lipoma is not available to the body in cases of starvation; in fact, as normal body fat undergoes wasting, the lipoma may actually increase in size.[20]

Additional varieties of fatty tumors are multiple symmetric lipomatosis (in which diffuse and symmetric distribution of lipomas is recognized), hibernoma and lipoblastomatosis (which are rare embryonal fatty tumors),[25-27] lipoma arborescens (in which fat collects beneath the synovial lining of the joint, especially the knee, producing swollen, villous projections),[28] macrodystrophia lipomatosa (which can lead to grotesque enlargement of a digit) (Fig. 85–7), and mesenchymoma (in which fatty, fibrous, vascular, smooth muscle, and osseous elements are evident).

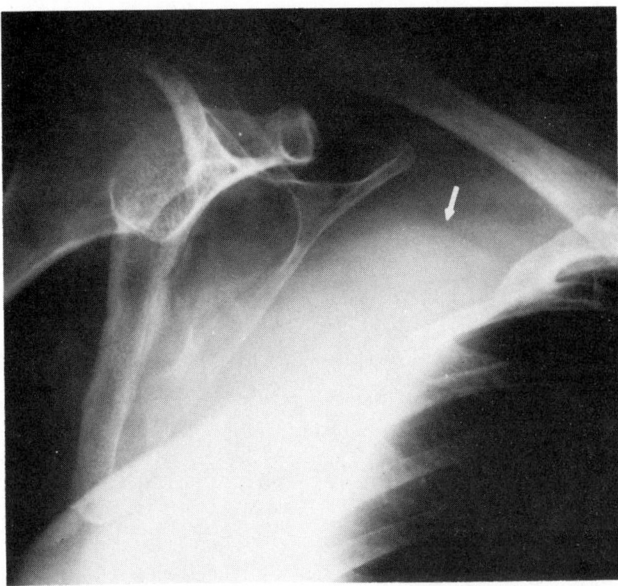

Figure 85–8. *Extra-abdominal desmoid tumor. This 55 year old woman presented with a mass in the area of the right scapula. The radiograph outlines lateral displacement of the scapula by a large, poorly defined soft tissue mass (arrow). Equivocal osseous changes are apparent. At surgery, the mass, weighing 1240 gm, was found to have infiltrated the chest wall between the ribs. Histologic analysis confirmed the diagnosis of fibromatosis. (Courtesy of Dr. A. Bonakdarpour, Temple University Hospital, Philadelphia, Pennsylvania.)*

Tumors of Fibrous Tissue

Fibrosarcomas occur in both adults and children, particularly men, and they predominate in the external soft tissues rather than the retroperitoneum, mediastinum, mesentery, or viscera.[20, 30, 31] The neoplasms lack any specific radiographic characteristics.

The classification of benign fibrous tissues is complicated. A *fibroma* represents a harmless pedunculated or filiform congenital malformation composed of the normal fibrous elements of the corium covered by epidermis.[20] Other varieties of benign fibrous proliferation are termed *fibromatoses*. In this latter group is a *desmoid tumor*, which arises in the abdominal and extra-abdominal musculature of men, women, and children and infiltrates the surrounding tissues in an insidious fashion, especially when located in extra-abdominal sites[32-36, 278] (Fig. 85–8). The shoulder area is not an uncommon site of extra-abdominal desmoid tumors.

Other types of fibromatoses are classified according to their location. *Recurring digital fibromas* of infancy represent a rare condition in which single or multiple fibromatous lesions arise from the fingers (and toes), affecting predominantly the dorsolateral aspect of the distal parts of adjacent digits.[37-39] They may reach considerable size but are usually painless. Their digital site of origin, their tendency to recur, and the presence of cytoplasmic inclusion bodies in some cases are characteristic features of this variety of fibromatosis. Furthermore, flexion contractures and hypoplastic or deformed metacarpals, metatarsals, or phalanges can be encountered. *Palmar* and *plantar fibromatoses* are terms applied to fibrous proliferations occurring in the palmar fascia (in association with Dupuytren's contracture) and plantar fascia. These lesions vary in size and commonly recur following local excision.

Juvenile aponeurotic fibroma is an aggressive variety of fibrous proliferation that arises in the aponeurotic tissues of the hands or feet of young children[40-42, 50] (Figs. 85–9 and 85–10). This lesion has a tendency to calcify, infiltrate adjacent tissues, and recur following incomplete excision. The aggressive histologic appearance and the recurrent nature of juvenile aponeurotic fibromatosis have raised the question of a low-grade malignancy in some cases. Lichtenstein and Goldman[43] have postulated that this tumor is an atypical cartilaginous growth that may appear in many areas of the body in both children and adults.

Additional types of fibrous proliferation include *fibromatosis colli*, which develops usually in the sternomastoid muscle of infants and children, *penile fibromatosis* (Peyronie's disease), which produces stiffening and deformity of the penis, *idiopathic retroperitoneal fibrosis*, in which fibrous proliferation of retroperitoneal tissues may lead to ureteral

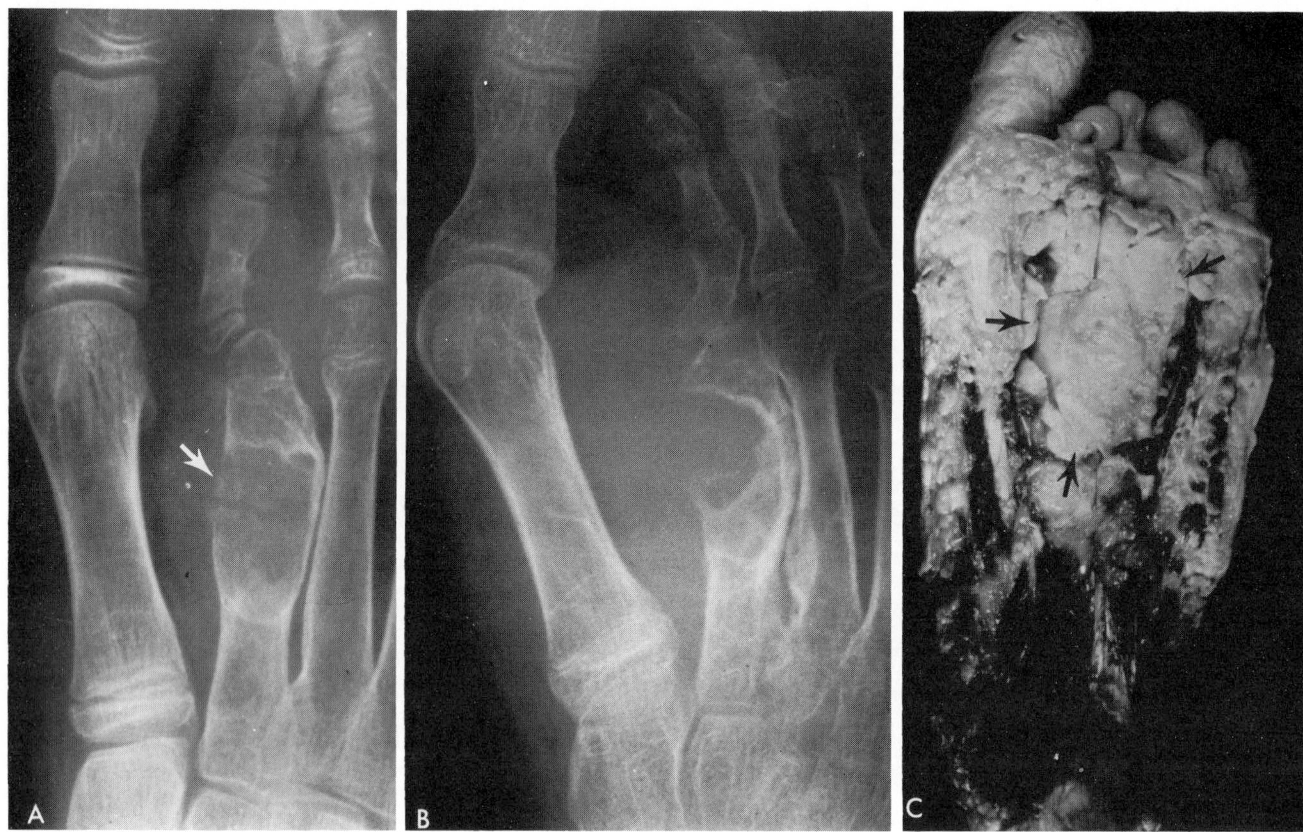

Figure 85–9. *Juvenile aponeurotic fibromatosis. This 13 year old girl developed a mass on the dorsum of the left foot.*

A *An initial radiograph reveals a soft tissue mass with adjacent osseous involvement and a pathologic fracture through a well-circumscribed lesion in the second metatarsal (arrow). There is displacement and deformity of the proximal phalanx in the same digit. Excisional biopsy resulted in a diagnosis of either neurofibroma or desmoplastic fibroma.*

B *Approximately 3 years after* **A**, *a recurrent mass has produced further destruction and distortion of the neighboring bones.*

C *After amputation, the specimen shows the extent of the fibrous tumor invading the metatarsals (arrows). Atypical fibrous tissue was demonstrated on histologic examination.*

(Courtesy of Dr. R. Freiberger, Hospital for Special Surgery, New York, New York, and Dr. J. Kaye, Vanderbilt University, Nashville, Tennessee.)

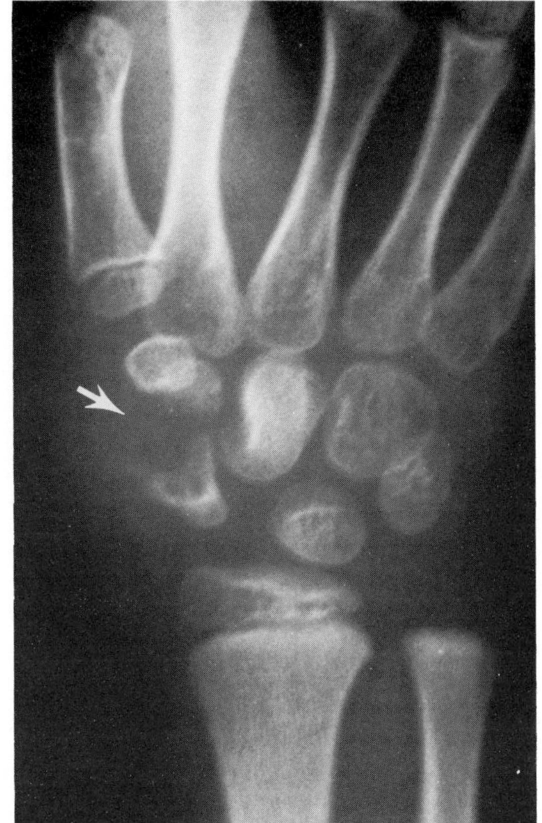

Figure 85–10. *Juvenile aponeurotic fibromatosis. This 5 year old girl developed progressive pain and swelling of the wrists. Several of the carpal bones are invaded (arrow) by an adjacent soft tissue mass. Biopsy confirmed the diagnosis of juvenile aponeurotic fibromatosis. (Courtesy of Dr. H. Hricak, Henry Ford Hospital, Detroit, Michigan.)*

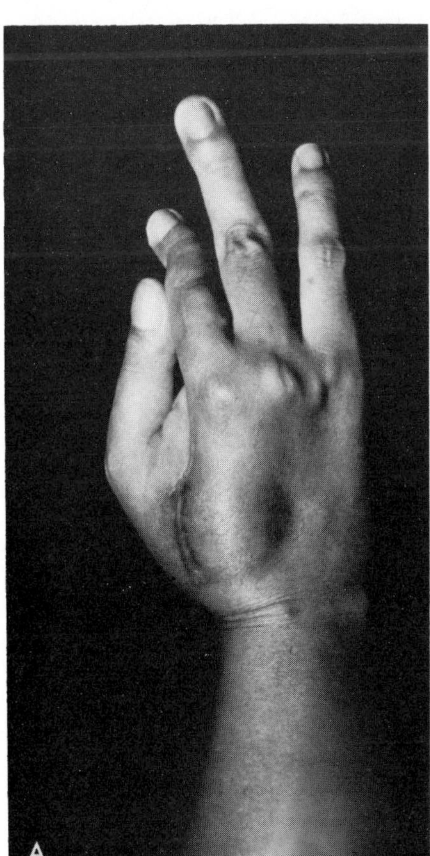

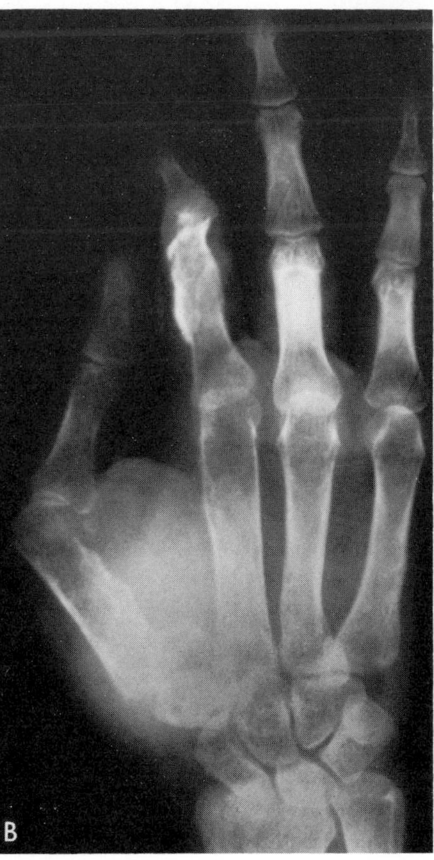

Figure 85–11. *Nodular fasciitis.*

A, B *This 35 year old woman had had long right index and middle fingers since birth. She developed swelling on the dorsum of the right hand over a 2 year period, which, following biopsy and amputation of the second digit, was diagnosed as nodular fasciitis. The mass recurred. A clinical photograph* **(A)** *demonstrates the soft tissue swelling over the dorsum of the hand and the scar from the previous biopsy and amputation of the second finger. A radiograph* **(B)** *outlines amputation of the second digit, a soft tissue mass, bony erosion, and infiltration of the first and third metacarpals. (***A, B,** *Courtesy of Naval Hospital, San Diego, California.)*

Illustration continued on the following page

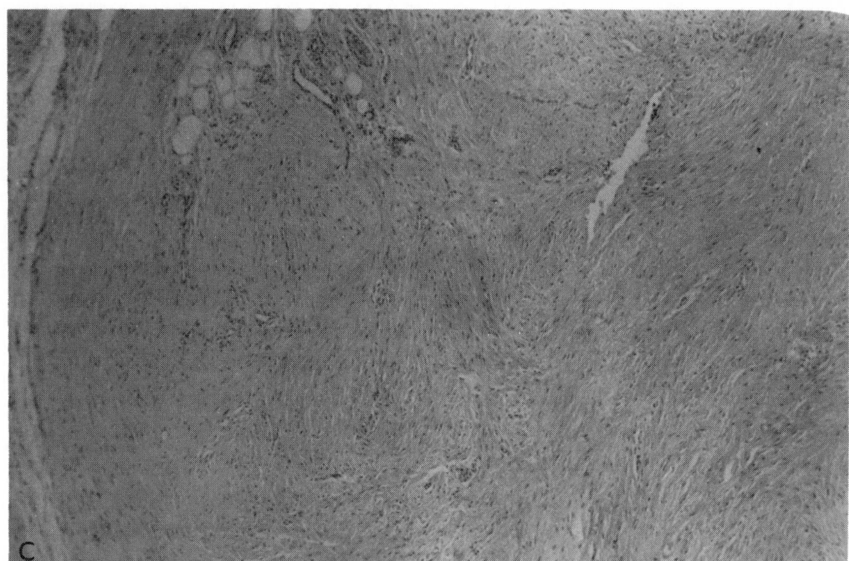

Figure 85–11. Continued

C *In this 51 year old woman with a mass over the right thumb, the histologic diagnosis of nodular fibromatosis is based upon irregularly defined, heavily collagenized bundles of occasionally plump and predominantly fibroblastic cells, with accompanying lymphocytic nests. Histiocytic clusters and fat are also identified (86×).*

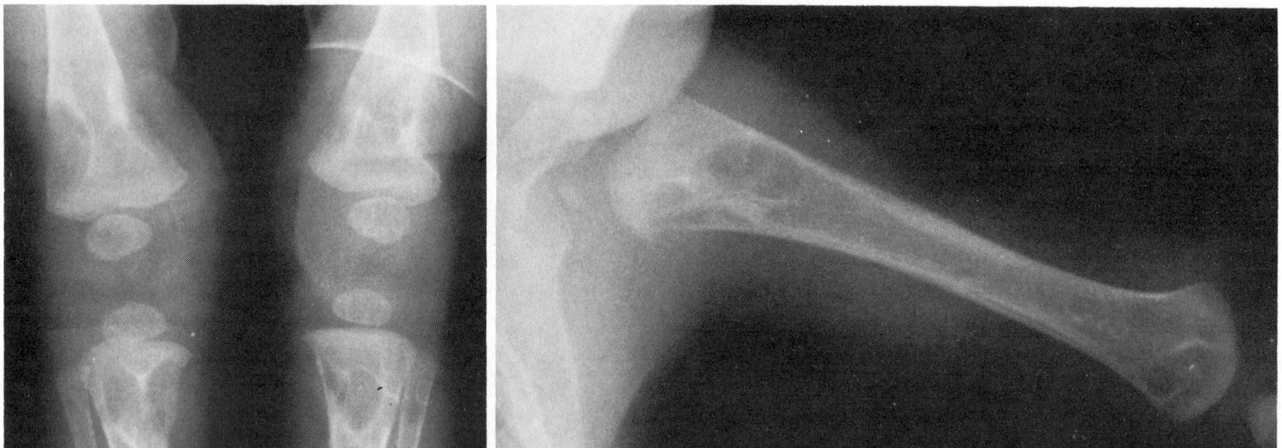

Figure 85–12. *Congenital generalized fibromatosis. Radiographs of this infant girl at the ages of 5 months* **(A, B)** *and 8 months* **(C, D)** *are shown. Multiple symmetrically distributed radiolucent foci, predominantly in the metaphyses of the tubular bones, represent sites of fibrous proliferation. Note the improvement in the later films. (Courtesy of Dr. D. Weissberg, Orange County, California.)*

obstruction, *irradiation fibromatosis*, in which local superficial soft tissue fibrous proliferation relates to heavy irradiation, *progressive myositis fibrosa* (hereditary polyfibromatosis), which represents an early stage of myositis ossificans before the development of bone formation, *elastofibroma*, in which unilateral or bilateral tumors containing elastinophilic fibers develop in middle-aged and elderly individuals, especially about the shoulders,[44-47] *pseudosarcomatous fasciitis*, related to fibroblastic proliferation in subcutaneous tissues, especially in the upper extremity, in children or men and women from infancy to old age[51] (Fig. 85–11), and *congenital generalized fibromatosis* affecting infants, in which fibrous proliferation occurs not only in the superficial soft tissues but also in viscera and bones[20] (Fig. 85–12). This latter condition may be familial and the tumors may disappear spontaneously.[48, 49]

Tumors of Muscle

Leiomyosarcomas are uncommon malignant neoplasms of soft tissues, primarily affecting adults[52] (Fig. 85–13*A*, *B*). *Leiomyomas*, the benign counterpart, can be found in the skin and subcutaneous tissue[53] (Fig. 85–13C). They arise at variable sites, are single or multiple, and may calcify, usually in association with necrosis of part of the tumor.[290]

Rhabdomyosarcoma can develop in a child or adult. In the pediatric age group, the tumors (juvenile rhabdomyosarcoma, embryonal rhabdomyosarcoma) predominate in the head, neck, and urogenital tract, and affect both boys and girls.[20, 54-57, 279] On radiographic examination, soft tissue masses, which rarely calcify or invade neighboring bone, are noted (Fig. 85–14). Skeletal metastasis can resemble neuroblastoma.[58] In adult rhabdomyosarcoma, many of the lesions are located in the deeper tissues of the extremities and torso, and few are found in the head and neck.

The *rhabdomyoma* is an extremely rare benign tumor composed of striated muscle cells.[20] In most cases, it is observed in the face and neck, although a special variety occurs in the heart. The *myoblastoma* (granular cell tumor) is a growth of mesenchymal origin that can be benign or malignant, arising in striated muscle, skin, mucous membranes, alimentary tract, and many other places.[20, 59, 60]

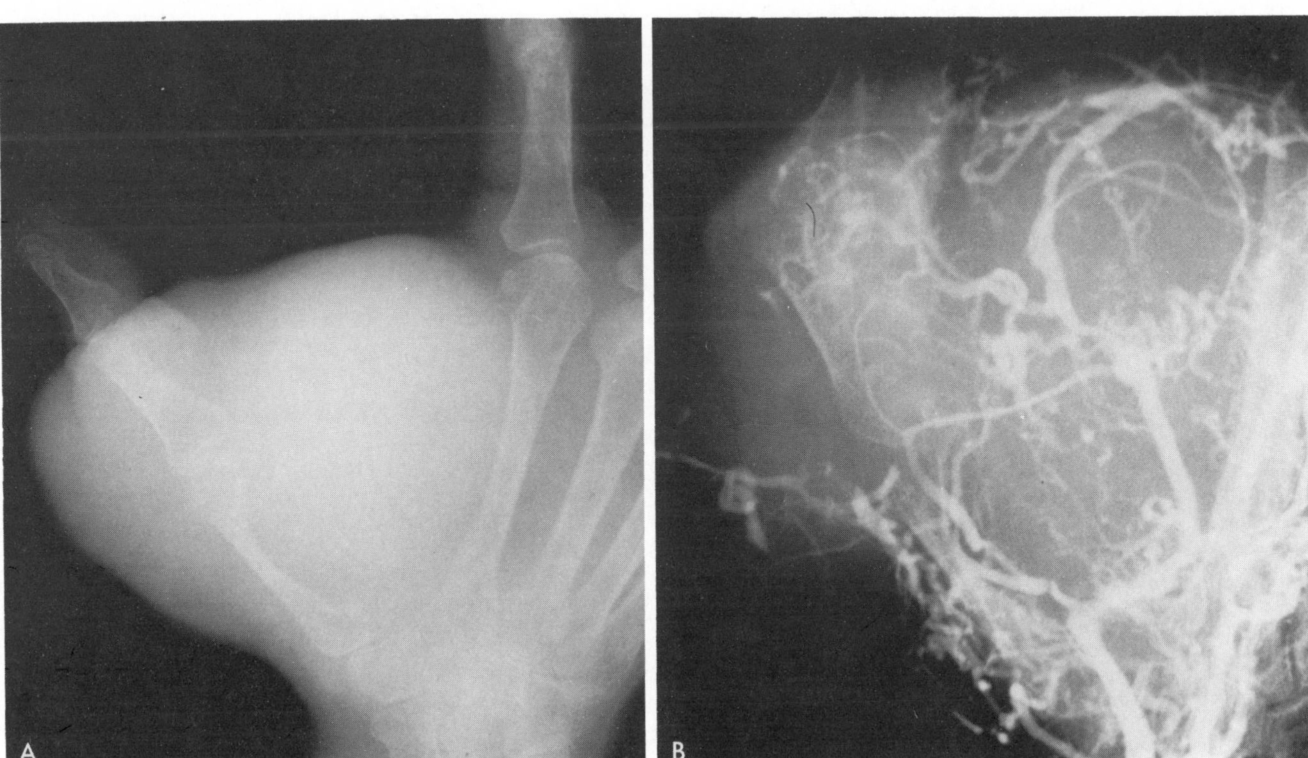

Figure 85–13. *Leiomyosarcoma and leiomyoma.*

A, B *Leiomyosarcoma. A 56 year old woman presented with a growing soft tissue mass in her hand and a pathologic fracture of the left femur. Observe the lobulated soft tissue mass in the thenar space, with pressure erosion of the first and second metacarpals and proximal phalanx of the thumb. The angiogram reveals irregular tumor vessels.* (**A, B,** *Courtesy of Dr. T. Staple, Memorial Hospital, Long Beach, California.*)

Illustration continued on the following page

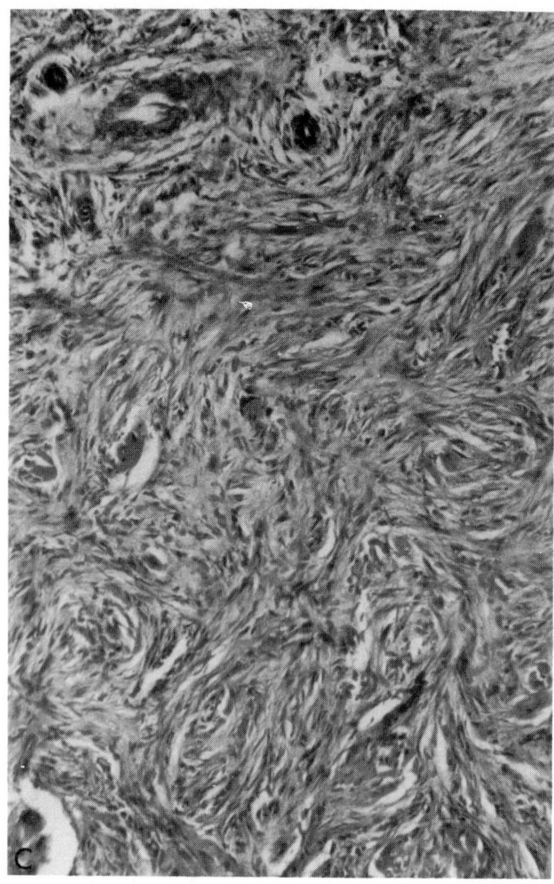

Figure 85–13. Continued

C *Leiomyoma. This 20 year old woman developed a mass on her back. Note the broad intertwining bands of spindled, swollen muscle cells admixed with collagenous fibers (trichrome stain, 215×).*

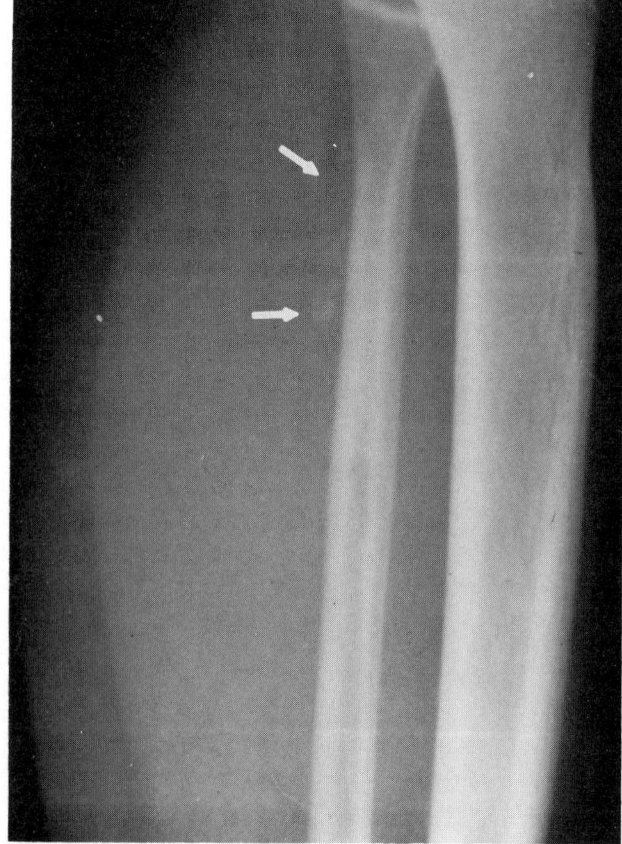

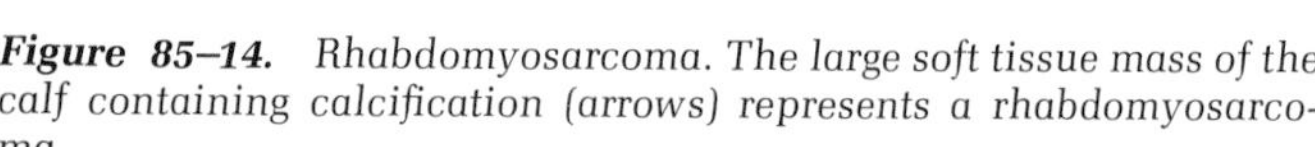

Figure 85–14. *Rhabdomyosarcoma. The large soft tissue mass of the calf containing calcification (arrows) represents a rhabdomyosarcoma.*

Myxomatoses

Neoplastic and non-neoplastic proliferation of myxoid tissue can be seen. The *ganglion* represents a cystic tumor-like lesion that is usually attached to a tendon sheath, particularly in the hands, wrists, and feet[20] (Fig. 85–15). It also arises from tendons, muscles, and semilunar cartilages. Unilocular or multilocular cystic swellings are observed, although their exact pathogenesis is not clear.[61] Synovial herniation and tissue degeneration are two suggested mechanisms for their development. Radiographic evaluation may reveal a soft tissue mass, surface bony resorption, and periosteal new bone formation, and arthrography or tenography may outline the communication of the mass with the underlying articular or tendinous structure.

The *myxoma* is a rare connective tissue tumor that may appear at any age.[62] It demonstrates an invasive manner of growth, particularly within striated muscle, and can recur[63] (Fig. 85–16). Solitary lesions of soft tissue outnumber multiple lesions. Rarely, they may calcify.[64] Myxomas of bone are almost exclusively limited to the jaws. However, multiple soft tissue myxomas have been reported in association with fibrous dysplasia of the adjacent bone.[65] The *myxosarcoma* is a rare malignant counterpart of the myxoma.

Tumors of Histiocytic Origin

Recent attention has been directed toward the soft tissue tumors dominated by the histiocyte.[66-73] A variety of malignant types has been recorded (*atypical fibrous histiocytoma, malignant histiocytoma, malignant fibrous histiocytoma,* and *epithelioid sarcoma*),[66, 71-73] which arise from the superficial or deep soft tissues in patients of all ages. The thigh and the extremities are common sites of involvement. Osseous invasion is seen. Local recurrence and metastases can be encountered.[292] An inflammatory type, the *inflammatory fibrous histiocytoma*, also reveals an aggressive and frequently lethal nature. A more benign variety, the *fibrous histiocytoma*, occurs in adults and children, and can lead to painful soft tissue masses, even in the fingers and toes[69, 70] (Fig. 85–17).

Xanthomatoses

Xanthomatoses consist of a group of tumor-like proliferations characterized by the presence of a variable number of foam cells.[20] Some of the tumors are associated with metabolic and endocrine disorders, such as hypercholesterolemia and diabetes mellitus[74-77] (see Chapter 57). Many varieties are

Text continued on page 3124

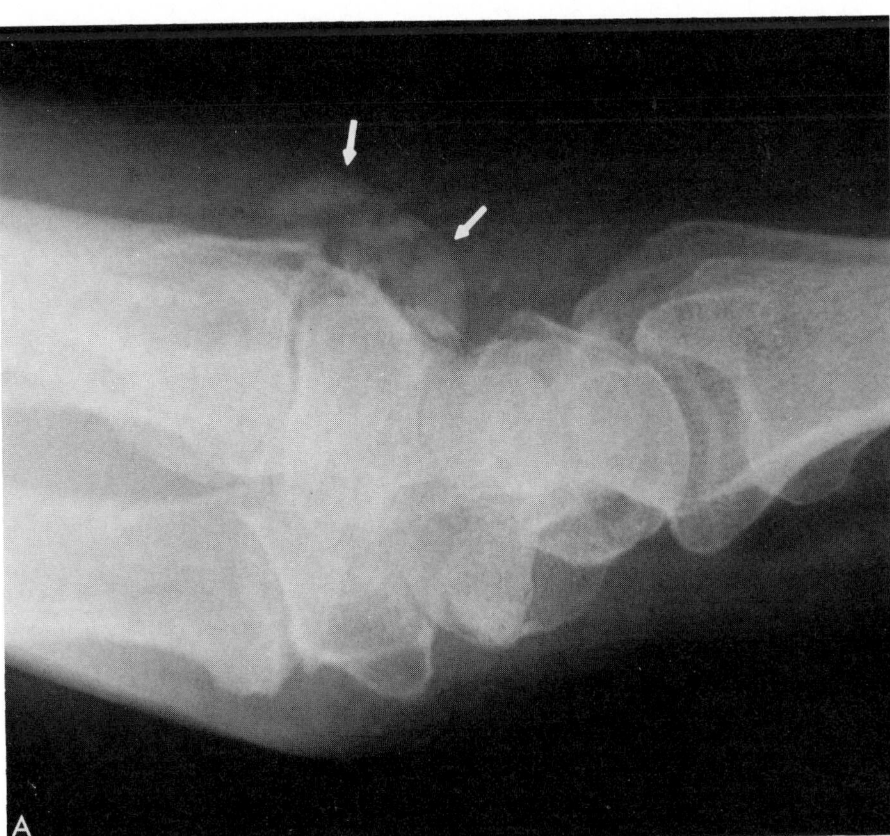

Figure 85–15. *Ganglion.*
A *An unusual example of a calcified ganglion on the dorsum of the hand (arrows) is shown.*

Illustration continued on the following page

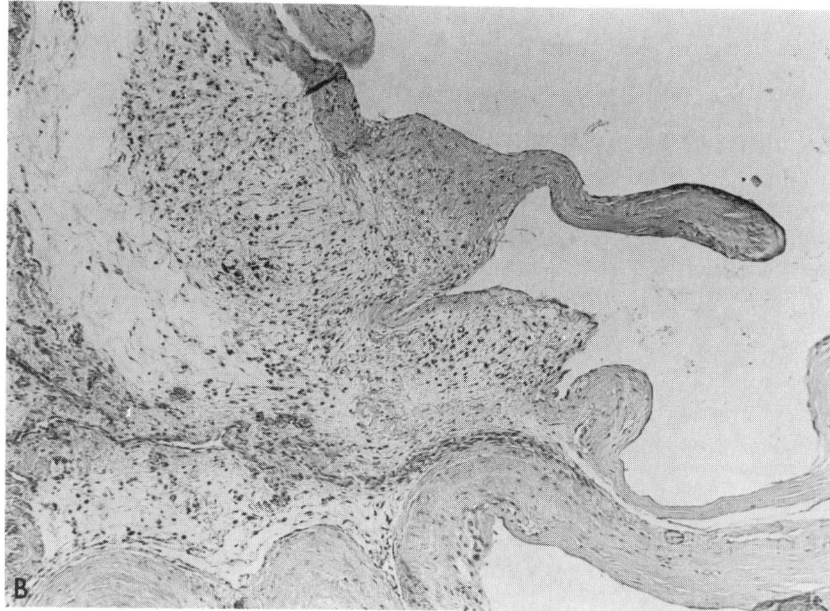

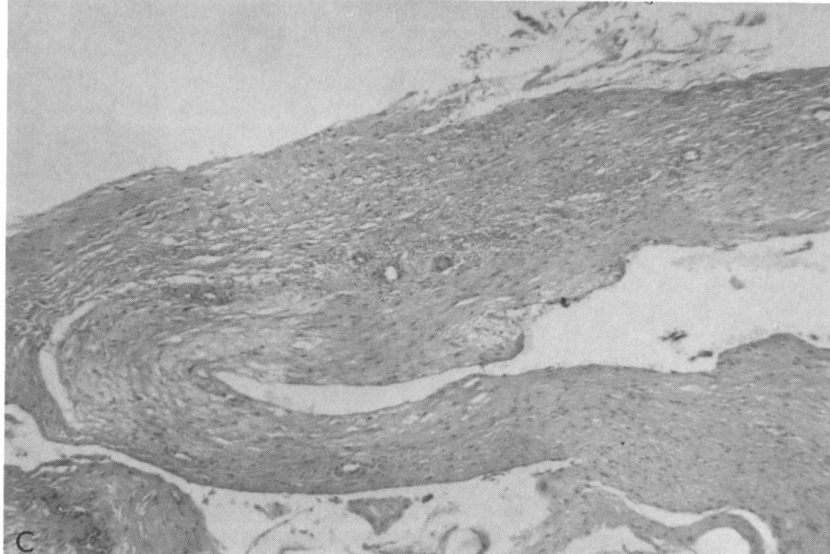

Figure 85–15. Continued

B *A photomicrograph (80×) reveals the cystic wall of a ganglion, consisting of adipose and fibrous tissue. The surface layer is composed of flat lining cells.*

C *In a 64 year old woman with a ganglion arising from a tendon sheath of the left index finger, note extensive myxoid degeneration, clefting, and cyst formation with some fibrin exudation (200×).*

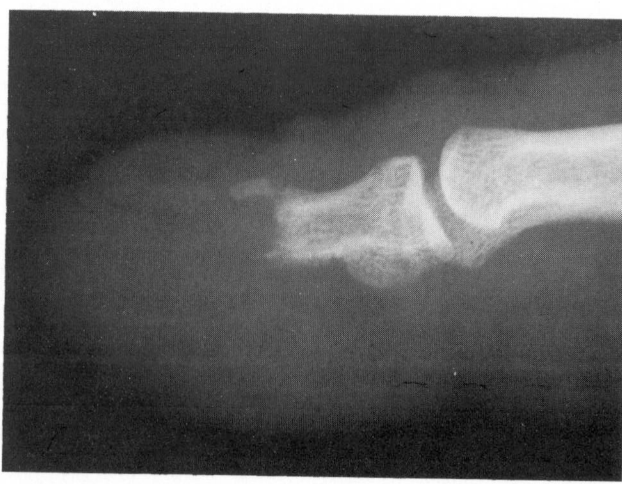

Figure 85–16. *Fibromyxoma. The soft tissue tumor invading the phalangeal tuft contained fibrous and myxomatous tissue on histologic evaluation.*

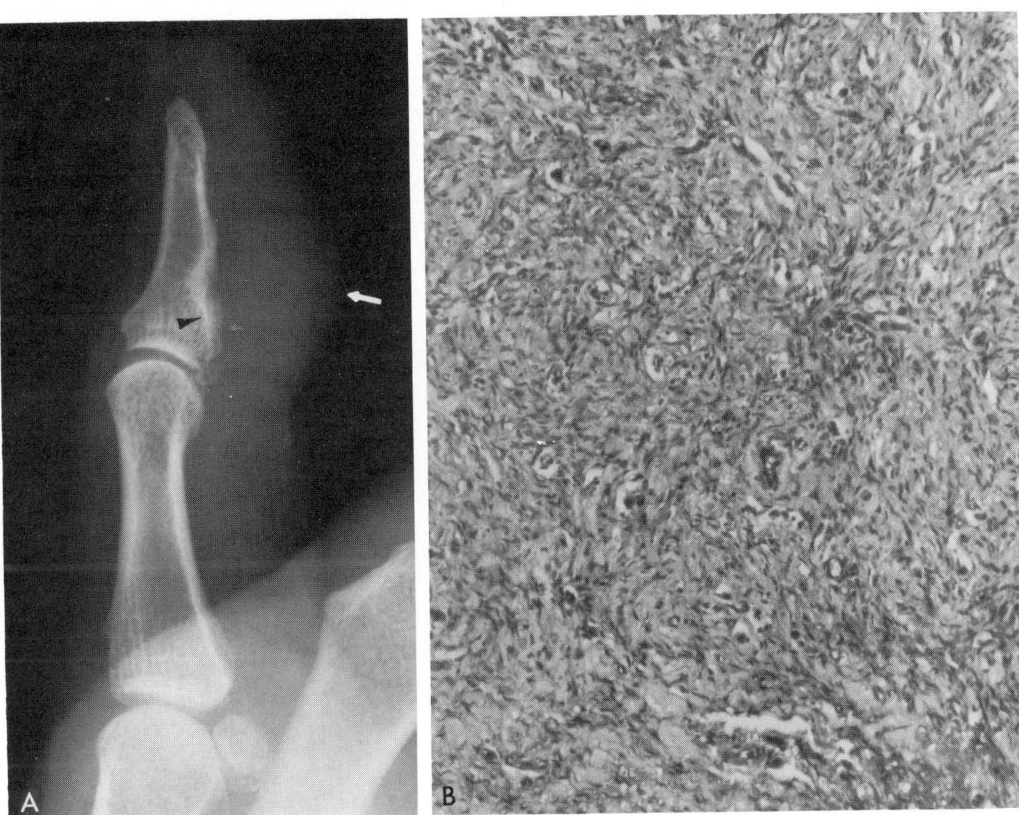

Figure 85–17. Fibrous histiocytoma.

A *This 44 year old woman had developed a mass on her thumb over a 1 year period. Biopsy revealed a fibrous histiocytoma. Note the soft tissue mass on the volar surface of the thumb (arrow), with underlying periosteal bone formation (arrowhead).*

B *Histologic examination of a fibrous histiocytoma of the skin reveals bundles of collagen arranged in multiple directions with entrapped fat. The nuclei of the connective tissue cells are small and spindly, and the cells have relatively sparse cytoplasm (215×).*

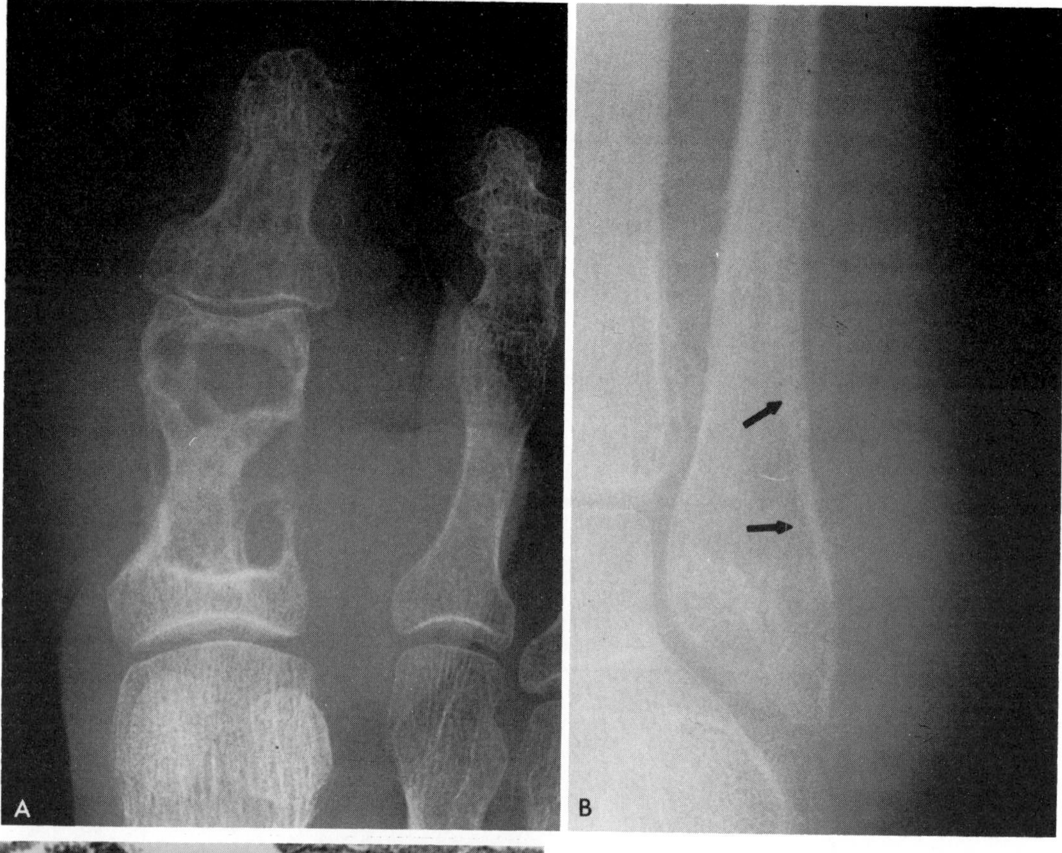

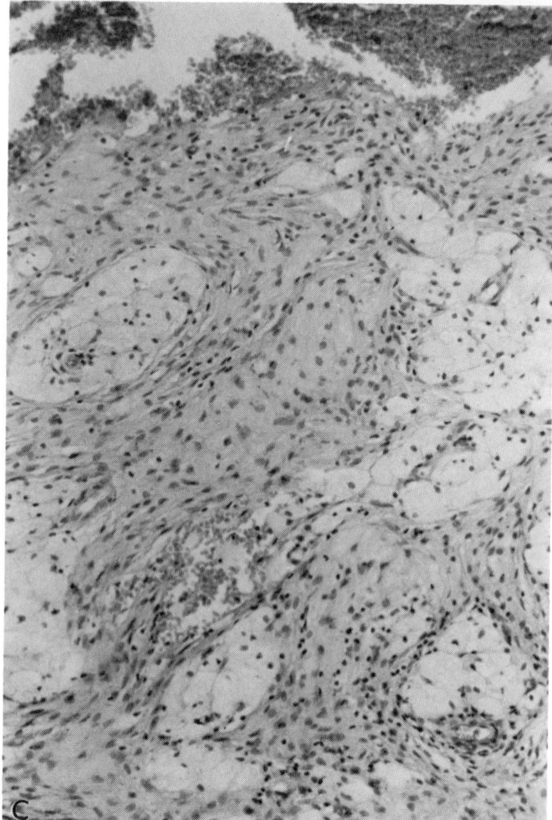

Figure 85–18. *Xanthoma.*

A *In this patient with cerebrotendinous xanthomatosis, note the large soft tissue mass with invasion of the proximal phalanx of the great toe.*

B *Tendinous xanthomatous deposits have produced lobulated swelling of the lateral aspect of the ankle, with resorption and erosion of the underlying fibula (arrows).*

C *Xanthomatous change, related to old hemorrhage, is revealed on this photomicrograph (200×).*

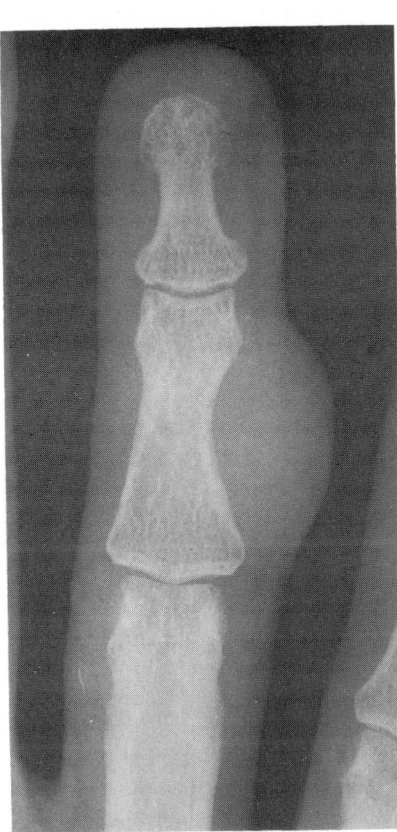

Figure 85–19. Fibrous xanthoma. A soft tissue mass adjacent to the middle phalanx has produced erosion of the adjacent bone. This pattern of bony resorption is indicative of pressure atrophy and is not a sign of malignancy.

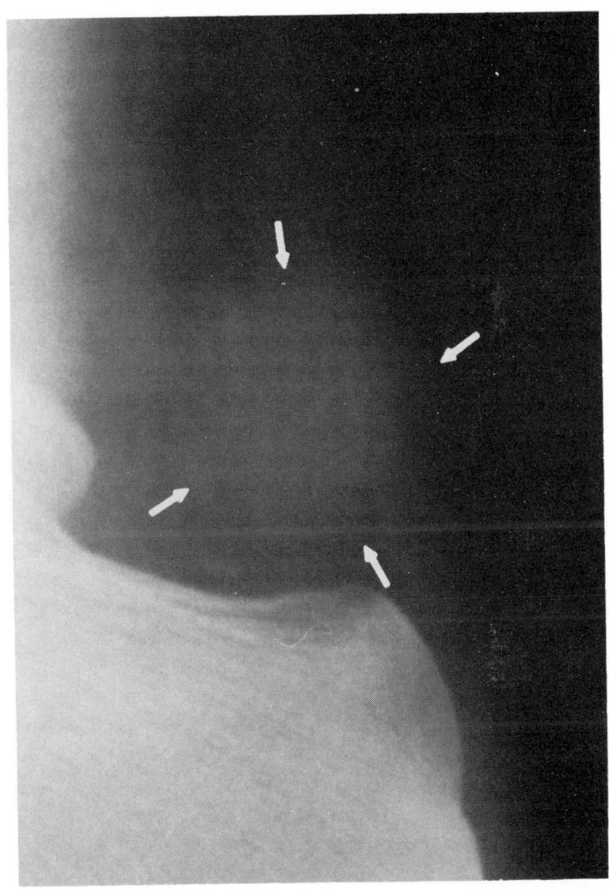

Figure 85–20. Sclerosing hemangioma. Observe the nodular soft tissue mass adjacent to the Achilles tendon (arrows).

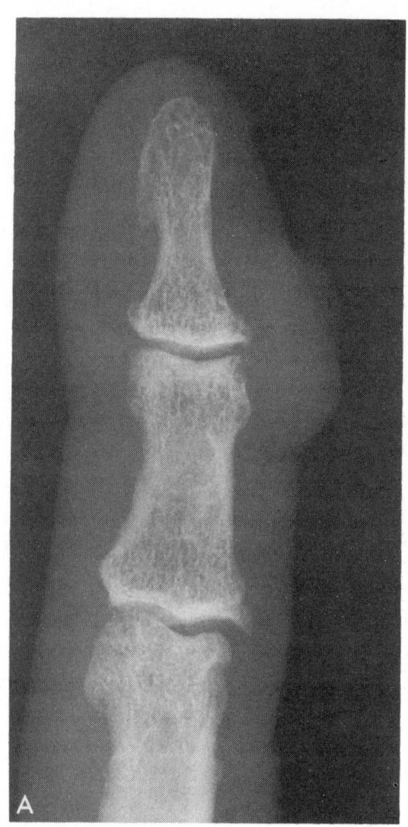

Figure 85–21. *Giant cell tumor of tendon sheath.*

A *The soft tissue mass about the distal interphalangeal joint in this 50 year old man represents a giant cell tumor of the tendon sheath.*

Illustration continued on the opposite page

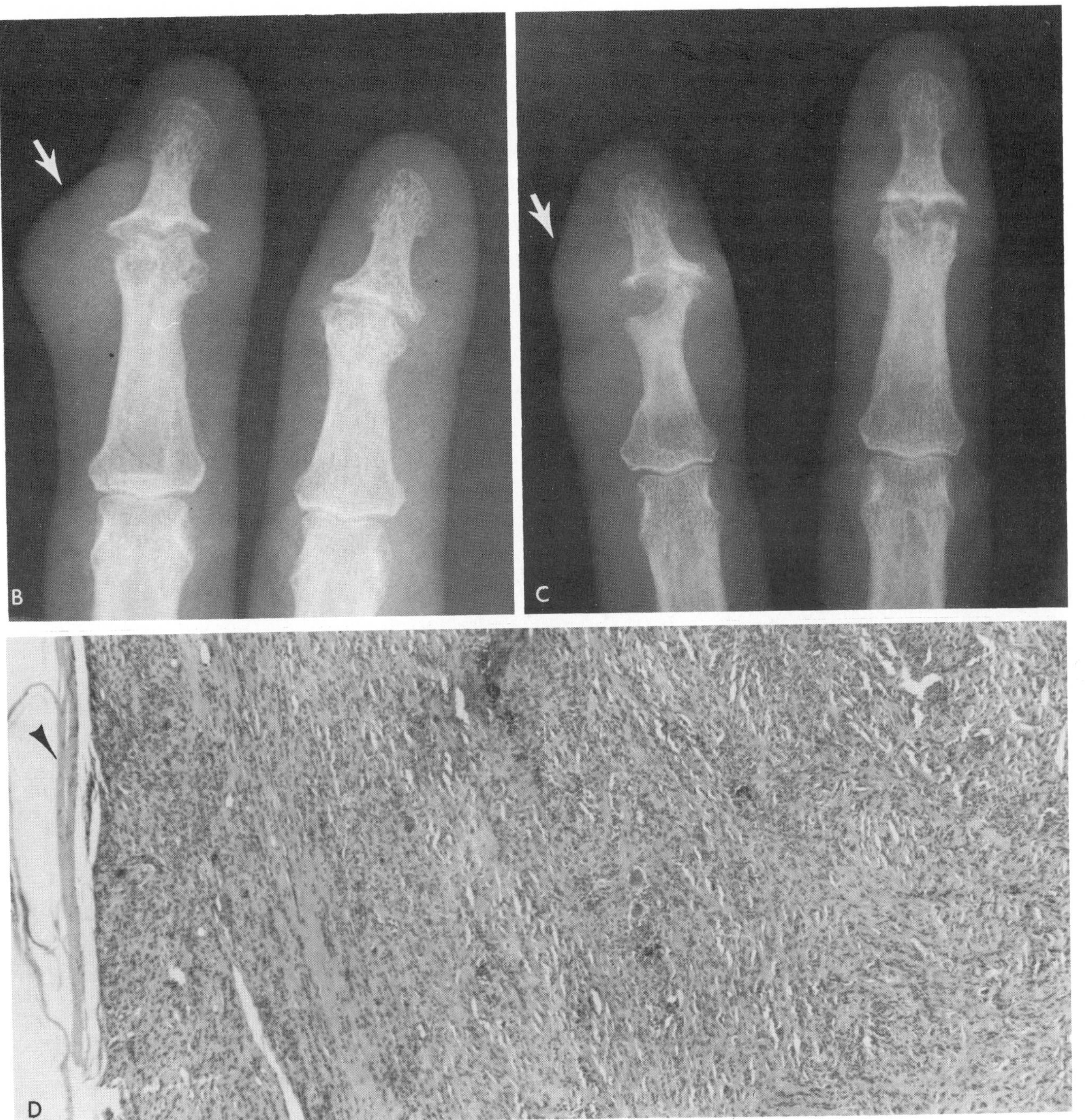

Figure 85–21. Continued

B, C *In a 55 year old woman with a 2 year history of pain and gradual swelling of the fingers, soft tissue masses (arrow) can be identified about two distal interphalangeal joints. Underlying inflammatory osteoarthritis of these articulations is evident, and the combination of findings would suggest that the masses represent mucous cysts. Biopsy of the affected joints demonstrated the findings of giant cell tumor of the tendon sheath.*

(**B, C,** From Crosby EB, et al: Radiology 122:671, 1977.)

D *A photomicrograph (86×) in a different case reveals a tendon capsule (arrowhead) with a tumor associated with moderately vascularized stroma, rather plump spindle-shaped or ovoid cells, and multinucleated giant cells.*

recognized (Fig. 85–18). *Tendinous xanthomas* are common about the fingers, heel, elbow, and knee, where they may erode subjacent bone. Calcification appears in 20 to 25 per cent of cases. A *fibrous xanthoma* (xanthofibroma) represents a small thickening of the corium covered by an intact epidermis (Fig. 85–19). Other types include *dermatofibrosarcoma protuberans*, located in the skin and deeper tissues, which may grow to considerable size, *sclerosing hemangioma*, which is a vascular lesion frequently found in the skin (Fig. 85–20), and *giant cell tumor of the tendon sheath*, which is detected in the hands and feet, attached to tendons, tendon sheaths, and fibrous capsules[291] (Fig. 85–21) (see Chapter 74). Rarely, *intraosseous xanthomas* are recognized producing nonspecific, well-defined radiolucent lesions. Malignant counterparts include *xanthosarcoma* and *fibrous xanthosarcoma* (Fig. 85–22).

Angiomatoses

Angiomatoses are classified according to their tissue composition.[20] A *capillary hemangioma* is composed solely of capillaries. If the capillaries are widely dilated, the tumor is called a *cavernous hemangioma*. If a vascular tumor has thicker walls and contains smooth muscle cells, it is called a *venous hemangioma*. Capillary hemangiomas with prominent proliferation of the endothelial layer are called *benign hemangioendotheliomas*, whereas

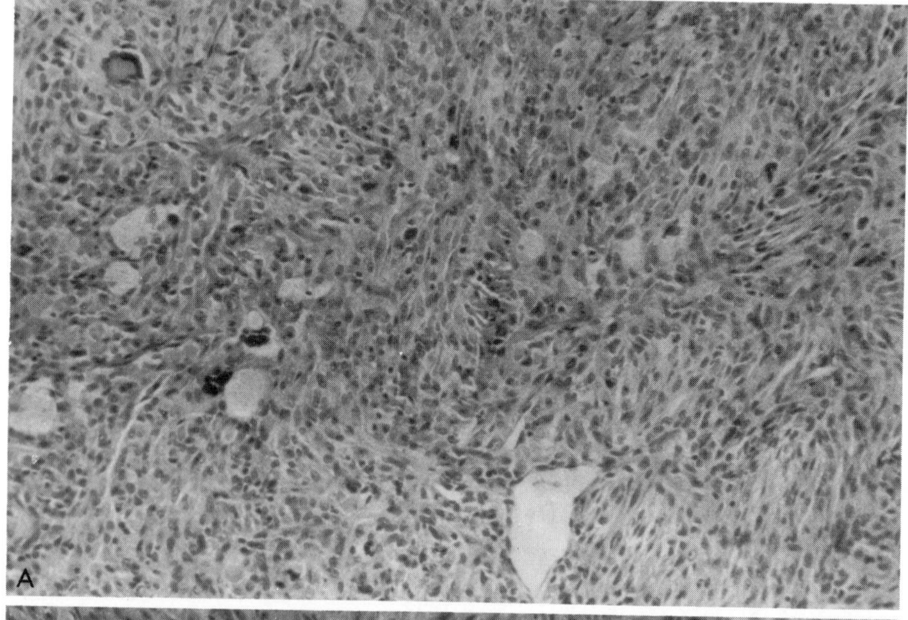

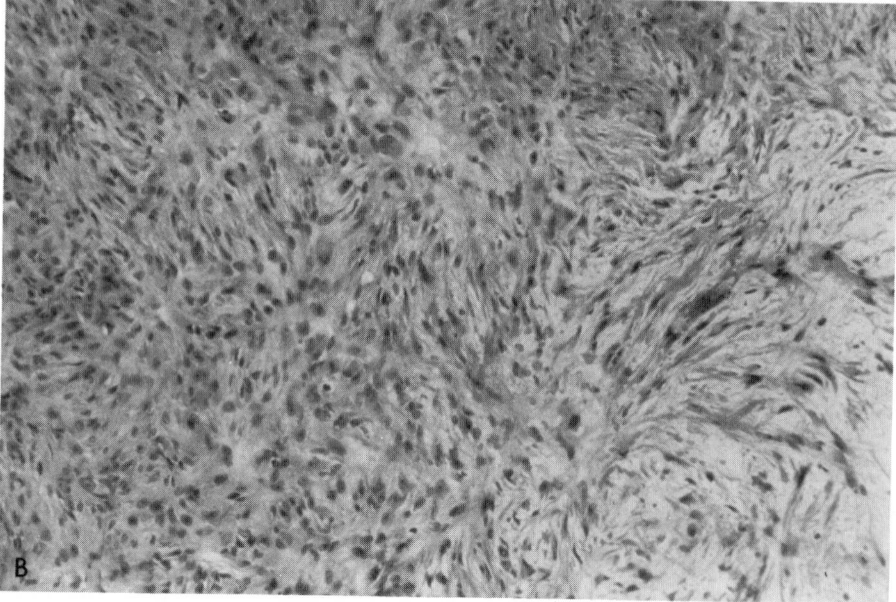

Figure 85–22. *Fibrous xanthosarcoma. A 59 year old man developed a mass in his left foot.*

A *The tumor consists of a variegated pattern of cells, some of which are plump or spindly, containing nuclei varying from round to oval in shape. Giant cells are seen, which reveal a peripheral rim of compact nuclei. Many large foam cells are evident (215×).*

B *In another area, peripheral pseudopod-like extensions radiate into the adjacent areolar tissue (215×).*

those with proliferation of pericytes are *benign hemangiopericytomas*. The most recognized variety of benign hemangiopericytomas is the *glomus tumor*, typically located beneath the fingernails but occasionally noted at other sites as well (Fig. 85–23). Other benign types of angiomatoses are the *cirsoid aneurysm*, a vascular malformation consisting of arterial vessels, the *venous racemose aneurysm*, a malformation consisting of venous structures, *diffuse angiomatosis* due to capillary proliferation, a *lymphangioma*, a proliferation of lymphatic vessels, and *lymphangiopericytomas*.

Radiographs of hemangiomas and related lesions may reveal evidence of soft tissue masses containing circular calcified collections, termed phleboliths; in addition, osseous involvement, overgrowth, and articular abnormalities due to accompanying synovial lesions may be encountered[78-81] (Figs. 85–24 and 85–25) (see Chapter 59). Arteriography may allow precise documentation of the pattern of vascular proliferation.

On the malignant end of the spectrum, angiosarcomatoses are much less frequent. These lesions are classified according to the dominant cell pattern.[20] If

Text continued on page 3130

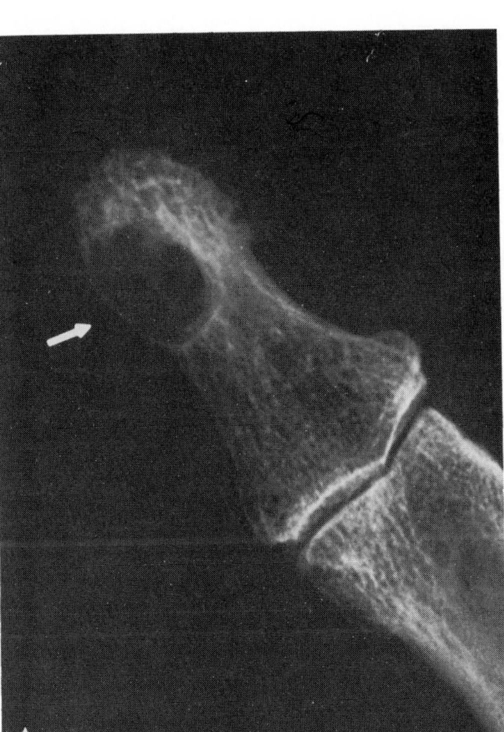

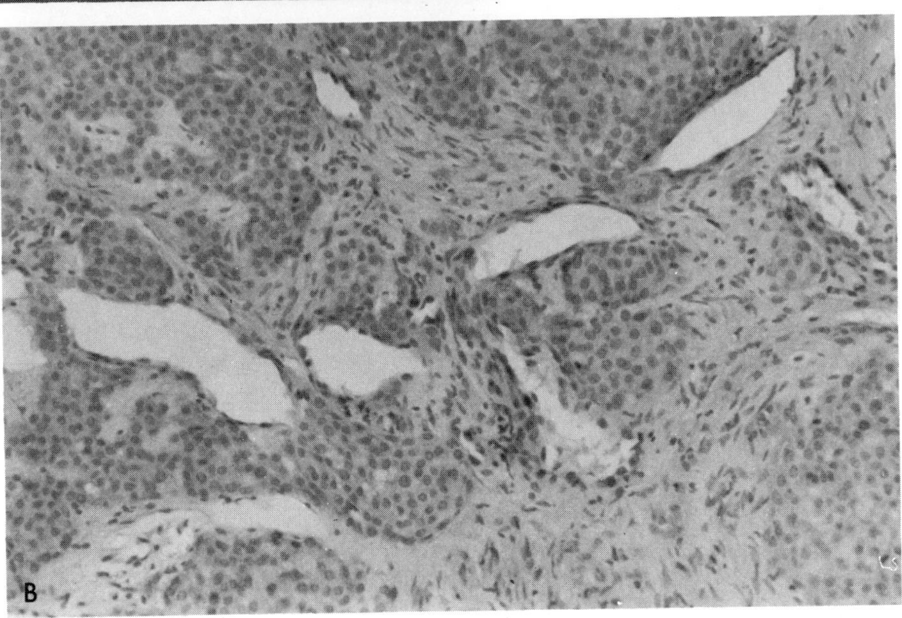

Figure 85–23. Glomus tumor.

A *A well-defined cystic lesion of a terminal tuft is seen (arrow).*

B *A photomicrograph (215×) reveals multiple vascular channels surrounded by irregular extensions of cells with eosinophilic cytoplasm and bland, somewhat monotonous nuclei.*

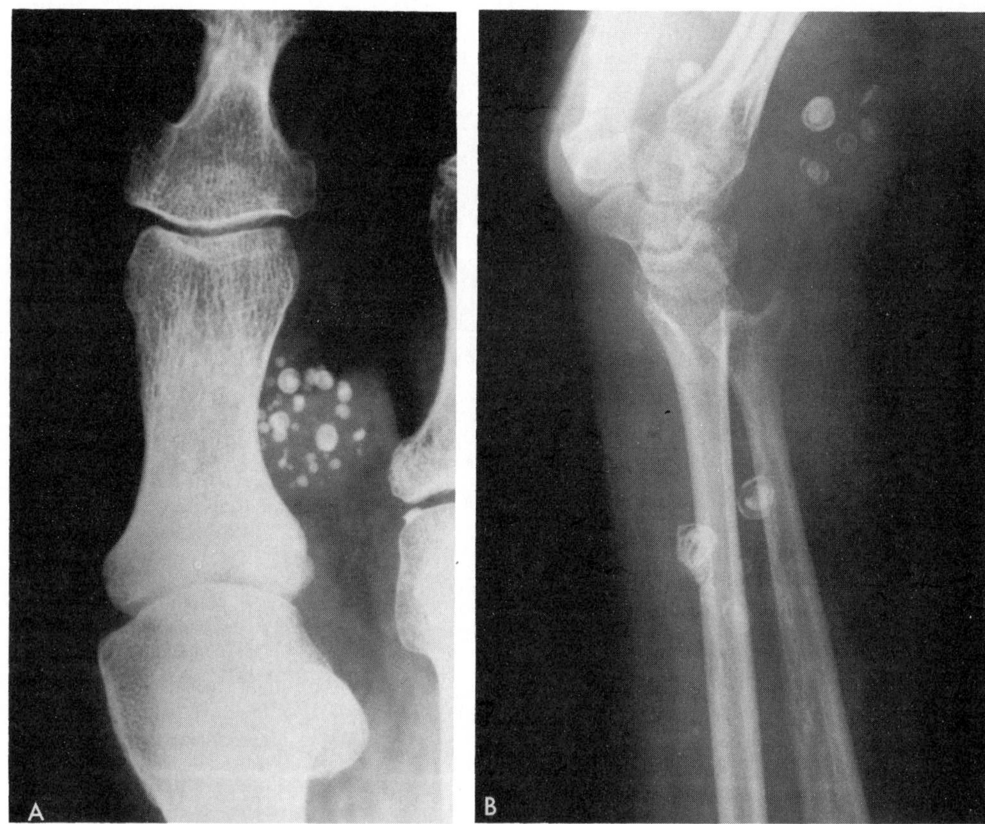

Figure 85–24. *Hemangioma.*

A *Circular calcifications, some of which contain lucent centers, within the mass of the great toe represent phleboliths.*

B *In a different patient, phleboliths of the forearm and hand are associated with soft tissue swelling and osseous involvement of the ulna, characterized by a coarsened trabecular pattern.*

Illustration continued on the opposite page

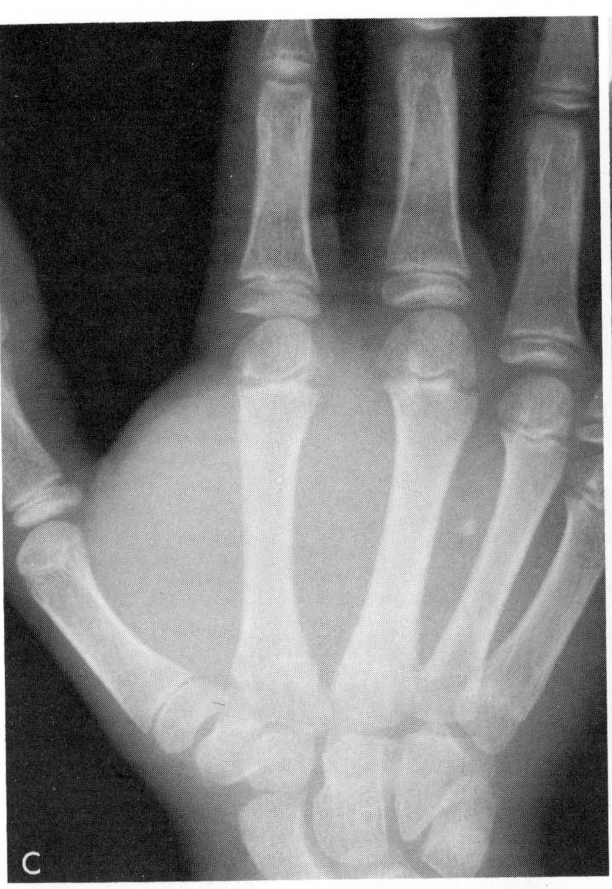

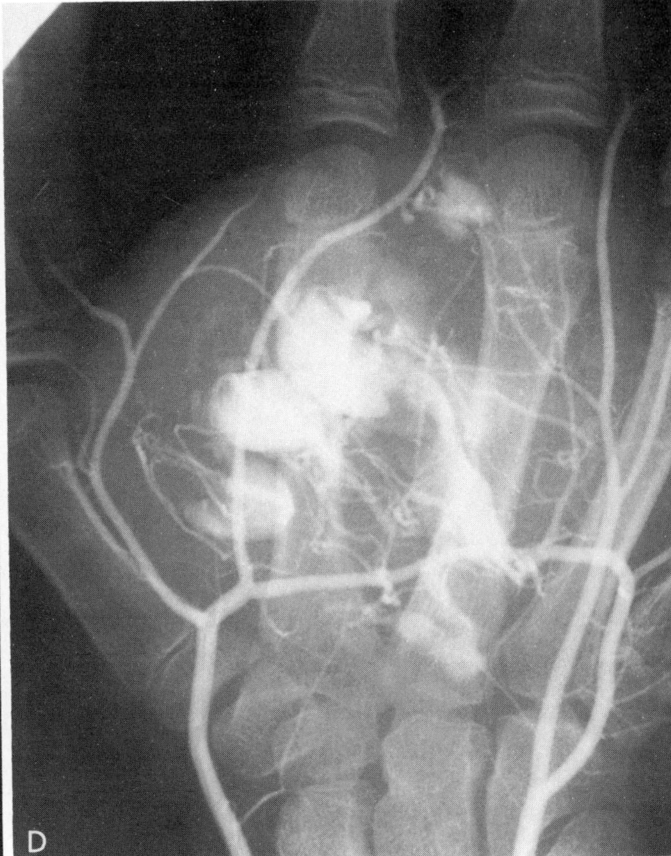

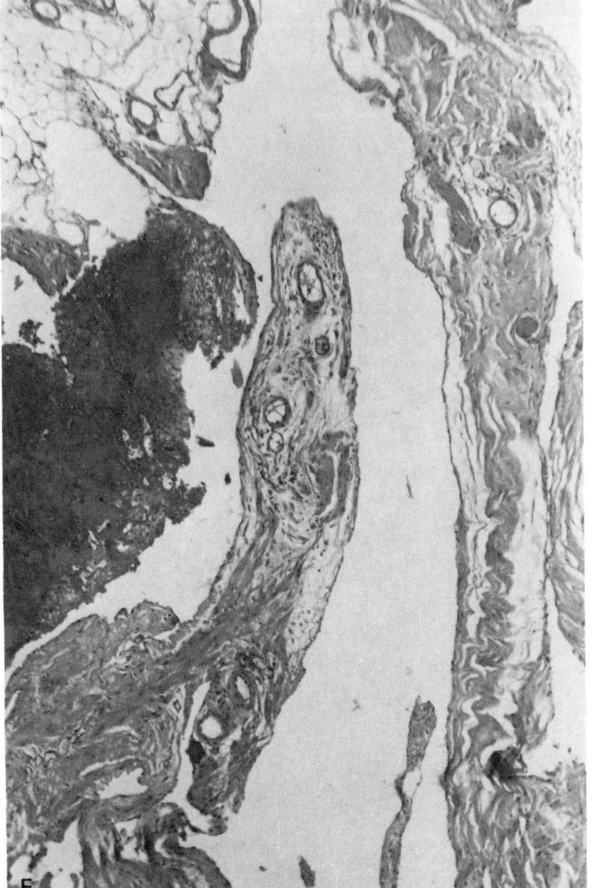

Figure 85–24. Continued

C–E *Cavernous hemangioma. An 11 year old black boy had a 1 year history of gradual swelling of the palm. The mass was soft and nontender. The radiograph* **(C)** *reveals soft tissue swelling of the thenar eminence as well as a phlebolith projected between the third and fouth metacarpals. Brachial arteriography* **(D)** *demonstrates large pools or lakes of contrast medium, which persisted late into the venous phase. A photomicrograph* **(E)** *from a patient with a similar lesion reveals dilated vascular channels and a recent thrombus.*

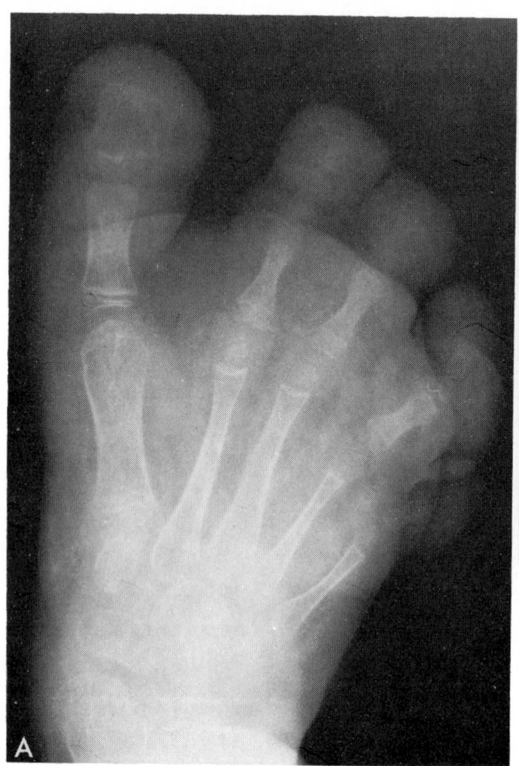

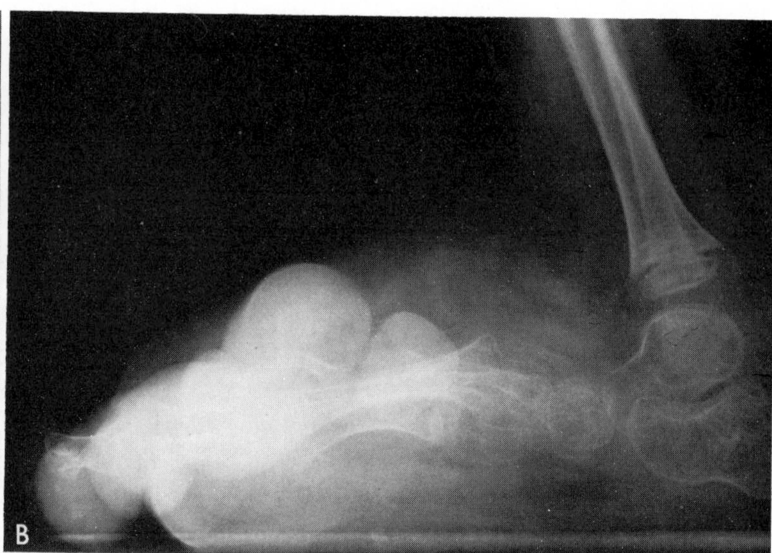

Figure 85–25. Lymphangioma. In this 4 year old boy, diffuse lymphangiomatosis of the tissues of the foot has produced nodular soft tissue enlargement. Osseous deformity is also present, but no phleboliths are apparent.

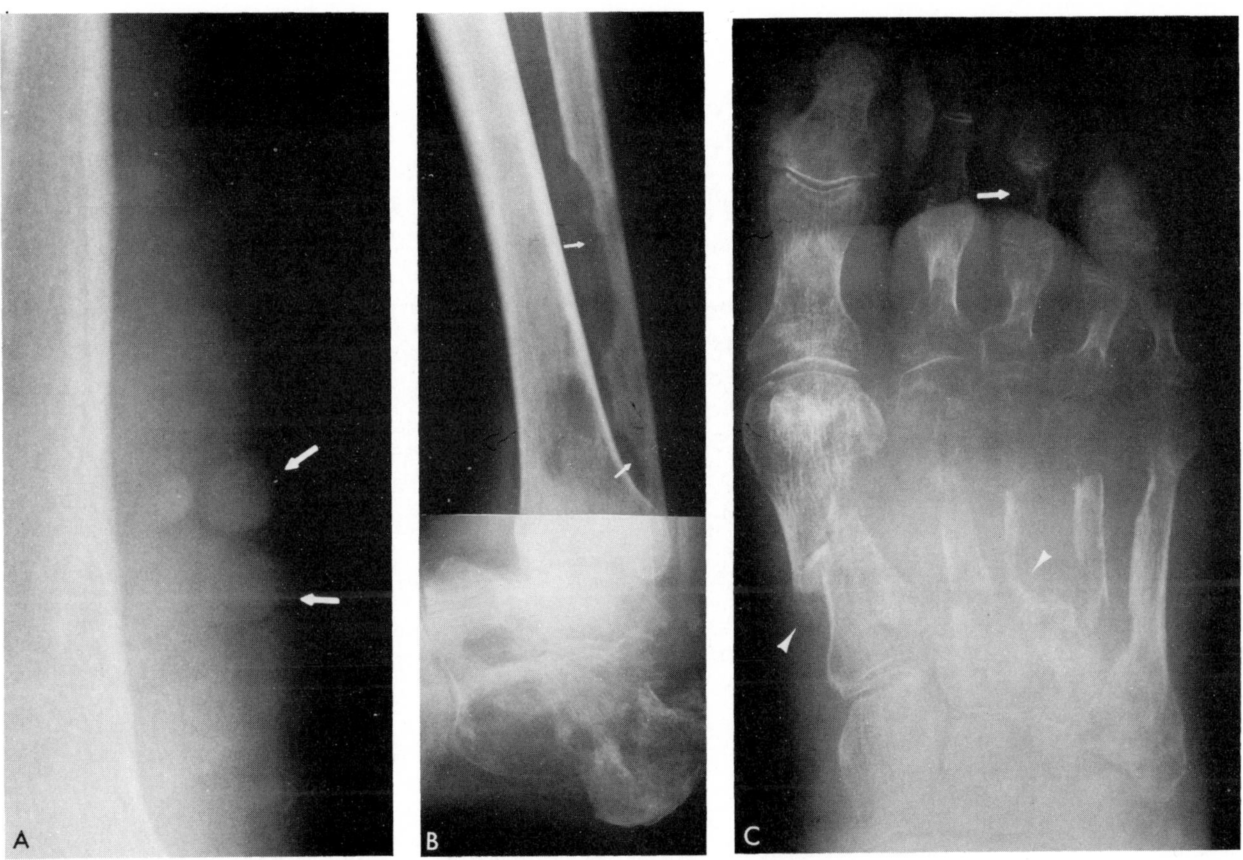

Figure 85–26. *Kaposi's sarcoma.*

A *Nodular lesions of the soft tissues (arrows) are apparent.*

B, C *This 77 year old man with Kaposi's sarcoma reveals lytic destruction of the tibia, fibula, tarsals, metatarsals, and phalanges. Observe the eccentric location of many of the erosions (arrows) and pathologic fractures (arrowheads).* (**B, C,** *Courtesy of Dr. P. Ellenbogen, Presbyterian Hospital, Dallas, Texas.*)

Illustration continued on the following page

endothelial cells predominate, a *malignant hemangioendolithelioma* is present. With pericytic proliferation, a *malignant hemangiopericytoma* is found. A malignant tumor composed of lymphatic endothelioblasts frequently associated with lymphedema is termed a *lymphangiosarcoma* (see Fig. 85–64).

Kaposi's sarcoma is a complex vascular growth consisting of both capillaries and fibrosarcoma-like cells.[82-86] This lesion predominates in adult men, and is especially common in blacks in certain parts of Africa. Cutaneous eruptions or nodules, frequently in the lower extremity, may lead to invasion of underlying bone (Fig. 85–26). Some patients also reveal evidence of malignant lymphoma, lymphatic leukemia, diabetes mellitus, and varicosities. The pathogenesis of Kaposi's sarcoma is not known.[307] Some investigators regard it as a neoplasm, whereas others suggest a vascular or infectious process. The prognosis is guarded; the survival time after diagnosis ranges from 5 to 20 years. Although individual lesions may heal, recurrences are the rule.

Cartilaginous and Osseous Tumors

Soft tissue *chondromas* are rare.[87] The tumors occur predominately in the third and fourth decades

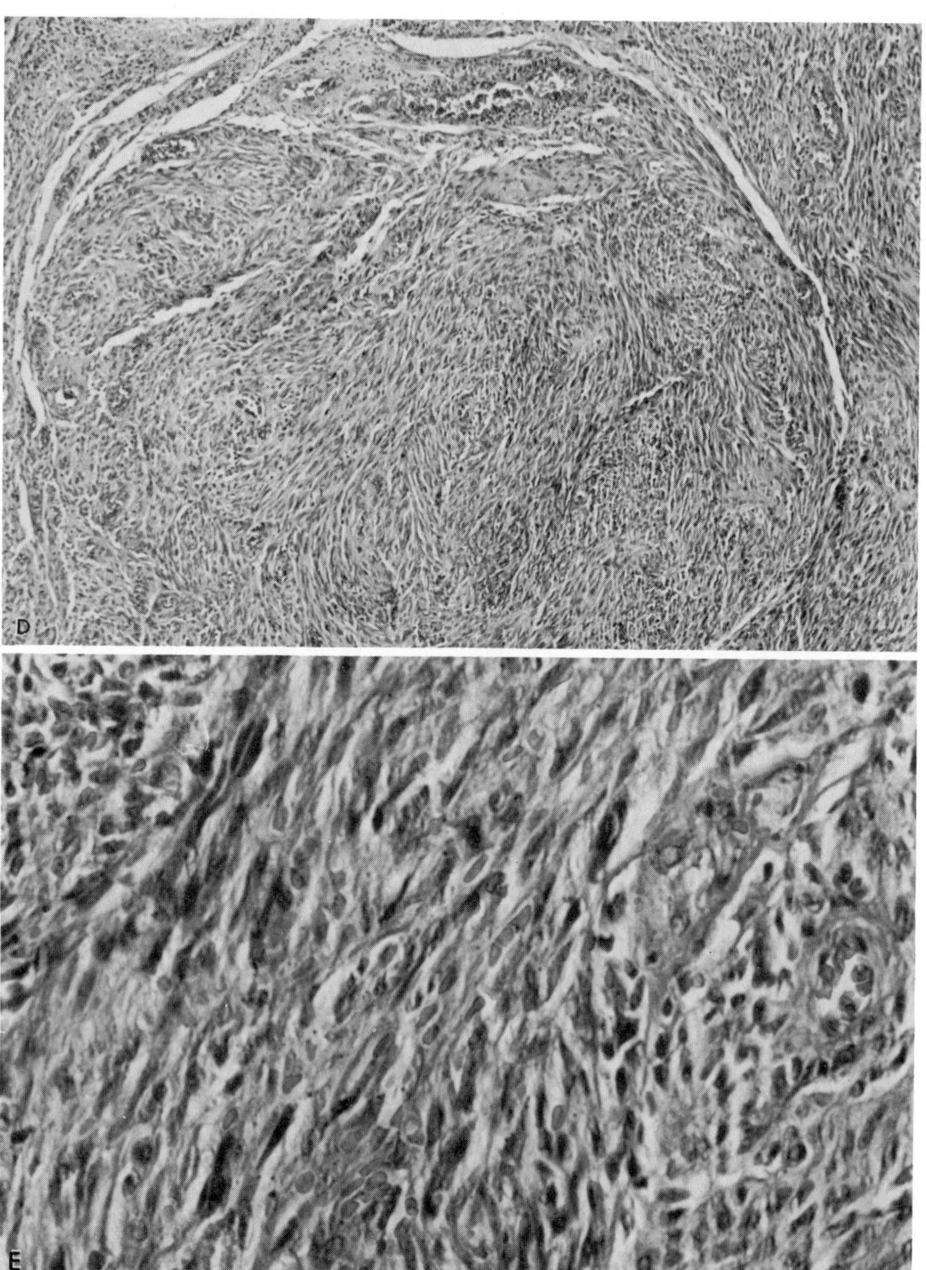

Figure 85–26. Continued
D, E *Photomicrographs (90×, 230×) demonstrate nodular masses composed of whorled spindle cells with occasional slits and vascular clefts. Cellular atypism and hemosiderin pigmentation are noted.*

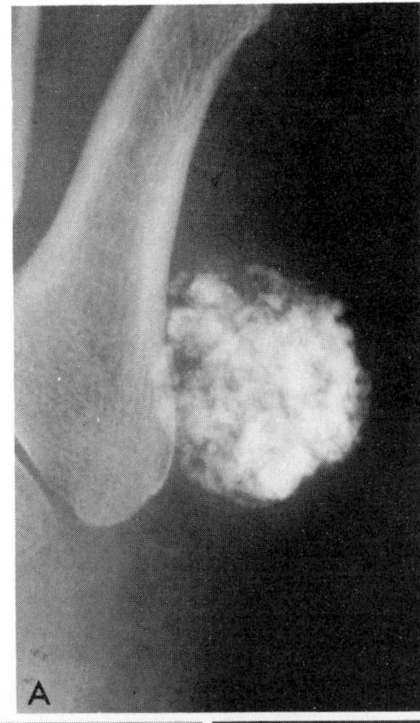

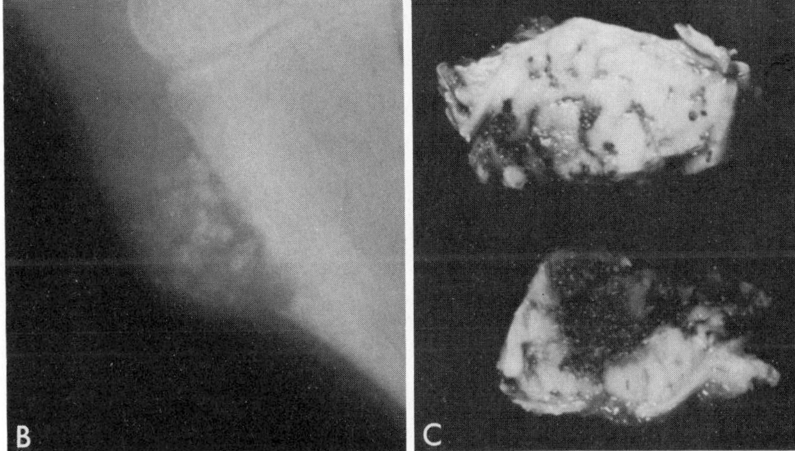

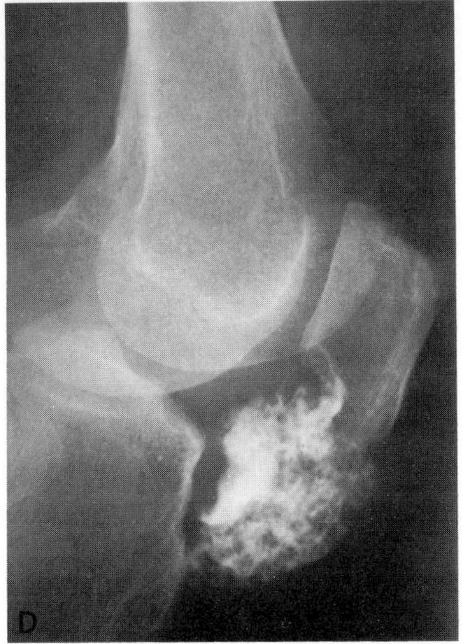

Figure 85–27. *Chondroma.*

A *Soft tissue chondroma. Observe the calcified soft tissue mass adjacent to the fifth metatarsal.*

B, C *Juxtacortical (periosteal) chondroma. This 8 year old boy had a lump below the knee. A radiograph reveals a partially calcified and ossified soft tissue mass in the region of the anterior tibial tubercle. Minimal erosion of the cortex is seen. The pathologic specimen demonstrates a calcified mass, and the diagnosis of a juxtacortical chondroma was established.*

*(**B, C,** From Kirchner SJ, et al: Am J Roentgenol 131:1088, 1978. Copyright 1978, American Roentgen Ray Society.)*

D *Intra-articular chondroma. This 65 year old woman developed knee pain and swelling. A radiograph reveals a large calcified lesion in the infrapatellar fat pad, producing erosion of the patella and tibia. Excision with histologic evaluation documented mature and metaplastic cartilage surrounded by fat and synovium. The consensus favored an intra-articular (intracapsular) chondroma.*

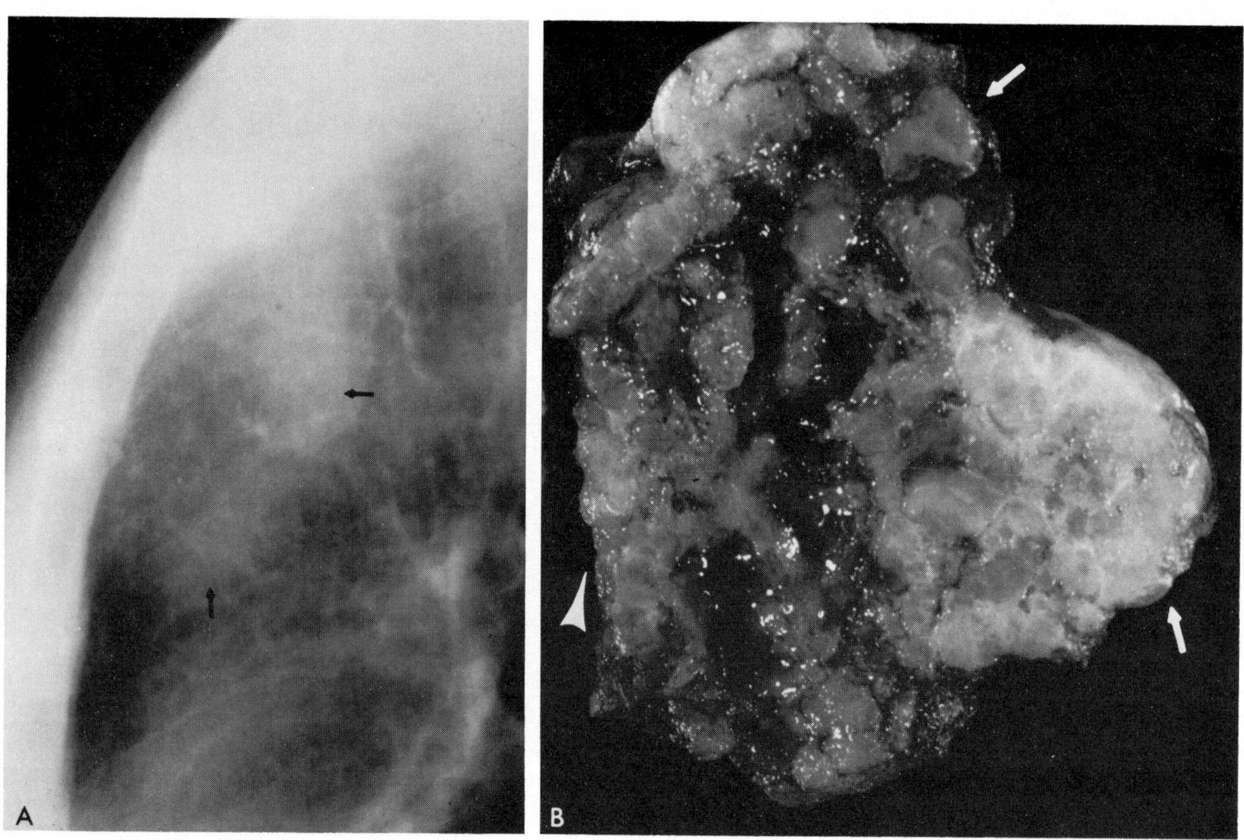

Figure 85–28. *Chondrosarcoma.*

A, B *An anterior mediastinal mass (arrows) containing small calcific foci represents a chondrosarcoma attached to the sternum (arrowhead).*

Illustration continued on the opposite page

of life, especially in the hands and feet. They enlarge slowly and are well-demarcated and lobulated. Radiographs reveal soft tissue masses frequently containing calcification (Fig. 85–27*A*). Subjacent cortical erosion and sclerosis may simulate the findings in a juxtacortical (periosteal) chondroma (Figs. 85–27*B*, *C*). Although local recurrences can be seen, metastasis is not evident, and the prognosis is good. Rarely, chondromas may arise within articulations or in tendon sheaths.[88, 89] The intracapsular chondroma is a rare and debated entity (Fig. 85–27*D*). It may represent a true benign neoplasm of cartilage, and may appear in the knee as a mass inferior to the patella.[281] In this location, the lesion may attach to the meniscus, be located in the infrapatellar fat pad, and produce pain and locking of the joint.[293]

Extraskeletal soft tissue *chondrosarcomas* are also very uncommon.[90-93] These lesions are distinguished from those arising in a bone or in the periosteum and perichondrium. The soft tissues of

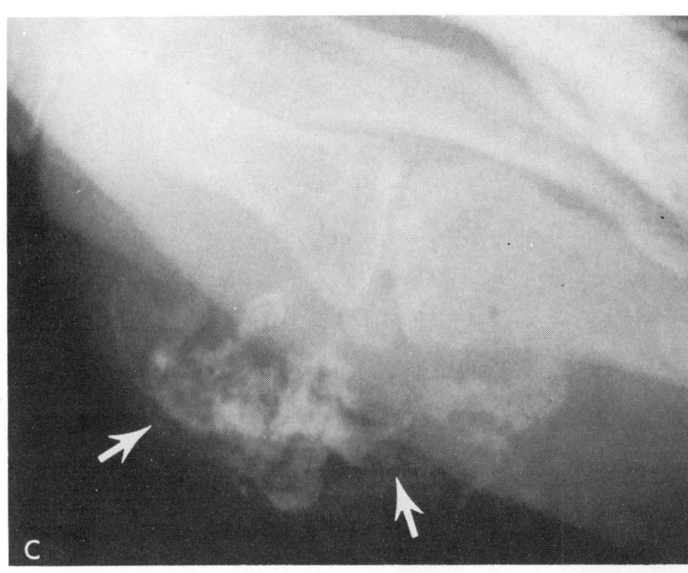

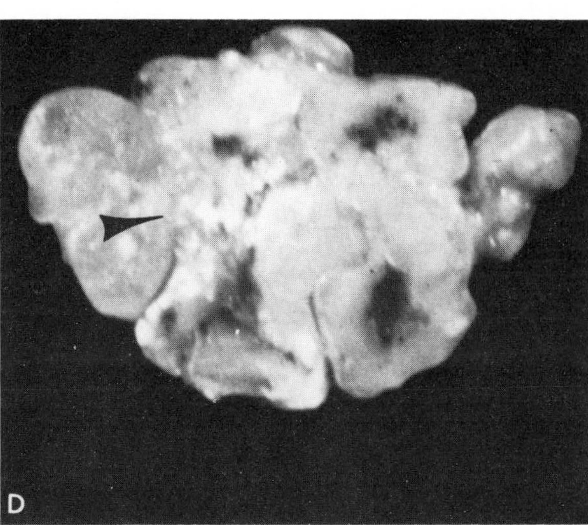

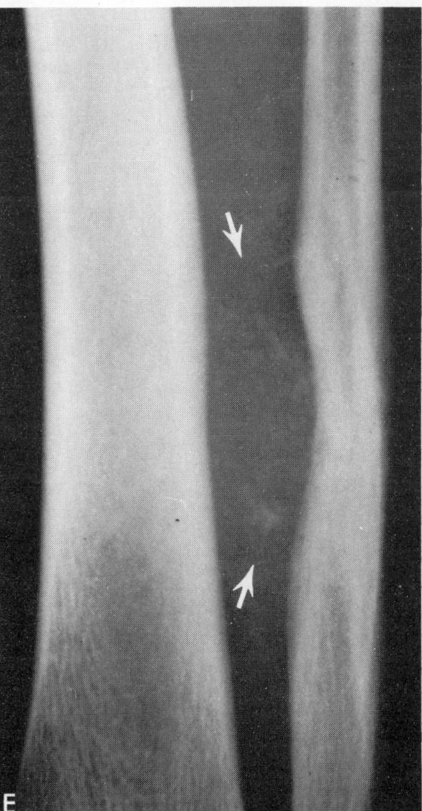

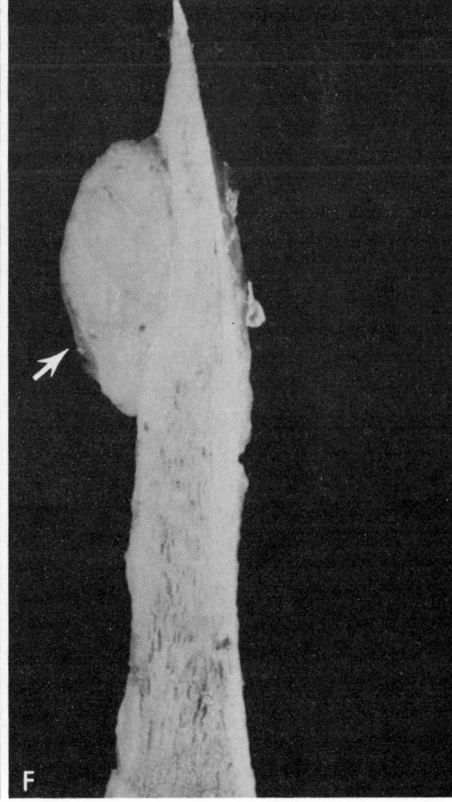

Figure 85–28. Continued

C, D *The lobulated mass on the palmar aspect of the hand (arrows) is a chondrosarcoma. Note the calcifications (arrowhead) in the mass.*

E, F *This 15 year old boy complained of swelling and pain. The radiograph reveals a soft tissue mass with calcification (arrows) between the tibia and fibula, with erosion of both bones. Note buttressing or thickening of the outer aspect of the fibula. A photograph of a longitudinal section of the fibula demonstrates the relationship of the mass to the bone (arrow). The final diagnosis was mesenchymal chondrosarcoma.*

*(***E, F***, Courtesy of Dr. R. Freiberger, Hospital for Special Surgery, New York, New York, and Dr. J. Kaye, Vanderbilt University, Nashville, Tennessee.)*

Illustration continued on the following page

the head and neck, extremities, shoulders, and buttocks are typically affected. Histologic features vary from well-differentiated cartilage proliferation to myxoid or mesenchymal elements.[306] A soft tissue mass with calcification and underlying osseous involvement can be detected on roentgenography (Fig. 85–28). The prognosis is variable; some lesions are highly aggressive, whereas others follow a more protracted course.

Soft tissue *osteogenic sarcomas* are rarely encountered.[94-97] These lesions are distinguished from medullary, periosteal, and parosteal osteogenic sarcomas of bone. They are usually evident in middle-aged and elderly patients, in the deeper tissues of the extremities, thighs, or shoulder region (Fig. 85–29). Patients may relate a history of significant trauma, suggesting to some investigators that the neoplasms arise in foci of myositis ossificans. Radiographically, a soft tissue mass with ossification can be seen. On histologic examination, the osteogenic sarcoma resembles the lesions that are encountered in bones.[294] The malignant potential of these tumors appears to be high.

Soft tissue neoplasms containing ossific and

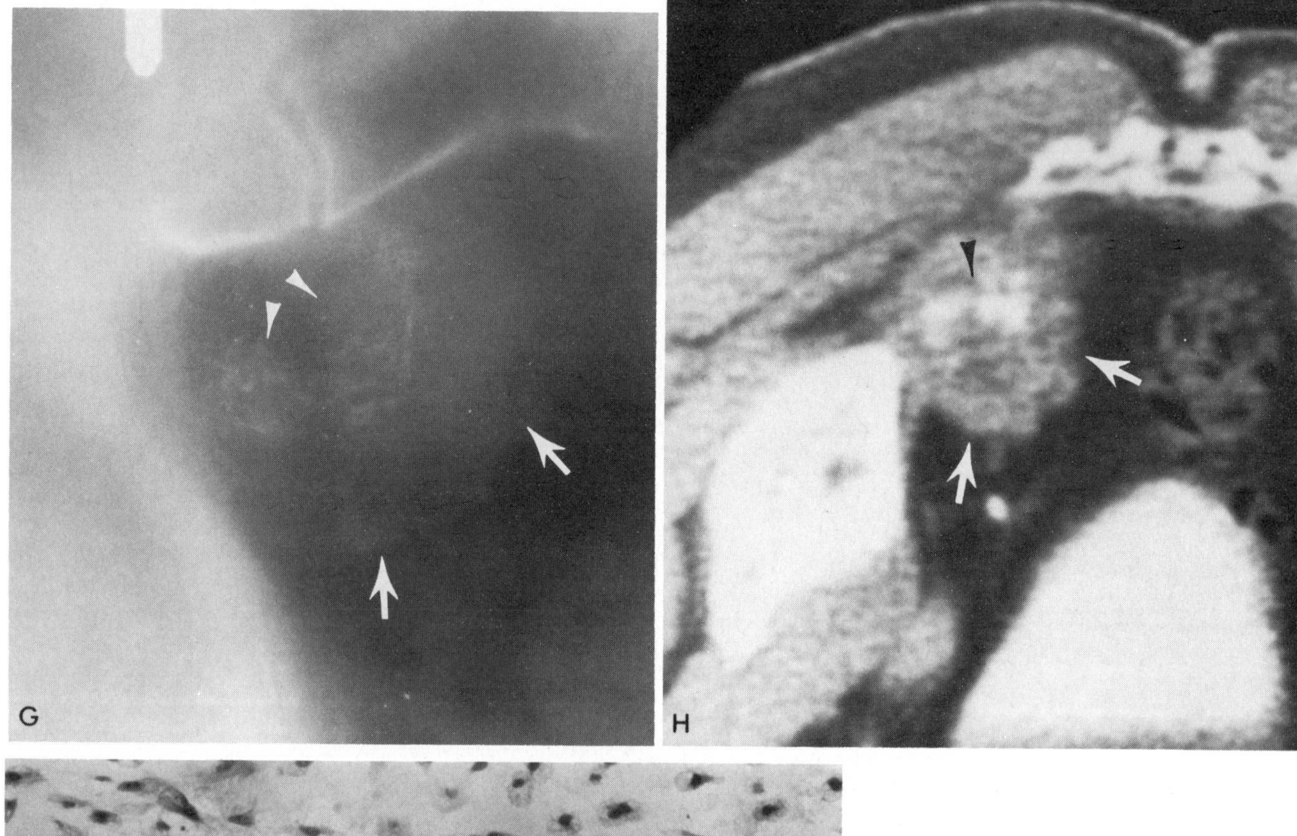

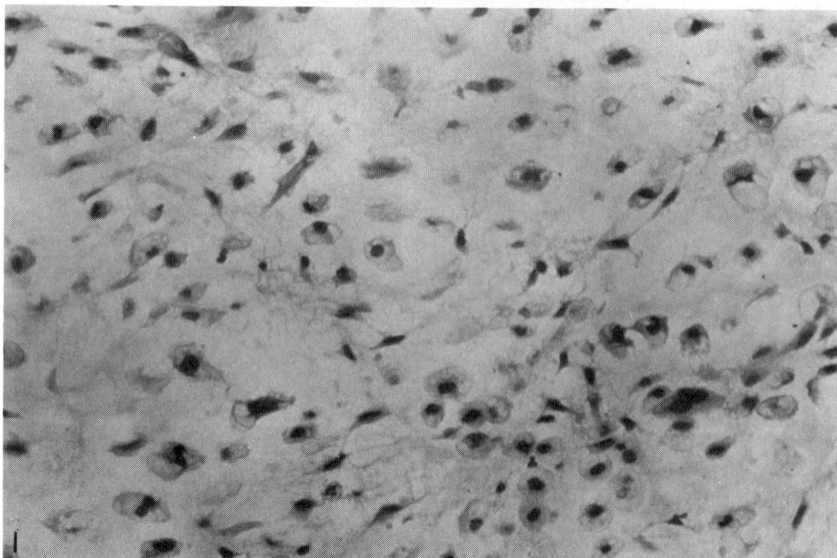

Figure 85–28. Continued

G, H *In this 67 year old man, a frontal tomogram of the pelvis reveals a soft tissue mass (arrows) with calcification (arrowheads) just below the right sacroiliac joint. The computed tomogram at a level through the mass shows the tumor (arrows) and calcification (arrowhead).*

*(**G, F,** Courtesy of Dr. V. Vint, Scripps Clinic, LaJolla, California.)*

I *A photomicrograph (430×) of a typical chondrosarcoma shows pleomorphic immature cartilage cells lying in a myxoid matrix. Binucleated cells and cells with giant nuclei are seen.*

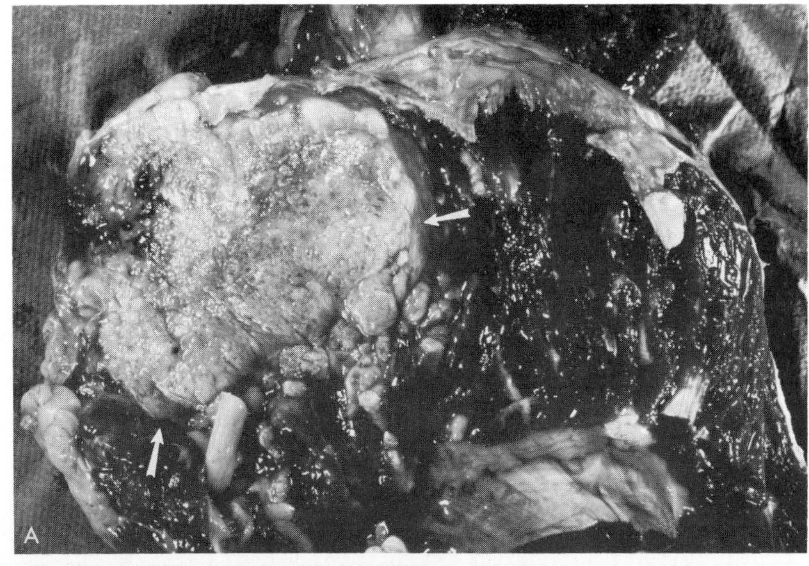

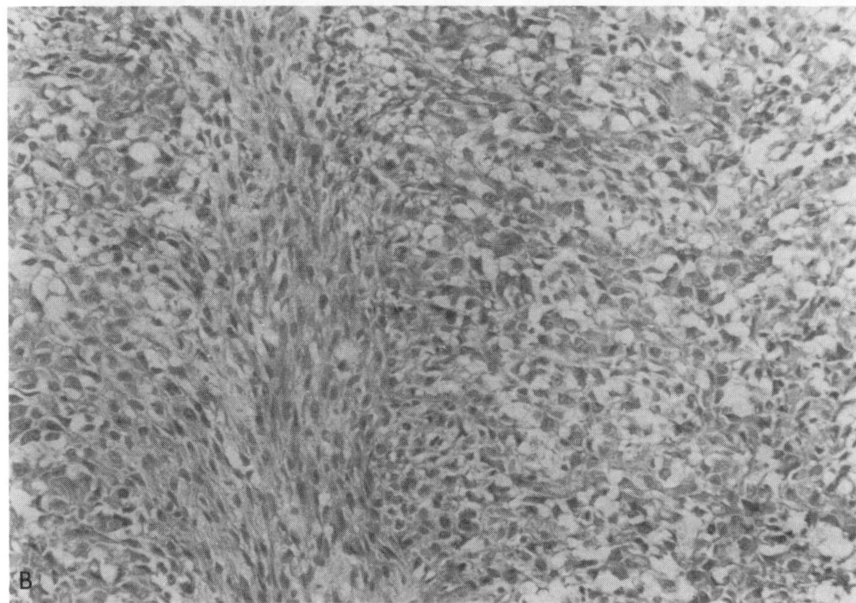

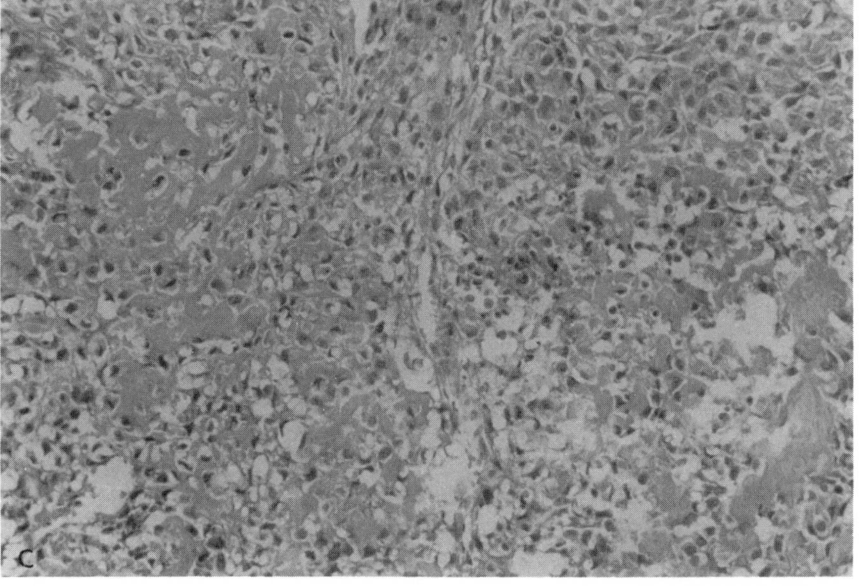

Figure 85–29. *Osteogenic sarcoma.*

A *A mass lesion in the gluteal muscles (arrows) in this patient was a soft tissue osteogenic sarcoma.*

B, C *Photomicrographs demonstrate poorly differentiated cells producing osteoid (200×).*

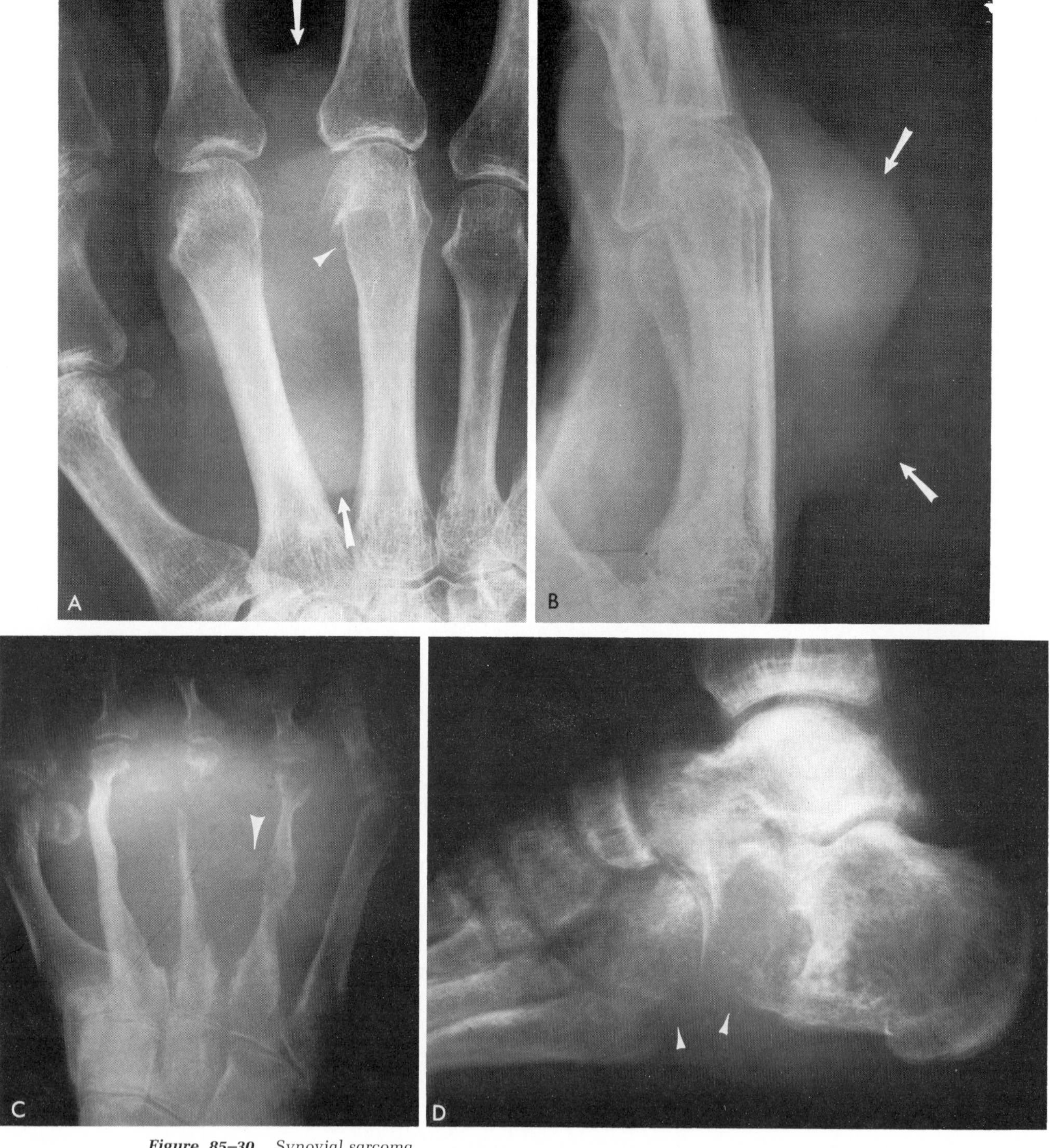

Figure 85–30. *Synovial sarcoma.*

A, B *The lobulated soft tissue mass (arrows) on the dorsum of the hand is eroding the second and third metacarpals (arrowhead).*

C *This 25 year old woman developed an extensive mass on the left foot. Observe the pressure erosion of multiple metatarsal shafts with fracture and soft tissue calcification (arrowhead).*

D *A 17 year old man had an enlarging mass of the foot. Destruction of the calcaneus and cuboid bones is seen (arrowheads). There is surrounding sclerosis, but the patient had previously received cobalt therapy. Osteoporosis is also evident.*

Illustration continued on the opposite page

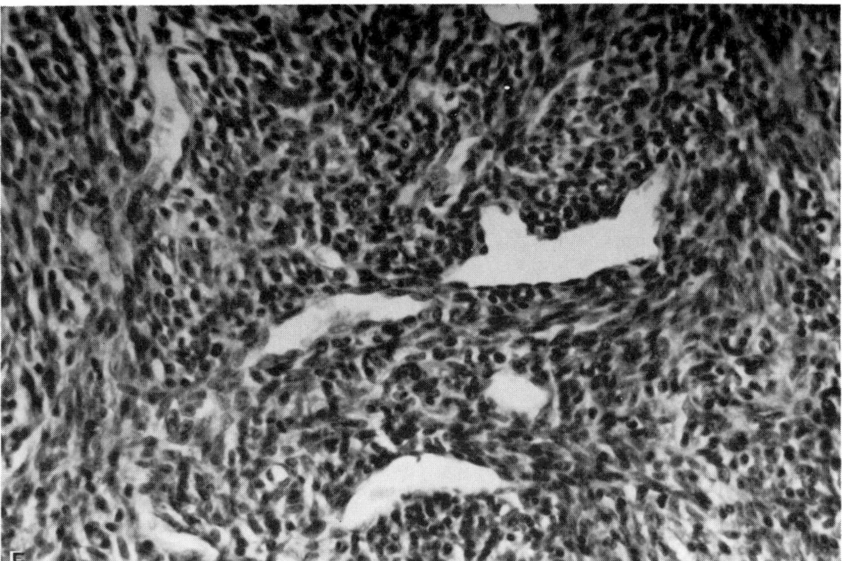

Figure 85–30. Continued
E *A photomicrograph (200×) demonstrates synovioblastic and spindle-cell fibroblastic elements with slit formation.*

calcific foci must be distinguished from "benign" lesions such as myositis ossificans traumatica, and pseudomalignant osseous tumors of soft tissue (see below).

Synovial Sarcomas

Synovial sarcomas are uncommon malignant neoplasms that can arise from within a joint but are more frequent in extraarticular locations.[98-103, 295] A distinct predilection exists for involvement of the thigh and lower extremity. Patients of all ages can be affected, although most are in the third and fourth decades of life. On radiographs, a soft tissue mass is seen, which may reveal evidence of calcification in 20 to 30 per cent of cases and of osseous erosion or invasion in 5 to 20 per cent of cases[104] (Fig. 85–30). Reactive sclerosis is unusual. On histologic examination, synovioblastic and spindle-cell fibroblastic elements are seen. The prognosis is poor. Sooner or later, metastatic deposits appear, especially in the lungs, that on rare occasions may calcify.[105] A benign variety of tumor, termed the *benign synovioma*, has been observed in the capsule of the knee.[20]

Other Tumors

Tumors of nerves and related tissue include the *neurinoma, neurilemoma, neurofibroma, malignant schwannoma,* and *neurofibrosarcoma* (see Chapter 14) (Fig. 85–31). A *Morton's neuroma* represents a condition produced by degenerative changes in one or more intermetatarsal nerves that can lead to paroxysms of pain.[106]

Additional benign neoplasms include a *mixed tumor* arising in the sweat glands of the corium, especially in the face and head, a *mesenchymoma* containing a mixture of fibrous and mesenchymal tissue (Fig. 85–32),[289] and a *mesothelioma,* usually apparent in the pleura; these tumors may have their malignant counterparts, such as the *malignant mesenchymoma* and the *malignant mesothelioma.*[20]

Clear cell sarcomas are malignant neoplasms that arise in the vicinity of tendons and aponeuroses of the upper and lower extremities.[107] The underlying bone may be affected.[108]

An *alveolar soft part sarcoma* (malignant granular cell myoblastoma) is usually found in muscles but may also appear in the orbit, retroperitoneum, and elsewhere, in both children and adults.[109-111] It grows slowly, may invade the underlying bone, and eventually may metastasize widely through the bloodstream. The histology resembles that of a paraganglioma, with subtle differences. The exact nature of the tumor remains uncertain.

Malignant lymphoid and reticuloendothelial tumors such as *reticulum cell sarcoma* and *extraosseous plasmacytoma* can rarely arise in the soft tissues.[20]

Malignant melanoma (melanosarcoma) is a neoplasm of contested origin containing fibroblast-like cells, some of which contain melanin. It can arise from the skin and produce local and distant osseous destruction (see Chapter 75).

Squamous cell carcinoma of the skin can invade subjacent bone. This tumor can arise at various sites and is not uncommon in areas of chronic cutaneous irritation, such as about a draining sinus in associa-

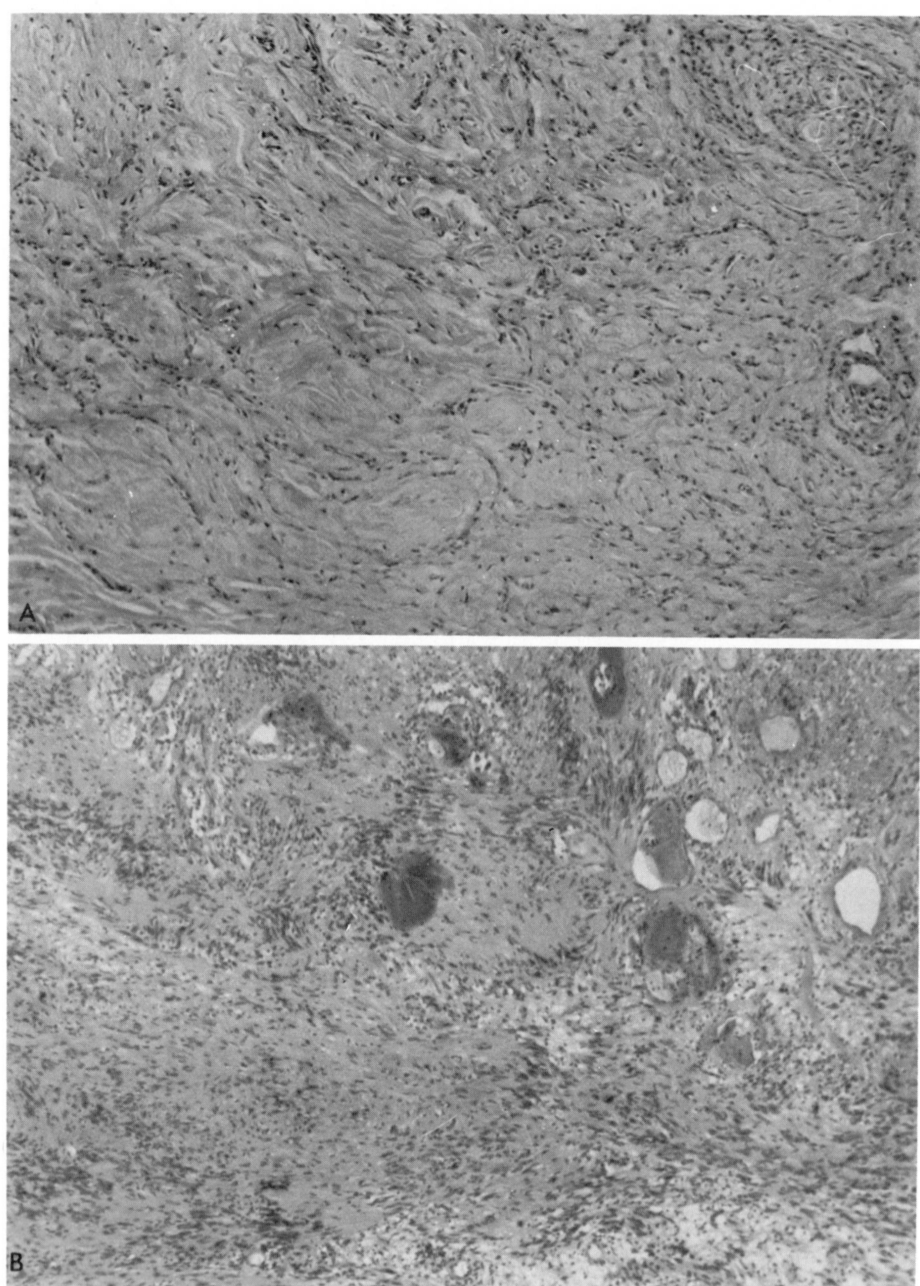

Figure 85–31. Neurogenic tumors.

A *Traumatic neuroma. Dense dermal collagen tissue with entrapped pockets of neurofibrils is seen (90×).*

B *Neurilemoma. Neural bundles of spindle cells show a focal palisading configuration (90×).*

Illustration continued on the opposite page

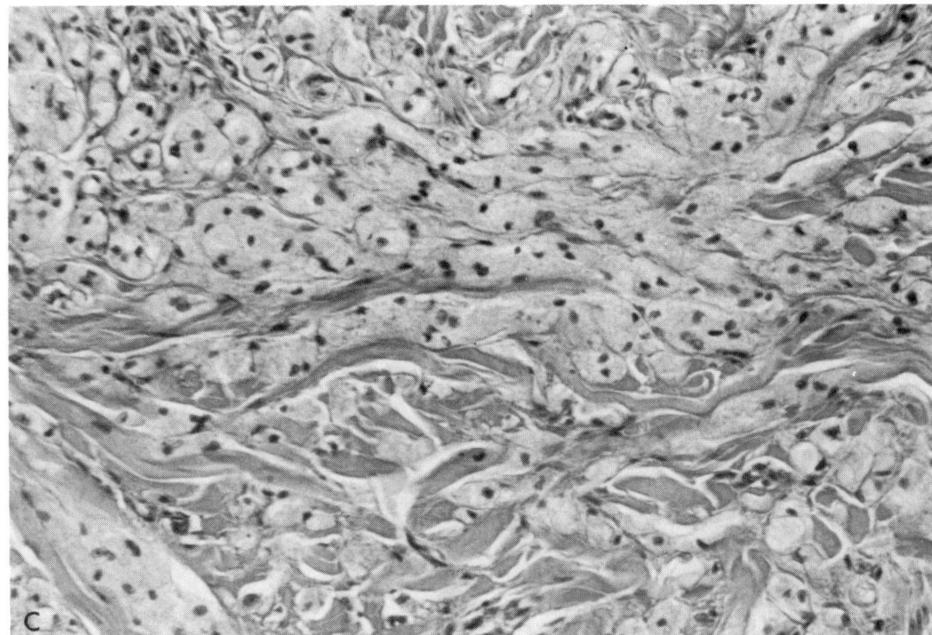

Figure 85–31. Continued
C *Granular cell schwannoma. The dermis contains a tumor composed of large cells with pink granular cytoplasm and cytologically benign nuclei. The tumor is not encapsulated, has an irregular outline, and extends into the subcutaneous tissue (230×).*

tion with osteomyelitis. *Pilomatrixomas* (calcifying epitheliomas) are benign soft tissue tumors occurring in the dermis or subjacent tissues, frequently in children.[112, 113] The lesions may be heavily calcified.

Metastases

Single or multiple soft tissue metastatic deposits can accompany a variety of primary malignant neoplasms. In general, a nonspecific soft tissue mass is produced. The underlying bone can be eroded, and the osseous defects may resemble a "cookie bite." In our experience, bronchogenic carcinoma frequently leads to such a roentgenographic appearance (Fig. 85–33).

Radiographic Approach

Considering the large number of soft tissue neoplasms that were noted earlier in this chapter, it is not surprising that the accurate preoperative radiographic diagnosis of the type of tumor is frequently difficult or impossible to accomplish. More feasible and more important, assessment of radiographic criteria may allow differentiation of a neo-

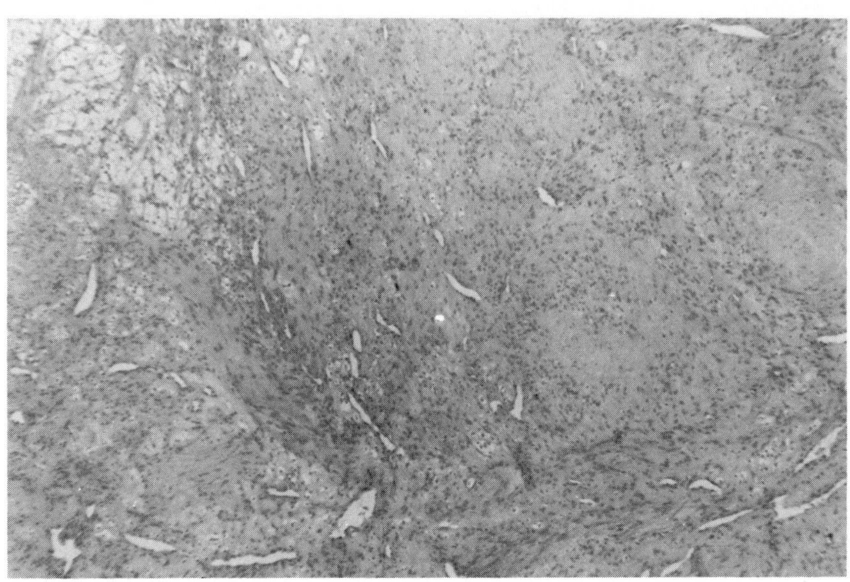

Figure 85–32. Benign mesenchymoma. A well-circumscribed, only partially encapsulated tumor is composed of a mixture of whorled and intersecting broad bands of dense fibrous connective tissue, with focal areas of foamy adipose tissue. Blood vessels within the tumor have a slit-like outline and hypertrophied fibromuscular walls (86×).

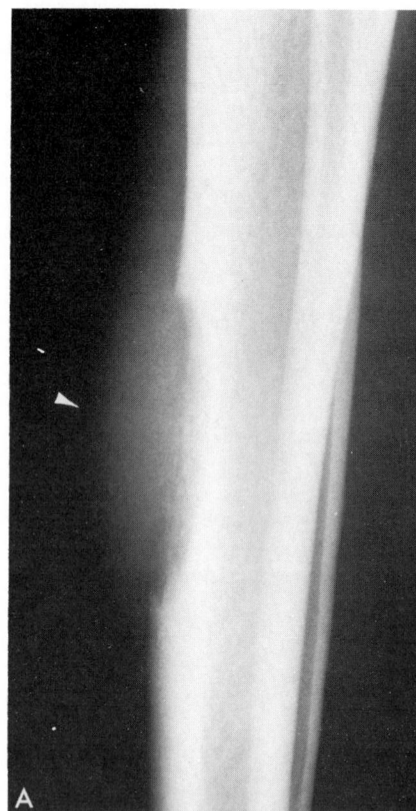

Figure 85–33. Skeletal metastasis: Bronchogenic carcinoma.

A *The "cookie-bite" appearance of a tibial shaft is the result of a metastatic deposit from bronchogenic carcinoma. Note the soft tissue swelling (arrowhead).*

B, C *In a different patient, an eccentric erosion of the cranial vault (arrowhead) has resulted from metastasis due to bronchogenic carcinoma. Note the soft tissue mass (arrow) on the computed tomogram.*

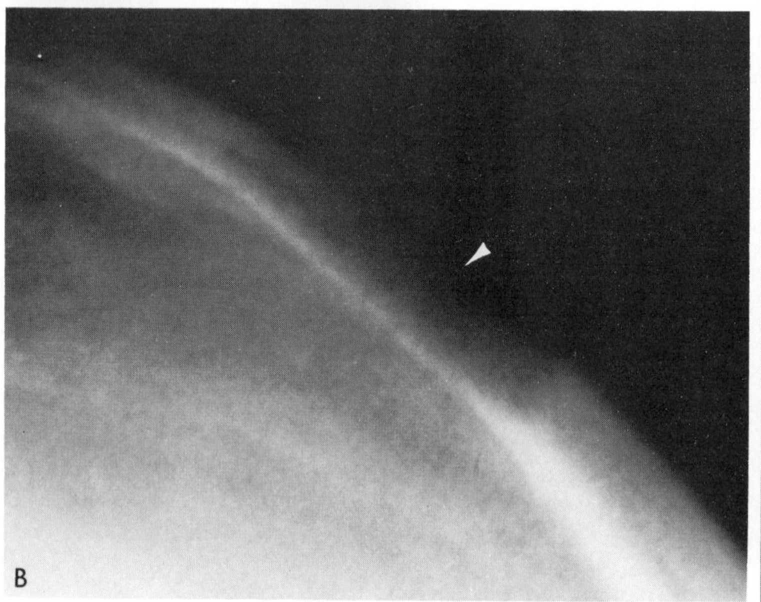

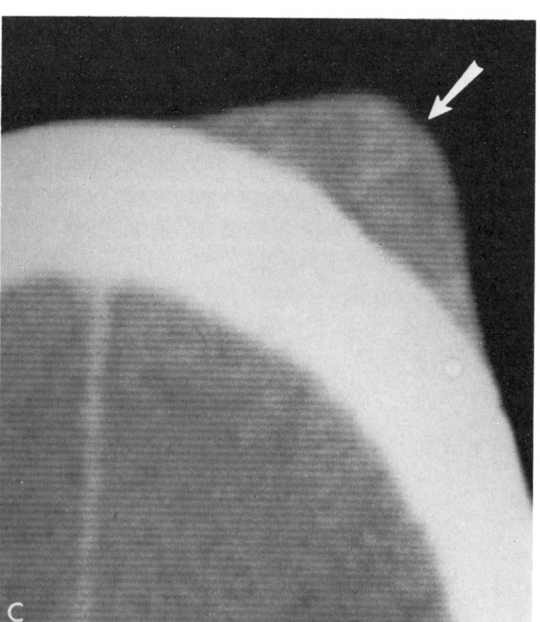

Table 85–1

RADIOGRAPHIC CHARACTERISTICS OF BENIGN AND MALIGNANT SOFT TISSUE TUMORS

	Benign Tumor	Malignant Tumor
Size	Variable	Variable
Rate of growth	Slow	Rapid[1]
Number	Single or multiple[2]	Single or multiple[3]
Radiodensity	Vary from lucent (lipoma) to soft tissue density	Soft tissue density
Calcification/ossification	Possible[4]	Possible[5]
Tumor interface	Sharply demarcated	Poorly or sharply demarcated[6]
Osseous involvement	Smooth pressure erosion with or without sclerosis	Smooth pressure erosion without sclerosis; cortical osteolysis due to hyperemia; cortical invasion

[1]Rapid growth can also indicate hemorrhage or infection.
[2]Examples of multiple lesions are lipomas, fibromas, hemangiomas, neurogenic tumors.
[3]Examples of multiple lesions are metastases, Kaposi's sarcomas.
[4]Examples of calcifying tumors are hemangiomas, xanthomas, myxomas, lipomas, pilomatrixomas, chondromas.
[5]Examples of calcifying or ossifying tumors are synovial sarcomas, rhabdomyosarcomas, malignant histiocytomas, chondrosarcomas, osteogenic sarcomas.
[6]Infection can also produce indistinctness of mass outline.

plastic from a non-neoplastic disorder, and a benign from a malignant process[2] (Table 85–1). However, this differentiation is not always possible, even with the utilization of certain roentgenographic characteristics, and an accurate diagnosis must frequently await evaluation by the pathologist.

Tumor Size and Rate of Growth. The actual size of a mass provides little information about its nature. Benign processes may be large and malignant processes may be small. More significantly, serial or comparison films will allow assessment of the rate of growth. Very rapid enlargement of a mass can indicate hemorrhage, inflammation, or perhaps a malignant neoplasm but is not characteristic of a benign tumor. Conversely, absent or slow growth is typical of benign neoplasm.

Tumor Location and Number. Some of the characteristic locations of certain tumors have been indicated. Examples include the predilection of specific fibromatoses to involve the hands and the feet (Fig. 85–9), of xanthomatoses to affect tendons about the hands, elbows, and heels (Fig. 85–2), and of synovial sarcomas to appear in the thighs or lower extremities (Fig. 85–30). Non-neoplastic processes also have typical locations, such as the popliteal regions for synovial cysts.

Certain masses are frequently multiple, including neurofibromas and other neurogenic tumors, Kaposi's sarcomas (Fig. 85–26), lipomas, and even metastases.[2]

Tumor Radiodensity. Lipomas produce radiolucent masses that are frequently well demarcated from the surrounding soft tissues (Fig. 85–6*D*). Liposarcomas are less radiolucent and, when poorly differentiated, may contain few if any lucent zones. Most of the other soft tissue neoplasms are of approximately the same radiodensity as the adjacent tissue unless they contain zones of calcification or ossification.

Tumor Calcification or Ossification. Calcification may appear in benign or malignant neoplasms (as well as in non-neoplastic masses). Of the benign neoplasms, hemangiomas may reveal typical circular calcifications with lucent centers (phleboliths) (Fig. 85–24), whereas other tumors may be associated with sharply circumscribed peripheral calcific collections (e.g., myxoma, xanthoma, hamartoma, lipoma)[114] (Fig. 85–34) or small or large foci of sand-like calcification (pilomatrixoma). Malignant neoplasms can lead to necrosis and hemorrhage, with secondary calcification that appears as irregular, faint amorphous zones of increased density on roentgenograms.[2] Such deposits are seen in synovial sarcomas[101, 104] (Fig. 85–30), malignant histiocytomas,[115] and rhabdomyosarcomas. In addition, calcification can appear in pseudosarcomatous fasciitis.[51]

Extraskeletal chondrosarcomas or osteogenic sarcomas may show irregular, poorly marginated calcific and ossific deposits that differ from the other patterns of calcification[2] (Fig. 85–28). The resulting radiographic picture must be differentiated from non-neoplastic ossifying processes of soft tissue, such as myositis ossificans traumatica, and lipomas.[116]

Tumor Interface (Fig. 85–35). Benign neoplasms are characteristically sharply demarcated, and the surrounding tissue planes are displaced but not obliterated.[2] However, malignant neoplasms can result in similar changes, although distortion and blurring of part of the interface between neoplasm and soft tissues can be seen in some cases. In inflammatory conditions, the entire interface may be obscured owing to fluid infiltration into the adjacent soft tissues.

Osseous Involvement (Fig. 85–36). Smooth resorption of cortical bone is more indicative of the proximity of a soft tissue process to subjacent bone than of its nature. Thus, benign and malignant neoplasms arising near bone can produce pressure scalloping of the periosteal surface. Hyperemia due to vascularity of a neoplasm may contribute to cortical osteolysis.[2] The presence of sclerosis about the osseous defect suggests a slowly evolving process and is more typical of benign neoplasm; the absence of such bone formation is suggestive but not diagnostic of malignancy. The presence of irregular cortical destruction with or without medullary involvement is strongly indicative of a malignancy or infection.

In the presence of a soft tissue mass and osseous

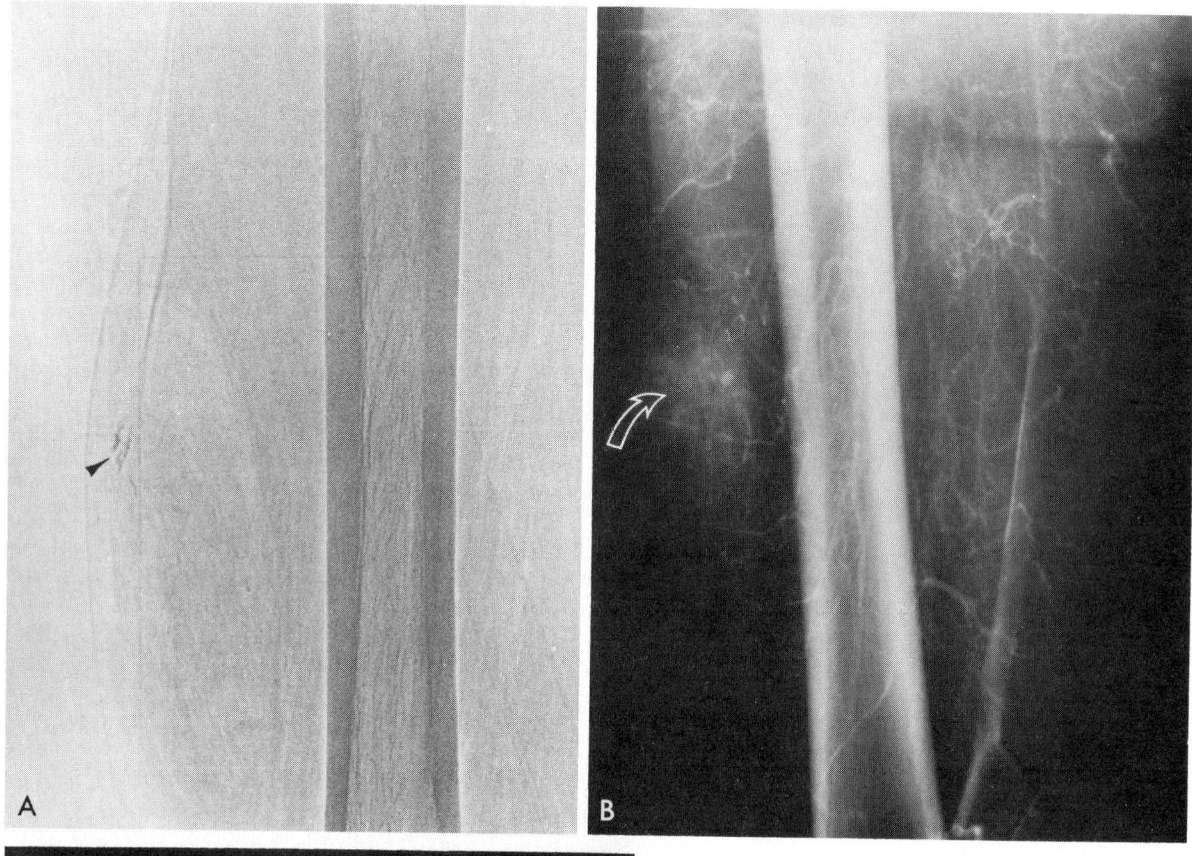

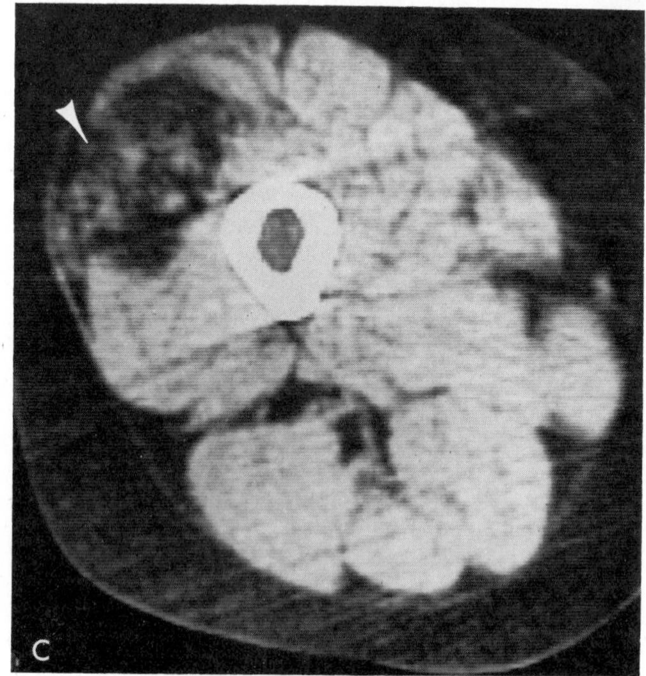

Figure 85–34. *Infiltrating angiolipoma. A 35 year old woman presented with a soft, slightly tender mass in the anterolateral aspect of the thigh.*

A *Xeroradiography reveals small, sharply defined calcific dense areas in the periphery of the mass (arrowhead).*

B *The late arterial phase of a right femoral angiogram shows a tangle of irregular vessels and a tumor stain (arrow).*

C *A computed tomogram without contrast administration demonstrates poorly defined margins and a heterogeneous mixture of fat and elements of water density (arrowhead). The CT numbers ranged from −60 to −30.*

Illustration continued on the opposite page

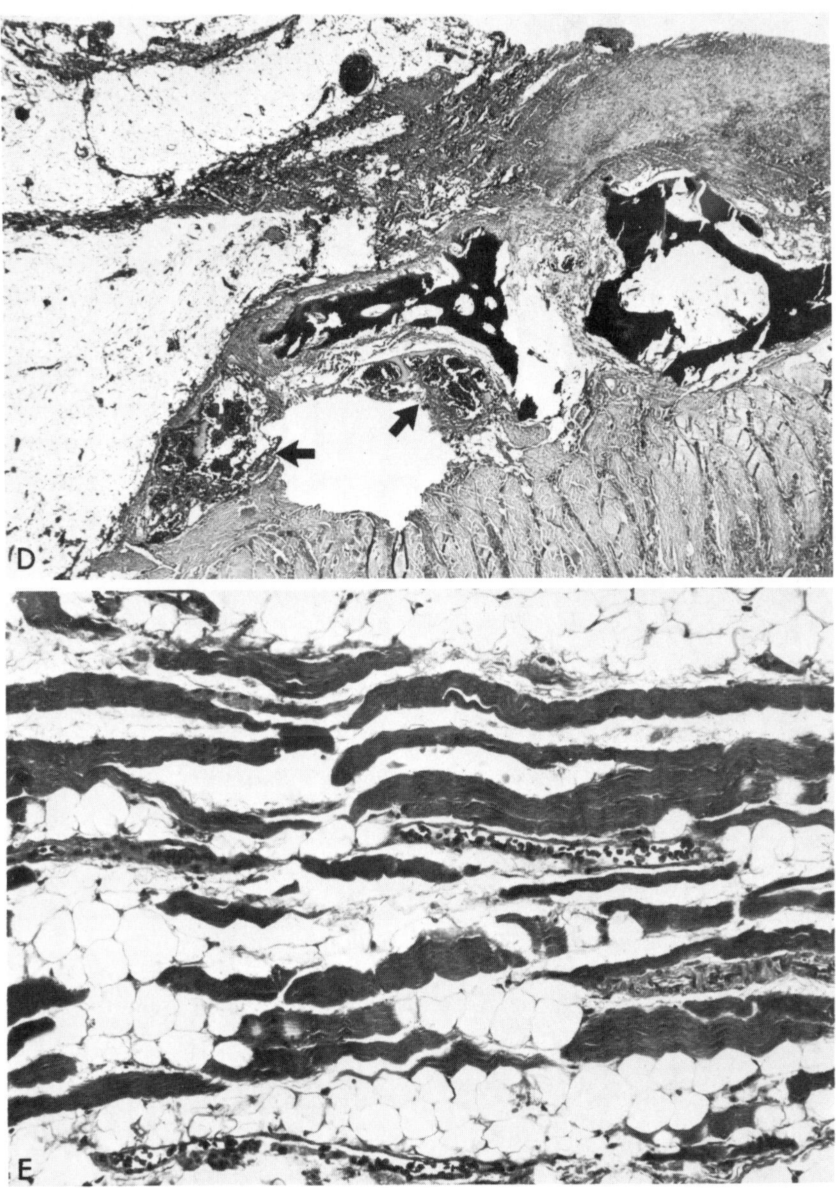

Figure 85–34. Continued

D *Mature adipose tissue on the left adjoins dense collagen on the right, which contains islands of darkly staining lamellar bone. Dilated vascular channels (arrows) in a pattern of cavernous hemangioma lie below the island of bone in the center of the photomicrograph (15×).*

E *Mature adipose tissue and longitudinally cut capillaries extend among darkly staining skeletal muscle fibers (150×).*

(From Hunter JC, et al: Skel Radiol 4:79, 1979.)

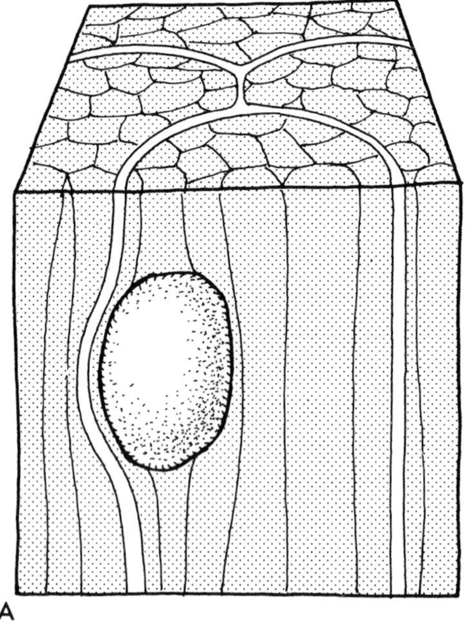

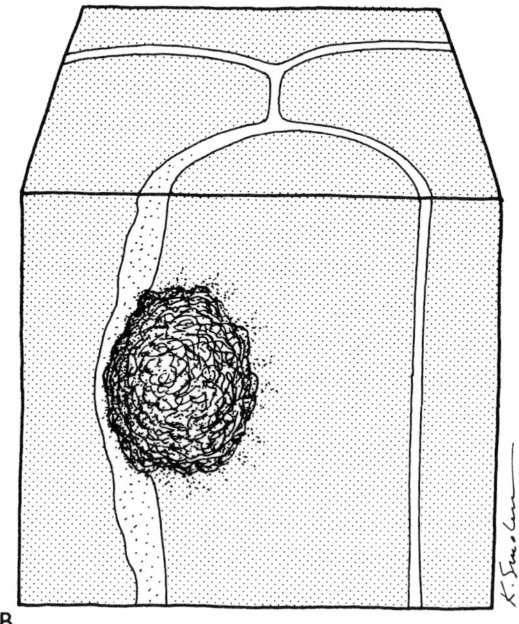

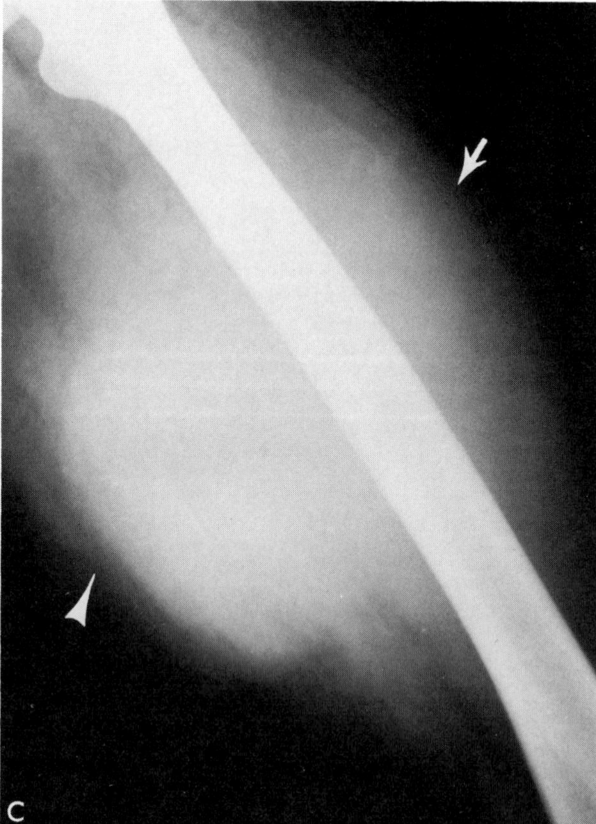

Figure 85–35. *Tumor interface.*

A *Benign neoplasms may displace tissue planes, but the planes are not obliterated. The tumors are frequently well defined or marginated.*

B *Malignant neoplasms can distort and obscure portions of the tissue planes. A poorly defined or irregular tumor outline can be seen.*

C *Undifferentiated sarcoma. Note the poorly defined soft tissue mass that is obliterating soft tissue planes in some areas (arrowhead) and displacing them in others (arrow).*

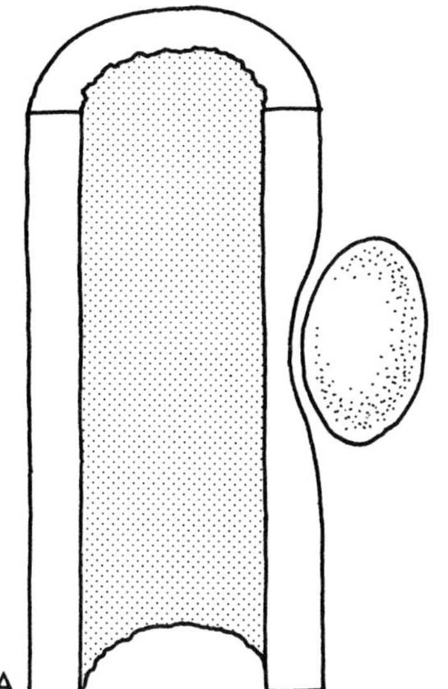

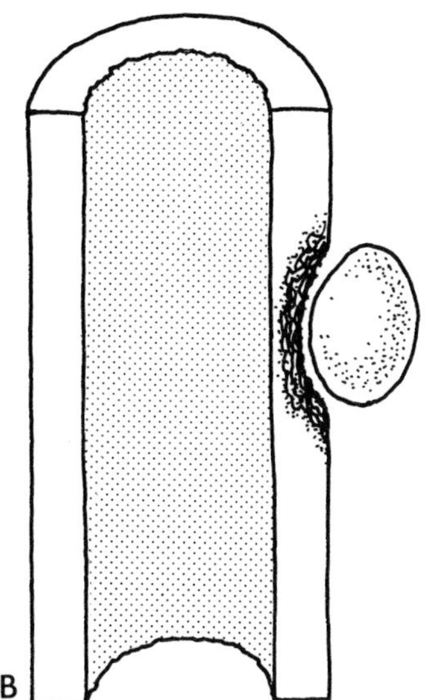

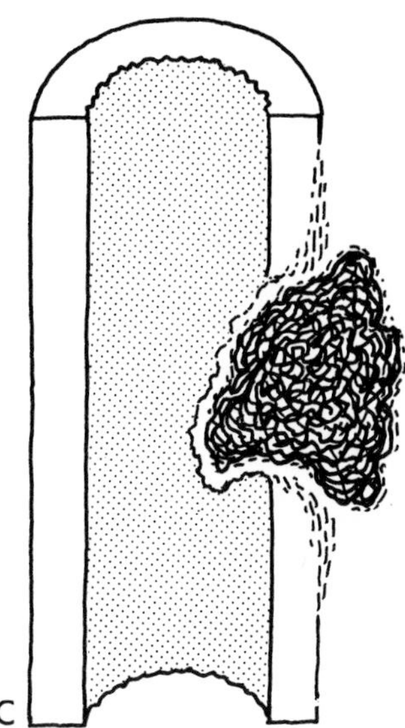

Figure 85–36. *Osseous involvement.*

A *Smooth resorption of the cortical surface of a bone indicates the presence of an adjacent soft tissue mass but provides little information regarding its benign or malignant nature.*

B *Cortical resorption associated with reactive sclerosis suggests a slowly evolving process and is more compatible with a benign neoplasm.*

C *Irregular cortical destruction with medullary involvement and periostitis is strongly indicative of a malignancy or infection.*

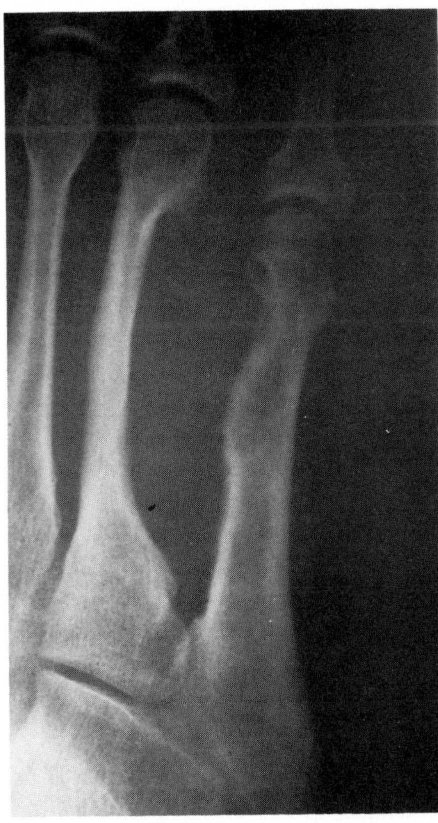

Figure 85–37. *Osseous involvement. The detection of resorption or invasion of more than one bone usually indicates the presence of a primary soft tissue process. In this case, scalloped erosion of the fourth and fifth metatarsals has resulted from a synovial sarcoma.*

abnormality, it may be difficult to differentiate a primary soft tissue tumor with osseous invasion from a bone tumor with soft tissue extension.[2] In general, the site of more extensive abnormality (bone versus soft tissue) represents the initial focus of the process. However, this rule is not without exception. Some osseous conditions, such as metastatic disease (thyroid, renal, bronchogenic, and prostatic carcinomas) and plasma cell myeloma, may produce extraordinary soft tissue components with minor bony destruction, whereas some soft tissue conditions, such as synovial sarcoma, may be present with a considerable amount of bony abnormality. The detection of a large soft tissue mass and resorption or destruction of more than one bone (e.g., metatarsals, metacarpals, radius and ulna, tibia and fibula) usually indicates the presence of a primary extraosseous neoplasm (Fig. 85–37).

SOFT TISSUE CALCIFICATION AND OSSIFICATION

The radiographic detection of calcification and ossification in the soft tissues provides an important clue to proper diagnosis. Although it is certainly helpful to distinguish between calcific and ossific radiodense lesions, this is not always possible, particularly if the collections are of small size. The documentation of ossification depends upon the recognition of a trabecular pattern within the dense areas, a pattern which is more easily identified when large ossific masses are encountered. Calcification appears as irregular punctate, circular, linear, or plaque-like radiodense areas that do not possess trabecular or cortical structure.

Calcification

Greenfield[117] has classified the conditions that lead to deposition of calcium within soft tissues into three types: metastatic calcification related to a disturbance in calcium or phosphorus metabolism; calcinosis due to the deposition of calcium in skin and subcutaneous tissue in the presence of normal calcium metabolism; and dystrophic calcification related to calcium deposits in damaged or devitalized tissue in the absence of a generalized metabolic derangement. Causes of metastatic calcification include hyperparathyroidism, hypoparathyroidism, renal osteodystrophy, hypervitaminosis D, milk-alkali syndrome, sarcoidosis, and processes associated with massive bony destruction, such as metastasis, plasma cell myeloma, and leukemia. In these disorders, collections of various sizes may appear in visceral and soft tissue locations; periarticular sites are frequently affected. The causes of generalized calcinosis include collagen vascular disorders, such as scleroderma and dermatomyositis, idiopathic tumoral calcinosis, and idiopathic calcinosis universalis. The disorders leading to dystrophic calcification are many; neoplastic, inflammatory, and traumatic conditions are prime considerations, although tissue injury from any cause may produce lower carbon dioxide concentration, local alkalinity, and calcium deposition (Fig. 85–38).

The radiographic appearance in cases of soft tissue calcification usually does not allow a specific diagnosis. The terms calcinosis universalis, tumoral calcinosis, and calcinosis circumscripta should be regarded as descriptive designations for widespread, mass-like, or localized calcific deposits, respectively, and not as a single disease entity. Thus, "universal," "tumoral," or "circumscribed" deposits can accompany several collagen vascular or additional disorders, or appear on an idiopathic basis.

In some conditions, the roentgenographic characteristics of the calcification are relatively diagnostic. Circular or elliptical calcific collections with radiolucent centers may represent the phleboliths in hemangiomas or varicosities (Fig. 85–39), the calcified fatty deposits in Ehlers-Danlos syndrome (Fig. 85–40), or cysticercosis. A reticulated pattern of calcification is frequent in dermatomyositis.

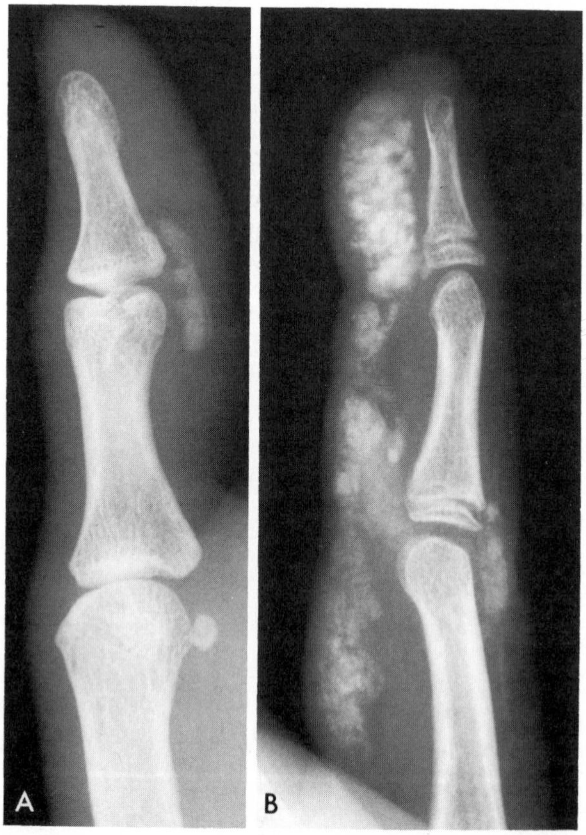

Figure 85–38. *Dystrophic soft tissue calcification. Calcific deposits in the fingers of these two patients followed local injuries.*

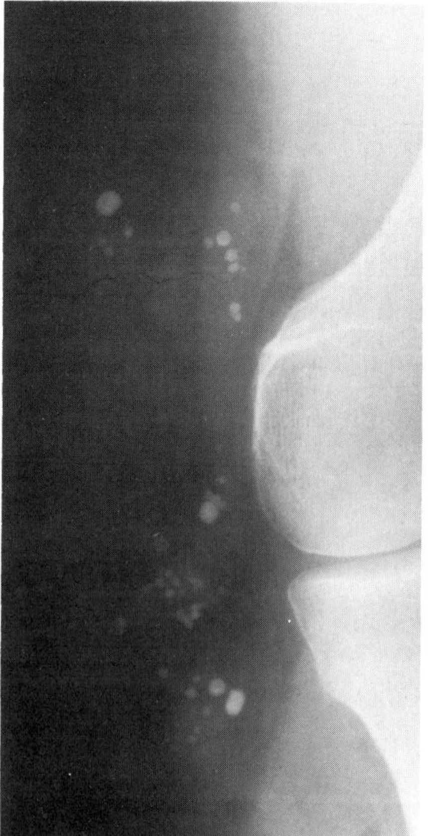

Figure 85–39. *Hemangioma. Circular calcifications with lucent centers are typical of hemangiomas.*

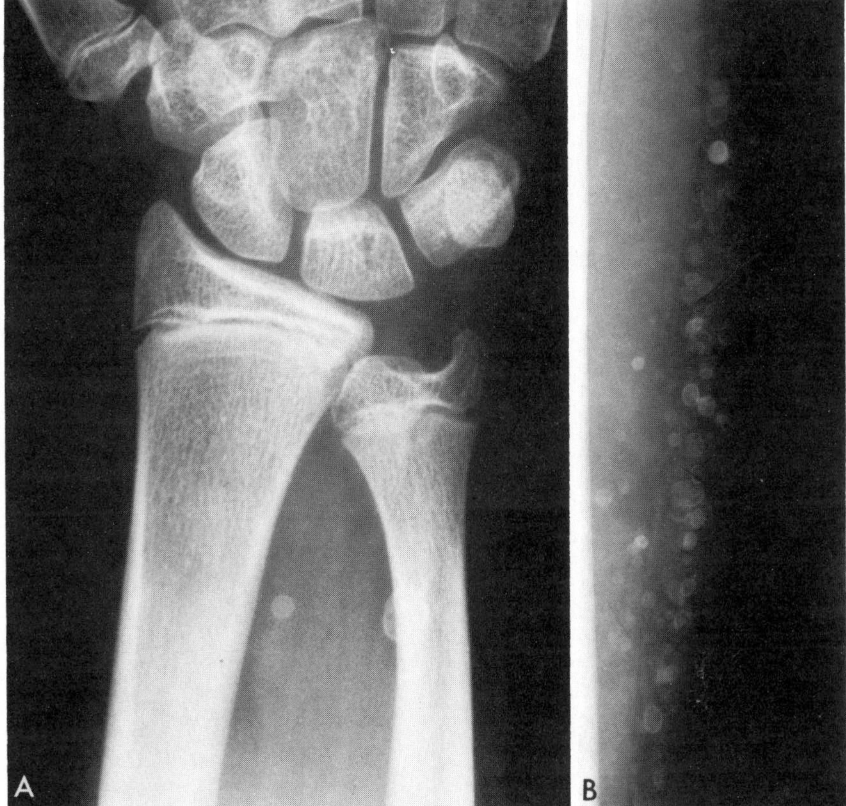

Figure 85–40. Ehlers-Danlos syndrome. Circular calcified fatty deposits with lucent centers can be seen in this syndrome. (Courtesy of Dr. M. Dalinka, University of Pennsylvania, Philadelphia, Pennsylvania.)

The site of calcification also provides a clue to the correct diagnosis.[117-119] Examples include the periarticular deposits of hyperparathyroidism, renal osteodystrophy, milk-alkali syndrome, hypervitaminosis D, and collagen vascular disorders; the calcified tendons or bursae of hydroxyapatite or calcium pyrophosphate dihydrate crystal deposition disease; the lymph node collections that may appear in various granulomatous infections; the arterial calcifications of renal osteodystrophy, diabetes mellitus, and hypervitaminosis D; the calcified nerves of leprosy; chondrocalcinosis that appears in idiopathic calcium pyrophosphate dihydrate crystal deposition disease, hemochromatosis, hyperparathyroidism, and, rarely, other crystal deposition diseases; the calcified intervertebral discs that may accompany alkaptonuria, idiopathic calcium pyrophosphate dihydrate crystal deposition disease, hyperparathyroidism, immobilization, and trauma; the fingertip deposits that are seen in scleroderma and other collagen vascular disorders; and calcification of the pinna of the ear, which may be evident in a variety of endocrine diseases, thermal or physical trauma, and perichondritis.

The uptake of ^{99m}Tc-labeled phosphate compounds by metastatic calcifications is a well recognized but nondiagnostic phenomenon.[303, 304] As the collections contain apatite, it has been suggested that such uptake is due to the same process of surface adsorption on the hydroxyapatite crystal that takes place in bone.[120] Alternative explanations suggest that the polyphosphate radical is metabolized in the same manner as ionic phosphate or that uptake is mediated by enzymatic receptors, such as the phosphatases. No matter what the cause, the abnormal scintigraphic pattern, although defining the location and extent of soft tissue calcification, provides little help in reaching a specific diagnosis.

Many of the disorders leading to calcific deposits in the soft tissue have been described in other sections of the book. Two additional entities are noted here.

Idiopathic Calcinosis Universalis. This rare disorder of unknown etiology affects infants and children.[121-123] The deposits initially appear in the subcutaneous fat of the extremities but subsequently involve other connective tissues, such as muscles, ligaments, and tendons, and other body regions. It appears that calcium phosphate and calcium carbonate are deposited about normal fat cells in the absence of infection, infarction, inflammation, or hemorrhage. A foreign body reaction occurs, leading to cellular infiltration, giant cell formation, and fibrosis. Calcareous nodules coalesce, becoming large masses that may violate the skin, producing fistulae. Internal organs are not affected. Serum calcium and phosphorus levels are normal.

Radiographs reveal discrete conglomerations of calcium that are arranged in longitudinal bands (Fig. 85–41). In the infant, the deposits are usually limited

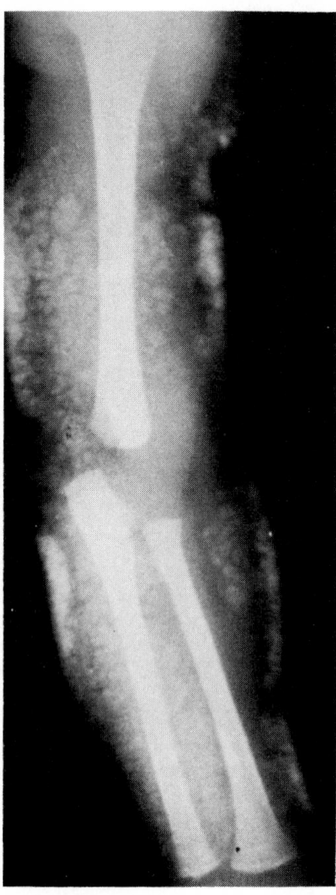

Figure 85–41. Calcinosis universalis. Longitudinal bands of calcification in the subcutaneous fat can be identified in this 3 month old male infant.

to the subcutaneous fat, whereas in the child, both fat and connective tissue are affected.[123]

The major differential diagnosis is dermatomyositis.[124] Other processes such as calcified subcutaneous fat necrosis,[125] extravasation of calcium gluconate injection solutions,[126, 296] and hyperparathyroidism must also be considered.

Idiopathic Tumoral Calcinosis. In 1943, Inclan and associates[127] first introduced the term tumoral calcinosis to describe the appearance of prominent periarticular calcified masses, especially about large joints such as the hip, the shoulder, and the elbow. Numerous descriptions of this entity now exist, although a variety of names has been utilized,[128] including lipocalcinogranulomatosis,[129] lipocalcinogranulomatous bursitis,[130] tumoral lipocalcinosis,[131, 132] calcifying collagenolysis,[133] and calcified bursae.[134] The designation of tumoral calcinosis is most widely encountered.[128, 135-141]

Tumoral calcinosis usually becomes manifest in the second and third decades of life. Men are more commonly affected than women, and blacks are especially susceptible. A family history is apparent in 30 to 40 per cent of cases. A previous episode of significant trauma is rarely reported. On clinical evaluation, firm, tumor-like painless swellings are evident, especially about the hip and the shoulders as well as the elbows, and these may interfere with joint motion. Solitary or multiple foci can be evident. The overlying skin is usually intact, although soft tissue ulcerations occasionally are apparent. The lesions may recur following incomplete excision.

Laboratory analysis usually indicates normal or slightly elevated levels of serum calcium and normal levels of serum electrolytes, phosphorus, urea, uric acid, and alkaline phosphatase. The observation in some individuals of (1) a slightly raised urinary level of hydroxyproline and hyperphosphatemia, (2) an increased intestinal absorption of dietary calcium coupled with radioactive studies with ^{47}Ca indicating rapid exchange of calcium between serum and masses, and (3) a family history of disease has suggested to some investigators that the disorder may be an inborn error of phosphorus metabolism.[143] Recent data have indicated that in patients with tumoral calcinosis and hyperphosphatemia, parathyroid hormone levels and renal responsiveness are normal and that parathyroid hormone–independent enhancement of phosphate reabsorption possibly in the proximal tubule may underlie the chronic hyperphosphatemia.[297]

Radiographs reveal circular or oval, well-demarcated masses of calcium about articulations (Fig. 85–42). A lobulated inhomogeneous appearance is characteristic. Radiolucent linear bands separate the calcific foci. The individual lesions vary from 1 to 20 cm in diameter and may reveal fluid levels on erect, decubitus, or cross-table roentgenograms.[136, 137, 142] Radionuclide studies with technetium compounds may outline increased accumulation in areas of calcinosis.[140, 147, 305] Pathologic examination reveals a lobulated soft tissue mass containing fibrovascular fronds dividing it into several loculi. Yellowish-white in color, the masses exude a purulent calcified material or a pasty, chalky liquid. Analysis of this material documents accumulations of calcium phosphate, calcium carbonate, or a mixture of these. Histologic characteristics include active areas consisting of large numbers of mononuclear cells, probably histiocytes, and multinucleated giant cells, and vascular indolent areas consisting of foci of edematous and granulomatous or dense collagenous tissue with chronic inflammatory cells.[128]

The exact nature of tumoral calcinosis is a mystery. The elevated serum phosphorus levels noted in some patients have been viewed as supporting the existence of an inborn error of metabolism,[143] perhaps related to an inherited reduction in renal tubular responsiveness to parathyroid hormone.[144] Traumatic or infectious (parasitic) causes have also been suggested as factors that might stimulate the proliferation of primitive mesenchymal cells.[138, 145] Others consider the disease a variant of calcinosis universalis, a reaction of surrounding soft tissue to ectopic synovial membrane, or a degradation of periarticular collagen with dystrophic calcification.

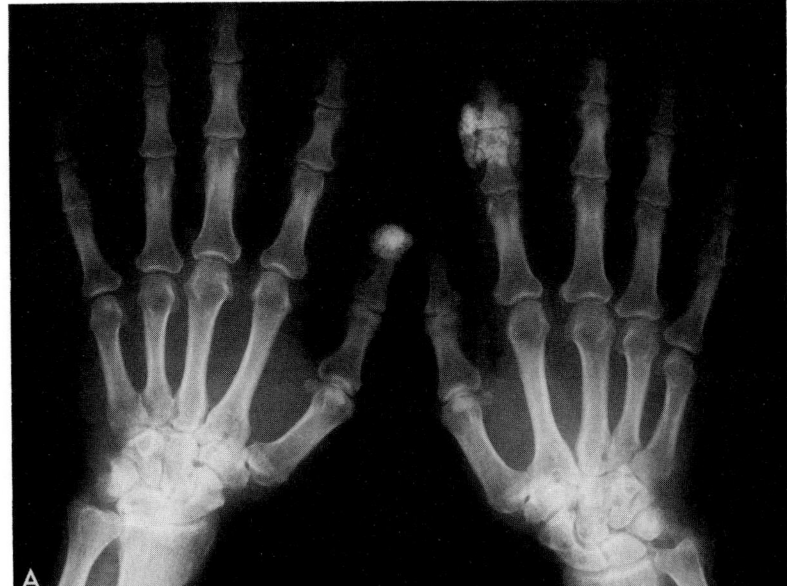

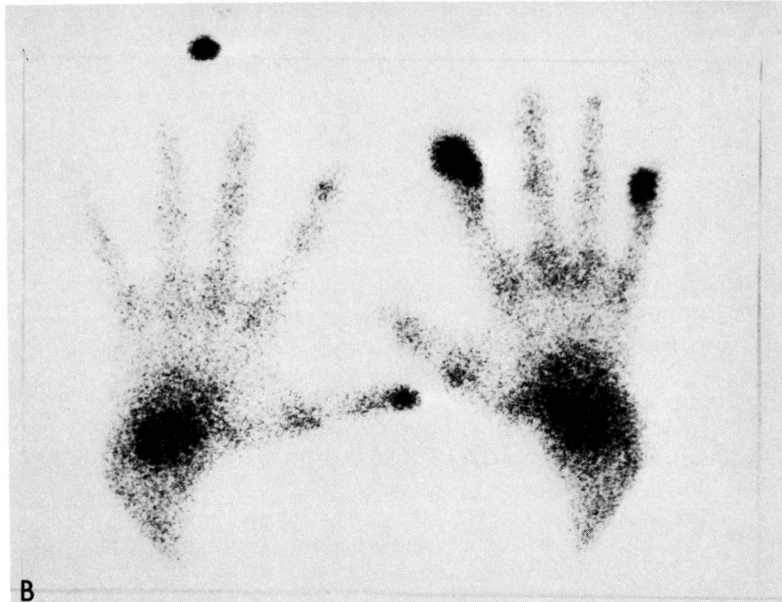

Figure 85–42. *Tumoral calcinosis. A 51 year old white man presented with tumoral calcific deposits about multiple joints, including the shoulders, the hips, the feet, and the fingers. Soft tissue ulcerations had developed.*

A *A radiograph of the hands reveals dense nodular calcific deposits about two distal interphalangeal joints and the terminal tuft of the thumb.*

B *Bone scan with ^{99m}Tc pyrophosphate delineates increased accumulation of radionuclide at sites of calcification.*

Illustration continued on the following page

Calcification may indeed represent a secondary phenomenon related to a genetically determined defect in collagenous tissue.[128] Tumoral calcinosis has been described in association with massive osteolysis[146] and Down's syndrome.[136]

The diagnosis of idiopathic tumoral calcinosis is one of exclusion. Other processes, such as collagen vascular disorders, hyperparathyroidism, hypervitaminosis D, milk-alkali syndrome, and chronic renal disease must first be eliminated by clinical, laboratory, and radiologic examinations.

Ossification

The disorders leading to ossification of soft tissues are more limited in number than those producing soft tissue calcification (Table 85–2). Heterotopic ossification appearing in association with neurologic disorders or problems (Fig. 85–43) (see Chapter 69), thermal burns (see Chapter 64), and venous insufficiency (see Chapter 81) has been discussed previously. In the first two situations, para-articular collections are frequent, which may lead to "ankylosis" of joints, whereas in the latter situation, small subcutaneous ossicles or a dense meshwork of osseous fibrils, usually in an edematous lower extremity, are observed. Ossification appearing in scars has also been reported, creating plaque-like radiodense areas, especially on abdominal radiographs. Soft tissue osteogenic sarcoma represents an additional cause of ossification, in this situation related to tumor production of bone (see earlier discussion).

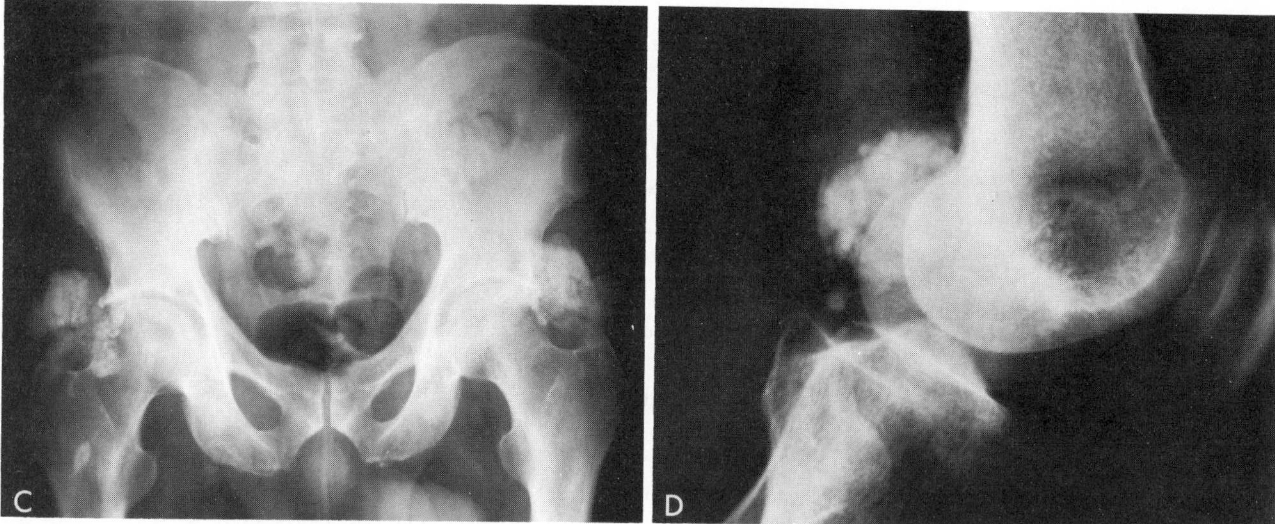

Figure 85–42. Continued
C, D *Additional deposits of calcification are evident about the hips, the ischial tuberosities, and the knee. The joint spaces are normal.*
(**A, B, D,** *From Brown ML, et al: Radiology 124:757, 1977.)*

In each of the situations mentioned previously, as well as those that are noted later in this chapter, radiographs may outline definite trabecular structure within the ossific collections, allowing differentiation of ossification from calcification. At certain times, serial roentgenograms will permit assessment of the maturity of the ossific deposit; initial cloud-like radiodense areas will mature into trabecular bone. Such an assessment is important, as removal of heterotopic bone prior to maturity in cases of burn or paraplegia may not afford long-term relief owing to rapid reaccumulation of the deposits. Unfortunately, roentgenographic changes and even serum alkaline phosphatase determinations do not adequately reflect the activity of the ossification process in many cases.[148, 149] Serial radionuclide studies utilizing strontium[150] or technetium[151] compounds may be more accurate in this regard (see Chapter 17) and can be supplemented with bone marrow scans to assess the maturity of heterotopic ossification appearing in the paralyzed or burned patient or even in the individual following local trauma, tetanus,[152, 157, 158] or carbon monoxide poisoning.[153]

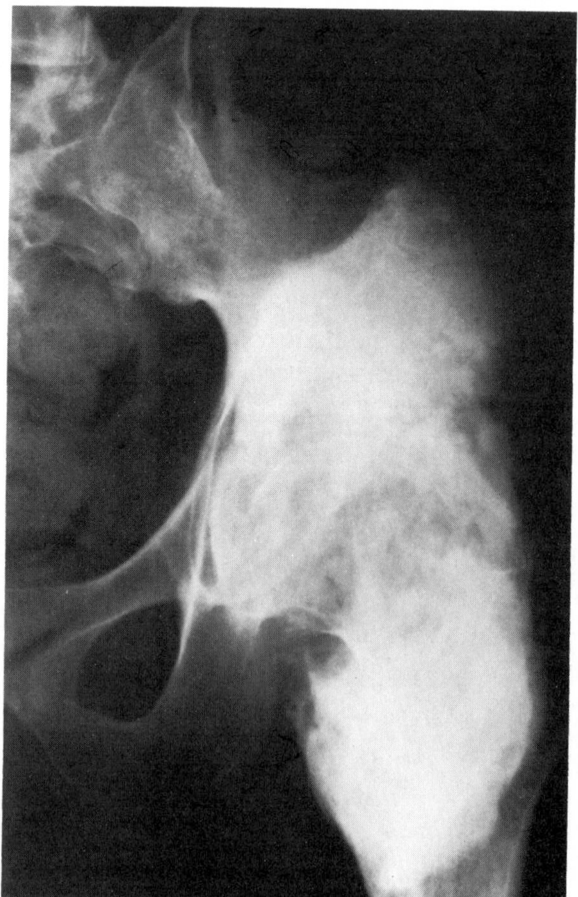

Figure 85–43. Neurologic disorders. *Following paralysis, extensive soft tissue ossification can appear, especially about the hip, the shoulder, and the knee. Here, the ossific deposits bridge the joint.*

Table 85–2

CAUSES OF SOFT TISSUE OSSIFICATION

Neurologic diseases
Physical and thermal injuries
Venous insufficiency
Neoplasms (e.g., parosteal osteosarcoma, extraskeletal osteosarcoma)
Pseudomalignant osseous tumor of soft tissue
Myositis ossificans progressiva
Melorheostosis
Surgical scars
Postoperative period

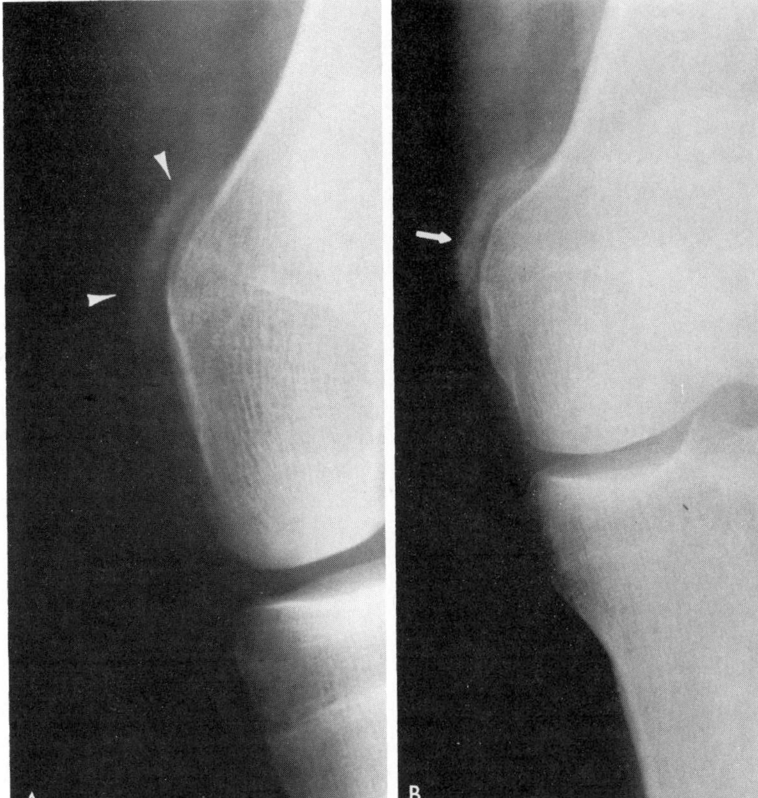

Figure 85–44. Pellegrini-Stieda syndrome. Two examples of posttraumatic ossification in the medial collateral ligament of the knee are given. Initially, the deposits may be arcuate or curvilinear in appearance (arrowheads). Subsequently, they mature and trabeculae can be recognized (arrow).

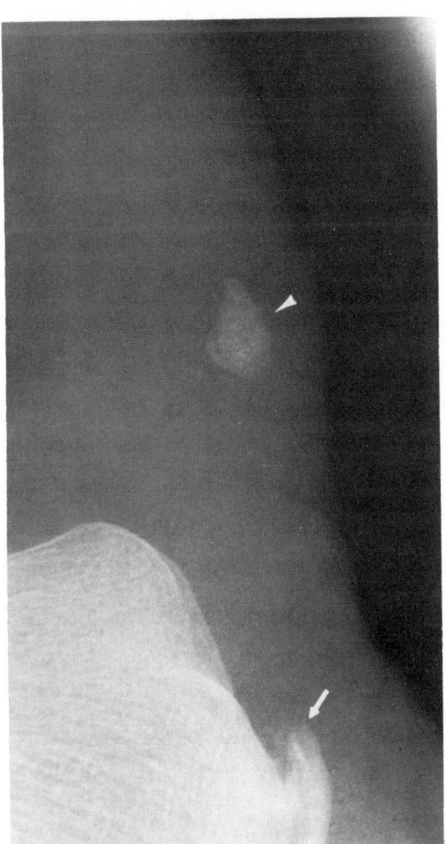

Figure 85–45. Ossification of the Achilles tendon. Idiopathic ossification of this tendon (arrowhead) developed in this patient. Note the enlarged tendinous outline and the excrescence (arrow) at the site of tendinous attachment to the calcaneus. A history of trauma was not elicited.

Ossification of Tendons. Although calcific tendinitis due to hydroxyapatite or calcium pyrophosphate dihydrate crystal deposition is common and well recognized (see Chapters 44 and 45), ossification within tendinous structures is relatively rare. Posttraumatic calcification and ossification of tendons or ligaments may be encountered at certain sites, such as the medial collateral ligament of the knee, where it is termed the Pellegrini-Stieda syndrome or disease, appearing as arcuate or curvilinear radiodense collections adjacent to the medial femoral condyle (Fig. 85–44). Ossification of the Achilles tendon has also been recognized,[154-156] although this, too, appears to be an unusual syndrome (Fig. 85–45). The deposits may originate in the body of the tendon or at its insertion into the calcaneus, producing a firm, nontender mass. A definite history of trauma or surgery is frequent but not invariable. Significant local symptoms and signs may indicate a fracture of the ossified deposit.[156]

Bony excrescences at sites of tendinous attachment should be differentiated from true tendinous ossification. These osseous outgrowths are frequent, especially in older patients, and may represent a manifestation of diffuse idiopathic skeletal hyperostosis (see Chapter 41). This disorder can also lead to true ossification of the substance of tendons and ligaments, a situation that may additionally be encountered in fluorosis (see Chapter 81).

Myositis Ossificans Traumatica. Sixty[159] to 75 per cent[160] of patients with localized soft tissue ossifications (myositis ossificans circumscripta) relate a clear history of trauma; the other individuals either suffer from one of the systemic problems associated with soft tissue ossification, such as neurologic conditions, burns, and tetanus, or develop the lesions spontaneously.[161, 280] The spontaneous cases are termed myositis ossificans nontraumatica or pseudomalignant osseous tumor of soft tissue (see discussion later in this chapter). The radiographic and pathologic features of myositis ossificans traumatica and pseudomalignant osseous tumor of soft tissue are virtually identical.

The accuracy of the designation "myositis ossificans" for this lesion has been challenged on numerous occasions. Indeed, the absence of inflammation as well as muscular involvement in some cases would indicate the inappropriateness of this name.[162] It has been postulated that the soft tissue ossification results from damage to the interstitium, not to the muscle.[162, 163] The presence of osteoblastosis on histologic examination is irrefutable, but the source of the osteoblasts remains a mystery; they may originate from damaged periosteum or pleuripotent cells already present in the connective tissue.[161, 164, 165]

Myositis ossificans traumatica usually appears in adolescents or young adults; rarely, infants or children are affected.[169] The sites of localization are areas susceptible to injury, such as the elbow, the thigh,[309] the buttocks, and, less often, the shoulder and the calf.[159] The appearance of ossification following elbow injuries[166] (Fig. 85–46) or about the region of the quadriceps[167] is well recognized although virtually any site can be affected, including the hand.[170] When there has been a history of injury, specific radiographic features can be correlated with the time that has elapsed following trauma, although in some individuals, the initiating injury may be of such minor nature as to be unrecognized or soon forgotten.[168]

Shortly after injury, a soft tissue mass or swelling becomes apparent, which may be associated with periosteal reaction in 7 to 10 days (Fig. 85–47). Flocculent dense lesions arise in the mass from 11 days to 6 weeks after the trauma.[161] The calcific dense areas gradually enlarge, and at 6 to 8 weeks a lacy pattern of new bone is sharply circumscribed about the periphery of the mass.[159] The soft tissue central core occasionally becomes encysted, and an enlarging central cavity combined with peripheral calcification and ossification resembles an eggshell. Maturity is reached in 5 to 6 months, and the mass then shrinks.

The recognition of a peripheral rim of calcification and ossification about a more lucent center

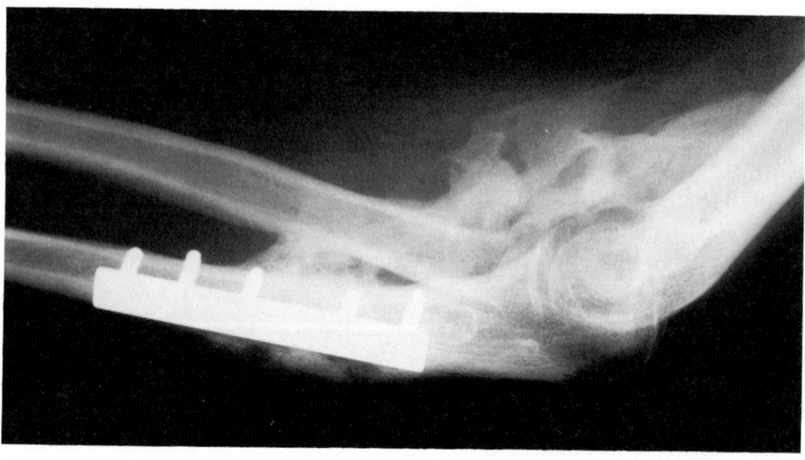

Figure 85–46. Myositis ossificans traumatica: Elbow. Heterotopic bone formation following elbow injuries is a well-recognized finding.

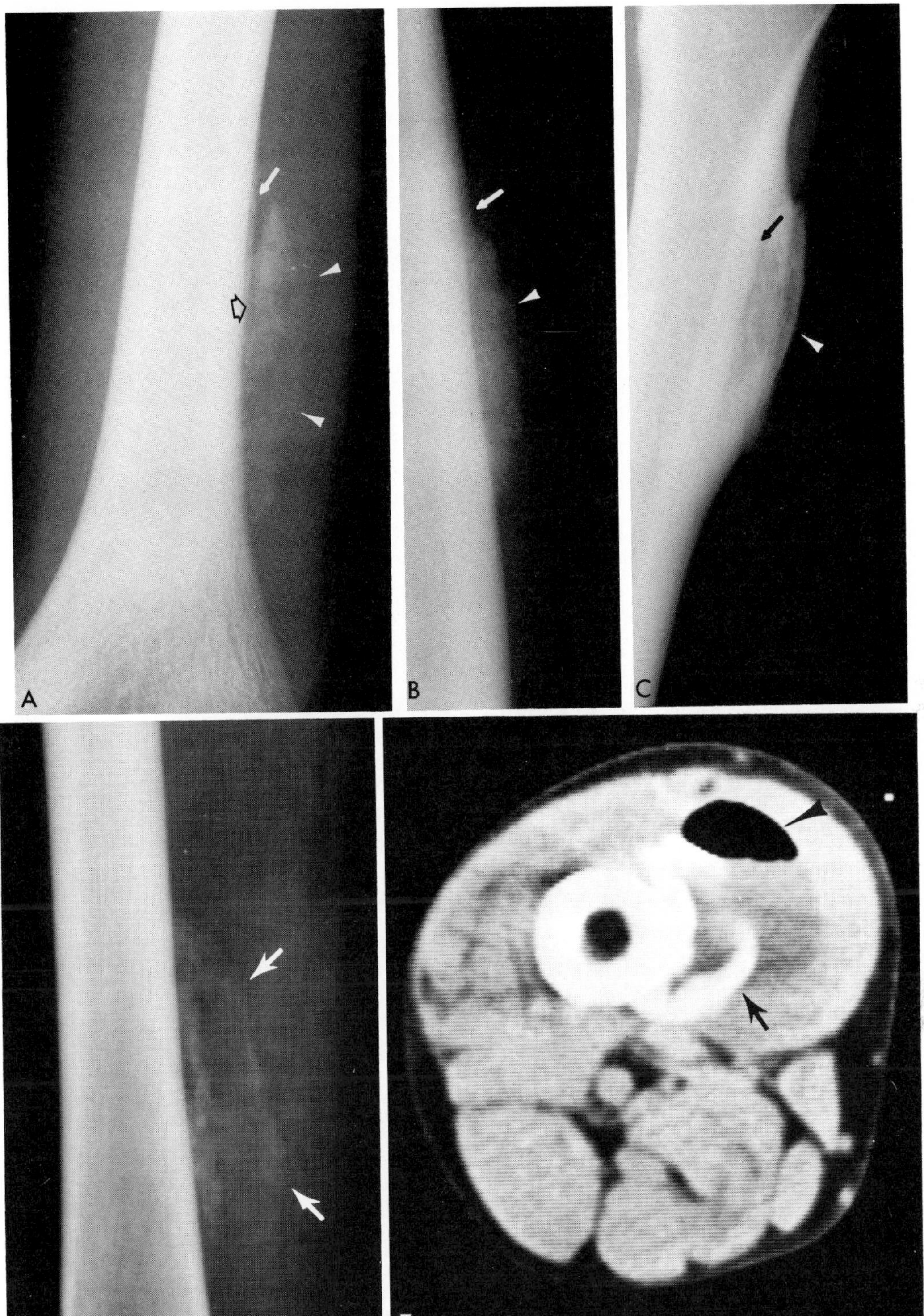

Figure 85–47. *Myositis ossificans traumatica: Sequential radiographic abnormalities (four different patients).*

A *Shortly after injury, a soft tissue swelling appears that may be associated with periostitis (arrow). Ill-defined osseous dense areas (arrowheads) appear within 2 to 6 weeks following the traumatic insult. Note the lucent area (open arrow) between the ossifications and the underlying bone.*

B *Subsequently, a trabecular architecture can be seen in the mass (arrowhead) and the subjacent lucent area is obliterated. More mature periostitis (arrow) is seen.*

C *Eventually, the mass of mature bone (arrowhead) merges with the underlying cortex, producing a localized osseous expansion that resembles an osteochondroma. However, the original cortical line (arrow) can be recognized.*

D, E *This 56 year old man with a history of occupational trauma to the thigh developed progressive pain and swelling for a period of 2 months. The radiograph* **(D)** *outlines an ill-defined mass adjacent to the femur with a peripheral rim of ossification (arrows). A computed tomogram* **(E)** *following intra-articular administration of air reveals the mass containing an ossific rim (arrow) and air within the suprapatellar pouch (arrowhead). Subsequent radiographs obtained over a 6 month period demonstrated maturation of the lesion, with relief of clinical findings.*

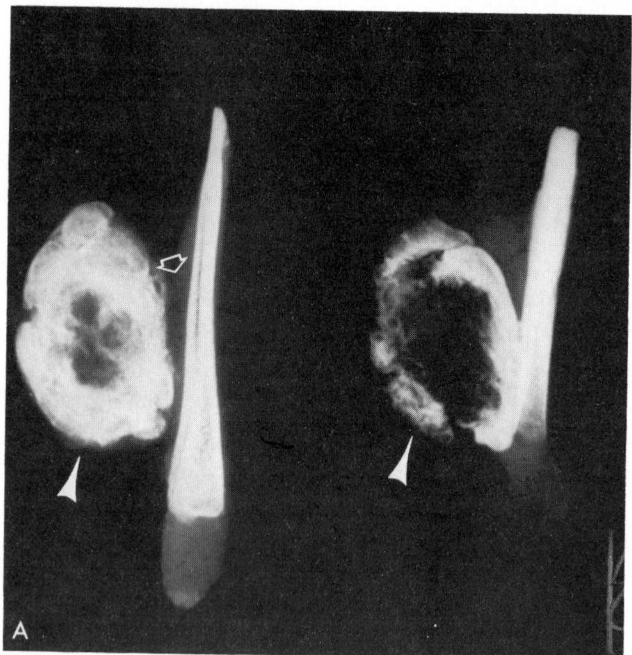

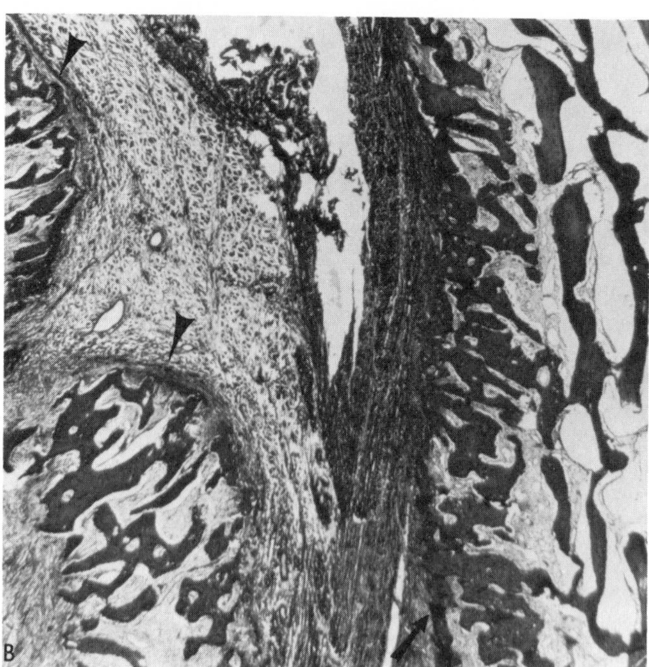

Figure 85–48. *Myositis ossificans traumatica: Radiographic-pathologic correlation.*

A *Serial sections through a focus of myositis ossificans delineate a well-encapsulated lesion possessing a peripheral zone of ossification and a lucent center (arrowheads). Note the separation or clear zone (open arrow) between the lesion and the underlying bone.*

B *Fibrous tissue separates the maturing foci of myositis ossificans (arrowheads) from the periosteal new bone (arrow) and is the basis for the zone of radiolucency observed between the lesion and the parent bone.*

(Courtesy of Dr. A. Norman, Hospital for Joint Diseases, New York, New York.)

cannot be overemphasized as an important radiographic manifestation of myositis ossificans (Fig. 85–48). Furthermore, a radiolucent band or zone between the lesion and the subjacent cortex is also a very important finding, reflecting the lack of intimacy between the ossified mass and neighboring bone, and allowing differentiation of myositis ossificans from parosteal osteosarcoma (see discussion later in this chapter). However, topographic variations in the ossifying process can lead to radiograpic alterations that may be more difficult to analyze.[161] Direct damage to the cambium layer of the periosteum from the traumatic insult can lead to an ossifying subperiosteal hematoma[168] or periosteoma, in which a sunburst periosteal reaction within the first 2 weeks may be easily misinterpreted as evidence of a malignant process. Second, a true hematoma of the muscle can create a soft tissue mass that is quite distant from the nearest bone and which may or may not ossify (ossifying hematoma) on subsequent examination.[171] In addition, a progressive variety of localized myositis ossificans has been recorded that does not recur following surgery.[172, 173]

The microscopic changes of myositis ossificans have been well documented[161] (Fig. 85–49). Mesenchymal proliferation results in the accumulation of focal masses of collagen in which calcium salts are deposited. Heterotopic osteoblasts appear, produce matrix, and create a well-defined lesion possessing a fibrous capsule. The developing lesion demonstrates three distinct zones, a phenomenon that allows differentiation from sarcomatous processes.[162, 174] The center of the lesion contains rapidly proliferating fibroblasts with areas of hemorrhage and necrosis. A middle zone contains osteoblasts with islands of immature bone. Biopsy of cellular inner and middle layers alone may result in an erroneous diagnosis of a sarcoma. It is the outer zone of the lesion that reveals the true benign nature of the process. In this region, mature trabeculae are discovered that are clearly demarcated from the surrounding connective tissue. Thus, a peripheral shell of maturing bone exists about a soft cellular center, and maturation proceeds in a centrifugal fashion with the center layer being the last to ossify. Pathologic criteria that are helpful in differentiation of myositis ossificans from sarcoma are a zone phenomenon, the lack of invasion of adjacent tissues, and the inclusion of viable muscle fibers, which would be destroyed by an advancing tumor.[161]

Based upon the clinical and radiologic findings, identification of myositis ossificans is usually possible (Fig. 85–50). Although other diagnostic modalities, such as arteriography,[175] ultrasonography,[176] scintigraphy, and computed tomography, may occasionally aid in the evaluation of this condition, they are usually not required. In questionable cases, his-

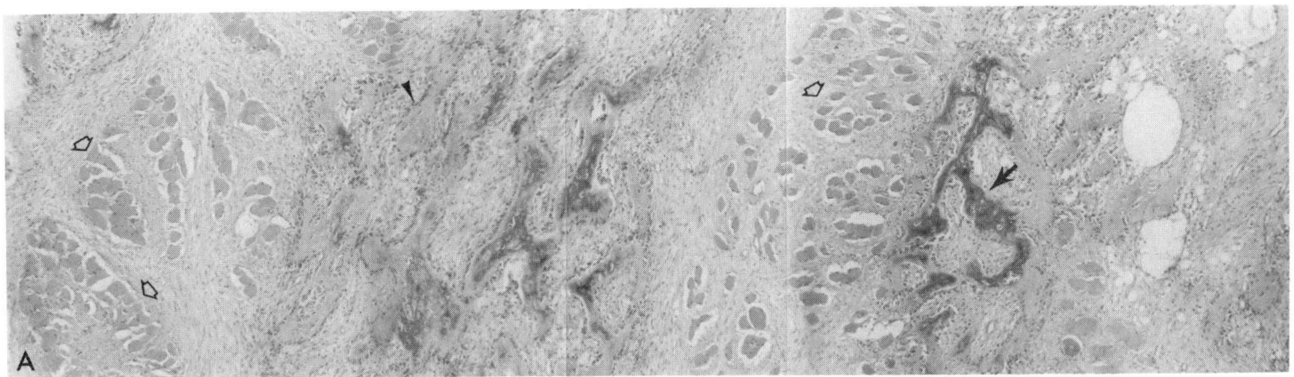

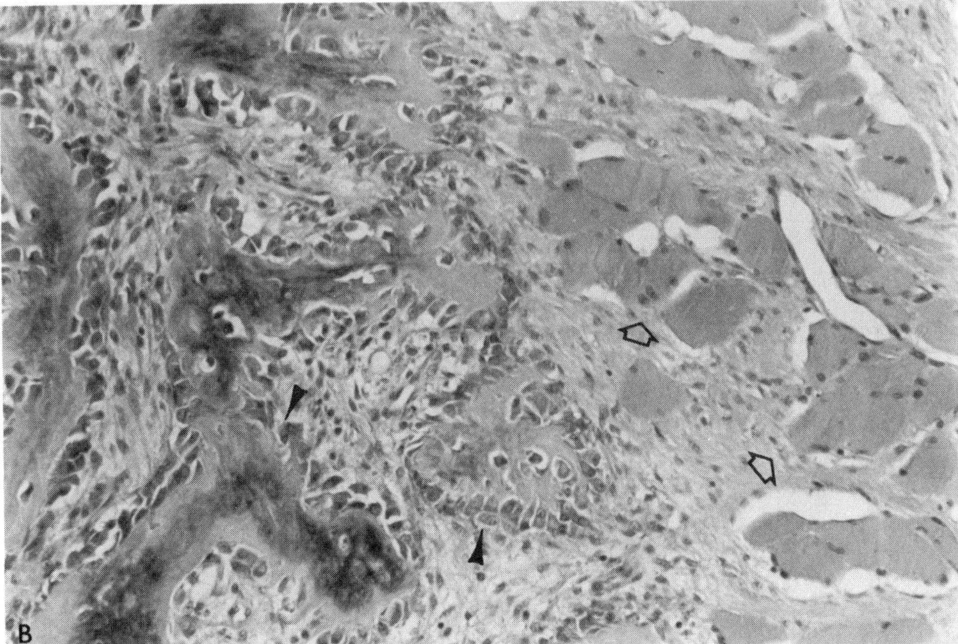

Figure 85–49. *Myositis ossificans traumatica: Pathologic abnormalities.*

A *Muscular tissue can be identified (open arrows). In certain areas (intermediate zone), osteoid and immature bone formation in cellular fibrous tissue is seen (arrowhead); elsewhere (outer zone), maturation of ossification is evident (solid arrow) (68×).*

B *Observe muscle bundles (open arrows) and newly formed bone trabeculae with prominent osteoblasts (arrowheads) (170×).*

tologic documentation may be necessary to establish a definite diagnosis; however, the pathologist must be wary of the "pseudomalignant" nature of the central portion of the lesion, which can complicate the evaluation. Furthermore, reports have been made of sarcomatous degeneration in foci of myositis ossificans, usually taking the form of fibrosarcoma[178, 179] or osteosarcoma,[94, 177] an occurrence that could further complicate accurate histologic appraisal. Fortunately, the incidence of sarcomatous change in myositis ossificans appears to be very small.

Myositis ossificans must be differentiated from parosteal osteosarcoma, periosteal osteosarcoma, extraskeletal (soft tissue) osteosarcoma or chondrosarcoma, osteochondroma, osteoma, and juxtacortical chondroma. *Parosteal osteosarcomas*[180-182] arise in the metaphysis of tubular bones, especially along the

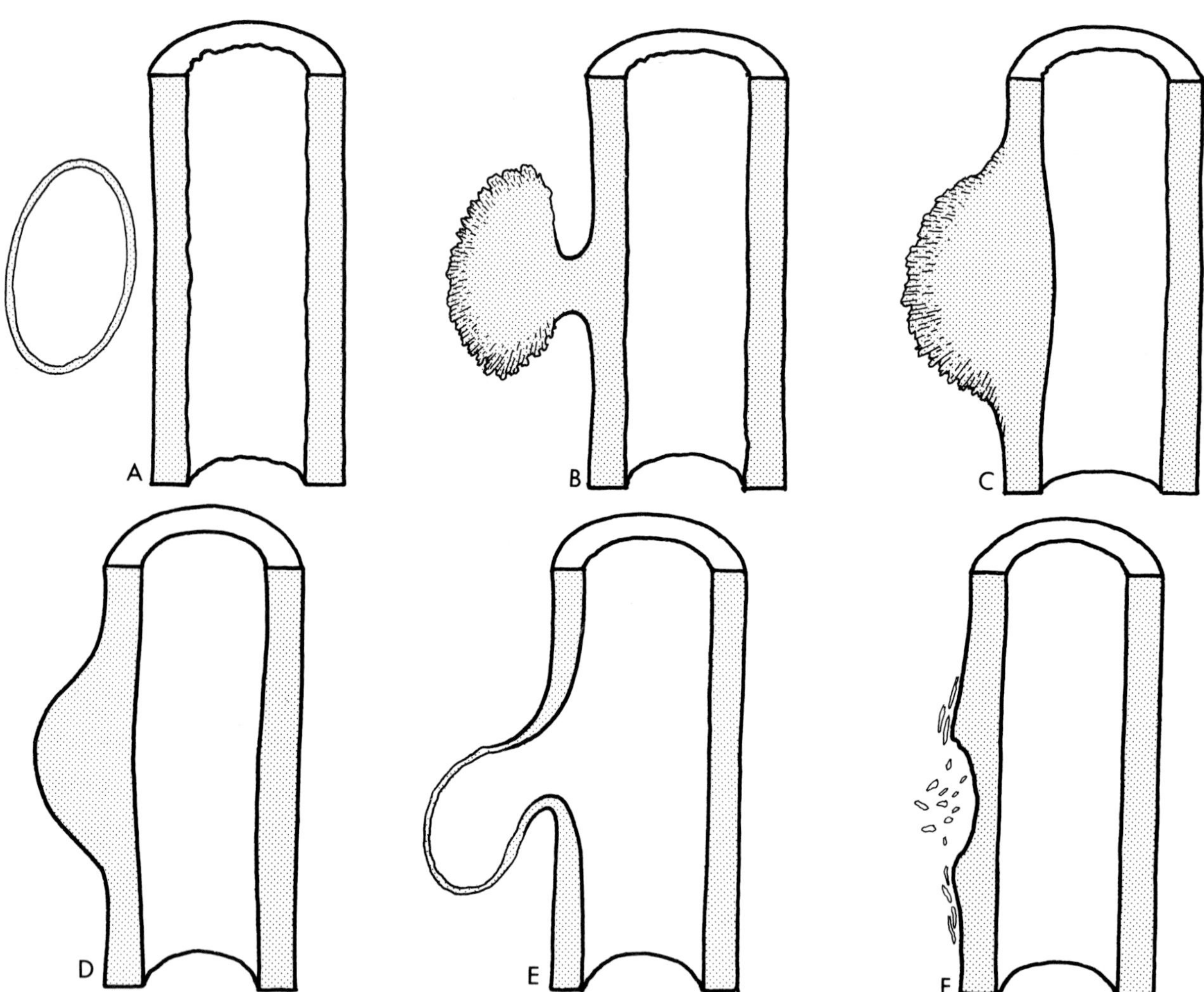

Figure 85–50. *Myositis ossificans traumatica: Differential diagnosis.*

A *Myositis ossificans traumatica. The shell-like configuration of the ossification with a clear zone between it and the underlying bone is typical of this condition.*

B *Parosteal osteosarcoma. These lesions appear as central ossifying foci with irregular outlines and may be connected to the underlying bone by a stalk.*

C *Periosteal osteosarcoma. These tumors arise in the cortex of a diaphysis of a tubular bone and produce cortical thickening and spiculated osteoid matrix.*

D *Osteoma. Characteristic of this lesion is a localized excrescence that produces bulging of the cortical contour.*

E *Osteochondroma. An exostosis protrudes from the cortical surface. Its medullary and cortical bone is continuous with that of the underlying osseous structure.*

F *Juxtacortical chondroma. These periosteal lesions produce localized excavation of the cortex with periostitis. They may contain calcification.*

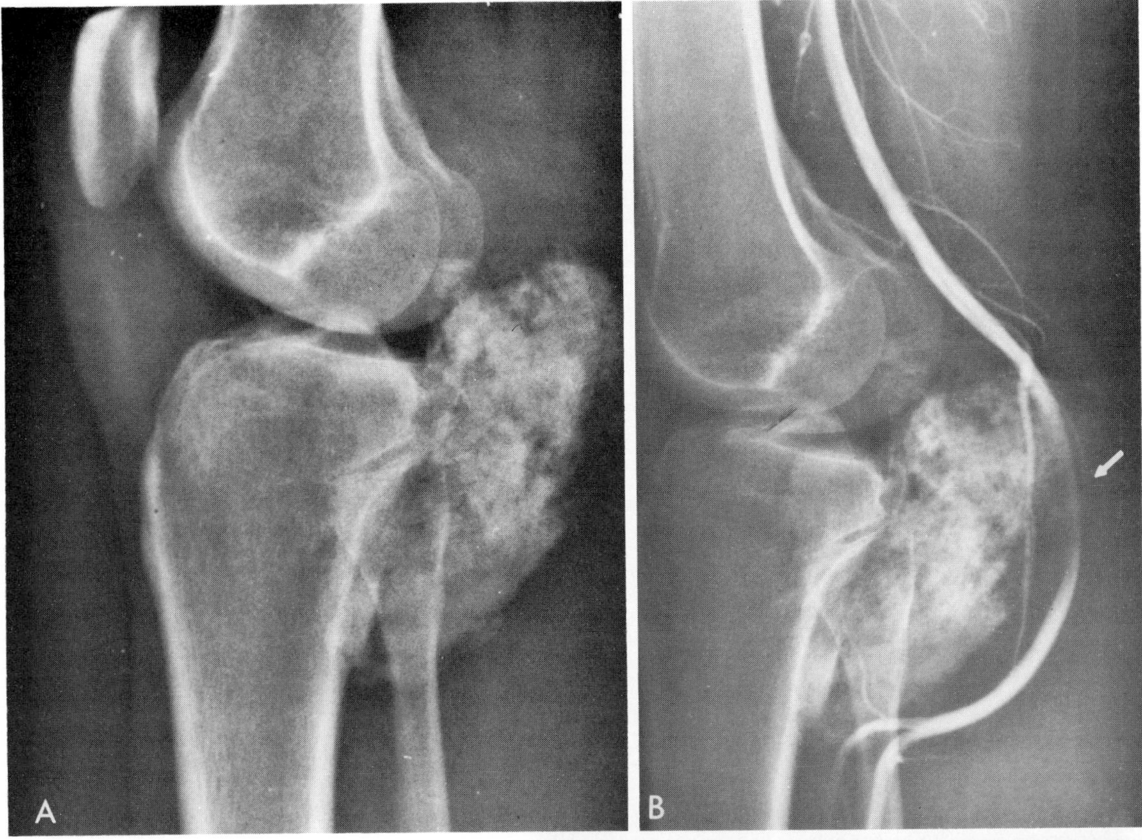

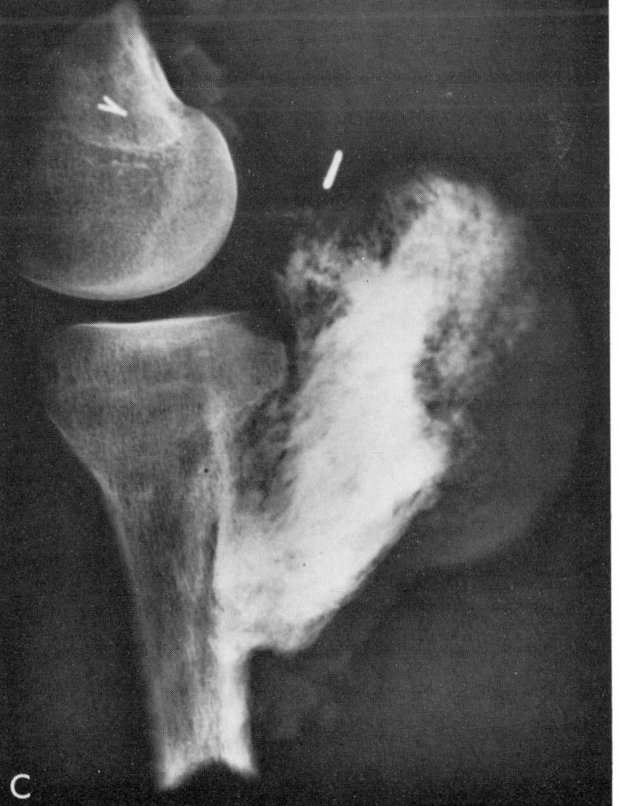

Figure 85–51. *Parosteal osteosarcoma.*

A *An ossified rectangular mass arises from the posterior aspect of the proximal tibia.*

B *Femoral arteriography delineates posterior displacement and stretching of the adjacent artery (arrow).*

C *A radiograph of the specimen reveals ossified and unossified portions of the tumor and its relationship to the tibia.*

(**A, B,** Courtesy of Dr. J. Smith, Memorial Hospital, New York, New York; **C,** From Ahuja SC et al: J Bone Joint Surg 59A:632, 1977.)

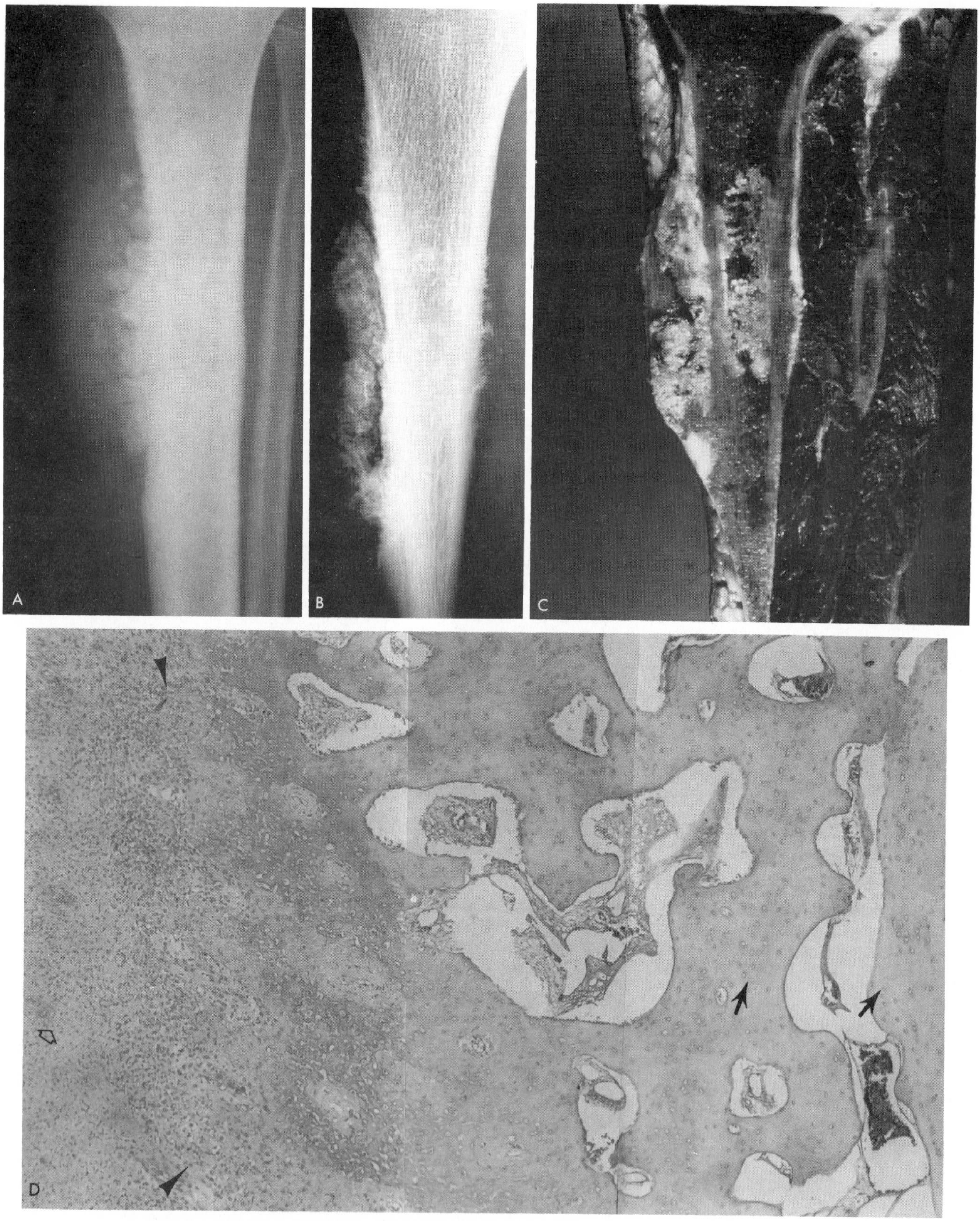

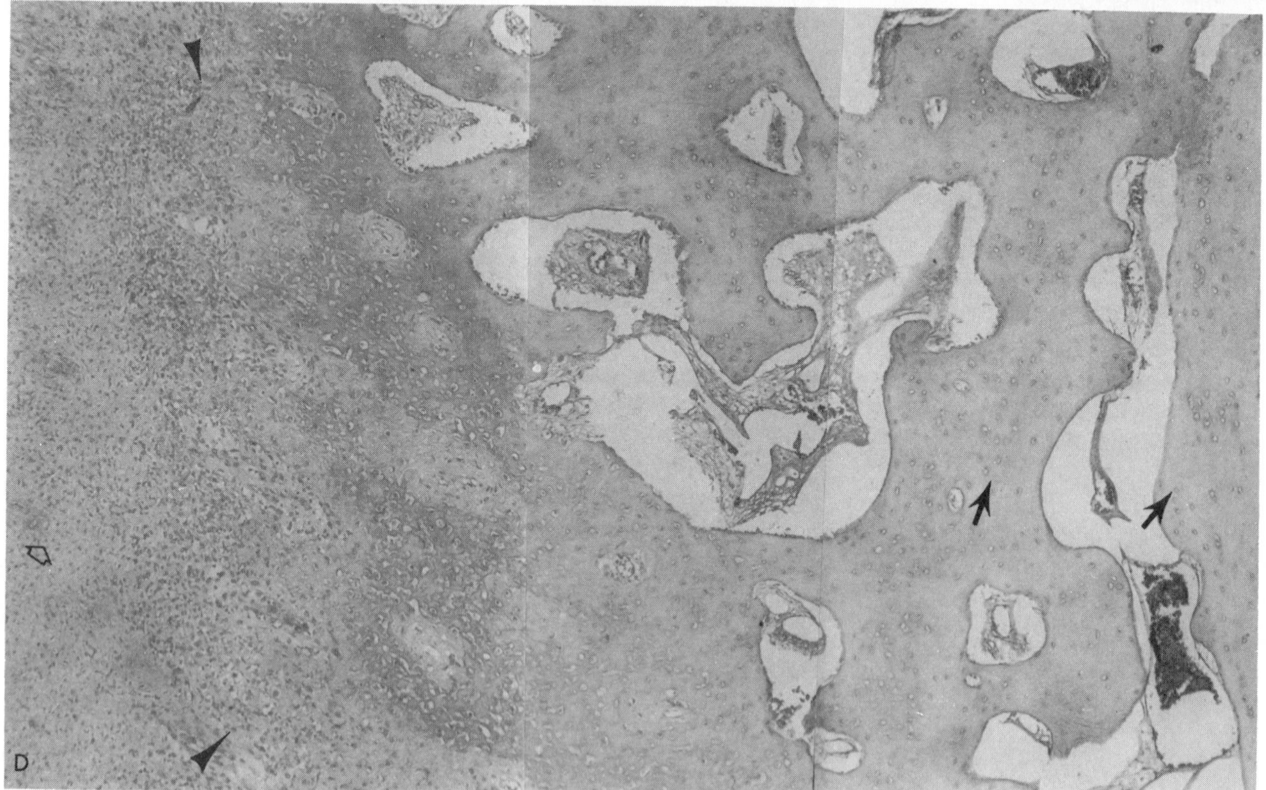

Figure 85–52. *Parosteal osteosarcoma. This 10 year old Mexican boy noted a slowly enlarging tender mass over a one year period following trauma to the tibia.*

A *A radiograph reveals a soft tissue mass containing central irregular ossification. The lesion in the fibula is a cortical defect.*

B, C *A radiograph and photograph of the specimen better demonstrate the location and nature of the lesion. Following considerable debate, the final diagnosis was parosteal osteosarcoma.*

D *Photomicrograph (76×) reveals hypertrophic trabeculae (solid arrows), chondromatous fibrous tissue with cellular atypia (open arrow), and atypical chondrocytes at the junction of fibrous and osseous tissues (arrowheads).*

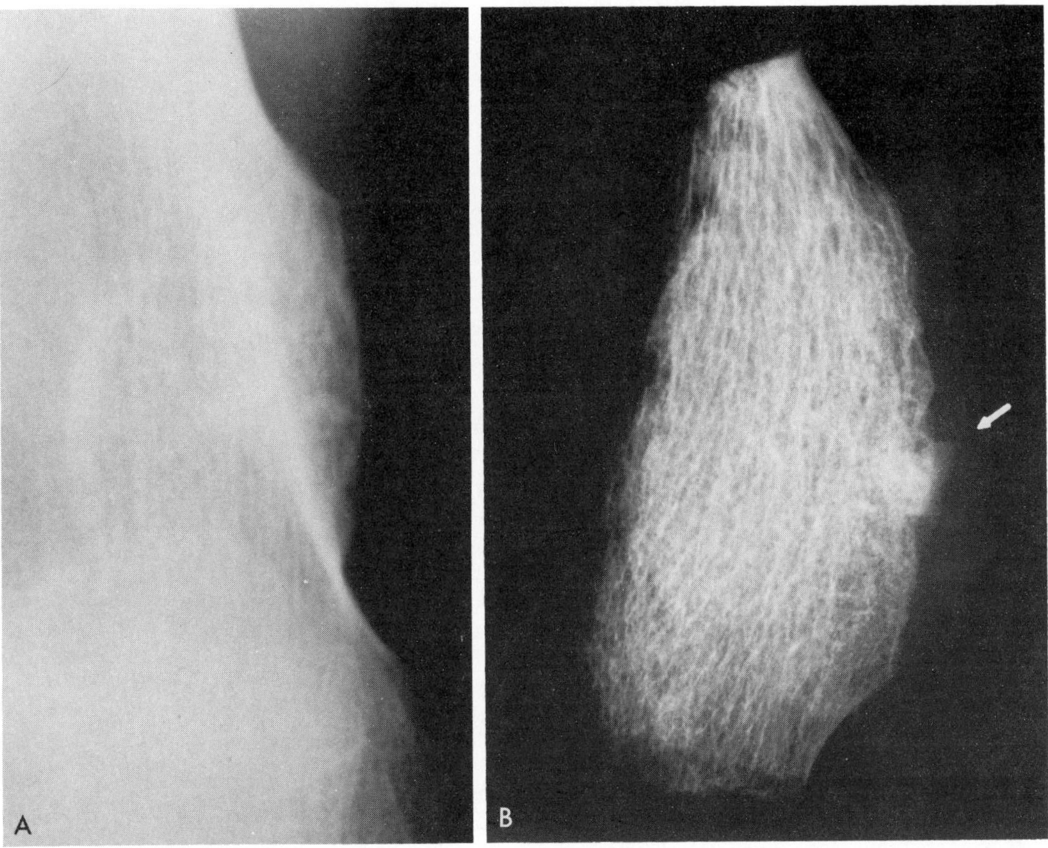

Figure 85–53. *Osteochondroma.*
A *A broad-based osteochondroma of the distal femur is evident.*
B *A radiograph of the removed specimen reveals its trabecular structure and cartilaginous cap (arrow).*

posterior aspect of the distal femur (Figs. 85–51 and 85–52). Although a lucent zone may exist between the tumor and underlying bone, the zone is usually incomplete, as a pedicle extends from the neoplasm to the subjacent osseous tissue. Furthermore, a parosteal osteosarcoma is more heavily calcified in its central portion and base of attachment, the periphery is less dense and poorly circumscribed, and the tumor enlarges with time. *Periosteal osteosarcomas*[183, 184] arise in the cortex of a diaphysis of a tubular bone and lead to cortical thickening and spiculated osteoid matrix that is progressively denser from the periphery to their cortical base. *Extraskeletal osteosarcomas*[94] are rare neoplasms that can cause difficulty in differential diagnosis. They grow slowly and affect older patients. An *osteochondroma* arises from and is connected to the subjacent bone; it possesses a cartilaginous cap (Figs. 85–53 to 85–55). Both the cortex and the spongiosa of the osteochondroma and parent bone are continuous. Occasionally, a mature focus of myositis ossificans may develop a cartilaginous cap and areas of cartilage,[162] whereas an osteochondroma may give rise to a chondrosarcoma. In these cases, differential diagnosis may be more difficult. An osteoma is an osseous excrescence extending from the outer surface of the cortex that is readily differentiated from myositis ossificans (see Chapter 81), whereas a *juxtacortical chondroma* produces soft tissue calcification, an excavation of the cortex, and adjacent periosteal proliferation (Fig. 85–56).

Pseudomalignant Osseous Tumor of Soft Tissue. The presence of a nonmalignant tumor of soft tissue exhibiting sarcoma-like histologic features in its central portion and mature-appearing bone in its periphery was defined by Fine and Stout in 1956,[94] although previous reports can be found in the literature.[185-187] These lesions, which are usually termed pseudomalignant osseous tumors of soft tissue,[94, 160, 161, 188-191] appear in patients who do not relate a history of antecedent trauma and are well circumscribed, nonaggressive, and compatible with long-term survival. Men and women are affected, and most individuals are in the second and third decades of life. Most tumors are located in the extremities or the gluteal regions, and they rarely are greater than 6 cm in diameter (Figs. 85–57 and 85–58). Soft tissue swelling with or without pain precedes the appearance of calcification and ossification by a short interval of approximately 2 to 3 weeks. Although previous trauma or infection is cited in some of the reports, this is an inconstant and

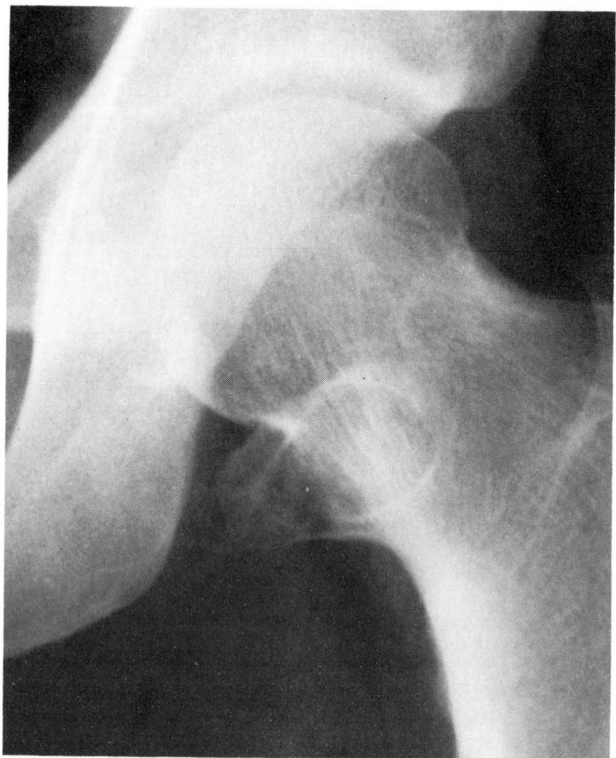

Figure 85–54. Osteochondroma. An overgrowth of the medial aspect of the femoral neck is evident.

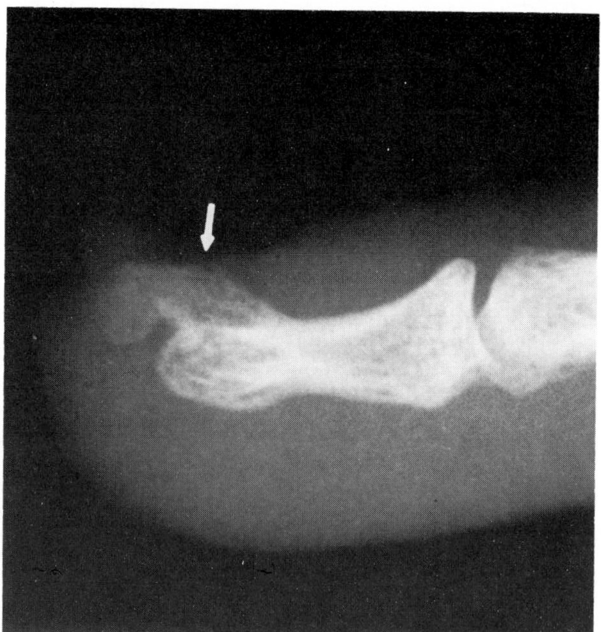

Figure 85–55. Subungual exostosis. An outgrowth of the distal aspect of the phalanx (arrow) can produce painful deformity of a nail.

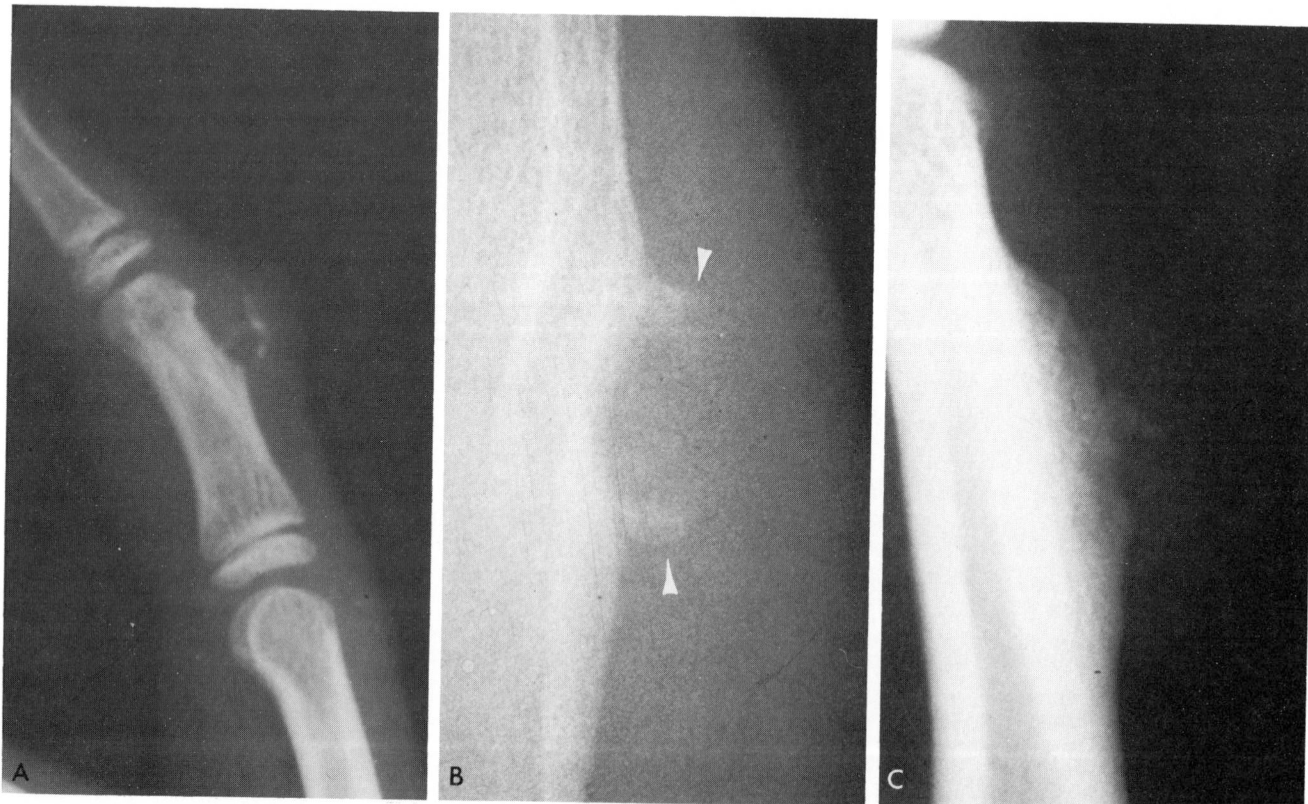

Figure 85–56. Juxtacortical chondroma. Three examples of this lesion are presented. The radiographs may reveal a soft tissue mass with or without calcification, with local excavation of the cortex and periostitis **(A)**, circumferential periosteal bone proliferation (arrowheads) **(B)**, or irregular, broad-based excrescences **(C)**.

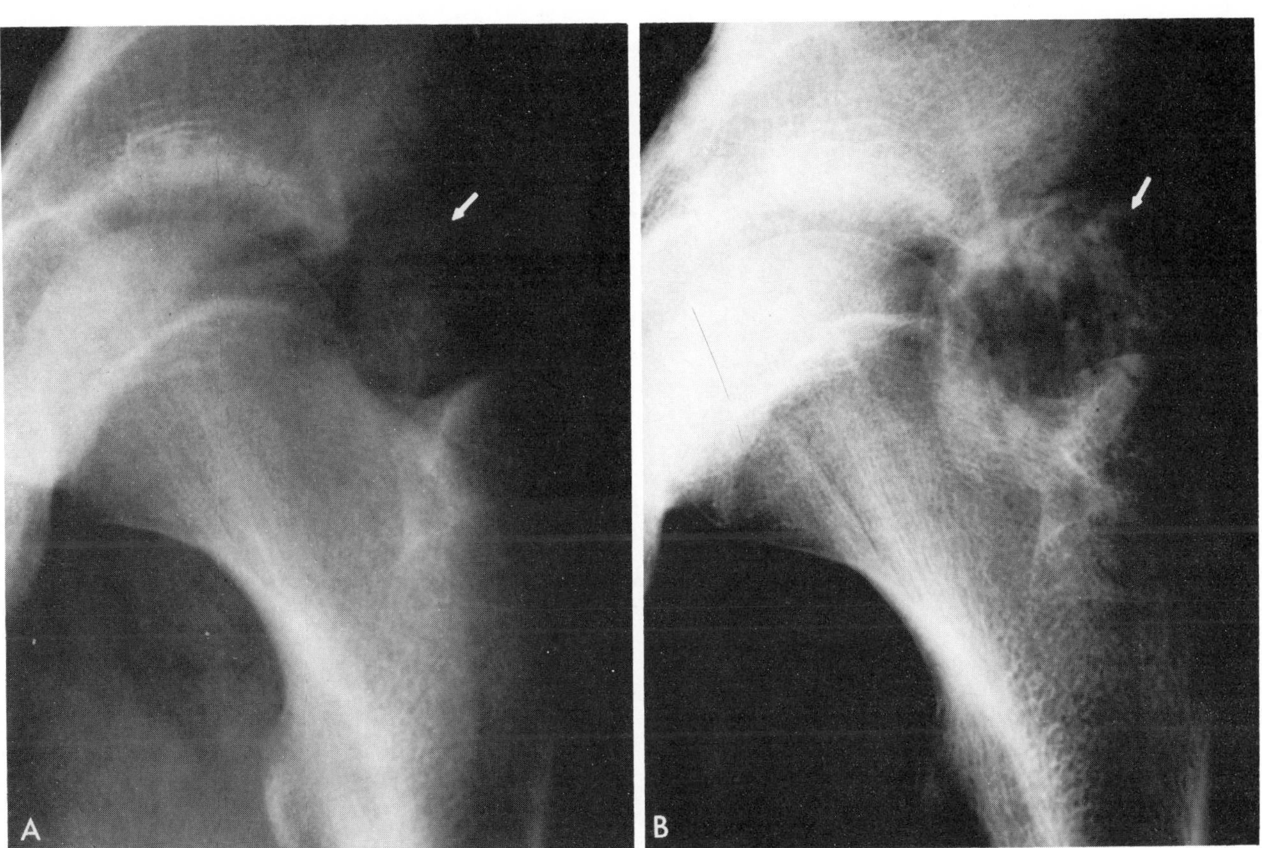

Figure 85–57. *Pseudomalignant osseous tumor of soft tissue. Ossification about the hip in this child appeared without antecedent trauma.*

A, B *Sequential stages in the ossifying process (arrow) are demonstrated on x-rays taken 4 weeks apart. On the later study, the shell-like configuration of the lesion is evident.*

Illustration continued on the following page

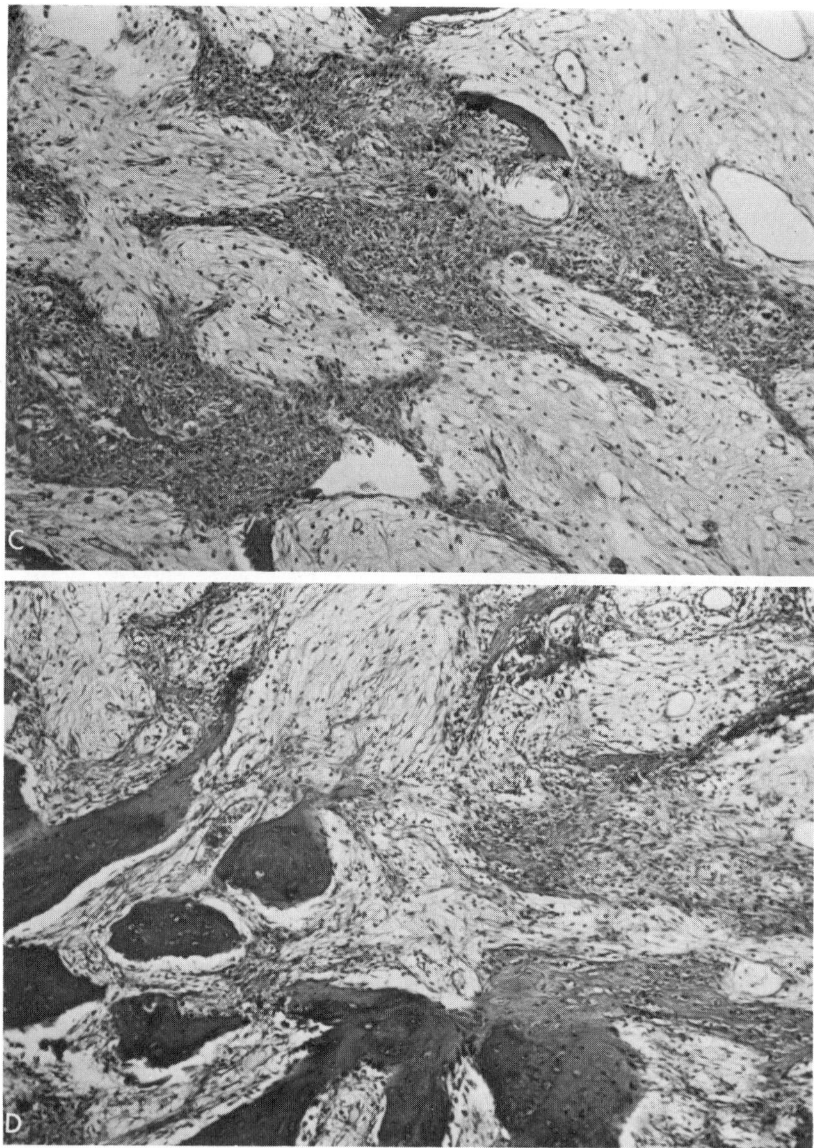

Figure 85–57. Continued

C *In the central portion of the lesion, concentrated collections of spindle cells are observed, especially in pericystic locations. Loosely arranged spindle cells are also noted.*

D *In the peripheral portion of the lesion, regularly arranged mature spongy bone is seen separated by loosely arranged connective tissue.*

(From Schulze K, et al: Fortschr Geb Roentgenstr Nuklearmed 129:343, 1978. Courtesy of Georg Thieme Verlag, Stuttgartt.)

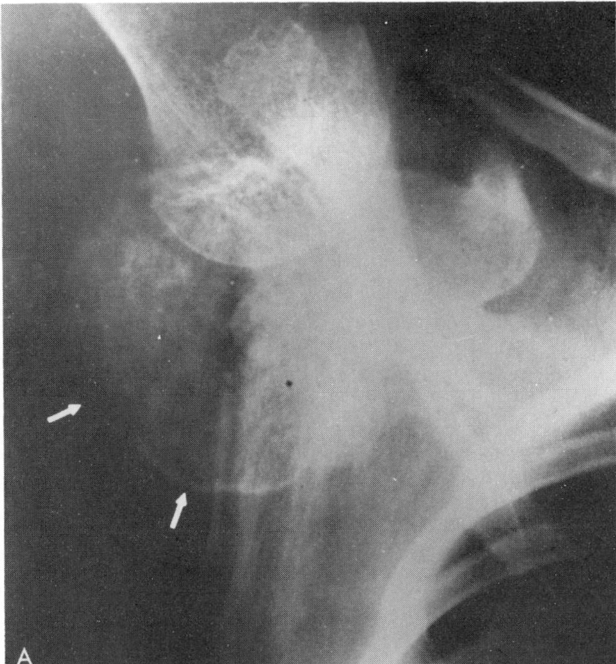

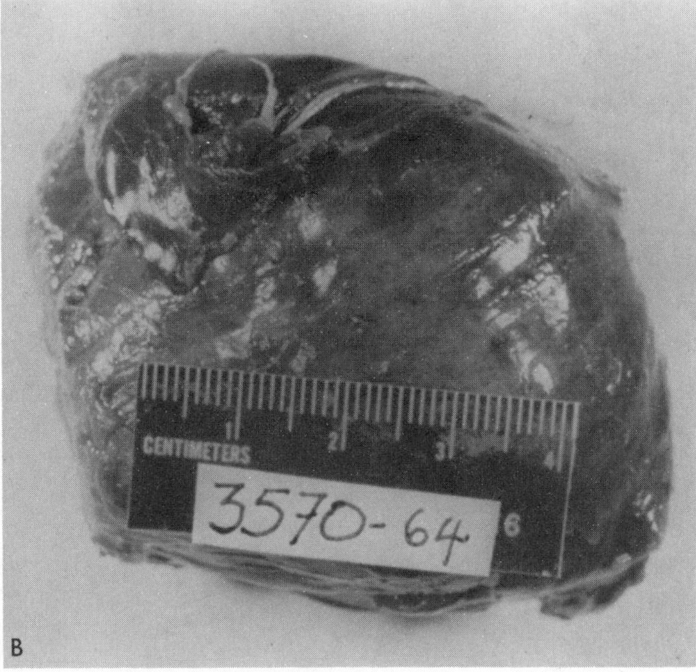

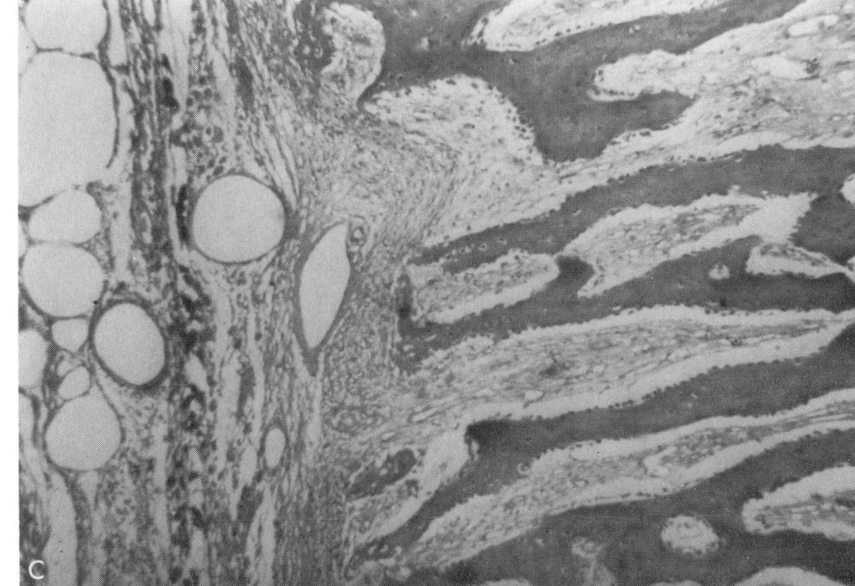

Figure 85–58. *Pseudomalignant osseous tumor of soft tissue. This 11 year old girl noted the onset of pain and swelling in the right shoulder. A history of trauma was not elicited, and the presumptive clinical diagnosis was a malignant tumor.*

A *A roentgenogram demonstrates an ossified soft tissue mass with a shell-like configuration (arrows).*

B *A photograph of the specimen reveals the nature of this mass.*

C *Although the inner and middle zones of the mass contained hemorrhage, necrosis, fibroblasts, osteoblasts, and immature bone, the outer zone or periphery of the lesion is composed of mature trabeculae.*

(Courtesy of Dr. A. Goldman, Hospital for Special Surgery, New York, New York.)

infrequent feature. The course is typically benign, and, in some cases, the lesions have become smaller or disappeared. The histologic characteristics include central connective tissue showing varying cell density with bundles of fibroblasts, cellular pleomorphism with giant cells, and occasional mitotic figures; in addition, there is peripheral mature trabecular bone with spicules of osteoid tissue radiating toward the central areas of the lesion.[189] These alterations resemble those in myositis ossificans traumatica, although muscle fibers, hematomas, and peripheral extension in the soft tissues are not found. The major importance of pseudomalignant osseous tumor of soft tissue is the fact that it must be distinguished from malignant processes, especially osteogenic sarcoma of soft tissue. The presence of the zone phenomenon, the peripheral location of the ossification, the limitation in size, and the absence of stromal cell atypism in pseudomalignant osseous tumor are helpful in this regard.

Myositis Ossificans Progressiva (Fibrodysplasia Ossificans Progressiva). This is a rare disorder of mesodermal tissue in which inflammatory foci initially appear and proliferate in fibrous tissue.[192-202] It is discussed in depth in Chapter 72, and only a few comments will be included here. The hallmark of the disease is soft tissue ossification. Primary changes occur in the fibrous tissue, and the

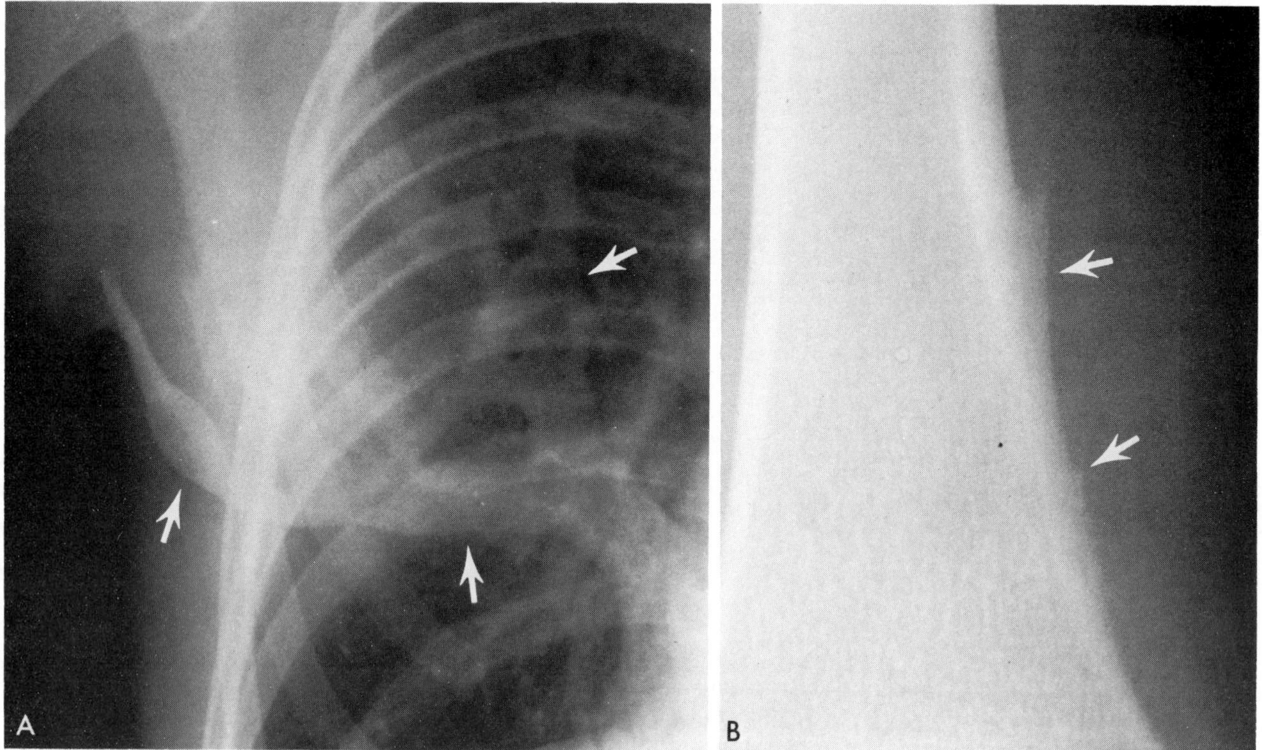

Figure 85–59. Myositis ossificans progressiva.
A Sheet-like ossified bridges about the shoulder girdle are typical (arrows).
B Broad-based excrescences (arrows) can be seen in the tubular bones.

muscles are affected secondarily from the contiguous fascial coverings. Histologic assessment of involved areas confirms ossified connective tissue and degenerating skeletal muscle. On roentgenograms, sheets of ossified tissue are encountered in the thoracic and abdominal walls and may bridge articulations, leading to contractures and "ankylosis"; osteophyte-like outgrowths of tubular bones can also be seen (Fig. 85–59). The findings can be striking, and in certain regions, such as the neck, a solid mass of bone may be found, associated with ossification of multiple intervertebral discs. A peculiar additional feature of the disease is the high incidence of associated congenital anomalies of the thumb and big toe that are present at birth and that are apparently unrelated to the ossifying diathesis. Among others, these include microdactyly or adactyly, hallux valgus, ankylosis of interphalangeal and metatarsophalangeal joints, and clinodactyly of fingers.

The major differential diagnosis is idiopathic calcinosis universalis. This disease is associated with linear calcification appearing in the extremities, differing from the ossification of the axial skeleton that predominates in myositis ossificans progressiva. In the latter disorder, para-articular osseous bridges may simulate the changes in neurologic illnesses or following burns, whereas the ossification about the spine can resemble the changes in ankylosing spondylitis or juvenile chronic arthritis. Accurate diagnosis generally is not difficult, especially when the anomalies of the toes and fingers are appreciated.

SOFT TISSUE BANDS AND CONTRACTURES

Amniotic (or Streeter's) constriction bands have been recognized for over 150 years.[203-208] These soft tissue grooves or depressions can affect any portion of a limb, but most frequently they involve the fingers. Their etiology is debated. Streeter[203] and Glessner[209] proposed that constriction rings could develop from defective germ plasm, perhaps related to an insult to the fetus at the time of differentiation of the limb buds.[203] Torpin and co-workers,[210] Blanc and associates,[206] and Latta[211] postulated that premature rupture of the fetal amnion could produce raw surfaces and strings that attach to and mechanically entrap the limb, leading to rings and amputations. Abbe[212] proposed that the central nervous system could exert a deficient control of the developing tissue that could result in congenital bands. The role of intra-amniotic infection or trauma[213] has also been emphasized.

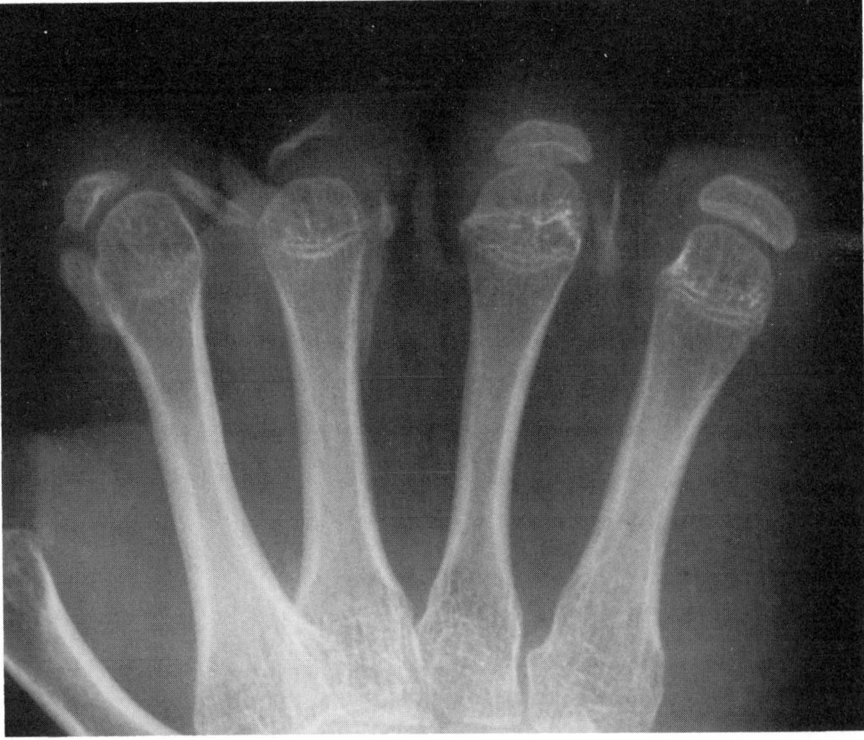

Figure 85–60. Amniotic (or Streeter's) constriction bands. Autoamputation of the fingers is presumably the result of amniotic bands, although the presence of small ossific foci about the metacarpal heads may indicate the occurrence of malformed phalanges and congenital defects of the hand.

The incidence of such bands is variously recorded as 1 in 5000 to 1 in 45,000 births.[206, 209, 214, 215] The cases are sporadic, as no familial history has been noted. Many of the patients are products of first pregnancies and of young mothers, and additional deformities of nails or other structures are frequent.[208] Common associated anomalies are clubbed feet and cleft lip and palate. Bleeding in the third trimester of pregnancy has also been associated with this condition.[216] On clinical examination, scarred rings encircle a digit or limb, and temperature gradients and sensory deficits may be evident across the constricted areas.[217] Multiple and symmetrically distributed lesions are typical. Radiographs delineate the soft tissue constrictions that extend for a variable depth and may contact the subjacent bone. It is the visualization of soft tissue deficit that allows differentiation of this condition from congenital defects.[216] The underlying bones may be poorly developed or absent, and distal to the lesions, lymphedema or fatty accumulation may be encountered. Syndactyly or amputation can also be evident (Fig. 85–60).

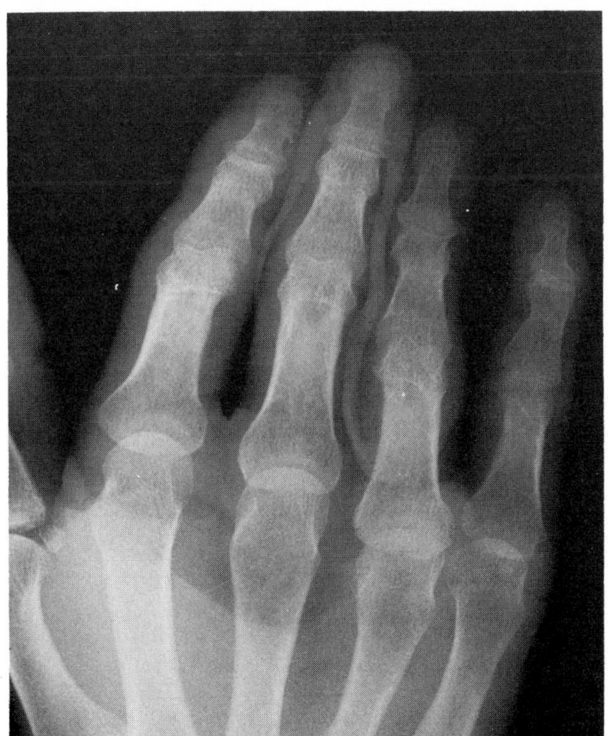

Figure 85–61. Dupuytren's contracture. Observe the flexion deformities about the metacarpophalangeal joints of the four ulnar digits.

Acquired rings may also occur, perhaps related to an encircling foreign object, such as a rubber band.[216] Ainhum (see Chapter 62) is a tropical disease in which a deep constricting band appears about the fifth toe on one or both feet.

Soft tissue contractures can accompany many congenital disorders, such as arthrogryposis multiplex congenita,[218] Leri's pleonosteosis,[219] and contractural arachnodactyly[220]; acquired conditions such as Volkmann's ischemic contracture,[221] thermal burns, and neurologic injury; and various rheumatologic diseases, such as rheumatoid arthritis and systemic lupus erythematosus. Additional well-known examples in the hand are Dupuytren's contracture of the palmar fascia (Fig. 85–61), camptodactyly, in

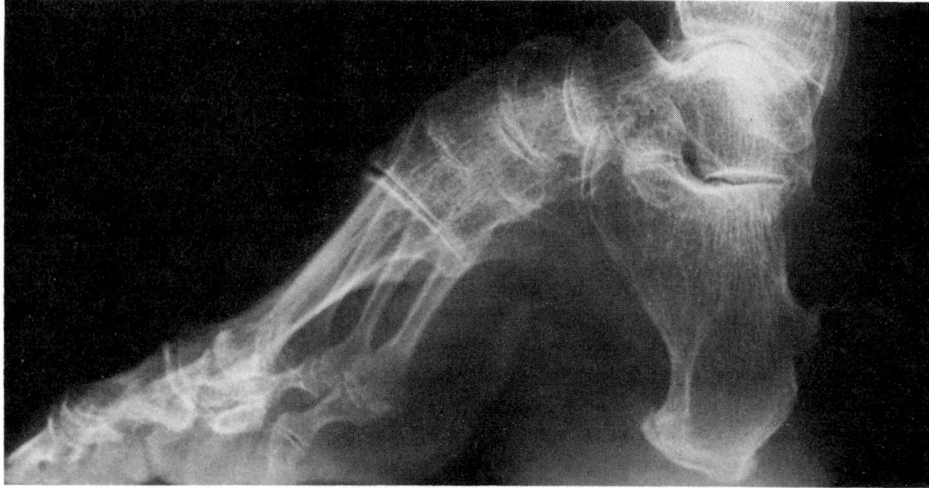

Figure 85–62. Bound foot of a Chinese woman. Observe the extreme calcaneus deformity of the hindfoot and pes cavus.

which a flexion contracture involves predominantly the proximal interphalangeal articulation of the fifth digit,[222] clinodactyly, in which a curvature of a finger occurs in a mediolateral plane,[223] and Kirner's deformity, in which palmar bending of the shaft of a terminal phalanx may be associated with epiphyseal separation.[224] In fact, many syndromes are associated with crooked fingers or crooked toes.[216] Furthermore, other skeletal sites can be affected, and the list of disorders associated with soft tissue contractures is extensive. One interesting example is the appearance of contracted and deformed soft tissues and bones associated with the former Chinese custom of binding women's feet (Fig. 85–62).

SOFT TISSUE EDEMA

Traumatic or inflammatory processes can lead to localized soft tissue edema. In addition, venous or lymphatic obstruction from many diverse causes

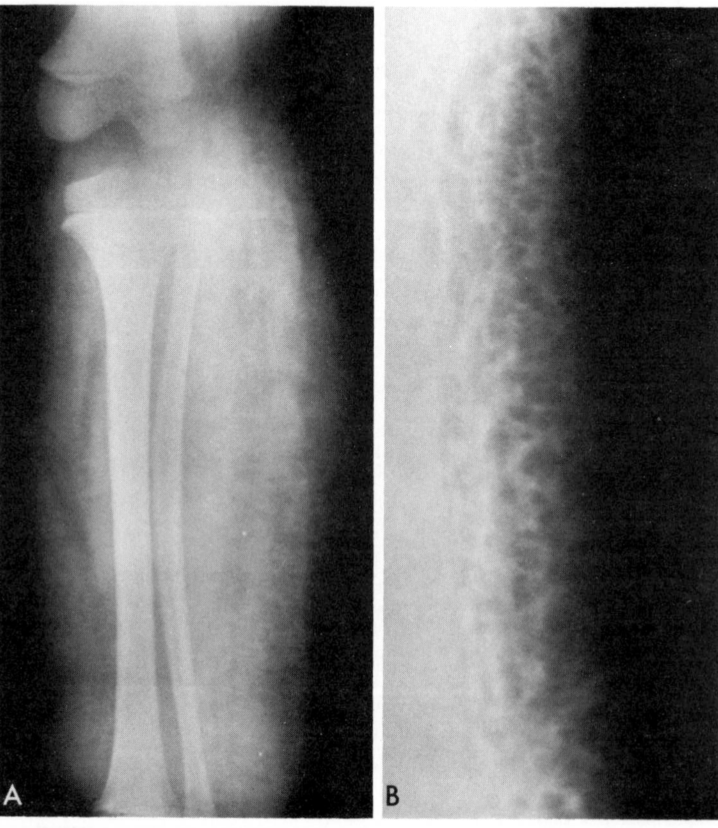

Figure 85–63. Lymphedema.

A A 5 year old boy with congenital lymphedema reveals the typical striated pattern in the enlarged soft tissues.

B A coned-down view in another patient delineates the reticular soft tissue pattern.

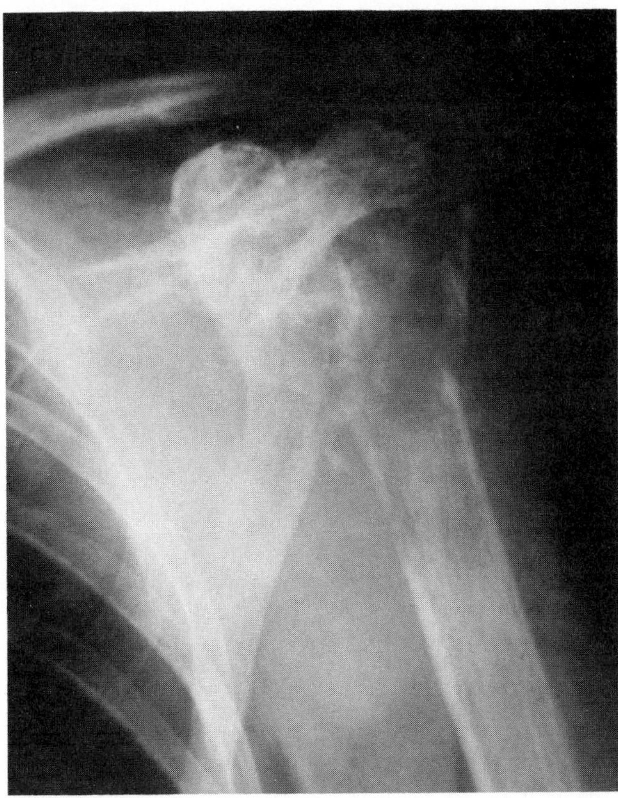

Figure 85–64. Lymphedema with lymphangiosarcoma. In this patient with breast carcinoma who had had a radical mastectomy, and who had lymphedema of the arm, a lymphangiosarcoma developed, which led to osseous destruction of the proximal humerus. Irradiation effect is also evident. (Courtesy of Dr. D. McEwan, Winnipeg, Manitoba, Canada.)

may produce edema that is recognized radiographically as enlargement of the soft tissue contour, obliteration of the fascial planes, and a fine or coarsened reticular pattern (Fig. 85–63). Special studies, such as phlebography or lymphangiography, can accurately define the nature of the obstructive lesion. Lymphedema itself may result from various processes, including primary or congenital disorders,[225] trauma, infection (filariasis), irradiation, tumor, and surgery (e.g., following mastectomy). Lymphedema may also accompany thyroid acropachy, melorheostosis, infantile cortical hyperostosis, and acromegaly. The occurrence of lymphangiosarcomas in areas of long-term lymphedema has been documented (Fig. 85–64).

SOFT TISSUE EMPHYSEMA

Collections of gas, including air, in the soft tissues can be caused by several mechanisms. Air can be introduced iatrogenically into the soft tissues or joints during puncture for diagnostic or therapeutic purposes. Air can also penetrate the soft tissues in cases of communicating wounds or fistulae. Gas formation by bacteria such as clostridia may lead to radiolucent streaks or bubbles in the subcutaneous or muscular tissues (see Chapters 60 and 62). This is not infrequent in diabetic patients (Fig. 85–65).

SPECIAL SYNDROMES OF SKIN AND SOFT TISSUE

Certain afflictions of the cutaneous and subcutaneous tissues can be associated with radiographic abnormalities. Some of the important afflictions are described here; however, others, such as ichthyosis, in which dry, scaly, thickened skin is observed, can produce soft tissue nodularity or irregularity (Fig. 85–66).

Epidermolysis Bullosa

This is a rare chronic skin disorder that results from poor adherence of the epidermis to the dermis, as a consequence of which vesicles, bullae, and ulcerations form either spontaneously or following minor traumatic insults.[226-230] The disorder is inherited in either a dominant or a recessive manner, and the latter form is more severe. Further division of the disease is based upon specific clinical manifestations. Four types are recognized: the simple type, an autosomal dominant trait; the hyperplastic dystrophic type, also an autosomal dominant; the dystrophic polydysplastic type, with recessive inheritance; and the lethal type, also with recessive inheritance.[230]

The simple variety is mild, becoming evident any time during the first year of life. Bullae appear in areas subjected to trauma, especially in the hands, feet, elbows, and knees, and they heal by epithelialization without scarring. Although new lesions may subsequently appear, the disease usually subsides after puberty. The hyperplastic dystrophic variety also is mild, becoming apparent before puberty. Bullae result from trauma, and the lesions heal with the development of hyperkeratosis and thin, atrophic scars. Fingernails and toenails may be lost, but the mucous membranes are rarely affected, and there is no interference with growth or development. The dystrophic polydysplastic type is severe. Bullae are noted at birth or shortly thereafter, developing after trauma or spontaneously. The mucous membranes of the eyes, nose, oropharynx, anus, and genital tract are always affected, and esophageal lesions may lead to dysphagia, spasm, scarring, and contractures. Malnourishment, retardation of physical development, thin, scarred atrophic skin, and hand deformities are encountered. The lethal type is rare, producing severe and widespread involvement with death in early infancy.

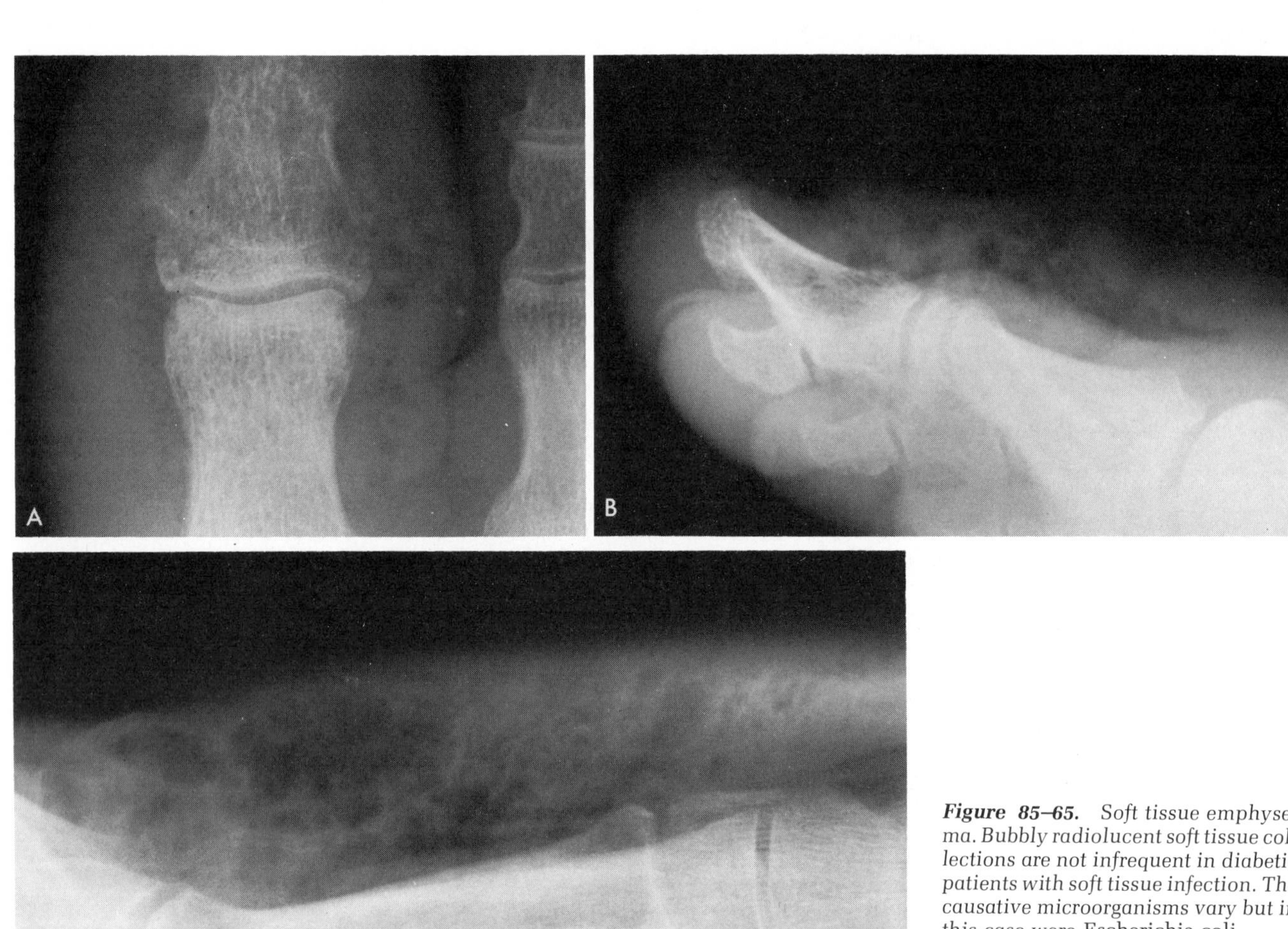

Figure 85–65. *Soft tissue emphysema. Bubbly radiolucent soft tissue collections are not infrequent in diabetic patients with soft tissue infection. The causative microorganisms vary but in this case were* Escherichia coli.

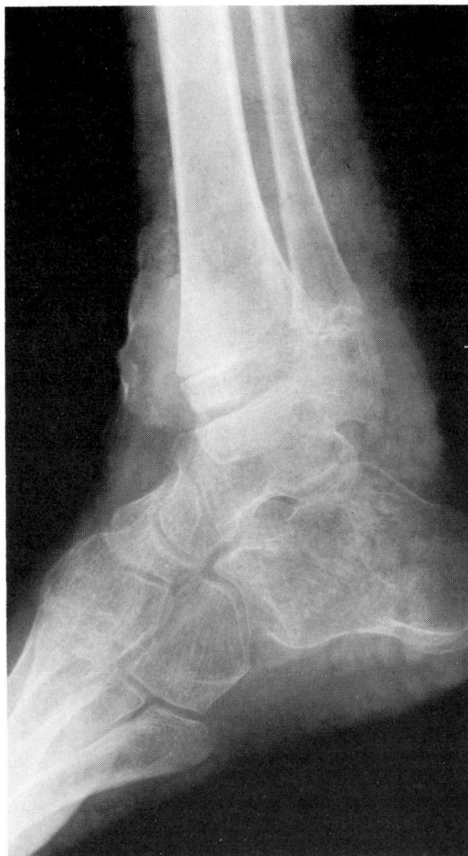

Figure 85–66. Ichthyosis. Observe the soft tissue nodularity due to the presence of irregular skin thickening.

Radiographic findings are characteristic but not specific. They vary with the type of disease that is present. Flexion contractures of the metacarpophalangeal and interphalangeal articulations, webbing between the fingers, and distal trophic changes can be encountered (Fig. 85–67). The terminal phalanges of the hands (and, less frequently, the feet) are distorted, becoming pointed or wedged-shaped, resembling the findings in scleroderma. This resemblance may be accentuated by the rare appearance of soft tissue calcification in epidermolysis bullosa.[226] The combination of flexion deformities of the fingers and toes and webbing is important in the diagnosis of this rare skin disease.[228] Osteoporosis, slender diaphyses of the tubular bones, perhaps due to chronic muscle atrophy, dental caries, periapical abscesses, loss of teeth, and esophageal strictures can be seen. The dental changes are presumably related to poor oral hygiene and extensive scarring in and around the mouth in early life, although an intrinsic dysplasia may also be important.[229, 231] As a result of scarring in the face and the jaw, underdevelopment of the mandible and maxilla, and an increase in the mandibular angle with prognathism can be noted.[226, 227, 232]

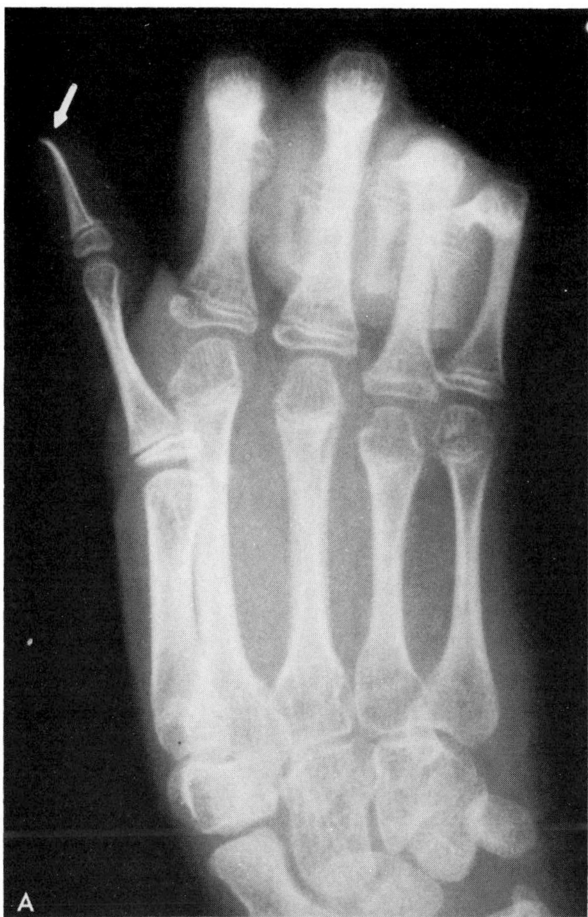

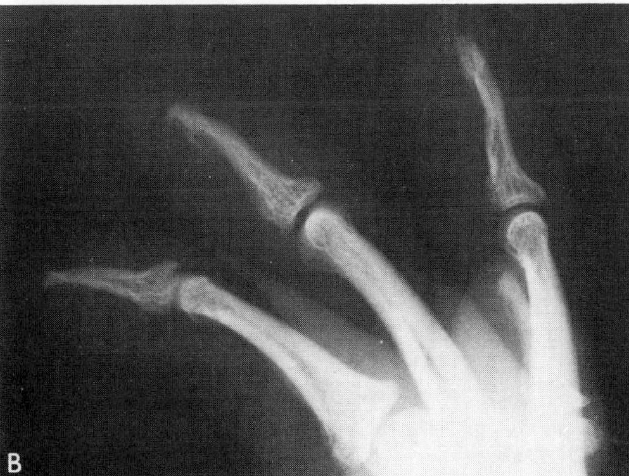

Figure 85–67. Epidermolysis bullosa.

A *Observe contractures of the interphalangeal articulations, webbing between the digits, skin and bone atrophy, osteoporosis, epiphyseal deformity, and pointing of the terminal tufts of the phalanges, most evident in the thumb (arrow).*

B *In another patient, the tapered resorption of the terminal phalanges is well seen.*

The pathologic findings have been well documented.[230] The bullae are tense, thin-walled structures filled with straw-colored fluid that occasionally is hemorrhagic or cloudy. The location of the bullae is variable. In the polydysplastic pattern, they are subepidermal; in other types, they are intraepidermal. Inflammation is not prominent. The characteristics of the healing stage also vary according to the pattern of disease. Scars are seen in those patients who do not have the simple variety of epidermolysis bullosa, and keloids, milia, and pigmentation can be evident.

A series of biochemical and histologic studies have been undertaken to define the etiology and pathogenesis of the disease as well as to differentiate among the various clinical patterns. The mechanism of blister formation seems to be related to an abnormal synthesis of collagen or a presence of abnormal collagen produced in some other fashion.[233-238] A primary role for the proteolytic enzyme collagenase has been suggested; bioassays and radioimmunoassays have revealed increased levels of collagenase in both blistered and clinically normal skin in some patients with epidermolysis bullosa.[236] A structural defect at the basement membrane zone may also be important; deficient or absent anchoring fibers have been reported in both blistered and clinically normal skin.[237] Such structural changes may produce an increased susceptibility of the basement membrane zone to proteolytic enzymes.[238] Other hypotheses regarding the etiology of the disease include a hereditary vascular anomaly of the skin[239] and a congenital defect in the hyaluronidase–hyaluronic acid system.[240]

Occasionally patients with epidermolysis bullosa develop skin cancer[241, 242] and a decreased tolerance to the effects of ionizing radiation.[243]

Congenital Cutis Laxa (Generalized Elastolysis)

This is an inherited disorder of connective tissue that becomes manifest at birth by a striking laxity of the skin, which hangs in pendulous folds over the entire body.[244-247] The cutaneous manifestations are associated with abnormalities of other organs and structures containing elastic tissue. Although the disorder may resemble Marfan's syndrome, Ehlers-Danlos syndrome, and pseudoxanthoma elasticum, it is a distinct entity. Autosomal dominant and recessive patterns exist. Children with the dominant variety of the disease reveal cutaneous abnormalities, a normal life span, and few complications. Patients with the recessive form are more severely affected and may die at an early age owing to pulmonary and cardiovascular involvement. The clinical manifestations combined with biopsy studies that indicate sparse, fragmented, disrupted elastic fibers and an accumulation of material that resembles acid mucopolysaccharide allow accurate diagnosis.

Radiographic manifestations include hernias, diverticula of the gastrointestinal and genitourinary tracts, pulmonary emphysema, and diaphragmatic elevation. Numerous pronounced skin folds may be evident. Hypermobility and instability of joints are not seen. Spontaneous rupture of patellar tendons and an association with plasma cell myeloma have been recorded.[248, 249] Arteriograms may reveal a tortuous, dilated aorta, peripheral pulmonary artery stenosis, and irregular and kinked peripheral vessels.

The etiology is unknown. An abnormality of elastin, elastase, and elastase inhibitor biochemical complex has been suggested.[247, 250]

Eosinophilic Fasciitis (Shulman Syndrome)

This is a newly recognized disorder consisting of a scleroderma-like appearance, eosinophilia, hypergammaglobulinemia, and muscle fascia inflammation in the presence of normal skin.[251-253, 298-300] Men and women are affected and the age of onset varies from childhood to the seventh decade of life. Painful, swollen, indurated skin and subcutaneous tissues, especially in the distal portions of the forearms or legs, may lead to restricted motion in the hands and feet. Raynaud's phenomena and visceral manifestations of scleroderma are lacking. Biopsies outline sclerosis of the dermis and inflammation and fibrosis of the panniculus and deep fascia. Within 6 to 12 months, marked skin hardness can develop, and histologic changes may be very similar to those of scleroderma. Dramatic improvement following steroid medication has been noted. Although articular abnormalities are unusual, some reports of patients with eosinophilic fasciitis have stressed polyarticular manifestations with synovitis, mildly inflammatory synovial fluid, and the carpal tunnel syndrome.[300]

Erythema Nodosum

Erythema nodosum is a relatively uncommon inflammatory disorder leading to nodular cutaneous eruptions, which are red, tender, and warm but do not ulcerate. Located primarily on the lower legs, the lesions can also affect the hands, arms, face, and thighs. Microscopy outlines a nonspecific cutaneous vasculitis with subcutaneous infiltration of lymphocytes, granulocytes, histiocytes, and eosinophils.[254]

Erythema nodosum occurs as an idiopathic disorder (60 to 70 per cent of cases) or as a cutaneous manifestation of many systemic illnesses (30 to 40 per cent of cases), including infections (streptococcal, meningococcal, fungal, mycobacterial), sarcoidosis, Behçet's syndrome, ulcerative colitis, Crohn's disease, and leprosy, as well as following administration of certain drugs (oral contraceptives, sulfonamides).[254, 255] When it is idiopathic, the disease has a benign course, subsiding in a period of weeks or months.

Women are affected more often than men. Patients of all ages are involved, many being in the third and fourth decades of life. Clinical manifestations include fever, skin eruption, and joint abnormalities. The latter are observed in 50 to 75 per cent of cases and frequently precede the cutaneous alterations. Symmetric arthralgias and arthritis are noted in the knees and ankles and, less commonly, the wrists, elbows, shoulders, fingers, and hips. Affected articulations are swollen and tender, and a joint effusion may be detected on clinical and radiologic examination. Typically, no cartilaginous or osseous destruction is seen, and the articular abnormalities decrease and disappear in a few weeks to 6 months.[256] Recurrences of joint manifestations can appear simultaneously with the development of additional cutaneous lesions. An associated radiographic finding in either idiopathic or nonidiopathic cases is bilateral hilar adenopathy.

Laboratory analysis may indicate an elevated erythrocyte sedimentation rate and, possibly, hypergammaglobulinemia as well as positive sensitized sheep cell tests in low titer.

Erythema nodosum is generally considered to represent a hypersensitivity reaction to some agent or an allergic cutaneous vasculitis.[257]

Nevoid Basal Cell Carcinoma Syndrome (Gorlin's Syndrome)

This syndrome is an inherited disorder that is characterized by multiple basal cell carcinomas, palmar pits, odontogenic keratocysts, rib and spine anomalies, brachydactyly, and various neurologic and ophthalmologic abnormalities.[258-265] The disorder is inherited in an autosomal dominant pattern with variable expressivity and appears with equal frequency in both sexes.

Basal cell epitheliomas usually are seen near puberty, although they can be evident as early as 2 years of age. The lesions are slightly raised, translucent, and 1 to 10 mm in diameter, and may reveal brown discoloration. Some are aggressive, with ulceration and local invasion. Typically affected sites are the face and trunk, although other regions can be involved. Less constant skin abnormalities include milia, comedones, sebaceous or epithelial cysts, and dyskeratosis.[260]

Dentigerous cysts of the mandible are common in this disorder but rarely produce clinical findings prior to the age of 6 to 7 years (Fig. 85–68). They may antedate the appearance of the skin lesions, and symptoms and signs related to these cysts may be the presenting manifestations of the disease. Swelling, pain, and spontaneous drainage are seen. Mandibular cysts can be single or multiple, vary in diameter from 1 or 2 mm to several centimeters, are located predominantly at the angle of the jaw, and appear as radiolucent lesions with ill-defined margins. Pathologic fractures and, rarely, ameloblastomas can develop from such lesions.[259, 266, 267] The cysts are follicular or dentigerous in type and are lined with epithelium that may be stratified squamous or abnormally keratinized. Their surgical removal may be followed by recurrence, perhaps related to activation of retained microcysts.

The common rib anomalies are splaying, synostosis, and bifid and cervical ribs[263] (Fig. 85–69). Unilateral or bilateral alterations in the first to fourth ribs are most typical. Shortening of the metacarpals, especially the fourth and fifth, is also a rather common finding, similar to that which occurs in pseudohypoparathyroidism, multiple hereditary exostosis, and other conditions. In the spine, kyphoscoliosis, spina bifida occulta, block vertebrae, and hemivertebrae can be seen. The list of additional skeletal manifestations in the basal cell nevus syndrome is impressive and includes shortened distal phalanges and notching of the inferior aspect of the scapula. In the skull, calcification of the falx cerebri (Fig. 85–69), dura, tentorium, and choroid, partial agenesis of the corpus callosum, hypertelorism, and anosmia[268] may occur. Mental retardation, congenital hydrocephalus, and changes in the eyes (dysgenesis oculi neuroblastica gliomatosa) have been noted. Several instances of medulloblastoma or meningioma in this syndrome have been recorded.[259, 262]

Gonadal abnormalities in the female include ovarian and uterine fibromas and in the male hypogonadism and cryptorchidism.[260, 266]

Two recent reports have emphasized the occurrence of small, flame-shaped, cystic lucent areas in the phalanges and tubular bones of the arms[264, 265] (Fig. 85–70). The lesions, which may also be observed in the metatarsals, are multiple, elongated, and frequently eccentric in location. They may appear as enclosed medullary or cortical foci or as scalloped defects on the external surface of the bone. The pathogenesis of these lucent areas is unknown, although they may relate to intraosseous epithelial cysts, lipomas, or fibromas, which do occur in other locations in this syndrome. The alterations may resemble those in sarcoidosis or tuberous sclerosis.

The presence of shortened metacarpals in as many as 50 per cent of patients with this syndrome, a finding that is also evident in pseudohypoparathyroidism and pseudo-pseudohypoparathyroidism, has raised the possibility of an association among these disorders. This possibility is strengthened by the fact that soft tissue calcification occasionally is

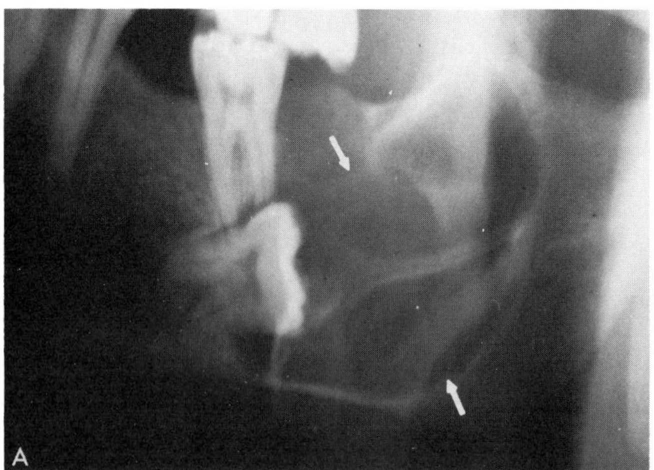

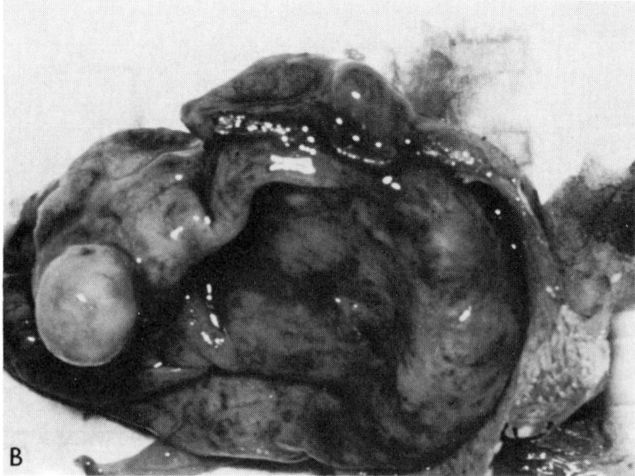

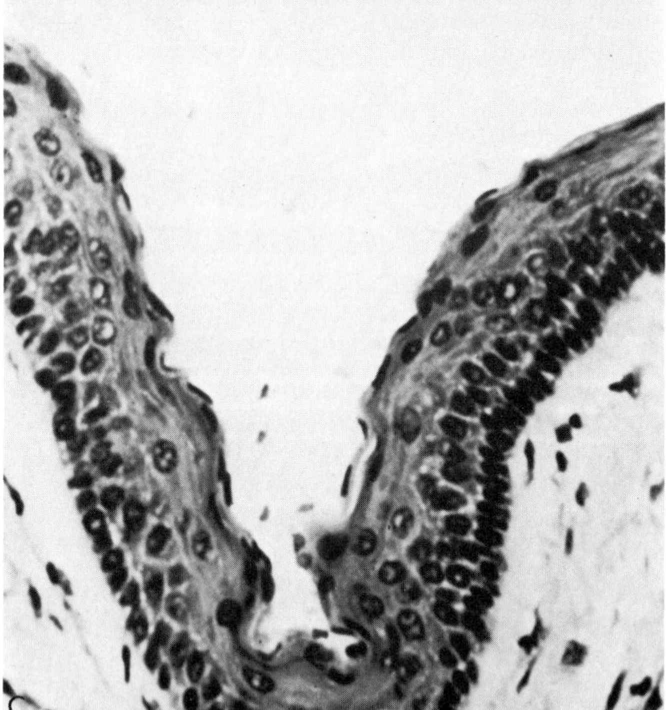

Figure 85–68. *Nevoid basal cell carcinoma syndrome (Gorlin's syndrome): Mandibular abnormalities.*

A *Dentigerous cysts (arrows) are common in this syndrome.*

B, C *The size of the dentigerous cysts is variable, but they may reach several centimeters in diameter. The lining of the cysts consists of epithelium that may be keratinized.* (**B, C,** *Courtesy of Dr. R. Smith, University of California, San Francisco.*)

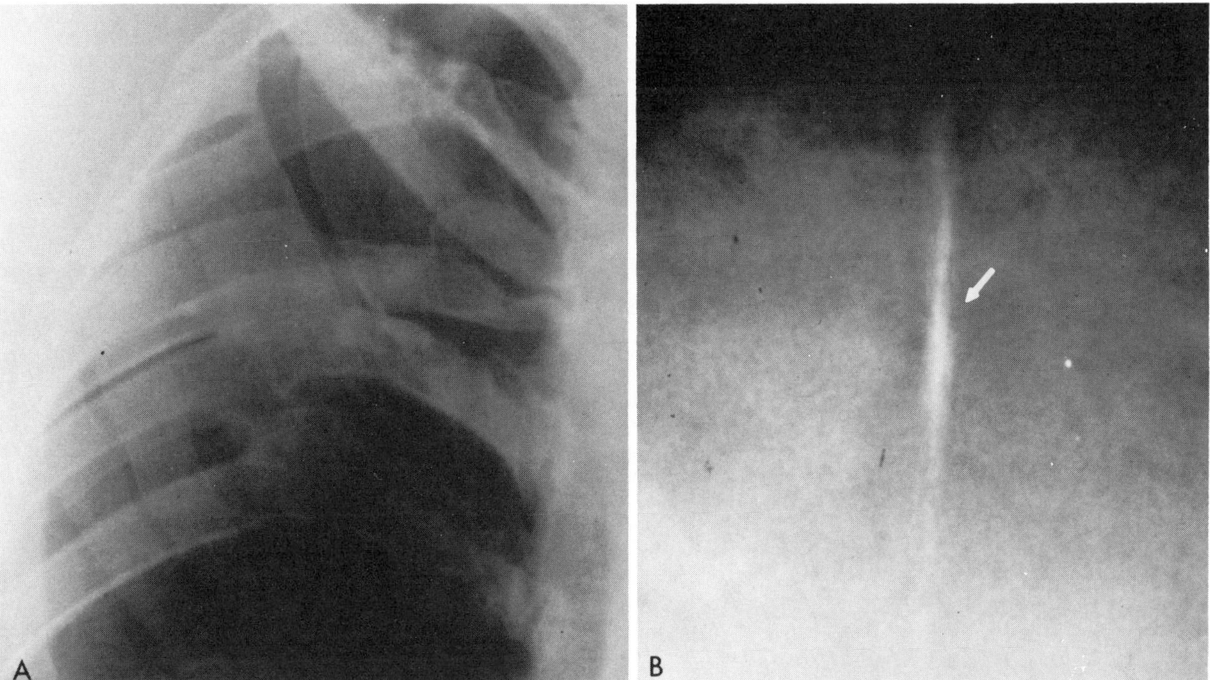

Figure 85–69. Nevoid basal cell carcinoma syndrome (Gorlin's syndrome): Other abnormalities.

A Typical rib anomalies are demonstrated.

B Calcification of the falx cerebri (arrow) is not unusual in this syndrome.

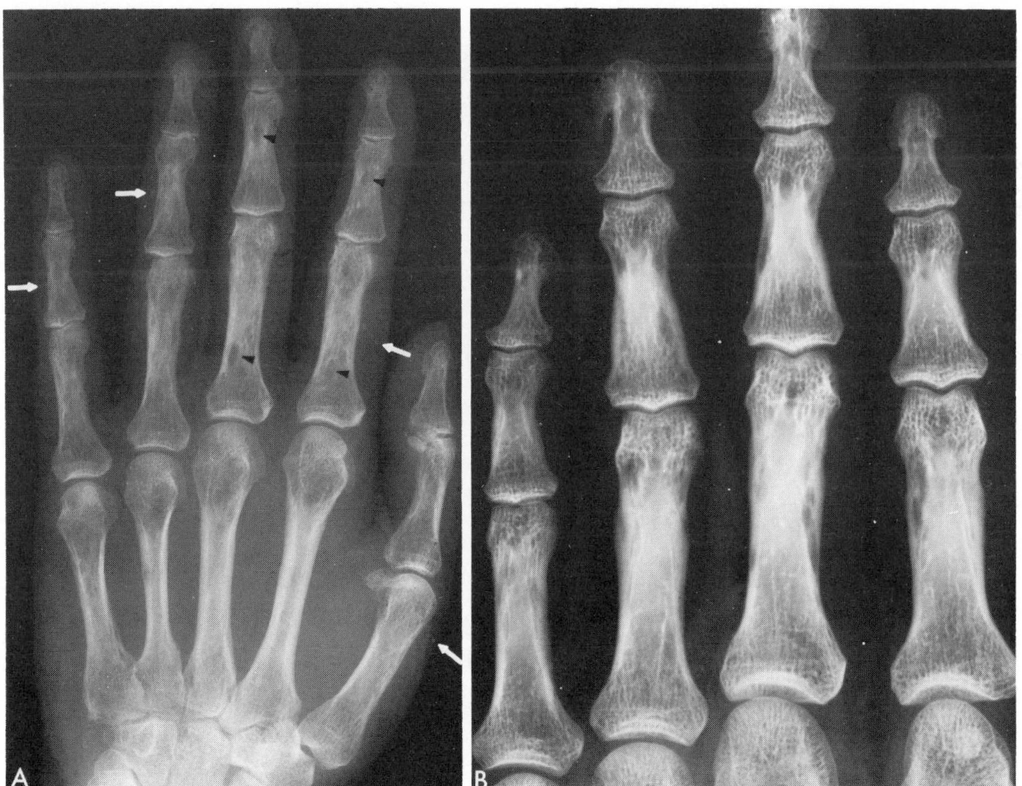

Figure 85–70. Nevoid basal cell carcinoma syndrome (Gorlin's syndrome): Cystic lesions of the hand.

A In this 65 year old woman, note multiple lucent lesions of the phalanges and the metacarpals (arrowheads), as well as small foci of soft tissue calcification (arrows).

B In a 25 year old man, note the flame-shaped configuration and eccentric location of many of the lucent lesions.

(From Dunnick NR, et al: Radiology 127:331, 1978.)

found in all of these diseases. Tissue response to parathyroid hormone has been reported to be less than normal in both the nevoid basal cell carcinoma syndrome and pseudohypoparathyroidism.[269] However, other investigations have failed to document an abnormal parathyroid hormone response in patients with the nevoid basal cell carcinoma syndrome.[270, 271] In addition, serum calcium and phosphorus levels are normal in individuals with this disease.[265] At this writing, the basic defect is not known.

Linear Nevus Sebaceus Syndrome

This is a recently recognized neurocutaneous syndrome characterized by an epidermal nevus, seizures, and mental retardation.[272-276] The syndrome may involve a variety of tissues of ectodermal and mesenchymal origin and, in this regard, resembles neurofibromatosis, tuberous sclerosis, the Sturge-Weber syndrome, and von Hippel–Lindau disease. Malformations of the brain, viscera, and skeleton can lead to various radiographic alterations. These include asymmetry of the skull and facial bones, premature fusion of sutures, cerebral atrophy with ventricular dilatation, hydrocephalus, scoliosis, kyphoscoliosis, and deformities of the pelvis and long bones. The findings are not specific. The diagnosis should be considered when a variety of cranial, cerebral, and skeletal manifestations are detected in a mentally retarded child with seizures and typical skin lesions.

Panniculitis and Related Syndromes

Panniculitides represent inflammatory disorders of subcutaneous fat. They are classified into patterns based upon the location of inflammation within the lobular arrangement of subcutaneous tissue: inflammation around the central arterial system leads to changes affecting the entire lobule (lobular panniculitis); inflammation about the venous system produces septal changes (septal panniculitis).[282] Erythema nodosum and subacute migratory panniculitis are examples of septal panniculitis; Weber-Christian disease, erythema induratum, and systemic vasculitis are examples of lobular panniculitis.[282]

Weber-Christian disease is a contested entity. Some investigators believe it is a distinct pathologic condition, whereas others regard this disorder as pancreatic in origin.[283] Typically, a woman in the fourth or fifth decade of life is affected, presenting with tender nodules in the trunk and buttocks. Some of the lesions may ulcerate. On histologic examination, the nodules are initially characterized by polymorphonuclear leukocytic infiltration in the fat and subsequently reveal fatty degeneration, macrophage accumulation, and lymphocyte and plasma cell infiltration.[282] Vascular changes and scar tissue may appear. Although radiographic changes are usually absent, we have observed one patient with peculiar structural changes in the hips resembling a combination of osteonecrosis and osteoarthritis (Fig. 85–71).

Other varieties of lobular panniculitis are erythema induratum or nodular vasculitis (occurring in middle-aged women as bilaterally distributed painful nodules on the calves) and systemic vasculitis (in which subcutaneous nodules may appear during the course of systemic lupus erythematosus, periarteritis nodosa, Behçet's syndrome, and other vasculitic disorders).[282]

Juxta-articular adiposis dolorosa or Dercum's disease is also a debated entity.[284] In this disorder,

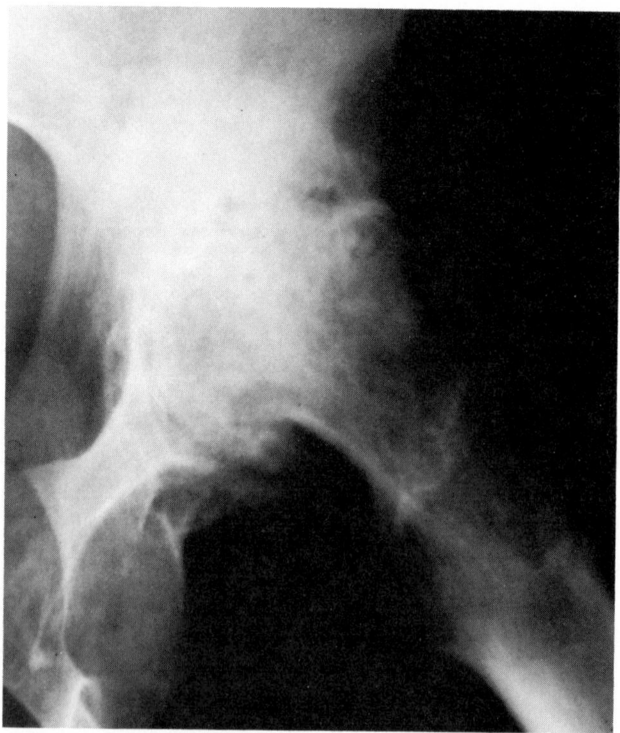

Figure 85–71. *Weber-Christian disease. This 52 year old man developed tender 2 to 4 cm nodules over both arms and legs without erythema or drainage. A biopsy was interpreted as showing Weber-Christian disease. Progressive hip and shoulder pain was also apparent. A radiograph outlines peculiar structural joint damage of the hip characterized by loss of articular space, collapse and sclerosis of the femoral head and acetabulum, and medial femoral osteophytosis. The nature of the articular abnormalities and their relationship to Weber-Christian disease are unclear.*

generalized obesity, weakness, fatigability, and emotional instability may be accompanied by painful, circumscribed or diffuse fatty deposits, frequently localized to the lower extremity. Although some reports emphasize additional abnormalities of various endocrine glands, others doubt this association. In some patients, an autosomal dominant pattern of inheritance is evident.

Miscellaneous Syndromes and Conditions

Keratodermia palmaris et plantaris is a rare autosomal inherited condition in which hyperkeratosis of the palms and soles develops in infancy or childhood. In occasional patients, clubbing and osteolysis or deformity of terminal phalanges has been noted.[285]

Other varieties of hyperkeratosis have been associated with destructive changes of bone.[286, 301]

SUMMARY

The radiographic alterations in soft tissue disorders include masses, increased lucency, calcification or ossification, bands, contractures, and edema. In most instances, the findings lack specificity, although at times, careful analysis may allow delineation of the "benign" or "malignant" nature of the process. Especially important is the differentiation of myositis ossificans traumatica from various malignant tumors, and the recognition that widespread skeletal abnormalities may accompany certain cutaneous syndromes. Utilization of other diagnostic modalities including xeroradiography, low KV radiography, computed tomography, angiography, and scintigraphy may be required to supplement the radiographic evaluation and provide more accurate information regarding the extent of the soft tissue process and its relationship to adjacent structures.

REFERENCES

1. Frantzell A: Soft tissue radiography. Technical aspects and clinical applications in the examination of limbs. Acta Radiol Suppl *85*:1, 1951.
2. Martel W, Abell MR: Radiologic evaluation of soft tissue tumors. A retrospective study. Cancer *32*:352, 1973.
3. Friedmann G, Mödder U, Tismer R: Xeroradiographicsche Befunde bei osteosynthetische versorgten Frakturen. Röentgenblaetter *27*:586, 1974.
4. Wolfe JN: Xeroradiography of the bones, joints and soft tissues. Radiology *93*:583, 1969.
5. Otto RC, Pouliadis GP, Kumpe DA: The evaluation of pathologic alterations of juxtaosseous soft tissue by xeroradiography. Radiology *120*:297, 1976.
6. Hermann G, Rose JS: Computed tomography in bone and soft tissue pathology of the extremities. J Comput Assist Tomog *3*:58, 1979.
7. Cohen WN, Seidelmann FE, Bryan PJ: Computed tomography of localized adipose deposits presenting as tumor masses. Am J Roentgenol *128*:1007, 1977.
8. Weinberger G, Levinsohn EM: Computed tomography in the evaluation of sarcomatous tumors of thigh. Am J Roentgenol *130*:115, 1978.
9. Wilson JS, Korobkin M, Genant HK, Bovill EG Jr: Computed tomography of musculoskeletal disorders. Am J Roentgenol *131*:55, 1978.
10. Hunter JC, Johnston WH, Genant HK: Computed tomography evaluation of fatty tumors of the somatic soft tissues: Clinical utility and radiologic-pathologic correlation. Skel Radiol *4*:79, 1979.
11. Ney FG, Feist HH, Altemus LR, Ordinario VR: The characteristic angiographic criteria of malignancy. Radiology *104*:567, 1972.
12. Levin DC, Watson RC, Baltaxe HA: Arteriography in diagnosis and management of acquired peripheral soft tissue masses. Radiology *104*:58, 1972.
13. Herzeberg DL, Schreiber MH: Angiography in mass lesions of the extremities. Am J Roentgenol *111*:541, 1971.
14. Cockshott WP, Evans KT: The place of soft tissue arteriography. Br J Radiol *37*:367, 1964.
15. Bliznak J, Staple TW: Radiology of angiodysplasias of the limb. Radiology *110*:35, 1974.
16. Bartley O, Wickbom I: Angiography in soft tissue hemangiomas. Acta Radiol *51*:81, 1959.
17. Levin DC, Gordon DH, McSweeney J: Arteriography of peripheral hemangiomas. Radiology *121*:625, 1976.
18. Richman LS, Gumerman LW, Levine G, Sartiano GP, Boggs SS: Localization of Tc^{99m} polyphosphate in soft tissue malignancies. Am J Roentgenol *124*:577, 1975.
19. Thrall JH, Ghaed N, Geslien GE, Pinsky SM, Johnson MC: Pitfalls in Tc^{99m} polyphosphate skeletal imaging. Am J Roentgenol *121*:739, 1974.
20. Stout AP, Lattes R: Tumors of the Soft Tissues. Atlas of Tumor Pathology, Series 2, Fascicle 1. Bethesda, Md, Armed Forces Institute of Pathology, 1967.
21. Edland RW: Liposarcoma. A retrospective study of fifteen cases, a review of the literature and a discussion of radiosensitivity. Am J Roentgenol *103*:778, 1968.
22. Pack GT, Pierson JC: Liposarcoma: A study of 105 cases. Surgery *36*:687, 1954.
23. Leffert RD: Lipomas of the upper extremity. J Bone Joint Surg *54A*:1262, 1972.
24. Lin JJ, Lin F: Two entities in angiolipoma. A study of 459 cases of lipoma with review of literature on infiltrating angiolipoma. Cancer *34*:720, 1974.
25. Chung EB, Enzinger FM: Benign lipoblastomatosis. An analysis of 35 cases. Cancer *32*:482, 1973.
26. Brines OA, Johnson MH: Hibernoma, a special fatty tumor; report of a case. Am J Pathol *25*:467, 1949.
27. Vellios F, Baez J, Schumacker HB: Lipoblastomatosis: A tumor of fetal fat different from hibernoma. Report of a case with observations of the embryogenesis of human adipose tissue. Am J Pathol *34*:1149, 1958.
28. Weitzman G: Lipoma arborescens of the knee. Report of a case. J Bone Joint Surg *47A*:1030, 1965.
29. Kaufman JH, Cedermark BJ, Parthasarathy KL, Didolkar MS, Bakshi SP: The values of ^{67}Ga scintigraphy in soft-tissue sarcoma and chondrosarcoma. Radiology *123*:131, 1977.
30. Stout AP: Fibrosarcoma: The malignant tumor of fibroblasts. Cancer *1*:30, 1948.
31. Stout AP: Fibrosarcoma in infants and children. Cancer *15*:1028, 1962.
32. Bonakdarpour A, Pickering JE, Resnick EJ: Case report 49. Skel Radiol *2*:181, 1978.
33. Enzinger FM, Shiraki M: Musculo-aponeurotic fibromatosis of the shoulder girdle (extra-abdominal desmoid). Analysis of thirty cases followed up for ten or more years. Cancer *20*:1131, 1967.
34. Greenfield GB, Rubenstone AI, Lo M: Case report 31. Skel Radiol *2*:43, 1977.
35. Barber HM, Galasko CSB, Woods CG: Multicentric extra-abdominal desmoid tumours. Report of two cases. J Bone Joint Surg *55B*:858, 1973.
36. Rosen RS, Kimball W: Extra-abdominal desmoid tumor. Radiology *86*:534, 1966.
37. Reye RDK: Recurring digital fibrous tumours of childhood. Arch Pathol *80*:228, 1965.
38. Bloem JJ, Vuzevski VD, Huffstadt AJC: Recurring digital fibroma of infancy. J Bone Joint Surg *56B*:746, 1974.
39. Lakhanpal VP, Yadav SS, Sastry VRK, Krishnamurthy CS: Recurring digital fibromas of infancy. A case report. Acta Orthop Scand *49*:147, 1978.

40. Keasbey LE: Juvenile aponeurotic fibroma (calcifying fibroma): A distinctive tumor arising in the palms and soles of young children. Cancer *6*:338, 1953.
41. Vatopoulos PK, Garofalakis EE, Papathanassiou BT: Juvenile aponeurotic fibroma. Report of a case. Acta Orthop Scand *45*:158, 1974.
42. Keller RB, Baez-Giangreco A: Juvenile aponeurotic fibroma. Report of three cases and a review of the literature. Clin Orthop Rel Res *106*:198, 1975.
43. Lichtenstein L, Goldman RL: The cartilage analogue of fibromatosis —a reinterpretation of the condition called juvenile aponeurotic fibroma. Cancer *17*:810, 1964.
44. Prete P, Thorne RP: Elastofibroma: A rare cause of periscapular pain. Arthritis Rheum *22*:792, 1979.
45. Renshaw TS, Simon MA: Elastofibroma. J Bone Joint Surg *55A*:409, 1973.
46. Deutsch GP: Elastofibroma dorsalis treated by radiotherapy. Br J Radiol *47*:621, 1974.
47. Javors BR, Katz MC, Kwon CS: Case report 73. Skel Radiol *3*:183, 1978.
48. Schaffzin EA, Chung SMK, Kaye R: Congenital generalized fibromatosis with complete spontaneous regression. J Bone Joint Surg *54A*:657, 1972.
49. Heiple KG, Perrin E, Aikawa M: Congenital generalized fibromatosis. A case limited to osseous lesions. J Bone Joint Surg *54A*:663, 1972.
50. Karasick D, O'Hara AE: Juvenile aponeurotic fibroma. A review and report of a case with osseous involvement. Radiology *123*:725, 1977.
51. Broder MS, Leonidas JC, Mitty HA: Pseudosarcomatous fasciitis: An unusual cause of soft tissue calcification. Radiology *107*:173, 1973.
52. Stout AP, Hill WT: Leiomyosarcoma of the superficial soft tissues. Cancer *11*:844, 1958.
53. Bulmer JH: Smooth muscle tumours of the limbs. J Bone Joint Surg *49B*:52, 1967.
54. Hornback NB, Shidnia H: Rhabdomyosarcoma in the pediatric age group. Am J Roentgenol *126*:542, 1976.
55. Moskowitz M, Rosenbaum HT, Sweet R, McLeod C: Calcified embryonal rhabdomyosarcoma with local bone invasion. An unusual case. Radiology *91*:121, 1968.
56. McDowell CL, Cardea JA: Embryonal rhabdomyosarcoma of the hand. A case report. Clin Orthop Rel Res *100*:238, 1974.
57. Bailey WC, Holaday WJ, Kontras SB, Clatworthy WW Jr: Rhabdomyosarcomas in childhood: A review of 14 cases. Arch Surg *82*:943, 1961.
58. Simmons M, Tucker AK: The radiology of bone changes in rhabdomyosarcoma. Clin Radiol *29*:47, 1978.
59. Crane AR, Tremblay RG: Myoblastoma (granular cell myoblastoma or myoblastic myoma). Am J Pathol *21*:357, 1945.
60. Bielejeski TR: Granular-cell tumor (myoblastoma) of the hand. Report of a case. J Bone Joint Surg *55A*:841, 1973.
61. Ghormley RK, Dockerty MB: Cystic myxomatous tumors about the knee: Their relation to cysts of the menisci. J Bone Joint Surg *25*:306, 1943.
62. Dutz W, Stout AP: The myxoma in childhood. Cancer *14*:629, 1961.
63. Stout AP: Myxoma; the tumor of primitive mesenchyme. Ann Surg *127*:706, 1948.
64. Milgram JW, Preininger RE: Calcifying myxoma. A case report. J Bone Joint Surg *55A*:401, 1973.
65. Ireland DCR, Soule EH, Ivins JC: Myxoma of somatic soft tissues. A report of 58 patients, 3 with multiple tumors and fibrous dysplasia of bone. Mayo Clin Proc *48*:401, 1973.
66. Soule EH, Enriquez P: Atypical fibrous histiocytoma, malignant fibrous histiocytoma, malignant histiocytoma, and epithelioid sarcoma. A comparative study of 65 tumors. Cancer *30*:128, 1972.
67. Kyriakos M, Kempson RL: Inflammatory fibrous histiocytoma. An aggressive and lethal lesion. Cancer *37*:1584, 1976.
68. Solomon MP, Sutton AL: Malignant fibrous histiocytoma of the soft tissues of the mandible. Oral Surg *35*:653, 1973.
69. Spencer D, Wrighton JD: Histiocytoma presenting as swelling on the toe. Arch Dis Child *47*:828, 1972.
70. Helal B, Currey HLF, Vernon-Roberts B: Fibrous histiocytoma of the thumb. Br J Surg *61*:909, 1974.
71. Lo HH, Kalisher L, Faix JD: Epithelioid sarcoma: Radiologic and pathologic manifestations. Am J Roentgenol *128*:1017, 1977.
72. Bryan RS, Soule EH, Dobyns JH, Pritchard DJ, Linscheid RL: Primary epithelioid sarcoma of the hand and forearm. A review of thirteen cases. J Bone Joint Surg *56A*:458, 1974.
73. DeLuca FN, Neviaser RJ: Epithelioid sarcoma involving bone. Clin Orthop Rel Res *107*:168, 1975.
74. Hamilton WC, Ramsey PL, Hanson SM, Schiff DC: Osseous xanthoma and multiple hand tumors as a complication of hyperlipidemia. Report of a case. J Bone Joint Surg *57A*:551, 1975.
75. Fahey JJ, Stark HH, Donovan WF, Drennan DB: Xanthoma of the Achilles tendon. Seven cases with familial hyperbetalipoproteinemia. J Bone Joint Surg *55A*:1197, 1973.
76. Yaghmai I: Intra- and extraosseous xanthomata associated with hyperlipidemia. Radiology *128*:49, 1978.
77. Gattereau A, Davignon J, Langelier M, Levesque HP: An improved radiological method for the evaluation of Achilles tendon xanthomatosis. Can Med Assoc J *108*:39, 1973.
78. Neviaser RJ, Adams JP: Vascular lesions in the hand. Current management. Clin Orthop Rel Res *100*:111, 1974.
79. McNeill TW, Ray RD: Hemangioma of the extremities. Review of 35 cases. Clin Orthop Rel Res *101*:154, 1974.
80. Ayella RJ: Hemangiopericytoma. A case report with arteriographic findings. Radiology *97*:611, 1970.
81. Carroll RE, Berman AT: Glomus tumors of the hand. Review of the literature and report on twenty-eight cases. J Bone Joint Surg *54A*:691, 1972.
82. Gorham LW: Kaposi's sarcoma involving bone: With particular attention to angiomatous components of the tumor in relation to osteolysis. Arch Pathol *76*:456, 1963.
83. Cox FH, Helwig EB: Kaposi's sarcoma. Cancer *12*:289, 1959.
84. Bluefarb SM, Webster JR: Kaposi's sarcoma associated with lymphosarcoma. Arch Intern Med *91*:97, 1953.
85. Aegerter EE, Peale AR: Kaposi's sarcoma. A critical survey. Arch Pathol *34*:413, 1942.
86. Glatt OS: Kaposi's sarcoma. J Am Geriat Soc *21*:469, 1973.
87. Chung EB, Enzinger FM: Chondroma of soft parts. Cancer *41*:1414, 1978.
88. Murphy AF, Wilson JN: Tenosynovial osteochondroma in the hand. J Bone Joint Surg *40A*:1236, 1958.
89. Strong ML Jr: Chondromas of the tendon sheath of the hand. Report of a case and review of the literature. J Bone Joint Surg *57A*:1164, 1975.
90. Smith MT, Farinacci CJ, Carpenter HA, Bannayan GA: Extraskeletal myxoid chondrosarcoma. A clinicopathological study. Cancer *37*:821, 1976.
91. Guccion JG, Font RL, Enzinger FM, Zimmerman LE: Extraskeletal mesenchymal chondrosarcoma. Arch Pathol *95*:336, 1973.
92. Angerval L, Enerbäck L, Knutston H: Chondrosarcoma of soft tissue origin. Cancer *32*:507, 1973.
93. Hernandez R, Heidelberger KP, Poznanski AK: Case report 63. Skel Radiol *3*:61, 1978.
94. Fine G, Stout AP: Osteogenic sarcoma of the extraskeletal soft tissues. Cancer *9*:1027, 1956.
95. Kauffman SL, Stout AP: Extraskeletal osteogenic sarcomas and chondrosarcomas in children. Cancer *16*:432, 1963.
96. Lorentzon R, Larsson SE, Boquist L: Extra-osseous osteosarcoma. A clinical and histopathological study of four cases. J Bone Joint Surg *61B*:205, 1979.
97. Adler CP: Case report 92. Skel Radiol *4*:107, 1979.
98. Thompson DE, Frost HM, Hendrick JW, Horn RC Jr: Soft tissue sarcomas involving the extremities and the limb girdles: A review. South Med J *64*:33, 1971.
99. Tillotson JF, McDonald JR, Janes JM: Synovial sarcomata. J Bone Joint Surg *33A*:459, 1973.
100. Pack GT, Ariel IM: Synovial sarcoma (malignant syniovoma). A report of 60 cases. Surgery *28*:1047, 1950.
101. Cadman NL, Soule EH, Kelly PJ: Synovial sarcoma. An analysis of 134 tumors. Cancer *18*:613, 1965.
102. Cameron HU, Kostuik JP: A long-term follow-up of synovial sarcoma. J Bone Joint Surg *56B*:613, 1974.
103. Murray JA: Synovial sarcoma. Orthop Clin North Am *8*:963, 1977.
104. Horowitz AL, Resnick D, Watson RC: The roentgen features of synovial sarcomas. Clin Radiol *24*:481, 1973.
105. Desantos LA, Lindell MM Jr, Goldman AM, Luna MA, Murray JA: Calcification within metastatic pulmonary nodules from synovial sarcoma. Orthopedics *1*:141, 1978.
106. Reed RJ, Bliss BO: Morton's neuroma. Regressive and productive intermetatarsal elastofibrositis. Arch Pathol *95*:123, 1973.
107. Enzinger FM: Clear-cell sarcoma of tendons and aponeuroses. An analysis of 21 cases. Cancer *18*:1163, 1965.
108. Radstone DJ, Revell PA, Mantell BS: Clear cell sarcoma of tendons and aponeuroses treated with bleomycin and vincristine. Br J Radiol *52*:238, 1979.
109. Smetana HF, Scott WF Jr: Malignant tumors of nonchromaffin paraganglia. Milit Surgeon *109*:330, 1951.
110. Christopherson WM, Foote FW Jr, Stewart FW: Alveolar soft-part sarcomas. Structurally characteristic tumors of uncertain histogenesis. Cancer *5*:100, 1952.
111. Dutt AK, Balasegaram M, Din OB: Alveolar soft-part sarcoma with invasion of bone. A case report. J Bone Joint Surg *51A*:765, 1969.
112. Forbis R Jr, Helwig EB: Pilomatrixoma (calcifying epithelioma). Arch Dermatol *83*:606, 1961.
113. Haller JO, Kassner EG, Ostrowitz A, Kottmeier K, Pertschuk LP: Pilomatrixoma (calcifying epithelioma of Malherbe): Radiographic features. Radiology *123*:151, 1977.

114. DuToit G, Rang M: Congenital calcific hamartoma. A resolving lesion producing gastrocnemius contracture — report of a case. Clin Orthop Rel Res *135*:79, 1978.
115. Feldman F, Norman D: Intra- and extraosseous malignant histiocytoma (malignant fibrous xanthoma). Radiology *104*:497, 1972.
116. Louis DS, Dick HM: Ossifying lipofibroma of the median nerve. J Bone Joint Surg *55A*:1082, 1973.
117. Greenfield GB: Radiology of Bone Diseases. 2nd Ed. Philadelphia, JB Lippincott Co, 1975, p 491.
118. Mathias K, Baumeister L: Röntgenologische Differentialdiagnose von Extremitäten-Verkalkungen. Radiologe *18*:129, 1978.
119. Weber U, Pfeifer G: Beitrag zur Differentialdiagnose kalkdichter Weichteilverschattungen der Extremitäten. Z Orthop *115*:256, 1977.
120. Epstein DA, Solar M, Levin EJ: Demonstration of long-standing metastatic soft tissue calcification by ^{99m}Tc diphosphonate. Am J Roentgenol *128*:145, 1977.
121. Bauer W, Marble A, Bennett G: Further studies in a case of calcification of the subcutaneous tissue ("calcinosis universalis") in a child. Am J Med Sci *182*:237, 1931.
122. Leistyna JA, Hassan HI: Interstitial calcinosis. Am J Dis Child *107*:96, 1964.
123. Caffey J: Pediatric X-ray Diagnosis, 7th Ed. Chicago, Year Book Medical Publishers, 1978, p 984.
124. Ozonoff MB, Flynn FJ Jr: Roentgenologic features of dermatomyositis of childhood. Am J Roentgenol *118*:206, 1973.
125. Shackelford GD, Barton LL, McAlister WH: Calcified subcutaneous fat necrosis in infancy. J Can Assoc Radiol *26*:203, 1975.
126. Harris V, Ramamurphy RS, Pildes RS: Late onset of subcutaneous calcifications after intravenous injections of calcium gluconate. Am J Roentgenol *123*:845, 1975.
127. Inclan A, Leon P, Camejo MG: Tumoral calcinosis. JAMA *121*:490, 1943.
128. Hacihanefioğlu U: Tumoral calcinosis. A clinical and pathological study of eleven unreported cases in Turkey. J Bone Joint Surg *60A*:1131, 1978.
129. Traca G, Hennebert P-N, Mazabraud A: Considérations sur un cas de lipocalcinogranulomatose. Presse Med *73*:543, 1965.
130. Bancale A: Lipo-calcino-granulomatous bursitis (Teutschlaender's disease). Minerva Ortop *12*:833, 1961.
131. Veress B, Malik MOA, El Hassan AM: Tumoural lipocalcinosis: A clinicopathological study of 20 cases. J Pathol *119*:113, 1976.
132. Hartofilakidas-Garofalidis G, Theodossiou A, Matsoukas J, Rigopoulos G, Papathanassiou B: Tumoral lipo-calcinosis. Acta Orthop Scand *41*:387, 1950.
133. Thomson JG: Calcifying collagenolysis (tumoral calcinosis). Br J Radiol *39*:526, 1966.
134. Ghormley RK: Multiple calcified bursae and calcified cysts in soft tissues. Trans West Surg Assoc *51*:292, 1942.
135. Barton DL, Reeves RJ: Tumoral calcinosis. Report of three cases and review of the literature. Am J Roentgenol *86*:351, 1961.
136. Sammarco GJ, Makley JT: Tumoral calcinosis and mongolism. A case report. Clin Orthop Rel Res *91*:164, 1973.
137. Kolawole TM, Bohrer SP: Tumoral calcinosis with "fluid levels" in the tumoral masses. Am J Roentgenol *120*:461, 1974.
138. Slavin G, Klenerman L, Darby A, Bansal S: Tumoral calcinosis in England. Br Med J *1*:147, 1973.
139. Wilson AL, Chater EH: Tumoral calcinosis — an obscure disease. A report of four cases. J Irish Med Assoc *69*:61, 1976.
140. Brown ML, Thrall JH, Cooper RA, Kim YC: Radiography and scintigraphy in tumoral calcinosis. Radiology *124*:757, 1977.
141. Currie H: Tumoral calcinosis. Br Med J *2*:120, 1969.
142. Baldursson H, Evans EB, Dodge WF, Jackson WT: Tumoral calcinosis with hyperphosphatemia. A report of a family with incidence in four siblings. J Bone Joint Surg *51A*:913, 1969.
143. Lafferty FW, Reynolds ES, Pearson OH: Tumoral calcinosis. A metabolic disease of obscure etiology. Am J Med *38*:105, 1965.
144. Wilber JF, Slatopolsky E: Hyperphosphatemia and tumoral calcinosis. Ann Intern Med *68*:1044, 1968.
145. Harkess JW, Peters HJ: Tumoral calcinosis. A report of six cases. J Bone Joint Surg *49A*:721, 1967.
146. Frame B, Herrera LF, Mitchell DC, Fine G: Massive osteolysis and tumoral calcinosis. Am J Med *50*:408, 1971.
147. Eugenidis N, Locher JT: Tumoral calcinosis imaged by bone scanning: Case report. J Nucl Med *18*:34, 1977.
148. Bolger JT: Heterotopic bone formation and alkaline phosphatase. Arch Phys Med Rehabil *56*:36, 1975.
149. Furman R, Nicholas JJ, Jivoff L: Elevation of the serum alkaline phosphatase coincident with ectopic-bone formation in paraplegic patients. J Bone Joint Surg *52A*:1131, 1970.
150. Muheim G, Donath A, Rossier AB: Serial scintigrams in the course of ectopic bone formation in paraplegic patients. Am J Roentgenol *118*:865, 1973.
151. Tanaka T, Rossier AB, Hussey RW, Ahnberg DS, Treves S: Quantitative assessment of para-osteo-arthropathy and its maturation on serial radionuclide bone images. Radiology *123*:217, 1977.
152. Gunn DR, Young WB: Myositis ossificans as a complication of tetanus. J Bone Joint Surg *41B*:535, 1959.
153. Bour H, Tutin M, Pasquier P, Quevauvilliers J: Les paraostéoarthropathies au décours des comas oxycarbonés graves. Sem Hôp Paris *42*:1912, 1966.
154. Ghormley JW: Ossification of the tendo Achillis. J Bone Joint Surg *20*:153, 1938.
155. Marottoli OR: Osificaciones en el tendon de Aquiles. Rev Ortop Traumatol *11*:53, 1941.
156. Lotke PA: Ossification of the Achilles tendon. Report of seven cases. J Bone Joint Surg *52A*:157, 1970.
157. Mitra M, Sen AK, Deb HK: Myositis ossificans traumatica: A complication of tetanus. Report of a case and review of the literature. J Bone Joint Surg *58A*:885, 1976.
158. Pitts NC: Myositis ossificans as a complication of tetanus. JAMA *189*:237, 1964.
159. Norman A, Dorfman HD: Juxtacortical circumscribed myositis ossificans: Evolution and radiographic features. Radiology *96*:301, 1970.
160. Paterson DC: Myositis ossificans circumscripta. Report of four cases without history of injury. J Bone Joint Surg *52B*:296, 1970.
161. Goldman AB: Myositis ossificans circumscripta: A benign lesion with a malignant differential diagnosis. Am J Roentgenol *126*:32, 1976.
162. Ackerman LV: Extra-osseous localized non-neoplastic bone and cartilage formation (so-called myositis ossificans): Clinical and pathological confusion with malignant neoplasms. J Bone Joint Surg *40A*:279, 1958.
163. Adams RD, Denny-Brown D, Pearson CM: Diseases of Muscle: A Study in Pathology, 2nd Ed. New Yrok, Harper & Row, 1962.
164. Mohan K: Myositis ossificans traumatica of the elbow. Int Surg *57*:475, 1972.
165. Flynn JE, Graham JH: Myositis ossificans. Surg Gynecol Obstet *118*:1001, 1964.
166. Thompson HC III, Garcia A: Myositis ossificans: Aftermath of elbow injuries. Clin Orthop Rel Res *50*:129, 1967.
167. Ellis M, Frank HG: Myositis ossificans traumatica with special reference to the quadriceps femoris muscle. J Trauma *6*:724, 1967.
168. Gilmer WS Jr, Anderson LD: Reactions of soft somatic tissue which may progress to bone formation: Circumscribed (traumatic) myositis ossificans. South Med J *52*:1432, 1959.
169. Dickerson RC: Myositis ossificans in early childhood. Report of an unusual case. Clin Orthop Rel Res *79*:42, 1971.
170. Johnson MK, Lawrence JF: Metaplastic bone formation (myositis ossificans) in the soft tissue of the hand. Case report. J Bone Joint Surg *57A*:999, 1975.
171. Zadek I: Ossifying hematoma in the thigh. A case report. J Bone Joint Surg *51A*:386, 1969.
172. Maini PS, Singh M: Localized myositis ossificans progressiva. A case report. J Bone Joint Surg *49A*:955, 1967.
173. Parkash S, Kumar K: Fibrodysplasia ossificans traumatica. A case report. J Bone Joint Surg *54A*:1306, 1972.
174. Johnson LC: Histogenesis of myositis ossificans (Abstr). Am J Pathol *24*:681, 1948.
175. Yaghmai I: Myositis ossificans: Diagnostic value of arteriography. Am J Roentgenol *128*:811, 1977.
176. Kramer FL, Kurtz AB, Rubin C, Goldberg BB: Ultrasound appearance of myositis ossificans. Skel Radiol *4*:19, 1979.
177. Shanoff L, Spira M, Hardy SB: Myositis ossificans: Evolution to osteogenic sarcoma. Report of a histologically verified case. Am J Surg *113*:537, 1967.
178. Huvos AG, Higinbotham NL: Primary fibrosarcoma of bone: A clinicopathologic study of 130 patients. Cancer *35*:837, 1975.
179. Kagan AR, Steckel RJ: Heterotopic new bone formation: Myositis ossificans versus malignant tumor. Am J Roentgenol *130*:773, 1978.
180. Dwinnell LA, Dahlin DC, Ghormley RK: Parosteal (juxtacortical) osteogenic sarcoma. J Bone Joint Surg *36A*:732, 1954.
181. Van der' Heul RO, von Ronnen JR: Juxtacortical osteosarcoma. Diagnoses, differential diagnoses, treatment, and an analysis of eighty cases. J Bone Joint Surg *49A*:415, 1967.
182. Smith J, Ahuja SC, Huvos AG, Bullough PG: Parosteal (juxtacortical) osteogenic sarcoma. A roentgenological study of 30 patients. J Can Assoc Radiol *29*:167, 1978.
183. Unni KK, Dahlin DC, Beabout JW: Periosteal osteogenic sarcoma. Cancer *37*:2476, 1975.
184. deSantos LA, Murray JA, Finklestein JB, Spjut HJ, Ayala AG: The radiographic spectrum of periosteal osteosarcoma. Radiology *127*:123, 1978.
185. Mayer L, Friedman M: Extraskeletal bone-forming tumor of the fascia resembling osteogenic sarcoma. Bull Hosp Joint Dis *2*:187, 1941.
186. Mallory TB: A group of metaplastic and neoplastic bone- and cartilage-containing tumors of soft parts. Am J Pathol *8*:765, 1933.

187. Rhoads CP, Blumgart H: Two osteoblastomas not connected with bone, histologically identical with osteogenic sarcoma, and clinically benign. Am J Pathol *4*:363, 1928.
188. Schulze K, Treugut H, Schmitt WG: Die nicht traumatische Myositis ossificans circumscripta. Fortschr Geb Roentgenstr Nuklear Med *129*:343, 1976.
189. Chaplin DM, Harrison MHM: Pseudomalignant osseous tumour of soft tissue. Report of two cases. J Bone Joint Surg *54B*:334, 1972.
190. Angervall L, Stener B, Stener I, Ahren C: Pseudomalignant osseous tumour of soft tissue. A clinical, radiological, and pathological study of five cases. J Bone Joint Surg *51B*:654, 1969.
191. Jeffreys TE, Stiles PJ: Pseudomalignant osseous tumour of soft tissue. J Bone Joint Surg *48B*:488, 1966.
192. Lutwak L: Myositis ossificans progressiva. Mineral, metabolic and radioactive calcium studies of the effects of hormones. Am J Med *37*:269, 1964.
193. Letts RM: Myositis ossificans progressiva: A report of two cases with chromosome studies. Can Med Assoc J *99*:856, 1968.
194. Smith DM, Zeman W, Johnston CC Jr, Deiss WP Jr: Myositis ossificans progressiva. Case report with metabolic and histochemical studies. Metabolism *15*:521, 1966.
195. Dixon TF, Mulligan L, Nassim R, Stevenson FH: Myositis ossificans progressiva. Report of a case in which ACTH and cortisone failed to prevent ossification after excision of ectopic bone. J Bone Joint Surg *36B*:445, 1954.
196. Smith R, Russell RGG, Woods CG: Myositis ossificans progressiva. Clinical features of eight patients and their response to treatment. J Bone Joint Surg *58B*:48, 1976.
197. Holmsen H, Ljunghall S, Hierton T: Myositis ossificans progressiva. Clinical and metabolical observations in a case treated with a diphosphonate (EHDP) and surgical removal of ectopic bone. Acta Orthop Scand *50*:33, 1979.
198. Hentzer B, Jacobsen HH, Asboe-Hansen G: Fibrodysplasia (myositis) ossificans progressiva treated with disodium etidronate. Clin Radiol *29*:69, 1978.
199. Eaton WL, Conkling WS, Daeschner CW: Early myositis ossificans progressiva occurring in homozygotic twins. A clinical and pathological study. J Pediatr *50*:591, 1957.
200. Bassett CAL, Donath A, Macagno F, Preisig R, Fleisch H, Francis MD: Diphosphonates in the treatment of myositis ossificans progressiva. Letter to Editor. Lancet *2*:845, 1969.
201. Russell RGG, Smith R, Bishop MC, Price DA, Squire CM: Treatment of myositis ossificans progressiva with a diphosphonate. Lancet *1*:10, 1972.
202. Weiss IW, Fisher L, Phang JM: Diphosphonate therapy in a patient with myositis ossificans progressiva. Ann Intern Med *74*:933, 1971.
203. Streeter GL: Focal deficiencies in fetal tissues and their relation to intra-uterine amputation. Contrib Embryol *22*:1, 1930.
204. Plotkin D: Congenital cicatrizing fibrous bands. Report of 2 cases. Arch Pediatr *68*:120, 1951.
205. Blackfield HM, Hause DP: Congenital constricting bands of the extremities. Plast Reconstr Surg *8*:101, 1951.
206. Blanc WA, Mattison DR, Kane R, Chauhan P: LSD, intrauterine amputations, and amniotic-band syndrome. Letter to Editor. Lancet *2*:158, 1971.
207. Field JH, Krag DO: Congenital constricting bands and congenital amputation of the fingers: Placental studies. J Bone Joint Surg *55A*:1035, 1973.
208. Moses JM, Flatt AE, Cooper RR: Annular constricting bands. J Bone Joint Surg *61A*:562, 1979.
209. Glessner JP Jr: Spontaneous intra-uterine amputation. J Bone Joint Surg *45A*:351, 1963.
210. Torpin R, Goodman L, Gramling ZW: Amnion string swallowed by the fetus. Am J Obstet Gynecol *90*:829, 1964.
211. Latta JS: Spontaneous intrauterine amputations. Am J Obstet Gynecol *10*:640, 1925.
212. Abbe T: Report of a case of congenital amputation of fingers. Am J Obstet Dis Women *73*:1089, 1916.
213. Kino Y: Clinical and experimental studies of the congenital constriction band syndrome, with an emphasis on its etiology. J Bone Joint Surg *57A*:636, 1973.
214. Chemke J, Graff G, Hurwitz N, Liban E: The amniotic band syndrome. Obstet Gynecol *41*:332, 1973.
215. Birch-Jensen A: Congenital Deformities of the Upper Extremities. Odense, Denmark, Andelsbogtrykkeriet, 1949.
216. Poznanski AK: The Hand in Radiologic Diagnosis. Philadelphia, WB Saunders Co, 1974.
217. Barenberg LH, Greenberg B: Intra-uterine amputations and constriction bands. Report of a case with anesthesia below the constriction. Am J Dis Child *64*:87, 1942.
218. Friedlander HL, Westin GW, Wood WL Jr: Arthrogryposis multiplex congenita. A review of forty-five cases. J Bone Joint Surg *50A*:89, 1968.
219. Rukavina JG, Falls HF, Holt JF, Block WD: Léri's pleonosteosis. A study of a family with a review of the literature. J Bone Joint Surg *41A*:397, 1959.
220. Beals RK, Hecht F: Congenital contractural arachnodactyly. A heritable disorder of connective tissue. J Bone Joint Surg *53A*:987, 1971.
221. Seddon JH: Volkmann's ischemia in the lower limb. J Bone Joint Surg *48B*:627, 1966.
222. Currarino G, Waldman I: Camptodactyly. Am J Roentgenol *92*:1312, 1964.
223. Poznanski AK, Pratt GB, Manson G, Weiss L: Clinodactyly, camptodactyly, Kirner's deformity and other crooked fingers. Radiology *93*:573, 1969.
224. Blank E, Girdany BR: Symmetric bowing of the terminal phalanges of the fifth fingers in a family (Kirner's deformity). Am J Roentgenol *93*:367, 1965.
225. Kinmonth JB, Taylor GW, Tracy GD, Marsh JD: Primary lymphedema. Clinical and lymphangiographic studies of a series of 107 patients in which the lower limbs were affected. Br J Surg *45*:1, 1957.
226. Hadley M, MacDonald AF: Epidermolysis bullosa. Br J Radiol *33*:646, 1960.
227. Alpert M: Roentgen manifestations of epidermolysis bullosa. Am J Roentgenol *78*:66, 1957.
228. Becker MH, Swinyard CA: Epidermolysis bullosa dystrophica in children. Radiologic manifestations. Radiology *90*:124, 1968.
229. Brinn LB, Khilnani MT: Epidermolysis bullosa with characteristic hard deformities. Radiology *89*:272, 1967.
230. Horner RL, Wiedel JD, Bralliar F: Involvement of the hand in epidermolysis bullosa. J Bone Joint Surg *53A*:1347, 1971.
231. Winstock D: Oral aspects of epidermolysis bullosa. Br J Dermatol *74*:431, 1962.
232. Moynahan EJ: Epidermolysis bullosa dystrophica with severe deformity of hands and pharyngeal stenosis, relieved by cortisone. Proc R Soc Med *54*:693, 1961.
233. Pearson RW, Spargo B: Electron microscope studies of dermal-epidermal separation in human skin. J Invest Dermatol *36*:213, 1961.
234. Pearson RW: Studies on the pathogenesis of epidermolysis bullosa. J Invest Dermatol *39*:551, 1962.
235. Sasai Y: A histochemical study on the mechanism of blister formation in epidermolysis bullosa group. Tohoku J Exp Med *85*:340, 1965.
236. Bauer EA, Gedde-Dahl T, Eisen AZ: The role of human skin collagenase in epidermolysis bullosa. J Invest Dermatol *69*:119, 1977.
237. Briggaman RA, Wheeler CE: Epidermolysis bullosa dystrophica-recessive: A possible role of anchoring fibrils in the pathogenesis. J Invest Dermatol *65*:203, 1975.
238. Mathias CGT, Daroczy J, Huttner I, Schopflocher P, Wilkinson R: Pityriasis rosea in a patient with epidermolysis bullosa dystrophica. J Cutan Pathol *6*:139, 1979.
239. Winer MN, Orman JM: Epidermolysis bullosa — a suggestion as to possible causation. Arch Dermatol *52*:317, 1945.
240. Lutowiecki J: Betrachtungen zur Klassifizierung und Differentzierung von bullösen Krankheiten. Hautarzt *15*:228, 1964.
241. Halpern LK: Development of squamous cell epithelioma in epidermolysis bullosa; report of a case. Arch Dermatol *56*:517, 1947.
242. Rasponi L: Il cancro sullepidermolisi bollosa distrofica. Arch Ital Dermatol Sif *23*:19, 1950.
243. Edland RW: Dystrophica epidermolysis bullosa. Tolerance of the bed and response of multifocal squamous cell carcinomas to ionizing radiation: Report of a case. Am J Roentgenol *105*:644, 1969.
244. Meine F, Grossman H, Forman W, Jackson D: The radiographic findings in congenital cutis laxa. Radiology *113*:687, 1974.
245. Lally JF, Gohel VK, Dalinka MK, Coren GS: The roentgenographic manifestations of cutis laxa (generalized elastolysis). Radiology *113*:605, 1974.
246. Merten DF, Rooney R: Progressive pulmonary emphysema associated with congenital generalized elastolysis (cutis laxa). Radiology *113*:691, 1974.
247. Harris RB, Heaphy MR, Perry HO: Generalized elastolysis (cutix laxa). Am J Med *65*:815, 1978.
248. Hashimoto K, Kanzaki T: Cutis laxa: ultrastructural and biochemical studies. Arch Dermatol *111*:861, 1975.
249. Scott MA, Kauh YC, Luscombe HA: Acquired cutis laxa associated with multiple myeloma. Arch Dermatol *112*:853, 1976.
250. Goltz RW, Hult AM, Goldfarb M, Gorlin RJ: Cutis laxa. A manifestation of generalized elastolysis. Arch Dermatol *92*:373, 1965.
251. Shulman LE: Diffuse fasciitis hypergammaglobulinemia and eosinophilia: a new syndrome? J Rheumatol *1* (Suppl 1):46, 1974.
252. Caperton EM, Hathaway DE: Scleroderma with eosinophilia and hyper-

gammaglobulinemia. The Shulman syndrome (Abstr). Arthritis Rheum *18*:391, 1975.

253. Rodnan GP, DiBartolomeo AG, Medsger TA Jr, Barnes EL Jr: Eosinophilic fasciitis: Report of 7 cases of a newly recognized scleroderma-like syndrome (Abstr). Arthritis Rheum *18*:422, 1975.
254. Blomgren SE: Erythema nodosum. Semin Arthritis Rheum *3*:1, 1974.
255. Sams WM Jr, Winkelmann RK: The association of erythema nodosum with ulcerative colitis. South Med J *61*:676, 1968.
256. Truelove LH: Articular manifestations of erythema nodosum. Ann Rheum Dis *19*:174, 1960.
257. Fine RM, Meltzer HD: Erythema nodosum — a form of allergic cutaneous vasculitis. South Med J *61*:680, 1968.
258. Gorlin RJ, Goltz RW: Multiple nevoid basal-cell epithelioma, jaw cysts, and bifid rib. A syndrome. N Engl J Med *262*:908, 1960.
259. Gorlin RJ, Vickers RA, Kelln E, Williamson JJ: The multiple basal-cell nevi syndrome. An analysis of a syndrome consisting of multiple nevoid basal-cell carcinoma, jaw cysts, skeletal anomalies, medulloblastoma, and hyporesponsiveness to parathormone. Cancer *18*:89, 1965.
260. Becker MH, Kopf AW, Lande A: Basal cell nevus syndrome: Its roentgenographic significance. Review of the literature and report of four cases. Am J Roentgenol *99*:817, 1967.
261. Kozlowski K, Baker P, Glasson M: Multiple nevoid basal cell carcinoma syndrome (report of five cases in a family). Pediatr Radiol *2*:185, 1974.
262. Stoelinga PJW, Peters JH, Van de Staak WJB, Cohen MM Jr: Some new findings in the basal-cell nevus syndrome. Oral Surg *36*:686, 1973.
263. Lile HA, Rogers JF, Gerald B: The basal cell nevus syndrome. Am J Roentgenol *103*:214, 1968.
264. Novak D, Bloss W: Röntgenologische Aspekte des Basalzell-naevus-syndroms (Gorlin-Goltz-Syndrom). Fortschr Geb Roentgenstr Nuklearmed *124*:11, 1976.
265. Dunnick NR. Head GL, Peck GL, Yoder FW: Nevoid basal cell carcinoma syndrome: Radiographic manifestations including cystlike lesions of the phalanges. Radiology *127*:331, 1978.
266. Davidson F: Multiple naevoid basal cell carcinomata and associated congenital abnormalities. Br J Dermatol *74*:439, 1962.
267. Binkley GW, Johnson HH Jr: Epithelioma adenoides cysticum: Basal cell nevi, agenesis of corpus callosum and dental cysts. A clinical and autopsy study. Arch Dermatol *63*:73, 1951.
268. Wallace DC, Murphy KJ, Kelly L, Ward WH: The basal cell naevus syndrome. Report of a family with anosmia and a case of hypogonadotrophic hypopituitarism. J Med Genet *10*:30, 1973.
269. Block JB, Clendenning WE: Parathyroid hormone hyporesponsiveness in patients with basal-cell nevi and bone defects. New Engl J Med *268*:1157, 1963.
270. Kaufman RL, Chase LR: Basal cell nevus syndrome: Normal responsiveness to parathyroid hormone. Birth Defects Original Article Series *7*:149, 1971.
271. Aurbach GD, Marcus R, Winickoff RN, Epstein EH Jr, Nigra TP: Urinary excretion of 3',5'-AMP in syndromes considered refractory to parathyroid hormone. Metabolism *19*:799, 1970.
272. Marden PM, Venters HD Jr: A new neurocutaneous syndrome. Am J Dis Child *112*:79, 1966.
273. Solomon LM, Fretzin DF, Dewald RL: The epidermal nevus syndrome. Arch Dermatol *97*:273, 1968.
274. Bianchine JW: The nevus sebaceous syndrome of Jadassohn. A neurocutaneous syndrome and a potentially premalignant lesion. Am J Dis Child *120*:223, 1970.
275. Lovejoy FH Jr, Boyle WE Jr: Linear nevus sebaceous syndrome. Report of two cases and a review of the literature. Pediatrics *52*:382, 1973.
276. Leonidas JC, Wolpert SM, Feingold M, McCauley RGK: Radiographic features of the linear nevus sebaceous syndrome. Am J Roentgenol *132*:277, 1979.
277. Kadir S, Athanasoulis CA, Waltman AC: Tolazoline-augmented arteriography in the evaluation of bone and soft-tissue tumors. Radiology *133*:792, 1979.
278. McDougall A, McGarrity G: Extra-abdominal desmoid tumours. J Bone Joint Surg *61B*:373, 1979.
279. Bergiron C, Markovits P, Benjaafer M, Piekarski JD, Garel L: Lymphography in childhood rhabdomyosarcomas. Radiology *133*:627, 1979.
280. Jajic I, Rulnjevic J: Myositis ossificans localisata as a complication of tetanus. Acta Orthop Scand *50*:547, 1979.
281. Sarmiento A, Elkins RW: Giant intra-articular osteochondroma of the knee. J Bone Joint Surg *57A*:560, 1975.
282. Morgan CJ Jr: Panniculitis and erythema nodosum. *In* WN Kelley, ED Harris Jr, S Ruddy, CB Sledge (Eds): Textbook of Rheumatology. Philadelphia, WB Saunders, 1981, p 1203.
283. Moore S: Relation of pancreatic disease to Weber-Christian disease. Can Med Assoc J *88*:1238, 1963.
284. Eisman J, Swezey RL: Juxta-articular adiposis dolorosa: What is it? Report of 2 cases. Ann Rheum Dis *38*:479, 1979.
285. Hedstrand H, Berglund G, Werner I: Keratodermia palmaris et plantaris with clubbing and skeletal deformity of the terminal phalanges of the hands and feet. Acta Dermatovenereol *52*:278, 1972.
286. Greenfield GB, Rosado W, Rothbart F: Benign proliferative skin lesions causing destructive and resorptive bone changes. Am J Roentgenol *97*:733, 1966.
287. Evans HL: Liposarcoma. Am J Surg Pathol *3*:507, 1979.
288. Chew FS, Hudson TM, Hawkins IF Jr: Radiology of infiltrating angiolipoma. Am J Roentgenol *135*:781, 1980.
289. Dorfman HD, Levin S, Robbins H: Cartilage-containing benign mesenchymomas of soft tissue. J Bone Joint Surg *62A*:472, 1980.
290. Ledesma-Medina J, Oh KS, Girdany BR: Calcification in childhood leiomyoma. Radiology *135*:339, 1980.
291. Myers BW, Masi AT, Feigenbaum SL: Pigmented villonodular synovitis and tenosynovitis: A clinical epidemiologic study of 166 cases and literature review. Medicine *59*:223, 1980.
292. Zazzaro PF, Bosworth JE, Schneider V, Zelenak JJ: Gallium scanning in malignant fibrous histiocytoma. Am J Roentgenol *135*:775, 1980.
293. Milgram JW, Dunn EJ: Para-articular chondromas and osteochondromas. Clin Orthop Rel Res *148*:147, 1980.
294. Wu KK, Guise ER: Extraosseous osteogenic sarcoma: A clinical analysis of ten cases. Orthopedics *3*:115, 1980.
295. Schiffman R: Epithelioid sarcoma and synovial sarcoma in the same knee. Cancer *45*:158, 1980.
296. Balsam D, Goldfarb R, Stringer B, Farruggia S: Bone scintigraphy for neonatal osteomyelitis; simulation by extravasation of intravenous calcium. Radiology *135*:185, 1980.
297. Mitnick PD, Goldfarb S, Slatopolsky E, Lemann J Jr, Gray RW, Agus ZS: Calcium and phosphate metabolism in tumoral calcinosis. Ann Intern Med *92*:482, 1980.
298. Nassonova VA, Ivanova MM, Akhnazarova VD, Oshilko TG, Bjelle A, Hofer P-A, Henriksson, K-G, Ström T: Eosinophilic fasciitis. Scand J Rheum *8*:225, 1979.
299. Moore TL, Zuckner J: Eosinophilic fasciitis. Semin Arthritis Rheum *9*: 228, 1980.
300. Rosenthal J, Benson MD: Diffuse fasciitis and eosinophilia with symmetric polyarthritis. Ann Intern Med *92*:507, 1980.
301. Sekkat A, Benhayoune TS: A propos d'un cas de kératodermie Aïnhumoïde et mutilante. Ann Dermatol Venereol *107*:447, 1980.
302. Kan WC, Wiley AL Jr, Wirtanen GW, Lange TA, Moran PR, Paliwal BR, Cashwell RJ: High Z elements in human sarcomata: Assessment by multi-energy CT and neutron activation analysis. Am J Roentgenol *135*:123, 1980.
303. Desai A, Eymontt M, Alavi A, Schaffer B, Dalinka MK: ^{99m}Tc-MDP uptake in nonosseous lesions. Radiology *135*:181, 1980.
304. Choy D, Murray IPC: Metastatic visceral calcification identified by bone scanning. Skel Radiol *5*:151, 1980.
305. Balachandran S, Abbud Y, Prince MJ, Chausmer AB: Tumoral calcinosis: Scintigraphic studies of an affected family. Br J Radiol *53*:960, 1980.
306. Pringle J, Stoker DJ: Case report 127. Skel Radiol *5*:263, 1980.
307. Safai B, Good RA: Kaposi's sarcoma: A review and recent developments. Clin Bull *10*:62, 1980.
308. Stephenson TF: Computerized tomography of soft tissue abnormalities. Computerized Tomography *4*:181, 1980.
309. Jones BV, Ward MW: Myositis ossificans in the biceps femoris muscles causing sciatic nerve palsy. A case report. J Bone Joint Surg *62B*:506, 1980.

GENERAL ORGAN SYSTEMS

by David S. Feigin, M.D., and Joel E. Lichtenstein, M.D.

86

Many of the rheumatic diseases have important nonarticular and nonosseous manifestations. Such manifestations may aid significantly in the differential diagnosis and may also be important in consideration of response to treatment and of prognosis. In many cases, the systemic manifestations are life-threatening.

This chapter will not describe diseases that are principally systemic, since such diseases are discussed completely in other works. Also excluded are diseases that are principally articular but which rarely manifest themselves by radiographically evident systemic disease. Discussions of Sjögren's syndrome and amyloidosis, however, have been included because their roentgenographic manifestations in various organ systems are not often found elsewhere.

RHEUMATOID ARTHRITIS

Pulmonary and Pleural Manifestations

Pleuritis and Pleural Effusions. Among the extra-articular manifestations of rheumatoid arthritis that are visualized roentgenographically, pleuritis is generally recognized as the most common[1] (Fig. 86–1). Bilateral or, less commonly, unilateral pleural effusions are usually the only roentgenographic evidence of this pleural disease. Although the onset is often unilateral, the effusions become bilateral in the vast majority of patients.[2]

As is the case with most extra-articular manifestations of rheumatoid arthritis, pleuritis is most common in individuals who already have severe rheumatoid joint disease.[3,4] Despite the fact that rheumatoid disease is more common in women than men, the pleural manifestations are found disproportionately in men, especially those of middle age.[5] Pericarditis with pericardial effusion is often found in those patients who also have pleuritis.

Clinical manifestations are usually mild. The effusions are often asymptomatic and are nearly always transient.[2] The onset may be heralded by the initial attack of arthritis or by an acute exacerbation of arthritic symptoms.[5] The effusions usually recur and become chronic.[3] Eventually, pleural thickening may be visualized in addition to pleural effusions, but true pleural masses are not seen in rheumatoid pleuritis despite the fact that rheumatoid nodules may be demonstrated in the pleura pathologically.[2]

Analysis of the pleural fluid generally reveals low glucose levels.[6] The glucose levels are even lower than those found in tuberculosis except when tuberculosis is accompanied by empyema. A method of distinguishing between the pleural fluid in these two

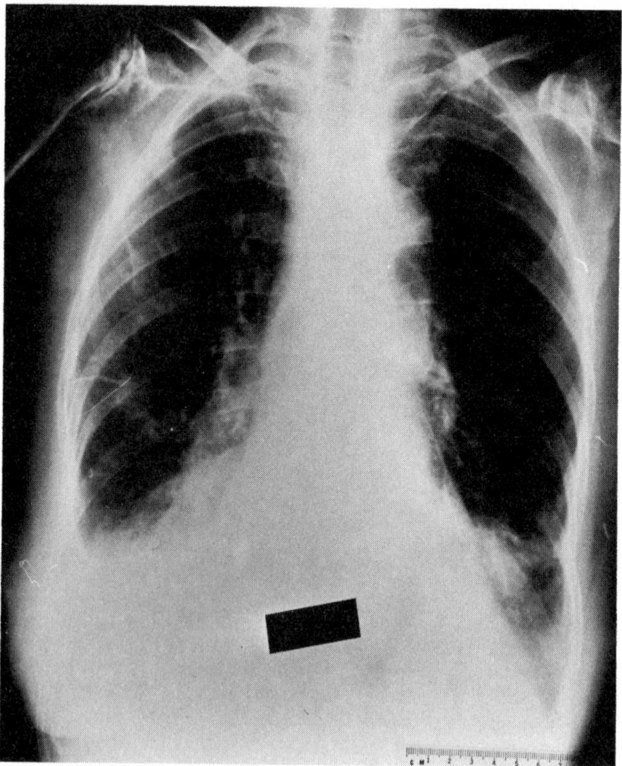

Figure 86–1. *Rheumatoid arthritis: Pleuritis and effusion. This 66 year old woman had severe, crippling rheumatoid arthritis since age 21 years. Chest film shows a large right pleural effusion and pleural thickening bilaterally over the costophrenic angles. Rheumatoid interstitial pulmonary disease is also present, especially evident in the right lower lung field. Rheumatoid articular disease is also seen, especially in the shoulders. (Armed Forces Institute of Pathology Neg. No. 77-8006.)*

diseases is to infuse glucose intravenously and subsequently resample the pleural fluid. The glucose level does not rise in rheumatoid effusions, as it generally does in tuberculous effusions.[6] Other chemical characteristics of the fluid include the facts that lipid may be present and that lactic dehydrogenase (LDH) levels are often elevated. Rheumatoid factor, especially as demonstrated by the sheep cell agglutination test, may be present in the fluid.[5] Eosinophils may be present and are rare in carcinoma and in chronic granulomatous infections, including tuberculosis and fungal disease.[3] Large numbers of leukocytes are usually found in the fluid, including polymorphonuclear leukocytes with dense black granules ("RA cells") that release rheumatoid factor when they disintegrate.[7]

Pneumothorax is sometimes associated with rheumatoid pleural disease but this is not considered common. Although the pneumothorax may be caused by pleuritis, it is often caused by the rupture of subpleural pulmonary nodules, leading to bronchopleural fistulae.[2, 8]

Treatment of rheumatoid pleuritis may include fluid aspiration, intrathoracic injection of agents such as tetracycline, and, rarely, decortication.[7] Corticosteroid therapy is effective in treating rheumatoid pleuritis. The transient nature of the effusions and the tendency for the pleural manifestations to be asymptomatic (although chronic) militate against the need for direct therapy.

NECROBIOTIC PULMONARY NODULES. Although pulmonary necrobiotic rheumatoid nodules are rare manifestations of rheumatoid disease, they are among the more common pulmonary manifestations.[2, 8] The nodules are round pulmonary lesions histologically identical to subcutaneous rheumatoid nodules; they consist of an area of central necrosis surrounded by a zone of fibroblasts in a palisade arrangement, which is in turn surrounded by a peripheral zone of mixed inflammatory cells, including plasma cells and lymphocytes.[9] The nodules were first described by Ellman and Ball in 1947 and 1948.[10, 11]

Roentgenographically, rheumatoid nodules are usually discrete, round, and possibly lobulated pulmonary masses, which may be tiny to several centimeters in diameter (Fig. 86–2). They are usually multiple, although solitary nodules have been reported.[2] There are no specific location preferences. These nodules may be found subpleurally, where their rupture may cause pneumothorax (see earlier discussion).[12] The nodules may increase or decrease in size rapidly and may disappear completely. Because the center of each lesion is necrotic, cavitation often occurs, leaving a cavitated mass in which the wall is usually thick because of the proliferation of inflammatory cells outside the region of necrosis. The walls are generally symmetric about the cavity.

Pulmonary rheumatoid nodules do not appear to be directly associated with other roentgenographically visible pleural or pulmonary manifestations of rheumatoid arthritis. Approximately half the described cases have evidence of rheumatoid interstitial pneumonitis pathologically,[2] but fewer cases demonstrate pneumonitis radiographically. As with other manifestations of extra-articular rheumatoid disease, this abnormality occurs disproportionally in men in comparison to the female predominance of articular rheumatoid disease. There does appear to be an association of incidence between pulmonary and subcutaneous rheumatoid nodules.[9]

No specific symptoms appear to be associated with rheumatoid pulmonary nodules, and no specific therapy appears useful. A few cases have been reported of rheumatoid nodules preceding the development of rheumatoid articular disease, and there are also a few cases of pathologically proved rheumatoid nodules in patients who never develop other clinical or pathologic evidence of rheumatoid disease.[8]

INTERSTITIAL INFLAMMATORY AND FIBROTIC PULMONARY DISEASE. It has been recognized[11] that pulmonary infiltrates of noninfectious etiology are associated with rheumatoid disease and have been called "rheumatoid lung" or "rheumatoid pulmonary fibrosis." The incidence of interstitial disease in patients with rheumatoid arthritis varies in different studies; the incidence is as low as 1 per cent of all rheumatoid arthritis patients[5] but as high as 30 to 40 per cent in patients with severe disease, especially those who are hospitalized.[7]

Rheumatoid lung disease is generally considered to be a nonspecific reaction similar to other forms of usual interstitial pneumonitis (UIP),[12] fibrosing alveolitis,[13] or idiopathic pulmonary fibrosis (IPF). Fibrosing alveolitis and IPF are terms used to describe a nonspecific chronic inflammatory reaction in the pulmonary interstitium that may lead to significant interstitial fibrosis. The fibrosis may be severe enough to form true honeycomb lung, also

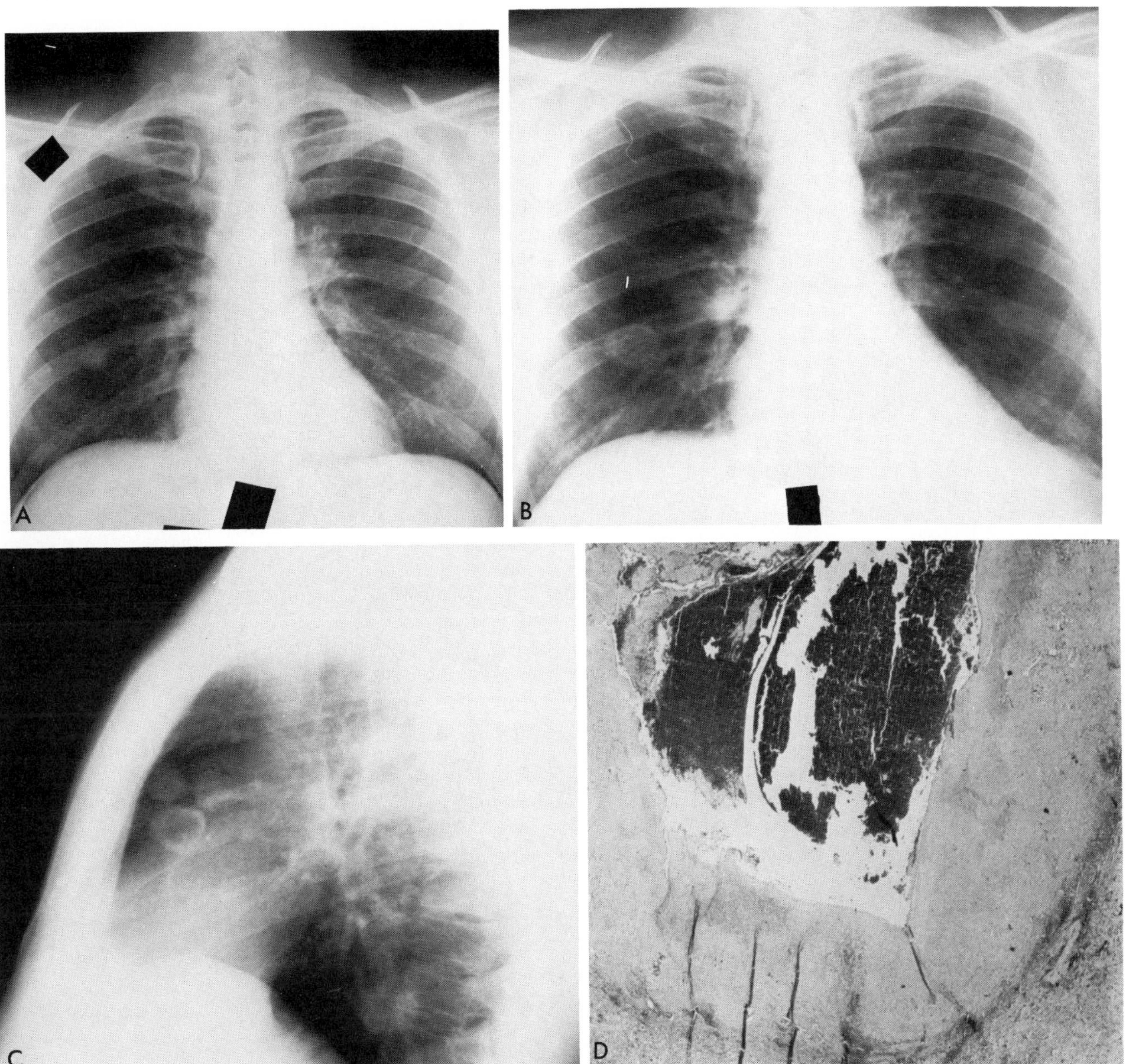

Figure 86–2. *Rheumatoid arthritis: Necrobiotic pulmonary nodules. In a 42-year-old man with a long history of rheumatoid arthritis with positive serology, pulmonary symptoms were absent.*

A *Initial frontal film shows a small noncavitary mass in right lower lung field.*

B, C *Three years later, the mass is much larger and is now cavitated. Other masses are also visible, especially on the lateral view.*

D *Low power photomicrograph of the cavitated nodule shows the thick inflammatory wall and necrotic center.*

(Armed Forces Institute of Pathology Neg. Nos. 66-6668-1,2,3,4.)

known as "end-stage lung."[14] Although there may be histologic differences between UIP caused by rheumatoid disease and that occurring on an idiopathic basis, the roentgenographic manifestations, natural history, and response to therapy do not differ significantly, except that the rheumatoid form is often less severe.[7] A histologic finding distinctive for rheumatoid lung disease is greater lymphocytic infiltration than that found in other forms of interstitial pneumonitis. The lymphocytes may be found as small nests rather than as diffuse collections spread throughout the interstitium.

The nonspecificity of the interstitial inflammation in rheumatoid lung disease has led some authors to believe that this is a diffuse form of the necrobiotic nodules described previously.[2, 15] Nevertheless, the two manifestations are more often seen separately than together, and regression of the nodules is more common than is regression or therapeutic response of the interstitial infiltrate. Although the development of arthritis generally precedes the development of interstitial pulmonary disease, cases have been reported in which rheumatoid lung involvement has been the first manifestation of rheumatoid disease.[2] There is no obvious relation between the severity of the joint manifestations and that of the interstitial disease.

Roentgenographically, rheumatoid pulmonary disease is not distinct from other forms of interstitial pneumonitis. The most common appearance is a bilateral, lower lung field linear or finely nodular infiltrate, which may be associated with Kerley B lines. The cardiac silhouette and hemidiaphragms may be indistinct because of superimposed interstitial thickening. Normal pulmonary markings, although they may be somewhat thickened, are usually less distinct because of the interstitial thickening. True honeycombing may be present in small areas and may become diffuse after many years of disease. Throughout the course of the disease, however, the lower lung field is generally more involved than the upper lung field (Figs. 86–3 to 86–5).

Clinical evidence of rheumatoid pulmonary disease generally consists of nonspecific respiratory symptoms, including cough and dyspnea, especially on exertion. Hemoptysis is an uncommon symptom in rheumatoid lung disease and when present suggests infective pulmonary disease in addition to rheumatoid disease. Pulmonary function tests show significant restrictive disease, which is often progressive; small airway disease is commonly present as well.[7] As with other extra-articular manifestations of rheumatoid disease, the numbers of men involved are out of proportion to the numbers affected by rheumatoid disease as a whole.[5] Although corticosteroid therapy is often prescribed in rheumatoid lung disease, it is generally ineffective or only briefly effective.[5, 16]

The etiology of rheumatoid pulmonary involvement is not known. Although, as mentioned above, some authors believe it to be a diffuse manifestation of rheumatoid nodular disease, others believe it is caused by vasculitis. This view is supported by the fact that histologically the disease is most severe

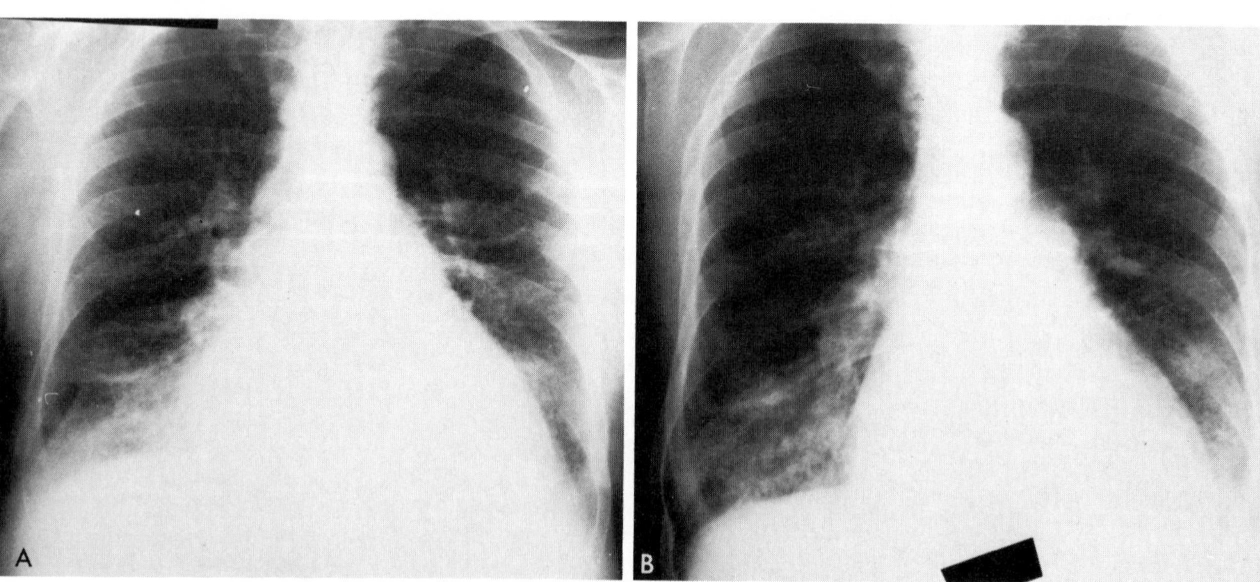

Figure 86–3. *Rheumatoid arthritis: Early interstitial disease, with rheumatoid carditis and pericarditis. This 65 year old woman had had rheumatoid arthritis for several years before becoming short of breath.*

A *Initial film shows bilateral lower lobe nonspecific interstitial infiltration. The pericardial silhouette is markedly enlarged and mild pulmonary venous hypertension is also presnt.*

B *Two years later, the cardiac silhouette is small but the interstitial pulmonary disease remains, and a left pleural effusion is also evident.*

(Armed Forces Institute of Pathology Neg. Nos. 77-2048-1,2.)

around vessels.[15] Despite the finding that inhaled substances such as silica are rarely found in association with diffuse changes, the role of environmental agents in causing this manifestation may be important, as rheumatoid disease may contribute an increased reactivity of lung tissue to inhaled substances.[15] An increased incidence of rheumatoid pneumonitis in cigarette smokers has recently been documented.[7] Nonpathogenic organisms, such as those involved in allergic alveolitis, may also be involved.[2]

A few authors have speculated that patients

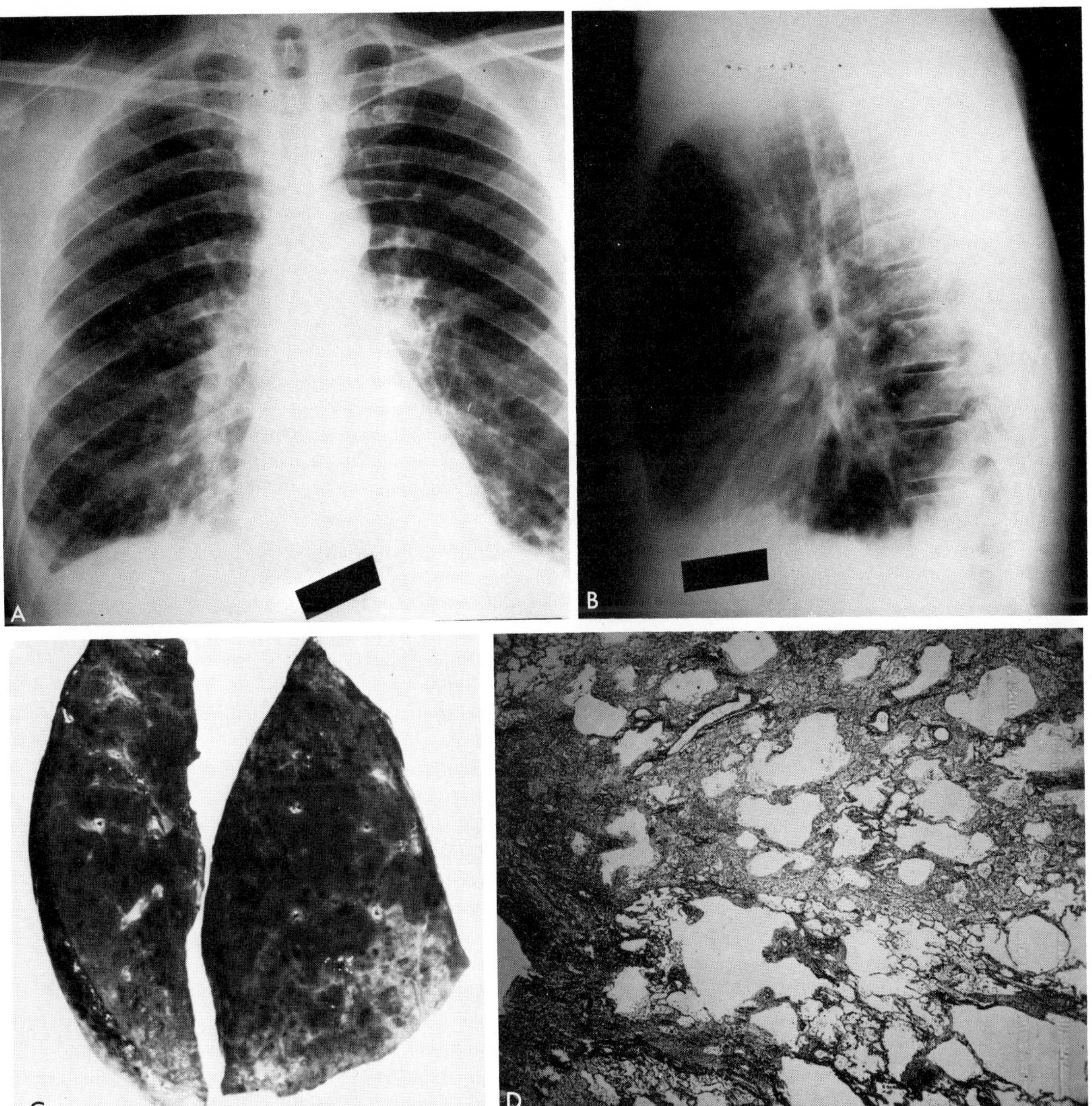

Figure 86–4. *Rheumatoid arthritis: Late interstitial pulmonary disease. This 45 year old man had a 1 year history of rheumatoid arthritis and nonspecific pulmonary symptoms.*

A, B *Chest film shows irregular interstitial infiltration of lower lung fields with bilateral pleural effusions.*

C *Photograph of gross lung specimen, from a different patient, shows similar diffuse irregular infiltration of lower lobes.*

D *Low power photomicrograph shows diffuse inflammatory infiltration of interstitium without alveolar filling or collapse.*

(Armed Forces Institute of Pathology Neg. Nos. 78-2906-1,2; 74-12844-2; 76-1776.)

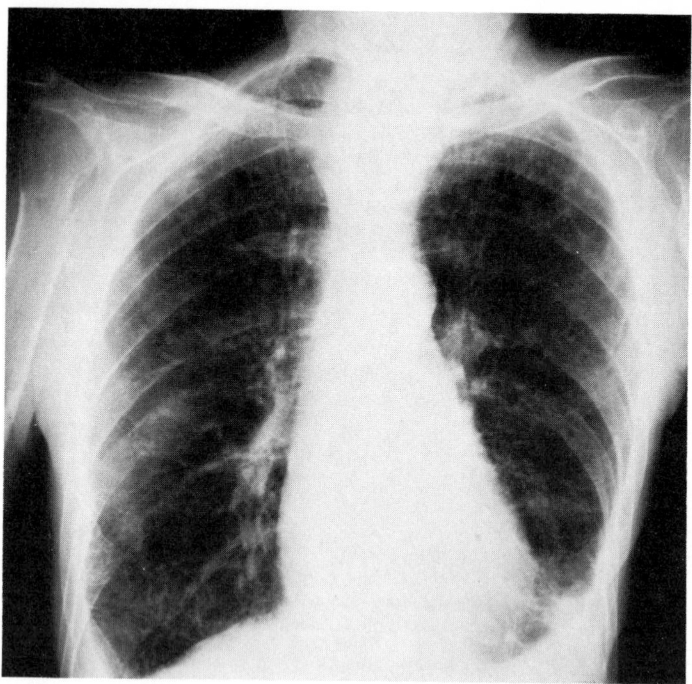

Figure 86–5. Rheumatoid arthritis: Interstitial pulmonary disease with end-stage lung disease. Chest film of an elderly man with long-standing rheumatoid arthritis shows irregular cystic changes throughout both entire lung fields and marked irregular interstitial infiltration. Pleuritis is demonstrated at both costophrenic angles and obvious articular changes are seen about the right humerus and distal clavicle.

with rheumatoid pulmonary disease may be more likely to develop pulmonary neoplasms than other people.[16, 17] All patients with bronchogenic carcinoma and rheumatoid lung disease, however, have been heavy smokers. It is possible that the hyperplasia of bronchiolar epithelium[16, 17] found in rheumatoid lung disease may be a factor in the development of bronchogenic carcinoma.

Pulmonary Arteritis and Hypertension. Pulmonary hypertension occurs rarely in patients with articular rheumatoid disease. Several cases have been reported sporadically.[5] The pulmonary hypertension is probably caused by vasculitis of pulmonary arterioles, causing gradually increasing pulmonary arterial pressure. It is possible that some cases of unexplained pulmonary hypertension without arthritis may also be secondary to rheumatoid vasculitis involving these arterioles. In any event, the manifestations of pulmonary hypertension are no different in rheumatoid disease than those that appear in association with other disorders. There does not seem to be any association between the presence of pulmonary hypertension and the appearance of other manifestations of rheumatoid disease in the lungs or pleurae, but pulmonary hypertension may occur in a patient who also has other manifestations visible roentgenographically.

Caplan's Disease. Caplan's disease is rheumatoid pulmonary disease, usually nodular, in association with pneumoconiosis. Caplan originally described a high incidence of rheumatoid arthritis in miners with conglomerate pneumoconiosis who also had nodular pulmonary disease. The pulmonary nodules often preceded the onset of arthritis. Caplan's original description of rheumatoid pneumoconiosis has been broadened[18, 19] to include nodular interstitial pneumonitis as well as larger pulmonary nodules as manifestations of the same basic disease process.

Caplan originally described rheumatoid pneumoconiosis as manifested by nodules 0.5 to 5 cm in diameter with frequent roentgenographic evidence of cavitation and calcification. Subsequently, he described the presence of smaller nodules (0.3 to 1 cm in diameter), which were similar in appearance to the nodules of simple silicosis. Caplan found that two thirds of patients with the classic nodules had rheumatoid arthritis, whereas only one third of those with smaller nodules or interstitial pneumonitis had clinical evidence of rheumatoid arthritis. However, all manifestations of rheumatoid pneumoconiosis were associated with serologic evidence of rheumatoid disease even if no arthritis was present.

Roentgenographically, rheumatoid pneumoconiosis may thus consist of nodular dense lesions of any size, often occurring in groups or nests, and often becoming confluent (Fig. 86–6). Mild to moderate interstitial pneumonitis may coexist with the nodules. In contrast to other manifestations of rheumatoid disease in the lungs, which principally involve the lower lung fields, rheumatoid pneumoconiosis more often involves the upper lung fields and may have a strikingly apical distribution similar to that of silicosis or coal worker's pneumoconiosis. This upper lobe predilection is even present in other pneumoconioses, such as asbestosis, in which the usual roentgenographic manifestations are predominantly in the lower lung fields.[13] In contrast to

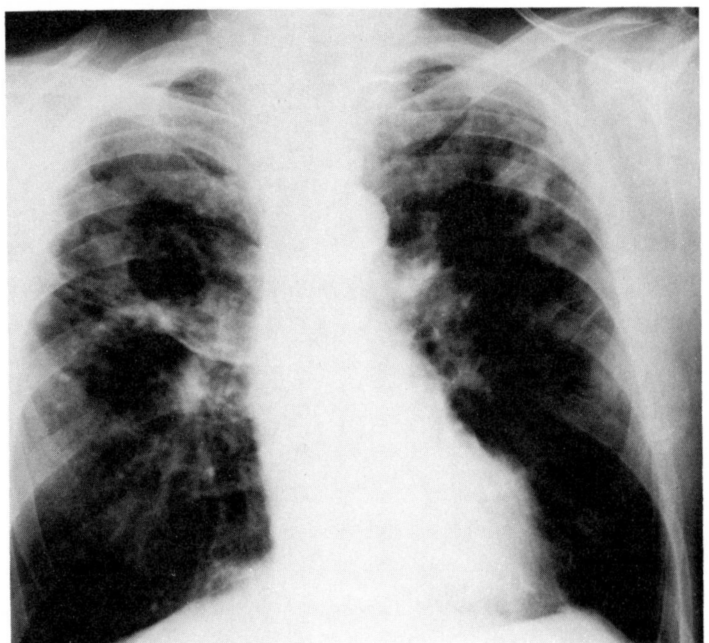

Figure 86–6. Caplan's disease. This middle-aged coal miner had symptoms of chronic lung disease. Clusters of nodules are present in the upper lung fields, especially in the periphery. There is also bilateral upper lobe loss of volume. Pencil-like thinning of the distal left clavicle is evident. (Armed Forces Institute of Pathology Neg. No. 68-10341-4.)

lesions of pulmonary massive fibrosis (PMF), rheumatoid pneumoconiotic lesions are generally rounder and more peripheral in location, although, as stated earlier, they may also coalesce.[13]

Although the disease was originally described in miners, several reports show similar roentgenographic manifestations in asbestosis, silicosis, exposure to soap abrasives, exposure to aluminum powder, and exposure to various other agents.[13] The incidence in Europe and Great Britain far exceeds that in the United States, for unknown reasons.[7] In contrast to the lesions in other pneumoconioses, rheumatoid pneumoconiotic lesions may increase in size very rapidly, often within a period of weeks, and have also been shown to disappear rapidly. Rheumatoid pneumoconiosis is most common when the more typical manifestations of pneumoconiosis are mild; UICC categories 0 and 1 are those most commonly associated.

The specific etiology of rheumatoid pneumoconiosis remains obscure. Miall[20] has shown that there is no increased incidence of rheumatoid arthritis in miners as a whole and thus that exposure to inhaled dust per se cannot be implicated as a cause of rheumatoid arthritis. The presence of rheumatoid disese, however, may increase the susceptibility of an individual to pulmonary reaction in response to an inhaled substance, including dust. This theory has also been used to explain the presence of necrobiotic nodules in the lungs of patients with rheumatoid arthritis implicating antigens other than inhaled dust as the direct stimulants.

Although the lesions of rheumatoid pneumoconiosis are roentgenographically indistinguishable from those of other forms of rheumatoid pulmonary disease (except for their distribution), there are pathologic differences between classic rheumatoid pneumoconiosis nodules and necrobiotic nodules. The classic rheumatoid pneumoconiosis nodule contains a pigmented ring of dust around the periphery of the lesion. Furthermore, palisading of fibroblasts just outside the area of central necrosis is far less marked in the pneumoconiotic nodule than in the typical necrobiotic nodule.[18]

Pericarditis and Carditis

Although pericarditis is found at autopsy in 30 to 50 per cent of patients with rheumatoid arthritis,[21] the manifestation is far less common roentgenographically during life. Evidence of other cardiac manifestations of rheumatoid arthritis is even less common than pericardial disease, although subclinical mitral valve changes may be common. These manifestations almost invariably occur in patients with known active rheumatoid articular disease. Other extra-articular manifestations are common, including subcutaneous nodules and pleural effusions. There may be a relationship between the carditis and pericarditis of rheumatoid disease and the presence of necrotizing arteritis elsewhere.[23]

The pericarditis of rheumatoid disease is generally heralded by left-sided chest pain. Symptoms of congestive heart failure are present in about half the patients and approximately two thirds have evidence of congestive failure on physical examination. Pericardial friction rubs are heard in approximately two thirds of patients.[21] As with other extra-articular manifestations of rheumatoid disease, the cardiac

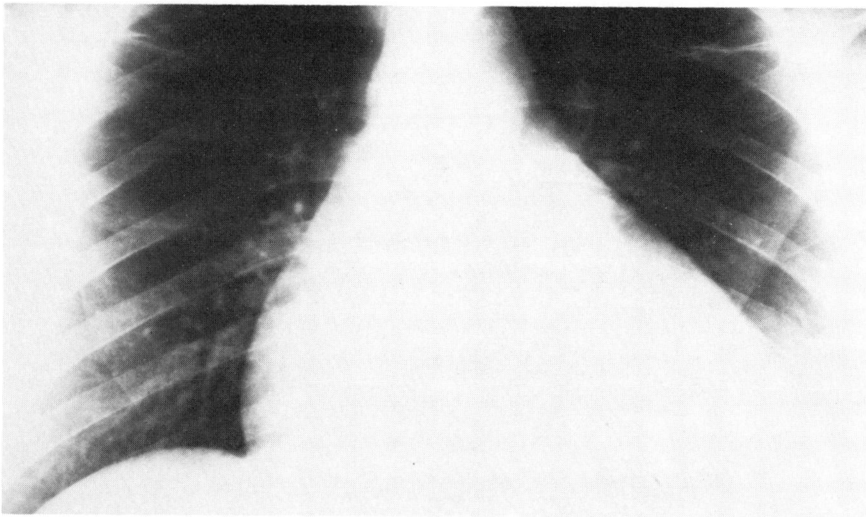

Figure 86–7. Rheumatoid arthritis: Pericarditis and carditis in a 35 year old man with documented rheumatoid joint disease. There is marked enlargement of the cardiopericardial silhouette, typical of pericardial effusion of any cause. A left pleural effusion is also noted. (Armed Forces Institute of Pathology Neg. No. 70-1291.)

manifestations occur disproportionately in men in comparison with the disease in general.[22]

The cardiac manifestations of rheumatoid disease are indistinguishable from the enlarged pericardial-cardiac silhouette that is seen in many other disorders (Figs. 86–3, 86–7, and 86–8). The presence of a pericardial effusion may easily be confirmed echographically, and it is often necessary to analyze the pericardial fluid to rule out infectious or neoplastic causes. Such analysis reveals chemical findings similar to those of pleural effusions, including especially a glucose level that is low in comparison with the serum glucose level.

Initially, the pericarditis of rheumatoid disease generally responds to corticosteroid therapy. Later, however, fibrous pericarditis may ensue, and approximately 15 per cent of patients with rheumatoid pericarditis may eventually develop cardiac tamponade, necessitating pericardiectomy.[21, 24] Pericardiocentesis is usually not helpful.[25]

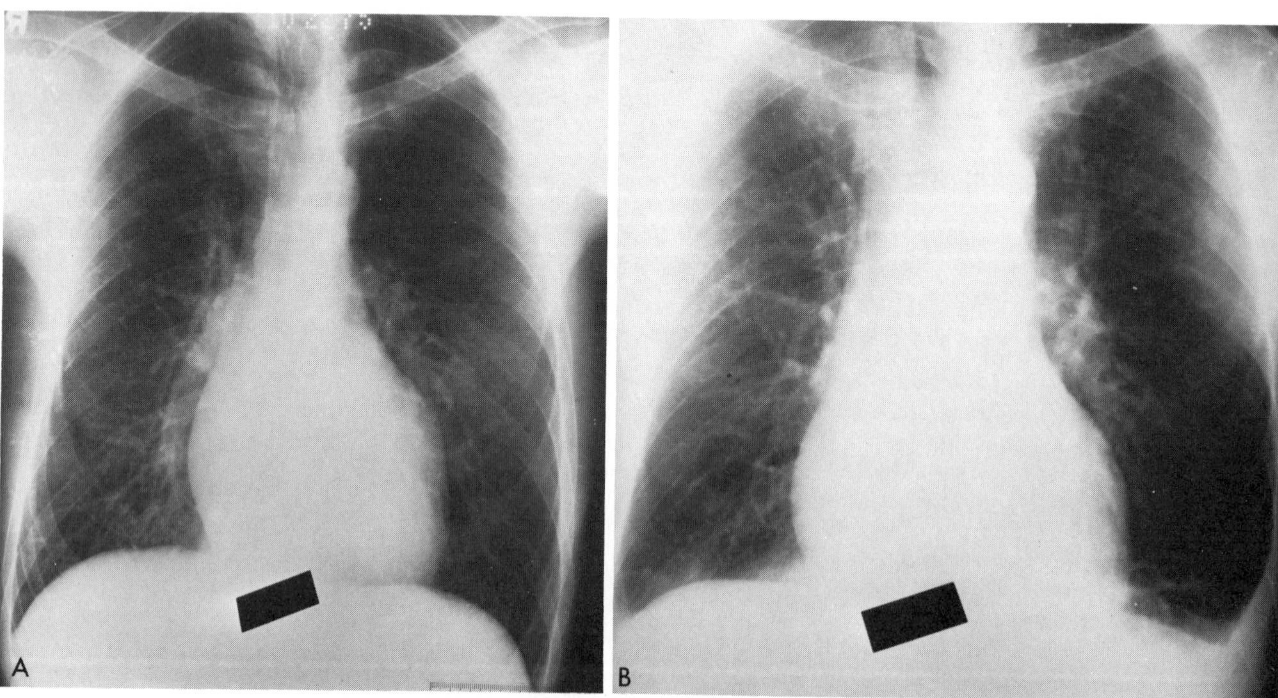

Figure 86–8. Rheumatoid arthritis: Pericardial effusion. This 46 year old man with long-standing rheumatoid arthritis presented with left anterior chest pain.

A Film 1 year prior to admission shows no significant abnormality.

B Admission film shows cardiopericardial enlargement and left pleural effusion.

Illustration continued on the opposite page

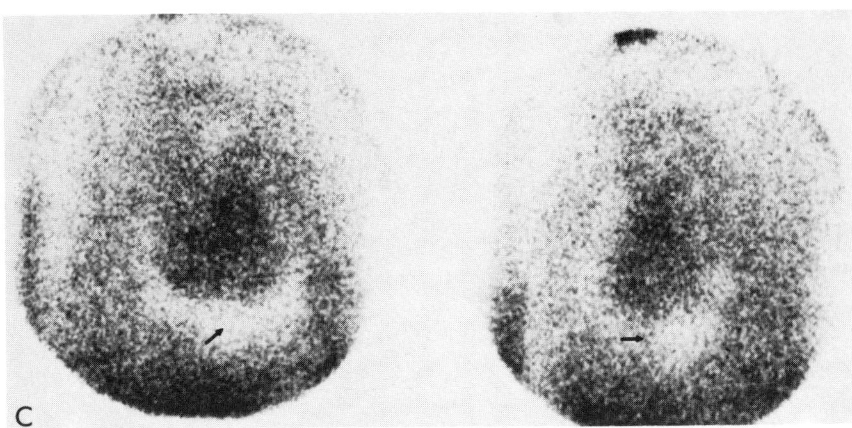

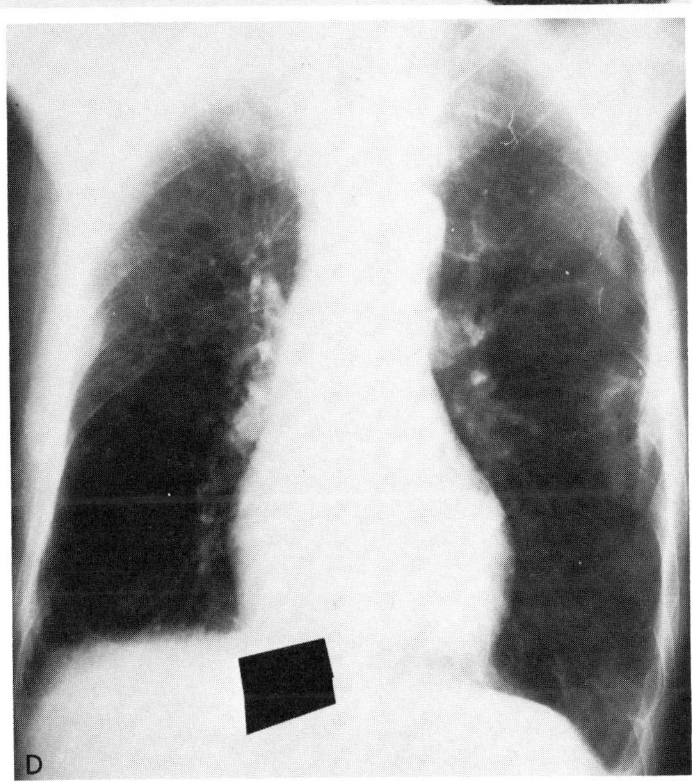

Figure 86–8. Continued
C *Combined blood pool lung scan shows large area of decreased activity corresponding to large pericardial effusion (arrows).*
D *Frontal film following pericardiectomy shows normal cardiac shadow and decreased pleural effusion.*
(Courtesy of Dr. Jack Rabinowitz, City of Memphis Hospital, Memphis, Tennessee, and Armed Forces Institute of Pathology Neg. Nos. 76-11562-1,2.)

Lymphadenopathy and Splenomegaly, Including Felty's Syndrome

Generalized lymphadenopathy and splenomegaly are often found in patients with rheumatoid articular disease.[4] The lymphadenopathy may occasionally be visible roentgenographically but is usually more obvious clinically. Splenomegaly may be detectable on films of the abdomen or chest.

Felty's syndrome consists of splenomegaly and neutropenia in patients, usually women, with rheumatoid arthritis. The white cell count is usually less than 3500 cells per cu cm, with fewer than 2000 cells per cu cm being polymorphonuclear leukocytes. The serologic test for rheumatoid factor usually yields positive results. Two thirds of patients have positive results on antinuclear antibody tests or lupus erythematosus preparation tests, but the syndrome is generally believed to be independent of systemic lupus erythematosus.[26] Lymphadenopathy is not considered a part of Felty's syndrome.

Rheumatoid pulmonary nodules and Sjögren's syndrome are commonly found in association with Felty's syndrome, but other nonarticular manifestations of rheumatoid disease are uncommon.

Pathologic changes in the spleen in Felty's syndrome are specific and differ from those found in the spleens of patients with other rheumatoid disorders. Portal hypertension commonly accompanies this syndrome, but the pathologic findings are not explainable on that basis alone. The hypersplenism that results generally causes anemia due to increased hemolysis. Corticosteroid therapy appears to have little effect on this hypersplenism.[27] If severe infection, severe anemia, or hemorrhage due to thrombocytopenia ensues, splenectomy is often indicated in Felty's syndrome. Splenectomy is generally not indicated in the presence of neutropenia alone.

Vasculitis and Ischemic Ulcers

Peripheral vasculitis is a rare extra-articular manifestation of rheumatoid arthritis. Three forms have been described: (1) subacute small vessel lesions, (2) severe, diffuse necrotizing arteritis similar to that in periarteritis nodosa, and (3) obliterative endarteritis in digits and viscera.

The vascular changes are most often visualized in the digital arteries.[28] Arteriography reveals irregularity, narrowing, or obliteration of the lumen of digital vessels and formation of collateral vessels. These changes may occur in any of the arteries of the hand and foot but are especially prominent in the digits. Hyperemia may also be visualized, especially adjacent to synovial disease.[29] Neuropathy may result from ischemia secondary to arteritis.

In elderly men with long-standing rheumatoid arthritis, vasculitis may result in leg ulcers. Trivial injury may trigger the onset of these ulcers, and chronic corticosteroid therapy is probably also a contributing factor.[30] Subcutaneous nodules are found in nearly all patients with leg ulcers. Although corticosteroids are usually effective in the treatment of the leg ulcers, grafts are occasionally needed, especially following recurrence of the ulcerations.

JUVENILE CHRONIC ARTHRITIS

Acute Carditis, Including Pericarditis

The extra-articular manifestations of juvenile chronic arthritis are most common in those patients with seronegative chronic arthritis. Patients with seropositive juvenile rheumatoid arthritis rarely have systemic manifestations but, when present, they resemble those of adult rheumatoid arthritis.[2, 31] Patients with juvenile ankylosing spondylitis and pauciarticular disease likewise rarely, if ever, manifest extra-articular disease. Systemic features are also rare in psoriatic arthritis occurring in childhood.

In seronegative chronic arthritis, the onset of acute disease (Still's disease) is generally heralded by polyarticular arthritis with fever and any combination of other systemic manifestations, including rash, generalized lymphadenopathy, splenomegaly, hepatomegaly, or pericarditis. At least half to two thirds of the reported patients are less than 5 years old at onset. Iridocyclitis does not usually occur in this group.

Systemic manifestations of juvenile chronic arthritis are generally present at the time of onset of illness if they appear at all.[32] The symptoms rarely last more than 6 months, although the polyarthritis often becomes chronic. In addition to the clinical findings noted above, most patients have leukocytosis, high sedimentation rate, increased IgG levels, and the presence of immune complexes detectable by many different techniques.[31]

Manifestations visible roentgenographically include lymphadenopathy, splenomegaly, and peri-

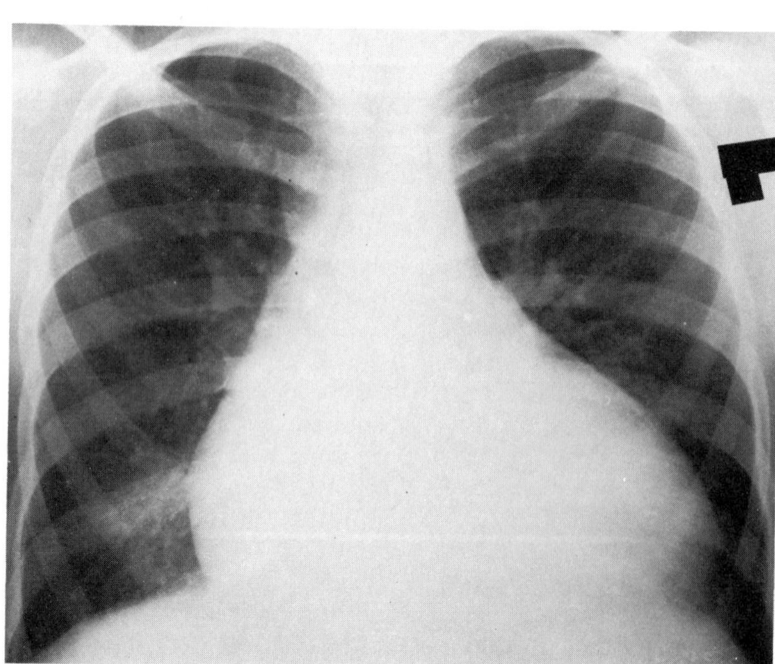

Figure 86–9. *Juvenile chronic arthritis: pericarditis. This 12 year old boy had a long history of seronegative chronic arthritis. The marked enlargement of the cardiopericardial silhouette is nonspecific.*

(Armed Forces Institute of Pathology Neg. No. 74-4343.)

carditis (Fig. 86–9). Pericarditis is not often clinically evident, but, according to some authors, its incidence may be underestimated.[31] In Schaller's series of 124 patients with juvenile rheumatoid arthritis, one third had pericarditis and one third had pleuritis manifested by pleural effusions.[32] Schaller also reported two patients with interstitial pulmonary disease.

An important distinction between Still's disease and acute rheumatic fever is that endocarditis, common in acute rheumatic fever, does not occur in juvenile chronic arthritis. Enlargement of the cardiopericardial silhouette does, of course, occur in both diseases.

ANKYLOSING SPONDYLITIS

Pulmonary Inflammatory and Fibrocystic Disease

The pulmonary disease associated with ankylosing spondylitis is characterized by upper lobe fibrotic scarring and infiltration with cavitation and large cystic spaces. It is generally believed that these abnormalities are secondary to impaired respiratory excursion and decreased ventilation of the apices secondary to immobility of the thoracic spine.[33]

The pulmonary fibrocystic disease occurs in only a small minority, probably less than 5 per cent, of patients with ankylosing spondylitis,[34] although there is wide variation in reported incidence throughout the literature. Men between 20 and 40 years of age are most commonly affected, and all have a history of spondylitis preceding the pulmonary changes, usually for long periods.[35]

The roentgenographic appearance consists most frequently of bilateral, coarse, linear and cystic dense shadows involving both upper lung fields, especially the apices. Cavitation and the formation of large cystic spaces are common (Fig. 86–10). Unilateral involvement occurs in fewer than one third of patients,[33] but it appears to be more common on the right side than on the left in such cases. The disease involves the midlung fields in a small minority of cases. The changes resemble those of chronic tuberculosis and other chronic granulomatous diseases.

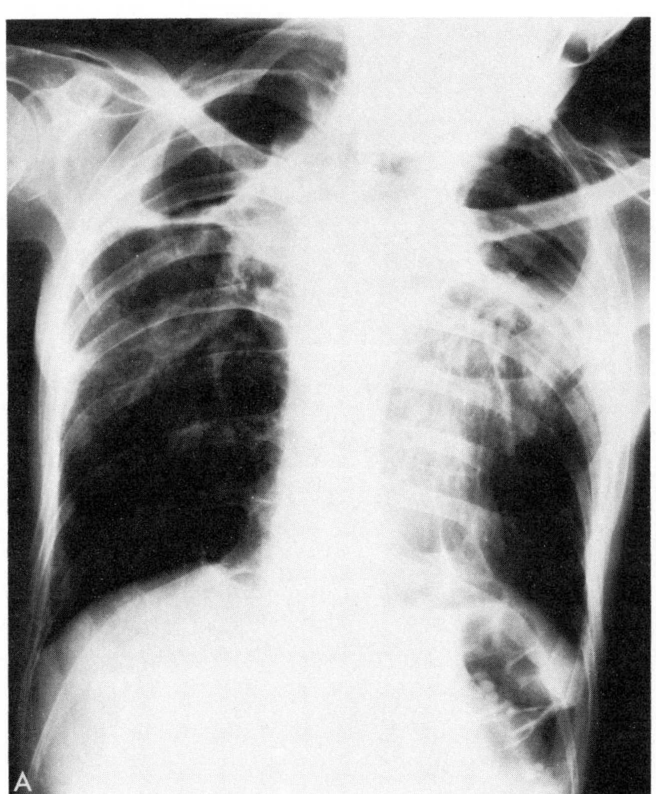

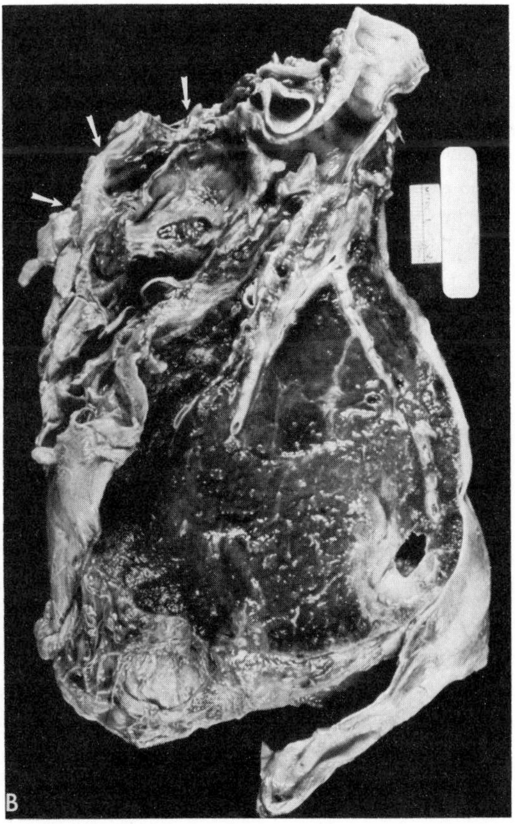

Figure 86–10. *Ankylosing spondylitis: Fibrocystic pulmonary disease. This 47 year old man had a long history of ankylosing spondylitis and severe pulmonary symptoms.*

A *Frontal film shows large fibrotic cysts in both upper lung fields with marked hilar retraction and mid–lung field scarring.*

B *Autopsy specimen of right lung shows large cavity in right upper lobe with severe upper lobe volume loss and diffuse scarring and pleural thickening (arrows).*

The earliest manifestation of the abnormality is thought to be bilateral apical scarring (also called apical pleural thickening by many authors), which is, of course, also seen in many individuals without ankylosing spondylitis. The dense lesions then progress downward as small bullae appear, which subsequently enlarge to involve both upper lung fields (Fig. 86–11). At this stage, bronchiectasis may also be evident roentgenographically.[34] Secondary infection may then ensue, especially the formation of fungus balls, which, in one series, occurred in 41 per cent of all patients with this pulmonary disease.[35] Aspergillus is the most common organism to cause this superinfection, and the agent may be visible roentgenographically as round or irregular dense areas within preexisting cavities. Bronchopneumonia and pleuritis may accompany the fibrocavitary disease at any stage.[36]

Pulmonary function studies show decreased respiratory excursion and decreased vital capacity. Most patients demonstrate increased diaphragmatic excursion, presumably in response to immobility of the chest wall and decreased thoracic wall compliance.[34] Ventilation studies have shown decreased uptake of xenon in the apical regions.[37] Since diaphragmatic movement is responsible for nearly the entire tidal volume in these patients, diaphragmatic failure can result in severe pulmonary disease, including cor pulmonale.[34]

The pathology is nonspecific, consisting of patchy inflammatory infiltration, progressing to extensive intra-alveolar fibrosis with dilated bronchi and thin-walled bullae.[35] These changes apparently resemble those that occur in the aorta of some patients with ankylosing spondylitis. The process, including the roentgenographic findings, does not appear to be reversible. There is no known effective therapy. Approximately one fourth of the affected patients eventually die of respiratory disease.[33]

Although most authors agree that the etiology of these pulmonary changes is the impaired respiratory excursion secondary to involvement of the vertebral column and costovertebral joints in ankylosing spondylitis,[33] other suggestions have included chronic aspiration pneumonitis from decreased esophageal function and infection alone.[38]

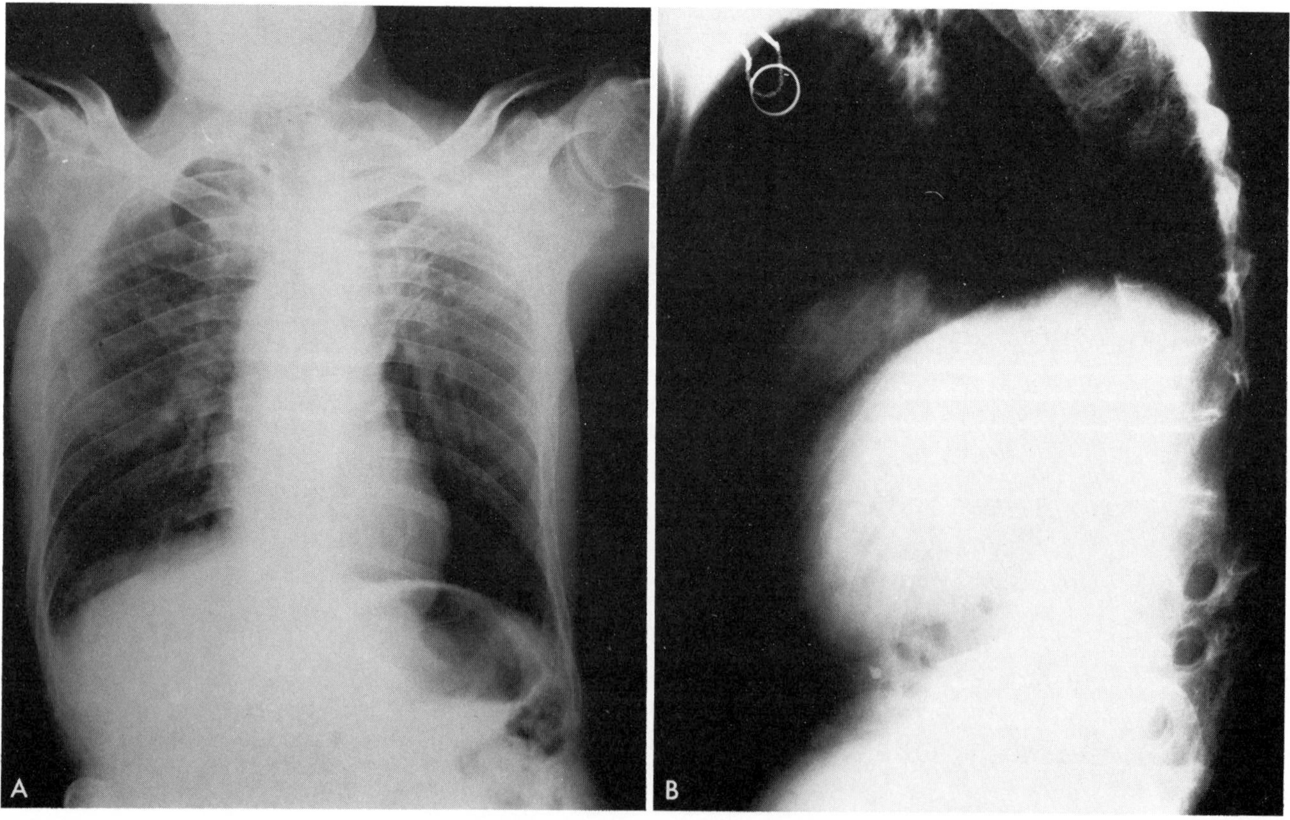

Figure 86–11. *Ankylosing spondylitis: Inflammatory and fibrocystic pulmonary disease. This middle-aged man had severe ankylosing spondylitis and nonspecific pulmonary symptoms.*

A *Frontal chest film shows bilateral upper lobe loss of volume, greater on the left than on the right side and typical of fibrosis. Cyst formation is not seen at this early stage. The overall pulmonary inflation appears normal.*

B *Lateral view shows severe ankylosing spondylitis of the thoracic spine.*

Endocardial and Myocardial Disease

Endocardial disease in ankylosing spondylitis is primarily manifested as isolated aortic insufficiency.[39] The largest reported series showed that approximately 2 per cent of patients with ankylosing spondylitis had valvular disease and, of these, 75 per cent had involvement of the aortic valve and 25 per cent, the mitral valve. Approximately 5 per cent of all cases of aortic insufficiency is found at surgery to be related to ankylosing spondylitis.[40] Histologically, chronic inflammation is found mainly at the base of the valve and not at the cusps and leaflets. Thus, leaflet fusion and valvular stenosis do not generally occur.[39]

Myocardial disease in ankylosing spondylitis is far less specific than the endocardial involvement but is considerably more common.[41] In one series of 55 patients,[41] 28 were found to have myocardial disease of unknown etiology after those with atherosclerotic heart disease and other known cardiac diseases were excluded. The nature of the myocardial involvement has not been documented pathologically to be a distinct entity.

Heart block is also associated with ankylosing spondylitis. Especially common is first degree arteriovenous block. This has been shown pathologically to be secondary to a fibrotic lesion, which is not granulomatous as it is in rheumatoid arthritis.[41] Fibrotic lesions have also been noted in vessels, especially the aorta, in which medial and intimal hypertrophy and intimal hyperplasia and fibrosis have been seen without evidence of rheumatoid lesions of any kind.[39]

The only characteristic cardiac roentgenographic abnormality associated with ankylosing spondylitis is left ventricular enlargement without overall cardiomegaly.[42] Pulmonary venous congestion may be present and can be documented in most of those patients who have clinical evidence of cardiomyopathy.[41] There does not appear to be any relation between the degree of thoracic spondylitis and the presence or severity of any of the cardiac manifestations of ankylosing spondylitis.

INTESTINAL ARTHROPATHIES

Ulcerative Colitis

Ulcerative colitis is a chronic, idiopathic, superficial inflammatory disease classically confined to the colon and involving the rectum. The disease frequently begins in teenagers and young adults, affecting both men and women equally. Relapses and remissions are common.

The radiographic appearance depends upon the stage of the disease at the time of observation. The earliest stages are characterized by edema and spasm. Radiographically, the mucosa assumes a diffuse, finely granular texture, becoming coarser and more stippled with progression toward frank ulceration.[43] Mucosal crypt ulcerations, although nonspecific, also occur in a characteristic diffuse pattern, frequently involving large areas of the bowel at approximately the same stage of disease simultaneously.[44, 45] The disease is classically limited to the layers of the bowel superficial to the muscle wall. Characteristic flat-bottomed, collar-button, or flask-shaped ulcers represent undermining of surrounding intact or edematous mucosa and are limited by the deeper muscle layers.[46] More extensive ulceration may result in isolated islands of edematous mucosa referred to as pseudopolyps. Where relatively more mucosa is preserved, an extensively polypoid pattern may predominate, although this pattern may be transient. Further extension of disease results in nearly total destruction of the superficial layers of the mucosa. With healing, granulation tissue and fibrosis appear, and there is loss of haustral markings and a tendency toward shortening of the left side of the colon. Reepithelialization of the bowel during remissions may be accompanied by the formation of hyperplastic polyps. Sometimes these become long and filamentous, forming mucosal bridges or growing into clumps simulating villous adenomas.[47-50] Such hyperplastic changes also are seen in the healing phases of other inflammatory diseases and thus are not specific for ulcerative colitis.[51-54]

There is a markedly increased incidence of carcinoma in patients with chronic ulcerative colitis, especially those with onset in childhood or adolescence.[45] For these patients, the incidence of carcinoma rises approximately 10 to 20 per cent per decade after the first decade of disease.[55, 56] Cancer in inflammatory bowel disease usually arises from dysplastic regenerating epithelium rather than from adenomatous polyps, limiting the usefulness of radiography in its early detection.[47] Total colectomy cures the underlying ulcerative colitis and is frequently advised as a cancer prophylactic measure.

A wide variety of extraintestinal manifestations of ulcerative colitis have been described. Joint manifestations probably occur in approximately 20 per cent of patients, although figures ranging from 4 to 50 per cent have been reported.[57-59] The higher figures tend to be associated with patients who have arthralgias in various joints and periarticular tissues rather than well-defined, or radiographically evident, arthritis.

Patients with arthritis can be divided into two major groups. Approximately 75 per cent of such patients have an arthritis of peripheral joints referred to as colitic arthritis.[57] The other 25 per cent have a condition indistinguishable from classic ankylosing spondylitis. Colitic arthritis involves mainly the large joints of the extremities, frequently in a migratory fashion. The onset usually follows the clinical presentation of the inflammatory bowel disease. The arthritis frequently flares coincidentally with exacerbations of the colitis and other systemic manifestations, particularly uveitis and erythema nodosum–like conditions. Rheumatoid factor, antinuclear antibody, and LE factor are negative, and this form of arthritis is not associated with human leukocyte A antigen (HLA B27). These points are useful in differential diagnosis from coincidental rheumatoid arthritis and related arthropathies. The peripheral arthritis seldom results in permanent joint deformity and is usually relieved by colectomy (see Chapter 32).

Spondylitis is more common in patients with inflammatory bowel disease than in the general population and is indistinguishable from classic ankylosing spondylitis.[59-61] However, the usual male predominance of ankylosing spondylitis is not noted in cases related to inflammatory bowel disease. Seventy-five per cent of patients with colitis-associated spondylitis do have the expected association with HLA B27 antigens.[62] The spondylitis appears to progress independently of the bowel disease, often predating the onset of colitis and continuing even after colectomy.[63] The HLA B27 antigen may be useful in predicting which patients with inflammatory bowel disease are at risk of developing spondylitis and a closely correlated uveitis,[58] and it may also have a similar predictive value in family members of colitis patients[64] (see Chapter 32).

Regional Enteritis

Regional enteritis (RE) is another chronic inflammatory disease of unknown etiology. It was originally described by Crohn and co-workers in 1932 as a disease involving the terminal ileum.[65] Although the distal small bowel is most commonly affected, it is now generally conceded that all parts of the gastrointestinal tract may be involved.[66] Approximately 40 per cent of cases involve the colon and in approximately 10 per cent of cases the colon alone is involved.[67] Classically, regional enteritis is a transmural inflammatory process involving all layers of the bowel wall with a noncaseating granulomatous inflammatory reaction.[44, 66] The earliest changes are thought to be scattered small, mucosal elevations that ulcerate centrally in a "punched-out" fashion.[43, 68] These lesions are referred to as aphthoid ulcers. More extensive crisscrossing linear ulceration gives a polypoid or nodular appearance to the bowel, classically described as a "cobblestone" pattern.[66] The transmural involvement eventually is manifested as asymmetric wall thickening and fibrosis leading to the stenotic phase of the disease (Fig. 86–12). The associated extramural masses frequently ulcerate or develop sharp fissures, forming fistulae and abscesses. Especially during the early, acute exacerbations, the colonic disease may be difficult to distinguish from ulcerative colitis, but usually this separation can be made as the disease progresses.[66, 69-71] Crohn's disease tends to be patchy or segmental, and when the colon is involved the rectal area is spared more frequently than in ulcerative colitis (Fig. 86–12).

Both sexes are affected with equal frequency, and persons of all ages may be involved, although RE tends to present somewhat earlier than ulcerative colitis.[67] The disease is said to be most common in Caucasians and especially in Jews. Family groupings are common, but no genetic transmission pattern has been defined.

Approximately 25 per cent of RE patients have joint manifestations.[72] As in ulcerative colitis, two forms of arthropathy have been described. The more common is a relatively mild peripheral form, which varies with the clinical severity of the bowel disease and is seen especially in patients with colonic involvement. A less common form is indistinguishable from ankylosing spondylitis, in which approximately 75 per cent of patients have associated HLA B27

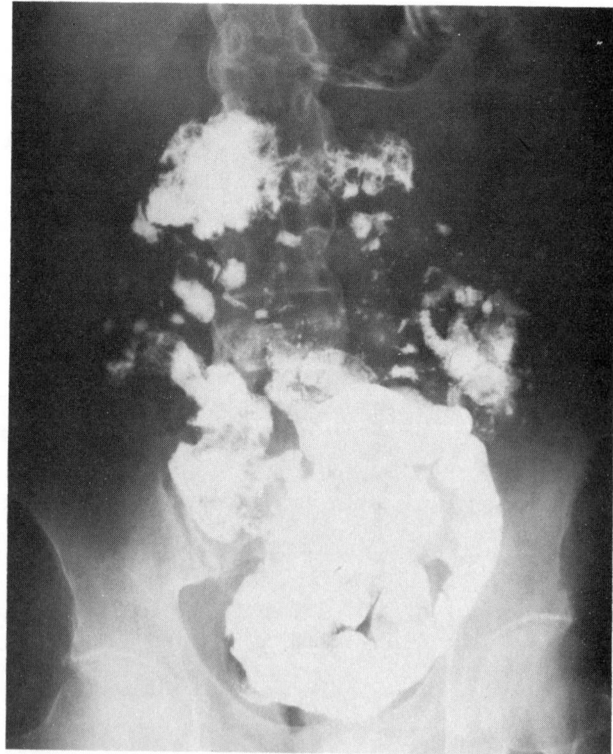

Figure 86–12. *Regional enteritis and spondylitis. Thirty minute film from a small bowel follow-through examination on a 44 year old man. The abnormal small bowel pattern, consisting of irregularly nodular narrowed areas, bowel wall thickening, and increased secretion, is consistent with the clinical history of regional enteritis. Bone changes consistent with ankylosing spondylitis are prominent in the lumbar spine. (Armed Forces Institute of Pathology Neg. No. 77-1107-7.)*

antigens.[62, 73] The ankylosing spondylitis seen with RE is not well correlated with colonic involvement or severity of bowel disease[63, 74] (Fig. 86–12). Thus, the associated arthropathies are not helpful in distinguishing between ulcerative colitis and RE[75] (see Chapter 32).

Extraintestinal manifestations such as erythema nodosum, iritis, clubbing of fingertips, periostitis, and pericholangitis are seen in both regional enteritis and ulcerative colitis.[45, 76-79] A granulomatous myositis and myopathy have been reported in association with Crohn's colitis.[80] An increased incidence of bowel malignancy has been reported in Crohn's disease, but this tendency is much less striking than in ulcerative colitis and is more likely to involve the small bowel.[81-84] Surgery is generally avoided in Crohn's disease because of a high recurrence rate and the chronic nature of the disease. The usual treatment includes steroids and certain antimetabolites. The success of such agents has been cited as evidence to support a possible autoimmune etiologic mechanism. Antibodies against bowel mucosal cells and against coliform bacteria have also been noted in some patients. Systemic antibiotic therapy has shown some efficacy, but the data are preliminary and an infectious etiology has never been proved.[85]

Whipple's Disease

Whipple's disease is an uncommon, chronic, multisystem disease characterized clinically by arthralgias, abdominal pain, diarrhea, and malabsorption. It was originally described in 1907 by Whipple, who considered it to be an intestinal lipodystrophy.[86] Men in the third to fifth decades are most commonly affected. Arthralgia is present in 70 to 90 per cent of patients and is usually the first symptom. It tends to involve the large joints in a migratory fashion and commonly persists throughout the course of the disease. Three stages of clinical progression have been described.[87] The first is characterized by the insidious onset of arthralgia, weight loss, fatigue, and anemia. Various abdominal symptoms, primarily diarrhea and steatorrhea, appear in the second phase. In untreated cases, a third, terminal stage, with severe steatorrhea, malnutrition, and cachexia, has been described. Death generally comes suddenly, with the immediate cause often being difficult to determine.[87]

Pathologically, the disease is characterized by PAS-positive particulate matter in macrophages and extracellular spaces throughout the body, but most

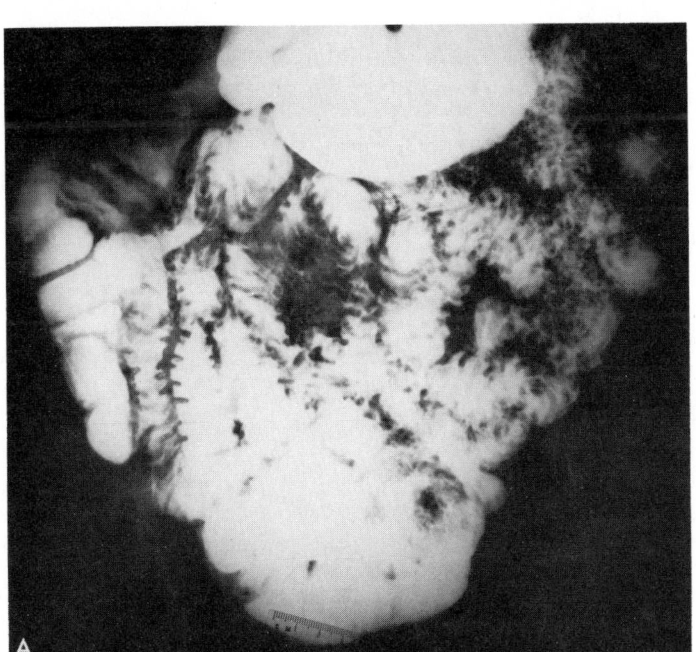

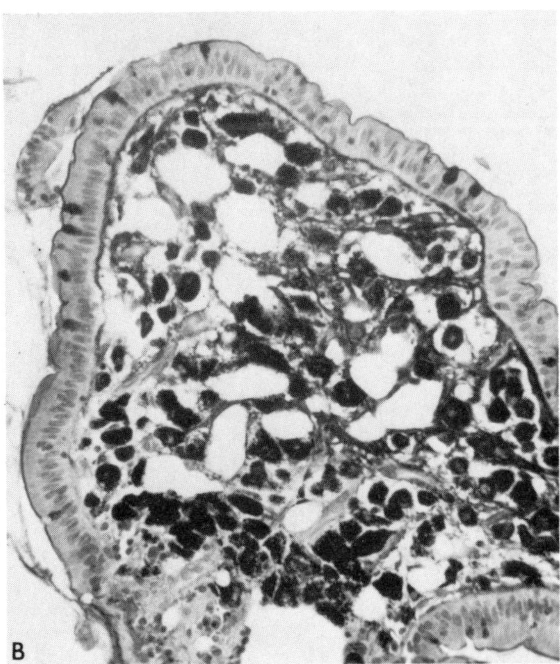

Figure 86–13. *Whipple's disease.*

A *Late film from a small bowel follow-through on a 56 year old man with malabsorption, diarrhea, and anemia, who had a long history of peripheral arthralgias. Grossly thickened valvulae conniventes are most evident in the proximal small bowel. There is a shaggy, somewhat bizarre appearance of the jejunum, and some areas show a superimposed granular pattern suggestive of villous distention as well as submucosal fold thickening. (Armed Forces Institute of Pathology Neg. No. 76-7632-1.)*

B *Photomicrograph of the tip of a small bowel villus in Whipple's disease. Dark staining cells are macrophages containing granular PAS-positive material, some of which is also seen in the extracellular spaces. Larger clear areas are dilated lymphatic channels contributing to the distention of the villus. (Armed Forces Institute of Pathology Neg. No. 79-12958.)*

prominently in the lamina propria of the small bowel and in mesenteric lymph nodes (Fig. 86–13). The lymphadenopathy causes partial obstruction of lymphatic channels with proximal dilatation, especially in the submucosa and mucosa of the bowel. The PAS-positive material, the dilated lymphatics, and the edema from hypoproteinemia secondary to malabsorption all contribute to thickening of small bowel folds with a superimposed distention of the villi. These changes are most evident in the jejunum (Fig. 86–13).

The PAS-positive material has been found in most of the organ systems of the body. Central nervous system involvement has been widely reported.[87-91] The myocardium may be infiltrated and a valvular endocarditis with vegetations containing PAS-positive particles has been described. Light and electron microscopy consistently demonstrates small, rod-shaped organisms approximately half the size of typical *Escherichia coli* within the macrophages, and histochemical studies support the probable bacterial origin of the PAS-positive material.[88, 90-94] Thus far, however, no single organism has been consistently isolated from cultures.[88] Wide-spectrum antibiotic therapy is frequently employed to eradicate the causative organisms and their breakdown products and is associated with clinical improvement. Central nervous system manifestations have disappeared, thus requiring long-term treatment.[88-90]

Roentgenographic findings in Whipple's disease are usually confined to the small bowel and are well correlated with the malabsorption and pathologic changes described earlier[95] (Fig. 86–13). Increased fluid in the lumen causes dilution of the barium column and sometimes the classic "malabsorption" changes of segmentation and fragmentation of the barium column. The small bowel folds are thickened, especially in the jejunum, often with the tips of the folds appearing thicker than their bases. The superimposed villous distention tends to give a fine, granular appearance to the fold pattern. This frequently results in a shaggy, bizarre appearance to the small bowel, which is seen most prominently in the jejunum, while the distal ileum may be nearly normal.

SYSTEMIC LUPUS ERYTHEMATOSUS (SLE)

Pulmonary and Pleural Manifestations

Pleuritis and Pleural Effusions. Over half of all patients with systemic lupus erythematosus manifest pleural thickening, pleural effusion, or both during the course of their disease[96, 97] (Fig. 86–14). Pleural thickening is generally considered the most common chest roentgenogram abnormality in SLE. The thickening is bilateral in approximately half the cases.[98] Effusions are less common than thickening and occur in approximately one fourth to one third of SLE patients.

The pleuritis of SLE is thought to be a manifestation of the same polyserositis that affects the joints.[96] It can be the presenting symptom of the disease, especially in men. The pleuritis may be associated with pulmonary infiltration, especially linear atelectasis (see discussion later in this chapter) secondary to splinting that results from pleuritic pain. Symp-

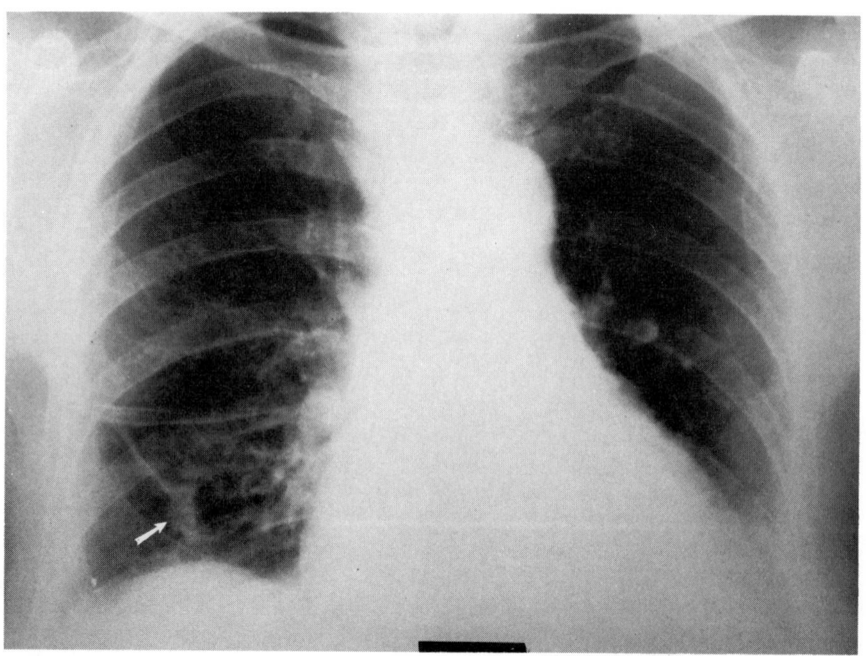

Figure 86–14. *Systemic lupus erythematosus: Pleuritis, pleural effusion, linear pulmonary disease, and pericarditis. This 73 year old woman had a 2 year history of pleuritic chest pain and arthralgias. The frontal chest film shows a left pleural effusion and thickening of the right lateral pleura. An irregular linear dense area (arrow) is noted in the right lower lung field below a prominent minor fissure. There is also enlargement of the cardiopericardial silhouette, which was subsequently confirmed as caused by pericarditis and pericardial effusion. (Armed Forces Institute of Pathology Neg. No. 71-12933.)*

toms, however, vary and the pleuritis, although often painful, may be asymptomatic or associated only with mild discomfort.[7]

Pleural effusions are usually recurrent. They may be massive and lead to severe pleural adhesions and fibrosis.[99] Chemical analysis of the pleural effusions shows that, in contradistinction to effusions in rheumatoid arthritis, the glucose level is normal. LE cells may be present.[96] Effusions in SLE may be secondary to lupus nephrosis and are distinguished from those secondary to pleuritis, since the former are painless.

Both pleuritis and pleural effusions generally abate with corticosteroid therapy.[100]

PULMONARY DISEASE. A multitude of different pulmonary abnormalities have been described in patients with systemic lupus erythematosus. Most of these abnormalities are either pulmonary infections or pulmonary manifestations of SLE involving other tissues, especially the kidneys or pleura. A primary pneumonitis does appear to occur in lupus erythematosus but is quite rare, involving far fewer than 5 per cent of all patients with SLE and, at least in some series, fewer than 1 per cent.[7]

"Lupus pneumonitis" has been recognized only in patients who have had documented systemic lupus erythematosus for long periods, usually several years.[101] A few patients have been found to have pulmonary symptoms at the time of original diagnosis. The vast majority of those affected are women, as is typical of systemic lupus erythematosus in general. The disease is characterized roentgenographically by diffuse or patchy dense areas involving the lower lung fields much more than the upper lung fields (Fig. 86–15). The dense areas are often linear or streaky and have thus been considered to be interstitial by most authors.[99-101] The infiltrate may also have the appearance of small nodules, which are usually poorly defined. Basilar volume loss has been described in approximately half the patients. The majority also have pleural thickening or effusions, as described earlier. The appearance most resembles the typical infiltrates of viral pneumonitis[96] or desquamative interstitial pneumonitis (DIP). The infiltrates are usually chronic, although some apparently respond to corticosteroid therapy.[97] Matthay and coworkers have suggested that abatement of the infiltrates with corticosteroid therapy may be useful in differentiating these infiltrates from infection.[102]

Pulmonary function tests show restrictive disease with decreased diffusion capacity. Matched ventilation and perfusion defects have been described in over half the patients in one series.[101] The pathology has not been well studied and appears to consist of only nonspecific chronic inflammatory changes. The changes most resemble those of usual interstitial pneumonitis (UIP), also known as idiopathic pulmonary fibrosis.

Other pulmonary parenchymal abnormalities described in lupus erythematosus include an acute alveolar infiltration, which is usually bilateral and also most severe in the lower lung fields. Matthay and associates reported 12 such patients, six of whom died and three of whom developed chronic changes similar to those described earlier.[102] These patients presented with acute symptoms, including tachypnea, dyspnea, cyanosis, tachycardia, and high fever. They responded favorably to corticosteroid administration but often had clinical exacerbations. Acute alveolar infiltration has been described by other authors as usually patchy and poorly defined.[99, 100] Some of these acute cases may be caused by uremic pneumonitis secondary to lupus nephritis. Such infiltrates are usually fluffy and symmetric, involving

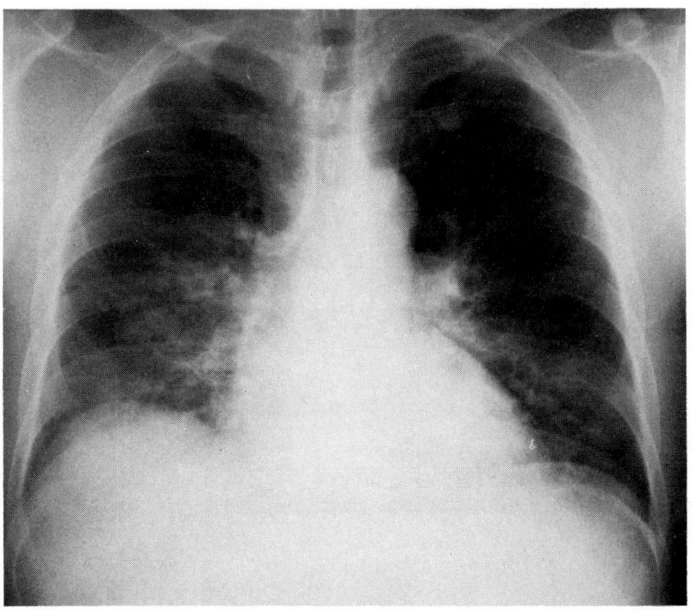

Figure 86–15. *Systemic lupus erythematosus: Lupus pneumonitis. This 45 year old man had positive test results for antinuclear antibodies, arthralgias, and increasing dyspnea. The frontal chest film shows mild hypoventilation with interstitial pneumonitis in both basilar regions, greater on the right. There is no evidence of pleural or pericardial disease from this study.*

the lower lung fields or perihilar regions. Evidence of vascular congestion may be present as well.[100]

Another pulmonary infiltrate seen in lupus erythematosus is horizontal linear infiltration, most common at the bases (Fig. 86–14). This change is often attributed to plate-like atelectasis[96, 98, 99, 101] and is often accompanied by loss of volume in the involved area of lung. Pleural thickening or effusion is also often present and may be the cause of plate-like atelectasis (see earlier discussion). Significant diaphragmatic dysfunction secondary to diffuse myopathy has been documented in systemic lupus erythematosus and may also contribute to atelectasis.[7]

The common presence of pulmonary vasculitis at autopsy[103] and the sporadic reports of pulmonary infarctions and thromboembolic disease occurring in lupus erythematosus have led some authors to question whether some of the linear dense areas may be "Fleischner lines" — thrombosed arteries or, more commonly, thrombosed veins with surrounding inflammation and, eventually, fibrosis.[104] A small region of indrawn, thickened pleura may be associated with these dense regions, as has been documented in scars secondary to infarcts. It is certainly possible that both plate-like atelectasis and thromboembolic disease may be the cause of linear dense shadows in patients with SLE.

Other uncommon pulmonary roentgenographic findings in SLE include nodular or even miliary infiltrations. Larger cavitary nodules, such as those seen in periarteritis nodosa and Wegener's granulomatosis, have also been reported.[99] These respond rapidly to corticosteroid therapy. Although nodular infiltrates may be manifestations of lupus pneumonitis in some cases, probably most are infectious in origin. Another recent report describes diffuse pulmonary hemorrhage causing bilateral ground-glass opacities but no hemoptysis.[105] The hemorrhage was found to be secondary to immune complexes at the alveolar basement membrane, with damage to papillary endothelium.

Thus, most pulmonary infiltrates seen in patients with SLE are probably secondary to infection, pulmonary thromboembolic disease, pleural disease, or nephritis. True lupus pneumonitis does occur but is quite rare.

Pericarditis and Cardiac Disease

Cardiac manifestations are more prominent in lupus erythematosus than in other connective tissue diseases and may cause the presenting symptoms.[97] The most common cardiac manifestation of lupus erythematosus is pericarditis, which is usually transient and may be asymptomatic; it can be documented clinically in approximately one third of patients with systemic lupus erythematosus.[97] There are rare reports of cardiac tamponade and constrictive pericarditis resulting from lupus pericarditis.[96] Like lupus pleuritis, lupus pericarditis is a manifestation of the polyserositis characteristic of the disease. Gross pericardial disease is usually not present upon pathologic examination of autopsy material.[98]

Myocardial involvement occurs less frequently than pericardial involvement in lupus erythematosus. It is difficult to document clinically but is generally characterized by tachycardia out of proportion to fever, congestive heart failure, typical electrocardiographic changes and gallop rhythm. Pathologically, there is fibrinoid degeneration of connective tissue with small vessel fibrinoid necrosis and inflammatory change leading to fine scars or extensive areas of myocardial degeneration.[106]

The endocarditis associated with lupus erythematosus is known as Libman-Sacks endocarditis. It is exceedingly rare for this atypical nonbacterial verrucous endocarditis to be clinically significant, and the vast majority of cases have been discovered only at autopsy.[96] There are unusual reports of clinically significant lesions causing mild disease.[98]

Lupus pericarditis and myocarditis are usually manifested roentgenographically only as enlargement of the cardiopericardial silhouette (Fig. 86–14). Pericardial effusion may be confirmed by cardiac ultrasonography.[107] It should be remembered, however, that involvement of other organs in lupus erythematosus may also cause cardiomegaly and congestive heart failure. This is especially true of the hypertension that may result from renal disease.

Lymphadenopathy and Splenomegaly

Lymphadenopathy and splenomegaly may occur in as many as half of all patients with systemic lupus erythematosus.[98, 108] Gould and Daves were able to identify 34 large spleens on plain films of the abdomen in 100 patients with SLE.[98] Lymphadenopathy most commonly involves the cervical, axillary, and inguinal regions. There are scattered reports of hilar and mediastinal lymphadenopathy in systemic lupus erythematosus[108-110] (Figs. 86–16 and 86–17). Hilar lymphadenopathy is so rare, however, that other causes should be strongly considered whenever hilar enlargement is seen in patients with SLE.

The lymphadenopathy of SLE is distinctive pathologically. Hematoxylin bodies are found in association with areas of necrosis and are thought to be specific for this diagnosis.[108]

Lupus Nephritis

The greatest source of morbidity and mortality in systemic lupus erythematosus is lupus renal dis-

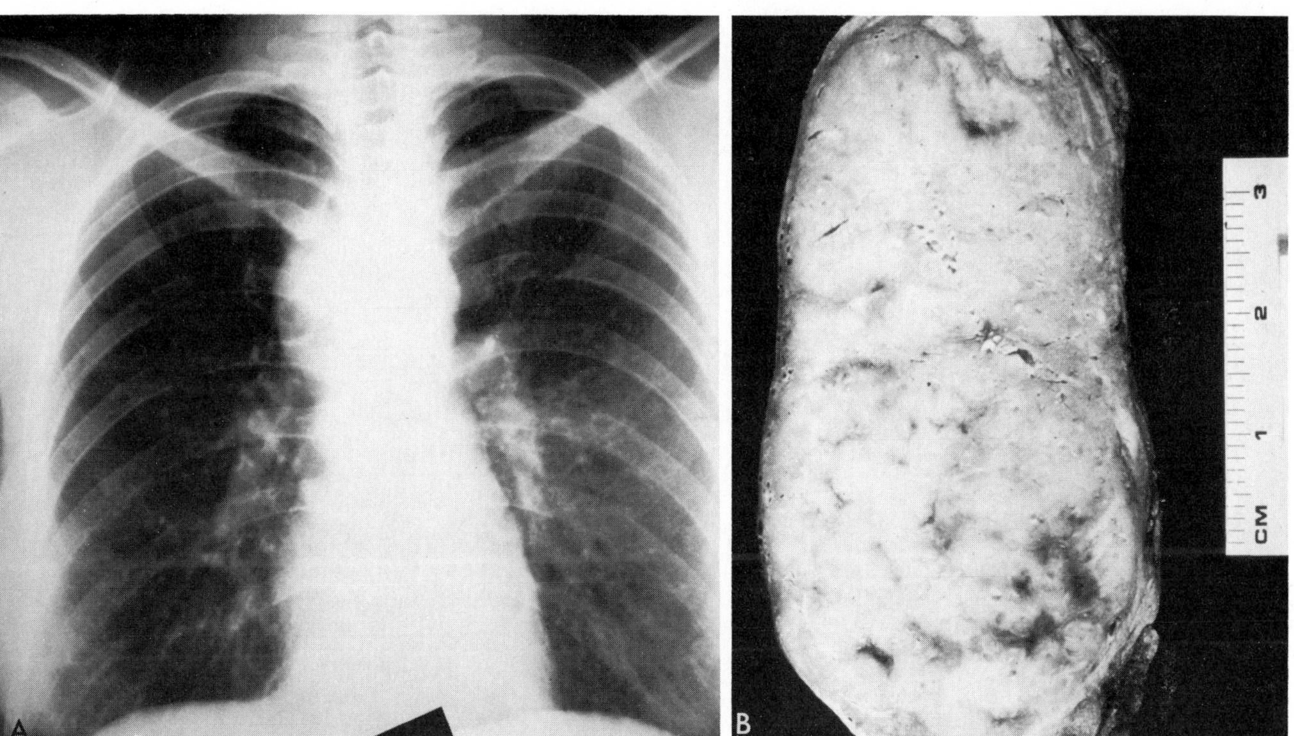

Figure 86–16. *Systemic lupus erythematosus: Mediastinal lymphadenopathy. This 42 year old woman had a 3 year history of varied systemic complaints and positive test results for antinuclear antibody. No symptoms were referable to the chest.*

A *Frontal chest film shows a right paratracheal mass typical of lymphadenopathy. Although pulmonary markings are minimally increased at the bases, there is no definite evidence of interstitial pneumonitis.*

B *Large hyperplastic lymph node removed from a patient with a similar condition shows diffuse enlargement with preservation of the normal architecture as in the other causes of lymphadenitis and giant lymph node hyperplasia.*

(Armed Forces Institute of Pathology Neg. Nos. 71-6155, 68-10358.)

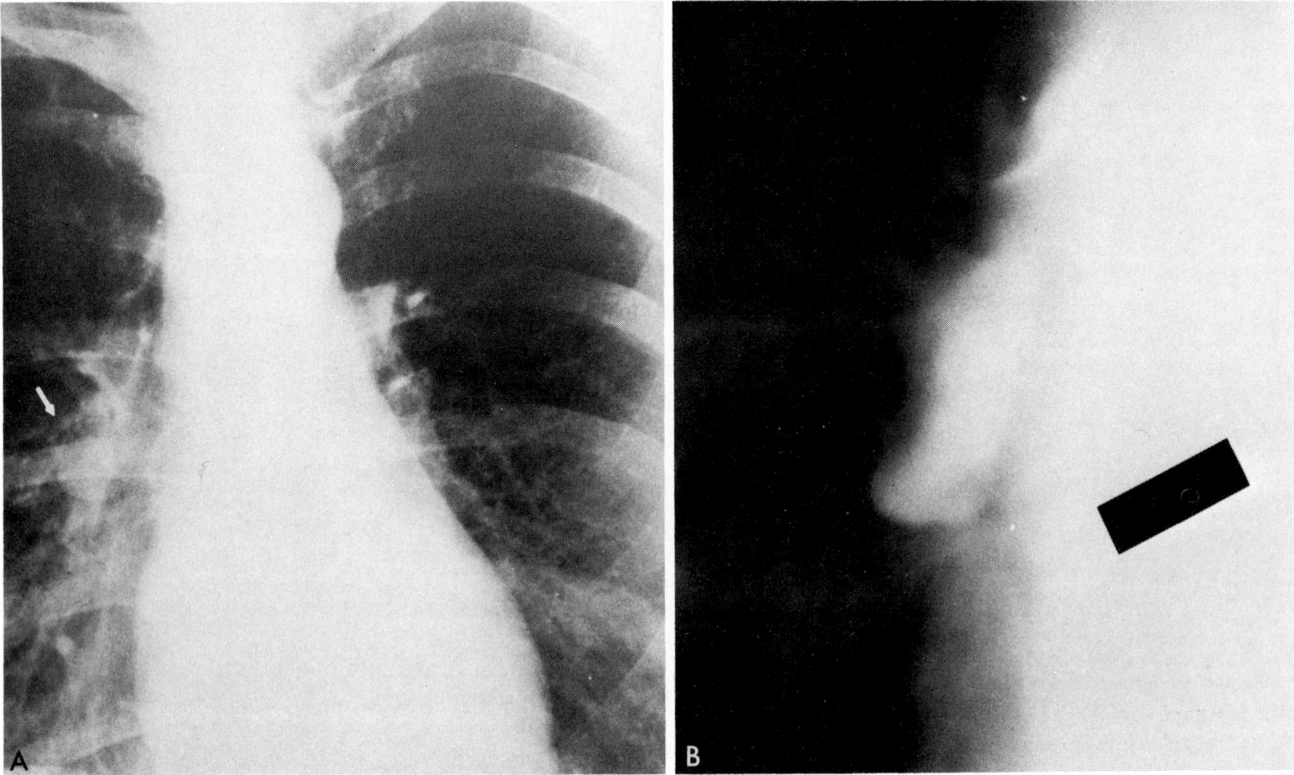

Figure 86–17. Systemic lupus erythematosus: Hilar lymphadenopathy and mild interstitial pneumonitis. This 42 year old woman had systemic symptoms and positive test results for antinuclear antibody.

A Frontal chest film shows enlargement of the right hilum suggestive of lymphadenopathy (arrow).

B The lymphadenopathy was confirmed with a frontal tomogram. Although there are no definitive findings of interstitial infiltration, biopsy revealed mild interstitial pneumonitis in the right lower lobe.

(Armed Forces Institute of Pathology Neg. Nos. 77-6130-1,3.)

ease.[96, 97] Renal involvement is the initial manifestation of disease in 4 to 8 per cent of patients and involves 35 per cent of patients within 1 year of diagnosis.[96] The renal involvement is usually seen early in the course of disease, if at all, and is more common in younger patients than in older ones. The manifestations include hypertension, edema, acute and chronic renal failure, hematuria, proteinuria, and the nephrotic syndrome.

Three forms of renal disease are associated with systemic lupus erythematosus.[111] Focal glomerulitis causes abnormal urine production, but renal insufficiency and the nephrotic syndrome are rare. Corticosteroid administration leads to prompt response, with no renal failure. The second form of renal disease, diffuse proliferative glomerulitis, produces the nephrotic syndrome, usually with renal insufficiency. Most patients with this form of nephritis relapse following therapy and eventually die of renal insufficiency. The third form of involvement is membranous lupus nephritis. This form also causes the nephrotic syndrome, and most patients eventually develop renal insufficiency. Most patients with the diffuse and membranous forms of nephritis develop hypertension, although steroid therapy may contribute to this finding. Renal involvement has not been shown to vary from one type to another in any one patient over the course of the disease.

The only roentgenographic evidence of any of the forms of lupus nephritis is generalized decreased renal function on intravenous pyelograms.[98] Characteristic findings are visible on arteriography.

Neurologic Manifestations

Neurologic abnormalities are common in lupus erythematosus, with the incidence ranging from 25 per cent in one large series[97] to nearly 60 per cent in other series.[112] In the era before widespread use of corticosteroid therapy, central nervous system phlebitis or arteritis was the second most frequent cause of death, after nephritis,[97] in systemic lupus erythematosus. Decker has divided the neurologic manifestations into six categories: (1) alterations of mental function; (2) transient or recurrent seizure activity; (3) paralysis secondary to ischemia or hemorrhage; (4) tremor and choreoathetoid or ataxic movements; (5) cranial neuropathy; and (6) peripheral neuropathy.[96]

The etiology of the alterations in mental function is often unclear, but in many cases the changes are caused by small vessel disease with microinfarctions.[113-115] Communicating hydrocephalus has been reported[116] and pseudotumor cerebri with papilledema has also been noted.[117] The brain scan is often abnormal if diffuse cerebritis is present.[112] The scan appearance may become normal rapidly as symptoms subside. Functional psychoses are often secondary to corticosteroid therapy and may abate rapidly when such therapy is tapered.[118] Altered mental function may also be caused by superimposed infection, leading to abscess or cerebritis.

Seizure activity in lupus erythematosus usually involves the motor areas. As with mental deterioration, the seizure activity may be secondary to microinfarctions.[114]

Gross motor abnormalities, including paresis and paralysis, are generally attributed to large infarcts or intracerebral hemorrhages.[113] The anatomic abnormalities may be visualized with brain scans, computed tomograms, and angiograms.[114] The lesions are caused by segmental vascular destructive and proliferative changes. True vasculitis is rare in lupus erythematosus.[113, 116] Inflammatory cells may be present, but they are more commonly perivascular than vascular in location.[114]

Angiography in hemiparesis may show stenosis or occlusion of major cerebral arteries, including the internal carotids.[115] The angiographic defects are smooth and localized, and they are easily differentiated from atherosclerotic plaque. Embolic phenomena have been reported, including one report of cerebral embolization from Libman-Sacks endocarditis.[115]

Pneumatosis Intestinalis

Pneumatosis intestinalis occurs in lupus erythematosus in the absence of necrotizing enterocolitis.[119] As in scleroderma, a mottled or bubbly appearance on plain abdominal films may be the only manifestation of pneumatosis. When intraluminal gas is seen as a curvilinear lucent area in a patient with lupus erythematosus, necrotizing enterocolitis is probably the cause, as large amounts of gas are not usually seen in systemic lupus erythematosus.[120] The presence of pneumatosis and acute abdominal pain should always suggest necrotizing enterocolitis in a patient with SLE.

The cause of pneumatosis intestinalis in systemic lupus erythematosus is probably vascular.[120] Ischemia secondary to arteritis also often causes paralytic ileus in this disease.[119]

Drug-Induced Lupus Erythematosus

The clinical manifestations and findings in drug-induced lupus (DIL) erythematosus are very similar to those of systemic lupus erythematosus. Differential diagnosis between these disorders may be difficult. Drug-induced lupus erythematosus becomes more likely if the patient is not a young woman, the individuals most often affected by SLE. Lee and Chase advise that criteria for diagnosis of DIL must include evidence that (1) the drug was administered before any sign or symptom of lupus erythematosus had been recognized, and (2) the disease process reversed promptly after withdrawal of the drug.[121] Serologic changes may require several weeks or months to revert to normal.

Drugs causing DIL are listed in Table 86–1. Hydralazine, phenytoin, sulfonamides, and procainamide have received the most attention. Many of the other agents listed cause serologic evidence of lupus erythematosus without clinical abnormalities.[122]

Differences between DIL and SLE include the finding that pulmonary disease is more common in DIL than in SLE.[122] This finding, however, may be secondary to the fact that patients with DIL are generally older than those with SLE and are therefore more likely to have pulmonary disease on that basis alone. DIL has not been shown to cause lymphadenopathy, nephritis, or central nervous system involvement, and it generally is a milder disease than SLE.

Serologic differences also occur between DIL and SLE. The type of anti-DNA antibody differs and no decrease in serum complement level occurs in

Table 86–1

DRUGS THAT INDUCE LUPUS ERYTHEMATOSUS*

Sulfonamides
Anticonvulsants
Phenytoin
Mephenytoin
Trimethadione
Ethosuximide
Cardiovascular Agents
Procainamide
Hydralazine
Practolol
Others
Thiouracils
Isoniazid
Chlorpromazine
D-Penicillamine
Allopurinol

*After Griesmer DA: Johns Hopkins Med J *138*:289, 1976.

DIL. Both DIL and SLE probably have multiple mechanisms of origin, accounting for the various similarities and differences between the manifestations of these diseases.

PROGRESSIVE SYSTEMIC SCLEROSIS (PSS)

Gastrointestinal Manifestations

Esophageal Dysfunction. About half of patients with progressive systemic sclerosis have alimentary tract symptoms.[123] Although the entire alimentary tract may be affected, esophageal involvement is by far the most frequent and characteristic and eventually occurs in 50 to 90 per cent of patients, but not all are symptomatic.[124-127]

The smooth muscle of the distal two thirds of the esophagus undergoes progressive atrophy in a patchy distribution frequently involving the lower esophageal sphincter mechanism. Collagen deposition, fibrous replacement of muscle tissue, and vasculitis tend to follow. There may also be a diffuse increase in collagen in the lamina propria and submucosa. Atony, disordered peristalsis, and lower esophageal sphincter incompetence are characteristic roentgenographic and manometric manifestations often seen even in the absence of esophageal symptoms. These abnormalities may even antedate histologically detectable changes.[128] Gastroesophageal reflux, frequently leading to erosive esophagitis, is common, producing distal esophageal stricture in about 40 per cent of patients[128] (Figs. 86–18 and 86–19). Retention of air in the esophagus related to reduced peristalsis may be a useful roentgenographic sign of PSS, having been reported in 12 to 75 per cent of patients, depending upon rigidity of criteria. It is best seen late in the disease, when large gaseous collections are found in association with pulmonary fibrosis, a combination highly suggestive of the diagnosis.[125, 129-131] Loss of the longitudinal

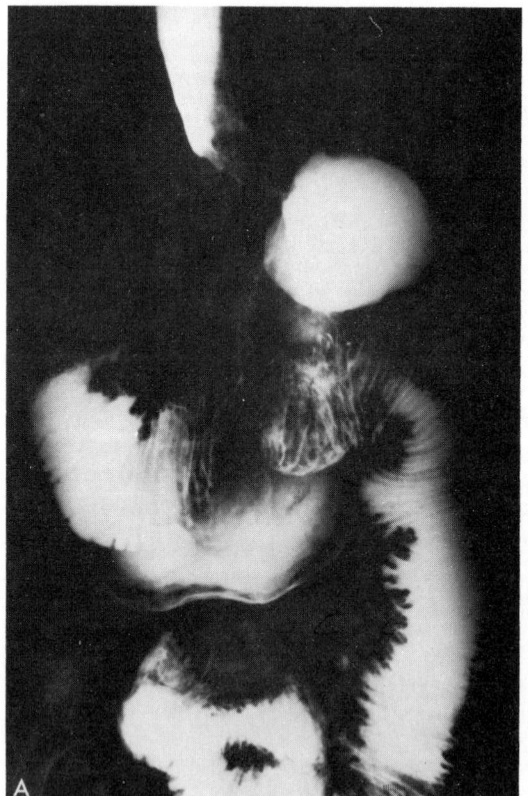

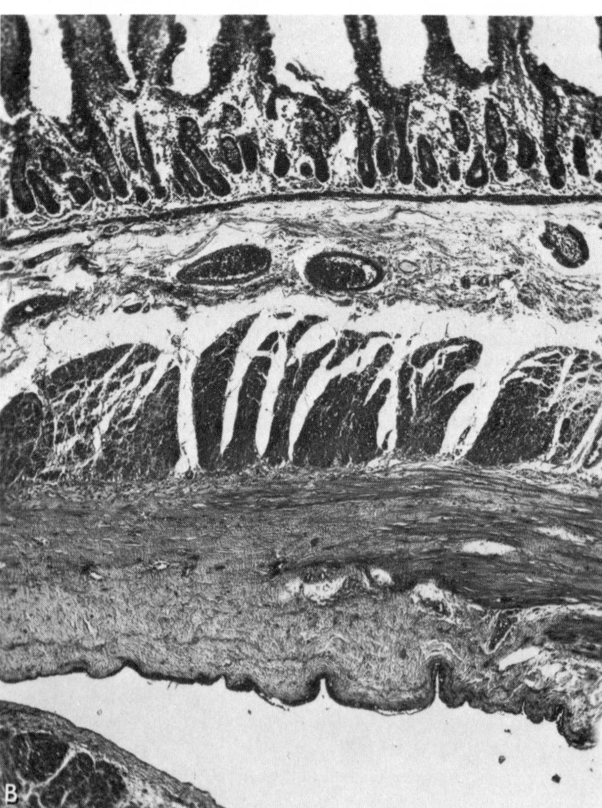

Figure 86–18. *Progressive systemic sclerosis: Esophageal and small bowel abnormalities.*

A *This 61 year old woman had known progressive systemic sclerosis. The esophagus is dilated above a distal stricture, and there is delayed clearing of barium from the esophagus. The small bowel is dilated, with a "hidebound" appearance. The third portion of the duodenum is compressed in the region of the superior mesenteric artery and is dilated proximal to this region. (From Olmsted WW, Madewell JE: Gastrointest Radiol 1:33, 1976. Armed Forces Institute of Pathology Neg. Nos. 74-4601-5.)*

B *Photomicrograph of the wall of the small bowel, from a patient with a similar condition, shows extensive replacement of the outer muscular layer by fibrous tissue. (Armed Forces Institute of Pathology Neg. No. 75-11074.)*

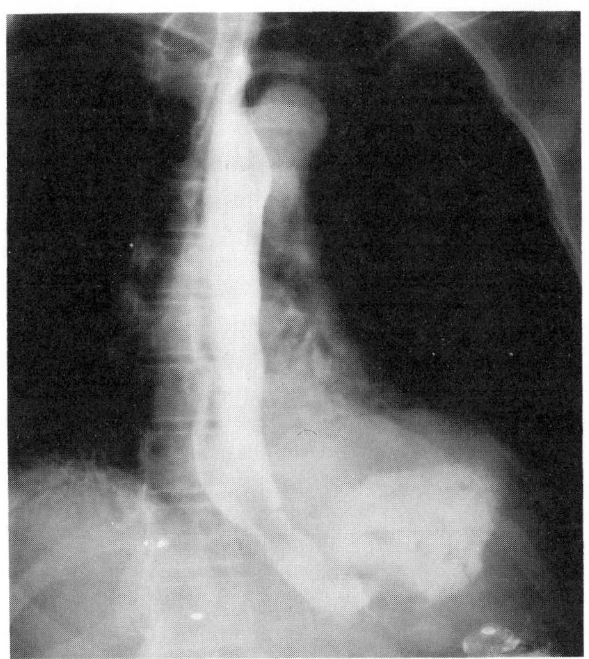

Figure 86–19. *Progressive systemic sclerosis: Esophageal dysfunction in an elderly man with long history of the disease. The esophagus is diffusely dilated and shows delayed emptying. Marked hypoperistalsis was demonstrated fluoroscopically. Fibrosis of the lung bases is also evident. (Armed Forces Institute of Pathology Neg. No. 66-13113-9.)*

mucosal fold pattern has been described as a reliable sign of muscular involvement,[132] and recently a corrugated or pleated appearance of the mucosa on double contrast studies has been noted in association with scleroderma.[133]

A very close association between esophageal dysfunction and Raynaud's phenomenon has been noted,[126, 128] suggesting that ischemia might play some role in the esophageal phenomena. The characteristic manometric patterns may also be seen in systemic lupus erythematosus, mixed connective tissue disease, and other conditions associated with Raynaud's phenomenon.

Intestinal Disorders. In addition to the esophagus, the duodenum, jejunum, and colon are involved in order of decreasing frequency. Significant stomach involvement is quite rare and usually limited to dilatation and delayed emptying.[125, 127, 134, 135]

The major bowel manifestations are patchy areas of atrophy associated with atony and dilatation. A pseudo-obstruction phenomenon is common.[136] Enlargement and hypomotility of the duodenum may simulate, or be associated with, superior mesenteric artery obstruction syndrome.[136, 137] Small bowel fold thickening is sometimes seen owing to inflammatory infiltration of the mucosa and submucosa, but usually the folds remain stretched and thin.

Progressive sclerosis is associated with scattered asymmetric collagen replacement of muscle. The resulting uneven binding together of the stretched folds causes the so-called "hidebound" appearance[138] (Fig. 86–18). This appearance is in contrast to the dilatation with uniform stretch-

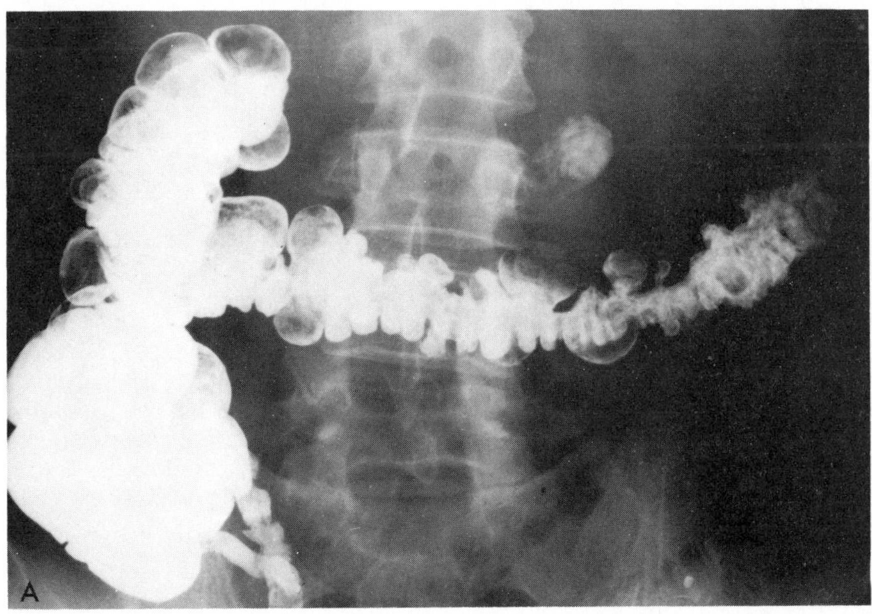

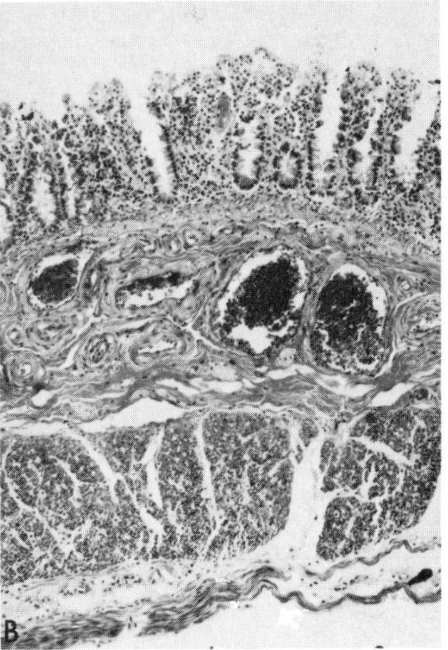

Figure 86–20. *Progressive systemic sclerosis: Colon abnormalities.*

A *Same patient as in Figure 86–19. Wide-mouthed or "kettle drum" sacculations involve all elements of the colonic wall. (From Olmsted WW, Madewell JE: Gastrointest Radiol 1:33, 1976.) Armed Forces Institute of Pathology Neg. No. 66-13113-7.)*

B *Photomicrograph of the wall of the colon, from a patient with a similar condition, shows marked deposition of wavy collagen fibers in the submucosa, especially involving the perivascular spaces. Muscle atrophy and infiltration by collagen are also present to a mild degree. (Armed Forces Institute of Pathology Neg. No. 79-12959.)*

ing and separation of folds that is seen in mechanical obstruction. Dense bowel wall fibrosis alternates with atonic areas, which are less infiltrated with collagen and which become asymmetrically dilated, resulting in the wide-mouthed or "kettle drum" sacculations that are especially common in the colon (Fig. 86–20). These outpouchings involve all layers of the bowel wall, in contrast to the usual type of acquired colonic diverticula.[125, 137, 139-141] Less frequently, loss of haustral markings and lengthening of the bowel are seen.[134, 142] Intussusception similar to that seen in sprue may be another manifestation seen with the patchy areas of atony and fibrosis.[138] Symptoms related to colonic involvement, however, are relatively uncommon.[139]

Submucosal and subserosal gas cysts in the bowel wall (pneumatosis intestinalis and pneumatosis coli) occur with increased frequency in connective tissue diseases, particularly progressive sclerosis[143-147] (Fig. 86–21). Pneumatosis has been seen in association with numerous conditions in which there is gross or prolonged distention of the gut. It is postulated that mucosal atrophy or effects of ischemia may allow gas to enter the bowel wall. Pneumatosis, when associated with collagen vascular disease, has been considered to be an ominous prognostic sign, but this has not been a uniform observation.[145, 146, 148]

In the small bowel, absorption is frequently abnormal and may be aggravated by bacterial overgrowth owing to stasis in areas of atony, resulting in deconjugation of bile salts. In some cases the malabsorption may be partially responsive to antibiotics.[149]

Hepatic and Pancreatic Involvement. Hepatic involvement in progressive systemic sclerosis is rare and nonspecific.[127] However, primary biliary cirrhosis has been reported in women with the CRST syndrome (cirrhosis, Raynaud's phenomenon, scleroderma, and telangiectasia).[150] Hepatosplenomegaly may be seen, but is usually related to heart failure.

Pancreatic secretion is abnormal in about one third of scleroderma patients.[151] Gross pancreatic insufficiency, however, is rare and malabsorption is usually better attributed to bowel stasis.

Pulmonary Fibrosis

Pulmonary abnormalities in systemic sclerosis are far less common clinically and roentgenographically than they are pathologically.[152, 153] The reported incidence of clinical and roentgenographic disease varies markedly (13 to 78 per cent). Higher values generally reflect abnormal pulmonary function test results in the absence of other clinical findings. It is important to realize that roentgenographic evidence of abnormality in systemic sclerosis usually implies considerable clinical severity of disease and is rarely the first indication of pulmonary involvement.[153, 154]

All described cases of "scleroderma lung" show histologic evidence of pulmonary fibrosis of the

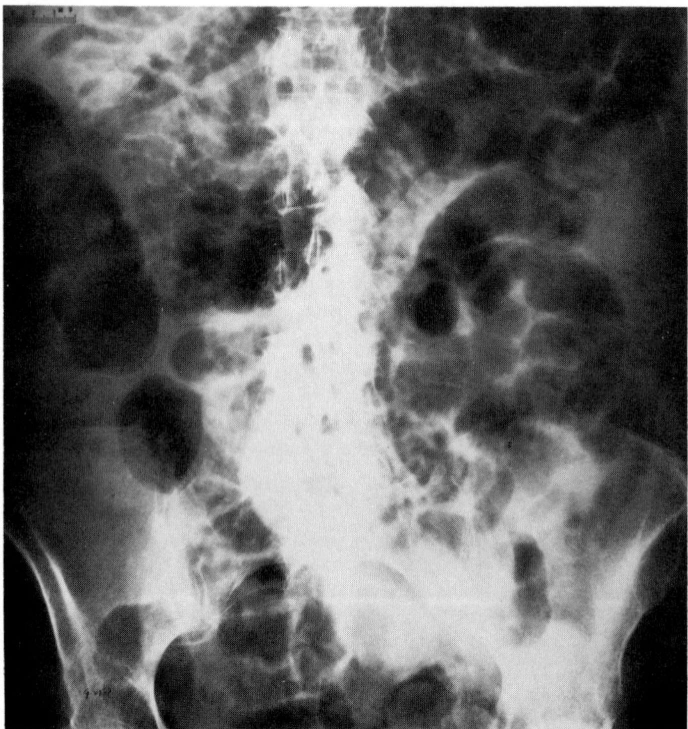

Figure 86–21. *Progressive systemic sclerosis: Pneumatosis cystoides intestinalis. Plain film of the abdomen in a patient with this disease shows extensive bubble-like accumulations of gas. (Armed Forces Institute of Pathology Neg. No. 78-2300-2.)*

interstitium, most marked at the bases of the lungs and always more severe in the lower two thirds of the lung than in the upper one third. Collagenosis of walls of blood vessels with intimal proliferation and medial hypertrophy is also commonly observed.[153] Abnormal small airways with increased thickness of the basement membrane and metaplasia of the lining epithelium are seen, often with inflammation and bronchiolectasis.[153] Small epithelium-lined cystic spaces are often observed, especially in the subpleural regions. These spaces range up to 1.5 cm in diameter.[125] The cysts are thought to represent either abnormal small airways or new spaces forming in the distorted architecture of fibrotic pulmonary interstitium.[155] In either case, they closely resemble cystic spaces seen in other forms of UIP and true "honeycomb lung."

Pulmonary function tests are the most important indicators of pulmonary abnormalities in scleroderma.[156-158] Decreased diffusion capacity is the single most sensitive indicator, with decreased vital capacity generally considered less sensitive.[159] DeMuth and co-workers[159] reported a good correlation between clinical evidence of dyspnea and decreased diffusion capacity. Other abnormalities of pulmonary function occur less consistently. Symptoms of pulmonary scleroderma are nonspecific, with dyspnea on exertion and cough being the most common in most series.

The severity of roentgenographic abnormality correlates with the overall severity of clinical pulmonary disease, but does not correlate with its duration.[153, 159] The appearance is characterized by bilateral, lower lung field, coarse interstitial infiltration, which often forms small regions of honeycombing (Figs. 86–22 and 86–23). The abnormalities are usually most marked just above the hemidiaphragms and rarely involve the upper one third of the lung fields. With increased severity, the periphery of the lower lung fields becomes more severely involved, and it is in this region that irregular cystic spaces may be observed, which correlate with those seen pathologically (see earlier discussion). The cysts may be as large as 1.5 cm in diameter. Some authors[125] believe that rupture of these cystic spaces may be the origin of the pneumothoraces that are occasionally reported in patients with scleroderma lung disease.[153] Pleural thickening and effusion are much less common in scleroderma than in other collagen vascular diseases that involve the chest.[7]

The etiology of pulmonary involvement in systemic sclerosis is unclear, although vascular fibrosis appears to be the principal cause, and vascular changes are universally present on pathologic examination. It is no longer widely believed that aspiration secondary to abnormal esophageal function plays a significant role in the origin of pulmonary disease, since Mahrer and associates showed that involvement of the esophagus was evident in only 62 per cent of 57 patients with scleroderma lung disease.[160] Another theory holds that fibrosis of skin, chest wall muscles, or pleura contributes to decreased pulmonary compliance, but this theory is not consistent with the observation that abnormal

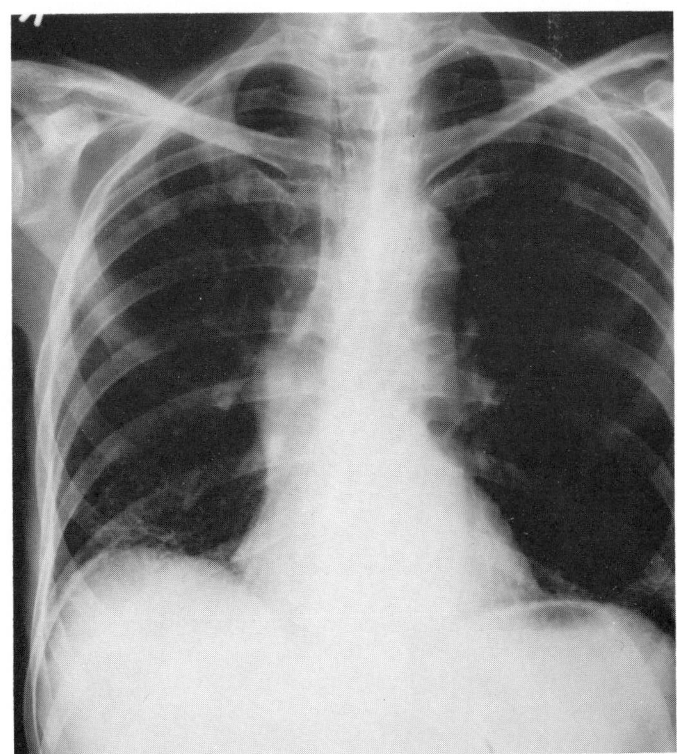

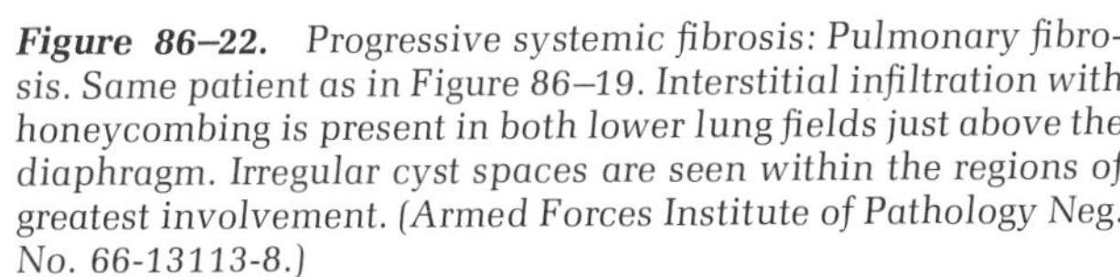

Figure 86–22. *Progressive systemic fibrosis: Pulmonary fibrosis. Same patient as in Figure 86–19. Interstitial infiltration with honeycombing is present in both lower lung fields just above the diaphragm. Irregular cyst spaces are seen within the regions of greatest involvement. (Armed Forces Institute of Pathology Neg. No. 66-13113-8.)*

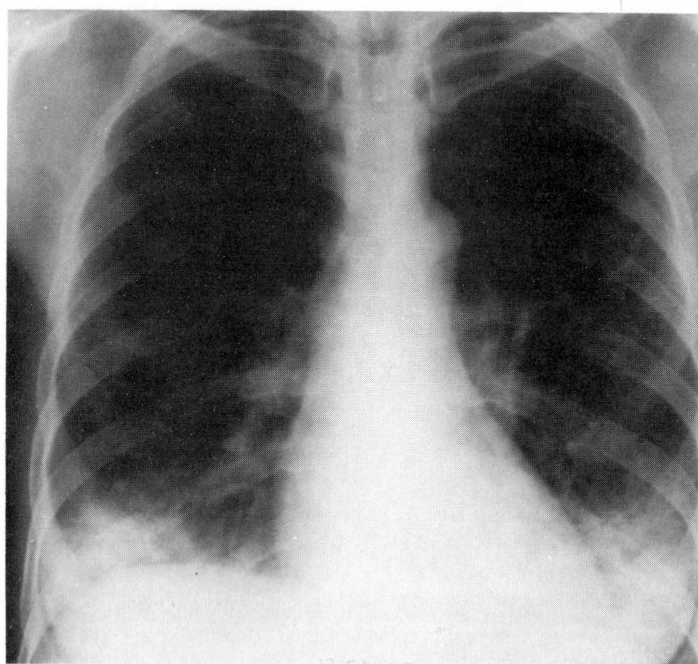

Figure 86–23. *Progressive systemic sclerosis: Pulmonary fibrosis. This middle-aged woman had had this disease for several years. There is more extensive infiltration of the lower lobes than is seen in Figure 86–22, and irregular cystic spaces are present, especially in the mid–lung field on the left. The appearance of alveolar filling in this patient shows the pleomorphism of interstitial fibrosis. (Armed Forces Institute of Pathology Neg. No. 68-10446.)*

diffusion capacity is the primary functional abnormality in patients with systemic sclerosis,[159] nor has diaphragmatic motion been shown to be significantly abnormal. Pericapsular fibrosis of costovertebral joints may contribute to restriction of chest motion. It appears probable that fibrosis of the pulmonary interstitium is the primary process, similar to fibrosis in many other organs in systemic sclerosis, and that vascular fibrosis, which may lead to pulmonary hypertension, contributes to the degree of architectural distortion of the pulmonary interstitium.

There are scattered reports of an increased incidence of bronchogenic carcinoma, especially bronchoalveolar cell carcinoma, in systemic sclerosis,[153, 155, 161] although no direct link has been shown to exist.

Myocardial Fibrosis

Direct cardiac involvement in systemic sclerosis consists of diffuse or patchy myocardial fibrosis that is not explainable on the basis of coronary atherosclerosis or any other cardiac disease. This pathologic finding is common in autopsies of patients with systemic sclerosis, having been found in 90 per cent of autopsies in one study.[152] Pericardial disease is not generally associated with systemic sclerosis, although occasional pericardial plaques may be present in autopsy material.

Clinical and roentgenographic evidence of "scleroderma heart disease" is far less common than autopsy evidence[156] but may be found in as many as 30 per cent of cases.[125] Roentgenograms show diffuse cardiac enlargement, and decreased pulsation may be visible on fluoroscopic evaluation. Echography can demonstrate increased ventricular wall thickness and decreased compliance.[162] The findings of all these studies are thus consistent with any type of myocardiopathy.

Congestive heart failure is a common cause of death in patients with systemic sclerosis.[153] The failure is often predominantly right-sided and is always refractory to therapy.[156] Sackner and colleagues[163] emphasized the role of pulmonary hypertension secondary to peripheral pulmonary vasculitis as the origin of congestive heart failure in many patients with systemic sclerosis. They stated that right ventricular myocardial fibrosis is probably secondary to pulmonary hypertension and that left ventricular fibrosis may similarly be caused by systemic hypertension secondary to renal sclerosis. They noted the exceeding rarity of patients presenting with heart disease who do not have severe systemic sclerosis of other organs.

Renal Involvement

Fifteen to 45 per cent of patients with progressive systemic sclerosis have clinical evidence of renal involvement, most frequently proteinuria and hypertension.[127, 164] Renal failure is the most common cause of death in this disease, followed by pulmonary insufficiency and heart failure.[164-167] Two clinical patterns have been described.[164] In one there is abrupt onset of malignant hypertension. In the other, hypertension is more mild and chronic, but it is frequently followed by the sudden development of rapidly progressive renal failure. Histologic evidence of renal involvement is seen in up to 90 per cent of PSS patients during autopsy examination and, thus, often is present even in the absence of clinical signs and symptoms.[127, 164, 166]

Pathologically, many of the changes seen in scleroderma, particularly in late cases, are similar to and frequently indistinguishable from those seen in malignant hypertension. Vascular intimal hyperplasia, onion-skinning, and fibrinoid necrosis may be detected especially in the interlobular arteries and afferent arterioles. In some cases there is an inflammatory necrotizing arteriolitis, and the necrosis may extend to the vascular tuft of the glomerulus. Arterial constriction or thrombus formation leads to patchy ischemia and small cortical infarcts. The glomeruli show thickening of the basement membrane, which may be localized or diffuse. This may give a "wire loop" appearance, as in lupus erythematosus, or may simulate diffuse membranous glomerulonephritis.

The predominance of interlobular artery involvement is characteristic of scleroderma and may allow its differentiation from the nephrosclerosis seen in the more common forms of hypertension. Perivascular fibrosis has been described as a distinguishing characteristic of PSS,[164] but it has not been widely reported.

Radiographically, plain films and excretory urograms are normal or nonspecific. The kidneys may be small but usually are of normal size. Decreased renal function, however, may impair urographic visualization.

The classic angiographic findings are irregularity and constriction of the interlobular arteries and decreased cortical blood flow[164, 168, 169] (see Chapter 16). The main renal arteries and the interlobar and arcuate arteries are relatively uninvolved, although they may show some irregularity, and a standing wave artifact may been seen centrally. Lack of filling of cortical arteries gives the arterial tree a "pruned" appearance. The patchy appearance of spasm, constriction, and, finally, obliteration of the interlobular arteries causes focal cortical ischemia. An inhomogeneous or spotty nephrogram results. Contrast transit through the kidney is markedly delayed, prolonging the arterial phase. The corticomedullary junction may be indistinct, or, in late cases, the angiographic nephrogram may be absent.

Decreased cortical blood flow may also be shown by radioisotope studies, even when angiography is still normal.[164] A drop in renal cortical perfusion coinciding with Raynaud's phenomenon induced by peripheral cutaneous cooling may be seen in PSS patients without other evidence of kidney abnormality.[164] This observation raises the speculation that changes in cortical perfusion regulation are related to the pathogenesis of the hypertension and the renal failure that later develop.

POLYMYOSITIS AND DERMATOMYOSITIS

Gastrointestinal Involvement

The entire gastrointestinal tract may be involved in dermatomyositis.[170] In the distal esophagus, stomach, small bowel, and colon, the changes, both pathologically and radiologically, are essentially indistinguishable from those of scleroderma. The sole difference is observed histologically; the involvement of the striated muscle of the esophagus that occurs in dermatomyositis usually is not seen in scleroderma. Dysphagia may thus be a prominent symptom because of involvement of the proximal esophageal muscles, as well as the muscles of the jaws, hypopharynx, and cervical esophagus. This involvement, together with stomatitis, may lead to difficulties in swallowing, and to the frequent and serious clinical problem of tracheal aspiration. Retention of barium within the valleculae may be a roentgenographic sign.[171-175]

Smooth muscle involvement of the remainder of the gastrointestinal tract is relatively uncommon, occurring in about 5 per cent of patients. When it occurs, dilatation and decreased transit time are common features as in PSS. Muscle atrophy and patchy fibrosis of the bowel wall are noted, sometimes with thickening secondary to edema and infiltration of the mucosa and submucosa by inflammatory cells. Mucosal ulceration and hemorrhage are clinically significant complications.[174] Pneumatosis intestinalis and benign, sometimes long-term, pneumoperitoneum may be evident in polymyositis as in progressive systemic sclerosis. Because of the poor surgical risk these patients present, it is very important to distinguish this condition from the more serious complication of bowel perforation, which may also occur.[176-178]

Pulmonary Interstitial Infiltration

The lung is another visceral organ that is sometimes involved in polymyositis.[179-181] In most patients the chest x-ray will be normal, but an interstitial or reticulonodular pattern may be seen, especially in the bases[180] (Fig. 86–24). The changes closely mimic those seen in scleroderma. Pathologically, there is an infiltration of lymphocytes and plasma cells. There may be an associated vasculitis,

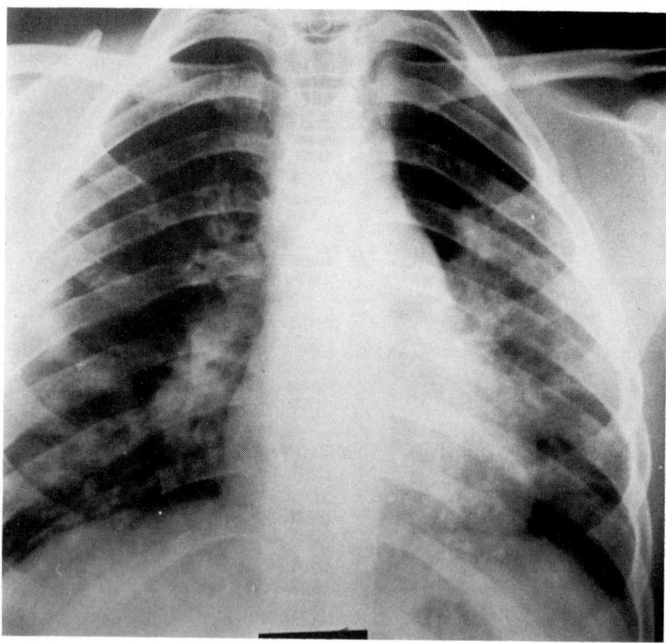

Figure 86–24. Dermatomyositis: Pulmonary infiltration. This teenage girl had a 2 year history of polyarthritis, episodic cutaneous ulceration, Raynaud phenomenon, and recent onset of chest symptoms. Frontal chest view shows nonspecific basilar and mid-lung interstitial infiltrates bilaterally. (Armed Forces Institute of Pathology Neg. No. 76-2074.)

especially in children, leading to thrombosis and multiple infarcts. Considerable interstitial fibrosis may result. Pulmonary symptoms may precede the myositis, and changes may be seen pathologically and roentgenographically, even when symptoms are not present. Corticosteroids may be effective in alleviation of symptoms.[247]

Secondary manifestations of the underlying disease also may result in pulmonary abnormalities. When the striated muscles of the chest wall and diaphragm are involved, plate-like atelectasis is a common finding. With significant pharyngeal involvement, it is not unusual to see aspiration pneumonia and its sequelae.

Associated Malignancy

An increased association of malignancy in dermatomyositis is cited frequently in the literature, the reported incidence varying considerably. The consensus is that approximately 15 per cent of patients develop neoplasms, with the stomach, breast, lung, and ovary being the most common sites of involvement.[182, 183] The risk of developing a tumor has been considered to be greatest in adult men. However, the reliability of the data upon which the association of dermatomyositis and neoplasm has been based is questioned, and if a true association exists, it has probably been greatly exaggerated.[171]

PERIARTERITIS NODOSA

Necrotizing vasculitis occurs in a wide variety of clinical settings, and several classifications have been suggested, depending upon the size and site of the involved vessels and the histology of the lesions.[184-189] The term periarteritis nodosa (PAN) is generally applied to a subacute or chronic focal necrotizing inflammation involving all of the layers of the walls of medium- and small-sized vessels. The vessels that are involved tend to be larger than those affected in systemic lupus erythematosus (SLE). Lesions are scattered in a random fashion throughout multiple organs.[190] This distribution accounts in part for the broad spectrum of clinical manifestations that occurs in this disease and for an overlap in classification systems. Relatively acute forms of PAN have sometimes been termed hypersensitivity angiitis.

There is at least a 2:1 male to female predominance in periarteritis nodosa, which is the opposite of that seen in SLE.[190-192] The disease can occur at any age but is most common in adulthood. Clinical manifestations include fever, weakness, weight loss, and myalgia in addition to joint manifestations (see Chapter 36). The kidney is affected in about 80 per cent of patients and is the organ that is most frequently involved.[191, 193] The resulting hypertension and renal failure are associated with a particularly poor prognosis.[192, 194] Renal infarcts and perirenal hematomas may be a source of acute pain.[195] Abdominal pain may also be related to ischemia and thromboembolism that in turn are secondary to mesenteric and gastrointestinal tract vasculitis. Necrotizing, ischemic enterocolitis and severe gastrointestinal bleeding may result[196, 197] and small bowel intussusception has been reported in children.[248] Mesenteric aneurysms may lead to intra- or retroperitoneal hemorrhage or, less commonly, to mesenteric hematoma.[198] Acute cholecystitis secondary to vasculitis is a common form of clinical presentation of PAN.[199, 200]

Myocardial disease is sometimes seen with involvement of the vessels of the heart. A peripheral neuropathy, or mononeuritis multiplex, is evident when the blood supply to nerves, the vasa vasorum, is affected. The lungs may be involved, either primarily, as a result of focal vascular lesions, or secondarily, by thromboembolism. Pulmonary involvement is relatively infrequent and may be associated with peripheral blood eosinophilia.[188] Whether or not the lungs are involved, however, seems to make little difference in the overall prognosis.[192]

An autoimmune phenomenon is frequently invoked as the etiology of the disease, based largely on indirect evidence. A strong association between polyarteritis and the hepatitis B surface antigen has been noted.[201, 202] Many cases follow upper respiratory infections and, particularly in children, an association with type A streptococcal infection has been seen.[203] Necrotizing angiitis has also been associated with drug therapy and drug abuse, although some of these cases might better be characterized as hypersensitivity angiitis.[204]

Laboratory studies show a consistent leukocytosis and thrombocytosis as well as an elevated erythrocyte sedimentation rate. Such studies may provide markers which can be utilized to follow the progress of the disease. Immunoglobulin concentrations are frequently abnormal, as are complement levels, particularly C3. Other laboratory manifestations depend on the degree of involvement of various organs, especially the liver and kidneys.[190]

The pathologic picture depends upon the duration of the disease and the organ under examination. The individual lesions tend to be focal but widely scattered. Acutely there is an intense infiltration of initially neutrophilic and later eosinophilic inflammatory cells. All layers of the vessel wall and the perivascular space are involved. Asymmetric degeneration of the muscular media and destruction of the inner lining of the intima result (Fig. 86–25). Small and medium-sized arteries are the main targets, particularly at sites of bifurcation. Adjacent arterioles and veins may be involved, but capillaries are usually spared. The acute lesions may not be apparent microscopically. Intravascular thrombosis is frequent and leads to ischemia of the neighboring areas. Organization of such thrombi leads to intravascular fibrosis. Fibrous proliferation and formation of granulation tissue also occur within the walls of the vessel, again frequently in an asymmetric

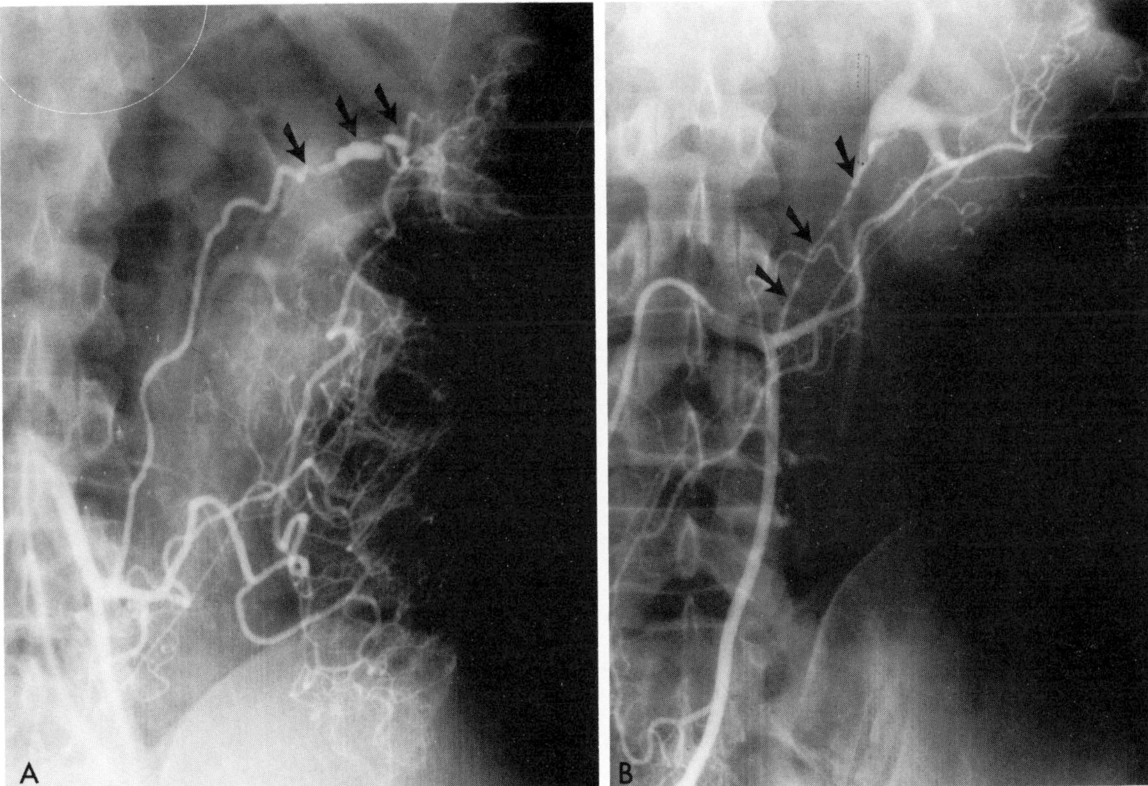

Figure 86–25. *Periarteritis nodosa (PAN): Vasculitis. Selective inferior mesenteric arteriograms from a patient with systemic PAN.*

A *A large fusiform aneurysm in the distal end of the left colic artery preceded by a small saccular aneurysm and associated with a more distal fusiform aneurysm is noted (arrows).*

B *Following surgery, the aneurysm has been removed. More extensive narrowing and beading of the proximal left colic artery is evident (arrows).*

Illustration continued on the following page

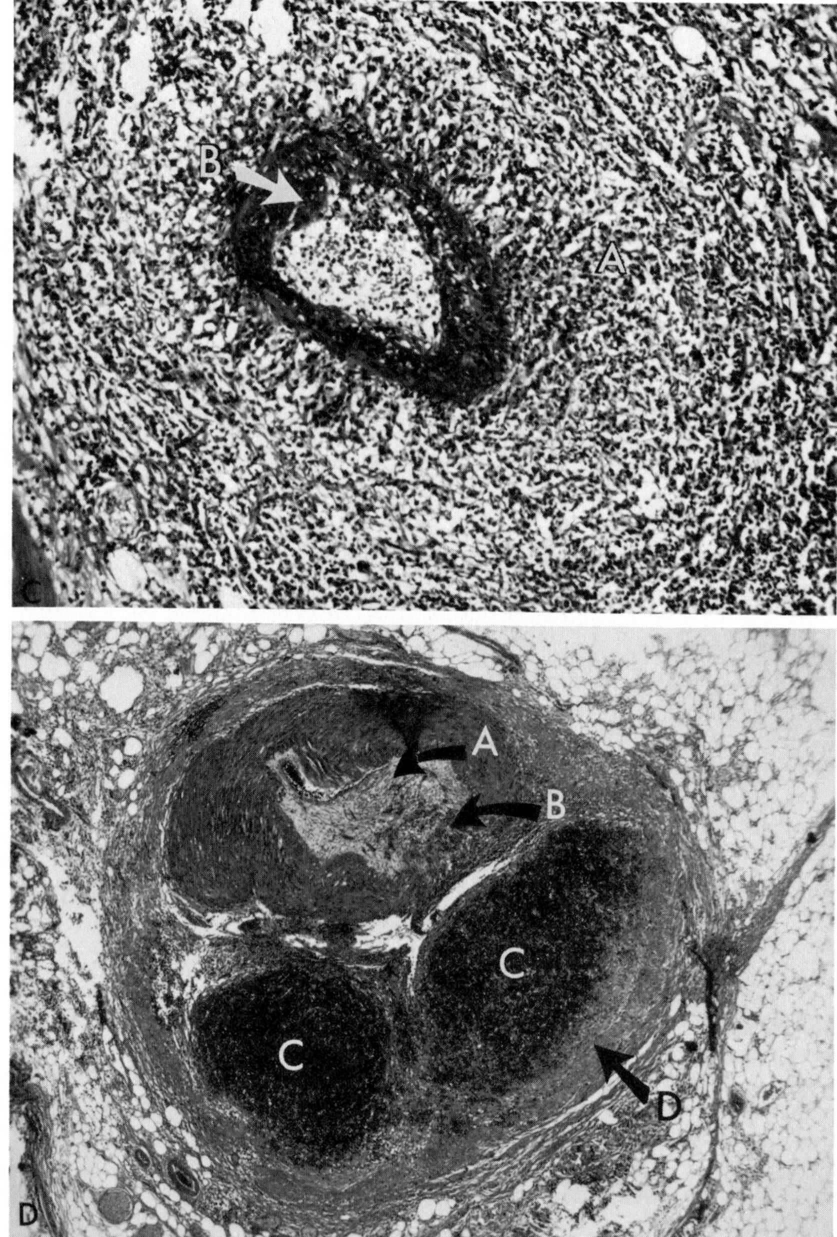

Figure 86–25. Continued

C *Photomicrograph shows intense perivascular inflammatory infiltrates (A) and inflammatory cells infiltrating the muscular medial wall of the artery, which is swollen and distorted (B) (60×).*

D *Photomicrograph showing the late effects of transmural arterial inflammation. The original artery is represented by the rounded structure in the upper part of the field. The lumen is largely replaced by the fibrotic material of an organizing thrombus, which incorporates portions of the intima (A). The media is thickened and partially destroyed in a localized area at B. The two large, darker staining areas (C) represent organizing hemorrhage in an area of pseudoaneurysm that has resulted from the destruction of the media at B. A new adventitial coating of fibrotic tissue surrounds the entire complex (D) (22 ×).*

(Armed Forces Institute of Pathology Neg. Nos. 77-8622-7,6; 79-12957; 79-12808.)

pattern. Aneurysm formation and rupture may lead to hematomas in the walls of vessels or in the perivascular space. The resulting clots then undergo further organization and fibrosis (Fig. 86–25). The more advanced lesions classically lead to microscopic nodules along the vessels, which sometimes have a beaded appearance.[190, 191] Pathologic diagnosis requires the identification of such lesions on biopsy. The scattered distribution of the lesions dictates the desirability of obtaining material from clinically involved sites.

Radiographic features vary with the site and the duration of involvement. The sine qua non is the angiographic demonstration of multiple scattered aneurysms of medium-sized and small arteries[191, 193, 195, 205, 206] (Figs. 86–25 and 86–26). Such aneurysms may be demonstrated angiographically in the majority of patients with PAN and have been outlined in most of the abdominal visceral arteries and their branches.[205] In some cases the angiographic appearance of vascular aneurysms may become less marked with time, but this radiographic improvement does not necessarily imply regression of the pathologic process.[207] Secondary changes, such as evidence of renal ischemia and infarction and of ischemic lesions of the bowel, including ulceration, bleeding, and stenosis, may be seen (Fig. 86–27). Pneumatosis intestinalis may be seen in necrotizing enterocolitis, which has been reported in systemic lupus erythematosus and periarteritis.[197]

Pulmonary changes in PAN usually consist of peripheral wedge-shaped or rounded alveolar infiltrates typical of pulmonary embolic disease. Interstitial lower lobe pneumonitis may also occur, possibly as the result of fibrotic scarring from previous infarcts or secondary to vasculitis, as in scleroderma. When severe renal disease is present, findings typical of alveolar edema may be seen, sometimes representing uremic pneumonitis (Fig. 86–28).

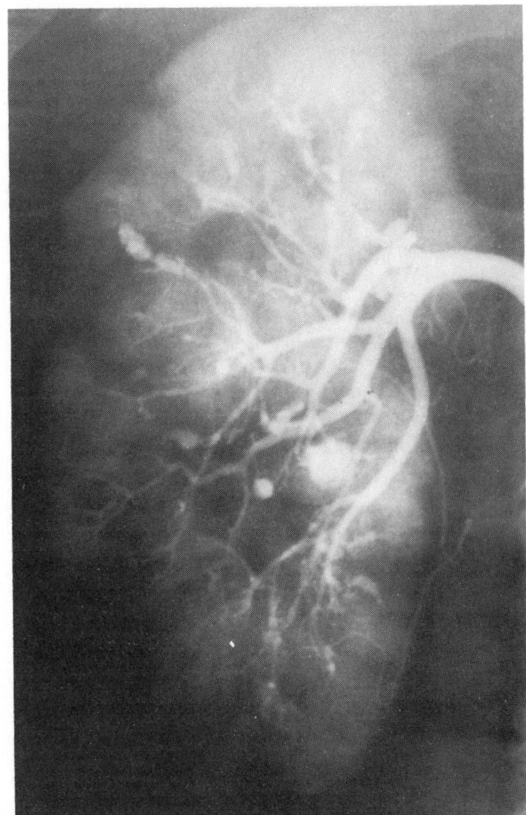

Figure 86–26. *Periarteritis nodosa: Renal vasculitis. Selective right renal arteriogram in a 55 year old man shows numerous aneurysms. The patient died of cerebral vascular involvement and, at autopsy, the kidneys showed multiple infarcts and thrombosis. (Armed Forces Institute of Pathology Neg. No. 71-6830.)*

Periarteritis nodosa, if untreated, tends to be progressive. Death may ensue in a matter of weeks or months, especially if there is hypertension and severe renal involvement. More commonly, the course

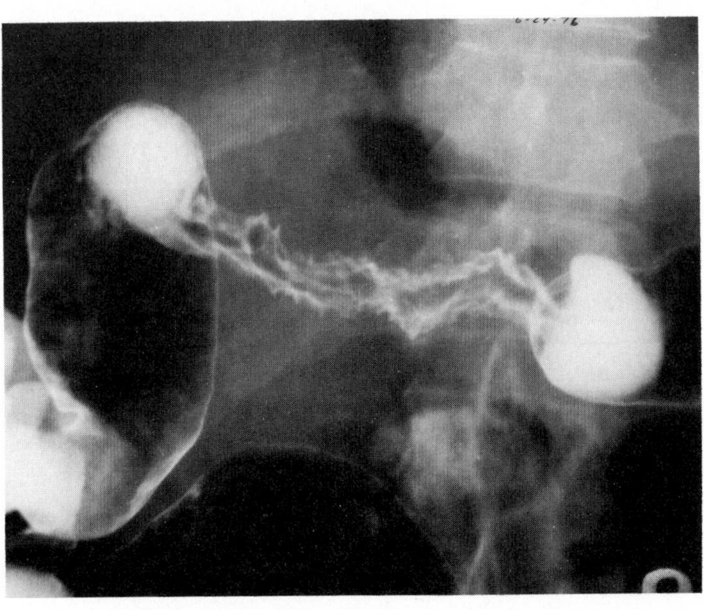

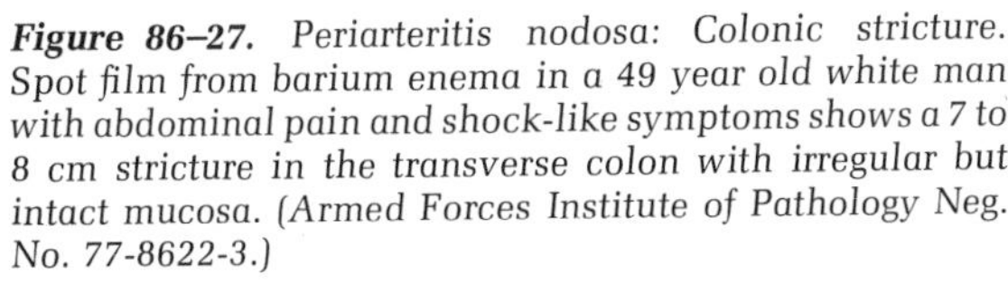

Figure 86–27. *Periarteritis nodosa: Colonic stricture. Spot film from barium enema in a 49 year old white man with abdominal pain and shock-like symptoms shows a 7 to 8 cm stricture in the transverse colon with irregular but intact mucosa. (Armed Forces Institute of Pathology Neg. No. 77-8622-3.)*

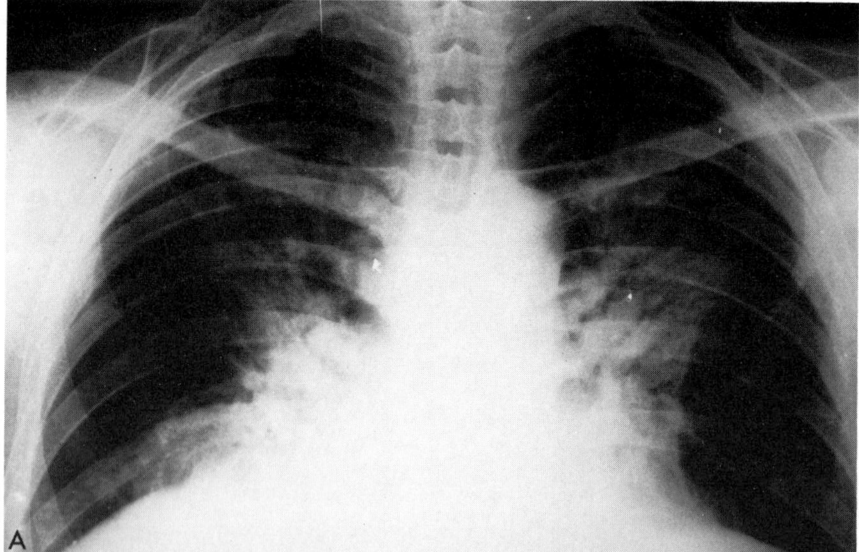

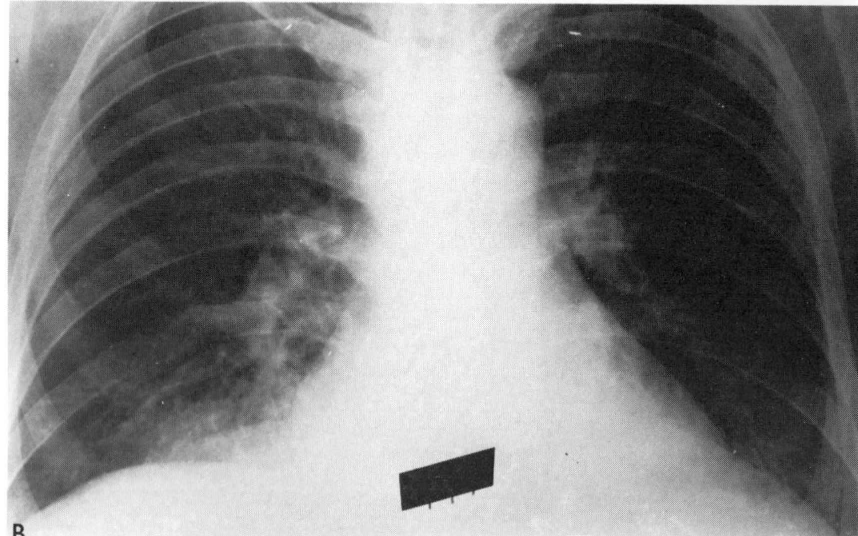

Figure 86–28. Periarteritis nodosa (PAN): Pulmonary infiltrates. This 30 year old man had PAN with severe renal disease.

A Frontal film shows perihilar alveolar infiltration caused by uremic pneumonitis.

B Film obtained 3 weeks later, following dialysis, shows small infiltrates at both bases. Autopsy showed bilateral basilar pulmonary infarcts.

(Armed Forces Institute of Pathology Neg. Nos. 77-3418-1,2.)

is protracted.[190] With steroid therapy, approximately half the patients may be expected to survive for 5 years or more.[192]

SJÖGREN'S SYNDROME

Salivary Gland Manifestations

Sjögren's syndrome is characterized by keratoconjunctivitis sicca and xerostomia. A connective tissue disorder is generally associated with Sjögren's syndrome and is usually rheumatoid arthritis, but the syndrome may also be associated with scleroderma, systemic lupus erythematosus, periarteritis nodosa, and dermatomyositis.[208, 209, 249] The syndrome is most common in women over the age of 50 years.[210] Approximately 90 per cent of patients have arthritis prior to the onset of ocular and oral symptoms. Many patients can be shown to have antibody against salivary and tear gland ducts. Such anti–salivary duct antibody is not found when keratoconjunctivitis sicca and xerostomia are present without connective tissue disease. This "sicca syndrome" is more often associated with a poor prognosis than is the complete syndrome with connective tissue component also present.

Clinical differences have recently been noted between the sicca syndrome alone and the complete syndrome with connective tissue disease.[211] Patients with the sicca syndrome alone reportedly have a higher frequency of recurrent parotitis, Raynaud's phenomenon, purpura, lymphadenopathy, myositis, and renal involvement. These clinical differences, coupled with the serologic differences noted previously and genetic differences that have also been

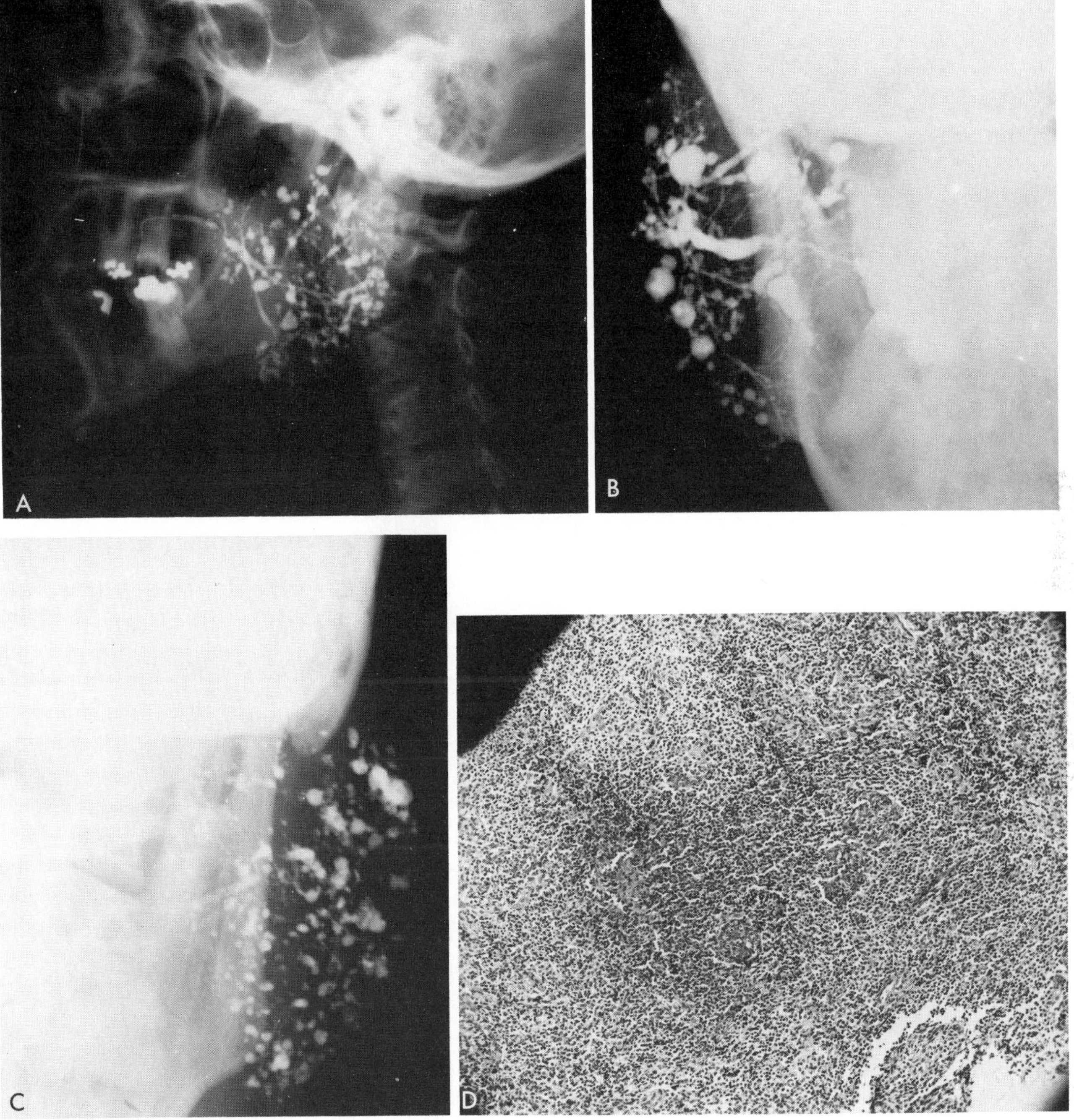

Figure 86–29. *Sjögren's syndrome: Sialography. This 37 year old woman had recurrent parotid swelling for 8 years with polyarticular inflammation.*

A–C *Sialograms (**A**, **B**, right gland; **C**, left gland) show dilatation of ductules and acini with ductal irregularity. Delayed clearance of contrast material was also observed. These findings are typical of inflammatory conditions, including Sjögren's syndrome.*

D *Low power photomicrograph of parotid gland biopsy shows diffuse infiltration by lymphocytes.*

(Armed Forces Institute of Pathology Neg. Nos. 60-11722-6,8,5,1.)

observed, have led some authors to believe that the sicca syndrome is a pathologic entity distinct from the complete Sjögren's syndrome.

The extra-articular symptoms of Sjögren's syndrome are caused by hyposecretion of salivary and lacrimal glands. Pathologically, the glands show a lymphocytic infiltrate that may also involve the lids, genital organs, and respiratory tract (see discussion later in this chapter).

The abnormal activity of the salivary glands may be studied by use of nuclear imaging and by sialography. Sequential salivary scintigraphy is a method by which an intravenous dose of ^{99m}technetium pertechnetate is administered and the region of the mouth is imaged at 2, 6, 10, 20, 40 and 60 min following injection. With normal salivary function there is progressive uptake of the radiopharmaceutical in the first 20 min, followed by prompt excretion and visualization in the oral cavity within 20 to 40 min. At the end of 1 hour, the oral cavity should contain most of the radiopharmaceutical. Patients with Sjögren's syndrome may show decreased uptake in the glands and fail to accumulate significant activity within the mouth. Milder forms of the disease may be manifested by a delay in uptake in the glands and a diminished concentration within the mouth. With very severe involvement, no significant activity above background levels will be found within the glands, and the oral cavity will show less activity than the surrounding tissues after 1 hour. Scintigraphy is a sensitive method of studying salivary gland function and can detect mild degrees of dysfunction of the gland, such as may be present in Sjögren's syndrome. The degree of abnormality correlates well with the severity of the symptoms.[209]

Sialography has also been used to study salivary gland function in Sjögren's syndrome (Fig. 86–29). The detected abnormalities are similar to those found in other inflammatory diseases, including infections[212, 213]; a "pruned tree" appearance, due to acinar edema within the gland, is the mildest detectable sign of such disease.[214] More severe manifestations include dilatation of ductules and acini, irregularity of ducts, dissection of contrast medium within the gland, and ductular obstruction.[213] Clearing of contrast material from the gland is often retarded. The sialographic findings in Sjögren's syndrome differ from those in infection only in that abscess formation is not visualized in Sjögren's syndrome. Other mass lesions, including neoplasms, can also be excluded by the absence of ductal displacement, encasement, or amputation, or the absence of areas of nonopacification within the gland parenchyma.

The salivary and lacrimal gland abnormalities in Sjögren's syndrome have often been compared with the synovial alterations of rheumatoid arthritis. In both diseases, lining cells synthesize and proliferate great quantities of immunoglobulins and rheumatoid factor. A common immunologic mechanism may underlie both Sjögren's syndrome and rheumatoid arthritis by interfering with the secretory ability to proliferate saliva or synovial fluid. Since viruses cause changes in secretory tissues that resemble the changes described in both diseases, viral infection could play a role in the origin of either Sjögren's syndrome or rheumatoid arthritis, or both.

Pulmonary Manifestations

Pulmonary abnormalities in Sjögren's syndrome are found in 10 to 15 per cent of patients.[210, 215] The pulmonary abnormalities can be divided into (1) manifestations of hyposecretion of tracheobronchial glands, (2) interstitial pneumonitis, and (3) lymphocytic pulmonary parenchymal infiltrates.

Manifestations of hyposecretion result from a reduction in the size and number of tracheal and bronchial submucous glands.[215] Pathologically, there is degeneration of glandular acini and infiltration of lymphocytes and plasma cells, with dilatation of secretory ducts. The hyposecretion may cause or exacerbate any of the following findings: chronic cough, bronchiectasis, chronic bronchitis and emphysema, recurrent pulmonary infection, focal atelectasis, lobar or segmental atelectasis, and obstructive (endogenous lipoid) pneumonitis. These abnormalities and their associated roentgenographic manifestations are neither specific nor diagnostic.

Interstitial pneumonitis with fibrosis, identical to that seen in rheumatoid arthritis, may be present in Sjögren's syndrome[210] (Fig. 86–3). As in rheumatoid lung, this finding is most prevalent in the lower lung fields. Many patients with this abnormality are positive for rheumatoid factor and have other evidence of rheumatoid arthritis. An immunologic basis is presumed for the interstitial infiltrate of Sjögren's syndrome.[210]

The third form of pulmonary disease in Sjögren's syndrome is lymphocytic infiltration of the pulmonary parenchyma, consisting of lymphocytic interstitial pneumonitis (LIP), pseudolymphoma, and pulmonary lymphoma. All of these forms have been observed in association with Sjögren's syndrome. The roentgenographic appearances do not differ from those observed when these diseases occur without Sjögren's syndrome.

Pseudolymphoma is most often manifested as a triangular perihilar infiltrate with hazy borders and an air bronchogram demonstrable on plain films or tomograms[109] (Fig. 86–30). Lymphadenopathy and pleural effusions generally are not seen. In some cases, a peripheral lesion rather than a central lesion may be present, but an air bronchogram will still be evident. Pseudolymphoma is not considered a premalignant lesion but is often difficult to differentiate histologically from pulmonary lymphoma. This manifestation is more common in patients with the sicca syndrome alone than in patients with all of the

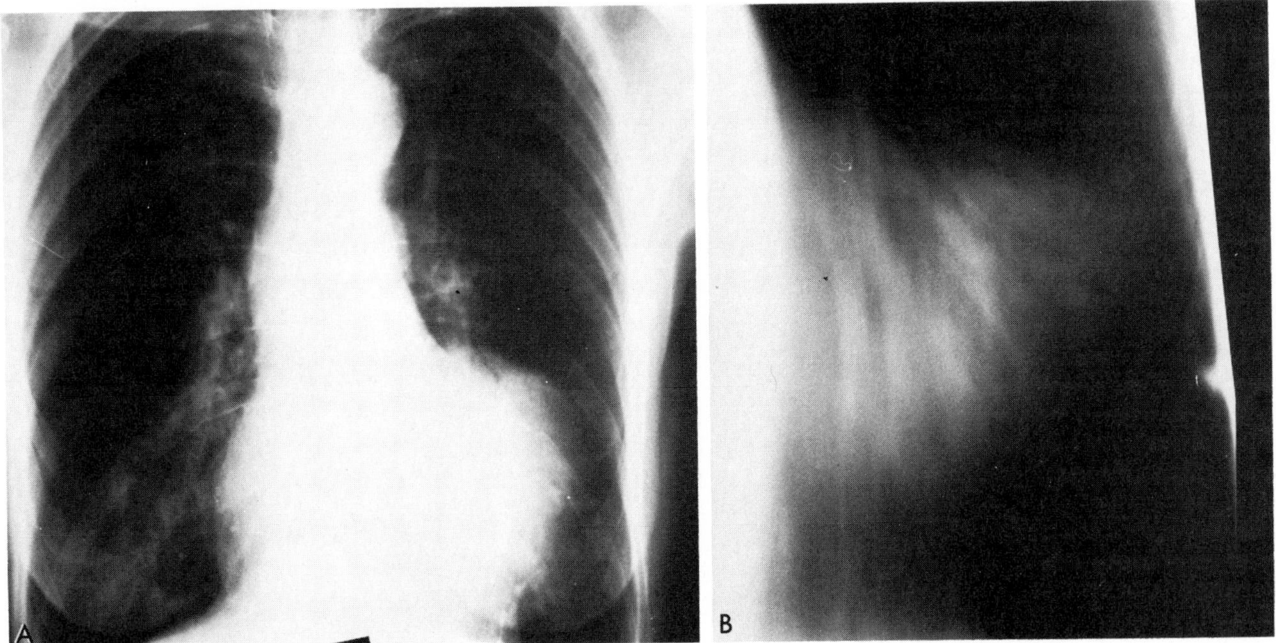

Figure 86–30. *Pseudolymphoma of lung. This 60 year old man had no symptoms referable to the chest.*

A *Frontal roentgenogram shows a left lower lobe infiltrate with an air bronchogram near its superior border.*

B *Tomogram shows triangular shape, hazy peripheral border and prominent air bronchogram.*

(Armed Forces Institute of Pathology Neg. Nos. 77-456-1,3.)

manifestations of Sjögren's syndrome. Elevated levels of IgM have been found in many patients with pseudolymphoma in Sjögren's syndrome.[210]

Lymphocytic interstitial pneumonitis (LIP) is often considered to be the pulmonary analogue of the lymphocytic infiltration of glands found in Sjögren's syndrome. LIP is most often manifest as a lower lobe bilateral interstitial infiltrate not

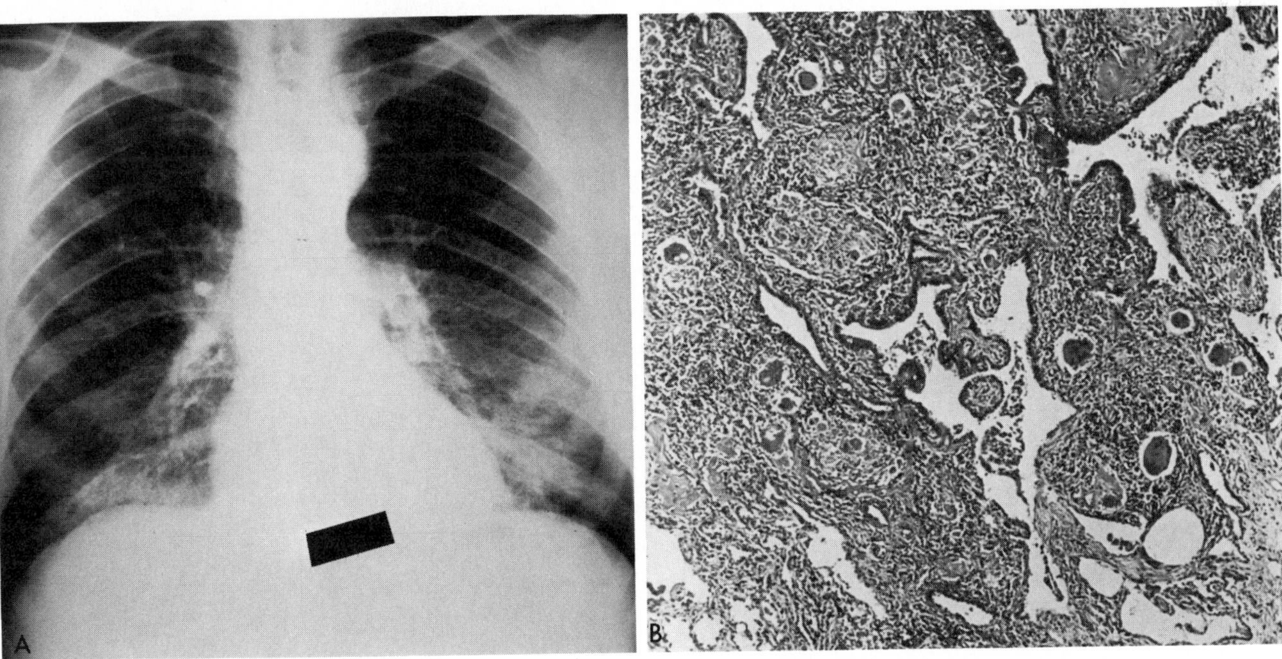

Figure 86–31. *Lymphocytic interstitial pneumonitis. This 51 year old man had increasing dyspnea of several months' duration.*

A *Frontal chest film shows irregular interstitial infiltration of both lower lung fields without lymphadenopathy.*

B *High power photomicrograph from a similar patient shows diffuse thickening of the pulmonary interstitium by lymphocytes and other chronic inflammatory cells.*

(Armed Forces Institute of Pathology Neg. Nos. 77-6231, 73-10535.)

roentgenographically distinguishable from usual interstitial pneumonitis (UIP) and other lower lobe interstitial infiltrations (Fig. 86–31). Lymphadenopathy is not an associated finding, but pleural effusions have been reported.[109] Patients with Sjögren's syndrome with LIP may manifest alveolar filling infiltration because of the secretion of amyloid or an amyloid-like material into the alveoli.[210] It is controversial whether LIP may occasionally progress to pulmonary lymphoma.

Malignant lymphoma of the lungs occurs in a small minority of patients with Sjögren's syndrome. Symptoms of the syndrome have usually been present for more than 15 years, and the incidence of pulmonary lymphoma appears highest when there is a low serum IgM level and absence of rheumatoid factor and when the sicca syndrome is present without collagen vascular disease. Lymphoma may be manifested by generalized lymphadenopathy or salivary gland enlargement with purpura, vasculitis, and neuropathy.[216] The lungs are nearly always involved when malignant lymphoma complicates Sjögren's syndrome.

Radiologically, any of the manifold pulmonary appearances of lymphoma may be evident in Sjögren's syndrome (Fig. 86–32). Generalized interstitial infiltrations, similar to those in LIP, may occur, or there may be a localized alveolar infiltrate resembling pneumonia. Hilar and mediastinal lymphadenopathy and pleural effusions are often present.[217] Multinodular infiltrates and pulmonary masses may also occur.[215]

It is impossible to differentiate roentgenographically between the benign and the malignant pulmonary infiltrations associated with Sjögren's syndrome. LIP and pulmonary lymphoma are often identical in their appearance, and lymphoma may perfectly mimic the roentgenographic appearance of pseudolymphoma. Open pulmonary biopsy is usually necessary for differentiation, as transbronchial and percutaneous needle biopsies do not provide sufficient pathologic material for this difficult differential diagnosis.

Other Lymphoid Disease

Although extraglandular lymphoid infiltration in Sjögren's syndrome is most common in the lungs, it also occurs in other organs. The infiltration may be benign ("pseudolymphoma") or malignant. In addition to the lymph nodes, the liver, spleen, upper respiratory tract, bones, kidneys, and genital organs may also be involved.[209, 210] Serologic changes in patients with benign infiltrations associated with Sjögren's syndrome may include increased production of IgM. Such patients may develop Waldenström's macroglobulinemia. A decrease in pro-

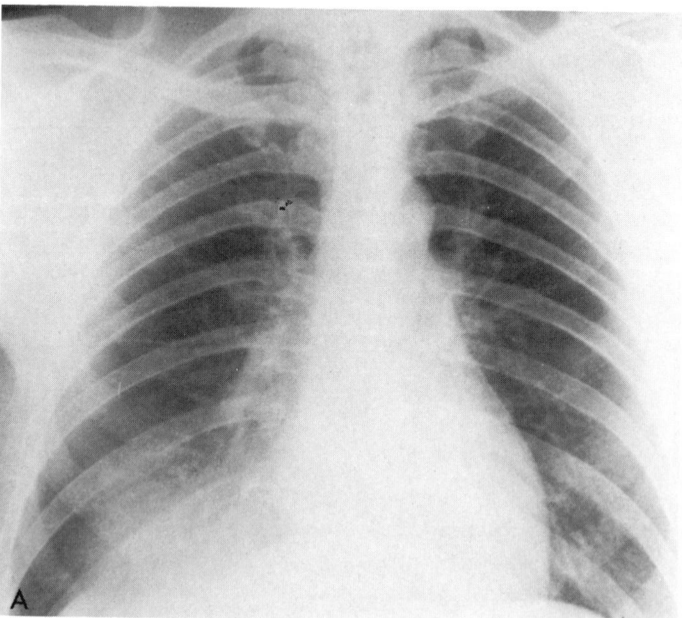

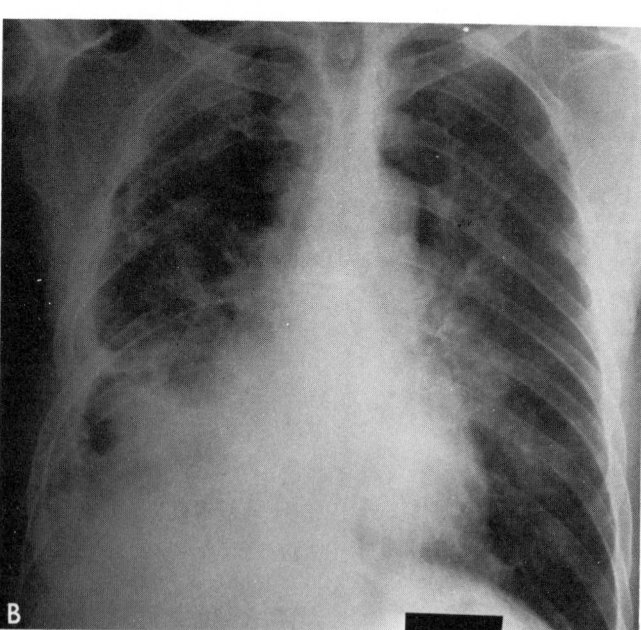

Figure 86–32. *Pulmonary lymphoma. This 38 year old man was originally admitted to the hospital for symptoms of pneumonia and a right lower lobe infiltrate.*

A *Frontal chest film on admission shows an infiltrate in the right lower lobe with an air bronchogram. Biopsy showed this lesion to be lymphoid but benign.*

B *Chest film obtained 15 years later shows diffuse infiltration of both lung fields, right pleural thickening and effusion, and mediastinal widening suggestive of lymphadenopathy. A repeat lung biopsy now demonstrated lymphoma.*

(Armed Forces Institute of Pathology Neg. Nos. 75-11568-1,2.)

duction of IgM may be associated with a change from benign to malignant forms of lymphoproliferative disease.[209]

In addition to Waldenström's macroglobulinemia and pulmonary lymphoma, lymphomas of lymph nodes or other extranodal tissues and reticulum cell sarcomas have been described in Sjögren's syndrome. Characteristic roentgenographic abnormalities include hepatosplenomegaly and diffuse lymphadenopathy in addition to the pulmonary abnormalities described previously.[218] The incidence of all lymphomas in Sjögren's syndrome is highest in patients with parotid gland enlargement, splenomegaly, and lymphadenopathy.[219]

AMYLOIDOSIS

Renal Infiltration

The kidney is the organ most frequently involved in amyloidosis, and renal failure is a common cause of death with severe amyloid infiltration.[220]

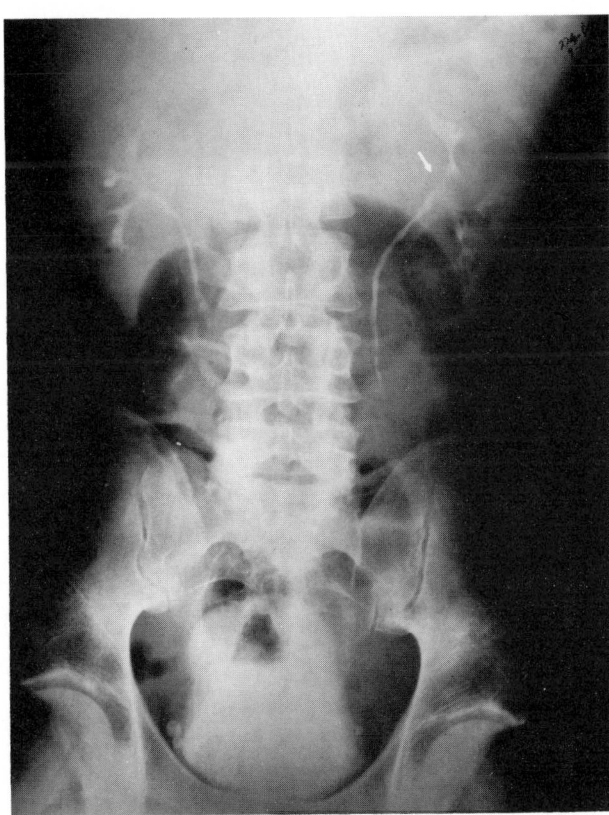

Figure 86–33. Amyloidosis: Kidneys. Excretory urogram from a 50 year old man with renal amyloidosis secondary to Waldenström's macroglobulinemia shows narrowing of renal pelves bilaterally, especially on the left (arrow). The left ureter is minimally irregular in caliber. The vertical elongation of the bladder was thought to be secondary to pelvic lymphadenopathy. (Armed Forces Institute of Pathology Neg. No. 75-15335-1.)

As in other organs, early involvement may be inapparent grossly or microscopically. Deposition is most prominent around the glomeruli, but perivascular deposition is also common, and deposition in the interstitial spaces around the tubules may also be present.

Severe involvement results in a pale, somewhat waxy appearance of the organ, which appears grossly nodular. The kidney becomes enlarged, but there is increasing evidence that this is a manifestation only of severe, acute involvement. Later, the involved kidney commonly becomes shrunken, probably because of vascular involvement and ischemia.[221]

Except for an eventual decrease in renal function, there is little to distinguish amyloidosis on excretory urography. Narrowing of the infundibula or the renal pelvis may be seen (Fig. 86–33). Renal angiograms are almost always abnormal, with irregular and narrowed interlobular arteries, distinct boundaries between the cortex and medulla, and nonvisualization of cortical arteries.[222, 223] Occasionally, renal amyloidosis is confined to the pelvis, in which case submucosal calcifications may be a striking finding.[224, 225] Localized amyloidosis has also been reported to cause strictures of the ureters.[226, 227]

Hepatomegaly, Splenomegaly, and Lymphadenopathy

Amyloid deposition in the liver is very common (up to 90 per cent of patients) in both primary and secondary amyloidosis.[221] The deposits may be grossly inapparent or, if more extensive, may result in an enlarged, pale, somewhat waxy-appearing liver that shows typical discoloration with iodine and sulfuric acid staining. Histologically, the deposits are extracellular in the spaces of Disse and in the perivascular areas.[228] Hepatic function remains surprisingly good for long periods,[228] but eventually the liver parenchyma may become severely compromised. Portal hypertension may develop and may lead to esophageal varices, but ascites is rare.[227] Nuclear scans with sulfur colloid usually demonstrate organomegaly and patchy decreased tracer accumulation.[229, 230]

Early splenic involvement may also be inapparent grossly, but eventual splenomegaly is common. Two patterns of deposition have been described. The first is the so-called "sago spleen," wherein the amyloid is deposited in the follicles, forming a globular appearance. In the other form, the pulp is affected rather than the follicles, resulting in the so-called "lardaceous spleen." Large, confluent, irregular areas of waxy amyloid deposits are late findings in this form.

Lymph node involvement with amyloidosis is frequently seen and may lead to gross lymphadenopathy (Fig. 86–33). Many investigators believe that the reticuloendothelial system is the ultimate source of the amyloid material seen in all cases. The lymphadenopathy often is visible on chest roentgenograms as it may involve either the hilum or the mediastinum, or both, and may be unilateral or bilateral.[231] Its appearance is nonspecific and most resembles granulomatous diseases, including histoplasmosis and sarcoidosis. Coarse calcifications may be present, similar to those seen in late histoplasmosis.[232] Diffuse lymphadenopathy appears especially common in Waldenström's macroglobulinemia, in which lymphography demonstrates a reticular pattern identical to that of lymphoma.[233] Hilar and mediastinal lymphadenopathy in any form of amyloidosis may be present with or without cardiac or pulmonary infiltration.

Pericardial and Myocardial Infiltration

Infiltration of the heart is common in all forms of amyloidosis. Pathologic evidence of myocardial infiltration is much more common than is clinically or radiologically significant disease. The incidence of clinically significant cardiac involvement ranges from 5 to 15 per cent and is highest in the primary form of amyloidosis.[228]

Primary amyloidosis, most often found in elderly individuals and possibly a result of the aging process alone, involves the heart more often than other organs. Familial forms of primary amyloidosis also often involve the heart, especially primary familial amyloidosis with polyneuropathy, in which conduction defects are common and may be fatal.[228] Familial Mediterranean fever with amyloidosis leads to infiltration of the heart as well as nearly all vessels throughout the body, and "familial primary amyloidosis" produces massive amyloidosis of the myocardium and endocardium, with little involvement of other organs.

Amyloidosis associated with multiple myeloma or Waldenström's macroglobulinemia causes diffuse myocardial infiltration of amyloid as well as infiltration of the liver, spleen, kidney, and lungs.[234] Congestive heart failure often ensues in these patients.

Secondary amyloidosis involves the gastrointestinal system and kidneys far more often than the heart.[228] Approximately 5 to 15 per cent of patients with rheumatoid arthritis, however, do develop cardiac amyloidosis, and this manifestation appears to be most common in patients with long-standing rheumatoid disease. Corticosteroid therapy does not appear to contribute to the development of amyloid in rheumatoid arthritis.[228] Secondary amyloidosis involving the heart also occurs in chronic rheumatic heart disease, dermatomyositis, scleroderma, and systemic lupus erythematosus.[228]

Cardiac amyloidosis consists principally of diffuse myocardial infiltration. Fibrils of amyloid are intermingled with myocardial fibers, resulting in a restrictive myocardiopathy that may be severe.[229] Nodular elevations of the pericardial and endocardial surfaces, including the valves, may also be present.[228] Clinically, the amyloid infiltration results in congestive heart failure and conduction disturbances, most commonly right bundle branch block.[229] The electrocardiogram shows diffuse low voltage. Cardiac arrhythmias are common, and an unusual sensitivity to digitalis is often present.[221]

Coronary artery disease may result from amyloid infiltration of these vessels and can lead to myocardial infarctions, which are usually anterior or anteroseptal in location.[228] The roentgenographic appearance of cardiac amyloidosis is nonspecific and may include a "water bottle"–shaped heart, as is seen in patients with large pericardial effusions.[231] Diffuse cardiomegaly is usually the sole roentgenographic finding (Fig. 86–34).

The cardiac manifestations of amyloidosis often mimic the clinical findings of constrictive pericarditis because the myocardium is firm, rubbery, and noncompliant. Angiography may be used to differentiate between amyloidosis and constrictive pericarditis; the most useful differential feature is the demonstration of restricted movement of the crista supraventricularis in amyloidosis. In addition, angiography in cases of amyloidosis may also demonstrate the ability of distal coronary vessels to reach the edge of the cardiac image and lack of motion of the ventricles during atrial systole. Neither of these features is demonstrable in constrictive pericarditis.[235]

There is no known treatment for any of the manifestations of cardiac amyloidosis. Digitalis should be used sparingly if at all because of the danger of arrythmias. Intractable congestive heart failure is thus a common cause of death in patients with severe systemic amyloidosis.

Pulmonary Interstitial Infiltration

There are three distinct types of pulmonary amyloidosis. Two of these types, solitary or multiple pulmonary nodules and localized or diffuse tracheobronchial infiltration, generally occur without systemic disease and without amyloidosis in other organs,[236] and therefore will not be discussed further here. The third type, diffuse parenchymal (or septal) infiltration, is often associated with multiple myeloma or Waldenström's macroglobulinemia but may also be associated with primary amyloidosis, invariably involving other organs, such as the heart, liver, and kidneys.[237] In addition, there are sporadic reports of diffuse parenchymal amyloidosis confined

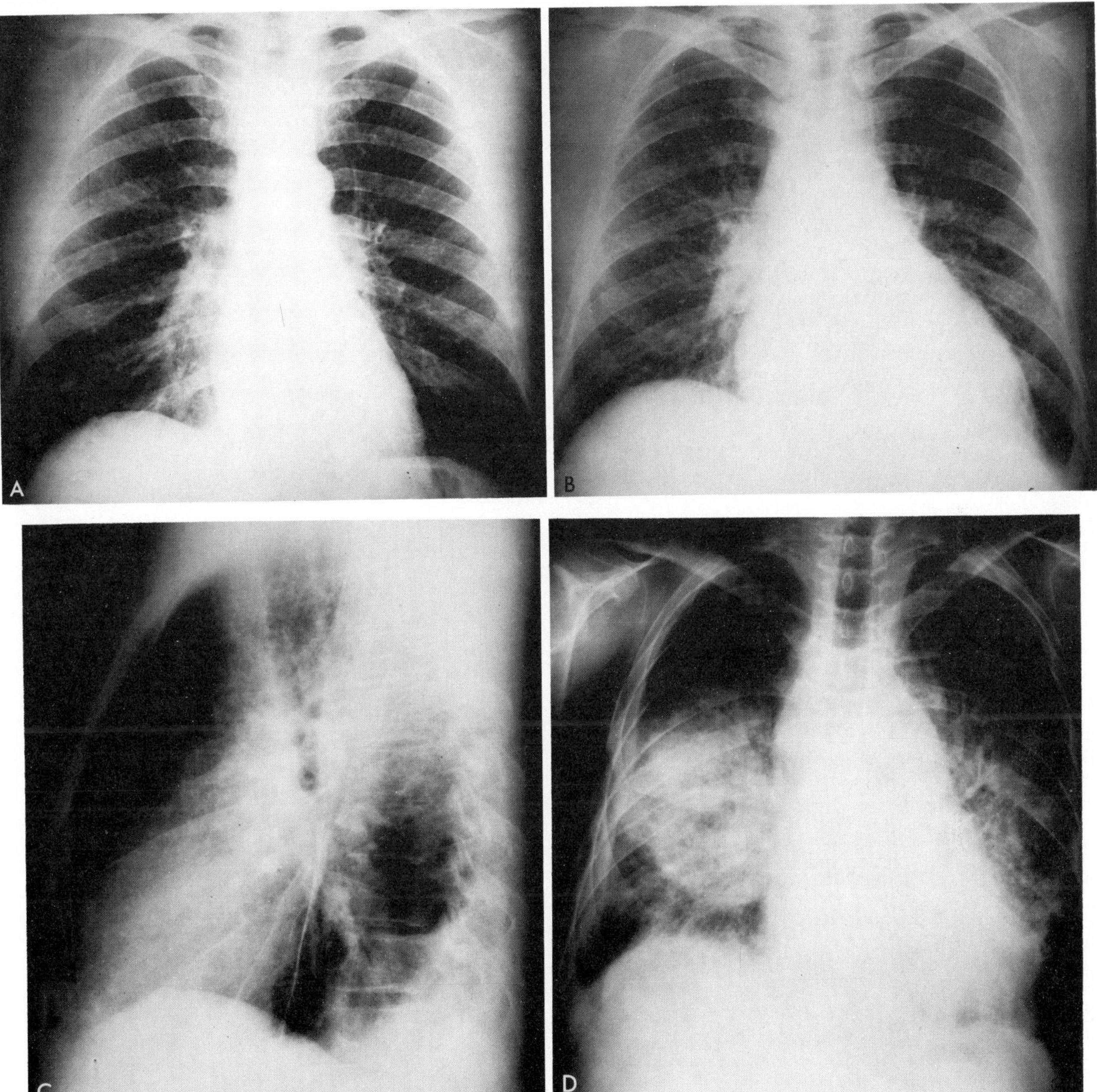

Figure 86–34. *Amyloidosis: Cardiac and diffuse septal pulmonary involvement. This 50 year old man (the same patient as in Figure 86–33) had Waldenström's macroglobulinemia with diffuse amyloidosis.*

A *Initial chest films show heart of normal size and very mild interstitial infiltration, especially in mid-lung fields.*

B, C *One year later, there is diffuse cardiomegaly and increasing interstitial infiltration by amyloid. There is no evidence of pulmonary venous hypertension, although a left pleural effusion is evident.*

D *Film obtained shortly before death shows severe interstitial involvement of mid-lung fields and diffuse pleural thickening. Alveolar infiltration is probably also present, especially in the right mid-lung field. Cardiomegaly is again noted.*

(Armed Forces Institute of Pathology Neg. Nos. 75-15335-3,4,2,6.)

to the lungs[238]; in some cases, amyloidosis may be associated with lymphocytic interstitial pneumonitis.[231]

Pulmonary amyloidosis is rarely encountered in cases of secondary amyloidosis. Minimal infiltration by amyloid may be found pathologically around bronchial glands and in pulmonary vessels, but clinically significant pulmonary amyloidosis has only been reported in two instances.[239]

Diffuse pulmonary amyloidosis consists of infiltration of the alveolar septa. The amyloid deposition may be relatively uniform or patchy and irregular.[239] In various series, the reported incidence of such pulmonary involvement ranges from 36 to 90 per cent of patients with primary systemic amyloidosis. Clinical symptoms, which vary depending on the extent and duration of amyloid infiltration, include severe dyspnea, cough, and hemoptysis.[228]

Diffuse, uniform interstitial infiltration occurs principally in men 40 to 60 years of age. The prognosis in such patients is very poor, and they usually succumb within 1 year of diagnosis. Radiologically, diffuse interstitial infiltration is seen, especially in the lower or midlung fields (Fig. 86–34). The diffuse interstitial infiltrate may evolve into a roentgenographic pattern of alveolar infiltration, as the amyloid may cause fluid exudation into the alveoli.[231] Severe restriction is always evident on pulmonary function tests, and some obstructive component may also be present.[239] Diffuse interstitial amyloidosis is often associated with severe involvement of other organs, especially the heart. Some cases of apparently intractable congestive heart failure secondary to cardiac amyloid may, in fact, represent a sequela of diffuse interstitial pulmonary amyloid, as the diffuse interstitial infiltration is often indistinguishable from interstitial edema.

Patchy, irregular septal amyloidosis, a less severe form of interstitial amyloidosis, is associated with a better prognosis than the diffuse form. Most patients survive 5 to 15 years.[239] Roentgenograms may show a nodular or reticulonodular pattern rather than the more uniform interstitial infiltration described earlier.

Gastrointestinal Infiltration

Amyloid may involve any portion of the gastrointestinal tract, from the tongue to the anus. Such involvement generally occurs more often in primary than in secondary forms.[240, 241] The earliest deposition is mainly perivascular, in the lamina propria beneath the basement membrane of the epithelial cells and between muscle cells of the lamina muscularis mucosae and wall (Fig. 86–35).[228, 242, 243] Later

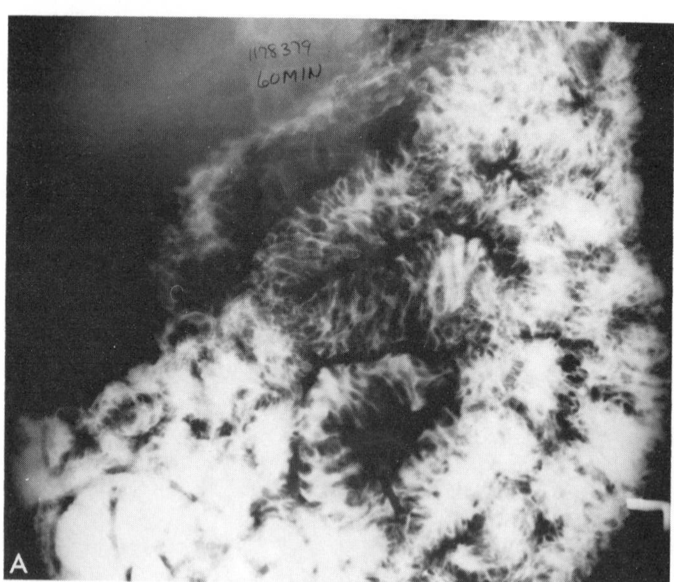

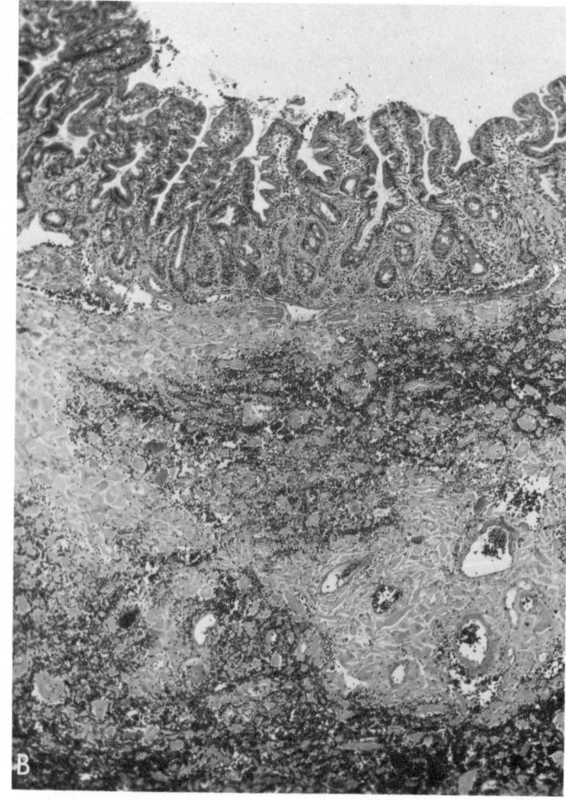

Figure 86–35. *Amyloidosis: Small bowel.*

A *Sixty minute film from the small bowel examination of a 70 year old man with systemic primary amyloidosis. There is marked thickening of the folds thoughout the small bowel, and secondary changes of increased fluid and dilatation are minimal.*

B *Photomicrograph of small bowel wall shows extensive pale-staining amyloid deposits in submucosa and lamina propria, especially in the perivascular spaces (50×).*

(Armed Forces Institute of Pathology Neg. Nos. 69-9700-2, 75-96947.)

there is extension to adjacent areas of the submucosa, muscularis, and subserosa. The tongue is classically involved, particularly in primary amyloidosis. It may be enlarged or stiffened, thus interfering with swallowing. Esophageal infiltration leads to dilatation and diminished peristalsis, resembling the findings in scleroderma.[227, 242]

The eventual diffuse infiltration of the bowel wall is usually assumed to account for the classic roentgenographic appearance. The hallmark is diffuse thickening of the submucosa in the absence of increased secretions, particularly in the small bowel, but also in the stomach and occasionally the colon[244] (Fig. 86–35). Many cases, however, show a more nonspecific pattern, with increased secretion and more irregularity of folds. Diarrhea is frequent, but prolonged transit time may also be seen.[242] Many of the changes found in the gut are probably attributable to ischemia secondary to vascular involvement in the mesentery and bowel wall and to the effects of mesenteric lymph node infiltration.[245]

Malabsorption is a consequence of amyloid deposition and may account in part for the increased fluid in the small bowel. Gallbladder and pancreatic infiltration may further contribute to such changes. Ulceration and bleeding, which are often more important clinically than is malabsorption, were seen in 50 per cent of patients in one series.[221] The pattern in the colon may resemble that seen in inflammatory bowel disease.[243] Intestinal stricture and obstruction resembling findings in carcinoma may occur but are relatively infrequent.[227, 228, 246]

Although the kidney is the most common site of involvement, and therefore the most fruitful source for biopsy to obtain diagnostic material, rectal biopsy is positive in approximately 75 per cent of cases of systemic amyloidosis, and the rectum is a more accessible site. Biopsy of the tongue or capsular biopsy of the small bowel may also yield material that is diagnostic on histochemical analysis.

SUMMARY

The discussion in this chapter has concentrated on specific systemic manifestations of musculoskeletal diseases. While following the course of a patient with such disease, it is important to monitor closely the systemic manifestations, especially those that can become life-threatening. The carditis and pericarditis of rheumatoid arthritis, the pulmonary fibrocystic disease of ankylosing spondylitis, lupus nephritis, and the diffuse arteritis of periarteritis nodosa are all examples of progressive and potentially fatal systemic manifestations of articular diseases. The choice of therapy for articular disease and the evaluation of response to such therapy can only be accomplished with cognizance of the systemic manifestations of the disorders.

REFERENCES

1. Hurd ER: Extraarticular manifestations of rheumatoid arthritis. Sem Arthritis Rheum *8*:151, 1979.
2. Martel W, Abell MR, Mikkelsen WM, Whitehouse WM: Pulmonary and pleural lesions in rheumatoid disease. Radiology *90*:641, 1968.
3. Campbell GD, Ferrington E: Rheumatoid pleuritis with effusion. Dis Chest *53*:521, 1968.
4. Gordon DA, Stein JL, Broder I: The extra-articular features of rheumatoid arthritis. A systemic analysis of 127 cases. Am J Med *54*:445, 1973.
5. Walker WC, Wright V: Pulmonary lesions and rheumatoid arthritis. Medicine *47*:501, 1968.
6. Carr DT, Mayne JG: Pleurisy with effusion in rheumatoid arthritis, with reference to the low concentration of glucose in pleural fluid. Am Rev Resp Dis *85*:345, 1962.
7. Hunninghake GW, Fauci AS: Pulmonary involvement in the collagen vascular diseases. Am Rev Resp Dis *119*:471, 1979.
8. Eraut D, Evans J, Caplin M: Pulmonary necrobiotic nodules without rheumatoid arthritis. Br J Dis Chest *72*:301, 1978.
9. Robertson JL, Brinkman GL: Nodular rheumatoid lung disease. Am J Med *31*:483, 1961.
10. Ellman P: The etiology of chronic rheumatism. Proc R Soc Med *40*:332, 1947.
11. Ellman P, Ball RE: "Rheumatoid disease" with joint and pulmonary manifestations. Br Med J *2*:816, 1948.
12. Doctor L, Snider GL: Diffuse interstitial pulmonary fibrosis associated with arthritis. With comments on the definition of rheumatoid lung disease. Am Rev Resp Dis *85*:413, 1962.
13. Morgan WKC, Wolfel DA: The lungs and pleura in rheumatoid arthritis. Am J Roentgenol *98*:334, 1966.
14. Genereux GP: The end-stage lung. Pathogenesis, pathology, and radiology. Radiology *116*:279, 1975.
15. Patterson CD, Harville WE, Pierce JA: Rheumatoid lung disease. Ann Intern Med *62*:685, 1965.
16. Stack BHR, Grant IWB: Rheumatoid interstitial lung disease. Br J Dis Chest *59*:202, 1965.
17. Levin DC, Scoggin CH, Ostroy P: Productive cough and hemoptysis in rheumatoid lung disease. Chest *69*:667, 1976.
18. Caplan A, Payne RB, Withey JL: A broader concept of Caplan's syndrome related to rheumatoid factors. Thorax *17*:205, 1962.
19. Portner MM, Gracie WA Jr: Rheumatoid lung disease with cavitary nodules, pneumothorax and eosinophilia. New Engl J Med *275*:697, 1966.
20. Miall WE: Rheumatoid arthritis in males. An epidemiological study of a Welsh mining community. Ann Rheum Dis *14*:150, 1955.
21. Franco AE, Levine HD, Hall AP: Rheumatoid pericarditis — report of 17 cases diagnosed clinically. Ann Intern Med *77*:837, 1972.
22. Nomeir AM, Turner RA, Watts LE: Cardiac involvement in rheumatoid arthritis. Followup study. Arthritis Rheum *22*:561, 1979.
23. Schmid FR, Cooper NS, Ziff M., McEwen C: Arteritis in rheumatoid arthritis. Am J Med *30*:56, 1961.
24. John JT Jr, Hough A, Sergent JS: Pericardial disease in rheumatoid arthritis. Am J Med *66*:385, 1979.
25. Burney DP, Martin CE, Thomas CS, Fisher RD, Bender HW Jr: Rheumatoid pericarditis. Clinical significance and operative management. J Thor Cardiovasc Surg *77*:511, 1979.
26. Barnes CG, Turnbull AL, Vernon-Roberts B: Felty's syndrome. A clinical and pathological survey of 21 patients and their response to treatment. Ann Rheum Dis *30*:359, 1971.
27. Ruderman M, Miller LM, Pinals RS: Clinical and serologic observations on 27 patients with Felty's syndrome. Arthritis Rheum *11*:377, 1968.
28. Scott JT, Hourihane DO, Doyle FH, Steiner RE, Laws JW, Dixon AS, Bywaters EGL: Digital arteritis in rheumatoid disease. Ann Rheum Dis *20*:224, 1961.
29. Laws JW, Lillie JG, Scott JT: Arteriographic appearances in rheumatoid arthritis and other disorders. Br J Radiol *36*:477, 1963.
30. Wilkinson M, Kirk J: Leg ulcers complicating rheumatoid arthritis. Scot Med J *10*:175, 1965.
31. Ansell BM: Chronic arthritis in childhood. Ann Rheum Dis *37*:107, 1978.

32. Schaller J, Wedgwood RJ: Juvenile rheumatoid arthritis: A review. Pediatrics *50*:940, 1972.
33. Vale JA, Pickering JG, Scott GW: Ankylosing spondylitis and upper lobe fibrosis and cavitation. Guys Hosp Rep *123*:97, 1974.
34. Rosenow ED III, Strimlan CV, Muhm JR, Ferguson RH: Pleuropulmonary manifestations of ankylosing spondylitis. Mayo Clin Proc *52*:641, 1977.
35. Davies D: Ankylosing spondylitis and lung fibrosis. Q J Med *41*:395, 1972.
36. Libshitz HI, Atkinson GW: Pulmonary cystic disease in ankylosing spondylitis: Two cases with unusual superinfection. J Can Assoc Radiol *29*:266, 1978.
37. Stewart RM, Ridyard JB, Pearson JD: Regional lung function in ankylosing spondylitis. Thorax *31*:433, 1976.
38. Zorab PA: The lungs in ankylosing spondylitis. Q J Med *31*:267, 1962.
39. Davidson P, Baggenstoss AH, Slocumb CH, Daugherty GW: Cardiac and aortic lesions in rheumatoid spondylitis. Mayo Clin Proc *38*:427, 1963.
40. Schilder DP, Harvey WP, Hufnagel CA: Rheumatoid spondylitis and aortic insufficiency. New Engl J Med *255*:11, 1956.
41. Takkunen J, Vuopale U, Isomäki H: Cardiomyopathy in ankylosing spondylitis. Part I. Medical history and results of clinical examination in a series of 55 patients. Ann Clin Res *2*:106, 1970.
42. Toone EC Jr, Pierce EL, Hennigar GR: Aortitis and aortic regurgitation associated with rheumatoid spondylitis. Am J Med *26*:255, 1959.
43. Laufer, I, Costopoulos L: Early lesions of Crohn's disease. Am J Roentgenol *130*:307, 1978.
44. Sommers SC: Ulcerative and granulomatous colitis. Am J Roentgenol *130*:817, 1978.
45. Wright R: Ulcerative colitis. Gastroenterology *58*:875, 1970.
46. Lichtenstein JE, Madewell JE, Feigin DS: The collar button ulcer. A radiologic-pathologic correlation. Gastrointest Radiol *4*:79, 1979.
47. Bartram CI: Radiology in the current assessment of ulcerative colitis. Gastrointest Radiol *1*:383, 1977.
48. Goldberger LE, Neely HR, Stammer JL: Large mucosal bridges. An unusual roentgenographic manifestation of ulcerative colitis. Gastrointest Radiol *3*:81, 1978.
49. Hammerman AM, Shatz BA, Susman N: Radiographic characteristics of colonic "mucosal bridges": Sequelae of inflammatory bowel disease. Radiology *127*:611, 1978.
50. Hinrichs HR, Goldman H: Localized giant pseudopolyps of the colon. JAMA *205*:248, 1968.
51. Ferrucci JT Jr, Vickery AL Jr: Right-lower-quadrant mass after 4 and a half years of ulcerative colitis. N Engl J Med *268*:147, 1972.
52. Jones B, Abbruzzese AA: Obstructing giant pseudopolyps in granulomatous colitis. Gastrointest Radiol *3*:437, 1978.
53. Wills JS, Han SS: Localized giant pseudopolyposis complicating granulomatous ileocolitis. Radiology *122*:320, 1977.
54. Zegal HG, Laufer I: Filiform polyposis. Radiology *127*:615, 1978.
55. Devroede GJ, Taylor WF, Sauer WG, Jackman RJ, Stickler GB: Cancer risk and life expectancy of children with ulcerative colitis. N Engl J Med *285*:17, 1971.
56. Truelove SC: Ulcerative colitis beginning in childhood. N Engl J Med *285*:50, 1971.
57. Clark RL, Muhletaler CA, Margulies SI: Colitic arthritis. Clinical and radiographic manifestations. Radiology *101*:585, 1971.
58. Wright R, Lumsden K, Luntz MH, Sevel D, Truelove SC: Abnormalities of the sacroiliac joints and uveitis in ulcerative colitis. Q J Med *34*:229, 1965.
59. Wright V, Watkinson G: Articular complications of ulcerative colitis. Am J Proctol *17*:107, 1966.
60. McEwen C, Lingg C, Kirsner JB: Arthritis accompanying ulcerative colitis. Am J Med *33*:923, 1962.
61. McEwen C, Ditata D, Lingg C, Porini A, Good A, Rankin T: Ankylosing spondylitis and spondylitis accompanying ulcerative colitis, regional enteritis, psoriasis and Reiter's disease. A comparative study. Arthritis Rheum *14*:291, 1971.
62. Morris RI, Metzger AL, Bluestone R, Terasaki PI: HL-A-W27 — A useful discriminator in the arthropathies of inflammatory bowel disease. N Engl J Med *290*:1117, 1974.
63. Schaller JG: The arthritis of inflammatory bowel disease in children. Clin Rheum Dis *2*:353, 1976.
64. Schumacher TM, Genant HK, Kellet MJ, Mall JC, Fye KH: HLA-B27 associated arthropathies. Radiology *126*:289, 1978.
65. Crohn BB, Ginzburg L, Oppenheimer GD: Regional ileitis. A pathologic and clinical entity. JAMA *99*:1323, 1932.
66. Marshak RH: Granulomatous disease of the intestinal tract (Crohn's disease). Radiology *114*:3, 1975.
67. Zetzel L: Granulomatous (ileo)colitis. New Engl J Med *282*:600, 1970.
68. Laufer I, Mullens JE, Hamilton J: Correlation of endoscopy and double-contrast radiography in the early stages of ulcerative and granulomatous colitis. Radiology *118*:1, 1978.
69. Glotzer DJ, Gardner RC, Goldman H, Hinrichs HR, Rosen H, Zetzel L: Comparative features and course of ulcerative and granulomatous colitis. N Engl J Med *282*:582, 1970.
70. Margulis AR, Goldberg HI, Lawson TL, Montgomery CK, Rambo, ON, Noonan CD, Amberg JR: The overlapping spectrum of ulcerative and granulomatous colitis: A roentgenographic-pathologic study. Am J Roentgenol *113*:325, 1971.
71. Margulis AR: Radiology of ulcerating colitis. Radiology *105*:251, 1972.
72. Greenstein AJ, Janowitz HD, Sachar DB: The extra-intestinal complications of Crohn's disease and ulcerative colitis: A study of 700 patients. Medicine *55*:401, 1976.
73. Haslock I, Wright V: The musculoskeletal complications of Crohn's disease. Medicine *52*:217, 1973.
74. Mueller CE, Seeger JF, Martel W: Ankylosing spondylitis and regional enteritis. Radiology *112*:579, 1974.
75. Palumbo PJ, Ward LE, Sauer WG, Scudamore HH: Musculoskeletal manifestations of inflammatory bowel disease. Mayo Clin Proc *48*:411, 1973.
76. Brom B, Bank S, Marks IN, Cobb JJ: Periostitis, aseptic necrosis, and arthritis occurring in a patient with Crohn's disease. Gastroenterology *60*:1106, 1971.
77. Strole WE Jr, Galdabini JJ: Pruritis and abnormal liver-function tests with inflammatory bowel disease. N Engl J Med *289*:964, 1973.
78. Farman J, Effmann EL, Grnja V: Crohn's disease and periosteal new bone formation. Gastroenterology *61*:513, 1971.
79. Farman J, Twersky J, Fierst S: Ulcerative colitis associated with hypertrophic osteoarthropathy. Am J Dig Dis *21*:130, 1976.
80. Ménard DB, Haddad H, Blain JG, Beaudry R, Devroede G, Massé S: Granulomatous myositis and myopathy associated with Crohn's colitis. N Engl J Med *295*:818, 1976.
81. Farmer RG, Hawk WA, Turnbull RB Jr: Clinical patterns in Crohn's disease: A statistical study of 615 cases. Gastroenterology *68*:627, 1975.
82. Nesbit RR Jr, Elbadawi NA, Morton JH, Cooper RA Jr: Carcinoma of the small bowel. A complication of regional enteritis. Cancer *37*:2948, 1976.
83. Valdes-Dapena A, Rudolph I, Hidayat A, Roth JLA, Laucks RB: Adenocarcinoma of the small bowel in association with regional enteritis. Four new cases. Cancer *37*:2938, 1976.
84. Weedon DD, Shorter RG, Ilstrup DM, Huizenga KA, Taylor WF: Crohn's disease and cancer. N Engl J Med *289*:1099, 1973.
85. Moss AA, Carbone JV, Kressel HY: Radiologic and clinical assessment of broad-spectrum antibiotic therapy in Crohn's disease. Am J Roentgenol *131*:787, 1978.
86. Whipple GH: A hitherto undescribed disease characterized anatomically by deposits of fat and fatty acids in the intestinal and mesenteric lymphatic tissues. Johns Hopkins Hosp Bull *18*:382, 1907.
87. Enzinger FM, Helwig EB: Whipple's disease. A review of the literature and report of fifteen patients. Virchows Arch Pathol Anat *336*:238, 1963.
88. Bayless TM, Knox DL: Whipple's disease: A multisystem infection. N Engl J Med *300*:920, 1979.
89. Feurle GE, Volk B, Waldherr R: Cerebral Whipple's disease with negative jejunal histology. N Engl J Med *300*:907, 1979.
90. Knox DL, Bayless TM, Pittman FE: Neurologic disease in patients with treated Whipple's disease. Medicine *55*:467, 1976.
91. Maizel H, Ruffin JM, Dobbins WO III: Whipple's disease: A review of 19 patients from one hospital and a review of the literature since 1950. Medicine *49*:175, 1970.
92. Davis TD Jr, McBee JW, Borland JL Jr, Kurtz SM, Ruffin JM: The effect of antibiotic and steroid therapy in Whipple's disease. Gastroenterology *44*:112, 1963.
93. Puppala AR, Singh S, Munaswamy M: Whipple's disease. Endoscopic documentation, light and electron microscopic features in an 80-year-old man. Am J Gastroenterol *70*:407, 1978.
94. Trier JS, Phelps PC, Eidelman S, Rubin CE: Whipple's disease: Light and electron microscope correlations of jejunal mucosal histology with antibiotic treatment and clinical status. Gastroenterology *48*:684, 1965.
95. Clemett A, Marshak R: Whipple's disease: Roentgen features and differential diagnosis. Radiol Clin North Am *7*:105, 1969.
96. Decker JL, Steinberg AD, Gershwin ME, Seaman WE, Klippel JH, Plotz PH, Paget SA: Systemic lupus erythematosus. Contrasts and comparisons. Ann Intern Med *82*:391, 1975.
97. Dubois EL, Tuffanelli DL: Clinical manifestations of systemic lupus erythematosus. Computer analysis of 520 cases. JAMA *190*:104, 1964.
98. Gould DM, Daves ML: Roentgenologic findings in systemic lupus erythematosus. An analysis of 100 cases. J Chron Dis *2*:136, 1955.
99. Castaneda-Zuniga WR, Hogan MT: Cavitary pulmonary nodules in systemic lupus erythematosus. Radiology *118*:45, 1976.
100. Levin DC: Proper interpretation of pulmonary roentgen changes in systemic lupus erythematosus. Am J Roentgenol *111*:510, 1971.
101. Eisenberg H, Dubois EL, Sherwin RP, Balchium OJ: Diffuse interstitial

lung disease in systemic lupus erythematosus. Ann Intern Med *79*:37, 1973.
102. Matthay RA, Schwarz MI, Petty TL, Stanford RE, Gupta RC, Sahn SA, Steigerwald JC: Pulmonary manifestations of systemic lupus erythematosus: Review of twelve cases of acute lupus pneumonitis. Medicine *54*:397, 1975.
103. Gross M, Esterly JR, Earle RH: Pulmonary alterations in systemic lupus erythematosus. Am Rev Resp Dis *105*:572, 1972.
104. Simon G: Further observations on the long line shadow across a lower zone of the lung. Br J Radiol *43*:327, 1970.
105. Gamsu G, Webb WR: Pulmonary hemorrhage in systemic lupus erythematosus. J Can Assoc Radiol *29*:66, 1978.
106. Brigden W, Bywaters EGL, Lessof MH, Ross IP: The heart in systemic lupus erythematosus. Br Heart J *22*:1, 1960.
107. Collins RL, Turner RA, Nomeir AM, Hunt R, Johnson AM, McLean RL, Watts JE: Cardiopulmonary manifestations of systemic lupus erythematosus. J Rheumatol *5*:299, 1978.
108. Kassan SS, Moss ML, Reddick RL: Progressive hilar and mediastinal lymphadenopathy in systemic lupus erythematosus on corticosteroid therapy. N Engl J Med *294*:1382, 1976.
109. Feigin DS, Siegelman SS, Theros EG, King FM: Nonmalignant lymphoid disorders of the chest. Am J Roentgenol *129*:221, 1977.
110. Gordonson J, Quinn M, Kaufman R, Van den Tweel JG: Mediastinal lymphadenopathy and undifferentiated connective tissue disease: Case report and review. Am J Roentgenol *131*:325, 1978.
111. Baldwin DS, Lowenstein J, Rothfield NF, Gallo G, McCluskey RT: The clinical course of the proliferative and membranous forms of lupus nephritis. Ann Intern Med *73*:929, 1970.
112. Bennahum DA, Messner RP, Shoop JD: Brain scan findings in central nervous system involvememt by lupus erythematosus. Ann Intern Med *81*:763, 1974.
113. Johnson RT, Richardson EP: The neurological manifestations of systemic lupus erythematosus. A clinical-pathological study of 24 cases and review of the literature. Medicine *47*:337, 1968.
114. Bilaniuk LT, Patel S, Zimmerman RA: Computed tomography of systemic lupus erythematosus. Radiology *124*:119, 1977.
115. Trevor RP, Sondheimer FK, Fessel WJ, Wolpert SM: Angiographic demonstration of major cerebral vessel occlusion in systemic lupus erythematosus. Neuroradiology *4*:202, 1972.
116. Kitching GB, Thompson JR, Hasso AN, Hirst AE: Angiographic demonstration of lupus cerebral phlebitis with communicating hydrocephalus. Neuroradiology *14*:59, 1977.
117. Carlow TJ, Glaser JS: Pseudotumor cerebri syndrome in systemic lupus erythematosus. JAMA *228*:197, 1974.
118. Sergent JS, Lockshin MD, Klempner MS, Lipsky BA: Central nervous system disease in systemic lupus erythematosus. Therapy and prognosis. Am J Med *58*:644, 1975.
119. Derksen OS: Pneumatosis intestinalis in a female patient with systemic lupus erythematosus. Radiologia Clin *47*:334, 1978.
120. Kleinman P, Meyers MA, Abbott G, Kazam E: Necrotizing enterocolitis with pneumatosis intestinalis in systemic lupus erythematosus and polyarteritis. Radiology *121*:595, 1976.
121. Lee SL, Chase PH: Drug-induced systemic lupus erythematosus: A critical review. Semin Arthritis Rheum *5*:83, 1975.
122. Griesemer DA, Ed.: Procainamide-induced lupus. Johns Hopkins Med J *138*:289, 1976.
123. Poirier TJ, Rankin GB: Gastrointestinal manifestations of progressive systemic scleroderma based on a review of 364 cases. Am J Gastroenterol *58*:30, 1972.
124. Bluestone R, Macmahon M, Dawson JM: Systemic sclerosis and small bowel involvement. Gut *10*:185, 1969.
125. Gondos B: Roentgen manifestations in progressive systemic sclerosis (diffuse scleroderma). Am J Roentgenol *84*:235, 1960.
126. Hurwitz AL, Duranceau A, Postlethwait RW: Esophageal dysfunction and Raynaud's phenomenon in patients with scleroderma. Am J Dig Dis *21*:601, 1976.
127. Tuffanelli DL, Winkelmann RK: Systemic scleroderma. A clinical study of 727 cases. Arch Dermatol *84*:359, 1961.
128. Cohen S: Motor disorders of the esophagus. N Engl J Med *301*:184, 1979.
129. Dinsmore RE, Goodman D, Dreyfuss JR: The air esophagram: A sign of scleroderma involving the esophagus. Radiology *87*:348, 1966.
130. House AJS, Griffiths GJ: The significance of an air esophagogram visualized on conventional chest radiographs. Clin Radiol *28*:301, 1977.
131. Martinez LO: Air in the esophagus as a sign of scleroderma (differential diagnosis with some other entities). J Can Assoc Radiol *25*:234, 1974.
132. Owen JP, Muston HL, Goolamali SK: Absence of esophageal mucosal folds in systemic sclerosis. Clin Radiol *30*:489, 1979.
133. Clements JL Jr, Abernathy J, Weens HS: Corrugated mucosal pattern in the esophagus associated with progressive systemic sclerosis. Gastrointest Radiol *3*:119, 1978.
134. Peachey RDG, Creamer B, Pierce JW: Sclerodermatous involvement of the stomach and the small and large bowel. Gut *10*:285, 1969.
135. Goldgraber MB, Kirsner JB: Scleroderma of the gastrointestinal tract: Review. Arch Pathol *64*:255, 1957.
136. Abrams HL, Carnes WH, Eaton J: Alimentary tract in disseminated scleroderma with emphasis on small bowel. Arch Intern Med *94*:61, 1954.
137. Heinz ER, Steinberg AJ, Sackner MA: Roentgenographic and pathologic aspects of intestinal scleroderma. Ann Intern Med *59*:822, 1963.
138. Horowitz AL, Meyers MA: The "hide-bound" small bowel of scleroderma: Characteristic mucosal fold pattern. Am J Roentgenol *119*:332, 1973.
139. Ballard JL, Snyder CR, Jansen GT: The gastrointestinal manifestations of generalized scleroderma. South Med J *62*:1243, 1969.
140. Olmsted WW, Madewell JE: The esophageal and small-bowel manifestations of progressive systemic sclerosis. Gastrointest Radiol *1*:33, 1976.
141. Queloz JM, Woloshin HJ: Sacculation of the small intestine in scleroderma. Radiology *105*:513, 1972.
142. Martel W, Chang SF, Abell MR: Loss of colonic haustration in progressive systemic sclerosis. Am J Roentgenol *126*:704, 1976.
143. Dodds WJ, Stewart ET, Goldberg HI: Pneumatosis intestinalis associated with hepatic portal venous gas. Am J Dig Dis *21*:992, 1976.
144. Freiman D, Chon H, Bilaniuk L: Pneumatosis intestinalis in systemic lupus erythematosus. Radiology *116*:563, 1975.
145. Gompels BM: Pneumatosis cystoides intestinalis associated with progressive systemic sclerosis. Br J Radiol *42*:701, 1969.
146. Marshak R, Lindner A, Maklansky D: Pneumatosis cystoides coli. Gastrointest Radiol *2*:85, 1977.
147. Mueller CF, Morehead R, Alter AJ, Michener W: Pneumatosis intestinalis in collagen disorders. Am J Roentgenol *115*:300, 1972.
148. Meihoff WE, Hirschfield JS, Kern F Jr: Small intestinal scleroderma with malabsorption and pneumatosis cystoides intestinalis. Report of three cases. JAMA *204*:854, 1968.
149. Kahn IJ, Jeffries GH, Sleisenger MH: Malabsorption in intestinal scleroderma. Correction by antibiotics. N Engl J Med *274*:1339, 1966.
150. Reynolds TB, Denison EK, Frankl HD, Lieberman FL, Peters RL: Primary biliary cirrhosis with scleroderma, Raynaud's phenomenon and telangiectasia. New syndrome. Am J Med *50*:302, 1971.
151. Dreiling DA, Soto JM: The pancreatic involvement in disseminated "collagen" disorders. Studies of pancreatic secretion in patients with scleroderma and Sjögren's "disease." Am J Gastroenterol *66*:546, 1976.
152. Piper WN, Helwig EB: Progressive systemic sclerosis. Visceral manifestations in generalized scleroderma. Arch Dermatol *72*:535, 1955.
153. Weaver AL, Divertie MB, Titus JL: Pulmonary scleroderma. Dis Chest *54*:490, 1968.
154. Olson DS, Kumar UN, Funahashi A: Progressive systemic sclerosis presenting as interstitial pulmonary fibrosis. Postgrad Med *64*:173, 1978.
155. Ashba JK, Ghanem MH: The lungs in systemic sclerosis. Dis Chest *47*:52, 1965.
156. Bianchi FA, Bistue AR, Wendt VE, Puro HE, Keech MK: Analysis of 27 cases of progressive systemic sclerosis (including two with combined systemic lupus erythematosus) and a review of the literature. J Chronic Dis *19*:953, 1966.
157. Barnett AJ: The systemic involvement in scleroderma. Med J Aust *2*:659, 1977.
158. Barnett AJ: Scleroderma (progressive systemic sclerosis): Progress and course based on a personal series of 118 cases. Med J Aust *2*:129, 1978.
159. DeMuth GR, Furstenberg NA, Dabich L, Zarafonetis CJD: Pulmonary manifestations of progressive systemic sclerosis. Am J Med Sci *255*:94, 1968.
160. Mahrer PR, Evans JA, Steinberg I: Scleroderma: Relation of pulmonary changes to esophageal disease. Ann Intern Med *40*:92, 1954.
161. Talbott JH, Barrocas M: Progressive systemic sclerosis (PSS) and malignancy, pulmonary and non-pulmonary. Medicine *58*:182, 1979.
162. Gottdiener JS, Moutsopoulos HM, Decker JL: Echocardiographic identification of cardiac abnormality in scleroderma and related disorders. Am J Med *66*:391, 1979.
163. Sackner MA, Heinz ER, Steinberg AJ: The heart in scleroderma. Am J Cardiol *17*:542, 1966.
164. Cannon PJ, Hassar M, Case DB, Casarella WJ, Sommers SC, LeRoy EC: The relationship of hypertension and renal failure in scleroderma (progressive systemic sclerosis) to structural and functional abnormalities of the renal cortical circulation. Medicine *53*:1, 1974.
165. Masi AT, D'Angelo WA: Epidemiology of fatal systemic sclerosis (diffuse scleroderma). A 15-year survey in Baltimore. Ann Intern Med *66*:870, 1967.
166. Oliveros MA, Herbst JJ, Lester PD, Ziter FA: Pneumatosis intestinalis in childhood dermatomyositis. Pediatrics *52*:711, 1973.
167. Kovalchik MT, Guggenheim SJ, Silverman MH, Robertson JS, Steiger-

wald JC: The kidney in progressive systemic sclerosis. A prospective study. Ann Intern Med *89*:881, 1978.
168. Lester PD, Koehler PR: The renal angiographic changes in scleroderma. Radiology *99*:517, 1971.
169. Winograd J, Schimmel DH, Palubinskas AJ: The spotted nephrogram of renal scleroderma. Am J Roentgenol *126*:734, 1976.
170. Feldman F, Marshak RH: Dermatomyositis with significant involvement of the gastrointestinal tract. Am J Roentgenol *90*:746, 1963.
171. Bohan A, Peter JB: Polymyositis and dermatomyositis. Parts I and II. N Engl J Med *292*:344, 403, 1975.
172. Kleckner FS: Dermatomyositis and its manifestations in the gastrointestinal tract. Am J Gastroenterol *53*:141, 1970.
173. O'Hara JM, Szemes G, Lowman RM: The esophageal lesions in dermatomyositis. A correlation of radiologic and pathologic findings. Radiology *89*:27, 1967.
174. Steiner RM, Glassman L, Schwartz MW, Vanace P: The radiological findings in dermatomyositis of childhood. Radiology *111*:385, 1974.
175. Cohen S: Motor disorders of the esophagus. N Engl J Med *301*:184, 1979.
176. Dodds WJ, Stewart ET, Goldberg HI: Pneumatosis intestinalis associated with hepatic portal venous gas. Am J Dig Dis *21*:992, 1976.
177. Mueller CF, Morehead R, Alter AJ, Michener W: Pneumatosis intestinalis in collagen disorders. Am J Roentgenol *115*:300, 1972.
178. Oliveros M, Herbst JJ, Lester PD, Ziter FA: Pneumatosis intestinalis in childhood dermatomyositis. Pediatrics *52*:711, 1973.
179. Camp AV, Lane DJ, Mowat AG: Dermatomyositis with parenchymal lung involvement. Br Med J *1*:155, 1972.
180. Frazier AR, Miller RD: Interstitial pneumonitis in association with polymyositis and dermatomyositis. Chest *65*:403, 1974.
181. Thompson PL, Mackay IR: Fibrosing alveolitis and polymyositis. Thorax *25*:504, 1970.
182. Pearson CM: Polymyositis. Ann Rev Med *17*:63, 1966.
183. Williams RC Jr: Dermatomyositis and malignancy: A review of the literature. Ann Intern Med *50*:1174, 1959.
184. Alarcón-Segovia D, Brown AL Jr: Classification and etiologic aspects of necrotizing angiitides: An analytic approach to a confused subject with a critical review of the evidence for hypersensitivity to polyarteritis nodosa. Mayo Clin Proc *39*:205, 1964.
185. Christian CL, Sergent JS: Vasculitis syndromes: Clinical and experimental models. Am J Med *61*:385, 1976.
186. DeShazo RD, Levinson AI, Lawless OJ, Weisbaum G: Systemic vasculitis with coexistent large and small vessel involvement. A classification dilemma. JAMA *238*:1940, 1977.
187. Moskowitz RW, Baggentoss AH, Slocumb CH: Histopathologic classification and periarteritis nodosa: A study of 56 cases confirmed at necropsy. Mayo Clin Proc *38*:345, 1963.
188. Rose GA: The natural history of polyarteritis. Br Med J *2*:1148, 1957.
189. Zeek PM: Periarteritis nodosa: A critical review. Am J Clin Pathol *22*:777, 1952.
190. Robbins SL, Cotran RS: Pathologic Basis of Disease. 2nd Ed. Philadelphia, WB Saunders Co, 1979, p. 312.
191. Evens RG, Dobry CA, Eckert JF: An exercise in radiologic-pathologic correlation. Radiology *91*:1028, 1968.
192. Frohnert PP, Sheps SG: Long-term follow-up study of periarteritis nodosa. Am J Med *43*:8, 1967.
193. Fleming RJ, Stern LZ: Multiple intraparenchymal renal aneurysms in polyarteritis nodosa. Radiology *84*:100, 1965.
194. Sack M, Cassidy JT, Bole GG: Prognostic factors in polyarteritis. J Rheumatol *2*:41, 1975.
195. Peterson C Jr, Willerson JT, Doppman JL, Decker JL: Polyarteritis nodosa with bilateral renal artery aneurysms and perirenal hematomas: Angiographic and nephrotomographic features. Br J Radiol *43*:62, 1970.
196. Han SY, Jander HP, Laws HL: Polyarteritis nodosa causing severe intestinal bleeding. Gastrointest Radiol *1*:285, 1976.
197. Kleinman P, Meyers MA, Abbott G, Kazam E: Necrotizing enterocolitis with pneumatosis intestinalis in systemic lupus erythematosus and polyarteritis. Radiology *121*:595, 1976.
198. Buranasiri S, Baum S, Nusbaum M, Finkelstein D: Periarteritis of the middle colic artery. Arteriographic, surgical and pathological correlation. Am J Gastroenterol *59*:73, 1973.
199. Fayemi AO, Ali M, Braun EV: Necrotizing vasculitis of the gallbladder and the appendix. Similarity in the morphology of rheumatoid arthritis and *Polyarteritis nodosa*. Am J Gastroenterol *67*:608, 1977.
200. LiVolsi VA, Perzin KH, Porter M: Polyarteritis nodosa of the gallbladder, presenting as acute cholecystitis. Gastroenterology *65*:115, 1973.
201. Duffy J, Lidsky MD, Sharp JT, Davis JS, Person DA, Hollinger FB, Min KW: Polyarthritis, polyarteritis and hepatitis B. Medicine *55*:19, 1976.
202. Gocke DJ, Hsu K, Morgan C, Bombardieri S, Lockshin M, Christian CL: Association between polyarteritis and Australia antigen. Lancet *2*:1149, 1970.
203. Blau EB, Morris RF, Yunis EJ: Polyarteritis nodosa in older children. Pediatrics *60*:227, 1977.
204. Halpern M, Citron BP: Necrotizing angiitis associated with drug abuse. Am J Roentgenol *111*:663, 1971.
205. Bron KM, Gajaraj A: Demonstration of hepatic aneurysms in polyarteritis nodosa by arteriography. N Engl J Med *282*:1024, 1970.
206. Herschman A, Blum R, Lee YC: Angiographic findings in polyarteritis nodosa. Report of a case. Radiology *94*:147, 1970.
207. Robins JM, Bookstein JJ: Regressing aneurysms in periarteritis nodosa. A report of 3 cases. Radiology *104*:39, 1972.
208. Alarcón-Segovia D, Ibáñez G, Velázquez-Forero F, Hernández-Ortíz J, Gonzáles-Jiménez Y: Sjögren's syndrome in systemic lupus erythematosus. Clinical and subclinical manifestations. Ann Intern Med *81*:577, 1974.
209. Cummings NA, Schall GL, Asofsky R, Anderson LG, Talal N: Sjögren's syndrome — newer aspects of research, diagnosis, and therapy. Ann Intern Med *75*:937, 1971.
210. Strimlan CV, Rosenow EC III, Divertie MB, Harrison EG Jr: Pulmonary manifestations of Sjögren's syndrome. Chest *70*:354, 1976.
211. Moutsopoulos HM, Webber BL, Vlagopoulos TP, Chused TM, Decker JL: Differences in the clinical manifestations of sicca syndrome in the presence and absence of rheumatoid arthritis. Am J Med *66*:733, 1979.
212. Rubin P, Holt JF: Secretory sialography in diseases of the major salivary glands. Am J Roentgenol *77*:575, 1957.
213. Yune HY, Klatte EC: Current status of sialography. Am J Roentgenol *115*:420, 1972.
214. Barone R, Wallace SL: Abrupt onset of Sjögren's syndrome. Letter to Editor. J Rheumatol *3*:437, 1976.
215. Baruch HH, Firooznia H, Sackler JP, Genieser NB, Rafii H, Golimbu C: Pulmonary disorders associated with Sjögren's syndrome. Rev Interam Radiol *2*:77, 1977.
216. Anderson LG, Talal N: The spectrum of benign to malignant lymphoproliferation in Sjögren's syndrome. Clip Exp Immunol *10*:199, 1972.
217. Faguet GB, Webb HH, Agee JF, Ricks WB, Sharbaugh AH: Immunologically diagnosed malignancy in Sjögren's pseudolymphoma. Am J Med *65*:424, 1978.
218. Talal N, Sokoloff L, Barth WF: Extrasalivary lymphoid abnormalities in Sjögren's syndrome (reticulum cell sarcoma, "pseudolymphoma," macroglobulinemia). Am J Med *43*:50, 1967.
219. Kassan SS, Thomas TL, Moutsopoulos HM, Hoover R, Kimberly RP, Budman DR, Costa J, Decker JL, Chused TM: Increased risk of lymphoma in sicca syndrome. Ann Intern Med *89*:888, 1978.
220. Kyle RA, Bayrd ED: Amyloidosis: Review of 236 cases. Medicine *54*:271, 1975.
221. Brandt K, Cathcart ES, Cohen AS: A clinical analysis of the course and prognosis of forty-two patients with amyloidosis. Am J Med *44*:955, 1968.
222. Ekelund L: Radiologic findings in renal amyloidosis. Am J Roentgenol *129*:851, 1977.
223. McCormick TL, and Cho KJ: Angiographic findings in renal amyloidosis. Am J Roentgenol *129*:855, 1977.
224. Brown J: Case of the spring season. Semin Roentgenol *12*:93, 1977.
225. Gardner KD Jr, Castellino RA, Kempson R, Young BW, Stamey TA: Primary amyloidosis of the renal pelvis. N Engl J Med *284*:1196, 1971.
226. Lee KT, Deeths TM: Localized amyloidosis of the ureter. Radiology *120*:60, 1976.
227. Pear BL: The radiographic manifestations of amyloidosis. Am J Roentgenol *111*:821, 1971.
228. Cohen AS: Amyloidosis. Parts I, II, and III. N Engl J Med *277*:522, 574, 628, 1967.
229. Barth WF, Willerson JT, Waldmann TA, Decker JL: Primary amyloidosis. Clinical, immunochemical and immunoglobulin metabolism studies in 15 patients. Am J Med *47*:259, 1969.
230. Sostre S, Martin ND, Lucas RN, Strauss HW: Scintigraphic findings in primary amyloidosis. An analysis of 7 cases. Radiology *115*:675, 1975.
231. Himmelfarb E, Wells S, Rabinowitz JG: The radiologic spectrum of cardiopulmonary amyloidosis. Chest *72*:327, 1977.
232. Wilson SR, Sanders DE, Delarue NC: Intrathoracic manifestations of amyloid disease. Radiology *120*:283, 1976.
233. Stevens DB, Whitehouse GH: Waldenström's macroglobulinemia with amyloidosis — lymphographic findings. Lymphology *9*:142, 1976.
234. Lewinsohn G, Bruderman I, Bohadana A: Primary diffuse pulmonary amyloidosis with monoclonal gammopathy. Chest *69*:682, 1976.
235. Chang LWN, Grollman JH Jr: Angiocardiographic differentiation of constrictive pericarditis and restrictive cardiomyopathy due to amyloidosis. Am J Roentgenol *130*:451, 1978.
236. Madewell JE, Feigin DS: Benign tumors of the lung. Semin Roentgenol *12*:175, 1977.
237. Poh SC, Tjia TS, Seah CH: Primary diffuse alveolar septal amyloidosis. Thorax *30*:186, 1975.
238. Rubinow A, Celli BR, Cohen AS, Rigden BG, Brody JS: Localized

amyloidosis of the lower respiratory tract. Am Rev Resp Dis *118*:603, 1978.

239. Celli BR, Rubinow A, Cohen AS, Brody JS: Patterns of pulmonary involvement in systemic amyloidosis. Chest *74*:543, 1978.
240. Dahlin DC: Secondary amyloidosis. Ann Intern Med *31*:105, 1949.
241. Symmers WS: Primary amyloidosis: A review. J Clin Pathol *9*:187, 1956.
242. Legge DA, Carlson HC, Wollaeger EE: Roentgenologic appearance of systemic amyloidosis involving gastrointestinal tract. Am J Roentgenol *110*:406, 1970.
243. Seliger G, Krassner RL, Beranbaum ER, Miller F: The spectrum of roentgen appearance in amyloidosis of the small and large bowel: Radiologic-pathologic correlation. Radiology *100*:63, 1971.
244. Marshak RH, Lindner AE: Radiology of the Small Intestine, 2nd Ed. Philadelphia, WB Saunders Co, 1976.
245. Schroeder FM, Miller FJ Jr, Nelson JA, Rankin RS: Gastrointestinal angiographic findings in systemic amyloidosis. Am J Roentgenol *131*:143, 1978.
246. Pandarinath GS, Levine SM, Sorokin JJ, Jacoby JH: Selective massive amyloidosis of the small intestine mimicking multiple tumors. Radiology *129*:609, 1978.
247. Songcharden S, Raju SF, Pennebaker JB: Interstitial lung disease in polymyositis and dermatomyositis. J Rheumatol *7*:353, 1980.
248. Fujioka, M, Bender T, Young LW, Girdany BR: Polyarteritis nodosa in children: Radiological aspects and diagnostic correlation. Radiology *136*:359, 1980.
249. Moutsopoulos HM, Chused TM, Mann DL, et al: Sjögren's syndrome (sicca syndrome): Current Issues. Ann Intern Med *92*:212, 1980.

SECTION XX

SYNOPSIS

THE "TARGET AREA" APPROACH TO ARTICULAR DISORDERS: A SYNOPSIS

by Donald Resnick, M.D.

87

An accurate radiologic diagnosis of joint disease is based upon evaluation of two fundamental parameters: the morphology of the articular lesions and their distribution in the body. Morphologic characteristics vary among the disorders in response to the underlying pathologic aberrations. For example, well known to the radiologist is the appearance of symmetric soft tissue swelling, periarticular osteoporosis, diffuse loss of interosseous space, and marginal and central osseous erosions in the presence of inflamed rheumatoid synovial tissue; of lobulated soft tissue swelling, mild loss of interosseous space, eccentric, well-defined osseous erosions, bony proliferation, and absence of osteoporosis in association with intra-articular and periarticular crystal deposition in gout; of localized joint space diminution, subchondral sclerosis, cyst formation, and osteophytosis in conjunction with altered stress across an articulation in degenerative joint disease; and of poorly defined osseous destruction in the infected articulation.

Equally important in the interpretation of the radiographs is the evaluation of the distribution of articular lesions. There is a remarkable proclivity of certain disorders to affect specific joints (and regions of those joints), which is largely unexplained, but it is this very characteristic that provides an important clue as to the nature of the underlying condition. Radiographic analysis of the distribution of articular lesions is termed the "target area" approach. The basic rules for this analysis in extraspinal locations are summarized in this chapter, but they must be interpreted cautiously with full knowledge of certain restrictions that prevent an overly enthusiastic or rigorous application of these rules to all cases of articular disease. For example, although a specific disorder may characteristically appear in one or two sites with relative sparing of other locations, one should *never* say that the condition *never* affects these other sites because, almost invariably, such a statement will lead to error. The "target area" approach dictates locations that are predominantly involved in a disease process, not those that are exclusively involved. If the radiographs are surveyed and the sites of more significant disease are recorded, the pattern of distribution when coupled with the morphology of the lesions assures a confident and precise diagnosis in most patients with articular disease.

HAND

The articulations of the hand consist of the distal interphalangeal, proximal interphalangeal, and metacarpophalangeal joints of the second to fifth digits and the metacarpophalangeal and interphalangeal joints of the thumb (Fig. 87–1). In many respects, the latter joint resembles a proximal interphalangeal articulation in that many disorders leading to osseous and cartilaginous destruction of proximal interphalangeal joints (e.g., rheumatoid arthritis) may also involve the interphalangeal articulation of the thumb.

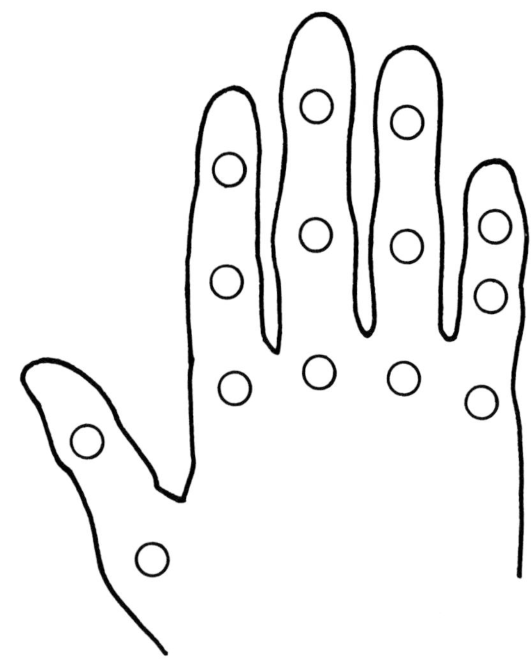

Figure 87–1. *Articulations of the hand.*

Rheumatoid Arthritis (Fig. 87–2)

Both hands are affected in a relatively symmetric fashion. Major alterations appear in all five metacarpophalangeal joints, the proximal interphalangeal articulations, and the interphalangeal joint of the thumb. Abnormalities in the distal interphalangeal articulations are infrequent and mild and, when present and severe, may indicate a second process (e.g., degenerative joint disease or psoriatic arthritis). The earliest changes are most frequently apparent in the second and third metacarpophalangeal joints and the third proximal interphalangeal joint. Fusiform soft tissue swelling, regional osteoporosis, diffuse loss of interosseous space, and marginal and central bony erosions are the observed findings.

Juvenile Chronic Arthritis (Fig. 87–3)

A symmetric or asymmetric distribution can be evident. As opposed to adult-onset rheumatoid arthritis, juvenile chronic arthritis can affect any articulation of the hand, including the distal interphalangeal joints, and its exact pattern is influenced by the specific type of disease that is present (juvenile-onset adult type rheumatoid arthritis, Still's disease,

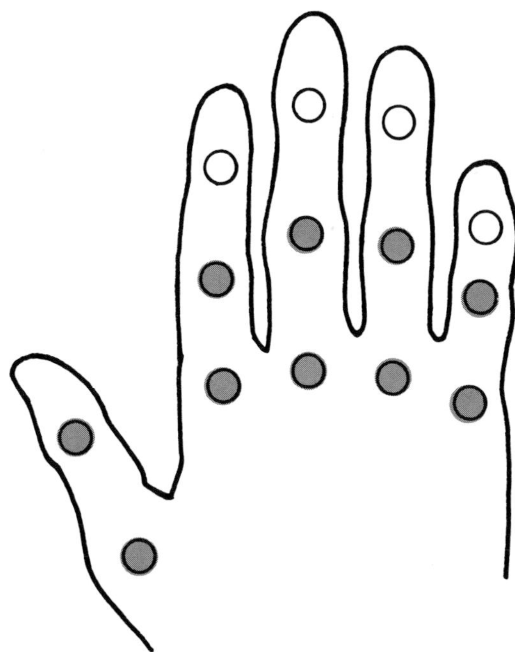

Figure 87–2. *Rheumatoid arthritis.*

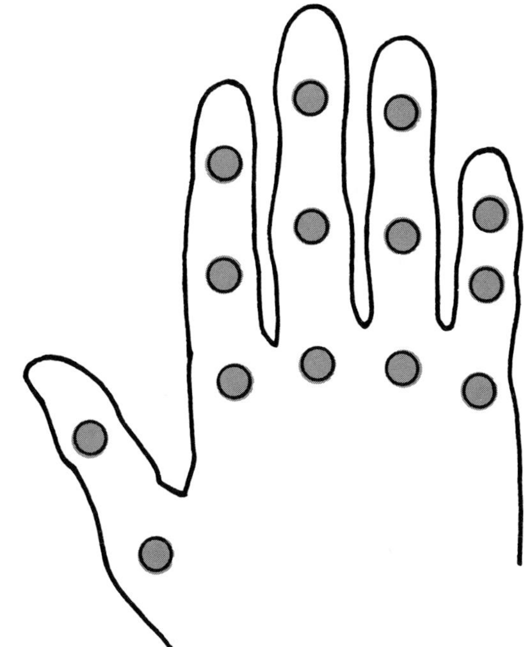

Figure 87–4. *Ankylosing spondylitis.*

and so forth). The degree of osteoporosis, joint space narrowing, and osseous erosion is variable, and bony proliferation (periostitis and intra-articular fusion) may be a prominent finding.

Ankylosing Spondylitis (Fig. 87–4)

Bilateral and asymmetric findings predominate. Distal interphalangeal, proximal interphalangeal, and metacarpophalangeal joints as well as the interphalangeal articulation of the thumb can be affected, although the findings in the distal interphalangeal articulations are generally less marked than in more proximal locations. Osteoporosis, joint space diminution, osseous erosions, and deformities are less striking in this disease than in rheumatoid arthritis. Osseous proliferation can be exuberant.

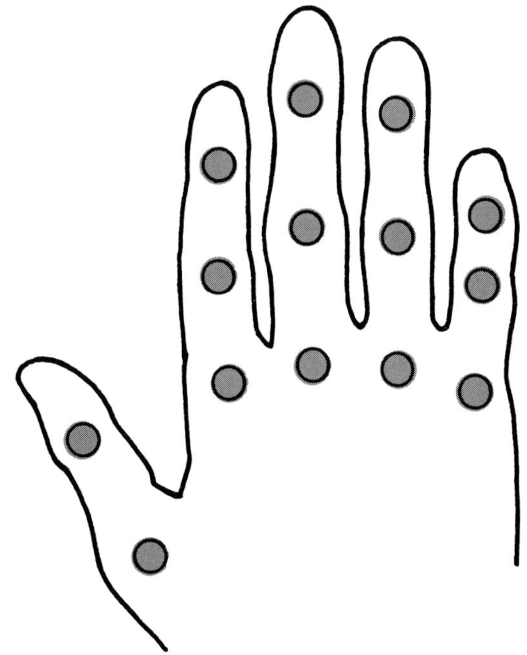

Figure 87–3. *Juvenile chronic arthritis.*

Psoriatic Arthritis (Fig. 87–5)

The distribution of this disease is widely variable. Bilateral asymmetric polyarticular changes are most characteristic, with predilection for the interphalangeal articulations. In many patients, the extent of distal interphalangeal joint abnormalities is striking and, when proximal interphalangeal and metacarpophalangeal articular changes are also present, a characteristic picture is produced. Osteoporosis may be absent and intra-articular osseous fusion and periarticular osseous excrescences can be evident, allowing differentiation from rheumatoid arthritis. In other psoriatic individuals, however, a symmetric polyarthritis can be identical to rheumatoid arthritis in its distribution.

Reiter's Syndrome (Fig. 87–6)

Asymmetric changes are most typical. Monoarticular or pauciarticular disease can affect any articulation of the hand, including the distal interphalangeal joints. Its features are virtually identical to those

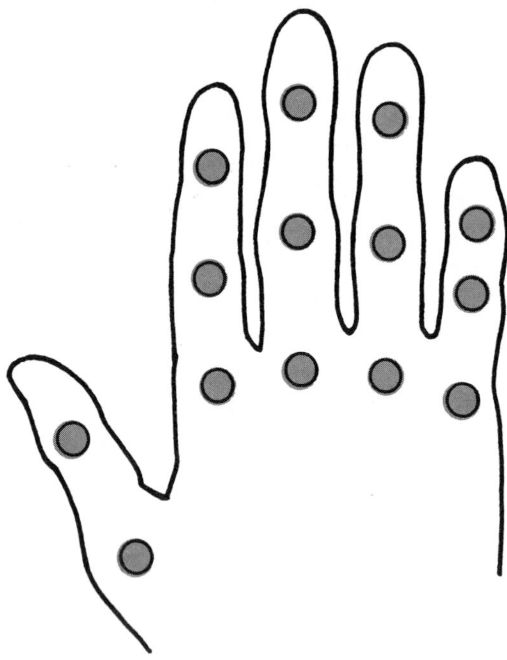

Figure 87–5. Psoriatic arthritis.

of psoriatic arthritis or ankylosing spondylitis, with lack of osteoporosis and presence of exuberant periostitis. Intra-articular osseous fusion and prominent soft tissue swelling (sausage digit) can also be noted.

Degenerative Joint Disease (Osteoarthritis) (Fig. 87–7)

Bilateral, symmetric, or asymmetric findings can be observed. Distal interphalangeal and proximal interphalangeal articulations are generally affected to a greater degree than metacarpophalangeal joints, although joint space narrowing is not infrequent at the latter location. Isolated abnormalities may appear at the distal interphalangeal or proximal interphalangeal joints, but changes are rarely isolated to the metacarpophalangeal joints. In interphalangeal articulations, loss of interosseous space, subchondral eburnation, marginal osteophytes, and small ossicles appear.

Inflammatory (Erosive) Osteoarthritis (Fig. 87–8)

A bilateral, symmetric, or asymmetric distribution is encountered. The distribution of this disorder is similar to that in nonerosive osteoarthritis, with distal interphalangeal and proximal interphalangeal joint abnormalities predominating over metacarpophalangeal joint changes. The morphologic aspects of the alterations can be indistinguishable from noninflammatory osteoarthritis, although the presence of centrally located osseous defects in combination with osteophytosis allows this specific diagnosis to be made.

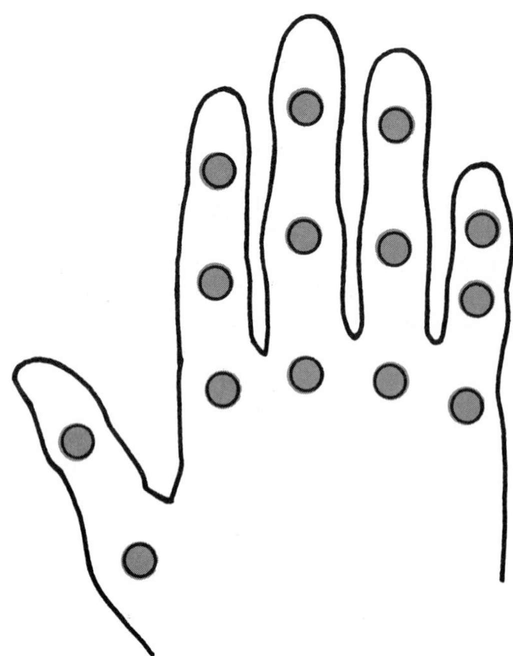

Figure 87–6. Reiter's syndrome.

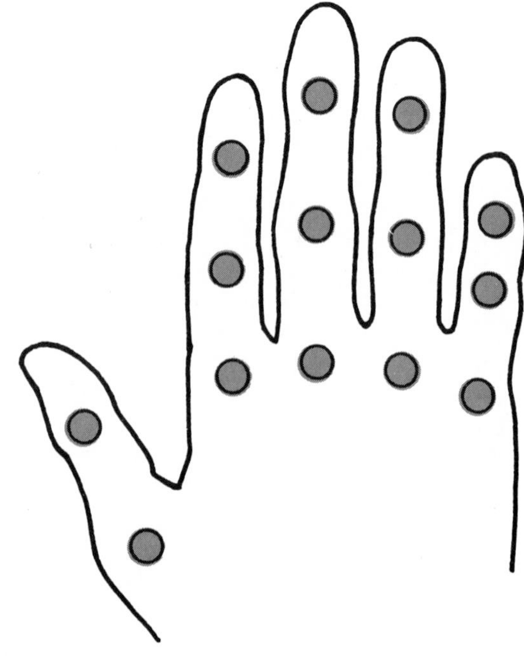

Figure 87–7. Degenerative joint disease (osteoarthritis).

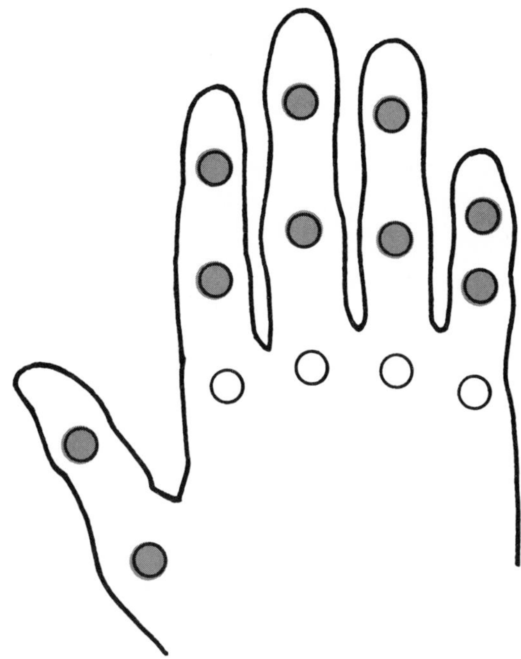

Figure 87–8. Inflammatory (erosive) osteoarthritis.

Systemic Lupus Erythematosus (Fig. 87–9)

A deforming, nonerosive arthropathy with a bilateral and symmetric distribution affecting metacarpophalangeal and interphalangeal articulations of all of the digits including the thumb characterizes one type of joint abnormality in this disease. Osteonecrosis at one or more metacarpophalangeal articulations is a second pattern of articular disease in systemic lupus erythematosus. Finally, some patients reveal a rheumatoid arthritis–like condition and may, in fact, have coexistent rheumatoid arthritis, mixed connective tissue disease, or an "overlap" syndrome.

Scleroderma and Polymyositis (Fig. 87–10)

A bilateral erosive arthritis showing predilection for the distal interphalangeal and, to a lesser extent, the proximal interphalangeal joints has been observed in some patients with scleroderma. Features may resemble psoriatic arthritis or inflammatory (erosive) osteoarthritis. A similar pattern of joint disease is rarely encountered in patients with polymyositis. In both of these diseases, more characteristic findings, such as soft tissue calcification and tuftal resorption, are usually evident.

Gouty Arthritis (Fig. 87–11)

A bilateral and asymmetric process predominates. Changes may appear in distal interphalangeal, proximal interphalangeal, or metacarpophalangeal joints, consisting of lobulated soft tissue masses, eccentric intra- and extra-articular osseous erosions, preservation of joint space, proliferation of bone

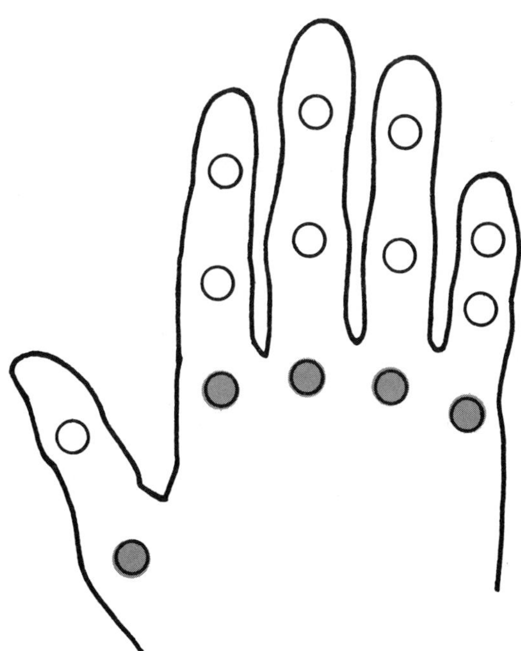

Figure 87–9. Systemic lupus erythematosus.

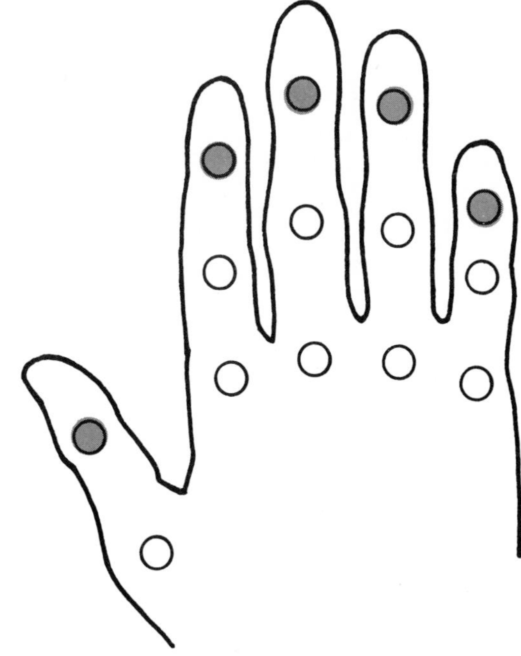

Figure 87–10. Scleroderma and polymyositis.

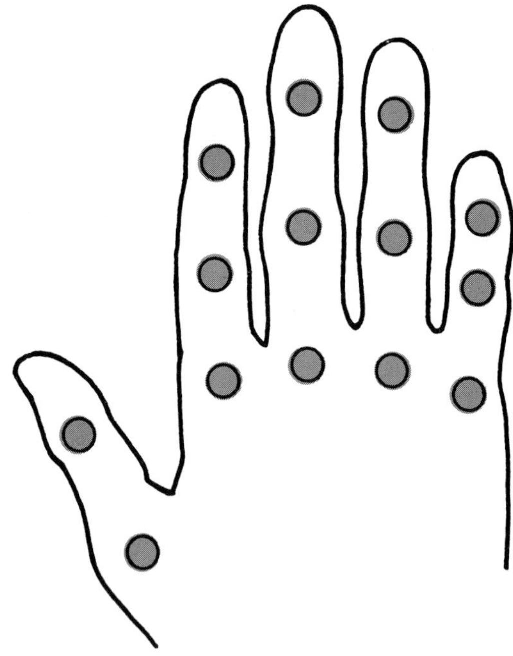

Figure 87–11. Gouty arthritis.

("mushrooming" or "overhanging edges"), and lack of osteoporosis.

Calcium Pyrophosphate Dihydrate Crystal Deposition Disease (Fig. 87–12)

Idiopathic calcium pyrophosphate dihydrate crystal deposition disease or that associated with hemochromatosis produces bilateral, relatively symmetric changes that predominate at the metacarpophalangeal articulations. Although findings may also be evident at distal interphalangeal and proximal interphalangeal joints, they are not specific and generally are mild in comparison with those of the metacarpophalangeal joints. The latter findings may resemble degenerative joint disease, but their isolation to the metacarpophalangeal articulations and the possible presence of intra-articular or periarticular calcification allow an accurate diagnosis.

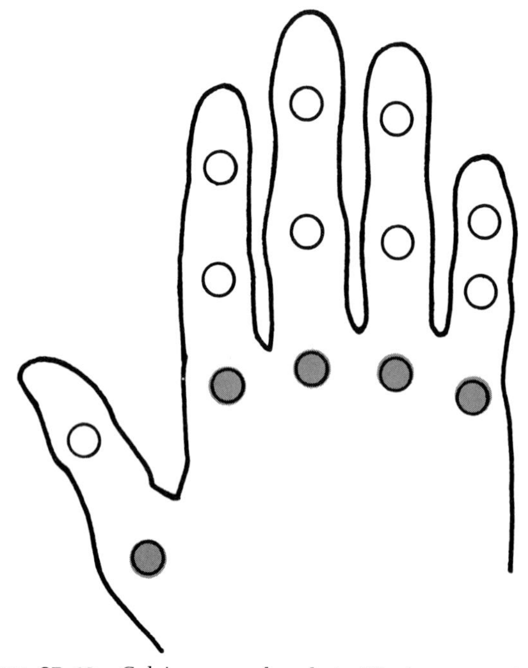

Figure 87–12. Calcium pyrophosphate dihydrate crystal deposition disease.

Other Diseases

Multicentric reticulohistiocytosis can lead to significant abnormalities of both hands that usually are most striking in the distal interphalangeal and, to a lesser extent, the proximal interphalangeal articulations. *Thermal injuries,* including frostbite and burns, may produce alterations that also predominate in distal locations. *Hyperparathyroidism* (and renal osteodystrophy) can lead to a peculiar "erosive" arthritis of the digits that affects distal interphalangeal, proximal interphalangeal, or metacarpophalangeal articulations of both hands. In most cases, the changes, which relate to subchondral resorption of bone, are combined with more widely recognized abnormalities, particularly subperiosteal resorption along the radial aspect of the proximal and middle phalanges and in the terminal tufts. In *rheumatic fever,* a deforming, nonerosive arthropathy (Jaccoud's arthropathy) predominates in the fourth and fifth digits. At this site, ulnar deviation of the metacarpophalangeal articulations may be associated with deformity of the proximal interphalangeal or distal interphalangeal articulations. *Septic arthritis* of the metacarpophalangeal joints may follow a fist fight in which the fist, when striking the opponent's teeth, is cut, allowing direct access of organisms into the joint cavity.

WRIST

The major joints or compartments of the wrist are the radiocarpal (between the distal radius and proximal carpal row), midcarpal (between the distal and proximal carpal rows), common carpometacarpal (between the distal carpal row and the bases of the four ulnar metacarpals), first carpometacarpal (between the trapezium and base of the first metacarpal), inferior radioulnar (between the distal radius and distal ulna, separated from the radiocarpal compartment by the triangular fibrocartilage of the wrist), and pisiform-triquetral (between the pisiform and triquetrum) compartments (Fig. 87–13).

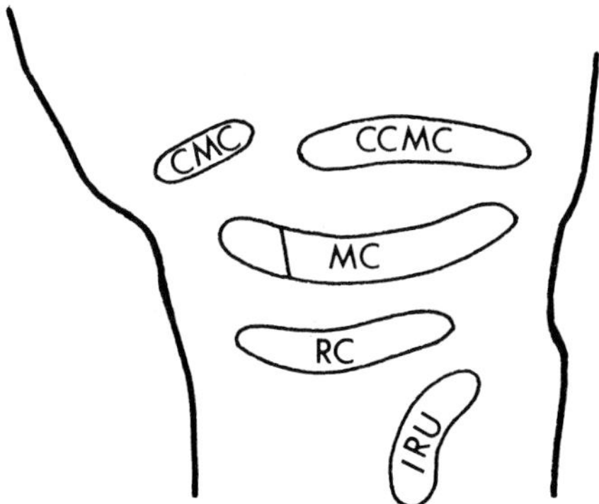

Figure 87–13. Articulations of the wrist. RC, Radiocarpal compartment; IRU, inferior radioulnar compartment; MC, midcarpal compartment; CCMC, common carpometacarpal compartment; CMC, first carpometacarpal compartment. The pisiform-triquetral compartment is not shown. The trapezioscaphoid region of the midcarpal joint is separated by a vertical line from the remainder of this joint.

Rheumatoid Arthritis (Fig. 87–14)

A bilateral and symmetric process is usually evident. Initial abnormalities predominate in the radiocarpal, inferior radioulnar, and pisiform-triquetral compartments and are associated with tenosynovitis, especially in the sheath of the extensor carpi ulnaris tendon. There is often simultaneous involvement of the midcarpal and common carpometacarpal compartments. It is unusual to note extensive changes in the radiocarpal, inferior radioulnar, and pisiform-triquetral compartments without the others being affected to some degree. Thus, early in the course of the disease, all the compartments of the wrist are affected. Above all else, this pancompartmental distribution is an important characteristic of the wrist involvement in rheumatoid arthritis.

Juvenile Chronic Arthritis (Fig. 87–15)

The pattern of wrist involvement is variable. In some forms of juvenile chronic arthritis, all the

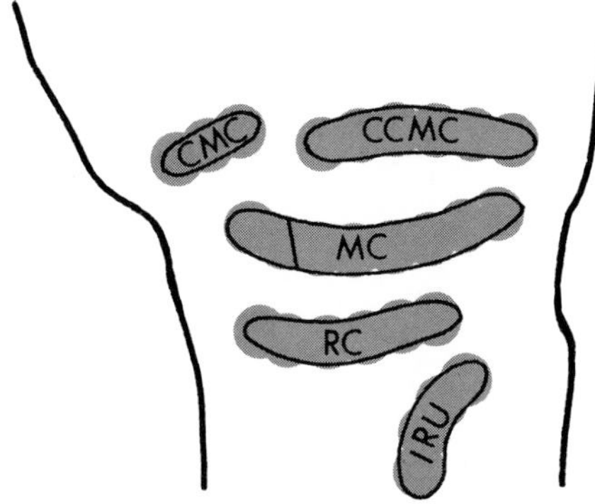

Figure 87–14. Rheumatoid arthritis.

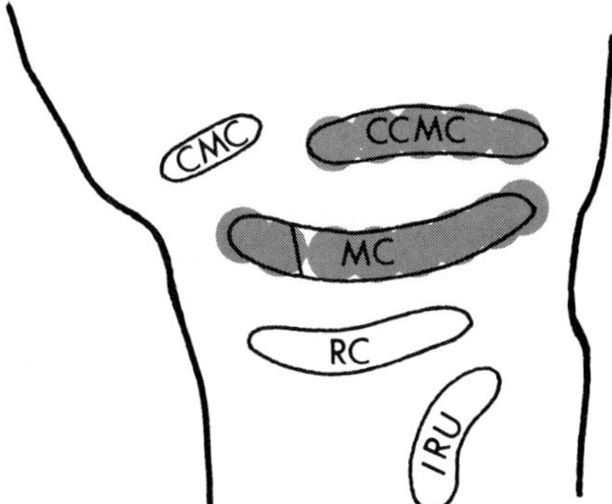

Figure 87–15. Juvenile chronic arthritis.

carpal bones migrate toward the bases of the metacarpals, reflecting joint space loss in the midcarpal and common carpometacarpal compartments. In fact, eventual osseous fusion of the proximal and distal carpal rows and bases of the four ulnar metacarpals may be seen, with relative sparing of the first carpometacarpal and radiocarpal compartments. A similar pattern of disease may be apparent in some patients with adult-onset Still's disease.

Ankylosing Spondylitis, Psoriatic Arthritis, and Reiter's Syndrome (Fig. 87–16)

Asymmetric findings in the wrist can appear during the course of any of these three disorders. Pancompartmental changes, especially in psoriatic arthritis and ankylosing spondylitis, can be seen. Although similar to rheumatoid arthritis, these disorders are associated with less frequent and extensive wrist disease, the absence of osteoporosis, and the presence of ill-defined osseous excrescences or "whiskers."

Degenerative Joint Disease (Osteoarthritis) (Fig. 87–17)

In the absence of significant accidental or occupational trauma, degenerative joint disease of the wrist is virtually limited to the first carpometacarpal and trapezioscaphoid areas. One or both wrists may be involved, and findings can be isolated to or predominate in either one of these two sites. At the first carpometacarpal joint, radial subluxation of the metacarpal base can be evident, whereas at the trapezioscaphoid area of the midcarpal compartment, joint space narrowing and eburnation may be the only findings.

In the presence of occupational or accidental trauma, more widespread alterations of the wrist may be detected. Thus, abnormalities of the radiocarpal and midcarpal compartments can follow a

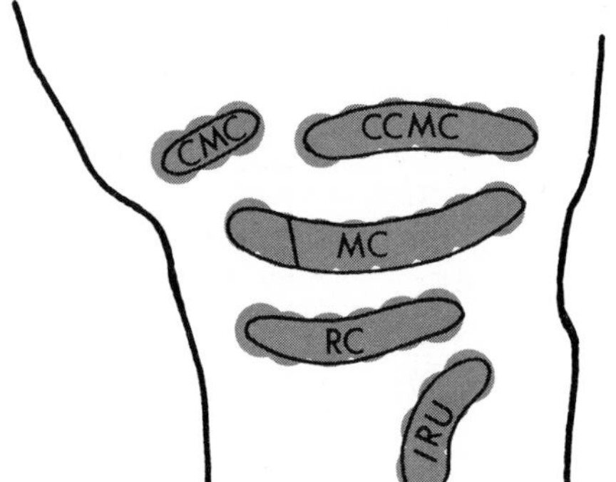

Figure 87–16. Ankylosing spondylitis, psoriatic arthritis, and Reiter's syndrome.

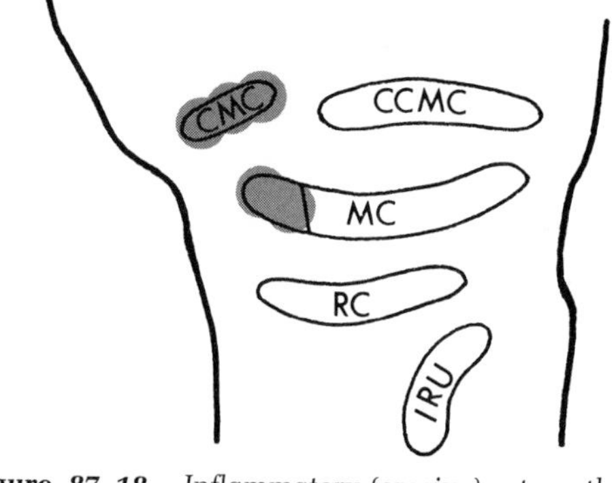

Figure 87–18. Inflammatory (erosive) osteoarthritis.

scaphoid fracture or Kienböck's disease, changes at the inferior radioulnar compartment can appear after a subluxation or dislocation about the distal ulna, and abnormalities of the radiocarpal and midcarpal areas can be observed in pneumatic tool operators or professional athletes.

Inflammatory (Erosive) Osteoarthritis (Fig. 87–18)

A bilateral symmetric or asymmetric appearance can be noted. Changes predominate along the radial aspect of the wrist at the first carpometacarpal and trapezioscaphoid areas, a distribution identical to that in noninflammatory osteoarthritis. At these sites, joint space narrowing and eburnation predominate, although, rarely, erosive abnormalities may be detected. More widespread involvement of the wrist in this condition, particularly when the radiocarpal or inferior radioulnar compartment, or both, are altered, may indicate the superimposition of rheumatoid arthritis or a crystal-induced arthropathy.

Scleroderma (Fig. 87–19)

Selective involvement of one or both first carpometacarpal and inferior radioulnar compartments has been noted in some patients with scleroderma. The changes at the first carpometacarpal articulations consist of scalloped erosions of the base of the metacarpal and adjacent trapezium and may relate to mechanical attrition caused by radial and proximal subluxation of the metacarpal. In fact, similar alterations of the first carpometacarpal joint can be encountered in other diseases in which tendinous and muscular imbalances are apparent, such as systemic lupus erythematosus, polymyositis, and Ehlers-Danlos syndrome. In scleroderma, intra-articular and periarticular calcification can frequently be observed about the altered articulation.

The involvement of the inferior radioulnar compartment in scleroderma consists of soft tissue swelling and erosion of the distal ulna.

Gouty Arthritis (Fig. 87–20)

In long-standing gouty arthritis, bilateral symmetric or asymmetric changes can be observed in the wrist. A pancompartmental distribution, similar to that in rheumatoid arthritis, may be apparent. Of diagnostic significance, the common carpometacarpal compartment may be the site of the most extensive abnormality in this disease. At this site, scal-

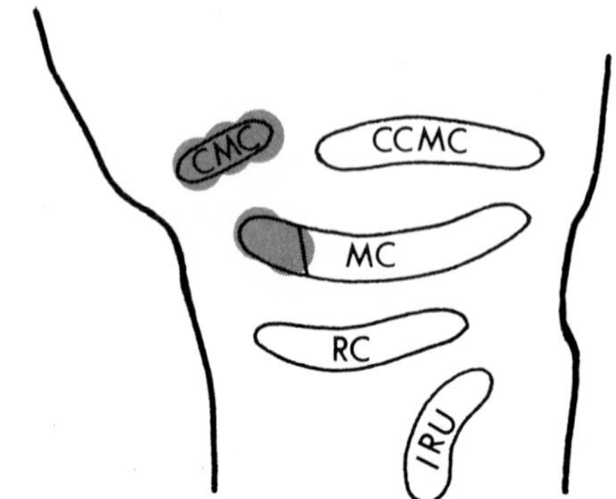

Figure 87–17. Degenerative joint disease (osteoarthritis).

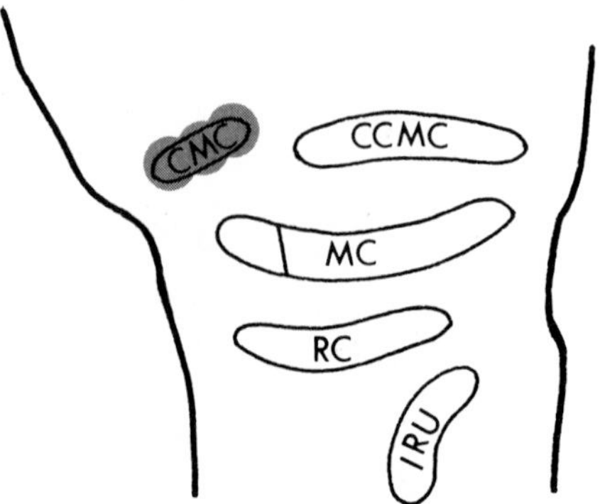

Figure 87–19. Scleroderma.

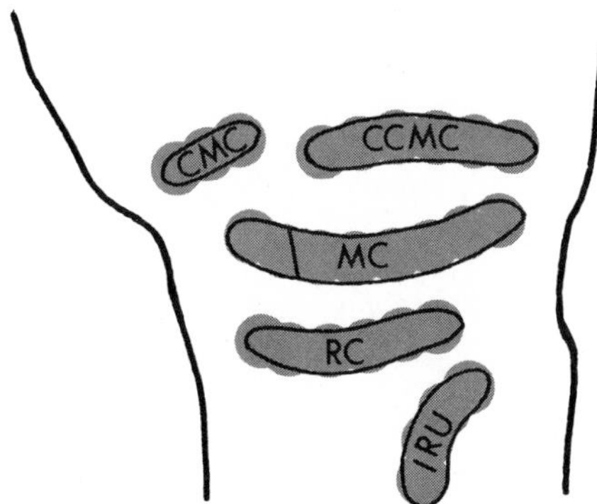

Figure 87–20. Gouty arthritis.

loped erosions of the bases of one or more of the four ulnar metacarpals are seen. Additional findings, such as the absence of osteoporosis and the presence of eccentric erosions with sclerotic margins, lobulated soft tissue masses, and preservation of joint space, also aid in the differentiation of gouty arthritis from rheumatoid arthritis.

Calcium Pyrophosphate Dihydrate Crystal Deposition Disease (Fig. 87–21)

This disorder leads to bilateral symmetric or asymmetric changes that reveal distinct predilection for the radiocarpal compartment of the wrist. At this site, extensive narrowing or obliteration of the space between the distal radius and scaphoid may be combined with sclerosis and fragmentation of apposing osseous surfaces, "incorporation" of the scaphoid into the articular surface of the distal radius, prominent cysts, and calcifications, especially of the triangular fibrocartilage. Elsewhere in the wrist, severe involvement of the trapezioscaphoid area of the midcarpal compartment and the first carpometacarpal compartment may be apparent. The inferior radioulnar compartment is relatively spared, although the progressive narrowing of the radiocarpal area may eventually lead to sclerosis of apposing portions of ulna and triquetrum.

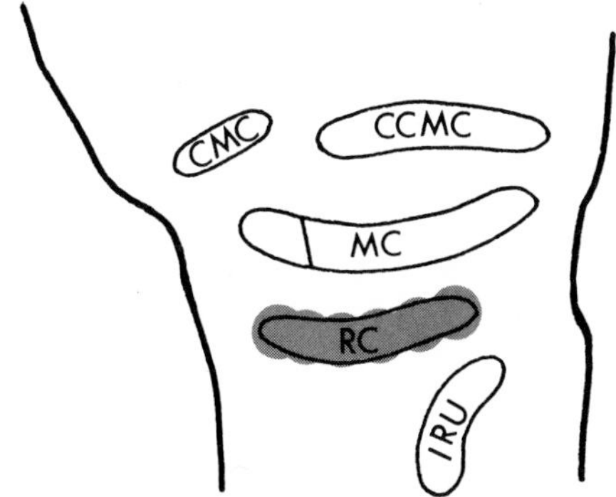

Figure 87–21. Calcium pyrophosphate dihydrate crystal deposition disease.

Other Diseases

Septic arthritis of the wrist, due to bacterial, mycobacterial, or fungal agents, leads to monoarticular disease. Although initially one compartment may be involved, pancompartmental disease is the rule in neglected infection. *Amyloidosis* can also affect one or both wrists. In this disease, localization to the inferior radioulnar compartment is not unusual. A peculiar variety of *osteolysis,* appearing in young individuals, can lead to progressive involvement of the carpus and tarsus. The resulting radiographic abnormalities may resemble those in juvenile chronic arthritis.

FOREFOOT

The articulations of the forefoot include the distal interphalangeal, proximal interphalangeal, and metatarsophalangeal articulations of the second to fifth digits and the interphalangeal and metatarsophalangeal articulations of the great toe (Fig. 87–22).

Rheumatoid Arthritis (Fig. 87–23)

A bilateral and symmetric process of the forefoot represents one of the earliest and most frequent

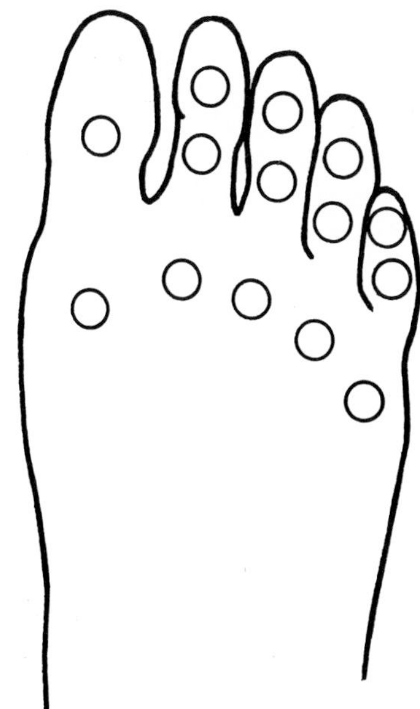
Figure 87–22. Articulations of the forefoot.

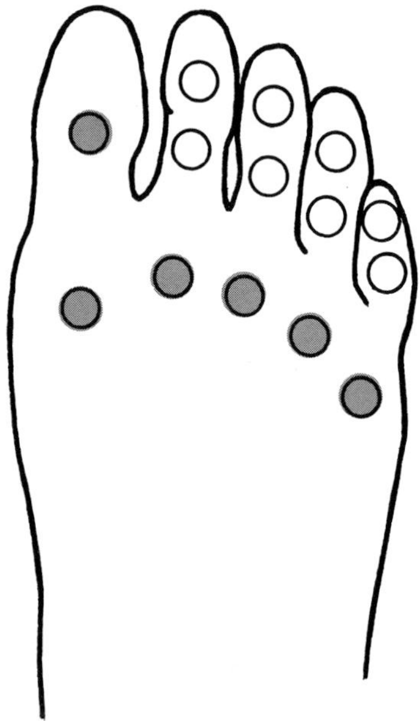

Figure 87–23. Rheumatoid arthritis.

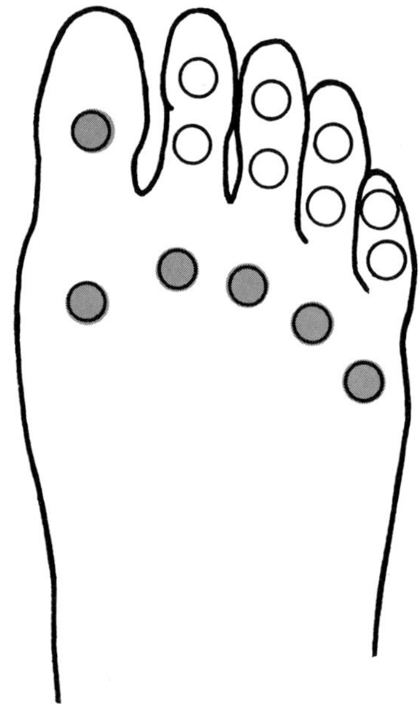

Figure 87–24. Ankylosing spondylitis.

radiographic findings in rheumatoid arthritis. Typically, the predominant changes occur at one or more metatarsophalangeal articulations and the interphalangeal joint of the great toe. Significant involvement of the proximal interphalangeal and distal interphalangeal articulations of the second to fifth toes is infrequent. At the metatarsophalangeal joints, abnormalities are most commonly encountered on the medial aspect of the metatarsal heads of the second to fifth digits and on the medial and lateral aspects of the metatarsal head of the fifth digit. In fact, the earliest radiographic sign of the disease may be a defect on the lateral aspect of the fifth metatarsal head. At the interphalangeal joint of the great toe, a typical erosion appears on the medial aspect of the distal portion of the proximal phalanx. Changes on the lateral aspect of this articulation are less frequent and less extensive; furthermore, widespread intra-articular destruction at this location is less common in rheumatoid arthritis than in psoriatic arthritis, Reiter's syndrome, or gouty arthritis.

Ankylosing Spondylitis, Psoriatic Arthritis, and Reiter's Syndrome (Figs. 87–24 and 87–25)

In ankylosing spondylitis, symmetric or asymmetric abnormalities may appear at the metatarsophalangeal articulations and the interphalangeal joint of the great toe. Findings in the proximal interphalangeal and distal interphalangeal joints of the second to fifth toes are infrequent and mild.

Psoriatic arthritis can be associated with a bilateral symmetric or asymmetric or unilateral process leading to considerable abnormalities of the forefoot. The most severe changes are commonly seen at the metatarsophalangeal articulations and the interphalangeal joint of the great toe. At the latter site, the degree of osseous destruction is greater in this disease than in any other articular disorder. Prominent erosions and intra-articular osseous fusion can be evident at other interphalangeal joints as well. In this fashion, the distribution of changes in psoriatic arthritis differs from that in rheumatoid arthritis.

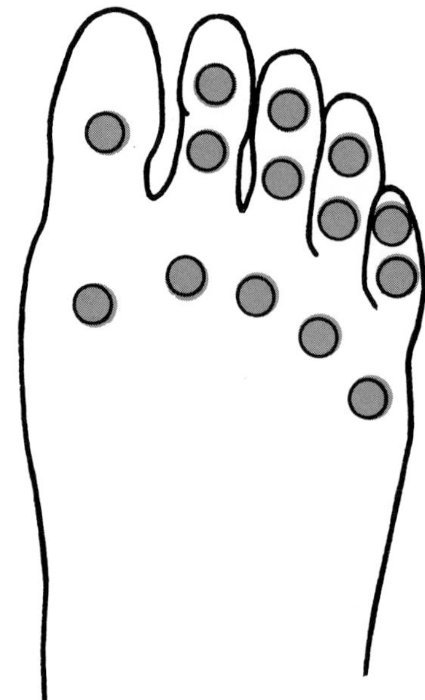

Figure 87–25. Psoriatic arthritis and Reiter's syndrome.

Asymmetric or unilateral abnormalities of the forefoot are frequent in Reiter's syndrome. Fewer articulations are affected in this disorder than in rheumatoid arthritis or psoriatic arthritis. However, any joint of the forefoot is a potential site of abnormality, including the distal interphalangeal, proximal interphalangeal, and metatarsophalangeal joints. Selective involvement of the interphalangeal articulation of the great toe can be encountered, similar to that seen in psoriatic arthritis.

Degenerative Joint Disease (Osteoarthritis) (Fig. 87–26)

Of all the joints of the forefoot, it is the first metatarsophalangeal articulation that is most frequently affected in degenerative joint disease. A unilateral or bilateral distribution can be evident, and changes include loss of interosseous space, eburnation, osteophytosis, and even hallux valgus deformity.

Gouty Arthritis (Fig. 87–27)

Bilateral symmetric or asymmetric changes in gouty arthritis can appear in any joint of the forefoot. The characteristic distribution includes the first metatarsophalangeal joint and, to a lesser degree, the interphalangeal articulation of the great toe. However, prominent changes about other metatarsophalangeal and interphalangeal articulations are not infrequent. At any involved site, a large soft tissue mass commonly indicates the presence of a tophus.

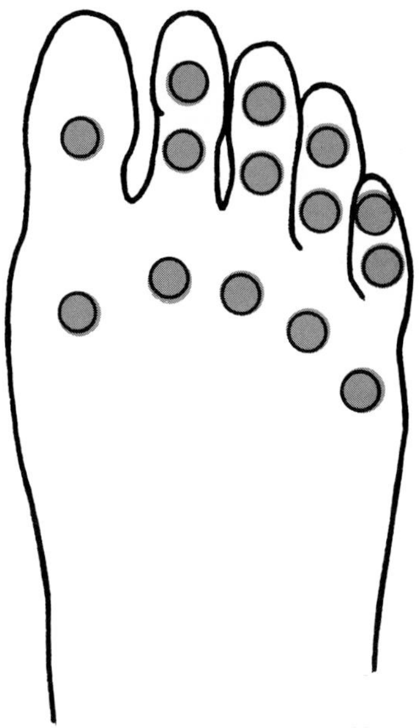

Figure 87–27. Gouty arthritis.

Neuroarthropathy (Fig. 87–28)

Neuropathic joint disease, particularly in diabetic patients, frequently affects the forefoot in a bilateral distribution. Metatarsophalangeal joint abnormalities predominate, although with progressive disease a great degree of phalangeal absorption can be evident. Other causes of neuroarthropathy, such as leprosy and alcoholism, can occasionally produce a similar pattern of disease.

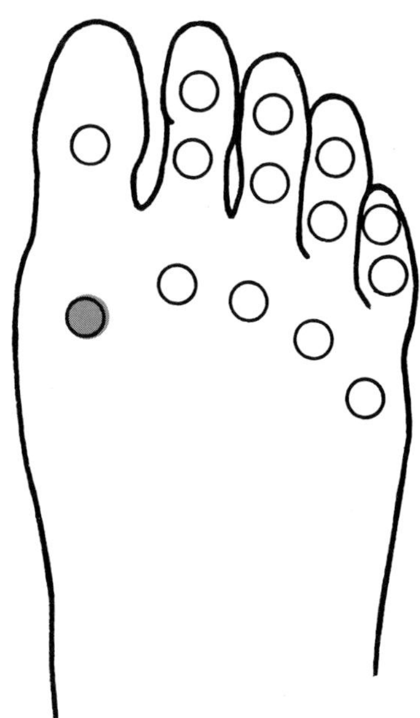

Figure 87–26. Degenerative joint disease (osteoarthritis).

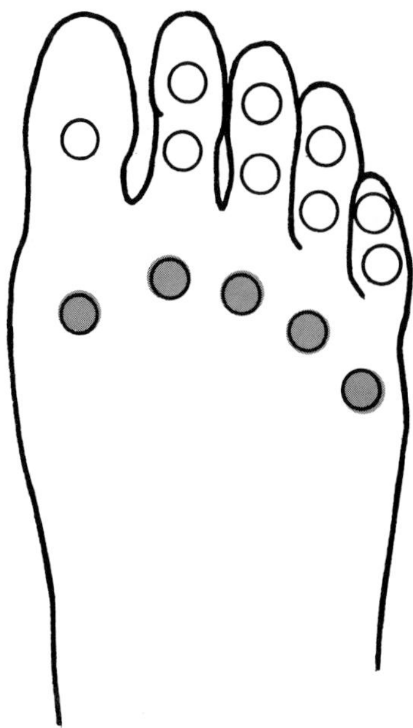

Figure 87–28. Neuroarthropathy.

Other Diseases

Infrequently, metatarsophalangeal joint abnormalities may be seen in *calcium pyrophosphate dihydrate crystal deposition disease, scleroderma, systemic lupus erythematosus,* and *Jaccoud's arthropathy.* Other findings usually assure accurate diagnosis in these cases. Similarly, *infectious processes* of the foot not infrequently follow diabetes mellitus and local puncture wounds.

MIDFOOT

The major articulations of the midfoot are the "posterior" subtalar, talocalcaneonavicular, calcaneocuboid, cuneonavicular, cuneocuboid, and medial, intermediate, and lateral tarsometatarsal joints (Fig. 87–29). Some of these joints communicate with each other and others are separated by only weak intervening connective tissues. They are best observed on the oblique rather than the anteroposterior view of the foot.

Rheumatoid Arthritis (Fig. 87–30)

As in the wrist, rheumatoid arthritis frequently affects all the compartments or articulations of the midfoot, commonly in association with changes at the metatarsophalangeal joints. Bilateral and symmetric abnormalities predominate. The most typical sites of involvement are the talonavicular portion of the talocalcaneonavicular joint, the tarsometatarsal joints, and the "posterior" subtalar joint. The changes become more extensive in long-standing disease. Initial abnormalities consist of superficial osseous erosions and diffuse joint space narrowing. These may eventually progress to the extent that the tarsus becomes a single ossified mass.

Juvenile Chronic Arthritis (Fig. 87–31)

Any of the articulations of the midfoot can be affected in this disease. Bony ankylosis of the tarsal bones and bases of the metatarsals of both feet may eventually be encountered.

Degenerative Joint Disease (Osteoarthritis) (Fig. 87–32)

Abnormalities of the first tarsometatarsal articulation in one or both feet represent the most typical pattern of degenerative joint disease in the midfoot. The findings, consisting of joint space narrowing, sclerosis, and osteophytosis, can simulate those of gout. Following injury, alterations at other tarsometatarsal or intertarsal joints may be apparent.

Gouty Arthritis (Fig. 87–33)

Although any of the compartments of the midfoot can be affected, predilection for the tarsometatarsal articulations exists. A bilateral symmetric or

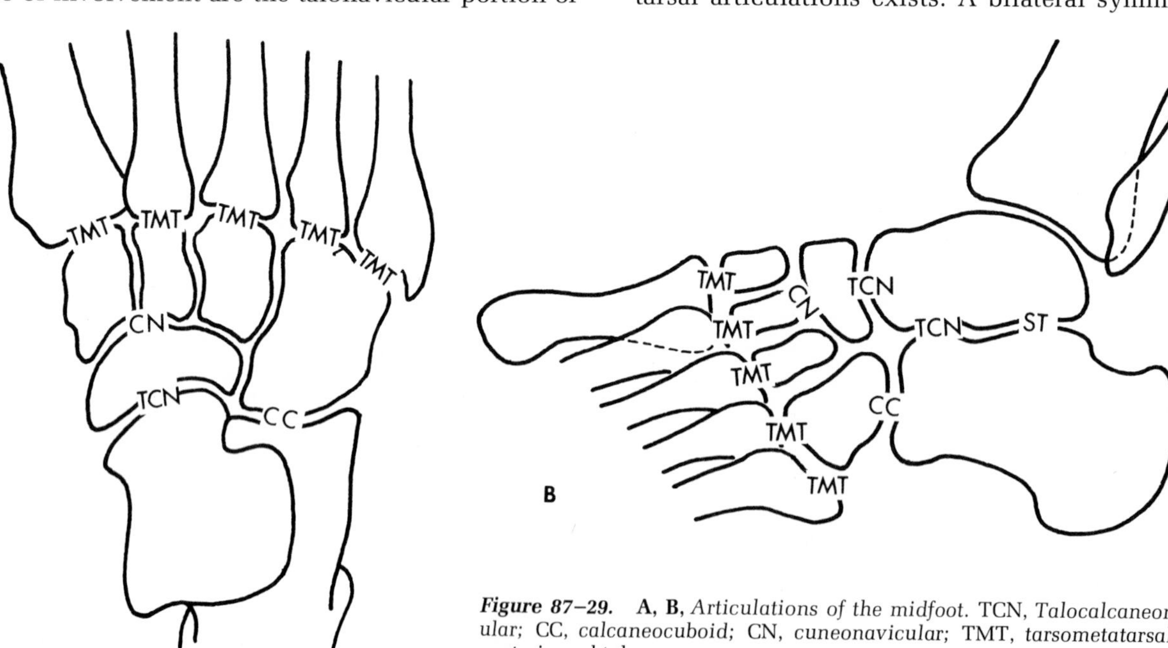

Figure 87–29. **A, B,** *Articulations of the midfoot.* TCN, *Talocalcaneonavicular;* CC, *calcaneocuboid;* CN, *cuneonavicular;* TMT, *tarsometatarsal;* ST, *posterior subtalar.*

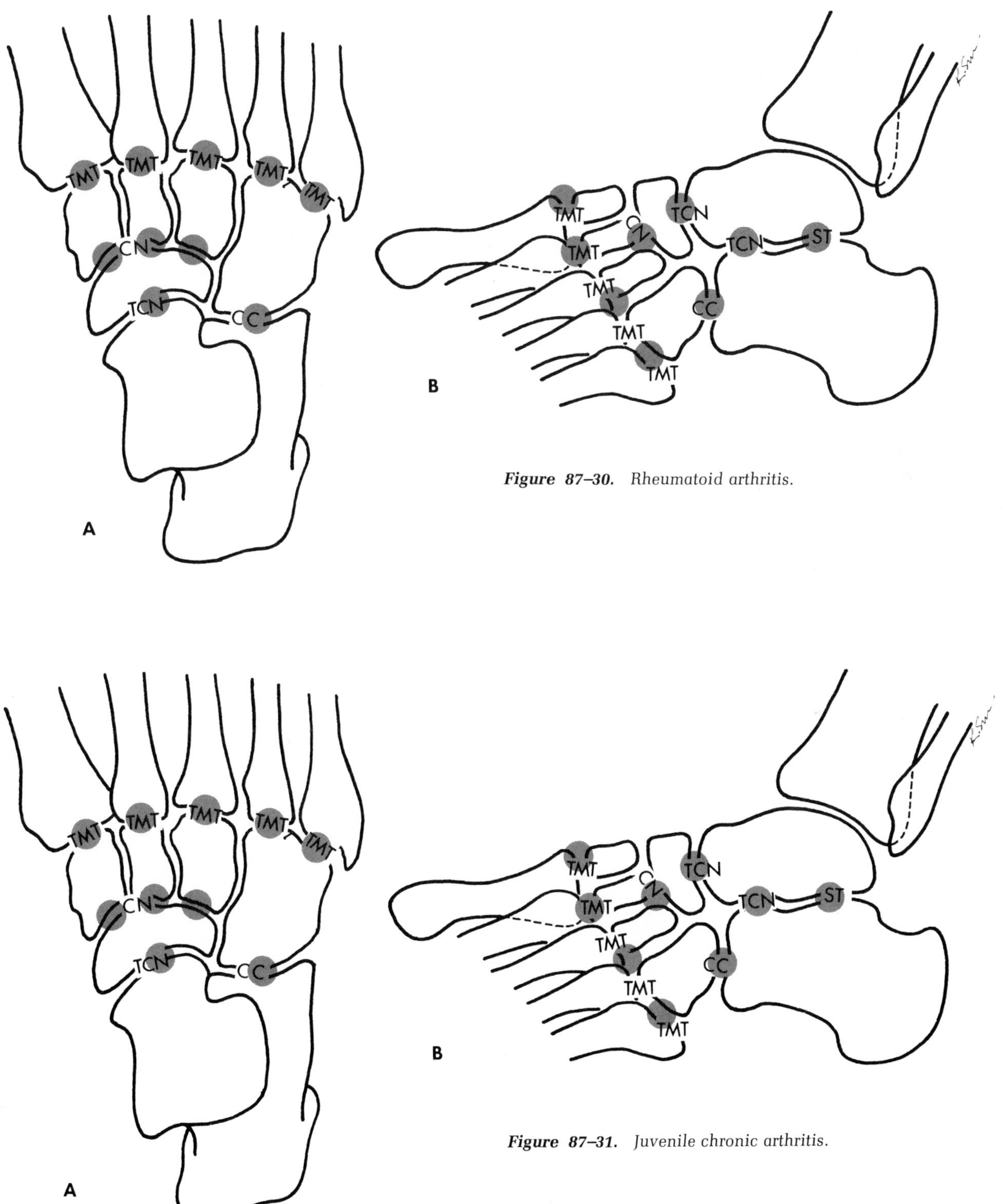

Figure 87–30. *Rheumatoid arthritis.*

Figure 87–31. *Juvenile chronic arthritis.*

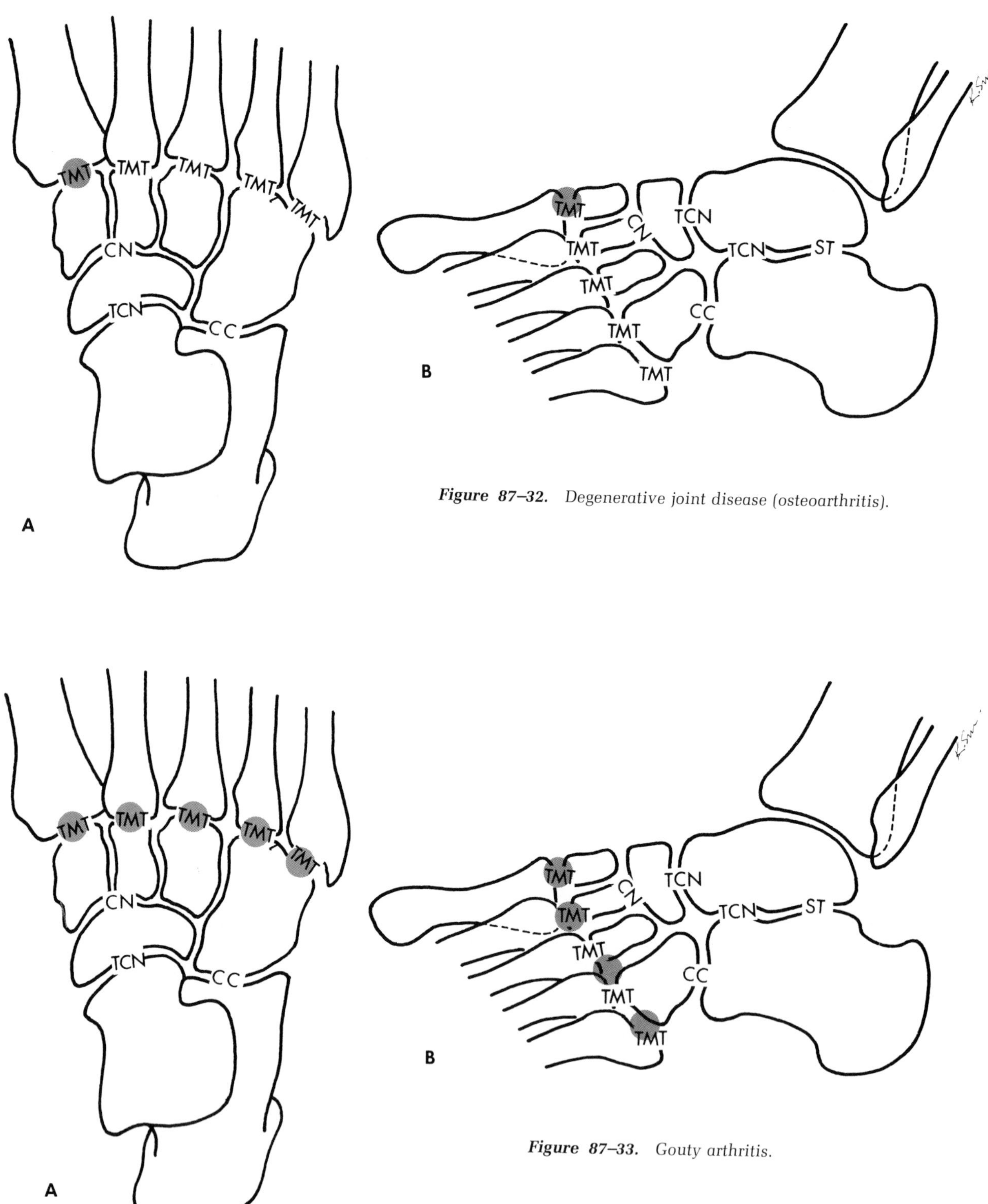

Figure 87–32. Degenerative joint disease (osteoarthritis).

Figure 87–33. Gouty arthritis.

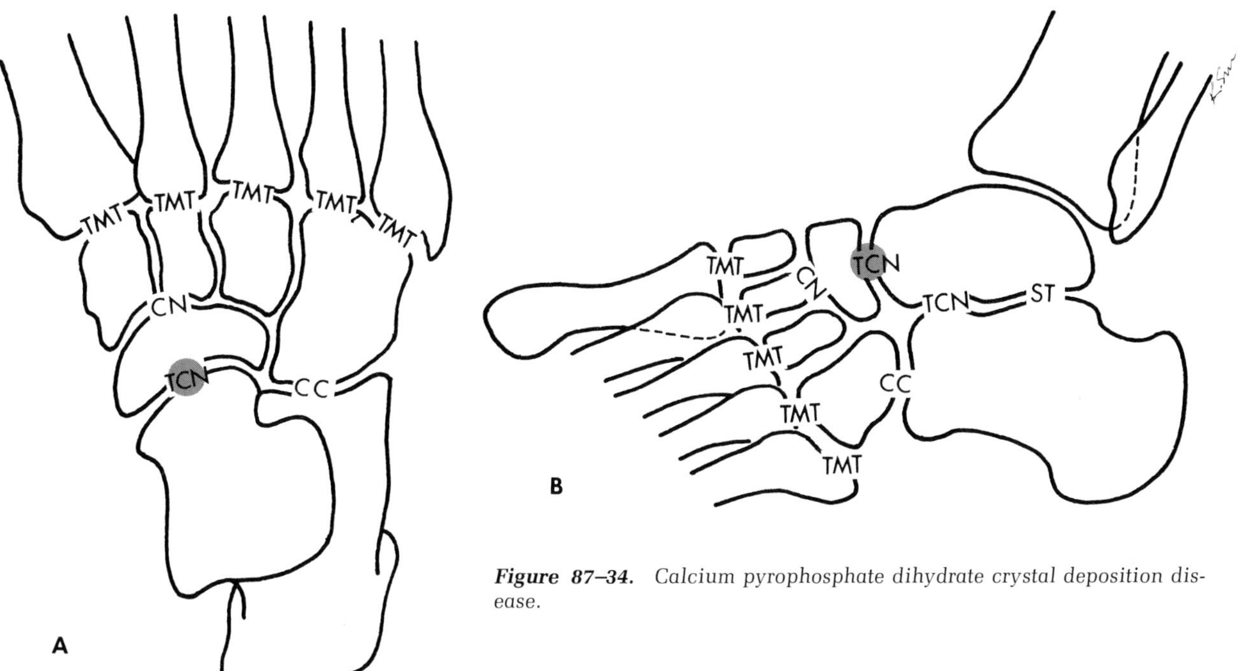

Figure 87–34. Calcium pyrophosphate dihydrate crystal deposition disease.

asymmetric process is most frequent. Prominent osseous erosions of the bases of one or more metatarsals are especially characteristic, usually combined with findings in more distal locations.

Calcium Pyrophosphate Dihydrate Crystal Deposition Disease (Fig. 87–34)

Considerable osseous destruction and fragmentation in a bilateral distribution about the talonavicular aspect of the talocalcaneonavicular joint represents an infrequent but distinctive pattern in this disorder. The apposing surfaces of the talus and the navicular are progressively destroyed and the appearance and distribution are difficult to distinguish from those accompanying the neuroarthropathy of diabetes mellitus.

Neuroarthropathy

The midfoot is not an infrequent site of involvement in certain disorders that lead to neuroarthropathy. Included in these disorders are diabetes mellitus and leprosy. Tarsal disintegration with extension to the bases of the metatarsals may be combined with changes at one or more metatarsophalangeal articulations. In some cases, fragmentation and subluxation at the tarsometatarsal joints simulate the appearance of a Lisfranc's fracture-dislocation.

CALCANEUS

Five potential target areas exist on the calcaneus: (1) the superior surface; (2) the posterior surface above the attachment of the Achilles tendon; (3) the posterior surface at the site of attachment of the Achilles tendon; (4) the plantar surface at the site of attachment of the plantar aponeurosis; and (5) the plantar surface anterior to the attachment of the aponeurosis (Fig. 87–35). Of fundamental importance is the intimate relationship of a synovium-

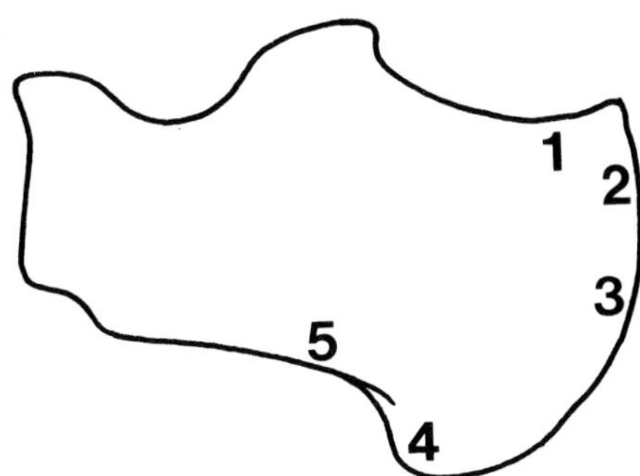

Figure 87–35. Target areas of the calcaneus (see text for identification of numbered areas).

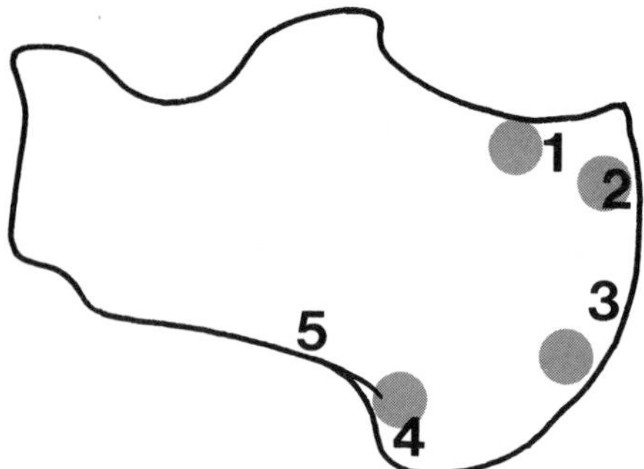

Figure 87–36. Rheumatoid arthritis.

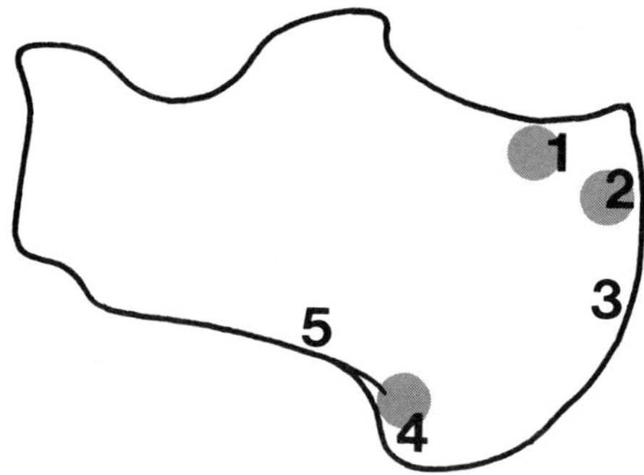

Figure 87–38. Reiter's syndrome.

lined sac, the retrocalcaneal bursa, to the posterosuperior aspect of the calcaneus as it lies between the Achilles tendon and the osseous surface.

Rheumatoid Arthritis (Fig. 87–36)

Retrocalcaneal bursitis leads to unilateral or bilateral calcaneal erosions in both site 1 and site 2. An adjacent soft tissue mass projecting into the pre-Achilles fat pad is frequently evident. Well-defined posterior (site 3) and plantar (site 4) calcaneal spurs are also typical. They are not specific, as identical abnormalities can be evident in "normal" individuals. Plantar osseous erosions of considerable size are distinctly unusual. Achilles tendinitis producing an enlarged or ill-defined tendinous outline can be seen.

Ankylosing Spondylitis and Psoriatic Arthritis (Fig. 87–37)

Similar abnormalities occur in both of these disorders, frequently in a bilateral distribution. Retrocalcaneal bursitis leads to osseous erosions that predominate at site 2. The changes, which may occasionally be combined with alterations at site 1, resemble the findings in rheumatoid arthritis, although reactive bone formation may be more prominent. Well-defined calcaneal spurs at the site of attachment of the Achilles tendon (site 3) can also be observed, a nonspecific finding. On the plantar aspect of the bone, at sites 4 and 5, poorly marginated erosions, reactive sclerosis, and ill-defined spurs may be detected. The outgrowths are more irregular and "fuzzy," and the degree of sclerosis is more prominent in these disorders than in rheumatoid arthritis. Achilles tendon thickening can be seen.

Reiter's Syndrome (Fig. 87–38)

In this disease, unilateral or bilateral alterations can be encountered. Retrocalcaneal bursitis produces erosions at sites 1 and 2 that resemble the findings in rheumatoid arthritis. Abnormalities at site 3, including well-defined calcaneal excrescences, are less frequent than in psoriatic arthritis, ankylosing spondylitis, and rheumatoid arthritis, probably reflecting the younger age of the patients. On the plantar aspect of the bone, osseous erosions and ill-defined bone formation predominate at site 4. The irregular spurs that develop may become better defined over an extended period of time.

Gouty Arthritis (Fig. 87–39)

Tophaceous nodules in and about the Achilles tendon can lead to erosions at sites 2 and 3. The findings are combined with other, more typical

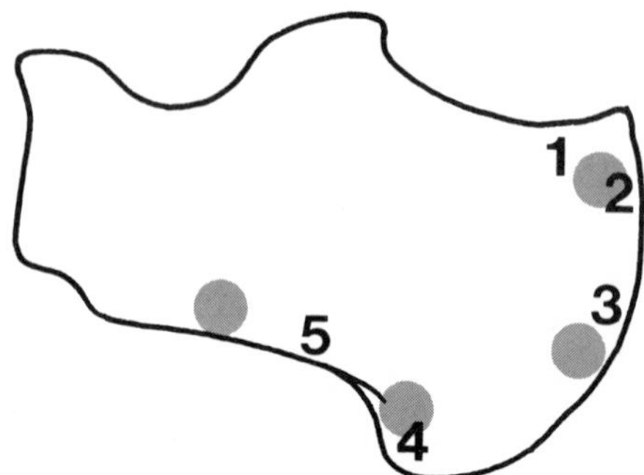

Figure 87–37. Ankylosing spondylitis and psoriatic arthritis.

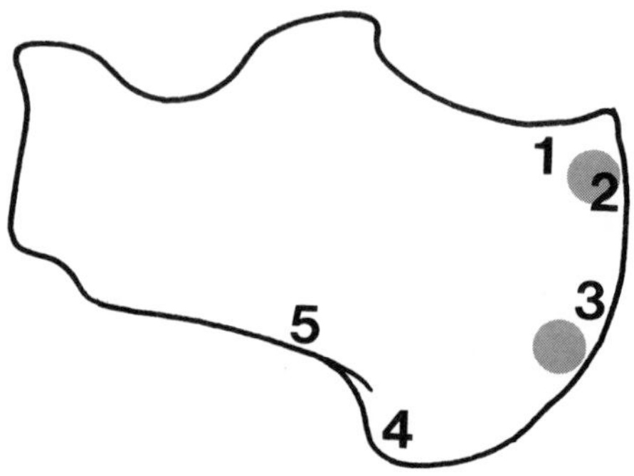

Figure 87–39. Gouty arthritis.

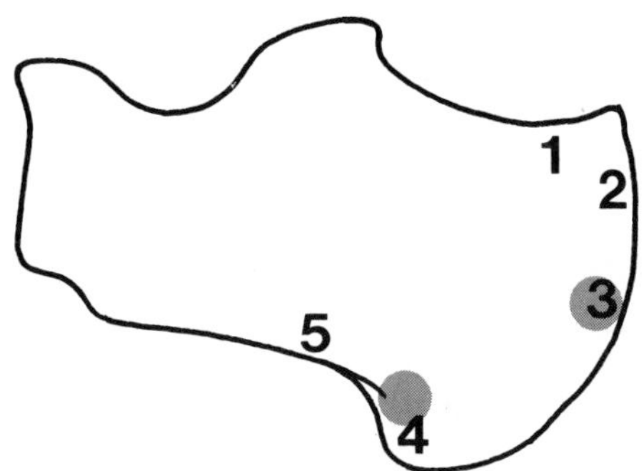

Figure 87–40. *Calcium pyrophosphate dihydrate crystal deposition disease.*

changes at the metatarsophalangeal and interphalangeal articulations.

Calcium Pyrophosphate Dihydrate Crystal Deposition Disease (Fig. 87–40)

Calcific collections consisting of calcium pyrophosphate dihydrate crystals can be deposited in the Achilles tendon and plantar aponeurosis of one or both feet in this disorder. The deposits are linear in configuration and may be of considerable length. Similar abnormalities may be seen in calcium hydroxyapatite crystal deposition disease.

Xanthomatosis (Fig. 87–41)

Tendinous xanthomas can appear in the Achilles tendon and the plantar aponeurosis in a unilateral or bilateral distribution. They produce eccentric soft tissue masses that do not calcify. On rare occasions, they may erode subjacent bone.

Diffuse Idiopathic Skeletal Hyperostosis (Fig. 87–42)

Well-defined outgrowths of variable size occur at the sites of bony attachment of the Achilles tendon and plantar aponeurosis (sites 3 and 4). Generally, both sides are affected in a relatively symmetric fashion and, in some cases, the excrescences may reach considerable size. Rarely, bony protuberances may appear on the anterior plantar aspect of the calcaneus (site 5).

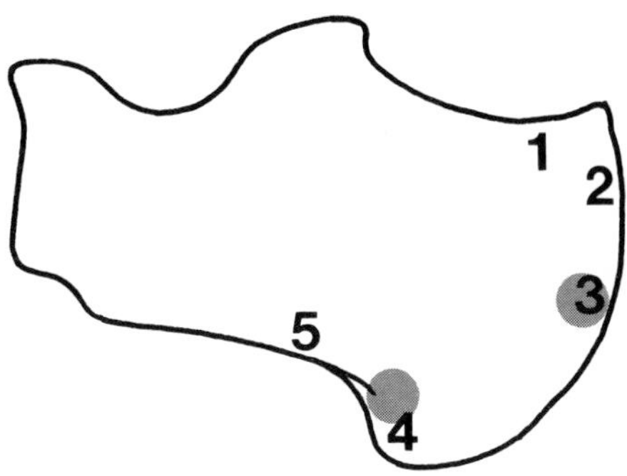

Figure 87–42. *Diffuse idiopathic skeletal hyperostosis.*

Other Diseases

Hyperparathyroidism can lead to subligamentous erosion at site 4, as well as subtle defects elsewhere in the calcaneus, including site 1 (Fig. 87–43). Both feet are usually affected and, in general, other findings are present elsewhere in the skeleton.

KNEE

It is useful to analyze separately three major areas or spaces of the knee: the medial femorotibial space, the lateral femorotibial space, and the patellofemoral space (Fig. 87–44). Processes within the knee can also extend into a fourth area, the proximal tibiofibular joint, although this latter articulation will not be considered here.

Anteroposterior radiographs allow analysis of the medial and lateral femorotibial compartments,

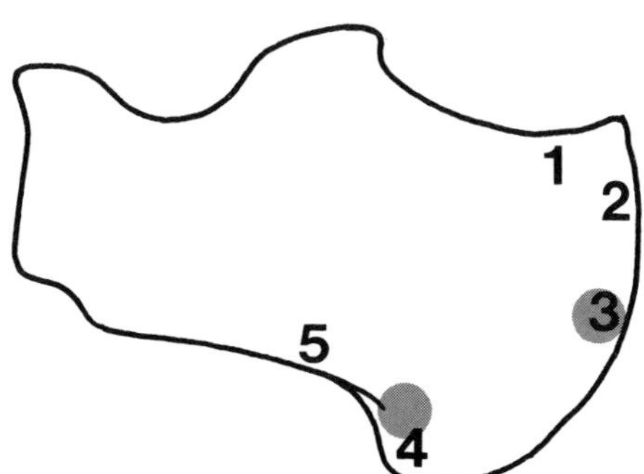

Figure 87–41. *Xanthomatosis.*

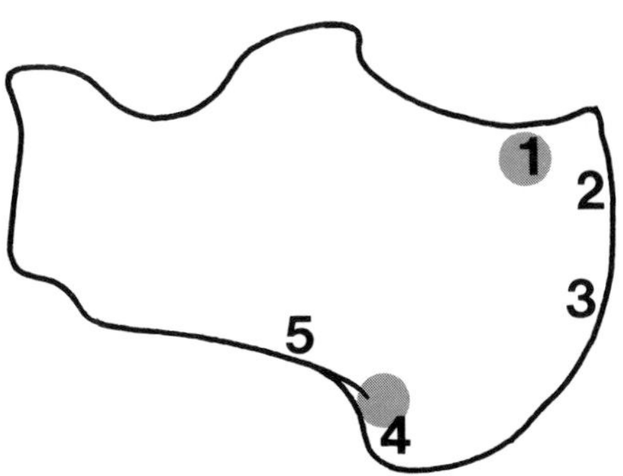

Figure 87–43. *Hyperparathyroidism.*

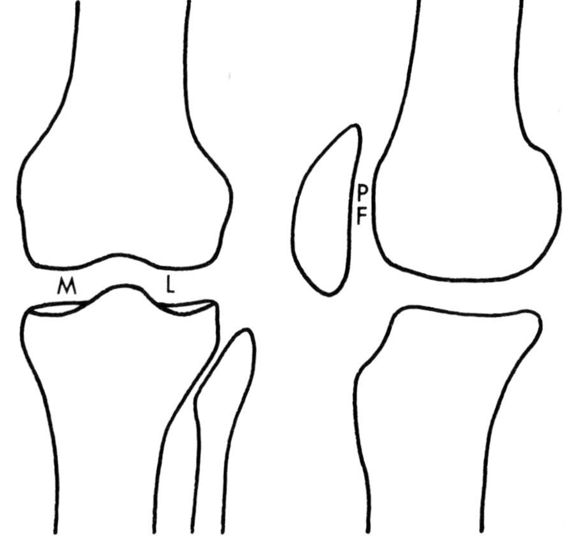

Figure 87–44. Compartments of the knee. (M, Medial femorotibial; L, lateral femorotibial; PF, patellofemoral.)

an analysis that can be improved by obtaining radiographs with the patient standing. Lateral and axial radiographs allow evaluation of the patellofemoral compartment.

Rheumatoid Arthritis (Fig. 87–45)

This disorder usually leads to alterations that are bilateral and symmetric in distribution and affect both medial and lateral femorotibial compartments to an equal degree. The appearance of diffuse loss of interosseous space in the medial and lateral compartments is of great aid in the diagnosis of this disease. This finding may be combined with osteoporosis, superficial and deep marginal or central osseous erosions, and subchondral sclerosis, especially in the tibia. Crumbling of the osteoporotic bone of the tibia in combination with ligamentous abnormalities may create varus or valgus angulation of the knee.

Involvement of the patellofemoral space is often combined with involvement of the other two compartments in the rheumatoid knee. Although not invariably present, tricompartmental abnormalities that are of equal severity are most suggestive of rheumatoid arthritis.

Ankylosing Spondylitis, Psoriatic Arthritis, and Reiter's Syndrome (Fig. 87–46)

Any of these three disorders can affect one or both knees. A tricompartmental distribution may be encountered, although the degree of joint space narrowing, osteoporosis, and osseous erosion is less than in rheumatoid arthritis, and the extent of periosteal proliferation or "whiskering" may be pronounced.

Degenerative Joint Disease (Osteoarthritis) (Fig. 87–47)

A unilateral or bilateral distribution can be seen. Asymmetric involvement of the medial and lateral femorotibial compartments predominates, frequent-

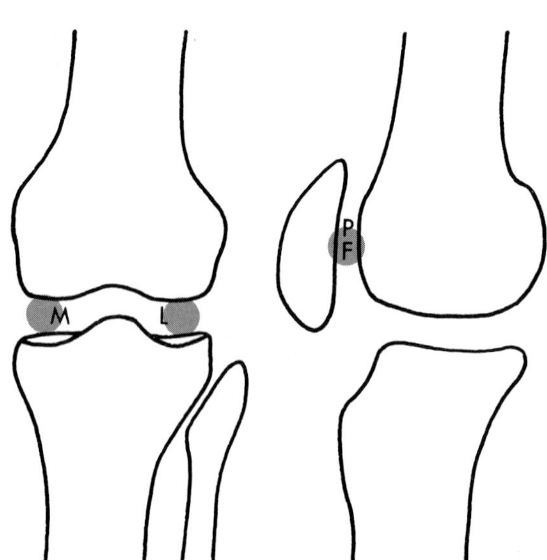

Figure 87–45. Rheumatoid arthritis.

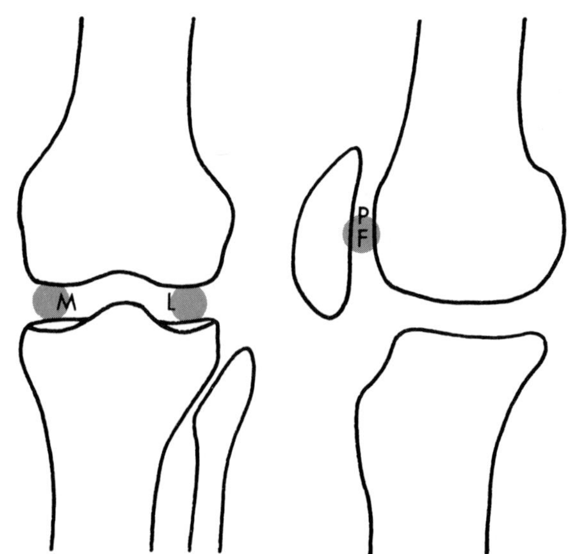

Figure 87–46. Ankylosing spondylitis, psoriatic arthritis, and Reiter's syndrome.

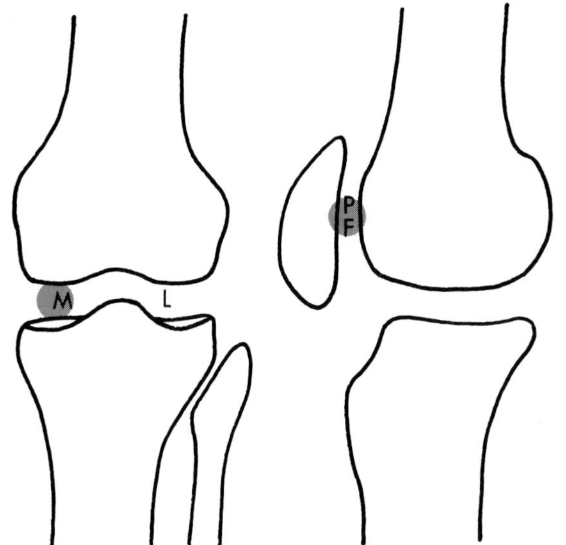

Figure 87–47. *Degenerative joint disease (osteoarthritis).*

ly in combination with significant patellofemoral compartmental disease. Thus, bicompartmental rather than tricompartmental findings are evident on the roentgenograms. In most instances, it is the medial femorotibial compartment that is more severely affected, and the asymmetric nature of the process may lead to moderate or severe varus deformity, especially in men. Severe alterations in the lateral femorotibial compartment and valgus deformity are far less common on roentgenograms of the osteoarthritic knee. However, radionuclide studies may indicate the presence of lateral compartmental changes when plain film roentgenograms are unimpressive.

Isolated abnormalities of the patellofemoral compartment are relatively unusual in degenerative joint disease of the knee. The detection of joint space narrowing, sclerosis, and osteophytosis in this location in the absence of similar changes in either the medial or lateral femorotibial space should initiate a search for other disease processes, such as calcium pyrophosphate dihydrate crystal deposition disease. Rarely, findings are restricted to the patellofemoral space in degenerative joint disease, perhaps representing a sequela of chondromalacia.

Calcium Pyrophosphate Dihydrate Crystal Deposition Disease (Fig. 87–48)

The distribution of abnormalities of the knee in patients with calcium pyrophosphate dihydrate crystal deposition disease is somewhat variable. Usually both knees are affected, although the changes may be asymmetric in extent and severity. The medial femorotibial and patellofemoral compartments are commonly affected simultaneously, a distribution that is identical to that in osteoarthritis. In these cases, the greater extent of osseous destruction and fragmentation may allow accurate differentiation of calcium pyrophosphate dihydrate crystal deposition disease from osteoarthritis. Lateral femorotibial compartmental changes with or without medial femorotibial compartmental abnormalities can also be encountered in this disease and, in some instances, may lead to impressive valgus deformity of the knee. Furthermore, findings isolated to the patellofemoral compartment are also observed in some patients. In fact, a "degenerative"-like arthropathy of the patellofemoral compartment appearing in the absence of significant medial or lateral femorotibial space alterations raises the possibility that this disease is present.

Other Diseases

In addition to subperiosteal resorption of bone along the medial aspect of the tibia, *hyperparathyroidism* can produce a peculiar variety of articular abnormality on knee roentgenograms. Subchondral resorption of bone may be evident in any compartment, usually in a bilateral but not necessarily symmetric distribution. The changes, consisting of ill-defined "erosion" and sclerosis, may be especially marked in the patellofemoral areas, and a concave posterior patellar surface may appear to "wrap" itself about the anterior portion of the femur (Fig. 87–49).

Septic arthritis affecting the knee can become initially evident in any compartment, although involvement of the medial or lateral femorotibial space is most typical, especially if the infection has arisen via hematogenous dissemination. As in rheumatoid arthritis, the alterations can spread to all areas of the joint (including the proximal tibiofibular space), producing tricompartmental disease. A unilateral distribution is most frequent.

Neuroarthropathy accompanying tabes dorsalis or, more rarely, other diseases with neurologic deficit can lead to involvement of one or both knees with sclerosis, fragmentation, subluxation, and disorganization of the joint.

HIP

In evaluating articular disorders that affect the hip, it is useful to define the nature or location of any accompanying joint space loss. With diminution of the articular space, the femoral head migrates in one of three basic directions with respect to the adjacent acetabulum. If the loss is confined to the superior

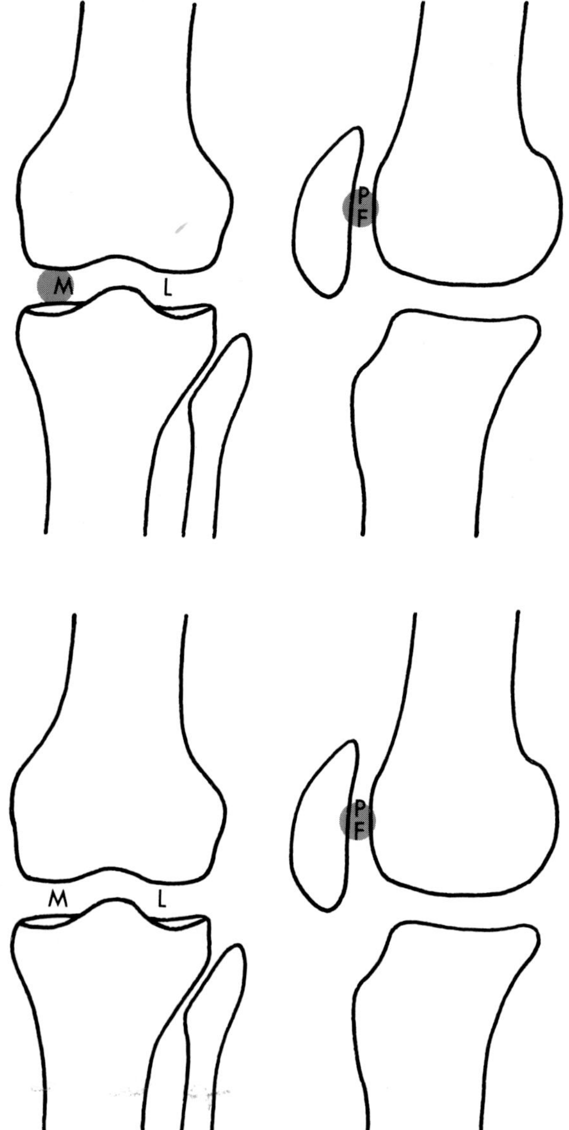

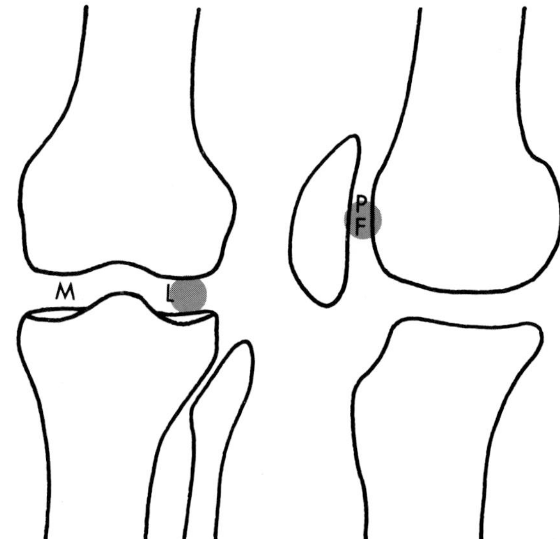

Figure 87–48. *Calcium pyrophosphate dihydrate crystal deposition disease.*

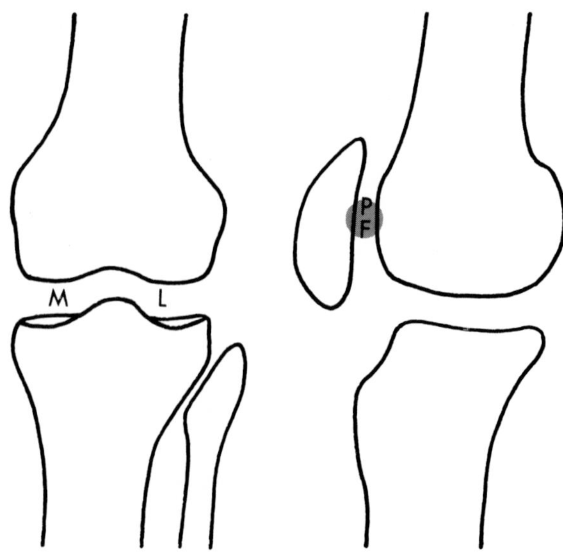

Figure 87–49. Hyperparathyroidism.

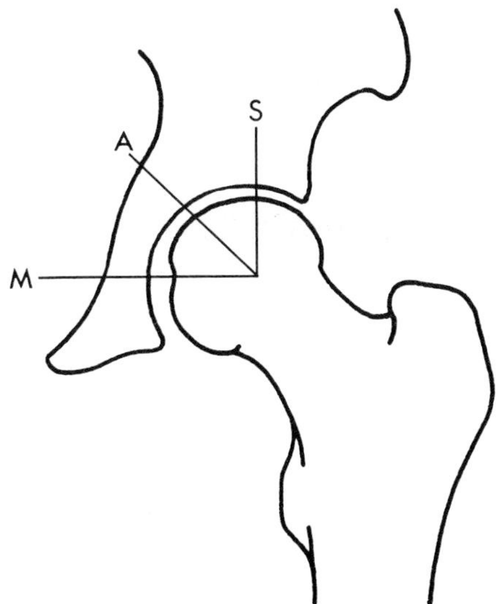

Figure 87–50. Patterns of migration of the femoral head. S, Superior migration; A, axial migration; M, medial migration.

aspect of the joint, the femoral head moves in an upward or superior direction; if the loss is confined to the inner third of the articulation, the femoral head migrates in a medial direction; and if the joint space loss involves the entire articulation, the femoral head migrates in an axial direction along the axis of the femoral neck (Fig. 87–50). Certain disorders are associated with characteristic patterns of femoral head migration.

Rheumatoid Arthritis (Fig. 87–51)

In this disease, the entire articular cartilaginous coat of the femoral head and acetabulum is typically affected in a bilateral and symmetric fashion. Thus, with progressive chondral destruction, symmetric loss of the interosseous space occurs with axial migration of the femoral head with respect to the acetabulum. This finding is usually accompanied by marginal and central osseous erosions and cysts and even localized sclerosis. Osteophytosis is not a prominent feature. It should be emphasized that such hip abnormalities in rheumatoid arthritis are not usually an early feature of the disease. Rather, they appear in long-standing cases, especially in patients receiving corticosteroid medications.

Juvenile Chronic Arthritis

The incidence and type of hip involvement in juvenile chronic arthritis are influenced by the specific variety of disease that is present (e.g., juvenile-onset adult type seropositive rheumatoid arthritis, Still's disease, juvenile-onset ankylosing spondylitis). In some patients, diffuse loss of joint space with concentric narrowing of the articulation results in axial migration of the femoral head and a roentgenographic picture that resembles that in adult-onset rheumatoid arthritis. In others, osseous erosions may be unaccompanied by loss of interosseous space. In patients with juvenile-onset ankylosing spondylitis, the radiographic findings are similar to those in adult-onset ankylosing spondylitis and may eventually be characterized by bony ankylosis of the joint.

Ankylosing Spondylitis (Fig. 87–52)

A bilateral and symmetric pattern consisting of axial migration of the femoral head due to diffuse

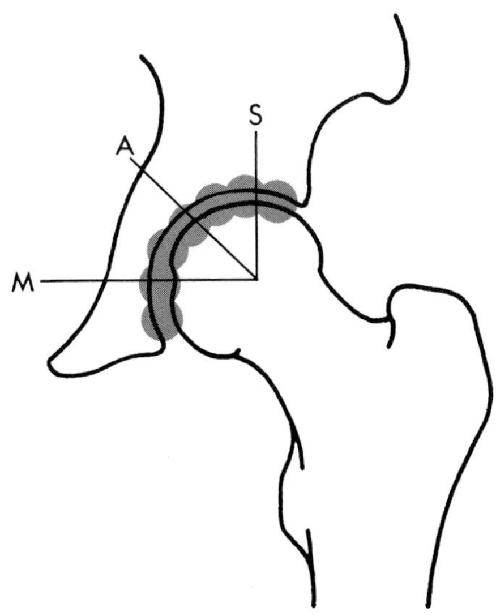

Figure 87–51. Rheumatoid arthritis.

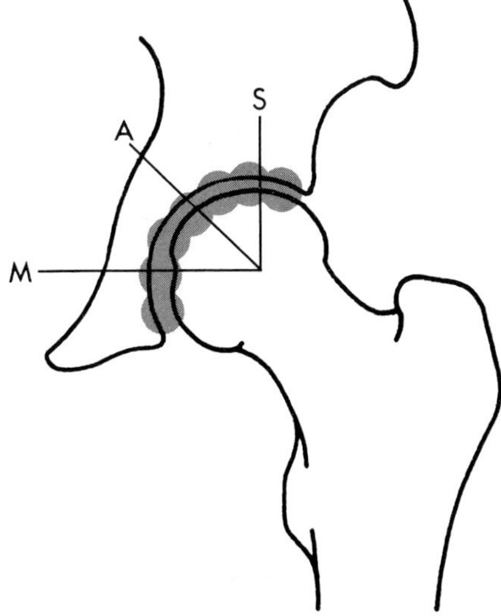

Figure 87–52. Ankylosing spondylitis.

loss of joint space is seen. Although this pattern is identical to that in rheumatoid arthritis, the presence of osteophytosis, commencing on the superolateral aspect of the femoral head and progressing as a collar about the femoral head–neck junction, is distinctive of ankylosing spondylitis. Such osteophytosis is not evident in rheumatoid arthritis, and the combination of axial migration of the femoral head and osteophyte formation is most characteristic of ankylosing spondylitis and calcium pyrophosphate dihydrate crystal deposition disease. Rarely, patients with degenerative joint disease may reveal symmetric loss of interosseous space, but the usual pattern in this latter disease is dominated by superior or medial loss of joint space. In ankylosing spondylitis, acetabular and femoral cysts, mild acetabular protrusion, and partial or complete intra-articular bony ankylosis can be observed.

Psoriatic Arthritis and Reiter's Syndrome

Hip involvement is unusual in both of these disorders. Occasionally a patient with either disease may reveal concentric loss of joint space resembling that in rheumatoid arthritis, and, rarely, patients with psoriatic arthritis will have more extensive osseous destruction leading to a blunted and eroded femoral head.

Degenerative Joint Disease (Osteoarthritis) (Fig. 87–53)

Unilateral or bilateral alterations can be delineated. Most commonly, loss of interosseous space is maximal on the upper aspect of the articulation, resulting in superior migration of the femoral head with respect to the acetabulum. Less frequently, medial loss of joint space is seen, which may be associated with mild protrusio acetabuli deformity. Rarely, axial migration of the femoral head indicates diffuse loss of the cartilaginous surfaces of the femur and acetabulum. In all cases of degenerative joint disease, femoral and acetabular osteophytes, sclerosis, and cyst formation are common, and thickening or buttressing of the medial femoral cortex is apparent.

Gouty Arthritis

Hip involvement is unusual in this disease. Rarely, osseous erosion or osteonecrosis can be seen, although the exact relationship of the second finding to gouty arthritis is speculative.

Calcium Pyrophosphate Dihydrate Crystal Deposition Disease (Fig. 87–54)

The arthropathy of calcium pyrophosphate dihydrate crystal deposition disease may involve one or both hips. It is characterized by symmetric loss of joint space with axial migration, sclerosis, cyst formation, and osteophytosis. The degree of osseous collapse and fragmentation may be extreme, and the resulting radiographic features may be misinterpreted as neuroarthropathy or osteonecrosis. Additional findings, such as chondrocalcinosis of the acetabular labrum and symphysis pubis detectable on pelvic roentgenograms, provide helpful clues to the correct diagnosis.

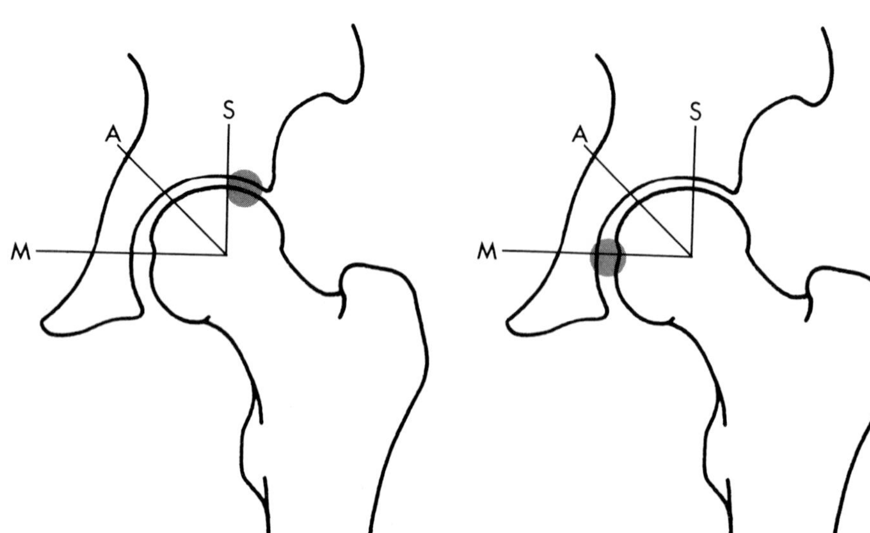

Figure 87–53. *Degenerative joint disease (osteoarthritis).*

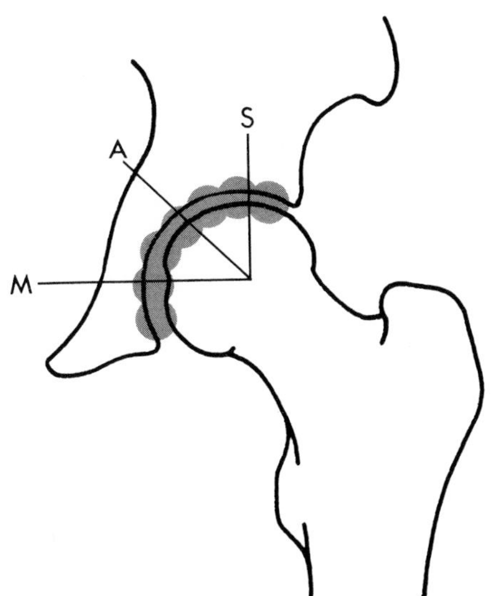

Figure 87–54. Calcium pyrophosphate dihydrate crystal deposition disease.

Osteonecrosis

Although osteonecrosis of one or both femoral heads can accompany a vast number of diseases, the joint space is remarkably preserved in most cases, even in the presence of significant bony collapse and fragmentation. In long-standing cases, secondary degenerative joint disease can result, owing to the incongruity of the apposing articular surfaces. In these instances, loss of joint space usually predominates in the superior aspect of the articulation, leading to superior migration of the femoral head with respect to the acetabulum. Occasionally, loss of joint space is more diffuse, involving the entire articulation. It is not clear whether this change is the result of degenerative joint disease or chondrolysis.

Neuroarthropathy

Disintegration of osseous and cartilaginous tissue in one or both hips can be a manifestation of neuroarthropathy. In these cases, tabes is the most typical underlying disorder, as changes in this articulation are unusual in diabetes mellitus and syringomyelia.

Other Diseases

In *Paget's disease*, involvement of para-articular osseous tissue can lead to secondary degenerative joint disease. The radiographic findings are influenced by the distribution of pagetic changes; the pattern of joint space loss may differ in cases in which the acetabulum is affected alone, in those in which both the acetabulum and femur are affected, and in those in which the femur is the only site of involvement. Because of these variations, any pattern of femoral head migration can appear in Paget's disease; instances of medial, axial, or superior migration are recognized. The diagnosis is facilitated by the recognition of Paget's disease in the adjacent bone.

Idiopathic chondrolysis of the hip is rare, but it is associated with diffuse loss of joint space and axial migration of the femoral head with respect to the acetabulum. The appearance may closely resemble that of infection.

Regional migratory osteoporosis and *transient osteoporosis of the hip* are self-limited conditions that can produce a periarticular osteoporosis that improves spontaneously over several months. A unilateral distribution is typical, and when transient osteoporosis affects a woman in the third trimester of pregnancy, the left hip is almost invariably involved. Preservation of joint space and the absence of significant defects in the subchondral bone plate are features of regional osteoporosis that allow its differentiation from infection.

Infections of the hip can have a bacterial, mycobacterial, or fungal etiology. The radiographic features and prognosis are influenced by the age of onset. In the infant, pyogenic arthritis of the hip requires immediate attention to prevent permanent epiphyseal damage. Joint space loss, which is generally diffuse in nature, is a fundamental finding in all infectious disorders, although the rapidity of the loss is influenced by the nature of the causative organism; rapid loss of interosseous space is characteristic of pyogenic (bacterial) infection, whereas slow loss is typical of tuberculosis and fungal disorders. Other findings, such as osteoporosis and marginal and central osseous erosions, are also influenced by the specific cause of the infection.

Pigmented villonodular synovitis and *idiopathic synovial osteochondromatosis* are two disorders that can produce monoarticular disease of the hip. In both conditions, soft tissue swelling and osseous erosions may appear in the absence of joint space narrowing and osteoporosis, although the latter findings are also evident in some cases. The presence of cystic erosions of the femoral neck on plain films and of intra-articular masses on arthrograms in both conditions and the detection of calcific or ossific foci in idiopathic synovial osteochondromatosis are important diagnostic clues.

SHOULDER

In the shoulder region, there are three potential target areas that can be affected in various articular disorders: the glenohumeral joint, the acromioclavicular joint, and the undersurface of the distal

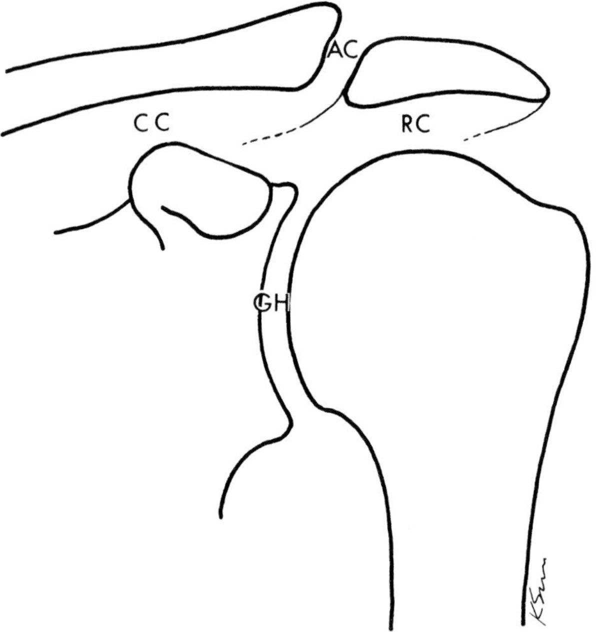

Figure 87–55. *Target areas of the shoulder. GH, Glenohumeral joint; AC, acromioclavicular joint; CC, coracoclavicular ligament; RC, rotator cuff.*

clavicle at the site of attachment of the coracoclavicular ligament (Fig. 87–55). One or more of these sites can be altered in one or both shoulders.

Rheumatoid Arthritis (Fig. 87–56)

All three target areas on both sides of the body can be involved in rheumatoid arthritis. Glenohumeral joint alterations consist of osteoporosis, symmetric loss of joint space, and marginal osseous erosions, predominantly on the superolateral aspect of the humeral head. Associated atrophy or tear of the rotator cuff may lead to slow or rapid elevation of the humeral head with respect to the glenoid process and narrowing of the acromiohumeral head distance.

Acromioclavicular joint erosion with widening of the articular space is a recognized manifestation of this disease. Bony defects appear on both the acromial and the clavicular aspect of the joint, and the margins of the distal clavicle may assume a tapered appearance. Similarly, scalloped erosion on the undersurface of the distal clavicle opposite the coracoid process is an additional manifestation of rheumatoid arthritis, although it is almost invariably recognized in the later stages of the disease, at a time when other manifestations are evident.

Ankylosing Spondylitis (Fig. 87–57)

The changes about the shoulder in this disease resemble those in rheumatoid arthritis. Glenohumeral joint involvement leads to joint space narrowing and osseous erosion. A large bony defect can appear on the superolateral aspect of the humeral head, the "hatchet" deformity, which is distinctive. The absence of osteoporosis and the presence of bony proliferation about the osseous erosions are additional characteristics of ankylosing spondylitis that are helpful in diagnosis.

Osseous erosions about the acromioclavicular

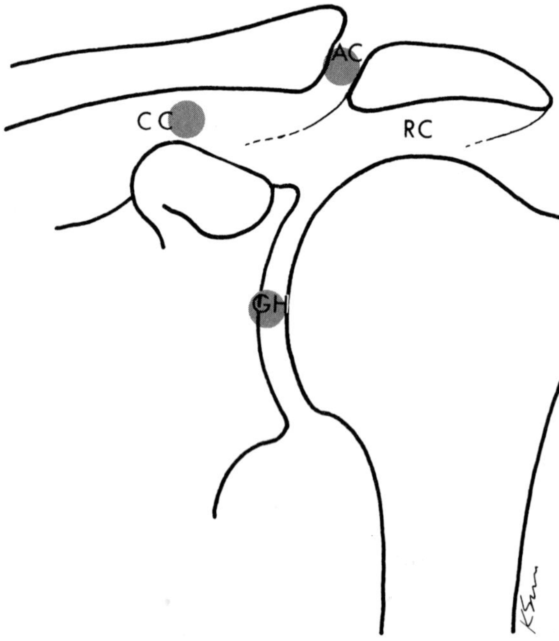

Figure 87–56. *Rheumatoid arthritis.*

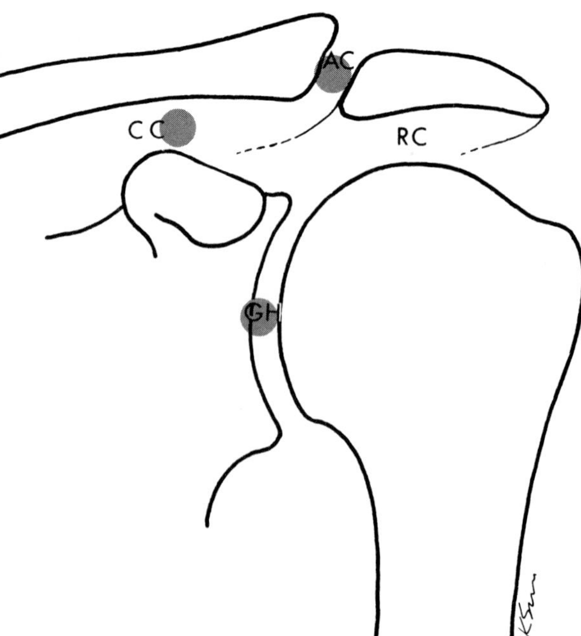

Figure 87–57. *Ankylosing spondylitis.*

joint and along the undersurface of the distal clavicle can also be noted in ankylosing spondylitis. Adjacent bony proliferation along the inferior clavicle is more common and exuberant in this disease than in rheumatoid arthritis.

Degenerative Joint Disease (Osteoarthritis) (Fig. 87–58)

The glenohumeral joint is an unusual site of osteoarthritis unless significant accidental or occupational trauma has occurred; in this latter situation, joint space narrowing, sclerosis, and osteophytosis are typical. On the other hand, degeneration and disruption of the rotator cuff are frequent in elderly individuals, producing elevation of the humeral head. Although the appearance may simulate that of rotator cuff injury in rheumatoid arthritis, the lack of significant glenohumeral joint involvement in association with degeneration of the cuff is noteworthy.

Acromioclavicular joint degeneration is frequent in middle-aged and elderly individuals. Changes are usually mild in nature, consisting of articular space narrowing and eburnation. Proliferative degenerative abnormalities along the inferior surface of the distal clavicle are not conspicuous in the absence of significant injury, especially subluxation or dislocation of the acromioclavicular joint.

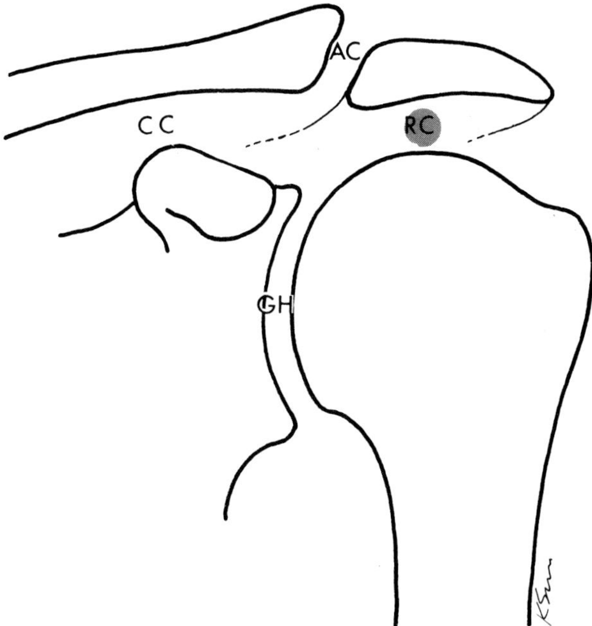

Figure 87–58. *Rotator cuff degeneration.*

Calcium Pyrophosphate Dihydrate Crystal Deposition Disease (Fig. 87–59)

Both the glenohumeral and acromioclavicular articulations can be affected in this disease, although the abnormalities are less extensive than changes in other articulations, such as the wrist, the metacarpophalangeal joints, and the knee. Fibrocartilage or hyaline cartilage calcification, articular space narrowing, sclerosis, and osteophytosis can appear at either shoulder location. Although the findings may be reminiscent of those in degenerative joint disease, the absence of a history of trauma and the presence of calcific deposits and extensive osseous alterations are features that suggest calcium pyrophosphate dihydrate crystal deposition disease.

Other Diseases

Alkaptonuria (ochronosis) can lead to an arthropathy resembling degenerative joint disease of the glenohumeral articulation in one or both shoulders. Similarly, in *acromegaly*, osteophytosis can be evident in this site, especially on the inferior aspect of the humeral head. *Hyperparathyroidism* leads to osseous resorption of the distal clavicle and adjacent acromion as well as of the inferior aspect of the clavicle at the site of attachment of the coracoclavicular ligament. *Posttraumatic changes* include osteolysis of the distal clavicle, and degenerative joint disease may be seen in association with recurrent posterior dislocation of the glenohumeral joint.

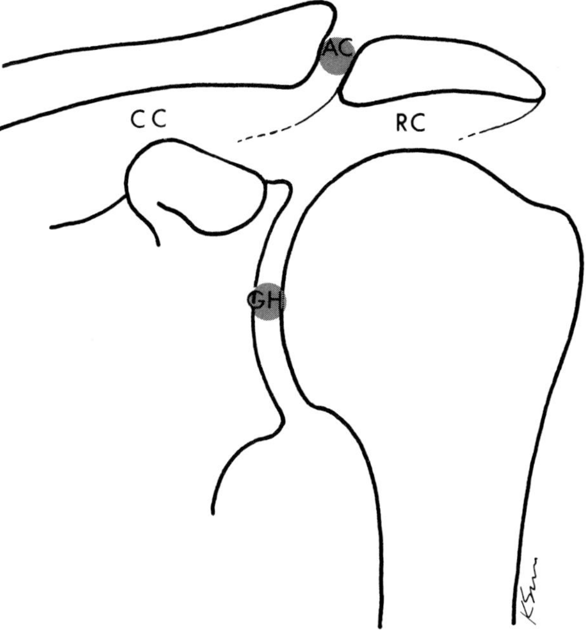

Figure 87–59. *Calcium pyrophosphate dihydrate crystal deposition disease.*

SACROILIAC JOINT

The most important aspect in the differential diagnosis of diseases that affect the sacroiliac joint is the distribution of the abnormalities. Findings can be bilateral and symmetric, bilateral and asymmetric, or unilateral (Fig. 87–60). In nearly every instance, the synovial portion of the joint (the lower one half or two thirds of the interosseous space between sacrum and ilium) is affected to a greater degree than the ligamentous portion (that area above the synovium-lined space).

Rheumatoid Arthritis (Fig. 87–60 *B, C*)

Abnormalities of the sacroiliac joint in rheumatoid arthritis are generally a minor feature of the disease. Bilateral asymmetric or unilateral changes predominate, consisting of joint space narrowing, superficial osseous erosions, minor sclerosis, and absence of widespread bony ankylosis. When a bilateral and symmetrically distributed process consisting of osseous erosions or bony ankylosis is evident, the possibility of superimposed ankylosing spondylitis must be considered.

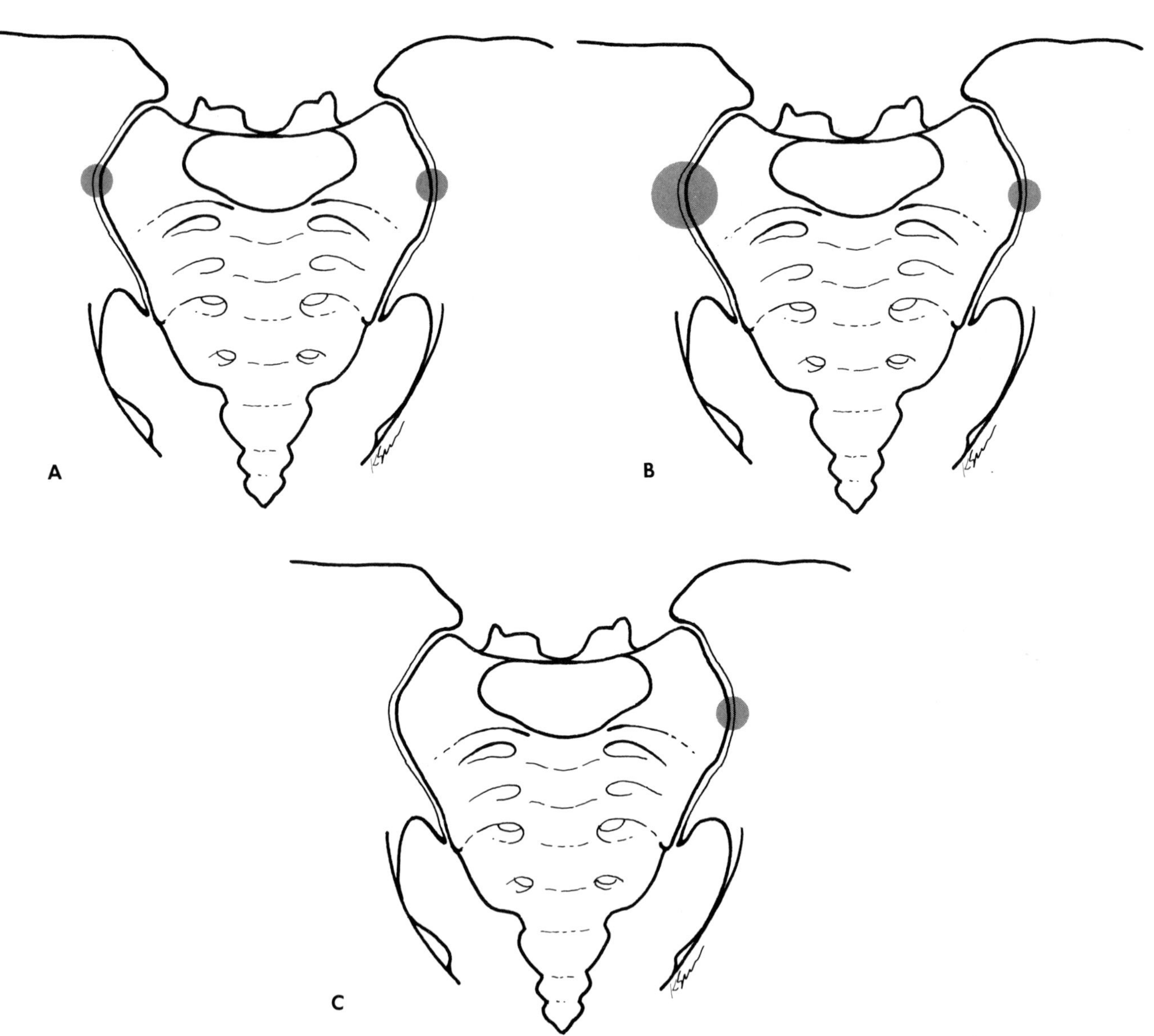

Figure 87–60. *Distribution of sacroiliac joint changes.*
A *Symmetric.*
B *Asymmetric.*
C *Unilateral.*

Juvenile Chronic Arthritis

The incidence and appearance of sacroiliac joint changes in juvenile chronic arthritis depend upon the subgroup of disease that is present. Changes are usually not prominent unless juvenile-onset ankylosing spondylitis is evident. In this case, a bilateral and symmetric distribution is encountered.

Ankylosing Spondylitis (Fig. 87–60*A*)

The classic findings in this disease are bilateral and symmetric in distribution. Erosions, sclerosis, and bony ankylosis of the synovial articulation are frequently combined with poorly defined osseous margins in the ligamentous aspect of the joint. Occasionally, initial radiographs will reveal asymmetric abnormalities. In all cases, iliac abnormalities predominate.

Psoriatic Arthritis and Reiter's Syndrome (Fig. 87–60 *A–C*)

The distribution of abnormalities is variable in these two diseases. Changes may be bilateral and symmetric, bilateral and asymmetric, or unilateral. Osseous erosion and bony sclerosis are similar to the findings in ankylosing spondylitis, although joint space narrowing and bony ankylosis occur with decreased frequency. Proliferation of bone in the ilium and sacrum above the synovial aspect of the joint may be prominent, particularly in Reiter's syndrome.

Degenerative Joint Disease (Osteoarthritis) (Fig. 87–60 *A–C*)

Osteoarthritis of the sacroiliac joint can be unilateral or bilateral in distribution. Unilateral abnormalities of the sacroiliac articulation in conjunction with osteoarthritis of the contralateral hip may be encountered. Findings include joint space narrowing, sclerosis, and osteophytosis. The bony excrescences predominate on the anterosuperior and anteroinferior aspects of the joint. Erosions are not prominent and para-articular rather than intra-articular ankylosis predominates.

Gouty Arthritis (Fig. 87–60 *A–C*)

Abnormalities of the sacroiliac joint can be seen in patients with long-standing tophaceous gout. Bilateral symmetric, bilateral asymmetric, or unilateral alterations consisting of large erosions and reactive sclerosis are found.

Other Diseases

Sacroiliitis accompanying *inflammatory bowel diseases* is bilateral and symmetric in distribution and cannot be differentiated from that seen in ankylosing spondylitis (Fig. 87–60*A*). In *hyperparathyroidism,* subchondral resorption of bone, especially in the ilium, produces bilateral and symmetric changes consisting of joint space widening and reactive sclerosis (Fig. 87–60*A*). Unilateral abnormalities are typical of sacroiliac joint *infection* (Fig. 87–60*C*). Such infection can be related to bacterial, mycobacterial, or fungal agents and is not infrequent in the drug abuser. *Osteitis condensans ilii* produces bilateral and symmetric alterations in young women consisting of well-defined triangular sclerosis of the inferior aspect of the ilium (Fig. 87–60*A*). Sacroiliac joint involvement may also accompany *familial Mediterranean fever, relapsing polychondritis, Behçet's syndrome, alkaptonuria, immobilization, or disuse.*

SUMMARY

The "target area" approach is a useful concept in the radiographic evaluation of articular diseases. The pattern of distribution of the lesions in each of the diseases is remarkably constant. Furthermore, because this pattern varies from one disorder to the next, it may be utilized for accurate differential diagnosis in many cases. Exceptions to the rules do exist, and the physician must guard against an overenthusiastic application of the "target area" approach.

APPENDIX 1
ARTHROSCOPY

by Donald Resnick, M.D.

Arthroscopy is a technique in which endoscopic evaluation of a joint cavity is accomplished. The procedure was originated in Japan by Professor Kenji Takagi and subsequently developed by one of his pupils, Dr. Masaki Watanabe.[1] Technologic efforts addressed the major problem of designing instrumentation that would permit adequate illumination of the joint cavity through a narrow arthroscope and that would contain an optic system capable of magnifying the images seen. With the incorporation of projected fiberoptics and fiber light, arthroscopes of superior design and performance have become available, so that currently arthroscopy is an important diagnostic modality available to the orthopedic surgeon.[2, 20, 21] Although originally designed to diagnose tuberculosis of the knee joint, the arthroscope is now utilized to investigate a variety of disorders in any of several articulations, including the knee, hip, elbow, ankle, and glenohumeral joint.

Arthroscopes of varying sizes are available. Small needle arthroscopes, possessing a diameter of 2 to 3 mm, can be introduced through tiny incisions under local anesthesia and can reach the deeper recesses of the articular cavity; however, they have less than optimal optical lighting capabilities, may not allow the introduction of surgical instruments, and can be broken rather easily when the joint is flexed or vigorous stresses are applied. Larger arthroscopes, possessing a diameter of 2 to 6.5 mm, provide better viewing ability and superior lighting, but general anesthesia and larger skin incisions are usually required, and the instrument may be too bulky to reach confined areas of the joint, necessitating additional punctures. Tourniquet application and joint aspiration and irrigation (usually with normal saline solution) are generally advised.[1]

The evaluation of internal derangements of the knee represents the prime indication for arthroscopy, although a debate has existed regarding the need for arthroscopy, arthrography, or both in this clinical setting.[3-11] The reported diagnostic accuracy of knee arthroscopy has varied from 85 to 99 per cent; this variation is related, in part, to the expertise and experience of the examiner as well as the type of injury being evaluated. The reported accuracy of knee arthrography has varied from about 75 to 98 per cent, depending again upon examiner expertise and the type of joint problem.[4, 10, 12] Although some investigators believe that arthroscopy or arthrography alone allows adequate visualization of all important intra-articular structures, it is generally recognized that certain "blind" areas exist within the joint that cannot be examined utilizing one diagnostic technique without the other.[12] An anterolateral approach during arthroscopy does not allow optimal identification of the posterior horns of the medial and lateral menisci and their peripheral attachments,[7, 12, 13] especially that area between the medial collateral ligament and the intercondylar attachment of the posterior horn of the meniscus.[4] This technique does provide good visualization of the anterior horns of the menisci and the anterior cruciate ligament, and arthroscopic evaluation utilizing multiple entrance sites may provide better visualization of the posterior structures of the knee. Knee arthrography, although accurate in the analysis of peripheral and midbody meniscal regions, may be less precise in identifying lesions in the central edge, anterior horn, and popliteal area of the lateral meniscus.[10] Arthrography is also less accurate than arthroscopy in outlining cruciate ligament abnormalities and chondromalacia, although special techniques, including arthrotomography, may improve this deficiency. These strengths and weaknesses of arthrography and arthroscopy in the diagnosis of internal derangements of the knee indicate that the procedures should be regarded as complementary in nature. The combined accuracy when both examinations are utilized may approach 97 or 98 per cent.[8, 10]

Knee arthroscopy is also useful in allowing direct visualization of the inflamed joint lining in a variety of disorders, such as rheumatoid arthritis, pigmented villonodular synovitis, and crystal-induced arthropathies.[14] In this fashion, the nature and extent of the articular process can be evaluated and, if needed, a synovial biopsy under visual control can be performed. The arthroscope can then be used to assess the natural history of the disease and its response to therapy. In osteoarthritis, arthroscopy allows direct inspection of the three compartments of the knee — the medial femorotibial, the lateral femorotibial; and the patellofemoral compartments — and the distribution of abnormalities that are uncovered may influence the choice of surgical technique.[15] Clinical improvement in some patients with osteoarthritis of the knee has been noted following arthroscopy, perhaps related to the beneficial effects of joint distention and irrigation.[2] Similar irrigation with disruption of adhesions and loculations may be helpful in the treatment of septic arthritis,[1, 17] although some regard joint sepsis as a contraindication to the procedure. Additional contraindications include joint stiffening and ankylosis; the ideal knee in which to perform arthroscopy is large, with normal laxity and a full range of motion.[1] In the joint with limited mobility, a small arthroscope is often required.

The utilization of arthroscopy of the knee as well as of other joints in the diagnosis and treatment of chondral and osteochondral fragments is especially noteworthy.[22] Plain film radiography may be unrewarding in this clinical setting, and arthrography, although perhaps identifying a defect of the cartilaginous surface, is commonly unsuccessful in delineating the presence and number of intra-articular bodies. Arthroscopy can demonstrate the cartilage surface lesion and, in addition, can locate loose or synovium-embedded osteocartilaginous fragments. These then may be removed by passing instruments through the arthroscope. Pieces of intra-

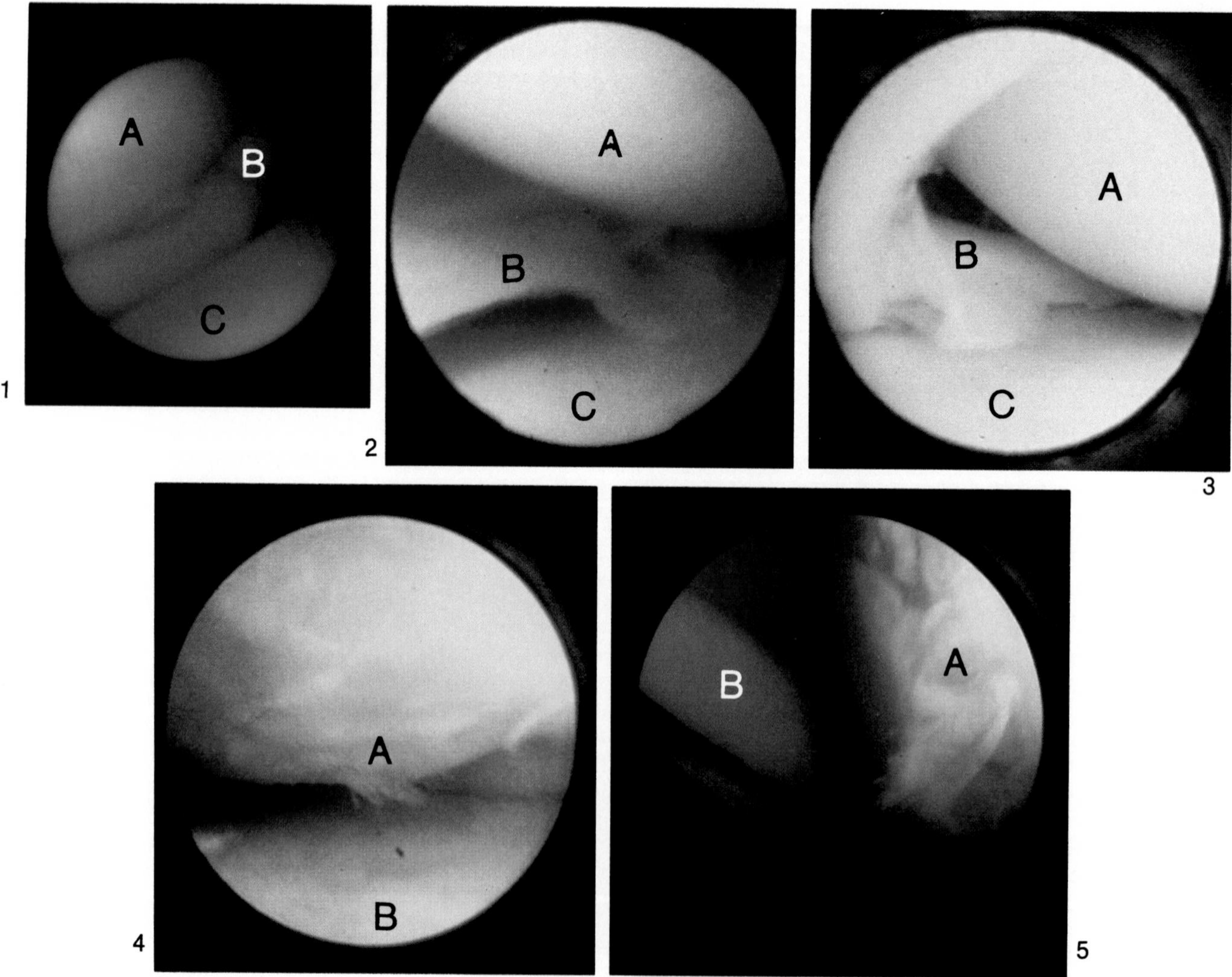

Figures 1 to 5. *See legends on opposite page.*

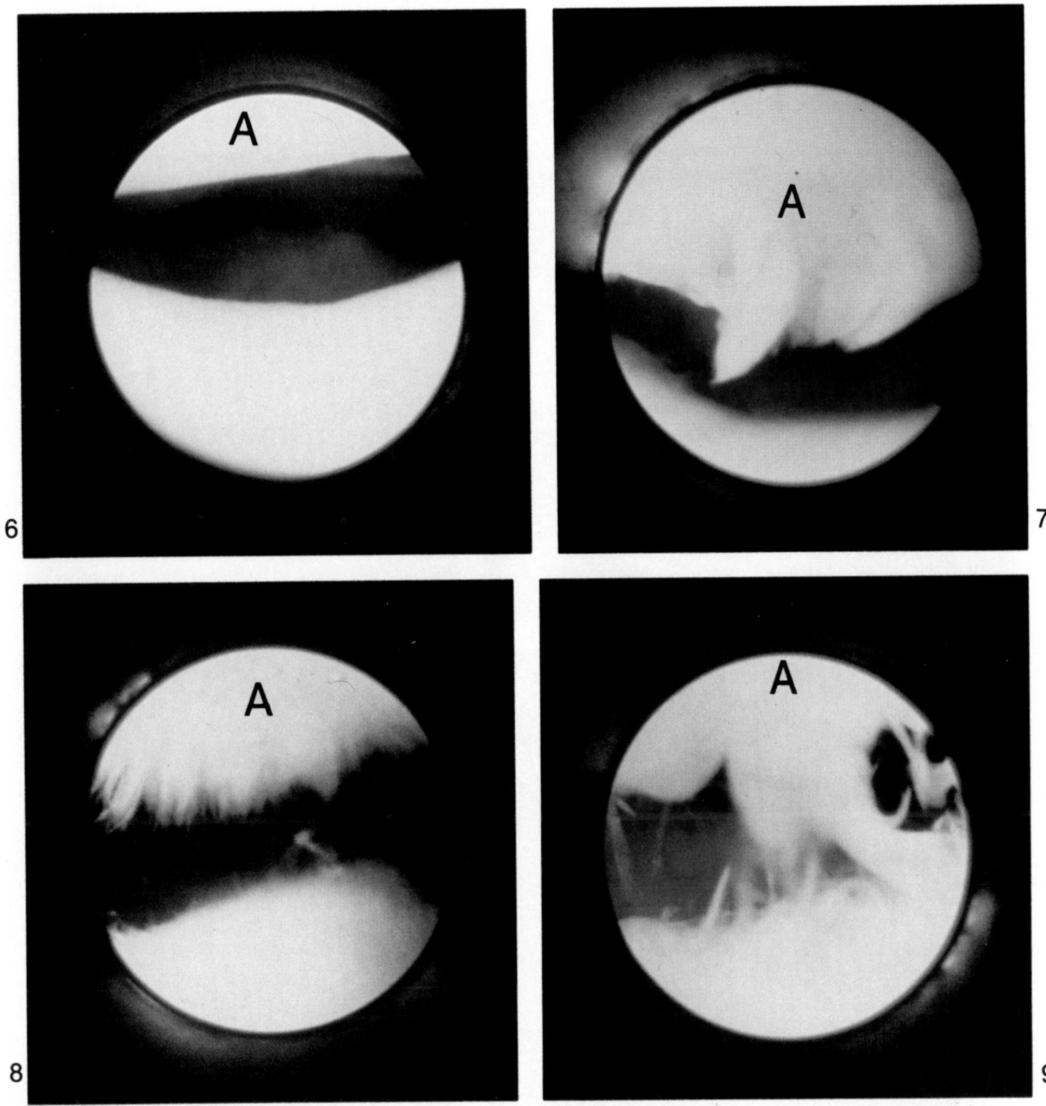

Figure 6. *Normal patellofemoral cartilage. A, Patella.*
Figure 7. *Chondromalacia (mild). A, Patella with cartilage fibrillation.*
Figure 8. *Chondromalacia (moderate). A, Patella with cartilage fibrillation.*
Figure 9. *Chondromalacia (severe). A, Patella with cartilage fibrillation.*

Figure 1. *Meniscal tear. A, Lateral femoral condyle. B, Bucket-handle fragment of meniscus in the intercondylar notch. C, Tibial plateau.*

Figure 2. *Meniscal tear. A, Femoral condyle. B, Torn meniscus. C, Tibial plateau.*

Figure 3. *Meniscal tear. A, Femoral condyle. B, Torn meniscus. C, Tibial plateau.*

Figure 4. *Articular cartilage degeneration. A, Femoral condyle cartilage fibrillation. B, Tibial plateau.*

Figure 5. *Articular cartilage degeneration (in the knee of a 14-year-old boy with sickle cell disease). A, Degeneration of medial femoral condyle. B, Meniscus.*

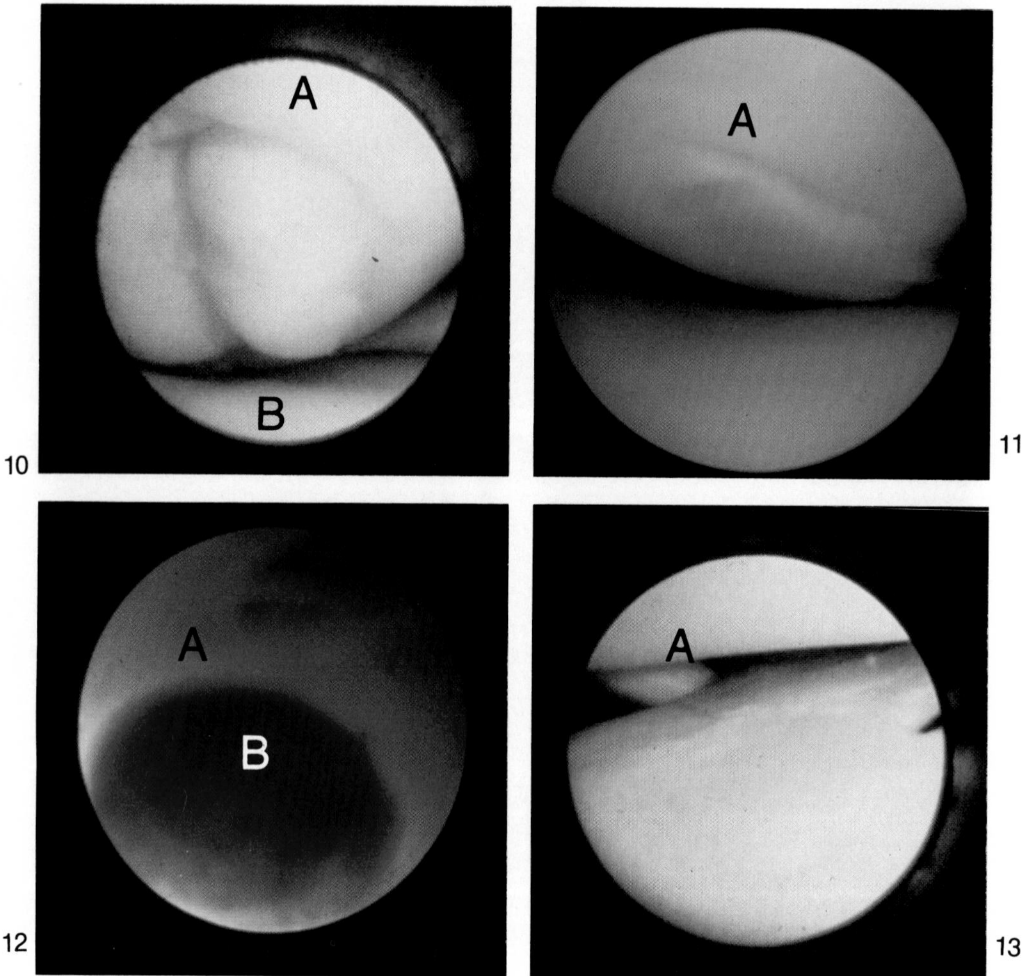

Figure 10. *Osteochondral defect of femoral condyle. A, Femoral condyle with defect. B, Tibial plateau.*

Figure 11. *Osteochondral defect of medial femoral condyle. In spite of intensive conservative treatment, this young woman continued to complain of pain. A, Defect in condyle.*

Figure 12. *Defect in medial femoral condyle caused by a 0.22 caliber bullet. Missile was removed with arthroscope. A, Medial femoral condyle. B, Defect.*

Figure 13. *Osteochondral body. A, Intraarticular body.*

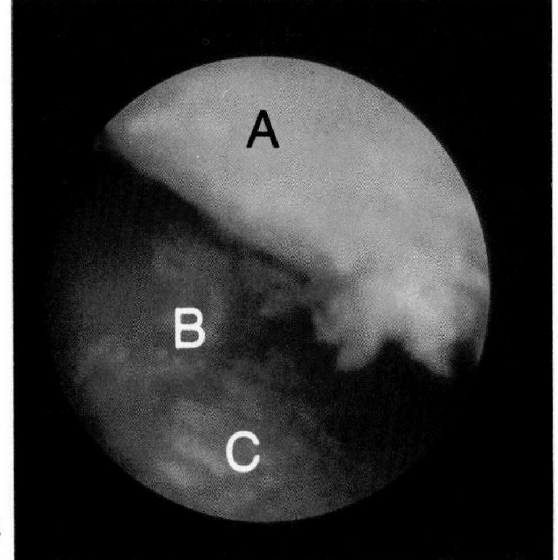

Figure 14. Gout. Monosodium urate crystal deposits in a middle-aged man. Clinical findings originally failed to yield a diagnosis. Specimen obtained arthroscopically supplied the correct answer. A, Medial femoral condyle with degenerative change.

Figures 15 and 16. *Synovial inflammatory changes.*

15

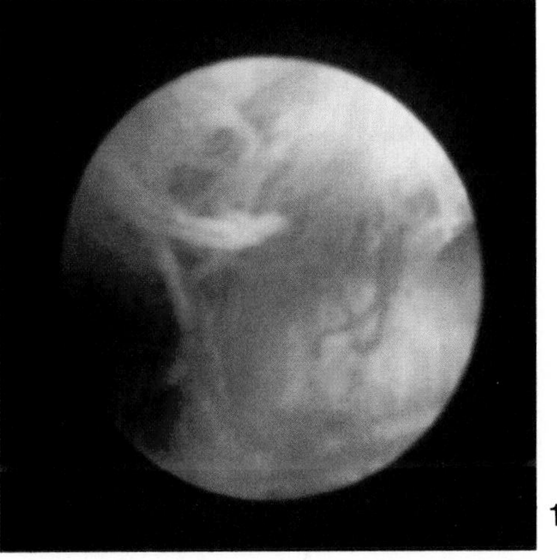

articular cement following arthroplasty can similarly be localized and removed in this fashion.[16] Furthermore, meniscal fragments may be excised making use of the arthroscope.

Arthroscopy of the glenohumeral joint has been advocated in patients with apparent historical evidence of recurrent dislocation in whom documentation by medical observation or by roentgenograms is lacking.[18] In this situation, a Hill-Sachs or glenoid lesion, or both may be demonstrated. Additional indications for glenohumeral joint arthroscopy may include the delineation of the degree and extent of synovial irritation, alterations or hypermobility of the bicipital tendon, and rotator cuff atrophy or tear. In the ankle and subtalar regions, arthroscopy may reveal osteochondritis dissecans, chondromalacia, synovial inflammation, and fibrosis or scar formation.[19, 20]

In addition to the difficulty of performing arthroscopy in the presence of restricted joint motion, another technical problem is the presence of exuberant synovium in patients with inflammatory or posttraumatic synovitis, which, because of hyperemia, may bleed with even gentle movement of the arthroscope.[1] The tourniquet should then be inflated and thorough irrigation should be employed to produce a clear field. Hemorrhage itself is not a contraindication to arthroscopy, although at the conclusion of the procedure, the joint should be irrigated with copious amounts of saline solution until the efflux is completely clear of blood.

Figures 1 to 16 demonstrate a spectrum of abnormalities of the knee that may be detected with arthroscopy. These illustrations were kindly supplied by Dr. Cliff Colwell, Scripps Clinic, LaJolla, California (Figs. 2 to 4, 6 to 10, 13, 15, 16), and Dr. John Joyce III, Philadelphia, Pennsylvania (Figs. 1, 5, 11, 12, 14).

REFERENCES

1. Jackson, RW, Dandy DJ: Arthroscopy of the Knee. New York, Grune & Stratton, 1976.
2. Combs JJ Jr, Hunder GG: Arthroscopy. *In* AS Cohen (Ed): Rheumatology and Immunology. New York, Grune & Stratton, 1979, p 110.
3. McGinty, JB, Freedman PA: Arthroscopy of the knee. Clin Orthop Rel Res *121*:173, 1976.
4. Dettaven KE, Collins HR: Diagnosis of internal derangements of the knee. The role of arthroscopy. J Bone Joint Surg *57A*:802, 1975.

5. Dandy DJ, Jackson RW: The impact of arthroscopy on the management of disorders of the knee. J Bone Joint Surg *57B*:346, 1975.
6. Korn MW, Spitzer, RM, Robinson KE: Correlations of arthrography with arthroscopy. Orthop Clin N Am *10*:535, 1979.
7. Gillies H, Seligson D: Precision in the diagnosis of meniscal lesions: A comparison of clinical evaluation, arthrography, and arthroscopy. J Bone Joint Surg *61A*:343, 1979.
8. Ireland J, Trickey EL, Stoker DJ: Arthroscopy and arthrography of the knee. A critical review. J Bone Joint Surg *62B*:3, 1980.
9. Jackson RW, Abe I: The role of arthroscopy in the management of disorders of the knee. J. Bone Joint Surg *54B*:310, 1972.
10. Levinsohn EM, Baker BE: Prearthrotomy diagnostic evaluation of the knee: Review of 100 cases diagnosed by arthrography and arthroscopy. Am J Roentgenol *134*:107, 1980.
11. Henry AN: Arthroscopy in practice. Br Med J *1*:87, 1977.
12. Freiberger RH, Killoran PJ, Cardona, G: Arthrography of the knee by double contrast method. Am J Roentgenol *97*:736, 1966.
13. Jackson RW: The role of arthroscopy in the management of the arthritic knee. Clin Orthop Rel Res *101*:28, 1974.
14. O'Connor RL: The arthroscope in the management of crystal-induced synovitis of the knee. J Bone Joint Surg *55A*:1443, 1973.
15. Thomas RH, Resnick D, Alazraki NP, Daniel D, Greenfield R: Compartmental evaluation of osteoarthritis of the knee. A comparative study of available diagnostic modalities. Radiology *116*:585, 1975.
16. Shifrin LZ, Reis ND: Arthroscopy of a dislocated hip replacement: a case report. Clin Orthop Rel Res *146*:213, 1980.
17. Jackson RW, Parson CJ: Distention-irrigation treatment of major joint sepsis. Clin Orthop Rel Res *96*:160, 1973.
18. Johnson LL: Arthroscopy of the shoulder. *In* RL O'Connor (Ed): Arthroscopy. Kalamazoo, Michigan, Upjohn Company, 1977, p 49.
19. O'Connor RL: Pathologic conditions within the knee. *In* RL O'Connor (Ed.): Arthroscopy. Kalamazoo, Michigan, Upjohn Company, 1977, p. 55.
20. O'Connor RL: Arthroscopy. Philadelphia, JB Lippincott Co, 1977.
21. American Academy of Orthopedic Surgeons: Symposium on Arthroscopy and Arthrography of the Knee. St Louis, CV Mosby Co, 1978.
22. Gilley, JS, Gelman MI, Edson M, Metcalf RW: Chondral fractures of the knee. Arthrographic, arthroscopic, and clinical manifestations. Radiology *138*:51, 1981.

APPENDIX 2
SYNOVIAL FLUID EXAMINATION

by Gen Niwayama, M.D., and Donald Resnick, M.D.

The technique of joint aspiration and direct examination of aspirated synovial fluid or synovial membrane is described in Chapter 23. Identification and characterization of crystals or organisms allow precise documentation of crystal-induced or septic arthritis. Less specific tests performed on the synovial fluid are summarized in Chapter 23 (Table 23–1), and are based upon the appearance and viscosity of the fluid as well as its protein content, biochemical characteristics, and cellular constituents. The cell content in the fluid, which may be composed of leukocytes and erythrocytes in addition to synovial and cartilage cells, is dependent upon the nature of the pathologic process leading to the joint effusion. Thus, careful cytologic examination of the synovial fluid provides an important clue to the nature of the synovial membrane aberrations and aids in accurate diagnosis of the joint disease.

SYNOVIAL FLUID

Total leukocyte counts are determined by examining undiluted synovial fluid or fluid containing a diluent (physiologic saline solution plus a small amount of 0.1 per cent methylene blue).[1] The reported upper limit of normal for the synovial leukocyte count has ranged from under 200 cells per cu ml[2] to under 750 per cu ml.[3] A phase contrast microscope is often useful for accurate distinction between leukocytes and erythrocytes. The differential cell count can be estimated by examination of undiluted synovial fluid or that concentrated by centrifugation.[4-7] Utilizing these methods, investigators have described the cellular morphology of the fluid, which may be dramatically influenced by the presence of synovial membrane pathology.[8] Light microscopic examination of normal synovial fluid may show scattered inflammatory cells (10 to 200 cu ml) containing many mononuclear histiocytes (65 per cent).[7] These histiocytes contain abundant foamy phagocytic cytoplasm with occasional azurophilic granules. The nuclei are centrally located and are round, oval, or moon-shaped, with prominent nucleoli. Variable numbers of leukocytes (10 per cent) and mature lymphocytes (25 per cent) are also seen. In addition, there are scattered single synovial cells in the smear, which cytologically resemble reactive mesothelial cells such as are seen in the serous cavities of the body. They have abundant cytoplasm, an elongated shape, and round or oval, eccentric basophilic nuclei with a fine, granular chromatin pattern. In the normal situation, no cartilaginous or inclusion-bearing cells are seen.

SYNOVIAL MEMBRANE

Under normal conditions, the synovial cells of the lining layer present four morphologic forms when examined with electron microscopy.[9]

1. The most common cell is the "synthetic" or B

cell, which has well-developed rough endoplasmic reticulum cisternae that contain amorphous material. Well-developed Golgi lamellae, vesicles, free ribosomes, and ribosomal rosettes are seen.

2. The second most common cell is the fibrocyte, which has a thin rim of cytoplasm, a few ribosomes in rosette form, cisternae of rough endoplasmic reticulum, few mitochondria, no Golgi apparatus, and rare lysosomes.

3. The third type of synovial cell is the intermediate or C cell, which has abundant rough endoplasmic reticulum, Golgi apparatus, and a few lysosomes, micropinocytotic vesicles, and filopodia on the surface.

4. The fourth cell is a "phagocytic" A cell. This type is infrequently seen and contains much rough endoplastic reticulum, Golgi apparatus, few lysosomes, and many filopodia.

When the synovial membrane is subjected to an injurious process of any nature — physical, chemical, or infectious — the synovial cells proliferate and become hypertrophic, and, in certain situations, the process may lead to cellular necrosis of the synovial membrane. Proliferation may create two to three rows of synovial cells. Fibroblasts in the subsynovial layer also frequently proliferate and are often difficult to distinguish from adjoining hypertrophic synovial cells on light microscopic examination. Traumatic or articular disorders (rheumatoid arthritis, osteoarthritis) producing disruption of the joint surface may lead to fragmentation of the hyaline cartilage and subchondral bone, and the fragments may be dislodged into the joint cavity or become embedded in the synovial membrane. Hemosiderin pigments, end products of hemorrhage, are often engulfed as granules by hypertrophic synovial cells and histiocytes. Synovial giant cells can also be seen in the synovial membrane.[8] They are ovoid or round in shape, with peripherally denser cytoplasm from which a few plump processes extend in all directions. The nuclei number from two to about 12, most commonly between three and eight, rarely as many as 30, and resemble those of hypertrophic synovial cells.

DISEASE STATES

Some characteristics of synovial fluid aspirates in various conditions have been described.

1. *Septic arthritis.* Gram's stain is positive in about 50 per cent of patients with articular sepsis, and culture may be positive in about 30 to 80 per cent of patients with septic arthritis.[10, 11] Articular infection may coexist with other types of arthritis so that cytologic evaluation and crystal identification cannot be neglected in establishing a definitive diagnosis.

2. *Traumatic arthritis.* Hemorrhagic or xanthochromatic fluid may be obtained. Variable numbers of degenerated synovial cells are often seen in large sheets rather than singly.[7] Similarly, large sheets of degenerative cartilaginous cells may be noted.

3. *Osteoarthritis.* The most remarkable feature of the synovial fluid is the presence of numerous, well-preserved normal-appearing multinucleated cartilaginous cells.[6, 7] These are frequently seen in sheets or clusters rather than singly, with an exceptionally clean background on the smear. Fragments of cartilage may appear birefringent under polarized light[12] but do not possess parallel margins. These fragments as well as collagen fibrils may be present in the synovial fluid in both osteoarthritic and traumatic disorders.

4. *Pigmented villonodular synovitis.* Foreign body giant cells with hemosiderin pigments and papillary aggregates of synovial cells are described as characteristic in this condition.[6, 7] The background of the smear is often clustered with erythrocytes and protein debris.

5. *Rheumatoid arthritis.* Cytologic studies reveal the presence of monolobulated or polylobulated neutrophils containing 2 to 15 round, dark inclusions (granules) in the cytoplasm (rheumatoid arthritis or RA cells).[7, 13] These cells are seen in about 95 per cent of patients, and the inclusions, which are present in 5 to 100 per cent of neutrophils,[5] are 0.5 to 2.0 micrometers in diameter. The inclusions can be clearly identified using phase contrast microscopy with oil immersion, and by immunofluorescent techniques that reveal immune complexes: IgG, IgM, complement, and rheumatoid factor. RA cells are not entirely specific for rheumatoid arthritis, as they may also be seen in other conditions, such as gout and septic arthritis.[14]

6. *Systemic lupus erythematosus.* The cytologic diagnosis is based upon the recognition of the presence of LE cells, which are mature, enlarged polymorphonuclear neutrophils with large, hyaline, pink, homogeneous inclusions distending the cytoplasm.[7] In some cases, LE cells are present in synovial fluid with a negative LE test on peripheral blood, and a few patients with rheumatoid arthritis also may have LE cells in the synovial fluid.[5] The nuclei of these neutrophils are usually compressed in the form of a crescent around the periphery of the inclusion. The synovial cells are few, single, and not remarkable.[7]

7. *Reiter's syndrome.* Large histiocytic cells with intracytoplasmic inclusions (chlamydial inclusions) have been described on Giemsa and Papanicolaou stains.[6, 7] Chlamydial agent may be isolated from the infected synovial membrane.[15] Large amounts of inflammatory cells (50,000 per cu ml) are usually present, with a predominance of monocytes, lymphocytes, and macrophages in the early phase of the lesion and of polymorphonuclear neutrophils in

the later stage.[7] No cartilage cells or crystals are seen.

8. *Neoplasm.* Articular involvement by primary or metastatic neoplasms has been studied cytologically.[7, 16] The diagnosis of tumor is established by the presence of sheets or clusters of neoplastic cells with features foreign to the lining membrane of the joint. In this fashion, osteogenic sarcoma cells have been detected in synovial fluid.[16] In cases of synovial sarcoma, the synovial fluid is serous, mucinous, or hemorrhagic and contains papillary structures in a pseudoglandular arrangement resembling the normal synovial cells except for their shape and size variation, nuclear hypertrophy, and hyperchromasia.[7]

9. *Crystal-induced arthritis.*

A. *Hydroxyapatite crystal deposition disease.* The apatite crystals appear as shining inclusions on wet preparations or dark cytoplasmic inclusions on Wright's stain.[17] Definitive diagnosis requires the utilization of electron microscopy.

B. *Monosodium urate crystal deposition disease (gout).* Monosodium urate crystals appear as negatively birefringent rods or needles under polarized light microscopy and vary from 1 to 20 micrometers in length.[18-20, 23] It should be noted that certain crystal and corticosteroid preparations appear morphologically similar to monosodium urate crystals.[21, 22] Definitive identification of needle-like crystals may be aided by incubation with uricase. During an acute attack of gout, the number of inflammatory cells may exceed 10,000 per cu ml with a preponderance of degenerative polymorphonuclear neutrophils.[7] The exfoliated cells are few and usually show advanced degenerative changes. There are occasional poorly preserved cartilaginous cells.

C. *Calcium pyrophosphate dihydrate crystal deposition disease.* Crystals of calcium pyrophosphate dihydrate (CPPD) appear as positively birefringent rods, rectangles, or rhomboids varying from 1 to 20 micrometers in length and to about 4 micrometers in width,[20] an appearance that may also be seen following intra-articular injection of corticosteroids or that may result from the presence of cholesterol crystals in chronic effusions.[22, 24] In CPPD crystal deposition disease,[7] the amount of inflammatory cells (80 per cent polymorphonuclear leukocytes) varies from 200 to 30,000 per cu mm, with an average of 10,000 cells per cu mm, depending upon the acuteness of the crisis. Rheumatoid arthritis cells may be noted, although their number will vary, usually being less than that found in rheumatoid arthritis.

D. *Talc-induced arthritis.* Talcum crystals can be introduced during articular surgery, producing a chronic arthritis. The crystals have a Maltese cross appearance

Text continued on page 3271

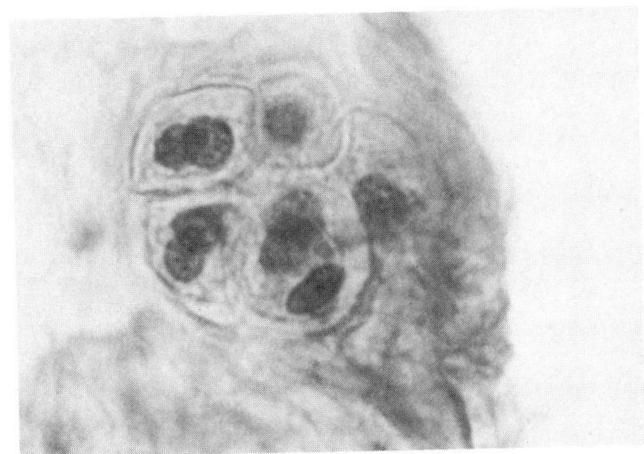

Figure 2. *An aggregate of chondrocytes. Two chondrocytes have double nuclei (Papanicolaou stain, 920×).*

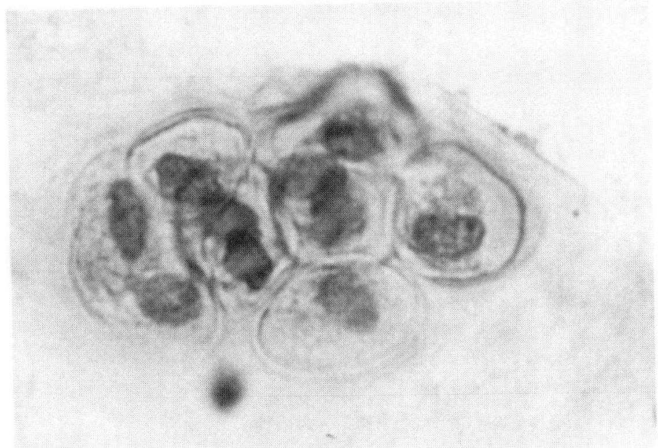

Figure 1. *An aggregate of chondrocytes with ovoid nuclei (Papanicolaou stain, 920×).*

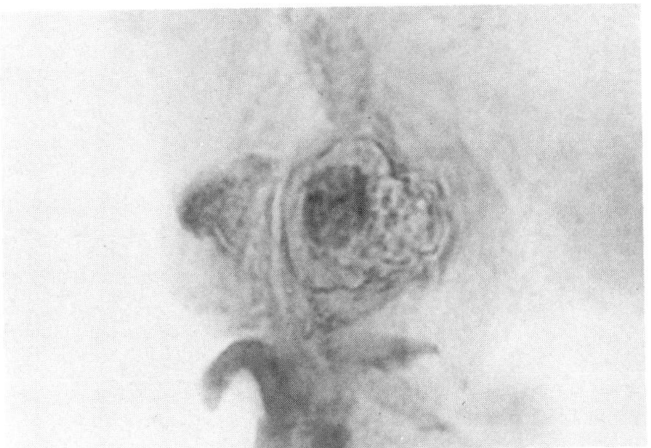

Figure 3. *A chondrocyte with fine cytoplasmic vacuoles (Papanicolaou stain, 920×).*

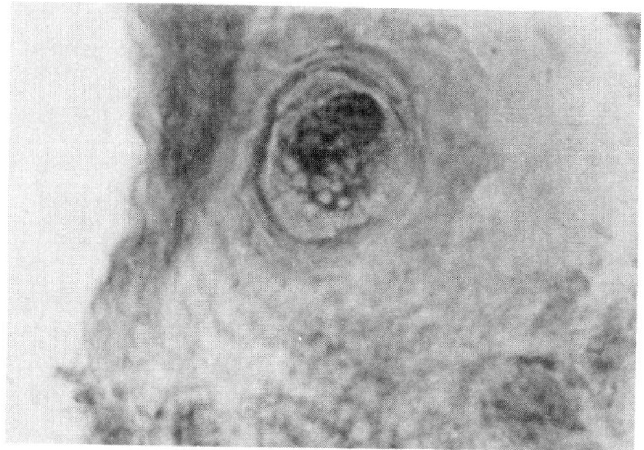

Figure 4. *A chondrocyte with an ovoid nucleus and fine cytoplasmic vacuoles (Papanicolaou stain, 920×).*

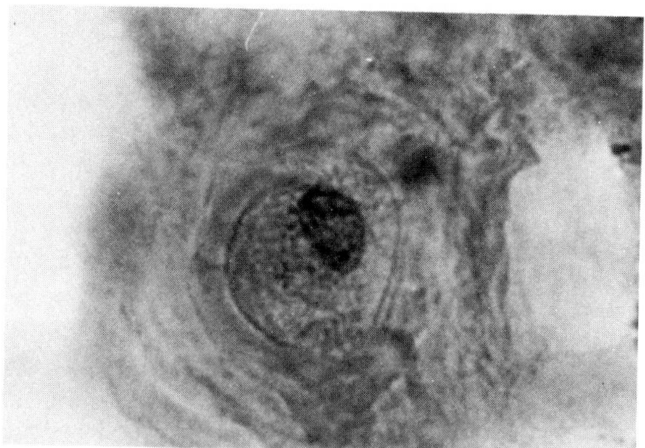

Figure 7. *A chondrocyte with a prominent nucleolus (Papanicolaou stain, 920 ×).*

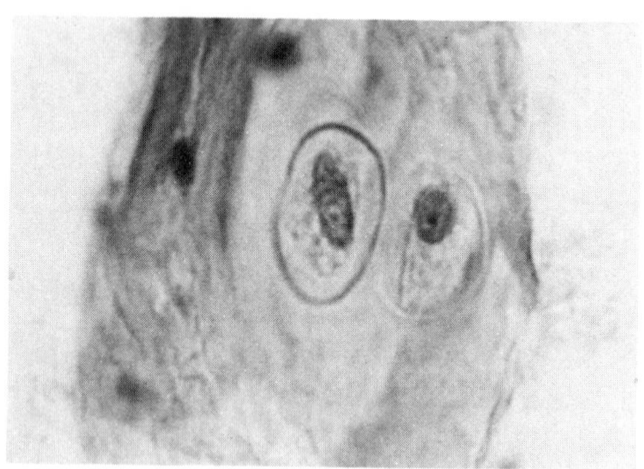

Figure 5. *Two chondrocytes with nucleoli (Papanicolaou stain, 920×).*

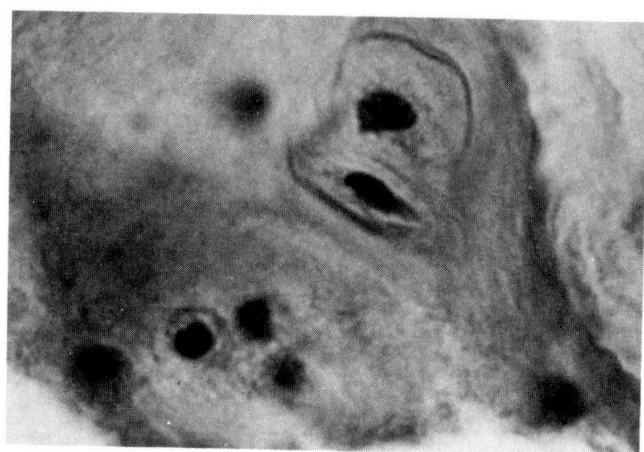

Figure 8. *Two chondrocytes with pyknotic nuclei (Papanicolaou stain, 920×).*

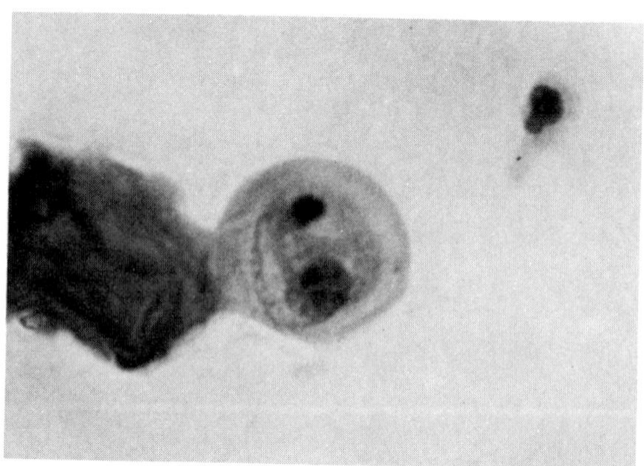

Figure 6. *A chondrocyte with an enlarged nucleolus (Papanicolaou stain, 920 ×).*

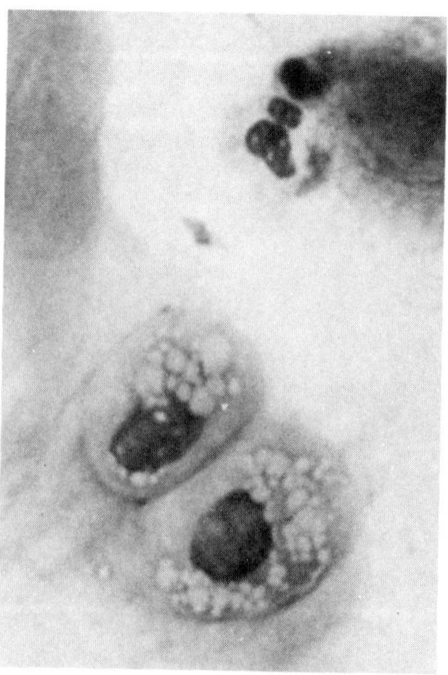

Figure 9. *Two chondrocytes (air-dried smear with Wright stain). Multiple fine cytoplasmic vacuoles are seen (920×).*

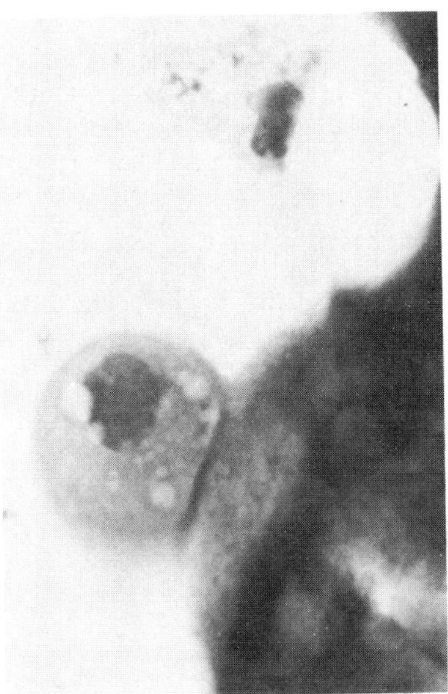

Figure 10. *A chondrocyte with slightly enlarged cytoplasmic vacuoles (air-dried smear with Wright stain) (920×).*

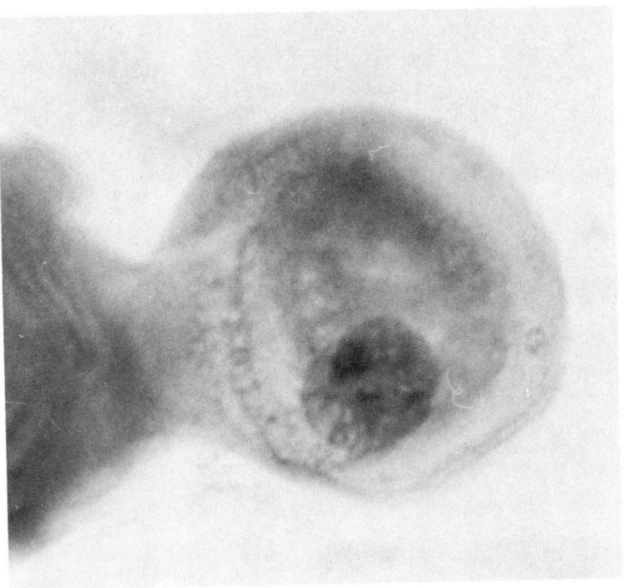

Figure 11. *A chondrocyte with enlarged nucleolus (Papanicolaou stain, 2300×).*

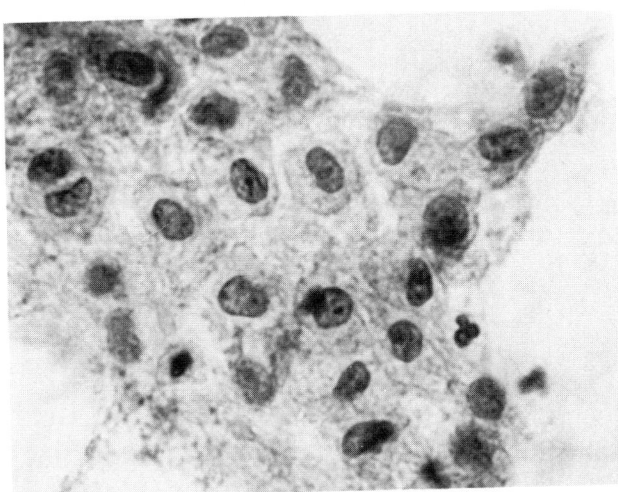

Fig. 12

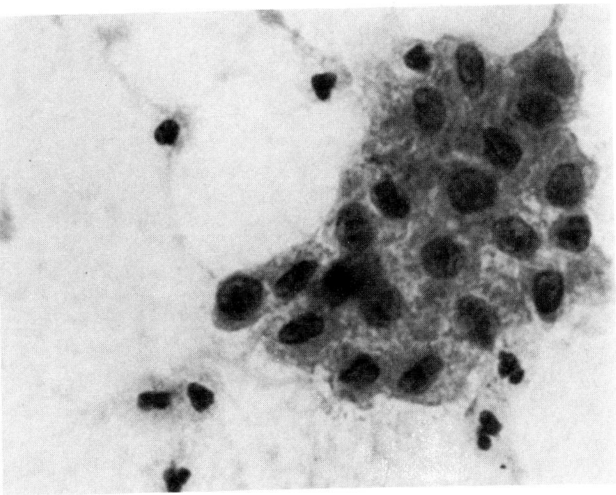

Fig. 13

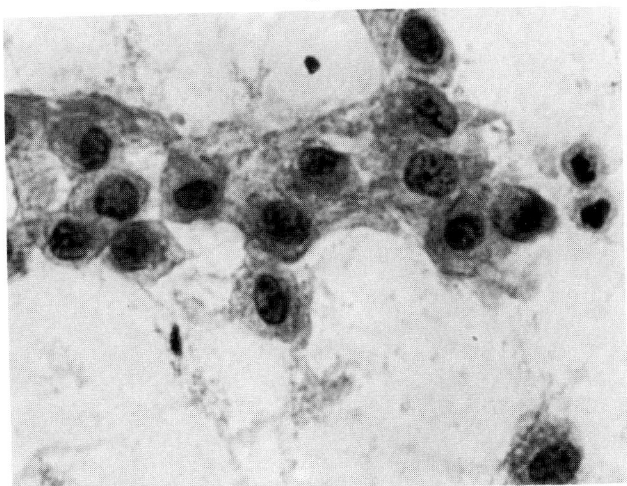

Fig. 14

Figures 12, 13, 14. *Sheets of synovial cells with round or ovoid nuclei and nucleoli. These cells resemble cytologically mesothelial cells of serous cavities (Papanicolaou stain, 920×).*

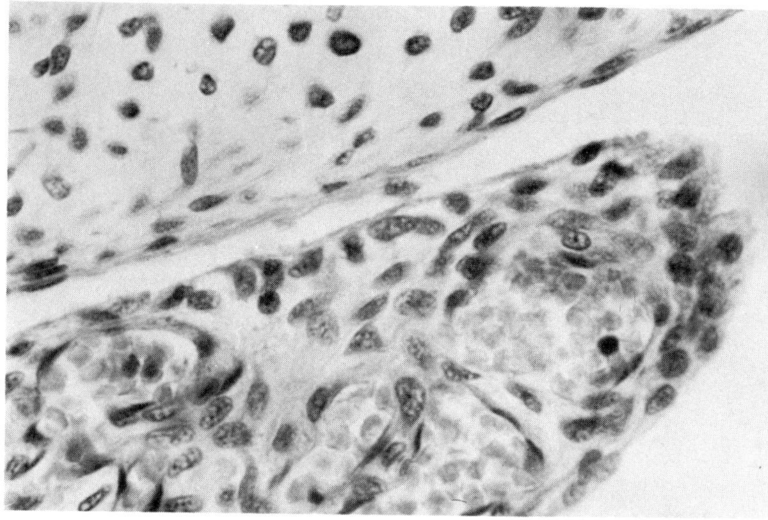

Figure 15. *Twenty-two week fetus: knee joint. Fetal cartilage (upper portion) and fetal synovial tissue are shown. Round or ovoid shaped synovial cells are seen. Fetal chondrocytes reveal round or ovoid nuclei and scanty neoplasm (hematoxylin and eosin stain, 860×).*

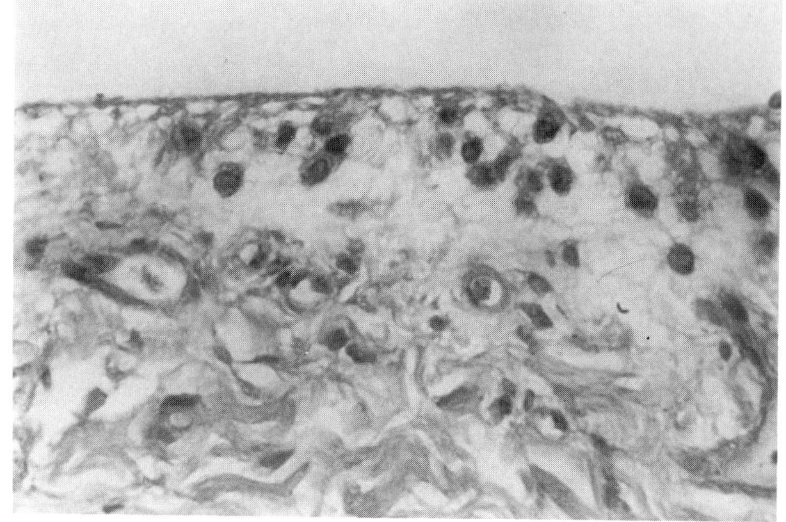

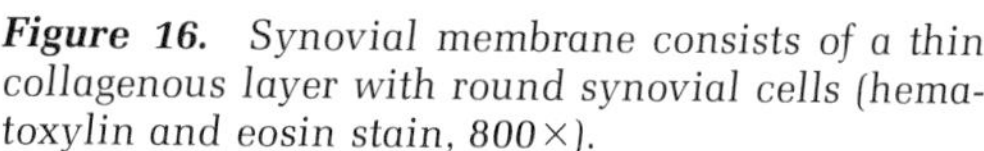

Figure 16. *Synovial membrane consists of a thin collagenous layer with round synovial cells (hematoxylin and eosin stain, 800×).*

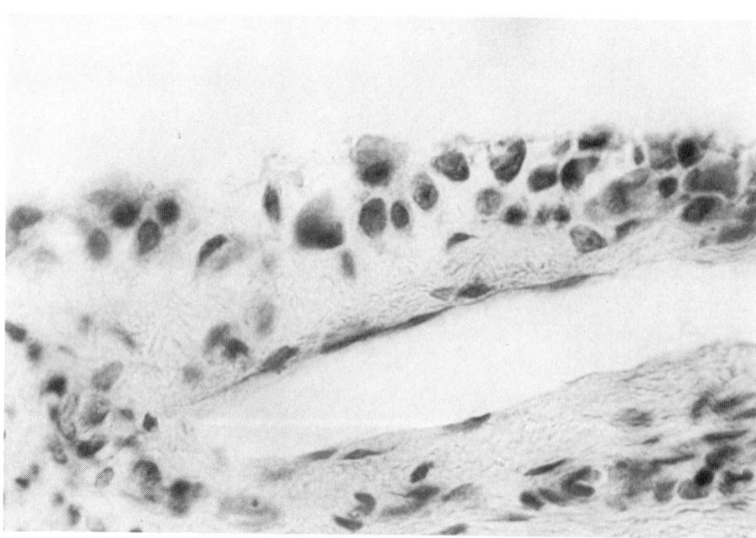

Figure 17. *Synovial cells show mild variation in nuclear size and cell size. This appearance suggests an irritation of the articular surface (hematoxylin and eosin stain, 800×).*

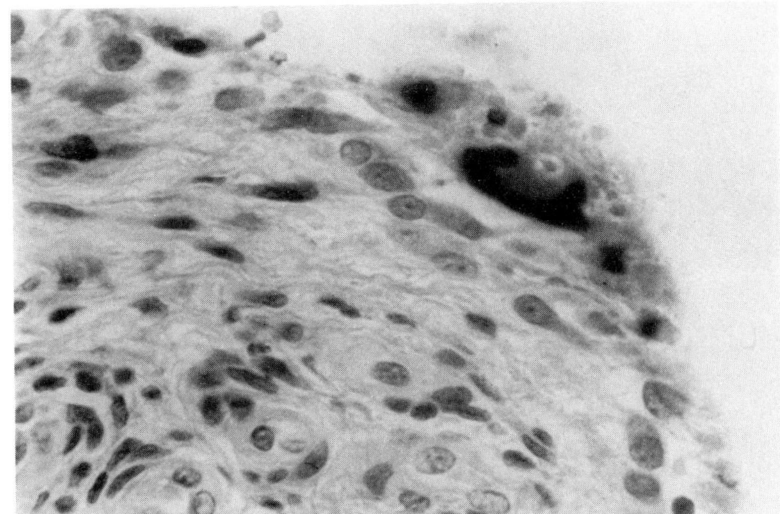

Figure 18. *A hyperchromatic multinuclear cell is seen on the surface. Other synovial cells reveal ovoid nuclei and ovoid or slightly elongated cytoplasm (hematoxylin and eosin stain, 800×).*

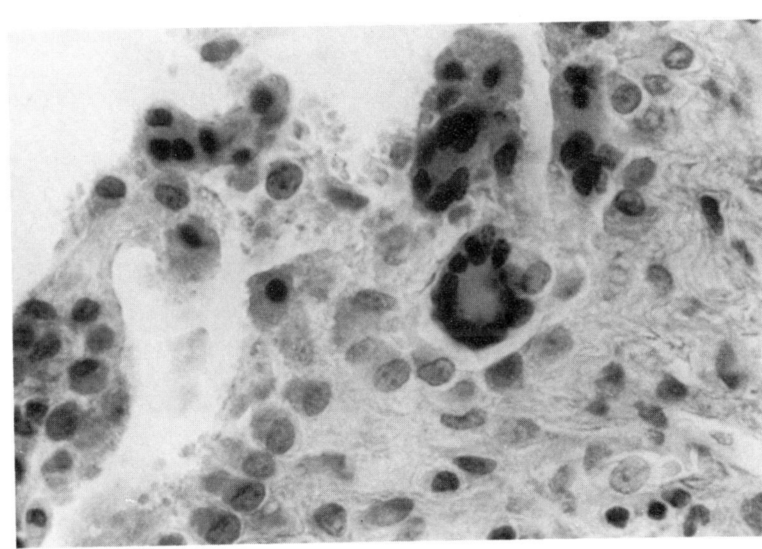

Figure 19. *A few multinucleated synovial cells are seen over the synovial surface. Other synovial cells show ovoid nuclei with small nucleoli. Synovial cells are increased in number (hematoxylin and eosin stain, 800×).*

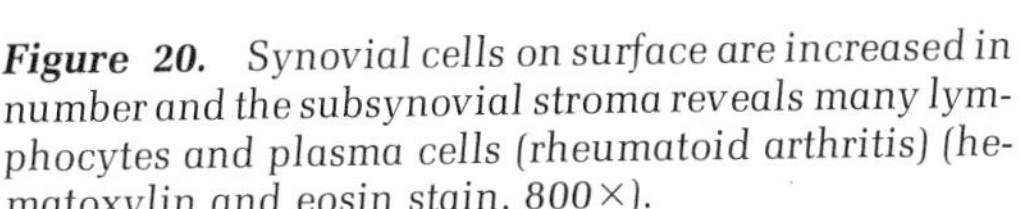

Figure 20. *Synovial cells on surface are increased in number and the subsynovial stroma reveals many lymphocytes and plasma cells (rheumatoid arthritis) (hematoxylin and eosin stain, 800×).*

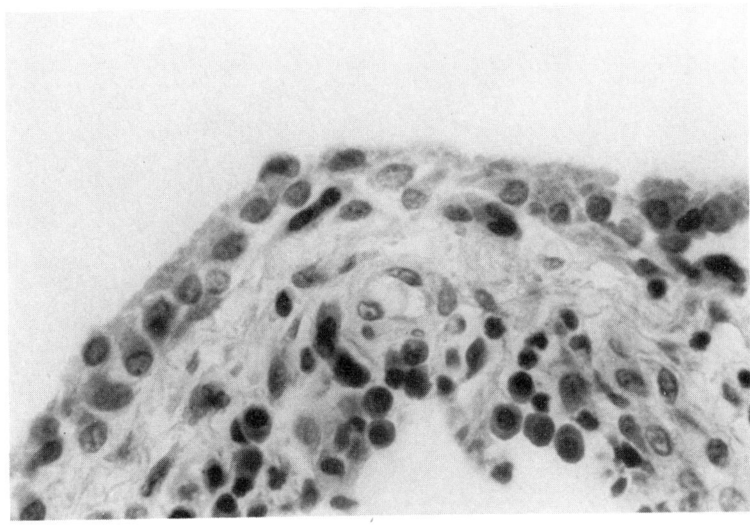

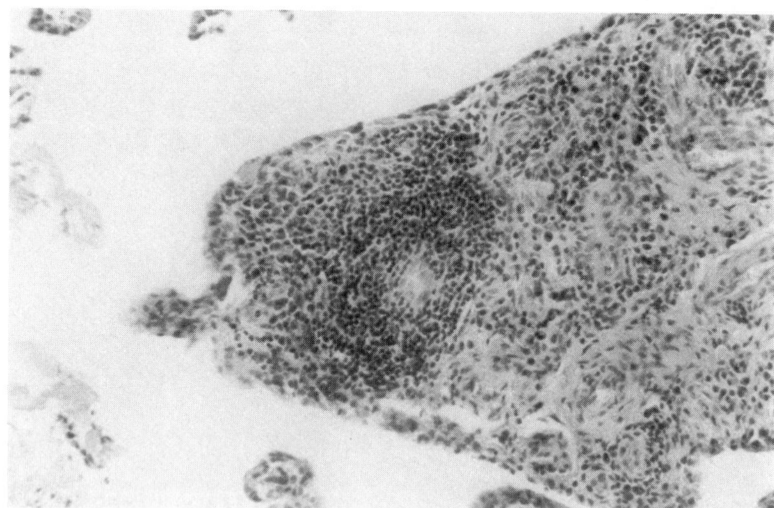

Figure 21. *Synovial tissue reveals marked cellular increase with lymphocytes (lymphoid follicle) and plasma cells (rheumatoid arthritis) (hematoxylin and eosin stain, 200×).*

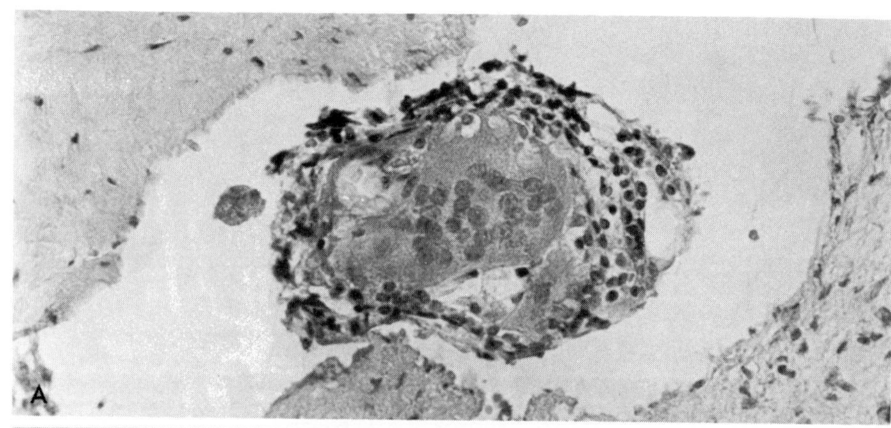

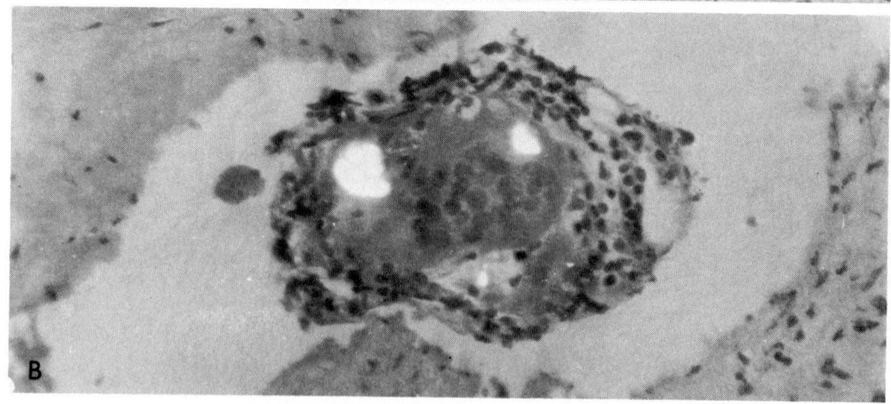

Figure 22. Nonpolarized **(A)** *and polarized* **(B)** *photomicrographs reveal multinucleated giant cells containing urate crystals (gouty arthritis) (hematoxylin and eosin stain, 600×).*

and may be as small as 5 to 10 micrometers.[7] Their presence should be reported since they can cause articular granulation tissue formation.

E. *Crystalline corticosteroid–induced arthritis.* Acute synovitis can be caused by intra-articular injection of crystalline corticosteroid preparations.[21] Crystals may be identified in synovial fluid for a month or longer after such intra-articular injection. The crystalline corticosteroids appear as long needles or rhomboids under polarized light, characteristics that may be confused with monosodium urate or calcium pyrophosphate dihydrate crystals. Short rods, plates, fragments, or clumps of crystals are also seen.

Representative cytologic preparations of synovial fluid and histologic preparations of synovial membrane from surgically resected specimens are demonstrated in Figures 1 to 22.

REFERENCES

1. Cohen AS, Brandt KD, Drey PR: Synovial fluid. *In* Cohen AS (Ed): Laboratory Diagnostic Procedures in the Rheumatic Diseases. Boston, Little, Brown & Co, 1975.
2. Ropes MW, Bauer W: Synovial Fluid Changes in Joint Disease. Cambridge, Harvard University Press, 1953.
3. Currey HLF, Vernon RB: Examination of synovial fluid. Clin Rheum Dis *2*:149, 1976.
4. Hollander JL, Reginato A, Torralba TP: Examination of synovial fluid as a diagnostic aid in arthritis. Med Clin North Am *50*:1281, 1966.
5. Krieg AF: Cerebral fluid and other body fluids. *In* Henry JB (Ed): Clinical Diagnosis and Management by Laboratory Methods. 16th Ed. Philadelphia, WB Saunders Co, 1979.
6. Broderick PA, Corvese N, Peirik MG, Pike RF, Mariorenzi AL: Exfoliative cytology interpretation of synovial fluid in joint disease. J Bone Joint Surg *58A*:396, 1976.
7. Naib ZM: Cytology of synovial fluids. Acta Cytol *17*:299, 1973.
8. Soren A: Histodiagnosis and Clinical Correlation of Rheumatoid and Other Synovitis. Philadelphia, JB Lippincott Co, 1978.
9. Wayne-Roberts CR, Anderson C: Light and electron microscopic studies of normal juvenile human synovium. Semin Arthritis Rheum *7*:279, 1978.
10. Cooke CL, Owen DS, Irby R, Toone E: Gonococcal arthritis. JAMA *217*:204, 1971.
11. McCord WC, Nies KM, Louie JS: Acute venereal arthritis. Arch Intern Med *137*:858, 1977.
12. Kitridou R, McCarty DJ, Prockop DJ, Hummeler K: Identification of collagen in synovial fluid. Arthritis Rheum *12*:580, 1969.
13. Hollander JL, McCarty DJ, Astorga G, Castro-Murillo E: Studies on the pathogenesis of rheumatoid joint inflammation. I. The "RA cell" and a working hypothesis. Ann Intern Med *62*:271, 1965.
14. Scott JT: The analysis of joint fluids. Br J Hosp Med *14*:653, 1975.
15. Schachter J, Barnes MG, Jones JP, Engleman EP, Meyer KF: Isolation of bedsoniae from the joints of patients with Reiter's syndrome. Proc Soc Exp Biol Med *122*:283, 1966.
16. Meisels A, Berebichez M: Exfoliative cytology in orthopedics. Can Med Assoc J *84*:957, 1961.
17. Schumacher HR, Smolyo AP, Tse RL, Maurer K: Arthritis associated with apatite crystals. Ann Intern Med *87*:411, 1977.
18. Schumacher HR, Jimenez SA, Gibson T, Paseual E, Tragcoff R, Dorwart BB, Reginato AJ: Acute gouty arthritis without urate crystals identified on initial examination of synovial fluid. Arthritis Rheum *18*:608, 1975.
19. Suprun H, Mansoor I: An aspiration cytodiagnostic test for gouty arthritis. Acta Cytol *17*:198, 1973.
20. McCarty DJ, Gatter RA, Brill JM, Hogan JM: Crystal deposition disease. JAMA *193*:123, 1965.
21. Kahn CB, Hollander JL, Schumacher HR: Corticosteroid crystals in synovial fluid. JAMA *211*:807, 1970.
22. Nye WHR, Terry R, Rosenbaum DL: Two forms of crystalline lipid in "cholesterol" effusions. Am J Clin Pathol *49*:718, 1968.
23. McCarty DJ, Hollander JL: Identification of urate crystals in gouty synovial fluid. Ann Intern Med *54*:452, 1961.
24. Wild JH, Zvaifler NJ: An office technique for identifying crystals in synovial fluid. Am Fam Physician *12*:72, 1975.

APPENDIX 3
SYNOVIAL MEMBRANE BIOPSY

by Donald Resnick, M.D., and Gen Niwayama, M.D.

Because the appearance of the synovial membrane can be an important indicator of the nature of an articular process, it is not surprising that efforts have been directed toward the development and refinement of synovial biopsy techniques. Synovial membrane biopsy can be performed by an open surgical technique, by a closed blind technique, or as an adjunct to arthroscopy during which direct visualization of the biopsy area can be provided. Open surgical biopsy procedure is especially helpful in the evaluation of processes affecting the hip, the sacroiliac or glenohumeral joint, and the small articulations of the hand and foot.[1] Large synovial membrane samples can be obtained from selected areas of the joint.

Although closed synovial membrane biopsy techniques were introduced about 50 years ago, their use was not feasible until small caliber biopsy needles became available. The first punch biopsy needle to receive wide acceptance was introduced by Polley and Bickel in 1951.[2, 3] The instrument was 5 mm in diameter and was most effective in sampling a portion of the synovial lining of the knee. In 1963, a small caliber needle was introduced by Parker and Pearson.[4] Because of its size, the Parker-Pearson needle can be used to obtain synovial tissue not only from the knee but also from the wrist, elbow, ankle, and other synovial sacs and bursae.[3, 5] Thorough cleaning of the skin is followed by the administration of a local anesthetic agent. The needle is then inserted into the articulation. For the knee, the needle is usually introduced into the suprapatellar pouch, a syringe is attached to the end of the needle, and any synovial fluid is removed and sent for appropriate cytologic, chemical, and microbiologic studies.[1] Saline injection may be used to distend the articulation prior to biopsy, although this technique is not uniformly performed. The trocar is then re-

Table 1

HISTOLOGIC ABNORMALITIES OF TISSUE OBSERVED BY SYNOVIAL MEMBRANE BIOPSY*

Disorder	Characteristics
Rheumatoid arthritis and seronegative spondyloarthropathies	Vascular congestion and edema, synovial cell proliferation, inflammatory cell infiltration
Systemic lupus erythematosus	Minimal synovial cell hyperplasia, dense surface fibrin deposits, mild inflammatory cell infiltration
Scleroderma	Marked superficial fibrin deposits, minimal vascular or synovial cell proliferation
Degenerative joint disease	Normal or mild fibrous atrophy and vascular congestion
Septic arthritis (bacterial)	Identification of organisms
Septic arthritis (tuberculosis)	Identification of organisms, caseating granulomas with giant cells
Sarcoidosis	Noncaseating granulomas
Hemochromatosis	Iron in synovial lining cells
Pigmented villonodular synovitis	Villous hypertrophy, giant cells, hemosiderin deposition
Idiopathic synovial osteochondromatosis	Islands of metaplastic cartilage in synovium and subsynovial connective tissue
Alkaptonuria (ochronosis)	Fragments of pigmented cartilage (shards)
Multicentric reticulohistocytosis	Foamy appearing giant cells
Amyloidosis	Minimal inflammatory cell infiltration or synovial lining cell proliferation, amyloid deposits on Congo red stain
Gout	Monosodium urate crystal deposition
Calcium pyrophosphate dihydrate crystal deposition disease	Calcium pyrophosphate dihydrate crystal deposition
Primary and secondary neoplasms	Malignant cells in synovium

*From Goldenberg CL: Synovial membrane biopsy. *In* AS Cohen (Ed): Rheumatology and Immunology. New York, Grune & Stratton, 1979, p 89.

moved and a biopsy needle is inserted. External pressure is applied with the examiner's finger in order to introduce synovial tissue into the hooked lip of the biopsy needle. Gentle suction can also be utilized to engage the synovial membrane. Multiple small biopsy specimens are obtained, which are fixed in formalin. If crystal-induced synovitis is suspected, a portion of the specimen is also fixed in absolute alcohol.[1]

The procedure is not difficult and is usually without significant complications. Mild pain and tenderness can be evident for a short period following synovial biopsy. Joint effusion or, very rarely, hemarthrosis may be seen. Strict antiseptic technique makes the development of a joint infection very unlikely. Rare reports describe additional complications of this procedure, including breaking of the needle itself.[7]

The results of synovial membrane biopsy can provide useful information in the accurate diagnosis of the joint affliction[1] (Table 1), although in many disorders the histologic findings are not specific.[6] Thus, the discovery of crystals in patients with gout or calcium pyrophosphate dihydrate crystal deposition disease, of bacteria in patients with pyogenic arthritis, and of lymphoid follicles in patients with rheumatoid arthritis provides precise diagnostic information, but microscopic characteristics, such as the amount of fibrin deposits on the synovial surface, vascular proliferation and edema, and inflammatory or synovial cellular proliferation, are less specific. The reported success of the procedure in obtaining adequate synovial tissue has varied with the specific joint being evaluated and the size of the biopsy needle; in general, the success rate has been between 75 per cent and 95 per cent.[8]

REFERENCES

1. Goldenberg CL: Synovial membrane biopsy. *In* AS Cohen (Ed): Rheumatology and Immunology. New York, Grune & Stratton, 1979, p 89.
2. Polley HF, Bickel WW: Punch biopsy of synovial membrane. Ann Rheum Dis *10*:277, 1951.
3. Yates DB: Arthroscopy, arthrography and synovial biopsy. *In* JT Scott (Ed): Copeman's Textbook of the Rheumatic Diseases. 5th Ed. Edinburgh, Churchill Livingstone, 1978, p 1022.
4. Parker RH, Pearson CM: A simplified synovial biopsy needle. Arthritis Rheum *6*:172, 1973.
5. Schumacher HR, Kulka JP: Needle biopsy of the synovial membrane — experience with the Parker-Pearson technique. N Engl J Med *8*:416, 1972.
6. Goldenberg DL, Cohen AS: Synovial membrane histopathology in the differential diagnosis of rheumatoid arthritis, gout, pseudogout, systemic lupus erythematosus, infectious arthritis, and degenerative joint disease. Medicine *57*:239, 1978.
7. Bocanegra TS, McClelland JJ, Germain BF, Espinoza LR: Intra-articular fragmentation of a new Parker-Pearson synovial biopsy needle. J Rheumatol *7*:248, 1980.
8. Moon M-S, Kim I, Kim J-M, Lee H-S, Ahn Y-P: Synovial biopsy by Franklin-Silverman needle. Clin Orthop Rel Res *150*:224, 1980.

APPENDIX 4
GROSS PATHOLOGIC SPECIMEN PREPARATION AND MACERATION

by Gen Niwayama, M.D., and Donald Resnick, M.D.

The specimens are first radiographed and photographed. They are then frozen at −40° to −60°C for 48 hours and serially sectioned in appropriate planes, usually at 0.5 cm levels. When histologic and cytologic diagnosis is required, sample sections should be obtained prior to freezing in order to avoid introducing artifactual cellular damage.

Tissue maceration is most simply accomplished by gently washing the specimen in warm running water. In this manner, cellular elements are removed and bony and soft tissue structures are reasonably well demonstrated. However, trabecular architectural detail may be inadequate with this method, requiring treatment of the tissue with chemical solution.

We prefer a simple chemical solution, commercial Clorox. The tissue section is placed in a pan or container containing Clorox for a variable length of time. If complete maceration is desired without the necessity of maintaining original anatomic relationships, the tissue is placed in the solution for several hours to days; if it is important that original anatomic relationships be preserved, more careful monitoring of the maceration process is essential. Furthermore, gentle handling of specimens is important during maceration and subsequent photography and radiography to maintain fine and delicate osseous and soft tissue structures.

The following photographs (Figs. 1 to 6) illustrate progressive stages of maceration of an amputated foot from a diabetic patient.

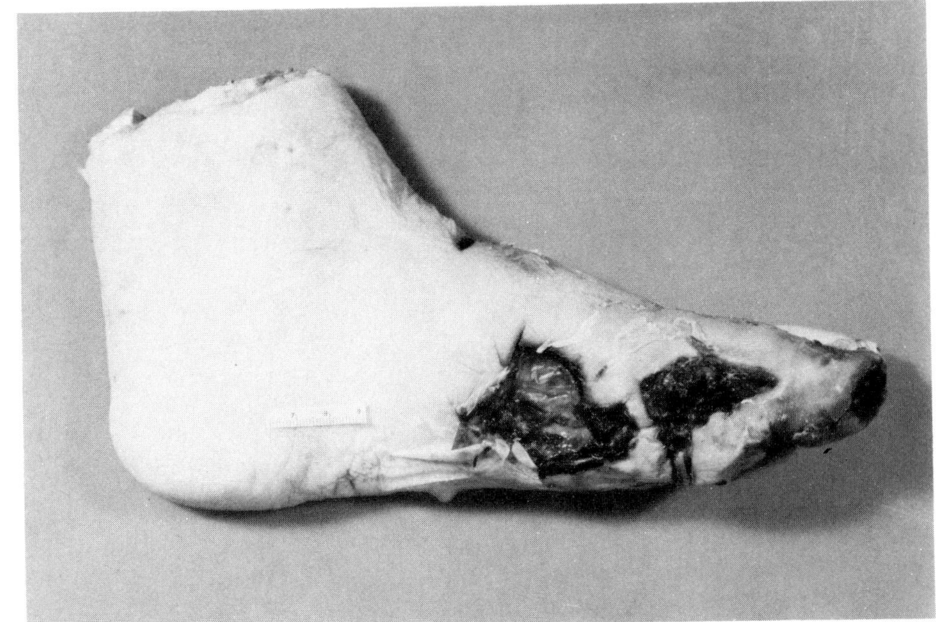

Figure 1. *The medial surface of the left foot is the site of two ulcerating gangrenous skin lesions.*

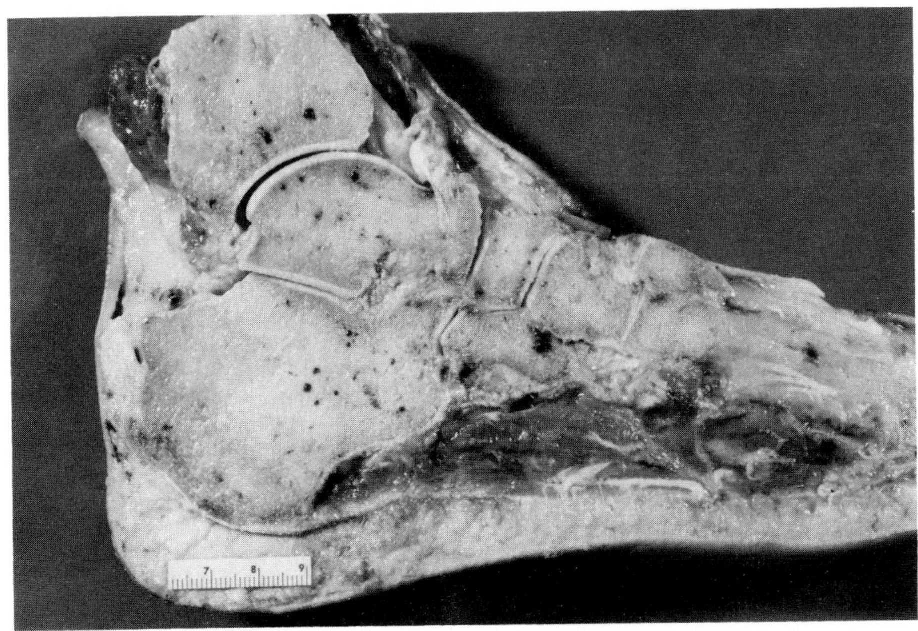

Figure 2. *Sagittal section of the left foot prior to tissue freezing.*

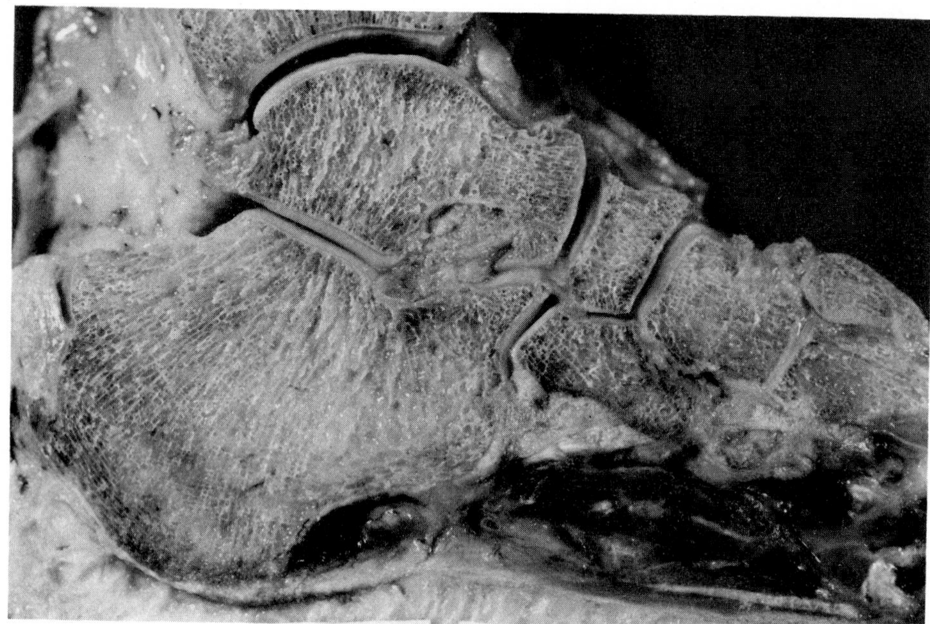

Figure 3. *Cut surface after 30 minutes of treatment in commercial Clorox solution.*

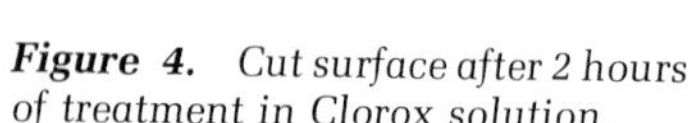

Figure 4. *Cut surface after 2 hours of treatment in Clorox solution.*

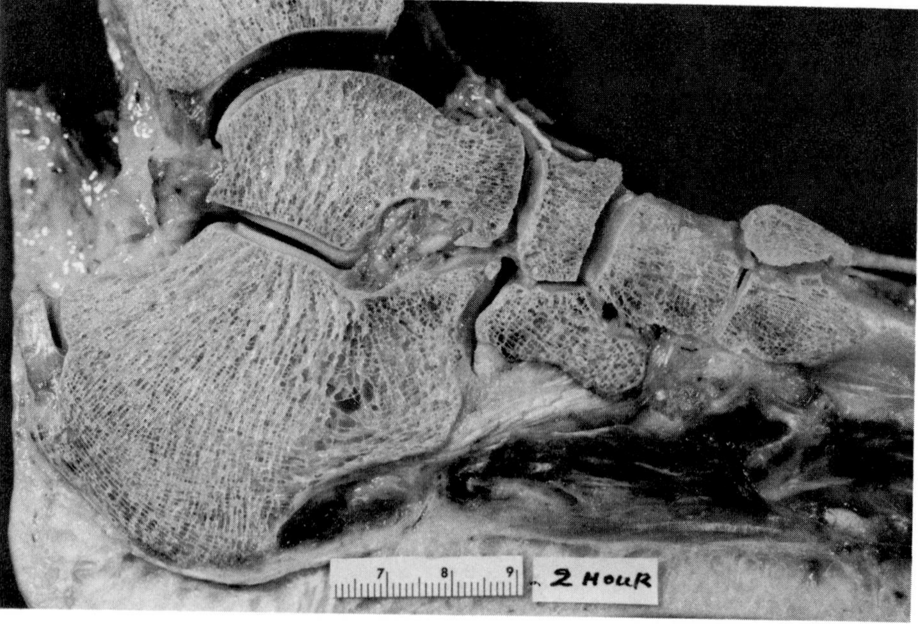

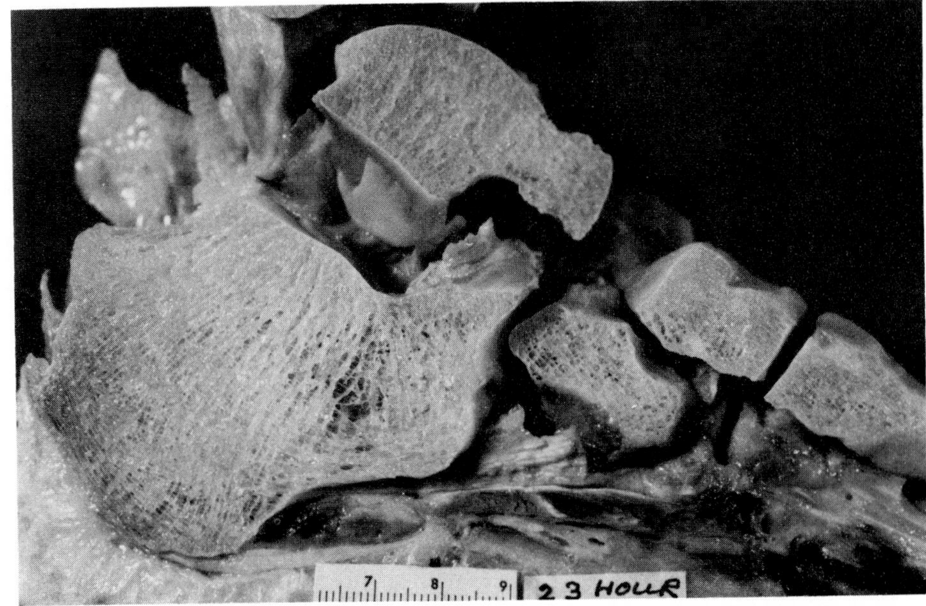

Figure 5. *Cut surface after 23 hours of treatment in commercial Clorox solution. Note disruption and loss of some of the osseous structures.*

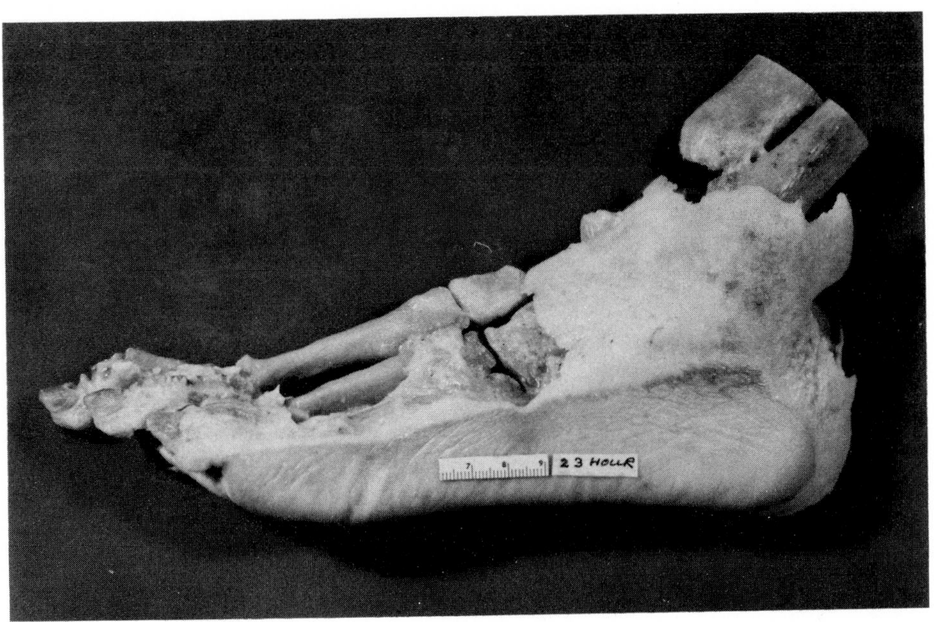

Figure 6. *The lateral external surface of the left foot after 23 hours of treatment in commercial Clorox solution. Although the cut surface of the specimen had been submerged during the maceration process, the external surface was macerated more slowly. Therefore, it is possible to obtain specimens in which osseous and soft tissue structures are both well delineated.*

INDEX

INDEX

Page numbers in *italics* indicate illustrations; (t) indicates tables.